Lumb & Jones'
Veterinary Anesthesia and Analgesia

Fourth Edition

Lumb & Jones'
Veterinary Anesthesia and Analgesia

Fourth Edition

Edited by

William J. Tranquilli

John C. Thurmon

Kurt A. Grimm

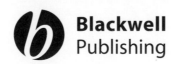

Blackwell Publishing Professional
2121 State Avenue, Ames, Iowa 50014, USA

Orders: 1-800-862-6657
Office: 1-515-292-0140
Fax: 1-515-292-3348
Web site: www.blackwellprofessional.com

Blackwell Publishing Ltd
9600 Garsington Road, Oxford OX4 2DQ, UK
Tel.: +44 (0)1865 776868

Blackwell Publishing Asia
550 Swanston Street, Carlton, Victoria 3053, Australia
Tel.: +61 (0)3 8359 1011

Authorization to photocopy items for internal or personal use, or
the internal or personal use of specific clients, is granted by
Blackwell Publishing, provided that the base fee is paid directly to
the Copyright Clearance Center, 222 Rosewood Drive, Danvers,
MA 01923. For those organizations that have been granted a
photocopy license by CCC, a separate system of payments has
been arranged. The fee code for users of the Transactional
Reporting Service is ISBN-13: 978-0-8138-1592-3.

First edition, © 1973 Lea & Febiger
Second edition, © 1984 Lea & Febiger
Third edition, © 1996 Williams & Wilkins
Fourth Edition, © 2007 Blackwell Publishing

Library of Congress Cataloging-in-Publication Data

Lumb & Jones' veterinary anesthesia and analgesia. —4th ed. /
edited by William J. Tranquilli, John C. Thurmon, and Kurt A.
Grimm.
        p. ; cm.
     Rev. ed. of: Lumb and Jones' veterinary anesthesia / edited by
John C. Thurmon, William J. Tranquilli, G. John Benson.
3rd ed. 1996.
     Includes bibliographical references and index.
     ISBN-13: 978-0-8138-1592-3 (alk. paper)
     ISBN-10: 0-8138-1592-4 (alk. paper)
     1. Veterinary anesthesia. 2. Analgesia. I. Tranquilli, William J.
II. Thurmon, John C. III. Grimm, Kurt A. IV. Veterinary anesthesia.
V. Lumb and Jones' veterinary anesthesia. VI. Title: Lumb and
Jones' veterinary anesthesia and analgesia. VII. Title: Veterinary
anesthesia and analgesia.
     [DNLM: 1. Anesthesia—veterinary. 2. Analgesia—veterinary.
SF 914 L9567 2007]
SF914.L82 2007
636.089'796—dc22

                                        2006025002

The last digit is the print number: 9 8 7 6 5 4 3 2 1

Disclaimer
The contents of this work are intended to further general
scientific research, understanding, and discussion only and are
not intended and should not be relied upon as recommending
or promoting a specific method, diagnosis, or treatment by
practitioners for any particular patient. The publisher and the
editor make no representations or warranties with respect to the
accuracy or completeness of the contents of this work and
specifically disclaim all warranties, including without limitation
any implied warranties of fitness for a particular purpose. In
view of ongoing research, equipment modifications, changes in
governmental regulations, and the constant flow of information
relating to the use of medicines, equipment, and devices, the
reader is urged to review and evaluate the information provided
in the package insert or instructions for each medicine,
equipment, or device for, among other things, any changes in
the instructions or indication of usage and for added warnings
and precautions. Readers should consult with a specialist where
appropriate. The fact that an organization or Website is referred
to in this work as a citation and/or a potential source of further
information does not mean that the editor or the publisher
endorses the information the organization or Website may
provide or recommendations it may make. Further, readers
should be aware that Internet Websites listed in this work may
have changed or disappeared between when this work was
written and when it is read. No warranty may be created or
extended by any promotional statements for this work. Neither
the publisher nor the editor shall be liable for any damages
arising herefrom.

Dedication

The fourth edition of this text is dedicated to the pioneering individuals instrumental in developing the specialty of veterinary anesthesiology and to the practitioners and scientists who continue to advance veterinary anesthesia and the evolving field of pain management. Every veterinarian, technician, and staff member who daily champions the humaneness of patient care in the academic, research, or clinical environment is to be appreciated. We owe much to members of the veterinary profession, as well as to those in allied medical fields, who have focused their life's work on discovering better and safer methods of achieving anesthesia and pain alleviation in the animals that we are privileged to attend and heal.

We dedicate our efforts in bringing this edition to publication to our parents for imparting the values of hard work, loyalty, and patience; to our teachers and colleagues for the belief that scientific knowledge gives us the best chance to know what is real; to our wives for their undying devotion and support of family; and to our children and students for making everything joyful and worthwhile.

William J. Tranquilli
John C. Thurmon
Kurt A. Grimm

Contents

VII. ANESTHESIA AND ANALGESIA OF PATIENTS WITH SPECIFIC DISEASE

VIII. ANESTHESIA AND ANALGESIA FOR SELECTED PATIENTS AND PROCEDURES

Contributors

Jon M. Arnemo, DVM, PhD
Department of Food Safety and Infection Biology
Section of Arctic Veterinary Medicine
Norwegian School of Veterinary Science
NO-9292 Tromsø, Norway

Richard M. Bednarski, DVM, MS, DACVA
Department of Veterinary Clinical Sciences
College of Veterinary Medicine
Ohio State University
Columbus, OH 43210

Keith R. Branson, DVM, MS, DACVA
Department of Medicine and Surgery
College of Veterinary Medicine
University of Missouri
Columbia, MO 65211

David B. Brunson, DVM, MS, DACVA
Department of Surgical Sciences
School of Veterinary Medicine
University of Wisconsin
Madison, WI 53711

Rachael E. Carpenter, DVM
Department of Veterinary Clinical Medicine
College of Veterinary Medicine
University of Illinois
Urbana, IL 61802

Gwendolyn Light Carroll, DVM, MS, DACVA
Department of Small Animal Clinical Sciences
College of Veterinary Medicine and Biomedical Sciences
Texas A&M University
College Station, TX 77843-4474

Nigel A. Caulkett, DVM, MVetSc, DACVA
Faculty of Veterinary Medicine
University of Calgary
Calgary, Canada T2N 4N1

Janyce L. Cornick-Seahorn, DVM, MS, DACVA, DACVIM
Equine Veterinary Specialists
Georgetown, KY 40324

Helio Autran de Morais, DVM, PhD, DACVIM
Department of Medical Sciences
School of Veterinary Medicine
University of Wisconsin
Madison, WI 53706

Dianne Dunning, DVM, MS, DACVS
College of Veterinary Medicine
North Carolina State University
Raleigh, NC 27606

Stephen J. Ettinger, DVM, DACVIM
California Animal Hospital Veterinary Specialty Group
Drs. Ettinger, Lusk, Barrett, Norman, Charette, and Sammut, A
    Veterinary Corporation
Los Angeles, CA 90025

A. Thomas Evans, DVM, MS, DACVA
Veterinary Clinical Center
Michigan State University
East Lansing, MI 48824

Anna D. Fails, DVM, PhD, DACVIM
Department of Biomedical Sciences
College of Veterinary Medicine and Biomedical Sciences
Colorado State University
Fort Collins, CO 80523

Paul A. Flecknell, VetMB, PhD, DECLAM, DECVA
Comparative Biology Centre
Newcastle University
Newcastle upon Tyne, UK NE2 4HH

James S. Gaynor, DVM, MS, DACVA
Animal Anesthesia and Pain Management Center
Colorado Springs, CO 80918

Elizabeth A. Giuliano, DVM, MS, DACVO
Department of Medicine and Surgery
College of Veterinary Medicine
University of Missouri–Columbia
Columbia, MO 65211

Maria Glowaski, DVM, DACVA
Department of Veterinary Clinical Sciences
College of Veterinary Medicine
Ohio State University
Columbus, OH 43210-1089

Gregory F. Grauer, DVM, MS, DACVIM
Department of Clinical Sciences
College of Veterinary Medicine
Kansas State University
Manhattan, KS 66506

Stephen A. Greene, DVM, MS, DACVA
Department of Veterinary Clinical Sciences
College of Veterinary Medicine
Washington State University
Pullman, WA 99164-6610

Jennifer B. Grimm, DVM, MS, DACVR
Veterinary Specialist Services, PC
Conifer, CO 80433-0504

Kurt A. Grimm, DVM, PhD, DACVA, DACVP
Veterinary Specialist Services, PC
Conifer, CO 80433-0504

Marjorie E. Gross, DVM, MS, DACVA
Department of Clinical Medicine
College of Veterinary Medicine
Oklahoma State University
Stillwater, OK 74078-2005

Tamara L. Grubb, DVM, MS, DACVA
Pfizer Animal Health
Uniontown, WA 99179

Elizabeth M. Hardie, DVM, PhD, DACVS
Department of Clinical Sciences
College of Veterinary Medicine
North Carolina State University
Raleigh, NC 27606

Sandee M. Hartsfield, DVM, MS, DACVA
Department of Small Animal Clinical Sciences
College of Veterinary Medicine and Biomedical Sciences
Texas A&M University
College Station, TX 77843-4474

Ralph C. Harvey, DVM, MS, DACVA
Department of Small Animal Clinical Sciences
College of Veterinary Medicine
University of Tennessee
C247 Veterinary Teaching Hospital
Knoxville, TN 37996-4544

Steve C. Haskins, DVM, MS, DACVA, DACVECC
Department of Surgical and Radiological Sciences
School of Veterinary Medicine
University of California
Davis, CA 95616

Darryl J. Heard, BVMS, PhD, DACZM
Department of Small Animal Clinical Sciences
College of Veterinary Medicine
University of Florida
Gainesville, FL 32610-0126

Peter W. Hellyer, DVM, MS, DACVA
College of Veterinary Medicine and Biomedical Sciences
Colorado State University
Fort Collins, CO 80523

John A. E. Hubbell, DVM, MS, DACVA
Department of Veterinary Clinical Sciences
College of Veterinary Medicine
Ohio State University
Columbus, OH 43210

Robert D. Keegan, DVM, DACVA
Department of Veterinary Clinical Sciences
College of Veterinary Medicine
Washington State University
Pullman, WA 99164

Carolyn L. Kerr, DVM, DVSc, PhD, DACVA
Department of Clinical Studies
Ontario Veterinary College
University of Guelph
Guelph, Canada N1G 2W1

Leigh A. Lamont, DVM, MS, DACVA
Department of Companion Animals
Atlantic Veterinary College
University of Prince Edward Island
Charlottetown, Canada C1A 4P3

B. Duncan X. Lascelles, BVSc, PhD, DECVS, DACVS
Department of Clinical Sciences
College of Veterinary Medicine
North Carolina State University
Raleigh, NC 27606

Kip A. Lemke, DVM, MS, DACVA
Department of Companion Animals
Atlantic Veterinary College
University of Prince Edward Island
Charlottetown, Canada C1A 4P3

Hui-Chu Lin, DVM, MS, DACVA
Department of Clinical Sciences
College of Veterinary Medicine
Auburn University
Auburn, AL 36849

John W. Ludders, DVM, DACVA
Department of Clinical Sciences
College of Veterinary Medicine
Cornell University
Ithaca, NY 14853

Victoria M. Lukasik, DVM, DACVA
Southwest Veterinary Anesthesiology
Southern Arizona Veterinary Specialty Center
Tucson, AZ 85705

Khursheed R. Mama, DVM, DACVA
Department of Clinical Sciences
College of Veterinary Medicine and Biological Sciences
Colorado State University
Fort Collins, CO 80523-1620

Sandra Manfra Marretta, DVM, DAVDC
Department of Veterinary Clinical Medicine
College of Veterinary Medicine
University of Illinois
Urbana, IL 61802

Steven L. Marks, BVSc, MS, DACVIM
Department of Clinical Sciences
College of Veterinary Medicine
North Carolina State University
Raleigh, NC 27606

David D. Martin, DVM, DACVA
Veterinary Operations
Companion Animal Division
Pfizer Animal Health
New York, NY

Elizabeth A. Martinez, DVM, DACVA
Department of Small Animal Clinical Sciences
College of Veterinary Medicine and Biomedical Sciences
Texas A&M University
College Station, TX 77843-4474

Karol A. Mathews, DVM, DVSc, DACVECC
Department of Clinical Studies
Ontario Veterinary College
University of Guelph
Guelph, Canada N1G 2W1

Nora S. Matthews, DVM, DACVA
Department Small Animal Clinical Sciences
College of Veterinary Medicine and Biomedical Sciences
Texas A&M University
College Station, TX 77843-4474

Wayne N. McDonell, DVM, PhD, DACVA
Department of Clinical Studies
Ontario Veterinary College
University of Guelph
Guelph, Canada N1G 2W1

James N. Moore, DVM, PhD, DACVS
Department of Large Animal Medicine
College of Veterinary Medicine
University of Georgia
Athens, GA 30602

William W. Muir, DVM, PhD, DACVA, DACVECC
Department of Veterinary Clinical Sciences
College of Veterinary Medicine
Ohio State University
Columbus, Ohio 43210

Robert R. Paddleford, DVM, DACVA, DACVECC
Department of Small Animal Clinical Sciences
College of Veterinary Medicine
University of Tennessee
Knoxville, TN 37996-4544
   and
Volunteer Veterinary Anesthesia Consulting Service
Rockford, TN 37853

Mark G. Papich, DVM, MS, DACVCD
Department of Molecular Biomedical Sciences
College of Veterinary Medicine
North Carolina State University
Raleigh, NC 27606

Glenn R. Pettifer, DVM, DVSc, DACVA
Veterinary Emergency Clinic and Referral Centre
Toronto, Canada M4W 3C7

Aleksandar Popovic, DVM, Cert LAS
Merck Frosst Centre for Therapeutic Research
Kirkland, Canada H9H 3I1

Marc R. Raffe, DVM, MS, DACVA, DACVECC
Department of Veterinary Clinical Medicine
College of Veterinary Medicine
University of Illinois
Urbana, IL 61802

Claire A. Richardson, BVM&S
Comparative Biology Centre
Newcastle University Medical School
Newcastle upon Tyne, UK NE2 4HH

Thomas W. Riebold, DVM, DACVA
Department of Clinical Sciences
College of Veterinary Medicine
Oregon State University
Corvallis, OR 97331

Sheilah A. Robertson, BVM&S, PhD, DACVA
Department of Small Animal Clinical Sciences
College of Veterinary Medicine
University of Florida
Gainesville, FL 32610

Michael Schaer, DVM, DACVIM, DACVECC
Department of Small Animal Clinical Sciences
College of Veterinary Medicine
University of Florida
Gainesville, FL 32610

David C. Seeler, DVM, MSc, DACVA
Department of Companion Animals
Atlantic Veterinary College
University of Prince Edward Island
Charlottetown, Canada, C1A 4P3

Charles E. Short, DVM, PhD, DACVA, DECVA
Department of Small Animal Clinical Sciences
College of Veterinary Medicine
University of Tennessee
Knoxville, TN 37996-4544

Roman T. Skarda, DMV, PhD (*deceased*), DACVA, DECVA
Department of Veterinary Clinical Sciences
College of Veterinary Medicine
Ohio State University
Columbus, OH 43210-1089

Geoffrey W. Smith, DVM, PhD, DACVIM
Department of Population Health and Pathobiology
College of Veterinary Medicine
North Carolina State University
Raleigh, NC 27606

Eugene P. Steffey, VMD, PhD, DACVA, DECVA
Department of Surgical and Radiological Sciences
School of Veterinary Medicine
University of California
Davis, CA 95616

Mark D. Stetter, DVM, DACZM
Disney's Animal Programs
Walt Disney World
Lake Buena Vista, FL 32830

William B. Thomas, DVM, MS, DACVM
Department of Small Animal Clinical Sciences
University of Tennessee
C247 Veterinary Teaching Hospital
Knoxville, TN 37996-4544

John C. Thurmon, DVM, MS, DACVA
Department of Veterinary Clinical Medicine
College of Veterinary Medicine
University of Illinois
Urbana, IL 61802

William J. Tranquilli, DVM, MS, DACVA
Department of Veterinary Clinical Medicine
College of Veterinary Medicine
University of Illinois
Urbana, IL 61802

Cynthia M. Trim, BVSc, DACVA, DECVA
Department of Large Animal Medicine
College of Veterinary Medicine
University of Georgia
Athens, GA 30602

Ann E. Wagner, DVM, MS, DACVP, DACVA
Department of Clinical Sciences
College of Veterinary Medicine and Biomedical Sciences
Colorado State University
Fort Collins, CO 80523

Deborah V. Wilson, BVSc, MS, DACVA
Department of Large Animal Clinical Sciences
College of Veterinary Medicine
Michigan State University
East Lansing, MI 48824

Foreword

Since the initial publication of *Veterinary Anesthesia* in 1973, the science and art of anesthesia and pain management have matured immeasurably. Today, a comprehensive book covering the entire field is beyond the capabilities of any one individual or area of study. As such, and as Founding Diplomates of the American College of Veterinary Anesthesiologists, it has been gratifying to see numerous authors, more than 65 in all, young and old alike, from a wide array of backgrounds and clinical specialties make contributions to this, the fourth edition and newly titled *Lumb and Jones' Veterinary Anesthesia and Analgesia*.

We are indebted to Drs. Tranquilli, Thurmon, and Grimm for assuming editorship of this challenging endeavor. We believe that the fourth edition will continue to serve students, academic colleagues, and practitioners alike as the world's most comprehensive source of information regarding the science and art of anesthesia and pain control in the numerous species that make up the animal world.

William V. Lumb
E. Wynn Jones

Preface

The first edition of *Veterinary Anesthesia* was published in 1973, followed by the second edition in 1984, and the third edition in 1996. The publishing of this, the fourth edition, in 2007 marks this text's thirty-fourth anniversary.

Many changes have occurred in veterinary medicine and anesthesia during this time, with each succeeding edition of this text attempting to update and document these advances. In recent years, the ever-increasing emphasis on the treatment of animal pain has placed veterinary anesthesiology and pain management in a central role in the delivery of humane veterinary care. Accordingly, several chapters focusing on recent advancements in animal pain management have been included in this revision and, most noticeably, are reflected in the new title, *Lumb and Jones' Veterinary Anesthesia and Analgesia*. Where possible, we have endeavored to conserve as much of the previous editions' text as possible so as to continue to provide information on older anesthetic drugs and techniques that might still be employed by veterinarians in various regions of the world. Nevertheless, given the volume of space required to discuss much of the new knowledge and contemporary issues pertinent to veterinary anesthesia and analgesia, retention of much of the previous editions' text was simply not possible. Fortunately, this information, much of which is of historical interest, will forever be available from earlier editions. It should be noted that some chapters' text has been retained from previous editions and, as such, the current authors of these chapters (if not the same) wish to acknowledge the continued valuable contributions of earlier authors to this edition, as well. As in previous editions, the fourth edition provides evidence of numerous advances in our scientific and clinical knowledge pertinent to the provision of anesthesia and analgesia in a multitude of animal species.

This Lumb and Jones' edition has more than 65 contributing authors, offering a wide array of scientific training and clinical experience. As would be expected, many contributors are anesthesiologists, but a number of new authors are specialized in other clinical areas, including clinical pharmacology, surgery, medicine, critical care, cardiology, neurology, urology, ophthalmology, dentistry, radiology, physical rehabilitation, and lab animal medicine. It is hoped that this increased diversity in authorship expertise will provide a comprehensive perspective to the management of anesthesia and pain in patients suffering from an array of clinical conditions and disease. All of the contributing authors have been encouraged to share their personal experiences in an effort to enhance the clinical utility of the information provided. The editors are indebted to the authors for the many hours devoted to the preparation of their individual chapters. Many of these authors have dedicated their careers to the field of veterinary anesthesiology and the humane treatment of animals. In so doing, these individuals have made numerous and, in some instances, monumental contributions to the advancement of veterinary medicine. Included among these individuals are Drs. W. Lumb, E. W. Jones, C. E. Short, W. W. Muir, W. N. McDonell, E. P. Steffey, R. T. Skarda, S. M. Hartsfield, S. C. Haskins, and P. A. Flecknell. Most recently, this dedication was best exemplified by Dr. Roman Skarda's insistence on his continued contribution to the fourth edition while battling debilitating and painful disease before his eventual passing. These individuals cannot help but provide inspiration to all who have contributed their time and expertise to the completion of this book and to all who benefit from its reading.

Similar to previous editions, this revision can be viewed both as a textbook and as a comprehensive source of scientific knowledge relevant to the clinical management of anesthesia and provision of analgesic therapy. Individuals requiring information on the immobilization and anesthesia of wild, zoo, and laboratory animals also will find chapters devoted to these unique circumstances. In addition to chapters on cardiovascular, respiratory, nervous system, and acid-base physiology, the pharmacology of various classes of drugs employed in the delivery of anesthesia and analgesia has been reviewed and updated. Chapters on anesthetic equipment, monitoring, mechanical ventilation, and regional analgesic techniques are provided. Chapters covering acupuncture, physical rehabilitation, and palliative analgesia of companion animals have been added. Chapters continue to be devoted to the anesthesia of specific species and classes of animals including dogs, cats, horses, swine, ruminants, lab animals, zoo animals, free ranging terrestrial and aquatic mammals, birds, reptiles, amphibians, and fish. Several chapters discussing the unique anesthesia and pain management requirements of companion animals with specific diseases have again been included, as have chapters on specific surgical patients and procedures. New chapters on dental, cancer, orthopedic, and equine colic patients have been included in this edition. As in the third edition, chapters have been organized into sections to aid readers in locating specific information rapidly.

In closing, the editors extend their thanks to all of the anesthesiology faculty and staff at the University of Illinois for their hard work and understanding. Without their support, time would not have been available for the editorial assignments required by such a task.

The editors are also deeply indebted to and thank Erin Gardner and the staff at Blackwell Publishing for their untiring support and encouragement.

William J. Tranquilli
John C. Thurmon
Kurt A. Grimm

Section I
GENERAL TOPICS

Chapter 1
History and Overview of Veterinary Anesthesia

John C. Thurmon and Charles E. Short

Introduction
History of Animal Anesthesia
Organized Veterinary Anesthesia in North America
Definitions
Reasons for Administering Anesthesia
Types of Anesthesia

Introduction

The earliest recorded attempts to induce anesthesia appeared to have been performed in humans. Drugs and techniques used included opiates, alcohol, and asphyxiation by compression of the carotid arteries to induce unconsciousness, thus alleviating the pain of surgery. In 1540, Paracelsus produced ether and reported it to have a soporific effect in birds. Despite this discovery, no further progress was made until chemistry was developed and carbon dioxide and several other gases, including oxygen, were discovered.

History of Animal Anesthesia

In 1800, Sir Humphrey Davy suggested that nitrous oxide might have anesthetic properties. Approximately 20 years later, H. H. Hickman (1824) demonstrated that pain associated with surgery in dogs could be alleviated by inhalation of a mixture of nitrous oxide and carbon dioxide. He reasoned that the latter increased the rate and depth of breathing, thus enhancing the effects of nitrous oxide. More recent studies have shown that unconsciousness can be induced in 30 to 40 s in piglets breathing carbon dioxide (50%) alone in oxygen (50%).[1]

It was not until 1842 that ether was used for human anesthesia. Two years later, a dentist, Horace Wells (1844), discovered the anesthetic properties of nitrous oxide. Although this finding was neglected for several years, nitrous oxide was reintroduced in humans in 1862. C. T. Jackson, a Boston physician, was the first to employ ether extensively in animals.[2]

Chloroform was discovered by Liebig in 1831, but it was not until 1847 that it was first used to induce anesthesia in animals by Flourens and in people by J. Y. Simpson of Edinburgh, Scotland. With the introduction of chloroform, reports began to appear in the veterinary literature of its use in animals. Dadd routinely used general anesthesia in animals and was the first in the United States to advocate humane treatment of animals and the application of scientific principles (i.e., anesthesia) in veterinary surgery.[3]

In 1875, Ore published the first monograph on intravenous anesthesia using chloral hydrate; 3 years later, Humbert described its use in horses. Pirogoff was the first to attempt rectal anesthesia with chloral hydrate in 1847. The rectal administration of chloral hydrate was used later in veterinary practice. Intraperitoneal injection was first used in 1892 in France. Thus, the various routes of administration of general anesthetics to animals were established by the end of the 19th century.

After the initial isolation of cocaine by Albert Niemann of Germany in 1860, Anrep, in 1878, suggested the possibility of using cocaine as a local anesthetic. In 1884, Kohler used cocaine for local anesthesia of the eye, and Halsted described cocaine nerve-block anesthesia a year later. Its use was popularized by Sir Frederick Hobday, an English veterinarian. Thereafter, G. L. Corning was credited for inducing cocaine spinal anesthesia in dogs in 1885. From his description, however, it would appear that he induced epidural anesthesia. In 1898, August Bier of Germany induced true spinal anesthesia in animals and then in himself and an assistant.[4]

While local infiltration was popularized by Reclus (1890) and Schleich (1892), conduction anesthesia was first introduced by Halsted and Hall in New York in 1884. These techniques increased in popularity with the discovery of local anesthetics less toxic than cocaine. These developments enabled Cuille and Sendrail (1901) of France to induce subarachnoid anesthesia in horses, cattle, and dogs. Cathelin (1901) reported epidural anesthesia in dogs, but it remained for Retzgen, Benesch, and Brook to apply this technique in large animal species in the 1920s. Although paralumbar anesthesia was employed in humans by Sellheim in 1909, it was not until the 1940s that Farquharson and Formston applied this technique in cattle. Despite these promising developments with local analgesic techniques in the latter half of the 19th century, and perhaps owing to unfavorable results, general anesthesia was not readily adopted by the veterinary profession until well into the 20th century. It is sad to say, but a "heavy hand," without analgesia/anesthesia, was the stock in trade of many practicing veterinarians.

In small domestic animals, ether and chloroform were commonly administered in the early part of the 20th century. However, general anesthesia became more widely accepted after discovery of the barbiturates in the late 1920s and, in particular, with the development of pentobarbital in 1930. Barbiturate anesthesia received an additional boost with the introduction of the thiobarbiturates and particularly with thiopental in 1934. Because of rough, prolonged recovery, the acceptance of general anesthesia in large animals was delayed until phenothiazine derivatives were introduced by Charpentier in France in 1950.

General anesthesia of large farm animals was further advanced by the discovery of fluorinated hydrocarbons and the development of large animal anesthetic equipment for their safe administration. Discovery of newer drugs (e.g., tranquilizers, opioids, α_2-adrenergic agonists, dissociatives, muscle relaxants, and inhalant anesthetics) has further advanced the utility of veterinary anesthesia in large and small animal species.[5]

Organized Veterinary Anesthesia in North America

During the late 1960s and early 1970s, a small group of physician anesthesiologists made it possible for a number of future diplomates of the American College of Veterinary Anesthesiologists (ACVA) to participate in their programs and to learn about the development of new anesthetic drugs and techniques. Among these physicians were Robert Dripps, University of Pennsylvania; Arthur Keats, Baylor University; Mort Shulman and Max Sadolv, University of Illinois; and Edmond I. Eger, University of California Medical College. During this same period, E. W. Jones (Oklahoma State University) and William Lumb (Colorado State University) were making significant contributions to the field of veterinary anesthesiology while at their respective institutions. Jerry Gillespie was also making a unique contribution through his work on respiratory function of anesthetized horses.

Even though there were a number of interested faculty within veterinary colleges and research laboratories, not until 1970 was a major thrust directed at organizing veterinarians. Initially, a society of veterinary anesthesia was perceived. Later this society became the American Society of Veterinary Anesthesia (ASVA). Membership in the ASVA was open to all individuals working in the veterinary profession who had an interest in veterinary anesthesiology. In 1970, the first organizational meeting was held in conjunction with the American Veterinary Medical Association (AVMA) to coordinate the efforts/interest of all those wishing to organize and develop the specialty of veterinary anesthesiology. Their primary goal was to improve anesthetic techniques and to disseminate knowledge whenever and wherever possible. Charles Short was elected the first president of the new society. The ASVA was designed expressly to promote dissemination of information on veterinary anesthesia irrespective of individual training or background. Of major interest was the selection of individuals to speak at the ASVA and other scientific and educational meetings (e.g., the AVMA, the American Animal Hospital Association [AAHA], and the American Association of Equine Practitioners [AAEP]). As the ASVA developed, publication of articles on anesthesiology seemed in order. Bruce Heath accepted editorial responsibilities of articles submitted for the ASVA journal. In 1971, John Thurmon chaired the Ad Hoc Committee to establish the American College of Veterinary Anesthesiologists. The AVMA had established guidelines for the selection of founding-charter diplomates of specialty organizations. The Ad Hoc Committee requirements for charter diplomate status included 10 years of active service in the specialty, significant publications,

intensive training, and being the head of an anesthesiology program or spending a major portion of one's professional time in anesthesia or a closely related subject area. Seven members of the ASVA were found to meet these qualifications. This group would later become the founding diplomates of the ACVA.

Between 1970 and 1975, the constitution and bylaws were drafted and formalized. In 1975, the AVMA Council on Education recommended preliminary approval of the ACVA. This was confirmed by the AVMA House of Delegates in that same year. Thus, the ACVA was officially established in North America. Of importance throughout this process were the insight and efforts of Drs. Lumb and Jones, after which this text is named. They greatly assisted in the establishment of the ACVA because of their sincere interest in the sound principles of veterinary anesthesiology. During this period, several didactic texts were published on animal anesthesiology that helped to establish anesthesia as a stand-alone discipline and specialty within veterinary medicine. The first edition of this text, *Lumb and Jones' Veterinary Anesthesia*, was published in 1973; *Clinical Veterinary Anesthesia*, edited by Charles Short, was published in 1974; and *Textbook of Veterinary Anesthesia*, edited by Larry Soma, was published in 1971.

During the late 1970s, many of the founding diplomates began to establish residency training programs in their respective veterinary colleges. From 1975 to 1980, the ACVA developed continuing education programs, programs in self-improvement, and programs for testing and certification of new diplomates. Along with residency training programs, new faculty positions were created for training veterinary anesthesiologists in a number of colleges of veterinary medicine across North America. In 1980, the ACVA sought and was granted full accreditation by the AVMA, an effort headed by Eugene Steffey, then president of the ACVA.

During the past 3 decades, a number of other organizations around the world have promoted and contributed greatly to the standing of veterinary anesthesia. They include the Association of Veterinary Anaesthetists of Great Britain and Ireland (AVA), as well as the Veterinary Anesthesia and Surgery Association in Japan. These associations were instrumental in organizing the first International Congress of Veterinary Anesthesiology with its stated objective of globally advancing the field of veterinary anesthesiology. The first International Congress of Veterinary Anesthesiology was held in Cambridge, England, in 1982, followed by congresses in Sacramento, California, in 1985; in Brisbane, Australia, in 1988; in Utrecht, the Netherlands, in 1991; in Guelph, Canada, in 1994; in Thessaloniki, Greece, in 1997; in Bern, Switzerland, in 2000; in Knoxville, Tennessee, in 2003; and in Santos, Brazil, in 2006.

Concurrently, organized veterinary anesthesiology was being advanced in Europe. Veterinary anesthesiologists in the United Kingdom established the Association of Veterinary Anaesthetists and awarded the Diploma of Veterinary Anaesthesia to those with specialty training. Later, interests in board specialization became evident in the United Kingdom and many European countries, resulting in the establishment of the European College of Veterinary Anesthesiologists (ECVA). Currently, a number of veterinary anesthesiologists are boarded by both the ACVA and the ECVA. For further information concerning the early history of anesthesia, the reader is referred to a number of sources.[6–9]

The establishment of the ACVA and the ECVA in recent decades has advanced veterinary anesthesia on a worldwide stage primarily through the increased availability of scientific meetings and literature. Both the ACVA and the ECVA have, as their official scientific publication, the *Journal of Veterinary Anaesthesia and Analgesia*.

Definitions

The term *anesthesia*, derived from the Greek term *anaisthaesia*, meaning "insensibility," is used to describe the loss of sensation to the entire or any part of the body. Anesthesia is induced by drugs that depress the activity of nervous tissue locally, regionally, or within the central nervous system (CNS). From a pharmacological viewpoint, there has been a significant redefining of the term *general anesthesia*.[10] Both central nervous stimulants and depressants can be useful general anesthetics.[11] Several terms are used in describing the effects of anesthetic drugs:

1. *Analgesia* refers to freedom from or absence of pain.
2. *Tranquilization* results in behavioral change wherein anxiety is relieved and the patient becomes relaxed but remains aware of its surroundings. In this state, it may appear to be indifferent to minor pain.
3. *Sedation* is a state characterized by central depression accompanied by drowsiness. The patient is generally unaware of its surroundings but responsive to painful manipulation.
4. *Narcosis* is a drug-induced state of deep sleep from which the patient cannot be easily aroused. Narcosis may or may not be accompanied by analgesia.
5. *Hypnosis* is a condition of artificially induced sleep, or a trance resembling sleep, resulting from moderate depression of the CNS from which the patient is readily aroused.
6. *Local analgesia* (anesthesia) is a loss of sensation in circumscribed body area.
7. *Regional analgesia* (anesthesia) is insensibility in a larger, though limited, body area (e.g., paralumbar nerve blockade).
8. *General anesthesia* is drug-induced unconsciousness that is characterized by controlled but reversible depression of the CNS and analgesia. In this state, the patient is not arousable by noxious stimulation. Sensory, motor, and autonomic reflex functions are attenuated.
9. *Surgical anesthesia* is the state/plane of general anesthesia that provides unconsciousness, muscular relaxation, and analgesia sufficient for painless surgery.
10. *Balanced anesthesia* is induced by multiple drugs. Drugs are targeted to specifically attenuate individual components of the anesthetic state; that is, consciousness, analgesia, muscle relaxation, and alteration of autonomic reflexes.
11. *Dissociative anesthesia* is induced by drugs (e.g., ketamine) that dissociate the thalamocortic and limbic systems. This form of anesthesia is characterized by a cataleptoid state in which the eyes remain open and swallowing reflexes remain intact. Skeletal muscle hypertonus persists unless a strong sedative, peripheral or central muscle relaxant, or other concurrent medications are administered.

Reasons for Administering Anesthesia

First and foremost, anesthetics alleviate pain and induce muscle relaxation, essential for safe surgery.[12] Other important uses include restraint, safe transportation of wild and exotic animals, various diagnostic and therapeutic procedures, euthanasia, and the humane slaughter of food animals.

Types of Anesthesia

The diverse uses for anesthesia (as it relates to immobilization, muscle relaxation, and analgesia) and the requirements peculiar to species, age, and disease state necessitate the use of a variety of drugs, drug combinations, and methods. Anesthesia is often classified according to the type of drug and/or method/route of drug administration:

1. *Inhalation:* Anesthetic gases or vapors are inhaled in combination with oxygen.
2. *Injectable:* Anesthetic solutions are injected intravenously, intramuscularly, and subcutaneously. Other injectable routes include intrathoracic and intraperitoneal. These latter two routes are not generally recommended.
3. *Oral or rectal:* These routes are ordinarily used for liquid anesthetics or suppositories.
4. *Local and conduction:* Anesthetic drug is applied topically, injected locally into or around the surgical site (field block), or injected around a large nerve trunk supplying a specific region (conduction or regional nerve block). In the latter instance, the injection may be perineural (nerve block) or into the epidural or subarachnoid space (true spinal analgesia).
5. *Electronarcosis, electroanesthesia, or electrosleep:* Electrical currents are passed through the cerebrum to induce deep narcosis. Even though there have been successful studies, this form of anesthesia has never gained popularity and is rarely used in veterinary practice. Electronarcosis should not be confused with the inhumane practice of electroimmobilization.
6. *Transcutaneous electrical nerve stimulation (TENS, TNS, or TES):* Local analgesia is induced by low-intensity, high-frequency electric stimulation of the skin through surface electrodes.
7. *Hypnosis:* A non–drug-induced trancelike state sometimes employed in rabbits and birds.
8. *Acupuncture:* An ancient Chinese system of therapy using long, fine needles to induce analgesia.
9. *Hypothermia:* Body temperature is decreased, either locally or generally, to supplement insensitivity and decrease anesthetic drug requirement and reduce metabolic needs. It is primarily used in neonates or in patients undergoing cardiovascular surgery.

References

1. Thurmon JC, Benson GJ. Anesthesia in ruminants and swine. In: Howard JL, ed. Current Veterinary Therapy, vol 3. Philadelphia: WB Saunders, 1993:58–76.

2. Jackson CT. Etherization of Animals. Report of the Commissioner of Patients for the Year of 1853. Washington, DC: Beverly Tucker, Senate Printer, 1853:59.

3. Dadd GH. The Modern Horse Doctor. Boston: JP Jewett, 1854.

4. Keys TE. The development of anesthesia. Anesthesiology 3:11–23, 1942.

5. Stevenson DE. The evolution of veterinary anesthesia. Br Vet J 119:477, 1963.

6. Clark AJ. Aspects of the history of anesthetics. Br Med J 2:1029, 1938.

7. Smithcors JE. The early use of anesthesia in veterinary practice. Br Vet J 113:284, 1957.

8. Lee JA. A Synopsis of Anesthesia, 4th ed. Baltimore: Williams and Wilkins, 1959.

9. Miller RD. Anesthesia, 2nd ed. New York: Churchill Livingstone, 1986.

10. Heavner JE. Veterinary anesthesia update. J Am Vet Med Assoc 182:30, 1983.

11. Winters WD, Ferrer AT, Guzman-Flores C. The cataleptic state induced by ketamine: A review of the neuropharmacology of anesthesia. Neuropharmacology 11:303–315, 1972.

12. Short CE. The management of animal pain: Where have we been, where are we now, and where are we going? Vet J 165:101–103, 2003.

Chapter 2

Considerations for General Anesthesia

William W. Muir

Pharmacology

Anesthesia is, of necessity, a reversible process. Knowledge of the factors underlying production of anesthesia, and those that may modify it, is essential to the success of the procedure. The dose of anesthetic and the techniques for its administration are based on the average normal healthy animal. Because of the many phenomena that modify the effect of an anesthetic, it is unlikely that any given animal will be exactly average.

Marked variations in response to a standard dose of anesthetic result from the interplay of many factors, especially those related to the central nervous system (CNS) status (excited or depressed) and metabolic activity of the animal, existing disease or pathology, and the uptake and distribution of the anesthetic.

Biological Variation

Since elimination of anesthetics depends on the species and the metabolic processes within the animal, conditions affecting the metabolic rate exert a marked influence on anesthetic effect. Small animals have a higher basal metabolic rate per unit of surface area than large animals; therefore, in general, the smaller the

animal, the larger is the dose per unit of body weight necessary for anesthesia. Animals with large quantities of fat, which is a relatively inactive nonmetabolizing tissue, have a lower basal metabolic rate per unit of body weight and usually require less anesthetic than lean muscular animals in good condition.[1] Animals in poorer condition may also require less anesthetic. Dogs kept on a low food intake causing weight losses of 10% to 20% showed a marked increase in duration of anesthesia after a single anesthetic injection.[2] In newborns, the basal metabolic rate is low. It gradually increases to its highest point at puberty through early adulthood and then gradually declines. Response to barbiturates varies in dogs of differing ages.[2] Very young animals and older adult animals are most sensitive, whereas dogs in the age range of 3 to 12 months are least sensitive. These age variations are also related to changes in liver enzyme activity.[3] Changes in metabolism with age are not as clear-cut as originally thought. This probably reflects that neither gross weight nor surface area are reliable measures of the active tissue mass of the body. In humans, at least, data on fat-free body weight indicate little change between young and aged adults.[4] The basal metabolic rate of males is approximately 7% higher than that of females. In females, a rise occurs during pregnancy, owing to the metabolic activity of the fetuses. Conflicting evidence regarding sex differences in susceptibility to anesthetics has been reported.[5] For example, pregnant rats were most susceptible, nonpregnant females less, and male rats least susceptible to anesthetic effect. In contrast, Kennedy[6] could find no sex variance in the response of mice to barbiturate anesthesia. Female rats have been shown to be more sensitive to muscle relaxants than males of a similar age.[7] Apparently, hormones may cause minor differences in an individual's response to an anesthetic.

Pharmacogenetic Differences

Variation in the dose response to drugs because of genetic-related factors can be found in the literature. As examples, the heritable difference in the ability of rabbits to hydrolyze atropine and cocaine,[8] genetic variations in response to pentobarbital in mice,[7] and strain sensitivity to nitrous oxide and to non-oxygen-dependent reductive biotransformation of halothane in rats have all been reported.[7,9] In a few people, plasma cholinesterase has been found to be completely absent or replaced by an inactive variant with resultant prolonged action of succinylcholine.[10] Some breeds of swine are susceptible to malignant hyperthermia.[11] Metabolic rate increases with activity; hence, active animals require relatively larger doses of anesthetic agents. Mice have been shown to be most sensitive to pentobarbital in the early morning. A seasonal response to morphine has been recorded in rabbits, and circadian rhythms have been shown to modify minimum alveolar concentrations for halothane and other inhalant anesthetics by 5% to 10% in rats.[7]

Pharmacokinetics

General anesthesia is produced by the action of an anesthetic on the brain and spinal cord. The agent must therefore achieve access to the central nervous tissue. Although Van Dyke and Chenoweth[12] demonstrated that significant quantities of some inhalation anesthetics are metabolized within the body, for practical purposes they are primarily exhaled. Small amounts are eliminated in feces and urine or diffused through the skin and mucous membranes. Thus, providing respiration and circulation are maintained, inhalants are readily eliminated from the body. In contrast, injectable agents depend on redistribution within the body, biotransformation, principally in the liver, and excretion via the kidneys. With injectable anesthetics, there is less control over the elimination process; for this reason, some consider them to be more dangerous than inhalant anesthetics.

Anesthetics are commonly administered by intravenous injection and occasionally by intramuscular, intrathoracic, intraperitoneal, subcutaneous, and even oral or rectal routes. Intravenous administration bypasses the absorption phase of the drug with the consequences that onset and intensity of action are less variable, titration of dose according to response is facilitated, and the risk of toxicity lessens quickly with the progressive decline of drug concentration in the plasma.[13]

The body may be considered to have multiple compartments (Table 2.1), which are differentiated by blood supply and tissue-blood partition coefficients. After initial intravenous injection, mixing and dilution rapidly occur, and an initial blood concentration of the drug is established. Blood thus becomes the medium by which the drug is delivered to and removed from its site of action. Factors affecting drug concentration and/or availability in the plasma also affect its concentration and availability at the site of action. Binding of drugs to plasma protein, in which form they cannot readily penetrate cellular membranes, and the removal of drugs by tissues that store, metabolize, and excrete them are both important factors that lower the effective concentration of drugs at their site of action.[13,14] Binding is a reversible fusion of small molecules, such as barbiturates, with protein or other macromolecules, thereby limiting penetration of cellular membranes by molecular size, ionization, and limited lipid solubility. Protein binding varies with the properties of the drug, its concentration, and plasma pH and protein concentration. The fraction of bound drug increases with decreasing drug concentration and vice versa, and is modified by the presence of other drugs that compete for available binding sites. The rate of clearance of drug from the blood, the drug's distribution to the tissues, and availability of drug to produce its desired effects thus may all be modified by the drug concentration, plasma pH and protein, state of body hydration, and minimally by the presence of other drugs.[14]

After initial dilution within the vascular system, the drug is distributed to the various tissue compartments according to their

Table 2.1. Body compartments based on tissue perfusion.

Group	Region	Mass (kg)	% Cardiac Output
Vessel rich	Brain	1.4	14
	Liver (splanchnic)	2.6	28
	Heart	0.3	5
	Kidney	0.3	23
Intermediate	Muscle	31.0	16
	Skin	3.6	8
Fat	Adipose tissue	12.5	6
Vessel poor	Residual tissue	11.3	—
Total		63.0	100

From Bard.[73] Data on adipose tissue and residual tissue have been added.

perfusion, their capacity for the drug (volume of tissue × tissue-blood partition coefficient), and the partial pressure gradient of drug between blood and tissue. The vessel-rich group of tissues achieves equilibrium with the blood more quickly than do other tissue groups (Table 2.2).[14] Although fat and muscle groups have similar tissue blood flows per unit of tissue, the higher solubility of most anesthetics (e.g., thiobarbiturates) in fat than in muscle accounts for the greater time required to achieve equilibrium for fat than for muscle. Changes in tissue blood flow, solubility, and blood-tissue partial pressure gradients thus influence uptake and distribution of intravenous anesthetics. Since the plasma concentration of an intravenous anesthetic falls rapidly (Fig. 2.1),[15] and its partial pressure is quickly exceeded by that in the vessel-rich tissues, anesthetic reenters the blood from these tissues to be redistributed to tissues that have greater time constants. This redistribution reduces anesthetic concentration in the brain, anesthesia lightens, and anesthetic accumulates in muscle, fat, and vessel-poor tissues.

The ultimate effect of any general anesthetic is contingent upon its ability to cross the blood-brain barrier. This barrier, like the placenta, has permeability characteristics of cellular membranes and therefore limits the penetration of nonlipophilic, ionized, or protein-bound drugs. Penetration of these barriers is, in fact, so slow that little or no drug of the aforementioned types enters the brain or fetus after a single intravenous bolus dose. The barriers are not, however, absolute, and slow penetration does occur, becoming significant when the level of drug is maintained over a prolonged period.[13] The high lipid solubility of thiopental relative to pentobarbital accounts for the more rapid onset of, and recovery from, anesthesia induced by the former.[16]

Within moments of tissue uptake and redistribution, elimination of the drug begins. The circulation distributes drug to vessel-rich organs able to biotransform and/or excrete it. The liver is the primary site of biotransformation, whereas the kidney is primarily responsible for excretion. Other organs may occasionally be involved, such as in the elimination of morphine via the gastrointestinal tract.[13] Biotransformation increases the rate of disappearance of the drug from active sites and converts most hypnotics

Table 2.2. Factors influencing rate of tissue equilibration of a drug such as thiopental.

Tissue	Blood Flow (L/min)	Tissue Volume (L)	Thiopental Tissue-Blood Partition Coefficient	Capacity[a]	Time Constant (min)[b]
Vessel-rich group	4.5	6	1.5	9	2
Muscle group	1.1	33	1.5	50	45
Fat group	0.32	14.5	11.0	160	500
Vessel-poor group	0.075	12.5	1.5	19	250

[a]Tissue volume × tissue-blood partition coefficient.
[b]Capacity/blood flow.
From Saidman.[14]

and anesthetics from lipophilic nonpolar compounds to polar water-soluble derivatives capable of excretion by the kidneys. Without such conversion, elimination of lipophilic nonvolatile drugs is markedly prolonged owing to reabsorption, after glomerular filtration, into the systemic circulation via the tubular epithelium. Although the metabolites produced by biotransformation are usually less active, in the case of prodrugs (e.g., chlo-

ral hydrate) toxic compounds may be produced.[17] The biotransformation rate is determined by the drug concentration at the site of metabolism (e.g., plasma concentration and hepatic blood flow) and by the intrinsic rate of the process. The latter is determined by such factors as enzymatic activity and cofactor availability (e.g., genetics, presence of other drugs, nutrition, or hypoxia).[13] Most drug metabolism follows first-order kinetics (a constant fraction is metabolized in a given period). In the event that the concentration exceeds the capacity of the biotransformation process (saturation), elimination assumes zero-order kinetics, where a constant amount of drug is eliminated,[13] and the pharmacological effect is disproportionately prolonged with increasing or multiple doses.[16] Species variations in biotransformation may also be encountered; for example, the duration and effects of lidocaine in humans, dogs, guinea pigs, and rats differ, and the glucuronide conjugation of drugs, such as morphine, salicylic acid, and propofol, in cats markedly differs from dogs.

Excretion subsequent to or independent of biotransformation is primarily a function of the kidney. Renal excretion is the principal process by which predominantly ionized drugs or those of limited lipid solubility are eliminated.[16] The excretion rate is determined by renal blood flow, glomerular filtration, and tubular secretion and reabsorption. Filtered drug passes through the glomerulus. Other drugs and metabolites may require the active transport processes of tubular secretion, which are sensitive to transport inhibitors and hypoxia. Reabsorption is efficient for those drugs (e.g., nonpolar lipophilics) able to penetrate cellular membranes and is modified by pH (drug ionization) and the rate of tubular urine flow.[13] Intravenous agents used to produce or facilitate anesthesia, such as barbiturates, narcotics, tranquilizers, and nondepolarizing relaxants, are excreted primarily by the kidneys.[15,18] Although inhalant anesthetics are primarily eliminated by exhalation, their metabolites are excreted largely by the kidney.

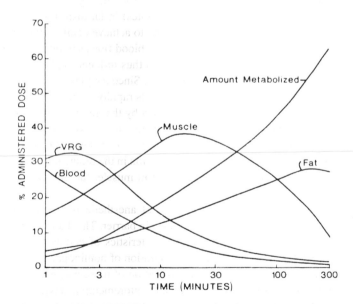

Fig. 2.1. Following an intravenous bolus, the percentage of thiopental remaining in blood rapidly decreases as the drug moves from the blood to the body tissues. Time to attainment of peak tissue levels is a direct function of tissue capacity for barbiturate relative to blood flow. Thus, a larger capacity or smaller blood flow is related to a longer time to reach a peak tissue level. Initially, most thiopental is taken up by the vessel-rich group (VRG) because of its high blood flow. Subsequently, the drug is redistributed to muscle and, to a lesser extent, to fat. Throughout this period, small but substantial amounts of thiopental are removed by the liver and metabolized. Unlike removal by the tissues, this removal is cumulative. Note that the rate of metabolism equals the early rate of removal by fat. The sum of this early removal by fat and metabolism is the same as the removal by muscle. From Eger.[15]

Factors Modifying Pharmacokinetics

It is thus apparent that many factors of common occurrence, such as rate of administration and concentration of anesthetic, physical status, muscular development, adiposity, respiratory and circulatory status, drug permeability coefficients, prior and/or concurrent drug administration, fear, recent feeding, and solubility of inhalant anesthetics in bags and hoses may all modify the uptake, distribution, and elimination of anesthetics. Concentration and rate of injection of a given dose affect anesthetic action, particularly with rapid-acting anesthetics. The more dilute the drug or slower the injection, the less is the effect produced.

Modification of cardiac output, ventilation, ventilation-perfusion ratios, and/or alveolar-capillary diffusion from any cause will influence both the uptake and elimination of inhalant drugs, most especially those of greater solubility. Some common examples causing these modifications include diaphragmatic hernia, pulmonary edema, pulmonary emphysema or atelectasis, and recumbency in large animals.

Permeation of the blood-brain barrier by narcotics and narcotic antagonists is contingent on partition coefficients, ionization, and protein binding, and is therefore influenced by hypocarbia and hypercarbia. For example, during hypocarbia (alkalemia), higher serum morphine concentrations, higher drug distribution in the lipid phase, and increased ratio of free base-acid salt of morphine facilitate penetration of morphine into the canine brain, despite decreased cerebral blood flow.[19]

Variation in distribution of blood to the vessel-rich and vessel-poor tissues, to fat, to muscle, and to the alveoli themselves will modify the pattern of induction and recovery. In shock, the proportion of the cardiac output flowing to the brain is increased, and the potential for redistribution is reduced. Owing to reduced blood volume, dilution of the drug is also diminished, as is hepatic and renal blood flow. The reduction in blood volume diminishes both biotransformation and renal excretion. Induction is thus rapid, the dose required is reduced, and recovery is delayed. Even removal of 2% of the body weight in blood tremendously prolongs dogs' recovery time from thiopental anesthesia.[2] It may thus be concluded that significant hemorrhage, such as might accompany a surgical bleed, will significantly increase sleeping time.

When fear, struggling, or fever occur, increases in cardiac output and decreases in circulation time prolong the time necessary for equilibration of inhalant anesthetic concentration between alveoli and pulmonary capillaries. Muscle and skin blood flow is increased, induction of inhalant anesthesia is delayed, and more anesthetic is required. It is well known that animals showing a period of excitement during induction of inhalant anesthesia always require more anesthetic. This causes a tendency toward overdosing, with its attendant dangers. For this reason, preanesthetic sedation is often advantageous.

Hounds such as the whippet, greyhound, Afghan, borzoi, wolfhound, and saluki have a low fat-to-body mass ratio, a low muscle-to-body mass ratio, and consequent increased blood levels of unbound drug when anesthetized with a barbiturate. Anesthesia with a barbiturate alone is thus characterized by increased sleep times, rougher recoveries, and occasional fatalities. Thin-type muscled or emaciated patients may have similar characteristics.[20]

According to Dukes,[21] a large meal of meat may increase the metabolic rate of dogs as much as 90% above the basal level (specific dynamic effect). Carbohydrate and fat also produce this elevation, though to a lesser extent. It is usually 12 to 18 h after the last meal before the basal metabolic rate is attained in carnivorous animals. In contrast, birds are more susceptible to starvation. A 6-h preanesthetic fast may induce hypoglycemia and marked sensitivity to depressant drugs in small birds.[22] Certainly it is important to consider that starvation induces low plasma glucose, mobilizes liver glycogen stores, and reduces circulating fatty acids, all of which may alter drug detoxification rates.[7] In addition to altering the metabolic rate, feeding increases chylomicrons in the blood. It has been shown that thiobarbiturates localize in these, which shortens the anesthesia time.[23] Feeding also increases blood flow to the abdominal viscera and influences overall anesthetic distribution.

With the exception of the gastrointestinal tract, nitrogen is the major gas constituent of closed internal body spaces. Owing to the high blood-gas partition coefficient of nitrous oxide relative to nitrogen and the gases of the intestinal tract, administration of nitrous oxide transfers this gas to internal gas spaces of the body. The volume or pressure of the gases within these spaces may thus increase. Volume increases in highly compliant spaces (e.g., intestinal, peritoneal, and thoracic) and pressure changes in noncompliant spaces (e.g., sinuses and middle ear).[15] In the intestinal loops of dogs anesthetized with halothane-oxygen and 75% nitrous oxide, the intestinal gas volume was shown to increase 1.8 times in 2 h and 2.5 times in 4 h, respectively. In experimental pneumothorax in dogs, the increase was more rapid: A 200-mL pneumothorax was doubled in 10 min, tripled in 45 min, and quadrupled in 2 h. In pneumoencephalograms in dogs, the inhalation of 75% nitrous oxide increased cisternal pressure by 60 torr in 10 min.[15] Consequently, the use of nitrous oxide is contraindicated in patients with pneumothorax, in those undergoing pneumoencephalograms, and in patients with intestinal obstructions requiring prolonged anesthesia.

Most noninhaled drugs are weak acids (barbiturates) or weak bases (narcotics, narcotic antagonists, and muscle relaxants). Once the drug is injected, equilibrium between ionized and nonionized forms of drug depends on the pH of the blood or tissues and the dissociation constant (pK_a) of the drug. A difference in pH between tissue and blood may thus cause a drug concentration difference. Plasma acidosis, for instance, increases intracellular barbiturate but decreases intracellular narcotic concentration.[14]

Drug availability at the site of action or of elimination is also modified by the degree of protein binding. Protein binding is diminished by uremia, hypoproteinemia, and minimally by administration of drugs competing for the binding sites. It may also be impaired by a change in pH or in the nature of the protein secondary to disease, or by dehydration. Decreased binding may make more drug available for specific action, with consequent increased sensitivity to a normal dose.[14]

Preanesthetic administration of opioid analgesics generally lowers the metabolic rate, whereas atropine administration causes a slight rise. When they are administered in combination, however, the metabolic rate is usually decreased. Generally speaking, tranquilizers can be expected to lower the metabolic rate.

It has been known for decades that administration of various drugs and pesticides can either stimulate or inhibit hepatic microsomal drug-metabolizing enzymes (enzyme induction and enzyme inhibition). More than 200 drugs are recognized as enzyme

Table 2.3. Examples of drugs capable of producing microsomal enzyme induction.

Hypnotics	Antihistaminics
Barbiturates	Diphenhydramine (Benadryl)
Glutethimide (Doriden)	Steroids
Ethanol	Cortisone
Chloral hydrate	Prednisone
Tranquilizers	Norethynodrel (Enovid)
Chlorpromazine (Thorazine)	Methyltestosterone
Promazine (Sparine)	Anesthetics
Meprobamate (Equanil)	Diethyl ether
Chlordiazepoxide (Librium)	Halothane (Fluothane)
Anticonvulsants	Insecticides
Diphenylhydantoin (Dilantin)	DDT
Methylphenylethylhydantoin (Mesantoin)	Chlordane

From Brown.[17]

Table 2.4. Interactions at tissue receptor sites.

The following agents have neuromuscular blocking properties. They may intensify the effects of nondepolarizing neuromuscular blocking agents (tubocurarine, gallamine, and dimethyl tubocurarine), or they may interact with each other:

Antibiotics	*General Anesthetics*
Bacitracin	Ether
Streptomycin, dihydro streptomycin	Halothane
	Methoxyflurane
Neomycin	
Kanamycin	*Other Agents*
Gentamicin	Muscle relaxants
Polymyxin B	Quinine
Oxytetracycline	Promethazine
Lincomycin	Magnesium sulfate
Other tetracyclines	Barbiturates
Colistimethate	Na citrate
Paronomycin	Organophosphorus insecticides
Vancomycin	

The following agents may intensify the neuromuscular blockade produced by succinylcholine:

Anticholinesterase agents
Magnesium sulfate

The following reactions occur at adrenergic receptor sites:

Drug 1	*Drug 2*	*Effect*
Epinephrine	Chloroform	Arrhythmias due to sensitization
Levarterenol	Halothane	of the heart to catechola-
Isoproterenol	Thiamylal	mines by Drug 2

From Abbitt.[74]

inducers (Table 2.3). Enzyme levels are maximally enhanced after approximately 5 days of administration of the inducing agent.[24] The nature of the induction varies with the type of drug, its dose, and the patient's age, thyroid function, and genetics, to name a few factors.[16,24] Enzyme induction with accelerated biotransformation reduces the pharmacological activity of drugs normally eliminated by biotransformation, such as certain barbiturates, tranquilizers, hypnotics, and anti-inflammatory drugs. Because inhalation anesthetics undergo minimal biotransformation, their elimination is influenced by enzyme induction less. Although this occurrence has little or no effect on the conduct of clinical anesthesia, it is of significance relative to viscerotoxicity. Inhalant anesthetics are variably metabolized to inorganic fluoride and hexafluoroisopropanol by cytochrome P-450, which, although produced in less than toxic concentrations ($<50 \mu m/L$), are potentially toxic to both the liver and the kidney.[25] The potential for such toxicity during anesthesia is enhanced by hypoxia. Toxicity associated with biotransformation is also enhanced by reduced liver antioxidants, such as glutathione or vitamin E. In all instances, toxicity of the organohalogens depends primarily on formation of reactive intermediates, especially those produced by non-oxygen-dependent (*reductive*) biotransformation,[25] and is contingent on the extent and type of biotransformation, and the metabolic and environmental drug pathways resulting from induction.[24] The extent to which such induced metabolic effects influence clinical animal anesthesia is unknown. Inhalant anesthetics (halothane, isoflurane, sevoflurane, and desflurane) are also known to form carbon monoxide and increase anesthetic circuit temperatures when they come in contact with soda lime or Barlyme.[26–28] The production of carbon monoxide is highest with desflurane and isoflurane and almost nonexistent with halothane and sevoflurane, although sevoflurane causes the greatest increases in anesthetic circuit temperature and can be degraded to a nephrotoxic vinyl ether (compound A).[29,30] Concentrations of compound A in the anesthetic circuit rarely reach nephrotoxic concentrations even during low-flow anesthesia unless the carbon dioxide–absorbant material has become desiccated.[30]

Hepatic microsomal enzymes may also be inhibited, with delay of biotransformation. Known inhibitors include organophosphorus insecticides, pesticide synergists of the methylenedioxyphenyl type, guanidine, carbon tetrachloride, chloramphenicol, tetracyclines, and certain inhalation anesthetics.[16,17] Inhibition has been illustrated by the prolonged plasma half-lives of barbiturates, narcotics, and local anesthetics during halothane anesthesia and by prolonged barbiturate anesthesia after a prior or concurrent chloramphenicol medication.[17,31]

Relevant drug interactions may also result from protein binding and interaction at receptor sites. To prevent or treat bacterial infections associated with surgery, antibiotics are often administered prior to, during, or immediately after general anesthesia. In many instances, little consideration is given to altered responses that may occur from the interaction between antibiotics and drugs commonly used in the operating room.[32] For example, a variety of antibiotics have been shown to cause neuromuscular blockage, the most notable of which are the aminoglycosides (Table 2.4).[32,33]

The effect of disease on the metabolic rate usually varies with its duration. In the early febrile stage, the rate may be increased;

however, as the disease progresses, toxemia may reduce the rate to low levels. Fever increases the metabolic rate in accordance with van't Hoff's law, which states that for each degree Fahrenheit the temperature rises, the metabolic rate increases by 7%. When animals suffer from toxemia or liver disease, liver functions are often impaired and the ability of the animal to detoxify anesthetics is depressed. Shock lowers the metabolic rate and, because of suppressed cardiovascular function, impairs uptake and distribution of anesthetic agents.

Hepatocellular disease causes reduced protein (primarily albumin) production with consequent limitation of protein binding, increased pharmacological activity of drugs, and unexpected sensitivity to such drugs as thiopental and propofol. Production of specific protein, such as pseudocholinesterase, may also be impaired, with consequent increased duration of action of succinylcholine. Hepatic disease may delay drug biotransformation because of enzyme inhibition or decreased hepatic blood flow.[34] Significant amounts of some drugs (e.g., morphine, chloramphenicol, and digitoxin) and/or their metabolites (polar, molecular weight > 300) are likely to be excreted in the bile.[16] Drugs dependent on hepatic elimination must therefore be administered with caution and modified by dose in the presence of hepatic disease.

Distribution and elimination of anesthetic and related drugs can also be impaired by renal disease with increased potential toxicity. Protein binding of organic acids is reduced in uremic patients, causing increased pharmacological activity (sensitivity); examples include pentobarbital, phenylbutazone, and cardiac glycosides. The increase in free-drug fraction in plasma of patients with renal disease correlates with the degree of hypoalbuminemia.[16] Renal disease may also limit excretion and thereby prolong activity of muscle relaxants, such as pancuronium.

The degree by which renal disease actually influences drug protein binding, and therefore overall drug activity and/or excretion, may be modified by fluid therapy (dilution or increased glomerular filtration) and by changes in plasma pH.[15]

Hyperthyroidism is accompanied by an elevated metabolic rate and may increase anesthetic requirement, whereas hypothyroidism is generally accompanied by a lowering of the metabolic rate and a reduced anesthetic requirement. Leukemia in some forms increases the metabolic rate, as does long-term severe pain, and thus these pathologies may likewise increase overall anesthetic requirement.[35]

Irradiation may affect (a) potency, onset, duration of action, and brain levels of injectable anesthetics, and (b) activity of the hepatic microsomal enzyme system.[36] Earlier onset of drug action can apparently be caused by radiation-induced modification of the blood-brain barrier. In adult animals, drug action is prolonged, which may be caused by (a) sensitization with a region-specific increase in brain serotonin and/or (b) partial inhibition of hepatic oxidase. Prenatal irradiation may impair the hepatic microsomal enzyme system. The anesthetic effects of barbiturates (thiopental and pentobarbital) decrease immediately after irradiation (1 to 3 h). Later, as irradiation sickness develops (days 10 to 15), sensitivity to anesthetics increases.[37]

Cellular Effects and Teratogenicity

Interest in mutagenic, carcinogenic, and teratogenic effects of anesthetics peaked after an increase in spontaneous abortions among anesthetists was noted in 1970.[38] It is assumed that this increased abortion rate was caused by chronic exposure to trace concentrations of anesthetics. Exposure to such anesthetic concentrations in the first trimester of pregnancy should be avoided. Exposure of rats to nitrous oxide on day 9 of gestation has been shown to cause fetal resorption and skeletal and soft tissue anomalies. Others have also demonstrated that inhalation anesthetics are teratogenic in animals, especially chicks.[38,39] Corresponding teratogenesis in humans has not been conclusively proved.

Epidemiological studies have suggested an increased incidence of cancer among women, but not men, who work in operating rooms.[34] Commonly used anesthetics, with the exception of fluroxene, have not been shown to be potential carcinogens by in vitro tests. Both general and local anesthetics can inhibit cell division. Anesthetics also affect such immune phenomena as cellular adherence, phagocytosis, lymphocyte transformation, chemotaxis, and the killing of tumor cells.[40]

Assessment of Anesthetic Actions

General anesthesia has simply been defined as complete unconsciousness.[41,42] When inducing this state, however, anesthetists require all the following components in patients: unconsciousness, insensitivity to pain, muscle relaxation, and absence of reflex response. The degree to which these are required for specific procedures varies. Anesthetists must therefore select the most suitable drugs and be able to assess the degree to which the varying effects are induced. Anesthesia depth is often difficult to assess, and several experimental measures, including minimum alveolar concentration (MAC) and minimum inhibitory concentration (MIC), have been developed for assessing and comparing anesthetic activity (Table 2.5).[41,42] Anesthetic drugs that induce adequate anesthesia in one species and operation may be insufficient at similar doses in another species. Signs characterizing a continuum of progressive increases in CNS depression and analgesia may not occur with some drugs and drug combinations. For example, the dissociatives do not induce the typical ocular signs of increasing CNS depression, and higher doses of propofol do not produce more insensitivity to pain commensurate with increased CNS depression. Consequently, veterinarians using modern anesthetic drugs must be familiar with their specific characteristics in order to use them effectively and safely.

Historically, the progressive changes produced by the administration of anesthetic drugs have been classified into four stages. Recognizing the signs characteristic of these stages following administration of most anesthetics enables anesthetists to determine whether the required CNS depression has been achieved or whether it is insufficient or too much.

Stages of General Anesthesia

For descriptive purposes, the levels of CNS depression induced by anesthetics have been divided into four stages depending on neuromuscular signs exhibited by patients (Table 2.6). It should

Table 2.5. Key terms.

Median alveolar concentration (MAC): The end-tidal concentration (in standardized pressure units) of inhaled anesthetic that ablates movement (e.g., withdrawal) in response to surgical incision in 50% of a test population. The MAC is synonymous with MAC immobility. The original acronym MAC stood for minimal alveolar concentration, an end point that measured the concentration of inhaled anesthetic required to block purposeful movement in an individual subject.

Median alveolar concentration awake (MAC-awake): The end-tidal concentration of inhaled anesthetic that prevents appropriate voluntary responses to spoken commands (e.g., to open one's mouth or to raise a hand) in 50% of a test population. This end point measures perceptive awareness rather than memory.

Median alveolar concentration for blunting autonomic responses (MAC-BAR): The end-tidal concentration of inhaled anesthetic that blocks changes in blood pressure and heart rate in response to surgical incision in 50% of a test population.

Minimum infusion rate (MIR): The minimum infusion rate of a drug, administered alone or in combination, required to eliminate reflexes commonly used to assess anesthetic depth (e.g., eyelid, laryngoscope, toe pinch, and tail clamp) in 50% of a test population.

Loss of righting reflexes (LORR): The failure of an animal to regain upright posture when placed on its back. Because this end point measures responses to nonnoxious stimuli, its dependence on anesthetic concentration is closely related to MAC-awake, which can be measured only in humans.

Potency: A measure of relative drug activity that is inversely related to the concentration required to produce a standard effect. A volatile anesthetic that produces a behavioral effect at half the concentration of another anesthetic is said to be twice as potent.

Hypnosis: There are various functional definitions of this term. We use it to connote drug-induced impairment of cognitive functions required for responding appropriately to environmental stimuli, including attention and perception. For a patient in the awake state, administration of inhaled anesthetics can produce a wide range of hypnotic depths, from mild inattention to unresponsiveness to noxious stimuli.

Sedation: There are various functional definitions of this term, which is sometimes used as a synonym for *hypnosis*. We use the term to connote drug-induced hypnosis with anxiolysis, diminished motor activity, and decreased arousal.

be emphasized that no clear division exists between stages, one blending into the next. In addition, variation in response among patients is to be expected. Preanesthetic medication, adequacy of oxygenation, carbon dioxide retention, and physical status of the patients all modify the signs. Patient response is also governed by the anesthetic that is being administered, considerable variation existing between anesthetics.

Stage I. This is termed the *stage of voluntary movement* and is defined as lasting from initial administration to loss of consciousness. Some analgesia may be present in the deeper phases of this stage. In any case, this stage is the most variable. Deviations are caused by the anesthetic used, from variations in the temperament and condition of the patient, from the manner in which the animal is restrained, and from the rate of induction. Nervous animals are bound to resist restraint. Should the anesthetic necessitate the use of a mask or be irritating to the upper airway, fear with consequent resistance by the patient will be accentuated. Excited, apprehensive animals may struggle violently and voluntarily hold their breath for short periods. Epinephrine release causes a strong, rapid heartbeat and pupillary dilation. Salivation is frequent in some species, as are urination and defecation. With the approach of stage II, animals become progressively ataxic, lose their ability to stand, and assume lateral recumbency. Initially, they can turn or lift the head without support.

Stage II. This is called the *stage of delirium or involuntary movement.* As the CNS becomes depressed, patients lose all voluntary control. This feature marks the change from stage I. By definition, this stage lasts from loss of consciousness to the onset of a regular pattern of breathing. As a result of anesthetic depression of the CNS, reflexes become more primitive and exaggerated. Patients react to external stimuli by violent reflex struggling, breath holding, tachypnea, and hyperventilation. Continued catecholamine release causes a fast, strong heartbeat, cardiac arrhythmias may occur, and the pupils may be widely dilated. Eyelash and palpebral reflexes are prominent. Nystagmus commonly occurs in horses. During this stage, animals may whine, cry, bellow, or neigh, depending on the species concerned. In some species, especially ruminants and cats, salivation may be excessive; in dogs, cats, and goats, vomiting may be evoked. The larynx of cats and pigs is very sensitive at this stage, and stimulation may cause laryngeal spasms. Jaw tone is still present, and attempts at endotracheal intubation are met with struggling and may initiate vomition in dogs and cats and active regurgitation in ruminants. In view of the exaggerated reflex responses during this stage, stimulation of any kind should be avoided.

Stage III. This is the stage of *surgical anesthesia* and is characterized by unconsciousness with progressive depression of the reflexes. Muscular relaxation develops, and ventilation becomes slow and regular. Vomiting and swallowing reflexes are lost.

In humans, this stage has been further divided into planes 1 to 4 for finer differentiation. Others have suggested the simpler classification of light, medium, and deep. Light anesthesia persists until eyeball movement ceases. Medium anesthesia is characterized by progressive intercostal paralysis, and deep anesthesia by diaphragmatic respiration.[43] A medium depth of unconsciousness or anesthesia has traditionally been considered a light plane of surgical anesthesia (stage III, plane 2) characterized by stable respiration and pulse rate, abolished laryngeal reflexes, a sluggish palpebral reflex, a strong corneal reflex, and adequate muscle relaxation and analgesia for most surgical procedures. Deep surgical anesthesia (stage III, plane 3) is characterized by decreased intercostal muscle function and tidal volume, increased respiration rate, profound muscle relaxation, diaphragmatic breathing, a weak corneal reflex, and a centered and dilated pupil. If CNS depression is allowed to increase further, patients will progress to stage IV.

Stage IV. In this stage, the CNS is extremely depressed, and

Table 2.6. Characteristics of the stages of general anesthesia.

System Affected	Characteristic Observed	Stage I	Stage II	Stage III — Plane 1 (Light)	Plane 2 (Medium)	Plane 3	Plane 4 (Deep)	Stage IV
Cardiovascular	Pulse[a]	Tachycardia			Progressive bradycardia			Weak or imperceptible
	Blood pressure[a]	Hypertension		Normal	Increasing hypotension			Shock level
	Capillary refill	1 s or less			Progressive delay			3 s or longer
	Dysrhythmia probability	++	+++	++	+		++	++++
Respiratory	Respiratory rate[a]	Irregular or increased		Progressive decrease			Slow irregular	Ceased; may gasp terminally
	Respiratory depth[a]	Irregular or increased		Progressive decrease			Irregular	Ceased
	Mucous membrane, skin color			Normal			Cyanosis	Pale to white
	Respiratory action	May be breath holding		Thoracoabdominal, abdominal			Diaphragmatic	Ceased
	Cough reflex	++++		+	Lost			
	Laryngeal reflex	++++ May vocalize		Lost				
	Intubation possible	No	Yes					
Gastrointestinal	Salivation	++++	++++	+	Diminished, absent, except in ruminants			Absent
	Oropharyngeal reflex	++++	++++	+	Lost			
	Vomition probability	+++	+++	+	Very slight			
	Reflux (regurgitation) potential	None		Increases with relaxation			++++	
	Tympany (rumen, cecum)	None		Potential increases with duration of anesthesia				
Ocular	Pupils	Dilated			Normal or constricted, progressive dilation			Acutely dilated
	Corneal reflex	Normal	+++		Diminishes, lost (horses may persist)			Absent
	Lacrimation	Normal	+++		Diminishes, absent			Absent
	Photomotor reflex	Normal	+++		Diminishes, absent			Absent
	Palpebral reflex	Normal	+++		Diminishes, absent			Absent
	Eyeball position	Normal	Variable		Ventromedial in dogs and cats or central			
	Nystagmus	++++ Especially horses and cows					+	None
Musculoskeletal	Jaw tone	++++			Decreased, minimal		Lost	
	Limb muscle tone	++++			Decreased, minimal		Lost	
	Abdominal muscle tone	++++		++	Decreased, minimal			Lost
	Sphincters (anus, bladder)	May void		Lost	Progressive relaxation		Control lost	Lost
Nervous	Sensorium	++	+	Lost				
	Pedal reflex	++++	++++	Decreased	Absent			
	Reaction to surgical manipulation	++++	++++	+	None			

[a]Surgical stimulation causes increased heart rate, blood pressure, and respiratory rate via autonomic responses that persist in plane 2. Vagal reflexes due to visceral traction persist in plane 3.

+ to ++++ = degree present.

respirations cease. The heart continues to beat only for a short time. Blood pressure is at the shock level, capillary refill of visible mucous membranes is markedly delayed, and the pupils are widely dilated. The anal and bladder sphincters relax. Death quickly intervenes unless immediate resuscitative steps are taken. If the anesthetic is withdrawn and artificial respiration is initiated before myocardial collapse, these effects may be overcome and patients will go through the various stages in reverse.

The stages just described are best seen when inhalant anesthetics are administered, probably because considerable time is required for an anesthetic concentration to accrue in the CNS. This allows the various signs to become apparent. With some intravenous anesthetics (e.g., dissociatives) or the concurrent use of preanesthetic sedatives, anesthetic-induced depression is difficult to assess, and signs of anesthetic depression are not uniformly apparent.

Signs of Anesthesia

Respiration

Respiratory minute volume typically increases during stage I especially if preanesthetic sedation is not used. As anesthetic depression increases to stage II, respirations become irregular, and breath holding commonly occurs. With the onset of stage III, breathing once again becomes regular. The respiration depth at this time depends on the respiratory threshold to stimulation; surgical manipulation, for instance, stimulates respiration, whereas premedication depresses it. If barbiturates or propofol are used for either preanesthetic sedation or induction, early respiratory depression occurs. During stage III, the intercostal muscles and the diaphragm weaken progressively.[44] The depth of respiration declines progressively, thoracic movement decreases, respiration becomes largely or entirely abdominal, and the respiration rate may increase. With an overdosage, respiration becomes entirely abdominal, and diaphragmatic contraction causes the abdomen to bulge during inspiration and the thorax to collapse. During expiration, the reverse occurs, the anterior excursion of the diaphragm causing the thorax to expand. With progressive overdosage, diaphragmatic movements become smaller, respiratory exchange diminishes further, and respirations are gasping and ultimately cease. In dogs, oral and cervical movements (tracheal tugging) may be observed during this stage.

Circulation

Although blood pressure may be monitored by indirect methods or by direct arterial catheterization, veterinarians often do not measure pressure, but must depend on the pulse rate or bleeding at the surgical site, and on induction of momentary blanching by compressing an exposed mucous membrane (such as the conjunctiva, oral mucosa, or tongue) to give some indication of the circulatory status of patients. The mucous membranes may show pallor as a result of hemorrhage or shock and cyanosis caused by hypoxia. In rodents, feet, ears, and muzzles are observed for such signs; in poultry, it is necessary to examine the comb and/or wattles; in rats and rabbits, the color of light reflected from the eye is helpful.

During stages I and II, the pulse is strong and accelerated. Arrhythmias sometimes occur during stage II. In stage III, the pulse rate is regular and usually slightly accelerated. During inhalant anesthesia, progressive bradycardia occurs. Pain stimulation in light stage III may induce tachycardia or even arrhythmias. As the anesthesia depth increases, blood pressure declines, and the pulse weakens.

Ocular Signs

These include eyeball position and movement, photomotor reflexes and pupillary size, lacrimation, and palpebral, corneal, and conjunctival reflexes. Although ocular signs are often helpful, they can be quite variable in most species and should never replace observation of respiratory and circulatory signs.[45] Eyeball movement is especially valuable in horses, in which nystagmus occurs with the onset of stage II and continues through light surgical anesthesia. In cattle, eyeball rotation is very consistent and a reliable indicator of anesthetic depth whether anesthesia is produced by inhalation anesthetics, barbiturates, or combinations of central muscle relaxants, dissociatives, and α_2-agonists (Fig. 2.2). In light and medium surgical anesthesia in dogs, cats, and pigs, their eyeballs are generally turned downward. The eyelids during this time are usually closed, and the third eyelid overlays the medial portion of the cornea. The palpebral reflex becomes sluggish in all species when surgical anesthesia is attained. The pupillary size is modified by the degree of light and by premedication with such drugs as morphine and atropine. The pupils are dilated during stage II but thereafter constrict. In deep (stage III, plane 4) anesthesia or stage IV, pupillary dilation indicates overdosage. Reflex constriction of the pupil on exposure to light stimuli (photomotor reflex) is lost on transition from light to medium surgical anesthesia.

Lacrimation is no longer observed in the deeper stages of surgical anesthesia. In horses, lacrimation is a consistent sign of light surgical anesthesia. Because the eyes may also be open in deep anesthesia, the cornea appears dull and is subject to the adverse effects of drying. To protect against this hazard, ointment should be applied to the eyes or they should be taped closed after anesthesia has been induced. The palpebral reflex, which is a blink induced by touching the eyelids, becomes sluggish or is lost as medium surgical anesthesia develops. Blinking induced by gently touching the cornea (corneal reflex) is variable, but is usually lost shortly after the palpebral reflex. In horses, the corneal reflex persists into deeper anesthesia.

Pharyngeal and Upper-Airway Reflexes

Suppression of these reflexes is of particular importance for endotracheal intubation and for induction of anesthesia in animals, such as ruminants, with full stomachs. Coughing and laryngospasm in response to intubation are lost in light surgical anesthesia, but may persist into medium anesthesia in cats. The intensity of these responses varies with the animal species concerned: especially intense in the cat, and relatively mild in cattle and horses. The swallowing and vomiting reflexes disappear with the onset of stage III; like the laryngeal reflexes, the swallowing reflex persists into medium anesthesia in cats.

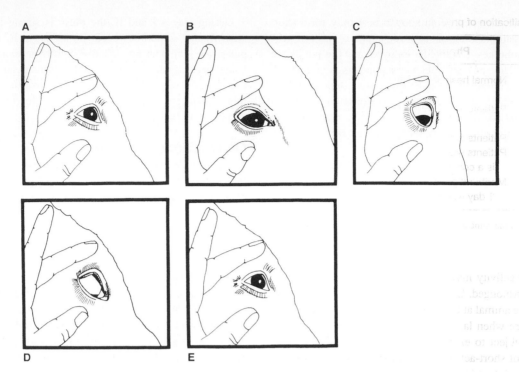

Fig. 2.2. Eyeball position during induction and maintenance of general anesthesia of cows. **A:** Position of the cow's eye when awake and positioned in lateral recumbency. Induction of anesthesia is accompanied by a progressive ventral rotation of the eyeball, becoming partially obscured by the lower eyelid. **B and C:** As the depth of anesthesia is increased, the cornea becomes completely hidden by the lower eyelid. **D:** At this time, surgical anesthesia is present. Applying traditional methods of assessing anesthetic depth, the cow would be in stage III, plane 2 to 3. Increasing the depth of anesthesia causes the eye to rotate dorsally, with the cornea becoming centered between the palpebra. **E:** At this time, deep surgical anesthesia with profound muscle relaxation and central nervous system depression is present. Eye reflexes have been lost, and the cornea will appear dry and wrinkled. Maintaining this extreme depth of anesthesia can rapidly end in death of the patient. Decreasing the depth of anesthesia is accompanied by eyeball rotation occurring in reverse order. From Thurmon and Benson.[75]

Other Signs of Anesthesia

After an initial increase during stage II, muscle tone progressively declines, as indicated by relaxation of the abdominal muscles, decreasing efficiency of the intercostal muscles, and reduced resistance to passive flexion of the limbs. In lean animals with shorthaired coats, abdominal muscle relaxation may be such that the profile of viscera is readily apparent. The contour of the rumen may become visible in some ruminants. In cats, detectable extensor tone, in response to passive flexion of the limb by pushing on the digits, persists into medium surgical anesthesia. Generally, limb muscles are relaxed in light anesthesia, whereas abdominal muscles are not well relaxed until anesthesia is deep. The tone of the anal sphincter of horses is a good indicator of relaxation in this species. During stage II, the sphincter is tight, but as anesthetic depth increases, the sphincter relaxes so that in deep surgical anesthesia it may gape to such an extent that feces can be observed in the anal canal. Concomitant with progressive dilatation, the anal sphincter gradually loses ability to contract in response to mechanical stimulation in medium to deep surgical anesthesia. Deliberate anal dilation induces an increase in respiratory rate; this respiratory reflex is lost during early stage III.

In dogs, response to opening the jaw is considered to be a useful sign by many veterinarians. During transition from stage II to stage III, passive opening of the mouth may elicit yawning, which is a response especially likely in barbiturate anesthesia. Resistance to opening the mouth fully is lost in medium anesthesia. The digital (pedal) reflex, in which the limb is flexed in response to painful stimulation of the digits or interdigital region, is also a useful guide to the depth of anesthesia in dogs, cats, and rats. This reflex is lost as the transition from light to medium surgical anesthesia occurs. Head shaking in response to ear pinching is a helpful sign in cats, rabbits, and guinea pigs, and is lost with the onset of surgical anesthesia. In cattle and cats, the ear-flick reflex in response to tactile stimulation of the hairs within the pinna remains until a medium level of anesthesia is present. Twitching of the whiskers in response to ear pinching is lost as light anesthesia progresses to medium. Response to painful stimulation by pinching the tail of rodents and snakes and the wattles or combs of birds is a useful indicator of the onset of surgical anesthesia. The anal reflex remains until a deeper plane of anesthesia is achieved in birds and is often referred to as the *vent reflex* in this species.

Signs of Anesthesia Recovery

As anesthetic drugs are eliminated from the CNS, the degree of anesthesia lightens and reverse progress through the stages of anesthesia occurs. Induction techniques are usually selected and performed to minimize the duration of stage II, in which excite-

Table 2.7. Classification of physical status[a].

Category	Physical Status	Possible Examples of This Category
I	Normal healthy patients	No discernible disease; animals entered for ovariohysterectomy, ear trim, caudectomy, or castration
II	Patients with mild systemic disease	Skin tumor, fracture without shock, uncomplicated hernia, cryptorchidectomy, localized infection, or compensated cardiac disease
III	Patients with severe systemic disease	Fever, dehydration, anemia, cachexia, or moderate hypovolemia
IV	Patients with severe systemic disease that is a constant threat to life	Uremia, toxemia, severe dehydration and hypovolemia, anemia, cardiac decompensation, emaciation, or high fever
V	Moribund patients not expected to survive 1 day with or without operation	Extreme shock and dehydration, terminal malignancy or infection, or severe trauma

[a]This classification is the same as that adopted by the American Society of Anesthesiologists.

ment and motor activity may occur. During recovery, however, stage II can be prolonged. Every effort should be made to avoid stimulation of the animal at this time. This stage of recovery is of particular concern when large animals are anesthetized. Horses are especially subject to excitement and struggling during this period. The use of short-acting anesthetics and postoperative sedation can do much to minimize recovery delirium.

During recovery, the question arises of how best to judge the recovery from anesthesia, particularly when so many modifying factors must be considered. Experienced anesthetists find themselves relying less on classic signs of anesthesia and more on a patient's response to stimuli. Needless to say, effective anesthesia is not only that which just obliterates a patient's response to painful stimuli without excessive depression of vital functions, but also that from which recovery is relatively rapid and uneventful.

Patient Evaluation and Preparation

A thorough history should be recorded and a complete physical examination performed before anesthesia. Every animal should be categorized regarding its physical health, pain and stress status, and anesthetic risk (Table 2.7). Appropriate medical and nursing issues should be reviewed and provided before producing anesthesia.

Preanesthetic Evaluation

The purpose of the preanesthetic patient evaluation is to determine a patient's physical status. In general, *physical status* refers to the presence or absence of disease, severity of pain (if present), and the level of stress. Specifically, the term refers to a patient's medical condition, including the degree of pain and stress and the overall efficiency and function of organ systems. The goal is to determine any deviations from the norm that will affect anesthetic uptake, action, elimination, and safety. Organ systems of greatest concern are the nervous, cardiopulmonary, hepatic, and renal. Knowledge of the physical status is an aid to selection of anesthetic drugs and techniques and arriving at a preanesthetic prognosis. Physical status is one of the best determinants of the likelihood of cardiopulmonary emergencies occurring during the anesthetic period. As such, it is much better than arbitrary predic-

tors such as age. It is axiomatic that the sicker a patient (the poorer the physical status) is, the greater is the likelihood of adverse events or death. Physical status is determined by (a) history, including an assessment of pain; (b) inspection (attitude, condition, conformation, temperament, stress, or distress); (c) palpation, percussion, and auscultation; and (d) laboratory determinations and special procedures (e.g., radiographs). Any abnormalities should be noted. Those that can be corrected should be. If no further improvement can be reasonably corrected by medical treatment, the patient's overall risk and prognosis can be determined.

The history and physical examination are the best determinants of the presence of disease. Laboratory tests should be done on the basis of the physical exam and history. The use of extensive laboratory screening of patients has not been found to improve the outcome of surgical patients in either human or veterinary medicine. Laboratory screenings frequently fail to uncover pathological conditions, they detect abnormalities that do not necessarily improve patient care or outcome, and they are inefficient in screening for asymptomatic disease. Moreover, abnormalities that are detected seldom have any impact on anesthetic protocol or surgical management.[46]

The use of multiple chemical and enzymatic analyses of blood and urine in surgical patients has become common with the advent of automated analyzers and their availability to veterinarians. Their use, as previously noted, has not appreciably improved the outcome of veterinary surgical patients. Frequently, when an abnormal value is reported, surgery is delayed and the test rerun, adding to the total cost of the procedure, with little patient benefit. It should be remembered that reference ranges compare the test result with a set of values from a group of similar animals in a defined state of health (determined by physical examination). The reference range, *normal*, is presumed to be within ±2 standard deviations of the mean. A common error, however, is to assume that the upper and lower limits of this presumed normal range represent a rigid cutoff point between a state of health and disease or normal and abnormal function. Indeed, 5% of normal animals fall outside this range. Furthermore, a test result in the normal range (within 2 standard deviations of the mean) implies that function is normal, but does not account for normoglycemic diabetics or animals with cirrhosis that have normal hepatic enzymes and bilirubin values. Because 5% of nondiseased animals fall outside the normal range as previously defined, 1 of 20 healthy animals tested will fall outside the range. If multiple tests are performed, the frequency of abnormal test results in nondiseased animals increases with the number of tests done. As the number of tests increases, the likelihood of an abnormal result in a nondiseased animal increases. In a ten-test profile of independent parameters, there is a 40% chance of at least one test result being outside the reference range. Reference ranges do provide useful standards by which extreme test values can be recognized. However, there is no consistent relationship between the extremeness of test results and the presence of a disease. Frequently, there is overlap in the distribution of measured test values between healthy and diseased populations. This is caused in part by the statistical nature of the reference ranges, the inherent spectrum of disease (latent to fulminant), and the variable rate of disease progression and host response that the test measures. Thus, test results must be carefully interpreted in light of the physical examination and the history and not rigidly interpreted on an empirical basis of simply being more than 2 standard deviations from the mean of the reference population.[47]

A thorough preanesthetic evaluation of patients is essential for successful anesthesia and subsequent surgery. Every effort should be made to detect factors that may modify anesthetic action and safety, emphasizing concurrent diseases, current or projected painful conditions, and stress status. Although such evaluation is important in all patients, it is especially important in critically ill patients. In addition to body weight and vital signs, the following should be included: The history should include previous and current health; presenting complaint, its severity, and its duration; concurrent symptoms of disease (e.g., diarrhea, vomiting, exercise intolerance, ascites, rales, dyspnea, and polyurea-polydipsia); pregnancy; exposure to drugs; prior anesthetic history; and recent feeding. Especially important to consider are the status of cardiopulmonary function, the potential of acid-base or electrolyte imbalance, the possibility of a full or distended stomach or of hepatic or renal disease, and the prior or concurrent administration of drugs (e.g., organophosphates, diuretics, digitalis preparations, anticonvulsants, corticosteroids, aminoglycoside antibiotics, sulfonamides, and nonsteroidal anti-inflammatory drugs).

All body systems should be examined and any abnormalities identified. The physical examination and medical history will determine the extent to which laboratory tests and special procedures are necessary. In all but extreme emergencies, packed cell volume and plasma protein concentration should be routinely determined. Contingent on the medical history and physical examination, additional evaluations may include complete blood counts; urinalysis; blood chemistries to identify the status of kidney and liver function, blood gases, and pH; electrocardiography; clotting time and platelet counts; fecal and/or filarial examinations; and blood electrolyte determinations. Tests should not be run unless it is suspected their results could cause a change in anesthetic management. Radiographic and/or fluoroscopic examination may also be indicated, especially in animals, such as primates, calves, sheep, and rodents, that are susceptible to chronic respiratory infections.

Following examination, the physical status of the patient should be classified as to its general state of health according to the American Society of Anesthesiologists (ASA) classification and the information recorded (Table 2.7). This mental exercise forces the anesthetist to evaluate the patient's condition and proves valuable in the proper selection of anesthetic drugs. Classification of overall health is an essential part of any anesthetic-record system. The preliminary physical examination should be done in the owner's presence, if possible, so that a prognosis can be given personally. This allows the client to ask questions and enables the veterinarian to communicate the risks of anesthesia and allay any fears regarding management of the patient.

Pain

Pain and the biological responses to it are part of a highly integrated warning system directed toward maintaining homeostasis and preventing further injury.[48] Pain, along with heart rate, respiratory rate, temperature, and blood pressure, should be considered the fifth clinical sign routinely assessed prior to medical treatment. The pain system includes sensors, neural pathways, and processing centers that are responsible for detecting, transmitting, and activating animals' biological and behavioral responses to noxious events. Pain warns animals of potential tissue damage and protects them from further injury. Animal pain has been defined as "an aversive feeling or sensation associated with actual or potential tissue damage," broadening the dictionary definition to include behavioral changes, neuroendocrine activation, and the "stress response."[48] The latter definition is the basis for why pain perception alone is not considered to fully represent the pain experience and helps to explain the relationship between painful experiences and pain behaviors in animals. Nociception is the neurophysiological process whereby noxious mechanical, chemical, or thermal stimuli are transduced into electrical signals (action potentials) by high-threshold pain receptors (nociceptors) located on the peripheral terminals of very thin, noninsulated or minimally insulated (myelinated) C and A-δ nerve fibers, respectively.[48] These electrical signals are subsequently transmitted to the superficial and deeper layers of the dorsal horn of the spinal cord, modified (modulated), and projected to the brain (perception). The free nerve endings of afferent sensory pain fibers encode noxious stimuli, depending on the modality, intensity, duration, and location of the stimulus. The intensity of the stimulus producing pain is considerably greater than that required to elicit innocuous sensations and is the most important factor determining the severity of pain. In the absence of tissue damage, pain is considered to be *physiological* or "ouch" pain, which warns and protects animals from tissue damage. *Pathological* pain occurs when tissues or nerves are damaged and has been "clinically" categorized based on the most likely mechanism responsible (e.g., inflammation, neuropathy, and cancer).[48] Unlike physiological pain, pathological pain can be produced by stimulation of large myelinated A-β nerve fibers, which normally do not transmit painful sensations. Severe injuries and chronic pathological pain states can change (dynamic plasticity) the intensity of the stimulus required to initiate pain (hypersensitivity). The development of tissue hypersensitivity (nociceptor sensitization) can be responsible for the development of increased sensitivity to noxious stimuli (hyperalgesia) and painful sensations arising from normally nonpainful perceptions (allodynia).

Tissue damage and inflammation can result in the activation and release of intracellular components from damaged cells, inflammatory cells (lymphocytes, neutrophils, and macrophages), and the primary nerve fiber itself. The local release and spread of ions (hydrogen and potassium), prostaglandins (prostaglandin E_2), bradykinin, cyclooxygenase, neurotrophic growth factors and cytokines (interleukin 1, interleukin 6, and tumor necrosis factor α [TNF-α]) sensitize pain fibers to subsequent painful and nonpainful stimuli.[48] Mast cell degranulation increases the local concentration of 5-hydroxytryptamine (5-HT or serotonin) and histamine. Together these substances produce a "sensitizing soup" that lowers the threshold of nociceptors and activates "silent" nociceptors (10% to 40% of the total nociceptor population), amplifying the pain response and producing a zone of primary hyperalgesia.[48] Local vasodilation and plasma extravasation further amplify the inflammatory response and spread hypersensitivity to surrounding tissues, and hypersensitivity to nonpainful stimuli occurs.

More severe tissue trauma or nerve damage produces electrical signals that continuously bombard dorsal horn neurons, producing a cumulative effect and activation of alternate receptors on dorsal horn neurons, resulting in central sensitization. Central sensitization occurs when the cumulative effects of frequent (chronic) or severe peripheral nociceptor input releases excessive quantities of CNS neurotransmitters (substance P, neurokinin A, and brain-derived neurotrophic factor), including glutamate, which activates N-methyl-D-aspartate and other receptors, resulting in an increase in sensitization (windup) of neurons in the dorsal horn of the spinal cord.[48] Sensitization of dorsal horn neurons can last for hours and is believed to be responsible for pain outside the area of tissue injury (secondary hyperalgesia) and allodynia. Central sensitization is fundamentally different from peripheral sensitization in that the former enables low-intensity stimuli to produce pain sensations. When pain is chronic, central sensitization enables sensory fibers that normally transmit nonpainful stimuli (low-threshold A-β fibers) to produce pain as a result of changes in sensory processing in the spinal cord. Central sensitization increases the responsiveness of dorsal horn neurons to sensory inputs (allodynia), expands receptive field, and is believed to be responsible for the discomfort and agony produced by severe injury. Chronic pain, therefore, can be responsible for activity-dependent plasticity and long-term structural changes (neuroplastic) within the CNS, leading to the development or modification of memory patterns that change animal behavior. Together the development of windup and central sensitization represent a process that exists as a consequence of continuous, unrelenting, and untreated pain causing stress and distress. The diagnosis and treatment of pain, therefore, require an appreciation of its consequences, a fundamental understanding of the mechanisms responsible for its production, and a practical appreciation of the analgesic drugs that are available. Semiobjective and objective behavioral, numerical, and categorical methods

Table 2.8. American Animal Hospital Association pain management standards (2003).

1. Pain assessment for all patients regardless of presenting complaint
2. Pain assessment using standardized scale/score and recorded in the medical record
3. Pain management is individualized for each patient
4. Practice utilizes preemptive pain management
5. Appropriate pain management is provided for the anticipated level and duration of pain
6. Pain management is provided for the anticipated level and duration of pain
7. Patient is reassessed for pain throughout potentially painful procedure
8. Patients with persistent or recurring disease are evaluated to determine their pain management needs
9. Analgesic therapy is used as a tool to confirm the existence of a painful condition when pain is suspected but cannot be confirmed by objective methods
10. A written pain management protocol is utilized
11. When pain management is part of the therapeutic plan, the client is effectively educated

have been developed for the diagnosis of pain and, among these, the visual analogue scale (VAS) has become popular. A trained observer rates pain along a 10-cm line from no pain to worst possible pain and, based on this rating, prescribes appropriate therapy. Ideally, pain therapy should be directed toward the mechanisms responsible for its production (multimodal therapy), with consideration, when possible, of initiating therapy before pain is initiated (preemptive therapy). The American Animal Hospital Association (AAHA) has developed standards for the assessment, diagnosis, and therapy of pain that should be adopted by all veterinarians (Table 2.8).

Stress

Animals feel pain, which affects their physiology, quality of life, and interactions with their environment. Pain normally serves a protective function by warning animals of real or impending tissue damage but, when severe or chronic, is responsible for temporary periods of dramatic increases in sympathoadrenal and neuroendocrine activity, which is commonly referred to as the *stress response*. Both acute and chronic pain can produce stress.[49] Untreated pain can initiate an extended and potentially destructive series of events characterized by neuroendocrine dysregulation, fatigue, dysphoria, myalgia, abnormal behavior, and altered physical performance. This type of response has been termed the *sickness syndrome*. Even without a painful stimulus, environmental factors (loud noise, restraint, or a predator) can produce a state of anxiety or fear that sensitizes and amplifies the stress response. *Distress*, an exaggerated form of stress, is present when the biological cost of stress negatively affects the biological functions critical to survival. Pain, therefore, should be considered in terms of the stress response and the potential to develop distress.

Normally, the stress response is an adaptive pattern of neural, behavioral, endocrine, immune, hematologic, and metabolic changes directed toward maintaining or restoring homeostasis.[49] Most stress is temporary because the stressor is removed. During threatening circumstances, the stress response prepares animals for an emergency reaction and fosters survival (fight or flight). Acute pain can produce significant stress in dogs and cats. Pain induced by surgical or accidental trauma evokes characteristic responses typified by activation of the sympathetic branch of the autonomic nervous system, secretion of glucocorticoids (primarily cortisol), hypermetabolism, sodium and water retention, and altered carbohydrate and protein metabolism (Table 2.9). Increased central sympathetic output causes increases in heart rate and arterial blood pressure, sweating, piloerection, and pupil dilatation. The secretion of catecholamines from the adrenal medulla and spillover of norepinephrine released from postganglionic sympathetic nerve terminals augment these central effects. Increased concentrations of circulating catecholamines augment glycogenolysis and gluconeogenesis and promote insulin resistance. Corticotrophin-releasing factor (CRF) is released from the hypothalamus, amplifying the startle response, anxiety, fear and, in some animals, rage. CRF serves as an excitatory neurotransmitter releasing cortical norepinephrine, dopamine, and 5-HT, with resultant behavioral changes, including hyperresponsiveness, hyperarousal, vigilance, and agitation. Mild to moderate acute pain caused by tissue trauma may activate the immune response. Severe acute pain produces behavioral, autonomic, neuroendocrine, and immunologic responses that upset homeostasis and can lead to self-mutilation and immune incompetence. Chronic pain produces sustained increases in circulating concentrations of cortisol, epinephrine, norepinephrine, and glucagon, suppressing both the humoral and cellular immune response. The systemic release of endogenous opioids (endorphin and enkephalin) may contribute to immunosuppression. The messengers of the immune system are cytokines (interleukin 1, interleukin 6, and TNF-α). The acute-phase response can be triggered by severe stress from any cause. The main feature of the acute-phase response is the release of proteins from the liver that act as inflammatory mediators and scavengers in tissue repair. They include C-reactive protein, fibrinogen, macroglobulin, and antiproteinases. Excessive production of these proteins can contribute to the development or maintenance of the systemic inflammatory-response syndrome (SIRS). The peripheral blood white cell count generally reflects a stress leukogram typified by an elevated number of immature polymorphonuclear leukocytes (left shift) and reduced numbers of lymphocytes. Stress induced by chronic pain often produces morphological changes that are typical of long-term aversive stimuli and include a failure to thrive, poor hair coat, weight loss, and acceleration of aging. Ultimately, changes in an animal's behavior may be the most noninvasive and promising method to monitor the severity of an animal's pain and associated stress.

Patient Preparation

Too often, operations are undertaken with inadequate preparation of patients. Some foresight here is beneficial. With most types of

Table 2.9. Consequences and indicators of the stress response.

Neurohumoral response
Pituitary
  Adrenocorticotropic hormone increases
  Growth hormone increases
  Vasopressin increases
  Thyroid-stimulating hormone increases
Adrenal cortex
  Cortisol increases
  Aldosterone increases
  Catecholamines increase
Pancreas
  Insulin often decreases
  Glucagon increases
Thyroid
  Thyroxine decreases

Systemic effects
Activation of CNS
  Hypothalamus, amygdala, and locus caeruleus
Increases in CNS sympathetic output
  Catecholamines
Endocrine "stress" response
  Pituitary hormone secretion
  Adrenal hormone secretion
Glucosemia
Insulin resistance
Cytokine production
Acute-phase reaction
Neutrophil leukocytosis
Immunologic and hematologic changes

Indicators of stress caused by pain
Reduced activity
  Quiet/loss of curiosity
  Less social
  Loss of appetite
  Stiff posture/gait
Refuses to move
  Vocalizes
  Stops grooming
  Guards
  Self-mutilation

CNS, central nervous system.

general anesthesia, it is best to have patients off feed for 12 h previously. It should be recalled that some species are adversely affected by fasting. Birds, neonates, and small mammals may become hypoglycemic within a few hours of starvation, and mobilization of glycogen stores may alter rates of drug metabolism and clearance. The latter may be a factor in ruminants. In contrast, feeding dogs increases their metabolic rate for up to 18 h. Induction of anesthesia in animals having a full stomach should be avoided, if at all possible, because of the hazards of aspiration. Distension of the rumen in sheep and larger ruminants has been shown to impair ventilation, with consequent hypoxemia and hypercapnia.[50] In horses, a full stomach may rupture during induction and casting. Although limitation of food does not empty the rumen, the possibility of regurgitation is perhaps reduced if water is withheld for 12 to 24 h prior to induction.

In most species, especially in the young and aged, water is usually offered up to the time that preanesthetic agents are administered. It should be remembered that many older animals suffer from renal disease. Although these animals remain compensated under ideal conditions, the stress of hospitalization, water deprivation, and anesthesia, even without surgery, may cause acute decompensation. To withhold water from these animals, even for short periods, may prove hazardous. Ideally, a mild state of diuresis should be established with intravenous fluids in nephritic patients prior to the administration of anesthetic drugs. In any case, it is good anesthetic practice to administer intravenous fluids during anesthesia to help maintain adequate blood pressure and urine production, and to provide an available route for drug administration.

Systemic administration of antibiotics preoperatively is a helpful prophylactic measure prior to major surgery or if contamination of the operative site is anticipated. However, the potential interaction of antibiotics with anesthetic or related drugs should receive careful consideration, and antibiotics ideally are given 1 or 2 h before anesthetic induction begins. In surgery of the colon, rectum, and anus, preoperative enemas administered 1 or 2 days prior to surgery will remove fecal material and facilitate manipulation. On the other hand, an enema just prior to surgery may complicate the situation, because feces will be fluid and the operative site may easily become contaminated.

Dehydrated animals should be treated with fluids and appropriate alimentation prior to operation; fluid therapy should be continued as required. The delay occasioned by administration of fluids is more than compensated for by the animal's increased ability to withstand the stress of anesthesia and surgical trespass. An attempt should be made to correlate the patient's electrolyte balance with the type of fluid that is administered. Anemia and hypovolemia, as determined clinically and hematologically, should be corrected by administration of whole blood or blood components and balanced electrolyte solutions. Patients in shock without blood loss or in a state of nutritional deficiency benefit by administration of plasma or plasma expanders.[51]

Several conditions may severely restrict effective ventilation. These include upper-airway obstruction by masses or abscesses, pneumothorax, hemothorax, pyothorax, chylothorax, diaphragmatic hernia, and gastric or rumen distention. Affected animals are often in a marginal state of oxygenation. Oxygen administration by nasal catheter or mask is indicated if the patient will accept it. Alternatively, a tracheotomy may be performed under local anesthesia prior to induction. Intrapleural air or fluid should be removed by aspiration prior to induction, because the effective lung volume may be greatly reduced and severe respiratory embarrassment may occur on induction. Although no attempt should be made to insert an endotracheal catheter in these patients prior to anesthesia, this must be done immediately after induction. Anesthetists should be prepared to carry out all phases of induction, intubation, and controlled ventilation in one continuous operation.

In laboratory animals, especially rats, guinea pigs, mice, and rabbits, chronic respiratory disease may be endemic. In calves, sheep, and swine, lung lesions are common. In primates, tuberculosis may be encountered. Animals having such infections should receive specific therapy prior to anesthesia, and, should resolution not occur, local or regional anesthesia should be strongly considered.

Decompensated heart disease is a contraindication for general anesthesia. If animals must be anesthetized, an attempt at compensation through appropriate inotropes, antiarrhythmic drugs, and diuresis should be made prior to anesthesia. If ascites is present, this fluid should be aspirated to reduce excessive pressure on the diaphragm.

In cases of hepatic or renal insufficiency—for instance, in many bacterial and viral infections of mice, dogs, or primates, or in parasitism of calves, sheep, and rabbits—the mode of anesthetic elimination should receive strong consideration, with inhalation anesthesia preferred. Under experimental conditions, animals with clinical or subclinical disease of any body system should be identified and treated before inclusion.

Just prior to induction, it is desirable to encourage defecation and/or urination by giving animals access to a run or exercise pen. If this attempt is unsuccessful, catheterization or bladder compression may be necessary prior to surgery. Once an animal is anesthetized, the bladder can be emptied by slow, steady compression through the abdominal wall or by catheterization. An empty bladder is an advantage in abdominal surgery because urine may contaminate the operative field.

During anesthesia, patients should, if possible, be restrained in a normal physiological position. Compression of the chest, acute angulation of the neck, overextension or compression of limbs, and compression of the posterior vena cava by large viscera can all lead to serious compromise. Complications include hypoventilation, nerve and/or muscle damage, and impaired venous return. Horses are especially susceptible to myopathy and/or neuropathy caused by excessive extension, abduction, or compression and ischemia of the muscles. Such complications are more likely to occur when good relaxation is achieved or when blood pressure is depressed and recumbency is prolonged in a lateral position. Such a position also adversely affects ventilation-perfusion ratios and thereby the efficiency of gas exchange within the lungs. The inefficiency of respiratory exchange may be greater in one position than another.[52] In some cases, a periodic change in position may be beneficial during long surgical procedures.

Tilting anesthetized patients alters the amount of respiratory gases that can be accommodated in the chest (functional residual capacity [FRC]) by as much as 26%.[53] In dogs subjected to hemorrhage, tilting them head-up was detrimental, producing lowered blood pressure, hyperpnea, and depression of cardiac contractile force.[54] When dogs were tilted head-down, no circulatory improvement occurred. In pentobarbital-anesthetized dogs lying on a horizontal table, sternal recumbency and left and right lateral recumbency positions consistently produced the least overall change in cardiopulmonary function (D. W. DeYoung and W. V. Lumb, unpublished data, 1971). The supine position was the least physiological of the level positions assessed. Prone and supine head-down positions (60°) produced the greatest physiological derangement.

In all species, the head should be extended to provide a free airway and to prevent kinking of the endotracheal tube. In ruminants, it is desirable to have the head tilted down to enable drainage of saliva. Downward tilting of the hindquarters and abdomen (below the thorax), with minimal compression of the abdomen, limits reflux of rumen contents. On induction, if active regurgitation begins with large volumes of ruminal contents flowing into the pharyngeal cavity, pressure should be applied immediately by externally grasping the esophagus dorsal to the trachea to prevent further flow. Alternatively, an endotracheal tube can be inserted into the esophagus and the cuff rapidly inflated, directing the flow through the tube away from the laryngeal opening while an endotracheal tube is properly placed to protect the airway from contamination. Precautions should also be taken to prevent accumulation of rumen gases during anesthesia. This may be done by passage of a large-bore stomach tube. During emergence from anesthesia, it is desirable to position ruminants in sternal recumbency. When large species are restrained in recumbency, viscera, restraining ropes, and bands may restrict respiration or compress nerves or muscle groups severely. During restraint in dorsal recumbency, abdominal viscera may compress the large veins and restrict venous return. In all instances, thorough padding beneath the animal is mandatory.

Selection of an Anesthetic

The ideal anesthetic is one that

1. Does not depend on metabolism for its termination of action and elimination
2. Enables rapid induction, quick alteration in anesthesia depth, and rapid recovery
3. Does not depress cardiopulmonary function
4. Does not irritate any tissue
5. Is inexpensive, stable, noninflammable, and nonexplosive
6. Requires no special equipment for administration

No anesthetic drug possesses all of these qualities. Therefore, selection of an anesthetic is a compromise based on appraisal of the situation. Factors to be considered include

1. The patient's species, breed, and age
2. The patient's physical status
3. The time required for the surgical (or other) procedure, its type and severity, and the surgeon's skill
4. Familiarity with the proposed anesthetic technique
5. Equipment and personnel available

In general, veterinarians will have greatest success with drugs they have used most frequently and with which they are most familiar. The art of administration is developed only with experience; therefore, change from a familiar drug to a new one is usually accompanied by a temporary increase in anesthetic risk. Clarke,[55] speaking of anesthesia in people, stated, "The outstanding fact is that thorough familiarity with a technique is equivalent at least to a 30 percent increase in efficiency and safety. If a person has mastered a technique, it is not worth his while changing to a new and unfamiliar one unless the change promises some big advantage."

Often the length of time required to perform a surgical procedure and the amount of help available during this period dictate the anesthetic that is used. Generally, short procedures are done with short-acting agents, such as thiobarbiturates, propofol, alphaxalone-CD, and etomidate, or with combinations using dissociative, tranquilizing, and/or opioid drugs. Where longer anesthesia is required, inhalation or balanced anesthetic techniques can usually be safely used.

Species differences may prevent the use of some drugs. For example, procaine is frequently lethal for parakeets and, in high doses, morphine can be excitatory in cats. On the other hand, once adjusted for species dose requirements, most agents can be used interchangeably among species. Anesthesia in the very young is attended with increased risk owing to size limitations, limited muscular and adipose tissue in which anesthetic may be redistributed, and immature metabolic and excretory mechanisms. For this reason, the use of barbiturates in very young patients is generally not recommended.

Aged animals are often poor anesthetic risks because of decreased vitality and the possibility of decreased cardiac, hepatic, and renal function (reserve), which may not be apparent on casual examination. Drugs should be chosen and administered in doses that minimally depress these systems and that can be easily metabolized and eliminated or reversed with specific antagonists. The same is true of patients in poor physical condition, because the liver and kidneys usually are somewhat affected.

General anesthesia is to be avoided, if at all possible, in animals with renal failure. Local, regional or epidural anesthesia should be used where possible. If general anesthesia must be used, induction with a short-acting anesthetic such as propofol or etomidate, a potent opioid, or very low doses of a thiobarbiturate and inhalant anesthetic is preferred.

A cardiac murmur per se is not a contraindication to general anesthesia unless the murmur is accompanied by untreated cardiac decompensation (no exercise tolerance). However, such patients may have less cardiac reserve and require more careful supervision during anesthesia. Patients with heartworm infestation and congenital lesions of the heart and great vessels also fall into this category. Balanced techniques using less depressant drugs such as dissociatives, opioids, etomidate and isoflurane are preferred.

Brachycephalic dogs, because of their pendulous soft palate and restricted respiratory passages, may have difficulty in breathing even when awake. This is particularly true in hot, humid weather. During anesthesia, the degree of airway obstruction is compounded, and these animals often have severe respiratory strider unless a patent airway is maintained via endotracheal intubation. It is wise to use short-lasting agents that are rapidly eliminated (e.g., propofol) so that a prolonged recovery period is avoided and patient control of the airway recovers rapidly.

In large animals such as horses and cattle, anesthetics should be selected to provide rapid recovery with minimal emergence struggling. Emergence struggling is usually more of a problem in equine anesthesia, whereas general anesthesia in ruminants is complicated by the hazards of rumen tympany, regurgitation, and aspiration. These latter complications make the use of regional anesthesia desirable where appropriate. In the event general anesthesia is used, endotracheal intubation is mandatory. Regional anesthesia with the patient in the standing position has the advantage of preventing compression of abdominal viscera and is therefore less likely to impede respiratory and cardiovascular function.

The overriding consideration in choosing an anesthetic protocol is patient safety. This is based on

1. Patient factors likely to influence responses to anesthesia, uptake, distribution, and elimination
2. The physical status of the animal
3. The specific needs of the species
4. The specific needs in the case, including the relative requirements for sedation, immobilization, analgesia, relaxation, and safety

Secondarily, the anesthetic protocol should be one that provides convenience to the surgeon so that the procedure can be completed efficiently, insures patient comfort, allows for appropriate monitoring, and can be administered with confidence by the veterinarian.

Operative Risk

Operative risk refers to uncertainty and the potential for misadventure or adverse outcome as a result of anesthesia and surgery. It should be emphasized that physical status, anesthetic risk, and operative risk are entirely different. To determine anesthetic risk, many factors must be considered, including the degree of skill of the anesthetist, the anesthetic to be employed, and the physical status of the patient. To determine operative risk, the foregoing must be appraised and, in addition, the operation to be performed and the skill of the surgeon must be taken into consideration. Operative risk, then, is determined by factors associated with the patient, anesthesia, and surgery.[55-59] Patient factors affecting risk include physical status, temperament, age, species and breed, and overall physical fitness. Perioperative morbidity and mortality increase with the severity of preexisting disease. Geriatric and pediatric patients are at increased risk because of limited ability to respond to stress because of decreased functional reserves in the former and incomplete development in the latter. Depressed or overly apprehensive or fractious patients are often unstable and difficult to safely induce and maintain. In such patients, careful consideration should be given to preanesthetic management and choice of drugs. Species and breed characteristics can contribute to operative risks. Examples include the increased risk of airway obstruction in brachycephalic dogs, malignant hyperthermia in some strains of swine, increased incidence and severity of myositis in heavy draft horses, and increased incidence of regurgitation and aspiration in ruminants.

Surgical factors that can increase risk include the nature of the procedure itself (i.e., duration, complexity, organ involvement,

operating conditions, and emergency). Major surgical procedures and procedures that are complex are associated with increased morbidity and mortality as compared with minor and simple procedures. Involvement of major organs increases risk; CNS, cardiac, and pulmonary procedures have the highest risk, followed by the gastrointestinal tract, liver, kidney, reproductive organs, muscles, bone, and skin. Emergency procedures are more risky because of poorer patient status, that is, unstable or severely compromised patients, decreased ability to prepare or stabilize the patient, and lack of preparation by the surgical and anesthetic team. *Operating conditions* refer to the physical facilities and equipment and support personnel available. The aggressiveness of the surgical team, experience with the procedure, and frequency of performance are also important. Lastly, the duration of the procedure and fatigue must be considered because patients cannot be operated on indefinitely. The incidence of morbidity and mortality increases with the duration of anesthesia and surgery. Thus, efficiency of the surgical team is important in reducing risk. A related factor is fatigue.[60]

Anesthetic factors that can affect risk include the choice of anesthetic drugs to be used, the anesthetic technique, and the duration of anesthesia. The choice of anesthetic can adversely affect the outcome, but more commonly the agents are not so much at fault as the manner in which they are given. Many adverse physiological effects of anesthesia and surgery are time related. Experience of the anesthetist with the protocol is important to its safe administration. Fatigue increases risk because it decreases vigilance. Thus, efficiency of patient monitoring and timely recognition and response to potentially life-threatening events are decreased. It is worth noting that human error remains the number one reason for anesthesia-related mishap and is a major contributor to anesthetic risk (Table 2.10).[61-71]

Record Keeping and Monitoring

"For every mistake that is made for not knowing, a hundred are made for not looking."

Anonymous

Death of a patient from any cause is always unpleasant, but a fatality during anesthesia and surgery is even more so because of the obvious practitioner involvement. One will occasionally hear a veterinarian state that he or she has never lost an animal because of anesthesia. This is conceivably true, though highly unlikely if a sizable number of animals have been anesthetized. Obviously, the criteria for anesthetic mortality in this instance must be defined. It is human nature for a veterinarian to forget the disagreeable and to excuse a fatality by blaming it on something over which he or she has no control. Not all deaths in the perioperative period are anesthetic deaths. Deaths may be caused by (a) anesthesia; (b) surgery; (c) anesthesia primarily, with only a minor surgical contribution; (d) surgery primarily, with only a minor anesthetic contribution; (e) the patient's disease primarily; or (f) indeterminate causes. Deaths related to anesthesia should be recognized and identified. Examples of deaths that are attributable to anesthetic management are (a) death during induction,

Table 2.10. Mortality rate in anesthesia of various species[56–72].

Year	Species	Mortality Rate %	Cause(s)	Reference
1973	Human	1.9	Physical status of patient Physician judgment	62
1975	Human	0.2[b]		63
1982	Human	0.6 0.01[b]		64
1990	Human	1.2 0.05 >0.1	0.05% of patients died during anesthesia >0.1% of patients died during the recovery period	65
1973	Equine	1.18	More gastrointestinal surgeries being performed	66
1983	Equine	2.7[a] 0.8[b]		67
1993	Equine	0.68	Ischemic myopathy Fracture of the cervical or long bones Cardiac arrest	60
1995	Equine	1.6 0.9[d] (foals excluded)	Anesthesia in third trimester of pregnancy Emergency abdominal surgery Orthopedic procedures involving internal fixation Administration of xylazine	68
1998	Equine	0.63[a] 0.08[b]	Elective surgery	69
1998	Equine	31.4 35.5[c] 15.3[d]	Cardiac arrest Uncontrollable massive hemorrhage Irreversible endotoxic shock	70
2000	Equine	1.9 7.9[c] 0.9[d]	Cardiac arrest Fractures Ischemic myopathy Cardiovascular collapse	71
1977	Feline	0.3	Inaccurate body weights of animals Inadequate and ineffective premedications Inability to intubate the trachea	72
1990	Canine Feline	0.23 0.29	Administration of xylazine	56
1992	Canine Feline	0.11 0.06	Cardiopulmonary arrest	57
1994	Canine Feline	0.43 0.43	Cardiac arrest	58
1998	Canine Feline	0.11 0.1	Cardiac arrest Cardiac arrest with xylazine administration (dogs)	59

[a]Mortality attributable to anesthesia and surgery.
[b]Mortality attributable to anesthesia only.
[c]Abdominal surgeries only.
[d]Abdominal surgeries excluded.

(b) explosion (rare at this time), (c) pulmonary aspiration, (d) failure to secure the airway, (e) hypoxia, (f) anesthetic overdose, (g) technical mismanagement of the anesthetic system, and (h) maladministration of fluids and air embolism.[72]

As long as anesthetics are administered, the hazard of death can never be eliminated completely; it can, however, be minimized, particularly if one is willing to investigate and to learn from mistakes. Once an anesthetic fatality has occurred, the sequence of the perioperative events preceding the death should be reviewed, their significance should be evaluated, and a necropsy should be performed to piece together its pathogenesis and etiology. Armed with this information, the practitioner can then take steps to prevent a recurrence of this tragedy.

Unfortunately, there is little recorded information concerning mortality in animals anesthetized in clinical practice. This may be because (a) busy practitioners do not have time to collect the necessary data, (b) there is no economic gain to be derived from such collection, or (c) there is lack of interest on the part of individuals best able to obtain these data. To obtain meaningful data concerning anesthesia, certain information must be collected and definite criteria established. A record must be made for each animal anesthetized, with the owner's name and the case number written on it. Among the items that should be recorded are

1. Species, breed, age, gender, weight, and physical status of the animal
2. Surgical procedure or other reason for anesthesia
3. Preanesthetic agents given
4. Anesthetic agents used and method of administration
5. Person administering anesthesia (veterinarian, technician, student, or lay personnel)
6. Duration of anesthesia
7. Supportive measures
8. Difficulties encountered and methods of correction

Tabulation of these data will provide not only extensive information on anesthesia, but also the incidence of surgical diseases in various species, age groups, and breeds.

Moribund patients are poor anesthetic risks, and if a single agent is used to anesthetize them, the mortality rate for this agent may appear to be disproportionately high. When one is discussing anesthetic mortality, therefore, it is necessary to categorize the physical status of a patient prior to anesthesia to assess risk. The ASA has developed a five-division classification of physical health and therefore anesthetic risk (Table 2.7). A modification of this classification of anesthetic risk can relate severity of patient disease to the occurrence of death. As expected, the mortality rate increases sharply as physical status deteriorates. There are various reasons that animals with poor physical status undergo anesthesia. In some instances, anesthesia and surgery are performed to secure diagnoses on animals that would likely have died within hours. Although data are available to define mortality based on patient disease and surgical procedure, percentage figures derived from large patient populations are not necessarily applicable to individual patients or hospitals.

It is necessary that each step of anesthetic administration, along with the patient's response, be recorded in an anesthetic record (Fig. 2.3). Minimally, the pulse and respiratory rate should be monitored at 5-min intervals and charted at 10-min intervals. Trends in these parameters thus become apparent before a patient's condition severely deteriorates, so that remedial steps may be taken.

The diplomates of the American College of Veterinary Anesthesiologists (ACVA) have proposed guidelines (1994) for anesthetic monitoring, with the intention of encouraging high-quality care of anesthetized veterinary patients (Table 2.11). The ACVA recognizes that some of the methods may be impractical in certain clinical settings and that anesthetized patients can be monitored and managed without specialized equipment. The ACVA does not suggest that using any or all of these methods can ensure successful patient outcome or that failure to use any or all of these methods causes poor outcome. These suggestions are offered only to assist veterinarians in determining priorities for monitoring and record keeping during anesthesia, surgery, and recovery. These suggestions may be revised as warranted by developing knowledge and technology. The aspects of anesthetic management addressed by the ACVA guidelines that deserve careful

attention include patient circulation, oxygenation, and ventilation. Methods of monitoring each of the physiological processes are listed in Table 2.11 in approximate order of simplest, most economic, and least invasive, to the most complex, expensive, and invasive. Circulation can be assessed by palpation of peripheral pulse, palpation of heartbeat by chest wall, auscultation of heartbeat (stethoscope, esophageal stethoscope, or other audible heart monitor), use of an electrocardiogram, use of noninvasive blood flow or blood pressure monitor (e.g., a Doppler ultrasonic flow detector or an oscillometric flow detector), or use of an invasive blood pressure monitor (an arterial catheter connected to a transducer or aneroid manometer). Oxygenation can be assessed by observation of mucous membrane color, pulse oximetry (noninvasive estimation of hemoglobin saturation), oxygen analyzer in the inspiratory limb of the breathing circuit, blood-gas analysis (arterial oxygen partial pressure), or hemoximetry (measurement of hemoglobin saturation in the blood). Ventilation can be assessed with observation of chest wall movement, observation of breathing-bag movement, auscultation of breath sounds, audible respiratory monitor, respirometry, capnography (measurement of carbon dioxide in end-expired gas), or blood-gas monitoring (arterial carbon dioxide partial pressure).

The ACVA further recommends that an anesthetic record should be compiled for each patient to maintain a legal record of significant events and to enhance recognition of trends in monitored parameters (Fig. 2.3). The record should include all drugs administered, noting the dose, time, and route of administration. Monitored parameters should be recorded regularly (at least every 10 min) during anesthesia. Responsible individuals should be aware of the patient status at all times during anesthesia and recovery and be prepared to alert the veterinarian about changes in the patient's condition. If a veterinarian, technician, or other responsible person cannot remain with the patient continuously, a responsible person should check the patient's status regularly (at least every 5 min) during anesthesia and recovery. The responsible person may be present in the same room although not necessarily solely occupied with the anesthetized patient (e.g., the surgeon may also be responsible for overseeing anesthesia). In either of these situations, the use of audible heart and respiratory monitors is suggested. In the best of situations, a person, solely dedicated to managing and caring for the anesthetized patient, remains with the patient continuously until the end of the anesthetic period.

Insurance Claims and Anesthesia Risk

Claims presented to the American Veterinary Medical Association Professional Liability Insurance Trust from 1976 through 1982 and from 1999 to 2003 based on anesthetic, surgical, and medical incidents reflect changing trends in veterinary practice and owner concern for optimal patient care (Table 2.12). It should be noted that the percentage of anesthesia claims decreased by over 50% for both dogs and horses from 1982 to 2003, reflecting the increasing sophistication and safety of veterinary anesthesia during the last 20 years. For more recent data on anesthetic-related claims, the reader is referred to the American Veterinary Medical Association Liability Insurance Trust.

ANESTHETIC RECORD

| PATIENT INFORMATION | Date: | Cage #: | Surgeon: |
| | Procedure(s): | | Anesthetist: |

Preanesthetic Values / Animal Status

	HR	RR	MM color	Temp	PCV	TP	Weight (kg / lb)	Hydration

Preanesthetic Drugs

Drug	Dose	Route	Time

Induction Drugs

Drug	Dose	Route	Time

Physical Status

1	2	3	4	5	E

PAIN Evaluation: No Pain I--I Worst Pain

| Time | 00 | 15 | 30 | 45 | 00 | 15 | 30 | 45 | 00 | 15 | 30 | 45 |

Anesthesia

_ Isoflurane

_ Sevoflurane

_ Other

Vaporizer Setting: 5.0 / 4.0 / 3.0 / 2.5 / 2.0 / 1.5 / 1.0 / 0

O_2 Flow (L/min)

CODES

A Anesthesia — 200

O Surgery — 180

D Drape — 160

R Recovery — 140

SYMBOLS — 120

X Pulse — 100

o Respirations — 80

∨ Systolic — 60

∧ Diastolic — 40

- Mean — 30

* SpO_2 — 20

Δ PCO_2 — 10

τ Temp — 0

Fluids type_____	mL
Total fluids_____	Extubation Time _____ Sternal Time _____ Temperature ≥98°F Time _____
Comments:	

PAIN Evaluation Post-Op: No Pain I--I Worst Pain

Fig. 2.3. Example anesthetic record. The anesthetic record provides written documentation of the anesthetic drugs and techniques used to produce general anesthesia and suggests methods for monitoring the patient throughout anesthesia. The patient's physical status and pain should be assessed before and after any procedure. Other drugs, fluids, surgical and medical techniques, and the personnel involved should be recorded.

Table 2.11. American College of Veterinary Anesthesiologists' suggestions for monitoring.

Circulation

Objective: to ensure that blood flow to tissues is adequate

Methods:

1. Palpation of peripheral pulse
2. Palpation of heartbeat through the chest wall
3. Auscultation of heartbeat (stethoscope, esophageal stethoscope, or other audible heart monitor)
4. Electrocardiogram (continuous display)
5. Noninvasive blood flow or blood pressure monitor (e.g., Doppler ultrasonic flow detector or oscillometric flow detector)
6. Invasive blood pressure monitor (arterial catheter connected to transducer/oscilloscope or to anaeroid manometer)

Oxygenation

Objective: to ensure adequate oxygen concentration in the patient's arterial blood

Methods:

1. Observation of mucous membrane color
2. Pulse oximetry (noninvasive estimation of hemoglobin saturation)
3. Oxygen analyzer in the inspiratory limb of the breathing circuit
4. Blood-gas analysis (arterial oxygen partial pressure)
5. Hemoximetry (measurement of hemoglobin saturation in the blood)

Ventilation

Objective: to maintain a legal record of significant events and to enhance recognition of trends in monitored parameters

Methods:

1. Observation of chest wall movement
2. Observation of breathing-bag movement
3. Auscultation of breath sounds
4. Audible respiratory monitor
5. Respirometry (measurement of tidal volume ± minute volume)
6. Capnography (measurement of carbon dioxide in end-expired gas)
7. Blood-gas monitoring (arterial carbon dioxide partial pressure)

Anesthetic Record

Objective: to maintain a legal record of significant events and to enhance recognition of trends in monitored parameters

Methods:

1. Record all drugs administered to each patient, noting the dose, time, and route of administration
2. Record monitored parameters (minimum: heart rate, respiratory rate) regularly (minimum: every 10 min) during anesthesia

Personnel

Objective: to ensure that a responsible individual is aware of the patient's status at all times during anesthesia and recovery, and is prepared either to intervene when indicated or to alert the veterinarian in charge about changes in the patient's condition

Methods:

1. If a veterinarian, technician, or other responsible person cannot remain with the patient continuously, a responsible person should check the patient's status regularly (at least every 5 min)
2. A responsible person may be present in the same room, although not necessarily solely occupied with the anesthetized patient (e.g., the surgeon may also be responsible for overseeing anesthesia)
3. In either of the foregoing situations, the use of audible heart and respiratory monitors is suggested
4. A responsible person, solely dedicated to managing and caring for the anesthetized patient during anesthesia, remains with the patient continuously until the end of the anesthetic period

Aftercare

Although in most instances recovery from anesthesia is uneventful, patients should be kept under observation during the recovery period to prevent untoward sequelae. In animal hospitals and laboratory-animal facilities, it is wise to have a recovery room for this purpose, because all of the necessary equipment, drugs, and materials can be kept in one place, and it is less difficult to observe several animals. In some instances, the prep room may also serve as the recovery room; alternatively, recovery and intensive care functions may be combined. Such facilities should be conveniently located for nursing staff.

Small Animals

Following removal from the operating room, the animal should be placed in its cage in lateral recumbency.

While the animal remains unconscious or immobile, monitoring deemed necessary in the operating room should be continued. In any case, vital signs should be recorded at 10-min intervals

Table 2.12. Trends in claims involving anesthesia, surgery, and medicine presented to the American Veterinary Medical Association (AVMA) Professional Liability Insurance Trust.

Species	Total No. of Claims	Anesthesia (%)	Surgery (%)	Medicine (%)
1976 to 1982				
Dogs	1225	13.1	42.5	44.4
Cats	216	6.5	45.8	47.7
Horses	542	13.8	41.7	44.5
Cattle	436	3.9	44.2	51.8
1999 to 2003				
Dogs	6892	5.1	40.7	41.8
Cats	2135	7.0	40.7	42.2
Horses	1521	4.5	37.2	42.3
Cattle	727	2.1	52.4	29.3

Courtesy of the AVMA Professional Liability Insurance Trust, Chicago, Illinois.

until the animal regains consciousness. Continued supervision is especially important until extubation and the return of coughing and swallowing reflexes. A blanket, pad, or even newspaper should be placed under and over the patient to conserve body heat. In very small or newborn animals, the ambient temperature should approximate body temperature. Incubators designed for babies are helpful in maintaining body temperature and are used routinely in many laboratories where birds, rodents, and primates are anesthetized. In newborn pigs, an environmental temperature of 90°F has been found desirable. Otherwise, shivering occurs with increased oxygen and energy requirements, and hypoglycemia may result. During recovery, birds should be housed at 100°F; mice, hamsters, and small primates at 95°F; rats, guinea pigs, and rabbits at 90°F; and cats, dogs, and similar carnivores at 77° to 86°F.[7] Depending on environmental temperatures, heat lamps, heating pads, or warm-water blankets may be required. If fluid therapy is used, fluids should be warmed to body temperature.

During recovery, the patient's tongue should be pulled forward to preclude its blocking the pharynx. In brachycephalic breeds or in animals in which respiratory function is compromised, an endotracheal tube should remain in place until upper-airway reflexes and jaw movements return. In such animals, sternal recumbency, if practical, is preferred. Care is necessary to assure freedom of the airway from blankets or paper. The water pan should always be removed from the cage to prevent accidental drowning in the event a semiconscious patient should place its nose and mouth or endotracheal catheter in the container. Food and water may be offered as soon as a patient can stand.

Predisposition to postoperative respiratory failure may result from continuing drug-induced respiratory depression, postextubation spasm or glottic edema, other respiratory obstructions, diffusion hypoxia, mechanical splinting associated with pain and/or dressings, and persistent hypoventilation and/or atelectasis during anesthesia. Careful evaluation of respiration during the immediate postanesthetic period is therefore essential. If hypoventilation is identified, predisposing causes should be corrected and, if necessary, supportive respiratory therapy should be initiated. Since postoperative hypotension may be caused by a

persistent drug effect, hemorrhage, and inadequate volume, adequacy of cardiovascular function should also be carefully and frequently evaluated.

Under no circumstances should an anesthetized animal be placed in the same cage with a conscious one, because the former cannot protect itself. Cannibalism has been known to occur (e.g., among pigs and rats), particularly where the anesthetized patient had an open wound!

When preanesthetic sedation has not been used, animals may thrash and struggle, bruising themselves severely and even breaking teeth during the recovery period. Coursing breeds, such as greyhounds, Russian wolfhounds, and Afghans, are particularly prone to this phenomenon. The judicious use of tranquilizers or opioids in small doses quiets animals in this condition. Plastic-covered sponge-rubber mats or other suitable pads in recovery cages also afford protection.

After administration of large doses of barbiturates, some animals will have a prolonged recovery period. Special attention must be given these animals to prevent hypostatic congestion and subsequent pneumonia. They should, of course, be kept warm and turned frequently. In addition, prophylactic antibiotic therapy may be desirable and a protective ophthalmic ointment placed in the eyes to prevent corneal drying. Intravenous electrolyte solutions in moderate amounts prevent dehydration.

Constrictive bandaging of the head or throat must be avoided because of the danger of asphyxiation. Occasionally, cats that have been tightly bandaged around the abdomen show evidence of posterior paralysis on recovery. This condition is apparently caused by decreased circulation to the hindquarters. Removal of the bandage may quickly resolve paralysis.

It is unwise to send anesthetized animals home, because owners generally cannot cope with any unusual situation that may arise. In addition, the owners may become alarmed by the signs of their animal's approaching consciousness and may demand service unnecessarily.

Large Animals

Like smaller animals, large animals should be removed to a recovery room (stall). The room should be padded to minimize injury during emergence from the anesthetic and recovery of righting reflexes. Availability of oxygen and suction is essential. If a padded floor and pads are unavailable and bedding material such as straw must be used, this should be covered with a tarpaulin so that it is kept clear of the external nares or end of the endotracheal tube and the eyes. Using pads beneath the head and limbs is essential. In horses especially, bony prominences must be protected from abrasion. It is an excellent practice to bandage and pad all limbs prior to anesthesia and to keep these protections in place until recovery is complete. A horse's head is especially subject to trauma during recovery, with resulting abrasions, edema, and even facial paralysis. It should therefore be protected with a pad or a padded hood. Halters or headstalls should be used when necessary and should be padded.

Whenever possible, horses should be allowed to lie quietly in a darkened environment neither restrained nor disturbed. The possibility of emergence struggling and of attempts to stand before coordination is fully recovered is thus less likely. If an endotracheal tube has been used, it should remain in situ until the return of upper-airway and swallowing reflexes necessitates its removal. Food and water should be removed from the stall until recovery is complete. If straw or other bedding material is used, the animal is observed to prevent it from eating. When eye reflexes have fully returned, and nystagmus is absent, horses are usually able to stand. While animals attempt to rise, a steady influence exerted by the handlers in holding up the head and in upward traction on the tail may be helpful.

Some horses, despite preanesthetic sedation, struggle during recovery from anesthesia. Additional sedation or manual restraint may be required. A tail rope or a halter to restrain the head and neck is usually sufficient. Alternatively, a sedative (e.g., xylazine) may be administered. Control by medication is preferable, although recovery may be prolonged with large doses. Small amounts of xylazine (100 mg per 1000-pound horse) have proved useful in alleviating pain and calming recovery without unduly lengthening it. Some veterinarians restrain a horse either on the operating table or by ropes and hobbles until they judge the animal is able to stand. Such a practice predisposes animals to struggling and injuries.

When recovery rooms are not available, it may be necessary to permit recovery in the operating room. Operating rooms having a padded floor, or a padded floor with table that lowers to floor level, are suitable. Restraint with straps on the operating table until recovery is complete is undesirable, especially for horses; struggling is likely, and abrasions and nerve injuries are common. Rupture of the colon has been attributed to such restraint in several instances. If a cart is available to transport the animal, a grassy plot is a desirable location for recovery.

Ruminants are handled in a manner similar to that used for horses. Struggling and resulting trauma are usually not problems. Instead, it is necessary to minimize possible regurgitation and aspiration of rumen contents, and ruminal tympany. The endotracheal tube with cuff inflated should therefore remain in position as long as possible. Use of a speculum to prevent damage to, or constriction of, the tube is helpful. During recovery, ruminants should be placed in sternal recumbency. If their flexed limbs are abducted slightly, the animals can usually be propped in this position. Padded bolsters, other supports, or even bales of hay can be used to assist in maintaining this position. The head should be down and extended and the end of the endotracheal tube unobstructed. When anterior epidural anesthesia has been used, the hind legs should be hobbled to a degree sufficient to prevent abduction until muscle control is regained.

Recovering large animals should be protected from temperature extremes. In the absence of heating or air conditioning, the use of blankets, heaters, or fans may be necessary. If an outside recovery area is used, animals should be shaded from direct sunlight in hot weather and blanketed in cold weather. When recovery is prolonged, animals should be turned frequently, and warmed fluids should be administered intravenously. Vital signs should be continually and routinely monitored until the return of coughing, swallowing, and righting reflexes.

References

1. Knight GC. Barbiturate anaesthesia in small animals. Proc R Soc Med 42:525, 1949.

2. De Boer B. Factors affecting pentothal anesthesia in dogs. Anesthesiology 8:375, 1947.

3. Kato R, Takanaka A. Metabolism of drugs in old rats. I. Activities of NADPH-linked electron transport and drug metabolizing enzyme systems in liver microsomes of old rats. Jpn J Pharmacol 18:381, 1968.

4. Keys A. Age and the Basal Metabolism: Guidelines to Metabolic Therapy, vol 2. Kalamazoo, MI: Upjohn, 1973.

5. Nicholas JS, Barron DH. The use of sodium amytal in the production of anesthesia in the rat. J Pharmacol Exp Ther 46:125, 1932.

6. Kennedy WP. Sodium salt of C-C-cyclohexenylmethyl-N-methyl barbituric acid (Evipan) anaesthesia in laboratory animals. J Pharmacol Exp Ther 50:347, 1934.

7. Green CJ. Animal Anaesthesia. London: Laboratory Animals, 1979.

8. Stormont C, Suzuki Y. Atropinesterase and cocainesterase of rabbit serum: Localization of the enzyme activity in isozymes. Science 167:200, 1970.

9. Gourlay GK, Adams JF, Cousins MJ, Hall P. Genetic differences in reductive metabolism and hepatotoxicity of halothane in three rat strains. Anesthesiology 55:96, 1981.

10. Jenkins J, Balinsky D, Patient DW. Cholinesterase in plasma: First reported absence in the Bantu—Half-life determination. Science 156:1748, 1967.

11. Jones EW, Nelson TE, Anderson IL, Kerr DD, Burnap TK. Malignant hyperthermia of swine. Anesthesiology 36:42, 1972.

12. Van Dyke RA, Chenoweth MB. Metabolism of volatile anesthetics. Anesthesiology 26:348, 1965.

13. Hug CC. Pharmacokinetics of anesthetics: Intravenous drugs. Annual Refresher Course Lectures, Lecture 225A. Park Ridge, IL: American Society of Anesthesiologists, 1978.

14. Saidman LJ. Uptake and distribution of intravenous agents: The thiopental model. Refresher Courses in Anesthesiology 3:141, 1975.

15. Eger EI II. Anesthetic Uptake and Action. Baltimore: Williams and Wilkins, 1974.

16. Baggot JD. Principles of Drug Disposition in Domestic Animals. Philadelphia: WB Saunders, 1977.

17. Brown BR. Enzymes of biotransformation as related to anesthesia. Refresher Courses in Anesthesiology 3:27, 1975.

18. Mazze RI. Renal toxicity of anesthetics. Refresher Courses in Anesthesiology 1:85, 1973.

19. Nishitateno K, Ngai SH, Finek AD, Berkowitz BA. Pharmacokinetics of morphine: Concentrations in the serum and brain of the dog during hyperventilation. Anesthesiology 50:520, 1979.

20. Rouse S. Effects of thiobarbiturate anesthetics on lean dogs. Vet Anesthesiol 5:22, 1978.

21. Dukes HH. The Physiology of Domestic Animals, 6th ed. Ithaca, NY: Comstock, 1947.

22. Arnall L. Aspects of anaesthesia in cage birds. In: Graham-Jones O, ed. Small Animal Anaesthesia. Oxford: Pergamon, 1964:137.

23. Anderson EG, Magee DF. A study of the mechanism of the effect of dietary fat in decreasing thiopental sleeping time. J Pharmacol Exp Ther 117:281, 1956.

24. Brown BR. Anesthetic hepatic toxicity: A scientific problem? Annual Refresher Course B Lectures, Lecture 106B. Park Ridge, IL: American Society of Anesthesiologists, 1979.

25. Brown BR. Pharmacogenetics and the halothane hepatitis mystery. Anesthesiology 55:93, 1981.

26. Wissing H, Kuhn I, Dudziak R. Heat production from reaction of inhalation anesthetics with dry soda lime. Anaesthetist 46:1064, 1997.

27. Baxter PJ, Garton K, Kharasch ED. Mechanistic aspects of carbon monoxide formation from volatile anesthetics. Anesthesiology 89:929, 1998.

28. Wissing H, Huhn I, Warnken U, Dudziak R. Carbon monoxide production from desflurane, enflurane, halothane, isoflurane and sevoflurane with dry soda lime. Anesthesiology 95:1205, 2001.

29. Steffey EP, Laster MJ, Ionescu P, Eger EI, Gong D, Weiskopf RB. Dehydration of Baralyme increases compound A resulting from sevoflurane degradation in a standard anesthetic circuit used to anesthetize swine. Anesth Analg 85:1382, 1997.

30. Muir WW, Gadawski J. Cardiorespiratory effects of low-flow and closed circuit inhalation anesthesia, using sevoflurane delivered with an in-circuit vaporizer and concentrations of compound A. Am J Vet Res 59:603, 1998.

31. Teske RH, Carter GG. Effect of chloramphenicol on pentobarbital-induced anesthesia in dogs. J Am Vet Med Assoc 159:777, 1971.

32. Adams HR, Teske RH, Mercer HD. Anesthetic-antibiotic interrelationships. J Am Vet Med Assoc 168:409, 1976.

33. Pittinger C, Adamson R. Antibiotic blockade of neuromuscular function. Annu Rev Pharmacol 12:169, 1972.

34. Stoelting RK. Estimation of hepatic function: Effects of anesthetic experience. Refresher Courses in Anesthesiology 4:139, 1976.

35. Adriani J. Anesthesia for patients with uncommon and unusual diseases. Anesth Analg 37:1, 1958.

36. Nair V. An ontogenic study of the effects of exposure to x-irradiation on the pharmacology of barbiturates. Chicago Med School Q 28:9, 1969.

37. Saksonov PO, Kozlov VA. Features of the pharmacological action of some anaesthetic drugs in radiation injury. Voen Med Zh 10:40, 1968.

38. Brown BR. Molecular toxicity of inhalation anesthetics. Refresher Courses in Anesthesiology 5:1, 1977.

39. Cullen BF. Cellular effects and toxicity of anesthetics. Refresher Courses in Anesthesiology 6:43, 1978.

40. Duncan PG, Cullen BF. Anesthesiology and immunology. Anesthesiology 45:552, 1976.

41. Urban BW, Bleckwenn M. Concepts and correlations relevant to general anaesthesia. Br J Anaesth 89:3, 2002.

42. Campagna JA, Miller KW, Forman SA. Mechanisms of actions of inhaled anesthetics. N Engl J Med 348:2110, 2003.

43. Lee JA, Atkinson RSA. Synopsis of Anaesthesia, 6th ed. Baltimore: Williams and Wilkins, 1968.

44. Gray TC. A reassessment of the signs and levels of anaesthesia. Irish J Med Sci 419:499, 1960.

45. Collins KB, Gross ME, Moore CP, Branson KR. Physiologic, pharmacologic, and practical considerations of anesthesia of domestic animals with eye disease. J Am Vet Med Assoc 207:220, 1995.

46. Roizen MF. Routine perioperative evaluation. In: Miller RD, ed. Anesthesia, 2nd ed. New York: Churchill Livingstone, 1986:225.

47. MacWilliams PS, Thomas CB. Basic principles of laboratory medicine. Semin Vet Med Surg (Small Anim) 7:253, 1992.

48. Muir WW, Woolf CJ. Mechanisms of pain and their therapeutic implications. J Am Vet Med Assoc 219:1346, 2001.

49. Muir WW. Pain and stress. In: Gaynor JS, Muir WW, eds. Handbook of Veterinary Pain Management, 1st ed. St Louis: CV Mosby, 2002:46.

50. Ungerer T, Orr JA, Bisgard GE, Will JA. Cardiopulmonary effects of mechanical distension of the rumen in nonanesthetized sheep. Am J Vet Res 37:807, 1976.

51. Kudnig ST, Mama K. Perioperative fluid therapy. J Am Vet Med Assoc 221:1112, 2002.

52. De Moor A, Desmet P, Verschooten F. Influence of change of body position on arterial oxygenation and acid-base status in the horse in lateral recumbency. Zentralbl Veterinarmed 21:525, 1974.

53. Kilburn KH, McDonald J, Piccinni FP. Effects of ventilatory pattern and body position on lung volume in dogs. J Appl Physiol 15:801, 1960.

54. Liu CT, Hoff HE, Huggins RA. Circulatory and respiratory responses to postural changes in the hemorrhagic dog. J Appl Physiol 27:460, 1969.

55. Clarke KC, Hall LW. A survey of anaesthesia in small animal practice: AVA/BSAVA report. J Assoc Vet Anaesth 17:4, 1990.

56. Dodman NH, Lamb LA. Survey of small animal anaesthetic practice in Vermont. J Anim Hosp Assoc 28:439, 1992.

57. Gaynor JS, Dunlop CI, Wagner AE, Wertz EM, Golden AE, Demme WC. Complications and mortality associated with anesthesia in dogs and cats. J Anim Hosp Assoc 35:13, 1994.

58. Dyson DH, Maxi MG. Morbidity and mortality associated with anesthetic management in small animal veterinary practice in Ontario. J Anim Hosp Assoc 35:325, 1998.

59. Young SS, Taylor PM. Factors influencing the outcome of equine anesthesia: A review of 1,314 cases. Equine Vet J 25:147, 1993.

60. Collins VJ. Preanesthetic evaluation and preparation. In: Collins VJ, ed. Principles of Anesthesiology, 2nd ed. Philadelphia: Lea and Febiger, 1976.

61. Marx GF, Mateu CV, Orkin LR. Computer analysis of postanesthetic deaths. Anesthesiology 39:54, 1973.

62. Bodlander FMS. Deaths associated with anaesthesia. Anaesthesia 47:36, 1975.

63. Lunn JN, Mushin WW. Mortality associated with anaesthesia. Anaesthesia 37:856, 1982.

64. Pedersen T, Eliasen K, Henriksen E. A prospective study of mortality associated with anaesthesia and surgery: Risk indicators of mortality in hospital. Acta Anaesthesiol Scand 34:176, 1990.

65. Lumb WV, Jones EW, eds. Euthanasia. In: Veterinary Anesthesia, 2nd ed. Philadelphia: Lea and Febiger, 1973:611.

66. Tevik A. The role of anesthesia in surgical mortality in horses. Nord Vet Med 35:175, 1983.

67. Johnston GM, Taylor PM, Holmes MA, Wood JLN. Confidential enquiry of perioperative equine facilities (CPEF-I): Preliminary results. Equine Vet J 27:193, 1995.

68. Mee AM, Cripps PJ, Jones RS. A retrospective study of mortality associated with general anesthesia in horses: Elective procedures. Vet Rec 142:275, 1998.

69. Mee AM, Cripps PJ, Jones RS. A retrospective study of mortality associated with general anesthesia in horses: Emergency procedures. Vet Rec 142:307, 1998.

70. Johnston GM. Equine anesthesia: A chance to cut is a chance to kill. In: Proceedings of the Association of Veterinary Anesthesiologists, 2000:1.

71. Dodman NH. Feline anesthetic survey. J Small Anim Pract 10:653, 1977.

72. Collins VJ. Records, mortality and medical legal considerations. In: Principles of Anesthesiology, 2nd ed. Philadelphia: Lea and Febiger, 1976.

73. Bard P. Blood supply of special regions. In: Medical Physiology, 11th ed. St Louis: CV Mosby, 1961:239.

74. Abbitt LE. Drug interactions. In: Abbitt LE, Davis LE, Farey SD, Scalley RD, eds. Drug Interactions, Incompatibilities and Adverse Reactions in Veterinary Practice. Fort Collins, CO: Colorado State University, 1975.

75. Thurmon JC, Benson EJ. Anesthesia in ruminants and swine. In: Howard JL, ed. Current Veterinary Therapy 3: Food Animal Practice. Philadelphia: WB Saunders, 1993.

Chapter 3
Pain and Its Management

Peter W. Hellyer, Sheilah A. Robertson, and Anna D. Fails

Introduction

The prevention and control of pain are central to the practice of anesthesia. It is essential that anesthetists have an understanding of the physiological processes leading to the perception of pain and the responses of patients to this process. Ultimately, *anesthetic patient management* is the control of pain and maintenance of homeostasis in the face of noxious stimuli. The perioperative analgesic protocol has an impact on patient well-being that often extends far beyond the immediate anesthetic period. Appropriate pain management is not only integral to an anesthetic plan; it is a fundamental component of good medical practice.

In human medicine, several organizations are dedicated to improving the understanding and treatment of acute and chronic pain. Despite the efforts of these organizations, it has taken an inordinate amount of time for the human medical profession to accept that pain is a matter to be taken seriously. A landmark paper by Marks and Sachar[1] exposed both the indifference of physicians to the pain of terminally ill people and the knowledge deficits of medical professionals about effective pain control. Unfortunately, it is still commonplace for physicians to be considered the individuals that effect a cure, while nurses care for patients and try to alleviate pain and suffering. The fact that many physicians and institutions have ignored the importance of patient pain has not been lost on the public or regulatory agencies, prompting the Joint Commission on Accreditation of Healthcare Organizations (JCAHO) to mandate in the year 2000 that human hospitals elevate pain to the fifth vital sign (along with temperature, pulse, respiration, and blood pressure). The new requirements for assessing and controlling pain in people assert that "appropriate pain management is good medicine because it results in quicker clinical recovery, shorter hospital stays, fewer readmissions, and improved quality of life, leading to increased productivity."[2] Thirty years have passed since Marks and Sachar put in print what ordinary people already knew: Despite all of our resources and the modern technology devoted to medical care, attention to pain management and patient comfort fell short of the mark. It took almost 30 years for JCAHO to finally regulate the delivery of appropriate pain management care.

The similarities between human and veterinary medicine are impressive. Numerous dedicated individuals over the last several decades have worked to improve our understanding and treatment of animal pain, yet the paradigm shift to comprehensive and effective perioperative analgesia has been slow. Lloyd Davis[3] had exposed the myth approximately 35 years ago that opioids could not be given to cats, yet it is still relatively common to hear that opioids will induce mania in cats. Bernie Rollin, 25 years ago, established the moral imperative to minimize and treat pain in research animals and has been speaking and writing about the issue ever since.[4] In what may be considered a watershed paper, Hansen and Hardie[5] blew the whistle on academic veterinary practice, much as Marks and Sachar did, by exposing the lack of provision of effective analgesics to dogs and cats that had undergone major surgical procedures. Several surveys from within the veterinary profession indicate that pain management is improving, but is far from ideal.[6–10] In 2003, the American Animal Hospital Association (AAHA) followed JCAHO's initiative and elevated pain to the fourth vital sign in animals (in addition to temperature, pulse, and respiration). Although the AAHA is a voluntary organization of small animal veterinary hospitals, the actions taken to improve the recognition and treatment of pain are a watershed in veterinary medicine. These 11 AAHA standards emphasize patient evaluation, appropriate treatment, and effective communication with clients about the degree of patient pain and discomfort, treatment options, and possible side effects. Pain is easy to overlook in animals; thus, efforts to increase our vigilance to assessing, preventing, and alleviating pain will serve to improve the quality of care that can be delivered to animals.

The Definition of Pain

Pain is an unpleasant sensory and emotional experience (perception) associated with actual or potential tissue damage or is described in terms of such damage. The inability to communicate in no way negates the possibility that an individual is experiencing pain and is in need of appropriate pain relieving treatment.

Pain arises from the activation of a discrete set of receptors and neural pathways by noxious stimuli that are actually or potentially damaging to tissues. Pain is a conscious awareness of acute or chronic discomfort occurring in varying degrees of severity resulting from injury, disease, or emotional distress as evidenced by biological or behavioral changes or both. It is a subjective experience accompanied by feelings of fear, anxiety, and panic. Pain elicits protective motor actions, results in learned avoidance, and may modify species-specific traits of behavior, including social behavior.[11,12] *Acute pain* is the result of a traumatic, surgical, or infectious event that begins abruptly and is relatively brief. It is generally alleviated by analgesic drugs. *Chronic pain* is pain that persists beyond the usual course of an acute disease or beyond a reasonable time for an injury to heal, or that is associated with a chronic pathological process that persists or recurs for months or years (e.g., osteoarthritis). Chronic pain is seldom permanently alleviated by analgesics, but may respond to a combination of analgesics, tranquilizers or psychotropic drugs, physical therapy, environmental manipulation, and behavioral conditioning. Acute pain is a symptom of disease, whereas chronic pain, in and of itself, is a disease.[13] Acute pain has a biological function in that it serves as a warning that something is wrong and leads to protective behavioral changes. Chronic pain does not serve a biological function and imposes severe detrimental stresses. Because pain is a perception, it is always subjective.

In people, pain experience has three dimensions—sensory-discriminative, motivational-affective, and cognitive-evaluative—which are subserved by physiologically distinct systems.[14,15] The *sensory-discriminative* dimension provides information on the onset, location, intensity, type, and duration of the pain-inducing stimulus. This aspect is subserved primarily by the lateral ascending nociceptive tracts, thalamus, and somatosensory cortex. The *motivational-affective* dimension disturbs the feeling of well-being of the individual, resulting in the unpleasant experience of pain and suffering, and triggers the organism into action. This dimension is closely linked to the autonomic nervous system, and cardiovascular, respiratory, and gastrointestinal responses are associated with it (although these can also occur reflexly). This dimension is subserved by the medial ascending nociceptive tracts and their input into the limbic system. The *cognitive-evaluative* dimension encompasses the effects of prior experience, social and cultural values, anxiety, attention, and conditioning. These activities are largely caused by cortical activity, although cortical activation is dependent on reticular activity. The cognitive-evaluative dimension of the pain experience in lower mammals may be the only one that differs significantly from that in people. To discuss pain physiology and its management requires a review of the definitions commonly used to describe this perception.

Definitions

Agology. The science and study of pain phenomena.

Allodynia. Pain caused by a stimulus that does not normally provoke pain.

Analgesia. The absence of pain in the presence of stimuli that would normally be painful.

Analgesics. Drugs that produce analgesia.

Anesthesia. The absence of all sensory modalities.

Anesthetics. Drugs that induce regional anesthesia (i.e., in one part of the body) or general anesthesia (i.e., unconsciousness).

Cancer pain. Pain that is caused by primary tumor growth, metastatic disease, or the toxic effects of chemotherapy and radiation, such as neuropathies caused by neurotoxic antineoplastic drugs.[16]

Causalgia. A syndrome of prolonged burning pain, allodynia, and hyperpathia after a traumatic nerve lesion, often combined with vasomotor and sudomotor (sweating) dysfunction and later trophic changes.

Central pain. Pain associated with a lesion of the central nervous system.

Chronic pain. Pain that persists for longer than the expected time frame for healing or pain associated with progressive nonmalignant disease (such as osteoarthritis).[16]

Deafferentation pain. Pain caused by loss of sensory input into the central nervous system, as occurs with avulsion of the brachial plexus or other types of peripheral nerve lesions, or caused by pathology of the central nervous system.

Dermatome. The sensory segmental supply to skin and subcutaneous tissue.

Distress. The external expression through emotion or behavior (i.e., fear, anxiety, hyperactivity, or aggression) of suffering.[17–19]

Dysesthesia. An unpleasant abnormal sensation, whether spontaneous or evoked.

Hyperalgesia. An increased response to a stimulation that is normally painful.

Hyperesthesia. An increased sensitivity to stimulation, excluding special senses.

Hypoalgesia. A diminished sensitivity to noxious stimulation.

Hypoesthesia. A diminished sensitivity to stimulation, excluding special senses.

Inflammatory pain. Spontaneous pain and hypersensitivity to pain in response to tissue damage and inflammation.[20]

Neuralgia. Pain in the distribution pathway of a nerve or nerves.

Neuritis. An inflammation of a nerve or nerves.

Neuropathic pain. Spontaneous pain and hypersensitivity to pain in association with damage to or a lesion of the nervous system.[20]

Neuropathy. A disturbance of function or a pathological change in a nerve.

Nociception. The reception, conduction, and central nervous processing of nerve signals generated by the stimulation of nociceptors. It is the physiological process that when carried to completion results in the conscious perception of pain.

Nociceptive pain. Transient pain in response to noxious stimuli.[20]

Nociceptor. A receptor preferentially sensitive to a noxious stimulus or to a stimulus that would become noxious if prolonged.

Nociceptor threshold. The minimum strength of stimulus that will cause a nociceptor to generate a nerve impulse.

Noxious stimulus. One that is actually or potentially damaging to body tissue. It is one of intensity and quality that are adequate to trigger nociceptive reactions in an animal, including pain in people.

Pain (detection) threshold. The least experience of pain that an individual can recognize. The point at which an individual just begins to feel pain when a noxious stimulus is being applied in an ascending trial or the point at which pain disappears in a descending trial. The pain-detection threshold is relatively constant among individuals and species. In most cases, it is higher than the nociceptor threshold.

Pain tolerance. The greatest level of pain that an individual will tolerate. Pain tolerance varies considerably among individuals, both human and animal. It is influenced greatly by the individual's prior experience, environment, stress, and drugs.

Pain-tolerance range. The arithmetic difference between the pain-detection threshold and the pain-tolerance threshold.

Paresthesia. An abnormal sensation, whether spontaneous or evoked. Paresthesias are not painful (as opposed to dysesthesias).

Radiculalgia. Pain along the distribution of one or more sensory nerve roots.

Radiculitis. An inflammation of one or more nerve roots.

Radiculopathy. A disturbance of function or pathological change in one or more nerve roots.

Reactions. A combination of reflexes designed to produce widespread movement in relation to the application of a stimulus. Reactions are mass reflexes not under voluntary control and therefore do not involve the cerebral cortex.

Reflexes. Involuntary, purposeful, and orderly responses to a stimulus. The anatomical basis for the reflex arc consists of a receptor, a primary afferent nerve fiber associated with the receptor, a region of integration in the spinal cord or brain stem (synapses), and a lower motor neuron leading to an effector organ such as skeletal muscles (somatic reflexes), smooth muscles, or glands (visceral reflexes).

Responses. Willful movement of the body or parts of the body. A response cannot occur without involvement of the somatosensory cerebral cortex. A decerebrate animal can give a reaction but not a response. Reflexes and reactions may or may not be perception linked (i.e., the stimulus perceived as painful). Because responses require a functioning somatosensory cortex, the initiating stimulus must first be perceived.

Somatic. Usually used to describe input from body tissues other than viscera.

Suffering. An unpleasant emotional state that is internalized and not expressed outwardly. It is described as an undesirable mental state or as an unpleasant emotion that people or animals would normally prefer to avoid. Suffering can refer to a wide range of intense and unpleasant subjective states, such as fear and frustration. It can be of either physical or psychological origin. Suffering can be provoked by pain or by pain-free non–tissue-damaging external stimuli such as denial of the fulfillment of an animal's natural instincts or needs, such as maternal deprivation, social contacts, and so on.

Neuroanatomy of Nociceptive Pathways

Nociceptors and Stimuli

Nociception is the reception of signals from activation of *nociceptors*, which are receptors that detect tissue-damaging (*noxious*) stimuli. *Pain* implies that noxious stimuli have been perceived at the cortical level. Activating stimuli for nociceptors can include mechanical, thermal, or chemical stimuli. Some nociceptors respond only to one of these modalities, whereas others are sensitive to a variety of them (polymodal nociceptors). Nociceptors are naked (nonencapsulated) nerve endings, widely distributed in skin and deep tissues. These represent the peripheral termini of nociceptive primary afferent neurons that possess lightly or unmyelinated, small-diameter axons. Activation of fast-conducting (5 to 30 m/s), *A-δ fibers* are associated with sharp, pricking pain (as reported by humans). Slow-conducting (0.5 to 2.0 m/s), unmyelinated *C fibers* are associated with a slower, burning type of pain.[21-23] Both types of nociceptive fibers innervate the skin (*superficial pain*) and deep somatic or visceral structures (*deep pain*). The distinction between superficial and deep pain is not just an arbitrary one based on "outside" and "inside." Each is associated with an anatomically and functionally segregated central pain pathway; they are differentially susceptible to injury, and they are examined separately in a neurological exam.

Pain research has revealed the presence of a particular functional type of nociceptor referred to as a *silent nociceptor*.[24-26] The high threshold of this nerve ending ensures that under normal circumstances it is relatively insensitive to any stimuli. Following release of tissue-inflammatory mediators, however, the threshold is markedly reduced, and these previously silent nociceptors can be activated by a variety of thermal and mechanical stimuli. The presence of silent nociceptors is one mechanism by which inflammation produces primary hyperalgesia.

Divergence in Nociceptive Pathways

In addition to the connections of ascending nociceptive pathways with somatosensory cortex for conscious perception, pain pathways exhibit variable degrees of connectivity with a number of subcortical regions of the brain and through these connections elicit a variety of nonconscious responses.[21,26-29]

A behaviorally important aspect of nociception (and other sensory modalities) is the degree to which it affects mental alertness. This relationship between sensation and consciousness is orchestrated in the *reticular formation* (RF), a loose aggregate of nuclei in the central core of the brain stem, extending from diencephalon through medulla oblongata. Functions of the RF include regulation of heart and respiratory rates, selective attention to stimuli, and maintenance of consciousness and cortical alertness. The RF is critical to the regulation of the level of consciousness through its rostral projections to the diencephalon, which, in turn, diffusely excites the cerebral cortex. The RF receives input from all afferent pathways, although the degree to which these connections are made is variable, depending on the pathway. Stimuli—but most especially noxious stimuli—increase alertness and autonomic functions, such as heart and respiratory rates.

Nociceptive information is simultaneously directed to the *hypothalamus*, which is the brain's coordinator of elaborate autonomic responses and the primary integrator of physiological and emotional responses. Input from nociceptive pathways to the hypothalamus produces activity in the sympathetic nervous system and the pituitary gland and thus increases circulating epinephrine/norepinephrine and glucocorticoids. The catabolic and other endocrinologic manifestations of this activation can have negative effects on health.

Both the hypothalamus and the RF have projections to other parts of the so-called *limbic system*, a group of cortical and subcortical regions that produce the behavioral, cognitive, and physiological changes that people describe as emotions. Comments on the role of emotion in pain responses are presented below.

Nociceptive pathways send collateral projections to the *mesencephalon (midbrain)*. One set of nuclear targets in the midbrain consist of motor neurons that coordinate orienting movements of the head and eyes toward the noxious stimulus (the visual grasp reflex. Other neurons that form the *periaqueductal grey matter* of the midbrain activate important descending pain modulatory systems.

Nociception: Ascending Spinal Pathways

Multiple nociceptive pathways that have been described in the spinal cord of domestic animals are present in all funiculi of the cord and with a confusing degree of overlap in their functions. None of these pathways are exclusive for transmission of nociception (all have fibers conducting tactile information). For clinical purposes, only two need be understood fully: the spinocervicothalamic and spinoreticular tracts.

The *spinocervicothalamic tract* is concerned with the transmission of *superficial pain* and tactile sensations and is regarded as the primary conscious pain pathway in carnivores.[30,31] The primary afferents of this pathway synapse in the dorsal horn, from which secondary afferents then mediate local reflexes and project craniad in an ipsilateral tract in the dorsal part of the lateral funiculus. The axons in this tract ascend to spinal cord segments C1 and C2, where they synapse in the *lateral cervical nucleus* (Fig. 3.1). The fibers arising from this nucleus will then decussate and project through the brain stem to the thalamus. Some collaterals of the ascending fibers will terminate in the RF. From the thalamus, fibers project to the somatosensory cortex.

The sensations transmitted by the spinocervicothalamic tract are *touch* and *superficial pain*. This pathway is *discriminative* in that the location of the painful stimulus can be precisely determined by the animal, which is a quality linked to the high degree of somatotopy exhibited by this pathway. Clinically, function of the spinocervicothalamic tract is tested by lightly pinching the skin with fingers or a mosquito hemostat. This stimulus is applied *lightly* and *briefly* so as to activate the spinocervicothalamic pathway preferentially.

The *spinoreticular tract* is primarily concerned with transmission of *deep-pain* and *visceral sensations*.[22,32,33] The primary afferents of this pathway enter the cord and immediately diverge to

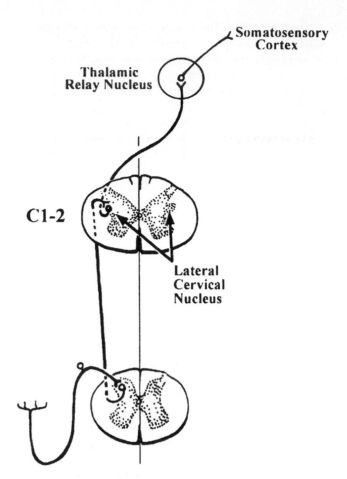

Fig. 3.1. Spinocervicothalamic tract.

send collaterals several segments rostral and caudal to the segment of entry. This spreading of information across several spinal cord segments enables these afferents to participate in intersegmental reflexes (various manifestations of withdrawal and postural reflexes in response to painful stimuli). Second-order neurons are found in the dorsal horn. Axons of projection neurons in this system are present diffusely in the lateral and ventral funiculi. These projections are *bilateral*; decussation of axons in this system occurs diffusely throughout the long axis of the spinal cord (Fig. 3.2).

Most ascending projections of the spinoreticular tract that reach the brain stem do not project directly to the thalamus; rather, they terminate in the RF. Therefore most deep pain that is consciously perceived arrives at the cortex via diffuse reticular projections to the thalamus. Activation of this pathway increases arousal and activates the limbic system, a connection that in humans is associated with emotional responses to pain. There is ample reason to believe that animals, too, experience emotional aspects of pain. As a consequence of the multisynaptic and diffuse nature of this pathway, somatotopy is not well defined, and sensations brought to consciousness by the spinoreticular tract are *poorly localized*: that is, the animal experiences pain and arousal, but cannot readily pinpoint the source.

Diencephalon

Brainstem

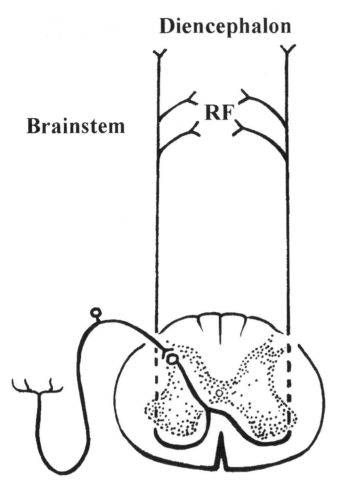

Fig. 3.2. Spinoreticular tract.

TRIGEMINAL SYSTEM
(dorsal view of brainstem)

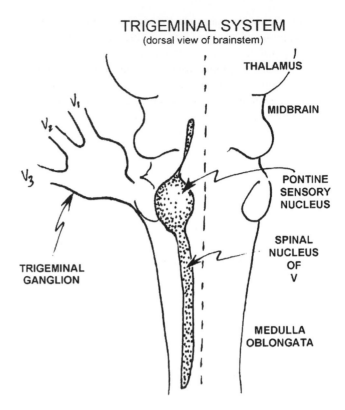

Fig. 3.3. Trigeminal afferent tract.

Visceral pain is particularly poorly localized (see the later comments on referred pain). Visceral afferent fibers travel in sympathetic nerves, have large overlapping receptor fields, and respond primarily to stretch, ischemia, dilation, or spasm (direct trauma to viscera—including surgical trauma—is a surprisingly ineffective stimulus for nociceptors).[22,34,35] Whereas in somatic structures the ratio of A-δ to C fibers is about 1:2, that ratio in viscera is about 1:10.[35] By extension, then, pain of visceral origin tends to be dull, aching, or burning. Primary afferents from viscera follow autonomic nerves (e.g., the vagus and sympathetic nerves) to the central nervous system (CNS).

The deep-pain pathway is tested in the neurological examination by application of a hemostats across the base of a toenail (taking care to exclude skin), a manipulation that stimulates nociceptors in the periosteum of the third phalanx.

Trigeminal System

For the head, nociception and tactile information are transmitted by the trigeminal system.[29,36] Cell bodies of primary afferent fibers reside within the *trigeminal* (semilunar) *ganglion*. Their central processes enter the pons with the trigeminal nerve and course caudal along the lateral surface of the medulla (Fig 3.3). A nuclear column lies medial to the spinal tract throughout its

length. At its rostral extent in the pons, this group of cell bodies comprises the *pontine sensory nucleus*. More caudally, the column is known as the *spinal nucleus of V*. The pontine and spinal nuclei of V contain somata of the second-order neurons in this system. There is a rostral-to-caudal segregation of function in these nuclei; the pontine nucleus is primarily concerned with discriminative tactile and proprioceptive stimuli, and the rostral part of the spinal nucleus of V sends somatosensory information to the cerebellum. The majority of neurons in the spinal nucleus of V, however, are concerned with nociception. Many of these will project to motor nuclei of cranial nerves to participate in reflex arcs (e.g., corneal and palpebral reflexes), and many more will project to the RF to affect autonomic responses and increase arousal. Fibers for conscious perception, however, cross the midline of the medulla diffusely and join the contralateral quintothalamic tract, adjacent to the medial lemniscus. The quintothalamic (aka trigeminal lemniscus) tract projects to the thalamus, and, from there, nociceptive information reaches the somatosensory cortex via the internal capsule.

Nociception: Concepts and Perception (Pain)

Human pain has been described as having three facets, each reflecting the different targets of this sensory information.[37] The sensory-discriminative aspect of pain is concerned with identifying its onset, location, intensity, and character, and is primarily a function of the somesthetic cortex. Behavioral, emotional, and autonomic responses constitute the motivational-affective facet of nociception, and arise in large measure from the connections nociceptive pathways make with the RF, hypothalamus, and the limbic system. Finally, responses to nociception that are a result of experience, attention, and cultural conditioning are described as cognitive-evaluative. These responses are generated by higher cortical functions (awareness, memory, and reasoning).

Painful stimuli are not emotionally neutral events. There is, after all, adaptive value in having an aversion to noxious stimuli; the strong connections of pain pathways to the limbic system ensure that the organism (whether human or animal) will have a negative emotional reaction to pain, which is a feature that is referred to as the *affective component of pain*. This may seem oddly obvious to normally functioning organisms like veterinarians—pain hurts, after all, so why wouldn't you want to avoid it? Reflect for a moment on the myriad of other stimuli constantly made available to the conscious brain; the majority of sensory experiences are emotionally neutral. Feel the surface of this paper: Your fingers relay a vast amount of sensory information, but unless you give yourself a paper cut (a noxious stimulus) or have developed a fetish for paper (resulting in pleasurable feelings as a result of learned associations), you don't have an emotional response to this sensation.

Pain *hurts*, then, because the nociceptive pathways make connections to the limbic system, which assigns an emotional value to it. There are, in fact, documented human cases where brain injury interrupts this valuation process; these patients can feel pain, can identify it, its character, and location accurately, and yet feel no aversion to the stimulus (an extraordinary condition called *asymbolia for pain*).

Suffering is the state of emotional distress associated with events that threaten an organism. Pain need not be the only cause of suffering, although it is probably safe to say that it is the primary one in nonhuman animals. It has been stated that animals do not suffer, because they cannot generate the same *anticipation* of pain and its outcome. Although the ability to anticipate a painful event and put it in a complex context (i.e., How bad is this going to hurt? How long will it hurt? Am I going to die? Who's going to take care of my family?) probably *is* limited in domestic animals, this ability very likely is only partly responsible for the emotional state people associate with suffering. Anticipation is really a feature of the cognitive-evaluative aspect of pain. That this aspect is not well developed in animals is probably defensible on a purely anatomical basis. However, suffering is clearly an *emotional* state. It is probably therefore firmly rooted in the connections between nociceptive pathways and the limbic system, the generator of behavior and emotion. Suffering is a part of the motivational-affective facet of nociception, and there is ample neuroanatomical evidence that the connections between nociceptive pathways and the limbic system are at least as well developed in animals as in people.

Pain Modulation

There is a tendency to conceive of somatosensory pathways as electrical circuits that respond to stimuli in predictable ways and that consistently produce a sensory perception that is a faithful recording of the stimulus in the periphery. This is a useful model, of course, but it grossly oversimplifies the actual condition, wherein activity in the CNS can *modulate* somatosensory processing. This ability to alter activity in sensory systems is especially well developed in nociceptive pathways. *The ability of a given stimulus to produce a perception of pain is a highly labile property and can be modified in the periphery, in the spinal cord, in the brain stem, and in higher centers.*

Modulation in the Periphery (Nociceptors)

Nociceptor threshold is not a constant. As was described above, the presence of so-called *silent nociceptors* is one example of how conditions in the cellular environment of the naked nerve ending can change the sensitivity of the receptor to stimulus. The high threshold of silent nociceptors ensures that, under normal circumstances, they are relatively insensitive to any stimuli, but, on exposure to inflammatory mediators, this threshold is markedly reduced, and previously silent nociceptors can be activated.[24–26]

Similarly, many inflammatory mediators (e.g., prostaglandins and leukotrienes), collectively referred to as *nociceptor sensitizers*, will lower the threshold of other populations of nociceptors.[24,38,39] Thus, in damaged or inflamed tissue, stimuli that would normally be subthreshold may produce activity in nociceptive afferents. Likewise, certain inflammatory mediators (e.g., bradykinin and serotonin) or substances released by damaged cells (e.g., potassium ions and adenosine triphosphate) directly stimulate nociceptors and can thus be considered *nociceptor activators*. Interestingly, stimulated free-nerve endings can release substances directly into the surrounding tissues. Notable among these is *substance P*. Substance P (which is also an important neurotransmitter in central nociceptive pathways) dilates blood vessels and degranulates mast cells, both of which contribute to inflammation and increased sensitization of local nociceptors. All of these events contribute to the development of *primary hyperalgesia* (resulting from the increased responsiveness of nociceptors to noxious stimuli) and a related phenomenon, *allodynia* (wherein normally nonnoxious stimuli, such as those that elicit a touch sensation, become capable of activating nociceptors). Administration of nonsteroidal anti-inflammatory drugs (NSAIDs) is intended to obviate the expression of hyperalgesia and allodynia in injured—and specifically *inflamed*—tissue.

Modulation in the Dorsal Horn

Considerable processing of nociceptive information occurs in the dorsal horn, although precisely what happens there is debated. One of the fundamental concepts of dorsal horn processing is that one population of second-order neurons is dedicated to nociception (nociceptive-specific cells) and an additional, smaller group receives input from primary afferents conducting both noxious and nonnoxious tactile information.[22,25,40] It is suspected that the nociceptive-specific neurons are primarily involved in discriminative nociception (i.e., localization). The second group, referred to as wide-dynamic-range or *WDR neurons*, responds both to noxious and nonnoxious stimuli, and is likely to be recruited in

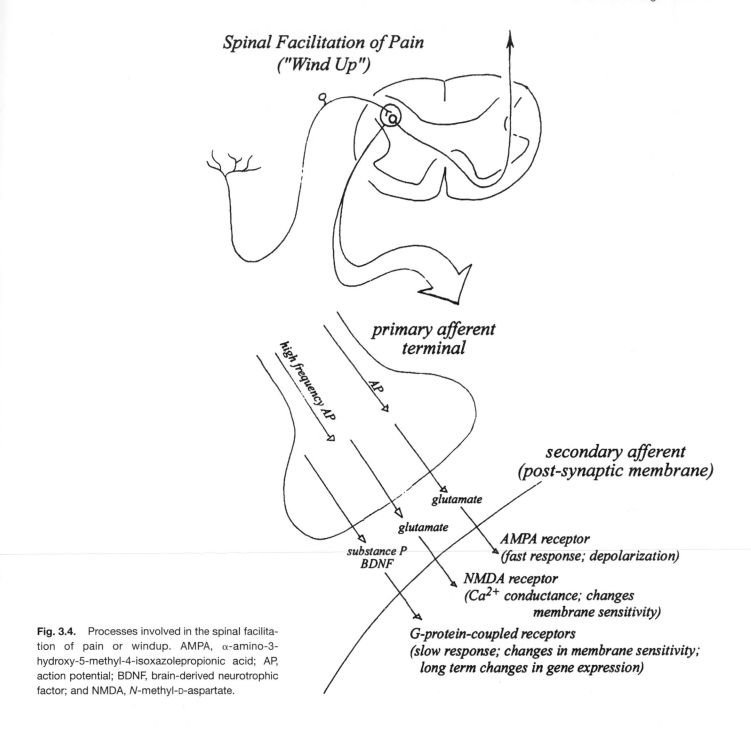

*Spinal Facilitation of Pain
("Wind Up")*

*primary afferent
terminal*

high frequency AP

AP

*secondary afferent
(post-synaptic membrane)*

glutamate

glutamate

*substance P
BDNF*

*AMPA receptor
(fast response; depolarization)*

*NMDA receptor
(Ca²⁺ conductance; changes
membrane sensitivity)*

*G-protein-coupled receptors
(slow response; changes in membrane sensitivity;
long term changes in gene expression)*

Fig. 3.4. Processes involved in the spinal facilitation of pain or windup. AMPA, α-amino-3-hydroxy-5-methyl-4-isoxazolepropionic acid; AP, action potential; BDNF, brain-derived neurotrophic factor; and NMDA, *N*-methyl-D-aspartate.

pathways that exhibit less somatotopy (i.e., are less discriminative). The WDR neurons appear to be relatively insensitive to tactile information, discharging at one rate in response to innocuous touch stimuli, while responding more vigorously (at a greater frequency) to noxious stimulation. These neurons also receive information from both somatic and visceral structures, which is a feature believed to underlie the phenomenon of *referred pain.*[41] In referred pain, noxious stimuli originating in viscera are perceived as originating instead from a somatic region (body wall or skin). This perception is thought to result from the fact that information from that region of viscera converges on WDR neurons and path-

ways that also convey information from somatic structures. Since we (and presumably other organisms) are much more familiar with sensations arising from our skin and body wall, the pain is interpreted to originate in these somatic structures.

The WDR neurons are probably the cells most important in the expression of *spinal facilitation of pain,* or *windup* (Fig. 3.4). Windup occurs with rapid, continuous firing of primary nociceptive afferents, probably most especially small-diameter, unmyelinated fibers (C fibers).[38,42,43] The high-frequency volley of action potentials in the primary afferent terminal stimulates release of increased amounts of glutamate and is also associated with release of substance P and brain-derived neurotrophic factor.[43,44] The increased exposure to glutamate in the synaptic cleft activates N-methyl-D-aspartate (NMDA) receptors (inactive except under conditions of persistent membrane depolarization) on the postsynaptic membrane. This particular variety of glutamate receptor is unique in that it exhibits a calcium conductance; its activation is therefore associated with influx of calcium ions onto the postsynaptic neuron, leading to a series of intracellular cascades that ultimately results in upregulation of receptors.[42,45] Substance P and brain-derived neurotrophic factor are neuromodulatory neurotransmitters that bind with G-protein–coupled receptors. These, too, activate intracellular signaling cascades that increase the membrane's sensitivity to subsequent stimulation.

The net effect of these events is that high-frequency action potentials in the primary afferent neuron "train" the second-order neurons to respond more vigorously to subsequent stimulation. This change can last from hours to days (and longer) after the causative event ends. Effectively, then, prolonged noxious stimuli produce greater sensitivity to subsequent stimuli. What is especially significant about this phenomenon is that general anesthesia does not prevent windup, as it does not prevent generation of action potentials in the primary afferents. This observation has been used as a compelling argument for the use of analgesics preoperatively or intraoperatively as a preemptive strike against the development of windup during surgeries (e.g., orthopedic procedures) likely to activate C fibers. In 1965, Melzack and Wall[46] developed a concept of spinal cord pain modulation that they called the *gate control theory*. The specifics of the neuronal interactions in the original gate control theory have since been shown to be inaccurate, and many contemporary pain researchers object to the continued use of the term "gate control theory." Nonetheless, the term is in very wide use among professionals educated in medicine, and the model, however inaccurate in its details, is useful as a basis for understanding the modulatory influences of tactile information on nociceptive information at the level of the spinal cord. The gate control theory was developed primarily to explain the common observation that nonnoxious tactile stimulation (e.g., vibration and massage) can reduce the perception of pain. That this is so is evident in our common pain experiences. For example, when you "bark your shin," your first impulse is to rub the injured region. To do so lessens the perceived pain.

In a simplified form, the gate control theory may be summarized as follows: Both nociceptive-specific C fibers and nonnociceptive (tactile) A-ß fibers converge on WDR neurons of the dorsal horn. The nonnociceptive fibers also make connections with interneurons whose effects on transmission neurons of the dorsal horn are inhibitory. When A-ß fibers are activated by tactile stimuli, they weakly stimulate the WDR projection neurons and simultaneously stimulate the inhibitory interneurons. These inhibitory neurons reduce transmission in the nociceptive pathways either by (a) inhibiting activity in the WDR projection neurons (postsynaptic inhibition) or (b) inhibiting release of neurotransmitter from the C-fiber terminals in an axoaxonic connection (presynaptic inhibition). Whatever the mechanism, the end result is that ascending transmission of nociception is decreased.[41]

The gate control theory, regardless of the exact circuitry, explains the observation that certain kinds of tactile stimuli can reduce perception of pain. These stimuli can take the form of heat or cold application, massage, vibration, or transcutaneous electrical nerve stimulation, a pain therapy used in human medicine, among others. Additionally, the described modulation at the level of the dorsal horn may be at least partly responsible for the effectiveness of acupuncture for relief of pain.

Suprasegmental Modulation

Activity in spinal nociceptive pathways is also strongly influenced by antinociceptive systems that originate in the brain stem.[21,41,44,47] The midbrain (mesencephalon) and medulla both possess a series of midline nuclei that modulate the transmission of nociception. Input from higher cerebral centers and collaterals from ascending nociceptive pathways, particularly those conveying deep pain (spinoreticular tract), activate these nuclei. Among the nuclei that give rise to descending pain modulatory pathways, of particular note are the mesencephalic *periaqueductal gray matter* (PAG) and the *nucleus raphe magnus* of the rostroventral medulla.

The PAG receives input from ascending nociceptive tracts and higher centers (including limbic structures and cerebral cortex) and sends axons to the nucleus raphe magnus, to other medullary reticular nuclei, and, to a much lesser extent, to the dorsal horn of the spinal cord. These axons release multiple neurotransmitters, most notably *endorphins*, which are transmitters with powerful antinociceptive properties. The PAG input to the nucleus raphe magnus activates (through disinhibition) the monoaminergic pathways that arise here and descend the cord to modulate nociception at the level of the dorsal horn (Fig. 3.5). The primary neurotransmitters of the nucleus raphe magnus and other medullary nuclei are serotonin and norepinephrine. Activity in these systems will recruit a pool of interneurons whose neurotransmitters (endorphin, enkephalin, and dynorphin) inhibit transmission in spinal cord pain pathways at the level of the dorsal horn.

Neuropathic Pain

This is pain that is caused by injury to the nervous system. Damage leading to neuropathic pain can result from a variety of insults, including trauma (e.g., amputation and crushing injury), vascular injury (e.g., thromboembolic disease), endocrinopathy (e.g., diabetes mellitus), or infection (e.g., postherpetic neuralgia). Neuropathic pain resulting from these many different causes is probably not a single uniform entity. Several mechanisms are thought likely to contribute to neuropathic pain; not all of these necessarily underlie any given case of neuropathic pain, although they are not mutually exclusive.[38,48,49]

Hyperalgesia and allodynia are both commonly associated with neuropathic pain. *Dysesthesias*, which are unpleasant, abnormal sensations often characterized as tingling or "electric," are sometimes described by affected people, although neuropathic pain is most usually described as having a burning, lancinating quality. In the peripheral nervous system, injury to pri-

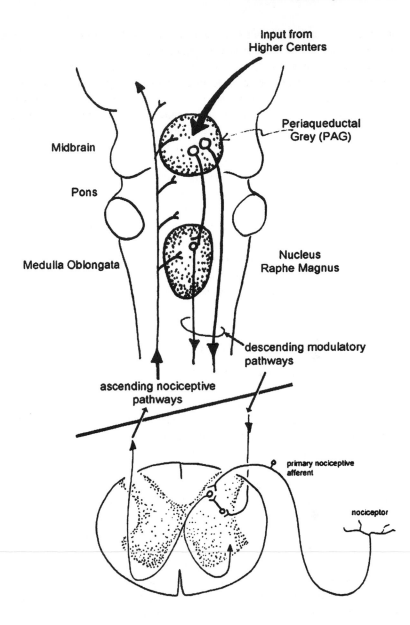

Fig. 3.5. Descending inhibitory pain pathways.

mary afferents (up to and including the dorsal root ganglia) can cause neuropathic pain. The pathomechanisms producing this pain are not clearly understood and, like all facets of neuropathic pain, are likely to be multiple. In at least some cases, the damaged primary afferent produces an increased frequency of spontaneous action potentials (most neurons do this to some extent, but normal nociceptive afferents typically do so at a very low rate), a phenomenon called *ectopic discharge*.[38,48] Damaged primary afferents are also apt to develop collateral sprouting, perhaps in response to neurotrophic factors released by damaged tissues. Aberrant collaterals of nociceptive neurons may spread into adjacent skin or other tissues, where their activation can produce an abnormal perception of pain.[38] One line of inquiry has revealed a phenomenon of electrical coupling between somatosensory and sympathetic fibers in the periphery (including the dorsal root ganglia). This coupling, called *sympathetically maintained pain*, activates nociceptive pathways (and pain perception) with activity in sympathetic neurons.[38,48]

Centrally, the alterations described in the discussion of windup (spinal facilitation of pain) are likely to play a role in the development of sustained, neuropathic pain, inasmuch as the upregulation of receptors on postsynaptic membranes can persist for a prolonged time.[43,45] Since activation of NMDA glutamate receptors is a key part of spinal facilitation of pain, use of NMDA antagonists shows potential as a therapy for neuropathic pain. Additionally, there is evidence that tactile (i.e., nonnociceptive) A-ß afferent fibers sprout collateral connections in the dorsal horn (again, probably in response to neurotrophic factors released by injured nervous tissue), making aberrant connections with projection neurons that are normally associated with nociception.[48] Activity in these fibers will therefore produce activity in nociceptive pathways, leading ultimately to the perception of increased pain.

There is also ample evidence that the repertoire of neurotransmitters and/or receptors within the dorsal horn undergoes changes in response to injury.[49,50] Some researchers have documented a decrease in γ-aminobutyric acid (an inhibitory neurotransmitter) in animal models of neuropathic pain. Experimental techniques that increase levels of γ-aminobutyric acid in the spinal cord are associated with an attenuation of allodynia, which is characteristic of neuropathic pain.

A particularly frustrating aspect of neuropathic pain is the extent to which it is refractory to opioids. This is likely because of a loss of opioid receptors, which is a phenomenon that has been reported in the dorsal root ganglion and the dorsal horn.[48] Simultaneously, cholecystokinin and its receptors appear to be upregulated by nervous tissue injury; cholecystokinin has documented opioid antagonist activity.[48]

Neuropathic pain is a well-recognized problem in human medicine, and there is observational evidence that it is a significant cause of postinjury morbidity in animals, as well. Therapies to effectively reverse the development of neuropathic pain will rely on a clear understanding of the cellular biology and neurophysiology that underlie it.

Response to Pain and Injury

Nociceptive stimulation of medullary centers of circulation and ventilation, hypothalamic centers of neuroendocrine function (primarily sympathetic), and limbic structures produces suprasegmental reflex responses. These include hyperventilation, increased hypothalamic neural sympathetic tone, and increased release of catecholamines and other endocrine hormones. Increased neural sympathetic tone and catecholamine secretion add to that induced segmentally to further increase cardiac output, peripheral resistance, blood pressure, cardiac work, and myocardial oxygen consumption. In addition, there is increased secretion of cortisol, adrenocorticotropic hormone, glucagon, cyclic adenosine monophosphate, antidiuretic hormone, growth hormone, renin, and other catabolic hormones, and a concomitant decrease in the anabolic hormones insulin and testosterone. These responses, characteristic of the stress response, cause increased blood glucose, free fatty acids, blood lactate, and ketones, as well as an increased rate of metabolism and oxygen consumption. These responses cause substrate mobilization to central organs and injured tissues, and lead to a catabolic state and negative nitrogen balance. The magnitude and duration of these changes parallels those of the degree of tissue damage and may last for days when weight loss and muscle wastage become clinically obvious.[17,51–54]

These nociceptive responses also occur in anesthetized or unconscious patients because the nociceptive neural activity is not obtunded at the spinal and brain-stem levels. Nevertheless, the patients are pain free because the nociceptive activity does not terminate or impinge on a functioning cerebral cortex. It has been proposed that these responses can be obtunded or largely prevented by the preoperative administration of analgesic agents (so-called preemptive analgesia).[55] More specifically, when evoked potential responses to somatic stimulation are abolished by epidural or intrathecal local anesthetics, the stress response is inhibited. Peripheral nerve blockade alone is not as effective at blocking the stress response. Systemic opioids have little effect on the stress response. Epidural or intrathecal opioids when used alone appear to obtund the stress response, but not nearly as effectively as do local anesthetics. Norepinephrine, epinephrine, adrenocorticotropic hormone, and cortisol increased intraoperatively corresponding to surgical manipulation in dogs anesthetized with isoflurane alone for ovariohysterectomy, and remained elevated postoperatively. These endocrine responses were prevented by the preoperative administration of the α$_2$-agonist medetomidine.[56] Administration of analgesics (e.g., morphine or xylazine) has been shown to decrease plasma catecholamine concentrations in cats after onychectomy.[57]

Intense anxiety and fear, which are an integral part of the pain experience and response, greatly enhance the hypothalamic responses through cortical stimulation. Pain-free anxiety can cause greater cortisol and catecholamine responses than those resulting directly from nociceptive impulses reaching the hypothalamus.[58,59] In addition, anxiety causes cortically mediated increases in blood viscosity, clotting time, fibrinolysis, and platelet aggregation.[60–63] Pain-induced responses are summarized in Table 3.1.[64]

These reflex responses induced by tissue damage and pain, although immediately protective for short-term survival of the organism, can be deleterious if prolonged. Indeed, in the hospital setting, and specifically in a surgical environment, they may be more deleterious than beneficial. More specifically, the stress response increases cardiac output, cardiac work, and oxygen consumption at a time when cardiac reserve is diminished. Intense vasoconstriction, especially of the splanchnic beds, leads to ischemia, tissue hypoxia, and release of myocardial toxins. Renal failure may ensue as a result of intense vasoconstriction and the release of arginine vasopressin (antidiuretic hormone) and aldosterone. In many patients with severe posttraumatic or postsurgical pain, these neuroendocrine responses are of sufficient magnitude to initiate and maintain shock.[65]

Attenuation of the stress response through adequate pain relief and supportive therapy should improve patient outcome and promote healing. For example, in a recent report, the continuous-rate infusion of butorphanol (13 μg/kg/h) for 1 day following abdominal surgery in horses decreased plasma cortisol concentrations and improved behavior scores when compared with horses that did not receive butorphanol.[66] Similarly, dogs undergoing forelimb amputation that received a constant-rate infusion of ketamine during and after surgery in addition to standard analgesics had significantly lower pain scores 12 and 18 h after surgery and were more active on postoperative day 3 as compared with dogs that did not receive ketamine.[67] Pain can be managed initially through systemic administration of analgesics, primarily opioids, α$_2$-adrenergic agonists, local anesthetic nerve blocks, lidocaine administered intravenously, ketamine, and NSAIDs. Long-term (up to 12 h) control of pain may include epidural or spinal administration of many of these agents in combination with local anesthetics. Local and regional nerve blocks (e.g., intercostal, brachial plexus, or intra-articular) can play an important role in the perioperative period and as a part of a balanced anesthetic protocol.[68] Preventive analgesia has been shown to be highly effective in preventing windup and in decreasing postoperative pain as measured by a reduced requirement for analgesics.[55,69]

Table 3.1. Neuroendocrine and metabolic responses to pain.

Segmental and suprasegmental reflexes
Increased sympathetic tone
Vasconstriction: skin and viscera
Increased systemic vascular resistance and preload
Increased stroke volume, heart rate, and cardiac output
Increased arterial pressure and myocardial work
Increased metabolic rate and oxygen consumption
Decreased gastrointestinal and urinary tone
Increased skeletal muscle tone
Endocrine responses
Increased adrenocorticotropic hormone, cortisol, antidiuretic
 hormone, and growth hormone
Cyclic adenosine monophosphate, catecholamines, renin, and
 angiotensin II
Aldosterone, glucagon, and interleukin I
Decreased insulin and testosterone
Metabolic responses
Hyperglycemia
Glycogenolysis and gluconeogenesis
Increased muscle protein metabolism
Increased lipolysis
Water and electrolytes
Retention of water and sodium ions
Increased potassium-ion excretion
Decreased extracellular fluid
Ventilation
Central hyperventilation
Segmental hypoventilation
Splinting and bronchospasm
Diencephalic and cortical responses
Anxiety and fear increase sympathetic responses
Blood viscosity and clotting time
Fibrinolysis and platelet aggregation
Psychological effects
Overall effects of pain
Prolonged recovery
Slower return to normal behaviors

Preemptive analgesia clearly has beneficial effects in the immediate perioperative period, including being able to maintain anesthesia with less inhalant agent (less cardiopulmonary depression) and improved recovery from anesthesia and surgery. Based on survey studies from human medicine, the overall impact of preemptive analgesia on patient pain and outcome variables is somewhat less clear.[70–74] Large-scale clinical studies evaluating the role of preemptive analgesia in overall patient outcome have not been published in the veterinary literature to date. Nevertheless, the clinical benefits of preemptive analgesia likely outweigh the costs. As such, analgesics should be administered to all animals undergoing a surgical or invasive diagnostic procedure unless there are compelling reasons to do otherwise. In addition, NSAIDs may be useful in relieving pain caused by the continued release of algogenic substances from injured and inflamed tissues. Nonpharmacological treatments, such as supportive bandages and splinting, should not be overlooked.

Communicating and Measuring Pain in Veterinary Patients

As previously mentioned, pain is an extremely complex multidimensional experience with both sensory and affective (emotional) elements. Obviously, there are distinct populations, including human neonates, nonverbal adults, and animals, that cannot express their pain overtly. However, all mammals possess the neuroanatomical and neuropharmacological components necessary for transduction, transmission, and perception of noxious stimuli; therefore, it is commonly assumed that animals experience pain even if they cannot exactly perceive or communicate it in the same way people do.[75]

All pain is subjective. No one can "feel" another person's pain. Even after identical surgical procedures, people do not experience the same quality and intensity of pain. In view of that, how can we determine with any degree of certainty what an animal feels? Put simply, in humans, pain is what the patient says it is; and, in animals, pain is what humans say it is. Clearly, there is more room for error when humans assess pain in an animal, because all judgments are subjective and, if the humans "get it wrong," a great disservice is done to the animal. It can be stated that pain has been treated effectively only if it can be measured. Veterinarians can measure many specifics in our patients, including blood pressure, temperature, and arterial oxygen partial pressure, all of which are expressed in quantifiable, completely objective units, but what is the unit of pain? There is none. Lord Kelvin stated in 1883, "I often say that when you can measure what you are speaking about and express it in numbers you know something about it; but when you cannot measure it, when you cannot express it in numbers, your knowledge is of a meager and unsatisfactory kind."[76]

With that in mind, there is presently no gold standard for assessing pain in animals. Many different scoring methods that include physiological variables (in an attempt to identify objective measures) and behavioral variables have been published, but few have been rigorously validated. The issue of pain assessment in animals is especially complex because consideration must include differences in gender, age, species, breed, strain, and environment. Assessment systems must also take into account the different types and sources of pain, such as acute versus chronic or neuropathic pain and visceral compared with somatic pain. For example, if a pain scale were developed to evaluate acute postoperative pain in dogs following routine abdominal surgery, such as ovariohysterectomy, then the scale might be inappropriate for assessing pain after orthopedic surgery or pain associated with chronic osteoarthritis in that species. There is no question that as more studies focus on species-specific pain behaviors and the different types of pain, the ability of the veterinary community to recognize and treat pain in animals will improve. Nevertheless, the assessment of pain in animals will remain a subjective and inaccurate undertaking for the foreseeable future. Despite that prediction, one fact remains certain: Ignoring pain simply because there is difficulty measuring it condemns animal patients to undue suffering.

Behavioral responses to pain vary greatly between species, and these differences may be linked to an animal's survival mechanisms. For example, because rats and mice are prey animals, overt signs of pain or injury draw the attention of predators, so the rodents have evolved to where they instinctively disguise their pain. The subtle signs of pain exhibited by these species, such as abdominal pressing and back arching, can be easily missed by an inexperienced observer.[77,78] Because of behavioral distinctions, pain-assessment tools must be species specific. There are also behavioral variations within a species: Few veterinarians would disagree that Labrador retriever dogs react differently from the Arctic breeds in the postoperative period!

It is now apparent that every animal is unique with respect to number, morphology, and distribution of opioid receptors; and these differences are genetically determined. This, as well as each individual's own endogenous ability to inhibit pain transmission and perception, may explain some of the variation in pain tolerance and the range of responses to analgesic drugs. From the work of Holton and others with dogs[79] and Roughan and Flecknell[78] with rats, it is obvious that creating meaningful pain-assessment tools is a painstaking and time-consuming task.

Pain-Assessment Tools in Veterinary Medicine

Acute Pain
Most studies in dogs and cats have focused on assessing acute postoperative pain. Not all of the systems used have been validated or rigorously tested, however; and the key question for a busy practitioner is "How well do these scoring systems perform in clinical practice?"

Objective Measures
In both cats and dogs, the correlation between easily measured physiological variables (heart rate, respiratory rate, blood pressure, and pupil diameter) and pain scores have been evaluated.[80–82] No study found a consistently reliable objective measure, which is not surprising as these parameters can be affected by many factors other than pain. For example, an opioid alone causes mydriasis in cats but miosis in dogs. Pupil size is also affected by fear and ambient light. In a tightly controlled research setting, blood pressure looked promising as an indirect indicator of pain in cats, but, in a clinical environment, this variable was an unreliable indicator of pain.[83,84]

Changes in plasma cortisol and ß-endorphins are components of the "stress response" to anesthesia and surgery, and much effort has been expended trying to correlate these hormones with pain in laboratory and clinical analgesia trials. Plasma cortisol was not a useful pain marker in dogs and is extremely unreliable in cats.[80,84–87] Mechanical nociceptive threshold testing with various devices (palpometers and algometers) has proved to be useful for evaluating both primary (wound) and secondary (remote area) hyperalgesia in cats and dogs.[81,88,89] Changes in wound sensitivity have correlated with visual analog scoring in cats, suggesting that assessing wound tenderness is a valuable tool and should be incorporated into an overall assessment protocol.[89] Force plate gait analyses have been widely used to assess lameness in dogs objectively. This technique has also been used to evaluate response to different surgical procedures and to assess the efficacy of a variety of analgesics. Conzemius et al.[90] have demonstrated that pressure platform gait analysis can be used successfully in cats and may provide a method of assessing pain after procedures such as onychectomy.

Scoring Systems
Because animals cannot self-report, all scoring systems that depend on a human observer must, by definition, be subjective to some degree and leave room for error, which could be either underassessment or overassessment of the animal's pain. Any system used must be valid, reliable, and sensitive.[91] Without strictly defined criteria and the use of well-trained and experienced observers, many scoring systems are too variable, which is one of the main criticisms of multicenter clinical trials. One scoring system may show an analgesic agent to be effective, and another shows that same analgesic to be ineffective. If a system is insensitive, then these differences are inevitable and result in large interobserver variability.

Simple descriptive scales. These are the most basic pain scales. These usually have four or five descriptors from which observers choose, such as *no pain*, *mild pain*, *moderate pain*, *severe pain*, or *very severe pain*. Although simple to use, these scales are extremely subjective and do not detect small changes in pain behavior.

Numerical rating scales. These are essentially the same as simple descriptive scales, but assign numbers for ease of tabulation and analyses; for example, absence of pain is assigned the number 0 and very severe pain the number 5. This system implies equal difference or weighting between each category, which is not the case. These are discontinuous scales; therefore, a dog experiencing pain that is "just in" category 2 is in quite different condition from a dog that is also in category 2 but almost in category 3. A further development of the simple descriptive and numerical rating systems is a categorized numerical rating system where certain behaviors are chosen and assigned a value. For example, vocalization can be divided into none (score = 0), crying but responsive (score = 1), and crying but nonresponsive (score = 2); other categories may include movement, agitation, and posture.[92]

Visual analog scale. In an attempt to improve on discontinuous scales, the visual analog scale (VAS) has been widely used in veterinary medicine (Fig. 3.6). This tool consists of a continuous line (usually 100 mm long) anchored at either end with a description of the limits of the scale, for example *no pain* or *no sedation* at one end and *severe pain* or *asleep* at the other end. An observer places a mark on the line at the point that he/she thinks correlates with the degree of pain in the animal under observation, and this point is later translated into a number by measuring the distance to the mark from zero. The VAS can be improved by adding a descriptor that says "Worst possible pain for *this* procedure," because the worst pain associated with a castration is likely to be different from the worst pain after a thoracotomy. Without training and experience, the VAS results in wide interobserver variation.

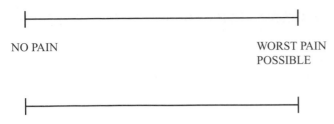

Fig. 3.6. The visual analogue scale used to assess pain in animals.

Holton and others[91] compared the use of simple descriptive, numerical rating, and visual analogue scales for assessing pain in dogs after surgery. The results showed significant observer variability—as high as 36%—with all three scales. These researchers suggested that the numerical rating scale was most suitable if a single, trained observer performed all assessments, which again emphasizes the difficulty in conducting reliable multicenter trials.

Lascelles and others[88] have reported the use of a dynamic and interactive visual analog scale (DIVAS) as an extension of the classic VAS system in dogs. With the DIVAS system, animals are first observed from a distance undisturbed and then approached, handled, and encouraged to walk. Finally, the surgical incision and surrounding area are palpated, and a final overall assessment of sedation and pain is made. This approach overcomes some of the deficiencies of purely observational systems; for example, a dog may lie very still and quiet *because* a wound is painful, and this would go undetected unless the observer interacted with the animal. The DIVAS system has also been used to assess postoperative pain in cats and, when performed by one individual unaware of treatments, it detected differences between analgesics (meperidine and carprofen) and between treated (analgesia) and untreated (no analgesia) cats.[93,94] So far, the scoring systems discussed in this section are regarded as *one-dimensional* in that they assess only intensity of pain.

Considering the complexity of pain, it is not surprising that simple, subjective, one-dimensional systems have not proven ideal. In humans, multidimensional systems, such as the McGill Pain Questionnaire, that account for not only intensity but also sensory and affective (emotional) qualities of pain have provided a more comprehensive assessment of a patient's pain. Multidimensional systems are particularly important when self-reporting is not possible, but reports must incorporate components that are proven to be sensitive and specific to pain (e.g., facial expressions in infants) in the species being studied.[95]

It is now accepted that quantitative measurements of behavior are the most reliable methods for assessing pain in animals and that, if the methodology used to develop and validate these systems is rigorous, they can be more objective with minimal observer bias.[96] Knowledge of normal behavior for the individual being evaluated is essential. Deviations from normal behavior suggest pain, anxiety, or some combination of stressors. Developing these quantitative systems is a daunting task; Fox et al.[97] identified 166 possible pain behaviors associated with ovariohys-

terectomy in bitches. The importance of noninteractive (videotaped in absence of caregivers) and interactive behaviors has also been demonstrated.[97,98] In these studies, dogs that had undergone surgery without analgesics spent more time sleeping than control animals did, but also showed increased cage-circling activity, lip licking, and flank gazing. These activities would be easy to miss in a busy clinical setting, however. Although reduced after surgery (with and without analgesics), tail wagging and positive interactions still occurred in the presence of a caregiver; and, during cursory examinations, the dog could easily be scored as *not painful*.

Sporadic observation of animal behavior may not reveal signs of pain. Some signs may be masked by behavior that is stereotypical of the species being observed. For instance, a dog may wag its tail and greet an observer at the cage door despite being in pain. Cats may simply hide in the back of their cages and demonstrate no behaviors that would suggest to a casual observer that they are painful. Behavioral changes indicating pain may not be what are expected. A cat sitting quietly in the back of the cage after surgery may be in pain; however, pain would not be recognized if the caregiver expects to see more active signs of pain, such as pacing, agitation, or vocalizing.

The University of Melbourne Pain Scale (UMPS) has been developed to incorporate objective physiological data (heart rate, respiratory rate, pupil size, and rectal temperature) and behavioral responses (activity, response to palpation, posture, mental status, and vocalization). By assigning numbers to each factor, a score between 0 and 27 is derived.[99] This scale has been tested on dogs following ovariohysterectomy and demonstrated good agreement between different assessors. It could differentiate between dogs that were anesthetized but not subjected to surgery and those undergoing surgery. With some refinement to detect smaller differences, the system shows promise for clinical use.

To date, the most vigorously validated scale for assessing acute postoperative pain in dogs is the Glasgow composite measures pain scale.[79] The original 279 words or expressions that could describe pain in dogs have been reduced to 47 well-defined words placed in one physiological category and seven behavioral categories. The behavioral categories comprise evaluations of

Posture
Comfort
Vocalization
Attention to the wound
Demeanor and response to humans
Mobility
Response to touch

Each descriptor is well defined to avoid misinterpretation. Assessment involves both observation from a distance and interaction with the patient (e.g., palpation of the wound). Frequent assessments are necessary because pain is not a static process, and the benefits of intervention with analgesics must be evaluated. In a busy practice, time-consuming assessments are the biggest drawbacks to effective pain management. For this reason, a short form of the Glasgow composite pain scale, which takes only a few minutes to perform, has been developed (Fig. 3.7).

SHORT FORM OF THE GLASGOW COMPOSITE PAIN SCALE

Dog's name _____

Hospital Number _____ Date / / Time

Surgery Yes/No (delete as appropriate)

Procedure or Condition_____

_____

In the sections below please circle the appropriate score in each list and sum these to give the total score.

A. Look at dog in Kennel

Is the dog?

(i)

Quiet	0
Crying or whimpering	1
Groaning	2
Screaming	3

(ii)

Ignoring any wound or painful area	0
Looking at wound or painful area	1
Licking wound or painful area	2
Rubbing wound or painful area	3
Chewing wound or painful area	4

In the case of spinal, pelvic or multiple limb fractures, or where assistance is required to aid locomotion do not carry out section **B** and proceed to **C**
Please tick if this is the case ☐ then proceed to C.

B. Put lead on dog and lead out of the kennel.

When the dog rises/walks is it?

(iii)

Normal	0
Lame	1
Slow or reluctant	2
Stiff	3
It refuses to move	4

C. If it has a wound or painful area including abdomen, apply gentle pressure 2 inches round the site.

Does it?

(iv)

Do nothing	0
Look round	1
Flinch	2
Growl or guard area	3
Snap	4
Cry	5

D. Overall

Is the dog?

(v)

Happy and content or happy and bouncy	0
Quiet	1
Indifferent or non-responsive to surroundings	2
Nervous or anxious or fearful	3
Depressed or non-responsive to stimulation	4

Is the dog?

(vi)

Comfortable	0
Unsettled	1
Restless	2
Hunched or tense	3
Rigid	4

Total Score (i+ii+iii+iv+v+vi) = _____

Fig. 3.7. Short-form pain questionnaire. The short-form composite measure pain score (CMPS-SF) can be applied quickly and reliably in a clinical setting and has been designed as a clinical decision-making tool that was developed for dogs in acute pain. It includes 30 descriptor options within 6 behavioral categories, including mobility. Within each category, the descriptors are ranked numerically according to their associated pain severity, and the person performing the assessment chooses the descriptor within each category that best fits the dog's behavior or condition. It is important to perform the assessment procedure as described on the questionnaire, following the protocol closely. The pain score is the sum of the rank scores. The maximum score for the 6 categories is 24, or 20 if mobility is impossible to assess. The total CMPS-SF score has been shown to be a useful indicator of analgesic requirement, and the recommended analgesic intervention level is 6/24 or 5/20.[170]

Suggestions for Creating an Acute-Pain Scoring System

Each practice should choose or design a pain-scoring system that meets its own specific needs, and finding one that suits may require trial and error. The system chosen should be user friendly and readily used by veterinarians and animal-care staff. It should also be an integral part of an animal's postoperative evaluation. After temperature, pulse, and respiration are checked, pain, which has been coined the "fourth vital sign," should also be assessed and treated, if necessary. A scale should include both non-interactive and interactive components and rely heavily on changes in behavior.

Considerations in Establishing a Pain Scale

Pain scales should not be used to deny analgesic therapy to an animal that is likely to be in pain following a procedure. Rather, the pain scale should be used to determine whether analgesic therapy needs to be increased or can be tapered off.

Therapy should not be based on rigid minimum scores.

Individual behaviors suggestive of animal pain or distress should overrule results of pain scoring.

If a procedure is likely to be painful, but the pain score is too low to prompt treatment, a test dose of analgesic should be administered and the patient's response observed.

Critically ill or compromised animals may be unable to show behaviors required to bring about treatment.

Consider low-dose opioid therapy in a painful animal that is slightly obtunded. Increased awareness of surroundings, but not agitation, suggests a beneficial effect of analgesic therapy.

If a practitioner is unsure that a patient is in pain, but tissue trauma has occurred, treat for pain conservatively and observe results.

How Often Should Animals Be Assessed?

Acute Pain

The health status of the animal, extent of surgery/injuries, and anticipated duration of analgesic drugs determine the frequency and interval of evaluations. In general, evaluations should be made at least hourly for the first 4 to 6 h after surgery, provided the animal has recovered from anesthesia, has stable vital signs, and is resting comfortably. Animals not recovering as anticipated from anesthesia/surgery and critically ill animals require much more frequent evaluations until they are stabilized. Patient response to analgesic therapy and expected duration of analgesic drug(s) administered help to determine frequency of evaluations. For example, if a dog is resting comfortably following the postoperative administration of morphine, it may not need to be reassessed for 2 to 4 h. Animals should be allowed to sleep following analgesic therapy. Vital signs can often be checked without unduly disturbing a sleeping animal. In general, animals are not awakened to check their pain status; however, that does not mean they should not receive their scheduled analgesics.

Continuous, undisturbed observations, coupled with periodic interactive observations (open the cage, palpate the wound, etc.) are likely to provide more information than occasionally observing the animal through the cage door. It is regrettable that continuous observations are not practical for most clinical situations. In general, the more frequent the observations, the more likely that subtle signs of pain will be detected.

Chronic Pain

Without doubt, chronic pain affects an animal's quality of life. Because of the nature of chronic pain, such as that associated with osteoarthritis in dogs and cats, the accompanying behavioral changes can be insidious and easily missed. Indeed, many owners assume these changes are inevitable with advancing age.

Preliminary data based on owner interviews revealed changes in 32 types of behavior in dogs with chronic pain.[100] This study also indicated that the owners are the best evaluators of their pet's pain. The Glasgow University Health-Related Dog Behavior Questionnaire has identified some key indicators of chronic pain, including, but not limited to, decreases in mobility, activity, sociability, and curiosity, and increases in aggression, anxiety, daytime sleeping, and vocalizing.[100]

Chronic pain is undoubtedly a clinical problem in cats, but is not well documented. Compared with dogs, very little is known about degenerative joint disease in cats, but radiographic evidence in geriatric cats suggests the incidence may be as high as 90%.[101] Because of a pet cat's lifestyle, lameness is not a common owner complaint; but changes in behavior, including decreased grooming, reluctance to jump up to favorite places, and soiling outside the litter box, should prompt veterinarians to look for sources of chronic pain. It is common for owners not to realize how debilitated their pet is until they see dramatic improvements following treatment. Radiographic lesions in the lumbosacral area have been correlated with neurological disease.[101]

Management and Control of Pain

Because the anatomical structures and neurophysiological mechanisms leading to the perception of pain (nociception) are remarkably similar in humans and animals, it is reasonable to assume that, if a stimulus is painful to a person, is damaging or potentially damaging to tissues, and induces escape and emotional responses in an animal, it must be considered to be painful to that individual.[102,103] That animals exhibit signs of distress and learned avoidance behavior, and vocalize in response to noxious (painful) stimuli, is further evidence of their capacity to suffer from pain. Pain may not always be overtly expressed and may be evidenced only by subtle changes in behavior or posture. A degree of anthropomorphism is appropriate and desirable, especially in situations that are known to cause pain in people.[104,105] A consensus statement from an international workshop on animal and human pain concluded that animals feel pain, but that it is unclear whether animals feel pain with the same qualities and intensities as humans. Furthermore, it is unclear at what taxonomic level noxious stimuli are associated with pain, but it is likely that all vertebrates and some invertebrates experience pain.[106] It is worth noting that humans have differing thresholds and sensitivities to pain, and it is likely that the experience of pain caused by given procedure or injury is quite varied. Thus, the consensus statement that it is unclear whether animals feel pain with the same quality or intensity as humans does nothing to minimize the importance or clinical relevance that animals feel pain. (Similarly, the variability in pain response between people does not negate the fact that pain exists and is unpleasant.)

Just as antibiotics are administered prophylactically to prevent infection, it is appropriate to administer analgesics to prevent pain where it is likely to occur. The commonly stated reasons for withholding analgesics (e.g., to avoid opioid-induced respiratory depression or because pain relief would increase activity leading to self-injury) are seldom valid and should be carefully examined before a decision is made to withhold analgesic drugs. Accurate selection and dosing of analgesic drugs provide relief of pain without severe respiratory depression. Where pulmonary function is compromised, monitoring for signs of respiratory depression and tailoring analgesic therapy to the individual patient will prevent hypoventilation or apnea. Appropriate splinting, bandaging, or confinement will prevent self-injury. Animals should not have to endure pain because of real or imagined sequelae to its relief. Pain-induced alterations in metabolism, endocrine, and cardiopulmonary function are well recognized and of serious consequence to animals.

Analgesia in the strictest sense is an absence of pain but clinically is the reduction in the intensity of pain perceived. The goal should not be to eliminate pain completely, but to make the pain as tolerable as possible without undue depression of patients. Analgesia in the clinical setting may be induced by obtunding or interrupting the nociceptive process at one or more points between the peripheral nociceptor and the cerebral cortex. Nociception involves four physiological processes that are subject to pharmacological modulation. *Transduction* is the translation of physical energy (noxious stimuli) into electric activity at the peripheral nociceptor. *Transmission* is the propagation of nerve impulses through the nervous system. *Modulation* occurs through the endogenous descending analgesic systems, which modify nociceptive transmission. These endogenous systems (opioid, serotonergic, and noradrenergic) modulate nociception through inhibition of the spinal dorsal horn cells. *Perception* is the final process resulting from successful transduction, transmission and modulation, and integration of thalamocortical, reticular, and limbic function to produce the final conscious subjective and emotional experience of pain.[107]

Transduction can be largely abolished by use of local anesthetics infiltrated at the site of injury or incision, or by intravenous, postthoracotomy intrapleural, or postlaparotomy intraperitoneal injection. NSAIDs will obtund transduction by decreasing production of endogenous algogenic substances such as prostaglandins at the site of injury. Transmission can be abolished by local anesthetic blockade of peripheral nerves or nerve plexuses or by epidural or subarachnoid injection. Modulation can be augmented by subarachnoid or epidural injection of opioids, and/or α$_2$-adrenergic agonists. Perception can be obtunded with general anesthetics or by systemic administration of opioids and α$_2$-agonists either alone or in combination with tranquilizer-sedatives.[107]

Balanced or multimodal analgesia results from the administration of analgesic drugs in combination and at multiple sites to induce analgesia by altering more than one part of the nociceptive process. Multimodal analgesia relies on the additive or synergistic effects of two or more analgesic drugs working through different mechanisms of action. When multimodal analgesia is used, doses of individual drugs can be reduced, thereby decreasing the potential for any one drug to induce adverse side effects. Thus, transduction could be reduced by NSAIDs, transmission decreased by epidural local anesthetics, and modulation increased by epidural or intrathecal opioids and/or α$_2$-agonists. Balanced analgesic techniques appear to offer several advantages in the management of postoperative pain. When used preemptively, this approach prevents nociceptive-induced neuroplasmic changes within the spinal cord (windup), prevents development of tachyphylaxis, and suppresses the neuroendocrine response to pain and injury more effectively than when single-drug regimens are used, and shortens convalescence through improved tissue healing and mobility. Preemptive analgesia refers to the application of balanced analgesic techniques prior to exposing patients to noxious stimuli (surgical trespass). By so doing, the spinal cord is not exposed to the barrage of afferent nociceptive impulses that induce the neuroplasmic changes leading to central hypersensitivity. This concept has gained acceptance as the most effective means of controlling postoperative pain.[55,108,109]

Analgesic Drugs

Analgesics consist of those classes of drugs whose primary effect is to suppress pain or induce analgesia (Table 3.2). Although actions and effects of most other drugs differ little among mammalian species, there are marked differences in response to selected analgesics (e.g., opioids) that are independent of pharmacokinetics among species.[110–112] The concentration of opioid receptors in the amygdala and frontal cortex of species that are depressed by opioids (e.g., dogs and primates) is nearly twice as great as in those species that become excited in response to opioids (e.g., horses and cats).[113] In contrast, μ opioid receptor binding in the frontal cortex, left somatosensory cortex, colliculus, and granule cell layer of the cerebellum was higher in horses than in dogs, whereas κ opioid receptors were higher in the frontal cortex of dogs as compared with horses and higher in the cerebellum of horses as compared with dogs.[114] Thus, the distribution of specific opioid receptors differs among species, which probably contributes to the clinical differences in mentation and efficacy when opioid analgesics are administered. Morphine doses of 100 to 170 μg/kg did not increase the risk of perioperative problems in horses undergoing general anesthesia and surgery as compared with horses that did not receive morphine.[115] Perhaps, by simply decreasing the dose, excitement can be avoided in those species prone to bizarre reactions. Excitement may result indirectly from increased release of norepinephrine and dopamine.[112] This may explain the mechanism whereby dopaminergic and noradrenergic blocking drugs such as phenothiazine and butyrophenone tranquilizers suppress clinical evidence of opioid-induced excitement. Xylazine and detomidine (α$_2$-agonists) are effective in preventing opioid-induced excitement in horses and ruminants. Because analgesia and excitement

Table 3.2. Classes of analgesic drugs commonly used in animals.

Classification	Examples
Opioids	Morphine, hydromorphone, fentanyl, meperidine, methadone oxymorphone, pentazocine, butorphanol, nalbuphine, and buprenorphine
Salicylates	Aspirin and salicylate
Para-aminophenol derivatives	Acetanilid, acetaminophen, and phenacetin
Nonopioid and nonsalicylate	Phenylbutazone, dipyrone, meclofenamic acid, flunixin, carprofen, ketoprofen, etodolac, meloxicam, tepoxaline, deracoxib, firocoxib, and piroxicam
Local anesthetic agents	Procaine, lidocaine, mepivacaine, tetracaine, and bupivacaine
α_2-Adrenergic agonists	Xylazine, detomidine, medetomidine, and romifidine

are mediated by different receptors (i.e., µ receptors for analgesia and phencyclidine for excitement), they can occur concurrently and are not mutually exclusive.

Opioid analgesics induce CNS depression accompanied by miosis, hypothermia, bradycardia, and respiratory depression in primates, dogs, rats, and rabbits. In horses, cats, ruminants, and swine, stimulation can be characterized by mydriasis, panting, tachycardia, hyperkinesis, and sweating.[111,112] Opioid-induced excitatory effects can occur in any species, but are uncommon when opioids are administered to animals in pain or are administered in combination with sedative/tranquilizing agents. Systemic effects of opioids include release of arginine vasopressin (antidiuretic hormone), prolactin, and somatotropin; inhibition of the release of luteinizing hormone; increased vagal tone; release of histamine and attendant hypotension; decreased motility and increased tone of the gastrointestinal tract; spasm of the biliary and pancreatic ducts; spasm of ureteral-smooth muscle and increased bladder tone; and decreased uterine tone.

Opioids raise the pain threshold or decrease the perception of pain by acting at receptors in the dorsal horn of the spinal cord and mesolimbic system (i.e., brain stem–nucleus raphe magnus and locus caeruleus), midbrain PAG, and several thalamic and hypothalamic nuclei. In the dorsal horn, opioids induce postsynaptic inhibition of nociceptive projection neurons (T cells). In addition, there is some evidence that opioids may act presynaptically to inhibit release of substance P from primary afferents. Centrally, at the level of the mesencephalon and medulla, opioids activate the descending endogenous antinociceptive system that modulates nociception in the dorsal horn via release of serotonin and perhaps norepinephrine. Opioids act at the limbic system to alter the emotional component of the pain response, thus making it more tolerable. The presence of opiate receptors in peripheral tissues has increased interest in using small doses of opioids for their peripheral effects. The density of opioid-binding sites in articular and periarticular tissues has been shown to be significantly increased 12 h after the induction of inflammation in the radiocarpal joints of dogs.[116] Immunohistochemical analysis and radioligand binding have demonstrated the presence of opioid receptors in the synovial membranes of horses.[117] These studies support the clinical practice of administering intra-articular opioids (morphine) for postoperative analgesia following arthroscopic surgery. The role of peripheral opioid receptors in pain re-

lief is intriguing because opioid receptors have traditionally been thought of as exerting their analgesic effects within the CNS. For example, morphine (5 mg) infiltrated into the donor bone graft site from the ileum for spinal fusion surgery significantly reduced the incidence of chronic pain at the donor site in people 1 year after surgery.[118] The reason why locally infiltrated morphine at the graft site exerted a significantly better analgesic effect as the same dose of morphine administered intramuscularly is not clear, but points to the ubiquitous role that opioid receptors play in both the peripheral and central nervous systems. Opioid growth factor and its specific receptors are present in the corneas of dogs, cats, and horses.[119] Although opioids have been theorized to inhibit corneal healing, the topical application of 1% morphine sulfate solution in dogs in one study provided analgesia without interfering with wound healing.[120]

Successful use of opioids requires appropriate selection of the drug and dose for the given species to avoid undesirable side effects. Opioids must be used with caution in animals that have impaired pulmonary function because they depress the respiratory and cough centers, decrease secretions, and may induce bronchospasm secondary to histamine release. In species that can freely vomit, nausea and vomiting may occur. Repeated doses can cause constipation, ileus, and urinary retention. Mice and rats rapidly develop tolerance to and physical dependence on opioid agonists.[121–123] Morphine decreases the number and phagocytic function of macrophages and polymorphonuclear leukocytes in mice and may alter their immune function. These side effects are typically managed successfully in clinical patients; thus, opioids are the analgesic drugs of choice for the treatment of all forms (mild to severe) of acute pain.

Whereas opioids induce analgesia by interfering with nociceptive neural transmission centrally, the nonopioid, nonsteroidal, anti-inflammatory analgesics (NSAIAs) act primarily in the periphery to decrease production of algogenic substances, primarily prostanoids, which facilitate generation and conduction of impulses that give rise to pain. When tissues are damaged, mediators are synthesized or released that activate nociceptors and primary afferent neurons, leading to the sensation of pain. When administered prior to tissue damage, the nonopioid analgesics induce analgesia by suppressing inflammation and the production and elaboration of kinins and prostaglandins. There is, however, evidence that NSAIAs may also act in the CNS. These drugs are effective primarily against pain of low to moderate intensity associated with inflammation.[124] They are generally regarded as being useful for treating chronic pain of somatic or integumental origin, but of little use for visceral pain. An exception is flunixin, which appears to blunt visceral pain effectively in horses.[125] The efficacy of NSAIAs has been investigated for acute postoperative pain. In dogs, the preemptive (preoperative) administration of carprofen has been shown to induce superior postoperative analgesia with less sedation than pethidine (meperidine) after orthopedic surgery.[126] Similarly, carprofen has been shown to induce profound analgesia as effective as that induced by papaveretum, but with quicker anesthetic recovery and less postrecovery sedation.[127] In horses, administration of carprofen, flunixin, and phenylbutazone at the end of surgery were equally effective at inducing postoperative analgesia, with flunixin providing the longest action and phenylbutazone the shortest.[128] In rats undergoing midline laparotomy, buprenorphine or carprofen administration results in greater food and water consumption and less weight loss than occur in rats receiving saline.[129] The optimal timing of NSAIA administration must be tailored to the individual patient in order to minimize side effects. In people, NSAIAs have been shown to exert a limited preemptive effect; however, the analgesic effects must be balanced against side effects, such as bleeding and impaired renal function.[74] Carprofen and meloxicam administered to healthy dogs prior to anesthesia had no adverse effects on renal function.[130–132] These studies used young, healthy dogs with normal renal function, and the degree of hypotension was moderate. Thus, caution should be used when considering the timing of NSAIA administration to clinical patients, particularly in older patients that may have subclinical renal compromise. Although NSAIAs are an integral part of many multimodal analgesic protocols, it is often safer to administer the NSAIAs postoperatively to avoid the concurrent potentially detrimental renal effects of NSAIAs and hypotension.

The pharmacokinetics of NSAIAs varies widely among species. Following oral administration, wide species variations in plasma concentration result in part from the size of the gastrointestinal tract and gastric emptying time, which affect the rate of absorption and the rate of metabolism and elimination.[133] Toxicity of the NSAIAs also varies widely among species and drugs and deserves some consideration.[125] The most common toxic side effects include gastric and intestinal ulceration, with secondary anemia and hypoproteinemia. Impaired platelet function and delayed parturition have been reported. Nephropathy can occur in patients with hypovolemia, congestive heart failure, or other cardiovascular impairment (anesthesia) caused by inhibition of renal prostaglandin function in the face of increased norepinephrine and angiotensin II. Chronic or repeated use has been associated with chronic interstitial nephritis and renal papillary necrosis. Phenylbutazone and dipyrone have been associated with blood dyscrasias.

α_2-Adrenergic agonists (e.g., xylazine, detomidine, medetomidine, dexmedetomidine, and romifidine) are generally regarded as sedative-hypnotics and are most commonly administered to induce sedation.[134,135] They possess some analgesic action, as well. Xylazine has been shown to be a more potent analgesic

agent in horses for the relief of both visceral and somatic pain than opioids and NSAIAs.[136,137] α_2-Agonists exert their sedative effects through stimulation of α_2-adrenoceptors in the brain, decreasing norepinephrine release. Sedation results from decreased activity of ascending neural projections to the cerebral cortex and limbic system.[121,122] Analgesia appears to be the result of both cerebral and spinal effects, possibly in part mediated by serotonin and the descending endogenous analgesia system.[123] α_2-Adrenergic and opioid receptors appear to interact in ways that are not fully understood.[123,134,138] Administration of α_2-agonists (i.e., clonidine) has been shown to relieve symptoms of withdrawal in opioid-dependent people.[139–142] They have also been used to "rescue" opioid-induced analgesia that has waned following chronic administration. The combination of an opioid and an α_2-agonist enhances and prolongs analgesia in dogs and cats, and these combinations have been used for some years in horses.[141–145]

Although xylazine is the most commonly used sedative-analgesic in veterinary medicine, its comparative pharmacokinetics have not been studied extensively.[135] When administered intravenously, xylazine has a rapid onset and brief action. There is a wide variation in species sensitivity and response to xylazine. Detomidine is more potent and longer acting than xylazine. Medetomidine use in small animal practice has been reviewed.[146] Medetomidine is the most potent and selective α_2-agonist in veterinary practice to date. In addition to having profound sedative and analgesic activity, α_2-agonists induce cardiovascular and metabolic responses also related to their peripheral adrenergic effects. Following their administration, arterial blood pressure increases and then decreases; cardiac output decreases.[147] Medetomidine (1 to 20 µg/kg intravenously) reduces cardiac index significantly in dogs, although the reduction is generally less with the use of lower doses (1 and 2 µg/kg).[148] Insulin release is inhibited, resulting in hyperglycemia.[149–151] Urinary output is increased as a result of decreased arginine vasopressin release and decreased water reabsorption by nephrons.[149,152–154] Analgesia can be induced by neural blockade of the nociceptive nerves or tracts by local infiltration, by regional nerve blocks, or by epidural or intrathecal injection of local anesthetic agents. Analgesia so induced is complete in the area blocked. Intercostal nerve blockade and intrapleural local anesthetic administration have been advocated to relieve pain following thoracotomy and presumably produce better alveolar ventilation postoperatively than when opioid-induced analgesia is present.[155,156] Digital nerve blocks or distal limb ring blocks with lidocaine and bupivacaine are an excellent means to control postoperative pain from declaw procedures in cats. Nonpharmacological methods of pain relief (rehabilitation therapy) can be used to good effect. These include immobilization and support with casts, splints, or bandages; appropriate use of hot or cold packs; and physical therapy such as massage and stretching.[157]

When pain is severe and acute, opioids are the most effective analgesics under most circumstances. These drugs do, however, have relatively short half-lives and thus require supplemental dosing. Most will provide analgesia within 30 min of administration. Duration of action varies but is usually on the order of 2 to 4 h. Surgically induced pain may require the use of opioids for 1 to 2 days postoperatively. Intra-articular morphine administration following joint surgery has been shown to relieve pain effectively for many hours postoperatively.[158] The NSAIDs generally are not sufficient by themselves to relieve severe postoperative pain. The NSAIDs can be used in combination with opioids postoperatively to good effect because these 2 classes of agents have differing mechanisms and sites of action. Further, NSAIDS can be continued when opioids are no longer necessary. Generally, NSAIDs provide good analgesia where pain is induced by inflammation or is chronic and of integumentary or musculoskeletal origin and are typically administered at 12- to 24-h intervals.

Although the foregoing discussion has focused on the use of analgesics to control pain in conscious patients, one must not ignore their use in patients that are chemically restrained. Animals are frequently anesthetized for diagnostic and manipulative procedures that are otherwise difficult or not possible in conscious patients. Where pain is not present or caused by the procedure (e.g., radiology), only muscle relaxation and hypnosis or sedation are required for patient management. However, when the procedure is painful or invasive, the protocol should be chosen to ensure that analgesia is sufficient to prevent the patient from perceiving pain. The phencyclidine derivatives ketamine and tiletamine induce a dissociative cataleptoid state, somatic analgesia, and altered consciousness. The patient is immobilized but not relaxed or fully unconscious, and analgesia is incomplete. The dissociative state is poorly understood, but it is believed that somatic analgesia results from the interruption or dissociation of ascending nociceptive input as painful stimuli traverse the thalamoneocortical system. The dissociative agents are excellent for chemical restraint and immobilization, but should be supplemented with an analgesic for invasive procedures and particularly those involving visceral manipulation. Several studies have assessed and documented the analgesic efficacy of epidurally administered ketamine; however, the safety of epidural ketamine has not been fully established.[159,160] Ketamine has long been known to induce analgesia for superficial pain (e.g., skin incisions) but not deep pain. Ketamine has been used to help prevent sensitization (windup) of the nociceptive pathways in the spinal cord. Ketamine blocks the effects of glutamate, an excitatory neurotransmitter, at the NMDA receptor. Stimulation of the NMDA receptor has been theorized to be a key component in sensitizing nociceptive pathways after surgery or trauma. The exact role that ketamine may play in preventing exaggerated pain states is not known at this time; however, ketamine might be doing more good than any of us realized.[161–167]

Recommended doses and dose intervals (where available) for selected analgesics used in common domestic species are listed in Tables 3.3 through 3.6. As with any therapeutic regimen, the response should be monitored, and where pain has not been adequately relieved, additional therapy should be considered. Extrapolation of data from one species to another should be avoided where specific information for pain therapy is available.

Table 3.3. Doses of analgesics for use in dogs.

Drug	Dose (mg/kg)	Route	Frequency/Duration
Opioid agonists			
Fentanyl[a]	0.001 to 0.002	IV	0.25 to 0.5 h
	0.001 to 0.006[b]	CRI (mg/kg/h)	Duration of infusion + ~0.5 h
	0.01 to 0.04[c]	CRI (mg/kg/h)	Duration of infusion + 0.5 to 1.0 h
Hydromorphone	0.02 to 0.1	IV, IM, SC	1 to 4 h
Methadone	0.1 to 1.0	IV, IM, SC	1 to 4 h
Oxymorphone	0.02 to 0.1	IV, IM, SC	1 to 4 h
Morphine[a]	0.05 to 1.0	IV, IM, SC	1 to 4 h
	0.1 to 0.3 mg/kg/h	CRI	Duration of infusion + 0.5 to 1.0 h
Preservative-free morphine	0.1 to 0.2	Epidural	6 to 24 h
Partial opioid agonist			
Buprenorphine	0.005 to 0.02	IV, IM	4 to 8 h
Opioid agonist-antagonist			
Butorphanol	0.1 to 0.5	IV, IM, SC	0.25 to 2.0 h
α_2-Agonists[e]			
Medetomidine	0.01 to 0.04	IM	0.5 to 2.0 h
(Postop: low dose)	0.001 to 0.002	IV	0.5 to 1.0 h
Xylazine	0.1 to 0.5	IM, SC	0.5 to 2.0 h
(Postop: low dose)	0.1 to 0.2	IV	0.5 to 1.0 h

(continued)

Table 3.3. Doses of analgesics for use in dogs (*continued*).

Drug	Dose (mg/kg)	Route	Frequency/Duration
Local anesthetics			
Bupivacaine	1.5 to 3.0	Local blocks	2 to 6 h
		Intrapleural	
	1.0 to 1.5	Epidural	4 to 6 h
	0.1 to 0.5[f]	Epidural	4 to 6 h
Lidocaine	1 to 2	Local blocks	1 to 2 h
		Prior to bupivacaine	
NMDA receptor antagonist			
Ketamine	0.25 to 0.5	IV	Loading dose
	0.01 to 0.02 mg/kg/h	CRI	Duration unknown
NSAIDs[g]			
Carprofen	2.2	SC, IM, PO	12 h
	4.4	SC, IM, PO	24 h
Deracoxib	3 to 4	PO (max. 7 days)	24 h
	1 to 2	PO	24 h
Firocoxib	5	PO	24 h
Ketoprofen	1 to 2	SC	24 h
Meloxicam	0.2	IV, SC, PO (once)	24 h
	0.1	IV, SC, PO	24 h

BID, twice a day; CRI, constant-rate infusion; IM, intramuscularly; IV, intravenously; NMDA, *N*-methyl-D-aspartate; NSAIDs, nonsteroidal anti-inflammatory drugs; PO, per os (orally); SC, subcutaneously; SID, once a day.

[a]Fentanyl doses may be increased incrementally above the recommended dose, provided the patient is monitored for respiratory depression and bradycardia.

[b]High doses of fentanyl are associated with bradycardia and hypoventilation, and usually decrease anesthetic gas requirements.

[c]Must be administered slowly to avoid side effects, such as hypotension and excitement.

[d]These doses have been compiled from many sources and reflect doses used by the authors. The wide variability of recommended doses appears related to the variety and severity of stimuli used to establish the individual drug's analgesic activity in a given species. Doses are intended as guidelines only. Clinical judgment must be exercised to provide effective analgesia in a given situation.

[e]Postsurgical doses and duration of effect have not been clearly established. Use cautiously to avoid profound cardiac depressant effects.

[f]Bupivacaine dose when combined with preservative-free morphine at 0.1 mg/kg.

[g]Do not use in the presence of hypovolemia, hypotension, renal disease, gastrointestinal bleeding, or coagulopathies.

Table 3.4. Doses of analgesics for use in cats.

Drug	Dose (mg/kg)	Route	Comments
Opioids			
Butorphanol	0.1 to 0.4	IV, IM	Short acting (less than 90 min). Increasing the dose does not provide more intense or longer periods of analgesia.
Buprenorphine	0.01 to 0.02	IV, IM, transmucosal	
Fentanyl	0.005 to 0.01	IV	May take up to 12 h to reach effective plasma concentration.
	25 µg/h patch	Transdermal	Uptake affected by body temperature.
Hydromorphone	0.05 to 0.1	IV, IM	SC route associated with vomiting. Doses of 0.1 mg/kg and higher can produce hyperthermia.
Meperidine	5 to 10	IM	Must not be given IV.
Morphine	0.2 to 0.5 mg/kg	IV, IM	May be less effective in cats compared with other species because of a lack of active metabolites.
Oxymorphone	0.05 to 0.01	IV, IM	
NSAIDs			Do not use in hypotensive or hypovolemic patients.
Carprofen	1 to 4	SC	Not licensed for cats in the United States. Should not be repeated.
Ketoprofen	1 to 2	SC	Not licensed for cats in the United States. Can be repeated with care (1 to 5 days at 1 mg/kg).
Meloxicam[a]	0.2 or 0.1	SC, IV, PO	One dose. Dose depends on degree of pain (e.g., orthopedic vs. soft tissue).
	0.1		Repeat once daily for 3 days.
	0.025 mg/kg (0.1 mg/cat) lean weight		Alternate day or twice weekly.
Local anesthetics			
Lidocaine	2 to 4	Local anesthetic blocks	Duration of action 1 to 2 h. Constant-rate infusions not recommended in cats because of cardiovascular depression.
Bupivacaine	2	Local anesthetic blocks	Duration of action 4 to 5 h.
α₂-Agonists			Use with great care in cats with cardiovascular disease.
Medetomidine	0.005 to 0.02	IV, IM, SC	Low doses combined with an opioid offer good sedation and analgesia.
	0.01	Epidural	
Other			
Ketamine	2	IV	No published data about cats on the efficacy of low-dose constant-rate infusions.

IM, intramuscularly; IV, intravenously; PO, per os (orally); SC, subcutaneously.

[a]The only licensed NSAID for cats in the USA. The oral formulation is off-label; however, this has been used in cats with *careful* attention to dose delivered.

Table 3.5. Doses of analgesics for use in horses[a]. [168]

Drug	Dose (mg/kg)	Route	Frequency/Duration
NSAIDs			
Phenylbutazone	2.2 to 4.4	IV, PO	SID-BID
Flunixin	1.1	IV, IM, PO	SID-BID
Ketoprofen	2.2	IV, IM	SID-BID
Carprofen	0.7	IV, PO	SID-BID
Opioids			
Butorphanol	0.01 to 0.02	IV	q 2 to 4 h
Morphine	0.02 to 0.1	IV	q 2 to 4 h
	0.1 to 0.2	Epidural	q 12 to 24 h
Preservative-free morphine (1 mg/mL)	5 to 10 mL	Intra-articular	Once
Fentanyl	0.001 to 0.002	IV	q 0.25 to 0.5 h
	0.001 mg/kg/h	CRI	
Fentanyl transdermal patch	1 to 3 patches per horse (10 mg or 100 µg/h patches)	72 h	
Local anesthetics			
Lidocaine	1 to 2	Infiltration	1 to 2 h
Lidocaine CRI	2	IV (loading dose administered over 20 min)	
	30 to 50 µg/kg/min	CRI	
Lidocaine patch	Undetermined at this time	Transdermal	
Bupivacaine	1 to 2	Infiltration	6 to 8 h
α_2-Agonists			
Xylazine	1.0 to 2.2	IM	0.5 to 2.0 h
	0.3 to 1.0	IV	0.5 h
	25-mg total dose	Epidural—added to morphine	
Detomidine	0.005 to 0.01	IV	1 to 2 h
	0.01 to 0.02	IV, IM	1 to 2 h
	0.03 to 0.06	Epidural	2 to 3 h
	0.01	Epidural—added to morphine	

BID, twice a day; CRI, constant-rate infusion; IM, intramuscularly; IV, intravenously; PO, per os (orally); SC, subcutaneously; SID, once a day.
[a]These doses have been compiled from many sources and reflect doses used by the authors. The wide variability of recommended doses appears related to the variety and severity of stimuli used to establish the individual drug's analgesic activity in a given species. Doses are intended as guidelines only. Clinical judgment must be exercised to provide effective analgesia in a given situation.

Table 3.6. Doses of analgesics for use in ruminants and swine[a]. [169]

Drug	Dose (mg/kg)	Route	Frequency	Species
NSAIDs				
Aspirin	50 to 100	PO	q 12 h	Cattle
	50 to 100	PO	q 12 h	Sheep/goat
	10	PO	q 4 h	Swine
Phenylbutazone	Not recommended			Cattle
	5	IV, PO	Daily	Sheep, llama
	4	IV, PO	Daily	Swine
Flunixin	1.1	IV	q 12 h	Cattle, llama
	2.2	IV	q 12 h	Sheep
Ketoprofen	1 to 3.3	IV, IM	Daily	Ruminants/llama
Opioids				
Butorphanol	0.044 to 0.07	IV	q 4 h	Cattle
	0.05 to 0.2	IV, IM	q 4 h	Camelid
	0.1 to 0.5	IV, IM, SC	q 4 h	Sheep
	0.1 to 0.2	IV, IM, SC	q 4 h	Goats
Buprenorphine	0.005 to 0.01	IV, IM, SC	q 12 h	Sheep, goats
Morphine	0.05 to 0.5	IV, IM, SC	q 4 to 6 h	Ruminants/camelids
	0.1	Epidural	q 12 h	Ruminants/camelids
	0.2	IV, IM	q 4 to 6 h	Swine
Fentanyl Patch	0.002 to 0.004	IV	q 0.25 to 0.5 h	Ruminants
	0.002	Transdermal	q 72 h	Sheep
	(equivalent to 15 mg/70-kg sheep)			
Local anesthetics				
Lidocaine	Do not exceed 10 mL (2% lidocaine)			Adult sheep/goats
	Do not exceed 1 mL (2% lidocaine)			Dehorning young kids
	4 to 5 mL (2%)	Epidural		Cattle
	1 to 2 mL (2%)	Epidural		Sheep
Bupivacaine	1 to 2 mg/kg	Infiltrations		Ruminants/camelids
α_2-Agonists				
Xylazine	0.1	IM	As needed	Cattle
	0.05 to 0.1	IM	As needed	Sheep
	1	IM	As needed	Swine
Detomidine	0.01	IV	As needed	Cattle

IM, intramuscularly; IV, intravenously; PO, per os (orally); SC, subcutaneously.

[a]These doses have been compiled from many sources and reflect doses used by the authors. The wide variability of recommended doses appears related to the variety and severity of stimuli used to establish the individual drug's analgesic activity in a given species. Doses are intended as guidelines only. Clinical judgment must be exercised to provide effective analgesia in a given situation.

References

1. Marks SM, Sachar EJ. Undertreatment of medical inpatients with narcotic analgesics. Ann Intern Med 78:173–181, 1973.
2. Phillips DM. JCAHO pain management standards are unveiled. J Am Med Assoc 284:428–429, 2000.
3. Davis LE, Donnelly EJ. Analgesic drugs in the cat. J Am Vet Med Assoc 153:1161–1167, 1968.
4. Rollin BE. The Unheeded Cry: Animal Consciousness, Animal Pain and Science. Oxford: Oxford University Press, 1989.
5. Hansen B, Hardie E. Prescription and use of analgesics in dogs and cats in a veterinary teaching hospital: 258 cases (1983–1989). J Am Vet Med Assoc 202:1485–1494, 1993.
6. Dohoo SE, Dohoo IR. Postoperative use of analgesics in dogs and cats by Canadian veterinarians. Can Vet J 37:546–551, 1996.
7. Dohoo SE, Dohoo IR. Factors influencing the postoperative use of analgesics in dogs and cats by Canadian veterinarians. Can Vet J 37:552–556, 1996.
8. Dohoo SE, Dohoo IR. Attitudes and concerns of Canadian animal health technologists toward postoperative pain management in dogs and cats. Can Vet J 39:491–496, 1998.
9. Capner CA, Lascelles BD, Waterman-Pearson AE. Current British veterinary attitudes to perioperative analgesia for dogs. Vet Rec 145:95–99, 1999.
10. Price J, Marques JM, Welsh EM, Waran NK. Pilot epidemiological study of attitudes towards pain in horses. Vet Rec 151:570–575, 2002.
11. Wright EM Jr, Marcella KL, Woodson JF. Animal pain: Evaluation and control. Lab Anim 14:20–36, 1985.

12. Zimmerman M. Behavioural investigations of pain in animals. In: Duncan IJH, Molony V, eds. Agriculture: Assessing Pain in Farm Animals. Luxembourg: Commission of the European Communities, 1986:16–27.

13. Siddall PJ, Cousins MJ. Persistent pain as a disease entity: Implications for clinical management. Anesth Analg 99:510–520, 2004.

14. Melzack R. Neurophysiological foundations of pain. In: Sternbach RA, ed. The Psychology of Pain. New York: Raven, 1986:1–24.

15. Melzack R, Casey KL. Sensory, motivational and central control determinants of pain. In: Kenshalo D, ed. The Skin Senses. Springfield, IL: Charles C Thomas, 1968:423–443.

16. Ashburn MA, Staats PS. Pain: Management of chronic pain. Lancet 353:1865, 1999.

17. Bonica JJ. General considerations of acute pain. In: Bonica JJ, Loeser JD, Chapman CR, Fordyce WE, eds. The Management of Pain, 2nd ed. Philadelphia: Lea and Febiger, 1990:159–179.

18. International Association for the Study of Pain. Pain terms: A list with definitions and notes on usage. Pain 6:249, 1979, and 14:205, 1982.

19. Kitchell RL, Guinan MJ. The nature of pain in animals. In: Rollan BE, Kesel ML, eds. The Experimental Animal in Biomedical Research, vol 1. Boston: CRC, 1990:185–204.

20. Woolf CJ. Pain: Moving from symptom control toward mechanism-specific pharmacologic management. Ann Intern Med 140:441–451, 2004.

21. Basbaum AI, Jessel TM. The perception of pain. In: Kandel ER, Schwartz JH, Jessel TM, eds. Principles of Neural Science, 4th ed. New York: McGraw-Hill, 2000:472–490.

22. Besson J-M, Chaouch A. Peripheral and spinal mechanisms of nociception. Physiol Rev 67:67–186, 1987.

23. Torebjörk E. Nociceptor activation and pain. Philos Trans R Soc Lond [Biol] 308:227–234, 1985.

24. Greenspan JD. Nociceptors and the peripheral nervous system's role in pain. J Hand Ther 10:78–85, 1997.

25. Sorkin LS, Wallace MS. Acute pain mechanisms. Surg Clin North Am 79:213–229, 1999.

26. Willis WD, Westlund KN. Neuroanatomy of the pain system and of the pathways that modulate pain. J Clin Neurophysiol 14:2–31, 1997.

27. Burt AM. Textbook of Neuroanatomy, 1st ed. Philadelphia: WB Saunders, 1993.

28. Craig AD, Dostrovsky JO. Medulla to thalamus. In: Wall PD, Melzack R, eds. Textbook of Pain, 4th ed. Philadelphia: Churchill Livingstone, 1999:183–214.

29. Warren S, Capra NF, Yezierski RP. The somatosensory system II: Non-discriminative touch, temperature, and nociception. In: Haines DE, ed. Fundamental Neuroscience. New York: Churchill Livingstone, 1996:237–253.

30. Ha H, Liu CN. Organization of the spino-cervico-thalamic system. J Comp Neurol 127:445–454, 1966.

31. Kennard MA. The course of ascending fibers in the spinal cord of the cat essential to the recognition of painful stimuli. J Comp Neurol 100:511–524, 1954.

32. Ammons WS, Girardot MN, Foreman RD. T2-T5 spinothalamic neurons projecting to medial thalamus with viscerosomatic input. J Neurophysiol 54:73–89, 1985.

33. Milne RJ, Foreman RD, Giesler GJ Jr, Willis WD. Convergence of cutaneous and pelvic visceral nociceptive inputs onto primate spinothalamic neurons. Pain 11:163–183, 1981.

34. Biamberardo MA, Vecchiet L. Visceral pain, referred hyperalgesia and outcome: New concepts. Eur J Anaesthesiol Suppl 10:61–66, 1995.

35. McMahon SB. Are there fundamental differences in the peripheral mechanisms of visceral and somatic pain? Behav Brain Sci 20:381–391, 1997.

36. De Lahunta A. Veterinary Neuroanatomy and Clinical Neurology. Philadelphia: WB Saunders, 1983.

37. Farina S, Tinazzi M, Le Pera D, Valeriani M. Pain-related modulation of the human motor cortex. Neurol Res 25:130–142, 2003.

38. Lamont LA, Tranquilli WJ, Grimm KA. Physiology of pain. Vet Clin North Am Small Anim Pract 30:703–728, 2000.

39. Woolf CJ. Dissecting out mechanisms responsible for peripheral neuropathic pain: Implications for diagnosis and therapy. Life Sci 74:2605–2610, 2004.

40. Devor M. Pain mechanisms. Neuroscientist 2:233–244, 1996.

41. Robinson AJ. Central nervous system pathways for pain transmission and pain control. J Hand Ther 10:64–77, 1997.

42. Dickenson AH. Central acute pain mechanisms. Ann Med 27:223–227, 1995.

43. Ren K, Dubner R. Central nervous system plasticity and persistent pain. J Orofac Pain 13:155–163, 1999.

44. Urban MO, Gebhart GF. Central mechanisms in pain. Med Clin North Am 93:585–596, 1999.

45. Eide PK. Wind-up and the NMDA receptor complex from a clinical perspective. Eur J Pain 4:5–15, 2000.

46. Melzack R, Wall PD. Pain mechanisms: A new theory. Science 150:971–979, 1965.

47. Sandkühler J. The organization and function of endogenous antinociceptive systems. Prog Neurobiol 50:49–81, 1996.

48. Bridges D, Thompson SWN, Rice ASC. Mechanisms of neuropathic pain. Br J Anaesth 87:12–26, 2001.

49. Ossipov MH, Lai J, Malan TP, Porreca F. Spinal and supraspinal mechanisms of neuropathic pain. Ann NY Acad Sci 909:12–24, 2000.

50. DeLeo JA, Winkelstein BA. Physiology of chronic spinal pain syndromes. Spine 27:2526–2537, 2002.

51. Melzack R, Wall PD. The Challenge of Pain. New York: Basic, 1982.

52. Kehlet H. Pain relief and modification of the stress response. In: Cousins MJ, Philips GD, eds. Acute Pain Management. New York: Churchill Livingstone, 1986:49–65.

53. Wilmore DW, Long JM, Mason AD, Pruitt BA. Stress in surgical patients as a neurophysiologic reflex response. Surg Gynecol Obstet 142:257–269, 1976.

54. Bessman FP, Renner VJ. The biphasic hormonal nature of stress. In: Crowley RA, Trump BF, eds. Pathophysiology of Shock, Anoxia and Ischemia. Baltimore: Williams and Wilkins, 1982:60–65.

55. Woolf CJ, Chong MS. Preemptive analgesia: Treating postoperative pain by preventing the establishment of central sensitization. Anesth Analg 77:362–379, 1993.

56. Benson GJ, Grubb T, Neff-Davis C, et al. Perioperative stress response in the dog: Effect of pre-emptive administration of medetomidine. Vet Surg 29:85–91, 2000.

57. Benson GJ, Wheaton LG, Thurmon JC, Tranquilli WJ, Olson WA, Davis CA. Postoperative catecholamine response to onychectomy in isoflurane-anesthetized cats: Effect of analgesics. Vet Surg 20:222–225, 1991.

58. Hume DM, Egdahl RH. The importance of the brain in the endocrine response to injury. Ann Surg 150:697–712, 1959.

59. Gann GS. The endocrine and metabolic response to injury. In: Schwartz SE, ed. Principles of Surgery. New York: McGraw-Hill, 1979:1–64.

60. Schneider RA. The relation of stress to clotting time, relative viscosity, and certain biophysical alterations of the blood in normoten-

sive and hypertensive subjects. In: Wolff HG, Wolff SG, Hare CC, eds. Life Stresses and Bodily Disease. Baltimore: Williams and Wilkins, 1950:818–831.

61. Dreyfuss F. Coagulation time of the blood, level of blood eosinophils and thrombocytes under emotional stress. J Psychosom Res 1:252–257, 1956.

62. Ogston D, McDonald GA, Fullerton HW. The influence of anxiety in tests of blood coagulability and fibrinolytic activity. Lancet 2:521, 1962.

63. Dreyfuss F, Zahavi J. Adenosine diphosphate–induced platelet aggregation in myocardial infarction and ischemic heart disease. Atherosclerosis 17:107–120, 1973.

64. Wright EM Jr, Woodson JF. Clinical assessment of pain in laboratory animals. In: Rollin BE, Kesel ML, eds. The Experimental Animal in Biomedical Research, vol 1. Boca Raton, FL: CRC, 1990:205–215.

65. Roizen MF. Should we all have a sympathectomy at birth? Or at least postoperatively? [Editorial]. Anesthesiology 68:482–484, 1988.

66. Sellon DC, Roberts MC, Blikslager AT, Ulibarri C, Papich MG. Effects of continuous rate intravenous infusion of butorphanol on physiologic and outcome variables in horses after celiotomy. J Vet Intern Med 18:555–563, 2004.

67. Wagner AE, Walton JA, Hellyer PW, Gaynor JS, Mama KR. Use of low doses of ketamine administered by constant rate infusion as an adjunct for postoperative analgesia in dogs. J Am Vet Med Assoc 221:72–75, 2002.

68. Kehlet H. Influence of epidural analgesia on the endocrine-metabolic response to surgery. Acta Anesthesiol Scand 70:39–42, 1978.

69. Woolf CJ. Recent advances in the pathophysiology of acute pain. Br J Anaesth 63:139–146, 1989.

70. Kelly DJ, Ahmad M, Brull SJ. Preemptive analgesia I: Physiological pathways and pharmacological modalities. Can J Anesth 48:1000–1010, 2001.

71. Kelly DJ, Ahmad M, Brull SJ. Preemptive analgesia II: Recent advances and current trends Can J Anesth 48:1091–1101, 2001.

72. Kissin I. Preemptive analgesia. Anesthesiology 93:1138–1143, 2000.

73. Møiniche S, Kehlet H, Berg J. A qualitative and quantitative systematic review of preemptive analgesia for postoperative pain relief. Anesthesiology 96:725–741, 2002.

74. Ochroch EA, Mardini IA, Gottschalk A. What is the role of NSAIDs in pre-emptive analgesia? Drugs 63:2709–2723, 2003.

75. Robertson SA, Hellyer PW. How do we know they hurt? In: Managing Medical, Surgical, Chronic, and Traumatic Pain: Protocols and Non-drug Approaches. Pfizer Proceedings, 2003.

76. Kelvin WTL. Electrical units of measurement. In: Constitution of Matter, 2nd ed. London: Macmillan, 1891:80–92.

77. Roughan JV, Flecknell PA. Effects of surgery and analgesic administration on spontaneous behaviour in singly housed rats. Res Vet Sci 69:283–288, 2000.

78. Roughan JV, Flecknell PA. Behavioural effects of laparotomy and analgesic effects of ketoprofen and carprofen in rats. Pain 90:65–74, 2001.

79. Holton L, Reid J, Scott EM, Pawson P, Nolan A. Development of behaviour-based scale to measure acute pain in dogs. Vet Rec 148:525–531, 2001.

80. Cambridge AJ, Tobias KM, Newberry RC, Sarkar DK. Subjective and objective measurements of postoperative pain in cats. J Am Vet Med Assoc 217:685–690, 2000.

81. Conzemius MG, Hill C, Sammarco J, Perkowski S. Correlation between subjective and objective measures used to determine severity of postoperative pain in dogs. J Am Vet Med Assoc 210:1619–1622, 1997.

82. Holton LL, Scott EM, Nolan AM, Reid J, Welsh E. Relationship between physiological factors and clinical pain in dogs scored using a numerical rating scale. J Small Anim Pract 39:469–474, 1998.

83. Smith JD, Allen SW, Quandt JE, Tackett RL. Indicators of postoperative pain in cats and correlation with clinical criteria. Am J Vet Res 57:1674–1678, 1996.

84. Smith J, Allen S, Quandt J. Changes in cortisol concentration in response to stress and postoperative pain in client-owned cats and correlation with objective clinical variables. Am J Vet Res 60:432–436, 1999.

85. Fox SM, Mellor JD, Lawoko CR, Hodge H, Firth EC. Changes in plasma cortisol concentrations in bitches in response to different combinations of halothane and butorphanol, with or without ovariohysterectomy. Res Vet Sci 65:125–133, 1998.

86. Roberston SA, Richter M, Martinez S. Comparison of two injectable anesthetic regimens for onychectomy in cats [Abstract]. In: Proceedings of the 20th Annual Meeting of the American College of Veterinary Anesthesiologists, Atlanta, Georgia, October 20, 1995:32.

87. Levy J, Lapham B, Hardie E, McBride MA. Evaluation of laser onychectomy in the cat. In: Proceedings of the 19th Annual Meeting of the American Society of Laser Machine and Surgery, Lake Buena Vista, Florida, 1999.

88. Lascelles B, Cripps PJ, Jones A, Waterman-Pearson AE. Efficacy and kinetics of carprofen, administered preoperatively or postoperatively, for the prevention of pain in dogs undergoing ovariohysterectomy. Vet Surg 27:568–582, 1998.

89. Lascelles B, Cripps PJ, Jones A, Waterman-Pearson AE. Use of a new finger-mounted device to compare mechanical nociceptive thresholds in cats given pethidine or no medication after castration. Res Vet Sci 70:243–246, 2001.

90. Conzemius M, Horstman CL, Gordon W, Evans R. Non-invasive, objective determination of limb function in cats using pressure platform gait analysis. In: Abstracts of the 30th Annual Conference of the Veterinary Orthopedic Society, Steamboat Springs, Colorado, 2003:21.

91. Holton LL, Scott EM, Nolan AM, Reid J, Welsh E, Flaherty D. Comparison of three methods used for assessment of pain in dogs. J Am Vet Med Assoc 212:61–66, 1998.

92. Vesal N, Cribb PH, Frketic M. Postoperative analgesic and cardiopulmonary effects in dogs of oxymorphone administered epidurally and intramuscularly, and medetomidine administered epidurally: A comparative clinical study. Vet Surg 25:361–369, 1996.

93. Lascelles BD, Cripps, Mirchandani S, Waterman AE. Carprofen as an analgesic for postoperative pain in cats: Dose titration and assessment of efficacy in comparison to pethidine hydrochloride. J Small Anim Pract 36:535–541, 1995.

94. Slingsby L, Waterman-Pearson A. Comparison of pethidine, buprenorphine and ketoprofen for postoperative analgesia after ovariohysterectomy in the cat. Vet Rec 143:185–189, 1998.

95. Stevens B. Pain in infants and children: Assessment and management strategies within the context of professional guidelines, standards and roles. In: Gaimberardino MA, ed. Pain 2002—An Updated Review: Refresher Course Syllabus. Seattle, WA: IASP, 2002:315–326.

96. Hansen B. Through a glass darkly: Using behavior to assess pain. Semin Vet Med Surg (Small Anim) 12:61–74, 1997.

97. Fox SM, Mellor DJ, Stafford KJ, Lawoko CR, Hodge H. The effects of ovariohysterectomy plus different combinations of halothane anaesthesia and butorphanol analgesia on behaviour in the bitch. Res Vet Sci 68:265–274, 2000.

98. Hardie E, Hansen B, Carrol G. Behavior after ovariohysterectomy in the dog: What's normal? Appl Anim Behav Sci 51:111–128, 1997.

99. Firth A, Haldane S. Development of a scale to evaluate postoperative pain in dogs. J Am Vet Med Assoc 214:651–659, 1999.

100. Wiseman ML, Nolan Am, Reid J, Scott EM. Preliminary study on owner-reported behaviour changes associated with chronic pain in dogs. Vet Rec 149:423–424, 2001.

101. Hardie E, Roe S, Martin F. Radiographic evidence of degenerative joint disease in geriatric cats: 100 cases (1974–1997). J Am Vet Med Assoc 220:628–632, 2002.

102. Rowan A, Tannenbaum J. Animal rights. Natl Forum 66:30–33, 1986.

103. Kitchell RL. Problems in defining pain and peripheral mechanisms of pain. J Am Vet Med Assoc 191:1195, 1987.

104. Soma LR. Behavioral changes and the assessment of pain in animals [Abstract]. In: Grady J, Hildebrand S, McDonnell W, eds. Proceedings of the Second International Congress of Veterinary Anesthesia, Sacramento, California, 1985:38–42.

105. Breazile JE, Kitchell RL, Naitok Y. Neural basis of pain in animals. In: Proceedings of the 15th Research Conference of the American Meat Institute Foundation, Chicago, 1963:53.

106. Paul-Murphy J, Ludders JW, Robertson SA, Gaynor JS, Hellyer PW, Wong PL. The need for a cross-species approach to the study of pain in animals. J Am Vet Med Assoc 224:692–697, 2004.

107. Katz N, Ferrante FM. Nociception. In: Ferrante FM, VadeBoncouer TR, eds. Postoperative Pain Management. New York: Churchill Livingstone, 1992:17–67.

108. Woolf CJ. Recent advances in the pathophysiology of acute pain. Br J Anaesth 63:139–146, 1989.

109. Woolf CJ, Thompson SWN. The induction and maintenance of central sensitization is dependent on N-methyl-D-aspartic acid receptor activation: Implications for the treatment of post-injury pain hypersensitivity states. Pain 44:293–299, 1991.

110. Davis LE, Neff-Davis CA, Wilke JR. Monitoring drug concentrations in animal patients. J Am Vet Med Assoc 176:1156–1158, 1980.

111. Jaffe JH, Martin WR. Opioid analgesics and antagonists. In: Gilman AG, Goodman LS, Rall TW, eds. The Pharmacologic Basis of Therapeutics, 7th ed. New York: Macmillan, 1985:491–531.

112. Booth NH. Neuroleptanalgesics, narcotic analgesics, and analgesic antagonists. In: Booth NH, McDonald LE, eds. Veterinary Pharmacology and Therapeutics, 5th ed. Ames, IA: Iowa State University Press, 1982:267–296.

113. Simon EJ. The opiate receptors. In: Smythes JR, Bradley RJ, eds. Receptors in Pharmacology. New York: Marcel Dekker, 1977:257–293.

114. Hellyer PW, Bai L, Supon J, et al. Comparison of opioid and alpha-2 adrenergic receptor binding in horse and dog brain using radioligand autoradiography. Vet Anaesth Analg 30:172–182, 2003.

115. Mircica E, Clutton RE, Kyles KW, Blissitt KJ. Problems associated with perioperative morphine in horses: A retrospective case analysis. Vet Anaesth Analg 30:147–155, 2003.

116. Keates HL, Cramond T, Smith MT. Intra-articular and periarticular opioid binding in inflamed tissue in experimental canine arthritis. Anesth Analg 89:409–415, 1999.

117. Sheehy JG, Hellyer PW, Sammonds GE, et al. Evaluation of opioid receptors in synovial membranes of horses. Am J Vet Res 62:1408–1412, 2001.

118. Reuben SS, Vieira P, Faruqi S, Verghis A, Kilaru PA, Maciolek H. Local administration of morphine for analgesia after iliac bone graft harvest. Anesthesiology 95:390–394, 2001.

119. Robertson SA, Andrew SE. Presence of opioid growth factor and its receptor in the normal dog, cat, and horse cornea. Vet Ophthalmol 6:131–134, 2003.

120. Stiles J, Honda CN, Krohne SG, Kazacos EA. Effect of topical administration of 1% morphine sulfate solution on signs of pain and corneal wound healing in dogs. Am J Vet Res 64:813–818, 2003.

121. Martin PR, Ebert MH, Gordon EK, Linnoila M, Kopin IJ. Effects of clonidine on central and peripheral catecholamine metabolism. Clin Pharmacol Ther 35:322–327, 1984.

122. Stenberg D. The role of alpha-adrenoceptors in the regulation of vigilance and pain. Acta Vet Scand 82:29–34, 1986.

123. Lewis JW, Liebeskind JC. Pain suppressive systems of the brain. Trends Pharmacol Sci 4:73–75, 1983.

124. Benson GJ, Thurmon JC. Species difference as a consideration in alleviation of animal pain and distress. J Am Vet Med Assoc 191:1227–1230, 1987.

125. Jenkins WL. Pharmacologic aspects of analgesic drugs in animals: An overview. J Am Vet Med Assoc 191:1231–1240, 1987.

126. Lascelles BD, Butterworth SJ, Waterman AE. Postoperative analgesic and sedative effects of carprofen and pethidine in dogs. Vet Rec 134:187–191, 1994.

127. Nolan A, Reid J. Comparison of the postoperative analgesic and sedative effects of carprofen and papaveretum in the dog. Vet Rec 133:240–242, 1993.

128. Johnson CB, Tailor PM, Young SS, Brearley JC. Postoperative analgesia using phenylbutazone, flunixin or carprofen in horses. Vet Rec 133:136–138, 1993.

129. Lyles JH, Flecknell PA. The comparison of the effects of buprenorphine, carprofen and flunixin following laparotomy in rats. J Vet Pharmacol Ther 17:284–290, 1994.

130. Bostrom IM, Nyman GC, Lord PF, Haggstrom J, Jones BE, Bohlin HP. Effects of carprofen on renal function and results of serum biochemical and hematologic analysis in anesthetized dogs that had low blood pressure during anesthesia. Am J Vet Res 63:712–721, 2002.

131. Ko JC, Miyabiyashi T, Mandsager RE, Heaton-Jones TG, Mauragis DF. Renal effects of carprofen administered to healthy dogs anesthetized with propofol and isoflurane. J Am Vet Med Assoc 217:346–349, 2000.

132. Crandell DE, Mathews KA, Dyson DH. Effect of meloxicam and carprofen on renal function when administered to healthy dogs prior to anesthesia and painful stimulation. Am J Vet Res 65:1384–1390, 2004.

133. Davis LE. Species differences in drug distribution vs. factors in alleviation of animal pain. In: Kitchell RL, Erickson HH, eds. Animal Pain: Perception and Alleviation. Bethesda, MD: American Physiological Society, 1983:161–173.

134. Short CE. Neuroleptanalgesia and alpha-adrenergic receptor analgesia. In: Short CE, ed. Principles and Practice of Veterinary Anesthesia. Baltimore: Williams and Wilkins, 1987:47–57.

135. Garcia-Villar R, Toutain PL, Alvineric M, Ruckebusch Y. The pharmacokinetics of xylazine hydrochloride: An interspecific study. J Vet Pharmacol Ther 4:87–92, 1981.

136. Pippi NL, Lumb WV. Objective tests of analgesic drugs in ponies. Am J Vet Res 40:1082–1086, 1979.

137. Muir WW, Robertson JT. Visceral analgesia: Effects of xylazine, butorphanol, meperidine, and pentazocine in horses. Am J Vet Res 46:2081–2084, 1985.

138. Browning S, Lawrence D, Livingston, Morris B. Interactions of drugs active at opiate receptors and drugs active at alpha 2-receptors on various test systems. Br J Pharmacol 11:487–491, 1982.

139. Bakris GL, Cross PD, Hammarstem JE. The use of clonidine for management of opiate abstinence in a chronic pain patient. Mayo Clin Proc 57:657–660, 1982.

140. Lal H, Fielding S. Clonidine in the treatment of narcotic addiction [Letter]. Trends Pharmacol Sci 70, 1983.

141. Benson GJ, Thurmon JC, Tranquilli WJ. Intravenous sedation-analgesia (neuroleptanalgesia?) induced by morphine or butorphanol and xylazine in pointer dogs [Abstract]. In: Proceedings of the American College of Veterinary Anesthesiologists, Las Vegas, Nevada, 1986.

142. Duke T, Komulainen A, Remedios A, Cribb PH. The analgesic effects of administering fentanyl or medetomidine in the lumbosacral epidural space of cats. J Vet Surg 23:143–148, 1994.

143. Branson K, Ko JCH, Tranquilli WJ, Thurmon JC. Duration of analgesia induced by epidurally administered morphine and medetomidine in dogs. J Vet Pharmacol Ther 16:369–372, 1993.

144. Klein LV, Baetjer C. Preliminary report: Xylazine and morphine sedation in horses. Vet Anesthesiol 1:2–6, 1974.

145. Tranquilli WJ, Thurmon JC, Turner TA, Benson GJ, Lock TF. A preliminary report: Butorphanol tartrate as an adjunct to xylazine-ketamine in the horse. Equine Pract 5:26–29, 1983

146. Sinclair MD. A review of the physiological effects of α_2-agonists related to the clinical use of medetomidine in small animal practice. Can Vet J 44:885–897, 2003.

147. Klide AM, Calderwood HW, Soma LR. Cardiopulmonary effects of xylazine in dogs. Am J Vet Res 36:931–935, 1975.

148. Pypendop BH, Verstegen JP. Hemodynamic effects of medetomidine in the dog: A dose titration study. Vet Surg 27:612–622, 1998.

149. Thurmon JC, Steffey EP, Zinkl JG, Woliner M, Howland D Jr. Xylazine causes transient dose-related hyperglycemia and increased urine volumes in mares. Am J Vet Res 45:224–227, 1984.

150. Thurmon JC, Neff-Davis CA, Davis LE, Stoker RA, Benson GJ, Lock TF. Xylazine hydrochloride-induced hyperglycemia and hypoinsulinemia in thoroughbred horses. J Vet Pharmacol Ther 5:241–245, 1982.

151. Benson GJ, Thurmon JC, Neff-Davis CA, et al. Effect of xylazine hydrochloride upon plasma glucose and serum insulin concentrations in adult pointer dogs. J Am Anim Hosp Assoc 20:791–794, 1984.

152. Thurmon JC, Nelson DR, Hartsfield SM, Rumore CA. Effects of xylazine hydrochloride on urine in cattle. Aust Vet J 54:178–180, 1978.

153. Greene SA, Thurmon JC, Tranquilli WJ, Benson GJ. Effect of yohimbine on xylazine-induced hypoinsulinemia and hyperglycemia in mares. Am J Vet Res 48:676–678, 1987.

154. Greene SA, Thurmon JC, Benson GJ, et al. ADH prevents xylazine-induced diuresis in mares [Abstract]. In: Veterinary Midwest Anesthesia Conference (VMAC), Urbana, Illinois, May 31, 1986.

155. Haskins SC. Use of analgesics postoperatively and in a small animal intensive care setting. J Am Vet Med Assoc 191:1266–1268, 1987.

156. Berg RJ, Orton EC. Pulmonary function in dogs after intercostal thoracotomy: Comparison of morphine, oxymorphone, and selective intercostal nerve block. Am J Vet Res 47:471–474, 1986.

157. Crane SW. Perioperative analgesia: A surgeon's perspective. J Am Vet Med Assoc 191:1254–1257, 1987.

158. Day TK, Pepper WT, Tobias TA, Flynn MF, Clarke KM. Comparison of intraarticular and epidural morphine administration for analgesia following stifle arthrotomy in dogs [Abstract]. In: Veterinary Midwest Conference (VMAC), Columbus, Ohio, June 17, 1995.

159. Klimscha W, Brinkmann H, Plattner O, et al. Epidural ketamine and clonidine for postoperative analgesia after lower limb surgery [Abstract]. Anesthesiology 79:A805, 1993.

160. Martin D, Tranquilli WJ, Thurmon JC, et al. Hemodynamic effect of the epidural injection of ketamine in isoflurane anesthetized dogs [Abstract]. In: Veterinary Midwest Anesthesia Conference (VMAC), Columbus, Ohio, June 17, 1995.

161. Bell RF. Low-dose subcutaneous ketamine infusion and morphine tolerance. Pain 83:101–103, 1999.

162. Dickenson AH. NMDA receptor antagonists: Interactions with opioids. Acta Anaesthesiol Scand 41(1 Pt 2):112–115, 1997.

163. Fu ES, Miguel R, Scharf JE. Preemptive ketamine decreases postoperative narcotic requirements in patients undergoing abdominal surgery. Anesth Analg 84:1086–1090, 1997.

164. Mao J, Price DD, Mayer DJ. Mechanisms of hyperalgesia and morphine tolerance: A current view of their possible interactions. Pain 62:259–274, 1995.

165. Menigaux C, Fletcher D, Dupont X, Guignard B, Guirimand F, Chauvin M. The benefits of intraoperative small-dose ketamine on postoperative pain after anterior cruciate ligament repair. Anesth Analg 90:129–135, 2000.

166. Stubhaug A, Breivik H, Eide PK, Kreunen M, Foss A. Mapping of punctuate hyperalgesia around a surgical incision demonstrates that ketamine is a powerful suppressor of central sensitization to pain following surgery. Acta Anaesthesiol Scand 41:1124–1132, 1997.

167. Pozzi A, Traverso F, Muir W. Prevention of central sensitization and pain by N-methyl-D-aspartate receptor antagonists. J Am Vet Med Assoc 228:53–60, 2006.

168. Moses VS, Pertone AL, Nonsteroidal anti-inflammatory drugs. In: Mama K, Hendrickson DA, eds. The Veterinary Clinics, Equine Practice. Philadelphia: WB Saunders, 2002:21–37.

169. George LW. Pain control in food animals. In: Steffey EP, ed. Recent Advances in Anesthetic Management of Large Domestic Animals. Ithaca, NY: International Veterinary Information Service, 2003. http://www.ivis.org.

170. University of Glasgow. Short Form Pain Questionnaire. Glasgow: Faculty of Veterinary Medicine, University of Glasgow. http://www.gla.ac.uk/vet/research/cascience/painandwelfare/cmps.htm.

Section II
PHYSIOLOGY

Chapter 4
Cardiovascular System

William W. Muir

Introduction

A fundamental understanding and appreciation of the role of the cardiovascular system and circulatory dynamics are paramount for safe anesthetic practice. The uptake, distribution, and elimination of anesthetic drugs depend on blood flow. The importance of the cardiovascular system to patient well-being and the diverse effects of drugs used in the practice of anesthesia on hemodynamics emphasize the need to have a working knowledge of hemodynamics to monitor patient status adequately. The cardiovascular system, which is composed of the heart, blood vessels, lymph vessels, and blood, is designed to supply a continuous flow of oxygen and nutrients to all tissues of the body. Oxygen

and nutrient supply and waste removal are facilitated by major exchange organs, including the lungs, where blood becomes oxygenated and carbon dioxide is removed; the gastrointestinal system, where nutrients are absorbed and solid and liquid wastes are eliminated; and the kidneys, where additional by-products of metabolism are excreted. More specifically, the principal function of the heart is to pump blood, of the vasculature to carry blood to and from the heart and facilitate exchange processes in the peripheral tissues, and of the blood to function as the transport medium, or solvent, for all the body homeostatic and exchange processes.

Oxygenated blood returning from the lungs enters the left ventricle via the left atrium and mitral valve, and is ejected into the aorta, which, through an elaborate array of major arteries, distributes blood to all the tissues of the body. The end branches of these major arteries—the arterioles—differentially regulate blood flow and give rise to a vascular bed of small vessels—the capillaries—where oxygen and nutrients are exchanged for the by-products of cellular metabolism. The capillaries, in turn, recombine to form venules and veins that return blood to the right atrium, right ventricle, and lungs (Fig. 4.1). Circulation of blood depends on a functional heart, normal blood vessels, and adequate blood volume, and serves to maintain a constant internal environment for all living cells.

This chapter reviews the physiology of the cardiovascular system. A stepwise approach is taken that describes the structure and function of the heart, blood vessels, lymphatic system, and blood. This is followed by a discussion of the neural, humoral, and local control mechanisms that regulate cardiovascular function. Methods for assessing cardiovascular function are briefly reviewed, followed by a general discussion of diseases of the cardiovascular system.

Functional Anatomy of the Heart and Circulation

Heart

The structure of the cardiovascular system is well suited for its function: the delivery of oxygen and nutrients to peripheral tissues and removal of the by-products of cellular metabolism. The heart, as one key component of the cardiovascular system, functions to pump blood throughout the body. The heart is composed of four chambers: two thin-walled atria separated by an interatrial septum, and two thick-walled ventricles separated by an interventricular septum. The boundaries of the various chambers

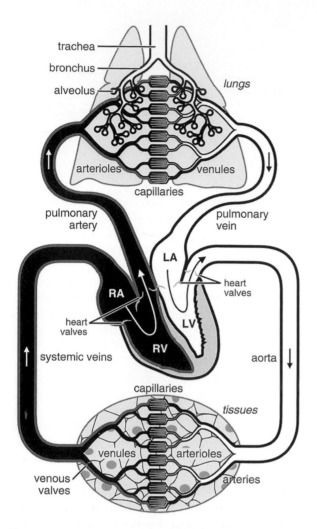

Fig. 4.1. The cardiovascular system is comprised of the heart, blood, and two parallel circulations (pulmonary and systemic). *Pulmonary circulation:* The pulmonary artery carries blood from the right ventricle (RV) to the lungs, where carbon dioxide is eliminated and oxygen is taken up. Oxygenated blood returns to the left atrium (LA) via the pulmonary veins. *Systemic circulation:* Blood is pumped by the left ventricle (LV) into the aorta, which distributes blood to the peripheral tissues. Oxygen and nutrients are exchanged for carbon dioxide and other by-products of tissue metabolism in capillary beds, after which the blood is returned to the right atrium (RA) through the venules and large systemic veins. Modified from Shepherd and Vanhoutte,[102] p. 3.

are easily defined by the great veins (cranial and caudal vena cava), which return blood to the right atrium; the smaller pulmonary veins, which return oxygenated blood from the lung to the left atrium; the coronary sulcus, which demarcates the atria from the ventricles; and the anterior and posterior interventricular (longitudinal) sulci, which separate the right and left ventricles (Fig. 4.2A).

The paraconal branch of the left main coronary artery, frequently referred to as the *left anterior descending coronary artery* in humans, provides the blood supply to the ventricular septum and left ventricular free wall. The subsinuosal coronary artery,

most frequently an extension of the left circumflex coronary artery (the other major branch of the left main coronary artery), but occasionally can branch off of the right coronary artery, provides the blood supply to the posterior left ventricle. The right coronary artery provides the blood supply to the right ventricular free wall and the posterior wall of the left ventricle (Fig. 4.2B). The left coronary artery is generally dominant in dogs and the right coronary artery is dominant in cats and horses. The atria receive blood returning from the systemic circulation (right atrium) and pulmonary circulation (left atrium), and to a limited degree act as storage chambers. The ventricles, the major pumping chambers of the heart, are separated from the atria by the tricuspid valve on the right side and the mitral valve on the left side. The ventricles receive blood from their respective atria and eject it across semilunar valves (the pulmonic valve between the right ventricle and pulmonary artery and the aortic valve between the left ventricle and aorta) into the pulmonary circulation (right ventricle) and systemic circulation (left ventricle). Once the process of cardiac contraction is initiated, almost simultaneous contraction of the atria is followed by nearly synchronous contraction of the ventricles, which results in pressure differences between the atria, ventricles, and pulmonary and systemic circulations. Cardiac contraction produces differential pressure changes that are responsible for atrioventricular and semilunar valve opening and closing and the production of heart sounds (S_1, S_2, S_3, and S_4). Chordae tendineae originating from papillary muscles located on the inner wall of the ventricular chambers are attached to the free edges of the atrioventricular valve leaflets and help to maintain valve competence and prevent regurgitation of blood into the atrium during ventricular contraction. Alteration in heart chamber geometry (e.g., stretch or hypertrophy) produced by changes in blood volume, deformation (pericardial tamponade), or disease can have profound effects on myocardial function, as do the effects produced by neurohumoral, metabolic, and pharmacological perturbations.

Blood Vessels

The principal role of blood vessels and the vascular network is to carry blood to and from oxygen-exchange and nutrient-exchange sites: the capillaries.[1] The large and small vessels of the pulmonary and systemic circulations facilitate the delivery of blood to the exchange sites in the pulmonary and systemic capillary beds and return blood to the heart. The aorta and other large arteries compose the high-pressure portion of the systemic circulation and are relatively stiff compared to veins, possessing a high proportion of elastic tissue in comparison to smooth muscle and fibrous tissues. This structural difference enables the aorta to stretch following ventricular contraction and the ejection of blood. The potential (stored) energy in the stretched aorta following cardiac contraction is returned as kinetic (motion) energy and blood flow during ventricular relaxation. The highly elastic architecture of the aorta facilitates the continuous, albeit nonuniform, flow of blood to peripheral tissues throughout the cardiac cycle (contraction-relaxation-rest) and has been termed the *Windkessel effect*. The Windkessel effect is believed to be responsible for as much as 50% of peripheral blood flow in most species during normal heart rates. Tachyarrhythmias and vascu-

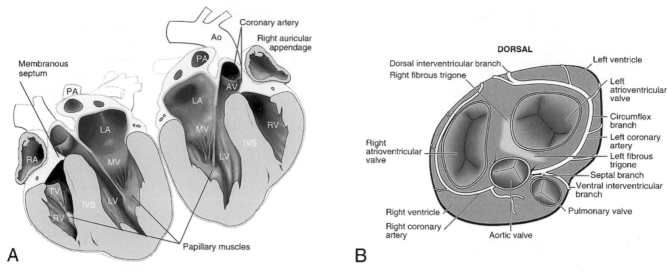

Fig. 4.2. **A:** The heart is a pump comprised of two thin-walled and two thick-walled chambers and a highly reactive and diffuse vascular network (coronary circulation). The thin-walled right atrium (RA) and left atrium (LA) are separated from each other by a membranous septum (between the right and left atria). The interventricular septum (IVS) lies between the right and left ventricles. The tricuspid valve (TV) and mitral valve (MV) lie between the RA and RV and the LA and LV, respectively. The pulmonary and aortic (AV) valves separate the RV and LV from the pulmonary artery (PA) and aorta (Ao), respectively. **B:** A fibrous trigone located at the center of the heart provides the scaffolding to which the heart valves, atria, and ventricles are attached. The right and left coronary arteries emerge from the base of the aorta and with the paraconal arteries to supply blood to all the chambers of the heart including the heart valves.

lar diseases (stiff nonelastic vessels) hamper the Windkessel effect and produce distinctive changes in the arterial pressure waveform. More distal larger arteries contain greater percentages of smooth muscle compared to elastic tissue and act as conduits for the transfer of blood under high pressure to tissues. The most distal small arteries, terminal arterioles, and arteriovenous anastomoses contain a predominance of smooth muscle, are highly innervated, and function as resistors that regulate the distribution of blood flow, aid in the regulation of systemic blood pressure, and modulate tissue perfusion pressure. The capillaries are the functional exchange sites for oxygen, nutrients, electrolytes, cellular waste products, and other substances. These vessels are generally no more than one or two cell layers thick and comprise that portion of the vasculature with by far the largest surface area. Capillaries are of three different types: continuous (lung and muscle), fenestrated (kidney and intestine), and discontinuous (liver, spleen, and bone marrow). All capillaries are highly porous and are found in varying numbers in different tissue beds, depending on tissue metabolism and the importance of fluid exchange. Postcapillary venules are composed of an endothelial lining and fibrous tissue and function to collect blood from capillaries. Some venules act as postcapillary sphincters, and all venules merge into small veins. Small and larger veins contain increasing amounts of fibrous tissue in addition to smooth muscle and elastic tissue, although their walls are much thinner than comparably sized arteries. Many veins contain valves that act in conjunction with external compression (contracting muscles and pressure differences in the abdominal and thoracic cavities) to facilitate the return flow of blood to the right atrium. The venous

system also acts as a major blood reservoir. Indeed, 60% to 70% of the blood volume may be stored in the systemic venous vasculature during resting conditions (Fig. 4.3).

Two additional structural components that are important during normal circulatory function are arteriovenous anastomoses and the lymphatic system. Arteriovenous anastomoses, as the name implies, bypass capillary beds. They possess smooth muscle cells throughout their entire length and are located in most, if not all, tissue beds. Most arteriovenous anastomoses are believed to be extremely important in regulating blood flow to highly vascular tissue beds (skin, feet, and hoofs). Their role in maintaining normal homeostasis, however, is speculative other than for thermoregulation.

The peripheral lymphatic system is not anatomically part of the blood circulatory system. Nevertheless, it is integrally involved in maintaining normal circulatory dynamics, especially interstitial fluid volume (approximately 10% of the capillary filtrate). Lymphatic capillaries collect interstitial fluid—lymph—which is eventually returned to the cranial vena cava and right atrium after passing through a series of lymph vessels, lymph nodes, and the thoracic duct. Lymph vessels have smooth muscle within their walls and contain valves similar to those in veins. Contraction of skeletal muscle (lymphatic pump) and lymph vessel smooth muscle, in conjunction with lymphatic valves, are responsible for lymph flow.

Blood

Blood is the fluid (approximately 60% plasma and 40% cells) responsible for carrying oxygen, nutrients, and other bloodborne

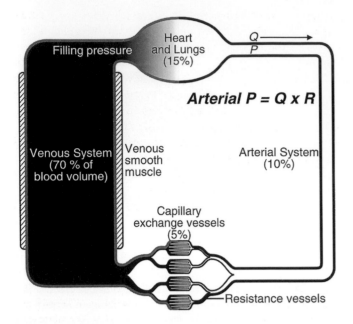

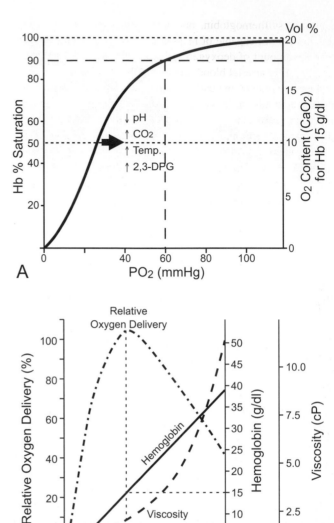

Fig. 4.3. Blood is unevenly distributed throughout the circulatory system. The largest portion of the blood volume is contained within the systemic veins. Relatively small changes in venous capacity can alter the heart's filling pressure dramatically, causing predictable changes in cardiac output (Q), peripheral vascular resistance (R), and arterial blood pressure (P). Decreases in filling pressure, for example, decrease Q and P and increase R. Modified from Shepherd and Vanhoutte,[102] p. 11.

substances to all the tissues of the body and for delivering carbon dioxide, the by-products of cellular metabolism, and foreign substances (e.g., anesthetic drugs) to the appropriate organs of elimination. This suspension of red and white blood cells and platelets in plasma is also responsible for maintaining a normal cellular environment (homeostasis), prevention of hemorrhage (clotting), and defense against foreign substances (immunity).[2] The most essential function of blood is to deliver oxygen to tissues. Oxygen is relatively insoluble in plasma (0.003 mL per 100 mL per 1 mm Hg partial pressure of oxygen [PO_2]; approximately 0.3 mL per 100 mL at PO_2 = 100 mm Hg). The erythrocytes (red blood cells [RBCs]) transport much larger amounts of oxygen than can be carried in solution, and the actual amount that can be carried depends on the amount of hemoglobin (Hb) in the erythrocytes. The balance between oxygen delivery by whole blood and oxygen partial pressure in the tissues and cells has evolved to incorporate a diverse group of regulatory processes designed to accommodate the encapsulation of Hb within RBCs. Hemoglobin exists as a tetramer (molecular weight, 64 kDa) consisting of two α and two β polypeptide chains. Each polypeptide chain contains heme and a central iron molecule that can bind oxygen.[3] The affinity of Hb for oxygen depends on the partial pressure of carbon dioxide (PCO_2), pH, body temperature, the intraerythrocyte concentration of 2,3-diphosphoglycerate and the chemical structure of Hb (Fig. 4.4A).[3] Heme must be in the reduced or ferrous state (Fe^{2+}) to bind oxygen. Methemoglobin is

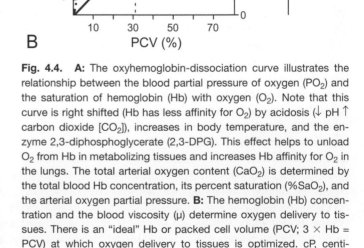

Fig. 4.4. **A:** The oxyhemoglobin-dissociation curve illustrates the relationship between the blood partial pressure of oxygen (PO_2) and the saturation of hemoglobin (Hb) with oxygen (O_2). Note that this curve is right shifted (Hb has less affinity for O_2) by acidosis ($\downarrow$ pH $\uparrow$ carbon dioxide [CO_2]), increases in body temperature, and the enzyme 2,3-diphosphoglycerate (2,3-DPG). This effect helps to unload O_2 from Hb in metabolizing tissues and increases Hb affinity for O_2 in the lungs. The total arterial oxygen content (CaO_2) is determined by the total blood Hb concentration, its percent saturation (%SaO_2), and the arterial oxygen partial pressure. **B:** The hemoglobin (Hb) concentration and the blood viscosity (μ) determine oxygen delivery to tissues. There is an "ideal" Hb or packed cell volume (PCV; 3 × Hb = PCV) at which oxygen delivery to tissues is optimized. cP, centi-Poise.

formed when the iron is oxidized to the ferric state (Fe^{3+}), and this form of Hb cannot bind oxygen. Hemoglobin is maintained in the Fe^{2+} state inside the RBC by reduced nicotine-adenine dinucleotide (NADH)–methemoglobin reductase. Carboxyhemoglobin, sulfhemoglobin, and cyanmethemoglobin are other Hbs that are not capable of reversible associations with oxygen. Once the amount of deoxygenated Hb (unsaturated Hb) exceeds 5 g/100 mL in arterial blood, the blood changes from red to blue (cyanosis). Some of the carbon dioxide produced by metabolizing tissues binds to deoxygenated Hb and is eliminated by the lungs during the Hb oxygenation process prior to the blood returning to the systemic circulation and the cycle repeating itself.

Encapsulation of Hb within RBCs has important biological consequences, including the rate of its saturation with oxygen, its intravascular half-life, prevention of renal toxicity, and maintenance of colloid osmotic pressure. The PO_2 at which Hb is half-saturated with oxygen is termed the P_{50}. The P_{50} varies among species (23 to 32 mm Hg), and free Hb (lysed RBCs and blood substitutes) has a lower P_{50} than does blood (Fig. 4.4A). The high intracellular concentration of 2,3-diphosphoglycerate compared to plasma facilitates the release of oxygen from Hb and helps maintain a physiologically relevant P_{50} (26 to 28 mm Hg). Once free in the plasma (hemolysis), Hb dissociates into $\alpha\beta$ dimers, which initially bind to haptoglobin and are removed by the liver. Depletion of haptoglobin leads to clearance of free Hb dimers by the kidneys. Renal clearance of large quantities of Hb dimers can result in their precipitation in the proximal tubules, leading to renal tubular damage and renal failure.[4] Free Hb also increases the colloid osmotic pressure of whole blood.

Blood is a nonhomogeneous suspension of particles (non-Newtonian fluid). Therefore, the concentration of RBCs, RBC interactions, and fluid characteristics of whole blood determine its fluidity, flow resistance, velocity, and local shear stress, which modifies cardiac output, cardiac work, blood flow distribution, and oxygen delivery to tissues. Oxygen delivery to tissues plays a very important role in determining microcirculatory autoregulatory responses, with increases in PO_2 causing vasoconstriction and vice versa. Changes in packed cell volume (PCV) require appropriate shifts in the viscosity (μ) of whole blood in order to optimize oxygen delivery to tissues. Small decreases impact PCV, and blood μ (hemodilution) generally increases blood flow velocity and decreases diffusional oxygen exit from the arterioles, thereby augmenting oxygen delivery to tissues (Fig. 4.4B). Intentional hemodilution (e.g., crystalloid or colloid administration) to improve oxygen delivery, however, is limited by the "transfusion trigger" (about 6 to 8 g/dL). When the Hb concentration decreases below this range, the decreased amount of oxygen carried by Hb may cause tissue hypoxia. Fortunately, increases in plasma μ induce vasodilatation, thereby helping to preserve capillary perfusion and functional capillary density, suggesting that the transfusion trigger is also a viscosity trigger and that both PCV and μ must be considered together when selecting fluid therapy.

Maintaining adequate tissue oxygenation depends on oxygen uptake by the lungs, oxygen delivery (DO_2) to and oxygen extraction (OE) by tissues, and oxygen use by the metabolic machinery within cells. The factors that determine the supply of oxygen to tissues are Hb concentration, the affinity of Hb for oxygen (P_{50}), the saturation of Hb with oxygen (SaO_2), the arterial oxygen partial pressure (PaO_2), the cardiac output (CO), and

the tissue oxygen consumption (VO_2). The Fick, or oxygen consumption, equation ($VO_2 = CO [CaO_2 - CvO_2]$) contains all the essential components of this relationship. The Fick equation can be used to derive oxygen delivery ($DO_2 = CO \times CaO_2$), oxygen extraction ($OE = CaO_2 - CvO_2$), and the oxygen extraction ratio ($OER = CaO_2 - CvO_2/CaO_2$), noting that all of the equations contain the term CaO_2 and are therefore mathematically coupled. Arterial blood oxygen content (CaO_2) is calculated by $CaO_2 = Hb \times 1.35 \times SaO_2 + PaO_2 \times 0.003$. Arterial blood (Hb = 15 g/dL; PCV = 45%), for example, contains approximately 20 to 21 mL of oxygen/dL of blood when the $SaO_2 = 100\%$ and the $PaO_2 = 100$ mm Hg (room air). The venous blood oxygen content (CvO_2) is generally 14 to 15 mL/dL yielding an OER of 0.2 to 0.3 (20% to 30%). Decreased hemoglobin concentrations (parasitism, hemorrhage, and hemodilution) cause oxygen extraction to increase to maintain the requisite oxygen delivery required by metabolizing tissues. The critical DO_2 and OER are approximately 5.0 mL/kg/min and 0.6 (60%) in normal healthy dogs, suggesting that most dogs and other mammals have significant reserve. An increase in arterial blood lactate concentration is the cardinal sign of inadequate oxygen delivery to metabolizing tissues and suggests that oxygen consumption has become delivery dependent or that some defect in tissue oxygen extraction or use has developed.

Hemorrheology

Hemorrheology is the study of blood flow in the vascular system.[5,6]

Pressure, Resistance, and Flow

In electric circuits, current flow (I) is determined by the electromotive force or voltage (E) and the resistance to current flow (R) according to Ohm's law:

$$I = E/R$$

The flow of fluids (Q) through nondistensible tubes depends on pressure (P) and the resistance to flow (R). Therefore, and in the most general terms,

$$Q = P/R$$

The resistance to blood flow is determined by blood viscosity (η) and the geometric factors of blood vessels (radius and length). The steady, nonpulsatile, laminar flow of Newtonian fluids (homogenous fluids in which viscosity does not change with flow velocity or vascular geometry), like water, saline, and, under physiological conditions, plasma, can be described by the Poiseuille-Hagen law, which states

$$Q = (P_1 - P_2) r^4\pi/8L\eta; R = 8L\eta/r^4\pi$$

where $P_1 - P_2$ is the pressure difference, r^4 is the radius to the fourth power, L is the length of the tube, η is the viscosity of the fluid, and $\pi/8$ is a constant of proportionality.[7] The maintenance of laminar flow is a fundamental assumption of the resistance offered to steady-state fluid flow in the Poiseuille-Hagen equation. This law, although frequently used for assessing blood flow in the vascular system, is descriptive only and must be kept in perspective when considering the real-life situation, because blood is not a homogenous fluid and blood flow is not steady, but pulsatile, and is not always laminar. These differences from the idealized steady laminar flow of Newtonian fluids through nondistensible tubes of constant radius have important consequences on the quantity of blood flow to peripheral tissue beds, oxygen delivery, and the distribution of blood flow between tissue beds.

The relationship between vessel (or chamber when describing the heart)-distending pressure, vessel diameter, vessel wall thickness, and vessel wall tension is described by Laplace's law:

$$P = 2Th/r \text{ or } T = Pr/2h$$

where T is wall tension, P is developed pressure, r is the internal radius, and h is the wall thickness. This relationship is extremely important because it relates pressure and vessel dimension to changes in developed tension, which is known to be an important determinant of ventricular-vascular coupling (afterload), myocardial work, and myocardial oxygen consumption.[8]

Viscosity

Since blood is a non-Newtonian fluid that is delivered through progressively narrowing blood vessels in a pulsatile nonlaminar or even turbulent manner, how can blood flow be accurately characterized? More specifically, how can the resistance (R) to blood flow be thought of in functional terms? First, the major factors influencing blood flow resistance (R_p) are blood viscosity (η) and impedance (Z), which collectively can be considered vascular hindrance:[9,10]

$$R_p = \eta \times Z$$

It should be noted that the term R_p is not the same as R in Ohm's law or the equivalent thereof in the Poiseuille-Hagen equation ($8L\eta/r^4\pi$), but represents the resistance to blood flow in a pulsatile (R_p; p = pulsatile) or oscillatory non–steady-state or, simply stated, more physiological system. The resistance (R) term in the two previous examples is more correctly thought of in terms of a nonpulsatile, nonoscillatory, and nonphysiological system.

The viscosity term (η), although of lesser importance than Z in determining R_p, depends on RBC concentration or hematocrit, RBC aggregability and deformability, plasma viscosity, temperature, and blood flow conditions.[6] The rheological term that characterizes blood flow conditions is shear rate, which is a function of blood flow velocity and vascular geometry. The viscosity of blood is shear rate dependent. Viscosity decreases as shear rate increases according to this equation:

$$\eta = \text{shear stress (dynes/cm}^2\text{)/shear rate (s}^{-1}\text{)}$$

where shear stress is the force applied during pulsatile blood flow between theoretic layers of blood in the blood vessel. It is interesting that shear rate gradually increases and η decreases as large arteries become smaller, and is greatest in the capillaries regardless of low flow rates and then decreases in venules and large veins. This phenomenon, known as the *Fahraeus-Lindquist effect*, is attributed to "plasma skimming" and RBC deformability; that is, viscosity in capillaries is low because RBCs may only be able to pass through capillaries single file, permitting the development of a cell-free layer of plasma next to the capillary wall that, in conjunction with RBC folding, increases the cell-free component of blood compared to the situation in larger blood vessels.[9] The smaller the vessel, the greater is the effect. Under normal circumstances, the most important variable in determining η is the hematocrit.

The optimum hematocrit for transporting the most oxygen per unit time to tissues varies among species (e.g., human, 47%; dog, 46%; cow, 32%; horse, 42%; and camel, 27%) because of differences in anatomy and circulatory dynamics. Dogs and horses also can contract their spleen, providing additional RBCs (raising the hematocrit) and oxygen-carrying capacity during times of stress or exercise. High hematocrits (polycythemia), low blood flow conditions (shock), increased RBC aggregability, rouleaux formation (sepsis), and hyperproteinemia (dehydration) can all cause η to increase, resulting in a decrease in oxygen delivery to tissues (Fig. 4.5). Hematocrits greater than 65% lead to sludging of blood in capillaries and venules and dramatically increase the work of pumping blood. Hemodilution (fluid administration) is often beneficial in treating these conditions and has been used during anesthesia to reduce RBC loss and improve oxygen delivery during low blood flow states.[11,12] Indeed, the optimum hematocrit for dogs subjected to hemorrhagic shock and an arterial blood pressure of 50 mm Hg is 20% to 25% (Fig. 4.5).[9] The advent and clinical use of hemoglobin-based oxygen-carrying solutions derived from human, bovine, or synthetic sources have provided an alternative method for oxygen delivery to tissues. Their development has markedly increased our understanding of oxygen uptake, delivery, and use and ushered in new ideas regarding the mechanisms responsible for the distribution of blood flow and the control of the microcirculation.

Impedance

The impedance (Z) term, the second key factor in determining blood flow in pulsatile systems, is a measure of the opposition to flow presented by pulsatile blood flow in an elastic vascular system.[10] Quantitatively, impedance is the relationship between pulsatile pressure and pulsatile flow in arteries:

$$Z_L = P_1 - P_2/Q \ (Z_L = R_P + R)$$

where Z_L represents longitudinal impedance, which is the sum of the pulsatile (R_p) and steady nonpulsatile resistive (R) components of longitudinal arterial resistance. Under normal (nonstressed) conditions, the steady nonpulsatile resistive component represents 90% of the total impedance to blood flow while the pulsatile component comprises 10%. This fact ($R = 90\%$ of Z_L) is the principal reason so many investigators and clinicians calculate vascular resistance from Ohm's law. The components of Z_L may change considerably, however, in diseased animals or during pharmacological manipulation, with R_p becoming much more important.

Impedance is determined by the various frequency components that comprise the arterial pressure and flow waveforms, is measured by applying a Fourier or harmonic analysis to these waveforms, and is expressed as a ratio or modulus and phase

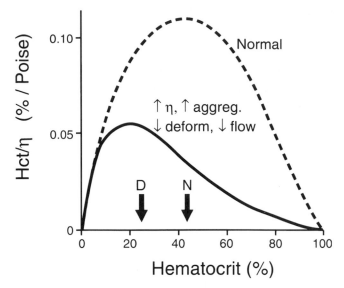

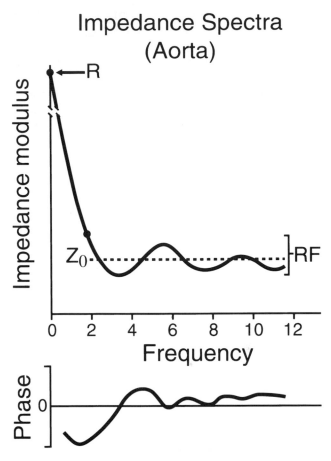

Fig. 4.5. The effects of changes in hematocrit (% Hct) on an index of oxygen transport (Hct/η). The *arrow marked N* represents a relatively normal Hct. The *arrow marked D* represents a patient with anemia or hemodilution. The *dashed line* represents the normal situation when Hct is the only variable. The *solid line* represents the response to changes in Hct when plasma viscosity (η) is increased, red cell aggregation (aggreg) is increased, red cell deformability (deform) is decreased, or blood flow rate is decreased. Modified from Lasala et al.,[6] p. 210.

Fig. 4.6. The impedance modulus and phase of a hypothetical aortic impedance spectra. The impedance modulus decreases from 0 Hz (*R*, peripheral vascular resistance) to a low value that oscillates around a characteristic value (Z_0) because of pulse-wave reflections (RF). Negative phase values indicate that flow harmonics lead pressure harmonics and vice versa.

(Fig. 4.6). A positive phase value indicates that flow harmonics lag behind pressure harmonics, and vice versa, the key point being that impedance is a frequency-dependent, not time-dependent, index. Input impedance (Z_i), the ratio of pressure and flow at an arterial site that is considered to be the input to the vascular tree (e.g., the aortic root), depends on local arterial properties (e.g., elastance or compliance), the properties of all the vessels beyond the point of measurement down to the points where pulsations and pulse-wave reflections from narrowing arteries (particularly arterioles) and vessel bifurcations disappear. Impedance to blood flow, therefore, is viewed as having a resistive (steady state) component due primarily to the arterioles and a reactive (pulsatile) component due to vessel wall properties (compliance, elastance, and pulse-wave reflection). Low systolic arterial pressure enables more complete ventricular ejection, maintains low myocardial oxygen demands, and provides little stimulus for hypertrophy. High diastolic pressure ensures adequate coronary blood flow and myocardial perfusion because the majority of myocardial blood flow occurs during ventricular relaxation. Increases in arterial stiffness increase pulse-pressure amplitude and systolic pressure, and decrease diastolic pressure. Poorly timed wave reflections generally increase diastolic pressure (increase Z). The totality of these effects increases myocardial work, oxygen consumption, and energy requirements, and decreases myocardial perfusion. Ideally, the best match between the heart's pumping activity and the vascular response to the ejection of blood (ventricular-vascular coupling) is obtained

when myocardial work is kept as low as possible (low systolic pressure) while adequate perfusion of the heart and peripheral tissues (high diastolic pressure) is maintained.[13–15] Within perfusing limits, a reduction in mean arterial pressure (a characteristic of most anesthetic drugs) improves arterial distensibility, delays pressure-wave reflections, and causes a smaller reduction in diastolic pressure than does hypovolemia. Anesthesia and anesthetic drugs also produce variable effects on hematocrit, RBC deformability, and plasma protein concentrations, leading to alterations in η, which, when combined with changes in Z, may favorably affect ventricular-vascular coupling, providing hypotension (mean, less than 50 to 60 mm Hg) does not occur.[9,16,17]

Turbulence

Pulsatile blood flow may be laminar with a longitudinal velocity that takes the form of a parabola or may be irregular or turbulent (Fig. 4.7). More pressure, myocardial release of energy, and work are required to pump blood when the flow is turbulent. The po-

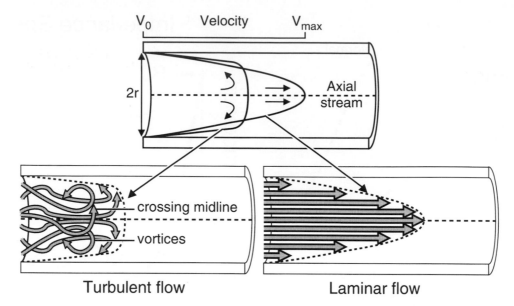

Fig. 4.7. Velocity profiles for laminar and turbulent blood flow. Note that during turbulent blood flow vortices develop and that both axial and mean velocities are lower than during laminar flow. V_{max}, maximum velocity.

tential for turbulence to develop in blood vessels can be predicted by a dimensionless number called the Reynolds number (RN):[18]

$$RN = pDv/\eta$$

where p is fluid density, D is vessel diameter, and v is the mean blood flow velocity. The blood viscosity (η) is inversely proportional to the Reynolds number and is an important determinant of turbulent blood flow. Turbulence usually produces periodic wave fluctuations and vibrations of the surrounding tissue structures, leading to murmurs and, with time, vascular dilation caused by weakening of the supporting elements of the vessel wall. Chronic or acute hemodilution (fluid therapy) reduces hematocrit; therefore, η, leading to an increase in Reynolds number and the production of "functional" cardiac murmurs. Furthermore, flow restriction caused by congenital disease (aortic or pulmonic stenosis) or blood vessel narrowing leads to an increase in the velocity of blood flow as predicted by the continuity equation which states that blood flowing through different areas of a continuous intact vascular system must be equal; therefore, blood flow through a narrowing or narrowed orifice must increase. The flow downstream from the obstruction or narrowing is usually turbulent with multiple velocities and directions. Cardiac diseases (pulmonic and aortic stenosis) and vascular diseases (thrombophlebitis) that narrow valve openings or blood vessels increase v and are important causes of murmurs. Blood flow velocity measurements can be assessed clinically by Doppler echocardiography and the Bernoulli equation, $\Delta P = 4v^2$, with the assumption that velocity distal to the obstruction is significantly greater than the velocity proximal to the obstruction and therefore may be ignored.

The Heart

The purpose of the heart is to pump blood in quantities sufficient to meet the body's metabolic and exercise demands. To achieve this function requires a highly integrated series of electric, mechanical, and metabolic events that culminate in repetitive contraction and relaxation of the myocardium.

Electrophysiology

Normal cardiac electric activity is essential for normal cardiac contractile function (excitation-contraction coupling). Indeed, myocardial contraction is preceded by, and will not occur without, electric activation, although normal or near-normal electric activity is possible without myocardial contraction (electric-mechanical uncoupling; electric-mechanical dissociation). The cardiac cell membrane (sarcolemma) is a highly specialized lipid bilayer that contains protein-associated channels, pumps, enzymes, and exchangers in an architecturally sophisticated, yet fluid (reorganizable and movable), medium. Most drugs and many anesthetic drugs produce important direct and indirect effects on the cell membrane and intracellular organelles, ultimately altering cardiac excitation-contraction coupling.

The molecular composition and fluidity of cardiac membranes determine their ion transport and membrane-associated electric properties. The unequal distribution of different ions, especially sodium, potassium, and chloride, is responsible for the development of the resting membrane potential of cardiac cells as predicted by the Nernst equation or, more accurately, the Goldman-Hodgkin-Katz constant-field equation.[19–21]

Nernst equation:

$$E = (RT/ZF) \ln(K_I/K_o)$$
$$-61 = 2.303 \, RT/F$$
$$E = -61 \text{ mV}/Z\log (C_i/C_o)$$

where

E = electromotive force
C_i and C_o = ion concentration inside (i) and outside (o) the cell membrane
Z = valence
R = gas constant
T = absolute temperature
F = Faraday constant
2.303 = conversion of ln to log 10
mV = millivolts at 37°C

Goldman-Hodgkin-Katz equation:

$$E_m = -61 \text{ mV} \log \frac{[K]_i + (P_{Na}/P_K) \, [Na]_i}{[K]_o + (P_{Na}/P_K) \, [Na]_o}$$

where

E_m = resting membrane potential
P_{Na}/P_K ratio = relative permeability of membrane Na to K, normally 0.04 in myocardial cells

The transmembrane electric potential generated by cardiac cells is the result of transmembrane ion fluxes (active properties) through "gated" membrane pores or channels (Table 4.1).[21] Ion channels are characterized by their ionic selectivity, conductance, gating characteristics, and density. The channel-gating mechanisms control ion passage and are composed of both activation

Table 4.1. Currents associated with the cardiac action potential

Current	Abbreviation	Qualities
Fast inward sodium current	I_{Na}	Responsible for upstroke of action potential; abolished by tetrodotoxin; inhibited by class I antiarrhythmic agents
Slow inward calcium current	I_{Ca} and I_{si}	Important for plateau phase of cardiac action potential; involved in excitation-contraction coupling; increased by ß stimulation; inhibited by calcium antagonist
Subtype T	$I_{Ca(t)}$	Transient calcium current, opening at low voltages (-60 to -50 mV); may be important in sinus node depolarization
Subtype L	$I_{Ca(l)}$	Long-duration calcium current; inhibited by calcium antagonists
Background potassium current (inward rectifier)	I_{K1} or I_{Kir}	Helps to maintain resting membrane potential
Voltage-gated delayed reactifier potassium currents	I_K (includes K_r and K_s)	Time-dependent outward potassium current; activated by depolarization (fully active at +10 mV) and deactivated by repolarization; voltage gated; responsible for repolarization in nodal cells and contributes to spontaneous depolarization; divided into I_{Kr} (r = rapid) and I_{Ks} (s = slow)
Early transient outward potassium current	I_{to}	Transient outward early potassium current, previously called *chloride current*; prominent in epicardial ventricular cells, Purkinje fibers, and atrial cells; causes phase 1; may also shorten action-potential duration
Other currents		
Diastolic pacemaker current in sinoatrial node and Purkinje fibers	I_f or I_h	Produces automaticity in sinoatrial node and Purkinje fibers
Sodium-calcium exchange current	$I_{NA/CA}$	Contributes to late phase of cardiac action potential
Chloride current	I_{Cl}	Activated by cAMP; shortens action-potential duration during adrenergic stimulation
Ligand-operated G-dependent K currents		
Acetylcholine sensitive	I_{KACh}	Activated by acetylcholine muscarinic receptors in nodal, Purkinje, and atrial cells; not in ventricles; time independent; when current switched on in nodal cells, spontaneous depolarization is delayed
Adenosine sensitive	I_{KADO}	Probably same as I_{KACh}; adenosine stimulates time-independent background potassium current
Adenosine triphosphate (ATP) regulated	I_{KATP}	Lack of ATP activates (e.g., ischemia); inhibited by sulfonylureas, activated by K-channel activators (pinacidil)

cAMP, cyclic adenosine monophosphate.
Modified from Opie.[106]

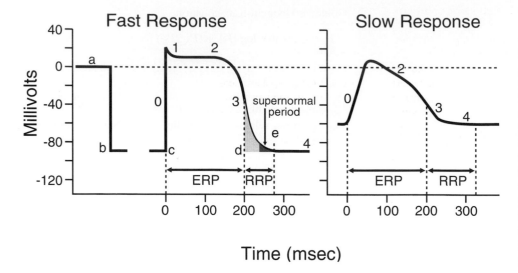

Fig. 4.8. Cardiac transmembrane potential changes associated with fast-response and slow-response action potentials. Note that slow-response action potentials originate from a less negative resting membrane potential and have a much slower rate of rise (phase 0). During the supernormal period, a subthreshold stimulus can elicit a normal action potential. See the text for an explanation of the action-potential phases 1 through 4. ERP, effective refractory period; and RRP, relative refractory period.

and inactivation gates, which are voltage and frequently time dependent. The functional configuration of the gates determines channel state: activated or open, inactivated or closed, and resting (capable of being activated). The directional movement (inward or outward) of the various ions ultimately depends on channel state and the electrochemical driving force (equilibrium potential minus membrane potential) for each ion. The electrochemical driving force, as illustrated by the Nernst equation, is composed of an electric force and a concentration gradient. It should be noted that in the presence of many anesthetic drugs, particularly local anesthetics (lidocaine or mepivacaine), and inhalation anesthetics (halothane, isoflurane, or sevoflurane), these same channels may demonstrate use-dependent block.[22,23] Use-dependent block is the phenomenon exhibited by cardiac cells wherein, in the presence of a drug, increases in stimulation rate (e.g., heart rate) produce a more pronounced drug effect on the electrophysiological properties of the heart than during slower rates of stimulation.

Excitability, or the ability of the cardiac cell membrane to generate an electric potential (action potential), is a fundamental intrinsic property of cardiac cells.[19] The action potential of cardiac muscle varies considerably from that of nerves and skeletal muscle. The cardiac action potential arises from a more negative membrane potential (90 vs. 65 mV), is greater in magnitude (130 vs. 80 mV), and is much longer in duration (150 to 300 vs. 1 ms). Five characteristic phases of the cardiac action potential are discernible in most cardiac cells: Phase 0, or the phase of rapid depolarization, is caused by the rapid and relatively large influx of sodium ions (fast inward current) into the cell; phase 1, the early phase of repolarization, is caused by the transient outward movement of potassium ions; phase 2, the plateau phase, is attributed to the continued, but decreased, entry of sodium ions and a large, but slow, influx of calcium ions (slow inward current) into cells; phase 3 is the phase of repolarization during which the membrane potential returns to its resting value because of potassium efflux (outward current) from the cell; and phase 4 is a resting phase in atrial and ventricular muscle cells prior to the initiation

of the next action potential (Fig. 4.8 and Table 4.2). The magnitude and rate of sodium influx into cardiac cells determine the magnitude and rate of change in membrane potential (dV/dt) during phase 0 of the cardiac action potential. The greater the dV/dt, the more rapid are the transmission and conduction of the cardiac impulse through cardiac tissue.[20] Cardiac cells that normally possess a more negative membrane potential (atrial and ventricular muscle cells, and Purkinje cells) demonstrate greater excitability and a more rapid conduction velocity than those with less negative membrane potentials (sinoatrial and atrioventricular nodes, and diseased myocardium).[23] Calcium entry into cardiac cells during phase 2 triggers intracellular calcium release, which is important for normal cellular contraction and, with potassium, determines action-potential duration in atrial and ventricular myocytes. Since calcium enters the cell slowly and at a less negative membrane potential, cardiac cells with a reduced resting membrane potential (sinoatrial and atrioventricular nodes) demonstrate a considerably decreased dV/dt and slow conduction velocity compared to atrial and ventricular muscle and Purkinje cells.[20] Potassium efflux from cardiac cells is controlled by a variety of mechanisms, including concentration differences across the membrane and the changing permeability (diffusional) characteristics of the cell membrane to potassium (Table 4.1). Collectively, the channels responsible for phase 3 repolarization are also the major determinants of cardiac action-potential duration, cardiac cell refractoriness, and the duration of the supernormal period (Fig. 4.8). The duration of the cardiac action potential has important clinical implications relative to the amount of calcium entry and the potential for arrhythmia development.[22] Longer cardiac action potentials permit more calcium entry into the cell and prolong cellular refractoriness. Arrhythmias develop if there are large disparities or inhomogeneities in the action-potential duration and refractoriness of adjacent cardiac cells because of reentry of electric impulses and reexcitation of the heart (see the Cardiac Arrhythmias section).[24] Reentry is one mechanism whereby the ultra-short-acting barbiturates and inhalation anesthetics are known to produce cardiac arrhythmias.

Table 4.2. Major ion fluxes during the cardiac action potential

Name	Ion	Movement	Current	Phase of Action Potential
I_{Na}	Na$^+$	In	Inward	0 Depolarization
I_{to}	K+	Out	Outward	1 (early repolarization)
I_{Cl}	Cl$^-$	In	Outward	1 Early repolarization
I_{Ca}	Ca^{2+}	In	Inward	2 Plateau
I_{K1}	K$^+$	Out	Outward	2 Plateau
I_k	K$^+$	Out	Outward	3 Repolarization
I_f	Na$^+$	In	Inward	4 Depolarization in automatic cells

Open I_{K1} channels in resting cells are the major contributors to the equilibrium responsible for the Nernst potential during phase 4 (resting potential).
Modified from Katz.[107]

Phase 4 diastolic depolarization (pacemaker potential) occurs in the sinoatrial and atrioventricular nodes and atrial and ventricular (Purkinje network) specialized tissues.[20,21] Diastolic depolarization imparts the unique property of automaticity to the heart. The resting membrane potential depolarizes toward a threshold potential in tissues with this property, which when reached triggers the development of an action potential. The ionic processes responsible for phase 4 or diastolic depolarization vary between the various specialized tissues of the heart primarily because of differences in their resting or maximum diastolic potential and cell type (e.g., sinoatrial node vs. atrioventricular node vs. Purkinje cell). Cells in the sinoatrial and atrial ventricular nodes have comparatively less negative maximum diastolic potentials (-65 mV) than do Purkinje cells and depend on the entry of calcium ion (slow inward current) and a progressive decrease in membrane permeability to potassium efflux for their automaticity (Fig. 4.9). Automatic cells in atrial specialized pathways and the ventricular Purkinje network have a more negative maximum diastolic potential (-90 mV) and depend on a hyperpolarizing-induced "funny" inward current, termed I_f, carried mainly by sodium ions and a decrease in potassium efflux for their automaticity (Table 4.1). Because potassium ions normally leave cardiac cells in order to restore or maintain the resting membrane potential, any decrease in potassium efflux facilitates depolarization. The principal mechanisms responsible for altering automaticity are changes in the threshold potential, the rate of phase 4 depolarization, and the maximum diastolic potential following repolarization. The cardiac tissue with the most rapid rate of phase 4 depolarization (normally the sinoatrial node) is termed the *pacemaker* and determines the heart rate. The cardiac pacemaker normally depresses the automaticity of slower or subsidiary pacemakers (overdrive suppression), preventing more than one pacemaker from controlling heart rate. In mechanical terms, overdrive suppression in subsidiary pacemakers is due to activation of the sodium ion–potassium ion (Na$^+$-K$^+$) pump, leading to membrane hyperpolarization and a longer time to reach threshold.[20,22] Subsidiary pacemakers are most suppressed at fast heart rates because the Na$^+$-K$^+$ pump is more active at faster rates, resulting in a more negative maximum diastolic potential. Automaticity is also influenced by local factors, including temperature, pH, and blood gases (PO$_2$ and PCO$_2$), extracellular potassium concentration, catecholamines, and various hormones (Fig. 4.9).

The algebraic sum of all the action potentials produced by each cardiac cell following activation by the sinoatrial node is responsible for the body surface electrocardiogram (ECG [Fig. 4.10]). Initiation of an electric impulse in the sinoatrial node is followed by rapid electric transmission of the impulse through

Fig. 4.9. The transmembrane potential of cardiac tissue within the sinoatrial node (pacemaker tissue) is characterized by a less negative maximum diastolic potential, which depolarizes toward threshold (phase 4 diastolic depolarization), a slow phase 0 caused primarily by activation of, and a relatively rapid repolarization due to, I_K. The rate of phase 4 diastolic depolarization (automaticity) can be increased by increases in heart rate, temperature, calcium, catecholamines, and thyroxine and decreases in oxygen tension and extracellular potassium concentration.

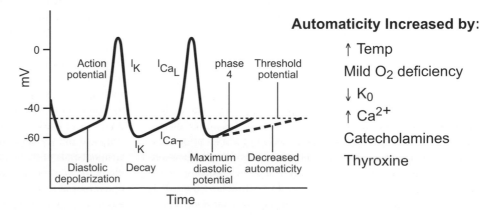

Automaticity Increased by:

↑ Temp

Mild O$_2$ deficiency

↓ K$_0$

↑ Ca^{2+}

Catecholamines

Thyroxine

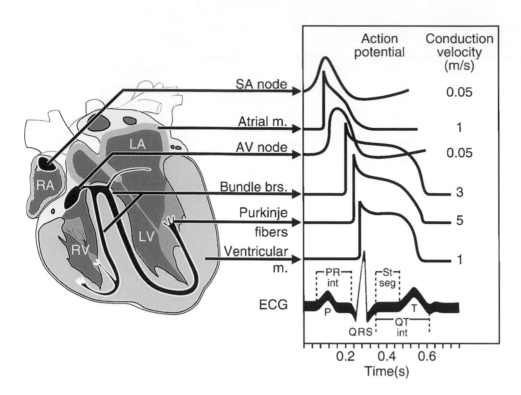

Fig. 4.10. The transmembrane potential (action potential) recorded from all the tissues of the heart (specialized tissue and muscle) summate to produce the P-QRS-T complex of the electrocardiogram (ECG) recorded at the body surface. AV, atrioventricular node; brs, branches; int, interval; LA, left atrium; LV, left ventricle; m, muscle; RA, right atrium; RV, right ventricle; SA, sinoatrial node; and seg, segment.

the atria, giving rise to the P wave. Repolarization of the atria gives rise to the Ta wave, which is most obvious in large animals (horses and cattle), where the total atrial tissue mass is substantial enough to generate enough electromotive force to be electrocardiographically recognizable. Repolarization of the atria in smaller species (dogs and cats) and depolarization of the sinoatrial and atrioventricular nodes do not generate a large enough electric potential to be recorded at the body surface except in cases of sinus tachycardia. Repolarization of the atria or Ta waves can be observed in dogs and cats with increased heart rates. Once the wave of depolarization reaches the atrioventricular node, conduction is slowed because of the atrioventricular node's low resting membrane potential (approximately −60 mV) and the relatively depressed rate of phase 0 (decremental conduction). Increased parasympathetic tone can produce marked slowing of atrioventricular nodal conduction, leading to first-degree, second-degree, and, rarely, third-degree heart block. Many drugs used in anesthesia, including opioids, α_2-adrenergic agonists, and occasionally acepromazine, increase parasympathetic tone, causing heart block and bradyarrhythmias (see the Cardiac Arrhythmias section). The use of antimuscarinic drugs atropine and glycopyrrolate is generally effective therapy in these situations unless the block is caused by structural disease (e.g., inflammation, fibrosis, or calcification).

Under normal conditions, conduction of the electric impulse through the atrioventricular node produces the PR or PQ interval of the ECG and provides time for the atria to contract prior to activation and contraction of the ventricles. This delay is functionally important, particularly at faster heart rates, because it enables atrial contraction to contribute to ventricular filling. It is worth remembering that cells of the atrioventricular node are ex-

tremely dependent on calcium ion for the generation of an action potential and conduction of the electric impulse. Thus, cells of the atrioventricular node are extremely sensitive to drugs that block transsarcolemmal calcium flux, like large doses of anesthetics (inhalant and injectable anesthetics) and the so-called calcium antagonists verapamil and diltiazem. These and other drugs and cardiac disease can produce atrioventricular block and post-repolarization refractoriness that are not responsive to anticholinergic drugs. Post-repolarization refractoriness is the phenomenon wherein cardiac cells remain refractory to electric activation after complete repolarization.[22,24] This phenomenon is most likely to produce atrioventricular block as the rate of atrial depolarization is increased. Increases in parasympathetic tone, therefore, particularly in the presence of drugs or disease (ischemia) that interfere with conduction of the electric impulse through the atrioventricular node, can lead to ECG evidence of first-degree (prolonged PR interval), second-degree (blocked P wave), or third-degree (dissociation of P and QRS complex) atrioventricular block.

Once the electric impulse has traversed the atrioventricular node, it is rapidly transmitted to the ventricular muscle by specialized muscle cells commonly referred to as *Purkinje fibers.* Bundles of Purkinje cells—the right and left bundle branches—transmit the electric impulses to the ventricular septum and the right and left ventricular free walls, respectively, via the moderator band in the right ventricle and the left anterior and posterior divisions of the left bundle branch in the left ventricle. Purkinje cells and the so-called M or midmyocardial cells located at the terminal ends of the ventricular bundle branches and in the middle of the ventricular walls, respectively, have the longest action potential and therefore serve as physiological "gates" preventing the reentry and recycling of electric impulses in the ventricular myocardium.[20] The relatively long duration of M cell action potential is believed to be, in part, responsible for the development of U waves in the ECG. Purkinje fibers conduct the electric impulse at relatively rapid speeds (3 to 5 m/s) based on their size and electric properties (Fig. 4.10). Their distribution accounts for differences in the pattern of the ECG (ventricular depolarization) among species. Purkinje fibers have much longer action potentials and refractory periods than do ventricular muscle cells, which normally prevents reentry of the electric impulse and reactivation of the ventricles (see the Cardiac Arrhythmias section).

It is important to remember that—although the transmission of the electric impulse has, by analogy, been compared to dropping a pebble in water, leading to a concentric wave front, or, in the case of the heart, a concentric wave of depolarization—the conduction of the electric impulse in the heart ultimately depends on uniform (isotropic) cell-to-cell resistive and capacitative (passive) membrane properties that are largely determined by low-resistance gap or nexus junctions between cells and the spatial variation in myocardial cell refractoriness.[25-27] The configuration and magnitude of the T wave vary considerably among species and are influenced by changes in heart rate, blood temperature, and the extracellular potassium concentration. Hyperkalemia, for example, produces an increase in membrane conductance to potassium. This shortens repolarization and produces T waves that are of large magnitude, generally spiked or pointed, and of short duration (short QT interval).

The interval beginning immediately after the S wave of the QRS complex (J point) and preceding the T wave is referred to as the *ST* or *ST segment* and is important clinically. Elevation or depression of the ST segment (±0.2 mV or greater) from the isoelectric line is usually an indication of myocardial hypoxia or ischemia, low cardiac output, anemia, pericarditis, or cardiac contusion, and suggests the potential for arrhythmia development. Rarely, U waves can be distinguished immediately following the completion of the T wave and are believed to represent repolarization of M cells and possible Purkinje cells.[20] Like Ta waves, U waves are more frequently observed in larger species (horses and cattle) during electrolyte imbalances (hypokalemia or hypocalcemia) or drug therapy (quinidine or digitalis) (Fig. 4.10).

In summary, the cardiac cell membrane possesses both active (ion movement) and passive (resistive and capacitive) properties that determine the heart's excitability, automaticity, rhythmicity, refractoriness, and ability to conduct an electric impulse. Anesthetic drugs, via their effects on both the active properties (e.g., lidocaine, a sodium-channel blocker; barbiturates and inhalants suppress calcium currents) and passive properties (e.g., volatile inhalant anesthetics change membrane fluidity and depress gap junctions) of the heart, can produce significant alterations in cardiac excitability and conduction of the electric impulse, ultimately predisposing patients to cardiac arrhythmias and mechanical contraction abnormalities.[28-33]

Excitation-Contraction Coupling

Excitation-contraction coupling refers to the process wherein electric activation of the heart is transformed to muscle contraction. The process begins with the cardiac action potential and depolarization, and ends with the interaction of the contractile proteins in the individual sarcomeres. The normal extracellular calcium-ion concentration is 10^{-3} M compared to an intracellular calcium-ion concentration of 10^{-7} M. The electric activation of the sarcolemma and transverse tubule (T tubule) membranes by the cardiac action potential causes an influx of a small quantity of calcium ions during phase 2 of the cardiac action potential, triggering the release of a much greater quantity of calcium (calcium-induced calcium release) from calsequestrin-bound calcium sources in the sarcoplasmic reticulum. Calcium-induced calcium release raises the intracellular calcium concentration from 10^{-7} to 10^{-5} M and causes cellular contraction (Fig. 4.11). The importance of calcium influx during phase 2 of the action potential in the contractile process of cardiac muscle compared to other muscles (skeletal and smooth) cannot be overemphasized, because cardiac contraction is more dependent on and responds instantaneously to changes in the extracellular calcium concentration. Most calcium ions entering the cardiac cell do so through voltage-dependent calcium channels, although some calcium ions enter via the calcium-sodium exchange reaction.[34] Calcium channels are located throughout the T-tubule system, which penetrates deep into the cell interior. The T tubules abut large terminal cisternae, which are the terminal portion of a diffuse intracellular longitudinal tubular system: the sarcoplasmic reticulum. Voltage-dependent calcium channels are of two types (Table 4.1): a slow, long-lasting (L type) channel that is opened by complete cellular depolarization, and a fast but transient (T type) channel that is activated earlier than L-type channels and at more negative potentials (Fig. 4.9). The exact mechanism whereby the calcium channels (both L type and T type) of the T tubules communicate with the calcium-release channels of the sarcoplasmic reticulum remains unresolved. It is generally accepted that the majority of calcium entering the cardiac cell during each action potential does so through the L-type channel, also termed the *dihydropyridine* (DHP) *receptor* because of its sensitivity to specific types of calcium antagonists (verapamil, diltiazem, and nifedipine-like compounds).[35] Whether or not the amount of calcium passing through the DHP receptor (L-type channel) is essential for initiating the series of events leading to cellular contraction, however, remains controversial, since it is known that the rate of change of intracellular calcium concentration is the most effective activator of intracellular calcium release from the sarcoplasmic reticulum. This latter observation suggests that the rapid T-type channels may be important in the excitation-contraction process. T-type channels activate at more negative potentials than L-type channels and are insensitive to sodium-channel blockers (e.g., lidocaine or tetrodotoxin) and calcium-antagonist drugs.[34] Taken together, these observations suggest that T-type channels account for the early phase of calcium-channel opening and may be important in initiating intracellular calcium release and electric depolarization of less polarized tissues, such as the sinoatrial and atrioventricular nodes.[21,22] The L-type (DHP receptor) channels are more prevalent in atrial and ventricular muscle cells than are T-type channels, open at less negative potentials, and may account for the latter phases of calcium-channel opening.[34] Both channels, however, are physio-

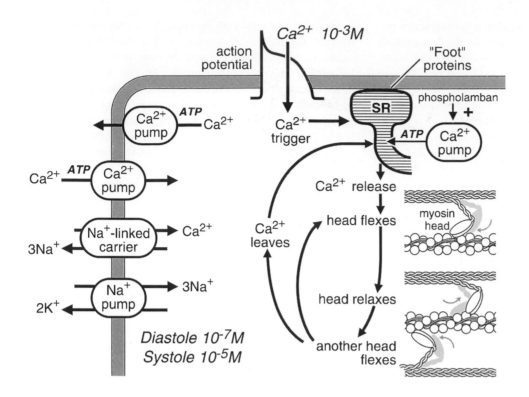

Fig. 4.11. Calcium can enter the cardiac cell during the cardiac action potential (slow response), via a calcium channel or in exchange for intracellular sodium. Increases in intracellular calcium trigger the release of calcium from the sarcoplasmic reticulum (SR) by a process termed *calcium-induced calcium release*. Increases in intracellular calcium (10^{-7} to 10^{-5} M) in the vicinity of the contractile proteins cause the myosin heads to flex, resulting in sarcomere shortening. The use of adenosine triphosphate (ATP) and formation of adenosine diphosphate and inorganic phosphate, in combination with reuptake of calcium by the SR, cause the myosin head to relax. Phospholamban modulates the pump responsible for the reuptake of calcium into the SR.

logically linked via specialized proteins termed *feet*, which are bridging or spanning proteins connecting them to the calcium-release mechanism in the sarcoplasmic reticulum. The foot proteins are a part of a high molecular weight protein complex in the sarcoplasmic reticulum, termed the *ryanodine receptor* because of its affinity for the insecticide ryanodine.[35] Low concentrations of ryanodine enhance calcium release, whereas large concentrations inhibit calcium release from the sarcoplasmic reticulum.

To summarize, the large extracellular (10^{-3} M) to intracellular (10^{-7} M) calcium-ion gradient facilitates the transsarcolemmal flux of calcium ions through calcium channels (T type and primarily L type) during the depolarization. The L-type channel can be blocked by DHP drugs and is therefore called a *DHP receptor*. The increase in intracellular calcium triggers the release of calcium from specialized calcium channels (ryanodine receptors in the sarcoplasmic reticulum), causing an increase in intracellular calcium-ion concentration (10^{-5} M), which causes myocardial cellular contraction.

Contraction and Relaxation

Contraction

Cardiac myocytes are composed of contractile units termed *sarcomeres*, which contain thick (myosin) and thin (actin) contractile proteins, regulatory proteins (troponin and tropomyosin), and various structural proteins. The thick myosin filaments are composed of approximately 300 molecules, each ending in a bilobed head. Half (150) of the myosin bilobed heads are located at each end of the sarcomere and project from the thick filament toward the thin filaments (crossbridges). The thin filaments are attached at one end to structural proteins (Z line) that separate each sar-

comere. Each thin filament contains two helical strands of actin intertwined with tropomyosin, which has periodic troponin complexes (Fig. 4.12). Increases in intracellular calcium initiated during phase 2 of the cardiac action potential and amplified by subsequent calcium-induced calcium release serve as the catalyst for actin-myosin interaction and sarcomere shortening. More specifically, calcium ions bind to the regulatory protein troponin C (C for calcium), which removes the inhibitory function of troponin I (I for inhibitor) on the chemical interaction between actin and myosin. Transformation of chemical energy into sarcomere shortening and mechanical work centers on adenosine triphosphate (ATP) hydrolysis by myosin ATPase. Hydrolysis of ATP to adenosine diphosphate (ADP) with the release of inorganic phosphate (P_i) produces a strong attachment between actin and myosin and a conformational change in the bilobed myosin head that causes the head to flex and the actin filaments to move centrally, resulting in sarcomere shortening and/or tension (Fig. 4.12). Increases in intracellular calcium facilitate this chemical process by increasing myosin ATPase activity. Therefore, by combining with troponin C and increasing intracellular myosin ATPase activity, calcium serves as the principal factor in determining the rate at which crossbridges attach and detach. The rate of crossbridge interaction is the basis for the force-velocity relationship in isolated tissue experiments studying cardiac muscle contractile activity (Fig. 4.13). The rate of crossbridge attachment determines the velocity of sarcomere shortening and has been termed *cardiac contractility*. Furthermore, by increasing the number of interacting crossbridges, intracellular calcium increases the maximum force attainable. Clinically, the rate of pressure change (*dP/dt*) and the rate of force development

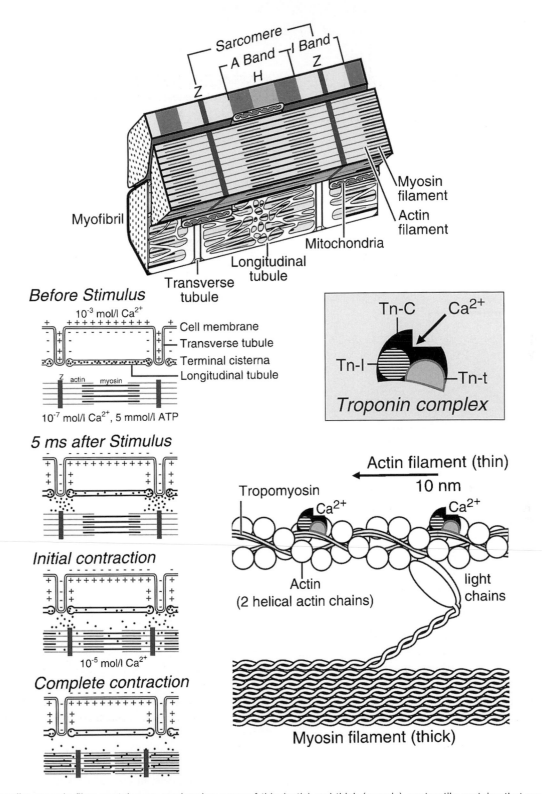

Fig. 4.12. A cardiac muscle fiber contains an overlapping array of thin (actin) and thick (myosin) contractile proteins that produces various bands (A, H, I, and Z) within each sarcomere when viewed microscopically. Note that both the transverse tubule (T tubule) and longitudinal tubule systems facilitate the presence of relatively large amounts of extracellular calcium (10^{-3} M) in the vicinity of the contractile proteins **(top)**. Membrane depolarization initiates calcium entry into the cardiac cell, contractile protein interaction, and sarcomere shortening **(left)**. More specifically, the binding of calcium with troponin C (Tn-C) removes the inhibitory function of troponin I (Tn-I) on actin-myosin interaction. Troponin t (Tn-t) links the troponin complex to tropomyosin **(right)**.

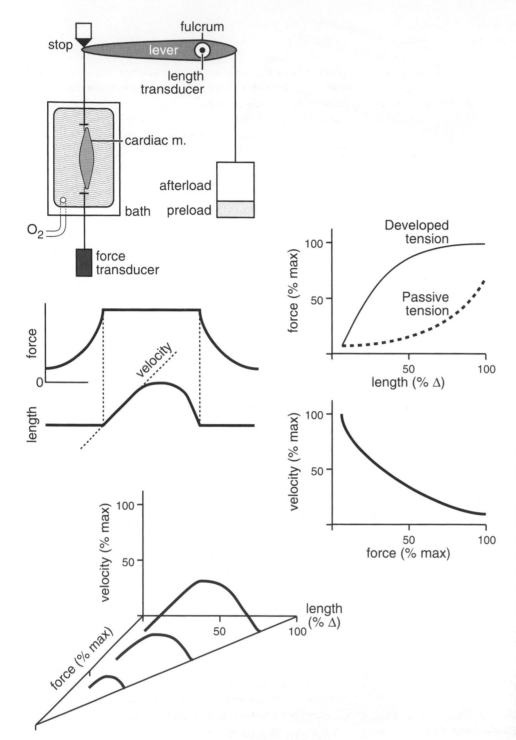

Fig. 4.13. The relationship between force development, velocity of muscle fiber shortening, and muscle length in an isolated cardiac muscle experiment. Within physiological limits, force and velocity increase as muscle length increases (Frank-Starling effect), and velocity decreases as developed force increases. Isolated muscle experiments are used to determine the direct effects of drugs upon cardiac mechanics without neurohumoral influences. Although preload is frequently equated to ventricular filling pressure and afterload is clinically thought of in terms of arterial blood pressure, the transfer of experimental data obtained from isolated muscle experiments to intact animals must be done knowledgeably and cautiously.

(dF/dt) in intact animals have been used as indirect, albeit crude, measures of cardiac contractility.[36,37]

Optimal sarcomere length for actin-myosin interaction is approximately 2.2 microns. Lengths shorter or greater than this were once thought to decrease the force of cardiac contraction by theoretically decreasing the number of available myosin heads for interaction with actin.[36] The concept of optimal sarcomere length relative to the velocity of sarcomere shortening serves as the explanation for the *Frank-Starling law of the heart*, which predicts an increase in contractile force when sarcomeres are stretched (increased ventricular volume) to their optimal length (Fig. 4.13). It is unlikely, however, that this explanation is totally correct, since sarcomeres rarely change in length (or only minimally so) when loaded, even during dilated forms of heart failure.[35] The more accepted and probable explanation for Starling's law of the heart is that sarcomere loading increases troponin-C affinity for calcium, leading to increased activation of the myofilament and sarcomere shortening without increases in sarcomere length or additional increases in intracellular calcium.[37] Many intravenous anesthetic drugs (e.g., barbiturates, ketamine, and propofol), and in particular the inhalation anesthetics, are known to decrease cardiac contractility by decreasing calcium influx through L-type channels, decreasing calcium release from the sarcoplasmic reticulum and decreasing troponin-C sensitivity to calcium.[38–46] This has led to the relatively routine use of positive inotropes (e.g., dopamine and dobutamine) to support cardiac contractile force and vascular tone in high-risk patients in order to increase cardiac output and arterial blood pressure.

Relaxation

Decreased interaction between actin and myosin filaments signals the beginning of the actin-myosin uncoupling process and myocardial relaxation, and is directly related to a decrease in intracellular calcium-ion concentration. Three principal mechanisms are important in reducing intracellular calcium-ion concentration and the subsequent decrease in cardiac contractile force. The depolarization-triggered increases in intracellular calcium increase the activity of the calcium regulatory protein calmodulin. Calmodulin serves as an intracellular calcium sensor and, when activated (calmodulin-calcium complex), stimulates the active extrusion of calcium by pumps in the sarcolemma, increases the activity of a phospholamban-modulated calcium pump (increasing calcium uptake by the sarcoplasmic reticulum), and enhances the activity of the sodium-calcium exchanger.[37] Notably, halothane (and other inhalants), ischemia, catecholamines, and acidosis interfere with the reuptake of calcium by the sarcoplasmic reticulum, thereby interfering with the relaxation process and ultimately leading to intracellular calcium depletion.[43,44] The calmodulin-calcium complex also inhibits the release of calcium from the sarcoplasmic reticulum. Mitochondrial uptake of calcium ion only minimally buffers increases in intracellular calcium concentration (Fig. 4.11). From this series of events, it is clear that increases in intracellular calcium first enhance (through the calcium-induced calcium-release mechanism) and then decrease (through the formation of the calmodulin-calcium complex and related mechanisms) the concentration of intracellular calcium, leading to cyclic sarcomere shortening and lengthening and ultimately myocardial contraction (systole), relaxation, and rest (diastole) before the next electric event triggers the mechanical process to repeat itself (Fig. 4.11).

The Cardiac Cycle and Pressure-Volume Loop

Historically, the cardiac cycle has been used as a diagrammatic attempt to describe the electric (ECG), mechanical (pressure, volume, and flow), and acoustic (heart sound) events associated with cardiac contraction and relaxation as a function of time (Fig. 4.14A). Just as important (but not as descriptive) as the time-varying cardiac cycle is the time-independent representation of the cardiac cycle: the ventricular pressure-volume loop (Fig. 4.14B). The advantage of the pressure-volume loop compared to the cardiac cycle is its ability to be used to assess load-independent indices of ventricular systolic and diastolic performance, ventricular vascular interaction (coupling), and myocardial energetics. Changes in the pressure-volume loop can also be used

to illustrate and quantitate the determinants of changes in cardiac function: preload, afterload, and cardiac contractility.[5,7,15,36] The various qualitative components of the cardiac cycle and pressure-volume loop are essentially identical for both the right and left ventricles, although the sequence of electric activation and the pressure changes is different.

Because electric activity precedes mechanical activity, the P wave of the surface ECG is a reasonable starting point to begin a description of the cardiac cycle (Fig. 4.14A). Electric activation of the atria produces the P wave of the ECG and causes almost simultaneous contraction of the atria. Atrial contraction increases intra-atrial pressure, producing the "a" wave of the atrial pressure curve. The atria (both right and left) normally function as blood reservoirs and conduits for blood transfer and, upon contraction, prime the ventricles by contributing approximately 10% to 30% (more at faster heart rates) of the blood volume that fills the ventricles. The atrial contribution to ventricular filling is frequently referred to as the *atrial kick*. The atrial kick brings the atrioventricular valves into relatively close apposition prior to ventricular contraction and is responsible for the fourth heart sound (S_4). Ventricular contraction is signaled by the R wave of the ECG and begins after a variable delay (PR interval) during which the electric impulse traverses the atrioventricular node and Purkinje network. Once the ventricular pressure increases to a value greater than that in the atrium, the atrioventricular valves close, actually bulging into their respective atria and giving rise to the "c" wave of the atrial pressure curve. The atrioventricular valves are prevented from completely prolapsing into the atrial chambers by chordae tendineae. The sudden development of tension in the contracting myocardium and tensing of the chordae tendineae coincident with atrioventricular valve closure are responsible for the first heart sound (S_1). The rapid increase in ventricular pressure while both the atrioventricular (mitral and tricuspid) and semilunar (aortic and pulmonic) valves are closed is termed *isovolumic contraction* because the volume of the ventricle remains constant (Fig. 4.14A and B). Once ventricular pressure exceeds that in the aorta or pulmonary artery, the semilunar valves open and ejection begins (Fig. 4.14A). The ejection phase of the cardiac cycle is characterized by a slowing of the increase in ventricular pressure after the semilunar valves open and an abrupt decrease in ventricular volume. These changes coincide with a large increase in aortic flow velocity and a decrease in the venous pressure curve as the atrioventricular valves are drawn toward the apex of the heart. Ventricular pressure exceeds aortic pressure during the first one-third of ventricular ejection (rapid ejection period), reaches equilibrium with aortic pressure, and thereafter, because of the onset of ventricular relaxation, declines more rapidly than aortic pressure. Blood continues to be ejected from the ventricle until the semilunar valves close. Closure of the semilunar valves marks the end of ventricular systole (by most definitions) and is associated with the development of the second heart sound (S_2). The second heart sound is composed of both aortic (A_2) and pulmonic (P_2) components and is frequently split (10 to 15 ms) during slow heart rates and in larger species (horses and cattle).[47] Rarely is the volume of blood ejected (stroke volume [SV]) by the normal

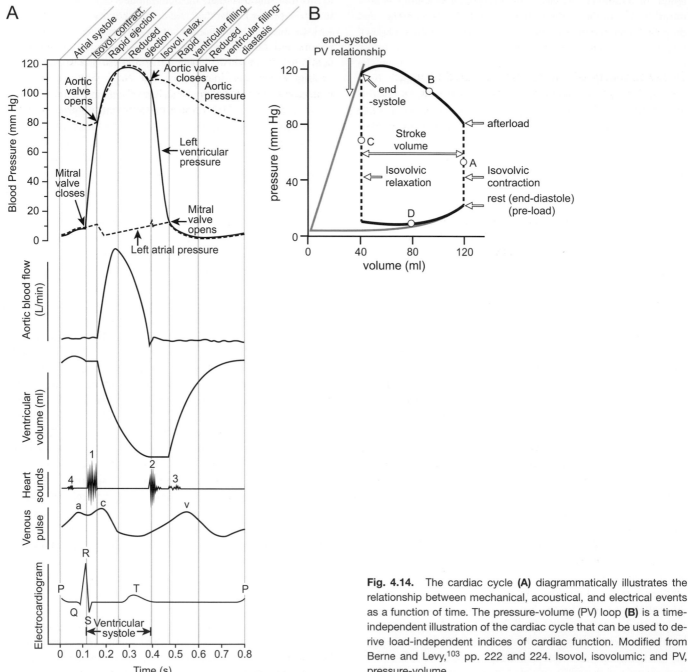

Fig. 4.14. The cardiac cycle **(A)** diagrammatically illustrates the relationship between mechanical, acoustical, and electrical events as a function of time. The pressure-volume (PV) loop **(B)** is a time-independent illustration of the cardiac cycle that can be used to derive load-independent indices of cardiac function. Modified from Berne and Levy,[103] pp. 222 and 224. Isovol, isovolumic; and PV, pressure-volume.

ventricle greater than 55% to 60% (ejection fraction [EF]) of its total volume.

The period between closure of the semilunar valves and opening of the atrioventricular valves is termed *isovolumic relaxation* and marks the beginning of ventricular relaxation (Fig. 4.14A and B). Isovolumic relaxation is characterized by a rapid decrease in ventricular pressure and no change in ventricular volume, and coincides with the V wave of the atrial pressure curve (Fig. 4.14A). Once ventricular pressure falls below atrial pressure, the atrioventricular valves open, initiating the phase of rapid ventricular filling (possibly facilitated by ventricular suction) and

producing the third heart sound (S_3). The third heart sound is believed to be caused by vibrations when the ventricular walls reach their elastic limit during ventricular filling, is relatively easily heard in larger species (horses and cattle), and gives rise to the characteristic ventricular gallop in dogs and cats with dilated forms of cardiac disease and increases in left atrial pressure.[48] Ventricular filling proceeds more gradually after the initial rapid filling phase, whereas ventricular pressure and volume increase nonlinearly during late diastole (Fig. 4.14B). The slope of the pressure-volume curve (*dP/dV*) during ventricular filling is an index of ventricular stiffness, and its inverse (*dV/dP*) is used to assess ventricular compliance.[49] The slow middiastolic ventricular-filling phase continues as blood returns to the atria from the systemic and pulmonary circulations until the cardiac cycle is reinitiated by the next electric impulse.[50]

Determinants of Performance and Output

The cardiac cycle and pressure-volume loop provide a picture of the temporal hemodynamic events that occur during cardiac contraction and relaxation. Clinically, M-mode echocardiography and color-flow Doppler echocardiography are used to assess ventricular function. These techniques provide a dynamic temporal representation of cardiac function and, when coupled with hemodynamic computer software analysis systems, a pictorial and quantitative assessment of cardiac performance (Fig. 4.15A to C). The oxygen requirements of tissues are met by the continuous adjustment of cardiac output (CO), which is the product of heart rate (HR) and stroke volume (SV):

$$CO = HR \times SV$$

Decreases in ventricular filling time and vascular autoregulatory effects limit cardiac output at faster heart rates.[7] Normal left ventricular ejection velocity is between 1.0 and 1.5 m/s. Many injectable anesthetics (barbiturates and propofol) and inhalant anesthetics (halothane, isoflurane, and sevoflurane) decrease ejection velocity and cardiac output. Stroke volume is the amount of blood ejected from the ventricle during contraction and therefore represents the difference between the end-diastolic and end-systolic ventricular volumes (SV = EDV − ESV [Fig. 4.14B]). Traditionally, stroke volume has been considered to be primarily determined by one intrinsic property, cardiac contractility, and two vascular coupling factors, preload and afterload.[15] The refinement and development of more descriptive methods for the assessment of cardiac function, however, have led to the consideration of relaxation (lusitropic) effects on stroke volume.[50,51] Lusitropic (compliance = 1/stiffness) properties are those that are responsible for ventricular chamber stiffness (dP/dV) or its inverse, compliance (dV/dP). Finally, ventricular wall motion abnormalities caused by ischemia, cardiac arrhythmias, myocardial inflammation, and space-occupying lesions (tumors or pericardial effusion) may influence stroke volume. It should be remembered that changes in preload, afterload, or myocardial contractile (inotropic) and relaxant (lusitropic) properties can influence one another and therefore influence stroke volume. These factors in turn are all influenced by heart rate, leading to a complex interplay of variables that collectively determine cardiac output (Fig. 4.16).[5,7,8]

The terms *preload* and *afterload*, described earlier in this section as two determinants of cardiac output, originated from isolated muscle experiments in which preload represented the original load, length, or stretch placed on the muscle prior to its stimulation and contraction, and afterload represented the force or tension developed before the ventricle ejects. Isolated cardiac muscle studies continue to be essential for understanding and describing cardiac muscle physiology, metabolism, and muscle responses to various perturbations (hypoxia, ischemia, and drugs), and are usually presented as three-dimensional plots of force, velocity, and length (Fig. 4.13). Cardiac function in intact animals is unlike isolated cardiac muscle, however, because ventricular performance is determined by intrinsic and vascular coupling factors and modulated by neurohumoral influences, the autonomic nervous system, pericardial and intrathoracic constraints, ventricular-vascular interaction, and atrial contraction.[13,52,53] Regardless, the terms *preload* and *afterload* remain popular jargon when describing ventricular performance in intact animals.

Preload

Preload in intact animals is usually explained in terms of the Frank-Starling relationship or as heterometric autoregulation: increases in myocardial fiber length (ventricular volume) (Figs. 4.16 and 4.17) increase the force of cardiac contraction and cardiac output.[8,15] Whether or not individual sarcomeres actually increase in length (stretch) with increases in ventricular volume is controversial (see the Contraction and Relaxation section); more likely, the myofilaments develop an increased sensitivity to calcium, resulting in an increase in contractile force.[35] Regardless of individual sarcomere length changes, the Frank-Starling relationship serves as an important compensatory mechanism for maintaining stroke volume when ventricular contractility and afterload are acutely changed. Because of the difficulty in accurately determining ventricular volume in the clinical setting, ventricular diameter, ventricular end-diastolic pressure, pulmonary capillary wedge pressure, and occasionally mean atrial pressure are used as estimates of preload.[50] The substitution of pressure for volume, although common, must be done with the understanding that there are many instances (open-chest procedures and stiff or noncompliant hearts) when pressure does not accurately represent changes in ventricular volume and therefore is not an accurate index of preload.

Afterload

The term *afterload* is used throughout the basic and clinical cardiology literature to describe the force opposing ventricular ejection.[7,15] One major reason for the great interest in this physiological determinant of cardiac function is its inverse relationship with stroke volume and its direct correlation with myocardial oxygen consumption (Fig. 4.16).[15,54] Although conceptually straightforward, clinical descriptions and use of the term *afterload* have suffered from an incomplete understanding of what the term actually represents. Afterload in isolated tissues is the force generated *after* the preload in order for the muscle to shorten. The total load in isolated muscle experiments is therefore represented by the preload plus the afterload. In contrast to isolated muscle, afterload in intact animals changes continuously throughout ventricular ejection and is more accurately described by the tension (stress) developed in the left ventricular wall during ejection or as the arterial input impedance (Z_i).[55] Ventricular wall stress or tension has traditionally been estimated from the Laplace relationship:

$$tension\ (T) = Pr/2h$$

It is noteworthy that using this assessment of ventricular afterload assumes a spherical ventricular geometry. A much more ac-

A. M-mode Echocardiography

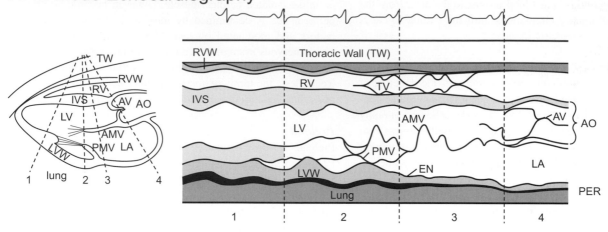

B. Pulsed-Wave Doppler Echocardiography

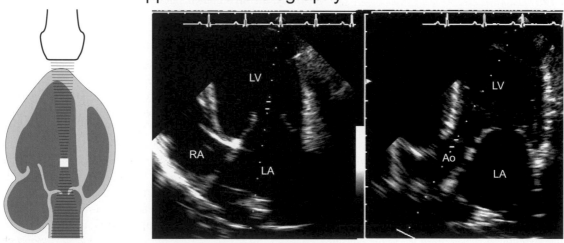

C. LVOT (Aortic) Velocity Profile

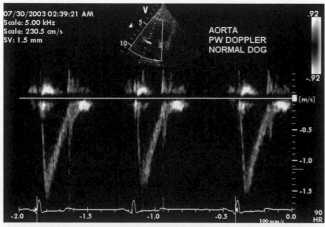

Fig. 4.15. M-mode **(A)** and color-flow Doppler echocardiography **(B and C)** are two popular clinical methods of assessing cardiac function in animals.

curate, yet technically more difficult, method for assessing afterload in intact animals is to measure ventricular-vascular coupling.[55] Arterial input impedance is an expression of the arterial system's response to pulsatile blood flow and is a function of arterial pressure, arterial wall elasticity, vessel dimensions down to

the point where pulsations are attenuated, and blood viscosity (see the section on Hemorrheology: Impedance). As such, arterial input impedance incorporates time-varying resistance components (pressure and flow) and reactance components (intrinsic vessel wall characteristics). The measurement of arterial input

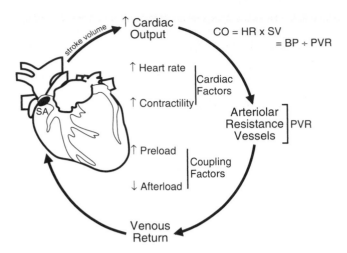

Fig. 4.16. Cardiac output is equal to heart rate (HR) times stroke volume (SV), or arterial blood pressure (BP) divided by peripheral vascular resistance (PVR). Increases in heart rate, cardiac contractility, and preload, and decreases in afterload can all increase cardiac output. Preload and afterload are considered to be coupling factors because they depend on vascular resistance, capacitance, and compliance.

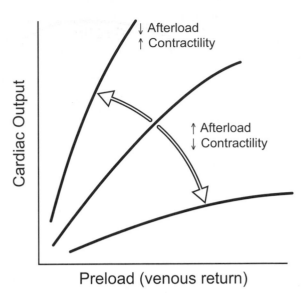

Fig. 4.17. Cardiac output increases as preload increases (Frank-Starling effect). The steepness of the Frank-Starling curve is also affected by changes in cardiac contractility and afterload.

impedance requires the simultaneous and instantaneous measurement of aortic root pressure and flow.[10,55] Both waveforms are subjected to a Fourier transformation from which a series of sine waves and frequencies are derived. The amplitude ratios of the pressure-flow components at each frequency are calculated and plotted versus frequency as impedance moduli. Any phase shift between pressure and flow (pressure leading flow or vice versa) occurring during the ejection phase is also plotted at each frequency (Fig. 4.6). From this relationship, the characteristic impedance (Z_o) can be determined by averaging the impedance moduli at high frequencies. The characteristic impedance is the pressure-flow relationship when pressure and flow waves are not influenced by wave reflection (it approximates input impedance during maximal vasodilation). Characteristic impedance is approximately 5% of the total arterial resistance and is generally an exquisitely sensitive indicator of vessel wall elasticity or compliance. The impedance modulus at zero frequency (nonpulsatile flow) is equivalent to vascular resistance (R) and is usually described as total peripheral resistance (TPR) or systemic vascular resistance (SVR). The SVR can be calculated (with appropriate values) by

$$SVR = 80 \times (MAP - CVP)/CO$$

where MAP is mean arterial pressure, CVP is central venous pressure, CO is cardiac output, and 80 is a conversion factor used to change measurements in L/min and mm Hg to dynes · s · cm^{-5}. Although much less accurate than the determination of impedance moduli, particularly when assessing the effects of progressive cardiac disease or drugs that change both cardiac and vascular properties simultaneously, the measurement of SVR is

used clinically as a measure of afterload and vascular tone because it is technically simple to obtain and intuitively easier to understand.

Inotropy

Cardiac contractility (inotropy) is the intrinsic ability of the heart to generate force and, as such, relates directly to physicochemical processes and the availability of intracellular calcium (see the section on Excitation-Contraction Coupling).[35,36] The term *homeometric autoregulation* is frequently applied to those factors other than muscle fiber length that influence the force of cardiac contraction.[7] Contractility is generally described in isolated muscle preparations by shifts of the force, velocity-length relationship (Fig. 4.13), or in intact animals by shifts in the ventricular function curve (e.g., shifts in the Frank-Starling relationship [Fig. 4.17]). A decrease in cardiac contractility is a key factor in heart failure in patients with cardiac disease or following the administration of potent negative inotropic drugs (e.g., anesthetics).[43,44,56–59]

Ideal indices of cardiac contractility should be independent of changes in heart rate, preload, afterload, and cardiac size—in other words, be load independent. Many indices of contractility have evolved in an attempt to develop a truly load-independent measure of cardiac contractile activity. These indices vary considerably in their load dependency, sensitivity, and specificity as measures of cardiac contractility, and generally fall into one of four broad categories: (1) isovolumic contraction phase indices, (2) ejection phase indices, (3) pressure-volume relationship indices, and (4) stress-strain relationship indices (Table 4.3).[49,59,60] Although many approaches for assessing cardiac contractility are

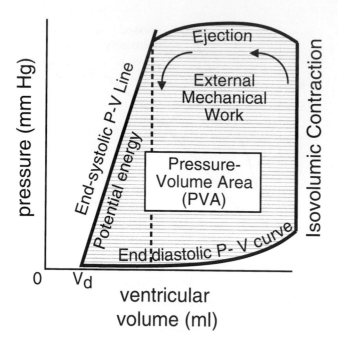

Fig. 4.18. The ventricular pressure-volume (P-V) loop and the end-systolic P-V line can be used to determine the pressure-volume area (PVA). The area within the pressure-volume loop (within the *dotted lines*) represents the external work done by the heart and is proportional to myocardial oxygen consumption. The *triangular area* between the end-systolic P-V line and isovolumic relaxation represents the end-systolic potential energy and is proportional to the oxygen consumed for basal metabolism.

Table 4.3. Hemodynamic indices of systolic and diastolic function

Systolic function
1. Isovolumic indices
   a. Echocardiographic assessment (M-mode, two-dimensional Doppler)
   b. dP/dt_{max}, dP/dt_{40}, and $dP/dt/V_{ed}$
   c. V_{max}
   d. Power; rate of charge of power
2. Ejection-phase indices
   a. Echocardiographic assessment (M-mode, two-dimensional Doppler)
   b. Cardiac output
   c. Ejection fraction, (EDV − ESV)/EDV
   d. Stroke work
   e. Maximum velocity of circumferential shortening
   f. Left ventricular ejection time
   g. Preejection period
3. Pressure-volume indices
   a. Echocardiographic assessment (M-mode, two-dimensional Doppler)
   b. E_{es} and E_{max}
   c. End-systolic pressure-volume ratios
   d. T_{max} (time to E_{max})
4. Stress-strain indices
   a. Elastic stiffness (stress/strain)
   b. End-systolic stress-volume ratio

Diastolic function
1. Isovolumic relaxation indices (pressure derived)
   a. Echocardiographic assessment (M-mode, two-dimensional Doppler)
   b. dP/dt_{min}
   c. Time constant of left ventricular pressure fall (T)
   d. Relaxation time
   e. $-dT/dt$ (tension fall)
2. Diastolic filling indices
   a. dP/dV
   b. Peak filling rate (dV/dt_{max})
   c. Chamber stiffness (dP/dV vs. P)
3. End-diastolic indices
   a. End-diastolic pressure
   b. End-diastolic P/V ratio
4. Interval-derived indices
   a. Echocardiographic assessment (M-mode, two-dimensional Doppler)
   b. Time to $-dP/dt_{min}$; time to 50% $-dP/dt_{min}$
   c. Diastolic filling time
   d. Isovolumic relaxation period
   e. Time from minimal left ventricular dimension to mitral valve opening

useful experimentally and clinically, only the isovolumic phase indices (because of their ease of measurement), the pressure-volume relationship indices (because of their load independence), and the ejection phase index (preload recruitable stroke work) have gained acceptance.[59] Additionally, the measurement of the pressure-volume relationship can be used to assess myocardial energetics.[15,49] This is because the amount of oxygen consumed by the heart for mechanical work is proportional to the area within the pressure-volume loop, while the oxygen consumed for basal metabolism is proportional to the area enclosed by the end-systolic pressure-volume relationship, the diastolic pressure-volume curve, and the isovolumic relaxation phase of the pressure-volume loop (Fig. 4.18).

Lusitropy

A description of the relaxation phases following cardiac contraction is often omitted from textbooks of cardiovascular physiology, but is fundamentally important to an understanding of cardiac performance.[50] Two reasons for the lack of attention are the inability to agree on a definition of when diastole begins and disagreement over acceptable indices for the assessment of the various phases of diastole. The most popular and clinically relevant definition of diastole states that relaxation begins with the closure of the aortic valve, which is heralded by the second heart sound (S_2 [Fig. 4.14A]).[50,51] Diastole is thereafter divided into four phases: (1) isovolumic relaxation, (2) early rapid ventricular

filling, (3) slow ventricular filling (diastasis), and (4) atrial systole (during sinus rhythm). Mechanical factors, loading factors, inotropic activity, heart rate, and asynchronicity (patterns of relaxation) are the major determinants of lusitropy. Factors and interventions that specifically alter the relationship of ventricular end-diastolic volume versus pressure, called lusitropic factors,

Table 4.4. Common hemodynamic effects of anesthetic drugs in animals

Drug	Heart Rate	Cardiac Output	Contractility	Blood Pressure	Right Atrial Pressure	Myocardial Oxygen Consumption
Anticholinergics	↑	↑	↑	NC or ↑	↓	↑
Phenothiazines	↑	↑	↓	↓	↓	NC or ↑
Butyrophenones	↑	NC or ↑	↓	Slight ↓	↓	NC or ↑
Benzodiazepines	NC	NC	NC	NC	NC	↓
α_2-Adrenergic agonists	↓	↓	NC or ↓	Initial ↑then↓	↑	↑
Opioids	↓	↓	NC or ↓	NC or ↓	NC	NC
Barbiturates	↑	↓	↓	↓	↓	NC or ↑
Propofol	NC or ↑	↓	↓	↓	↓	NC or ↑
Etomidate	NC or ↑	NC or ↓	NC or ↓	NC or ↓	NC or ↓	NC or ↑
Dissociative drugs	↑	↑	↑ or ↓	↑	↓	↑
Inhalation anesthetics	↓	↓	↓	↓	↓	↓
Skeletal muscle relaxants						
1. Pancuronium	↑	↑	NC	↑	NC	↑
2. Atracurium	NC or ↑	NC	NC	May ↓ (histamine)	NC	NC
3. Vecuronium	NC	NC	NC	NC	NC	NC

↑, increase; ↓, decrease; NC, no change.

are of special interest because of their importance in determining ventricular compliance or stiffness. A partial list of methods used to quantitatively describe relaxation includes pressure, volume-derived, and interval indices (Table 4.3). All of these indices provide useful information, but must be carefully applied in order to properly analyze the appropriate phase of relaxation. Indices of isovolumetric relaxation (rate of ventricular pressure decline $[-dP/dt]$ and the time constant for relaxation) are useful for measuring the active phase of relaxation and reflect the dissociation of actin-myosin linkages because of reuptake of cytoplasmic calcium by the sarcoplasmic reticulum (Fig. 4.11). These indices are particularly influenced by myocardial systolic function, ventricular loading conditions (preload and afterload), and heart rate. Indices of diastasis or slow ventricular filling (chamber stiffness, $-dP/dV$, and myocardial stiffness) are used to determine the passive properties of diastolic function and are principally influenced by viscoelastic properties, ventricular interaction, coronary blood flow, and pericardial restraint.

Regardless of the care in picking an index to evaluate cardiac systolic or diastolic performance, it is clear that even greater thought must be given to the factors (determinants of performance) that influence the index. Drugs used as preanesthetic medication or for intravenous or inhalation anesthesia can produce profound effects on indices of cardiac performance and are often much more complex in their actions than originally surmised (Table 4.4).[50,56,61–63]

Ventricular-Vascular Coupling

The concept of ventricular-vascular coupling is not new, but is rarely discussed or adequately described by most textbooks.[14] The principal reason for inadequate treatment is the historical focus on pressure-derived measurements and the cardiac cycle, which stems from the relative ease with which pressure can be measured. Sphygmomanometry-based measurements and their derivations are undoubtedly important, but by themselves lead to an overly simplistic and often erroneous understanding of cardiovascular function. New technologies (M-mode and two-dimensional Doppler echocardiography) and theory have made it possible to expand our understanding of cardiac mechanical activity and begin to appreciate the relevance, dependence, and importance of both the venous and the arterial systems and their coupling to the heart (Fig. 4.15A to C).[5,52] The clinical relevance of this understanding is increasingly apparent from the new and improved theories of cardiovascular disease (congenital or acquired), myocardial metabolic disturbances (ischemia and hypoxia), and the mechanisms of drug effects (anesthetics, etc.) on the cardiovascular system. Indeed, the clinical application of the principles of ventricular-vascular coupling has resulted in new and improved therapies for cardiovascular disease.[13,16]

Ventricular-vascular coupling, as the name implies, concerns the interrelationship or coupling of the heart to the venous and arterial systems. Thus, loading conditions (preload and afterload) and vascular dynamics (resistive, reactance, and viscoelastic properties) ultimately influence ventricular performance and blood flow.[14,49] Coronary blood flow and myocardial perfusion are also important components of ventricular-vascular coupling because normal function and the viability of the heart depend on adequate myocardial perfusion, which occurs almost exclusively during diastole.

Vascular Function Curve

The modern concept of ventricular-vascular coupling has been popularized by Guyton, who used the vascular function curve, and more precisely the venous-return curve and cardiac (ventricular) function curve, to predict changes in cardiac output (Fig. 4.19A).[5] Guyton's ventricular-vascular coupling diagrams emphasize that the important independent variables in the determination of cardiac output are the sums of vascular resistances and capacitances and cardiac contractility. The venous-return curve describes an inverse relationship between venous return and cardiac output. The horizontal (abscissa) intercept of the venous-return curve or the venous pressure at zero cardiac output is the mean circulatory filling pressure, which is a function of venous capacitance and the total blood volume and has been directly correlated with survival from hemorrhagic and septic shock. Variations in the venous-return curve can be produced by altering venous resistance, capacitance, or blood volume (Fig. 4.19B). Equilibrium of the venous-return–ventricular function curve is reached when venous return at a given pressure is matched by the ability of the ventricle, when distended to the same pressure, to pump the venous return. Thus, an increase in venous pressure increases cardiac output during the next cardiac cycle, as defined by the ventricular function curve. Increases in cardiac output in turn transfer blood from the venous to the arterial circulation, thus decreasing venous pressure. This process continues in progressively decreasing steps until a new equilibrium for cardiac output and venous return is reached, realizing that only one equilibrium point for cardiac output and venous return exists. Similar rationalizations can be used for other perturbations: changes in blood volume, arterial resistance, and cardiac contractility.[8,52] It can be argued that this type of presentation of hemodynamics and cardiovascular function results in circular reasoning, since a change in cardiac output can be used to explain the change in venous return and vice versa. Indeed, since both venous return and cardiac output are equal to the flow around the circuit, the point that a given cardiac output is obtained is determined by a myriad of venous-return and ventricular function curves and their determinants (venous and arterial capacitance and resistance, blood volume, and cardiac contractility).[5,7,8]

Ventricular-Arterial Coupling

More recent evaluations of ventricular-vascular coupling have focused on the left ventricular pressure-volume relationship and the ejection of blood into the ascending aorta (ventricular-arterial coupling) (Fig. 4.20A).[13] This approach, first popularized and validated by Suga and Sunagawa in isolated and intact dog hearts, has been applied clinically using noninvasive (echocardiographic) techniques.[15,49,53,64] The power of this approach stems from its clinical applicability and the ability to derive a multitude of important indices for assessing cardiovascular function in intact animals.[49]

The inscription of the instantaneous pressure-volume loop enables the calculation of load-dependent and independent indices of cardiac contractility, myocardial oxygen requirements, and myocardial efficiency.[15] For example, the ratio of ventricular pressure to ventricular volume (dP/dV) varies throughout the cardiac cycle (time-varying elastance) and inscription of the pressure-volume loop. Acute reductions in preload are used to produce progressively smaller pressure-volume loops and construct

a straight line by connecting all of the end-systolic points. This line is known as the *end-systolic pressure-volume relationship*, the slope of which is the end-systolic ventricular elastance (E_{es}), a load-independent index directly proportional to ventricular contractility (Figs. 4.18 and 4.20A). The mechanical work (stroke work [SW]) performed by the heart is proportional to the pressure-volume area (PVA), which is linearly related to myocardial oxygen consumption (MVO_2), and which, when plotted against the end-diastolic volume, derives another sensitive and load-independent index of cardiac contractility termed *preload recruitable stroke work* (PRSW). Mechanical efficiency (ME) of the heart is the ratio of SW to MVO_2 and is derived by dividing SW by PVA (ME = SW/PVA).

The ejection of blood into the ascending aorta is governed by the same resistive and reactive (viscoelastic) properties that govern venous return. These arterial loading properties (afterload) influence stroke volume.[55] The difference between the end-diastolic and end-systolic volumes of the pressure-volume relationship is stroke volume, which, when plotted versus end-systolic pressure (P_{es}) during decreases in stroke volume, renders a line, the slope of which is the effective arterial elastance (E_a). In practice, E_a is generally approximated by the ratio of P_{es} to stroke volume ($P_{es}/SV = E_a$). This parameter is particularly powerful because it incorporates the principal elements of vascular load (afterload), including peripheral resistance, total vascular compliance, characteristic impedance (see the section on Determinants of Cardiac Performance and Cardiac Output), and alterations induced by heart-rate changes. It is noteworthy that the purely resistive components of vascular load are adequately accounted for by determining the steady-state or nonpulsatile parameter, total peripheral resistance, which accounts for approximately 90% of vascular load under normal conditions. The pulsatile or dynamic component of vascular load generally accounts for approximately 10% of vascular load under normal conditions, adds to the resistive component, and becomes increasingly important during cardiovascular disease, changes in blood volume, or following the administration of drugs (e.g., anesthetics) that affect the cardiovascular system.[49,57,58,60] Other methods for accurately analyzing arterial afterload have been described (see the section Determinants of Cardiac Performance and Cardiac Output).

Because both E_{es} and E_a have the measurement of P_{es} and ventricular volume in common, they can be plotted on a single graph to yield the "ideal" ventricular-arterial coupling point for any set of cardiovascular circumstances (Fig. 4.20B). Stated another way, if end-diastolic volume (preload), E_a, and E_{es} are known, stroke volume and therefore cardiac output (CO = SV × HR) can be predicted. Furthermore, this analysis predicts that SW should be maximized when this relationship is equal to 1 ($E_{es} = E_a$) and that maximal mechanical efficiency (ME) is attained when $E_a = E_{es}/2$, since ME = SW/PVA = $1/(1 + E_a/E_{es}/2)$.

The ideal ventricular-arterial coupling point in intact animals occurs when mean arterial pressure is adequate for organ flow (approximately 60 to 70 mm Hg) and, as stated earlier, systolic pressure is low while diastolic pressure is high (small pressure pulse). Low systolic pressure facilitates maximal ventricular

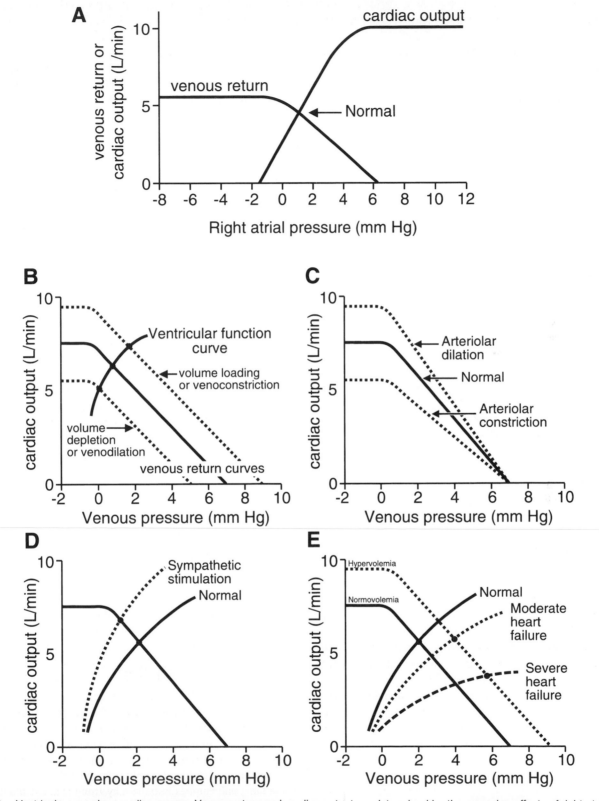

Fig. 4.19. Ventricular-vascular coupling curves. Venous return and cardiac output are determined by the opposing effects of right atrial pressure **(A)**. For example, increases in right atrial pressure increase cardiac output, but decrease venous return. Alterations in blood volume **(B)**, sympathetic tone **(C)**, vascular tone **(D)**, and cardiac function **(E)** produce predictable effects upon the coupling of venous return to cardiac output at a given venous pressure. Note that, during heart failure **(E)**, cardiac output is preserved at the expense of increases in venous pressure. Modified from Berne and Levy.[103]

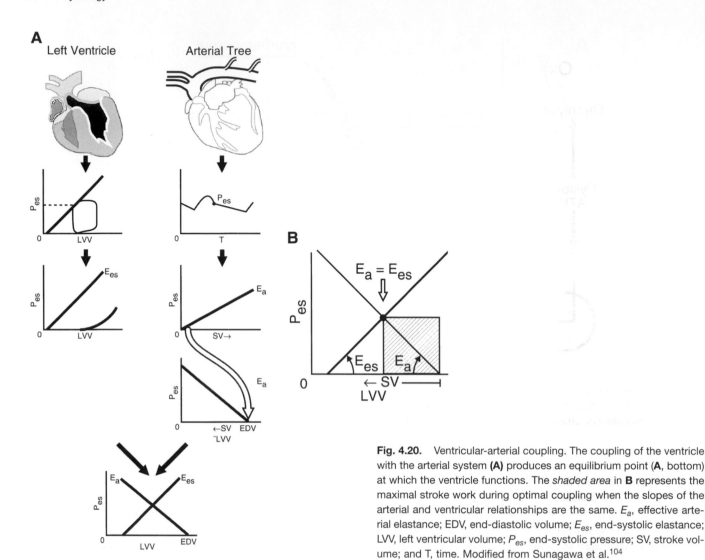

Fig. 4.20. Ventricular-arterial coupling. The coupling of the ventricle with the arterial system (**A**) produces an equilibrium point (**A**, bottom) at which the ventricle functions. The *shaded area* in **B** represents the maximal stroke work during optimal coupling when the slopes of the arterial and ventricular relationships are the same. E_a, effective arterial elastance; EDV, end-diastolic volume; E_{es}, end-systolic elastance; LVV, left ventricular volume; P_{es}, end-systolic pressure; SV, stroke volume; and T, time. Modified from Sunagawa et al.[104]

ejection and low oxygen demands by the myocardium, whereas high diastolic pressure ensures adequate coronary perfusion. Ideal ventricular arterial interaction is impaired by anything that decreases cardiac contractility (decreased E_{es}) or increases arterial stiffness (increased E_a). Increases in arterial stiffness increase pulse amplitude, increasing systolic pressure and thereby decreasing stroke volume for a given cardiac contractility while increasing MVO_2. Diastolic pressure usually falls, thereby reducing coronary blood flow and myocardial perfusion. Furthermore, alterations in the timing of pulse-wave reflection, principally initiated by increases in arteriolar tone, could augment systolic pressure and reduce diastolic pressure, exacerbating the situation.[10,55,65]

Cardiac Metabolism

The maintenance of normal cardiac activity depends on the metabolic pathways by which ATP is generated. Even a superficial description of these pathways is far beyond the scope and purpose of this chapter and is more appropriately described in texts specifically designed to discuss this subject.[54] Suffice it to say

that the heart generates ATP by two primary methods: glycolysis and oxidative phosphorylation. These processes are continually modified by the energy requirements of the cell and by neural and hormonal inputs. The ATP produced supplies energy for cardiac contraction, relaxation, and related activities (Fig. 4.21).

The Vascular System

The purpose of the vascular system (arteries, capillaries, and veins) is to transport and facilitate the exchange of a wide range of nutrients and waste products. Originating from the heart, the circulatory system consists of two separate circulations connected in series (Fig. 4.1). The pulmonary circulation receives the majority of its blood supply from the right ventricle, perfuses the lung, and empties into the left atrium. The systemic circulation receives its blood supply from the left ventricle, perfuses most of the body's organs and tissues, and empties into the right atrium. More specifically, the systemic circulation (like the pulmonary) undergoes repeated division into smaller and smaller parallel vascular beds that terminate in the arterioles (the smallest arteries), which further subdivide to form the capillary bed.[7]

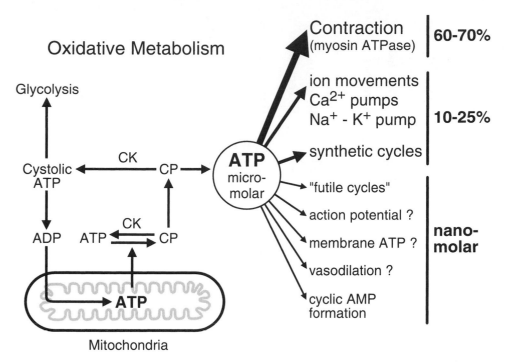

Fig. 4.21. Oxidative metabolism produces adenosine triphosphate (ATP), which supplies energy for cardiac contraction and other cellular activities. Note that over 60% of the ATP generated by oxidative metabolism is used for contraction. ADP, adenosine diphosphate; AMP, adenosine monophosphate; CK, creatine kinase; and CP, creatine phosphokinase.

During repeated division, the overall cross-sectional area of the circulation increases dramatically, reaching a maximum in the capillaries (Fig. 4.22).[1,66]

Structurally, all blood vessels contain an endothelial layer (tunica intima) on their inner surface that provides a smooth surface and prevents clotting. All but capillaries also contain varying proportions of elastic fibers, smooth muscle, and collagen (Fig. 4.23). These three tissue types comprise the tunica media, which is composed mostly of smooth muscle and elastic connective tissue, and the tunica externa (adventitia), which contains fibrous collagen fibers. The proportion of elastic connective tissue to smooth muscle determines the vessel's principal function (i.e., conduit, resistive, or capacitive). The amount of smooth muscle also determines the vessel's resting tone, myogenic basal tone (spontaneous contractions), and the amount of stress relaxation (delayed capacitance), and reverse stress relaxation exhibited by the vessel. Stress relaxation is characterized as a rapid initial increase in resting tone caused by an increase in vascular volume that declines gradually during the next several minutes. Pressure decreases because of smooth muscle myofilament rearrangement. Reverse stress relaxation is the reverse of this process.

Smooth Muscle Contraction

Vascular smooth muscle is considerably different from cardiac muscle, both structurally and functionally.[37] Vascular smooth muscle cells are small, 5 to 10 μm in diameter, and spindle shaped. They do not contain regular sarcomeric units or Z bands, or possess the same key regulatory proteins (absence of troponin

C and troponin N) as cardiac cells. Functionally, depolarization is not essential for initiation of muscle contraction in vascular smooth muscle. The contraction process is slow and tonic, is prolonged, and intracellular increases in cyclic adenosine monophosphate (cAMP) cause vascular smooth muscle cells and vessels to dilate, not contract. One thing that is similar between cardiac and vascular smooth muscle cells is that they both depend on increases in intracellular calcium for contraction.

A multitude of pathways are available by which vascular smooth muscle cells can increase intracellular calcium-ion concentration and contract, including calcium influx through voltage (slow calcium channels) and receptor-operated ion channels, calcium release from the sarcoplasmic reticulum by calcium (calcium-induced calcium release) or some other activator (inositol triphosphate [IP$_3$]), and reversal of the sodium-calcium exchange mechanism. Regardless of the mechanism responsible, increases in intracellular calcium serve as the second messenger for smooth muscle actin-myosin interaction. Once intracellular calcium concentration increases beyond a critical threshold, calcium ions combine with the ubiquitous calcium-binding protein calmodulin, forming a calcium-calmodulin complex, which in turn binds to myosin light-chain kinase and activates ATP-dependent phosphorylation of myosin, causing actin-myosin interaction (Fig. 4.24). The formation of the actin-myosin crossbridge in vascular smooth muscle (in contrast to cardiac muscle) produces a sustained tonic type of contraction. The slow-cycling or noncycling crossbridges formed in vascular smooth muscle are called *latchbridges*. Relaxation occurs when myosin light-

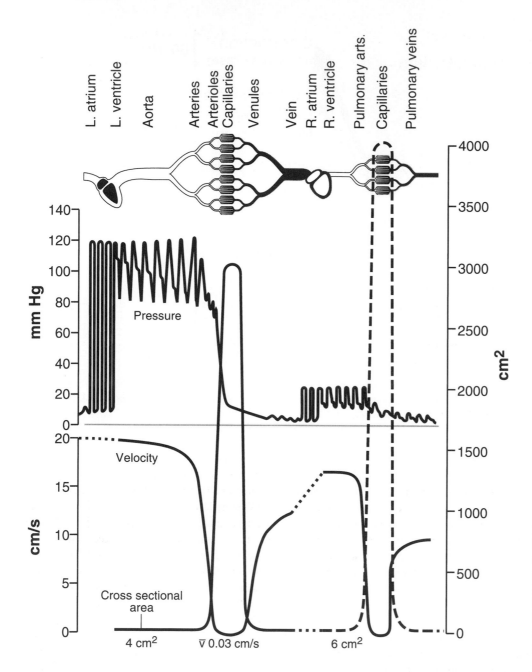

Fig. 4.22. The relationship between blood pressure, blood flow velocity, and cross-sectional area of the cardiovascular system. Note that, as blood approaches the capillaries, blood pressure and blood flow velocity decrease and cross-sectional area increases. v, average velocity. Modified from Witzleb,[68] p. 408.

chain kinase is dephosphorylated by the enzyme myosin light-chain phosphatase. The regulation of myosin light-chain phosphatase is poorly understood, but is probably affected by many drugs used to produce chemical restraint and anesthesia.[37,67] Other mechanisms that facilitate relaxation of vascular smooth muscle center around decreases in intracellular calcium concentration due to reuptake of calcium ion by the sarcoplasmic reticulum, exchange of intracellular calcium for extracellular sodium, stimulation of the calcium-ATPase calcium pump, and termination of calcium influx into the cell (Fig. 4.24). Increases in intracellular cAMP and cyclic guanosine monophosphate produce vasodilatory, not contractile, effects in vascular smooth muscle. Cyclic AMP inhibits myosin light-chain phosphorylation. The effects of cyclic guanosine monophosphate are incompletely understood, but it may produce an effect similar to cAMP or accelerate the ejection of calcium ions from vascular smooth muscle cells. Finally, vascular smooth muscle contraction can occur without an initial influx of extracellular calcium or the release of intracellular calcium.[37] α-Adrenoreceptor stimulation, for example, can act through a G protein to form diacylglycerol (DAG) and IP$_3$. IP$_3$ causes the release of calcium from the sarcoplasmic reticulum, initiating the contraction process. DAG can also activate a protein kinase, which may phosphorylate myosin light-chain kinase to initiate tonic contractions.

Vessel Types

From a purely functional standpoint, vessels can be categorized as primarily elastic Windkessel types or conduits (large arteries),

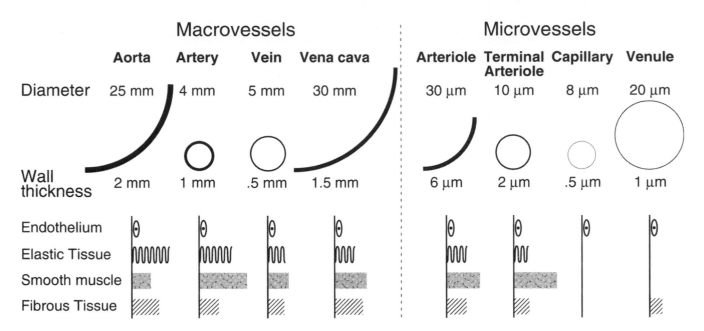

Fig. 4.23. The relative amounts of the various components (elastic, smooth muscle, and fibrous tissue) of macrovessels and microvessels are illustrated. Note the differences with changes in vessel diameter and between arteries and veins. Modified from Berne and Levy,[103] p. 195.

resistance vessels (small arteries), sphincter vessels (arterioles), exchange vessels (capillaries), capacitance vessels (venules and veins), and shunt vessels (arteriovenous anastomoses).[1,68]

Large Arteries

Large arteries near the heart and throughout the extremities are highly elastic tubes that serve as conduits through which blood is transported to the periphery. The elasticity of large arteries opposes the stretching effect that the blood pressure produces following ventricular contraction. The initial stretching of the aorta produced by ventricular ejection, for example, is opposed by the elastic tissue in the vessel walls, which returns the aorta and large arteries to their original dimension (Fig. 4.23). As was previously mentioned, this squeezing phenomena of large arteries is termed the *Windkessel effect* and helps to convert the discontinuous (cyclic or phasic) flow of arterial blood associated with ventricular pumping into a continuous, although somewhat nonuniform, flow to the peripheral arteries. The degree to which the larger arteries can be stretched depends on the ratio of elastic to collagen fibers. Systemic arteries are in general six to ten times less distensible than systemic veins. The pulmonary artery, by contrast, is about half as distensible as systemic or pulmonary veins (Fig. 4.25).[69]

Blood pressure in arteries (arterial pulse pressure and blood pressure), whether measured directly or indirectly, is frequently assessed during anesthesia. Arterial blood pressure measurement in particular is one of the fastest and most informative means of assessing cardiovascular function and, when done correctly and frequently, provides an accurate indication of drug effects, surgical events, and hemodynamic trends. The most important vascular determinant of arterial blood pressure is arteriolar tone, which can be modified by almost all drugs used to produce anesthesia.[5,7,68] The factors that determine arterial blood pressure are

heart rate, stroke volume, vascular resistance, arterial compliance, and blood volume. Blood volume is one of the major variables affecting the *mean circulatory pressure*, which is defined as the equilibrium pressure of the circulation when blood flow is zero. The mean circulatory filling pressure is approximately 7 mm Hg when blood volume is normal (90 mL/kg). Increases in mean circulatory filling pressure augment ventricular filling and cardiac output. From the mechanical analogue of Ohm's law ($E = IR$), we know that $P = QR$. This formula predicts that if either cardiac output (Q) or peripheral vascular resistance (R) increase either individually or together, so will arterial blood pressure. Arterial blood pressure is a key component in determining perfusion pressure (upstream minus downstream pressure) and the adequacy of tissue blood flow. Perfusion pressures greater than 60 mm Hg are generally thought to be adequate for perfusion of tissues. Structures like the heart (coronary circulation), lung (pulmonary circulation), kidneys (renal circulation), and the fetus (fetal circulation) contain special circulations where changes in perfusion pressure can have immediate effects on organ function. In the coronary circulation, for example, if perfusion pressure (determined by the difference between arterial diastolic and ventricular end-diastolic pressures) decreases, subendocardial ischemia develops.[7]

Clinically, arterial blood pressure is generally measured as mean arterial pressure. When mean arterial blood pressure cannot be directly assessed, it is estimated by this formula:

$$P_m = P_d + 1/3\ (P_s - P_d)$$

where P_m, P_s, and P_d are mean (*m*), systolic (*s*), and diastolic (*d*) blood pressures, respectively (Fig. 4.26).[4,5] Both P_s and P_d can be measured indirectly using either Doppler or oscillometric techniques. Most drugs used to produce anesthesia decrease car-

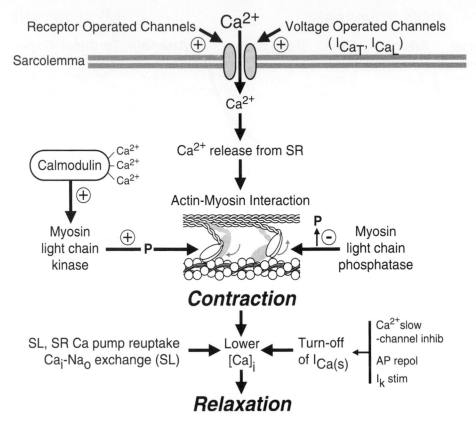

Fig. 4.24. The excitation-contraction coupling process in vascular smooth muscle. Calcium enters cardiac cells through two types of voltage-dependent calcium channels (L and T) and several types of receptor-operated channels, which triggers the release of intracellular calcium (calcium-induced calcium release) from the sarcoplasmic reticulum (SR). Not shown is that some agonists act on smooth muscle membrane receptors to stimulate phosphatidylinositol turnover and the production of inositol triphosphate (IP_3) and diacylglycerol (DAG). IP_3 releases calcium from the SR and DAG activates protein kinase C, which stimulates the activity of the voltage-dependent slow calcium channels. Increases in intracellular calcium also interact with calmodulin to form a calcium-calmodulin complex stimulating myosin light-chain kinase, which together with intracellular calcium facilitates actin-myosin interaction. Contraction terminates when myosin light-chain phosphatase dephosphorylates the myosin light chain and intracellular calcium is reduced by sarcolemmal (SL) and SR reuptake, intracellular calcium–extracellular sodium exchange, and the turning off of the slow calcium channels.

diac output and peripheral vascular resistance. It should be remembered that if peripheral vascular resistance is elevated, the arterial blood pressure may be within normal limits, regardless of low blood flow to peripheral tissues. Several sedative and anesthetic drugs (α_2-adrenergic agonists, ketamine, and low doses of thiobarbiturates) can increase peripheral vascular resistance (producing no change or increases in arterial blood pressure) while decreasing cardiac output (Table 4.4).

The arterial pulse pressure ($P_s - P_d$) and pulse-pressure waveform can provide valuable information regarding changes in vascular compliance and vessel tone. Generally, drugs (phenothiazines) or diseases (endotoxic shock) that produce marked arterial dilating effects increase vascular compliance, causing a rapid rise, short duration, and rapid fall in the arterial waveform while increasing the arterial pulse pressure. Situations that produce vasoconstriction decrease vascular compliance, producing a longer-duration pulse waveform and a slower fall in the systolic blood pressure to diastolic values.[68] The pulse pressure may con-

tain secondary and sometimes tertiary pressure waveforms, particularly if the measuring site is in a peripheral artery some distance from the heart.[65] Secondary and tertiary pulse waves are an indication of normal or elevated vascular tone in response to sympathetic nervous system stimulation or the vascular effects of drugs (e.g., ketamine, medetomidine, or catecholamines).

Resistance Vessels
These include the terminal (small) arteries, arterioles, and metarterioles, and to a much lesser extent the capillaries and venules. Under normal conditions, the arterioles provide over 50% of the total systemic vascular resistance, whereas large and small arteries account for 20%, capillaries 25%, and veins 5%. As indicated earlier, the Hagen-Poiseuille equation describes resistance as

$$R = 8\, L\eta/\pi r^4$$

where L is length, η is blood viscosity, π is the constant 2.13, and r is the vessel radius. From this relationship, it should be clear

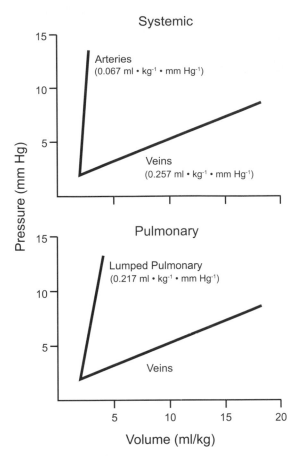

Fig. 4.25. Compliance (volume-pressure) curves for systemic arteries and veins and the lumped pulmonary vascular beds. Note that a small increase in volume causes a much larger increase in arterial pressure than venous pressure, suggesting a much lower compliance. Modified from Green,[69] pp. 66 and 67.

that as vessel radius decreases and vessel length and blood viscosity increase, vascular resistance increases.

Sphincter Vessels

Sphincter vessels represent a specific type of resistance vessel that is anatomically the absolute terminal portion of the precapillary arteriole. Functionally, sphincter vessels help to regulate the number of open capillaries and therefore the size of the capillary bed that is available for exchange processes. The relatively thick-walled muscular arterioles and sphincter vessels are influenced by a variety of neural, humoral, and local metabolic factors, and are the principal determinants for the regulation of both the volume and the distribution of blood flow to all tissues of the body (Table 4.5).

Arteriovenous Shunts

Arteriovenous anastomoses (AVAs) are a relatively poorly understood group of vessels that contain large amounts of vascular smooth muscle and function as pathways by which blood can bypass the capillaries and return to the venous circulation. These vessels can reduce or totally interrupt blood flow to capillaries.

AVAs are found in the greatest numbers in the skin and extremities (ears, feet, and hooves) of most species and were originally thought to be primarily involved in thermoregulation. More recently, their identification and verification in the intestinal wall, kidney, liver, and skeletal muscles have increased interest in their role as a separate blood flow regulatory mechanism for controlling nutrient blood flow to these tissues. The influence of anesthetic drugs on AVAs is poorly understood and largely unknown.[68,70]

Capillaries

These are functionally the most important portion of the circulatory system, because they are the exchange units between the blood and interstitial fluid. They penetrate nearly every tissue of the body, their numbers per gram of tissue and ultrastructure being dependent on tissue metabolic rate and tissue function. Structurally, capillaries are one layer of endothelial cells surrounded by reticular fibers. There are three types of capillaries. Capillaries located in striated and smooth muscle, connective tissue, and the pulmonary circulation are uninterrupted or continuous, although they contain a large number of pores. Capillaries in the glomeruli of the kidney and in the intestine are fenestrated because of the high levels of metabolism and importance of active exchange of fluids. Capillaries in the liver, spleen, and bone marrow are discontinuous, containing intercellular gaps through which fluid and blood cells can easily pass.[68] Regardless of the type of capillary examined, the exchange of fluid, nutrients, and cellular waste products between blood and interstitial fluid is their primary function. Capillary exchange is governed by two primary processes: *diffusion* and *filtration*. Fick's law of *diffusion* describes solute exchange (J_s) as

$$J_s = DA/M_T \Delta C$$

where D is the diffusion coefficient, A is the capillary surface area, M_T is the membrane thickness, and ΔC is the concentration gradient or difference. The diffusion coefficient is determined by the diffusion medium and qualities characteristic of the diffusion particle such as molecular weight, ionic charge, and lipid solubility. Exchange by *filtration* is determined by four primary factors (P_c, P_i, π_c, and π_i) according to a dynamic equilibrium equation, first proposed by Starling and Landis and modified by Pappenheimer and Soto-Rivera, wherein

$$Q_c = K_f(P_c - P_i) + \sigma(\pi_c - \pi_i)$$

where Q_c is fluid flow across the capillary (positive for filtration, and negative for reabsorption), P_c and P_i are capillary and interstitial hydrostatic pressures, π_c and π_i are the plasma in the capillary and interstitial colloid osmotic pressures of proteins, K_f is the capillary filtration coefficient, and σ is the osmotic reflection coefficient for all plasma proteins (Fig. 4.27).[71,72] The filtration coefficient (K) indicates the resistance of the capillary wall to fluid flow and is determined by the exchange surface area, the number and radius of capillary pores, the capillary wall thickness, and the viscosity of the filtering fluid. The osmotic reflection coefficient (σ) is an indicator of transvascular protein transport and is usually assumed to be 1, or close to 1, in normal

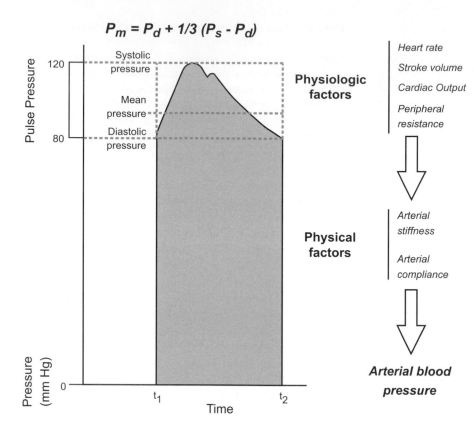

$$P_m = P_d + 1/3 (P_s - P_d)$$

Physiologic factors

Heart rate

Stroke volume

Cardiac Output

Peripheral resistance

Physical factors

Arterial stiffness

Arterial compliance

Arterial blood pressure

Fig. 4.26. Arterial blood pressure is determined by both physiological and physical factors. The mean arterial pressure (P_m) represents the area under the arterial pressure curve divided by the duration of the cardiac cycle and can be estimated by adding one-third the difference between the systolic arterial pressure (P_s) and diastolic arterial pressure (P_d) to P_d. P_s minus P_d is the pulse pressure. Modified from Berne and Levy,[103] p. 259.

animals, since most capillary beds are impermeable to colloids. Providing all factors can be measured, calculated, or estimated in Starling's equation, net fluid flux across the capillary wall can be quantitated accurately.[71] Under normal conditions, these factors are responsible for fluid filtration at the arterial end of the capillary and fluid reabsorption at the venous end of the capillary (Figs. 4.27 and 4.28). Lymph vessels carry excess fluid away. Increases in P_c (volume overload, venous obstruction, and heart failure) and K_f (histamine, cytokines, and kinins) or decreases in π_p (hypoproteinemia) cause excess fluid to accumulate in the interstitial space, resulting in edema. Excessive fluid accumulation in the lung, intestine, and liver (so-called overflow organs) can cause fluid collection in the alveoli, intestinal lumen, and peritoneal cavity.[72] Decreases in P_c (hypotension and hypovolemia) and increases in π_p (hyperproteinemia and dehydration) induce a net reabsorption of fluid from the interstitial space and an increase in plasma volume. Anesthesia, anesthetic drugs, quantity and type of fluid administered, and the type of anesthetic techniques used can have important effects on the Starling forces.[72] For example, most anesthetic drugs and anesthetic techniques decrease P_c, causing net fluid reabsorption from the interstitial space and hemodilution. If the anesthetic drug or technique produces significant cardiac depression, P_c may increase, resulting in edema (e.g., pulmonary edema). Finally, several drugs, including some opioids (e.g., morphine and meperidine), can cause histamine release, thereby increasing K_f, and interstitial fluid accumulation (Table 4.6).[68]

Table 4.5. Distribution of cardiac output to peripheral tissues

Organ	% of Total
1. Heart	4
2. Brain	14
3. Kidneys	20
4. Gastrointestinal tract	22
5. Resting skeletal muscle	20
6. Skin	8
7. Other organs	12

Veins and Venules

The veins and venules comprise the final component of the vascular system and, although structurally similar to arteries, are relatively devoid of elastic tissue and possess comparatively less smooth muscle (Fig. 4.23). Veins in general have a greater radius and thinner walls than arteries and functionally serve to return blood to the heart and as capacitance (volume storage) vessels (Fig. 4.3). The relationship between vascular volume (V) and vascular transmural pressure (P) is termed *vascular compliance* ($C = \Delta V/\Delta P$), which is the inverse of elasticity and for the low-pressure veins is several orders of magnitude greater than most arteries (Fig. 4.25).[69] The lumped compliance of the pulmonary vascular bed is less than that of the systemic circulation, imply-

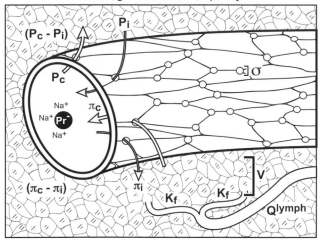

Starling's Law of the Capillary

Table 4.6. Causes of increased interstitial fluid volume and edema

Increased filtration pressure
  Arteriolar dilation
  Venule constriction
  Increased venous pressure (heart failure, incompetent valves, venous obstruction, increased total extracellular fluid volume, effect of gravity, etc.)
Decreased osmotic pressure gradient across capillary
  Decreased plasma protein level
  Accumulation of osmotically active substances in interstitial space
Increased capillary permeability
  Substance P
  Histamine and related substances
  Kinins, etc.
Inadequate lymph flow

Fig. 4.27. Starling's law of the capillary suggests that fluid (plasma) flux (exchange) across the capillary wall (J_v) and into the interstitium depends on transmural (capillary [c] − interstitial [i]) hydrostatic pressure ($P_c − P_i$), transmural protein colloid osmotic pressure (π; $\pi_C − \pi_I$), the fluid filtration coefficient or porosity (κ_F), and the reflection coefficient for the movement of proteins (σ). Increases in P_c and κ_F and decreases in P_i, π_C, and σ increase J_v and vice versa.

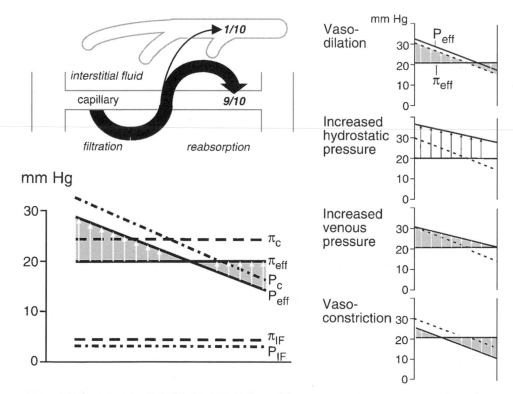

Fig. 4.28. Starling's law of the capillary suggests that fluid movement between the capillary and the interstitial space can be predicted by changes in capillary (P_c) and interstitial (P_i) hydrostatic pressures and capillary (π_c) and interstitial (π_i) colloid osmotic pressures. The algebraic sum of these pressures produces an effective transmural filtration pressure (P_{eff}) and effective colloid osmotic pressure (π_{eff}), which determine capillary filtration and reabsorption. Only about 10% of the plasma filtrate enters the lymphatic system under normal conditions. Filtration-reabsorption is shifted toward increased filtration during vasodilation and increased hydrostatic and venous pressure, and toward increased reabsorption during vasoconstriction. These diagrams assume the filtration coefficient and the osmotic reflection coefficient (see the text) are minimally affected. Modified from Witzleb,[68] pp. 419 and 420.

ing that the blood storage capability of the lungs compared to the systemic circulation, particularly the systemic small veins and venules, is small (Fig. 4.25). Venous return is facilitated by venous one-way valves, contraction of skeletal muscle (muscle pump), the negative intrathoracic pressure during breathing (respiratory pump), increases in intra-abdominal pressure (abdominal pump), and the suction effect of the heart during atrial relaxation, ventricular contraction, and rapid ventricular filling.[68] Hydrostatic pressure (gravity), increased intrathoracic pressure (intermittent positive-pressure ventilation [IPPV] and positive end-expiratory pressure [PEEP]), and venous occlusion or obstruction initially impair or inhibit venous return. The capacious venous vessels of the liver, splanchnic viscera, and skin (in many species), together with the sinusoids of the spleen, can be considered blood reservoirs, as are the pulmonary vessels, although to a much lesser extent.

Lymphatics

The lymphatic system constitutes a closed-ended, separate, yet parallel drainage system through which interstitial fluid (normally <10% of filtered fluid) is returned to the blood vascular system (Fig. 4.28).[72] Lymphatic channels are thin-walled vessels (generally one cell layer thick) that contain one-way valves that facilitate the transfer of lymph (interstitial fluid) via lymph vessels of increasing size first to lymph nodes and eventually to the thoracic lymphatic duct and heart. Skeletal muscle contraction facilitates lymph flow (lymphatic pump) to the heart similar to its effect on venous blood flow.[68]

Nervous, Humoral, and Local Control

The regulatory control of the cardiovascular system is integrated through the combined effects of the central and peripheral nervous systems, the influence of circulating (humoral) vasoactive substances, and local tissue mediators that modulate vascular tone.[73–77] These regulatory processes maintain blood flow at an appropriate level while distributing blood flow to meet the needs of tissue beds that have the greatest demand.

Tissue blood flow is regulated by the integration of supraregional (central nervous system [CNS]), regional and local factors. Together these factors coordinate immediate and long-term adjustments in cardiac output, total peripheral vascular resistance, vascular capacitance, and blood volume. Higher brain centers, including the hypothalamus (pain and temperature) and cerebral cortex (emotions: vigilance and fear), facilitate or modify cardiovascular responses. Continuous adjustments in cardiovascular system function help to buffer significant changes in arterial blood pressure and intravascular volume and sustain oxygen and nutrient delivery to tissues (Table 4.7). The autonomic nervous system exerts a major influence on the regulation of cardiovascular function.[76] Peripheral receptors, including baroreceptors, mechanoreceptors, and chemoreceptors, respond to changes in blood pressure, volume, or gas tensions, respectively, and send information to the CNS through afferent nerves. These sensory signals are integrated, in "control centers" located in the hypothalamus, pons, and medulla, into responses carried by efferent sympathetic or parasympathetic nerves to the periphery (Fig. 4.29). The autonomic nervous system also modulates the release of various peptides providing a generalized humoral influence on cardiac contractile performance and vascular tone.[66] Minute-to-minute changes in blood flow are regulated by local control mechanisms, which are somewhat independent from nervous system input. Vasodilator substances, primarily the by-products of tissue metabolism, act on small vessels, producing vasodilation proportional to the amount of metabolite produced. In addition, the vascular endothelium is known to modulate both local and neural control mechanisms through the release of prostaglandins and endothelium-derived factors, such as nitric oxide. Anesthetic drugs can and do interfere with the sensory (input), neural integration (processing), and effector (output) mechanisms that control cardiovascular function.[78–82] Decreases in arterial blood pressure from any cause (blood loss, bradycardia, or poor cardiac performance) are sensed by a variety of central and peripheral vascular baroreceptors, which are the most important short-term determinants of arterial blood pressure. Output from these receptors triggers readjustments in CNS autonomic output, which compensates for small changes in arterial blood pressure (Fig. 4.30). Local myogenic autoregulation also helps to protect the brain, heart, liver, mesentery, and skeletal muscle from small changes in blood pressure. If arterial blood pressure is reduced to a point that tissue blood flow is negatively affected, CNS centers are activated, leading to substantial increases in heart rate, cardiac contractility, and vascular tone. Epinephrine and norepinephrine are released from the adrenal gland, which, combined with increases in sympathetic tone and activation of the renin-angiotensin system, intensify vasoconstriction (Table 4.7). Blood flow is redistributed to the lungs, heart, and brain and away from the skin, skeletal muscle, and kidney and splanchnic viscera. Additionally, peripheral chemoreceptors sense changes in the blood oxygen tension (PO_2) and pH. The acute onset of hypoxemia or hypercarbia (acidemia) in conjunction with hypotension can induce peripheral vasoconstriction. If blood pressure is not restored, capillary hydrostatic pressure decreases, promoting the movement of fluid from the interstitial space into the capillaries, thus increasing intravascular volume. The intravascular shift of extravascular fluid can restore up to 50% of the intravascular volume in a relatively short period (hours). The constriction of the peripheral vasculature, centralization of blood volume, redistribution of the blood flow, and increase in cardiac output and arterial blood pressure are generally capable of restoring tissue perfusion, providing the episode of hypotension or blood loss does not exceed the body's compensatory capabilities.

Normally, neural, humoral, local myogenic, and metabolic autoregulatory mechanisms combine to adjust vascular resistance and tissue blood flow continuously to meet tissue requirements. The partial pressure of oxygen is chief among the local factors regulating tissue blood flow. Decreases in the arterial partial pressure of oxygen (i.e., ischemia or hypoxemia) cause vasodilatation and vice versa. Similarly, sustained increases in the local concentration of carbon dioxide, hydrogen ions, potassium, lac-

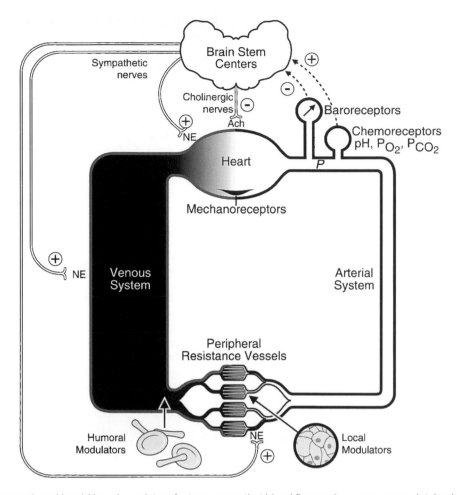

Fig. 4.29. Nervous, humoral, and local (tissue) regulatory factors ensure that blood flow and pressure are maintained within physiological limits. Mechanoreceptors and chemoreceptors sense changes in wall tension (stretch) and pH and blood gases (arterial oxygen partial pressure [PaO₂] and partial pressure of carbon dioxide [PaCO₂]), respectively. Substances produced in peripheral tissues and released into the circulation by endocrine glands also modulate blood vessels and the distribution of blood flow. Nervous impulses generated by the heart, vasculature, and peripheral sensors are transmitted to and integrated in the brain stem, which alters sympathetic and parasympathetic tone in order to make appropriate adjustments. The release of norepinephrine (NE) by sympathetic nerves stimulates the heart and constricts blood vessels. The release of acetylcholine (Ach) by parasympathetic nerves depresses the heart. PCO₂, partial pressure of carbon dioxide; PO₂, partial pressure of oxygen; +, stimulatory; and −, inhibitory. Modified from Shepherd and Vanhoutte,[102] p. 12.

tic acid, and/or adenosine induce arteriolar (the chief resistance vessels) vasodilatation. It is noteworthy that acid-base (pH < 7.20) and electrolyte disturbances ($\uparrow$ K⁺), relatively short periods (longer than 8 to 10 min) of hypoxemia (PaO₂ < 40 mm Hg) or ischemia (<25% of normal blood flow), and prolonged or excessive exposure to drugs (most anesthetics) can blunt or abolish baroreceptor and chemoreceptor reflex activity and the vascular response to sympathetic stimulation, leading to a poor compensatory response and a delay in normal tissue blood flow.

Neural Control of Cardiovascular Function

Nervous system regulation of the cardiovascular system and blood volume depends on three components within the nervous system: afferent input, central integration and processing, and efferent output.[76,83] Neural and hormonal factors, including osmoreceptors in the hypothalamus, antidiuretic hormone released by neurons in the supraoptic and paraventricular nuclei, aldos-

terone and renin produced by the kidney, and the release of atrial natriuretic peptide (ANP) by atrial receptors sensitive to stretch, are all integrally involved in maintaining plasma and therefore blood volume. The one mechanism above all others, however, that dominates the control of plasma and blood volume is the effect of blood volume on arterial blood pressure and the consequences of arterial blood pressure on the urinary excretion of sodium and water (Fig. 4.30A).[4] Alterations in arterial blood pressure, therefore, can have profound effects on fluid exchange and blood volume (natriuresis and pressure diuresis). The interplay of these mechanisms ultimately controls hemodynamics, blood volume, extracellular fluid volume, and renal excretion of salt and water (Fig. 4.30B).

Afferent Input

Afferent input to the CNS is received from peripheral sensors that respond to acute changes in blood pressure, blood volume,

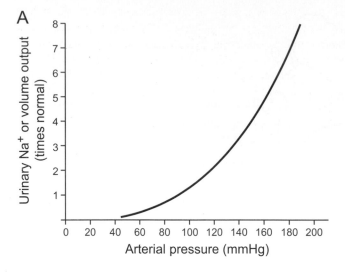

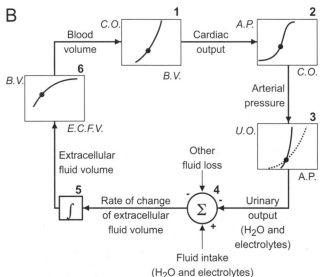

Fig. 4.30. The effect of arterial blood pressure on the urinary excretion of Na^+ and urine volume **(A)**, and a scheme for a basic feedback mechanism that controls blood volume and extracellular fluid volume **(B)**. A.P., arterial blood pressure; B.V., blood volume; C.O., cardiac output; E.C.F.V., extracellular fluid volume; and U.O., urine output. Modified from Guyton,[105] 321.

Table 4.7. Factors that regulate arterial blood pressure and tissue perfusion

Immediate (short term)
1. Autonomic nervous system (sympathetic and parasympathetic)
   Regulates heart rate and vessel tone and capacity
2. Vascular baroreceptor or pressoreceptor reflexes (stretch receptors)
   Regulate heart rate and vessel tone and capacity
3. Cardiac stretch receptors
   Regulate heart rate and vessel tone and capacity
4. Chemoreceptor reflexes (sense changes in oxygen and carbon dioxide (hydrogen ions)
   Regulate heart rate and vessel tone
5. Bloodborne (humoral) responses (epinephrine and norepinephrine)
   Regulate heart rate, vessel tone, and cardiac contractility
6. Local factors
   Arteriolar oxygen partial pressure
      Decreased oxygen produces vasodilatation and vice versa
   Local metabolites
      Increased production of carbon dioxide, hydrogen ions, and lactate
   Myogenic autoregulation
      Adjusts vessel tone to changes in blood pressure

Intermediate
1. Transcapillary fluid shifts (Starling's law of the capillary)
   Regulate fluid filtration and reabsorption
2. Hormonal responses (renin and angiotensin)
   Regulate vessel tone and salt and water retention

Long term
1. Oral fluid consumption
   Regulates net fluid intake
2. Renal control system (vasopressin [ADH], aldosterone, and atrial natriuretic peptide)
   Regulates total body water and renal fluid output

and tissue metabolism. These peripheral sensors are the first step in a reflex arc in which the effector organs are the heart and vasculature. The reflex arc generally operates as a negative-feedback system designed to maintain a variable blood pressure at a fixed value, or *set point*.[83]

Arterial baroreceptors are stretch receptors (mechanoreceptors) located in the carotid sinus and aortic arch that respond to increases in arterial blood pressure by incremental increases in the firing rate of sensory fibers, which are carried by the glossopharyngeal and vagus nerves.[76] These impulses travel to the nucleus tractus solitarius within the CNS, are processed, and initiate an effector response that returns blood pressure to its normal range (Fig. 4.29). This response is accomplished by parasympathetic activation, which decreases heart rate and inhibition of sympathetic vasoconstrictor output to arterioles and veins. Baroreceptors become inoperative at an arterial blood pressure below 60 mm Hg, but the frequency of nerve impulses increases progressively as pressure rises above 60 mm Hg, reaching a maximum at approximately 180 mm Hg.[4,83] Most baroreceptors have a set point of approximately 100 mm Hg. However, if arterial blood pressure changes to a new value and remains static, the baroreceptors can "reset" to this new set point within 24 to 48 h. This is why baroreceptors are only effective for short-term control of blood pressure. Most, if not all, anesthetic drugs interfere with baroreceptor responsiveness. Inhalation anesthetics in particular depress normal baroreflex responsiveness and diminish sympathetic output from the CNS. The degree of baroreceptor depression depends on both the depth of anesthesia and the patient's physical status.[84,85]

Cardiac mechanoreceptors are located in the right and left atria and ventricles and help to minimize changes in systemic blood pressure in response to changes in blood volume. These cardiac stretch receptors differ from the baroreceptors in that the stretch receptors respond to comparatively small changes in stretch or pressure as do pressure receptors within the pulmonary circulation. The atria contain two types of receptors located at the venoatrial junctions.[83] Atrial *A* receptors react primarily to changes in heart rate, whereas *B* receptors respond to short-term changes in atrial volume. An increase in atrial volume activates both the A and B atrial mechanoreceptors, sending impulses to the medulla via vagal afferents. Depending on the prevailing heart rate and arterial blood pressure, heart rate may increase (Bainbridge reflex) or decrease (baroreflex and activation of atrial depressor *C* fibers). Atrial distension also decreases sympathetic output to renal afferent arterioles, resulting in vasodilation, while the hypothalamus receives neural input, which decreases the release of vasopressin (antidiuretic hormone) that acts to increase urine flow.[76] A rapid loss of free water into the urine helps return circulating blood volume to normal values. In addition to these neural responses, ANP and brain natriuretic peptide (BNP) are released into the bloodstream.[73] ANP is produced in atrial cardiocytes in response to atrial distension and increases sodium excretion by the kidney with an accompanying increase in water loss.[74] Similarly, BNP, produced by ventricular muscle cells, depends on increases in ventricular filling pressures and myocardial stretch and becomes elevated during myocardial dysfunction.[73]

Ventricular mechanoreceptors located in the ventricular endocardium discharge in parallel with changes in ventricular pressure and produce effects that help to regulate systemic blood pressure and myocardial work. Ventricular distension, however, also stimulates powerful depressor reflexes that decrease heart rate and peripheral vascular resistance, resulting in bradycardia and hypotension (Bezold-Jarisch reflex).[83] The activation of ventricular nonmyelinated C fibers serves as the basis for this reflex response. Impulses initiated by either ventricular distention or the injection of certain chemicals (e.g., capsaicin or serotonin) into the coronary arteries can produce the Bezold-Jarisch reflex, which is also called the *coronary chemoreflex.*[83]

The carotid artery and aortic arch contain specialized sensory chemoreceptors termed the *carotid and aortic bodies* (Fig. 4.29).[76] The carotid and aortic bodies receive the highest blood flow per gram of tissue weight of any organ within the body. These chemoreceptors are sensitive to changes in arterial oxygen and carbon dioxide tension, hydrogen-ion concentration (pH), and temperature. The chemoreceptors of the carotid and aortic bodies help to regulate respiratory function in response to decreases in pH and the arterial partial pressure of oxygen and increases in the arterial partial pressure of carbon dioxide. Afferent activity from the carotid body is carried by the glossopharyngeal nerve and from the aortic body by the vagus. These sensors are most sensitive to changes in hydrogen-ion concentration and respond proportionally to the magnitude of the change from their set point. The set point for activation is a pH below 7.40. The approximate set point for carbon dioxide is 40 mm Hg and for oxygen 80 mm Hg. Increases in afferent activity from the chemoreceptors increase minute ventilation, restoring arterial blood pH, carbon dioxide, and/or oxygen to normal. Hypoxia, hypercarbia, and nonrespiratory acidosis may cause bradycardia, coronary vasodilation, and an increase in systemic arteriolar resistance. This effect is pronounced if the normal increase in ventilation is prevented, for example, during anesthesia. Chemoreceptors located in the ventricular epicardium respond to hypoxia or ischemia by initiating the coronary chemoreflex (Bezold-Jarisch reflex), producing bradycardia and hypotension (Table 4.8).

Central Nervous System Integration

No single brain nucleus or center controls cardiovascular function; rather, multiple regions modulate the autonomic nervous system. When afferent impulses from peripheral sensors arrive in the brain, they are integrated to produce a neural and/or humoral response. The nucleus tractus solitarius (NTS) in the medulla is the relay station for afferent impulses from peripheral sensors (Fig. 4.31). Neurons originating in the NTS send information to the vagal nucleus and to various regions collectively referred to as the *vasomotor center.* Vagal nuclei send nerve fibers directly to the heart. Nerve cell bodies for the sympathetic nervous system are located in the thoracolumbar spinal cord and are linked to the NTS through axons traveling in the bulbospinal tract (Fig. 4.32). The bulbospinal tract contains both excitatory and inhibitory axons that cause either increases or decreases in sympathetic output. Centers in the hypothalamus link the somatic and autonomic responses necessary for animals to adapt to their environment. The centers initiate adrenergic constriction of resistance and capacitance vessels and cholinergic dilation of vessels supplying skeletal and cardiac muscle during the fight-flight response. Hypothalamic centers modulate the cardiovascular response (cutaneous vasoactivity) to body temperature changes during shivering, sweating, or panting. The hypothalamus also modulates the cardiovascular response to exercise and may be involved in blood pressure regulation.[76] Finally, the cerebral cortex influences cardiovascular function by modulating the cardiovascular response to exercise, emotion, ischemia, and hypoxia.[83]

Efferent Output

The autonomic nervous system, which is the efferent link between the CNS and the cardiovascular system, provides rapid control of both blood pressure and blood flow.[76] Efferent impulses are carried by sympathetic and parasympathetic nerves. Adrenergic and cholinergic receptors in target organs initiate the intracellular changes that produce a cellular response to the signals arriving from the CNS (Table 4.9).

Sympathetic Nervous System

Sympathetic pathways originate in the intermediolateral columns of the thoracolumbar segments of the spinal cord.[74,76] Both inhibitory input and excitatory input arrive at preganglionic sympathetic nerve cell bodies via axons traveling in the bulbospinal tract (Fig. 4.32). Descending inhibitory pathways are serotoninergic; descending excitatory pathways are adrenergic. The balance between these two types of input determines the prevailing level of sympathetic tone to the periphery.

Table 4.8. Cardiovascular and pulmonary reflexes and signs

1. Branham's sign: slowing of the heart rate following compression or excision of an arteriovenous fistula (e.g., patent ductus arteriosus ligation).
2. Bainbridge reflex: an increase in heart rate caused by a rise in blood pressure in the great veins as they enter the right atrium.
3. Bezold-Jarisch reflex: afferent and efferent pathways in the vagus nerve—stimulation of cardiac, primarily ventricular, chemoreceptors or stretch receptors (mechanoreceptors), induce sinus bradycardia, hypotension, and peripheral vasodilation. Stretch of ventricular mechanoreceptors are responsible for syncope when standing.
4. High-pressure baroreceptor or pressoreceptor reflex: decreases in heart rate initiated by increases in arterial blood pressure. A decrease in arterial pressure produces hyperventilation, and an increase in arterial blood pressure causes respiratory depression and ultimately apnea.
5. Atrial stretch-receptor reflex: atrial distension causes the release of atrial natriuretic peptide (ANP) from the atria, resulting in diuretic activity, vasodilation, inhibition, and aldosterone secretion. ANP is an endogenous antagonist of angiotensin II. This response was previously considered to be a low-pressure baroreceptor response, but has since been demonstrated to be dependent on atrial stretch, not pressure. Sinus and supraventricular tachycardias are common stimuli for this response.
6. Vasovagal reflex: initiated by a decrease in venous return to the heart (e.g., hypovolemia, orthostasis, compression of the inferior vena cava, and regional analgesia), causing sinus bradycardia and vasodilation. The term has come to include neurocardiogenic syncope, carotid sinus syndrome, and micturition syncope in human patients.
7. Craniocardiac reflex: stimulation of cranial nerves (olfactory, ophthalmic, and trigeminal), resulting in bradycardia and hypotension (depressor effects).
8. Abdominocardiac reflex: mechanical stimulation of the abdominal viscera causes changes in heart rate, usually slowing; rarely causes extrasystoles.
9. Oculocardiac reflex (Aschner's reflex): compression of the eyeball causes slowing of sinus heart rate.
10. Hering-Breuer reflex: effects of the vagus in the control of respiration—lung inflation arrests inspiration, and lung deflation initiates inspiration.
11. Pulmonary chemoreflex: stimulation of C-fiber endings (juxtapulmonary capillary receptors [J receptors]) by tissue damage. Fluid accumulation of cytokines produces sinus bradycardia, hypotension, shallow breathing and apnea, bronchoconstriction, and mucous secretion (e.g., isoflurane administration).
12. Venorespiratory reflex: increases in right atrial pressure stimulate increases in respiration.
13. Cough reflex: stimulation of the larynx, trachea, or main bronchi or chemical stimulation throughout the respiratory tree result in cough.
14. Vagovagal reflex: afferent and efferent pathways in the vagus nerve—stimulation or irritation of the larynx or trachea by a laryngoscope or endotracheal tube precipitates bradycardia.

Preganglionic sympathetic nerves send axons via the ventral roots of the spinal cord to paravertebral ganglia located just outside of the vertebral column. Many of the preganglionic fibers ascend the paravertebral chains and synapse with postganglionic neurons in the cranial, middle, and caudal (stellate) cervical ganglia (Fig. 4.33). Here they synapse with postganglionic sympathetic neurons, which send their fibers to the heart, blood vessels, and viscera. Postganglionic cardiac sympathetic nerve fibers innervate the sinoatrial node, the atrioventricular node, the atria, and the myocardium (Fig. 4.32). Postganglionic sympathetic fibers release the neurotransmitter norepinephrine, which binds to adrenoreceptors on cardiac cell membranes (Table 4.9).

Postganglionic sympathetic nerve fibers also leave the paravertebral ganglia via spinal nerves to innervate vessels throughout the body. Normally, sympathetic tone maintains a partial state of contraction in vascular smooth muscle, providing the resistance necessary to maintain adequate systemic blood pressure and aid in the control of the fractional distribution of cardiac output to body tissues.[73,76] The extent of innervation to the resistance vessels (arterioles) varies with tissue type. The kidney, spleen, gastrointestinal tract, and skin are extensively innervated by the sympathetic nervous system. Redistribution of blood flow away from these tissues during times of crisis preserves blood flow to the brain, heart, and skeletal muscle.

Sympathetic Neurotransmission
The vast majority of sympathetic postganglionic fibers are adrenergic, releasing norepinephrine at their neuroeffector junctions. The amino acid tyrosine is the substrate used by these nerves to produce norepinephrine. Tyrosine is actively transported across the nerve cell membrane into the neural axoplasm, where it is converted by tyrosine hydroxylase and decarboxylation to dopamine, which is stored in vesicles within the nerve. Inside the storage vesicles, a final hydroxylation step takes place to produce the neurotransmitter norepinephrine. Nerve action potentials increase intracellular calcium, causing the vesicles to fuse with the nerve cell membrane and release norepinephrine into the synaptic cleft, where it binds to a variety of adrenoreceptors (Table 4.9). There are presynaptic receptors on the nerve cell membrane and postsynaptic receptors on the effector organ. Postsynaptic receptor binding of norepinephrine triggers a cascade of intracellular events that ultimately produce a cellular action. The effective half-life of norepinephrine after release into the synaptic cleft is very short. Norepinephrine is degraded locally at the neuroeffector junction by the enzymes, monamine oxidase (MAO) and catechol-*O*-methyltransferase (COMT). Most of the norepinephrine released into the synaptic cleft undergoes reuptake into adrenergic nerve terminals, where it reenters storage vesicles. This neuronal amine-uptake system is designated *uptake 1* and has a high affinity for norepinephrine, a lower affinity for epinephrine, and little affinity for the synthetic β-adrenergic agonist isoproterenol. Norepinephrine may rapidly diffuse out of the synaptic cleft, where it undergoes reuptake at extraneuronal sites or is carried into the venous blood and metabolized in the lung. The extraneuronal reuptake pathway has been designated *uptake 2* and has a low affinity for norepinephrine, a higher affinity for

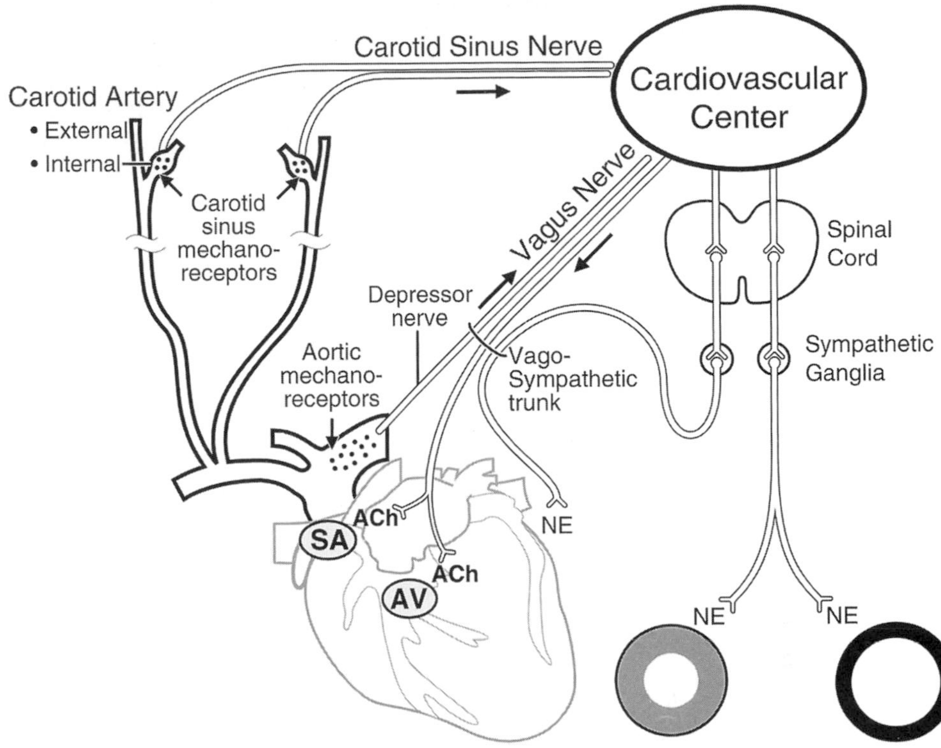

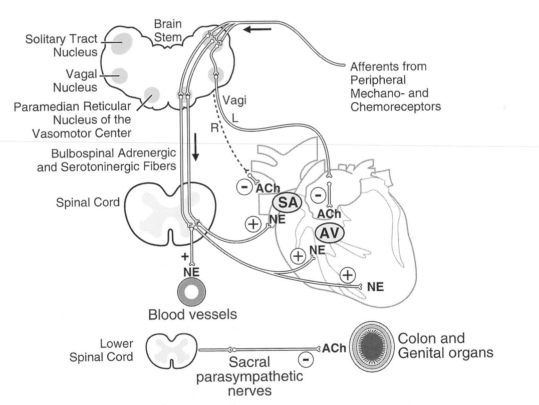

Fig. 4.31. Mechanoreceptors in the carotid sinus and aortic arch send impulses via the carotid sinus nerve, a branch of the glossopharyngeal nerve, and the vagosympathetic trunk, respectively, to the solitary tract nucleus in the brain stem (cardiovascular centers). Changes in the activity of these mechanoreceptors caused by changes in arterial blood pressure result in adjustments in sympathetic and parasympathetic outflow to the heart and resistance (arterial) and capacitance (veins) vessels. Ach, acetylcholine; AV, atrioventricular node; NE, norepinephrine; and SA, sinoatrial node. Modified from Shepherd and Vanhoutte,[102] p. 132.

Fig. 4.32. Distribution of sympathetic and parasympathetic nerves to the cardiovascular system. The solitary-tract nucleus is the main receiving point in the brain stem for afferent input arriving from peripheral sensors and higher centers in the brain. Interneurons connect the solitary-tract nucleus to the vasomotor center, from which bulbospinal tract fibers descend to the spinal cord and synapse with preganglionic sympathetic nerves to the heart and blood vessels. Interneurons also connect the solitary-tract nucleus to the vagal nucleus in the brain stem, where neurons synapse with preganglionic parasympathetic nerve fibers, which are carried by the vagus nerve to the heart. Parasympathetic nerve fibers to the blood vessels of the colon and genital organs arise from centers in the sacral portion of the spinal cord. Ach, acetylcholine; AV, atrioventricular node; L, left vagus; NE, norepinephrine; R, right vagus; and SA, sinoatrial node. Modified from Shepherd and Vanhoutte,[102] p. 124.

Table 4.9. Mechanism of action of selected neurotransmitters

Transmitter	Receptor	Second Messenger	Net Channel Effects
Acetylcholine	N_G and N_s	—	↑Na^+, other small ions
	m_1	↑IP_3, DAG	↑CA^{2+}
	m_2 (cardiac)	↓cAMP	↓Ca^{2+}, ↑K^+
	m_3	↑IP_3, DAG	
	m_4 (glandular)	↓cAMP	
	m_5	↑IP_3, DAG	
Dopamine	D_1	↑cAMP	
	D_2	↓cAMP	↑K^+, ↓Ca^{2+}
Norepinephrine[a]	α_1	↑IP_3, DAG	↓K^+
	α_2	↓cAMP	↑K^+, ↓Ca^{2+}
	β_1	↑cAMP	
	β_2	↑cAMP	
	β_3	↑cAMP	
5HT	$5HT_{1A}$	↓cAMP	↑K^+
	$5HT_{1B}$	↓cAMP	
	$5HT_{1C}$	↑IP_3, DAG	
	$5HT_{1D}$	↓cAMP	↓K^+
	$5HT_2$	↑IP_3, DAG	↓K^+
	$5HT_3$	—	↑Na^+
	$5HT_4$	↑cAMP	
Adenosine	A_1	↓cAMP	
	A_2	↑cAMP	
Glutamate, aspartate	NMDA	—	↑Na^+, Ca^{2+}
	AMPA	—	↑Na^+
	Quisqualate	↑IP_3, DAG	—
	Kainate	—	↑Na^+
GABA	$GABA_A$	—	↑Cl^-
	$GABA_B$	↑IP_3, DAG	↑K^+, ↓Ca^{2+}

5HT, 5-hydroxytryptamine [serotonin]; AMPA, α-amino-3-hydroxy-5-methyl-4-isoxazolepropionic acid; cAMP, cyclic adenosine monophosphate; DAG, diacylglycerol; GABA, γ-aminobutyric acid; IP_3, inositol triphosphate; NMDA, N-methyl-D-aspartate.
[a]Three subtypes of α_1 and three subtypes of α_2 receptors have been identified.
Modified from Ganong.[108]

epinephrine, and a very high affinity for isoproterenol. Uptake 2 is of the greatest physiological significance in the elimination of circulating catecholamines, primarily epinephrine, released by the adrenal gland, and has little physiological significance for norepinephrine released at postganglionic sympathetic nerve terminals.

Adrenoreceptors

The sequence of intracellular events initiated by receptor binding of norepinephrine is determined by the type of adrenoreceptor stimulated. The classification of adrenoreceptors continues to evolve based on both pharmacological and molecular criteria.[83–87] All adrenoreceptors have a similar homology of structure and produce intracellular events by binding to membrane guanine nucleotide–regulatory proteins (G proteins).[88] The structure of the G-protein–coupled receptor consists of a single-subunit protein with seven hydrophobic transmembrane segments, three hydrophilic extracellular sequences, and three hydrophilic intracytoplasmic loops. These membrane-associated regulatory proteins

serve to convert the signal arriving at the cell membrane into a specific enzyme system response or ion-channel activity that produces a cellular response. Autonomic transmission in the cardiovascular system is initiated by stimulation of three different G proteins: G_s stimulates adenylate cyclase, causing a rise in intracellular cAMP. G_i inhibits adenylate cyclase, decreasing the concentration of intracellular cAMP (Table 4.9). G_p activates phospholipase C, which hydrolyzes phosphoinositol to inositol triphosphate (IP_3) and diacylglycerol (DAG). IP_3 causes the release of calcium ions (Ca^{2+}) from the sarcoplasmic reticulum. DAG activates protein kinase C, which phosphorylates contractile proteins in the myocardium and vascular smooth muscle.

β-Adrenoreceptors are classified pharmacologically into three types—β_1, β_2, and β_3—based on their relative affinities for various agonists.[87] The physiological significance of the β_3 receptor is unclear, but appears to be involved in regulation of metabolism and energy regulation. The β_1- and β_2-adrenoreceptor subtypes, when activated by norepinephrine, epinephrine, or other β-

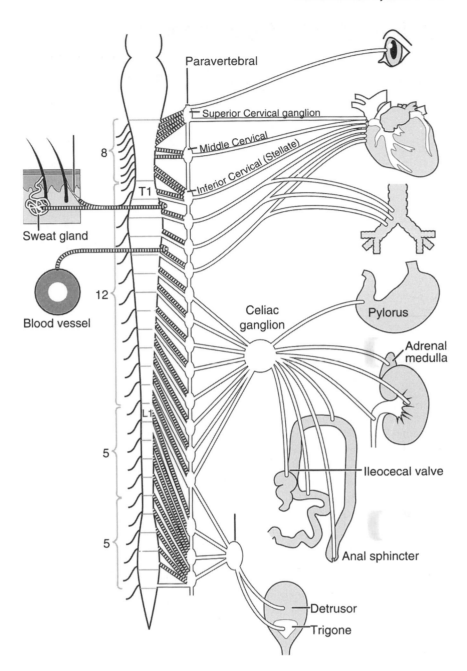

Fig. 4.33. The sympathetic nervous system. Note the location of the stellate and hypogastric ganglia. m, muscle. Modified from Guyton,[105] p. 668.

adrenergic agonists, stimulate the formation of the enzyme adenylate cyclase through the G_s protein, causing an increase in intracellular cAMP. β-Adrenoreceptors also activate L-type Ca^{2+} channels in myocardial and vascular tissue, thereby increasing intracellular calcium concentration (Table 4.9). Both $β_1$- and $β_2$- adrenoreceptors are found in the heart and are responsible for increases in heart rate and contractility during sympathetic stimulation (Table 4.10). β-Adrenoreceptor stimulation increases the slope of phase 4 diastolic depolarization in pacemaker tissues and subsidiary automatic cells. Increases in intracellular cAMP and Ca^{2+} increase cardiac contractility and facilitate cardiac relaxation. Although both $β_1$- and $β_2$-adrenoreceptors are present in the heart, $β_1$-adrenoreceptors predominate during health, especially in the ventricular myocardium.

$β_2$-Adrenoreceptors relax smooth muscle in vascular, bronchial,

gastrointestinal, and genitourinary tissues. $β_2$-Adrenoreceptors in the vasculature are not innervated and therefore produce vasodilation in response to circulating catecholamines or drugs. Their location in specific vascular beds suggests a role in the distribution of blood flow, especially during exercise.

Three $α_1$-receptor subtypes have been classified according to their affinity to adrenergic agonists.[86,87] The receptor subtypes are designated $α_{1A}$, $α_{1B}$, and $α_{1C}$, but their distribution is not universal across species or within specific tissue beds. All $α_1$- adrenoreceptor subtypes currently identified produce their intracellular effect by activation of the enzyme phospholipase C via the G_p protein. Phospholipase C hydrolyzes phosphoinositol and releases Ca^{2+} from intracytoplasmic stores, causing the contractile response seen in myocardial or vascular smooth muscle cells (Tables 4.9 and 4.10).

Table 4.10. G-protein–coupled receptor superfamily of genes and gene products in cardiac tissue[a]

Receptor Type and Subtype	Location	G Protein	Biological Response
Adrenergic			
β_1	Myocardium	G_s	AC stimulation, positive inotropic and chronotropic responses
	Coronary vascular	G_2	AC stimulation, vasodilation(?)
β_2	Myocardium	G_s	AC stimulation, positive inotropic and chronotropic responses
	Coronary vasculature(?)	G_s	AC stimulation, vasodilation(?)
α_1	Myocardium	G_p	PI hydrolysis stimulation, positive inotropic response(?)
	Coronary vasculature	G_p	PI stimulation, vasoconstriction
Muscarinic			
m_2	Myocardium	G_i	Shorten atrial action potential; slow sinus rate; slow AV conduction; AC inhibition, negative inotrope, and chronotrope
m_3	Coronary smooth muscle	G_p(?)	PI stimulation, vasoconstriction
m_3	Coronary endothelium	G_p(?)	EDRF production, GC stimulation, vasodilation

[a]AC, adenylate cyclase; EDRF, endothelium-derived relaxing factor or nitric oxide; GC, guanylate cyclase; PI, phosphatidylinositol. Modified from Opie,[106] p. 164.

Three subtypes of α_2-adrenoreceptors—α_{2A}, α_{2B}, and α_{2C}—have been identified by pharmacological studies, although the tissue distribution of these subtypes is unclear.[89] α_2-Adrenoreceptors inhibit adenylate cyclase through the G_i protein. Inhibition of adenylate cyclase attenuates cAMP production in target cells. This mechanism is important in platelets and renal tubules; however, in vascular smooth muscle, an alternative signal transduction mechanism is responsible for the vasoconstrictor response. α_2-Adrenoreceptors are located presynaptically and extrasynaptically in vascular smooth muscle. Stimulation of extrasynaptic α_2-adrenoreceptors by α-adrenergic agonists activates a receptor-operated calcium channel that increases the concentration of calcium intracellularly, producing vascular smooth muscle contraction that complements the contractile effect of α_1-adrenoreceptors activated by stimulation of sympathetic nerves. Because of their extrasynaptic location, α_2-adrenoreceptors respond to circulating catecholamines, such as epinephrine and norepinephrine, and aid in maintaining generalized sympathetic vasoconstriction in response to catecholamine output from the adrenal gland. This later response is important in the fight-flight response that occurs in crisis situations such as trauma or hemorrhage.

The α_1- and α_2-adrenoreceptors coexist in the vasculature as described earlier.[87] There is a greater response to α_2 stimulation on the venous side of the circulation compared to the arterial side. Therefore, α_2-adrenoreceptor–mediated vasoconstriction may be most important in mobilizing blood volume from veins, leading to an increase in cardiac filling, which is an important first step in increasing cardiac output during stress situations such as exercise or hemorrhage. Receptor-operated calcium channels in vascular smooth muscle can be blocked by calcium antagonists (e.g., verapamil, diltiazem, or nifedipine).[89]

The α_1- and α_2-adrenoreceptors can cause complementary or antagonistic responses, depending on their location. For example, norepinephrine stimulates α_1-adrenoreceptors located on the postsynaptic cell membrane, causing contraction of vascular smooth muscle and vasoconstriction. Norepinephrine also binds to presynaptic α_2-adrenoreceptors, producing a negative-feedback effect that decreases the release of norepinephrine from the nerve terminal. Thus, α_2-adrenoreceptors help to modulate the vasoconstrictor response initiated by α_1-postsynaptic-receptor stimulation. The α_2-adrenoreceptors help to ensure that only a short-term vasoconstrictor response occurs after sympathetic nerve stimulation.

Dopamine is the immediate metabolic precursor of norepinephrine in adrenergic nerves and functions as a neurotransmitter in the CNS (Table 4.9).[90] Disorders of dopamine transmission in the CNS are recognized clinically in human patients as Parkinson's disease. Peripheral dopamine receptors (DA_1 and DA_2) are particularly important in regulating blood flow to the mesenteric and renal vascular beds. Postsynaptic DA_1 receptors in the renal and mesenteric vascular beds cause vasodilation, increasing perfusion to renal and splanchnic tissues. DA_2 receptors, located presynaptically on postganglionic sympathetic nerves, inhibit the release of norepinephrine, much like the presynaptic α_2-adrenoreceptors.

Stimulation of postganglionic sympathetic fibers supplying vascular smooth muscle causes not only the release of the neurotransmitter norepinephrine, but also the release of the cotransmitter neuropeptide Y.[90,91] Neuropeptide Y is present in vesicles contained in postganglionic sympathetic nerve terminals, is synergistic with the effects of norepinephrine on the peripheral vasculature, and produces vasoconstriction. Neuropeptide Y is also found in the adrenal medulla. Circulating levels of neuropeptide Y inhibit renin release and stimulate the release of ANP. The role of neuropeptide Y in cardiovascular regulation has not been fully characterized; however, it may be an important mediator in the central control of blood pressure.

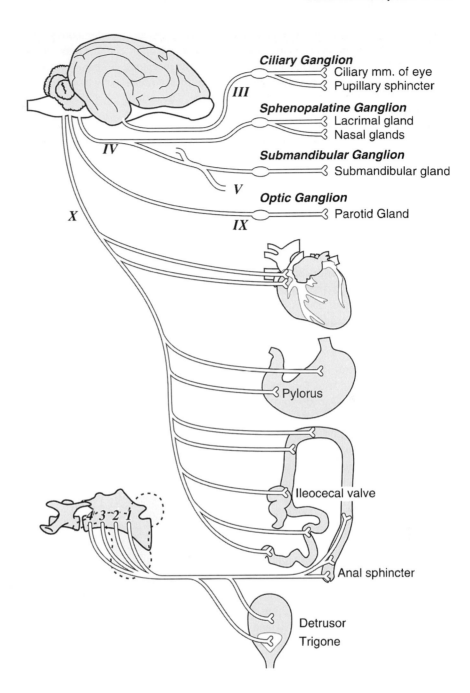

Fig. 4.34. The parasympathetic nervous system. Note the distribution of cranial nerves III, IV, V, IX, and X. mm, muscles. Modified from Guyton,[105] p. 669.

Sympathetic cholinergic nerve fibers originate in the cerebral cortex and send descending fibers to the spinal cord. These nerve fibers synapse in the sympathetic ganglia and send postganglionic fibers to precapillary vessels in skeletal muscle.[83] Postganglionic cholinergic sympathetic nerve fibers are activated only during times of high sympathetic tone (fear, pain, or exercise) and release acetylcholine, which produces vasodilation in skeletal muscle.

Parasympathetic Nervous System

The parasympathetic nervous system (PNS) originates from two sites within the CNS: cervical spinal cord and sacral spinal cord (Fig. 4.34). Long preganglionic parasympathetic nerve fibers located in the CNS synapse with relatively short postganglionic parasympathetic neurons in ganglia located in the target organ. The cranial portion of the parasympathetic nervous system originates in the medulla oblongata. Axions travel via the vagus nerve to synapse with postganglionic parasympathetic nerves that terminate in the heart and blood vessels.[76,83]

Parasympathetic Neurotransmission

Acetylcholine is the neurotransmitter released at autonomic ganglia and from postganglionic parasympathetic nerves. Cholinergic nerves actively transport choline from the extracellular fluid into the neural axoplasm, where it is acted upon by the enzyme choline acetyltransferase, combined with acetyl coenzyme A, and converted to acetylcholine, which like norepinephrine is stored in vesicles within the nerve. Cholinergic nerve action potentials increase intracellular calcium, causing vesicular and nerve cell membrane fusion and the release of acetylcholine into the synaptic cleft. Acetylcholine binds to specific receptors, mediating a cellular response that varies with the tissue innervated and the type of cholinergic receptor involved. The actions of acetylcholine are rapidly terminated by hydrolysis into choline and acetic acid by the enzyme acetylcholinesterase. The acetylcholine that diffuses out of the synaptic cleft and into the extracellular fluid or plasma is hydrolyzed by plasma butyrylcholinesterase (pseudocholinesterase). The choline produced from this metabolism is rapidly taken up by the nerve cell and used in the resynthesis of acetylcholine.

Cholinoreceptors

Cholinergic receptors are either nicotinic or muscarinic and are totally unrelated in location, structure, and function (Tables 4.9 and 4.10). Nicotinic receptors are located in autonomic ganglia, in the adrenal medulla, and at the neuromuscular junction of skeletal muscle. Muscarinic receptors are located at postganglionic parasympathetic nerve terminals.[92]

Nicotinic receptors are pentameric membrane proteins that form a nonselective ion channel in the cell membrane. Postsynaptic nicotinic receptors, located in the autonomic ganglia or the neuromuscular junction, when stimulated by acetylcholine, open their ion channel, allowing the flow of cations into the nerve or muscle cell, resulting in depolarization and ultimately nerve cell transmission of an electric impulse or muscular contraction. Nicotinic receptors are subclassified into N_G receptors, located at autonomic ganglia, and N_S receptors, located in the neuromuscular junction and within the CNS.

Muscarinic receptors are located in the autonomic effector organs of the parasympathetic nervous system, for example, the heart, smooth muscle, and the exocrine glands.[92] They are G protein coupled and show more homology to adrenergic and dopaminergic receptors than to the nicotinic cholinergic receptors. Five different cholinergic receptors have been distinguished through molecular binding techniques. Muscarinic receptors m_1, m_3, and m_5 are functionally similar and, when bound to their respective G proteins, stimulate phosphoinositol hydrolysis through activation of phospholipase C (Table 4.10). Muscarinic receptors m_2 and m_4 show similarity in that they both attenuate the actions of adenylate cyclase intracellularly.

The vagus nerve innervates the sinoatrial node, the atrial myocardium, the atrioventricular node, and to a much lesser extent the ventricular myocardium. Stimulation of m_2 receptors by acetylcholine activates several different membrane G proteins, resulting in inhibition of adenylate cyclase, activation of potassium channels, and activation of phospholipase C, which hydrolyzes phosphoinositol. These effects cause a decrease in the slope of phase 4 diastolic depolarization in pacemaker and subsidiary automatic tissues, and hyperpolarization of cardiac cell membranes through activation of membrane potassium channels. Heart rate is decreased, as are the rate of conduction of impulses through the atrioventricular node and cardiac contractility. High levels of parasympathetic tone can produce atrioventricular block (first-degree, second-degree, and third-degree heart block) and

temporary cardiac asystole. Stimulation of the parasympathetic nervous system produces minimal effects on most peripheral blood vessels. Acetylcholine binds to m_2 receptors in vessels, which mediates an endothelium-dependent vasorelaxation (Fig. 4.35).

The sacral division of the parasympathetic nervous system has preganglionic nerve cell bodies located in the intermediolateral column of the spinal cord.[76,83] Parasympathetic nerves in this region congregate to form the nervi erigentes or pelvic nerves that innervate the intestines, colon, rectum, bladder, and genitalia (Fig. 4.34). Stimulation of the parasympathetic nerves also causes increased blood flow to salivary glands and genital erectile tissue.

Humoral Mechanisms

The autonomic nervous system functions to produce acute changes in cardiovascular function that can be large in magnitude, but are generally brief. Sustained changes in cardiopulmonary function are produced by humoral mechanisms (Table 4.7).[75–77] The adrenal medulla is a modified sympathetic ganglion innervated by preganglionic sympathetic fibers and is part of the sympathetic nervous system. The neuronal cells of the adrenal medulla, rather than sending axons to target organs, release the neurotransmitters, epinephrine and norepinephrine, into the circulation. Precipitating factors for the release of catecholamines from the adrenal medulla include pain, trauma, hypovolemia, hypotension, hypoxia, hypothermia, hypoglycemia, exercise stress, and fear (fight-flight). Circulating catecholamines produce a variety of effects, including increases in metabolic rate, glycogenolysis in the liver and skeletal muscle, gluconeogenesis in the liver, and an increase in the availability of free fatty acids, an important nutrient source for the myocardium. Circulating catecholamines increase heart rate and cardiac contractility, dilate vascular beds in skeletal and cardiac muscle, and constrict splanchnic and cutaneous arterioles, diminishing blood supply to organs that are less essential during a fight-flight response.[66] The actions of the adrenal medulla are complementary to the effects of sympathetic nerve stimulation. Together the autonomic nervous system and humoral mechanisms provide both rapid (nervous system) and sustained (humoral) responses to stressful situations.[75,76,83]

The kidney is the major site for activation of the renin-angiotensin system.[75] Renin is produced in the kidney during sodium depletion, decreases in extracellular fluid volume, or increases in sympathetic output (Table 4.11). Secretion of renin into the systemic circulation converts circulating angiotensinogen, produced by the liver, to angiotensin I. Angiotensin I is converted to angiotensin II by an angiotensin-converting enzyme that is present in pulmonary vascular endothelium. Angiotensin II produces arteriolar constriction, producing increases in blood pressure, and stimulates the adrenal cortex to release aldosterone, a hormone that causes renal reabsorption of Na^+ and water, effectively increasing thirst and the extracellular fluid volume (Fig. 4.36).

The hypothalamus is directly involved in the central neural

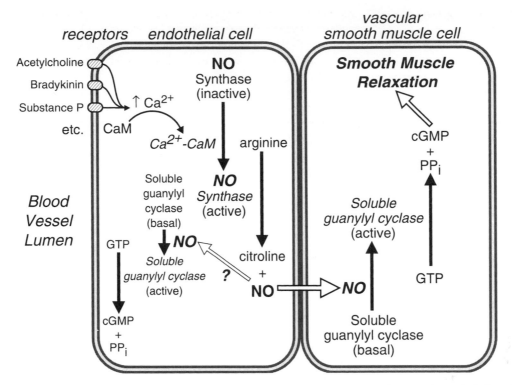

Fig. 4.35. Various agonists (acetylcholine, bradykinin, and substance P) stimulate receptors on the vascular endothelium, leading to the formation of nitric oxide (NO), which modulates the formation of soluble guanylyl cyclase, which in turn facilitates the formation of cyclic guanosine monophosphate (cGMP) and smooth muscle relaxation. Ca^{2+}, calcium; CaM, calmodulin; GTP, guanosine triphosphate; and PP_i, free phosphate. Modified from Guyton.[105]

Table 4.11. Stimuli that increase renin secretion

Increased sympathetic activity
Sodium depletion
Diuretics
Hypotension
Hemorrhage
Upright posture
Dehydration
Constriction of renal artery or aorta
Cardiac failure

control of cardiovascular responses, but it also plays an important role in the humoral regulation of cardiovascular function. Arginine vasopressin (antidiuretic hormone [ADH]) is produced in the hypothalamus and is transported through nerve cell axons to the posterior pituitary.[75] Under normal circumstances, the pituitary releases vasopressin in response to increases in plasma solute, resulting in an increase in circulating vasopressin. Vasopressin acts on the collecting ducts of the kidney, where it stimulates water conservation, thereby returning plasma osmolality (and volume) to normal. Vasopressin is a vasoconstrictor, especially in mesenteric vessels; therefore, the presence of circulating vasopressin is influential in the redistribution of systemic

blood flow. Vasopressin release by the pituitary can also occur in the absence of changes in plasma osmolality. Examples of nonosmotic stimuli that cause the release of vasopressin are pain, stress, hypoxia, heart failure, and vascular volume depletion. A number of anesthetic drugs are associated with increased circulating levels of arginine vasopressin, including opioids (morphine and meperidine) and barbiturates.[75]

Local Control Systems in the Vasculature

Autoregulation is the ability of blood vessels to adjust blood flow in accordance with metabolic need and to maintain blood flow despite extreme changes in tissue perfusion pressure (Fig. 4.37).[66] Most tissues can regulate their own blood flow during physiological changes in perfusion pressure.[68]

Neurogenic basal tone exists in many vessels. Nonneurogenic (intrinsic) basal tone is additive to neurogenic basal tone and is present in vessels of the skin and skeletal muscle. A reduction in vasomotor tone in these vessels usually represents a reduction in the neurogenic component. *Active dilation* is a term applied when vascular tone decreases below the nonneurogenic basal level and is the result of two components, a pressure-sensitive mechanism termed the *myogenic component* and a metabolic mechanism that is influenced by local oxygen tension.[66,68] Both mechanisms are linked to the release of local vasodilatory mediators. This phe-

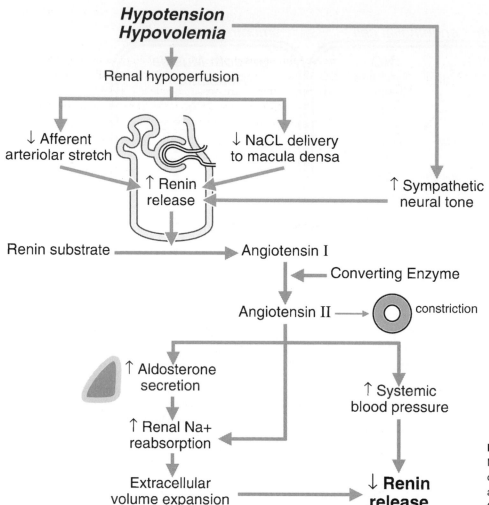

Hypotension
Hypovolemia

Renal hypoperfusion

↓ Afferent
arteriolar stretch

↓ NaCL delivery
to macula densa

↑ Renin
release

↑ Sympathetic
neural tone

Renin substrate ⟶ Angiotensin I

⟵ Converting Enzyme

Angiotensin II ⟶ ⬤ constriction

↑ Aldosterone
secretion

↑ Systemic
blood pressure

↑ Renal Na+
reabsorption

Extracellular
volume expansion ⟶ ↓ **Renin release**

Fig. 4.36. The renin-angiotensin system. Note that either hypotension or hypovolemia can cause renal hypoperfusion and activation of the sympathetic nervous system, which increase renal renin release.

nomenon, also termed *reactive hyperemia*, occurs in arterioles less than 25 μm in diameter. The myogenic mechanism is responsible for reactive hyperemia after short occlusion periods (<30 s). As flow returns to the previously occluded arteriole, blood flow velocity increases, which increases wall shear stress, causing the release of nitric oxide from the vascular endothelium.[93] The metabolic component of reactive hyperemia occurs after longer periods of occlusion (30 s). Decreases in oxygen tension release a vasodilatory prostaglandin that maintains blood flow until normal oxygen tension is reestablished. Endothelial damage in small arterioles eliminates the reactive hyperemic response altogether, since both nitric oxide and prostaglandins are products of vascular endothelial cells.[66,79,82,93] Hyperbaric oxygen conditions also eliminate the metabolic component of reactive hyperemia by maintaining elevated oxygen tensions in tissues despite vascular occlusion. Stretch of vascular smooth muscle opposes the myogenic vasodilator response seen in larger vessels (Bayliss effect).[66] The proposed mechanism for the Bayliss effect is a pressure-induced depolarization of the endothelial cell mediated through an inwardly rectifying potassium channel. The effects of anesthetic drugs on reactive hyperemia and the Bayliss effect are incompletely understood and highly variable.

Capillary blood flow is linked to the rate of tissue metabolism and oxygen tension. The exact mechanism involved in this linkage is not completely understood, although a number of mechanisms may be responsible for regulating capillary blood flow.[68] The number of open precapillary sphincters is approximately proportional to the level of metabolic activity in the tissue supplied. As metabolic activity increases, the local oxygen tension decreases until a critical level of tissue hypoxia occurs, inducing vasodilation. Precapillary sphincters are also responsive to mediators that are released as by-products of tissue metabolism, such as lactic acid, carbon dioxide, and potassium.

Peptides and other substances are important in regulating tissue blood flow (Table 4.12). The actions of local enzymes produce kinins such as bradykinin from the substrate kallikrein. Kinins produce vasodilatory effects that are short-lived because of rapid inactivation by peptidases in the plasma. Arachidonic acid metabolism produces a variety of prostaglandins that tend to be compartmentalized and produce very specific local effects. Stimulation of arachidonic acid metabolism in the pulmonary vasculature results in the production of the vasodilatory prostaglandin prostacyclin (prostaglandin I_2 [PGI_2]). Renal hypoperfusion initiates the production of PGI_2, which acts to re-

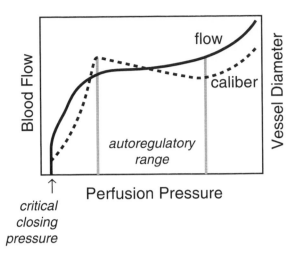

Fig. 4.37. The relationship between blood flow and perfusion pressure in peripheral vascular beds is characterized by an autoregulatory range over which blood flow changes very little regardless of increases or decreases in perfusion pressure. The normal autoregulatory range for most vascular beds is between 60 and 180 mm Hg. Some vascular beds (brain, gut, and skeletal muscle) acutely collapse when the perfusion pressure approximates 15 to 30 mm Hg (critical closing pressure). Modified from Shepherd and Vanhoutte,[102] p. 95.

store renal blood flow, urine volume, and sodium excretion. The preanesthetic administration of nonsteroidal anti-inflammatory analgesics (NSAIAs) may interfere with the production of these important prostaglandins by cyclooxygenase enzyme inhibition. There are specific receptor sites on vascular endothelium for a variety of agonists (including acetylcholine, bradykinin, and histamine) that when bound by the appropriate agonist induce the formation and release of nitric oxide. Nitric oxide is rapidly deactivated by hemoglobin and therefore is only important as a local mediator. Nitric oxide relaxes vascular smooth muscle through stimulation of guanylate cyclase, increasing intracellular cGMP (Fig. 4.35). Vascular endothelial cells also produce a po-

tent vasoconstrictor substance known as *endothelin* that acts upon endothelin receptors on vascular smooth muscle cells.[66,83] Endothelin is released by the endothelium in response to increased intraluminal pressure, contributing to the Bayliss effect, and is selective for certain vascular beds, including coronary vessels, renal afferent arteries, and venous capacitance vessels. It is both a positive inotrope and a chronotrope. Endothelin increases plasma levels of other humoral mediators, such as atrial natriuretic factor, renin, aldosterone, and circulating catecholamines. Endothelin receptors have been located in several areas of the brain involved in modulation of autonomic nervous system efferent activity (Table 4.12).

Diseases of the Cardiovascular System

Heart Disease

Historically, heart disease has been categorized based on cause, structural defect, and functional changes. Heart disease can produce heart failure, which is characterized by neurohumoral activation, sodium retention, and tissue proliferation (cardiac hypertrophy). One clinically useful method for categorizing heart disease is based on clinical signs (exercise intolerance, ascites, edema, cough, etc.). *Acute* and *chronic heart failure* are differentiated on the basis of the rapidity of development of clinical signs. Chronic heart failure usually takes many months to years to develop and is associated with a variety of compensatory neuroendocrine, physiological, and pathophysiological adjustments. *Congenital* or *acquired* heart disease identifies the condition as being present since birth or developing in association with a specific developing cardiac lesion. Congenital or acquired heart disease can be acute or chronic. *Right-sided* or *left-sided heart failure* identifies the right or left ventricle as the primary cause of heart failure. *Systolic dysfunction* and *diastolic dysfunction* refer to the phase of the cardiac cycle that is most severely compromised. *Forward heart failure* refers to cardiac diseases that cause a low cardiac output secondary to an impediment to ventricular ejection (increased afterload), decreased inotropy, or both. *Backward failure* refers to situations that cause pulmonary and

Table 4.12. Summary of factors affecting the caliber of the arterioles

Constriction	Dilation
Increased noradrenergic discharge	Decreased noradrenergic discharge
Circulating catecholamines (except epinephrine in skeletal muscle and liver)	Circulating epinephrine in skeletal muscle and liver
Circulating angiotensin II	Circulating atrial natriuretic peptide
Circulating arginine vasopressin (ADH)	Activation of cholinergic dilators in skeletal muscle
Locally released serotonin	Bradykinin
Endothelin I	Histamine
Neuropeptide Y	Substance P (axon reflex)
Circulating Na^+-K^+ ATPase inhibitor	Nitric oxide and endothelium-derived relaxing factor
Decreased local temperature	Prostacyclin and prostaglandin E_2
	Increased carbon dioxide tension
	Decreased pH
	Lactate, potassium ions, adenosine, etc.
	Increased local temperature

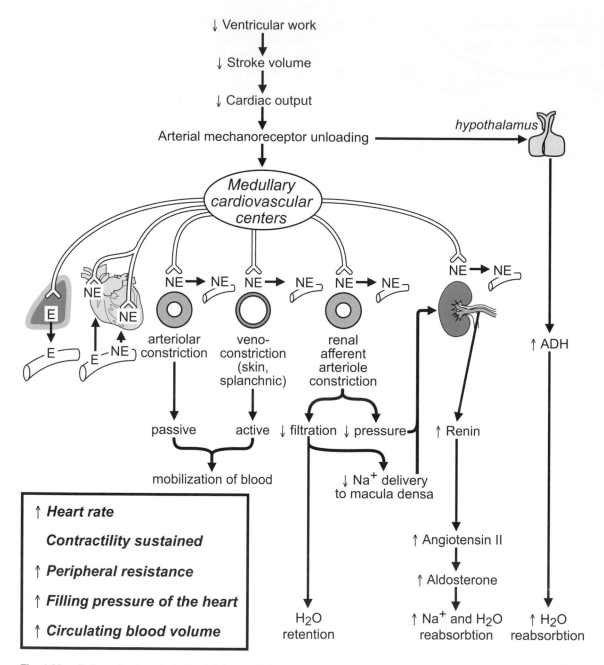

Fig. 4.38. Reflex adjustments to heart failure and decreased ventricular work include increases in heart rate, peripheral vascular resistance, vascular capacity, filling pressure of the heart, and circulating blood volume. Cardiac contractility is sustained by increases in sympathetic tone. These changes help to maintain cardiac output. ADH, antidiuretic hormone; E, epinephrine; and NE, norepinephrine. Modified from Shepherd and Vanhoutte,[102] p. 259.

systemic venous congestion (congestive heart failure). *Low output failure* occurs when cardiac output is below normal and *high output failure* when (and regardless of cardiac contractile function) cardiac output is above normal (e.g., septic shock). It should be clear that the terms that have evolved to categorize heart failure (acute, chronic; right-sided, left-sided; systolic, diastolic; forward, backward; and low output or high output) are for the most part descriptive and that an appreciation of their meaning must be considered in association with the pathophysiological compensatory changes that occur.

Heart disease from any cause usually progresses through three phases: overload (excessive work), compensatory, and pathological.[94] Whatever the inciting cause, ventricular overload brought about by excessive work leads to increases in both the oxygen and the nutrient requirements of the heart. Initial compensatory changes include increases in sympathetic tone and a variety of neurohumoral responses that act to sustain or increase cardiac inotropy and promote the retention of salt and water (Fig. 4.38). These responses are usually followed by compensatory ventricular hypertrophy associated with decreases in both the rate of ventricular pressure development and the rate of relaxation. The pathological phase of heart failure exists when an abnormality in cardiac function and excessive or maladaptive compensatory responses become responsible for a decrease in cardiac output to a degree that is insufficient to meet the oxygen and nutrient requirements of metabolizing tissues or exercising muscle. It is important to realize that this definition incorporates situations in which the heart may be contracting normally or be hypercontractile. For example, cardiac output may be decreased during sinus tachycardia or bradycardia, cardiac arrhythmias, and the initial stages of valvular insufficiency (mitral insufficiency). Decrease in cardiac contractile performance is only one potential cause for a decrease in cardiac output and should be differentiated from other potential causes of heart failure in order to provide appropriate therapy and prevent drug-induced complications.

Ultimately, failure of the ventricular myocardium is caused by pressure overload, volume overload, or primary myocardial disease (cardiomyopathy). The cardiomyopathies have been further categorized as hypertrophic, dilated, restrictive (infiltrative myocardial disease), or constrictive (pericardial disease).[94] The cause for many forms of hypertrophic and dilated cardiomyopathy remains unknown. The signal for ventricular hypertrophy, although uncertain, is probably multifactorial, involving stretch-activated ion channels, increased ventricular tension, adrenergic factors, increased oxygen consumption (oxygen supply/demand imbalance), and ATP use or increases in the quantity of metabolic breakdown products. Regardless of stimulus, increased work initiates the production of growth factors that, through various proto-oncogenes (*c-fos* and *m-myc*) and in conjunction with the production of heat-shock proteins (HSP-70), stimulate transcription, variably change myofibrillar isoform ratios from fast to slow (V_1 to V_3), and increase cell growth.[94,95] Clinically and experimentally, diseases that produce sustained pressure overload (aortic and pulmonic stenosis and hypertension) cause concentric ventricular hypertrophy, which is characterized by marked increases in ventricular wall thickness without increases in ventricular volume. Heart disease that is caused by volume overload is generally the result of valvular regurgitation (aortic or mitral incompetence) or congenital defects (atrial or ventricular septal defect or patent ductus arteriosus) and produces longitudinal or so-called eccentric hypertrophy. Longitudinal hypertrophy is characterized by increases in chamber volume without an increase in wall thickness. The type of ventricular hypertrophy that develops is governed by processes that minimize myocardial oxygen consumption and work and maintain or maximize ventricular efficiency. Regardless, myocardial hypertrophy produces cellular changes that interfere with normal cellular metabolism and predisposes patients to systolic and diastolic dysfunction (Table 4.13). These intracellular changes and resultant abnormalities in ventricular function are further exacerbated by a decrease in capillary surface area to cell volume (capillary inadequacy), thereby limiting oxygen delivery, which increases myocardial fibrosis. Decreases in oxygen delivery, whether brought about by capillary inadequacy, low cardiac output, or anemia, can result in myocardial ischemia, tissue hypoxia, and lactic acidosis (Fig. 4.39). Subendocardial ischemia is particularly common in pa-

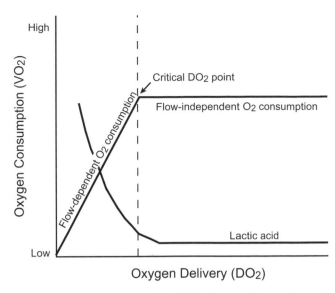

Fig. 4.39. Oxygen consumption (VO_2) is normally not limited by oxygen delivery ($DO_2 = CO \times CaO_2$) and oxygen extraction ($OE = CaO_2 - CvO_2$). However, decreases in cardiac output (blood flow) to critically low values (e.g., hemorrhagic shock or heart failure) produce situations where VO_2 can become DO_2 dependent. Oxygen deprivation (anaerobic metabolism) generates lactic acid, resulting in metabolic acidosis. CaO_2, arterial oxygen content; CO, cardiac output; and CvO_2, venous oxygen content.

Table 4.13. Receptors and signaling systems in heart failure

1. Receptors
   β_1-Adrenergic receptors downgraded, i.e., density decreased
   β_2-Adrenergic receptor density unchanged, function uncoupling
   α_1-Adrenergic receptors have increased activity
   These receptors actually decrease in density, but affinity is considerably increased
2. G proteins
   G_i increased with inhibition of adenylate cyclase
   G_s normal or decreased
3. Adenylate cyclase
   Decreased cyclase activity with less production of cAMP, related to G_i increase; still responds directly to forskolin
4. cAMP
   Production impaired, presumably due to adenylate cyclase inhibition
5. Calcium transients
   Transients with low peak and delayed fall in diastole
   Calcium uptake by sarcoplasmic reticulum unchanged or decreased in situ
   Calcium release by sarcoplasmic reticulum increased
   Decreased myofibrillae
   Sensitivity to calcium ion
   Activity of single calcium channels is normal
   Amount of calcium entry via calcium channel may be abnormal

cAMP, cyclic adenosine monophosphate.
Modified from Opie,[106] p. 409.

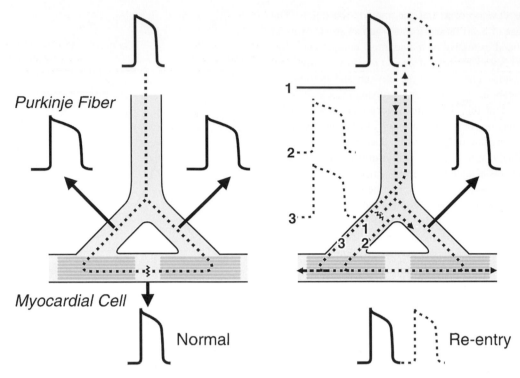

Fig. 4.40. During normal conditions, the cardiac action potential is transmitted through modified muscle fibers (specialized fibers) to the atrial and ventricular muscle cells, causing depolarization followed by repolarization. The action potential is not perpetuated because the surrounding tissues at the end point of activation remain refractory to reactivation (normal). During various disease processes (ischemia, hypoxia, inflammation, or fibrosis) and in the presence of some drugs (intravenous and inhalation anesthetics), the action potential may be blocked (unidirectional block) as it travels in an antegrade direction through cardiac tissue (*1*). If the electrical impulse is delayed (conduction delay) as it travels through adjacent tissue, it may reenter and be conducted in a retrograde direction (retrograde conduction), thereby reactivating the same tissue segment (*2*) or more peripheral tissue segments (*3*). The longer the conduction delay, the more likely is it that the electric impulse will find the tissue to be reentered excitable (not refractory) and the greater the likelihood for reentry (*dotted lines*). Continuous reentry of cardiac tissue is called *circus movement* and can lead to sustained cardiac rhythm disturbances, including ventricular fibrillation. Reentry involving a small amount (several square millimeters) of cardiac tissue is called *microreentry*, whereas reentry that incorporates the specialized conducting system of the heart is called *macroreentry*.

tients with heart failure, because subendocardial perfusion is influenced by the difference between aortic diastolic pressure and ventricular end-diastolic pressure and the ventricular wall tension. Myocardial ischemia in turn causes abnormal cellular calcium cycling, intracellular calcium overload, oxygen wastage, cardiac arrhythmias, sarcomere contracture, and eventually cell death. Familiarity with the pathophysiological mechanisms of heart failure and cellular metabolism during heart failure and ischemia aids in the selection of appropriate preanesthetic and anesthetic drugs and suggests potential approaches for therapy.[44]

Cardiac Arrhythmias

Cardiac arrhythmias include abnormalities in cardiac rate, rhythm, site of origin of the cardiac impulse, or pattern of atrial or ventricular depolarization. The cause for cardiac arrhythmias in intact hearts is attributed to abnormalities in automaticity, conduction, or both (Table 4.14). Ultimately, all changes in cardiac electric activity can be thought of in terms of alterations in one or more of the active or passive electrophysiological properties of the cell membrane.[24] Increases or decreases in normal automatic-

ity in spontaneously beating hearts, for example, result from changes in phase 4 depolarization, which is electrically initiated by calcium (I_{Ca}) and sodium (I_f) currents in sinoatrial and atrioventricular node or sodium (I_f) and potassium (I_{K1}) currents in Purkinje tissue. The ECG appearance of abnormal impulses due to abnormal automaticity, however, are most likely caused by changes in I_K or I_{Ca}. Abnormal electric impulses that occur as a direct result of prior electric activity are referred to as "triggered" and are in most instances caused by defects in I_{Ca}, leading to the development of both early (prior to repolarization) or delayed (after repolarization) afterpotentials arising from the cell membrane.[22] Abnormal heart rhythm caused by abnormal conduction and random or ordered reentry can be caused by spatial differences in membrane refractory periods or discontinuous anisotropic (dissimilar in all directions) propagation (Fig. 4.40). The latter electrophysiological abnormality can occur as a result of cellular uncoupling owing to a decreased number of effective cellular connections (gap junctions) caused by fibrosis, ischemia, or drug effects.[24,26,27] Regardless of cause, changes in either the active properties (ion-current movements) or the passive proper-

Table 4.14. Classification of arrhythmogenic mechanisms at the cellular level in terms of vulnerable parameters

Mechanisms of Arrhythmia	Vulnerable Parameter (Antiarrhythmic Effect)	Ionic Currents Most Likely to Modulate Vulnerable Parameter
Automaticity		
A. Enhanced normal automaticity	Phase 4 depolarization (decrease)	I_f; $I_{Ca\text{-}T}$ (block)
B. Abnormal automaticity	Maximum diastolic potential (hyperpolarize) or phase 4 depolarization (decrease)	I_{KACh} (activate) I_X; I_{KACh} (activate) $I_{Ca\text{-}L}$; I_{Na} (block)
Triggered activity		
A. Early afterdepolarizations (EADs)	Action-potential duration (shorten) or EADs (suppress)	I_X; (activate)
B. Delayed afterdepolarizations (DADs)	Calcium overload (unload) or DADs (suppress)	$I_{Ca\text{-}L}$; INa (block) $I_{Ca\text{-}L}$ (block) $I_{Ca\text{-}L}$; INa (block)
Conduction		
Reentry dependent on sodium channels		
A. Primary impaired conduction (long excitable gap)	Excitability and conduction (decrease)	I_{Na} (block)
B. Conduction encroaching on refractoriness (short excitable gap)	Effective refractory period (prolong)	I_K (block)
Other mechanisms		
A. Reentry dependent on calcium channels	Excitability and conduction (decrease)	$I_{Ca\text{-}L}$ (block)
B. Reflection	Excitability (decrease)	I_{Na}; $I_{Ca\text{-}L}$ (block)
C. Parasystole	Phase 4 depolarization (decrease)	I_f (block)

Modified from the Task Force of the Working Group on Arrhythmias of the European Society of Cardiology.[24]

ties (membrane characteristics) of the cardiac cell membrane can produce a wide array of cardiac rate or rhythm disturbances that are recordable at the body surface. Anesthetic drugs and various anesthetic techniques produce marked changes in cardiac cellular active and passive electrophysiological properties, resulting in the development of cardiac arrhythmias (Table 4.15). The inhalation anesthetics in particular are known to shorten the action potential and decrease refractoriness, thereby predisposing patients to conduction abnormalities and reentry. Halothane sensitizes the myocardium to catecholamines. Both α_1- and β_1-adrenoreceptors are involved in the cardiac sensitization phenomena.[96] Finally, most anesthetic drugs can produce pronounced effects on cardiac rate and rhythm because of their general membrane-depressant effects.

Vascular Disease

Primary diseases of the vascular system are not well recognized in veterinary medicine.[97] Arterial hypertension occurs in dogs and cats secondary to renal disease or endocrine disorders. Systemic hypertension is defined as a systolic blood pressure above 160 mm Hg and a diastolic blood pressure above 95 mm Hg. Chronic renal disease, especially glomerular disease, can be associated with systemic hypertension secondary to a decrease in renal blood flow and activation of the renin-angiotensin system, release of aldosterone, and an increase in sympathetic efferent activity.[75] Systemic vasoconstriction and renal retention of

sodium water contribute to the elevation of arterial blood pressure. Hyperadrenocorticism may cause systemic hypertension because mineralocorticoids cause retention of sodium and water, expanding the circulating blood volume. Pheochromocytomas secrete an excess of circulating catecholamines and perhaps neuropeptide Y, which induces systemic vasoconstriction, elevating blood pressure. No matter what the cause of systemic hypertension, myocardial work increases and can induce left ventricular hypertrophy and a decrease in cardiovascular reserve.

Canine heartworm disease can affect dogs and, rarely, cats.[97] Myointimal proliferation occurs in the pulmonary arteries, narrowing their lumen. Cellular debris from dying worms initiate the formation of thromboemboli that obstruct pulmonary arteries. Pulmonary vascular endothelial damage causes pulmonary vasoconstriction secondary to the loss of endothelium-derived relaxant factors. Right-sided congestive heart failure often develops secondary to the elevated pulmonary vascular resistance. Oxygen therapy (preoxygenation) and cardiovascular support may be required for heartworm patients prior to anesthesia.

Arteriovenous malformations cause an elevation in venous pressure that ultimately contributes to dilation and tortuosity of the vein. The arterial pressure downstream from the fistula may be decreased, impairing tissue perfusion. Arteriovenous malformations increase myocardial work by producing volume overload, similar to a ventricular septal defect or mitral insufficiency. The surgical correction of an arteriovenous fistula can produce reflex bradycardia (Branham's sign) at the time of shunt ligation.

Table 4.15. Cardiac arrhythmias produced by preanesthetic and anesthetic drugs

Drugs	Arrhythmia
Anticholinergics	
Atropine	Sinus tachycardia
Glycopyrrolate	Sinus tachycardia
Phenothiazine	
Acepromazine	Sinus tachycardia
	Sinus bradycardia (rarely)
α_2-Adrenergic agonists	
Xylazine	Sinus bradycardia, first-degree and second-degree atrioventricular
Detomidine	block, third-degree atrioventricular block (rarely), and sinus
Medetomidine	arrest (rarely)
Romifidine	
Opioids	Sinus bradycardia
Morphine	First-degree and second-degree atrioventricular block
Oxymorphone	
Hydromorphone	
Fentanyl	
Benzodiazepines	
Diazepam	Arrhythmias rarely observed; sinus bradycardia and temporary
Midazolam	cardiac arrest
Intravenous anesthetics	
Thiobarbiturates (thiamylal and thiopental)	Bradyarrhythmias
Ketamine	Premature ventricular depolarizations
Other injectables (propofol, etomidate, and alfaxolone are	Ventricular tachycardia
most likely to cause bradycardias)	Sinus tachycardia and ventricular arrhythmias
	Sinus tachycardia and bradyarrhythmias (rarely)
Inhalation anesthetics	
Halothane	Sinus bradycardia
Isoflurane	Bradyarrhythmias
Sevoflurane	Premature ventricular depolarizations
Desflurane	Ventricular tachycardia
	Ventricular fibrillation or cardiac arrest
	(Note: Halothane sensitizes the myocardium to catecholamines.)

The same phenomenon can be seen at the time of ligation of a patent ductus arteriosus due to the sudden increase in arterial pressure and the bradycardia induced by arterial baroreceptors. The administration of antimuscarinics can minimize or prevent bradycardia at this critical time.

Blood Components and Volume

Preservation of the integrity of the circulation is a responsibility that many humoral factors share. The effects of drugs used for chemical restraint and anesthesia (phenothiazines, butyrophenones, barbiturates, inhalation anesthetics) on clotting time and bleeding time are incompletely understood, but generally considered to be important in most animals. Exaggeration of bleeding disorders most frequently occurs in animals with thrombocytopenia or hereditary coagulation-factor deficiencies (von Willebrand's disease). Many drugs inhibit platelet aggregation, which normally contributes significantly to hemostasis.[98] Phenothiazines, barbiturates, and halothane decrease platelet numbers and inhibit platelet aggregation, although little change in gross

hemostasis occurs. Decreases in platelet and other circulating cell (red and white cells) numbers have been attributed to hemodilution secondary to hypotension, margination of white blood cells along vessel walls, and sequestration of RBCs in the spleen. Finally, it should be recognized that most intravenous and inhalation anesthetics are known to suppress the immune system, which is an effect that is generally short-lived but may become clinically relevant in immunosuppressed animals.[99]

The most important function of the cardiovascular system is to deliver oxygen and nutrients to metabolizing tissues.[3] The blood volume and hematocrit are of primary concern in maintaining adequate oxygen delivery, providing cardiac output and the distribution of blood flow are maintained within normal limits. The importance of adequate oxygen delivery (DO_2) cannot be overemphasized, because reduced oxygen consumption (VO_2) is known to be the common denominator in all forms of shock, including hemorrhagic and anemic shock (Fig. 4.39). There are multiple reasons for this: First, oxygen transport is the major function of the cardiovascular system; second, oxygen is the most flow-dependent blood constituent because it has the highest extraction ratio of any substance carried in the blood; third, oxygen cannot be stored; and, finally, oxygen transport and consumption are related to survival. Indeed, mortality is virtually 100% assured when the cumulative VO_2 deficit following hypoxemia, hemorrhage, or anemia exceeds 140 mL/kg.

Experimentally, hemorrhagic and anemic shock models are used to mimic clinical conditions where DO_2 and VO_2 are decreased. Popular models include a 50% to 75% decrease in blood volume (40 to 60 mL/kg; fixed-volume model), withdrawal of blood to a predetermined blood pressure (e.g., 40 mm Hg) and maintenance of this pressure for 2 h (fixed-pressure or Wigger's model), and a decrease of the hematocrit to 8% to 12% by acute exchange transfusion with crystalloid (lactated Ringer's) or colloidal (6% dextran 70) solutions (normoxic isovolemic hemodilution). These models produce acute reductions in DO_2 and a marked reduction in VO_2, which, if not treated, result in death (irreversible shock). Reductions in VO_2 therefore can be viewed as the ultimate regulatory factor responsible for cardiovascular compensatory responses, including increases in heart rate, cardiac contractility, cardiac output, and vascular tone. Other changes in cardiovascular function are determined by the primary precipitating event. Hemodilution, for example, produces a marked decrease in blood viscosity, increases in stroke volume, and a redistribution of blood flow to the coronary and cerebral blood vessels.[17] A decrease in blood viscosity facilitates capillary blood flow and can increase cardiac output by decreasing afterload. These hemodynamic changes have encouraged the clinical use of mild to moderate normovolemic hemodilution prior to anesthesia and surgery (Hb = 6 to 10 g/dL) in order to improve cardiac output, peripheral perfusion, and DO_2. The effects of anesthetic and inotropic drugs on VO_2, DO_2, cardiac output, and the distribution of blood flow should be considered prior to their use in any hypovolemic, anemic, or normovolemic anemic patients.[100,101] Fortunately, during anesthesia most patients' overall VO_2 is reduced because of decreasing body temperature and metabolism.

References

1. Mulvany MJ, Aalkjaer C. Structure and function of small arteries. Physiol Rev 70:921–961, 1990.
2. Burton AC. Composition of blood. In: Burton AC, ed. Physiology and Biophysics of the Circulation, 2nd ed. Chicago: Year Book, 1972:15–21.
3. Snyder JV. Oxygen transport: The model and reality. In: Snyder JV, Pinsky MR, eds. Oxygen Transport in the Critically Ill. Chicago: Year Book, 1987:3–15.
4. Vandergriff KD, Winslow RM. A theoretical analysis of oxygen transport: A new strategy for the design of hemoglobin-based red cell substitutes. In: Winslow RM, Vandergriff KD, Intaglieta M, eds. Blood Substitutes: Physiological Basis of Efficacy. Boston: Birkhauser, 1995:143–154.
5. Guyton AC. Overview of the circulation, and medical physics of pressure, flow, and resistance. In: Textbook of Medical Physiology, 8th ed. Philadelphia: WB Saunders, 1991:150–158.
6. Lasala PA, Chien S, Michelsen CB. Hemorrheology: What is the ideal hematocrit? In: Askanasi J, Starker RM, Weissman C, eds. Fluid and Electrolyte Management in Critical Care. Boston: Butterworth, 1986:203–213.
7. Berne RM, Levy MN. Hemodynamics. In: Principles of Physiology. St Louis: CV Mosby, 1990:245–254.
8. Berne RM, Levy MN. Control of cardiac output: Coupling of the heart and blood vessels. In: Principles of Physiology. St Louis: CV Mosby, 1990:287–299.
9. Burton AC. Viscosity and the manner in which blood flows. In: Physiology and Biophysics of the Circulation, 2nd ed. Chicago: Year Book, 1972:39–48.
10. Nichols WW, O'Rourke MF. Vascular impedance. In: Nichols WW, O'Rourke MF, eds. McDonald's Blood Flow in Arteries: Theoretical, Experimental and Clinical Principles, 3rd ed. Philadelphia: Lea and Febiger, 1990:283–329.
11. Chapler CK, Cain SM. The physiologic reserve in oxygen carrying capacity: Studies in experimental hemodilution. Can J Physiol Pharmacol 64:7–12, 1986.
12. Leone BJ, Spahn DR. Anemia, hemodilution, and oxygen delivery. Anesth Analg 75:651–653, 1992.
13. Little WC, Cheng C. Left ventricular-arterial coupling in conscious dogs. Am J Physiol 261 (1 Pt 2):H70–H76, 1991.
14. Shroff SG, Weber KT, Janicki JS. Coupling of the left ventricle with the systemic arterial circulation. In: Nichols WW, O'Rourke MF, eds. McDonald's Blood Flow in Arteries: Theoretical, Experimental and Clinical Principles, 3rd ed. Philadelphia: Lea and Febiger, 1990:343–359.
15. Suga H, Igarashi Y, Yamada O, Goto Y. Mechanical efficiency of the left ventricle as a function of preload, afterload, and contractility. Heart Vessels 1985:1:3–8.
16. Nichols WW, O'Rourke MF, Avolio AP, et al. Age-related changes in left ventricular/arterial coupling. In: Yin FCP, ed. Ventricular/ Vascular Coupling: Clinical, Physiological, and Engineering Aspects. New York: Springer-Verlag, 1987:79–114.
17. Bowens C, Spahn DR, Frasco PE, Smith R, McRae, RL, Leone BJ. Hemodilution induces stable changes in global cardiovascular and regional myocardial function. Anesth Analg 76:1027–1032, 1998.
18. Burton AC. Kinetic energy in the circulation; streamline flow and turbulence; measurement of arterial pressure. In: Burton AC, ed. Physiology and Biophysics of the Circulation, 2nd ed. Chicago: Year Book, 1972:104–114.
19. Berne RM, Levy MN. Electrical activity of the heart. In: Principles of Physiology. St Louis: CV Mosby, 1990:197–213.
20. Antzelevitch C, Shimizu W, Yan GX, et al. The M cell: Its contribution to the ECG and to normal and abnormal electrical function of the heart. J Cardiovasc Electrophysiol 10:1124–1152, 1999
21. Opie LH. Channels, pumps, and exchangers. In: Opie LH, ed. The Heart: Physiology and Metabolism, 2nd ed. New York: Raven, 1991:67–101.
22. Boyden PA. Cellular electrophysiologic basis of cardiac arrhythmias. In: Tilley LP, ed. Essentials of Canine and Feline Electrocardiography: Interpretation and Treatment, 3rd ed. Philadelphia: Lea and Febiger, 1992:274–286.
23. Turner LA, Polic S, Hoffmann RG, Kampine JP, Bosnjak ZJ. Actions of volatile anesthetics on ischemic and nonischemic Purkinje fibers in the infarcted canine heart: Regional action potential characteristics. Anesth Analg 76:726–733, 1993.
24. Task Force of the Working Group on Arrhythmias of the European Society of Cardiology. The "Sicilian gambit": A new approach to the classification of antiarrhythmic drugs based on their actions on arrhythmogenic mechanisms. Eur Heart J 12:1112–1131, 1991.
25. Burt JM, Spray DC. Volatile anesthetics block intercellular communication between neonatal rat myocardial cells. Circ Res 65:829–837, 1989.

26. Spach MS, Dolber PC. Discontinuous anisotropic propagation. In: Rosen MR, Janse MJ, Wit AL, eds. Cardiac Electrophysiology: A Textbook. Mount Kisco, NY: Futura, 1990:517–534.

27. Spach MS, Dolber PC, Heidlage JF. Influence of the passive anisotropic properties on directional differences in propagation following modification of the sodium conductance in human atrial muscle: A model of re-entry based on anisotropic discontinuous propagation. Circ Res 62:811–832, 1988.

28. Baum VC. Distinctive effects of three intravenous anesthetics on the inward rectifier (I_{K1}) and the delayed rectifier (I_K) potassium currents in myocardium: Implications for the mechanism of action. Anesth Analg 76:18–23, 1993.

29. Boban M, Atlee JL, Vicenzi M, Kampine JP, Bosnjak ZJ. Anesthetics and automaticity in latent pacemaker fibers. IV. Effects of isoflurane and epinephrine or norepinephrine on automaticity of dominant and subsidiary atrial pacemakers in the canine heart. Anesthesiology 79:555–562, 1993.

30. Eskinder H, Supan FD, Turner LA, Kampine JP, Bosnjak Z. The effects of halothane and isoflurane on slowly inactivating sodium current in canine cardiac Purkinje cells. Anesth Anal 77:32–37, 1993.

31. Hatakeyama N, Ito Y, Momose Y. Effects of sevoflurane, isoflurane, and halothane on mechanical and electrophysiologic properties of canine myocardium. Anesth Analg 76:1327–1332, 1993.

32. Polic S, Bosnjak ZJ, Marijic J, Hoffmann RG, Kampine JP, Turner LA. Actions of halothane, isoflurane, and enflurane on the regional action potential characteristics of canine Purkinje fibers. Anesth Analg 73:603–611, 1991.

33. Turner LA, Polic S, Hoffmann RG, Kampine JP, Busnjak ZJ. Actions of halothane and isoflurane on Purkinje fibers in the infarcted canine heart: Conduction, regional refractoriness, and reentry. Anesth Analg 76:718–725, 1993.

34. Balke CW, Gold MR. Calcium channels in the heart: An overview. Heart Dis Stroke 1:398–403, 1992.

35. Opie LH. Intracellular calcium fluxes and sarcoplasmic reticulum. In: Opie LH, ed. The Heart: Physiology and Metabolism, 2nd ed. New York: Raven, 1991:127–146.

36. Katz AM. Contractile proteins: Mechanisms and control of the cardiac contractile process, series elasticity, active state, length-tension relationship and cardiac mechanics. In: Katz AM, ed. Physiology of the Heart. New York: Raven, 1977:119–136.

37. Paul RJ, Ferguson DG, Heiny JA. Muscle physiology: Molecular mechanisms. In: Sperelakis N, Banks RO, eds. Physiology. Boston: Little, Brown, 1993:189–208.

38. Blanck TJJ, Chiancone E, Salviati G, et al. Halothane does not alter Ca^{2+} affinity of troponin C. Anesthesiology 76:100–105, 1992.

39. Bosnjak ZJ, Supan FD, Rusch NJ. The effects of halothane, enflurane, and isoflurane on calcium current in isolated canine ventricular cells. Anesthesiology 74:340–345, 1991.

40. Bosnjak ZJ, Aggarwal A, Turner LA, Kampine JM, Kampine JP. Differential effects of halothane, enflurane, and isoflurane on Ca^{2+} transients and papillary muscle tension in guinea pigs. Anesthesiology 76:123–131, 1992.

41. Frazer MJ, Lynch C. Halothane and isoflurane effects on Ca^{2+} fluxes of isolated myocardial sarcoplasmic reticulum. Anesthesiology 77:316–323, 1992.

42. Kongsayreepong S, Cook DJ, Housmans PR. Mechanism of the direct, negative inotropic effect of ketamine in isolated ferret and frog ventricular myocardium. Anesthesiology 79:313–322, 1993.

43. Pagel PS, Kampine JP, Schmeling WT, Warltier DC. Reversal of volatile anesthetic–induced depression of myocardial contractility by extracellular calcium also enhances left ventricular diastolic function. Anesthesiology 8:141–154, 1993.

44. Rusy BF, Komai H. Anesthetic depression of myocardial contractility: A review of possible mechanisms. Anesthesiology 67:745–766, 1987.

45. Schmidt U, Schwinger RHG, Uberfuhr P, et al. Evidence for an interaction of halothane with the L-type Ca^{2+} channel in human myocardium. Anesthesiology 79:332–339, 1993.

46. Wilde DW, Davidson BA, Smith MD, Knight PR. Effects of isoflurane and enflurane on intracellular Ca^{2+} mobilization in isolated cardiac myocytes. Anesthesiology 79:73–82, 1993.

47. Welker FH, Muir WW. An investigation of the second heart sound in the normal horse. Equine Vet J 22:403–407, 1990.

48. Ettinger SJ, Suter PF. Heart sounds and phonocardiography. In: Canine Cardiology. Philadelphia: WB Saunders, 1970:12–39.

49. Sagawa K. The end-systolic pressure-volume relation of the ventricle: Definition, modifications and clinical use. Circulation 63:1223–1227, 1981.

50. Brutsaert DL, Rademakers FE, Sys SU, Gillebert TC, Housmans PR. Analysis of relaxation in the evaluation of ventricular function of the heart. Prog Cardiovasc Dis 28:143–163, 1985.

51. Little WC, Downes TR. Clinical evaluation of left ventricular diastolic performance. Prog Cardiovasc Dis 32:273–290, 1990.

52. Freeman GL, Colston JT. Role of ventriculovascular coupling in cardiac response to increased contractility in closed-chest dogs. J Clin Invest 86:1278–1284, 1990.

53. Hayashida K, Sunagawa K, Noma M, Sugimachi M, Ando H, Nakamura M. Mechanical matching of the left ventricle with the arterial system in exercising dogs. Circ Res 71:481–489, 1992.

54. Opie LH. Ventricular function. In: The Heart: Physiology and Metabolism, 2nd ed. New York: Raven, 1991:301–338.

55. Nichols WW, O'Rourke FO, Auolio AP, et al. Age-related changes in left ventricular/arterial coupling. In: Yin CP, ed. Ventricular/Vascular Coupling: Clinical, Physiological, and Engineering Aspects. New York: Springer-Verlag, 1987:79–714.

56. Bonow RO, Udelson JE. Left ventricular diastolic dysfunction as a cause of congestive heart failure: Mechanisms and management. Ann Intern Med 117:502–510, 1992.

57. Pagel PS, Kampine JP, Schmeling WT, Warltier DC. Comparison of end-systolic pressure-length relations and preload recruitable stroke work as indices of myocardial contractility in the conscious and anesthetized, chronically instrumented dog. Anesthesiology 73:278–290, 1990.

58. Pagel PS, Kampine JP, Schmeling WT, Warltier DC. Ketamine depresses myocardial contractility as evaluated by the preload recruitable stroke work relationship in chronically instrumented dogs with autonomic nervous system blockade. Anesthesiology 76:564–572, 1992.

59. Swanson CR, Muir WW. Simultaneous evaluation of left ventricular end-systolic pressure-volume ratio and time constant of isovolumic pressure decline in dogs exposed to equivalent MAC halothane and isoflurane. Anesthesiology 68:764–770, 1988.

60. Pagel PS, Kampine JP, Schmeling WT, Warltier DC. Comparison of the systemic and coronary hemodynamic actions of desflurane, isoflurane, halothane, and enflurane in the chronically instrumented dog. Anesthesiology 74:539–551, 1991.

61. Moffitt EA, Sethna DH. The coronary circulation and myocardial oxygenation in coronary artery disease: Effects of anesthesia. Anesth Analg 65:395–410, 1986.

62. Pagel PS, Kampine JP, Schmeling WT, Warltier DC. Alteration of left ventricular diastolic function by desflurane, isoflurane, and

halothane in the chronically instrumented dog with autonomic nervous system blockade. Anesthesiology 74:1103–1114, 1991.

63. Pagel PS, Schmeling WT, Kampine JP, Warltier DC. Alteration of canine left ventricular diastolic function by intravenous anesthetics in vivo: Ketamine and propofol. Anesthesiology 76:419–425, 1992.

64. Asanoi H, Sasayama S, Kameyama T. Ventriculoarterial coupling in normal and failing heart in humans. Circ Res 65:483–493, 1989.

65. Milnor WR. The normal hemodynamic state: Vascular impedance and wave reflection. In: Milnor WR, ed. Hemodynamics, 2nd ed. Baltimore: Williams and Wilkins, 1989:142–224.

66. Bevan JA, Bevan RD. Changes in arteries as they get smaller. In: Vanhoutte P, ed. Vasodilatation: Vascular Smooth Muscle, Peptides, Autonomic Nerves and Endothelium. New York: Raven, 1988:55–60.

67. Tsuchida H, Namba H, Yamakage M, Fujita S, Notsuki E, Namiki A. Effects of halothane and isoflurane on cytosolic calcium ion concentration and contraction in the vascular smooth muscle of the rat aorta. Anesthesiology 78:531–540, 1993.

68. Witzleb Z. Functions of the vascular system. In: Schmidt RF, Thews G, eds. Human Physiology. New York: Springer-Verlag, 1983:397–455.

69. Green JR. Circulatory mechanics. In: Fundamental Cardiovascular and Pulmonary Physiology, 2nd ed. Philadelphia: Lea and Febiger, 1987:59–80.

70. Yano H, Takaori M. Effect of hemodilution on capillary and arteriolovenous shunt flow in organs after cardiac arrest in dogs. Crit Care Med 18:1146–1151, 1990.

71. Pappenheimer JR, Soto-Rivera A. Effective osmotic pressure of the plasma proteins and other quantities associated with the capillary circulation in the hindlimbs of cats and dogs. Am J Physiol 152:471–491, 1948.

72. Taylor AE. Capillary fluid filtration: Starling forces and lymph flow. Circ Res 49:557–575, 1981.

73. Valli N, Gobinet A, Bordenave L. Review of 10 years of the clinical use of brain natriuretic peptide in cardiology. J Lab Clin Med 134:437–444, 1999.

74. Levy MN. Neural and reflex control of the circulation. In: Garfein O, ed. Current Concepts in Cardiovascular Physiology. San Diego: Academic, 1990:133–207.

75. Mirenda JV, Grissom TE. Anesthetic implications of the renin-angiotensin system and angiotensin-converting enzyme inhibitors. Anesth Analg 72:667–683, 1991.

76. Shepherd JT, Vanhoutte PM. Neurohumoral regulation. In: The Human Cardiovascular System: Facts and Concepts. New York: Raven, 1979:107–155.

77. Oparil S, Katholi R. Humoral control of the circulation. In: Garfein O, ed. Current Concepts in Cardiovascular Physiology. San Diego: Academic, 1990:210–287.

78. Arimura H, Bosnjak ZJ, Hoka S, Kampine JP. Modifications by halothane of responses to acute hypoxia in systemic vascular capacitance, resistance, and sympathetic nerve activity in dogs. Anesth Analg 73:319–326, 1991.

79. Hart JL, Jing M, Bina S, Freas W, Van Dyke RA, Muldoon SM. Effects of halothane on EDRF/cGMP-mediated vascular smooth muscle relaxations. Anesthesiology 79:323–331, 1993.

80. McCallum JB, Stekiel TA, Bosnjak ZJ Kampine JP. Does isoflurane alter mesenteric venous capacitance in the intact rabbit? Anesth Analg 76:1095–1105, 1993.

81. Toda H, Nakamura K, Hatano Y, Nishiwada M, Kakuyama M, Mori K. Halothane and isoflurane inhibit endothelium-dependent relaxation elicited by acetylcholine. Anesth Analg 75:198–203, 1992.

82. Uggeri MJ, Proctor GJ, Johns RA. Halothane, enflurane, and isoflurane attenuate both receptor- and non-receptor-mediated EDRF production in rat thoracic aorta. Anesthesiology 76:1012–1017, 1992.

83. Kinsella SM, Tuckey JP. Perioperative bradycardia and asystole: Relationship to vasovagal syncope and the Bezold-Jarisch reflex. Br J Anaesth 86:859–868, 2001

84. Greisheimer FM. The circulatory effects of anesthetics. In: Hamilton WF, ed. Handbook of Physiology Circulation, sect 2, vol 3. Washington, DC: American Physiological Society, 1965: 2477–2510.

85. Hellyer PW, Bednarski RM, Hubbell JAE, Muir WW. Effects of halothane and isoflurane on baroreflex sensitivity in horses. Am J Vet Res 50:2127–2134, 1989.

86. Harrison JK, Pearson WR, Lynch KR. Molecular characterization of alpha-1 and alpha-2 adrenoceptors. Trends Pharmacol Sci 12:62–67, 1991.

87. Van Zwieten PA. Adrenergic and muscarinic receptors: Classification, pathophysiological relevance and drug target. J Hypertens 9(Suppl 6):S18–S27, 1991.

88. Schulz S, Yuen PST, Garbers DL. The expanding family of guanylyl cyclases. Trends Pharmacol Sci 12:116–120, 1991.

89. Maze M, Tranquilli W. Alpha-2 adrenoceptor agonists: Defining the role in clinical anesthesia. Anesthesiology 74:581–605, 1991.

90. Lokhandwala MF, Hegde SS. Cardiovascular pharmacology of adrenergic and dopaminergic receptors: Significance in congestive heart failure. Am J Med 90(Suppl 5B):2S–9S, 1991.

91. Walker P, Grouzmann E, Burnier M, Waeber B. The role of neuropeptide Y in cardiovascular regulation. Trends Pharmacol Sci 12:111–115, 1991.

92. Hosey MM. Diversity of structure, signaling and regulation within the family of muscarinic cholinergic receptors. FASEB J 6:845–852, 1992.

93. Zanzinger J. Role of nitric oxide in the neural control of cardiovascular function. Cardiovasc Res 43:639–649, 1999.

94. Drexler H. Reduced exercise tolerance in chronic heart failure and its relationship to neurohumoral factors. Eur Heart J 12:21–28, 1991.

95. Opie LH. Ventricular overload and heart failure. In: The Heart: Physiology and Metabolism, 2nd ed. New York: Raven, 1991: 396–424.

96. Brock WJ, Rusch GM, Trochimowicz HJ. Cardiac sensitization: Methodology and interpretation in risk assessment. Regul Toxicol Pharmacol 38:78–90, 2003.

97. Bonagura J, Stepien R. Vascular diseases. In: Birchard SJ, Sherding RG, eds. Saunders Manual of Small Animal Practice. Philadelphia: WB Saunders, 1993:494–499.

98. Barr SC, Ludders JW, Looney AL, Gleed RD, Erb HN. Platelet aggregation in dogs after sedation with acepromazine and atropine and during subsequent general anesthesia and surgery. Am J Vet Res 1992:53:2067–2070.

99. Lewis RE, Cruse JM, Hazelwood J. Halothane-induced suppression of cell-mediated immunity in normal and tumor-bearing C3Hf/He mice. Anesth Analg 59:666–671, 1988.

100. Van der Linden P, Gilbart E, Engelman E, Schmartz D, Vincent JL. Effects of anesthetic agents on systemic critical O_2 delivery. J Appl Physiol 71:83–93, 1994.

101. Pascoe PJ, Ilkiw JE, Pypendop BH. Effects of increasing infusion rates of dopamine, dobutamine, epinephrine, and phenylephrine in healthy anesthetized cats. Am J Vet Res 67:1491–1499, 2006.

102. Shepherd JT, Vanhoutte PM. The Human Cardiovascular System: Facts and Concepts, 1st ed. New York: Raven, 1979.

103. Berne RM, Levy MN. Principles of Physiology, 1st ed. St Louis: CV Mosby, 1990.

104. Sunagawa K, Maughan WL, Burkhoff D, Sagawa K. Left ventricular interaction with arterial load studied in isolated canine ventricle. Am J Physiol 245(5 Pt 1):H733–H780, 1983.

105. Guyton AC. Textbook of Medical Physiology, 8th ed. Philadelphia: WB Saunders, 1991.

106. Opie LH. The Heart: Physiology and Metabolism, 3rd ed. Philadelphia: Lippincott-Raven, 1998:91–97.

107. Katz AM. Physiology of the Heart, 3rd ed. Philadelphia: Lippincott Williams and Wilkins, 2001.

108. Ganong WF. Review of Medical Physiology, 16th ed. East Norwalk, CT: Appleton-Lange, 1993.

Chapter 5
Respiratory System

Wayne N. McDonell and Carolyn L. Kerr

Introduction

Maintenance of adequate respiratory function is a prime requirement for safe anesthesia. Inadequate tissue oxygenation may lead to an acute cessation of vital organ function, especially of the brain or myocardium, and an anesthetic fatality. Excessive elevations in arterial carbon dioxide (CO_2) tensions (arterial CO_2 partial pressure [$PaCO_2$]) or sustained moderate hypoxemia may produce some level of organ dysfunction, which contributes to a less than optimum postanesthetic recovery. Delayed recovery of consciousness, postanesthetic myopathy in large animals, and postanesthetic renal, hepatic, or cardiac insufficiency can all originate from inadequate respiratory function during anesthesia.

During general anesthesia, there is always a tendency for arterial oxygen tensions (arterial oxygen partial pressure [PaO_2]) to be less than observed with the same species while conscious and breathing the same fraction of inspired-oxygen concentration (F_IO_2).[1-5] There is also a tendency for $PaCO_2$ to be elevated above the conscious resting values if the anesthetized animal is breathing spontaneously, and for increases in airway resistance to occur unless an endotracheal tube is used. Some differences are seen, depending on the actual anesthetic regimen used, but the depth of anesthesia is often more of a factor. Species and breed differences exist, and some of these are illustrated in this chapter. Positioning during anesthesia, concurrent drug use, and the magnitude of preanesthetic cardiorespiratory dysfunction all affect respiratory function.

Respiratory dysfunction during general anesthesia and the postoperative period is caused by the disruption of many physiological mechanisms and, in the larger species especially, an exaggeration of anatomical and mechanical factors.[1,2,4] An understanding of respiratory function as it relates to anesthesia requires consideration of (a) the neural control of respiration and its effect on alveolar ventilation (V_A); (b) the influence of anesthesia on the airway, chest wall, and lung volumes; and (c) the alterations in ventilation-perfusion (*V/Q*) relationships during anesthesia.[4-6]

It is assumed that the readers are already reasonably knowledgeable regarding basic pulmonary physiology, which is considered in detail elsewhere.[5-7] The review by Robinson[7] is particularly useful for undergraduate readers. Much of the information that is available about the effects of anesthesia on respiration comes from studies in humans, and this information is summarized in a recent review at a level of complexity suitable for individuals in a specialist training program.[6] There are important differences, however, in the manner by which veterinarians generally administer anesthetics to animals when compared with anesthesia of people. In veterinary practice, intravenous anesthetics are often used without oxygen supplementation, at least under field conditions. There is much less use of peripheral-acting muscle relaxants in veterinary anesthesia, and, generally, intermittent positive-pressure ventilation (IPPV) is used on a "need to" rather than routine basis. During general anesthesia with inhalants, 100% oxygen is usually used as the carrier gas, whereas a 2:1 mixture of nitrous oxide and oxygen is commonly used as the carrier gas in human anesthesia. Dogs and cats have frequently been used for investigations of neural control and mechanical alterations associated with anesthesia, but often under experimental situations that differ quite markedly from how anesthetics are administered to veterinary patients. In addition, the range of body weight and size and, in many instances, unique physiological adaptations of domestic and nondomestic animals undergoing anesthesia mean that the respiratory response to anesthesia may well be different than as classically described for people.

Definitions

Respiration is the total process whereby oxygen is supplied to and used by body cells and carbon dioxide is eliminated by means of gradients. *Ventilation* is the movement of gas in and out of alveoli. The ventilatory requirement for homeostasis varies with the metabolic requirement of animals, and it thus varies with body size, level of activity, body temperature, and depth of anesthesia. Pulmonary ventilation is accomplished by expansion and contraction of the lungs. Several terms are used to describe the various types of breathing that may be observed:

1. *Eupnea* is ordinary quiet breathing.
2. *Dyspnea* is labored breathing.
3. *Tachypnea* is increased respiratory rate.
4. *Hyperpnea* is fast and/or deep respiration, indicating "over-respiration."
5. *Polypnea* is a rapid, shallow, panting type of respiration.
6. *Bradypnea* is slow regular respiration.
7. *Hypopnea* is slow and/or shallow breathing, possibly indicating "underrespiration."
8. *Apnea* is transient (or longer) cessation of breathing.
9. *Cheyne-Stokes respirations* increase in rate and depth, and then become slower, followed by a brief period of apnea.
10. *Biot's respirations* are sequences of gasps, apnea, and several deep gasps.
11. *Kussmaul's respirations* are regular deep respirations without pause.
12. *Apneustic respiration* occurs when an animal holds an inspired breath at the end of inhalation for a short period before exhaling.

To describe the events of pulmonary ventilation, air in the lung has been subdivided into four different volumes and four different capacities (Fig. 5.1). Only tidal volume and functional residual capacity can be measured in conscious uncooperative animals:

1. *Tidal volume* (V_T) is the volume of air inspired or expired in one breath.
2. *Inspiratory reserve volume* (IRV) is the volume of air that can be inspired over and above the normal tidal volume.

3. *Expiratory reserve volume* (ERV) is the amount of air that can be expired by forceful expiration after a normal expiration.
4. *Residual volume* (RV) is the air remaining in the lungs after the most forceful expiration.

Another term frequently used is the minute respiratory volume or *minute ventilation* (V_E). This is equal to V_T times the *respiratory frequency* (*f*). Occasionally, it is desirable to consider two or more of the aforementioned volumes together. Such combinations are termed *pulmonary capacities*:

1. *Inspiratory capacity* (IC) is the tidal volume plus the inspiratory reserve volume. This is the amount of air that can be inhaled starting after a normal expiration and distending the lungs to the maximum amount.

2. *Functional residual capacity* (FRC) is the expiratory reserve volume plus the residual volume. This is the amount of air remaining in the lungs after a normal expiration. From a mechanical viewpoint, at FRC the inward "pull" of the lungs due to their elasticity equals the outward "pull" of the chest wall.

3. *Vital capacity* (VC) is the inspiratory reserve volume plus the tidal volume plus the expiratory reserve volume. This is the maximum amount of air that can be expelled from the lungs after first filling them to their maximum capacity.

4. *Total lung capacity* (TLC) is the inspiratory reserve volume plus the tidal volume plus the expiratory reserve volume plus the residual volume, or the maximum volume to which the lungs can be expanded with the greatest possible inspiratory effort (or by full inflation to 30 cm H_2O airway pressure when a patient is anesthetized).

Ventilation and Gas Exchange in Conscious Animals

From an anesthetist's viewpoint, it is useful to consider the ventilatory system in terms of its major components: neural control, the bellows mechanism (chest wall and diaphragm), upper airway, and lung parenchyma (Fig. 5.2). Alterations of (a) the neural control of ventilation by sedative, opioid, or anesthetic depression; (b) upper-airway or lower-airway patency by muscle

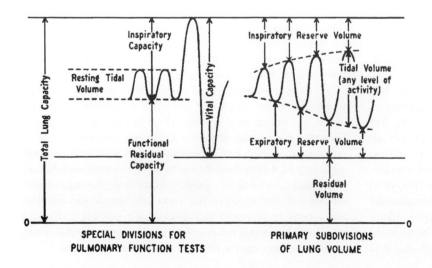

SPECIAL DIVISIONS FOR PULMONARY FUNCTION TESTS

PRIMARY SUBDIVISIONS OF LUNG VOLUME

Fig. 5.1. Lung volumes and capacities. From Pappenheimer.[206]

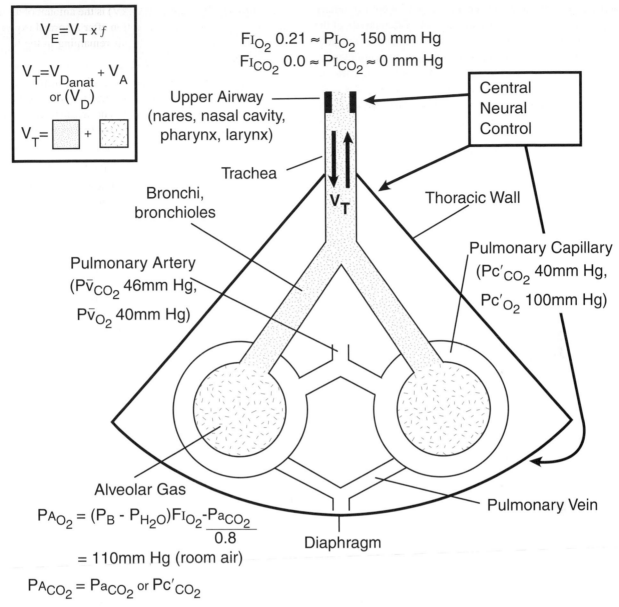

$$V_E = V_T \times f$$

$$V_T = V_{D\,anat} + V_A$$
or (V_D)

$$V_T = \boxed{} + \boxed{}$$

$F_{I_{O_2}}$ 0.21 ≈ $P_{I_{O_2}}$ 150 mm Hg
$F_{I_{CO_2}}$ 0.0 ≈ $P_{I_{CO_2}}$ ≈ 0 mm Hg

Upper Airway
(nares, nasal cavity,
pharynx, larynx)

Central
Neural
Control

Trachea

V_T

Thoracic Wall

Bronchi,
bronchioles

Pulmonary Artery
$(P\bar{v}_{CO_2}$ 46mm Hg,
$P\bar{v}_{O_2}$ 40mm Hg)

Pulmonary Capillary
$(Pc'_{CO_2}$ 40mm Hg,
Pc'_{O_2} 100mm Hg)

Alveolar Gas

$$P_{A_{O_2}} = (P_B - P_{H_2O})F_{I_{O_2}} - \frac{P_{a_{CO_2}}}{0.8}$$

= 110mm Hg (room air)

$$P_{A_{CO_2}} = P_{a_{CO_2}} \text{ or } Pc'_{CO_2}$$

Diaphragm

Pulmonary Vein

Fig. 5.2. Diagrammatic representation of the neural control, bellows mechanism (diaphragm and thoracic wall), and matching of pulmonary artery blood and alveolar gas in the lung. F_I refers to fraction of inspired gases, and f is respiratory frequency. Tidal volume (V_T), anatomical dead space ($V_{D\,anat}$), alveolar volume (V_A), and representative inspired (P_I), alveolar (P_A), pulmonary arterial or mixed venous ($P_{\bar{v}}$), and end-capillary (P_c') partial pressures of oxygen and carbon dioxide are also illustrated. See the text for a detailed explanation.

relaxation or spasm; or (c) the bellows mechanism of the thorax through neuromuscular paralysis, space-occupying lesions of the thorax, or a change in the diaphragm shape, location, or function may all appreciably affect ventilatory adequacy and the efficiency of gas exchange. Within the parenchyma, less than optimum matching of fresh alveolar gas with pulmonary capillary blood will produce blood-gas alterations, particularly in regard to PaO_2.

Control of Respiration

With the aid of the circulation, respiration regulates the oxygen, CO_2, and hydrogen-ion environment of the cell. Respiratory function is controlled by central respiratory centers, central and peripheral chemoreceptors, pulmonary reflexes, and nonrespiratory neural input. Control of respiration has been described as an integrated feedback control system.[6,7] The central neural "controller" includes specialized groups of neurons located in the cerebrum, brain stem, and spinal cord that govern both voluntary and automatic ventilation through regulation of the activity of the respiratory muscles. The respiratory muscles by contracting produce alveolar ventilation, and changes in alveolar ventilation affect blood-gas tensions and hydrogen-ion concentration. Blood-gas tensions and hydrogen-ion concentrations are monitored by peripheral and central chemoreceptors that return signals to the central controller to provide necessary adjustments in ventilation. Mechanoreceptors in the lungs and stretch receptors in the respiratory muscles monitor, respectively, the degree of expansion or stretch of the lungs and the "effort" of breathing, feeding back information to the central controller to alter the pattern of breathing. Adjustments also occur to accommodate nonrespiratory activities such as thermoregulation and vocalization.

Overall, this complex control system produces a combination of respiratory frequency and depth that is best suited for optimum ventilation with minimal effort for the particular species, and that adjusts oxygen supply and CO_2 elimination so as to maintain homeostasis (reflected by stable arterial blood-gas levels) over a wide range of environmental and metabolic situations. Sedatives, analgesics, anesthetics, and the equipment used for inhalational anesthesia may profoundly alter respiration and the ability of an animal to maintain cellular homeostasis.

Mechanical Factors

Transfer of gases to and from the lungs depends on developing a pressure gradient between the atmosphere and the alveoli, and is modified by the resistance to flow between these two regions and the elasticity of the lungs and chest wall. With spontaneous respiration, during inspiration active muscular effort serves to enlarge the pleural cavity through expansion of the thoracic wall and contraction of the diaphragm (Fig. 5.2). Intrapleural pressure is thereby reduced to a more subatmospheric pressure, and a mouth/nostril–alveolar pressure gradient is established. In contrast to inspiration, expiration is normally passive and depends on the return of the chest wall and lungs to a resting position, that is, to FRC. The horse is a notable exception in that abdominal muscle contraction plays a part in normal expiratory activity, producing a biphasic mode of exhalation.[7] As the size of the pleural space decreases, intrapleural and consequently alveolar pressures are elevated, and the pressure gradient is reversed so that air flows from the alveoli to the atmosphere. Thus, fluctuating pressure gradients between the atmosphere and the alveoli cause air to flow in and out of the lungs. The factors that contribute to these pressure gradients and the measurement of their magnitude are referred to as *pulmonary mechanics*.

During assisted or controlled artificial or mechanical ventilation, atmospheric to alveolar pressure gradients also occur, but mouth pressure is more positive than alveolar pressure on inspiration: hence the term *positive pressure ventilation*. This has important circulatory consequences. Both the lungs and chest wall provide an elastic resistance to expansion on inspiration. The relationship between the pressure gradient (P) and the resultant volume (V) increase in liters (L) of the lungs and thorax is known as *total compliance* (C_T).[6]

$$C_T \text{ (L/cm } H_2O) = \Delta V \text{ (L)}/\Delta P \text{ (cm } H_2O)$$

The relationship of C_T to the individual compliance of the lungs (C_L) and chest wall (C_{CW}) is additive, because the lungs and chest wall are arranged concentrically and can be expressed as

$$1/C_T = 1/C_L + 1/C_{CW}$$

To measure C_T, V and the transthoracic pressure (that is, the pressure at the alveolus minus ambient pressure) must be known. In anesthetized animals, this is often determined by measuring the inspiratory volume delivered from a ventilator bellows or rebreathing bag while recording the change in airway (taken to be alveolar) pressure between end exhalation and end inspiration. If the lungs and/or chest wall are less compliant (i.e., stiffer), then higher transthoracic pressures are required to deliver a given tidal volume. Experienced anesthetists can often sense this change as an increased force required to mechanically squeeze a set volume from a rebreathing bag by hand. This may provide the first clue that an animal is developing a space-occupying problem in the thorax or abdomen (e.g., accumulation of air or blood), or that the end of the endotracheal tube has become repositioned in one main bronchus and is inflating only one lung.

Dynamic C_T is the volume change divided by the transthoracic pressure change at the point of zero airflow (end inspiration) when the previous inflow of air has been sufficiently rapid for dynamic factors to influence the distribution of air throughout the lung. For practical purposes, dynamic C_T is equal to the tidal volume divided by the peak airway pressure. *Static C_T* is determined when the preceding inflow of air has been sufficiently slow for distribution throughout the lung to be solely in accord with regional elasticity. Under these conditions, gas distribution to alveoli with faster and slower filling rates is equivalent, and as a result the static C_T (or C_L) value is usually greater than dynamic C_T (or C_L).

To determine the elasticity of the lung per se (C_L), V and the transpulmonary pressure gradient (that is, pressure at the alveolus minus pressure at the pleural space) must be known. This measurement is harder to determine accurately. In practice, the transpulmonary pressure gradient is generally determined by using a differential pressure transducer to determine mouth (considered equal to alveolar) and pleural pressure changes simultaneously. Pleural pressure changes are estimated from intrathoracic esophageal pressure swings recorded with a balloon-tipped catheter. Lungs develop a low compliance (become stiffer) with a reduction in lung volume or regional atelectasis; as a result of pulmonary edema or fibrosis; and, in the case of dynamic C_L, with regional differences in airway resistance.

For air to flow into the lungs, a pressure gradient must also be developed to overcome the nonelastic (airway) resistance to airflow. The relationship between the pressure gradient across the pulmonary system (P_L) and the rate of airflow is known as *airway resistance* (R_L):[6]

$$R_L \text{ (cm } H_2O/L/s) = \Delta P_L \text{ (cm } H_2O)/(L/s)$$

The caliber of the airway and the rate and pattern of airflow all contribute to the pressure gradient along the airway. According to the Hagen-Poiseuille law, laminar gas flow through a tube is proportional to the pressure gradient across the tube, the fourth power of the diameter of the tube, and inversely to the viscosity:

pressure loss = constant × viscosity × length of tube × flow rate/diameter^4 × flow rate

The significance of this equation relative to anesthesia is to realize that changes in airway (or apparatus) diameter may markedly affect the resistance to airflow. If the diameter of the airway is reduced by 50%, for instance, by using too small an endotracheal tube, the resistance goes up 16-fold.

At higher flow rates that exceed the critical velocity of the system, or in the face of sudden changes in airway diameter, airflow will no longer be laminar and becomes turbulent. The significance of a transition from laminar to turbulent flow is illustrated by the fact that, at rates approximating critical flow, the resistance to flow increases by about 50% if the flow becomes turbulent. Airway resistance is measured by a variety of methods, most of which involve the simultaneous determination of instantaneous airflow with a pneumotachograph and of transpulmonary pressure (P_L), as described earlier.

Airway resistance increases with the rate of respiration and with narrowing of the airway by reflex contraction of the bronchiolar muscles, with small airway disease where there is edema of the airway wall and mucous accumulation, with a reduction in lung volume, or through aspiration of foreign material. Airway resistance during anesthesia can be minimized by using an airway that is as wide as possible and in which sudden alterations in direction or diameter are minimized.

Pulmonary Ventilation

The important factor in pulmonary ventilation is the rate at which *alveolar air* is exchanged with atmospheric air. This is not equal to the minute ventilation volume because a large portion of inspired air is used to fill the respiratory passages, rather than alveoli, and no significant gaseous exchange occurs in this air (Fig. 5.2). The *respiratory frequency* (*f*) and volume of each breath, *tidal volume* (V_T), determine the *minute ventilation* (V_E). The portion of each V_T that reaches only the upper airway and tracheobronchial tree fills the *anatomical dead space* and is referred to as *dead-space volume* ($V_{D\ anat}$). The $V_{D\ anat}$ is fairly constant; therefore, slow, deep breathing is more effective than rapid, shallow breathing. This is especially so during general anesthesia and with IPPV. The "effective" volume, or portion of V_T that contributes to gas exchange, is the *alveolar volume* (V_A), usually referred to as *minute alveolar ventilation* (V_A). Nonperfused alveoli do not contribute to gas exchange and constitute *alveolar dead space* (V_{DA}). In conscious healthy animals V_{DA} is minimal, whereas during general anesthesia it may increase owing to a fall in cardiac output (Q) and/or pulmonary artery blood pressure. *Physiological dead space* (V_D) includes $V_{D\ anat}$ and V_{DA} (Fig. 5.2), and is usually expressed as a minute value (V_D) along with V_A, or as a ratio of V_D/V_T. In unsedated tracheostomized dogs breathing quietly through a standard endotracheal tube, V_D was 5.9 mL/kg and the ratio of V_D/V_T was 35%.[8] This ratio of V_D/V_T is similar to that found in humans, but the V_D figure is larger, reflecting the in-

creased $V_{D\ anat}$ in dogs on a body-weight basis. During methoxyflurane anesthesia with spontaneous respiration, V_D increased very little (about 0.5 mL/kg), but V_D/V_T increased to over 50% because V_T decreased. Others have shown similar results with other anesthetics. In larger species such as horses and cows, the V_D/V_T ratio in conscious animals is about 50%.[9] Higher proportions of dead space have been reported, but such values probably reflect a tachypneic state or failure to subtract the added dead space associated with the use of the mask in gas collection. In unsedated cows, V_D is about 3.7 mL/kg and, in horses, about 5.2 mL/kg.[9] Representative normal ventilation, blood-gas, and acid-base values for a range of species are listed in Tables 5.1 and 5.2.

Lung Volumes

The subdivisions of lung volume are shown in Fig. 5.1. Most of these volumes cannot be measured in conscious animals, because to do so requires cooperation of the test subject. Measurements of V_T and FRC can be obtained in conscious animals; TLC is generally estimated by inflation of the lung to above 30 cm H_2O inflation pressure in anesthetized animals. Values for TLC are reasonably similar among the domestic species when compared on a body-weight basis, but the total volume varies from less than 2.0 mL in mice to over 45 L in horses and cows (Table 5.3). This factor and the variation in V_T observed across species (Table 5.1) have quite significant implications relative to the design of suitable inhalant anesthetic apparatus and the relative importance of added mechanical dead space. A liter of apparatus dead space in a healthy conscious horse or cow constitutes only a small portion of the V_T and has little effect on V_A or blood gases,[38] whereas a dead space of even 15 mL in a cat amounts to 50% of V_T and will quite likely alter alveolar ventilation and $PaCO_2$ levels. In the smallest mammals, virtually all mask systems will lead to some rebreathing of CO_2 during anesthesia, unless a loose-fitting mask is used with a flow-through system.

The volume of gas remaining in the lungs at the end of a normal expiration (i.e., the FRC) varies considerably as the position of the diaphragm, in particular, changes. Abdominal tympany from any source (e.g., near-term gravid uterus, bowel distension, obesity, or tumor) will tend to move the diaphragm forward and lessen the FRC. Few actual measurements have been made of this phenomenon in relation to animals, but the consequences on ventilation and respiratory function during anesthesia are consistent with a decrease in FRC.

Intrapulmonary Matching of Blood and Gas

Matching of alveolar gas and pulmonary capillary blood flow is influenced by gravitational factors and by the pulmonary artery circulation being a low-pressure system. Intrapleural pressure is more subatmospheric in the uppermost part of the thorax than in the lowermost portion,[39] partly because of the weight of the lung in the thorax. Alveolar size is largest in the uppermost areas of the lung and smallest in the ventral regions. Since the larger alveoli have a lower compliance (they are less distensible), they expand less on inspiration, and air preferentially enters the more compliant lower alveoli, producing a vertical gradient of ventilation in standing animals breathing quietly.[40,41] This tendency for

Table 5.1. Breathing frequency (f), tidal volume (V_T), and minute ventilation (APV_E) of various species.

Species	Mean Body Wt (kg)	n	Conditions[b]	f (breaths/min)	V_T mL	V_T mL/kg	APV_E mL/min	APV_E mL/kg/min	Refs.
Mice	0.02	NS[a]	Awake, prone	163.4	0.15	7.78	24.5	1239	10
	0.032	NS	Anesthetized	109	0.18	5.63	21.0	720	10
Rats	0.113	NS	Awake, prone	85.5	0.87	7.67	72.9	646	10
	0.305	NS	Awake, pleth	103	2.08	6.83	213	701	10
Cats	3.8	4	Unanesthetized, pleth	22	30	7.9	664	174	11
	3.7	NS	Anesthetized	30	34	9.2	960	310	10
Dogs	18.6	6	Awake, prone, chronic trach, intubated	13	309	16.6	3818	205	12
	18.8	8	Awake, standing, chronic trach, intubated	16.5	314	16.9	4963	264	8
Sheep	32–37	4	Awake, standing, mask	38	289	8.3	10,400	297	13
Goats	36.3	3	Awake, standing mask	13.6	470	12.9	6313	174	14
	46.4	6	Awake, standing mask	26	483	10.4	11,900	256	15
	47.6	6	Awake, standing mask	17.6	602	12.6	10,540	221	16
Pigs	12.9	4	Awake, standing	13.1	209	15.9	2731	208	17
Cows	517 Holstein	7	Awake, standing mask	23.7	3676	7.1	85,977	166	9
	405 Jersey	11	Awake, standing mask	28.6	3360	8.3	94,870	234	18
Calves	43–73 Hereford	8	4–6 weeks old, standing, sling	26.7	403	15.1	10,290	385	19
Horses	402	6	Awake, standing mask	11.8	4253	10.6	49,466	123	9
	483	6	Awake, standing mask	15.5	4860	10.1	74,600	154	20
	486	15	Awake, standing, mask (some sedated) (mask V_D not removed)	10	7300	15.0	79,000	163	21
Ponies	147	19	Awake, standing, mask	19.0	1370	9.3	26,380	180	22

[a]Not specified.
[b]Pleth, whole body plethysmograph; trach, tracheostomy.

preferential ventral ventilation in the lung may also be associated with regional chest wall and diaphragmatic movement. During anesthesia, the distribution of ventilation becomes more uneven and may even reverse so that the uppermost lung of a laterally recumbent horse is receiving most of the ventilation.

The major effect of gravity on the lung in most animals is to produce a vertical perfusion gradient in the pulmonary circulation, with the lower region being perfused more. The distribution of these gravitational effects on lung perfusion is commonly divided and functionally described as a three-zone or four-zone system.[41,42] At rest, the uppermost alveoli may be minimally perfused (Fig. 5.3, zone I), with alveolar pressure (P_A) greater than pulmonary artery (P_{pa}) and vein (P_{pv}) pressures. In zone II, P_{pa} is greater than P_A, and the difference between the two is the driving pressure for blood flow at the front end of the capillaries. The relationship between P_A and P_{pv} governs flow through the terminal aspect of the capillaries. In zone III, P_{pa} and P_{pv} both exceed P_A, and the vessels are fully distended, with the perfusion being determined by the pressure difference between P_{pa} and P_{pv}. In zone IV, the lung weight increases the interstitial pressure to a point that blood flow is reduced toward that of zone II, or less. These factors are important during anesthesia in that cardiac output is often reduced and P_{pa} may fall. Moreover, when the body position is altered and an animal becomes recumbent, the pulmonary blood flow is thought to realign along gravitational lines consistent with the new body position.[2,6] However, these relationships are not necessarily straightforward, especially in the larger species, perhaps because of the large decrease in FRC that accompanies recumbency and the generation of a larger zone IV area in the thorax.

It is also now apparent that gravitational effects may not be the dominant factor influencing regional pulmonary blood flow in conscious quadrupeds.[43,44] There appears to be a preferential distribution of blood flow to the dorsal region of the lung in these animals, especially during exercise. It is not known whether this species tendency is universal in quadrupeds or whether the phenomenon persists during general anesthesia.

A simplified diagrammatic representation of altered V/Q is shown in Fig. 5.4.[45] One extreme is to have a perfused alveolus or area of the lung with no ventilation so that the blood is not oxygenated while passing the region. Other extremes are for the alveolus to be ventilated but not perfused, or alternately for an alveolus or region to be neither ventilated nor perfused. Often the alteration of V/Q within the lung is somewhere in between these extremes and is characterized by alveoli throughout the lung that are only relatively underventilated or underperfused, producing

Table 5.2. Arterial blood-gas and acid-base values for various species.

Species	Mean Body Wt (kg)	n	Conditions	pH$_a$	PaCO$_2$	PaO$_2$	HCO$_3^-$	Refs.
Rats	0.207	10	Awake, chronic catheter	7.44	32.7		21.5	23
	0.305	8	Awake, prone, chronic catheter	7.467	39.8		28.7	24
Rabbits	3.1	NS[a]	Awake, catheter	7.388	32.8	86	21	25
	3.5	20	Awake, catheter	7.47	28.5	89.2	20.2	26
Cats	2.5–5.1	8	Unsedated, chronic catheter, prone	7.41	28.0	108	18	27
	3–8	10	Unsedated, not restrained, chronic catheter	7.426	32.5	108	22.1	28
Dogs	18.8	8	Chronic tracheostomy, catheter, unsedated, standing	7.383	39.0	103.8	22.1	8
	12.2	22	Chronic catheters lateral recumbency	7.40	35	102	21	29
Sheep	33	NS	Awake, catheter	7.44	40.9	96	27.6	25
	24.5	11	Unsedated, prone, carotid loop	7.48	33	92		30
Goats	18	6	Unsedated, standing	7.46	36.5	101		14
	47.6	6	Unsedated, standing, catheter	7.45	35.3	94.5	24.1	16
	46.6	6	Unsedated, standing	7.45	41.1	87.1	27.6	15
Calves	31–57	4	Standing, unsedated, aortic catheter	7.39	40	81	24	31
	48–66	20	Unanesthetized, catheter	7.37	42.8	93.6	23.6	32
Cows	517	7	Awake, unsedated, standing	7.40	39.6	83.1	24.4	9
	641	7	Awake, unsedated, standing	7.435	38.7	95.1	25.5	6
Horses	402	6	Awake, unsedated, standing	7.39	41.1	80.7	24.5	9
Ponies	147	19	Standing, aortic catheter	7.40	40	88.7	24.4	22

PaCO$_2$, arterial carbon dioxide partial pressure; PaO$_2$, arterial oxygen partial pressure; HCO$_3^-$, carbonic acid.
[a]Not specified.
[b]R. Warren and W. McDonell, unpublished observations.

Table 5.3. Lung volumes of various mammalian species: total lung capacity (TLC), functional residual capacity (FRC), and residual volume (RV).

Species	Mean Body Wt (kg)	n	Condition	TLC mL	TLC mL/kg	FRC (mL/kg)	RV (mL/kg)	Refs.
Mice	0.020	NS[a]	Anesthetized	1.57	78.5	25.0	19.5	10
Rats	0.31	NS	Anesthetized, prone	12.2	39.4	6.8	4.2	10
Rabbits	3.14	NS	Anesthetized, supine	111	35.4	11.6	6.4	10
Cats	3.7	4	Anesthetized			17.8		33
Dogs	18.6	6	Awake, prone	2090	112.4	53.6	16.7	12
	9.2	140	Unsedated, 1 year old			44.8		34
Sheep	24.5	4	Unsedated, prone, nasal endotracheal tube			45.3		30
Goats	46.4	6	Unsedated, standing, face mask			49.6		15
Cows	517	7	Awake, standing			39.4		35
	537	5	Anesthetized, prone	45,377	84.5	31.9	16.1	35
Horses	485		Anesthetized, prone	44,800	92.4	36.3	19.0	36
	402	6	Awake, standing			51.3		35
	394	4	Anesthetized, prone, lung inflated to 35–40 cm H$_2$O, starved 18 h	45,468	115.4	37.9		35
	450–822	6	Conscious, standing			35.6		37
Ponies	164–288	8	Conscious, standing			39.9		37

[a]Not specified.

an increase in the alveolar–arterial oxygen gradient. Since CO$_2$ is more diffusible across the alveolar capillary membrane, diffusion and V/Q problems commonly lead to decreased PaO$_2$ levels before there is a change in PaCO$_2$ levels. It is possible to compensate for nonventilation of portions of the lung through increased ventilation of the rest of the lung in terms of CO$_2$ clearance, as occurs with tachypneic pneumonic animals. However, the same increase in ventilation of "good" lung areas will never compensate completely for areas where there is inadequate oxygen uptake. The hemoglobin oxygen-saturation curve is sigmoid shaped

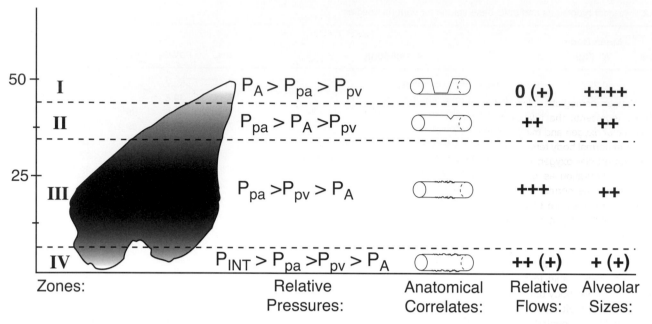

Fig. 5.3. Diagrammatic illustration of pulmonary artery (P_{pa}), pulmonary vein (P_{pv}), pulmonary interstitial (P_{INT}), and alveolar (P_A) pressure-flow relationships in the lung. Modified from Porcelli (p. 243),[42] with permission. See the text for a detailed explanation.

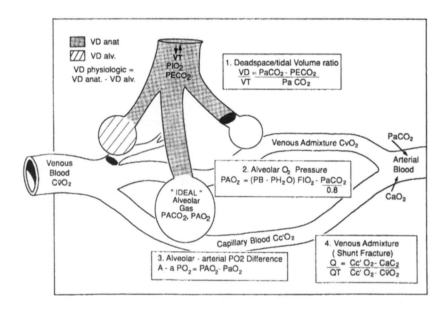

Fig. 5.4. Schematic of uneven ventilation and blood flow. The alveolus on the left is ventilated, but not perfused, and thus is considered to be alveolar dead space, whereas the alveolus on the right is perfused, but not ventilated, and thus contributes to venous admixture or so-called shunt flow. The center alveolus is perfused and ventilated equally and thus would have a V/Q ratio of 1.0. Relevant equations are shown respectively as Eqs. 1 to 4 for calculation of the dead space–tidal volume ratio, the alveolar partial pressure of oxygen (P_AO_2), the alveolar-to-arterial partial pressure of oxygen (A-a PO_2) difference, and the venous admixture (Q/QT) fraction. Reproduced from Robinson (p. 8),[45] with permission by Elsevier.

(Fig. 5.5), and hemoglobin is nearly fully saturated with oxygen at a PaO_2 of 90 to 100 mm Hg. Consequently, an increase in ventilation to the "good" areas of the lung cannot increase the oxygen content of blood very much, even though the alveolar partial pressure of oxygen (P_AO_2) increases. The clinical significance of this is that many pulmonary problems present as hypoxemia rather than hypercapnia.

Effect of Altered Alveolar Ventilation

For any given metabolic output, $PaCO_2$ and V_A are directly and inversely related: if V_A falls by 50%, $PaCO_2$ doubles; whereas, if V_A is increased by 100% (say, by IPPV), $PaCO_2$ levels will fall by 50% once equilibrium is established (Fig. 5.6). This is an important concept to grasp in that it explains how an experienced anesthetist can make fairly good approximations about the resultant $PaCO_2$ level he or she will produce when an animal is put on a volume-limited ventilator at a particular f and V_T setting. For instance, in most anesthetized dogs with a body weight that is average for the breed, $PaCO_2$ will be near eucapnic levels when f is set at 8 to 10/min and V_T at 20 mL/kg. In anesthetized adult horses and cows, a comparative eucapnic setting would be f at 5/min and V_T at 15 mL/kg.

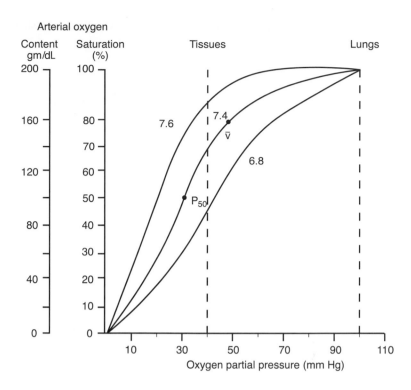

Fig. 5.5. Oxygen-hemoglobin dissociation curves. The center curve represents the relationship between the partial pressure of oxygen and the percentage hemoglobin saturation at normal body temperature and blood pH, and shows the arterial oxygen partial pressure (PaO_2) and percentage saturation as blood goes through the lungs and tissues. The normal mixed venous PO_2 and oxygen saturation values are shown ($\bar{v}$) along with the P_{50} value, which is the PO_2 at which the hemoglobin of a particular species is 50% saturated with oxygen. There is a shift of the hemoglobin dissociation curve to the right with acidemia (e.g., pH 6.8) or an increase in temperature, whereas there is a shift to the left with alkalemia (e.g., pH 7.6) or a lower body temperature. The oxygen-content values on the left represent the blood oxygen content that would be expected if the hemoglobin concentration was the theoretical normal level of 15 gm/dL and body temperature and pH levels were also normal.

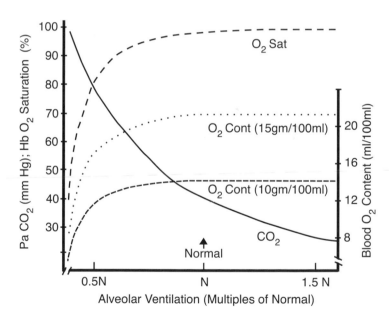

Fig. 5.6. Effect of altered alveolar ventilation on hemoglobin saturation, blood oxygen content, and arterial carbon dioxide partial pressure ($PaCO_2$) levels. As alveolar ventilation is halved, the $PaCO_2$ level doubles, illustrating the inverse and direct relationship between alveolar ventilation and carbon dioxide clearance. Note the difference in oxygen content with anemia (hemoglobin 10 g/100 mL instead of 15 g/100 mL), and the eventual sharp drop in hemoglobin oxygen saturation and oxygen content as alveolar ventilation decreases to less than 50% of the normal value. (See the text for further explanation.)

Hyperventilation occurs when V_A is excessive relative to metabolic rate; as a result, $PaCO_2$ is reduced. Hyperventilation may or may not be accompanied by an increased respiratory rate, referred to as *tachypnea*. *Hypoventilation* is present when V_A is small relative to metabolic rate, and $PaCO_2$ rises: hypoventilation may be accompanied by a slow (bradypnea), normal, or rapid *f*. A lowered $PaCO_2$ level is referred to as *hypocapnia* and an elevated level as *hypercapnia*, whereas normal $PaCO_2$ is termed *eucapnia*. Most, but not all, of the common mammalian species have a normal resting $PaCO_2$ level close to 40 mm Hg (Table 5.2). Hypercapnia and hypocapnia produce *respiratory acidosis*

and *alkalosis*, respectively, because CO_2 in the body is in dynamic equilibrium with carbonic acid (H_2CO_3) and, ultimately, hydrogen-ion concentration [H^+]:

$$CO_2 + H_2O \leftrightarrow H_2CO_3 \leftrightarrow H^+ + HCO_3^-$$

Acidemia and *alkalemia* are respectively defined as a plasma pH significantly below or above the normal arterial or venous value for the species in question. Concurrent metabolic acid-base disturbances and the presence or absence of compensation through renal excretion will determine the actual degree of pH change accompanying hypocapnia or hypercapnia. During general anesthesia, hypoventilation and hypercapnia are far more likely to occur in spontaneously breathing animals, whereas hyperventilation and hypocapnia most often occur when tidal volumes are too large in smaller animals during IPPV.

The relationship between V_A and oxygen saturation (and, in turn, the oxygen content of arterial blood) is not linear because of the sigmoid shape of the hemoglobin-saturation curve (Fig. 5.5). This factor has important clinical applications for anesthetists. With a 50% decrease in V_A, hemoglobin is still 80% saturated, and the actual oxygen content of blood (if hemoglobin concentration is 15 g/dL) will have fallen only from 21.2 to 16.8 mL/dL. Such an animal would not likely demonstrate cyanotic mucous membranes or even cardiovascular signs (tachycardia/bradycardia or increased/decreased blood pressure) associated with respiratory insufficiency. However, as the level of V_A decreases further, there is a sharp and potentially catastrophic decrease in the oxygen content of arterial blood so that, at a V_A that is 40% of normal, hemoglobin saturation is 50% and the oxygen content has fallen to 7.04 mL/dL. This degree of hypoxemia may well lead to cardiorespiratory collapse quite suddenly. An understanding of this nonlinear effect of V_A deficiency on oxygen content helps to explain why an apparently "okay" animal on an intravenous general anesthetic and breathing room air can suddenly stop breathing or go into cardiovascular collapse without any apparent change in the depth of anesthesia.

Figure 5.6 illustrates the important interrelationship between a lower hemoglobin level (e.g., 10 g/dL) and blood oxygen content with altered ventilatory homeostasis. The blood oxygen content is reduced by nearly 7 mL/dL with a decrease in hemoglobin from 15 to 10 g/dL even when hemoglobin saturation is 100%, and dangerously low blood oxygen contents occur with further ventilatory depression.

Hypoxia refers to any state in which the oxygen in the lung, blood, and/or tissues is abnormally low, resulting in abnormal organ function and/or cellular damage. *Hypoxemia* refers to insufficient oxygenation of blood to meet metabolic requirement. In spontaneously breathing animals, hypoxemia is characterized by PaO_2 levels lower than the normal for the species. Resting PaO_2 levels in domestic species generally range from 80 to 100 mm Hg in healthy, awake animals (Table 5.2). Some clinicians consider a PaO_2 below 70 mm Hg (ca. 94% hemoglobin saturation) as hypoxemia in animals at or near sea level, although the clinical significance of this degree of blood oxygen tension would vary depending on factors such as the health and age of an animal, hemoglobin concentration, and the duration of low oxygen tension in relation to the rate of tissue metabolism (e.g., hypothermic patients would be at less risk).

Oxygen Transport

Under normal conditions, oxygen is taken into the pulmonary alveoli and CO_2 is removed from them at a rate that is sufficient to maintain the composition of alveolar air at a relatively constant concentration. In the lung, gas is exchanged across both the alveolar and the capillary membranes.[7] The total distance across which exchange takes place is less than 1 μm; therefore, it occurs

Table 5.4. Composition of respiratory gases in humans.

Gas	Inspired Air (%)	Expired Air (%)	Alveolar Air (%)
Oxygen	20.95	16.1	14.0
Carbon dioxide	0.04	4.1	5.6
Nitrogen[a]	79.0	79.2	80.0

[a]There is no change in the absolute concentration of nitrogen. The change in percentage occurs because more oxygen is used than carbon dioxide produced.

rapidly. Other than at high exercise levels, equilibrium almost develops between blood in the lungs and air in the alveolus, and the partial pressure of oxygen (PO_2) in the blood almost equals the PO_2 in the alveolus. While diffusion of oxygen across the alveolar-capillary space is a theoretical barrier to oxygenation, it is seldom a practical problem during veterinary anesthesia unless considerable pulmonary edema is present.

There is a relatively steep concentration or *partial pressure gradient* of oxygen from room air to the various body tissues: nasal air = 160 mm Hg; alveolar air = 100 mm Hg; arterial blood = 90 to 95 mm Hg; interstitial fluid = 30 mm Hg; intracellular fluid = 10 mm Hg; and venous blood = 40 mm Hg. Little oxygen is lost in large blood vessels, and normally a continuous pressure gradient is present from the alveolus to the tissue cell.

The normal average alveolar composition of respiratory gases in humans is listed in Table 5.4. At body temperature, alveolar air is saturated with water vapor, which has a pressure at 37°C of 48 mm Hg. If the barometric pressure in the alveolus is 760 mm Hg (sea level), then the pressure due to dry air is 760 − 48 = 712 mm Hg. Knowing the composition of alveolar air, one can calculate the partial pressure of each gas in the alveolus:

$$O_2 = (760 - 48) \times 0.14 = 100 \text{ mm Hg}$$
$$CO_2 = (760 - 48) \times 0.056 = 40 \text{ mm Hg}$$
$$N_2 = (760 - 48) \times 0.80 = 570 \text{ mm Hg}$$

Oxygen partial pressure in the lungs at sea level is thus approximately 100 mm Hg at 37° to 38°C. Under these conditions, 100 mL of plasma will hold 0.3 mL of oxygen in physical solution. Whole blood, under the same conditions, will hold 20 mL of oxygen, or about 60 times as much as plasma. CO_2 is similarly held by blood. Thus, it is apparent that oxygen and CO_2 in blood are transported largely in chemical combination, since both are carried by blood in much greater quantities than would occur if simple absorption took place. At complete saturation, each gram of hemoglobin combines with 1.36 to 1.39 mL of oxygen. This is the total carrying capacity of hemoglobin, or four oxygen molecules combined with each hemoglobin molecule. The ability of hemoglobin to combine with oxygen depends on the PO_2 in the surrounding environment. The degree to which it will become saturated at various oxygen partial pressures varies considerably (Fig. 5.5). It is adjusted so that, even when ventilation is inefficient or the supply of oxygen is sparse as at higher altitudes, the degree of saturation still approaches 100%. For instance, although it is probably not fully saturated until it is exposed to a

PO_2 of 250 mm Hg, hemoglobin is approximately 94% saturated when the PO_2 is only 70 mm Hg.

Although there is relatively little change in hemoglobin saturation between 70 and 250 mm Hg PO_2, a marked change occurs between 10 and 40 mm Hg, a PO_2 characteristic of actively metabolizing tissues. Thus, as hemoglobin is exposed to tissues having partial pressures of oxygen within this range, it will yield its oxygen to the tissues. The lower the PO_2 of these tissues, the greater is the amount of oxygen that hemoglobin will yield. The degree to which hemoglobin yields its oxygen is influenced by environmental pH, PCO_2, and temperature—all mechanisms that protect the metabolizing cell. As the pH decreases and the PCO_2 and local temperature increase, at any given PO_2 value, especially in the range of 10 to 40 mm Hg, hemoglobin releases oxygen to the surrounding environment more readily (Fig. 5.5). It is also interesting to note that nature has adapted for the relatively lower oxygen environment of the fetus, because fetal hemoglobin carries a greater percentage of oxygen at a lower partial pressure.

Certain enzyme systems aid dissociation of oxygen from hemoglobin, the most completely studied being the enzyme system producing 2,3-diphosphoglycerate (2,3-DPG). This system enhances dissociation of oxygen from hemoglobin by competing with oxygen for the binding site. A lowered level of this enzyme, as occurs with stored blood used for transfusion, increases the affinity of hemoglobin for oxygen and thus acts as though the dissociation curve is shifted to the left. The oxygen tension at which 50% saturation of hemoglobin is achieved (P_{50}) is used to measure affinity of hemoglobin for oxygen. P_{50} is reduced in septic patients and in carbon monoxide poisoning. The reverse has been encountered in chronic anemia. Since tissues require a given volume of oxygen per unit of time, the hemoglobin concentration of blood has a significant influence on oxygen content and delivery to the tissues.

Although an increase in the P_AO_2 above normal causes only a small increase in the oxygen-carrying capacity of hemoglobin, plasma carries oxygen in an amount directly proportional to the PO_2 in the alveoli. At normal atmospheric pressure, when the animal is breathing air at 38°C, 0.3 mL of oxygen is carried in solution in 100 mL of blood. If pure oxygen is administered, the PO_2 in the alveoli is raised from 100 to almost 650 mm Hg. Plasma oxygen is thus elevated almost seven times, that is, from 0.3 to 1.8 mL per 100 mL of blood. The result is an increase of about 10% in oxygen content of the blood. This is of some importance, because oxygen transfers from blood to tissues by diffusion, and the process occurs at a rate proportional to the difference in oxygen tension between plasma and body tissues.

A common misconception is that oxygenation of patients can be improved by increasing the physical (airway) pressure at which oxygen is administered. Except in hyperbaric chambers, oxygenation of patients is improved not by increasing the barometric pressure of the gas mixture, but by increasing the *proportion* or PO_2 in the mixture. At a positive alveolar pressure exceeding 40 mm Hg, the capillary circulation in the lungs is inhibited; therefore, it is not practical to administer oxygen at a pressure exceeding this pressure. During anesthesia, hypoxemic episodes are best handled by reducing the level of inhalant anesthetic in the mask or rebreathing bag along with ensuring there is a high inspired-oxygen concentration, while instituting IPPV at a normal f, V_T, and inflation pressure (12 to 15 mm Hg in small animals, and 20 to 25 mm Hg in horses and cows).

In conscious, healthy animals, there is considerable capacity to increase the rate of oxygen supply to, and CO_2 removal from, the body tissues, with up to 30-fold increases seen in exercising horses. The gas transport is increased in conscious horses by a fivefold increase in cardiac output, a 50% increase in hemoglobin concentration, and a fourfold increase in the extraction of oxygen from the blood traversing skeletal muscle capillaries.[7] The capacity for increasing oxygen supply is considerably less in more sedentary species.

During general anesthesia, these adaptive mechanisms to increase systemic oxygen supply are markedly compromised. Anesthetized animals are not likely to be able to appreciably increase their V_E or cardiac output, the spleen is often dilated and incapable of contracting to increase hemoglobin levels, and a key muscle (myocardial) cannot extract a greater proportion of oxygen from the blood going through the capillaries in response to an increase in demand or decrease in oxygen supply.

Carbon Dioxide Transport

Arterial CO_2 levels are a function of both CO_2 elimination and production, and under normal circumstances $PaCO_2$ levels are maintained within narrow limits. During severe exercise, the production of CO_2 is increased enormously, whereas, during anesthesia, production likely decreases. Elimination of CO_2 depends on pulmonary blood flow (cardiac output) and V_A. Normally, the production of CO_2 parallels the oxygen consumption according to the respiratory quotient: $R = VCO_2/VO_2$. Although the value varies depending on the diet, usually R is 0.8 at steady state. Because of the blood buffer systems, CO_2 transport to the lungs for excretion is effected with little change in blood pH. The importance of the lungs in excreting this volatile acid is illustrated by the fact that, in humans, the kidneys eliminate 40 to 80 mEq of hydrogen ions per day, while the lungs eliminate 13,000 mEq per day as CO_2.

A CO_2 pressure gradient, opposite to that of oxygen and much smaller, exists from the tissues to the atmospheric air: tissues = 50 mm Hg (during exercise, this may be higher); venous blood = 46 mm Hg; alveolar air = 40 mm Hg; expired air = 32 mm Hg; atmospheric air = 0.3 mm Hg; and arterial blood = 40 mm Hg (equilibrium with alveolar air). CO_2 is carried from the mitochondria to the alveoli in a number of forms (Fig. 5.7).[45] In the plasma, some CO_2 is transported in solution (5%), and some combines with water and forms *carbonic acid*, which in turn dissociates into *bicarbonate* and *hydrogen ions* (5%). Most (ca. 90%) of the CO_2 diffuses into the red cells, where it is either bound to hemoglobin or transformed (reversibly) to bicarbonate and hydrogen ions through the action of the enzyme *carbonic anhydase*. The formation of bicarbonate in the red blood cell is accompanied by the chloride shift (this accounts for approximately 63% of the total CO_2 transport). The excellent buffering capacity

Equine Anesthesia

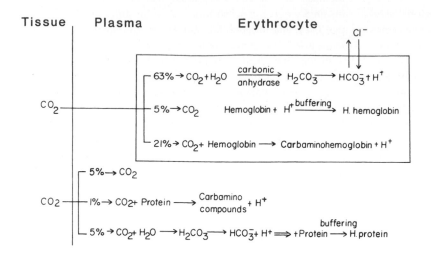

Fig. 5.7. Transport of carbon dioxide in the blood. Carbon dioxide diffuses out of the tissues into the plasma and erythrocytes, undergoing a variety of reactions that result in the production of bicarbonate and hydrogen ions. The hydrogen ions are then buffered either by proteins in the plasma or by hemoglobin, minimizing the pH change. In the lung, all of the reactions that are shown in this figure are reversed. Reproduced from Robinson (p. 30),[45] with permission by Elsevier.

of hemoglobin enables changes in hydrogen-ion content to occur during this process with minimal change in pH. Under ordinary circumstances, the pH of venous blood is only 0.01 to 0.03 pH units lower than that of arterial blood. CO_2 is also carried in the red cell in the form of carbamino compounds. Amino acids and aliphatic amines combine with CO_2 to form unstable carbamino compounds. Hemoglobin (Hb) is the main protein acting in this manner, though many can do so. The efficiency of this reaction is greater with Hb than with hemoglobin-bound oxygen. Thus, as hemoglobin and oxygen dissociate, hemoglobin's capacity to carry CO_2 increases.

The mechanisms of CO_2 and oxygen transport are integrated in the blood in at least three ways: (a) The acidity of carbonic acid produced in the tissues favors release of oxygen without a change in oxygen tension, whereas the release of CO_2 in the lungs favors oxygen uptake (Bohr effect). (b) Release of oxygen favors CO_2 uptake and vice versa in the carbamino mechanism. Upon the release of oxygen, hemoglobin becomes a weaker acid and is more capable of accepting hydrogen ions, thereby facilitating its buffering effect (Haldane effect). (c) The two acid forms of the hemoglobin molecule favor dissociation by shifting from one form to the other. Oxygen uptake favors CO_2 loss and vice versa.

Just as the amount of oxygen transported by the blood depends on the PO_2 to which the blood is exposed, so is CO_2 transport likewise affected; however, the CO_2 dissociation curve is more or less linear. Thus, in contrast to the minimal effects on oxygen content (Fig. 5.6), hyperventilation and hypoventilation may have marked effects on CO_2 content of blood and tissues.

Upper-Airway Obstruction

With the onset of general anesthesia, the nasal alar and pharyngeal musculature relax and, in deeper planes, the cough reflex is abolished. The net effect is to predispose patients toward upper-airway obstruction. This is particularly evident in brachycephalic dogs suffering from stenotic nares, an elongated soft palate,

everted lateral laryngeal ventricles, and/or a hypoplastic trachea. In these animals, the onset of general anesthesia may produce serious and potentially fatal upper-airway obstruction unless the trachea is intubated. Experience has shown that it is preferable to perform endotracheal intubation in all anesthetized dogs, partly to protect against upper-airway obstruction, but also to protect against possible aspiration of secretions or refluxed gastric contents from the stomach. It is important, however, that the endotracheal intubation be done atraumatically. Routine use of a laryngoscope reduces trauma during intubation. In many domestic and laboratory species, the decision as to whether to use an endotracheal tube is a risk-benefit decision that must be determined based on the species involved, the anesthetic regimen employed and the experience of the anesthetist, the intended operation, the health of the animal, and the duration of anesthesia.

In ruminants, endotracheal intubation is required for all but the shortest-acting anesthetics, such as diazepam premedication with low-dose ketamine in sheep, calves, and goats, which only lasts about 5 min. The prime reason for endotracheal intubation is to protect against aspiration of rumen contents after active or passive regurgitation. In swine, endotracheal intubation is comparatively difficult and requires considerable experience if trauma is to be avoided. Swine have inherently small airways and are more likely to develop apnea than other domestic species. Nevertheless, for most brief surgeries (e.g., hernia repair or cryptorchidectomy) the risk-benefit balance is better served by not intubating swine, but instead by paying careful attention to the depth of anesthesia and to the character of respiration and head position so as to minimize the chance of serious upper-airway obstruction. In most species, the best airway is provided when the head is kept in a somewhat extended position: Pigs are unusual in that the best airway is provided with the head at a normal angle to the neck.

If significant upper-airway obstruction occurs in any species, and the depth of anesthesia is not excessive, the animal usually develops an exaggerated respiratory effort that is primarily abdominal in character. The chest wall may even move inward on inspiration (paradoxical respiration) if the degree of upper-airway obstruction is moderate or severe. The only other clinical situation that produces this subtle, but distinctive, change in the character of respiration is extremely deep anesthesia. This usually occurs at an anesthetic plane just before complete cessation of respiratory drive—that is, apnea—ensues.

In rodents—such as mice, gerbils, hamsters, and guinea pigs—and in rabbits, endotracheal intubation may be difficult unless the anesthetist is experienced with the technique and has special equipment. In these species, longer, well-controlled periods of anesthesia for experimental purposes may well require endotracheal intubation. Shorter procedures in a veterinary practice may often be performed without using an endotracheal tube. A suitable face-mask and non-rebreathing administration system may be used for oxygen administration (in the case of injectable anesthesia) or for administration of an oxygen-inhalant regimen using a precision vaporizer. When the anesthetist is capable of performing atraumatic endotracheal intubation and has suitably small tubes (3 to 4 mm), it is preferable to intubate ferrets and rabbits, because surgical anesthetic planes produce considerable respiratory depression in both species, and it is much easier to deal with apnea if an endotracheal tube is already in place.

There is some controversy as to whether an endotracheal tube should always be placed in cats for shorter procedures (e.g., neutering). Cats tend to maintain a patent airway somewhat more effectively than do other species, unless drugs are used (e.g., ether) that increase the incidence of secretions and/or laryngospasm. Laryngospasm is comparatively rare when halothane, isoflurane, or sevoflurane are administered by mask, or when ketamine or propofol are used along with diazepam, acepromazine, or low-dose α_2-agonist sedation for injectable anesthesia. Moreover, endotracheal intubation requires a deeper level of anesthesia than is needed for some minor surgical or diagnostic procedures. Laryngospasm is more likely to occur after anesthesia when the larynx has been traumatized during intubation or when the endotracheal tubes have been cleaned with some sort of detergent or disinfectant between animals without adequate rinsing. In a large morbidity and mortality study conducted in the United Kingdom, postanesthetic airway obstruction was one of the more frequently encountered problems in cats,[46] and the suspicion is that this might well be associated with trauma during insertion of an endotracheal tube into the airway. On the other hand, there can be no denying the many advantages associated with endotracheal intubation in cats, as with other species. A patent airway is immediately available if the animal needs IPPV because of apnea or respiratory insufficiency, the risk of aspiration of gastric contents is markedly reduced, and it is easier to scavenge anesthetic waste gases if an inhalant anesthetic is being used. In cats, laryngeal desensitization with lidocaine will help to reduce spasm and trauma associated with the placement of a tube. Endotracheal tube placement for shorter procedures is not mandatory, providing that emergency airway and oxygen are readily available and the patency of the airway is being continuously monitored.

Veterinary anesthesia textbooks have hitherto placed little emphasis on the need to provide for a secure airway in horses, primarily because regurgitation is very rare. Although it is true that short-duration, injectable, field anesthetic techniques have been performed for many years without the use of an endotracheal tube, a considerable degree of upper-airway obstruction does occur in horses (Fig. 5.8), primarily because their nostrils no longer flare during inspiration. Therefore, placement of an endotracheal tube may be considered desirable in most circumstances.[47]

This tendency toward upper-airway obstruction increases when a horse has been anesthetized for longer than 1 or 2 h, especially when in dorsal recumbency. It is thought that passive congestion and tissue swelling occur because the nasopharynx structures are lower than the heart in anesthetized animals, and that this predisposes animals to airway obstruction in the recovery period when the endotracheal tube is removed. As a result, many equine anesthetists now secure an orotracheal, nasotracheal, or nasopharyngeal airway during the recovery process whenever horses have been anesthetized for any extended length of time (e.g., over 30 to 45 min).[48,49] Clinically, it appears that ensuring an adequate diameter patent airway while a horse is trying to stand up (and is breathing vigorously) prevents the panic associated with partial or complete airway obstruction and leads to more controlled recoveries. There is still a need for large-scale morbidity and mortality studies that address the issue of when and where endotracheal tubes should be used during routine veterinary anesthesia, especially in a practice setting.

Anesthetic Alteration of the Control of Respiration

Respiratory drive and the adjustment of f, V_T, and V_A are achieved in conscious animals through a complex neural regulatory mechanism. Respiratory rhythm originates in the medulla and is modified by inputs from higher brain centers and the activity of chemoreceptor, pulmonary, and airway receptors. The central neural control mechanisms regulate the activity of the primary and accessory respiratory muscles, producing gas movement into and out of the lung and tracheobronchial tree. These control mechanisms are described in detail elsewhere.[5–7,50] Although there is certainly a similarity in the respiratory control mechanism between species, it is important to realize that various components may assume greater importance in different species.

Normal Control Mechanisms

As important as the detailed information referred to earlier is in helping us understand the respiratory adaptations to high altitude, disease, and exercise, for the successful management of clinical anesthesia a much simplified understanding of the control of respiration will suffice (Fig. 5.9). In conscious animals, V_E and V_A are primarily determined by central chemoreceptor responsiveness to $PaCO_2$ levels. The *central chemoreceptors*, located on the ventral surface of the medulla and bathed by cerebrospinal fluid, are exquisitely sensitive to changes in $PaCO_2$ levels because CO_2 is readily diffusible into cerebrospinal fluid and the central chemoreceptor cell. The changes in $PaCO_2$ are probably ultimately detected as a change in the pH within the chemoreceptor

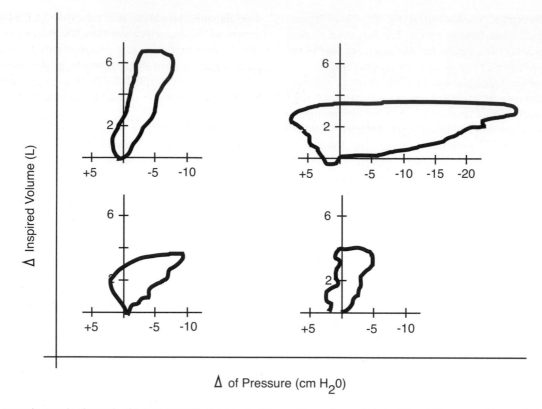

Fig. 5.8. Changes in nonelastic work of breathing with the onset of general anesthesia (thiobarbiturate) in a spontaneously breathing horse. The change in transpulmonary pressure (airway opening to esophageal balloon) is shown as the *abscissa*, and the change in volume (tidal volume) is shown on the *ordinate* scale. The area within the loops is a measure of the nonelastic work of breathing and is a reflection of the airway resistance, as well as a small component of tissue resistance. The *top left loop* was obtained from a conscious horse breathing quietly; the *top right loop* was obtained after 15 min of anesthesia with the horse in lateral recumbency and breathing without an endotracheal tube in place; the *bottom left loop* is after the horse was intubated with a 25-mm tube; and the *bottom right loop* was obtained once the horse stood in recovery with the tube removed. Note the large increase in nonelastic work of breathing during anesthesia until an endotracheal tube is inserted, and that fairly large negative pressures (10 to 15 cm H_2O) must be generated before there is an appreciable volume of inspired gas. This is indicative of upper-airway obstruction (W. McDonell, unpublished observations).

cell. This ventilatory response to CO_2 is often presented as a response curve wherein V_A or V_E is plotted against the $PaCO_2$, the alveolar partial pressure of carbon dioxide (P_ACO_2), the end-tidal CO_2 partial pressure ($P_{ET}CO_2$), or the inspired-CO_2 level (Fig. 5.10A). An increase in $PaCO_2$ of 3 to 5 mm Hg will produce a rapid doubling or tripling of V_A in an effort to return $PaCO_2$ to eucapnic levels. This response is a little less sensitive in horses[51,52] and a lot less sensitive in burrowing and diving mammals.[53] In ruminants, the gas produced in the rumen may consist of more than 60% CO_2, and when it is eructated a significant proportion of this gas is inhaled, contributing to a cyclic breathing pattern.[50] A fall in arterial pH will also stimulate respiration through the central and peripheral chemoreceptors, as seen with metabolic acidosis: This response is slower. The central chemoreceptors are not responsive to alterations in PaO_2 levels.

The *peripheral chemoreceptors*, which are located in the carotid and aortic bodies, generally play a significant part in respiratory drive only when PaO_2 levels fall below 60 mm Hg.[6,52] This is illustrated in Fig. 5.10B, drawn from a study on conscious horses.[54] As the F_IO_2 was decreased from 1.0 (100% inspired

oxygen) down to 0.16, there was no change in V_E. At an F_IO_2 of 0.16, the alveolar oxygen tension (P_AO_2) would be 60 to 65 mm Hg at sea level. In sheep, goats, calves, and ponies, however, carotid body denervation causes some hypoventilation, hypoxemia, and hypercapnia, and it is estimated that carotid body receptor activity is responsible for up to 30% of the resting V_A drive in calves at sea level[55] and up to 40% in miniature pigs.[17]

The activity of the central neural systems and the level of ventilatory drive are also influenced by the general level of central nervous system activity, especially by traffic through the reticular activating system (RAS). This is evidenced by the decrease in V_A and small increase in $PaCO_2$ that accompany sleep, and by the fact that exercising animals commonly become hypocapnic even if tissue oxygen delivery is adequate. Anesthetists make good use of this link between RAS activity and respiratory drive by using an increase in sensory stimulation (limb flexion, twisting a horse's ear, rolling a dog or cat over, or vigorously rubbing the body surface) to increase ventilatory drive during emergence from inhalation anesthesia, thereby speeding inhalant drug elimination and recovery.

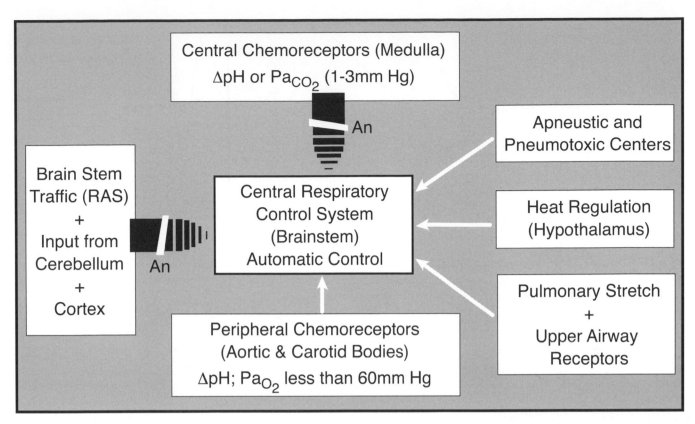

Fig. 5.9. Schematic diagram of the control of ventilation in conscious and anesthetized animals. In conscious animals, the level of alveolar ventilation is primarily determined by the arterial carbon dioxide partial pressure ($PaCO_2$) level (as sensed by the central chemoreceptors) and the level of brain-stem traffic, with the apneustic and pneumotaxic centers and the stretch receptors governing the relationship between tidal volume and frequency to achieve the required alveolar ventilation. General anesthesia (An) reduces brain-stem traffic and the chemoreceptor response to carbon dioxide, leading to an increase in $PaCO_2$. In most species, the peripheral chemoreceptors begin to influence the level of alveolar ventilation if PaO_2 falls below 60 mm Hg. ΔpH, change in PH; and RAS, reticular activating system.

The apneustic and pneumotaxic centers, and pulmonary and airway receptors, are primarily responsible for adjusting the balance between f and V_T to achieve a given level of V_A, usually in a way that minimizes the energy cost of breathing. Although the function of these receptors is generally not considered to be greatly influenced by the action of anesthetic and perianesthetic agents, they may play a part in some of the species differences we see in response to a particular drug or group of drugs. For instance, as the inhaled dose of isoflurane is increased, f remains stable or increases in ferrets,[56,57] whereas f decreases in rats[56] and rabbits.[57] In dogs and cats, as the dose of an inhalant agent increases, f often remains constant or increases,[58,59] although there is some variation in response between drugs.[60] In horses, f remains more or less constant with increasing inhalant anesthetic doses.[61–63] Respiratory rate is usually less with isoflurane, sevoflurane, or desflurane than with halothane at an equipotent dose, whereas V_T is larger.[61,63] The barbiturates usually decrease f and V_T as the dose is increased, whereas the primary response to increasing inhalant doses is to reduce V_T (ether is an exception). In ruminants, general anesthesia is often associated with tachypnea and very shallow breathing.[64,65] All of these differences might well originate from species and/or drug differences in the central inspiratory-expiratory switching mechanisms or

lung receptor activity (stretch receptors, irritant receptors, and C fibers), but so far the evidence is primarily speculative. Irritant airway receptor activity, especially in the larynx and tracheal regions, appears to differ quite markedly between species. Horses, for instance, have a weak laryngeal reflex, so it is rather easy to insert a nasoendotracheal tube in a conscious horse, even without the aid of local anesthesia. In contrast, swine and cats have a strong laryngeal reflex, and fairly deep anesthesia is required for easy endotracheal intubation unless local desensitization is produced using a topical anesthetic. The response of dogs is intermediate.

Apneic Threshold

The *apneic threshold* is the $PaCO_2$ level at which ventilation becomes zero; that is, where spontaneous ventilatory effort ceases (Fig. 5.10A). A $PaCO_2$ reduction of 5 to 9 mm Hg from normal values through voluntary hyperventilation (a conscious human), or by artificial ventilation of sedated or anesthetized animals, produces apnea. The distance between the resting $PaCO_2$ level and the apnea threshold is relatively constant (i.e., 5 to 9 mm Hg) irrespective of the anesthetic depth.[66] Veterinary anesthetists use the apneic threshold to control respiration (i.e., abolish spontaneous efforts) when putting an animal on a ventilator, or to tem-

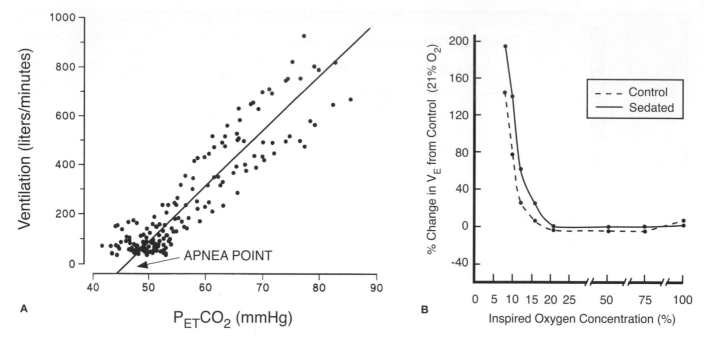

Fig. 5.10. **A:** This carbon dioxide response curve for six horses shows individual data points, the regression line, and the theoretical apnea point. Minute ventilation is plotted against end-tidal carbon dioxide. The horses were permitted to rebreathe carbon dioxide from a large spirometer filled with 30% oxygen. Data modified from Gauvreau et al.,[51] with permission. **B:** An oxygen response curve for unsedated horses and horses sedated with acepromazine. The percentage change in ventilation is plotted against the inspired-oxygen concentration. Data modified from Muir and Hamlin,[54] with permission.

porarily provide for a quiet surgical field without having to resort to the use of muscle relaxant drugs.

Drug Effect on Control of Ventilation

Anesthetics and some perianesthetic drugs alter the central and peripheral chemoreceptor response to CO_2 and oxygen in a dose-dependent manner.[66–68] This has important clinical implications in terms of maintaining homeostasis during the perioperative period. There will also be a diminution in external signs in hypoxemic or hypercarbic anesthetized animals. Whereas unsedated animals usually demonstrate obvious tachypnea and an increase in V_T or respiratory effort in response to serious hypoxemia or hypercapnia, these external signs of an impending crisis may well be absent or greatly diminished in anesthetized animals.

Inhalants and Injectable Drugs

All of the general anesthetic agents in current use produce a dose-dependent decrease in the response to CO_2.[5,24,67] With commonly used inhalant agents, the CO_2 response is almost flat at a minimum alveolar concentration of 2.0 (Fig. 5.11).[69] The reduced sensory input and central sensitivity to CO_2 produce a marked fall in V_A, usually through a dose-related fall in V_T, with f being reasonably well maintained. A proportional increase in V_D/V_T occurs, because $V_{D\ anat}$ is more or less constant. As a result of these changes, $PaCO_2$ levels increase as the anesthetic dose is increased when animals breathe spontaneously (Fig. 5.12A).[58,70,71] In light anesthetic planes (e.g., minimum alveolar concentration of 1.2), $PaCO_2$ will generally remain moderately elevated, but stable, over

many hours of anesthesia, whereas, at higher concentrations or in ruminants, $PaCO_2$ increases progressively over time. The degree of hypercarbia at equipotent doses of inhalant (and intravenous) anesthetic agents varies with the species and the degree of surgical stimulation (Fig. 5.12B).[61,72–74] Of the commonly used inhalant anesthetics, halothane produces the least increase in $PaCO_2$ during spontaneous respiration, whereas, at equipotent doses, isoflurane, sevoflurane, and desflurane produce somewhat higher and similar $PaCO_2$ levels in most species.[57,60–63,75]

In ruminants, the degree of hypercarbia is greater with equipotent inhalant anesthetic doses than for horses, and horses show more respiratory depression than monkeys or dogs (Fig. 5.12B). Clinically, swine, ferrets, and rabbits also seem to be more prone to hypercarbia, whereas deep-diving seals may become totally apneic during light levels of anesthesia or even just opioid sedation.[76]

During surgery the level of respiratory depression is usually less and the differences between drugs may disappear. For example, in dorsally recumbent, spontaneously breathing pregnant mares induced with xylazine and thiamylal sodium and maintained on halothane or isoflurane for laparotomy surgery, $PaCO_2$ levels increased from 53.8 to 58.3 mm Hg during halothane anesthesia and were 60.7 to 60.5 mm Hg during isoflurane anesthesia. There was no significant difference in $PaCO_2$ (or PaO_2) levels with the two agents from 30 to 90 min, although f was lower (4 to 5/min) with isoflurane than with halothane (8 to 10/min).[77]

Barbiturates, propofol, and the cyclohexamines (ketamine, phencyclidine, and tiletamine) also produce a similar dose-

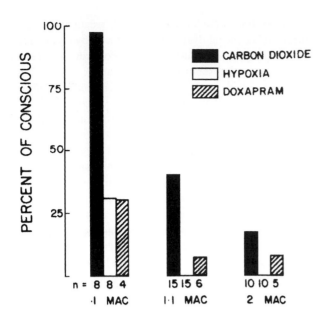

Fig. 5.11. Effect of halothane sedation (0.1 minimum alveolar concentration [MAC]) and anesthesia (1.1 and 2.0 MAC) on depression of the ventilatory response to hypoxia, hypercapnia, and doxapram expressed as a percentage of the awake control response. Reproduced from Knill and Gelb,[69] with permission.

related alteration in the CO_2 response, which may, in the case of barbiturates, outlast the period of actual anesthesia by some time.[78] Although it is generally considered that ketamine is not as much of a respiratory depressant as the barbiturates,[68] clinical

experience and survey studies have shown that safe, clinically effective doses of ketamine may induce apnea in some susceptible individuals.[46] The typical response to increasing doses of barbiturates is for both V_T and f to decrease. When injectable anesthetics are used before inhalation agents, as is commonly done in clinical veterinary anesthesia, the respiratory-depressant effects of both drugs are at least additive.[78]

Although the control of ventilation during anesthesia is primarily determined by central CO_2 responsiveness (albeit reduced), during very deep barbiturate anesthesia CO_2 ventilatory drive may disappear and the drive may become hypoxic. Hypoxic drive sensitivity is also lessened appreciably by general anesthetics (at least inhalants) in a dose-related manner (Fig. 5.11).[69] It is interesting to note that, although the peripheral chemoreceptor response to PaO_2 at physiological levels (80 to 110 mm Hg) is virtually nonexistent in conscious animals, in anesthetized horses and ducks the $PaCO_2$ levels are greater at F_IO_2 1.0 than at F_IO_2 0.3.[79,80] Therefore, the high oxygen levels used in most inhalant regimens might contribute somewhat to depression of ventilation while helping to ensure that the level of oxygenation is adequate.

Opioids
When given alone, opioids shift the CO_2 response curve to the right with little change in slope, except at very high doses. This means that the resting $PaCO_2$ level might be a little higher in an animal receiving a therapeutic dose of an opioid for premedication or postoperative recovery, but that the response to further CO_2 challenge (from metabolism, airway obstruction, etc.) will not be abolished. Clinically, when opioids are used at high doses

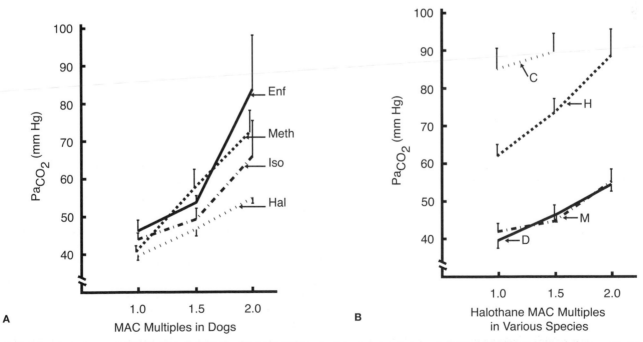

Fig. 5.12. **A:** Influence of increasing anesthetic dose (multiples of minimum alveolar concentration [MAC]) on arterial carbon dioxide partial pressure ($PaCO_2$) in spontaneously breathing dogs anesthetized with enflurane (Enf), methoxyflurane (Meth), isoflurane (Iso), or halothane (Hal). Data compiled from a series of studies done by Steffey and coworkers,[58,70,71] with permission. **B:** Differences in the $PaCO_2$ with spontaneous breathing and increasing halothane levels (multiples of MAC) in calves (C), horses (H), monkeys (M), and dogs (D). Data compiled from a series of studies done by Steffey and coworkers,[71–74] with permission.

as part of a balanced anesthetic regimen, there is an additive effect of the opioid depression of the respiratory center and the general anesthetic, and considerable hypercarbia or even apnea may be produced.[81,82] In addition, the μ opioids in particular tend to produce rapid, shallow breathing in dogs,[83] which may interfere with the subsequent uptake of an inhalant anesthetic.

At the doses commonly employed for routine opioid premedication or postoperative analgesia in veterinary practice, significant respiratory depression is very rarely seen, at least in terms of producing hypercapnia.[83–85] Frequency of ventilation may decrease owing to a decrease in apprehension. In fact, effective alveolar ventilation may well improve when opioid analgesics are employed for postoperative pain relief.[86] The postoperative use of opioids has been implicated in the development of an increased incidence of postoperative atelectasis and hypoxemia in human patients, especially during sleep.[87] Clinical evidence would suggest that the incidence of similar problems in veterinary patients is rare, but it is an area that warrants further study.

The historical tendency to minimize the use of opioids for postoperative analgesia because of the fear of serious respiratory problems is simply not based on facts, as is now well recognized.[88] There is a ceiling effect and less respiratory depression associated with opioid agonists/antagonists (e.g., pentazocine, butorphanol, nalbuphine, and buprenorphine) when used at high doses than with the pure μ-agonists (meperidine, morphine, and oxymorphone).[89] Using the epidural route of administration helps to ensure that there is minimal postoperative respiratory depression with high-risk cases.[90,91]

Tranquilizers

The phenothiazine and benzodiazepine sedatives often reduce the respiratory rate, especially if an animal is somewhat excited prior to administration, but they do not appreciably alter arterial blood-gas tensions.[84,92,93] There are few studies of the effect of these drugs on CO_2 responsiveness, especially in animals. Horses sedated with acepromazine (0.65 mg/kg intravenously [IV]) responded similarly, in terms of V_E change, to unsedated horses until the level of hypoxia or hypercapnia was quite severe (F_IO_2 of 0.1 or F_ICO_2 of 0.06), at which time the response was lessened.[54] When used alone, diazepam (0.05 to 0.4 mg/kg IV) does not produce significant changes in PaO_2 or $PaCO_2$ in horses.[94] The respiratory-protective nature of these drugs is such that when they are combined with a general anesthetic, and the required dose of the general anesthetic is thereby lessened, ventilation is better than when an equipotent higher concentration of the general anesthetic (barbiturate or inhalant) is used alone. This may be one of the reasons why phenothiazine and benzodiazepine tranquilizers are widely employed as preanesthetic drugs in clinical practice.

Sedatives and Hypnotics

The α_2-adrenoceptor agonists (α_2-agonists) produce a more complicated effect on respiration. The usual clinical doses of xylazine and detomidine produce laryngeal relaxation in horses and alter pulmonary mechanics (dynamic compliance and pulmonary resistance).[95,96] Some, but not all, of this effect is produced by the change in position of the horse's head with sedation.[97] Certainly, the degree of laryngeal dysfunction produced by α_2-agonist sedation in horses precludes using this type of sedation when carrying out diagnostic examination of the larynx. Although most studies have failed to demonstrate a significant increase in $PaCO_2$ levels after sedation of horses with xylazine, detomidine, or romifidine,[98,99] a fall in PaO_2 of 10 to 20 mm Hg is often observed.[95,97,98]

In sheep, it is apparent that clinically useful sedative doses of xylazine and other α_2-agonists produce significant hypoxemia, as illustrated in Fig. 5.13, without producing hypoventilation.[100,101] Sheep remain eucapnic or even become hypocapnic from the hypoxic stimulus. This response is associated with tachypnea, a fall in dynamic compliance of the lung (i.e., an increased stiffness), and an increase in the maximum change in transpulmonary pressure and pulmonary resistance during tidal breathing.[100–102] This response can occur with even subsedative doses,[102] and the hypoxemia can last longer than the period of sedation.[100,101] On conventional and electron-microscopic histological examination, the initial response appears to be associated with internalization of the surface coat and activation of the pulmonary intravascular macrophages found in sheep (and all other ruminants).[103] It is hypothesized that these reactive cells release inflammatory mediators that lead to the rapid onset of bronchoconstriction and to leakage of the pulmonary vascular bed. By 10 min, there is obvious evidence of intra-alveolar edema and hemorrhage after clinical sedative doses of xylazine (Fig. 5.14) or medetomidine, and even after administration of the peripherally acting nonsedative α_2-agonist ST-91.[103]

It is unclear whether this toxic response also occurs in other ruminants, partly because the effect of a change in body position or the concurrent use of other drugs is hard to differentiate. In calves, PaO_2 levels decreased from 88 to 55 mm Hg after xylazine sedation[104] and, in goats, a fall from 90 to 65 mm Hg was observed.[105] When seven healthy adult Holstein cows positioned in left lateral recumbency (on a tilt table) were given 0.2 mg/kg xylazine IV, mean PaO_2 levels decreased from 79.0 ± 4.5 mm Hg (SEM) to 54.5 ± 2.7 mm Hg at 5 min and to 58.4 ± 2.6 mm Hg at 15 min after xylazine administration. $PaCO_2$ levels also increased significantly from 34.9 ± 2.0 mm Hg to more normal levels of 45.0 ± 2.1 and 45.6 ± 1.4 mm Hg at 5 and 15 min (R. Warren and W. McDonell, unpublished data).

Hypoxemia is a significant problem when wild deer, bison, and wapiti are immobilized using drug combinations containing α_2-agonists (or opioids).[106–108] Treatment with supplemental oxygen is recommended and will increase PaO_2 to safer levels.[108]

When used alone at sedative doses, the α_2-agonists exhibit little evidence of true respiratory depression in healthy dogs or cats.[109–113] There may be a decrease in respiratory rate and perhaps a small increase in $PaCO_2$ levels, but PaO_2 levels are well maintained. The peripheral cyanosis that has been reported in up to one-third of dogs sedated with medetomidine is believed to be caused by the low blood flow through peripheral capillary beds and venous desaturation, rather than a fall in arterial saturation.[114]

It is important to appreciate, however, that the degree of respiratory depression produced by any α_2-agonist will be increased

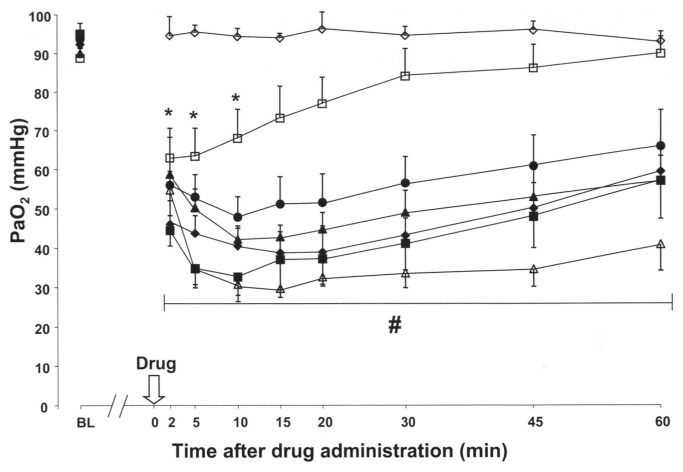

Fig. 5.13. Arterial oxygen tension (arterial oxygen partial pressure [PaO_2]) in sheep after intravenous saline, diazepam, or α_2-adrenergic agonist sedative administration in healthy adult sheep maintained in sternal recumbency. Baseline (BL) values over 1 h are shown for saline ($\diamond$), diazepam ($\square$, 0.4 mg/kg), xylazine ($\blacksquare$, 150 µg/kg), romifidine ($\triangle$, 50 µg/kg), detomidine ($\blacktriangle$, 30 µg/kg), medetomidine ($\blacklozenge$, 10 µg/kg) and the peripheral acting experimental nonsedative α_2-agonist ST-91 ($\bullet$, 30 µg/kg). Significant differences ($P \leq 0.05$) from placebo treatment for diazepam (*) and all other α_2-agonists (#) are shown. Note the marked degree of hypoxemia with arterial oxygen partial pressure (PaO_2) values well below normal venous levels, and also the persistence of the hypoxemia over the full 1 h. This was well past the actual duration of sedation for a number of the agents. Data modified from Celly et al.,[100,101] with permission.

(often substantially) when the agonist is given along with other sedatives or anesthetic agents. A number of studies have clearly demonstrated that medetomidine produces elevated $PaCO_2$ levels and PaO_2 levels in the mildly hypoxic range (i.e., 60 to 70 mm Hg) when combined with either µ or κ opioids, or with propofol or ketamine, at clinical doses in healthy animals. The decrease in PaO_2 levels is due in part to some degree of hypoventilation and to an increase in *V/Q* scatter, as described in the next section. Therefore, it is recommended that oxygen should be administered by face mask or endotracheal intubation whenever α_2-agonists are used in combination with other sedatives or injectable anesthetics.[114] This is especially true when dealing with geriatric or ill animals.

Ventilation-Perfusion Relationships During Anesthesia

The onset of general anesthesia[3,5,6] or, in the case of larger animals, even a change in body position[115–118] often produces lower PaO_2 levels than expected for the delivered concentration of in-

spired oxygen. This change can occur even without hypoventilation and during both spontaneous and controlled breathing. Lower PaO_2 is produced by altered ventilation-perfusion ratios within the lung. Much of what we know about this phenomenon of altered gas exchange is derived from studies of the human response to anesthesia, some experiments in dogs, and many studies on anesthetized horses. It is obvious when one looks at the collective results that there are important species differences, although the reason(s) for these differences are not always obvious.

Ventilation-Perfusion Scatter Under Normal Conditions

To understand how anesthesia alters ventilation-perfusion (or *V/Q*) relationships, it is first necessary to appreciate the scatter of *V/Q* ratios in the normal lung of unanesthetized animals and to appreciate the mechanisms by which regional matching of pulmonary blood flow and alveolar ventilation is optimized.[7,41] Figure 5.15 is a schematic representation of *V/Q* relationships in conscious and anesthetized animals.

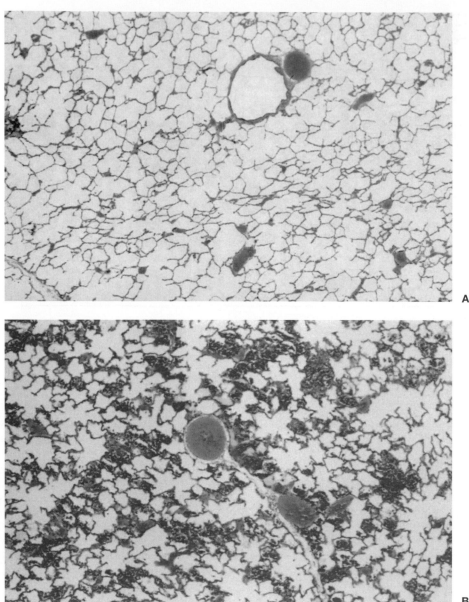

Fig. 5.14. Histology of sheep lungs 10 min after intravenous saline administration **(A)** or 150 µg/kg of xylazine **(B)**. Note the degree of alveolar hemorrhage and edema present after xylazine administration. Euthanasia and fixation as reported elsewhere.[103] Images courtesy of C. Celly, with permission.

Intrapleural pressure is more subatmospheric over the uppermost areas of the lung than adjacent to dependent regions because of the "weight" of the lung within the thoracic cavity.[39,119] Partly because of differences in lung density among species and partly because of differences in chest wall configuration, the total vertical gradient of intrapleural pressure over the whole lung apparently does not differ much among species, despite large differences in lung size and height. This is fortuitous, because otherwise there would be a tendency for too great a discrepancy between the size of the uppermost and lowermost alveoli. The gradient of intrapleural pressure means that in unanesthetized animals the uppermost alveoli (A in Fig. 5.15) are larger than alveoli in the middle and lower regions of the lung (C and D). Since the pressure-volume curve of the lung is sigmoid, the larger alveoli tend to be on the flat part of the curve and thus distend less for any given change of intrapleural pressure during inspira-

tion.[6,120] Thus, the more dependent alveoli (D) receive proportionally more of an inspired tidal volume, unless a disease process (e.g., chronic airway obstruction or pneumonia) or a decrease in lung volume leads to intermittent or complete airway closure (E and F) or actual atelectasis (G).

At the same time, there is a vertical gradient of pulmonary blood flow, because the pulmonary artery is a low-pressure system affected by hydrostatic pressure.[42,121] Some alveoli may receive no perfusion (A in Fig 5.15) and constitute an alveolar dead space, whereas alveolus D receives more perfusion than alveolus B. In most species, the increased ventilation of alveolus D is not sufficient to match the higher perfusion, and the V/Q ratio of alveolus D is 0.7, compared with the V/Q ratio of 1.7 for alveolus B. Overall, the collective scatter of V/Q ratios for the normal lung in resting individuals is 0.8 to 0.9.

Based on radioisotope-distribution evidence, the vertical gra-

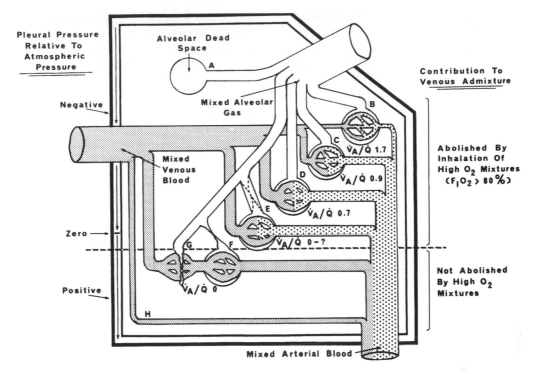

Fig. 5.15. Schematic diagram of ventilation-perfusion (*V/Q*) relationships in the lung and the primary mechanisms whereby venous admixture and the alveolar-to-arterial gradient ($P_{(A-a)}O_2$) increases during anesthesia. The gradient of pleural pressure is shown with the uppermost aspect of the pleural space more subatmospheric than the dependent region, which may even become positive relative to atmosphere if lung volume decreases enough. The inflow of gas is represented by the *nonshaded area* in the tracheobronchial tree. This inspired gas may reach alveoli that are not perfused (*A*), may reach alveoli that are variably perfused (*B* to *D*), or may intermittently reach alveoli (*E*) through airways that open only later during the inspiration. Nonventilated alveoli (*F*) will usually become atelectatic (*G*), especially when high inspired-oxygen levels are used. The *finely shaded area* represents the flow of mixed venous blood from the pulmonary artery, and the *coarsely shaded area* represents postcapillary oxygenated blood. Blood flow from alveoli with low *V/Q* ratios (*E*), from nonventilated alveoli, or from anatomical shunt areas (*H*) will all contribute to the venous admixture effect and increase the alveolar-to-arterial gradient ($P_{(A-a)}O_2$). The venous admixture effect of low *V/Q* areas is abolished when high-oxygen mixtures are inhaled, because even poorly ventilated alveoli will have sufficient oxygen to oxygenate the blood going past.

dient of perfusion and ventilation is minimal in standing dogs with a horizontal lung,[122] and matching of vertical perfusion and ventilation gradients in conscious horses is such that there is little difference in *V/Q* in different lung regions.[123] More recent studies using a multiple inert-gas washout method in horses suggest the scatter of *V/Q* ratios in conscious horses is very similar to that seen in people.[124] No regions of low *V/Q* were identified, but a minor shunt component (less than 3% of cardiac output) was observed. A high *V/Q* area was observed (constituting 3% to 17% of the total), and the extent of this area was correlated with lower pulmonary artery pressures.[124]

When pulmonary artery blood flows through vascular channels not adjacent to alveoli (H in Fig. 5.15) or passes nonventilated alveoli (G and F), unoxygenated blood will pass from the right side of the circulation into the left side, leading to a lower PaO_2.

In conscious animals, if regional ventilation is decreased, a local vasoconstriction (hypoxic pulmonary vasoconstriction [HPV]) tends to divert blood flow away from underventilated areas of the lung.[121] There is an apparent difference in the strength of the HPV response to whole lung hypoxia in various species,[125] based on high-altitude and excised lung studies.[126,127] Cattle and swine have a strong reflex, whereas ponies, cats, and rabbits have an intermediate response. Sheep, cats, and dogs show less response. It appears, however, that under normal conditions even species with a weak hypoxic pulmonary reflex are capable of considerable blood flow diversion in response to regional areas of low alveolar oxygen content.[125,128]

Measurement of V/Q Mismatch

When the barometric pressure, inspired-oxygen concentration, $PaCO_2$, and respiratory quotient are known, the $P_{A}O_2$ can be calculated by using one form of the alveolar air equation (Figs. 5.2 and 5.4). The difference between this value and the PaO_2 (i.e., the alveolar-to-arterial gradient [$P_{(A-a)}O_2$]) provides a convenient and practical measure of the relative efficiency of gas exchange. This measurement is commonly used in anesthetic studies. The measured $P_{(A-a)}O_2$ value increases as F_IO_2 goes up for any given *V/Q* situation, and it is imperative that the F_IO_2 level be taken into account when comparisons are made. In practice, most

$P_{(A-a)}O_2$ determinations are made at oxygen concentrations of 21% or near 100%.

The amount of venous admixture or pulmonary-shunt flow can be determined if mixed venous (pulmonary artery) and arterial blood oxygen contents are obtained along with a measurement of cardiac output and calculated P_AO_2. The terms *venous admixture* and *shunt flow* do not mean exactly the same thing, although they are often used interchangeably in the literature, which causes some confusion. *Venous admixture* refers to the degree of admixture of mixed venous blood with pulmonary end-capillary blood that would be required to produce the observed difference between the arterial and the end-capillary PO_2.[5,6] The end-capillary PO_2 is assumed to equal the alveolar PO_2. Venous admixture is a calculated amount (i.e., a proportion of cardiac output) and includes the PaO_2-lowering effect of low $\dot{V}/\dot{Q}$ areas, blood flow past nonventilated areas, and true *anatomical shunt flow* (bronchial and thebesian venous blood flow). When the inspired-oxygen level is high, blood passing low-$\dot{V}/\dot{Q}$ areas will be oxygenated (Fig. 5.15), and the $P_{(A-a)}O_2$ gradient and determination of venous admixture is a measure of all the total blood flow not contributing to gas exchange; hence the term *pulmonary-shunt flow*. Note that this flow includes both anatomical shunt flow and flow past nonventilated or collapsed alveoli.

If one knows the inspired-oxygen concentration and the PaO_2, and assumes that the arterial-venous oxygen extraction is normal, an isoshunt diagram can be used to provide a convenient and reasonably accurate estimate of the magnitude of pulmonary-shunt flow (Fig. 5.16).[129] Figure 5.16 is a diagram that illustrates the poor response, in terms of improving PaO_2, that will occur with increased inspired-oxygen concentrations when shunt flows are over 30%.

Effect of Positional Changes

Very few thorough studies of the respiratory consequences of positional changes in conscious domestic animals have been carried out because of the technical difficulties in doing such studies with uncooperative animals. In conscious human patients positioned in lateral recumbency, there is proportionately more ventilation to the lowermost lung.[130] There is a slight fall in FRC, but in individuals with normal lungs and body confirmation there is little change in PaO_2. Conscious dogs positioned in sternal (prone), lateral, and dorsal (supine) recumbency showed no positional change in FRC (Fig. 5.17).[131] Unsedated sheep,[115] cattle,[118] and ponies[116] develop some degree of hypoxia when put into lateral recumbency, although this finding was not present in another group of ponies.[132] Mean PaO_2 levels in unsedated adult cattle positioned in dorsal recumbency are in the range of 60 to 70 mm Hg, with some animals experiencing marked hypoxemia.[117,118]

Although the evidence in conscious animals is mainly circumstantial and meager, it does appear that the main determinant of FRC is a decrease in lung volume in recumbent animals (Fig. 5.18), as has been reported in anesthetized animals.[36,37] When conscious, sedated, 1400- to 4000-kg elephants voluntarily moved from a standing position to left lateral recumbency, PaO_2 levels decreased only from 96.2 to 83.8 mm Hg (at 10 min).[133] This relative protection against positional hypoxemia may be related to anatomical differences in the lung parenchyma, chest wall, and lung adhesion to the chest wall.[134]

In standing cows and sheep, rumen distension and the associated increase in abdominal pressure produce a decrease in PaO_2, and at very high rumenal pressures a reduction in V_E and cardiac output.[135,136] In four standing ponies (two starved for 18 h and two nonstarved), FRC as measured by helium dilution decreased

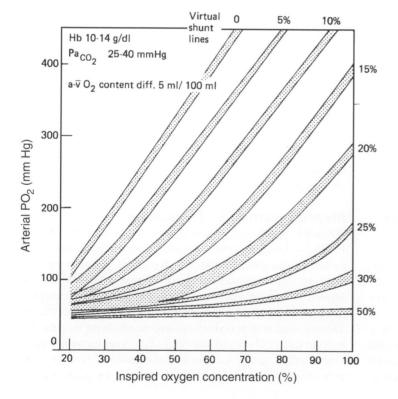

Fig. 5.16. An isoshunt diagram depicting the relationship between inspired-oxygen concentration, partial pressure of oxygen (PO_2), and various degrees of venous admixture or pulmonary shunt. Shunt flow is expressed as a percentage of cardiac output. The arteriovenous (a-v) oxygen-content difference is assumed to be 5.0 mL per 100 mL of blood, reflecting a normal cardiac output. The shunt bands have been drawn to include the range of hemoglobin (Hb) and arterial carbon dioxide partial pressure ($PaCO_2$) levels shown. Redrawn from Benetar et al. (p. 713),[129] with permission.

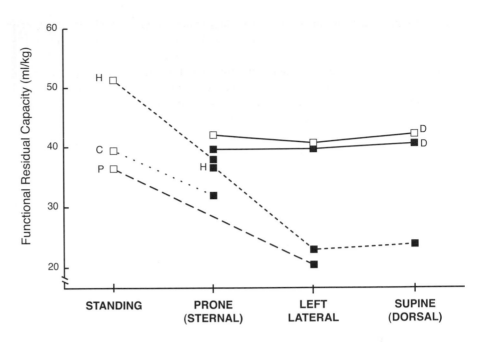

Fig. 5.17. Effect of positional changes and general anesthesia on functional residual capacity (FRC) in dogs (*D*), cattle (*C*), ponies (*P*), and horses (*H*). FRC in the conscious state is shown by the open squares and in the anesthetized state by the solid squares. All measurements were obtained during barbiturate anesthesia. Note that FRC does not change appreciably in anesthetized dogs with positional changes and decreases markedly with the onset of anesthesia and recumbency in the larger species. In horses, FRC is markedly less in dorsal or lateral recumbency, compared with sternal recumbency. Data taken from various studies.[35–37,117]

by 13.4% (range, 11.6% to 14.7%) after sedation with 0.04 mg/kg of acepromazine given intramuscularly. In another study, overnight starvation increased the FRC of five standing, unsedated ponies by about 16%.[37]

Species Differences

As mentioned earlier, deep sedation and general anesthesia commonly produce a fall in PaO_2 levels even in healthy animals. Some of this decrease can be associated with hypoventilation (Fig. 5.6), but even when $PaCO_2$ levels are eucapnic, PaO_2 is generally decreased. The anesthetic-induced change in PaO_2 is associated with increases in the scatter of *V/Q* ratios, the $P_{(A-a)}O_2$ gradient, and the level of venous admixture.[3,5,6] In the case of larger mammals, there may even be gross *V/Q* mismatch.[1,137] It is generally appreciated that $P_{(A-a)}O_2$ gradients are always increased during general anesthesia in horses.[1,2,138,139] Healthy horses may have low PaO_2 levels when anesthetized with injectable drugs.[140] In horses with diseased lungs or depressed cardiopulmonary function (e.g., anesthesia), it may be impossible to maintain PaO_2 levels above 70 mm Hg even with 100% inspired oxygen.[141] The same response to 100% oxygen administration may be observed in adult cattle.[65]

Recumbency per se does not produce significant hypoxemia in healthy dogs, cats, or people, and in the case of larger mammals produces less of an increase in the $P_{(A-a)}O_2$ gradient than is seen after the onset of anesthesia. What are the factors that produce hypoxemic changes in anesthetized animals? Research on the respiratory effects of anesthetics has focused on their influence on (a) HPV; (b) lung volume, chest wall, and pulmonary mechanical factors; and (c) the resultant distribution of regional pulmonary blood and gas flow.

Hypoxic Pulmonary Vasoconstriction

It appears that this important protective mechanism to optimize *V/Q* in the lung is obtunded by many anesthetics. Investigations

in intact animals and with excised lungs have established that most, if not all, inhalational agents reduce HPV, and that none of the injectable agents examined (narcotics, barbiturates, or benzodiazepines) have any detectable effect.[121] There is at least one report that HPV is better maintained with sevoflurane and desflurane,[142] but the practical importance of this finding is not yet clear. The onset of the interference with HPV is rapid with inhaled anesthetics and persists throughout anesthesia. The end result of this interference with HPV is that, for any given level of altered intrapulmonary gas distribution caused by reduced lung volume, intermittent airway closure, or regional atelectasis, a greater degree of hypoxemia exists. With an animal breathing 100% oxygen and HPV abolished, PaO_2 has been estimated to be only 100 mm Hg with 30% of the lung atelectatic, compared with a PaO_2 level of over 400 mm Hg with the same degree of atelectasis and an intact HPV response.[121] No clinically relevant, controlled comparisons of $P_{(A-a)}O_2$ gradients have been performed using intravenous anesthesia compared with inhalational anesthesia in veterinary patients. There is some evidence that PaO_2 is better maintained in horses when a xylazine-ketamine-guaifenesin infusion is used instead of halothane to maintain anesthesia.[143]

In anesthetized horses, there is evidence that pulmonary perfusion does not linearly increase from the uppermost lung areas to the lowermost areas solely on a gravitational basis, even when HPV is abolished.[144,145] It has been demonstrated that the gravity-dependent pulmonary blood flow of conscious horses is altered when they are positioned in sternal, lateral, or dorsal recumbency during halothane anesthesia.[146] There was a reduction in blood flow to the cranioventral areas of the lung and a proportional increase in flow to dorsocaudal regions, irrespective of body position. A nongravitational pulmonary blood flow pattern in pentobarbital anesthetized ponies has been demonstrated.[147] At least some of this diversion of pulmonary blood flow from the most dependent areas of the horse lung might be related to creation of a zone IV area of blood flow from reduced lung volume and an increase in interstitial fluid pressure (Fig. 5.3). This sort of diversion has been observed in persons at low lung volumes,[148] and in dogs when interstitial fluid pressures were elevated.[149] Whatever the cause, in laterally recumbent horses, the redistribution of pulmonary blood flow away from relatively nonventilated lower lung to better-ventilated upper lung has a beneficial effect in reducing the degree of venous admixture.[145] It is important to appreciate that redistribution is far from complete, and venous admixture or shunt flows in horses often exceed 20%.

Functional Residual Volume

In recumbent humans, FRC is reduced by about 0.5 L with the induction of general anesthesia,[120] which is 15% to 20% of the normal FRC. The mechanisms underlying this reduction in FRC remain unclear. Atelectasis, increased thoracic or abdominal blood volume, and loss of some inherent tone in the diaphragm at end exhalation all seem to be involved.[3,87,120,130] Irrespective of the cause, there is evidence of a correlation between changes in FRC and the $P_{(A-a)}O_2$ gradient after induction of anesthesia.[150] Airway closure, atelectasis, and dependent regions of poorly aerated lung tissue have been demonstrated by using inert-gas elimination and computed tomographic techniques.[151,152]

There is little information regarding FRC changes in dogs and cats, but in one well-controlled study the onset of general anesthesia did not alter FRC significantly in sternal, lateral, or dorsally recumbent dogs (Fig. 5.17).[131] These were medium-sized mongrel dogs (13 to 28 kg), and larger dogs might show a different response. Differences in V/Q ratios during anesthesia have been noted between beagles and greyhound-type dogs.[153]

In horses and cows, the decrease in FRC with the onset of recumbency and general anesthesia may be quite marked, as much as 50% to 70% (Fig. 5.17). This has been radiographically demonstrated[154,155] and directly measured by helium dilution[37,156] and nitrogen washout.[36] This change in FRC seems to be primarily related to the positional change from an upright posture to recumbency (Fig. 5.18) and, in horses at least, is greater in lateral or dorsal recumbency than when prone (Fig. 5.17).[36] In laterally recumbent animals, the dependent lung is poorly aerated radiographically[154,155] and has a smaller FRC (as measured by helium dilution) (Fig. 5.19). Studies using nuclear scintigraphy[137] and computed tomography[157] have clearly demonstrated that there is markedly less ventilation of the dependent lung of horses in lateral recumbency during anesthesia. This reduction in lower lung volume is accompanied by actual atelectasis (Fig. 5.20) and may be influenced by the degree of obesity or body conformation.[158]

The FRC of anesthetized horses can be increased and the $P_{(A-a)}O_2$ gradient reduced through the use of high (20 to 30 cm H_2O) positive end-expiratory pressure (PEEP).[141,159,160] If PEEP of this magnitude is introduced, there is a marked decrease in venous return to the heart and in cardiac output. The mechanism by which PEEP reduces the $P_{(A-a)}O_2$ gradient and venous admixture is likely through increasing total and/or regional FRC, with subsequent prevention of the intermittent airway closure and rever-

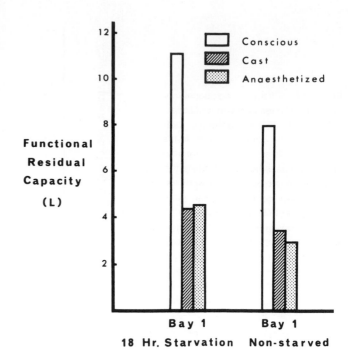

Fig. 5.18. Functional residual capacity (FRC) in a xylazine-sedated pony (273 kg) while standing (conscious), after positioning in left lateral recumbency with hobbles (cast), and after induction of anesthesia with thiopental (anesthetized). The study was done twice: once after an 18-h period of starvation and once without starvation. FRC was measured by helium dilution.[156]

sal of the atelectasis that is represented diagrammatically by alveoli F and G in Fig. 5.15. Moens and colleagues[161] used a double-lumened endotracheal tube and differential IPPV (higher V_T and PEEP of 10 to 20 cm H_2O) to the lowermost lung of quite large laterally recumbent horses (420 to 660 kg). This technique increased PaO_2 levels by over 100% and decreased pulmonary-shunt perfusion by 33%. Similar beneficial effects have been reported using PEEP and selective mechanical ventilation of dependent areas of the lungs in dorsally recumbent horses (Fig. 5.21).[162] With the onset of general anesthesia and positioning in lateral recumbency, PaO_2 levels were elevated to only about 250 mm Hg, rather than the expected above 500 mm Hg that should have occurred if there was no problem with gas exchange. When the horses were moved into dorsal recumbency, their mean PaO_2 level fell to below 100 mm Hg. Conventional IPPV of the whole lung did little to improve PaO_2, whereas selective mechanical ventilation of the dependent areas of the lung with 20 cm H_2O restored PaO_2 to the level measured in lateral recumbency.

Chest Wall and Pulmonary Mechanics Changes

The evidence implicating alteration of chest wall (including diaphragm) and lung mechanical factors as causative agents in the increase in $P_{(A-a)}O_2$ during anesthesia is often conflicting. Certainly, there is a difference in the chest wall mechanics between people and dogs during general anesthesia.[120] It appears that most dog breeds (and probably cats) have a more compliant lateral chest wall that tends to contribute relatively little to the in-

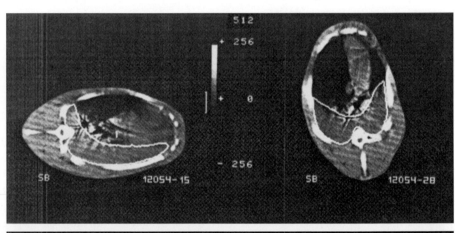

Fig. 5.19. Functional residual capacity (FRC) of the left and right lungs, and both lungs, in a horse positioned in dorsal and right and left lateral recumbency. The horse was maintained under stable intravenous anesthesia, and FRC was determined by helium dilution using a double-lumen endotracheal tube to separate the two lungs.[156] Note that the FRC of the dependent lung decreases from the proportion measured during dorsal recumbency and becomes a small percentage of the total FRC, irrespective of which lung is dependent.

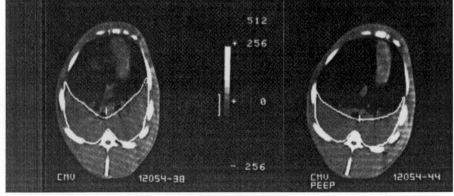

Fig. 5.20. Transverse computed tomographic scans of the thorax of a pony during anesthesia with thiopental/halothane in left lateral recumbency **(top left)** and in dorsal recumbency during spontaneous respiration **(top right)**, mechanical ventilation **(bottom left)**, and mechanical ventilation with positive end-expiratory pressure (PEEP) of 10 cm H_2O **(bottom right)**. Note the appearance of large dense areas encircled by a white line in dependent lung regions. The heart is visible as a white area in the middle of the thorax. Reproduced from Nyman et al.,[157] with permission.

spiratory effort, compared with the diaphragm, with clinical doses of most anesthetics. In all species, dangerously deep planes of anesthesia are commonly associated with flaccidity of the thoracic wall and paradoxical inward movement during inspiration (paradoxical inspiration). If one watches closely, this same type of respiration may be seen in cats, ferrets, and other small mammals, even with light levels of anesthesia.

In horses and cows, with the onset of anesthesia and movement into lateral recumbency, there is radiographic evidence of a marked change in the two-dimensional lung silhouette and the

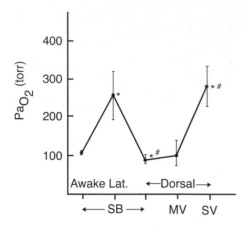

Fig. 5.21. Arterial oxygen tension (arterial oxygen partial pressure [PaO₂], mean ± SEM) in an awake standing horse ($F_1O_2 = 0.21$), and during anesthesia in the lateral (Lat.) and dorsal recumbent positions ($F_1O_2 > 0.92$). SB, spontaneous breathing; MV, general mechanical ventilation; SV, selective mechanical ventilation of dependent lung regions with positive end-expiratory pressure (PEEP) of 20 cm H_2O; *, significantly different from awake value; #, significantly different from the previous value. Reproduced from Nyman et al.,[162] with permission.

position of the diaphragm.[154,155] In ponies anesthetized with halothane, the diaphragmatic outline moved forward rather uniformly in sternal (prone) or lateral recumbency, but the forward shift was considerably greater in lateral recumbency.[154] When the ponies were positioned in dorsal (supine) recumbency, the diaphragmatic outline sagged toward the now-dependent spine region. With minor variations, observations by Watney[155] in studying 315- to 400-kg cattle were very similar. The positional alteration of the diaphragmatic silhouette agrees nicely with the reduction in FRC noted by Sorenson and Robinson[36] when ponies were moved from sternal to lateral or dorsal recumbency. In lateral recumbency, the dorsal areas of the diaphragm moved more during inspiration than did the more ventral sternal area, while the uppermost crural movement exceeded that of the lowermost crural segment.[163] This is in contrast to awake and anesthetized recumbent persons, where the most dependent portions of the diaphragm are most active.[164] The tonic activity of the lateral chest wall, especially that provided by the serratus ventralis muscle, is greatly decreased in anesthetized horses, and it is postulated that this reduces the stabilization of the lateral chest wall.[165]

Although it is generally accepted that halothane and isoflurane produce bronchodilation in humans,[6,166,167] general anesthesia produces an apparent increase in the elastic recoil of the lung.[120] In anesthetized ponies, halothane, isoflurane, and enflurane had a mild bronchodilating effect,[168] whereas, in cows[169,170] and in standing horses at subanesthetic concentrations,[171] halothane did not produce bronchodilation. Interpretation of measurements of pulmonary resistance and compliance during anesthesia are made difficult because changes in lung volume per se will alter these values,[6,169] as was demonstrated when nonstarved cows were studied over a 3-h anesthetic period.[172] It would appear, however, that the chest wall and lung volume changes play a

much larger part in the generation of increased $P_{(A-a)}O_2$ gradients during anesthesia than any true alteration of lung mechanics.

Clinical Implications of Altered Respiration During Anesthesia

The complexity of the respiratory response to anesthesia in veterinary patients may seem more than a little daunting to novice anesthetists and to veterinary practitioners of necessity functioning without the benefit of appreciable advanced training in the discipline. This is made so, in part, because of the variety of species that we attend to, as well as the wide range of drugs and environments in which veterinarians find that they must sedate, chemically restrain, or anesthetize animals. In this section, we summarize the most important clinical considerations relative to respiratory management on a species basis for typical patients. This overview is based to a large extent on personal experience and on discussions over the years with academic colleagues and practicing veterinarians. Unfortunately, there are exceedingly few morbidity and mortality surveys of relevant case material upon which one might base more objective conclusions. It is important to appreciate that exceptions to these generalizations may exist, based on the inherent health of the animal being treated, and because the anesthetic response in an individual animal is not always "typical." There is simply no safe alternative other than ongoing careful monitoring of the respiratory system during anesthesia.

Humans

Since so much of our knowledge of the altered physiology of anesthesia is derived from the literature on human patients, it helps to understand how human anesthesia differs from veterinary anesthesia. In anesthetized humans, alveolar dead space increases by about 70 mL, and venous admixture constitutes approximately 10% of the cardiac output, compared with 2% to 3% in unanesthetized individuals.[173] With this degree of venous admixture, an inspired-oxygen concentration of about 35% will usually restore a normal PaO₂ (Fig. 5.16). Thus, the upper limit for nitrous oxide in an oxygen–nitrous oxide mixture is commonly 66%, that is, a 1:2 ratio of O_2/N_2O. Muscle relaxants and comparatively high doses of opioids (on an "effect," not milligram per kilogram, basis) are commonly incorporated into the anesthetic regimen, so IPPV is very commonly employed.[5,6] The target when ventilating anesthetized patients is usually to produce eucapnia or slight hypocapnia. This was originally done because of an apparent potentiation effect of the anesthetic dose, but now is done primarily to prevent sympathetic stimulation with resultant tachycardia and hypertension, both of which are dangerous in a patient population prone to atherosclerotic disease. Eucapnia also minimizes the risk of increased intracranial or intraocular pressure, which is especially important in trauma patients, the elderly, or those with ocular and/or central nervous system disease.

Some form of airway protection (oropharyngeal or endotracheal tube) is almost always used, and continuous monitoring of airway pressure is employed to ensure that there is no inadvertent

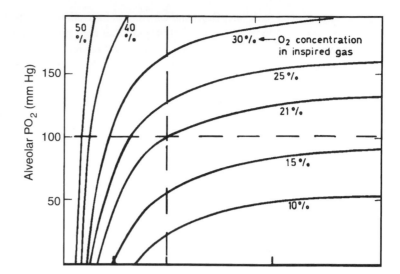

Fig. 5.22. Protective effect of increased inspired-oxygen concentrations with various degrees of alveolar hypoventilation and hyperventilation. With 30% inspired oxygen, alveolar partial pressure of oxygen (alveolar PO_2) levels are above 100 mm Hg even when alveolar ventilation is half normal. Modified from Nunn (p. 111),[207] with permission.

disconnection from the anesthetic circuit of a paralyzed patient that cannot breathe spontaneously. Continuous end-tidal CO_2 and hemoglobin-saturation monitoring is now widely employed, using capnography and noninvasive pulse oximetry, respectively.[174] The reasons for the increased use of these monitoring devices are that the equipment is now cost-effective and user-friendly, provides medicolegal protection, and provides an early warning system of cardiorespiratory failure that decreases the mortality rate associated with general anesthesia.[175,176]

Over the past decade in the field of human anesthesia, there has been considerable interest in the relationship between variable oxygen mixtures used for preoxygenation and during anesthesia and the development of atelectasis in the lung.[177,178] The usefulness of PEEP and/or forced vital capacity maneuvers (sighs or purposeful expansion of the lung) are being evaluated and debated in terms of the effect on the circulation of compromised patients, efficacy, and duration of effect.[179–183] The applicability of these findings is likely to vary among species, especially those that differ markedly in body mass from humans, or with increased communication (e.g., dogs) or decreased communication (e.g., ruminants) between alveoli through alveolar ducts or pores of Kohn.[125] In particular, it would be of great interest to know the highest F_IO_2 possible to administer during general anesthesia in cattle and horses without contributing to additional atelectasis beyond that produced by positional related changes in FRC.

Dogs and Cats

In reasonably healthy dogs and cats, the $P_{(A-a)}O_2$ gradient and the degree of venous admixture are less than in humans. Perhaps this is owing to the smaller lungs in these species or to the difference in the chest wall changes during anesthesia,[120] or perhaps because there is excellent collateral pulmonary ventilation in these species.[125] A high degree of collateral ventilation means that if an alveolus is not ventilated via the airway, it may well receive gas exchange through passages (pores of Kohn) leading to other alveoli that are ventilated.

Despite the relatively favorable situation in regard to V/Q mismatch in these species, a minimum inspired-oxygen level of 30% to 35% is still recommended. For the first few minutes after a barbiturate induction, PaO_2 may be as low as 50 mm Hg in nonventilated healthy dogs,[184] with less change in cats.[185] The degree of hypoxemia is somewhat less after a ketamine induction, but venous admixture still may be 20% to 25% for a few minutes after induction.[92,93] Obese, deeply anesthetized animals, animals with a distended abdomen (e.g., pregnancy or bowel obstruction), or those with pulmonary disease or space-occupying lesions of the thorax (tumor, pneumothorax, hemothorax, or diaphragmatic hernia) are particularly at risk. Oxygen supplementation is needed nearly as much in deeply sedated animals as in those receiving a general anesthetic (intravenous or inhalant). As can be seen in Fig. 5.22, increasing the inspired-oxygen level also provides protection against hypoxemia caused by hypoventilation and, again, adequate protection is generally achieved with a venous admixture of 30% to 35%. This is why simple maneuvers such as placing a face mask with oxygen on a high-risk patient before and during induction or use of a nasal oxygen catheter in the postoperative period are beneficial.

When 100% oxygen mixtures are used with the common inhalant anesthetics in dogs and cats free of serious cardiopulmonary disease, the arterial PaO_2 level is generally 450 to 525 mm Hg whether the animal is breathing spontaneously or being ventilated[58,70,186,187] and irrespective of body position. With such high inspired-oxygen levels, hypoxemia usually occurs only through disconnection of the animal from the anesthetic machine, or with faulty placement of the endotracheal tube, cardiac arrest, or total apnea for over 5 min. Nevertheless, even with such high PaO_2 levels, tissue hypoxia can occur if hemoglobin levels are low or circulation is inadequate (low cardiac output).

The decision to institute assisted or controlled IPPV is generally made to prevent or treat hypercapnia, rather than to achieve oxygenation. Nearly all spontaneously breathing dogs and cats show some degree of hypoventilation and hypercapnia ($PaCO_2$ of 45 to 55 mm Hg). The clinical importance of this in nonneurological cases is open to debate. Dogs and cats do not have atherosclerosis, and over the years hundreds of thousands of dogs and cats have been successfully anesthetized in practice while breathing spontaneously. From a practical viewpoint, with short-duration anesthetics (anesthesia of less than 1 h) in relatively healthy animals, the important aspects are to ensure that the airway is patent, that the animal is oxygenated, and that the animal does not become apneic; the development of moderate levels of hypercapnia is likely to be well tolerated. The need for IPPV increases as the depth of anesthesia has to be increased for certain types of surgery (e.g., hip replacement) unless local supplementation is used (e.g., epidural opioid or local anesthetic). It also increases when opioids are used as a major component of the anesthetic regimen; for obese, neonate, geriatric, or neurological patients; with certain body positions (e.g., perineal hernia repair or dorsal laminectomy); with prolonged operations; or when dealing with poor-risk patients.

Here are a few guidelines relative to the respiratory component of anesthesia for dogs and cats:

1. Nearly all canine anesthetics are better done with an endotracheal tube in place, and in many situations cats should be intubated.

2. Use at least 30% to 35% inspired oxygen in all anesthetized dogs and cats, even those on an injectable anesthetic mixture, or when deeply sedated.

3. Hypoxemia is rare in spontaneously breathing dogs and cats if breathing an oxygen mixture approaching 100%.

4. After a prolonged period of anesthesia in cats and smaller dogs, and with shorter anesthetics in larger dogs with deep chests, it is advisable to inflate the lungs to 30 cm H_2O of airway pressure (i.e., to "sigh" the lungs) periodically and at the end of anesthesia.

5. Prolonged immobility and excessive fluid administration can lead to increased venous admixture and a fall in PaO_2 in addition to that produced by anesthesia per se.[188]

Small Ruminants and Swine

Ruminants are especially prone to develop regurgitation and aspiration, along with tachypnea and hypoventilation, during general anesthesia.[64,65] For shorter procedures (45 to 60 min) hypoventilation and hypercapnia often may be safely ignored if an adequate oxygen supply is maintained. Sedation and local analgesia techniques are often used for anesthesia as a means of maintaining a secure airway and adequate respiration.[189] During clinical anesthesia in pigs, especially if a barbiturate is used in a field situation, particular care must be taken to ensure that the airway is patent and that apnea does not occur.

The degree of ventilation-perfusion mismatch and venous admixture is intermediate in these animals, and of such a magnitude that virtually all anesthetized animals breathing room air will have PaO_2 levels somewhat below normal. In dorsally recumbent, ventilated sheep anesthetized with pentobarbital-halothane, atelectasis of the dependent lung regions developed quite quickly.[190] The magnitude of this atelectasis was much less than the same group of researchers observed in ponies.[157] Pulmonary

disease is not uncommon in small ruminants and swine, and will lead to *V/Q* mismatch in addition to that induced by anesthesia, lowering PaO_2 levels further. Abdominal distension caused by the development of rumenal tympany or, in the case of swine, a full stomach will add to the degree of pulmonary dysfunction.

During inhalation anesthesia with 100% oxygen, PaO_2 is usually in the range of 200 to 350 mm Hg—well within safe limits.[72,191] In spontaneously breathing sheep, changes in body position (dorsal and left and right lateral) do not seem to alter the PaO_2 appreciably, and the $P_{(A-a)}O_2$ gradient is rather constant when the sheep are sighed every 3 to 5 min.[191] Clinical experience would suggest the situation is similar in goats and pigs. The following are guidelines for respiratory management during anesthesia:

1. General anesthesia in sheep, goats, and calves with a developed rumen (i.e., by 2 to 4 weeks) requires placement of an endotracheal tube if protection against regurgitation and aspiration is to be ensured. This is best done for all but the shortest and lightest anesthetics.

2. Endotracheal intubation is not advised for swine unless the operation is complex or prolonged, or the operator is skilled with the technique.

3. During intravenous anesthesia of more compromised animals, application of a face mask or insertion of a nasal or tracheal oxygen catheter and insufflation of 2 to 5 L oxygen/min will help to ensure that hypoxemia does not occur.

4. Ketamine-based anesthesia is less likely to lead to apnea or severe respiratory depression than is propofol or barbiturate anesthesia.

5. Prolonged inhalation anesthesia (longer than 45 to 60 min) may require IPPV to prevent hypercapnia and may be required to maintain a stable plane of anesthesia because of the tachypneic breathing pattern.

6. Mild to moderate hypercapnia is well tolerated, and serious hypoxemia is rare if inhalation anesthesia with 100% oxygen is used.

7. The combination of progressive abdominal tympany (even in animals starved for up to 24 h) and the rapid, shallow respiration tend to produce a progressive increase in $P_{(A-a)}O_2$ gradients. Periodic sighing of the lungs (every 10 to 15 min) by inflating them to 30 cm H_2O seems to minimize the progressive increase in venous admixture and is particularly advisable at the end of an operation before extubation and return to a room-air environment. Placement in sternal recumbency during recovery benefits pulmonary function and, in the case of ruminants, helps to protect against regurgitation and aspiration.

Adult Cattle and Horses

Adult cattle[172,192] and horses[1,2,139,193] develop very significant increases in $P_{(A-a)}O_2$ gradients and venous admixture when they are anesthetized and become recumbent. On the basis of inspired-oxygen concentration and PaO_2 levels, it can be calculated that spontaneously breathing halothane-anesthetized horses have pulmonary-shunt flows of 20% to 25%, with a reduction to about 15% in ventilated horses.[194] These were healthy horses, posi-

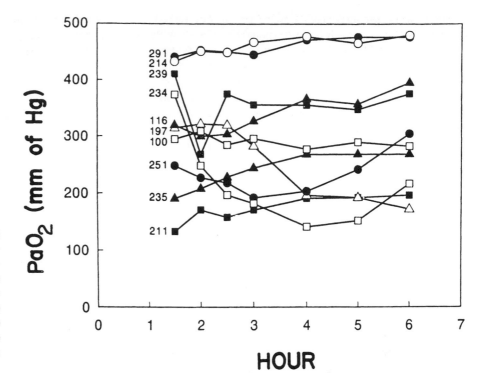

Fig. 5.23. Arterial oxygen partial pressure (PaO₂) values in ten spontaneously breathing, normal horses anesthetized with halothane over 5 h in lateral recumbency. Note the wide variability in the PaO₂ levels between horses and the relative stability of the value for an individual horse over time. The horses were starved overnight before the onset of anesthesia. Reproduced from Steffey et al.,[196] with permission.

tioned in lateral recumbency and subjected to no surgery. Over the intervening 25 years, others have reported PaO₂ levels and $P_{(A-a)}O_2$ gradients from many studies in other healthy horses that are reflective of pulmonary-shunt flows of at least the same magnitude.[157,195–198] The degree of *V/Q* mismatch is greater in dorsal than in lateral recumbency,[195,198–201] in larger horses, and perhaps in older horses.[195] Researchers have consistently noted that the actual variability between PaO₂ levels in similar horses receiving similar anesthetics is quite large (Fig. 5.23).[196] The reasons for this variability are not clear, but probably relate to

body conformation and perhaps the level of abdominal distension caused by obesity, gas distension, or ingesta in the large bowel. The $P_{(A-a)}O_2$ gradient in healthy starved animals does not generally increase over time,[196,200] but the PaO₂ will fall progressively if the degree of abdominal distension increases. This was clearly illustrated in an interesting study of fed and nonfed cows, where the failure to starve the cows before the general anesthetic led to a progressive increase in $P_{(A-a)}O_2$ and pulmonary resistance, and a decrease in PaO₂ and dynamic compliance (Figs. 5.24A and B).[172]

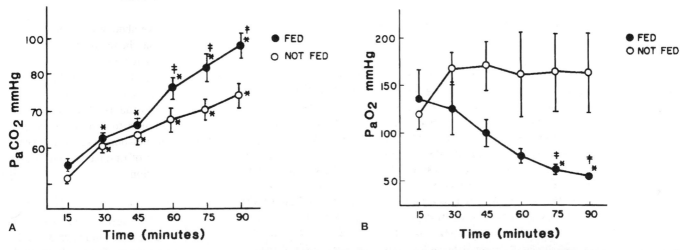

Fig. 5.24. Change in arterial carbon dioxide partial pressure (PaCO₂) **(A)** and arterial oxygen partial pressure (PaO₂) **(B)** levels in spontaneously breathing cows with and without prior starvation. Note the greater degree of hypercapnia in the fed animals and the progressively lower PaO₂. This change was accompanied by an increase in the alveolar-to-arterial gradient ($P_{(A-a)}O_2$), an increase in airway resistance, and a decrease in compliance. These changes were probably associated with a decrease in lung volume from the development of abdominal tympany. Reproduced from Blaze et al.[172] with permission.

When an anesthetized horse (usually during colic surgery or cesarean section) inhales 100% oxygen and has a resultant PaO_2 value of less than 70 mm Hg, it is clear from Fig. 5.16 that over 50% of the cardiac output is being shunted through the lungs without contributing to gas exchange. Although adult cattle also demonstrate fairly large $P_{(A-a)}O_2$ gradients during inhalational anesthesia, serious hypoxemia seems to be confined to very large animals, especially if they must be positioned in dorsal recumbency. Chronic pulmonary disease and lung consolidation are relatively common in cattle as an aftermath of juvenile respiratory disease. It is surprising that such animals do not demonstrate large increases in $P_{(A-a)}O_2$ levels during inhalant anesthesia, perhaps because pulmonary blood flow is also decreased in the nonventilated lung areas.

When adult cattle are positioned in dorsal recumbency by using rope restraint, with or without sedation, some of them become quite hypoxemic.[117,118] Horses anesthetized with the common injectable mixtures for brief field anesthesia also commonly have PaO_2 levels in the 55- to 65-mm Hg range.[202] Admittedly, the vast majority of animals so anesthetized survive with no obvious adverse after effects. This is more a credit to the inherent safety reserve that the animals have relative to oxygen supply and to the underlying good health status of most patients than to the anesthetic regimens per se. Nasal or nasotracheal oxygen insufflation (15 L/min) markedly improves the safety factor in restraining and anesthetizing such animals, and is always desirable if circumstances permit such treatment. Some guidelines relative to respiratory support of anesthetized adult cattle and horses include the following:

1. General anesthesia requires endotracheal intubation in adult cattle because the risk of regurgitation and aspiration is high, even with prior starvation. There is some risk of regurgitation and aspiration when cattle are restrained in a recumbent position with sedatives, including xylazine. The incidence of regurgitation, however, is fairly low, and routine intubation of nonanesthetized cattle is not practical.

2. Longer anesthesia in horses is better performed with an endotracheal tube in place, and this also facilitates oxygen insufflation.

3. Oxygen insufflation with 15 L/min, especially if the tip of the oxygen catheter tube is placed in the trachea, will usually prevent any serious hypoxia in relatively healthy horses and cattle during general anesthesia or recovery. This flow rate down the trachea will even maintain sufficient oxygenation to keep apneic animals alive for at least 10 min.[193]

4. If oxygen supplementation is not possible, adult cattle and horses are better positioned in lateral than in dorsal recumbency (if the surgery permits the choice).

5. When preoperative starvation can be used, it is desirable, because it improves ventilation and oxygenation after the induction of anesthesia.

6. Nitrous oxide use is generally not advisable for cattle or in dorsally recumbent horses and, if used to supplement analgesia for orthopedic surgery in laterally recumbent horses, should not exceed an inspired concentration of 50% (e.g., 4 L of oxygen per 4 L of nitrous oxide).[203]

7. Inhalant general anesthetics lasting longer than 45 min in cattle almost always require IPPV to prevent excessive $PaCO_2$ elevations. In horses, operations lasting over 1 or 2 h will generally need IPPV if the need has not developed earlier. It should be appreciated that in dorsally recumbent horses breathing spontaneously, arterial hypoxemia is not always improved with initiation of IPPV, which may actually decrease PaO_2 and seriously decrease oxygen delivery to tissues.[204] Moderate increases in $PaCO_2$ levels may actually produce useful hemodynamic stimulation without apparent adverse effects and seem to be well tolerated.[205]

8. Treatment of low PaO_2 levels with high levels of PEEP (20 to 30 cm H_2O) is feasible if the blood volume is adequate and inotropic support is used.[141,155] Although differential lung ventilation with PEEP reduces hypoxemia experimentally,[161,162] it is hard to see how this can be used clinically on those animals that actually need treating.

9. Periodic sighing of the lungs in adult cattle and horses probably does no harm, nor does it probably do much good. Full inflation of the lungs after the abdomen has been decompressed surgically, or when animals are positioned in sternal recumbency in recovery, can be quite useful in restoring adequate PaO_2 levels.

Exotic Species

It is very difficult to generalize how best to optimize respiratory function during anesthesia for the diverse range of exotic animals. Even if not used routinely, supplemental oxygenation and the means to establish an airway should be available, if at all possible. Chemical stimulation of respiration (e.g., with doxapram) or the availability of receptor-specific antagonist drugs can be lifesaving in the case of an inadvertent anesthetic overdose. Respiration is generally better supported with dissociatives than with propofol or barbiturate anesthetics. The larger the species, the more likely recumbency and positional changes may seriously interfere with cardiopulmonary homeostasis, although exceptions may exist (e.g., elephants). In general, it is desirable to keep larger terrestrial mammals in sternal rather than lateral or dorsal recumbency during restraint and/or anesthesia, unless such positioning is going to lead to excessive pressure on the limbs for a prolonged period.

References

1. Hall LW. General anesthesia: Fundamental considerations. Vet Clin North Am Large Anim Pract 1981;3:3–15.
2. Wagner AE. The importance of hypoxemia and hypercapnia in anaesthetized horses. Equine Vet Educ 1993;5:207–211.
3. Hedenstierna G. Gas exchange during anaesthesia. Br J Anaesth 1990;64:507–514.
4. McDonell WN. Respiratory system. In: Thurmon JC, Tranquilli WJ, Benson GJ, eds. Lumb and Jones Veterinary Anesthesia, 3rd ed. Baltimore: Williams and Wilkins, 1996:115–147.
5. Lumb AB. Nunn's Applied Respiratory Physiology, 5th ed. London: Butterworth-Heinemann, 2002.
6. Wilson WC, Benumof JL. Respiratory physiology and respiratory function during anesthesia. In: Miller RD, ed. Miller's Anesthesia, 6th ed. Philadelphia: Elsevier, Churchill Livingstone, 2005: 679–722.

7. Robinson NE. Respiratory function. In: Cunningham JG, ed. Textbook of Veterinary Physiology, 3rd ed. Philadelphia: WB Saunders, 2002:468–514.

8. McDonell WN. Ventilation and acid-base equilibrium with methoxyflurane anesthesia in dogs [MSc thesis]. Guelph, Canada: University of Guelph, 1969.

9. Gallivan GJ, McDonell WN, Forrest JB. Comparative ventilation and gas exchange in the horse and cow. Res Vet Sci 1989;46:331–336.

10. Lai Y-L. Comparative ventilation of the normal lung. In: Parent RA, ed. Treatise of Pulmonary Toxicology, vol 1: Comparative Biology of the Normal Lung. Boca Raton, FL: CRC, 1992:219–224.

11. Fordyce WE, Tenney SM. Role of carotid bodies in ventilatory acclimation to chronic hypoxia by the awake cat. Respir Physiol 1984;58:207–221.

12. Gillespie DJ, Hyatt RE. Respiratory mechanics in the unanesthetized dog. J Appl Physiol 1974;35:98–102.

13. Hales JRS, Webster MED. Respiratory function during thermal tachypnoea in sheep. J Physiol (Lond) 1967;190:241–260.

14. Bakima M, Gustin P, Lekeux P, Lomba F. Mechanics of breathing in goats. Res Vet Sci 1988;45:332–336.

15. Mesina JE, Bisgard GE, Robinson GM. Pulmonary function changes in goats given 3-methylindole orally. Am J Vet Res 1984;45:1526–1531.

16. Forster HV, Bisgard GE, Klein JP. Effect of peripheral chemoreceptor denervation on acclimatization of goats during hypoxia. J Appl Physiol 1981;50:392–398.

17. Verbrugghe C, Laurent P, Bouvert P. Chemoreflex drive of ventilation in the awake miniature pig. Respir Physiol 1982;47:379–391.

18. Keith IM, Bisgard GE, Manohar M, Klein J, Bullard YA. Respiratory effects of pregnancy and progesterone in Jersey cows. Respir Physiol 1982;50:351–358.

19. Bisgard GE, Ruis AV, Grover RF, Will JA. Ventilatory control in the Hereford calf. J Appl Physiol 1973;35:220–226.

20. Willoughby RA, McDonell WN. Pulmonary function testing in horses. Vet Clin North Am Large Anim Pract 1979;1:171–196.

21. Gillespie JR, Tyler WS, Eberly VE. Pulmonary ventilation and resistance in emphysematous and control horses. J Appl Physiol 1966;21:416–422.

22. Orr JA, Bisgard GE, Forster HV, Rowlings CA, Buss DD, Will JA. Cardiopulmonary measurements in nonanesthetized, resting normal ponies. Am J Vet Res 1975;36:1667–1670.

23. Libermann IM, Capano A, Gonzalez F, Bruzzana H. Blood acid-base status in normal albino rats. Lab Anim Sci 1973;23:862–865.

24. Lai Y-L, Tsuya Y, Hildebrandt J. Ventilatory response to acute CO_2 exposure in the rat. J Appl Physiol 1978;45:611–618.

25. Lahiri S. Blood oxygen affinity and alveolar ventilation in relation to body weight in mammals. Am J Physiol 1975;229:529–536.

26. Neutze JM, Wyler F, Rudolph AM. Use of radioactive microspheres to assess cardiac output in rabbits. Am J Physiol 1968;215:486–495.

27. Dyson DH, Allen DG, Ingwersen W, Pascoe PJ, O'Grady M. Effects of Saffan on cardiopulmonary function in healthy cats. Can J Vet Res 1987;51:236–239.

28. Herbert DA, Mitchell RA. Blood gas tensions and acid-base balance in awake cats. J Appl Physiol 1971;30:434–436.

29. Horwitz LD, Bishop VS, Stone HL, Stegall HF. Cardiovascular effects of low-oxygen atmospheres in conscious and anesthetized dogs. J Appl Physiol 1969;27:370–373.

30. Wanner A, Reinhart ME. Respiratory mechanics in conscious sheep: Response to methacholine. J Appl Physiol 1978;44:479–482.

31. Bisgard GE, Vogel JHK. Hypoventilation and pulmonary hypertension in calves after carotid body excision. J Appl Physiol 1971;31:431–437.

32. Donawick WJ, Baue AE. Blood gases, acid-base balance, and alveolar-arterial oxygen gradient in calves. Am J Vet Res 1968;29:561–567.

33. Crosfill ML, Widdicombe JG. Physical characteristics of the chest and lungs and the work of breathing in different mammalian species. J Physiol (Lond) 1961;158:1–14.

34. Mauderly JL. Effect of age on pulmonary structure and function of immature and adult animals and man. Fed Proc 1979;38:173–177.

35. Gallivan GJ, McDonell WN, Forrest JB. Comparative pulmonary mechanics in the horse and the cow. Res Vet Sci 1989;46:322–330.

36. Sorenson PR, Robinson NE. Postural effects on lung volumes and asynchronous ventilation in anesthetized horses. J Appl Physiol 1980;48:97–103.

37. McDonell WN, Hall LW. Functional residual capacity in conscious and anaesthetized horses. Br J Anaesth 1974;46:802–803.

38. Gallivan GJ, Bignell W, McDonell WN, Whiting TL. Simple nonrebreathing valves for use with large mammals. Can J Vet Res 1989;53:143–146.

39. Derksen FJ, Robinson NE. Esophageal and intrapleural pressures in the healthy conscious pony. Am J Vet Res 1980;41:1756–1761.

40. Amis TC, Pascoe JR, Hornof W. Topographic distribution of pulmonary ventilation and perfusion in the horse. Am J Vet Res 1984;45:1597–1601.

41. West JB. Ventilation-perfusion relationships. Am Rev Respir Dis 1977;116:919–943.

42. Porcelli RJ. Pulmonary hemodynamics. In: Parent RA, ed. Treatise on Pulmonary Toxicology, vol 1: Comparative Biology of the Normal Lung. Boca Raton, FL: CRC, 1992:241–270.

43. Hlastra MP, Bernard SL, Erikson HH, et al. Pulmonary blood flow distribution in standing horses is not dominated by gravity. J Appl Physiol 1996;81:1051–1061.

44. Pelletier N, Robinson NE, Kaiser L, Derksen FJ. Regional differences in endothelial function in horse lungs: Possible role in blood flow distribution? J Appl Physiol 1998;85:537–542.

45. Robinson NE. The respiratory system. In: Muir WW, Hubbell JE, eds. Equine Anesthesia: Monitoring and Emergency Therapy. St Louis: Mosby Year Book, 1991:7–38.

46. Clarke KW, Hall LW. A survey of anesthesia in small animal practice: AVA/BSAVA report. J Assoc Vet Anaesth 1990;17:4–10.

47. Daunt DA. Supportive therapy in the anesthetized horse. Vet Clin North Am Equine Pract 1990;6:557–573.

48. Kelly AB, Steffey EP. Inhalation anesthesia: Drugs and techniques. Vet Clin North Am Equine Pract 1981;3:59–71.

49. McDonell WN, Dyson DH. Management of anesthetic emergencies. In: White NA, Moore JN eds. Current Practice of Equine Surgery. Philadelphia: JB Lippincott, 1990:103–114.

50. Lekeux P, Rollin F, Art T. Control of breathing in resting and exercising animals. In: Lekeux P, ed. Pulmonary Function in Healthy, Exercising and Diseased Animals. Gent, Belgium: Flemish Veterinary Journal (Special Issue) 1993:123–145.

51. Gauvreau GM, Wilson BA, Schnurr DL, Young SS, McDonell WN. Oxygen cost of ventilation in the horse. Res Vet Sci 1995;59:168–171.

52. Muir WW, Moore CA, Hamlin RL. Ventilatory alterations in normal horses in response to changes in inspired oxygen and carbon dioxide. Am J Vet Res 1975;36:155–159.

53. Boggs DF. Comparative control of respiration. In: Parent RA, ed. Treatise on Pulmonary Toxicology, vol 1: Comparative Biology of the Normal Lung. Boca Raton, FL: CRC, 1992:314–315.

54. Muir WW, Hamlin RL. Effects of acetylpromazine on ventilatory variables in the horse. Am J Vet Res 1975;36:1439–1442.

55. Bisgard GE, Vagel JH. Hypoventilation and pulmonary hypertension in calves after carotid body excision. J Appl Physiol 1971;31: 431–437.

56. Imai A, Steffey EP, Farver TB, Ilkiw JE. Assessment of isoflurane-induced anesthesia in ferrets and rats. Am J Vet Res 1999;60: 1577–1583.

57. Imai A, Steffey EP, Ilkiw JE, Farver TB. Comparison of clinical signs and hemodynamic variables used to monitor rabbits during halothane- and isoflurane-induced anesthesia. Am J Vet Res 1999;60:1189–1195.

58. Steffey EP, Farver TB, Woliner MJ. Circulatory and respiratory effects of methoxyflurane on dogs: Comparison of halothane. Am J Vet Res 1984;45:2574–2579.

59. Gautier H, Bonora M, Zaoui D. Influence of halothane on control of breathing in intact and decerebrated cats. J Appl Physiol 1987; 63:546–553.

60. Mutoh T, Nishimura R, Kim HY, Matsunga S, Sasak N. Cardio-plumonary effects of sevoflurane, compared with halothane, enflurane, and isoflurane, in dogs. Am J Vet Res 1997;58:885–890.

61. Steffey EP, Howland D. Comparison of circulatory and respiratory effects of isoflurane and halothane anesthesia in horses. Am J Vet Res 1980;41:821–825.

62. Grosenbaugh DA, Muir WW. Cardiorespiratory effects of sevoflurane, isoflurane, and halothane in horses. Am J Vet Res 1998;59: 101–106.

63. Steffey EP, Woliner MJ, Puschner B, Galey FD. Effects of desflurane and mode of ventilation on cardiovascular and respiratory function and clinicopathologic variables in horses. Am J Vet Res 2005;66:669–677.

64. Trim CM. Sedation and general anesthesia in ruminants. Calif Vet 1981;35:29–36.

65. Steffey EP. Some characteristics of ruminants and swine that complicate management of general anesthesia. Vet Clin North Am Food Anim Pract 1986;2:507–516.

66. Hornbein TF. Anesthetics and ventilatory control. In: Covino BG, Fozzard HA, Rehder K, Strichartz G, eds. Effects of Anesthesia. Bethesda, MD: American Physiological Society, 1985:75–90.

67. Pavlin EG, Hornbein TF. Anesthesia and the control of ventilation. In: Fishman AP, ed. Handbook of Physiology, sect 3: The Respiratory System, vol 11: Control of Breathing, part 2. Bethesda, MD: American Physiological Society, 1986:793–813.

68. Hirshman CA, McCullough RE, Cohen PJ, Weil JV. Hypoxic ventilatory drive in dogs during thiopental, ketamine, or pentobarbital anesthesia. Anesthesiology 1975;43:628–634.

69. Knill RL, Gelb AW. Ventilatory response to hypoxia and hypercapnia during halothane sedation and anesthesia in man. Anesthesiology 1978;49:244–251.

70. Steffey EP, Howland D. Isoflurane potency in the dog and cat. Am J Vet Res 1977;38:1833–1836.

71. Steffey EP, Howland D. Potency of enflurane in dogs: Comparison with halothane and isoflurane. Am J Vet Res 1978;39:573–577.

72. Steffey EP, Howland D. Halothane anesthesia in calves. Am J Vet Res 1979;40:372–376.

73. Steffey EP, Gillespie JR, Berry JD, Eger EI, Rhode EA. Cardiovascular effects of halothane in the stump-tailed macaque during spontaneous and controlled ventilation. Am J Vet Res 1974;35: 1315–1319.

74. Steffey EP, Howland D, Giri S, Eger EI. Enflurane, halothane, and isoflurane potency in horses. Am J Vet Res 1977;38:1037–1039.

75. Steffey MA, Bresnan RJ, Steffey EP. Assessment of halothane and sevoflurane anesthesia in spontaneously breathing rats. Am J Vet Res 2003;64:470–474.

76. McDonell W. Anesthesia of the harp seal. J Wildl Dis 1972;8: 287–295.

77. Daunt DA, Steffey EP, Pascoe JR, Willits N, Daels PF. Actions of isoflurane and halothane in pregnant mares. J Am Vet Med Assoc 1992;201:1367–1374.

78. Brandstater B, Eger EI, Edelist G. Constant depth halothane anesthesia in respiratory studies. J Appl Physiol 1965;20:171–174.

79. Cuvelliez SG, Eicker SW, McLauchlin C, Brunson DB. Cardiovascular and respiratory effects of inspired oxygen fraction in halothane-anesthetized horses. Am J Vet Res 1990;51:1226–1231.

80. Seaman GC, Ludders JW, Erb HN, Gleed RD. Effects of low and high fractions of inspired oxygen on ventilation in ducks anesthetized with isoflurane. Am J Vet Res 1994;55:395–398.

81. Nolan AM, Reid J. The use of intraoperative fentanyl in spontaneously breathing dogs undergoing orthopaedic surgery. J Vet Anaesth 1991;18:30–39.

82. Steffey EP, Eisele JH, Baggot JD. Interactions of morphine and isoflurane in horses. Am J Vet Res 2003;64:166–175.

83. Copeland VS, Haskins SC, Patz DJ. Oxymorphone: Cardiovascular, pulmonary, and behavioral effects in the dog. Am J Vet Res 1987;48:1626–1630.

84. Turner DM, Ilkiw JE, Rose RJ, Warren JM. Respiratory and cardiovascular effects of five drugs used as sedatives in the dog. Aust Vet J 1974;50:260–265.

85. Berg RJ, Orton EC. Pulmonary function in dogs after intercostal thoracotomy: Comparison of morphine, oxymorphone, and selective intercostal nerve block. Am J Vet Res 1986;47:471–474.

86. Katz J, Kavanagh BP, Sandler AN. Preemptive analgesia: Clinical evidence of neuroplasty contributing to post-operative pain. Anesthesiology 1992;77:439–446.

87. Jones JG, Sapsford DJ, Wheatley RG. Post-operative hypoxaemia: Mechanisms and time course. Anaesthesia 1990;45:566–573.

88. Taylor PM, Houlton JEF. Post-operative analgesia in the dog: A comparison of morphine, buprenorphine, and pentazocine. J Small Anim Pract 1984;25:437–451.

89. Jacobson JD, McGrath CJ, Smith EP. Cardiorespiratory effects of induction and maintenance of anesthesia with ketamine-midazolam combination, with and without prior administration of butorphanol or oxymorphone. Am J Vet Res 1994;55:543–550.

90. Popilskis S, Kohn D, Sanchez JA, Gorman P. Epidural versus intramuscular oxymorphone analgesia after thoracotomy in dogs. Vet Surg 1991;20:462–467.

91. Pascoe PJ, Dyson DH. Analgesia after lateral thoracotomy in dogs: Epidural morphine versus intercostal bupivacaine. Vet Surg 1993;22:141–147.

92. Haskins SC, Farver TB, Patz JD. Cardiovascular changes in dogs given diazepam and diazepam-ketamine. Am J Vet Res 1986;17:795–798.

93. Farver TB, Haskins SC, Patz JD. Cardiopulmonary effects of acepromazine and of the subsequent administration of ketamine in the dog. Am J Vet Res 1986;47:631–635.

94. Muir WW, Sams RA, Huffman RH, Noonan JA. Pharmacodynamic and pharmacokinetic properties of diazepam in horses. Am J Vet Res 1982;43:1756–1762.

95. Reitemeyer H, Klein HJ, Deegen E. The effect of sedatives on lung function in horses. Acta Vet Scand 1986;82:111–120.

96. Lavoie JP, Pascoe JR, Kurpershoek CJ. Effects of xylazine on ventilation in horses. Am J Vet Res 1992;53:916–920.

97. Lavoie JP, Pascoe JR, Kurpershoek CJ. Effect of head and neck position on respiratory mechanics in horses sedated with xylazine. Am J Vet Res 1992;53:1653–1657.

98. Wagner AE, Muir WW, Hinchcliff KW. Cardiovascular effects of xylazine and detomidine in horses. Am J Vet Res 1991;52:651–657.

99. Clarke KW, England GCW, Goossens L. Sedative and cardiovascular effects of romifidine, alone and in combination with butorphanol, in the horse. J Vet Anaesth 1991;18:25–29.

100. Celly CS, McDonell WN, Young SS, Black WD. The comparative hypoxaemic effect of four alpha 2 adrenoceptor agonists (xylazine, romifidine, detomidine and medetomidine) in sheep. J Vet Pharmacol Ther 1997;20:461–464.

101. Celly CS, McDonell WN, Black WD, Young SS. Cardiopulmonary effects of clonidine, diazepam, and the peripheral α_2 adrenoceptor agonist ST-91 in conscious sheep. J Vet Pharmacol Ther 1997;20:472–478.

102. Celly CS, McDonell WN, Black. Cardiopulmonary effects of the alpha 2-adrenoceptor agonists medetomidine and ST-91 in anesthetized sheep. J Pharmacol Exp Ther 1999;289:712–720.

103. Celly CS, Atwal OS, McDonell WN, Black WD. Histopathological alterations induced by alpha$_2$ adrenoceptor agonists in the lungs of sheep. Am J Vet Res 1999;60:154–161.

104. Doherty TJ, Ballinger JA, McDonell WN, Pascoe PJ, Vallient AE. Antagonism of xylazine induced sedation by idazoxan in calves. Can J Vet Res 1987;51:244–248.

105. Kumar A, Thurmon JC. Cardiopulmonary, hemocytologic and biochemical effects of xylazine in goats. Lab Anim Sci 1979;29:486–491.

106. Caulkett NA, Cattet MR, Cantwell S, Cool N, Olsen W. Anesthesia of wood bison with medetomidine-zolazepam/tiletamine and xylazine-zolazepam/tiletamine combinations. Can Vet J 2000;41:49–53.

107. Caulkett NA, Cribb PH, Haigh JC. Comparative cardiopulmonary effects of carfentanil-xylazine and medetomidine-ketamine used for immobilization of mule deer and mule deer/white-tailed deer hybrids. Can J Vet Res 2000;64:64–68.

108. Read MR, Caulkett NA, Symington A, Shury TK. Treatment of hypoxemia during xylazine-tiletamine-zolazepam immobilization of wapiti. Can Vet J 2001;42:861–864.

109. Allen DG, Dyson DH, Pascoe PJ, O'Grady MR. Evaluation of a xylazine-ketamine hydrochloride combination in the cat. Can Vet Res 1986;50:23–26.

110. Nguyen D, Abdul-Rasool I, Ward D, et al. Ventilatory effects of dexmedetomidine, atipamezole, and isoflurane in dogs. Anesthesiology 1992;76:573–579.

111. Ko JCH, Bailey JE, Pablo LS, Heaton-Jones TG. Comparison of sedative and cardiorespiratory effects of medetomidine and medetomidine-butorphanol combination in dogs. Am J Vet Res 1996;57:535–540.

112. Ko JCH, Fox SM, Mandsager RE. Sedative and cardiorespiratory effects of medetomidine, medetomidine-butorphanol, and medetomidine-ketamine in dogs. J Am Vet Med Assoc 2000;216:1578–1583.

113. Lamont LA, Bulmer BJ, Grimm KA, Tranquilli WJ, Sisson DD. Cardiopulmonary evaluation of the use of medetomidine hydrochloride in cats. Am J Vet Res 2001;62:1745–1749.

114. Sinclair M. A review of the physiological effects of α_2-agonists related to the clinical use of medetomidine in small animal practice. Can Vet J 2002;44:885–897.

115. Mitchell B, Williams JT. Respiratory function changes in sheep associated with lying in lateral recumbency and with sedation by xylazine. Proc Assoc Vet Anaesth Gr Br Ir 1977;6:32–36.

116. Hall LW. Cardiovascular and pulmonary effects of recumbency in two conscious ponies. Equine Vet J 1984;16:89–92.

117. Klein L, Fisher H. Cardiopulmonary effects of restraint in dorsal recumbency on awake cattle. Am J Vet Res 1988;49:1605–1608.

118. Wagner AE, Muir WW, Grospitch BJ. Cardiopulmonary effects of position in conscious cattle. Am J Vet Res 1990;51:7–10.

119. Agostoni E. Mechanics of the pleural space. Physiol Rev 1972;52:57–128.

120. Rehder K. Anesthesia and the mechanics of respiration. In: Covino BG, Fozzard HA, Rehder K, Strichartz G, eds. Effects of Anesthesia. Bethesda, MD: American Physiological Society, 1985:91–106.

121. Marshall BE, Marshall C. Anesthesia and pulmonary circulation. In: Covino BG, Fozzard HA, Rehder K, Strichartz G, eds. Effects of Anesthesia. Bethesda, MD: American Physiological Society, 1985:121–136.

122. Amis TC, Jones HA, Hughes JMB. A conscious dog model for study of regional lung function. J Appl Physiol 1982;53:1050–1054.

123. Amis TC, Pascoe JR, Hornof W. Topographic distribution of pulmonary ventilation and perfusion in the horse. Am J Vet Res 1984;45:1597–1601.

124. Hedenstierna G, Nyman G, Kvart C, Funkquist B. Ventilation-perfusion relationships in the standing horse: An inert gas elimination study. Equine Vet J 1987;19:514–519.

125. Robinson NE. Some functional consequences of species differences in lung anatomy. Adv Vet Sci Comp Med 1982;26:1–33.

126. Tucker A, McMurtry IF, Reeves JT, Alexander AF, Will DH, Grover RF. Lung vascular smooth muscle as a determinant of pulmonary hypertension at high altitude. Am J Physiol 1975;228:762–767.

127. Elliott AR, Steffey EP, Jarvis KA, Marshall BE. Unilateral hypoxic pulmonary vasoconstriction in the dog, pony and miniature swine. Respir Physiol 1991;85:355–369.

128. Marshall BE, Marshall C, Benumof J, Saidman LJ. Hypoxic pulmonary vasoconstriction in dogs: Effects of lung segment size and oxygen tension. J Appl Physiol 1981;51:1543–1551.

129. Benetar SR, Hewlett AM, Nunn JF. The use of iso-shunt lines for control of oxygen therapy. Br J Anaesth 1973;45:711–718.

130. Froese AB. Effects of anesthesia and paralysis on the chest wall. In: Covino BG, Fozzard HA, Rehder K, Strichartz G, eds. Effects of Anesthesia. Bethesda, MD: American Physiological Society, 1985:107–120.

131. Lai YL, Rodarte JR, Hyatt RE. Respiratory mechanics in recumbent dogs anesthetized with thiopental sodium. J Appl Physiol 1979;46:716–720.

132. Rugh KS, Garner HE, Hatfield DG, Herrold D. Arterial oxygen and carbon dioxide tensions in conscious laterally recumbent ponies. Equine Vet J 1984;16:185–188.

133. Honeyman VL, Pettifer GR, Dyson DH. Arterial blood pressure and blood gas valves in normal standing and laterally recumbent African (*Loxodonta Africana*) and Asian (*Elephas maximus*) elephants. J Zoo Wildl Med 1992;23:205–210.

134. Engel S. The respiratory tissue of the elephant (*Elephas indicus*). Acta Anat (Basel) 1963;5:105–111.

135. Ungerer T, Orr JA, Bisgard GE, Will JA. Cardiopulmonary effects of mechanical distension of the rumen in nonanesthetized sheep. Am J Vet Res 1976;37:807–810.

136. Musewe VO, Gillespie JR, Berry JD. Influence of ruminal insufflation on pulmonary function and diaphragmatic electromyography in cattle. Am J Vet Res 1979;40:26–31.

137. Hornof WJ, Dunlop CI, Prestage R, Amis TC. Effects of lateral recumbency on regional lung function in anesthetized horses. Am J Vet Res 1986;47:277–282.

138. Thurmon JC. General clinical considerations for anesthesia in the horse. Vet Clin North Am Equine Pract 1990;6:485–494.

139. Stegman GF. Pulmonary function in the horse during anesthesia: A review. J S Afr Vet Assoc 1986;57:49–53.

140. Wan PY, Trim CM, Mueller PO. Xylazine-ketamine and detomidine-tiletamine-zolazepam anesthesia in horses. Vet Surg 1992;21: 312–318.

141. Wilson DV, McFeely AM. Positive end-expiratory pressure during colic surgery in horses: 74 cases (1986–1988). J Am Vet Med Assoc 1991;199:917–921.

142. Levsitsky MA, Davis S, Murray PA. Preservation of hypoxic pulmonary vasoconstriction during sevoflurane and desflurane anesthesia compared to the conscious state in chronically instrumented dogs. Anesthesiology 1998;89:1501–1508.

143. Young LE, Bartram DH, Diamond MJ, Gregg AS, Jones RS. Clinical evaluation of an infusion of xylazine, guaifenesin and ketamine for maintenance of anaesthesia in horses. Equine Vet J 1993;25:115–119.

144. Staddon GE, Weaver BMQ. Regional pulmonary perfusion in horses: A comparison between anesthetized and conscious standing animals. Res Vet Sci 1981;30:44–48.

145. Stolk PWT. The effect of anesthesia on pulmonary blood flow in the horse. Proc Assoc Vet Anaesth Gr Br Ir 1982;10:119–129.

146. Dobson A, Gleed RD, Meyer RE, Stewart BJ. Changes in blood flow distribution in equine lungs induced by anesthesia. Q J Exp Physiol 1985;70:283–297.

147. Jarvis KA, Steffey EP, Tyler WS, Willits N, Woliner M. Pulmonary blood flow distribution in anesthetized ponies. J Appl Physiol 1992;72:1173–1178.

148. Hughes JMB, Glazier JB, Maloney JE, West JB. Effect of lung volume on the distribution of pulmonary blood flow in man. Respir Physiol 1968;4:58–72.

149. Hughes JMB, Glazier JB, Maloney JE, West JB. Effect of extra-alveolar vessels on distribution of blood flow in the dog lung. J Appl Physiol 1968;25:701–712.

150. Hewlett AM, Hulands GH, Nunn JF, Milledge JS. Functional residual capacity during anesthesia. III. Artificial ventilation. Br J Anaesth 1974;46:495–503.

151. Reber A, Engberg G, Sporre B, et al. Volumetric analysis of aeration in the lungs during general anesthesia. Br J Anaesth 1996;76:760–766.

152. Rothen U, Sporre B, Engberg G, Wegenius G, Hedenstierna G. Airway closure, atelectasis and gas exchange during general anaesthesia. Br J Anaesth 1998;81:681–686.

153. Clerex C, Van den Brom WE, de Vries HW. Comparison of inhalation-to-perfusion ratio in anesthetized dogs with barrel-shaped thorax vs dogs with deep thorax. Am J Vet Res 1991;52:1097–1103.

154. McDonell WN, Hall LW, Jeffcott LB. Radiographic evidence of impaired pulmonary function in laterally recumbent anaesthetized horses. Equine Vet J 1979;11:24–32.

155. Watney GCG. Radiographic evidence of pulmonary dysfunction in anesthetized cattle. Res Vet Sci 1986;41:162–171.

156. McDonell WN. The effect of anesthesia on pulmonary gas exchange and arterial oxygenation in the horse [PhD dissertation]. Cambridge: University of Cambridge, 1974.

157. Nyman G, Funkquist B, Kvart C, et al. Atelectasis causes gas exchange impairment in the anaesthetised horse. Equine Vet J 1990;22:317–324.

158. Moens Y, Lagerweij E, Gootjes P, Poortman J. Distribution of inspired gas to each lung in anaesthetized horses and influence of body shape. Equine Vet J 1995;27:110–116.

159. Wilson DV, Soma LR. Cardiopulmonary effects of positive end-expiratory pressure in anesthetized, mechanically ventilated ponies. Am J Vet Res 1990;51:734–739.

160. Moens Y, Lagerweij E, Goottjes P, Poortman J. Influence of tidal volume and positive pressure on inspiratory gas distribution and gas exchange during mechanical ventilation in horses positioned in lateral recumbency. Am J Vet Res 1998;59:307–312.

161. Moens Y, Largerweij E, Gootjes P, Poortman J. Differential artificial ventilation in anesthetized horses positioned in lateral recumbency. Am J Vet Res 1994;55:1319–1326.

162. Nyman G, Frostell C, Hedenstierna G, Funkquist B, Kvart G, Blomqvist H. Selective mechanical ventilation of dependent lung regions in the anesthetized horse in dorsal recumbency. Br J Anaesth 1987;59:1027–1034.

163. Benson J, Manohar M, Kneller SK, Thurmon JC, Steffey EP. Radiographic characterization of diaphragmatic excursion in halothane-anesthetized ponies: Spontaneous and controlled ventilation systems. Am J Vet Res 1982;43:617–621.

164. Froese AB, Bryan AC. Effects of anesthesia and paralysis on diaphragmatic mechanics in man. Anesthesiology 1974;41:242–255.

165. Hall LW, Aziz HA, Groenendyk J, Keates H, Rex MAE. Electromyography of some respiratory muscles in the horse. Res Vet Sci 1991;50:328–333.

166. Aviado DM. Regulation of bronchomotor tone during anesthesia. Anesthesiology 1975;42:68–80.

167. Heneghan CPH, Bergman NA, Jordan C, Lehane JR, Catley DM. Effect of isoflurane on bronchomotor in man. Br J Anaesth 1986;58:24–28.

168. Watney GCG, Jordan C, Hall LW. Effect of halothane, enflurane and isoflurane on bronchomotor tone in anaesthetized ponies. Br J Anaesth 1987;59:1022–1026.

169. Watney GCG. Effects of xylazine/halothane anaesthesia on the pulmonary mechanics of adult cattle. J Assoc Vet Anaesth 1986/87; 14:16–28.

170. Watney GCG. Effect of halothane on bronchial caliber of anaesthetized cattle. Vet Rec 1987;20:9–12.

171. Hall LW, Young SS. Effect of inhalation anesthetics on total respiratory resistance in conscious ponies. J Vet Pharmacol Ther 1992; 15:174–179.

172. Blaze CA, LeBlanc PH, Robinson NE. Effect of withholding feed on ventilation and the incidence of regurgitation during halothane anesthesia of adult cattle. Am J Vet Res 1988;49:2126–2129.

173. Nunn JF. Anesthesia and pulmonary gas exchange. In: Covino BG, Fozzard HA, Rehder K, Strichartz G, eds. Effects of Anesthesia. Bethesda, MD: American Physiological Society, 1985: 137–147.

174. Barker SJ, Tremper KK. Respiratory monitoring, blood-gas measurement, oximetry, and pulse oximetry. Curr Opin Anaesthesiol 1992;5:816–825.

175. Cullen DJ, Nemeskal AR, Cooper JB, Zaslavsky A, Dwyer MJ. Effect of oximetry, age, and ASA physical status on the frequency of patients admitted unexpectedly to a postoperative intensive care

unit and severity of their anesthetic-related complications. Anesth Analg 1992;74:181–188.

176. Cote CJ, Rolf N, Lui LM, et al. A single blind study of combined pulse oximetry and capnography in children. Anesthesiology 1991;74:980–987.

177. Hedenstierna G, Rothen HU. Atelectasis formation during anesthesia: Causes and measures to prevent it. J Clin Monit Comput 2000;16:329–335.

178. Edmark L, Kestova-Aherdan K, Enlund M, Hedenstierna G. Optimal oxygen concentration during induction of general anesthesia. Anesthesiology 2003;98:28–33.

179. Rothen HU, Sporre B, Enberg G, Wegenius G, Hogman M, Hedenstierna G. Influence of gas composition on recurrence of atelectasis after a reexpansion maneuver during general anesthesia. Anesthesiology 1995;82:832–842.

180. Rothen HU, Neumann P, Berglund JE, Valtysson J, Magnusson A, Hedenstierna G. Dynamics of re-expansion of atelectasis during general anaesthesia. Br J Anaesth 1999;82:551–556.

181. Magnusson L, Tenling A, Lemoine R, Hogman M, Tyden H, Hedenstierna G. The safety of one, or repeated, vital capacity maneuvers during general anesthesia. Anesth Analg 2000;91:702–707.

182. Oczenski W, Schwarz S, Fitzgerald RD. Vital capacity manoeuver in general anaesthesia: Useful or useless? Eur J Anaesthesiol 2004;21:253–254.

183. Neumann P, Rothen HU, Berglund JE, Valtysson J, Magnusson A, Hedenstierna G. Positive end-expiratory pressure prevents atelectasis during general anaesthesia even in the presence of high inspired oxygen concentrations. Acta Anaesthesiol Scand 1999;43:295–301.

184. Turner DM, Ilkiw JE. Cardiovascular and respiratory effects of three rapidly acting barbiturates in dogs. Am J Vet Res 1990;51:598–604.

185. Dyson DH, Allen DG, Ingwersen W, Pascoe PJ. Evaluation of acepromazine/meperidine/atropine premedication followed by thiopental anesthesia in the cat. Can J Vet Res 1988;52:419–422.

186. Steffey EP, Farver TB, Woliner MJ. Cardiopulmonary function during 7 h of constant-dose halothane and methoxyflurane. J Appl Physiol 1987;63:1351–1359.

187. Ingwersen W, Allen DG, Dyson DH, Pascoe PJ, O'Grady MR. Cardiopulmonary effects of a halothane/oxygen combination in healthy cats. Can J Vet Res 1988;52:386–391.

188. Ray JF, Yost L, Moallem S, et al. Immobility, hypoxemia, and pulmonary arteriovenous shunting. Arch Surg 1974;109:537–541.

189. Ewing KK. Anesthesia techniques in sheep and goats. Vet Clin North Am Food Anim Pract 1990;6:759–778.

190. Hedenstierna G, Lundquist H, Lundh B, et al. Pulmonary densities during anaesthesia: An experimental study on lung morphology and gas exchange. Eur Respir J 1989;2:528–535.

191. Fujimoto JL, Lenchan TM. The influence of body position on the blood gas and acid-base status of halothane anesthetized sheep. Vet Surg 1985;14:169–172.

192. Semrad SD, Trim CM, Hardee GE. Hypertension in bulls and steers anesthetized with guaifenesin-thiobarbiturate-halothane combination. Am J Vet Res 1986;47:1577–1582.

193. Blaze CA, Robinson NE. Apneic oxygenation in anesthetized ponies and horses. Vet Res Commun 1987;11:281–291.

194. Hall LW, Gillespie JR, Tyler WS. Alveolar-arterial oxygen tension differences in anaesthetized horses. Br J Anaesth 1968;40:560–568.

195. de Moor A, van den Hende C. Inspiratory concentrations of O_2, N_2, and N_2O, arterial oxygenation and acid-base status during closed system halothane anaesthesia in the horse. Zentralbl Veterinarmed [A] 1972;19:1–7.

196. Steffey EP, Kelly AB, Woliner MJ. Time-related responses of spontaneously breathing, laterally recumbent horses to prolonged anesthesia with halothane. Am J Vet Res 1987;48:952–957.

197. Nyman G, Hedenstierna G. Comparison of conventional and selective mechanical ventilation in the anaesthetized horse. J Vet Med 1988;35:299–315.

198. Gleed RD. Improvement in arterial oxygen tension with change in posture in anaesthetized horses. Res Vet Sci 1988;44:255–259.

199. Nyman G, Funkquist B, Kvart C. Postural effects on blood gas tension, blood pressure, heart rate, ECG and respiratory rate during prolonged anaesthesia in the horse. J Vct Med 1988;35:54–62.

200. Steffey EP, Kelly AB, Hodgson DS, Grandy JL, Woliner MJ, Willits N. Effect of body posture on cardiopulmonary function in horses during five hours of constant-dose halothane anesthesia. Am J Vet Res 1990;51:11–16.

201. Stegmann GF, Littlejohn A. The effect of lateral and dorsal recumbency on cardiopulmonary function in the anaesthetized horse. J S Afr Vet Assoc 1987;58:21–27.

202. Kerr CL, McDonell WN, Young SS. A comparison of romifidine and xylazine when used with diazepam/ketamine for short duration anesthesia in the horse. Can Vet J 1996;37:601–609.

203. Young LE, Richards DLS, Brearly JC, Bartram DH, Jones RS. The effect of a 50% inspired mixture of nitrous oxide on arterial oxygen tension in spontaneously breathing horses anaesthetized with halothane. J Vet Anaesth 1992;19:37–40.

204. Day TK, Gaynor JS, Muir WW, Bednarski RM, Mason DE. Blood gas values during intermittent positive pressure ventilation and spontaneous ventilation in 160 anesthetized horses positioned in lateral and dorsal recumbency. Vet Surg 1995;24:266–276.

205. Wagner AE, Bednarski RM, Muir WW. Hemodynamic effects of carbon dioxide during intermittent positive-pressure ventilation in horses. Am J Vet Res 1990;51:1922–1928.

206. Pappenheimer JR. Standardization of definitions and symbols in respiratory physiology. Fed Proc 1950;9:602–605.

207. Nunn JF. Applied Respiratory Physiology, 3rd ed. London: Butterworth, 1987.

Chapter 6
Nervous System

Kurt A. Grimm and Anne E. Wagner

Introduction

Anesthetic and analgesic drugs alter the nervous system; therefore, an understanding of normal nervous system anatomy, physiology, and function is important to anesthetists. Generally, the nervous system can be separated into central and peripheral divisions, although they are integrated and function together. The central division, composed of the brain and spinal cord, contains all of the important nuclei and is essential for integrating sensory and motor functions. The peripheral division is composed of nerves (including cranial nerves) and ganglia that connect the organs and tissues to the central nervous system (CNS).

Functionally, the nervous system can be divided into somatic and autonomic portions, each with efferent and afferent fibers. The somatic afferent fibers convey three sensory modalities from the periphery: pain, temperature, and pressure. In addition, specialized somatic afferents conduct impulses arising in the eye and ear to provide sight and hearing. The somatic efferent fibers have primarily motor functions and terminate in the motor end plates of skeletal muscle.

Autonomic afferent fibers transmit encoded information from specialized receptors in the mucous membranes and tissue of organs stimulated by distension or ischemia or by chemical compounds located in the lumen or tissues. Specialized autonomic afferent fibers mediate the sensations of smell and taste. Autonomic efferent fibers innervate glandular tissue, smooth muscle, cardiac muscle, and the involuntary muscles of the pharynx and larynx.

In summary, the somatic division controls superficial sensations and voluntary movement, whereas the autonomic system maintains visceral organ function and homeostasis, including regulation of heart rate, blood pressure, tissue perfusion, glandular secretion, peristalsis, sphincter tension, and pupil size, as well as thermoregulation. Anesthetic and analgesic drugs can alter function in both divisions.

Brain Anatomy

The brain is divisible into five regions based on embryological development: telencephalon, diencephalon, mesencephalon, metencephalon, and myelencephalon. Grossly, it can be divided into the cerebrum and the brain stem. The cerebrum consists of telencephalic and diencephalic portions. The telencephalic portion can be further divided into the cerebral hemispheres and basal ganglia (also known as the basal nuclei). Together, the right and left hemispheres comprise the cerebral cortex, which is organized into an outer cortical layer of gray matter that contains a high density of nerve cell bodies and an inner medulla of white matter consisting mainly of myelinated nerve fibers. The basal ganglia (corpus striatum, amygdaloid, and claustrum) are large masses of gray matter at the base of each cerebral hemisphere. The functions of the corpus striatum and claustrum are poorly understood, but they appear to contribute to the extrapyramidal motor system through inhibition of motor function and maintenance of balance between opposing muscle groups. The amygdaloid nucleus is a component of the olfactory and limbic systems.

The cerebral cortex is where sensory, motor, and associational activity occurs. The white matter of the cerebrum consists of corticocortical and projection fibers. The corticocortical fibers connect different functional areas located in the same hemisphere (association fibers) and in the opposite hemisphere (commissural fibers). Fibers connecting the cortical areas of the two hemispheres cross the midline in a large commissure: the corpus callosum. Projection fibers originate or terminate in the cortex and connect it with the basal ganglia, brain stem, or spinal cord. The fibers passing between the cortex and subcortical centers converge to form a compact organized group of fibers: the internal capsule.

The diencephalic portion of the cerebrum, which is located below and between the cerebral hemispheres, is the central area through which most of the information traveling into and out of the hemispheres must traverse. It consists of the thalamus, subthalamus, epithalamus, and hypothalamus, and is positioned be-

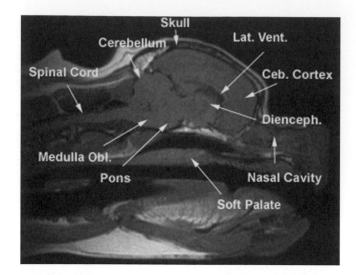

Fig. 6.1. Magnetic resonance image sagittal view of a canine brain and spinal cord. Lat. Vent., lateral ventricle; Ceb. Cortex, cerebral cortex; Dienceph., diencephalon; and Medulla Obl., medulla oblongata. Image courtesy of Igor Kuriashkin.

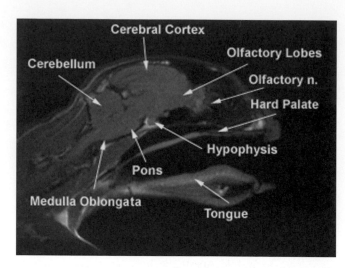

Fig. 6.2. Magnetic resonance image sagittal view of a feline brain and spinal cord. n., nerve. Image courtesy of Igor Kuriashkin.

tween the telencephalon and the brain stem. Magnetic resonance images of the sagittal view of the canine and feline brain are shown in Figs. 6.1 and 6.2. The thalamus receives fibers from all sensory systems except olfactory and projects to sensory areas of the cerebral cortex. Evolutionarily and developmentally, the cerebral cortex is an outgrowth of the lower centers, especially the thalamus. As a result, for each area of the cortex, there is a smaller corresponding area within the thalamus. Thalamic nuclei participate in neural circuits related to emotional aspects of brain function (limbic system), are part of the ascending reticular activating system, and are incorporated into motor pathways from the cerebellum and corpus striatum to the motor cortex.

The subthalamus is comprised of a motor nucleus, sensory tracts that terminate in the thalamus, and tracts that project from the cerebellum and corpus striatum to the thalamus. The epithalamus is composed of the pineal gland and tracts mediating autonomic responses to olfactory and emotional changes. The hypothalamus is the primary center for integrative control of the autonomic nervous system. Parasympathetic responses—including slowing of the heart rate, vasodilation, decreased blood pressure, salivation, increased gastrointestinal peristalsis, contraction of the urinary bladder, and sweating—are elicited by stimulation of the anterior hypothalamus. Stimulation of the posterior and lateral hypothalamus elicits sympathetic responses, including increased heart rate and blood pressure, cessation of gastrointestinal peristalsis, dilation of the pupils, and hyperglycemia. The hypothalamus plays a major role in maintaining homeostasis through control of temperature, thirst, and appetite. Nervous system control of the endocrine system is via the hypothalamic neurohypophyseal hormones. One exception is the adrenal medulla, which is regulated by direct nervous system connections (i.e., the preganglionic sympathetic fibers).

The brain stem is comprised of the portion of the brain caudal to the telencephalon excluding the cerebellum (e.g., the mid-

brain, pons, and medulla oblongata) (Figs. 6.1 and 6.2). The midbrain contains sensory and motor pathways, the nuclei of the third and fourth cranial nerves (oculomotor and trochlear), and two major motor nuclei: the red nucleus and the substantia nigra. The dorsal part of the midbrain is primarily involved with auditory function and visual reflex movements of the eyes and head. The cerebellum is connected to the midbrain by the superior cerebellar peduncles.

The pons consists of two distinct parts. The dorsal portion, like the rest of the brain stem, has both sensory and motor tracts. In addition, the dorsal pons contains nuclei associated with the fifth, sixth, seventh, and eighth cranial nerves (trigeminal, abducens, facial, and vestibulocochlear). The ventral pons functions as a large synaptic region, providing a connection between the cerebral motor cortex and the contralateral cerebellar hemisphere via the middle cerebellar peduncles.

Caudal to the pons is the medulla oblongata, and posterior to it is the spinal cord. In addition to nerve tracts, the medulla contains vital nerve centers that regulate respiration and circulation. Four pairs of cranial nerves connect to it: the glossopharyngeal (ninth), vagus (tenth), spinal accessory (eleventh), and hypoglossal (twelfth). The cerebellum is connected to the medulla by the inferior cerebellar peduncles.

The cerebellum, which lies dorsal to the brain stem, is formed by two hemispheres separated by a central portion: the vermis. The cerebellum receives input from the sensory systems and the cerebral cortex. The cerebellum modulates muscle tone in relation to equilibrium, locomotion, posture, and nonstereotyped movements based on experience. It is chiefly involved with muscular coordination.

Brain Physiology

The energy-consuming processes of the brain are divided into those of neuroprocessing and maintenance of cellular integrity.

Oxygen requirements for the conscious, healthy canine brain are approximately 5.5 mL $\cdot$ 100 g^{-1} $\cdot$ min^{-1}, with 60% needed for neuroprocessing and 40% for maintenance of brain cell integrity.[1] If cardiovascular function is normal, adequate oxygen delivery and normal electroencephalogram (EEG) function is expected with a PaO$_2$ of approximately 100 mm Hg and cerebral blood flow (CBF) of 50 mL $\cdot$ 100 g^{-1} $\cdot$ min^{-1}. Irreversible cerebral tissue damage is likely when PaO$_2$ drops below 20 to 23 mm Hg and CBF below 10 mL $\cdot$ 100 g^{-1} $\cdot$ min^{-1}.[1] In humans, normal function of the awake brain requires approximately 3.5 mL O$_2$ $\cdot$ 100 g^{-1} $\cdot$ min^{-1}, or a total of about 50 mL $\cdot$ min^{-1} extracted from an average normal CBF of 57 mL $\cdot$ 100 g^{-1} $\cdot$ min^{-1}. In the awake state, most of the brain's cellular energy stores are depleted within 2 to 4 min after oxygen delivery is interrupted. During the anoxic period, cellular lactate concentrations can increase three- to fivefold. Anesthesia, hypothermia, or brain injury can alter cerebral metabolic requirements for oxygen (CMRO$_2$) and must be considered when interpreting the adequacy of monitored cardiopulmonary parameters during anesthesia.

The mature brain in nonfasted animals uses oxidative metabolism of glucose as the primary source of energy. Under normal conditions, 95% of the glucose is metabolized by oxidative phosphorylation. The remaining 5% is metabolized by anaerobic pathways to lactate. Inadequate or marginal oxygen delivery to the brain will cause a rapid increase in anaerobic metabolism reflected by increased glucose consumption and lactate production.[1] Approximately 70 mg $\cdot$ min^{-1} of glucose are required for the adult human brain. Normal metabolism requires 5.5 mmol of oxygen for each millimole of glucose. The effects of analgesics and anesthetics on cerebral metabolism, CBF, and CMRO$_2$ are critical factors in producing safe reversible depression of the CNS in healthy and diseased animals.

Effects of Anesthetics on Brain Physiology

Anesthetic management of patients undergoing surgery on the nervous system requires that CBF be maintained at a level sufficient to meet the brain's metabolic demands. Autoregulation enables maintenance of a constant CBF over a wide range of systemic blood pressures. Autoregulation is not immediate; when systemic blood pressure changes, it takes about 2 min for CBF to return to normal.[2] There have been many studies on the effects of anesthetics on CBF and autoregulation, and the results have sometimes been confusing. All potent inhaled anesthetics tend to decrease cerebral metabolism and increase CBF and intracranial pressure (ICP), but vary in degree. Hyperventilation may prevent or reduce the increase in CBF and ICP associated with halothane or enflurane anesthesia, but only if instituted prior to induction. By comparison, hyperventilation may be effective in reversing the increase in CBF and ICP associated with isoflurane anesthesia, even if instituted after induction. For several years, isoflurane has been the preferred inhalant for use in neurological patients, because it apparently has the least negative effect on ICP and cerebral blood volume.[3] Sevoflurane seems to compare favorably with isoflurane in maintaining satisfactory CBF and cerebral perfusion pressure, with minimal to no change in ICP.[4] It is thought that desflurane also is similar to isoflurane in its effects on CBF,

cerebral metabolism, and responsivity to carbon dioxide, in both normal patients and those with intracranial masses. The effects of desflurane on ICP are less clear: Low doses (0.5 minimum alveolar concentration [MAC]) do not seem to change ICP, whereas higher doses (1.0 MAC) have been associated with increased ICP in some patients.[5] A study of pigs anesthetized at 0.5 and 1.0 MAC desflurane, isoflurane, or sevoflurane indicated that the three anesthetics did not differ much in their cerebral vasodilating effects at the lower dose, but, at the higher dose, desflurane induced more cerebral vasodilation than did the other two anesthetics.[6] The use of sevoflurane and desflurane, being less soluble in blood than isoflurane, may be somewhat advantageous in that rapid recovery from anesthesia may facilitate early neurological assessment after diagnostic or surgical procedures.

Cranial Nerves

These consist of a peripheral segment, a nuclear center in the brain stem (except olfactory and optic nerves), and communicating connections with other parts of the brain (Fig. 6.3). All 12 cranial nerves are paired. Functionally, cranial nerves can be divided into motor (efferent), sensory (afferent), and mixed. Sensory and motor cranial nerves are associated with at least one nuclei, and mixed cranial nerves are associated with at least two nuclei (Table 6.1).

The *olfactory*, *optic*, and *vestibulocochlear* nerves serve the senses of smell, sight, and hearing and balance respectively. The *oculomotor* nerve innervates most muscles of the eye: dorsal, medial, and ventral rectus muscles; ventral oblique; levator palpebrae superioris; ciliary muscle; and the sphincter pupillae. The *trochlear* nerve innervates the dorsal oblique muscle of the eye, and the *abducens* nerve supplies the lateral rectus and retractor oculi muscles. Like most cranial nerves, the *spinal accessory* nerve arises from the medulla, but it also has fibers from all seven cervical nerves that course cranially to combine with the medullary roots. The spinal accessory nerve contributes fibers to the vagus nerve before coursing caudally to innervate the muscles of the neck and shoulder. The *hypoglossal* nerve innervates the muscles of the pharynx and the larynx, and the intrinsic muscles of the tongue.

The *trigeminal* nerve carries sensory information from most of the rostral structures and surfaces of the head and motor impulses to the muscles of mastication. It has three main branches: the ophthalmic, maxillary, and mandibular nerves. The ophthalmic is sensory to skin of the forehead, the eyeball (corneal and palpebral reflexes), and the skin of the lower eyelid. The maxillary is sensory to the skin of the muzzle, nose, and upper lip; the mucous membranes of the nose, nasopharynx, the hard and soft palate, and the teeth of the upper jaw. The mandibular branch supplies sensation to the lower part of the face, side of the head, lower lip, and teeth, ear, and tongue, and is motor to the muscles of mastication.

The *facial* nerve is motor to all the cutaneous muscles of the face, lips, nose, cheeks, ears, and ventral neck, and to the submandibular and sublingual salivary glands and the lacrimal gland. It is sensory to the taste buds and to the skin of the exter-

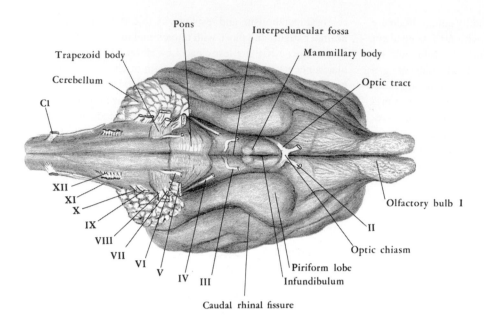

Fig. 6.3. Ventral view of a canine brain and cranial nerves. From Jenkins.[40]

Table 6.1. Sensory, motor, and mixed cranial nerves

Afferent Nerves	Efferent Nerves	Mixed Nerves
1. Olfactory	3. Oculomotor	5. Trigeminal
2. Optic	4. Trochlear	7. Facial
8. Vestibulocochlear	6. Abducens	9. Glossopharyngeal
	11. Spinal accessory	10. Vagus
	12. Hypoglossal	

nal ear. The *glossopharyngeal* nerve is motor to the stylopharyngeus muscle and to the parotid and zygomatic salivary glands. It is sensory to the pharynx, tonsil, tongue (touch, temperature, pain, and taste), carotid bodies, and sinuses (chemoreceptors and baroreceptors).

The *vagus* nerve innervates organs and muscles in the neck, thorax, and abdomen. Long preganglionic parasympathetic fibers are supplied to the heart and to the smooth muscles and glands of the thorax and abdominal viscera. Motor innervation is also supplied to the pharynx, cricothyroideus muscle of the larynx, intrinsic muscles of the larynx, and striated muscle of the esophagus. The sensory fibers of the vagus nerve innervate the base of the tongue (touch, temperature, pain, and taste), pharynx, esophagus, stomach, intestines, larynx, trachea, bronchi, lungs, heart, aortic baroreceptors, and other viscera.

Spinal Cord

Caudal to the medulla, the CNS continues as the spinal cord, which is contained in the spinal canal. The spinal cord is a complex collection of fibers organized into ascending and descending tracts, interneurons, neuron-supporting cells, blood vessels, and connective tissue. The cord is surrounded by the meninges, which support and protect it. From superficial to deep, they are the dura mater, arachnoid, and pia mater (Fig. 6.4).

The spinal cord is segmental in that it has paired spinal nerves that enter and leave it at each intervertebral space. The spinal nerves divide inside the vertebral canal: afferent fibers enter the cord via the dorsal root, and efferent fibers leave as the ventral motor root (Bell-Magendie law). In the fetus, all spinal nerves exit at right angles to the spinal cord. In the adult, however, owing to differential growth rates between the spinal cord and the bony vertebral canal, the nerves must run posteriorly to reach their respective intervertebral foramina. The cauda equina is composed of descending spinal nerves caudal to the termination of the cord (Fig. 6.5). In dogs, the cord and associated subarachnoid structures usually terminate at the level of L6-L7; in horses, ruminants, and swine, the cord terminates in the midsacrum; and, in cats, the cord terminates variably between L6 and the sacrum. Inadvertent subarachnoid administration of anesthetic or analgesic drugs is more likely in these noncanine species when the needle is inserted at the lumbosacral space.

The spinal cord has an H-shaped central core of gray matter containing nerve cell bodies. The gray matter functions as the ini-

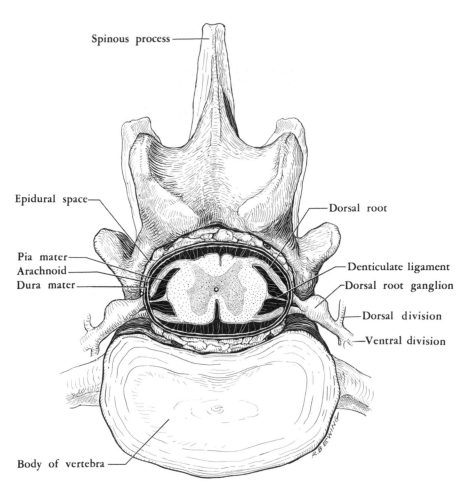

Spinous process

Epidural space

Pia mater
Arachnoid
Dura mater

Dorsal root

Denticulate ligament

Dorsal root ganglion

Dorsal division

Ventral division

Body of vertebra

Fig. 6.4. Transverse section of spinal cord within the vertebral canal. Note the adipose tissue and blood vessels in the epidural space. From Jenkins.[40]

tial site for processing of incoming sensory information and as a relay for transmission of these signals to the brain. It also serves as the final site for processing descending motor impulses from the brain to the skeletal muscles. The gray matter can be divided into dorsal, ventral, and lateral horns. The dorsal horn is the "gate" through which impulses in sensory nerve fibers are passed or blocked before initiating impulses in ascending tracts. According to the *gate control theory of pain*, incoming sensory information as well as descending modulating signals can control the gate, thus modulating incoming afferent information.[7] The lateral horns of the thoracolumbar segments contain the cell bodies of the preganglionic sympathetic nerves. The ventral horn of the gray matter contains the alpha and gamma motor neurons, which leave the cord via the ventral nerve roots to innervate the skeletal muscles.

There are three types of cells in the gray matter. Internuncial cells, which are the smallest, are most prevalent in the dorsal and intermediate zones. Internuncial cells receive afferents from dorsal root fibers and fibers in descending tracts of the white matter. Axons of internuncial cells terminate on motor and tract cell bodies and modulate their activity by releasing inhibitory or excitatory neurotransmitters. Motor nerve cell bodies are found in the ventral horn and consist of alpha and gamma motor neurons.

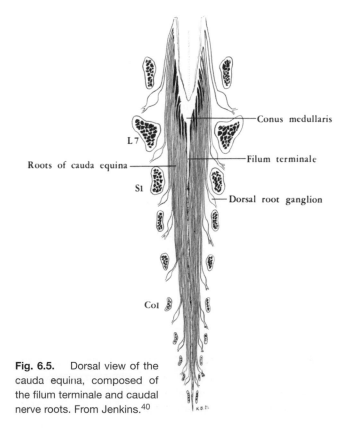

Conus medullaris

L7

Roots of cauda equina

S1

Filum terminale

Dorsal root ganglion

Co1

Fig. 6.5. Dorsal view of the cauda equina, composed of the filum terminale and caudal nerve roots. From Jenkins.[40]

Axons of tract cells constitute the ascending fasciculi of the lateral and ventral white columns. Tract cells (transmitter cells) are located primarily in the dorsal and intermediate zones of the gray matter. Cells of the lateral horn and the sacral autonomic nucleus are preganglionic neurons of the sympathetic and parasympathetic systems, respectively.

In contrast to the brain, spinal cord gray matter is surrounded by white matter, which is comprised of myelinated axons of intermediate longitudinally running nerve fibers. This outer white matter is divided into three major columns: dorsal, lateral, and ventral. Within these columns are ascending and descending tracts. The nerve fibers of the white matter are organized into ascending afferent tracts that convey sensory information to the brain and descending efferent tracts that convey impulses to peripheral effector organs. The spinal cord also contains nerves that subserve important spinal reflexes. Afferent fibers arriving at the cord through the dorsal nerve roots carry sensory impulses, which can initiate spinal reflexes and/or be transmitted to the brain stem and cerebellum, where they enter various pathways.

Efferent fibers, originating within the ventral horn of the cord, transmit motor impulses from higher centers or from reflex centers within the cord to muscles and glands. Ascending and descending tracts within the cord connect the higher centers and the various cord segments with one another. For a more complete description of the spinal tracts in dogs, readers are referred to the work by Hoerlein.[8]

Similar to the brain, the meninges (dura mater, arachnoidea, and pia mater) surround the spinal cord (Fig. 6.4). Various spaces are associated with the meninges and are important in understanding spinal anesthesia and its nomenclature. The dura mater has two layers within the cranial vault: an inner or visceral layer and an outer layer adherent to the cranial periosteum. The inner or visceral layer invests the spinal cord and ventral and dorsal nerve roots; the outer layer is absent in the vertebral canal of some species. The epidural (also referred to as the extradural or peridural) space is that space within the spinal canal outside the visceral layer of the dura mater. In those species having both layers of dura, "epidural" drug administration is actually into the *intradural space*. The dura mater adheres to the periosteum of the foramen magnum, thereby preventing communication between the cranial and vertebral epidural spaces. The epidural space is not an empty cavitary space, but instead contains blood vessels, lymphatics, and epidural fat, and communicates with the paravertebral tissues via the intervertebral foramina. This communication may be interrupted in older animals by fibrous connective tissue and bony malformations associated with spinal arthritis, and in obese patients by fat. This is of clinical significance because epidural injection volumes are often reduced in older or obese animals to prevent excessive cranial spread of drugs.

The subarachnoid space is located between the arachnoidea and pia mater. The subarachnoid space contains cerebrospinal fluid (CSF) and is continuous between the cranial and vertebral segments. There is no direct communication between the epidural and subarachnoid spaces; however, drugs (especially lipophilic drugs) can diffuse across the arachnoidea and enter the CSF after epidural administration. The pia mater, which is one cell layer thick, lies directly on the brain and spinal cord. The pia probably does not present a significant barrier to drug diffusion. The meninges cover the dorsal and ventral spinal nerve roots until they fuse, at which point they merge with the spinal nerve and extend no farther peripherally.

Cerebrospinal Fluid and Intracranial Pressure

Within the calvarium, CSF is found in both an internal (ventricular) system and an external (subarachnoid) system. The internal system consists of the bilaterally symmetrical lateral ventricles within the cerebral hemispheres, the third ventricle medially between the thalamus and hypothalamus, and the fourth ventricle, lying beneath the cerebellum and within the medulla (Figs. 6.6 and 6.7). CSF is produced by the choroid plexus, a fringelike fold of pia mater found on the floor of both lateral ventricles, in the fourth ventricle, and also by the ependymal lining of the ventricles.[8] Figure 6.8 depicts a magnetic resonance image of a choroid plexus tumor following contrast intensification in the area of the third ventricle. CSF is formed from the blood by secretory and filtration processes. Fluid in the lateral ventricles empties into the third ventricle through the paired foramina of Monro. The third ventricle, in turn, empties into the fourth through the aqueduct of Sylvius. The central canal of the spinal cord is continuous with the fourth ventricle. The external or subarachnoid system overlies the brain and spinal cord. The bilateral foramina of Luschka enable fluid to pass between the ventricular and subarachnoid systems. In most primates, the unpaired foramen of Magendie is present and enables an additional connection between the fourth ventricle and the subarachnoid space. The foramen of Magendie is not found in most common veterinary species.

CSF is absorbed at the arachnoid villi located primarily in the subdural venous sinuses. The arachnoid villi are fingerlike projections of the arachnoidal membrane that penetrate the venous sinuses. Their endothelium is porous and highly permeable, al-

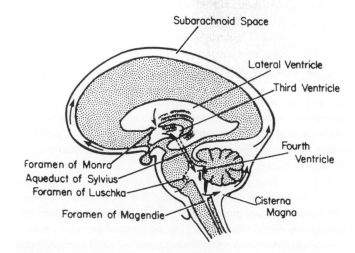

Fig. 6.6. Circulation of cerebrospinal fluid in the human and subhuman primates. Nonprimate mammals do not have the foramen of Magendie. From Stoelting.[41]

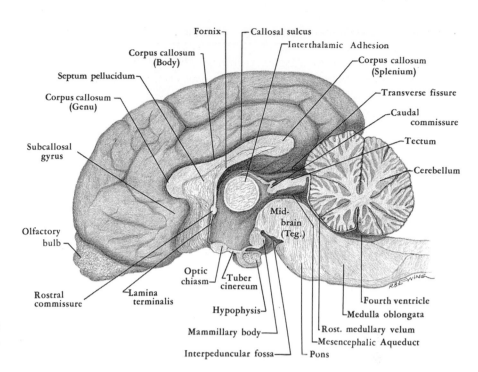

Fig. 6.7. Sagittal section of the canine brain. Rost., rostral; and Teg., tegumen. From Jenkins.[40]

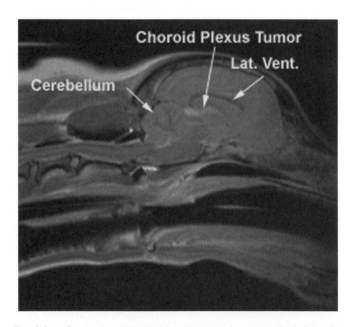

Fig. 6.8. Postcontrast magnetic resonance image sagittal view of a canine brain and spinal cord. Note the area of contrast intensification in the area of the third ventricle. Imaging diagnosis was choroid plexus tumor. Lat. Vent., lateral ventricle. Image courtesy of Igor Kuriashkin.

lowing free passage of water, electrolytes, proteins, and even red blood cells.

CSF cushions the brain and spinal cord. CSF normal pressure is approximately 10 mm Hg but can fluctuate within a narrow range. The composition of the CSF remains different from plasma because of the blood-brain barrier. The barrier is as much an enzymatic and cellular transporter barrier as an anatomical separation. The concentration of sodium is equal to that of plasma, the concentration of chloride in the CSF is 15% greater, and the concentration of potassium and glucose is 40% and 30% less than in plasma, respectively. The specific gravity of CSF is 1.002 to 1.009.

The pH of CSF is closely maintained at 7.32. Carbon dioxide, but not hydrogen ions, readily crosses the blood-brain barrier. Bicarbonate ions are actively transported. As a result, the pH of CSF is rapidly altered by changes in $PaCO_2$ but not by changes in arterial pH. The pH of CSF, not the PCO_2 directly, is the major mechanism regulating ventilation in most mammals. The choroid plexus and the capillary membranes are highly permeable to water, oxygen, carbon dioxide, and most lipid-soluble substances, such as anesthetics. It is only slightly permeable to electrolytes, such as sodium, potassium, and chloride, and nearly impermeable to plasma proteins and large organic molecules. This is clinically significant because fluid therapy in patients with CNS disease and intracranial hypertension must not deliver free water (which rapidly equilibrates across the blood-brain barrier) leading to increased pressure. Instead, hypertonic saline solutions, osmotic diuretics, and colloid solutions are often used to limit fluid influx or move fluid out of the brain tissue and decrease ICP. Glucose is actively transported across the capillary endothelium (blood-brain barrier) to provide a source of cellular energy. The pia mater, which covers the brain and spinal cord, and the ependyma, which lines the ventricles, are freely permeable to many substances; therefore, drugs that cannot gain access to CNS tissues when delivered by the blood may penetrate nervous tissues when administered into the subarachnoid space.

The skull forms a noncompliant chamber filled with brain parenchyma, blood, and CSF. An increase in volume of one com-

Table 6.2. Classification of nerve fibers

		Terminology	Fiber Diameter	Conduction Speed (m/s)
Myelinated somatic fibers	A	Alpha Beta Gamma Delta Epsilon	20 μm ↓ (3–4 μm) 2 μm	120 ↓ (6–30)→pain fibers 5
Myelinated visceral fibers (preganglionic autonomic)	B			3–15
Nonmyelinated somatic fibers	C			0.5–2.0→pain fibers

From Wylie and Churchill-Davidson[38] and Gasser.[39]

ponent must be accompanied by a compensatory decrease in the others or the ICP will increase (Monro-Kellie hypothesis). Normal ICP is less than 15 mm Hg. As the ICP increases, blood flow to the brain will decrease unless an increase in mean arterial pressure occurs to maintain cerebral perfusion pressure (cerebral perfusion pressure = mean arterial pressure − ICP). Arterial blood pressure should always be measured in animals suspected of having intracranial hypertension, because anesthetic-induced decreases in mean arterial blood pressure can lead to catastrophic cerebral ischemia even though arterial blood pressures were maintained above acceptable levels for healthy animals (e.g., mean arterial pressure of 60 mm Hg). Increased cerebral or spinal fluid pressure produces a reflex increase in heart rate and blood pressure (Cushing's response).[9] It has been hypothesized that the increase in CSF pressure creates ischemia of neurons, and that this is the stimulus for increased sympathetic activity.

Drugs that reduce cerebral metabolic activity or CBF, osmotic diuretics, hypothermia, and mechanical normoventilation or hyperventilation may all be used to decrease ICP. It is imperative that anesthetic management focus on maintaining adequate cerebral perfusion pressure rather than on reducing CBF or ICP alone. Administration of analgesic drugs, especially opioids, must be carefully monitored in animals with intracranial disease, because of their potential to increase $PaCO_2$, which could lead to increased CBF and ICP. Ventilatory support may be required if respiratory depression occurs.

Peripheral Nervous System

Spinal Nerves

These supply efferent and afferent innervation to most of the body, with the exception of the head and viscera. They also form part of the autonomic nervous system, which controls homeostatic functions. Spinal nerves vary in number, depending on species. Nerves can be classified by their size and degree of myelination, which determine speed of impulse transmission. Large, heavily myelinated fibers have the highest conduction velocities, whereas small nonmyelinated fibers have lower conduction rates (Table 6.2). The largest fibers, type A, are subclassified as A-alpha, A-beta, A-gamma, and A-delta fibers. A-alpha fibers in-

nervate skeletal muscles and also subserve proprioception. A-beta fibers normally subserve innocuous touch and pressure, but can be involved in nervous system "windup" that can result in hyperalgesia and/or allodynia following chronic nociceptor stimulation. A-gamma fibers innervate the skeletal muscle spindles to maintain muscle tone. A-delta fibers subserve temperature, fast pain, and touch. Type B fibers are preganglionic autonomic fibers. Type C fibers are small nonmyelinated fibers responsible for postganglionic sympathetic innervation and transmission of visceral and slow pain, touch, and temperature sensations. Abnormal nociceptive C fiber activity causes many chronic pain syndromes best described in humans, with diabetic neuropathy and postherpetic neuralgia being two examples. Similar C-fiber dysfunction is likely in a variety of chronic pain conditions in other mammalian species.

After leaving the intervertebral foramen, each spinal nerve divides into dorsal and ventral branches. The dorsal branches generally supply the muscles and skin of the back, whereas the ventral branches supply the muscles and skin of the thorax, abdomen, and extremities (Fig. 6.9). Branches from several spinal nerves may combine to form plexuses such as the brachial plexus or major nerves such as the sciatic nerve (Figs. 6.10 and 6.11). A *myotome*, which is the mass of musculature innervated from one ventral spinal nerve root, is derived from the somite of an embryonic segment and forms the skeletal musculature originating from that segment. The area supplied by a single dorsal nerve root is called a *dermatome*. There is considerable overlap of areas supplied by adjacent roots. Knowledge of myotomes and dermatomes is essential for performing a neurological examination and performing regional anesthesia of the thorax, abdomen, and limbs.

Branching off the spinal nerves in the thoracic and lumbar areas are rami communicantes, which connect the spinal nerves with a chain of ganglia lying lateral to the vertebral bodies, termed the *vertebral sympathetic ganglia*.

Autonomic Nervous System

In contrast with the somatic nervous system supplying the striated muscles, the autonomic nervous system requires no conscious control. The autonomic nervous system is composed of

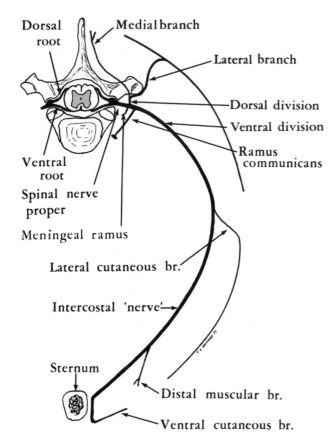

Fig. 6.9. Diagram of the anatomic components of a typical spinal nerve. br., branch. From Jenkins.[40]

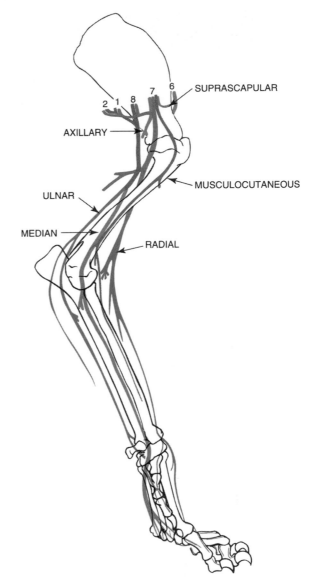

Fig. 6.10. A medial view of the canine front limb illustrating the relative course and distribution of the major nerves to the leg. Note the spinal nerves making up the brachial plexus, C6-7-8 and T1-2. From Hoerlein.[8]

the efferent and afferent nerves innervating the viscera, glands, and other tissues required for homeostasis and the fight-or-flight response. Its primary homeostatic role is control of circulation, breathing, and excretion, and maintenance of body temperature. These regulatory functions are subject to modification by input from higher brain centers, especially as a result of reactions to the environment.

Visceral autonomic efferent pathways consist of two neurons rather than a single motor neuron as occurs in the somatic system. The cell body of the first neuron is in the brain stem or spinal cord. Its axon terminates on the cell body of the second, located in an autonomic ganglion. The axon of the ganglion cell terminates in the effector cell.

Autonomic visceral afferents are primarily sensory neurons similar to those in somatic tissues, although they tend to have wider receptive areas, leading to less ability to discriminate the anatomic origin of the afferent signals. They elicit reflex responses in viscera and a feeling of fullness of hollow organs, such as the stomach, large intestine, and bladder. Afferent impulses contribute to feelings of well-being or malaise and transmit signals from nociceptors. Specialized visceral afferents transmit encoded signals that are perceived as the senses of taste and smell. In general, visceral afferents have their cell bodies in the sensory ganglia of the cranial and spinal nerves that include the autonomic outflow. These neurons are of two types: physiologi-

cal afferents and pain afferents. Physiological afferents are present in both sympathetic and parasympathetic divisions, whereas pain afferents are almost exclusively associated with the sympathetic. The most important visceral physiological afferents are associated with the parasympathetic division and mediate cardiovascular, respiratory, and gastrointestinal reflexes (e.g., baroreceptor, chemoreceptor, Hering-Breuer, emptying of the rectum and bladder subject to conscious control, and feelings of fullness or hunger).

Visceral pain afferents are associated with the sympathetic division. Cell bodies are located in the thoracolumbar dorsal root ganglia. Their peripheral processes reach the sympathetic trunk via the white rami communicantes, run in the sympathetic trunk, and reach the viscera through the cardiac, pulmonary, or splanch-

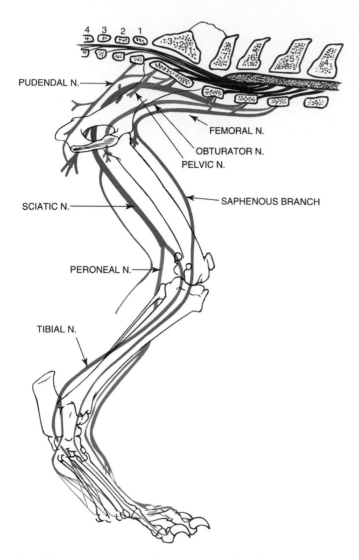

Fig. 6.11. A medial view of the canine hind limb illustrating the relative course and distribution of the major nerves. Note the spinal nerves making up the sciatic nerve. N., nerve. From Hoerlein.[8]

nic nerves. Central terminations are on transmitter cells in the substantia gelatinosa. Because the visceral pain afferents can travel cranially or caudally within the sympathetic trunk, the well-defined receptive fields seen with A-delta fiber–mediated pain are absent. Visceral nociceptor stimulation usually produces pain that is poorly localized. However, within the spinal cord, the ascending pathway for visceral nociception coincides at least in part with that for somatic nociception.

The hypothalamus is the primary area of the brain that controls the autonomic nervous system. The autonomic system can be subdivided into the craniosacral or parasympathetic system and the thoracolumbar or sympathetic system (Fig. 6.12). A characteristic of the autonomic nervous system is that both divisions are constantly active, resulting in a basal level of sympathetic and parasympathetic activity. Thus, each division can increase or decrease its effect at a given organ to regulate function more closely.

Parasympathetic System

This system functions to conserve and restore energy. Acetylcholine (ACh) is the neurotransmitter at both preganglionic and postganglionic neurons activating nicotinic receptors at the ganglion and usually muscarinic receptors on the effector cells. Each preganglionic fiber synapses with one to three postganglionic neurons, which terminate on a limited number of effector cells. ACh is normally rapidly inactivated by acetylcholinesterase at the synapse, resulting in a brief discharge and highly localized activity. However, with exposure to acetylcholinesterase inhibitors such as organophosphates or carbamates, prolonged and excessive parasympathetic nervous system activity ensues. Because of this, administration of antimuscarinic agents such as atropine prior to antagonism of competitive neuromuscular junction blockers with acetylcholinesterase-inhibiting drugs such as neostigmine is recommended.

Preganglionic fibers of the parasympathetic system arise in three areas: the midbrain (tectal outflow), the medulla (medullary outflow), and the sacral spinal cord (sacral outflow) (Fig. 6.12). These efferent fibers generally are long and synapse with one or two postganglionic fibers in a ganglion on or within the organ supplied. The tectal outflow originates in the Edinger-Westphal nucleus of the third cranial nerve (oculomotor) and synapses at the ciliary ganglion in the orbit to innervate the pupillary sphincter and ciliary muscles. The medullary outflow is comprised of the parasympathetic components of the seventh (facial), ninth (glossopharyngeal), and tenth (vagus) cranial nerves. The facial nerve parasympathetic fibers synapse at the submandibular ganglion to supply the submaxillary and sublingual glands, and at the pterygopalatine ganglion to innervate the lacrimal and nasal glands. The parasympathetic fibers of the glossopharyngeal nerve travel to the otic ganglion, where they synapse to innervate the parotid and orbital salivary glands.

The vagus nerves contain approximately 80% of the parasympathetic nerve fibers in the body. The preganglionic fibers are long and synapse in small ganglia that lie directly on or in the viscera of the thorax and abdomen. Efferent fibers are supplied to the heart, lungs, esophagus, stomach, small intestine, proximal colon, liver, gallbladder, pancreas, kidneys, and upper ureters. In the heart, they are distributed to the sinoatrial and atrioventricular nodes and, to a lesser extent, to the atria. There are few or no vagal parasympathetic fibers in the ventricles. In the intestinal wall, they form the plexuses of Meissner and Auerbach. The vagus also carries afferent fibers, arising from the nodose ganglion, that produce visceral reflexes but apparently not pain.

The sacral outflow originates in the second, third, and fourth sacral segments of the spinal cord. Preganglionic fibers form the pelvic nerves (nervi erigentes), which synapse in ganglia near the bladder, distal colon, rectum, and sexual organs. The vagus and pelvic nerves thus provide secretory, vasodilator, and motor fibers for the thoracic, abdominal, and pelvic organs.

Autonomic nerve endings in the effector organ may terminate within cells or on the cell membrane. Smooth muscle cells may have protoplasmic bridges so that neural stimulus of one causes many to react. No distinctive nerve ending exists comparable to somatic nerve endings within the myoneural junction.

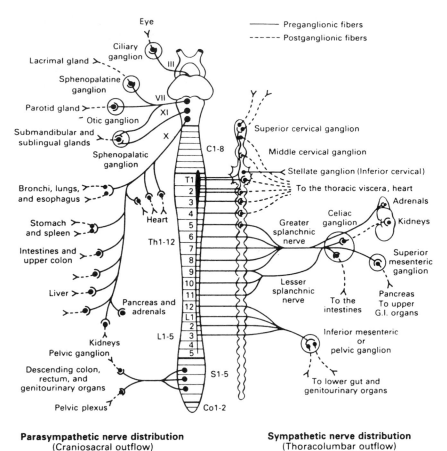

Preganglionic fibers
------ Postganglionic fibers

Parasympathetic nerve distribution
(Craniosacral outflow)

Sympathetic nerve distribution
(Thoracolumbar outflow)

Fig. 6.12. Schematic distribution of the craniosacral (parasympathetic) and thoracolumbar (sympathetic) nervous system. Parasympathetic preganglionic fibers pass directly to the organ that is innervated. Their postganglionic cell bodies are situated near or within the innervated viscera. This limited distribution of parasympathetic postganglionic fibers is consistent with the discrete and limited effect of parasympathetic function. The postganglionic sympathetic neurons originate in either the paired sympathetic ganglia or one of the unpaired collateral plexi. One preganglionic fiber influences many postganglionic neurons. Activation of the sympathetic nervous system produces a more diffuse physiologic response rather than discrete effects. G.I., gastrointestinal. From Barash et al.[42]

Sympathetic System

This mediates activities that accompany expenditures of energy, such as the *fight-or-flight response*. Thus, sympathetic activity is greatest during stress or times of emergency. Sympathetic activity in response to short-lived threats or pain is necessary for normal responses to these external stimuli (stressors). However, long-term stress, such as that seen with untreated pain, can lead to pathological changes, such as impaired immune system function and catabolic metabolism. As in the parasympathetic system, ACh acting on nicotinic receptors is the neurotransmitter between preganglionic and postganglionic neurons. However, the neurotransmitter between postganglionic neurons and effector cells is norepinephrine, which can act as an agonist at α_1-, α_2-, β_1-, or β_2-adrenergic receptors. An exception is the sweat gland, whose sympathetic terminals are cholinergic, except in horses, where sweat glands are under β_2 control.[10] In contrast to the parasympathetic division, strong sympathetic stimulation produces generalized effects, because each preganglionic neuron synapses with 20 to 30 postganglionic neurons, each of which terminates on many effector cells, leading to a divergence of effect. In addition, norepinephrine at postganglionic synapses and epinephrine secreted by the adrenal medulla are deactivated slowly relative to ACh.

Sympathetic preganglionic fibers arise from cells in the intermediolateral columns of the first thoracic to the fourth or fifth lumbar cord segments (canine) (Fig. 6.12). Their axons pass through the ventral spinal roots and synapse in sympathetic gan-

glia with postganglionic nerve cells. There are three types of sympathetic ganglia: vertebral, prevertebral, and terminal. *Vertebral ganglia* are paired and lie in the lateral sympathetic chains paralleling the vertebral column. They are connected to one another by nerve trunks and to the spinal cord and spinal nerves by rami communicantes. White rami carry the preganglionic outflow from the spinal cord in myelinated fibers. These synapse with nonmyelinated fibers in the vertebral ganglia. The nonmyelinated fibers exit via the gray rami to join the spinal nerves supplying the blood vessels of skeletal muscle and the sweat glands, pilomotor muscles, and blood vessels of the skin.

Prevertebral ganglia, which are located in the abdomen and pelvis, consist mainly of the celiac, aorticorenal, and anterior and posterior mesenteric ganglia. The bladder and rectum are supplied by *terminal ganglia* located close to these organs. Since visceral nociceptive afferents can colocalize with these sympathetic fibers, neuroblockade at the sympathetic ganglion (e.g., celiac plexus block) has been used to treat difficult-to-manage visceral pain, such as that associated with cancer. Blockade does not result in loss of somatic sensations, but may interfere with regional sympathetic control of vasomotor or visceral functions.

Preganglionic fibers from the upper thorax form the cervical sympathetic chain and synapse with postganglionic fibers to form the sympathetic supply to the head and neck (sudomotor, pilomotor, vasomotor, secretory, and pupillodilator innervation) (Fig. 6.12). The upper thoracic chain supplies postganglionic fibers that form the cardiac, esophageal, and pulmonary plexuses. The splanchnic nerves are formed from preganglionic fibers, which do not synapse until they reach the celiac ganglion. Postganglionic fibers from this and other prevertebral ganglia ramify widely to supply the abdominal viscera.

The adrenal medulla is unique in that it is embryologically, anatomically, and functionally homologous to the sympathetic ganglia. Chromaffin cells within the medulla originate from the neural crest and are innervated by preganglionic fibers. Activation of the sympathetic nervous system releases epinephrine and norepinephrine (approximately 80% and 20%, respectively), which act as systemic hormones, from the adrenal medulla. The response is similar to, but longer than (10 to 30 s), that which occurs with release from nerve terminals. Circulating norepinephrine causes vasoconstriction, inhibits gastrointestinal function, increases cardiac activity, and dilates the pupils. Circulating epinephrine has greater cardiac and metabolic effects than norepinephrine and, because of its increased ß$_2$-adrenergic receptor activity, induces vasodilation in skeletal muscle and bronchodilation. In addition, circulating norepinephrine and epinephrine have generalized metabolic effects in tissues that do not receive sympathetic innervation. Basal sympathetic tone is caused in part by adrenal medullary activity.

Nonadrenergic Noncholinergic Nervous System

A third division of the autonomic nervous system has been termed the *nonadrenergic noncholinergic* (NANC) nervous system. The NANC system (previously known as the enteric nervous system) is thought to regulate visceral organ function locally. It was first described with respect to the intestinal tract; thus, the name *enteric nervous system*. However, it has since been associated with some regulatory processes within other organs, such as the lung, and is therefore best termed *nonadrenergic noncholinergic nervous system*.

Neuron Function

Axonal Conduction

Nerve impulses are electrochemical currents that pass along the axon to the presynaptic membrane. From a pharmacological standpoint, there is an important distinction between electric *conduction* of a nerve impulse along an axon and chemical *transmission* of this signal across the synapse. Using electrodes, it can be shown that the internal resting potential of an axon is approximately 70 millivolts (mV) negative to the exterior of the axon. This is termed the *internal resting potential* and is caused by a relatively higher internal concentration of potassium and selective permeability of the resting axonal membrane to potassium.

When a resting axon is stimulated electrically, a nerve action potential is produced that travels the full length of the neuron in either direction. Most general anesthetics have little effect on nerve conduction velocity.[11,12]

Neuroregulators

These play a key role in communication among nerve cells (Table 6.3) and may be subdivided into two groups. Small mole-

Table 6.3. Neuroregulators and modulators

Small-molecule, rapidly acting neurotransmitters
Class I
  Acetylcholine
Class II: amines
  Norepinephrine
  Epinephrine
  Dopamine
  Serotonin
  Histamine
Class III: amino acids
  γ-Aminobutyric acid (GABA)
  Glycine
  Glutamate
  Aspartate

Neuropeptide, slowly acting transmitters
  Hypothalamic-releasing hormone
  Thyrotropin-releasing hormone
  Luteinizing-releasing hormone
  Somatostatin

Pituitary peptides
  Andrenocorticotropic hormone (ACTH)
  ß-Endorphin
  α-Melanocyte–stimulating hormone
  Prolactin
  Luteinizing hormone
  Thyrotropin
  Growth hormone
  Vasopressin
  Oxytocin

Peptides that act on gut and brain
  Leucine enkephalin
  Methionine enkephalin
  Substance P
  Gastrin
  Cholecystokinin
  Vasoactive intestinal polypeptide
  Neurotensin
  Insulin
  Glucagon

Peptides that act on other tissues
  Angiotensin II
  Bradykinin
  Carnosine
  Sleep peptides
  Calcitonin

---

cule neurotransmitters are synthesized in the cytosol of the presynaptic terminal, absorbed into the transmitter vesicles, and released into the synaptic cleft in response to the arrival of an action potential at the nerve ending. Release of neurotransmitters is voltage dependent and requires calcium influx into the presynaptic terminal. Following its release, the transmitter binds with the postsynaptic receptor. The postjunctional membrane is excited by increased sodium conductance and inhibited when potassium or chloride conductance is enhanced. Some transmitters bind to receptors that activate enzymes, thus altering cellular function.

Neuropeptide modulators are synthesized in the neuronal cell body and transported to the nerve terminal by axonal streaming. They are released in response to an action potential, but in much smaller quantities than are the small molecule transmitters. The neuropeptides induce prolonged effects to amplify or dampen neuronal activity. They exert their effects through a variety of mechanisms, including prolonged closure of calcium channels, alteration of cellular metabolism, activation or inactivation of specific genes, and prolonged alteration in the numbers of excitatory or inhibitory receptors. Although usually only a single small molecule neurotransmitter is released by each type of neuron (Dale's law), the same neuron may release one or more neuropeptide modulators at the same time. The latter can be released from within the brain or from other parts of the body to act on neurons distant from the release site.[13] In terms of anesthesia, many neuroregulators are known to be of great importance, whereas the significance of others may not be appreciated at this time.

In terms of chronic pain, little is known about the roles of neuromodulators involved in windup and sensitization. However, it is becoming more widely accepted that the pathological processing of nociceptive input in the brain and spinal cord involves more than simple changes in "wiring" of neurons. Recent evidence suggests an important role for the glia. Glia cells are traditionally thought of as serving only a supporting role as the glue that holds nervous structures in their correct orientation. However, microglia are now recognized to have immune system roles and the ability to secrete modulating substances, such as tumor necrosis factor, interleukins, and nitric oxide, that can alter neighboring cell physiology.[14,15] Future treatment strategies for chronic pain syndromes will likely address the role of immune cells like microglia (the resident CNS macrophages) in overall nervous system function and alteration.[16]

Transmission at the Neuromuscular Junction

The motor nerve axon terminates opposite the muscle cell at the presynaptic terminal membrane. Facing it is a second membrane: the postjunctional membrane. The two are separated by the subneural synaptic space. The area where the nerve meets the muscle is termed the *motor end plate* (Fig. 6.13).

The postjunctional membrane is preferentially permeable to sodium and potassium ions. The interior of the muscle cell is negatively charged, whereas the exterior, facing the nerve, is positively charged. This polarity is caused by an excess of sodium ions outside and potassium ions inside. The electromotive difference in potential between sides is approximately 90 mV. When a nerve impulse reaches the end of the axon, it initiates the release of ACh from its bound form in the synaptic vesicles. It diffuses across the synapse and is reversibly bound on the nicotinic cholinergic receptors of the postjunctional membrane. This changes the allosteric configuration of proteins in the membrane and its ion permeability. Sodium ions flow inward and potassium

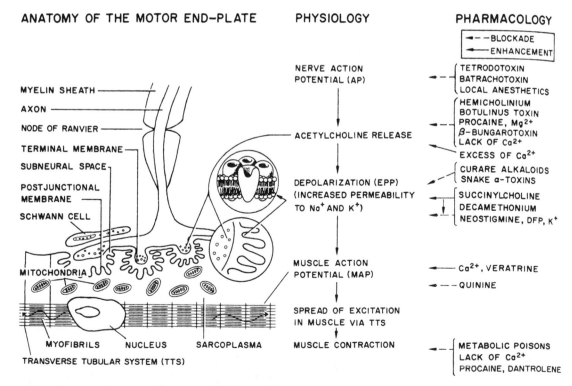

Fig. 6.13. The anatomy of the motor end plate and the sequence of events from the nerve action potential to the contraction of a muscle fiber. EPP, end-plate potential. From Gilman et al.[43]

outward, resulting in a decrease in electronegativity within the postjunctional membrane termed *depolarization*. From −90 to −45 mV, nothing occurs. This range is termed the *end plate potential*. Beyond the threshold potential, −45 mV, electrical depolarization spreads to the muscle around the end plate and is termed the *action potential*. This reaches a value of up to +30 mV.

Depolarization requires 0.2 to 0.4 ms, during which ACh is hydrolyzed to acetic acid and choline by ACh esterase present in the postjunctional membrane. As ACh is hydrolyzed, membrane permeability is restored to its normal state by sodium-potassium ATPase and the ions return to their respective resting sides (repolarization). Muscle contraction is delayed 2 to 3 ms; hence, repolarization is already complete when contraction occurs. Excess choline is taken up by the presynaptic nerve terminal and, through action of choline-*O*-acetyltransferase, acetic acid and choline recombine to re-form ACh. During rest, small quantities, or quanta, of ACh are continuously released from the nerve terminal, diffuse across the synaptic cleft, and bind to postsynaptic ACh receptors, causing small end-plate potentials. These miniature end-plate potentials do not cause muscle contraction, but are necessary for normal neuromuscular junction physiology. In contrast, when a nerve action potential arrives at the terminal, large quantities of ACh are released and motor end-plate depolarization and muscle contraction occur. The amount of ACh released with an action potential is about 10 times the amount required for muscle contraction. Extra ACh provides a safety margin in neuromuscular transmission and explains why more than 70% to 80% of postsynaptic junctional receptors need to be blocked before twitch tension is noticeably reduced. Most muscle fibers have one neuromuscular junction per fiber, although some muscles (e.g., extraocular muscles) may have more than one.

The three types of nicotinic cholinergic receptors at the neuromuscular junction are (a) junctional postsynaptic receptors located at the end plate that are responsible for neuromuscular transmission, (b) extrajunctional (i.e., extrasynaptic) postsynaptic receptors that do not normally participate in neuromuscular transmission but that may proliferate if the muscle is damaged or denervated, and (c) prejunctional receptors that modulate neurotransmitter mobilization from the nerve terminal. The adult postsynaptic junctional nicotinic receptor is composed of five subunits (two alpha subunits, and one each of beta, gamma, and delta) that are arranged to form an ion channel through the cellular membrane. When two ACh molecules bind to both alpha subunits, the channel opens and calcium and sodium enter, while potassium exits the cell.

Postsynaptic extrajunctional receptors, which are located on the muscle membrane away from the synaptic cleft, are present in low numbers in normal individuals but proliferate following denervation or muscle damage. When present in high numbers, extrajunctional receptors play an important role in the development of the exaggerated, and sometimes dangerous, response seen after administration of a depolarizing neuromuscular junction blocker.

Presynaptic junctional receptors are located on motor nerve terminals and modulate the mobilization and availability of neurotransmitters. Antagonism of presynaptic receptors does not appear to inhibit the release of ACh directly but may reduce synthesis or vesicular transport within the nerve terminal. Depletion of ACh stores following repeated or tetanic nerve stimulation noticeably reduces twitch tension. The role of the presynaptic receptor in the development of neuromuscular junction blockade is not completely understood.

Evaluation of Neurological Function During Anesthesia

Although the primary effect of anesthetics and anesthetic adjuncts is to reversibly alter CNS function, detailed studies of their neurophysiological effects have received comparatively limited attention. Traditionally, CNS activity has been evaluated subjectively by using classic signs of anesthesia (Guedel's stages of ether anesthesia) because interpretation of standard EEG recordings has required extensive training.

Electroencephalography

Historically, the electric activity of the CNS has been used in diagnostics of CNS disorders, especially seizures. The EEG has not gained widespread popularity as a clinical tool for evaluation of analgesia and anesthesia. Standard EEG tracings, using a Grass polygraph or other raw signal recorder, have required a degree of subjective interpretation. However, computer analyses of standard EEG tracings are now widely used to evaluate the effects of anesthetic adjuncts on neurological function.

The diagnostic EEG is usually used as a quantitative measure for spontaneous brain electrical activity. For intraoperative monitoring, amplitude, frequency, and bilateral symmetry over the two hemispheres are observed. When nutrient delivery to the brain is reduced, neurons sacrifice function before losing the ability to maintain their structure. The decrease in function can be detected as a change in the distribution of the EEG frequencies from higher to lower frequencies. Severe ischemia or very deep levels of anesthesia with some anesthetics produces irregular EEG signals and a phenomena termed *burst suppression* characterized as periods of electrical silence alternating with periods of activity. Eventually, with extreme anesthetic depression, the EEG will become completely silent (isoelectric) as neuron electrical activity ceases. Changes are reversible if anesthetic depression is lessened.

Hypothermia, hypotension, and hypercarbia can each alter the EEG and must be accounted for when interpreted clinically. Hypothermia will slow human EEG frequency in temperature-related fashion. Intermittent burst suppression will begin around 26°C, and isoelectricity will follow. Similarly, cerebral perfusion pressure below 50 mm Hg results in EEG slowing. It is important to note that significant changes in systemic blood pressure may not be accompanied by changes in EEG activity until a threshold level of hypoperfusion is reached.

Alternative methods for earlier detection of cerebral insult or increasing anesthetic depression use monitor-created stimuli, such as sound (brain-stem auditory evoked responses), light (visual), or noxious electrical pulses (somatosensory). These evoke a CNS response that can be detected with proper EEG processing and can be indicative of the status of the nervous system during anesthesia and surgery. Additionally, the evoked somatosensory potentials can be applied to distant regions of the body and used to assess total nervous system function, such as in monitoring of spinal cord function during spinal surgery. Evoked potentials are usually averaged to remove the cyclical changes in background EEG. The resulting EEG changes are temporally associated with the stimulus and latency and amplitude can be compared with normal or baseline values. Motor evoked potentials can be used to measure peripheral motor nerve function by measuring nerve or muscle responses.

The development of spectral analysis and computer-assisted analysis of EEG recordings enabled a quantitative comparison of the effects of various anesthetic agents and dosages over time.[17-23] Spectral edge analysis of the EEG has been correlated with anesthetic depth.[24] This system converts signals recorded in sequential epochs into numerical values for display of EEG amplitude and frequency distribution. Shifts in the 80% power spectral edge enable investigators to determine shifts objectively in electric frequencies as influenced by drugs.[17-22,25] Some investigators have used 95% spectral edge for analysis.[23] The spectral edge frequency is defined as that frequency below which a certain percentage (80% or 95%) of the total power (amplitude^2) is located. Concurrent analysis of airway, blood, or tissue drug concentrations, anesthetic depth, and spectral edge frequency provides a method of gauging the correlation of neurological responses to anesthetics and analgesics.[21,22]

In addition to the recording of raw EEGs, the mean frequencies and amplitudes for delta, theta, alpha, beta$_1$, and beta$_2$ frequency bands can be determined. These frequency bands correspond to below 3.9, 4.0 to 7.9, 8.0 to 12.9, 13.0 to 23.9, and 24.0 to 31.75 Hz, respectively. The summation for all activity is recorded at frequencies up to 31.75 Hz. The response curve for each frequency and the duration of drug effect can be determined at each dosage of anesthetic to assess actions on overall CNS activity. Details of the use of computerized spectral analysis of the EEG to assess anesthetic depression have been published.[17-27]

Bispectral Index Monitor

The bispectral index (BIS) monitor is a commercially available human monitor designed to enable anesthetists to conveniently measure an EEG-derived index of hypnotic level. The monitor records EEG activity from a pair of recording electrodes. The EEG signal is automatically processed, and a statistically derived index (the bispectrum) is reported. Electromyographic activity occurs with a frequency that overlaps with the EEG and can be problematic, especially in conscious animals or at light planes of anesthesia. Newer BIS monitors report the higher electromyographic frequencies and notify users of potential false elevation in the BIS number. Deep levels of anesthesia or neurological injury can result in EEG burst suppression. The BIS monitor reports a suppression ratio as well as displaying a continuous EEG waveform, enabling users to detect erroneous BIS values caused by isoelectric EEG activity.

In humans, BIS monitoring has been used as an indicator of hypnosis level. The BIS value best correlates to a patient's likelihood of response to verbal or physical stimulation. When delivering gas anesthetics to a patient, the BIS value should not be used as a "MAC meter." The BIS value is a processed signal, and changes are delayed 30 to 60 s from the change in EEG and physical status following an acute stimulus like a skin incision or a loud sound. This delay makes it difficult to use the BIS as an indication of CNS response to stimuli or changes in neurological status. The advantage of BIS evaluation lies in its approximation of the level of sedation. When coupled with the knowledge of the time of drug administration, the occurrence of surgical stimulation, and underlying patient physiology, the safety and quality of altered mentation can be crudely assessed.

In humans, a BIS index above 80 indicates a high probability of response to a command. For sedative agents, the likelihood of response drops dramatically to a very low probability as the BIS index nears 50. The index may also correlate with the incidence of recall, but since the index was statistically derived for movement, the values for recall and movement are different. Appropriate BIS values during anesthesia in veterinary patients are more difficult to determine. Since the index is derived using response to commands as the pharmacodynamic effect, veterinary publications reporting correlation of BIS values to MAC multiples are more difficult to interpret. Several studies have been performed to evaluate the usefulness of BIS in dogs.[28,29] In general, BIS was found to be useful in measuring depth of anesthesia, and values have been correlated with MAC multiples. Some species, such as cats, have unusually low BIS values when unstimulated, such as when being prepared for surgery, resulting in apparently poor correlation to depth, but noxious stimulation appears to raise values and result in a useful correlation.[30-32] Usefulness of BIS in swine is of interest because of their use as laboratory models. Early reports of BIS use indicated poor correlation with anesthetic depth; however, subsequent work using swine with individually measured MAC values had improved correlation with BIS and anesthetic depth.[33,34] Other species have been examined using BIS as an index of anesthetic depth.[35,36]

Functional Magnetic Resonance Imaging

Functional magnetic resonance imaging (fMRI) was developed in the early 1990s as a technique to localize brain activity. Its main advantages are its noninvasiveness and the spatial and temporal resolution it provides. fMRI uses the correlation between neuronal activity and regional CBF.[37] Currently, its use in animals has been limited to the research setting.

References

1. Michenfelder JD. Anesthesia and the Brain. New York: Churchill Livingstone, 1988.
2. Van Aken H. Influence of anaesthetics on cerebral metabolism and cerebral blood flow. Minerva Anestesiol 1993;59:809–815.
3. Hormann C, Kolbitsch C, Benzer A. The role of sevoflurane in neuroanesthesia practice. Acta Anaesthesiol Scand Suppl 1997;111: 148–150.
4. Duffy CM, Matta BF. Sevoflurane and anesthesia for neurosurgery: A review. J Neurosurg Anesthesiol 2000;12:128–140.

5. Young WL. Effects of desflurane on the central nervous system. Anesth Analg 1992;S32–S37.

6. Holmstrom A, Akeson J. Cerebral blood flow at 0.5 and 1.0 minimal alveolar concentrations of desflurane of sevoflurane compared with isoflurane in normoventilated pigs. J Neurosurg Anesthesiol 2003;15:90–97.

7. Melzack R, Wall PD. Pain mechanisms: A new theory. Science 1965;150:971–979.

8. Hoerlein BF. Canine Neurology: Diagnosis and Treatment, 3rd ed. Philadelphia: WB Saunders, 1978.

9. Evans AF, Geddes LA. Vasomotor response to increased cerebrospinal fluid pressure in the spinal animal. Cardiovasc Res Cent Bull 1969;7:100–110.

10. Scott CM, Marlin DJ, Schroter RC. Quantification of the response of equine apocrine sweat glands to beta2-adrenergic stimulation. Equine Vet J 2001;33:605–612.

11. De Jong RH, Hershey WN, Wagman IH. Nerve conduction velocity during hypothermia in man. Anesthesiology 1966;27:805–810.

12. De Jong RH, Nace RA. Nerve impulse conduction and cutaneous receptor responses during general anesthesia. Anesthesiology 1967;28:851–855.

13. Barchas JD, Akil H, Elliott GR, Holman RB, Watson SJ. Behavioral neurochemistry: Neuroregulators and behavioral states. Science 1978;200:964–973.

14. McCleskey EW. Neurobiology: New player in pain. Nature 2003;424:729–730.

15. Watkins LR, Milligan ED, Maier SF. Spinal cord glia: New players in pain. Pain 2001;93:201–205.

16. Marchand F, Perretti M, McMahon SB. Role of immune system in chronic pain. Nat Rev Neurosci 2005;6:521–532.

17. Gehrmann JE, Killam KF. Assessment of CNS drug activity in rhesus monkeys by analysis of the EEG. Fed Proc Fed Am Soc Exp Biol 1976;35:2258–2263.

18. Young GA, Steinfels GF, Khozan N, Glaser EM. Cortical EEG power spectra associated with sleep-awake behavior in the rat. Pharmacol Biochem Behav 1978;8:89–91.

19. Steinfels GF, Young GA, Khazan N. Opioid self-administration and REM sleep EEG power spectra. Neuropharmacology 1979;19:69–74.

20. Kareti S, Moreton JE, Khaza N. Effects of buprenorphine, a new narcotic agonist-antagonist analgesic on the EEG, power spectrum and behavior of the rat. Neuropharmacology 1980;19:195–201.

21. Scott JC, Ponganis KV, Stanski DR. EEG quantitation of narcotic effect: The comparative pharmacodynamics of fentanyl and alfentanil. Anesthesiology 1985;62:234–241.

22. Rampil IJ, Weiskopf RB, Brown JG, et al. I653 and isoflurane produce similar dose-related changes in the electroencephalogram of pigs. Anesthesiology 1988;69:298–302.

23. Stone DJ, DiFazio CA. Anesthetic action of opiates: Correlations of lipid solubility and spectral edge. Anesth Analg 1988;67:663–666.

24. Rampil IJ, Sasse FJ, Smith NT, Hoff BH, Flemming DC. Spectral edge frequency: A new correlation of anesthetic depth. Anesthesiology 1990;73:152.

25. Mathia A, Moreton JE. Electroencephalographic EEG, EEG power spectra, and behavioral correlates in rats given phencyclidine. Neuropharmacology 1986;25:763–769.

26. Zouridakis GZ, Papanicolaou AC. A Concise Guide to Intraoperative Monitoring. New York: CRC, 2001.

27. Otto K, Short CE. EEG power spectrum analysis as a monitor of anesthetic depth in horses. Vet Surg 1991;20:362–371.

28. Muir WW III, Wiese AJ, March PA. Effects of morphine, lidocaine, ketamine, and morphine-lidocaine-ketamine drug combination on minimum alveolar concentration in dogs anesthetized with isoflurane. Am J Vet Res 2003;64:1155–1160.

29. Greene SA, Benson GJ, Tranquilli WJ, Grimm KA. Relationship of canine bispectral index to multiples of sevoflurane minimal alveolar concentration, using patch or subdermal electrodes. Comp Med 2002;52:424–428.

30. Lamont LA, Greene SA, Grimm KA, Tranquilli WJ. Relationship of bispectral index to minimum alveolar concentration multiples of sevoflurane in cats. Am J Vet Res 2004;65:93–98.

31. March PA, Muir WW III. Use of the bispectral index as a monitor of anesthetic depth in cats anesthetized with isoflurane. Am J Vet Res 2003;64:1534–1541.

32. March PA, Muir WW III. Minimum alveolar concentration measures of central nervous system activation in cats anesthetized with isoflurane. Am J Vet Res 2003;64:1528–1533.

33. Martin-Cancho MF, Lima JR, Luis L, et al. Bispectral index, spectral edge frequency 95%, and median frequency recorded for various concentrations of isoflurane and sevoflurane in pigs. Am J Vet Res 2003;64:866–873.

34. Greene SA, Benson GJ, Tranquilli WJ, Grimm KA. Effect of isoflurane, atracurium, fentanyl, and noxious stimulation on bispectral index in pigs. Comp Med 2004;54:397–403.

35. Haga HA, Dolvik NI. Evaluation of the bispectral index as an indicator of degree of central nervous system depression in isoflurane-anesthetized horses. Am J Vet Res 2002;63:438–442.

36. Antognini JF, Wang XW, Carstens E. Isoflurane anaesthetic depth in goats monitored using the bispectral index of the electroencephalogram. Vet Res Commun 2000;24:361–370.

37. Di Salle F, Esposito F, Elefante A, et al. High field functional MRI. Eur J Radiol 2003;48:138–145.

38. Wylie WD, Churchill-Davidson HC. A Practice of Anaesthesia. London: Lloyd-Luke, 1966.

39. Gasser HS. Pain producing impulses in peripheral nerves. Res Assoc Res Publ Nerv Dis 1943;23:44.

40. Jenkins TJ. Functional Mammalian Neuroanatomy, 2nd ed. Philadelphia: Lea and Febiger, 1978.

41. Stoelting RK. The Pharmacology and Physiology in Anesthetic Practice, 2nd ed. Philadelphia: JB Lippincott, 1991.

42. Barash PG, Cullen BF, Stoelting RK. Clinical Anesthesia. Philadelphia: JB Lippincott, 1989.

43. Gilman AG, Goodman LS, Gilman A, eds. The Pharmacological Basis of Therapeutics, 6th ed. New York: Macmillan, 1980.

Chapter 7
Acid-Base Physiology

William W. Muir and Helio S. A. de Morais

Introduction

Probably the most fundamental and important principle of physiology is *homeostasis*: the maintenance of constant conditions through dynamic equilibrium of the internal environment of the body. One of the many processes that maintain homeostasis is the regulation of *acid-base balance*, a term introduced by L. J. Henderson (1909). Central to all schemes of acid-base balance is the understanding that normal oxygen-dependent metabolism of food (carbohydrates, lipids, and proteins) results in the predictable production of work, heat, and waste. Indeed, normal metabolic processes are responsible for the production of thousands of millimoles of carbon dioxide (CO_2; volatile acid) and potentially hundreds of milliequivalents of nonvolatile hydrogen ions (fixed acid) daily. Individual differences in the amount of CO_2 and hydrogen ion (H^+) produced are influenced by diet, cellular basal metabolic rate, and body temperature. Animals consuming high-protein diets, for example, produce CO_2 and excess quantities of H^+ precursors, whereas animals consuming diets high in plant material produce CO_2 and excess quantities of bicarbonate ion (HCO_3^-) precursors. The CO_2 that is produced is combined with water and is catalyzed by carbonic anhydrase (CA) to form carbonic acid (H_2CO_3). The formation of carbonic acid from CO_2 and water (H_2O) (Eq. 7.1) and the subsequent generation of H^+ and HCO_3^- (Eq. 7.2) serves as the focal point for almost all discussions of acid-base balance because (a) Henderson's studies highlighted that large quantities of CO_2 are produced by all metabolizing cells, (b) CO_2 is in equilibrium with H^+ and HCO_3^- ion, and (c) in the 1950s the plasma CO_2 content was the only relevant acid-base quantity that could be conveniently determined.

$$CO_2 + H_2O \rightarrow H_2CO_3 \tag{7.1}$$

$$H_2CO_3 \leftrightarrow H^+ + HCO_3^- \tag{7.2}$$

Combining Eqs. 7.1 and 7.2 yields

$$CO_2 + H_2O \overset{ca}{\leftrightarrow} H_2CO_3 \leftrightarrow H^+ + HCO_3^- \tag{7.3}$$

Although current understanding and appreciation for the many processes responsible for acid-base homeostasis have expanded considerably since Henderson's introduction of the term *acid-base balance*, the central importance of H^+ regulation to cell function and animal health cannot be overemphasized. This led A. B. Hastings (1961) to state: "Tiny though it is, I suppose no constituent of living matter has so much power to influence biological behavior."

Acid-base homeostasis ([H^+] regulation) involves the integrated normal activity of the lungs, kidney, and liver (Fig. 7.1). The lung removes CO_2, the kidneys remove H^+ as fixed acid, and the liver metabolizes protein, generating 1 mmol H^+/kg body weight daily. Following is a review of basic principles of acid-base balance and their integration into both the traditional and independent-variable (Stewart) approach to understanding and interpreting acid-base abnormalities in animals. Other more specific texts should be consulted for a more comprehensive review of the subject.[1–8]

Acids, Bases, pH, p*K*, and the Henderson-Hasselbalch Equation

Most formal definitions of acids or bases when applied to biological solutions universalize the Bronsted-Lowery concept, which classifies acids as proton donors and bases as proton acceptors. A more appropriate working definition, however, may be that acids are substances that increase H^+ concentration ([H^+]), a term used synonymously with *protons* in aqueous solutions. The strength of an acid and resultant acidity of a solution are determined by its activity coefficient, a factor influenced by temperature that determines the degree of dissociation. Since, by definition, a base is

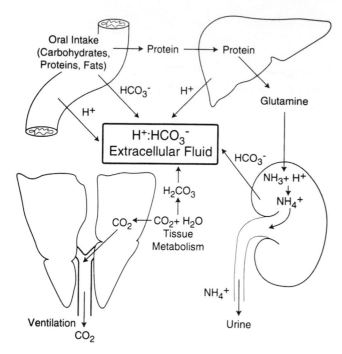

Fig. 7.1. Integration of the gut, liver, lung, and kidney in acid-base balance. HCO_3^-, sodium bicarbonate ion.

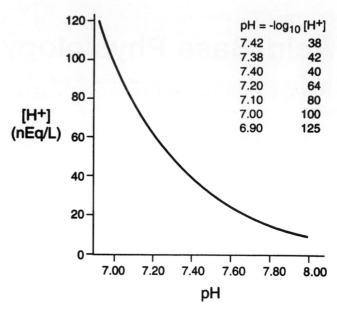

pH = $-\log_{10}$ [H⁺]	
7.42	38
7.38	42
7.40	40
7.20	64
7.10	80
7.00	100
6.90	125

Fig. 7.2. Relationship between [H⁺] and pH. Note that the relationship is exponential and not linear.

an H⁺ (proton) acceptor, each acid dissociates into H⁺ and a potential H⁺ acceptor or conjugate base. For example, H_2CO_3 in aqueous solution dissociates into H⁺ and its conjugate base HCO_3^-. Substances that are strong acids have weak conjugate bases and vice versa. Interestingly, water, the most abundant solvent in the body, can function as both an acid (H_3O^+; proton donor) or a base (H_2O; proton acceptor) depending on local conditions ($H^+ + H_2O \leftrightarrow H_3O^+$). At normal pH (7.40) and temperature (37° to 38°C), water is the most abundant base in the body.

In acid-base physiology, the formation of acids and therefore H⁺ production are emphasized because the end product of oral intake, tissue metabolism, and many pathophysiological disease processes is the production and release of hydrogen ion. Sorensen (1909) developed the concept of pH ($-\log_{10}[H^+]$) in order to simplify the notation necessary to describe the large changes of [H⁺] observed in nature and chemical experiments. This notation, although cumbersome mathematically and somewhat misleading because of nonlinearity, converts [H⁺] to pH by the formula (Fig. 7.2)

$$pH = -\log_{10} [H^+] = \log_{10} (1/[H^+]) \quad (7.4)$$

Regardless of the relatively narrow range (20 to 150 nEq/L) over which changes in [H⁺] occur in biological fluids, the concept of pH persists and is routinely reported on most pH and blood-gas machines. Conversion formulas for pH to [H⁺] have been developed:

$$pH > 7.40 \ [H^+] = (pH_m - 7.40) \ (40) \ (0.8) \quad (7.4a)$$

$$pH < 7.40 \ [H^+] = (7.40 - pH_m) \ (40) \ (1.25) \quad (7.4b)$$

where pH_m is the measured pH. The development of the pH concept by Sorensen combined with the theory of acid-base balance proposed by Henderson (1909) and the introduction of methods to measure pH in blood by Hasselbalch (1912) led to the development of the Henderson-Hasselbalch equation and the characterization of acid-base disturbances as being either respiratory or nonrespiratory (metabolic) in origin. Application of the law of mass action to body fluids produces many potential equilibrium equations that could be used to explain acid-base balance. The reasons why the carbonic acid equilibrium equation (Eqs. 7.1 and 7.2) was chosen to describe acid-base balance are (a) historical (method of assay development) factors; (b) the finding that, other than water, HCO_3^- is the major base in the extracellular fluid and H_2CO_3 the major acid; and (c) that the carbonic acid equation incorporates both volatile and nonvolatile substances. The law of mass action states that the rate (velocity) of a reaction is proportional to the concentration of the reactants and the dissociation constant (K) for the reaction. The rate of dissociation (r) for an acid can be characterized by

$$[HA] \rightarrow [H^+] + [A^-] \quad (7.5)$$

Using the dissociation constant K_1,

$$r_1 = K_1 [HA] \quad (7.6)$$

Similarly,

$$[H^+] + [A^-] \rightarrow [HA] \quad (7.7)$$

and

$$r_2 = K_2 [H^+] [A^-] \quad (7.8)$$

which at equilibrium results in $r_1 = r_2$, or

$$K_2/K_1 = K_a = [H+][A-]/[HA] \quad (7.9)$$

where K_a is the dissociation constant for the acid HA. Applying this law to carbonic acid, Henderson derived

$$[H+] = K_a[CO_2]/HCO_3^- \qquad (7.10)$$

Henderson used the concentration of dissolved molecular CO_2 instead of H_2CO_3 because H_2CO_3 could not be measured. Hasselbalch then introduced PCO_2 into Henderson's equation and put the equation into logarithmic form, producing the now universally applied Henderson-Hasselbalch equation:

$$pH = pK_a + \log_{10}\{[HCO_3^-]/[s \times PCO_2]\} \qquad (7.11)$$

where pH is $-\log_{10}[H^+]$, pK_a is $= \log_{10}K_a$, and s is the solubility of CO_2. This equation is frequently rewritten for explanatory purposes as

$$pH = pK_a + \log\left\{\frac{[base]}{[acid]}\right\} = \frac{kidney}{lung} \qquad (7.12)$$

Henderson deliberately applied the law of mass action to the equilibrium of carbonic acid. The Henderson-Hasselbalch equation indicates the amount of H^+ (protons) available to react with bases. Since acids and bases are charged particles, the application of this equation to biological fluids assumes that

1. Mass is conserved: The concentration of all substances can be accounted for as the sum of the concentrations of dissociated and undissociated forms.
2. All dissociation constants for all incompletely dissociated substances (weak acids or bases) are satisfied.
3. Electroneutrality is preserved: All positive charges must equal all negative charges.

These assumptions have particular relevance to the application of acid-base principles and to the interpretation of acid-base imbalance and are the basis for always integrating electrolyte (Na^+, K^+, Cl^-, etc.) abnormalities into the evaluation of acid-base balance.

Body Buffering Systems

The body uses three principal mechanisms to minimize or buffer changes in H^+.[6,7] *Chemical buffers* act within seconds to resist or reduce changes in $[H^+]$ and are the first line of defense against changes in pH. The *respiratory system* responds within minutes to resist changes in $[H^+]$ by regulating the partial pressure of CO_2 (physiological buffering) and eliminating excess CO_2 molecules caused by an increase in H^+ production (chemical buffering).

$$\uparrow H^+ + HCO_3^- \rightarrow H_2CO_3 \rightarrow H_2O +$$
$$CO_2 \text{ (increased minute volume)} \qquad (7.13)$$

Finally, H^+ that is produced by nonrespiratory mechanisms (metabolic or nonrespiratory acidosis) is excreted by the *kidney* in the urine over a period of hours or days (Fig. 7.3).

Chemical Buffers

These are compounds that minimize changes in the $[H^+]$ or the pH of a solution when an acid or base is added. A buffer solution consists of a weak acid and its conjugate base and is most effec-

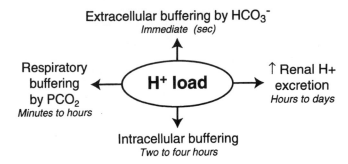

Fig. 7.3. Rate of response of the different buffering mechanisms in the body.

tive when the pH is within 1.0 pH units of its dissociation constant (pK_a) (Table 7.1). Alterations in blood, interstitial, and intracellular $[H^+]$ are immediately modified by chemical buffer systems. The ratio of the anion $[A^-]$ form of the buffer to its conjugate acid $[HA]$ is a function of its dissociation constant (pK_a) and the $[H^+]$. For weak acids, as $[H^+]$ increases, $[A^-]$ decreases and $[HA]$ increases by equal amounts, keeping the total amount of $A_{tot}(A_{tot} = HA + A^-)$ the same. The principle chemical buffers for excess H^+ production are the bicarbonate (HCO_3^-/H_2CO_3), phosphate (HPO_4^-/H_2PO_4), and protein ($Prot^-/H\ Prot$) buffer systems. Bone can contribute calcium carbonate and calcium phosphate to the extracellular fluid, thereby increasing the buffering capacity. Indeed, bone may account for up to 40% of the buffering of an acute acid load. Functionally, anytime there is an increase in $[H^+]$ in the body, the anion form of the buffer (HCO_3^-, HPO_4^-, and $Prot^-$) accepts the excess proton, converting the buffer to its conjugate acid (H_2CO_3, H_2PO_4, and $H\ Prot$). Because the body can have only one $[H^+]$, the ratio of the acid to salt forms of the various buffer pairs in solution can always be

Table 7.1. pK_a values of important chemical buffers[a]

Compound	pK_a
Lactic acid	3.9
3-Hydroxybutyric acid	4.7
Creatinine	5.0
Organic phosphates	6.0–7.5
Carbonic acid	6.1
Imidazole group of histidine	6.4–6.7
Oxygenated hemoglobin	6.7
Inorganic phosphates	6.8
α-Amino (amino terminal)	7.4–7.9
Deoxygenated hemoglobin	7.9
Ammonium	9.2
Bicarbonate	9.8

[a]Compounds with pK_a values in the range of 6.4 to 8.4 are most useful as buffers in biological systems. The pK_a values for the imidazole group of histidine and for α-amino (amino terminal) groups are for those side groups in proteins. The pK_a range for organic phosphates refers to such intracellular compounds as ATP, ADP, and 2,3-DPG.

Table 7.2. Major body buffers

	pK_a	Compartment pH	Basis of Effectiveness	Weakness
ECF				
HCO_3^-	6.1	7.4	CO_2 removal by the lungs	Distance of pH from pK
ICF[a]			Quantity	Depends on lungs
Imidazole	Close to 7	7.0	Exceedingly large quantity	Changes charge on ICF proteins[b]
HCO_3^-	6.1	7.0	Relatively large quantity	Depends on lungs for CO_2 removal
Urine				
Inorganic phosphate	6.8	5–7	pK higher than urine pH	Little capacity to increase excretion rate

ECF, extracellular fluid; ICF, intracellular fluid; and HCO_3^-, sodium bicarbonate ion.
[a]Although ICF creatine phosphate is not a buffer, during acidemia it is hydrolyzed, rendering it capable of H^+ binding.
[b]This change in charge on ICF proteins can have important effects on enzyme activities, transporters, and ICF volume.

predicted by the Henderson-Hasselbalch equation (isohydric principle), providing their concentration and their dissociation constant (pK_a) are known. With knowledge of the behavior of one buffer pair, one can predict the behavior of all the other buffer pairs in solution. The HCO_3^-/H_2CO_3 buffer pair is most frequently used to determine acid-base status in clinical practice because it is the most prominent chemical buffer in the extracellular fluid. Another important reason why the HCO_3^-/H_2CO_3 buffer pair is used to express acid-base status is that, in the presence of carbonic anhydrase, carbonic acid forms CO_2, which is eliminated by alveolar ventilation. Thus, the body can be considered an "open" system.

Approximately 60% of the body's chemical buffering capacity occurs by intracellular phosphates and proteins. Inorganic and organic (ATP, ADP, and 2,3-DPG) phosphates possess pK_a values that range from 6.0 to 7.5, making them ideal chemical buffers over a wide range of potential intracellular pH values. Inorganic phosphate (pK_a 6.8) is the major buffer in urine because renal tubular pH (6.0 to 7.0) includes the pK_a of the HPO_4^-/H_2PO_4 buffer pair.

Intracellular pH regulation depends on the activity of two cell membrane ion-transport systems: the Na^+-H^+ antiporter and the $Cl^-HCO_3^-$ antiporter (chloride pump), and intracellular proteins. Proteins are by far the most important intracellular buffers. Hemoglobin contributes approximately 80% of the nonbicarbonate buffering capacity of whole blood and with other intracellular proteins is responsible for three-fourths of the chemical buffering power of the body. The most important intracellular protein-dissociable group is the imidazole ring of histidine (pK_a 6.4 to 6.7). The α-amino groups of proteins (pK_a 7.4 to 7.9) play a secondary but important role in intracellular buffering. Plasma proteins, particularly albumin, also contain histidine and α-amino groups, and collectively are responsible for 20% of the nonbicarbonate buffering capacity of whole blood (Table 7.2).

Respiratory System

This offers an alternative route by which $[H^+]$ can be regulated by varying the partial pressure of carbon dioxide (PCO_2) (Fig. 7.1). Chemoreceptors throughout the body, but particularly those located in the medulla and carotid body, monitor changes in $[H^+]$ and PCO_2 and adjust breathing (tidal volume and frequency) to maintain a normal $[H^+]$. The association of H^+ with HCO_3^- and the subsequent formation of CO_2 and H_2O is an example of chemical buffering (closed system), and the elimination of CO_2 by the lung (open system) constitutes a physiological buffering mechanism. Changes in blood CO_2 also have important consequences for hemoglobin affinity for oxygen and its buffering capacity. Increases in PCO_2 increase blood $[H^+]$ and decrease hemoglobin affinity for oxygen (Bohr effect). This change in the oxygen affinity of hemoglobin is advantageous in tissues, allowing hemoglobin to release more oxygen for metabolism. Unoxygenated hemoglobin in turn can transport more CO_2 in the form of hemoglobin carbamino compounds (H^+ Prot) to the lungs (Haldane effect). It is important to realize that anytime there is a change in the PCO_2, there is a relatively much greater change in $[H^+]$ than $[HCO_3^-]$, because $[HCO_3^-]$ is measured in milliequivalents per liter and $[H^+]$ in nanoequivalents per liter. Maintenance of $[H^+]$ within a narrow range is vital to normal tissue enzyme activity.

Renal System

The synthesis of new HCO_3^- and excretion of excess H^+ emphasize the role of the kidneys as both a chemical and physiological buffer system (Fig. 7.1). Although relatively slow (hours or days), compared with the lungs (minutes) and chemical buffering (seconds), the kidney serves as the principal means by which acids that are produced by metabolic processes (not owing to CO_2 production but rather fixed acids) are ultimately eliminated (Fig. 7.3). All hydrogen ions produced by metabolic processes are excreted in the urine in combination with weak anions (titratable acidity), primarily phosphate and ammonium salts. The term *titratable acidity* may be considered synonymous with *urinary phosphate concentration* but actually represents all weak acids, including creatinine and urate. Net acid excretion by the kidney includes the titratable acidity and ammonium minus the HCO_3^- eliminated in the urine. Ammonium (NH_4^+) is produced in the proximal tubule primarily from glutamine metabolism to α-ketoglutarate and NH_3, a process that simultaneously gener-

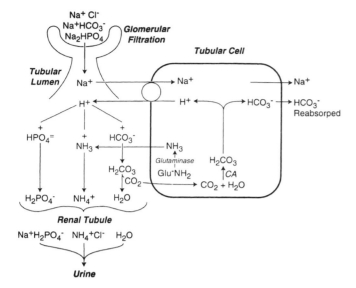

Fig. 7.4. Reabsorption and regeneration of sodium bicarbonate ion (HCO_3^-) in the renal tubules. Bicarbonate reabsorption in the proximal tubule coincides with H^+ secretion. Bicarbonate regeneration in the renal tubules coincides with titration of phosphate by H^+ and ammonium formation.

Table 7.3. Effect of temperature on PO_2, PCO_2, and pH

Temp °C	PO_2	PCO_2	pH
20	27	19	7.65
25	37	24	7.58
30	51	30	7.50
35	70	37	7.43
36	75	38	7.41
37	80	40	7.40
38	85	42	7.39
39	91	44	7.37
40	97	45	7.36

ates HCO_3^-. Increases in H^+ production can increase the rate of ammonium salt excretion by fivefold during severe metabolic acidosis (Fig. 7.4).

It is important to note that potassium loss from cells can lead to intracellular H^+ or Na^+ accumulation in order to maintain electric neutrality. This effect in renal tubular cells can lead to increased H^+ excretion (aciduria) and HCO_3^- reabsorption (alkalemia and "paradoxical aciduria"). Renal tubular cell acidosis may also augment glutamine metabolism and NH_3 production, leading to enhanced NH_4^+ excretion. Alkalemia and paradoxical aciduria is known to occur in people, rats, and ruminants. Its importance in dogs and cats is questionable.

Temperature Effects on Acid-Base Balance

Increases and, more routinely, decreases in body temperature are frequently encountered in patients undergoing anesthesia and surgery. Increases in body temperature may be associated with stress, increases in skeletal muscle activity (inadequate relaxation), systemic disease, and/or infectious and genetic disorders (malignant hyperthermia). Decreases in body temperature are

much more common than increases during anesthesia and surgery. Hypothermia may be much more profound in smaller patients (<8 to 10 kg) because of their larger body surface area to body mass ratio and is exaggerated by cleaning solutions (water or alcohol), cold exposure (steel tables), illness (shock), drugs that cause vasodilation (phenothiazine, barbiturates, or isoflurane), and toxicity. Changes in body temperature affect the $[H^+]$ of all body fluids. Increases in body temperature decrease pH and vice versa such that blood pH changes by 0.015 to 0.02 units/°C. Changes in pH with body temperature are expected because of known temperature-induced changes on dissociation constants (pK_a) and the solubility of CO_2 in blood. For example, as body temperature decreases, the pK_a and blood solubility of CO_2 increase, producing an increase in pH and decrease in PCO_2 (Table 7.3). These temperature-dependent changes in both intracellular and extracellular pH are believed to be important in maintaining an OH^-/H^+ (relative alkalinity) ratio of 16:1 throughout the body. A constant relative alkalinity of 16:1 for OH^- and H^+ is known to be optimal for cellular enzyme systems to function normally. The most important of the dissociable groups responsible for maintenance of a constant ratio between $[H^+]$ and $[OH^-]$ is the imidazole ring of the histidine residues of hemoglobin. Indeed, the fractional dissociation of imidazole-histidine remains constant as temperature changes and varies with pH during isothermal conditions. This regulation of the functional imidazole-histidine dissociation to maintain acid-base balance is termed *alpha-stat regulation* in contrast to *pH stat regulation*, in which pH values are maintained constant (Table 7.4).[7,9]

Both the alpha-stat and pH-stat concepts of acid-base balance have been used clinically when interpreting pH and blood gases

Table 7.4. Comparison of pH-stat and alpha-stat acid-base regulation

Concept	Purpose	Total CO_2	pH and $PaCO_2$ Maintenance	Intracellular State	α-Imidazole and Buffering	Enzyme Structure and Function
pH-stat	Constant pH	Increases	Normal corrected values	Acidotic (excess H^+)	Excess (+) charge, buffering decreased	Altered and activity decreased
Alpha-stat	Constant OH^-/H^+	Constant	Normal uncorrected values	Neutral ($H^+ = OH^-$)	Constant net charge, buffering constant	Normal and activity maximal

Table 7.5. Characteristics of primary acid-base disturbances

Disorder	pH	[H⁺]	Primary Disturbance	Compensatory Response
Nonrespiratory acidosis	↓	↑	↓ [HCO$_3^-$]	↓ PCO$_2$
Nonrespiratory alkalosis	↑	↓	↑ [HCO$_3^-$]	↑ PCO$_2$
Respiratory acidosis	↓	↑	↑ [PCO$_2$]	↑ [HCO$_3^-$]
Respiratory alkalosis	↑	↓	↓ [PCO$_2$]	↓ [HCO$_3^-$]

Nonrespiratory is used in preference to metabolic. HCO$_3^-$, sodium bicarbonate ion.

in patients with body temperatures higher or lower than normal.[7,9] Proponents of the pH-stat hypothesis argue that it is important to maintain a constant pH of 7.40 and PCO$_2$ of 40 mm Hg at any temperature, whereas proponents of the alpha-stat strategy attempt to keep a constant ratio of [H⁺] to [OH⁻] of 1:16. Proponents of the pH-stat strategy realize that if the pH and PCO$_2$ were kept constant at pH of 7.40 and PCO$_2$ of 40 mm Hg during hypothermia, the patient would be acidotic, but they argue that pH-stat–oriented therapy reduces morbidity. Proponents of alpha-stat–oriented therapy argue similarly and point out that blood flow to vital organs, particularly cerebral blood flow, becomes pressure dependent with pH-stat management. More research is required to resolve all of the controversies regarding the potential benefits of either strategy. From a practical standpoint, however, pH and PCO$_2$ need not be corrected for temperature. Measuring a blood sample taken from a hypothermic patient at 37° or 38°C (the temperature at which most blood-gas machines are calibrated) enables appropriate therapeutic decisions and eliminates the need to know the patient's precise body temperature for interpretation of acid-base abnormalities.

Clinical Acid-Base Terminology

Descriptions of acid-base balance and acid-base abnormalities have been based on familiarity with the Bronsted-Lowery definition of an acid and base, the Henderson-Hasselbalch equation, and standard medical terms describing body fluids or fluid compartments. The terms *acidosis* and *alkalosis*, for example, are used to describe the abnormal or pathological (-osis) accumulation of acid [H⁺] or alkali [OH⁻] in the body.[5] The terms *acidemia* and *alkalemia* are used to describe whether the blood pH is acid or alkaline, respectively. The Henderson-Hasselbalch equation characterizes all acid-base disturbances as being either respiratory or metabolic because of the body's production and elimination of volatile (dissolved CO$_2$; H$_2$CO$_3$) and nonvolatile or fixed (e.g., lactic and phosphoric) acids, respectively. Therefore, only four primary acid-base abnormalities are possible: respiratory acidosis, metabolic acidosis, respiratory alkalosis, and metabolic alkalosis (Table 7.5). Clinically, the terms *respiratory* and *metabolic* have been used to imply the involvement of the lung and kidney in acid-base regulation:

$$pH = HCO_3^-/PaCO_2 = \frac{\text{kidney function (fixed acids)}}{\text{lung function (volatile acids)}} \quad (7.14)$$

The term *nonrespiratory* frequently replaces *metabolic* in many discussions of acid-base imbalance because the term *metabolic* is not totally descriptive and is somewhat misleading (because it implies that all fixed acids are produced by cellular metabolism). The term *nonrespiratory* incorporates all mechanisms responsible for acid-base imbalance other than the production of CO$_2$ and carbonic acid (H$_2$CO$_3$). These mechanisms include alterations in the concentrations of strong (fully dissociated) ions and strong ion difference (SID), nonvolatile plasma buffers (primarily serum proteins; A$_{tot}$), and the ionic strength (dissociation constants; pK_a) of the solution (Fig. 7.5). The four factors used to describe changes in [H⁺] caused by respiratory and nonrespiratory imbalances are collectively referred to as *independent variables* (PCO$_2$, SID, A$_{tot}$, and pK_a) because each of them is regulated or changed independently of the others.[10–12] It should be noted, however, that changes in temperature can affect all the independent variables, a consideration that has special importance during surgery and anesthesia.

Primary abnormalities in acid-base balance can arise from disturbances in any one or several of the independent variables. Simple acid-base abnormalities are said to occur only when one independent variable is responsible for the acid-base disturbance. Mixed acid-base abnormalities are caused by disturbances in two or more of the independent variables. Mixed acid-base abnormalities may be additive (respiratory and nonrespiratory acidosis) or offsetting (respiratory alkalosis and metabolic acidosis) with regard to their ability to influence [H⁺] measured as pH. Offsetting mixed acid-base abnormalities occur when two primary acid-base abnormalities produce opposite effects on plasma [H⁺]. Patients with offsetting mixed acid-base abnormalities have both acidosis and alkalosis but do not necessarily demonstrate acidemia or alkalemia, because blood pH may be normal. These are some observations that should lead to suspicions of a mixed acid-base disturbance when evaluating blood-gas results:[2,13,14]

1. The presence of a normal pH with abnormal PCO$_2$ and/or [HCO$_3^-$]
2. A pH change in a direction opposite that predicted for the known primary disorder
3. PCO$_2$ and [HCO$_3^-$] changing in opposite directions

Mixed acid-base disorders can be classified based on the origin of the primary disturbances as mixed respiratory disturbances, mixed nonrespiratory and respiratory disturbances, mixed nonres-

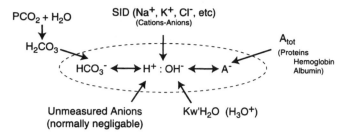

Fig. 7.5. Influence of independent variables on acid-base balance. The dependent variables (H⁺ and OH⁻) are enclosed by the dashed line. SID, strong ion difference.

piratory disturbances, and triple disorders. They also can be classified based on their effect on a patient's pH in additive combinations, offsetting combinations, and triple disorders (Table 7.6).[2] In additive combinations, both primary disorders tend to change pH in the same direction (e.g., respiratory acidosis and nonrespiratory acidosis), whereas, in offsetting combinations, the primary disorders tend to change the pH in opposite directions (e.g., respiratory alkalosis and nonrespiratory acidosis). The final pH reflects the dominant of the two offsetting disorders in offsetting combinations.[2] Detailed reviews of mixed acid-base disorders in domestic animals have been presented elsewhere.[2,13–15]

Secondary or compensatory (adaptive) acid-base changes frequently occur in response to most primary acid-base abnormalities and aid in buffering or minimizing changes in plasma [H⁺]. Respiratory acid-base abnormalities, for example, are generally compensated for by controlled, oppositely directed changes in nonrespiratory function. In simple acid-base abnormalities such as primary respiratory acidosis caused by hypoventilation, the kidney compensates by producing nonrespiratory alkalosis.

Respiratory compensation in metabolic acid-base disorders is obtained by changing alveolar ventilation and therefore changing CO_2 excretion by the lungs. Nonrespiratory acidosis is characterized by an increase in [H⁺], a decrease in blood [HCO_3^-] and pH, and a decrease in PCO_2, caused by secondary hyperventilation; whereas nonrespiratory alkalosis is characterized by a decrease in [H⁺], increase in blood [HCO_3^-] and pH, and an increase in PCO_2, owing to compensatory hypoventilation.

In respiratory acid-base disorders, the compensation occurs in two phases. The first phase consists of titration by nonbicarbonate buffers, and the second phase reflects renal compensation of the acid-base disorder, by increasing or decreasing HCO_3^- and Cl^- excretion in the urine. Respiratory acidosis is characterized by increased PCO_2, increased [H⁺], decreased pH, and a compensatory increase in blood [HCO_3^-]. CO_2 accumulation is caused by alveolar hypoventilation. Renal compensation occurs by titration of nonbicarbonate buffers, increase in net acid and Cl^- excretion, and increase in HCO_3^- reabsorption by the kidneys.[6,14] Respiratory alkalosis is characterized by decreased PCO_2, decreased [H⁺], increased pH, and a compensatory decrease in blood [HCO_3^-]. The initial compensation in respiratory alkalosis is caused by release of H⁺ from nonbicarbonate buffers within cells. The second phase is mediated by a compensatory decrease in net acid excretion by the kidneys.[14]

When analyzing secondary changes in a given acid-base disorder, it is important to remember the following:

1. With the exception of chronic respiratory alkalosis, compensation does not return the pH to normal.
2. Overcompensation does not occur.
3. Sufficient time must elapse for compensation to reach a steady state, at which time the expected compensation can be estimated using the formulas in Table 7.7.

Table 7.6. Classification of mixed acid-base disorders

Classification	Effect on the pH
Mixed respiratory disorders	
Acute and chronic respiratory acidosis	Additive
Acute and chronic respiratory alkalosis	Additive
Mixed respiratory and nonrespiratory disorders	
Respiratory acidosis and nonrespiratory acidosis	Additive
Respiratory acidosis and nonrespiratory alkalosis	Offsetting
Respiratory alkalosis and nonrespiratory acidosis	Offsetting
Respiratory alkalosis and nonrespiratory alkalosis	Additive
Mixed nonrespiratory disorders	
Nonrespiratory acidosis and nonrespiratory alkalosis	Offsetting
Normal plus high anion gap nonrespiratory acidosis	Additive
Mixed high anion gap nonrespiratory acidosis	Additive
Mixed normal anion gap nonrespiratory acidosis	Additive
Triple disorders	
Nonrespiratory acidosis, nonrespiratory alkalosis, and respiratory acidosis	Final pH is function of relative dominance of acidifying and alkalinizing processes
Nonrespiratory acidosis, nonrespiratory alkalosis, and respiratory alkalosis	

Table 7.7. Expected compensatory responses in primary acid-base disorders

Disorder	Primary Change	Expected Range of Compensation
Nonrespiratory acidosis	↓ [HCO_3^-]	PCO_2 = last 2 digits of pH × 100 $\Delta PCO_2 = 1 - 1.13\ (\Delta[HCO_3^-])$ $PCO_2 = [HCO_3^-] + 15$ $PCO_2 = 0.7\ [HCO_3^-] \pm 3$ (dogs)
Nonrespiratory alkalosis	↑ [HCO_3^-]	PCO_2: variable increase PCO_2 = increases of 0.6 mm Hg for each new 1 mEq/L increase in [HCO_3^-] $PCO_2 = 0.7\ [HCO_3^-] \pm 3$ (dogs)
Respiratory acidosis		
Acute	↑ PCO_2	Acute [HCO_3^-] increases 1 mEq/L and pH decreases 0.05 units for every 10 mm Hg increase in PCO_2 [HCO_3^-] = 0.15 PCO_2 ± 2 (dogs)
Chronic	↑ PCO_2	[HCO_3^-] increases 3.5 mEq/L and pH decreases 0.07 units for every 10 mm Hg increase in PCO_2 [HCO_3^-] = 0.35 PCO_2 ± 2 (dogs)
Respiratory alkalosis		
Acute	↓ PCO_2	[HCO_3^-] falls 2 mEq/L and pH increases 0.1 units for each 10 mm Hg fall in PCO_2 [HCO_3^-] = 0.25 PCO_2 ± 2 (dogs)
Chronic	↓ PCO_2	[HCO_3^-] falls 5 mEq/L and pH increases 0.15 units for each 10 mm Hg fall in PCO_2 [HCO_3^-] = 0.55 PCO_2 ± 2 (dogs)

HCO_3^-, sodium bicarbonate ion.

Care should be exercised when dealing with cats because they may not be able to compensate for nonrespiratory acidosis as well as dogs.

The question that often arises when analyzing simple acid-base abnormalities that demonstrate both respiratory acidosis and nonrespiratory alkalosis is, "Which is the primary problem and is there a secondary and/or compensatory event?" The answer is not always obvious, although simple primary acid-base abnormalities change pH in the direction of the primary disorder. For example, a patient with respiratory acidosis and compensatory nonrespiratory alkalosis would have a pH that tended to be acidotic (e.g., a pH of 7.31). Mixed respiratory and nonrespiratory acid-base abnormalities are much more difficult to decipher, and like simple acid-base abnormalities must be carefully evaluated in the context of a patient's signs, symptoms, and other available diagnostic information.

Because nonrespiratory acidosis is so frequently associated with disease processes in animals, indices of acid-base balance have evolved that enable the nonrespiratory component of acid-base abnormalities to be evaluated quantitatively. The *standard bicarbonate* is the concentration of bicarbonate in plasma after the whole blood sample has been equilibrated to a PCO_2 of 40 mm Hg at 38°C. This index quantifies the nonrespiratory component of any acid-base abnormality, because differences in the standard bicarbonate from normal (approximately 25 mEq/L) cannot be caused by changes in PCO_2, which is held constant at 40 mm Hg at 38°C. Similarly, the base excess (BE) quantitates the number of milliequivalents per liter of acid or base required to titrate 1 L of blood to pH 7.40 while the PCO_2 is held constant at 40 mm Hg at 38°C. Both the standard bicarbonate and BE (or

deficit) can be determined from nomograms. The BE has a normal value of zero (±3) and is changed only by nonvolatile acids, thereby indicating nonrespiratory acidosis. The numerical magnitude of the BE is a guide to therapy:

$$\text{Base (Na}^+\text{HCO}_3^-\text{) needed} = (0.3) \times (\text{BE}) \times (\text{body weight [kg]}) \tag{7.15}$$

where 0.3 = % body weight that is extracellular water.

Anion Gap

The anion gap (AG) is a useful tool to assess mixed acid-base disorders.[10,11,14] Chemically, there is no AG because electroneutrality must be maintained and the "anion gap" actually is the difference between the unmeasured anions (UA$^-$) and unmeasured cations (UC$^+$). Following the electroneutrality law,

$$([\text{Na}^+] + [\text{K}^+] + [\text{UC}^+]) - ([\text{Cl}^-] + [\text{HCO}_3^-] + [\text{UA}^-]) = 0 \tag{7.16}$$

or, when applied clinically,

$$\text{AG} = ([\text{Na}^+] + [\text{K}^+]) - ([\text{Cl}^-] + [\text{HCO}_3^-]) = [\text{UA}^-] - [\text{UC}^+] \tag{7.17}$$

Based on Equation 7.16, every time there is a decrease in [HCO_3^-], either [Cl^-] or [UA$^-$] must increase to maintain electroneutrality. When titrated HCO_3^- is replaced by Cl^- in nonrespiratory acidosis, the difference ([UA$^-$] − [UC$^+$]; and consequently the AG) will remain the same (called *hyperchloremic* or *normal AG acidosis*). When titrated HCO_3^- is replaced by UA$^-$, the difference ([UA$^-$] − [UC$^+$]; i.e., the AG) will increase

Table 7.8. Simple primary nonrespiratory acid-base disorders[a]

Nonrespiratory Disorder	Na⁺ Cl⁻		AG	TCO₂	Respiratory Compensation	Biochemical Profile
Alkaloses						
Hypoalbuminemia	N		N, ↓	↑	No	↓ Albumin
Hypochloremia	↑		N	↑	No	↓ [Cl⁻] corrected
Concentration	↑		N	↑	Yes	↑ [Na⁺]
Acidoses						
Hyperalbuminemia	N		N, ↑	↓	No	↑ Albumin
Hyperphosphatemia	N		N, ↑	↓	No	↑ Inorganic phosphate
Hyperchloremia	↓		N	↓	Yes	↑ [Cl⁻] corrected
Dilution	↓		N	↓	Yes	↓ [Na⁺]
Organic	N		↑	↓	Yes	Specific assays required

[a]Na⁺ − Cl⁻ difference between sodium and chloride concentration; AG, anion gap; TCO₂, total CO₂; ↑, increase; N, normal; and ↓, decrease. See the text for limitations in using Na⁺ − Cl⁻ difference and AG.
From de Morais and Muir.[11]

while [Cl⁻] remains the same (called *normochloremic* or *high AG acidosis*).[2,15]

Negatively charged proteins, phosphates, sulfates, and organic acids (e.g., lactate, ß-hydroxybutyrate, acetoacetate, and citrate) constitute the UA^-.[16] Usually an increase in AG implies an accumulation of organic acids in the body.[17] An increase in AG also occurs in alkalemia caused by an increase in the net negative charge on serum proteins or in situations where concomitant nonrespiratory alkalosis or respiratory alkalosis overrides a high-AG nonrespiratory acidosis.[18,19] Hypoalbuminemia probably is the only important cause of a decrease in AG, and each decrease in albumin concentration by 1 g/dL generally produces a decrease of approximately 3 mEq/L in the AG.

The AG concept has some limitations. The summation of [Cl⁻] and [HCO₃⁻] is not acceptable based on principles of chemistry.[20] Each of these anions has a different activity coefficient partially because they are present in extracellular fluid at concentrations that differ by a factor of more than 5 (i.e., [Cl⁻] = 110 mEq/L vs. [HCO₃⁻] = 21 mEq/L).[20] Regardless, this simplification of the AG is helpful clinically (Table 7.8). The AG also can change because of excessive exposure of serum to air, resulting in changes of 6.5 ± 2.3 mEq/L after 2 h.[21] These changes are more pronounced in patients with respiratory acidosis.[20]

[NA⁺] − [Cl⁻] Difference

Plasma Cl⁻ and HCO₃⁻ concentrations have a tendency to change in the opposite direction in nonrespiratory alkalosis and hyperchloremic acidosis, whereas sodium concentration tends to remain normal in acid-base disturbances unless the primary disorder also affects water balance. The difference between sodium and chloride concentrations ([Na⁺] − [Cl⁻]) is therefore useful in the assessment of those nonrespiratory disturbances not associated with an increase in unmeasured anions. The [Na⁺] − [Cl⁻] is approximately 36 mEq/L. If [Na⁺] is normal, an increase in this value is caused by hypochloremia and is an indication of

Table 7.9. Relative changes in [Na⁺]₀ and [Cl⁻]₀ as an index of disorders in hydration or acid-base balance or both

a. Proportionate change in [Na⁺]₀ and [Cl⁻]₀ are always due to the disturbances of hydration alone.
   Dehydration
   [Na⁺]₀ ↑ and [Cl⁻]₀ ↑
   Overhydration
   [Na⁺]₀ ↓ and [Cl⁻]₀ ↓
b. Changes in [Cl⁻]₀ without any change in [Na⁺]₀ is always due to disturbances of acid-base alone.
   Respiratory acidosis or nonrespiratory alkalosis
   [Na⁺]₀ and [Cl⁻]₀ ↓
   Respiratory alkalosis or hypercholemic acidosis
   [Na⁺]₀ and [Cl⁻]₀ ↑
c. Disproportionate changes in [Na⁺]₀ and [Cl⁻]₀ are due to disturbances in both hydration and acid-base balance.
   Dehydration plus respiratory acidosis or nonrespiratory alkalosis
   [Na⁺]₀ ↑ and [Cl⁻]₀
   Dehydration plus respiratory alkalosis or nonrespiratory acidosis
   [Na⁺]₀ ↑ and [Cl⁻]₀ ↑↑
   Overhydration plus respiratory alkalosis or hyperchloremic acidosis
   [Na⁺]₀ ↓ and [Cl⁻]₀
   Overhydration plus respiratory acidosis or nonrespiratory alkalosis
   [Na⁺]₀ ↓ and [Cl⁻] ↓↓

Modified from Emmett and Seldin.[30]

metabolic alkalosis, whereas a decrease in the [Na⁺] − [Cl⁻] gradient is an indication of hyperchloremic acidosis.[8] This difference, used in association with the AG, can be useful in identifying the presence of a mixed metabolic process (Table 7.9).

Strong Ion Difference

A new theory of acid-base regulation was proposed in the early 1990s.[8] According to this theory, $[HCO_3^-]$ and pH ($[H^+]$) depend on PCO_2, the total concentration of plasma weak nonvolatile acids ($[A_{tot}]$, composed mostly of albumin and inorganic phosphates), and the difference between the strong cations and the strong anions (called the *strong ion difference* or SID) (Fig. 7.5).[4,8] As was previously pointed out, strong ions are substances that are completely dissociated in plasma at body pH. The most important strong ions in plasma are Na^+, K^+, Ca^{2+}, Mg^{2+}, Cl^-, lactate, ß-hydroxybutyrate, acetoacetate, and sulfate. The influence of strong ions on pH and $[HCO_3^-]$ can always be expressed in terms of the SID. An increase in SID correlates with nonrespiratory alkalosis, whereas a decrease in SID correlates with nonrespiratory acidosis. Body homeostatic mechanisms indirectly regulate $[H^+]$ (and pH) and $[HCO_3^-]$ by changing PCO_2 (by changes in alveolar ventilation relative to CO_2 elimination rate) and SID (by differential reabsorption of Na^+ and Cl^- in the kidneys). Although changes in $[A_{tot}]$ will change $[HCO_3^-]$ and $[H^+]$, control of albumin production and inorganic phosphate concentration is not primarily directed at acid-base homeostasis.

Simple acid-base disturbances occur when an abnormality in one of the principal determinants of $[H^+]$ (e.g., PCO_2, SID, or $[A_{tot}]$) is present.[3,11,12] A simple acid-base disturbance includes both the primary process and the compensatory response: That is, if a sustained primary disturbance occurs in PCO_2, a compensatory change of regulated magnitude normally occurs in the SID and vice versa. If the primary disturbance results from a change in $[A_{tot}]$, however, renal or ventilatory compensation does not occur.[3]

Clinical Disturbances

One method of classifying acid-base disturbances provides a mechanistic view of the causative disturbances and integrates serum electrolytes and albumin concentration into the interpretation of acid-base balance.[7] Based on the preceding discussion, the following conclusions can be made: (a) acid-base homeostasis in body-fluid compartments is established based on the regulation of independent variables, including PCO_2, SID, and $[A_{tot}]$; (b) acid-base disturbances are primarily caused by changes in one or more of the independent variables; (c) acid-base status is best determined by analysis of the independent variables; and (d) the fundamental basis for therapeutic success or failure depends on interventions that adjust the independent variables.[3,22–25]

Disorders of PCO2

Primary respiratory disturbances result from increases (respiratory acidosis) or decreases (respiratory alkalosis) in PCO_2. CO_2 tension can be changed by alveolar ventilation, which has a profound effect on $[HCO_3^-]$ and $[H^+]$. Approximately 50% of daily variability of $[HCO_3^-]$ in normal dogs can be attributed to changes in PCO_2 alone. Because arterial PCO_2 ($PaCO_2$) is inversely related to alveolar ventilation, measurement of $PaCO_2$ provides clinicians with direct information about the adequacy of alveolar ventilation. Respiratory acidosis is therefore caused by and synonymous with hypoventilation, whereas respiratory alkalosis is caused by and synonymous with hyperventilation. The principal disorders associated with respiratory acidosis are airway obstruction, respiratory-center depression (e.g., drugs or neurological disorders), cardiopulmonary arrest ($PaCO_2$ may be below normal during cardiopulmonary resuscitation), neuromuscular diseases, diaphragmatic hernia, chest wall trauma, and inadequate mechanical ventilation. Therapy for respiratory acidosis should be directed toward the elimination of the underlying cause of alveolar hypoventilation. Ventilatory assistance should be provided when necessary. Respiratory acidosis is not an indication for bicarbonate therapy. Administration of sodium bicarbonate ($NaHCO_3$) will decrease $[H^+]$ and decrease ventilatory drive, thus worsening hypoxemia and hypercapnia. The underlying cause of hypercapnia in patients with chronic pulmonary disease cannot usually be removed, but appropriate treatment of the underlying disease should be attempted.

The principal causes of respiratory alkalosis are hypoxia, low cardiac output, severe anemia, pulmonary disease (stimulation of peripheral reflexes, e.g., pneumonia), hyperventilation mediated by the central nervous system (e.g., drugs, central nervous system inflammation or tumor, liver disease, fear, or pain), and overzealous mechanical ventilation. Hypocapnia itself is not a major threat to the well-being of patients with respiratory alkalosis. The arterial pH in chronic primary respiratory alkalosis is usually normal or slightly alkalemic owing to efficient renal compensation in this setting. Therapy for the underlying disease responsible for hypocapnia should be the primary focus in patients with respiratory alkalosis.

Increases in Alveolar-Arterial Oxygen Difference

The alveolar-arterial oxygen difference [$P(A-a)O_2$ gradient] may be useful in differentiating intrinsic pulmonary disease from extrapulmonary disease in animals with hypoxemia. The (A-a) gradient estimates the difference between the PO_2 in the alveoli (PAO_2) and the arterial blood (PaO_2). It can be calculated clinically as (A-a) gradient = $(150 - 1.25 \cdot PaCO_2) - PaO_2$. In normal animals at sea level, the $P(A-a)O_2$ gradient should be less than 15 mm Hg, although values up to 25 mm Hg have been considered normal.

Hypoxia can be caused by hypoventilation, decreased partial pressure of inspired O_2 (PiO_2), diffusion impairment, ventilation-perfusion mismatch, and right-to-left shunts. The $P(A-a)O_2$ gradient will be normal in patients with either hypoventilation or decreased PiO_2 (e.g., residence at high altitude) because they still have normal lung function. Patients with hypoventilation have an increase in PCO_2, whereas patients breathing air with a low PiO_2 have a below-normal PCO_2 (hyperventilating). In contrast, the $P(A-a)O_2$ gradient is increased in patients with diffusion impairment (rarely recognized in veterinary medicine), ventilation-perfusion mismatch, and right-to-left shunt. Administration of 100% oxygen will usually improve hypoxemia in patients with ventilation-perfusion mismatch, but not in patients with significant right-to-left shunt.

Table 7.10. Disorders in strong ion difference

Free-water abnormalities	
Increase in [Na$^+$]	→ Concentration alkalosis
Decrease in [Na$^+$]	→ Dilution acidosis
Chloride abnormalities	
Decrease in [Cl$^-$] corrected	→ Hypochloremic alkalosis
Increase in [Cl$^-$] corrected	→ Hyperchloremic acidosis
Unmeasured strong anion abnormalities	
Increase in [XA$^-$]	→ Organic acidosis

[XA$^-$], unidentified strong anions.

Table 7.11. Principal causes of free-water abnormalities

Concentration alkalosis (↑ [Na$^+$])
　Pure-water deficit
　　Primary hypodipsia
　　Diabetes Insipidus
　　Fever
　　Inadequate access to water
　　High environmental temperature
　Hypotonic fluid loss
　　Vomiting
　　Peritonitis
　　Pancreatitis
　　Nonoliguric renal failure
　　Postobstructive diuresis
　Sodium gain
　　Salt poisoning
　　Hypertonic fluid administration (e.g., hypertonic saline, sodium bicarbonate)
　　Hyperaldosteronism
　　Hyperadrenocorticism
Dilution acidosis (↓ [Na$^+$])
　Severe liver disease
　Nephrotic syndrome
　Advanced renal failure
　Congestive heart failure
　Psychogenic polydipsia
　Excessive sweating in horses
　Hypotonic fluid administration (e.g., 0.45% sodium chloride solution)
　Vomiting
　Diarrhea
　Uroabdomen
　Hypoadrenocorticism
　Diuretic administration

Adapted from de Morais and Muir.[11]

Disorders in [A$_{tot}$]

Albumin and inorganic phosphate are nonvolatile weak acids and collectively are the major contributors to [A$_{tot}$] (Fig. 7.5).[24] Consequently, changes in their concentrations will change [H$^+$]. Hypoalbuminemia will tend to decrease [A$_{tot}$] and cause a nonrespiratory alkalosis. Although rare, an increase in albumin concentration can cause nonrespiratory acidosis, owing to an increase in [A$_{tot}$]. Phosphate is the second most important component of [A$_{tot}$] and is normally present in plasma at a low concentration. Severe hyperphosphatemia can cause a large increase in [A$_{tot}$], which can result in nonrespiratory acidosis. The treatment for hyperphosphatemic acidosis, hyperalbuminemic acidosis, and hypoalbuminemic alkalosis should be directed at the underlying cause. The administration of sodium bicarbonate shifts phosphorus into cells and can be used as adjuvant therapy in patients with hyperphosphatemic acidosis.[25]

Disorders in Strong Ion Difference

Changes in SID usually are recognized by changes in [HCO$_3^-$] or BE.[26] A decrease in SID is associated with nonrespiratory acidosis, whereas an increase in SID is associated with nonrespiratory alkalosis. There are three general mechanisms by which SID can change (Table 7.10): (a) changing the free-water content of plasma, (b) changing the Cl$^-$ concentration, and (c) increasing the concentration of unidentified strong anions (XA$^-$).

Free-Water Abnormalities

Changing the water content of the various body-fluid compartments will dilute or concentrate both strong anions and cations. Consequently, SID will change by the same proportion. Changes in free water can be identified by evaluating the [Na$^+$]. An increase in SID caused by increases in [Na$^+$] results in concentration alkalosis, whereas a decrease in SID caused by decreases in [Na$^+$] results in dilution acidosis. It has been suggested that changes in extracellular fluid (ECF) volume alone lead to acid-base disturbances. However, change in ECF volume by itself does not change SID, PCO$_2$, or [A$_{tot}$] and therefore cannot change acid-base status.[4] The so-called contraction alkalosis believed to be caused by a decrease in ECF volume is in reality caused by a primary decrease in [Cl$^-$].[10,27] The principal causes of concentration alkalosis and dilution acidosis are listed in Table 7.11.

Therapy for dilution acidosis and concentration alkalosis should be directed at treating the underlying cause responsible for changing [Na$^+$]. If necessary, [Na$^+$] and osmolality should be corrected.[1] Nonrespiratory acidosis should be treated only in patients with more severe acidemia (pH < 7.2).

Isonatremic Chloride Abnormalities

If there is no change in the water content of plasma, plasma [Na$^+$] will be normal. Other strong cations (e.g., K$^+$) are regulated for purposes other than acid-base balance, and their concentration never changes sufficiently to affect SID substantially.[4] Consequently, SID changes only as a result of changes in strong anions when water content is normal. If [Na$^+$] remains constant, changes in [Cl$^-$] can substantially increase or decrease SID.[21,22,28] Evaluation of [Cl$^-$] must be considered in conjunction with measurement of [Na$^+$] because [Cl$^-$] can change for reasons other than a change in water balance.[21,28] Patient [Cl$^-$] is therefore "corrected" for changes in [Na$^+$], applying a formula developed for use in people and adapted for use in small and large animals:[11,27,29]

$$[Cl^-] \text{ corrected} = [Cl^-] \times [Na^+] \text{ normal}/[Na^+] \quad (7.18)$$

where $[Cl^-]$ and $[Na^+]$ are the patient Cl^- and Na^+ concentrations. The normal $[Na^+]$ is the normal Na^+ concentration for the species being evaluated. Suggested values for $[Na^+]$ in dogs are 146 and 147 mEq/L, whereas for cats they range from 150 to 156 mEq/L.[11,28] In large animals, normal $[Na^+]$ is approximately 136 mEq/L in horses and 144 mEq/L in cattle.[24] Normal $[Cl^-]$ is approximately 107 to 113 mEq/L for dogs, 117 to 123 mEq/L for cats, 97 to 103 mEq/L for horses, and 101 to 107 mEq/L for cattle.[10,24,28] These values may vary for different laboratories and different analyzers. An increase or decrease in corrected $[Cl^-]$ indicates that Cl^- is responsible at least in part for the changes in SID. An increase in corrected $[Cl^-]$ (i.e., an increase in $[Cl^-]$ relative to $[Na^+]$) results in a hyperchloremic nonrespiratory acidosis, whereas a decrease in corrected $[Cl^-]$ (i.e., a decrease in $[Cl^-]$ relative to $[Na^+]$) results in hypochloremic nonrespiratory alkalosis. A $[Cl^-]$ corrected to normal in the presence of abnormal observed $[Cl^-]$ indicates that SID changes are caused by dilution acidosis or concentration alkalosis.

The principal causes of hyperchloremic acidosis and hypochloremic alkalosis are listed in Table 7.12. Treatment of hyperchloremic acidosis should be directed at correction of the underlying disease. Administration of $NaHCO_3$, when needed, will tend to correct hyperchloremic acidosis because this solution has an SID greater than plasma.

Chloride-responsive hypochloremic alkalosis can be caused by excessive loss of Cl^- relative to Na^+ or by administration of substances containing more Na^+ than Cl^- compared with ECF (e.g., $NaHCO_3$). The former can occur following the administration of diuretics that cause Cl^- wasting (e.g., furosemide) or when the lost fluid has a low or negative SID, as in the case of vomiting of stomach contents. Chloride administration is essential in the treatment of chloride-responsive hypochloremic alkalosis. Renal Cl^- conservation is ordinarily enhanced in hypochloremic states and renal Cl^- reabsorption does not return to normal until plasma Cl^- concentration is restored to normal or near normal.[22] In cases where expansion of extracellular volume is desired, intravenous infusion of 0.9% NaCl is the treatment of choice. This solution has an SID of 0 and will decrease plasma SID.[4] If hypokalemia is present, KCl should be added to the fluid. When volume expansion is not necessary, Cl^- can be administered using salts without Na^+ (e.g., ammonium chloride, potassium chloride, calcium chloride, and magnesium chloride. These salts will correct the alkalosis because Cl^- is given together with cations that are regulated within narrow limits for purposes unrelated to acid-base balance.[4] Chloride-resistant hypochloremic alkalosis can be caused in animals by hyperadrenocorticism and primary hyperaldosteronism. In these diseases, increased mineralocorticoid activity causes sodium retention and urinary chloride loss, both of which will increase SID. Because of the increased chloruresis, administration of chloride will not correct the metabolic alkalosis. Fortunately, metabolic alkalosis in these patients is usually very mild.

Table 7.12. Principal chloride disorders

Hypochloremic alkalosis[a] ($\downarrow$ $[Cl^-]$ corrected)
  Excessive loss of chloride relative to sodium
    Vomiting of stomach contents
    Gastric reflux in horses with ileus
    Abomasum torsion (ruminants)
    Vagal indigestion with internal vomiting (ruminants)
    Therapy with thiazides or loop diuretics
    Hyperadrenocorticism
  Excessive gain of sodium relative to chloride
    Sodium bicarbonate therapy
Hyperchloremic acidosis[b] ($\uparrow$ $[Cl^-]$ corrected)
  Excessive loss of sodium relative to chloride
    Diarrhea
  Excessive gain of chloride relative to sodium
    Fluid therapy (e.g., 0.9% NaCl, KCl supplemental fluids)
    Salt poisoning
    Total parenteral nutrition
    Ammonium chloride or potassium chloride therapy
  Chloride retention
    Renal failure
    Renal tubular acidosis
  Hypoadrenocorticism
  Diabetes mellitus
  Drug induced (e.g., acetazolamide, spironolactone)

[a]Chronic respiratory acidosis will cause a compensatory decrease in corrected $[Cl^-]$.
[b]Chronic respiratory alkalosis will cause a compensatory increase in corrected $[Cl^-]$.
Adapted from de Morais and Muir.[11]

Isonatremic Organic Acid Abnormalities

Accumulation of metabolically produced organic anions (e.g., lactate, acetoacetate, citrate, or ß-hydroxybutyrate) or addition of exogenous organic anions (e.g., salicylate, glycolate from ethylene glycol poisoning, and formate from methanol poisoning) will cause nonrespiratory acidosis because these strong anions decrease SID.[22] Addition of some inorganic strong anions (e.g., SO_4^{2-} during renal failure) will resemble organic acidosis because these substances decrease SID without changing electrolytes.[1,11] The most frequently encountered causes of organic acidosis are listed in Table 7.13.

Treatment of organic acidosis should be directed toward the primary disorder and stabilization of the patient.[1] Sodium bicarbonate should be used cautiously because metabolism of accumulated organic anions will normalize SID and increase $[HCO_3^-]$. The initial goal in patients with severe organic acidosis is to raise systemic pH to 7.2.

Estimation of Strong Anion Concentration

Organic acidosis increases the AG, whereas hyperchloremic acidosis does not. The AG is used clinically to estimate the concen-

Table 7.13. Principal disorders of the unidentified strong anions in organic acidosis ($\uparrow$[XA$^-$])

Disorder	Strong Anions Decreasing Strong Ion Difference
Uremic acidosis	SO$_4^{2-}$ and other anions of renal failure
Diabetic ketoacidosis, ketosis, pregnancy toxemia	Acetoacetate, ß-hydroxybutyrate
Lactic acidosis	Lactate
Salicylate intoxication	Salicylate
Ethylene glycol toxicity	Glycolate
Methanol toxicity	Formate

[XA$^-$], unidentified strong anions.
Adapted from de Morais and Muir.[11]

Table 7.14. Simplified estimation of change in base excess associated with strong ion difference and [A$_{tot}$]

Free-water abnormalities: $0.3([Na^+] - 140) = \uparrow$
Chloride abnormalities: $102 - [Cl^-]_{corr} = \uparrow$
Protein abnormalities: $3(6.5 - [P_{tot}]) = \uparrow$
Unidentified anions make up the balance $= \uparrow$
Total is the observed (reported) base excess $= \uparrow$

$[Cl^-]_{corr} = [Cl^-]_{obs} \cdot 140/[Na^+]$.
For [Alb] instead of [P$_{tot}$], use $3.7(4.5 - [Alb])$.
Modified from Fencl and Leith.[31]

tration of "unmeasured anions" (UA$^-$). Unfortunately, UA$^-$ includes the strong anions (XA$^-$) and weak (variable charges of albumin and phosphates) unmeasured anions. The AG is therefore influenced by the concentration of plasma proteins, and changes in albumin concentration significantly change AG.[4] Hyperphosphatemia may also increase the AG. The AG will change secondarily to changes in PCO$_2$, SID, or [A$_{tot}$].[3] Thus, changes in AG do not always reflect a stoichiometric change in UA$^-$ even in the presence of organic acidosis. Two mathematical models have been developed for estimation of XA$^-$ in humans.[16,22,26] One of these models has been used in evaluating acid-base disorders in veterinary medicine.[10,11,28] Both models, however, still need to be validated in domestic animals. The history (e.g., ingestion of ethylene glycol); the clinical condition (e.g., shock); increases in serum creatinine concentration, blood urea nitrogen, or serum glucose; and the presence of ketonuria may help in establishing a diagnosis of organic acidosis. The measurement of plasma lactate concentration may be attempted in patients with suspected lactic acidosis.

Evaluations of Acid-Base Balance

A stepwise approach should be followed in all animals with suspected acid-base disorders.[1,29] After obtaining the samples, the first step is to determine the pH and the nature of the primary disorder from the blood-gas analysis results. The possibility of a mixed respiratory and nonrespiratory acid-base disorder should be assessed by calculating the expected compensation (Table 7.7). If a nonrespiratory acid-base disorder is present, it should be determined whether it is caused by a change in [A$_{tot}$], SID, XA$^-$, or a combination of these factors. Unfortunately, evaluation of changes in SID caused by increases in [XA$^-$] is not straightforward. An increase in [XA$^-$] may be suspected in acidotic patients with diseases known to be associated with organic acidosis (e.g., renal failure and diabetic ketoacidosis). Measurement of lactate concentration enables one of the many XA$^-$ to be quantified. When blood-gas results are not available, the bio-

chemical profile may help in determining the nonrespiratory abnormalities present (Tables 7.8 and 7.14).[12,29]

Two quantitative clinical approaches for assessment of nonrespiratory acid-base disturbances have been proposed, one based on the use of BE and the other based on a mathematical relationship to estimate SID. BE has been used to assess changes in the nonrespiratory component because *SID* is synonymous with *buffer base*. BE is a measurement of the deviation of buffer base (and therefore SID) from normal values. It should be pointed out, however, that Siggaard-Andersen studied blood, not plasma, and protein was not considered an acid-base variable. The BE has been used clinically for decades to assess the nonrespiratory acid-base status in humans.[3,4] Formulas to estimate changes in BE due to changes in SID and [A$_{tot}$] are presented in Table 7.14. These formulas are helpful in understanding complex acid-base disorders in domestic animals.[11,24,29] In the 1990s, a new mathematical approach was developed to evaluate nonrespiratory acid-base disorders.[15] The XA$^-$ obtained by using this mathematical model is not constrained by the limitations mentioned earlier for the AG and UA$^-$. Despite being very promising for assessment of nonrespiratory acid-base disorders, this model and the BE model were developed by using protein behavior of human albumin. However, calculation of SID$_{eff}$ in this model is not simple and may be clinically impractical.[15]

References

1. Dibartola SP. Metabolic acidosis. In: Dibartola SP, ed. Fluid Therapy in Small Animal Practice. Philadelphia: WB Saunders, 1992:216–275.
2. Emmet M, Narins RG. Mixed acid-base disorders. In: Maxwell MH, Kleeman CR, Narins RG, eds. Clinical Disorders of Fluid and Electrolyte Metabolism. New York: McGraw-Hill, 1987:743–758.
3. Fencl V, Rossing TH. Acid-base disorders in critical care medicine. Annu Rev Med 40:17–29, 1989.
4. Jones NL. Blood Gases and Acid-Base Physiology. New York: Thieme, 1987.
5. Rose BD. Clinical Physiology of Acid-Base and Electrolyte Disorders, 3rd ed. New York: McGraw-Hill, 1989.
6. Seldin DW, Giebisch G. The Regulation of Acid-Base Balance. New York: Raven, 1989.
7. Stewart PA. How to Understand Acid-Base: A Quantitative Acid-Base Primer for Biology and Medicine. New York: Elsevier, 1981.

8. Nattie EE. The alphastat hypothesis in respiratory control and acid-base balance. J Appl Physiol 69:1201–1207, 1990.

9. de Morais HSA. Chloride ion in small animal practice: The forgotten ion. J Vet Emerg Crit Care 2:11–24, 1992.

10. de Morais HSA. A non-traditional approach to acid-base disorders. In: DiBartola SP, ed. Fluid Therapy in Small Animal Practice. Philadelphia: WB Saunders, 1992:297–320.

11. de Morais HSA, Muir WW. Strong ions and acid-base disorders. In: Bonagura JD, Kirk RW, eds. Kirk's Current Veterinary Therapy, 12th ed. Philadelphia: WB Saunders, 1995:121–127.

12. Bia M, Thier SO. Mixed acid-base disturbances: A clinical approach. Med Clin North Am 65:347–361, 1981.

13. de Morais HSA, DiBartola SP. Mixed acid-base disorders. Part I: Clinical approach. Part II: Clinical disturbances. Compend Contin Educ Pract Vet 15:1619–1626, 1993 (Part I); and 16:477–488, 1994 (Part II).

14. Adams LG, Polzin DJ. Mixed acid-base disorders. Vet Clin North Am Small Anim Pract 19:307–326, 1989.

15. Figge J, Mydosh T, Fencl V. Serum proteins and acid-base equilibria: A follow-up. J Lab Clin Med 120:713–719, 1992.

16. Narins RG, Emmett M. Simple and mixed acid-base disorders: A practical approach. Medicine 56:38–54, 1980.

17. Gabow PA. Disorders associated with high altered gap. Kidney Int 27:472–483, 1985.

18. Goodkin DA, Krishna GG, Narins RG. The role of the anion gap in detecting and managing mixed metabolic acid-base disorders. Clin Endocrinol Metab 13:333–349, 1984.

19. Natelson S. On the significance of the expression "anion-gap." Clin Chem 29:283–284, 1988.

20. Constable PD. Clinical assessment of acid-base status: Comparison of the Henderson-Hasselbalch and strong ion approaches. Vet Clin Pathol 29:115–128, 2000.

21. Nanji A, Blank D. Spurious increases in the anion gap due to exposure of serum to air. N Engl J Med 307:190–191, 1982.

22. Constable PD. Hyperchloremic acidosis: The classic example of strong ion acidosis. Anesth Analg 96:919–922, 2003.

23. Staempfli HR, Constable PD. Experimental determination of net protein charge and A(tot) and Ka of nonvolatile buffers in human plasma. J Appl Physiol 95:620–630, 2003.

24. McCullough SM, Constable PD. Calculation of the total plasma concentration of nonvolatile weak acids and the effective dissociation constant of nonvolatile buffers in the plasma for use in the strong ion approach to acid-base balance in cats. Am J Vet Res 64:1047–1051, 2003.

25. Barsotti G, Lazzeri M, Cristofano C, Cerri M, Lupetti S, Giovannetti S. The role of metabolic acidosis in causing uremic hyperphosphatemia. Miner Electrolyte Metab 12:103–106, 1986.

26. Galla JH, Gifford JD, Luke RG, Rome L. Adaptations to chloride-depletion alkalosis. Am J Physiol 261(4 Pt 2):R771–R781, 1991.

27. Leith DE. The new acid-base: Power and simplicity. In: Proceedings of the Ninth ACVIM Forum. Lakewood, CO: American College of Veterinary Internal Medicine, 1991:611–617.

28. Whitehair KJ, Haskins SC, Whitehair JG, Pascoe PJ. Clinical applications of quantitative acid-base chemistry. J Vet Intern Med 9:1–11, 1995.

29. Story DA, Morimatsu H, Bellomo R. Strong ions, weak acids and base excess: A simplified Fencl-Stewart approach to clinical acid-base disorders. Br J Anaesth 92:54–60, 2004.

30. Emmett M, Seldin DW. Evaluation of acid-base disorders from plasma composition. In: Seldin DW, Giebisch G, eds. The Regulation of Acid-Base Balance. New York: Raven, 1989:259–268.

31. Fencl V, Leith DE. Stewart's quantitative acid-base chemistry: Applications in biology and medicine. Respir Physiol 91:1–15, 1993.

Section III
PHARMACOLOGY

Chapter 8
Fluid, Electrolyte, and Blood Component Therapy

David C. Seeler

Body-Fluid and Electrolyte Composition

At birth, total body water is more than 75% of body weight. Maturational changes result in reductions of total body-water content to 60%–66% of adult body weight.[1–5] Lower water content can be anticipated to exist in older or obese patients. Total body water is comprised of intracellular and extracellular compartments. The intracellular fluid volume increases slightly with age, and in mature animals it is equivalent to approximately 40% of body weight. The volume of the extracellular fluid compartment decreases with maturation and accounts for 20% of the weight of adult animals.[2] The extracellular fluid compartment is further divided into the interstitial, plasma or intravascular, and transcellular fluid compartments. The water volume in the interstitial compartment accounts for 15% of a mature animal's weight, whereas plasma water volume approximates 5%. Plasma consists of water, electrolytes, proteins, nutritive substances, and metabolites. Plasma water volume constitutes 5% of the body weight and approximately 50% of the total blood volume (Table 8.1). The transcellular fluid compartment consists of joint and cerebrospinal fluid (CSF) in addition to water located within the eye and pleural, peritoneal, and pericardial spaces and approximates 1.0% to 3.0% of body weight.

Constituents of the various fluid compartments are listed in Table 8.2. Chemical substances that dissociate in solution to form electrically charged particles or ions are *electrolytes*. Their concentrations in solution are generally expressed in millimoles per liter (mmol/L) or as milliequivalents per liter (mEq/L). Sodium is the most important extracellular cation, whereas chloride and bicarbonate are the primary extracellular anions. Together, these ions form more than 90% of the total solute within the extracellular fluid compartment.[6–8] Plasma proteins, which at a vascular pH of 7.4 have a net negative charge, play a key role in the maintenance of intravascular fluid volume. The primary intracellular ions are potassium, magnesium, and phosphate. Cytoplasmic proteins play a role in the maintenance of intracellular electric neutrality. Even though the cell membrane is freely permeable to sodium and potassium, the sodium-potassium pump maintains a concentration gradient for each cation across the cell membrane. Thus, sodium salts serve as an osmotic skeleton for the extracellular fluid volume while potassium salts serve the same function in the intracellular space. In addition to maintaining electric neutrality, ionic concentration differences on either side of the semipermeable cell membrane perform a key role in the normal physiological function of excitable cells.

Movement of body water throughout, and between, compartments occurs by *osmosis*, which is the process by which the net movement of water occurs due to concentration gradients across a semipermeable membrane. The pressure required to prevent water movement across semipermeable membranes is defined as the *osmotic pressure*, which depends on the number of nondiffusible, nondifferentiable particles such as ions or molecules in solution, and not their mass. To express the concentration of these particles in terms of their numbers, the unit called the *osmole* (osm) is used: 1 osm is equivalent to 1 g mol of nondiffusible and nonionizable substance. *Osmolality* is the osmolal concentration of a solution when the concentration is expressed in osmoles per kilogram (osm/kg) of water. In contrast, *osmolarity* is the concentration of a solution when expressed in osmoles per liter (osm/L) of water. Both terms are often used interchangeably in respect to discussions of fluid balance and therapy: 1 milliosmole (mOsm) per liter exerts an osmotic pressure of 19.3 mm Hg.

Total body water is determined by the number of osmotically active agents in both compartments.[9] Water distribution across the intracellular and extracellular compartments depends on osmotic equilibrium between the two compartments. More than 80% of the osmolality of the extracellular fluid compartment is determined by sodium and its associated anions.[10] As a result, sodium regulation plays a major role in extracellular fluid osmolality and extracellular fluid volume. The various cardiovascular, renal, and neurohormonal mechanisms that function in an integrated fashion to maintain and preserve sodium and water homeostasis are discussed elsewhere.[11,12] Of the intracellular fluid compartment's osmolality, 50% is determined by potassium, whereas the remainder is exerted by other intracellular constituents. Disturbance in osmolality of either compartment results in

Table 8.1. Approximate vascular fluid volumes (mL/kg) in mature species.

Species	Plasma Volume	Total Blood Volume
Bovine	38	57–60
Canine	50	88
Caprine	53	70
Equine		
Thoroughbred	61	100
Other		72
Feline	47	68
Ovine	50	60
Porcine	47	50

Table 8.2. Electrolyte distribution across fluid compartments (mEq/L).

Ion	Plasma	Interstitial	Intracellular
Na^+	142	145	13
K^+	5	4	155
Ca^{2+}	5	3	2
Mg^{2+}	2	2	35
Cl^-	106	115	2
HCO_3^-	24	30	10
Phosphates	2	2	113
Sulfates	1	1	20
Organic	5	5	0
Protein	16	1	60

a rapid shift in water balance in order that equilibrium between the two compartments is reestablished. For example, increases in extracellular osmolality, owing to either pure water loss or the gain of osmotically active agents, result in water movement from the intracellular compartment into the extracellular fluid space until an osmotic equilibrium is reached. Plasma electrolyte and osmolality values for the various domestic species are listed in Table 8.3.

Within the extracellular fluid space, plasma water communicates directly with water in the interstitial space at the level of the capillary beds. The direction and magnitude of water movement between the interstitial and intravascular spaces are determined by the algebraic sum of hydrostatic and osmotic forces in each compartment as originally described by Starling.[13,14] The capillary walls are freely permeable to sodium, chloride, and glucose. As a result, these substances are osmotically inactive across capillary membranes. However, plasma proteins are limited in their ability to cross capillary membranes. Blood or plasma volume ultimately is maintained by the colloid osmotic pressure or plasma oncotic pressure exerted by plasma proteins. Colloid osmotic pressure is approximately 23 mm Hg and results in a plasma osmolarity of 1.5 mOsm/L greater than that found in the interstitial or intracellular fluid spaces.[7] Despite that, the net forces in the

capillary beds lead to a net filtration of a small amount of fluid into the interstitial space. This loss is balanced by fluid return to the intravascular space through the lymphatic system.[9,13]

Alterations in volume or composition of either the extracellular or intracellular fluid compartments are readily assessed if a number of basic principles are followed. It is important to remember that the osmolalities of both compartments are at equilibrium except for a brief period (minutes) after a change in one of the compartments. Fluids are defined as isotonic, hypotonic, or hypertonic based on their effect on erythrocyte size or volume. *Isotonic solutions* exert no volume changes on erythrocytes, whereas *hypotonic solutions* increase erythrocyte size and *hypertonic solutions* decrease erythrocyte size. Administration of isotonic solutions to the intravascular space does not alter the osmolality of the extracellular fluid. As a result, there is no net osmotic effect, and only the volume of the extracellular fluid compartment is expanded. Parenteral administration of hypotonic solutions, however, reduces extracellular fluid osmolality and results in the osmotic movement of water into the intracellular compartment. Similarly, hypertonic solutions increase the osmolality of extracellular fluids, which causes a fluid shift out of the intracellular compartment.

Secondly, the number of osmotically active agents in either compartment remains constant unless one of the substances moves from one to the other compartment or is added or lost from either of the compartments. In this instance, sodium or potassium imbalances or acid-base or metabolic disorders can induce compositional changes that affect fluid balance between compartments.

Composition of Parenteral Solutions

Crystalloid Preparations

The term *crystalloid* refers to any solution of crystalline solids that are dissolved in water, such as sodium-based electrolyte solutions or solutions of dextrose in water. If the electrolyte composition of the prepared solution approximates that of the extracellular fluid, then the parenteral fluid is referred to as a *balanced electrolyte solution*. Multiple or balanced electrolyte solutions are formulated based on the concept that the amount of water and electrolytes that a patient retains depends on intact regulatory mechanisms in the body, not on the amount of water and electrolytes received. Commercial preparations are available as inexpensive sterile nonpyrogenic isotonic, hypotonic, or hypertonic solutions. The composition of each solution varies according to its intended purpose. Parenteral fluids provide water, electrolytes, and, in some instances, alkalinizing agents or a source of calories or both. Solutions that are polyelectrolytic have value in maintaining or replenishing electrolytes. Those preparations that contain lactate, acetate, or gluconate produce an alkalinizing effect when the anion is metabolized to carbon dioxide and water.

Maintenance Solutions

Daily water loss includes the insensible loss through evaporation from the respiratory system and skin, as well as sensible losses in which there is an associated obligatory loss of electrolytes. For

Table 8.3. Fluid and electrolyte panel: Normal values for chemistry and hematologic data at the Atlantic Veterinary College.

	Units[a]	Canine	Feline	Bovine	Equine	Porcine	Ovine
Sodium	mmol/L	144–162	150–160	135–151	135–148	140–150	143–151
Potassium	mmol/L	3.6–6.0	4.0–5.8	3.9–5.9	3.0–5.0	4.7–7.1	4.6–7.0
Chloride	mmol/L	106–126	118–128	96–110	98–110	100–105	102–116
Calcium	mmol/L	2.24–3.04	2.23–2.80	2.11–2.75	2.80–3.44	1.80–2.90	2.30–2.86
Phosphorus	mmol/L	0.82–1.87	1.03–1.92	1.08–2.76	1.00–1.80	1.30–3.55	0.82–2.66
Magnesium	mmol/L	0.70–1.16	0.74–1.12	0.80–1.32	0.74–1.02	0.78–1.60	0.9–1.26
Urea	mmol/L	3.0–10.5	5.0–11.0	3.0–7.5	3.5–7.0	3.0–8.5	2.0–10.0
Creatinine	μmol/L	60–140	90–180	67–175	105–170	90–240	69–105
Glucose	mmol/L	3.3–5.6	3.3–5.6	1.8–3.8	3.6–5.6	3.6–5.3	1.2–3.6
Total protein	g/L	51–72	68–80	66–78	60–77	34–60	61–81
Albumin	g/L	22–38	22–38	23–43	25–36	18–22	27–39
Albumin-globulin ratio	—	0.60–1.50	0.60–1.50	0.66–1.30	0.60–1.50	0.60–1.50	0.54–1.22
Hemoglobin	g/L	120–180	80–150	80–150	110–190	100–160	80–160
Hematocrit	L/L	0.37–0.55	0.24–0.45	0.24–0.46	0.32–0.52	0.32–0.50	0.24–0.50
Red blood cells	$\times 10^{12}$/L	5.5–8.5	5.0–10.0	5.0–10.0	6.5–12.5	5.0–8.0	8.0–16.0
Reticulocytes	%	0–1.5%	0–1%	0%	0%	0–1%	0%
Platelets	$\times 10^{9}$/L	200–900	300–700	100–800	100–600	310–510	250–750
Calculated osmolality	mOsm/kg	280–320	280–320	274–306	280–320	280–320	283–307
Anion gap	mmol/L	14–26	13–26	14–26	10–25	10–25	12–24

[a]Factors used to convert SI units to conventional units are listed in Table 8.6.

many domestic species and birds, the daily maintenance water requirement ranges from 40 to 60 mL/kg/day, whereas, in calves, it ranges from 80 to 100 mL/kg/day.[15–20] The daily requirement for nonlactating dairy cows and lactating cows has been estimated at 29 L/day and 56 L/day, respectively.[21] The net daily loss of sodium in small animals ranges from 35 to 50 mmol/L (35 to 50 mEq/L), whereas daily potassium losses are 20 to 30 mmol/L (20 to 30 mEq/L).[15]

Maintenance solutions are designed to meet the water and electrolyte requirements of patients that are not taking in adequate amounts sufficient to meet their daily requirements. To meet these specific requirements, maintenance solutions have lower sodium and chloride concentrations and an increased potassium concentration when compared with extracellular fluid. If the concentration of potassium in the parenteral solution is less than 20 mmol/L (20 mEq/L), then the maintenance fluid may be supplemented with additional potassium.

Infusion rates up to 15 mL/kg/h are safe as long as the potassium concentration in the parenteral solution is less than 30 mmol/L (30 mEq/L).[22] Hypotonic preparations, or solutions that contain dextrose, provide free water. Isotonic salt solutions provide osmolar water instead of free water. In the case of solutions containing dextrose, free water is not available to all body compartments until the dextrose has been metabolized. Maintenance fluids are generally administered over a 24-h period. These solutions should not be used in situations where large volumes are to be rapidly infused, because this could result in significant electrolyte abnormalities in the extracellular fluid.

Replacement Solutions

The composition of isotonic, balanced electrolyte solutions such as lactated Ringer's USP closely approximates the electrolyte composition of extracellular fluid. These solutions may be administered rapidly in large volumes to reexpand the extracellular fluid volume without inducing changes in its electrolytic composition. Since they are isotonic, their use does not induce fluid shifts between the intracellular and extracellular compartments. Balanced electrolyte solutions will rapidly equilibrate across the intravascular and interstitial fluid compartments. As a result, only 20% to 25% of the administered volume remains within the intravascular space after 1 h.[10] This must be considered when using replacement fluids to replenish intravascular volume losses. To replace the vascular deficit, it is necessary to administer a volume equivalent to at least three- to fourfold the volume of blood lost.[23] Many of the preparations presently available contain lactate, acetate, or gluconate, which serve as alkalinizing agents. Acid-base considerations in situations in which patients require acute care are discussed in Chapter 7.

Replacement solutions are often used as maintenance fluids. In this situation, normal renal function should be present to ensure that electrolytes in excess of daily requirements are eliminated. Long-term management of a patient's maintenance requirements with a replacement solution may cause hypokalemia. In this instance, replacement solutions should be supplemented with potassium chloride to provide a final potassium concentration of 20 mmol/L (20 mEq/L). Replacement fluids that have been supplemented with potassium chloride should not be used in clinical situations where large volumes may be rapidly infused.

Other Parenteral Solutions

Isotonic and Hypotonic Saline Isotonic saline, which is prepared as a 0.9% solution that contains 154 mmol/L (154 mEq/L) each of sodium and chloride ions and has an osmolarity of 308 mOsm/L, is often referred to as normal or physiological saline. However, only the sodium-ion concentration of the preparation matches that of extracellular fluid. The use of 0.9% sodium chloride solutions has been advocated for maintenance and replacement purposes. Isotonic saline does not meet the patient's free-water and electrolyte needs for maintenance purposes. It may be used for rapid expansion of the extracellular fluid volume despite the possibility of inducing a hyperchloremic acidosis in patients.[24–26] Similar to other crystalloid solutions, intravenously administered saline solutions rapidly distribute throughout the extracellular fluid space. However, their composition does not match that of extracellular fluid, and excessive use of isotonic saline for replacement purposes could lead to the unnecessary dilution of other extracellular electrolytes and buffers. Isotonic saline may also be used to correct hyponatremia or a metabolic alkalemia.

Hypotonic saline solutions are available in a number of strengths. Commercial preparations of 0.45% saline are hypotonic (osmolarity, 154 mOsm/L) and may be used as a hydrating solution. Hypotonic saline preparations may be used for maintenance purposes, particularly when they are supplemented with dextrose, potassium chloride, or both. When 2.5% dextrose is added to 0.45% saline, the resultant solution is isotonic. Upon metabolism of the dextrose, free water is made available for distribution across all fluid compartments.

Hypertonic Saline Traditionally, solutions of 3% and 5% saline have been used to treat patients who have severe hyponatremia where rapid sodium replacement is considered necessary. More recently, hypertonic saline solutions have been used successfully to manage severe shock, particularly hemorrhagic shock.[27–33] In situations in which a patient is moribund or critically ill, the infusion of small volumes of hypertonic saline enables the clinician to obtain the time required to institute other lifesaving measures. Hypertonic saline solutions of 7.5% have been used for this purpose. The osmolarity of 7.5% saline is 2400 mOsm/L. To prepare 7.5% saline, it is necessary to purchase 5% saline in 500-mL bags and 23.4% saline in 30-mL bottles (American Reagent Labs, Shirley, NY; Lyphomed Canada, Markham, Canada). Remove 120 mL of 5% saline from the 500-mL bag and inject 60 mL of the 23.4% saline solution into the bag to make a 7.5% solution.[27]

The mechanisms by which hypertonic saline exerts its physiological effects are still subject to some debate.[33–38] Overall changes attributed to hypertonic saline in the past included improved cardiac output and aortic blood pressure, reduced peripheral vascular resistance, an increase in plasma volume with hemodilution, and an increase in interstitial fluid volumes. These overall improvements in cardiovascular function and tissue perfusion were attributed to the direct and indirect effects of the infused hypertonic saline solution.[16,30,31,35,36,39–41] It had also been postulated that the sodium administered in the hypertonic solution stimulates pulmonary osmoreceptors or chemoreceptors,

thus activating a pulmonary vagal reflex. However, it has been pointed out that pulmonary reflexes have not been induced by using hypertonic saline in any species other than dogs anesthetized with pentobarbital.[33] Selective activation of sympathetic pathways was also thought to occur, resulting in venoconstriction of capacitance vessels, leading to improved cardiac filling along with selective precapillary vasoconstriction in skin and muscle, thus redistributing blood volume within the vascular space.[36]

It is now apparent that hypertonic saline exerts its beneficial effects through plasma volume expansion coupled with a transient decrease in afterload. Vasodilation occurs in some vascular beds because of the direct hyperosmotic effect of the solution. This reduces total peripheral resistance and enhances perfusion of vital organs.[30,36,39] Upon administration, hypertonic saline equilibrates rapidly throughout the extracellular fluid space. Because of the increase in extracellular fluid osmolality caused by the hypertonic solution, water moves out of the intracellular fluid compartment. As a result, the extracellular fluid compartment volume is expanded. Solutions of 7.5% saline, when infused intravenously into dogs, have been demonstrated to increase plasma volume 2 to 4 mL for 1 mL of solution administered.[30] The maximum vascular volume expansion occurs within 30 min of the administration of the hypertonic saline solution. These fluid shifts produce an intracellular water debt and an eventual decrease in total body water because of the obligatory water loss associated with natriuresis.[35,42]

The intravenous administration of 4 to 8 mL/kg in dogs or 1 to 4 mL/kg in cats of 7.5% saline over 3 to 5 min results in a rapid restoration of hemodynamic parameters with subsequent improvements in tissue perfusion.[15,28,34,43,44] It has been suggested that in dogs an infusion rate of 2 mL/kg/min be used to reduce the possibility of inducing acute hypotension.[39] In conscious horses, 5 mL/kg of 7.5% saline was infused at rates of 80 mL/min with no adverse effects noted.[45] In ruminants, it has been suggested that the rate of administration of 4 to 5 mL/kg of hypertonic saline not exceed 1 mL/kg/min.[33,46] Since relatively small volumes are infused, clinicians need not worry about fluid overload or the development of interstitial edema in patients. However, hypertonic saline solutions should not be used in situations where cardiac dysrhythmias exist, if hemorrhage is not controlled, or if a patient is hypernatremic, has coagulation disorders, or is significantly dehydrated.[27,40,47]

The hemodynamic effects of 7.5% hypertonic saline are not sustained.[28,30,40–42,48] The duration of effect in cats was found to be approximately 60 min in one study, whereas another study found improved hemodynamic function over a period of 180 min.[49] This concern has led to a number of studies that have demonstrated the feasibility of prolonging the beneficial effects of hypertonic saline by adding hyperoncotic preparations such as dextran 70 to the mixture.[35,41,42,50–56] Regardless of the eventual outcome of these and similar studies, it is advisable to use hypertonic saline solutions in the initial resuscitative management of moribund patients and to follow this initial treatment with more traditional therapeutic measures. When hypertonic saline is administered over a prolonged period, serum sodium and osmolality should be monitored.

Dextrose Solutions These are commercially available in a wide range of concentrations ranging from 2.5% to 50% dextrose in water; 5% dextrose in water contains 50 g of dextrose monohydrate per 1 L of water and exerts an osmolarity of 252 mOsm/L. Dextrose solutions provide a source of free water for total body distribution once the carbohydrate is metabolized. An additional 0.6 mL of water is made available for each gram of dextrose that is metabolized. The volume of water administered eventually distributes across all fluid compartments, so dextrose solutions are not effective for use as plasma volume expanders. However, they are effective in replenishing primary total body-water deficits (e.g., dehydration).

The 5% dextrose solutions contain 171 calories per liter, which does not meet the energy requirements of domestic animal species. Hypertonic dextrose solutions are generally used for caloric supplementation of parenteral maintenance fluids.[57] Long-term infusions of 5% dextrose or the infusion of hypertonic dextrose solutions may cause thrombophlebitis. Care should be taken to ensure that the hypertonic preparations in particular are infused via the caudal or cranial vena cava.[57] The administration rate of dextrose solutions should be less than 0.5 g/kg/h so as not to induce glucosuria.[22]

Alkalinizing Agents

Sodium Bicarbonate This solution is a hypertonic (1500 mOsm/L) preparation of sodium bicarbonate ($NaHCO_3$) in sterile water for injection. Solutions contain 5.0%, 7.5%, or 8.4% sodium bicarbonate in 50-mL ampules or vials and 500-mL bottles. The solution is administered intravenously, either in another parenteral solution or undiluted in emergencies. An isotonic solution results when a 50-mL vial of 7.5% sodium bicarbonate is added to 200 mL of sterile water for injection; with a 50-mL vial of 8.4% solution, 224 mL of sterile water is required. Alternatively, three 50-mL ampules of 8.4% solution may be added to 1 L of 5% dextrose.

Sodium bicarbonate is indicated in the treatment of metabolic acidosis. It is also indicated in barbiturate intoxication in order to facilitate dissociation of barbiturate-protein complex. Overcorrection of the bicarbonate deficit produces metabolic alkalosis with a rise in blood pH. From a clinical standpoint, alkalosis is seldom encountered. However, administration of sodium bicarbonate is generally contraindicated in patients losing chloride through vomiting or in those with hypokalemia. Sodium bicarbonate administration produces sodium retention and should be used with caution in patients with congestive heart failure or other conditions causing edema. Doses of up to 2 mEq/kg in cats induce minimal changes in the electrolyte status of the animal. Sodium bicarbonate doses in excess of 4 mEq/kg can induce hyperosmolality, hypernatremia and hypokalemia.[58]

The dose of sodium bicarbonate is determined by the base deficit of blood and the clinical symptoms of the patient. Quantitative estimation of the bicarbonate dose may be calculated from this formula:

$$base\ deficit \times 0.3 \times body\ weight\ (kg) = mEq\ of\ NaHCO_3$$

The factor 0.3 × body weight is an approximation of the acute volume of distribution of infused HCO_3^- and approximates the volume of the extracellular fluid compartment. Distribution to interstitial fluid requires approximately 30 min to be 98% complete. Although the factor 0.6 has been used in the formula, the use of 0.6 × body weight assumes that the volume of HCO_3^- distribution is total body water. About 18 h are required for complete distribution. When the 0.6 factor is used, the dose of HCO_3^- may be too high and, if given, must be administered slowly. The amount of HCO_3^- needed to correct the base deficit in metabolic acidosis varies widely depending on the cause of the acidosis and variations in distribution of HCO_3^- into intracellular spaces. Overtreatment should be avoided. Acid-base measurements should be made frequently, because changes with anesthesia and disease processes are dynamic. Usually half the calculated dose is administered, and a second base-deficit determination made. Should alkalosis result from sodium bicarbonate administration, the use of bicarbonate should be discontinued, and the patient should be treated according to the degree of alkalosis. Sodium chloride injection (0.9%) intravenously is usually sufficient to correct plasma chloride. If the alkalosis is severe enough to be accompanied by hyperirritability or tetany, ammonium chloride (NH_4Cl) may be given intravenously as a 1:6 molar solution (167 mEq/L). Calcium gluconate may also be useful in controlling tetany.

To correct for the acidity inherent in acid citrate dextrose (ACD)–preserved blood, the contents of 1 ampule added to 250 mL of sterile water for injection may be given for every 4 units (1600 mL) of blood administered.

Intravenous sodium bicarbonate administration leads to increased CO_2 levels in blood and CSF. Because plasma HCO_3^- enters the CSF slowly, a paradoxical acidosis in the brain may result. General depression of the central nervous system, including the medullary centers, may develop, reducing respiratory drive. Patients thus must be ventilated adequately to prevent these adverse side effects. When given in large quantities, sodium bicarbonate has been shown to cause hyperosmolality of blood. Experimental and clinical observations indicate that increases in plasma osmolality to levels exceeding 350 mOsm are potentially fatal. Detrimental effects of alkalemia include an increase in the affinity of hemoglobin for oxygen with an unfavorable effect on oxygen release. Routine measurement of plasma osmolality, in addition to acid-base determinations, is recommended prior to administration of additional doses of an alkalinizing agent. Another detrimental effect associated with the use of sodium bicarbonate is prolongation of thrombin clotting and prothrombin times.

Tromethamine Tromethamine (THAM) is a slightly hypertonic (380 mOsm/L) 0.3 M solution with the pH adjusted to 8.6 with acetic acid. This organic amine buffer is used for correction of severe systemic respiratory or metabolic acidosis, such as that which occurs during shock, cardiac arrest, or massive transfusions of ACD-preserved blood.[59] Given intravenously, it acts as an amine proton acceptor, attracting hydrogen ions to form salts that are then excreted by the kidneys. The buffering capacity of THAM is equivalent to that of sodium bicarbonate, yet it does not cause hypernatremia or hypercapnia.[59,60]

THAM also acts as an osmotic diuretic, increasing urine flow, urine pH, and excretion of electrolytes, fixed acids, and carbon dioxide. Approximately 30% of THAM at a pH of 7.4 is not ionized. As a result, THAM is an effective intracellular and extracellular buffer.[61]

The intravenous dose may be estimated from the buffer base deficit:

THAM (mL, of 0.3 M) required = body weight (kg) × base deficit (mEq/L) × 1.1

In treatment of cardiac arrest, THAM should be given at the same time that other standard resuscitative measures, including cardiac massage, are being applied. Intravenous doses of 3.5 to 6 mL/kg have been administered in these circumstances. Additional amounts may be required to control the systemic acidosis that persists after the cardiac arrest is reversed. The intravenous lethal dose of THAM in dogs is 500 mg/kg when given at 50 mg/kg/min.

The use of THAM is contraindicated in patients with anuria or uremia. Large doses may depress respiration, owing to pH change and CO_2 reduction with subsequent increase in blood lactate. Rapid infusion may produce electrocardiogram (ECG) changes similar to those of hyperkalemia. Hypoglycemia may also occur. For these reasons, blood pH, PCO_2, bicarbonate, glucose, and electrolyte levels should be determined during administration of large quantities of this drug. Although significant clinical coagulation abnormalities do not appear to be a problem when THAM is used in dogs with normal coagulation indices, care should be taken as coagulation time is increased.

Colloid Preparations

Colloids are a suspension of large molecular weight particles. If the average molecular weight of the particles in solutions exceeds 50,000, they will tend to remain within the vascular compartment. This increases intravascular colloid osmotic pressure, which not only limits further water movement out of the intravascular space but may also cause water movement from the interstitial space to the intravascular space. Colloid preparations are thus effective when used to expand vascular volume. To ensure that an effective vascular volume is maintained, colloids are also used in acute hypoproteinemic states where plasma albumin levels are less than 15 g/L (1.5 g/dL) or total serum protein levels are less than 35 g/L (3.5 g/dL). Natural colloids include plasma, albumin preparations, and whole blood. Artificial colloids include dextran, gelatin, and hydroxyethyl starch preparations. The effectiveness of the artificial colloids is determined by their physiochemical characteristics, such as average molecular weight, colloid content, and biodegradability. Artificial colloids exert a vascular effect similar to that of plasma. When using artificial colloids, the clinician's therapeutic goal is to maintain plasma oncotic pressure above 17 mm Hg.[10] They are more expensive than plasma, but under certain circumstances, such as during intraoperative procedures in large animals, they may be more readily available.

Plasma

Plasma proteins play a predominant role in establishing plasma oncotic pressure, which is ultimately responsible for maintaining vascular volume at the level of the capillary beds. The albumin fraction of total serum protein ranges from 35% to 50% (Table 8.3), and albumin accounts for 75% of the plasma oncotic pressure exerted by plasma proteins. Reductions in serum albumin levels to 15 g/L (1.5 g/dL), or total serum protein levels to 35 g/L (3.5 g/dL) or lower, result in a net water loss from the vascular compartment to the interstitial space. If untreated, vascular volume diminishes and interstitial edema occurs.

Plasma is harvested from whole blood and either used as fresh plasma for the treatment of coagulopathies or stored at −70°C as fresh-frozen plasma.[62] There is evidence to suggest that canine plasma may be stored for up to 30 days at 2°C with no significant effect on hemostatic parameters.[63] Each gram of albumin will retain approximately 17 to 18 mL of water within the vascular space. In the perioperative period, plasma is used to treat vascular volume deficits or hypoproteinemia. Plasma must be gradually warmed to 37°C prior to being administered. Plasma should not be thawed using temperatures higher than 37°C. A blood administration set with an in-line 18-micron micropore filter should be used when plasma is to be infused. It has been recommended that, for dogs, the recipient should receive 28 to 33 mL/kg of plasma to administer 1 g/kg of albumin when the protein concentration of plasma of the donor is 30 to 35 g/L (3.5 g/dL).[62] Alternatively, one may estimate the amount of donor plasma required:[64]

$$\begin{matrix} \text{amount donor} \\ \text{plasma required} = \\ \text{(mL)} \end{matrix} \left[\frac{\text{desired TP} - \text{actual TP}}{\text{donor plasma TP}} \right] \begin{matrix} \text{Recipient} \\ \text{Plasma} \\ \text{Volume} \\ \text{(mL)} \end{matrix}$$

Care should be taken to ensure that there are no allergic reactions to the transfusion or that the patient is not volume overloaded.

Whole Blood

Patients who are severely anemic or who have had a significant decrease in their packed cell volume (PCV) from normal (Table 8.3) are candidates for whole blood transfusion or the administration of packed red cells if plasma protein levels are within normal limits. In the perioperative period, acute blood loss exceeding 10% to 15% of the patient's blood volume should be replaced with whole blood. Chronic reductions in hematocrit to 15% in healthy nonexercising animals does not necessarily result in clinical signs of oxygen debt. However, when one considers the cardiopulmonary effects of most anesthetic agents, it is advisable to maintain a hematocrit of at least 21% to 25% or a hemoglobin concentration of at least 70 g/L (7 g/dL) in surgical patients.[64,65] This helps ensure that adequate oxygen is delivered to the peripheral tissues in the perioperative period.[66,67]

Whole blood is collected from donors in an anticoagulant such as ACD, citrate phosphate dextrose (CPD), citrate phosphate dextrose adenine (CPDA-1), sodium citrate, or heparin. Once collected, plasma may be harvested and stored separately, if desired. Whole blood and packed red cells are stored at 1° to 6°C.[68,69] Details regarding the collection and storage of whole blood or blood components may be obtained elsewhere.[68,69]

The duration of storage that is considered acceptable in terms of red cell viability depends on the anticoagulant used and the use of appropriate storage procedures.[70] Transfused red cell viability of previously stored blood should exceed 70% at 24 h after the transfusion. Nonviable transfused red cells are removed from the circulation within 24 h. Whole blood or packed cells that are properly stored in ACD may be used for up to 21 days after collection, whereas CPD and CPDA-1 maintain adequate red cell viability for up to 4 weeks.[68] Storage of red blood cells dramatically reduces DPG (2,3-diphosphoglycerate), which shifts the oxygen hemoglobin dissociation curve to the left in dogs.[70] In cats, the release of oxygen is independent of DPG.[71] Left shifts of the oxygen hemoglobin dissociation curve decrease oxygen availability to peripheral tissues. In humans, DPG returns to 50% of normal levels within 24 h of transfusion. If oxygen delivery to peripheral tissues is of significant concern in the perioperative period, then the use of freshly collected blood or blood that has been stored for a minimum period in CPD or CPDA-1 should be considered.

The number and type of clinically significant blood groups with respect to transfusion reactions vary among the domestic animal species (Table 8.4). Normal red blood cell viability or circulation half-life also varies significantly among the various species (Table 8.5). Where possible, all donors should be typed and all potential transfusion recipients should be typed and crossmatched with the donor.[62,68,69,72] Canine blood donors should be at least dog erythrocyte antigen 1.1 and 1.2 negative.[68] In cats, there are significant variations among breeds as to the predominant blood group, and naturally occurring isoagglutinins exist.[68,72–74] As a result, it is recommended that all feline donors and recipients be typed, donors of each blood group be available, and a crossmatch be performed on the first transfusion.

If donors are not typed, then fresh blood collected from the donor and recipient should be crossmatched. This enables the clinician to determine whether the recipient has been previously sensitized or has naturally occurring isoantibodies to the donor's red blood cells. A minor crossmatch would indicate whether the donor has antibodies against the recipient's red blood cells. It should be noted that the crossmatch tests only for isoagglutinins. In cattle and horses, isohemolysins play a major role in transfusion reactions.[69,75,76] As a result, the crossmatch in these species may not provide an adequate indication of the potential for a transfusion reaction, so alternative tests may be necessary.

Whole blood and packed red cells, like plasma, must be slowly rewarmed to 37°C prior to being transfused into the patient. Temperatures higher than 37°C should not be used to rewarm whole blood or blood products. Packed red cells may be diluted with 0.9% saline to facilitate the transfusion process by reducing the viscosity of the suspension. Under no circumstances should rewarmed whole blood, or red cells, be re-refrigerated if unused. Intravenous administration sets used for transfusion purposes should contain in-line filters with a pore size of 80 microns so that cellular debris and blood clots are not transfused into the patient. In cats, where blood is often collected into a syringe, syringe filters (Hemo-nate; Gesco International, San Antonio, TX) may be used to accomplish the same purpose. All blood transfu-

Table 8.4. Major blood groups of domestic animal species.

Species Groups	Number of Major Groups	Clinically Significant
Bovine	12	B, J
Canine	9	DEA 1.1, 1.2, 7
Caprine	5	?
Equine	9	A, C, Q
Feline	2	A, B
Ovine	7	B, R
Porcine	16	?

Table 8.5. Red blood cell survival times.

Species	Days
Bovine	140–160
Canine	110–120
Caprine	125
Equine	140–150
Feline	75–80
Ovine	64–94
Porcine	75–95

sions should be administered through a separate intravenous access, and other therapeutic agents should not be administered to the patient via the blood administration set.

The volume of blood to be administered may be set empirically at 10 to 40 mL/kg in dogs and 5 to 20 mL/kg in cats or calculated.[77] In species where the blood volume approximates 7% of total body weight, the following formulas may be used to calculate the required volume of whole blood or packed red cells for transfusion purposes. If the hematocrit of the donor's blood is 40%, then administration of 1.75 mL/kg will raise the recipient's hematocrit by 1%. Similarly, if the hematocrit of the packed cell solution is 70%, then administration of 1.0 mL/kg will raise the recipient's hematocrit by 1%.[78] Alternatively, in small animals, the following formulas may be used:[62,79]

For cats,

$$mL \text{ blood required} = BW_{kg} \times 70 \left[\frac{desired \text{ PCV} - patient \text{ PCV}}{donor \text{ PCV}} \right]$$

For dogs,

$$mL \text{ blood required} = BW_{kg} \times 90 \left[\frac{desired \text{ PCV} - patient \text{ PCV}}{donor \text{ PCV}} \right]$$

Whole blood, or suspensions of packed red cells, may be administered at rates of 5 to 10 mL/kg/h. In critical situations, where rapid restoration of blood volume is of concern, administration rates of 22 mL/kg/h in dogs and 40 mL/kg/h in cats may be used.[69] Rates of 10 to 40 mL/kg/h in cattle and 20 to 30 mL/kg/h in horses have been suggested.[69,80] Transfusions are best completed within 4 h to avoid bacterial contamination and functional loss of blood components. If more than 50 mL/kg of blood is administered, then consideration should be given to the administration of calcium chloride or gluconate to counteract the effects of the anticoagulant.[64]

Patients must be continuously monitored for clinical signs that suggest an acute adverse reaction to the transfusion. Adverse reactions may be caused by prior bacterial contamination of the donor's blood, allergic or immunologic reactions to the transfusion itself, circulatory overload, or citrate-induced hypocalcemia.[81] The nature of the observed clinical signs of acute transfusion reaction varies. In some species, hemolysis as opposed to agglutination occurs. Clinical signs may include tachycardia, dysrhythmias, hypotension, tachypnea, dyspnea, tremors, emesis, wheals, urticaria, transient fever, hemolysis, hemoglobinemia, and hemoglobinuria.[64,69,72,79,81] It is important to remember that a number of these clinical signs may not occur in anesthetized patients. Therefore, any unexpected changes in the clinical status of an anesthetized patient that is receiving a transfusion must be critically evaluated. If a transfusion reaction is suspected, then the transfusion must be terminated and supportive therapy instituted.[81,82] Sepsis, circulatory overload, and hypocalcemia are detected by careful monitoring of anesthetized patients and treated accordingly.

Dextran Solutions

Dextrans are low to average molecular weight polysaccharides that are produced as a result of bacterial enzymatic action on sucrose. Dextran 40 is a low molecular weight polysaccharide with an average molecular weight of 40,000 and a molecular weight range of 10,000 to 70,000. Dextran 70 and dextran 75, respectively, consist of glucose polymers with an average molecular weight of 70,000 and 75,000. Both preparations have a molecular weight range of 20,000 to 200,000, and as a result their clinical effects are similar. Polymers with a molecular weight less than 50,000 are eliminated from the circulation by glomerular filtration and renal excretion. Polysaccharides with a molecular weight greater than 50,000 are eventually stored in the reticuloendothelial system and subsequently metabolized.

Dextran solutions are used for plasma volume expansion when hematogenous products are not available. They are not a substitute for whole blood and possess no oxygen-carrying capacity. Therefore, to ensure that a patient's hematocrit is not reduced to critical levels, care should be exercised when dextran is used in the treatment of severe hemorrhage. Dextran may be used in situations where hypoproteinemia has been induced by the infusion of a large volume of a crystalloid solution and plasma is not available.

Dextran 70 and 75 are slightly hyperoncotic when compared with plasma, and they induce a water shift of approximately 20 to 25 mL/g from the interstitial fluid space into the vascular system. Dextran 70 and 75 increase the plasma volume by an amount that is slightly greater than the colloidal volume administered. The maximum increase in plasma volume occurs within 1 h of the termination of the infusion and lasts for up to 6 h. The duration of effect depends on the volume infused and rate of clearance from the vascular system.

Dextran 40 is used for vascular volume expansion. The 10% solution is significantly hyperoncotic when compared with plasma, so dextran 40 should be administered with an equal volume of a crystalloid solution to minimize fluid shifts from the interstitial space. The improvement in vascular volume that results from the administration of dextran 40 is equivalent to twice that of the volume infused. The peak volume effect occurs quickly but is brief, lasting only 2 to 3 h. Of the administered dose of dextran 40, 50% is excreted within 3 h, and 75% is excreted within 24 h. Low molecular weight dextran has been advocated for the treatment of impaired microcirculation or capillary sludging during low-flow states induced by hypovolemia or shock. The capability of dextran 40 to enhance blood flow in the microcirculation is attributed to (a) volume expansion and subsequent hemodilution, (b) maintenance of red cell electronegativity, (c) coating of red blood cells and platelets, (d) decreased blood fibrinogen levels, (e) subsequent reductions in blood viscosity, and (f) an increased suspension stability of blood. Dextran 40 has been associated with renal dysfunction, so the use of dextran 70 is preferable for volume expansion.

The primary concerns with respect to the use of dextran solutions relate to the potential for allergic reactions or interference with the normal hemostatic mechanisms of blood. The recommended dose for dextran 40, 70, or 75 is 10 to 20 mL/kg/day in dogs and 5 to 10 mL/kg/day in cats to reduce the possibility of adverse reactions. Infusion rates of 5 mL/kg/h may be used in noncritical situations. Administration rates of up to 20 mL/kg/h have been recommended in situations where the vascular volume must be quickly restored.[83] This rate of infusion induced minimal hemostatic abnormalities in clinically normal animals, but bleeding may be precipitated in dogs with deficiencies in hemostatic function.[83]

Hydroxyethyl Starch

Hydroxyethyl starch is a synthetic polymer that is synthesized from a waxy starch composed primarily of amylopectin. Hydroxyethyl ether groups are introduced into the glucose units of the starch compound to retard degradation of the compound by serum amylase. *Hetastarch*, a commercially available preparation, is a sterile, nonpyrogenic solution of 6% hetastarch in 0.9% saline. The oncotic pressure of hetastarch is 30 mm Hg, and its osmolarity is 310 mOsm/L. The number average molecular weight of hetastarch is 70,000, and the molecular weight of the polymers ranges from 10,000 to 1,000,000. The smaller particles are eliminated through glomerular filtration and renal excretion. Approximately 40% is excreted in urine within 24 h in patients with normal renal function.[84] The larger molecules are slowly degraded by serum amylase until they are small enough to be excreted or taken up into the reticuloendothelial system. This results in a sustained ability of hetastarch to maintain vascular volume expansion as compared with dextran preparations.

Hetastarch may be used for the same purposes as dextran solutions. The colloidal properties of hetastarch are similar to that of albumin. One gram of hetastarch causes a fluid shift into the vascular space of approximately 14 mL of water from the interstitial space.[84] The infusion of hetastarch expands plasma volume only slightly in excess of the volume infused. The volume expansion lasts less than 12 h in dogs and up to 24 h in horses.[85,86] As a result, multiple doses may be required in patients with ongoing protein losses. Hetastarch should not be used in normovolemic patients because of the potential for volume overload. Other complications associated with the infusion of hetastarch solutions include anaphylactoid reactions and coagulopathies.[15,84] A dose of 10 mL to 20 mL/kg/day of 6% hetastarch has been recommended for administration to dogs and 5 to 10 mL/kg/day in cats.[15,87] Rudloff and Kirby have recommended specific infusion rates based on the underlying disease process being treated.[44] Rapid infusion of hetastarch in cats may induce moderate reactions such as nausea and vomiting.[88]

Pentastarch is an isotonic, hyperoncotic solution of 10% pentastarch in 0.9% saline, with an osmolarity of 326 mOsm/L. The number average molecular weight of pentastarch is 35,000. Like hetastarch, pentastarch is indicated for plasma volume expansion when fresh-frozen plasma is not available. The infusion of 500 mL of pentastarch will expand the plasma volume by 700 mL. Pentastarch is more rapidly eliminated than is hetastarch and is less likely to cause coagulopathies. Based on clinical requirements, doses of 10 to 25 mL/kg/day in dogs and 5 to 10 mL/kg/day in cats for up to 3 days has been suggested.[87]

Considerations for Fluid Therapy

Perioperative recognition and management of fluid and electrolyte disturbances are important components of the anesthetic management of surgical patients. Patients that are presented for anesthesia and surgical or diagnostic procedures vary in size, age, metabolic requirements, and physical condition, in addition to the nature of the ongoing disease process. Anesthesiologists must consider each patient's current fluid and electrolyte status in addition to changes that are anticipated to occur during the immediate perioperative period.

In all but the most critical emergencies, clinically significant fluid and electrolyte imbalances in patients should be identified, assessed, and corrected prior to the induction of anesthesia. Many anesthetic protocols require that patients be kept off food and water for varying time lengths in the preoperative period. The use of non per os (NPO) orders causes varying degrees of total body-water deficits, which should be taken into account by the anesthesiologist during the anesthetic procedure. Furthermore, anesthetic agents and many surgical procedures have a significant effect on the cardiovascular stability of patients. There is a net loss of vascular volume during the surgical procedure because of hemorrhage, redistribution, and sequestration of fluids into traumatized tissues at the surgical site. Increased water loss owing to evaporation from the surgical site as well as the respiratory system also becomes important in surgical patients. Postoperatively, fluid and electrolyte imbalances may continue to occur, requiring that the patient be continuously assessed and treated.

Preoperative Considerations

A thorough history should be obtained from the owner. This should provide the clinician with information relating to the type, volume, and duration of fluid losses that have been experienced by the patient. This information, in conjunction with a detailed physical examination, should enable the clinician to estimate the degree of dehydration and the type of electrolyte disturbance that might exist. The degree of dehydration can be estimated by assessing the patient's skin turgor and correlating that information with the other clinical findings. Age of the animal, its nutritional status, and individual variations make skin turgor difficult to assess. In small animals, skin turgor is tested by pinching a skinfold over the torso and twisting it while the animal is in lateral recumbency. Skin turgor is tested in large animals by pinching and twisting the skin of the upper eyelid or the neck. Skin turgor can also be used to determine the hydration status of avian patients.[89] Total body-water deficits in liters are calculated in terms of percentage of body weight measured in kilograms. A patient that is estimated to be 10% dehydrated has lost a volume of water in liters equivalent to 10% of the animal's weight.

Patients with a history of water loss but that have no obvious clinical signs associated with dehydration are generally assumed to be less than 5% dehydrated. Clinical signs do occur in neonatal calves that are 4% dehydrated.[90] The skin tent persists for less than 2 s in these animals. An animal is assumed to be 6% to 8% dehydrated if, on clinical examination, the eyes are mildly sunken in their orbits, the mucous membranes are sticky to dry, and the skin tent persists for more than 3 s. Clinical signs are very pronounced when an animal is 10% to 12% dehydrated. The eyes will be deeply sunken into the orbits, with as much as a 2- to 4-mm gap between the eyeball and bony orbit. The mucous membranes are dry and possibly cold to the touch. The skin tent and twist will persist indefinitely. Animals that are dehydrated more than 15% are generally moribund.

The initial clinical assessment is confirmed by collecting baseline samples from the patient for laboratory analysis. These data confirm the diagnosis and provide a reference point for subsequent therapeutic measures. The information also ensures that the clinician can later assess the patient's response to therapy. Analysis of whole blood, plasma, and serum samples enables the clinician to determine hematologic values, plasma osmolality, serum electrolyte concentrations, and serum glucose, urea, or creatinine values. The measured parameters are then evaluated in relation to the patient's current condition and to expected normal values of each (Table 8.3). Table 8.6 lists the conversion factors required to convert from SI to conventional units. Although serial measurements of body weight have been recommended as aids in determining a patient's response to therapy, these data should be interpreted with care.[90,91]

Hematocrit and total protein values are commonly used to determine the degree of hemoconcentration or hemodilution in patients. Normally, hematocrit values vary widely in some species, whereas, in others, the spleen plays a major role in altering PCV.[33,92] The hematocrit should not be permitted to decrease below 21% to 25% in anesthesia candidates. Normovolemic reductions in PCV to 25% in dogs result in optimal delivery of oxy-

Table 8.6. Conversion of system international units to conventional units.

Constituent	SI Unit	Factor	Conventional Unit
Sodium	mmol/L	1	mEq/L
Potassium	mmol/L	1	mEq/L
Chloride	mmol/L	1	mEq/L
Calcium	mmol/L	4.0080	mg/dL
Magnesium	mmol/L	2.4307	mg/dL
Phosphorus	mmol/L	3.0969	mg/dL
Creatinine	μmol/L	0.0113	mg/dL
Glucose	mmol/L	18.0148	mg/dL
Urea nitrogen	mmol/L	2.8011	mg/dL
Hematocrit	L/L	100	mL/dL, %
Hemoglobin	g/L	0.1	g/dL
Albumin	g/L	0.1	g/dL

gen to peripheral tissues.[65,67,93] Stable, healthy surgical patients will tolerate normovolemic reductions in hematocrit to 21% or hemoglobin levels of 70 g/L if cardiac output is maintained and arterial oxygenation is ensured in the perioperative period.[94] Further reductions in hematocrit increase the potential for inadequate oxygen delivery to the peripheral tissues of anesthetized patients. This is of particular importance to patients with hemodynamic instability or pulmonary disease. Polycythemia, on the other hand, increases blood viscosity and reduces capillary flow, which can reduce the oxygen-delivery capacity of blood with respect to peripheral tissues.[67] Patients, particularly large animal patients, with PCVs in excess of 50% should be treated with fluids to restore the hematocrit to more normal levels.[92]

Total protein levels may represent a more effective index of plasma volume variations than does PCV. Serum protein levels should be maintained above 35 g/L (3.5 g/dL) and albumin levels above 15 g/L (1.5 g/dL) to ensure that there is not a net loss of water from the vascular compartment, resulting in interstitial edema. It has been recommended that, in large animals, fluid therapy is indicated if total serum protein exceeds 80 to 100 g/L (8 to 10 g/dL).[92]

Measurement of serum electrolytes enables clinicians to calculate or measure plasma osmolality and determine whether there are significant life-threatening compositional changes within the extracellular fluid. Plasma osmolality may be calculated as follows:

SI units:

$$mOsm/L = 1.86 \, (NA^+ + K^+) + glucose + BUN + 9$$

Conventional units:

$$mOsm/L = 1.86 \, (NA^+ + K^+) + \left[\frac{glucose}{18} \right] + \left[\frac{BUN}{2.8} \right] + 9$$

Differences between measured and calculated plasma osmolality indicate the presence of unmeasured osmotically active substances in plasma. Determination of plasma osmolality may also aid in the assessment of the degree of dehydration of patients. The fluid deficit in liters may be calculated as follows:[95]

$$fluid \ deficit \ (L) = (0.6) \, BW_{kg} \left[\frac{(mOsm \ plasma - 300)}{300} \right]$$

Urine should be collected and its specific gravity, osmolality, and pH determined. In addition, the sample should be tested for the presence of protein, red blood cells, and glucose.

Once a clinician has assessed a patient's fluid and electrolyte status, a plan for therapeutic intervention, if required, is initiated. Selection of the appropriate fluid for replacement purposes depends on the nature of the disease process and the composition of the fluid lost from the patient. The following criteria have been used in determining the appropriate therapeutic intervention: (a) volume deficit, (b) PCV and total serum protein concentrations, (c) plasma osmolality, (d) electrolyte concentrations, (e) acid-base status, (f) caloric requirements (water-soluble vitamins, carbohydrates, and amino acids), and (g) trace-element concentrations.[96] In those situations where it is necessary to correct fluid and electrolyte deficits prior to surgery, consideration is given to the replacement of previous and continuing losses as well as the provision of maintenance requirements if the animal is not currently ingesting food or water. It is preferable to replenish total body water and correct electrolyte deficits over a 24- to 48-h period. Patients may be stabilized over the first 4 to 6 h, with 50% of the estimated deficit being corrected during that period. Of the deficit, 75% may be corrected within 24 h, in addition to the replacement of concurrent losses and the administration of maintenance requirements. The remainder of the deficit, in conjunction with maintenance requirements, may be administered over the next 24 h. Continuing losses should be estimated and replaced, if necessary, over this period, as well.

In critically ill or moribund patients, vascular and interstitial volume deficits must be corrected as rapidly as is necessary to ensure survival. In the treatment of shock, initial fluid-administration rates of 50 to 90 mL/kg/h in dogs or 50 to 60 mL/kg/h in cats are recommended. Once the crisis has been averted, fluid-administration rates may be reduced to 10 to 12 mL/kg/h in dogs and 5 to 6 mL/kg/h in cats.[97] Lower administration rates in noncrisis situations help ensure adequate expansion of extracellular space before diuresis is induced. In large animal species, administration rates of 60 (equine), 80 (calves), and 40 mL/kg/h (cattle) may be used in the initial stages of shock therapy.[46,98–100]

Fluid Administration

Fluids may be administered orally, subcutaneously, or directly into the vascular space by the intravenous or intraosseous routes. Oral administration of fluids is recommended unless an animal is in critical condition or has severe gastrointestinal disease. Isotonic, nonirritating maintenance solutions may be administered subcutaneously if time and the clinical condition of the patient permit. In critically ill patients, where a rapid response to therapy is desired, fluids and electrolytes should be administered directly into the intravascular compartment. Fluids that are administered intravenously, particularly if administered rapidly or in large volumes, should be warmed to 37°C before being infused or transfused.

Venipuncture, for fluid-administration purposes, is best accomplished with intravenous butterfly sets or catheters. Butterfly infusion sets are not suitable for unsupervised fluid-therapy procedures because of the potential for extravascular infusion of fluids. Similarly, they should not be used routinely for perioperative venous access in surgical patients because they cannot be relied upon to remain intravascular. Short-term venous access for anesthetic procedures and fluid or drug administration is best accomplished with the use of over the needle–type catheters. Angiocath (Deseret Medical, Sandy, UT) intravenous catheters are available in sizes of 24-gauge × 1.9 cm to 10-gauge × 7.6 cm and are made of Teflon (polytetrafluoroethylene). Insyte catheters are constructed of Vialon (Deseret Medical) to increase wall strength that facilitates their passage through the tough skin of domestic and exotic animal species with which veterinarians deal. Catheters made of Vialon have been associated with a 46% lower incidence of thrombophlebitis when compared with catheters made of Teflon.[97] Another product, the Streamline intravenous catheter (Menlo Care, Menlo Park, CA), is made of an elastomeric hydrogel that is hydratable and enlarges after being intravenously placed. One study has demonstrated an increase in flow through a 20-gauge catheter of 26% within 1 h of its intravenous placement.[101] The 20-gauge catheter expanded in size to approximate an 18-gauge catheter.[101] Such products may be of value in establishing an intravenous access quickly when larger catheters may not be easily placed. Through the needle–type intravenous catheters (I-Cath; Delmed, New Brunswick, NJ) are ideal for long-term fluid therapy, although similar catheter styles and lengths are available as over-the-needle catheter placement units (E-Z Cath; Deseret Medical). The length of these intravenous placement units ensures that they are less likely to become dislodged from the intravenous space. This is of concern particularly in large animal patients.

Selection of the venous access site depends on the species involved, the physical condition of the patient, the volume and type of fluid to be administered, the rate of fluid administration, and the accessibility of a peripheral or central vein. The jugular and saphenous veins may be catheterized in most species. The cephalic vein is commonly used in small animal patients, and the auricular vein may be used in some large animal species. The saphenous or jugular veins may be used in larger birds, whereas the cutaneous ulnar vein may be used in small avian patients.[102,103] In situations where large volumes are to be infused quickly, the jugular vein is often the best choice. Catheterization of the jugular vein with a multiport catheter enables the clinician to administer fluids, monitor central venous pressure, and collect blood samples for laboratory analysis. There is a reduced chance of thrombophlebitis if dextrose or hypertonic solutions are infused into the jugular vein as opposed to infusions into smaller peripheral veins.

The rate at which fluids may be intravenously administered is determined by factors such as (a) viscosity of the fluid, (b) internal diameter of the catheter and intravenous administration sys-

tem, (c) length of the intravenous administration system, and (d) the height at which the fluid reservoir is hung above the patient.[104] Of these, the internal diameter of the catheter and the fluid-administration set is the most important factor in determining the maximum rate of flow through the system. In situations where rapid administration of fluid is required, the use of multiple large-bore catheters should be considered. A 20-gauge catheter will permit up to 75 mL/min to flow into the cephalic vein of a canine patient with a gravity feed of 1.75 m. However, if an 18-gauge catheter and a gravity feed of 1.0 to 1.75 m are used, the flow rate would increase to 114 mL/min.[82] Similarly, increasing catheter size to a 16-gauge device increases flow to 160 to 210 mL/min.[98,104] Flow through a 14-gauge catheter is 50% greater than that through a 16-gauge catheter.[105] Further flow increases of up to 21% may be obtained by using a blood administration set as opposed to a traditional intravenous fluid-administration set. In large animals, flow rates can be dramatically improved upon by modifying a Y Type TUR/Bladder Irrigation Set (Baxter, Toronto, Canada) to end in a standard luer lock connector. Fluid-administration rates can be increased further by using pressure-infusor sets, accommodating a 1-L fluid bag (Baxter) up to a 5-L fluid bag (Disposable Pressure Infusor; Biomedical Dynamics, Minneapolis, MN). More rapid rates of fluid administration may be achieved by using mechanized intravenous fluid pumps and multiple intravenous catheter sites.

The intraosseous space provides an alternative route for the parenteral administration of fluids and therapeutic agents into the vascular space. This method of fluid administration should be used whenever intravenous access cannot be established for the treatment of critically ill patients. Therapeutic agents and fluids that are administered into the intraosseous space rapidly reach the systemic circulation via the bone marrow.[106,107] In small animals, the intraosseous space may be accessed through the tibial tuberosity, the trochanteric fossa of the femur, or the flat media surface of the proximal tibial just distal to the tibial tuberosity. In the avian species, the distal end of the ulna is cannulated, because pneumatic bone must be avoided. The details with respect to cannula placement, maintenance, and use of intraosseous administration techniques in small animals have been described.[64,108–110]

Assessment

Once the fluid-therapy regimen is initiated, the clinician should continue to reevaluate the patient to determine its response to therapy. Serial measurements of weight and laboratory values in conjunction with frequent physical examinations enable the clinician to alter the therapeutic regimen according to the patient's changing status. Additional data are obtained in respect to the patient's status and response to therapy through monitoring systemic blood pressure, central venous pressure, volume of urine production, colloid oncotic pressures, and the ECG. These parameters are commonly monitored by the veterinarian in the perioperative period and are discussed in detail elsewhere (Chapter 19).

Intraoperative Considerations

The most common changes during the intraoperative period are alterations to the volume or composition of the extracellular fluid. These alterations result from increased evaporative losses of free water, sequestration of plasma water in traumatized tissues (third spacing), and hemorrhage. Maintenance deficits in anesthetized patients occur in the preoperative period, owing to NPO orders, and continue throughout the intraoperative and recovery periods. Consideration should be given to the fact that intraoperative losses of free water by evaporation exceed values commonly estimated for routine maintenance purposes. The perioperative free-water deficit can be estimated to be at least 2.0 to 2.5 mL/kg for each hour that an animal is not eating or drinking. Ideally, free-water deficits should be replaced using a hypotonic solution, 5% dextrose in water, or a maintenance solution. However, replacement solutions, such as lactated Ringer's, are often used for this purpose to simplify the intraoperative fluid-therapy regimen.

Third-space losses occur through translocation of plasma and intracellular water into surgically traumatized tissues.[94] The degree to which the vascular volume is reduced is directly related to the extent of the surgical trauma to the patient. These losses lead to a hemoconcentration effect and in some instances may be estimated as follows:

$$\text{plasma deficit (mL)} = \left[\text{normal blood volume} - \left[\frac{\text{normal blood volume} \times \text{initial PCV}}{\text{measured PCV}}\right]\right]$$

Third-space losses are replaced with balanced electrolyte solutions at administration rates of up to 2 mL/kg/h for superficial procedures, 3 to 5 mL/kg/h for mildly traumatic procedures, 5 to 10 mL/kg/h for moderately traumatic surgeries, and up to 15 mL/kg/h for severely traumatic procedures. Rates up to 15 mL/kg/h have minimal impact on the PCV of healthy dogs. In avian species, intraoperative fluid-administration rates of 10 mL/kg/h for the first 2 h and 5 to 8 mL/kg/h for subsequent hours have been recommended.[17] Third-space loss is replaced in addition to that volume of fluid being administered for maintenance purposes.

Acute, intraoperative losses of blood in excess of 15% of total blood volume in normal patients or 10% in critically ill patients should be replaced with whole blood or packed red cells. A hemoglobin-based, oxygen-carrying solution such as Oxyglobin (bovine hemoglobin glutamer 200) may be of value in instances where whole blood or packed red cells are not available. There is some debate as to the clinical utility of regular use of such solutions, and readers are directed to other sources for additional information.[111–116] The manufacturer's recommended dose of Oxyglobin in dogs is 30 mL/kg infused at a rate of 10 mL/kg/h. A lower infusion rate of 3 to 5 mL/kg/h should be used if the solution is administered to cats. The lower infusion rate in cats may prevent the development of pulmonary edema, pleural effusion, or both.[115] Blood loss that does not exceed the limits previously mentioned may be replaced with balanced electrolyte or replacement solutions. As already mentioned, crystalloid solutions equilibrate across the extracellular fluid space, and it is necessary to administer a volume of fluid up to five times the volume of blood that has been lost from the vascular space.[23] As they occur, whole blood losses are replaced with the appropriate volume of colloid or balanced electrolyte solution.

Finally, consideration must also be given to the administration of fluids to maintain cardiovascular stability and organ perfusion, which might be altered by the direct hemodynamic effects of the anesthetic drugs used. The total volume of fluid administered to patients in the perioperative period should be adjusted to ensure that vital signs such as blood pressure and urine production are maintained above critical levels. It is important to remember that perioperative release of alcohol dehydrogenase can reduce the volume of urine produced. This will complicate the ability to assess or use urine production as a prognostic indicator of volume expansion.

The intraoperative administration of large volumes of replacement fluids can lead to hemodilution and the interstitial accumulation of fluids. Although some degree of hemodilution can be beneficial, the hematocrit should be maintained above 21% in healthy patients and at 25% at least in critically ill patients. Total serum protein levels should not be permitted to decrease to below 35 g/L (3.5 g/dL) or albumin to levels below 15 g/L (1.5 g/dL).[65] It has been suggested that hypertonic saline and dextran 70 solutions may be of value for the intraoperative management of hemorrhagic episodes in maintaining hemodynamic function and reducing the possibility of inducing a fluid volume overload.[50]

Continual assessment of the patient is necessary to maintain cardiovascular stability postoperatively. If ongoing blood losses are not of concern, then the clinician's attention should be directed toward replacing continuing third-space losses and maintenance requirements of the patient. Care should be exercised when administering crystalloid solutions in the postoperative period. Overt fluid overloading may not be readily apparent in patients until 24 to 72 h after the surgical procedure. Postsurgical alterations in aldosterone and alcohol dehydrogenase activity result in reduced free-water clearance in the postoperative period. Once the neurohormonal responses to the surgical procedure abate, third-space fluid and the excess fluid in the interstitial space are mobilized and returned to the vascular space. This can cause a volume overload that might be detrimental to critically ill patients (e.g., those with pulmonary edema).[40]

Electrolyte Disturbances

Compositional changes in the extracellular fluid during the perioperative period may be caused by previous or ongoing disease processes or they may be iatrogenic in origin. Clinically significant disturbances in electrolyte balance should be corrected in the preoperative period. Acute, life-threatening, intraoperative alterations in sodium, calcium, or magnesium concentrations are uncommon unless iatrogenically induced.

Sodium

This is the osmolar skeleton of the extracellular fluid. Sodium balance may be altered by depletion or retention of water, sodium, or both. Sodium regulation and diseases that result in sodium imbalances are discussed elsewhere.[11,15,117]

Hyponatremia exists when the serum sodium concentration is less than 136 mmol/L (136 mEq/L). Clinical signs relating to neurological dysfunction occur when the sodium concentration is less than 120 mmol/L (120 mEq/L) and become marked when serum sodium is less than 110 mmol/L (110 mEq/L). Clinical signs include anorexia, lethargy, weakness, vomiting, muscle cramping, myoclonus, seizures, tachycardia, shock, and coma. In complicated cases, the ECG may reveal a widened QRS complex with an elevated ST segment. A nonrespiratory dilutional acidosis may also develop. Ventricular tachycardia or fibrillation can occur when serum sodium levels are below 100 mmol/L (100 mEq/L). Severe hyponatremia may be corrected with the careful administration of 3% saline over 24 h. It has been recommended that the amount of sodium to be administered during this period be calculated as follows:[15]

$$\text{mmol Na}^+ = 0.2\ \text{BW}_{kg}\,(\text{normal }[\text{Na}^+] - \text{patient's }[\text{Na}^+])$$

In less severe situations, free-water restriction, correction of the underlying cause, and intravenous administration of 0.9% saline may be considered.

Hypernatremia occurs most commonly owing to water loss in excess of the sodium loss in small animal patients. Those animals that do not have free access to water are prone to develop hypernatremia if they have increased water losses such as would occur from heat prostration, burns, and so forth. Salt poisoning occurs commonly in cattle and swine.[117] Serum sodium concentrations above 156 mmol/L (156 mEq/L) in dogs and 160 mmol/L (160 mEq/L) in cats and large animal species constitute hypernatremia. Severe hypernatremia may lead to nonrespiratory concentration alkalosis. Clinical signs include lethargy, confusion, muscle weakness, myoclonus, seizures, and coma. The severity of the clinical signs depends on the rate of onset and the degree of the hypernatremia. Treatment depends on the initial cause of the hypernatremia and the chronicity of the electrolyte imbalance. Significant sodium imbalances should be medically managed and corrected prior to any anesthetic or surgical procedure. Details regarding the medical management of hypernatremic states are readily available from a number of sources.[11,15,118]

Calcium

This ion plays a major role in the physiology of neuromuscular function, cell membrane permeability, muscle contraction, and hemostasis. With respect to total body content, up to 99% of calcium is located within bone. Total serum calcium consists of an ionized portion, a protein-bound portion, and a portion that is complexed to divalent anions such as phosphate and bicarbonate. Close to 50% of total serum calcium is bound to proteins, primarily albumin. Although the ionized portion (40%) is the physiologically active fraction, it is rarely measured. Serum ionized calcium levels are pH dependent, with alkalemia reducing and acidemia increasing ionized serum calcium levels. In dogs, formulas have been developed to adjust calcium measurements to account for alterations in serum protein or albumin concentrations.[119] In cats, at least one study has recommended that similar adjustments not be made.[120]

Symptomatic hypocalcemia can be caused by hypoparathyroidism and eclampsia in small animals or parturient paresis in large animal species. Intraoperative hypocalcemia, induced by the administration of large volumes of citrated whole blood, reduces ventricular function and systemic blood pressure.[121] Hypocalcemia exists when serum calcium levels are below 1.75 mmol/L (7 mg/dL) in small animals and below 2.0 mmol/L (8 mg/dL) in large animal species. Hypoalbuminemia may induce hypocalcemia of 1.75 to 2.0 mmol/L (7 to 8 mg/dL) in small animals. Serum calcium concentrations below 1.62 mmol/L (6.5 mg/dL) are generally the result of a metabolic disorder. Small animals with hypocalcemia may show clinical signs of restlessness, muscle fasciculations, tetany, or convulsions. The ECG may show prolonged QT and ST segments because of prolonged myocardial action potentials. Recently calved, mature cattle with parturient paresis often have serum calcium levels less than 1.25 mmol/L (5 mg/dL). These cows become recumbent when serum calcium levels are less than 1.5 mmol/L (6 mg/dL). Serum calcium levels less than 1.0 mmol/L (4 mg/dL) are fatal.

Acute, intraoperative, hypocalcemic episodes that are iatrogenic in origin may be treated with 10% calcium chloride or calcium gluconate: 10% calcium chloride contains 1.4 mEq/mL of calcium, whereas calcium gluconate contains 0.45 mEq/mL of calcium. The dose to be administered depends on the severity of the situation and ranges from 5 to 15 mg/kg administered over 1 h. If more than 50 mL/kg of whole blood or packed red cells is administered, then calcium supplementation should be considered in order to counteract the effects of the anticoagulant. Up to 6 mL of calcium chloride/gluconate per unit of blood may be administered via a separate intravenous route. The ECG should be observed for evidence of toxicity during the infusion, and additional laboratory data should be assessed prior to administering subsequent calcium salts.

Hypercalcemia can result from hyperparathyroidism or malignancies in small animals, whereas in large animals it is often iatrogenic in origin—in many instances the result of excessive dietary supplementation. Hypercalcemia has been reported to occur in horses with chronic renal failure.[117] Hemoconcentration that results in increased serum albumin levels may increase serum calcium levels to 3.2 mmol/L (13 mg/dL). Serum calcium concentrations above 3 mmol/L (12 mg/dL) in dogs and 2.74 mmol/L (11 mg/dL) in cats are indicative of hypercalcemia. Clinical signs include anorexia, vomiting, and gastrointestinal dysfunction. Generalized locomotor weakness may also be evident. Bradycardia, with a prolonged PR interval and a shortened ST segment, may be observed. Rapid increases in serum calcium levels in excess of 3.74 mmol/L (15 mg/dL) may lead to vagal stimulation and severe bradycardia, whereas severe, but less acute, increases may lead to ventricular dysrhythmias.[122,123]

Potassium

This is the primary intracellular cation, and at least 90% of the total body potassium content is located within the intracellular compartment. Extracellular fluid potassium content represents approximately 2% of the total body content. As a result, serum potassium levels may not accurately represent the extent or severity of a potassium disorder, particularly in chronic disease processes. Potassium is highly labile, and serum levels are significantly altered in the presence of acidemia, alkalemia, or extracellular fluid osmolality changes or by alterations in serum insulin, glucagon, or catecholamine concentrations. Changes in extracellular fluid pH cause rapid and significant alterations in the potassium concentration of extracellular fluid. Acute reductions in $PaCO_2$ of 10 mm Hg have been shown to increase plasma pH by 0.1 unit and decrease plasma potassium by 0.4 mmol/L (0.4 mEq/L) in dogs.[124] Similarly, in cats, serum potassium concentrations change on an order of 0.6 to 0.7 mmol/L (0.6 to 0.7 mEq/L) per 0.1 unit change in pH.[58] Intraoperative ventilatory or metabolic acid-base disturbances are common, particularly in critically ill patients. Anesthesiologists must monitor patients for, and respond to, significant alterations in plasma potassium levels before they become life-threatening.

Hypokalemia results from reductions in dietary intake or increased losses through the urinary or gastrointestinal systems. Increased losses through the urinary system can be caused by osmotic diuresis, chronic steroid therapy, or the use of loop or thiazide diuretics. Alkalemia will reduce serum potassium levels as extracellular potassium moves intracellularly in exchange for hydrogen ions. The degree to which clinical signs become apparent depends on the rapidity of the electrolyte alteration and the chronicity of the disease process. An acute reduction in serum potassium levels to less than 3.0 mmol/L (3 mEq/L) results in clinical signs that may include reduced gastrointestinal motility and generalized muscle weakness. Rapid reductions in extracellular potassium levels disrupt the normal intracellular to extracellular potassium ratio and hyperpolarize myocardial cells. The ECG demonstrates evidence of prolonged repolarization times, with prolonged PR, QRS, and QT intervals, depression of the ST segment, and a flattened or inverted T wave. Severe cardiac manifestations of hypokalemia may include sinus bradycardia, heart block, paroxysmal atrial tachycardia, and atrioventricular dissociation.[118] Clinical signs may not be apparent until the potassium concentration approaches 2.5 mmol/L (2.5 mEq/L) in chronic conditions.

Patients in which serum potassium levels have been acutely reduced to below 3.0 mmol/L (3 mEq/L) should have their serum potassium levels corrected, if at all possible, before inducing anesthesia. Moderate to severe reductions in serum potassium levels (2.5 mEq/L) may require the intravenous administration of potassium chloride. It is important that the clinician assess the patient's cardiac and renal function and that the fluid volume and acid-base status of the patient be determined. Volume deficits and acid-base disturbances should be corrected early to ensure adequate renal perfusion and to enable the clinician to determine the plasma potassium levels in a more normalized situation with respect to the patient's acid-base status. Potassium chloride may be infused at a rate of 0.5 mmol/kg/h (0.5 mEq/kg/h) to a maximum daily dose of 2 to 3 mmol/kg (2 to 3 mEq/kg).[118] Patient status must be monitored continually during this period. In addition to serial potassium determinations, the patient should be monitored with an ECG so that early signs of potassium toxicity can be detected.

In situations where the potassium imbalance is caused by a chronic disease process, anesthesia and surgery should be delayed, if possible, and the imbalance corrected and medically managed over 3 to 5 days. In this situation, the goal is to replenish the total body potassium deficit without inducing clinical signs of potassium toxicity. This may be accomplished through the oral administration of potassium supplements or the parenteral administration of a maintenance solution in which the potassium level has been adjusted to at least 20 to 30 mmol/L (20 to 30 mEq/L). Again, it is imperative to assess the patient's status continually and alter the therapeutic regimen accordingly.

If the surgical procedure cannot be delayed, then it may be prudent not to correct serum potassium levels that have been reduced to values between 2.5 to 3.0 mmol/L (2.5 to 3.0 mEq/L) by a chronic process. Rapid corrections of plasma potassium levels in this instance may acutely disturb the intracellular to extracellular potassium ratio and induce alterations in cell membrane stability. In humans, chronic reductions of serum potassium levels to 2.6 mmol/L (2.6 mEq/L) were not associated with, or predictive of, intraoperative dysrhythmias. Instead, intraoperative dysrhythmias were better correlated with the incidence of preoperative dysrhythmias.[125]

Hyperkalemia is not as common in large animals as in small animals, but it does occur with acidemia and equine hyperkalemic periodic paralysis. In small animals, increases in plasma potassium levels in excess of 6.5 mmol/L (6.5 mEq/L) may be iatrogenic or result from renal failure, urethral obstruction, hypoadrenocorticoidism, or acidemia. Postoperatively, increased plasma potassium levels may occur owing to increased tissue catabolism or acidemia. Neonates, Akitas, and English springer spaniels are known to have a high potassium content (20 mEq/L) within their red blood cells, and hemolysis may cause hyperkalemia.[126] In most instances, there is no total body excess of potassium, and the increase in potassium content is limited to the extracellular fluid compartment.

Increases in extracellular fluid potassium concentrations decrease the magnitude of cell membrane polarization, which subsequently enhances membrane excitability. Clinical signs become apparent once the plasma potassium concentration exceeds 6.5 mmol/L (6.5 mEq/L). Myocardial contractility decreases and bradycardia develops. As the plasma potassium concentration approaches 8 mmol/L (8 mEq/L), the ECG will show peaked T waves and a decrease in the P-wave amplitude. Plasma potassium concentrations above 8 mmol/L (8 mEq/L) have a significant effect on myocardial activity. The PR interval is prolonged, and the P wave may be absent. As the potassium level increases, the QRS complex widens until it assumes a sine-wave appearance, and atrioventricular dissociation occurs. Eventually, asystole or ventricular fibrillation ensues. Patients with a plasma potassium concentration above 6.5 mmol/L (6.5 mEq/L) should not be anesthetized unless the patient's life is immediately threatened by some other process.

Severe potassium-induced cardiotoxicity may be initially antagonized by the intravenous administration of 10% calcium chloride or gluconate at a dose of 0.2 to 0.3 mEq/kg. If the dysrhythmias persist, the dosage may be repeated in 5 min. Additional doses of calcium salts after this point are unlikely to be of benefit. Calcium will help restore cell membrane potentials, and although its effect will last only for 10 to 20 min, this will provide time to institute other therapeutic measures. Rapid decreases in plasma potassium concentration may also be achieved by instituting controlled ventilation and reversing respiratory acidosis rapidly.[94]

Fluid volume deficits and acid-base disturbances should be assessed and corrected: 5% dextrose or 0.9% saline may be used to correct the fluid deficit, promote diuresis, and functionally dilute the extracellular potassium. Dextrose solutions not only provide free water for volume-replacement purposes but enhance the cellular uptake of potassium as part of the normal mechanisms of glucose metabolism. In situations where plasma potassium levels are significantly increased, glucose may be administered at a dose of 0.5 to 1.0 g/kg to enhance the intracellular movement of potassium. The effect of this therapeutic measure should last for a few hours. The effect of glucose on serum potassium concentration may be facilitated by administering 0.5 unit/kg of regular insulin combined with dextrose at a ratio of 2 g of dextrose per unit of administered insulin.[118] Correction of acidemia will result in an intracellular shift of potassium in exchange for hydrogen ions. Considerations for therapeutic measures in acid-base disturbances are discussed in Chapter 7. Patients should be continually assessed and care taken to ensure that the therapeutic measures undertaken do not cause hypokalemia or other functional disturbances.

References

1. Spurlock SL, Furr M. Fluid therapy. In: Koterba AM, Drummond WH, Kosch PC, eds. Equine Clinical Neonatology. Philadelphia: Lea and Febiger, 1990:671–685.
2. Carlson GP. Fluid, electrolyte and acid-base balance. In: Kaneko JJ, Harvey JW, Bruss B, eds. Clinical Biochemistry of Domestic Animals, 5th ed. Boston: Academic, 1997:485–516.
3. Ruckebusch Y, Phaneuf L-P, Dunlop R, eds. Physiology of Small and Large Animals. Philadelphia: BC Decker, 1991:8–18.
4. Carlson GP. Blood chemistry, body fluids and hematology. In: Gillespie JR, Robinson N, eds. Equine Exercise Physiology 2. Davis, CA: ICEEP, 1987:393–425.
5. Wagstaff AJ, Maclean I, Michell AR, et al. Plasma and extracellular volume in calves: Comparison between isotopic and cold techniques. Res Vet Sci 53:271–273, 1992.
6. Turner DAB. Fluid, electrolyte and acid-base balance. In: Aitkenhead AR, Smith G, eds. Textbook of Anaesthesia, 2nd ed. New York: Churchill Livingstone, 1990:389–403.
7. Stoelting RK. Pharmacology and Physiology in Anesthetic Practice. Philadelphia: JB Lippincott, 1987.
8. Saxton CR, Seldin DW. Clinical interpretation of laboratory values. In: Kokko JP, Tannen RL, eds. Fluids and Electrolytes. Philadelphia: WB Saunders, 1986:3–62.
9. Rose BD. Clinical Physiology of Acid-Base and Electrolyte Disorders, 2nd ed. New York: McGraw-Hill, 1984:4–41.
10. Kirby R, Rudloff E. The critical need for colloids: Maintaining fluid balance. Compend Contin Educ 19:705–717, 1997.
11. Scott RC. Disorders of sodium metabolism. Vet Clin North Am Small Anim Pract 12:375–397, 1982.
12. Hardy RM. Disorders of water metabolism. Vet Clin North Am Small Anim Pract 12:353–373, 1982.
13. Goudsouzian N, Karamanian A. Physiology for the Anesthesiologist, 2nd ed. Norwalk, CT: Appleton-Century-Crofts, 1984.
14. Guyton AC, Coleman TC. Regulation on interstitial fluid volume and pressure. Ann NY Acad Sci 150:537–547, 1968.
15. Garvey MS. Fluid and electrolyte balance in critical patients. Vet Clin North Am Small Animal Pract 19:1021–1056, 1989.
16. Schaer M. General principles of fluid therapy in small animal medicine. Vet Clin North Am Small Anim Pract 19:203–213, 1989.
17. Steinohrt LA. Avian fluid therapy. J Avian Med Surg 13:83–91, 1999.
18. Rose RJ. A physiological approach to fluid and electrolyte therapy in the horse. Equine Vet J 13:7–14, 1981.
19. Barragry TB. Some aspects of fluid and electrolyte imbalances in animals. Ir Vet J Aug 28:153–159, 1974.
20. Tremblay RRM. Intravenous fluid therapy in calves. Vet Clin North Am Food Anim Pract 6:77–101, 1990.
21. Reece WO. Physiology of Domestic Animals. Philadelphia: Lea and Febiger, 1991.
22. Mitchell AR. Small animal fluid therapy 1: Practice principles. J Small Anim Pract 35:559–565, 1994.
23. Tollofsrud S, Elgjo GI, Prough DS, et al. The dynamics of vascular volume and fluid shifts of lactated Ringer's solution and hypertonic-saline–dextran solutions infused in normovolemic sheep. Anesth Analg 93:823–831, 2001.
24. Scheingraber S, Rehm M, Sehmisch C, et al. Rapid saline infusion produces hyperchloremic acidosis in patients undergoing gynecologic surgery. Anesthesiology 90:1265–1270, 1999.
25. Ho AM, Karmakar MK, Contardi LH, et al. Excessive use of normal saline in managing traumatized patients in shock: A preventable contributor to acidosis. J Trauma 51:173–177, 2001.
26. Prough DS. Acidosis associated with perioperative saline administration. Anesthesiology 93:1167–1169, 2000.
27. Gibbons G. Hypertonic solutions in the treatment of shock. In: Proceedings of the Eighth Annual Veterinary Medical Forum. Madison, WI: Omnipress, 1990:69–72.
28. Prough DS, Whitley JM, Olympio MA, et al. Hypertonic/hyperoncotic fluid resuscitation after hemorrhagic shock in dogs. Anesth Analg 73:738–744, 1991.
29. Zoran DL, Jergens AE, Riedesel DH, et al. Evaluation of hemostatic analytes after use of hypertonic saline solutions combined with colloids for resuscitation of dogs with hypovolemia. Am J Vet Res 53:1791–1796, 1992.
30. Muir WW, Sally J. Small volume resuscitation with hypertonic saline solution in hypovolemic cats. Am J Vet Res 50:1883–1888, 1989.
31. Schmall LM, Muir WW, Robertson JT. Haemodynamic effects of small volume hypertonic saline in experimentally induced haemorrhagic shock. Equine Vet J 22:273–277, 1990.
32. Schmall LM, Muir WW, Robertson JT. Haematological, serum electrolyte and blood gas effects of small volume hypertonic saline in experimentally induced haemorrhagic shock. Equine Vet J 22:278–283, 1990.
33. Constable PD. Hypertonic saline. Vet Clin North Am Food Anim Pract 15:559–585, 1999.
34. Muir WW. Small volume resuscitation using hypertonic saline. Cornell Vet 80:7–12, 1990.
35. Muir WW. Comparative aspects of hypertonic saline resuscitation. In: Proceedings of the Seventh Annual Veterinary Medical Forum. Madison, WI: Omnipress, 1989:836–839.
36. Rocha e Silva M, Velasco IT. Hypertonic saline resuscitation: The neural component. Prog Clin Biol Res 299:303–310, 1989.
37. Hellyer PW, Meyer RE. Effects of hypertonic saline on myocardial contractility in anaesthetized pigs. J Vet Pharmacol Ther 17:211–217, 1994.
38. Constable PD, Muir WW, Binkley PF. Effect of hypertonic saline solution on left ventricular afterload in normovolemic dogs. Am J Vet Res 56:1513–1521, 1995.

39. Kien ND, Kramer GC, White DA. Acute hypotension caused by rapid hypertonic saline infusion in anesthetized dogs. Anesth Analg 73:597–602, 1991.

40. Shackford SR. Hypertonic saline and dextran for intraoperative fluid therapy: More for less. Crit Care Med 20:160–162, 1992.

41. Kramer GC, English TP, Gunther RA, et al. Physiological mechanisms of fluid resuscitation with hyperosmotic/hyperoncotic solutions. Prog Clin Biol Res 299:311–320, 1989.

42. Gala GJ, Lilly MP, Thomas SE, et al. Interaction of sodium and volume in fluid resuscitation after hemorrhage. J Trauma 31:545–556, 1991.

43. Hinchcliff KW, Schmall LM, McKeever KH, et al. Effect of hypertonic saline administration on blood and plasma volume of normal horses. In: Proceedings of the Ninth Annual Veterinary Medical Forum. Madison, WI: Omnipress, 1991:387–388.

44. Rudloff E, Kirby R. Fluid therapy: Crystalloids and colloids. Vet Clin North Am Small Anim Pract 28:297–328, 1998.

45. Bertone JJ, Shoemaker KE. Effect of hypertonic and isotonic saline solutions on plasma constituents of conscious horses. Am J Vet Res 53:1844–1849, 1992.

46. Constable P. Fluid and electrolyte therapy in ruminants. Vet Clin North Am Food Anim Pract 19:557–597, 2003.

47. Rabinovici R, Krausz MM, Feuerstein G. Control of bleeding is essential for a successful treatment of hemorrhagic shock with 7.5 percent sodium chloride solution. Surg Gynecol Obstet 173:98–106, 1991.

48. Prough DS, Whitley JM, Olympio MA, et al. Hypertonic/hyperoncotic fluid resuscitation after hemorrhagic shock in dogs. Anesth Analg 73:738–744, 1991.

49. Rocha e Silva M, Negraes GA, Soares AM, et al. Hypertonic resuscitation from severe hemorrhagic shock: Patterns of regional circulation. Circ Shock 19:165–175, 1986.

50. Pascual JMS, Watson JC, Runyon AE, et al. Resuscitation of intraoperative hypovolemia: A comparison of normal saline and hyperosmotic/hyperoncotic solutions in swine. Crit Care Med 20:200–210, 1992.

51. Allen DA, Schertel ER, Muir WW, et al. Hypertonic saline/dextran resuscitation of dogs with experimentally induced gastric dilatation-volvulus shock. Am J Vet Res 52:92–96, 1991.

52. Horton JW, Walker PB. Small-volume hypertonic saline dextran resuscitation from canine endotoxin shock. Ann Surg 214:64–73, 1991.

53. Moon PF, Synder JR, Haskins SC, et al. Effects of a highly concentrated hypertonic saline–dextran volume expander on cardiopulmonary function in anesthetized horses. Am J Vet Res 52:1611–1618, 1991.

54. Sondeen JL, Gunther RA, Dubick MA. Comparison of 7.5% NaCl/6% dextran-70 resuscitation of hemorrhage between euhydrated and dehydrated sheep. Shock 3:63–68, 1995.

55. Okrasinski EB, Krahwinkel DJ, Sanders WL. Treatment of dogs in hemorrhagic shock by intraosseous infusion of hypertonic saline and dextran. Vet Surg 21:20–24, 1992.

56. Anaya C, Drace C, Myers T, et al. Less net volume loading with hypertonic saline dextran resuscitation of intraoperative hypovolemia [Abstract]. Anesthesiology 75:A1122, 1991.

57. Remillard RL, Thatcher CO. Parenteral nutritional support in the small animal patient. Vet Clin North Am Small Anim Pract 19:1287–1306, 1989.

58. Chew DJ, Leonard M, Muir WW. Effect of sodium bicarbonate infusion on serum osmolality, electrolyte concentrations, and blood gas tensions in cats. Am J Vet Res 52:12–17, 1991.

59. Moon PF, Barr SC, Erb HN. Effects of tromethamine buffer on coagulation variables and ionized calcium concentration in dogs. Am J Vet Res 58:777–780, 1997.

60. Moon PF, Gabor L, Gleed RD, et al. Acid-base, metabolic, and hemodynamic effects of sodium bicarbonate or tromethamine administration in anesthetized dogs with experimentally induced metabolic acidosis. Am J Vet Res 58:771–776, 1997.

61. Robin ED, Wilson RJ, Bromberg PA. Intracellular acid-base relationships and intracellular buffers. Ann NY Acad Sci 92:539–546, 1961.

62. Wolfsheimer KJ. Fluid therapy in the critically ill patient. Vet Clin North Am Small Anim Pract 19:361–378, 1989.

63. Iazbik C, Couto CG, Gray TL, et al. Effect of storage conditions on hemostatic parameters of canine plasma obtained for transfusion. Am J Vet Res 62:734–735, 2001.

64. Wagner A, Dunlop CI. Anesthetic and medical management of acute hemorrhage during surgery. J Am Vet Med Assoc 203:40–45, 1993.

65. Sunder-Plassmann L, Klovekorn WP, Holper K, et al. The physiological significance of acutely induced hemodilution. In: Ditzel R, Lewis D, eds. Proceedings of the Sixth European Conference on Microcirculation, 1970. Basel: S Karger, 1971:23–28.

66. Messmer K, Kreimeier U, Intaglietta M. Present state of intentional hemodilution. Eur Surg Res 18:254–263, 1986.

67. Messmer K. Hemodilution. Surg Clin North Am 55:659–677, 1975.

68. Lanevschi A, Wardrop KJ. Principles of transfusion medicine in small animals. Can Vet J 42:447–454, 2001.

69. Hunt E, Moore JS. Use of blood and blood products. Vet Clin North Am Food Anim Pract 6:133–147, 1990.

70. Ou D, Mahaffey E, Smith JE. Effect of storage on oxygen dissociation of canine blood. J Am Vet Assoc 167:56–58, 1975.

71. Harvey JW. The erythrocyte: Physiology, metabolism and biochemical disorders. In: Kanenko JJ, Harvey JW, Bruss B, eds. Clinical Biochemistry of Domestic Animals, 5th ed. Boston: Academic, 1997:157–203.

72. Giger U, Bucheler J. Transfusion of type-A and type-B blood to cats. J Am Vet Med Assoc 198:411–418, 1991.

73. Giger U, Kilrain CG, Filippich LJ, et al. Frequencies of feline blood groups in the United States. J Am Vet Med Assoc 195:1230–1232, 1989.

74. Griot-Wenk ME, Callan MB, Casal ML, et al. Blood type AB in the feline AB blood group system. Am J Vet Res 57:1438–1442, 1996.

75. Kallfelz FA, Whitlock RH, Schultz RD. Survival of 59Fe-labeled erythrocytes in cross-transfused equine blood. Am J Vet Res 39:617–620, 1978.

76. Stormont CJ. Blood groups in animals. J Am Vet Med Assoc 181:1120–1124, 1982.

77. Kirk RW, Bistner SI, Ford RB, eds. Handbook of Veterinary Procedures and Emergency Treatment. Philadelphia: WB Saunders, 1990.

78. Cassady JF, Patel RI, Epstein BS. Calculations for predicting blood transfusion needs [Letter to the editor]. Anesthesia 59:491, 1983.

79. Hammer AS, Couto CG. Disorders of hemostasis and principles of transfusion therapy. In: Allen DG, ed. Small Animal Medicine. Philadelphia: JB Lippincott, 1991:173–194.

80. Slovis NM. How to approach whole blood transfusions in horses. Am Assoc Equine Pract Proc 47:266–269, 2001.

81. Harrell K, Parrow J, Kristensen A. Canine transfusion reactions. Part I. Causes and consequences. Compend Contin Educ 19:181–200, 1997.

82. Harrell K, Parrow J, Kristensen A. Canine transfusion reactions. Part II. Prevention and treatment. Compend Contin Educ 19:193–201, 1997.

83. Concannon KT, Haskins SC, Feldman BF. Hemostatic defects associated with two infusion rates of dextran 70 in dogs. Am J Vet Res 53:1369–1375, 1992.

84. Fritsch R. A review of plasma substitutes. Proc Assoc Vet Anaesth Gr Br Ir 10:170–179, 1982.

85. Moore LE, Garvey MS. The effect of hetastarch on serum colloid oncotic pressure in hypoalbuminemic dogs. J Vet Intern Med 10:300–303, 1996.

86. Jones PA, Bain FT, Byars TD, et al. Effect of hydroxyethyl starch infusion on colloid oncotic pressure in hypoproteinemic horses. J Am Vet Med Assoc 218:1130–1135, 2001.

87. Mathews KA. The various types of parenteral fluids and their indications. Vet Clin North Am Small Anim Pract 28:483–513, 1998.

88. Rudloff E, Kirby R. The critical need for colloids: Selecting the right colloid. Compend Contin Educ 19:811–825, 1997.

89. Murray MJ. Use of subcutaneous fluids in the avian patient. J Assoc Avian Vet 3:194–195, 1989.

90. Constable PD, Walker PG, Morin DE, et al. Clinical and laboratory assessment of hydration status of neonatal calves with diarrhea. J Am Vet Med Assoc 212:991–996, 1998.

91. Hansen B, DeFrancesco T. Relationship between hydration estimate and body weight change after fluid therapy in critically ill dogs and cats. J Vet Emerg Crit Care 12:235–243, 2002.

92. Blood DC, Radostits OM, eds. Veterinary Medicine: A Textbook of the Diseases of Cattle, Sheep, Pigs, Goats and Horses, 7th ed. Philadelphia: Balliere Tindall, 1989:58–76.

93. Messmer K. Compensatory mechanisms for acute dilutional anemia. Bibl Haematol 47:31–42, 1981.

94. Njoku MJ, Matjasko MJ. Intraoperative fluid management. Surv Anesth 38:120–123, 1994.

95. Genetzky RM, Loparco FV, Ledet AE. Clinical pathologic alterations in horses during a water deprivation test. Am J Vet Res 48:1007–1011, 1987.

96. Haskins SC. Fluid and electrolyte therapy. Compend Contin Educ Pract Vet 6:244–260, 1984.

97. Goodwin JK, Schaer M. Septic shock. Vet Clin North Am Small Anim Pract 19:1239–1258, 1989.

98. Berchtold J. Intravenous fluid therapy of calves. Vet Clin North Am Food Anim Pract 15:505–531, 1999.

99. Roussel AJ Jr. Fluid therapy in mature cattle. Vet Clin North Am Food Anim Pract 6:111–123, 1990.

100. McDonell WN. General anesthesia for equine gastrointestinal and obstetric procedures. Vet Clin North Am Large Anim Pract 3:163–194, 1981.

101. Jones BR, Scheller MS. Flow increases with an enlarging intravenous catheter. J Clin Anesth 4:120–122, 1992.

102. Abou-Madi N. Avian fluid therapy. In: Proceedings of the Ninth Annual Veterinary Medical Forum. Madison, WI: Omnipress, 1991:495–497.

103. Redig PT. Fluid therapy and acid-base balance in the critically ill avian patient. In: Proceedings of the International Conference on Avian Medicine. Toronto: American Association of Avian Veterinarians, 1984:487–500.

104. Fulton RB, Hauptman JG. In vitro and in vivo rates of fluid flow through catheters in peripheral veins of dogs. J Am Vet Med Assoc 198:1622–1624, 1991.

105. Stoneham MD. An evaluation of methods of increasing the flow rate of i.v. fluid administration. Br J Anaesth 75:361–365, 1995.

106. Aeschbacher G, Webb AI. Intraosseous infusion during cardiopulmonary resuscitation. Vet Surg 20:159, 1991.

107. Hoelzer MF. Recent Advances in Intravenous Therapy. Emerg Med Clin North Am 4:487–500, 1986.

108. Otto CM, Crow DT. Intraosseous resuscitation techniques and applications. In: Kirk RW, Bonagura JD, eds. Current Veterinary Therapy XI: Small Animal Practice. Philadelphia: WB Saunders, 1992:107–112.

109. Golenz MR, Kuesis BS, Carlson GP. Intraosseous infusion of fluids and medications to a neonatal foal with septicemia: A case report. J Equine Vet Sci 14:152–154, 1994.

110. Hughes D, Beal MW. Emergency vascular access. Vet Clin North Am Small Anim Pract 30:491–507, 2000.

111. Muir WW, Wellman ML. Hemoglobin solutions and tissue oxygenation. J Vet Intern Med 17:127–135, 2003.

112. Day TK. Current development and use of hemoglobin-based oxygen-carrying (HBOC) solutions. J Vet Emerg Crit Care 13:77–93, 2003.

113. Muir WW, de Morais HSA, Constable PD. The effects of a hemoglobin-based oxygen carrier (HBOC-301) on left ventricular systolic function in anesthetized dogs. Vet Surg 29:449–455, 2000.

114. Driessen B, Jahr JS, Lurie F, et al. Inadequacy of low-volume resuscitation with hemoglobin-based oxygen carrier hemoglobin glutamer-200 (bovine) in canine hypovolemia. J Vet Pharmacol Ther 24:61–71, 2001.

115. Gibson GR, Jahr JS, Lurie F, et al. Use of hemoglobin-based oxygen-carrying solution in cats: 72 cases (1998–2000). J Am Vet Med Assoc 221:96–102, 2002.

116. Meyer RE. Current topics in fluid therapy: Oxyglobin. In: Gleed RD, Ludders JW, eds. Recent Advances in Veterinary Anesthesia and Analgesia: Companion Animals. Ithaca, NY: International Veterinary Information Service. http://www.ivis.org, 2001; document NO.A 1407.0501.

117. George LW. Diseases of the nervous system. In: Smith BP, ed. Large Animal Internal Medicine. Philadelphia: CV Mosby, 1990:948–950.

118. Schaer M. Disorders of serum potassium, sodium, magnesium and chloride. J Vet Emerg Crit Care 9:209–217, 1999.

119. Meuten DJ, Chew DJ, Capen CC, et al. Relationship of serum total calcium to albumin and total protein in dogs. J Am Vet Med Assoc 180:63–67, 1982.

120. Flanders JA, Scarlett JM, Blue JT, et al. Adjustment of total serum calcium concentration for binding to albumin and protein in cats: 291 cases (1986–1987). J Am Vet Med Assoc 194:1609, 1989.

121. Cote CJ, Drop LJ, Daniels AL. Treatment of citrate-induced hypocalcemia in dogs: Comparative response to calcium chloride and calcium gluconate. Anesth Analg 64:203, 1985.

122. Armstrong J, Meuten DJ. Parathyroid disease and calcium metabolism. In: Ettinger SJ, ed. Textbook of Veterinary Internal Medicine: Diseases of the Dog and Cat, 3rd ed. Philadelphia: WB Saunders, 1989:1610–1631.

123. Yates DJ, Hunt E. Disorders of calcium metabolism. In: Smith BP, ed. Large Animal Internal Medicine. Philadelphia: CV Mosby, 1990:1315–1322.

124. Muir WW, Wagner AE, Buchanan C. Effects of acute hyperventilation on serum potassium in the dog. Vet Surg 19:83–87, 1990.

125. Vitez TS, Soper LE, Wong KC, et al. Chronic hypokalemia and intraoperative dysrhythmias. Anesthesia 63:130–133, 1985.

126. DiBartola SP, Green RA, Autran de Morais HS, et al. Electrolyte and acid-base disorders. In: Willard MD, Tvedten H, eds. Small Animal Clinical Diagnosis by Laboratory Methods, 4th ed. Philadelphia: WB Saunders, 2004:117–134.

Chapter 9
Anticholinergics and Sedatives

Kip A. Lemke

Introduction

Anticholinergics and sedatives are two of the most widely used—and misused—classes of anesthetic adjuncts in veterinary medicine. Anticholinergics are used perioperatively to manage bradycardia and atrioventricular (AV) block associated with surgical manipulation (oculovagal and viscerovagal reflexes) or with the administration of other anesthetic adjunctive drugs (e.g., α_2-agonists or opioids). Occasionally, they are also used to control excessive oral and airway secretions. Anticholinergics are often combined with sedatives and opioids as part of a preanesthetic combination. Intraoperatively, anticholinergics are used primarily to manage sinus bradycardia and other vagally mediated arrhythmias. Sedatives are used perioperatively to induce sedation, provide restraint, and reduce the amount of injectable and inhalational anesthetics required to induce and maintain anesthesia. Some sedatives suppress or prevent vomiting (phenothiazines and butyrophenones), others provide muscle relaxation (benzodiazepines), and still others provide analgesia and muscle relaxation (α_2-agonists). Sedatives can also be used to promote a smooth recovery from anesthesia, and some sedatives (α_2-agonists, opioids, and benzodiazepines) have specific antagonists that can be administered after short diagnostic and minor surgical procedures.

Anticholinergics and sedatives should not be administered perioperatively on an indiscriminate basis. Rather, the risks and benefits associated with administration of different drugs should be assessed, and the safest drugs chosen for each patient. Most injectable and inhalational anesthetics that are used currently do not cause the dramatic autonomic responses (salivation and bradycardia) that occurred with some older anesthetics (ether). Further, the tachycardia induced by anticholinergic administration may be contraindicated in some patients with cardiovascular disease (e.g., hypertrophic cardiomyopathy). Therefore, anticholinergics should be administered only when there is a clear indication for their use (prevention or treatment of bradycardia). Similarly, most sedatives have significant cardiovascular side effects. The phenothiazines can contribute to the development of significant intraoperative hypotension. The α_2-agonists consistently cause bradycardia and a decrease in cardiac output. Alternately, the benzodiazepines are relatively free of cardiovascular side effects, but may not be reliable sedatives in some patients. The following patient-related factors should be considered when selecting anticholinergics and sedatives for perioperative use: age, species, temperament, concurrent disease, medications, and previous response to anesthetic drugs. Several procedure-related factors also play a practical role in drug selection. These include the type of procedure (inpatient or outpatient, diagnostic or surgical, and elective or emergency), as well as the duration of the procedure. Availability and clinical experience with the use of anticholinergics and sedatives in different species must also be considered.

Anticholinergics

Anticholinergics are often called parasympatholytic drugs because they block the effects of the parasympathetic nervous system on other body systems—especially the cardiovascular and gastrointestinal systems. Atropine and glycopyrrolate are the anticholinergics used most commonly in veterinary medicine. These two drugs do not block nicotinic cholinergic receptors and are more accurately classified as antimuscarinics. There are three major types of muscarinic receptors: M_1, M_2, and M_3 (Table 9.1). M_1 receptors are located on neurons in the central nervous system (CNS) and on autonomic ganglia. M_2 receptors are located in the sinoatrial (SA) and AV nodes and in the atrial myocardium. M_3 receptors are located in secretory glands, vascular endothelium, and smooth muscle. The cellular response to activation of these muscarinic receptors is mediated by several different molecular mechanisms (Table 9.1). Anticholinergics can also produce indirect sympathomimetic and parasympathomimetic effects. Presynaptic muscarinic receptors (heteroceptors) located on sympathetic nerve terminals normally inhibit release of norepinephrine, and blockade of these receptors by muscarinic antagonists facilitates release of norepinephrine. Similarly, presynaptic muscarinic receptors (autoreceptors) located on parasympathetic nerve terminals normally inhibit release of acetylcholine, and blockade of these receptors by muscarinic antagonists facilitates release of acetylcholine.

Atropine and glycopyrrolate are relatively nonselective mus-

Table 9.1. Anatomical location, cellular response, and physiological response associated with different muscarinic receptor subtypes

Receptor (G Protein)	Anatomical Location	Cellular Response	Physiological Response
M_1 ($G_{q/11}$)	Neurons and autonomic ganglia	Activate PLC and increase IP_3, DAG, and cytosolic calcium	Depolarization of neurons and autonomic ganglia
M_2 ($G_{i/o}$)	Sinoatrial node, atrioventricular node, and atrial myocardium	Increase potassium conductance Inhibit AC and decrease cAMP Decrease calcium conductance	Decreased sinus rate, conduction velocity, and contractile force
M_3 ($G_{q/11}$)	Secretory glands, smooth muscle, and vascular endothelium	Activate PLC and increase IP_3, DAG, and cytosolic calcium Generation of nitric oxide	Increased secretion and smooth muscle activity, and vasodilation

AC, adenylate cylase; cAMP, cyclic adenosine monophosphate; DAG, diacylglycerol; IP_3, inositol triphosphate; PLC, phospholipase C.

Table 9.2. Comparative effects of atropine and glycopyrrolate

	Sedation	Decrease in Oral Secretions	Increase in Heart Rate	Decrease in Gastrointestinal Motility	Ocular Effects	Increase in Gastric pH
Atropine	+	+	+++	++	++	0
Glycopyrrolate	0	++	+++	++	0	+

0, none; +, mild; ++, moderate; +++, marked.
Modified from Stoelting.[324]

carinic antagonists, but despite this lack of selectively the effectiveness of muscarinic blockade varies considerably from tissue to tissue (Table 9.2). Salivary and bronchial glands are the most sensitive to muscarinic blockade. Cardiac tissues and smooth muscle are intermediate in sensitivity, and gastric parietal cells are the least sensitive to muscarinic blockade. Cardioselective muscarinic (M_2) antagonists that prevent bradycardia and have limited effects on gastrointestinal smooth muscle activity have become available.[1,2]

Perioperatively anticholinergics are usually administered to prevent or treat severe bradycardia caused by surgical manipulation (vagal reflexes) or by administration of other anesthetic drugs (e.g., α_2-agonists and opioids). The incidence and severity of bradyarrhythmias can be reduced by preoperative administration of atropine or glycopyrrolate, but significant arrhythmias can still occur, and anticholinergic administration should never be used as a substitute for diligent patient monitoring. Anticholinergic administration routinely causes sinus tachycardia, which is problematic for many patients with cardiovascular disease. Tachycardia associated with administration of anticholinergics leads to an increase in myocardial work and a decrease in myocardial perfusion. Further, coadministration of anticholinergics and ketamine has been associated with the development of myocardial infarcts in, and the death of, young cats undergoing routine surgical procedures.[3] Anticholinergic administration also has dramatic effects on gastrointestinal function. At therapeutic doses, nonselective muscarinic antagonists like atropine and glycopyrrolate reduce lower esophageal sphincter tone and have little effect on gastric pH.[4] These two factors increase the incidence

of gastroesophageal reflux and esophagitis in anesthetized dogs.[5] Perioperative administration of anticholinergics also reduces intestinal motility and can lead to gastrointestinal complications postoperatively.[6]

Atropine

This agent is a racemic mixture of the l (−) and d (+) isomers of hyoscyamine. The l (−) isomer is at least 100 times more potent than the d (+) isomer. Chemically, atropine consists of two components (tropic acid and an organic base) that are bound by an ester linkage (Fig. 9.1). Atropine has approximately the same affinity for all three major types of muscarinic receptors. Relative to other synthetic muscarinic antagonists, atropine is very selective for muscarinic receptors and has little effect on nicotinic receptors.

Pharmacokinetics and Pharmacodynamics

Atropine is rapidly absorbed after intramuscular (IM) administration. Onset of cardiovascular effects occurs within 5 min, and peak effects occur within 10 to 20 min. After intravenous (IV) administration at a dose of 0.03 mg/kg, onset of cardiovascular effects occurs within 1 min, peak effects occur within 5 min, and heart rate increases by 30% to 40% for approximately 30 min (Fig. 9.2).[1] The effects of atropine on other body systems subside within a few hours, but ocular effects can persist for 1 to 2 days. Atropine is rapidly cleared from the blood after parenteral administration. Some of the drug is hydrolyzed to inactive metabolites (tropine and tropic acid), and some of it is excreted unchanged in the urine. Rabbits and some other species (cats and

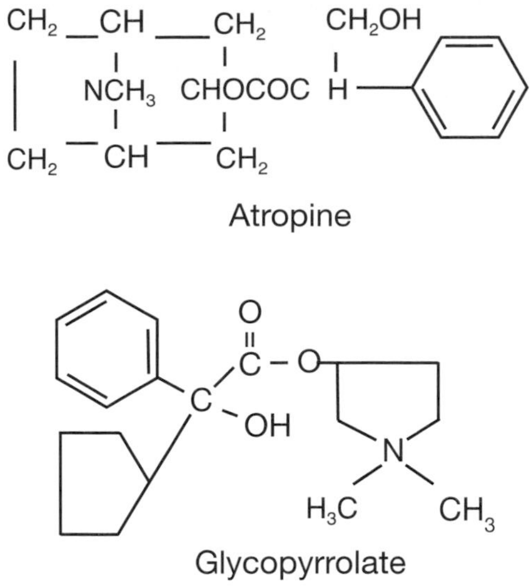

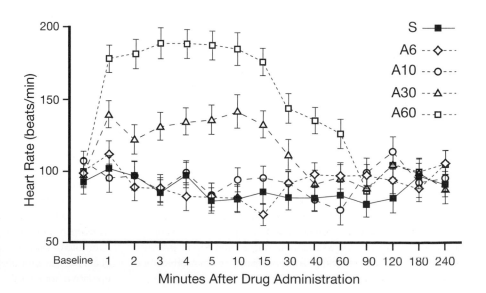

Fig. 9.1. Chemical structures of muscarinic antagonists
With permission from Stoelting.[324]

rats) have a plasma enzyme (atropine esterase) that accelerates metabolism and clearance of the drug.[7]

At therapeutic doses, atropine administration produces limited effects on the CNS. A mild sedative effect may be observed, and the incidence of vomiting mediated by the vestibular system may be reduced. Blockade of the pupillary constrictor muscle and the ciliary muscle produces long-lasting mydriasis and cycloplegia, respectively. Lacrimal secretions are also reduced, which may contribute to corneal drying during anesthesia unless artificial tears are applied concurrently.[8–10] Atropine should be used with discretion in animals with acute glaucoma and increased intraocular pressure because its mydriatic effect may impede drainage from the anterior chamber.

Atropine administration produces very dramatic effects on heart rate and rhythm.[11–13] The SA and AV nodes and the atrial myocardium all receive vagal parasympathetic input. Muscarinic receptors are located both presynaptically and postsynaptically in the SA and AV nodes. The typical response to IV or IM administration of therapeutic doses (0.02 to 0.04 mg/kg) of atropine is blockade of postsynaptic muscarinic receptors that leads to an increase in sinus rate, an acceleration of AV nodal conduction, and an increase in atrial contractility. At lower doses, a transient decrease in sinus rate and slowing of AV nodal conduction (AV blockade) can occur.[11,12] This response appears to be due to blockade of presynaptic muscarinic receptors that normally inhibit acetylcholine release.[14] Once postsynaptic muscarinic blockade is established, this paradoxical increase in vagal tone usually resolves.

Airway smooth muscle and secretory glands also receive parasympathetic input from the vagus nerves. Blockade of M_3 receptors by therapeutic doses of atropine decreases airway secretions and increases airway diameter and anatomical dead space. In the past, atropine was given before administration of noxious inhaled anesthetics (ether) to reduce airway secretions and the potential for laryngospasm. Modern inhaled anesthetics do not cause the same degree of airway irritation, and routine preoperative administration of atropine for this reason is difficult to justify.

Atropine administration also produces very dramatic effects on the gastrointestinal system. Blockade of M_1 and M_3 receptors in the gastrointestinal tract reduces secretory activity and motility. In dogs, administration of atropine reduces smooth muscle contractile activity, and administration of selective M_2 antagonists has limited effects on intestinal motility.[1] Atropine is not usually administered perioperatively to large animals. Although it can be given to horses intraoperatively to manage severe bradycardia associated with administration of α_2-agonists, gastrointestinal motility is reduced and colic can occur postoperatively.[6,15]

Clinical Uses

Atropine can be given subcutaneously (SC), IM, or IV, but the IM and IV routes are preferred because uptake from subcutaneous sites can be erratic in patients with altered hydration and peripheral

Fig. 9.2. Effect of intravenous administration of atropine (6 to 60 μg/kg) on heart rate in dogs. With permission from Hendrix and Robinson.[1]

circulation. Doses for dogs and cats range from 0.02 to 0.04 mg/kg. Atropine is also effective when given endotracheally or endobronchially to dogs for cardiopulmonary resuscitation.[16] Doses for ruminants and swine range from 0.04 to 0.08 mg/kg, but salivation may not be completed obtunded in these species. Atropine is not usually given perioperatively to horses because of its gastrointestinal side effects. Atropine can also be used to control muscarinic side effects when anticholinesterases (e.g., edrophonium) are administered to reverse neuromuscular blockade produced by nondepolarizing muscle relaxants (e.g., atracurium).

Glycopyrrolate

This is a synthetic quaternary ammonium muscarinic antagonist. Like atropine, the drug consists of two components (mandelic acid and an organic base) bound together by an ester linkage (Fig. 9.1). Glycopyrrolate is four times as potent as atropine and has approximately the same affinity for all three major types of muscarinic receptors. The drug's polar structure (quaternary amine) limits diffusion across lipid membranes and into the CNS and fetal circulation.[17]

Pharmacokinetics and Pharmacodynamics

Absorption, metabolism, and elimination of glycopyrrolate are similar to that of atropine. Absorption is rapid after IM administration. Onset of cardiovascular effects occurs within 5 min, peak effects occur within 20 min, and heart rate remains elevated for approximately 1 h.[18] Glycopyrrolate is rapidly cleared from the blood after parenteral administration, and most of the drug is excreted unchanged in the urine.

At therapeutic doses, glycopyrrolate produces few, if any, effects on the CNS. Unlike atropine administration, sedation is not observed, and recovery times are not prolonged. Administration of glycopyrrolate to conscious dogs with normal intraocular pressure does not alter pupil diameter and intraocular pressure, and intraoperative administration of glycopyrrolate to dogs with glaucoma and increased intraocular pressure appears to be safe.[19] Similarly, pupil diameter and light reflexes are unaffected when conscious horses are administered glycopyrrolate IV.[20]

Glycopyrrolate administration produces effects on the heart that are comparable to those of atropine.[12] Studies in people suggest that glycopyrrolate produces less tachycardia than atropine, but the two drugs produce similar increases in heart rate when administered IV to sedated or anesthetized dogs.[12,21] The typical response to IV or IM administration of therapeutic doses (5 to 10 µg/kg) of glycopyrrolate is an increase in sinus rate, acceleration of AV nodal conduction, and an increase in atrial contractility. At lower doses, a transient decrease in sinus rate and slowing of AV nodal conduction can occur.[12] Glycopyrrolate can also be given intraoperatively to correct bradycardia in both small and large animals. Dogs weighing less than 10 kg require a higher dose of glycopyrrolate (10 µg/kg IV) to correct bradycardia, and those over 10 kg require a lower dose (5 µg/kg IV).[22] Glycopyrrolate is given to horses at a lower dose (2.5 to 5.0 µg/kg IV) to correct bradycardia and to increase cardiac output and blood pressure (Fig. 9.3), but the potential for postoperative gastrointestinal complications (colic) must be considered.[23,24]

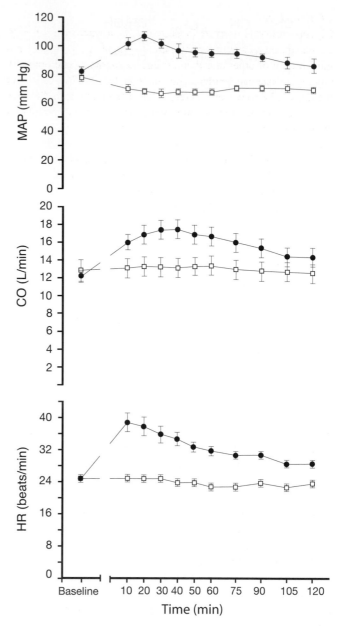

Fig. 9.3. Effect of intravenous administration of glycopyrrolate (2.5 to 7.5 µg/kg) on heart rate (HR), cardiac output (CO), and mean arterial blood pressure (MAP) in horses anesthetized with halothane and xylazine. With permission from Teixeira Neto et al.[24]

Like atropine, glycopyrrolate produces dramatic effects on the gastrointestinal system. Intestinal motility is reduced for at least 30 min in anesthetized dogs.[21] In conscious horses, gastrointestinal motility is reduced for 2.4 and 6.4 h after IV administration of glycopyrrolate at doses of 2.5 and 5.0 µg/kg, respectively.[20] Further, when these doses were given intraoperatively to 17 horses undergoing routine surgical procedures, only one horse developed signs of colic postoperatively.[23] Although well-controlled comparative studies are lacking, glycopyrrolate appears to be a safer choice than atropine for the treatment of intraoperative bradycardia in horses.

Clinical Uses

Glycopyrrolate is used perioperatively to prevent severe bradycardia caused by surgical manipulation (vagal reflexes) or by administration of other anesthetic drugs (α_2-agonists and opioids). Glycopyrrolate can be given subcutaneously (SC), IM, or IV, but the IM and IV routes are preferred because uptake from SC sites can be erratic in patients with altered hydration and peripheral circulation. Doses for dogs and cats range from 5 to 10 µg/kg. Intravenous doses for horses range from 2.5 to 5.0 µg/kg, but gastrointestinal side effects can occur. Like atropine, glycopyrrolate can be used to control muscarinic side effects when anticholinesterases (e.g., edrophonium) are given to reverse neuromuscular blockade produced by nondepolarizing muscle relaxants (e.g., atracurium).

Sedatives

Behavioral responses to different classes of sedatives vary considerably among species. The phenothiazines and α_2-agonists are effective sedatives in dogs and cats but are not reliable sedatives in swine. Conversely, the benzodiazepines are effective sedatives in ferrets, rabbits, swine, and birds but are not reliable sedatives in cats and young dogs. Dose requirements also vary considerably among species. For example, the α_2-agonists are effective sedatives in horses and cattle, but the xylazine dose requirement for horses is approximately ten times that for cattle. Because of this variability, accurate classification of these drugs as tranquilizers, sedatives, or hypnotics is problematic. Therefore, the drugs discussed in this chapter are simply referred to as sedatives, with the knowledge that their effects will vary with species and with dose.

In North America, only a limited number of sedatives are approved for use in animals. All of these sedatives are classified as phenothiazines (acepromazine), butyrophenones (azaperone), or α_2-agonists (xylazine, medetomidine, detomidine, and romifidine). Despite the widespread use of benzodiazepines (diazepam and midazolam) as sedatives, muscle relaxants, and anticonvulsants in veterinary medicine, none are approved and marketed for use in animals. In the United States, the benzodiazepine zolazepam is available in combination with a dissociative anesthetic (tiletamine) and is approved for use in cats and dogs as an anesthetic. Only acepromazine and xylazine are approved for use in cats, dogs, and horses. Medetomidine is approved for use in dogs, detomidine and romifidine are approved for use in horses, and azaperone is approved for use in swine. In Canada, acepromazine and xylazine are also approved for use in ruminants.

Selection of sedatives for different species and for animals with different behavioral and medical problems can be difficult without a thorough understanding of the physiological effects of the different classes of sedatives. In cats and dogs, administration of acepromazine or an α_2-agonist is associated with significant cardiovascular side effects (hypotension or bradycardia, respectively). Therefore, these sedatives are probably best reserved for use in young healthy animals. If a sedative is needed for pediatric, geriatric, or sick patients, administration of diazepam or midazolam should be considered. In horses, acepromazine and the α_2-agonists are the only reliable sedatives, and doses must be carefully individualized for each patient. Although midazolam is not widely used in animals, it is an excellent sedative for swine and some exotic species (rabbits, ferrets, and birds).

Phenothiazines and Butyrophenones

Phenothiazines and, to a lesser extent, butyrophenones produce a wide variety of behavioral, autonomic, and endocrine effects. The behavioral effects of these drugs are mediated primarily by blockade of dopamine receptors in the basal ganglia and limbic system. At therapeutic doses, phenothiazines and butyrophenones inhibit conditioned avoidance behavior and decrease spontaneous motor activity. At higher doses, extrapyramidal effects (tremor, rigidity, and catalepsy) can occur. These sedatives also have significant binding affinity for autonomic (adrenergic and muscarinic) and other types of receptors (Tables 9.3 and 9.4). For example, phenothiazines bind with greater affinity to α_1 recep-

Table 9.3. Relative receptor-binding affinities of phenothiazines and butyrophenones

	D_1	D_2	α_1	5-HT$_2$	M_3	H_1
Phenothiazines	+	++	+++	+++	+	+
Butyrophenones	++	+++	+	+	+	+

α_1, alpha receptor; D, dopamine receptor; H, histamine receptor; 5-HT$_2$, 5-hydroxytryptamine (serotonin) receptor; M$_3$, muscarinic receptor; +, weak; ++, moderate; +++, strong.

Table 9.4. Adverse effects of phenothiazines and butyrophenones

	Pharmacological Effects	Mechanism
Central nervous system	Catalepsy, tremor, and rigidity	Dopaminergic blockade
	Seizure activity	Electroencephalographic slowing and synchronization
Autonomic nervous system	Decreased blood pressure and hematocrit	α-Adrenergic blockade
	Decreased glandular secretions	Muscarinic blockade
Endocrine system	Galactorrhea, abnormal cycles, and altered libido	Dopaminergic blockade and increased prolactin secretion

tors than to dopaminergic receptors. Blockade of α_1 receptors is responsible for the hypotension that is typically associated with perioperative use of these drugs. Blockade of these receptors may also be responsible for the ability of phenothiazines and butyrophenones to protect against the development of malignant hyperthermia in susceptible animals anesthetized with halothane.[25] Dopamine receptors in the hypothalamus are responsible for tonic inhibition of prolactin secretion. Blockade of these receptors increases prolactin secretion and is responsible for most of the endocrine effects associated with administration of these drugs. Blockade of dopamine receptors in the chemoreceptor trigger zone of the medulla produces an antiemetic effect, and depletion of catecholamines in the thermoregulatory center of the hypothalamus leads to a loss of thermoregulatory control. Phenothiazines and butyrophenones also produce slowing and synchronization of the electroencephalogram, which can facilitate the development of seizures in predisposed animals.[26]

Dopamine is largely an inhibitory neurotransmitter and is responsible for regulation of behavior, fine motor control, and prolactin secretion. Dopamine receptors are G-protein–coupled receptors and are divided into two major families of receptors: Dopamine 1 (D_1) receptors are located postsynaptically, and dopamine 2 (D_2) receptors are located both presynaptically and postsynaptically. Activation of the D_1 family of receptors increases adenylate cyclase activity and intracellular levels of cyclic adenosine monophosphate (cAMP). Activation of the D_2 family of receptors decreases adenylate cyclase activity and intracellular levels of cAMP, and can also activate other presynaptic signal transduction pathways (decrease calcium conductance) and postsynaptic signal transduction pathways (increase potassium conductance). Most behavioral effects are mediated by the D_2 family of receptors.

Acepromazine

This is one of the most widely used sedatives in veterinary medicine. The chemical name of acepromazine is 2-acetyl-10-(3-dimethylaminopropyl) phenothiazine (Fig. 9.4). The drug is more potent than other phenothiazine derivatives and produces sedation at relatively low doses. Acepromazine administration produces some muscle relaxation but has no analgesic effect. In North America, the drug is sold as acepromazine maleate and is approved for use in both small and large animals.

Pharmacokinetics and Pharmacodynamics   Onset of sedation after parenteral administration of acepromazine to cats, dogs, and horses is relatively slow, and sedation persists for several hours. In dogs given acepromazine and an opioid IM, onset of sedation is observed within 15 min, peak effects are observed within 30 min, and sedation lasts for 2 to 3 h.[27,28] In horses given acepromazine IV, peak effects are observed within 30 min and sedation lasts for 1 to 2 h.[29,30] The pharmacokinetics of IV administration of acepromazine have been determined in horses at relatively high doses. At a dose of 0.3 mg/kg, acepromazine is widely distributed (V_d = 6.6 L/kg), is extensively protein bound (>99%), and has an elimination half-life of 3 h.[29] At a dose of 0.15 mg/kg, acepromazine has a smaller volume of distribution (V_d = 4.5

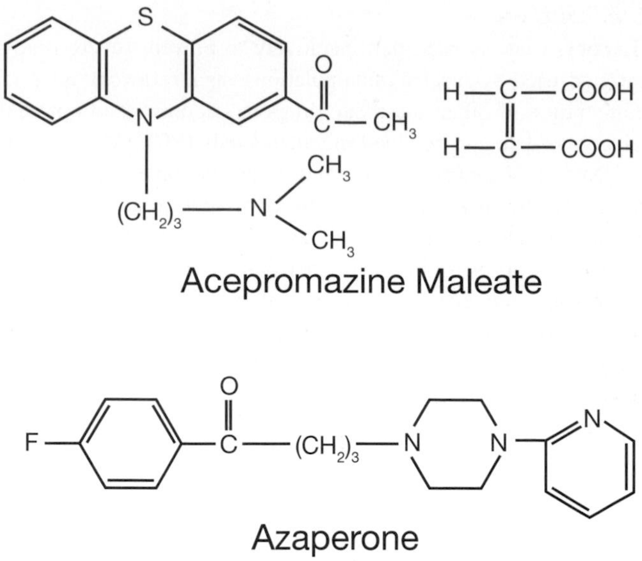

Fig. 9.4. Chemical structures of acepromazine and azaperone. With permission from Gross.[325]

L/kg) and shorter elimination half-life (1.6 h).[30] The drug is metabolized by the liver, and unconjugated and conjugated metabolites are excreted in the urine.[31]

Acepromazine administration decreases halothane and isoflurane requirements in several species. In dogs anesthetized with halothane, IM administration of acepromazine at doses of 0.02 and 0.2 mg/kg decreases the minimum alveolar concentration (MAC) by 34% and 44%, respectively.[32] In a comparative study, IM administration of acepromazine (0.2 mg/kg) to dogs anesthetized with halothane or isoflurane decreased the MAC by 28% and 48%, respectively.[33] Administration of acepromazine (0.05 mg/kg IV) also decreases the MAC of halothane in ponies by 37% and the MAC of isoflurane in goats by 44%.[34,35] Given the 30% to 40% reduction in halothane and isoflurane requirements that occurs when acepromazine is given perioperatively, patients should always be monitored closely and vaporizer settings reduced accordingly.[36]

Acepromazine administration produces dramatic effects on the cardiovascular system in both conscious and anesthetized animals. In conscious dogs, stroke volume, cardiac output, and mean arterial pressure decrease 20% to 25% after IV administration of acepromazine (0.1 mg/kg), and mean arterial pressure is reduced for at least 2 h.[37,38] In conscious cats, IM administration of acepromazine (0.1 mg/kg) decreases mean arterial pressure by 30% within 10 min of injection.[39] In dogs anesthetized with halothane, IV administration of acepromazine at doses of 0.05, 0.125, and 0.25 mg/kg decreases mean arterial pressure by 2.3%, 9.4%, and 16.8%, respectively.[40] Preanesthetic administration of acepromazine (0.1 mg/kg IM) also decreases mean arterial pressure by 24% in dogs anesthetized with isoflurane (Fig. 9.5).[41] In conscious horses, administration of acepromazine (0.1 mg/kg IV) decreases mean aortic pressure by 20% to 30% and decreases cardiac output by 10% to 15%.[42] In horses anesthetized with

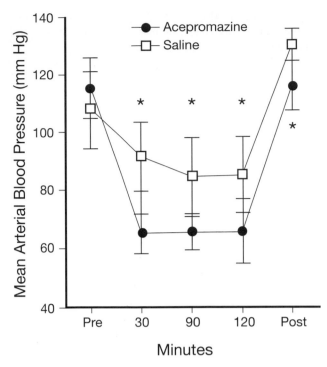

Fig. 9.5. Effect of acepromazine (0.1 mg/kg intramuscularly) on mean arterial pressure in dogs anesthetized with isoflurane (2%). With permission from Bostrom et al.[41]

halothane, IV administration of acepromazine (0.03 mg/kg) decreases mean arterial pressure by 25%.[43] When acepromazine is given preoperatively to animals anesthetized with halothane, a modest decrease in arterial pressure occurs. However, when acepromazine is given to animals anesthetized with isoflurane, a dramatic decrease in arterial pressure occurs. Currently, the widespread practice of administering acepromazine preoperatively, maintaining anesthesia with isoflurane, and failing to monitor arterial pressure contributes to the high incidence of intraoperative hypotension in small animals.

Heart rate does not change appreciably in conscious dogs and horses administered acepromazine (0.1 mg/kg IV).[37,42] Increases in heart rate and sinus tachycardia can occur in some patients. At very high doses (1 mg/kg), bradycardia and SA block can occur in dogs given acepromazine, but these arrhythmias are not usually observed at lower doses.[44] Heart rate decreases after administration of acepromazine in dogs anesthetized with halothane but does not change in horses anesthetized with halothane.[43,45] Premedication with acepromazine also increases the dose of epinephrine required to induce ventricular arrhythmias in dogs anesthetized with halothane.[46,47] Blockade of myocardial α_1 receptors by acepromazine may prevent the development of ventricular arrhythmias in anesthetized animals—provided that adequate diastolic pressure is maintained.[48]

Administration of acepromazine to conscious or anesthetized animals has little effect on pulmonary function. In conscious dogs and horses, respiratory rate decreases, but arterial pH, partial pressure of carbon dioxide (PCO_2), partial pressure of oxy-

gen (PO_2), and hemoglobin saturation do not change after IV administration of acepromazine.[42,44] In horses anesthetized with halothane, respiratory rate and arterial blood-gas values do not change after IV administration of acepromazine.[43]

Acepromazine administration produces significant gastrointestinal and urogenital effects. In dogs, administration of acepromazine 15 min before administration of morphine, hydromorphone, or oxymorphone lowers the incidence of vomiting from 45% to 18%.[49] However, administration of acepromazine alone or in combination with an opioid reduces lower esophageal sphincter tone, delays gastric emptying, and may increase the incidence of gastric reflux.[50–52] In horses, acepromazine administration delays gastric emptying and reduces intestinal motility.[53,54] Glomerular filtration is maintained in dogs premedicated with acepromazine and anesthetized with isoflurane.[41] Acepromazine also decreases urethral pressure by 20% in cats already anesthetized with halothane.[55]

Acepromazine administration can produce significant hematologic side effects in animals. In dogs and horses, hematocrit decreases by 20% to 30% within 30 min of acepromazine administration and remains well below baseline values for at least 2 h.[29,30,56] Acepromazine administration also inhibits platelet aggregation but does not appear to alter hemostasis in normal dogs.[57] Bradycardia and hypotension can occur in boxers and other breeds of dogs after acepromazine administration. These animals usually respond to fluid loading with isotonic crystalloids and administration of an anticholinergic to correct the bradycardia. Acepromazine administration produces penile protrusion in horses, and both the degree and duration of protrusion are dose dependent.[29] At a dose of 0.04 mg/kg, protrusion is 60% of the maximum length within 30 min and is below 30% after 90 min. At a dose of 0.4 mg/kg, protrusion is over 90% of the maximum length within 30 min and is still over 80% after 4 h. Although uncommon, prolonged prolapse or priapism can occur, and amputation may be required.[58] Low doses of acepromazine can be used safely in geldings but should be avoided in breeding stallions.

Clinical Uses Clinical uses of acepromazine are usually restricted to healthy animals. The drug is administered alone as a sedative for nonpainful diagnostic procedures or in combination with an opioid for painful diagnostic and minor surgical procedures. Acepromazine is also given alone and in combination with opioids as a preanesthetic to facilitate placement of IV catheters and to reduce the dose of injectable and inhalational anesthetics required to induce and maintain anesthesia. Small doses of acepromazine can also be given postoperatively to smooth recovery—provided that patients are hemodynamically stable and that pain has been managed effectively. Administration of acepromazine postoperatively to quiet patients in the absence of effective analgesic therapy makes accurate assessment of pain impossible and is inhumane. The drug is used in several species, including cats, dogs, and horses, but is not a reliable sedative in swine. Acepromazine can be given SC, IM, or IV, but the IM and IV routes are preferred because uptake from SC sites can be erratic in patients with altered peripheral circulation. Intramuscular doses for cats and small dogs range from 0.05 to 0.2 mg/kg, and those for larger dogs range from 0.04 to 0.06 mg/kg. Intravenous doses for horses range from 0.02 to 0.04 mg/kg.

Azaperone

This agent is a butyrophenone derivative (Fig. 9.4). The chemical name of the drug is 4-fluoro-4-(4-[2-pyridyl]-1-piperazinyl) butyrophenone. In North America, azaperone is approved for use in swine to produce sedation and control aggression when groups of animals are mixed. The drug produces some muscle relaxation but has no analgesic effect. Like acepromazine, azaperone can be used alone or in combination with other drugs (e.g., opioids and ketamine).

Pharmacokinetics and Pharmacodynamics   In pigs, sedation begins within 10 min after IM administration of azaperone at the label dose (2 mg/kg). Ideally, animals should be left undisturbed in a quiet environment for approximately 20 min. Peak sedation is reached within 15 min in young pigs and within 30 min in mature animals, and sedation persists for 2 to 3 h. Excitement has been observed in other species when azaperone is administered IV.[59] Limited pharmacokinetic data are available for azaperone, but the drug is metabolized by the liver and is rapidly cleared from tissues.

Azaperone administration produces dramatic effects on the cardiovascular system. Heart rate and cardiac output decrease by 20% to 40% in young pigs given azaperone IM at a dose of 2.5 mg/kg.[60] Arterial pressure decreases in pigs given azaperone IM at doses ranging from 0.3 to 3.5 mg/kg, and the pressure decrease is not dose dependent.[61]

As with acepromazine, azaperone administration has little effect on pulmonary function, but thermoregulation is impaired. Small increases in respiratory rate and decreases in arterial PCO_2 occur in pigs given azaperone IM at doses of 1 to 3.5 mg/kg.[61] Rectal temperature decreases 1° to 2°C over 4 h after IM administration of azaperone at a dose of 5 mg/kg.[62] Intramuscular administration of azaperone at a low dose (0.5 mg/kg) prevents serious fighting in breeding boars, but penile prolapse occurs in a small percentage of animals (<4%).[60]

Clinical Uses   Clinical uses of azaperone are usually restricted to healthy swine. The drug is used alone as a sedative for nonpainful diagnostic procedures or in combination with an opioid for painful diagnostic and minor surgical procedures. Azaperone is also used alone and in combination with opioids as a preanesthetic to facilitate placement of IV catheters and to reduce the dose of injectable and inhalational anesthetics. Intramuscular administration of azaperone at a dose of 1 to 2 mg/kg produces a mild to moderate sedative effect in most swine. Azaperone is also given in combination with ketamine to immobilize or anesthetize animals for various diagnostic and surgical procedures. In swine, administration of azaperone (1 mg/kg IM) and ketamine (5 to 10 mg/kg IM) will immobilize most animals, and administration of azaperone and ketamine at twice these doses will anesthetize most animals. Injections should always be made with needles long enough to reach the target muscle groups. In small pigs,

1-inch needles are adequate, but longer needles must be used in mature animals. In Canada, animals given azaperone must not be slaughtered for food for at least 1 day.

α_2-Agonists

α_2-Agonists are the most widely used class of sedatives in veterinary medicine. In most species, these drugs induce reliable dose-dependent sedation, analgesia, and muscle relaxation that can be readily reversed by administration of selective antagonists.

Xylazine has been used in both small and large animals for over two decades, and detomidine has been used in horses for over a decade.[63,64] In small animals, medetomidine has been used for several years in North America and in Europe.[65–67] Romifidine has also been used in horses in North America and in Europe.[64] Selective antagonists (tolazoline, yohimbine, and atipamezole) are available for use in both small and large animals in several countries. α_2-Agonists and their antagonists are also used to facilitate capture and handling of many exotic species.[68,69]

The α_2 receptors are located in tissues throughout the body, and norepinephrine is the endogenous ligand for these receptors. The α_2 receptors exist presynaptically and postsynaptically in neuronal and nonneuronal tissues, and extrasynaptically in the vascular endothelium and in platelets. Within the nervous system, α_2 receptors are located presynaptically on noradrenergic neurons (autoreceptors) and on nonnoradrenergic neurons (heteroceptors). The sedative and anxiolytic effects of α_2-agonists are mediated by activation of supraspinal autoreceptors or postsynaptic receptors located in the pons (locus ceruleus), and the analgesic effects are mediated by activation of heteroceptors located in the dorsal horn of the spinal cord.[70] Supraspinal α_2 receptors located in the pons also play a prominent role in descending modulation of nociceptive input.

Three distinct α_2-receptor subtypes (A, B, and C) have been identified.[71–73] The cellular response to activation of these receptor subtypes is mediated by several different molecular mechanisms (Table 9.5). Physiological responses have been determined in transgenic or "knockout" animals, but specific cellular responses associated with each of the receptor subtypes have not been clearly defined. The α_{2A} receptors mediate sedation, supraspinal analgesia, and centrally mediated bradycardia and hypotension, whereas the α_{2B} receptors mediate the initial surge in vascular resistance and reflex bradycardia. The α_{2C} receptors mediate the hypothermia that accompanies administration of α_2-agonists. Neurotransmitter release is modulated primarily by presynaptic α_{2A} receptors, and spinal analgesia appears to be mediated by both α_{2B} and α_{2C} receptors. Subtype selective agonists are not currently available, but α_{2A} selective agonists with fewer vascular side effects could potentially be developed.

In contrast to the physiological effects mediated by α_2 receptors, activation of α_1 receptors produces arousal, excitement, and increased locomotor activity in animals.[74,75] These behaviors are also observed after administration of excessive doses of less selective α_2-agonists and after accidental intracarotid injection. Excitement and muscle rigidity occur in dogs administered xylazine IM at high doses (4 to 8 mg/kg).[76] Similarly, excitement,

Table 9.5. Anatomical location, cellular response, and physiological response associated with different α_2-receptor subtypes

Receptor (G Protein)	Anatomical Location	Cellular Response	Physiological Response
α_{2A} ($G_{i/o}$)	Cerebral cortex, locus caeruleus, and platelets	Inhibit AC activity and decrease cAMP Increase potassium conductance Decrease calcium conductance	Sedation and supraspinal analgesia Centrally mediated bradycardia and hypotension
α_{2B} ($G_{i/o}$)	Spinal cord (dorsal root ganglia) and vascular endothelium	Activate PLC and increase IP_3, DAG, and cytosolic calcium	Spinal analgesia Vasoconstriction and peripherally mediated reflex bradycardia
α_{2C} ($G_{i/o}$)	Spinal cord (dorsal root ganglia)		Spinal analgesia Hypothermia and modulation of dopaminergic activity

AC, adenylate cylase; cAMP, cyclic adenosine monophosphate; DAG, diacylglycerol; IP_3, inositol triphosphate; PLC, phospholipase C.

seizures, and muscle rigidity occur in horses after intracarotid injection of xylazine.[77] This paradoxical response appears to be more common after administration of α_2-agonists that have some affinity for α_1 receptors (xylazine), but can occur in animals given toxic doses of more selective agonists.[78] Activation of central α_1 receptors can also antagonize the sedative effects of selective α_2-agonists.[79,80] Receptor binding or selectivity ratios (α_2/α_1) for xylazine, detomidine, romifidine and medetomidine are 160:1, 260:1, 340:1, and 1620:1, respectively.[81,82]

As with acepromazine, the clinical use of α_2-agonists is usually restricted to healthy animals. α_2-Agonists can be used alone or in combination with opioids to provide sedation for diagnostic and minor surgical procedures. α_2-Agonists can also be used in combination with ketamine to provide anesthesia for brief surgical procedures. Perioperatively, α_2-agonists are used at lower doses, alone or in combination with opioids, to produce sedation and analgesia required for catheter placement, to reduce the amount of injectable anesthetic (e.g., ketamine, thiopental, or propofol) required to induce anesthesia, and to reduce the amount of inhalational anesthetic (e.g., halothane or isoflurane) required to maintain anesthesia.[67] α_2-Agonists also potentiate the effects of other analgesic drugs (opioids and local anesthetics) and attenuate the stress response associated with surgical trauma. Postoperatively, low doses of α_2-agonists can be used to facilitate recovery from anesthesia in both small and large animals.

In small animals, the perioperative use of α_2-agonists has been controversial.[83,84] Certainly, the initial vasoconstriction and reflex bradycardia induced by administration of α_2-agonists are problematic. However, at low doses, these cardiovascular effects are not as pronounced nor as long in duration and are well tolerated by healthy animals. Preoperatively, anticholinergics can be administered with α_2-agonists to prevent bradycardia. α_2-Agonists also dramatically reduce the amount of thiopental or propofol required to induce anesthesia, and the amount of isoflurane required to maintain anesthesia.[85–87] Given that all of these anesthetics have a very narrow therapeutic range and produce dramatic effects on myocardial function, the reduction in dose achieved by administering α_2-agonists preoperatively significantly reduces the adverse cardiovascular effects associated with administration of most general anesthetics. Isoflurane administration also produces marked vasodilation and significant reductions in arterial pressure at concentrations normally required to induce and maintain anesthesia.[88] In dogs, concurrent administration of α_2-agonists initially increases vascular tone and attenuates the vasodilation and reduction in arterial pressure induced by high concentrations of isoflurane.[89,90] As a result, perioperative administration of α_2-agonists attenuates the vasodilatory effects of isoflurane by enhancing vascular tone. In sharp contrast, administration of acepromazine exacerbates vasodilation and the reduction in arterial pressure induced by isoflurane (Fig. 9.5).[41]

Some patients may be refractory to the sedative effects of α_2-agonists. Failure to achieve optimal sedation with α_2-agonists is often due to preexisting stress, fear, excitement, and pain. All of these conditions increase endogenous catecholamine levels and can interfere with reductions in excitatory neurotransmitter release induced by administration of α_2-agonists. Sedation is consistently achieved when xylazine or another α_2-agonist is given to calm patients in quiet surroundings with minimal environmental stimuli. In most species, sedation is even more reliable when α_2-agonists are administered in combination with opioids.

Concerns have been raised about the potential for α_2-agonists to sensitize the myocardium to epinephrine-induced arrhythmias.[48] Initial studies reported that high doses of xylazine facilitate the development of reentrant ventricular arrhythmias (premature depolarizations and tachycardia) in dogs anesthetized with thiopental and halothane—two drugs that dramatically sensitize the myocardium to epinephrine.[46,91] Subsequent studies in dogs anesthetized with halothane or isoflurane and administered lower doses of xylazine or medetomidine showed that α_2-agonists do not facilitate the development of reentrant ventricular arrhythmias.[47,92–94] Further, the decrease in sympathetic tone and increase in parasympathetic tone induced by the administration of selective α_2-agonists appear to attenuate the development of epinephrine-induced arrhythmias in dogs.[95]

In a 1998 survey of veterinarians in Ontario, an increase in the incidence of anesthetic complications was associated with the use of xylazine in small animals.[96] Failure to appreciate the dramatic reduction in anesthetic requirements produced by preoperative administration of xylazine and subsequent administration of a relative overdose of injectable or inhalational anesthetic may have contributed to the increased risk reported in this study. Given that patient monitoring standards were extremely lax a decade ago, failure to recognize and treat significant bradyarrhythmias could have been a factor, as well. More recent studies have found that administration of relatively low doses of medetomidine alone or in combination with opioids is associated with occasional bradyarrhythmias (sinus bradycardia and AV block) and a low incidence of severe anesthetic complications. Glycopyrrolate administration decreases the incidence and severity of bradyarrhythmias in healthy older (≥5 years old) dogs given medetomidine and butorphanol IM as preanesthetics, and only 1 of 88 dogs developed complications severe enough to require reversal with atipamezole.[97] Similarly, no anesthetic deaths and only 13 protocol modifications were recorded after repeated sedation of 136 geriatric cats (1862 procedures) and 541 geriatric dogs (6329 procedures) with medetomidine, butorphanol, and glycopyrrolate to facilitate radiation therapy.[98] Based on the latter studies, it appears that low doses of α_2-agonists can be used safely in older dogs and cats, provided that cardiopulmonary function is evaluated carefully before drug administration and monitored closely afterward.

Xylazine

Although its mechanism of action was unknown at the time of its introduction into clinical practice, xylazine was the first α_2-agonist to be used by veterinarians. The drug was synthesized in West Germany in 1962 for use as an antihypertensive in people but was found to have potent sedative effects in animals. The chemical name for xylazine is 2(2,6-dimethylphenylamino)-4H-5,6-dihydro-1,3-thiazine hydrochloride (Fig. 9.6). Initially, the drug was used as a sedative in cattle and other ruminants in Europe. In the early 1970s, reports of xylazine's utility as an anesthetic adjunct began appearing in American and European veterinary literature.[99–109] These reports documented the effectiveness of xylazine in eliminating muscular hypertonicity in dogs and cats given ketamine, and in producing rapid, predictable sedation, analgesia, and muscle relaxation in horses and cattle after IV administration. It was also evident that there was tremendous variation in the dose of xylazine required to produce equivalent levels of sedation and analgesia in different species. In 1981, the sedative and analgesic effects of xylazine were definitively linked to activation of central α_2-adrenergic receptors.[110,111]

Pharmacokinetics   The pharmacokinetics of xylazine have been determined in cattle, horses, and dogs after its IV and IM injection at doses of 0.2, 0.6, and 1.4 mg/kg, respectively.[112] After IV administration, the elimination half-life is 36, 50, and 30 min in cattle, horses, and dogs, respectively. After IM administration, peak plasma concentrations are reached within 15 min, and the elimination half-life is 58 and 35 min in horses and dogs, respectively. In cattle given xylazine IM (0.35 mg/kg), the drug and its metabolites are undetectable in tissues after 3 days and in milk after 12 h.[113] Despite the rapid clearance of xylazine from tissues

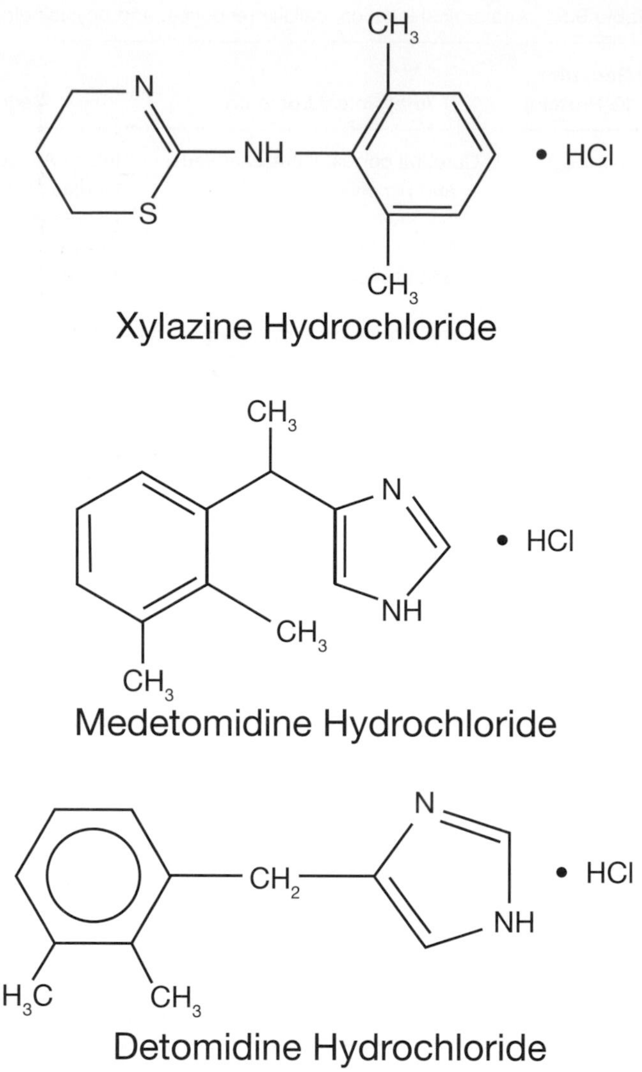

Fig. 9.6.   Chemical structures of α_2-receptor agonists. With permission from Gross.[325]

and milk, the United States Food and Drug Administration has refused to approve its use in food-producing animals.[114] This refusal underscores the failure to address animal-welfare issues associated with performing surgical procedures in the absence of appropriate sedation and analgesia, and legitimate human-safety concerns associated with restraint and handling of unsedated animals. Xylazine is approved for use in ruminants in Canada and several other countries around the world.

Pharmacodynamics   In most species, the onset of sedation and analgesia is rapid after parenteral administration of xylazine. In dogs, peak sedation and analgesia develop within 15 min and persist for 1 to 2 h after administration of xylazine (2.2 mg/kg IM).[115] In horses, peak sedation and analgesia develop within 5 min, persist for the next 30 min, and then subside over the next 30 min after administration of xylazine (1.1 mg/kg IV).[82,103,108,116] At a lower dose of xylazine (0.4 mg/kg IV), peak sedation develops

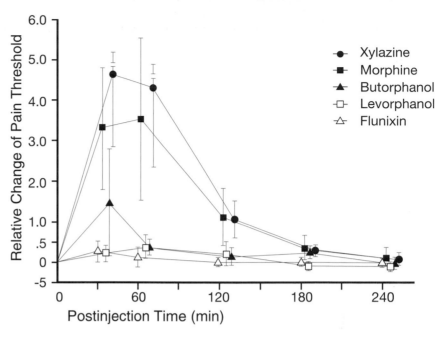

Superficial Pain

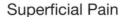

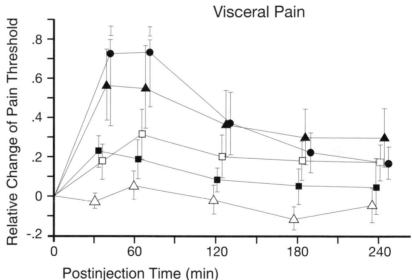

Visceral Pain

Fig. 9.7. Somatic and visceral analgesic effects of xylazine, morphine, butorphanol, levorphanol, or flunixin in ponies. With permission from Kalpravidh et al.[119]

with 10 min and then subsides over the next 20 min.[117] Most clinical studies show that the sedative and analgesic effects of xylazine are comparable in duration and do not support the "conventional wisdom" that the analgesic effect is significantly shorter than the sedative effect. Further, xylazine has been reported to be more effective than either opioid agonists (meperidine, methadone, morphine, oxymorphone, or fentanyl), agonist-antagonists (pentazocine, butorphanol, or levorphanol), or nonsteroidal anti-inflammatories (flunixin) in relieving somatic and visceral pain in horses (Fig. 9.7).[118,119]

Xylazine administration decreases injectable and inhalational anesthetic requirements dramatically in several species. Intramuscular administration of xylazine (2.2 mg/kg) decreases the dose of thiopental required to induce anesthesia in and cats and

dogs by 80%.[120,121] Although this dose of xylazine is relatively high and not recommended, this study illustrates the striking reduction in thiopental requirements that can be achieved when large doses of α_2-agonists are given as preanesthetics. Similarly, administration of xylazine (0.8 mg/kg IM) decreases the dose of propofol required to induce anesthesia in dogs by over 50%.[86,122] Perioperative administration of xylazine also reduces halothane and isoflurane requirements in animals. In dogs, administration of xylazine (1.1 mg/kg IV) decreases the MAC of halothane by 38%, an effect that was reversed by administration of an α_2-antagonist (tolazoline).[123] In horses, administration of xylazine (0.5 mg/kg IV) decreases the MAC of halothane and isoflurane by 20% and 25%, respectively (Fig. 9.8).[124,125] Given the results of these studies, doses of injectable and inhalational anesthetics

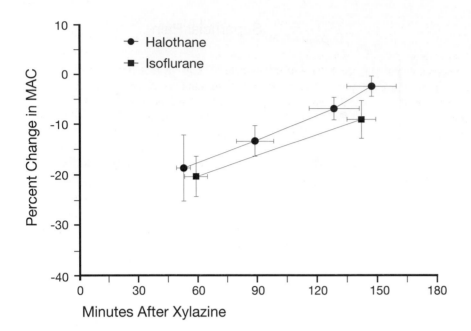

Fig. 9.8. Effects of xylazine (0.5 mg/kg intravenously) on the minimum alveolar concentration (MAC) of halothane or isoflurane in horses. With permission from Bennett et al.[124]

should be significantly reduced when xylazine is administered perioperatively to both small and large animals.

Intravenous administration of xylazine induces a brief period of hypertension and reflex bradycardia, followed by a longer-lasting decrease in cardiac output and arterial pressure. In most species, cardiac output decreases by 30% to 50% and arterial pressure by 20% to 30%.[42,103,126,127] The initial hypertensive phase is caused by activation of peripheral postsynaptic α_2 receptors, which produces vascular smooth muscle contraction and vasoconstriction. In horses, administration of a low dose of xylazine (0.4 mg/kg IV), produces less dramatic changes in arterial pressure, heart rate, and cardiac output.[117] Pretreatment with a calcium-channel blocker such as nifedipine dampens the initial increase in arterial pressure in dogs anesthetized with halothane.[128] In dogs, xylazine administration is associated with a decrease in splenic weight, which suggests a decrease in systemic vascular capacity.[129] Subsequent reductions in arterial pressure are due to decreases in sympathetic tone resulting from activation of central and peripheral (presynaptic autoreceptors) α_2 receptors. Xylazine administration also decreases heart rate by enhancing vagal tone and baroreceptor reflexes.[130] In contrast to the cardiovascular effects observed after IV injection, increases in arterial pressure and vascular resistance are not as dramatic after IM administration of xylazine in dogs and horses.[109,126] In calves given xylazine IM, hemodynamic effects are characterized by a 20% to 30% decrease in heart rate and cardiac output, and a 10% decrease in arterial pressure—without an initial increase in pressure.[131] These results suggest that IM administration of xylazine in calves does not cause transient vasoconstriction and an increase in arterial pressure to the same degree as it does in dogs and horses.

When xylazine is administered with ketamine, decreases in heart rate and cardiac output are partially offset. Ketamine administration increases heart rate and cardiac output, but arterial pressure, systemic vascular resistance, and myocardial oxygen con-

sumption increase, as well.[127,132] Because of these acute cardiovascular changes, xylazine-ketamine combinations should be reserved for use in healthy patients and not be used in patients with myocardial disease or reduced cardiopulmonary reserve.[127,132,133]

Sinus bradycardia and AV block are the arrhythmias that are encountered most commonly after xylazine administration.[126,127] Development of these arrhythmias is a normal physiological response to the increase in vagal tone induced by xylazine. Several studies have also assessed the ability of xylazine, administered alone or in combination with other anesthetic drugs, to sensitize the myocardium to the development of epinephrine-induced arrhythmias.[48] This is usually accomplished by measuring the amount of epinephrine required to induce premature ventricular depolarizations, and this amount is called the *arrhythmogenic dose of epinephrine* (ADE). In an initial study using a more severe test (the epinephrine fibrillation threshold), premedication with xylazine decreased the dose of epinephrine required to induce fibrillation in dogs anesthetized with thiamylal and halothane, whereas premedication with acepromazine had the opposite effect.[46] In a later study, ketamine administration reportedly decreased the ADE more than did xylazine administration, and coadministration decreased the ADE more than either drug alone.[134] Studies using a saline-controlled ADE model to reduce experimental error associated with repeated epinephrine administration demonstrated no change in the ADE after IM administration of xylazine or medetomidine in dogs anesthetized with halothane or isoflurane.[92,93] From these studies, it is clear that, if anesthetic-induced changes in the ADE (arrhythmogenicity) are a concern, selection of the inhalational anesthetic (halothane vs. isoflurane) is far more critical than selection of an α_2-agonist as the preanesthetic.

Although respiratory rate decreases after administration of clinically recommended doses of xylazine, arterial pH, PO_2, and PCO_2 remain virtually unchanged in cats, dogs, and horses.[42,103,117,126,127,135] Decreases in respiration rate are accompanied by increases in tidal volume, which keep alveolar ventilation and arterial blood-gas values relatively constant.[127,136] In horses suffering from recurrent obstructive pulmonary disease (heaves), xylazine administration decreases pulmonary resistance, increases dynamic compliance, and may have some therapeutic value.[137] In contrast, when a large dose of xylazine (1.0 mg/kg IV) is administered to healthy dogs, minute ventilation, physiological dead space, oxygen transport, venous PO_2 and oxygen content, and oxygen consumption decrease, and tidal volume increases.[127] Xylazine administration also increases airway resistance and resonant frequency in calves.[138] Intravenous administration of xylazine to horses (0.5 to 1.0 mg/kg) and sheep (0.02 to 0.05 mg/kg) anesthetized with halothane increases airway pressure and decreases arterial PO_2.[43,139] Similarly, arterial PO_2 decreases after administration of xylazine (0.05 to 0.3 mg/kg IV) to conscious sheep.[140–142] The results of these studies suggest that the decrease in arterial PO_2 is produced by activation of peripheral α_2 receptors and a perfusion-related imbalance between ventilation and the pulmonary circulation. Additionally, the dramatic decrease in arterial PO_2 observed in sheep after administration of xylazine may be primarily caused by a pulmonary inflammatory response that is confined to ruminants with a unique population of intravascular macrophages.[143,144] Thus, although the bulk of the evidence indicates a minimal detrimental effect on respiratory function in most domestic animals, caution is advised when administering xylazine or other α_2-agonists to small ruminants, when administering high singular or cumulative doses to any species, or when combining α_2-agonists with injectable or inhalational anesthetics that produce significant cardiopulmonary depression.

Alterations in gastrointestinal function after xylazine administration have been reported in several species. Excessive salivation can occur in animals that have not been given anticholinergics. In dogs, gastroesophageal sphincter pressure decreases, which may increase the incidence of gastroesophageal reflux.[50] Most cats and 10% to 20% of dogs vomit shortly after IM administration of xylazine. Emesis may be linked to activation of central α_2 receptors because prior administration of yohimbine—but not cholinergic, dopaminergic, histaminergic, serotonergic, or opioid receptor antagonists—prevents emesis.[145] Occasionally, acute gastric distension can occur in large dogs (>25 kg) given xylazine IV or IM.[146] This distension may be caused by aerophagia or by the parasympatholytic effects of xylazine on the gastrointestinal tract, leading to atony and accumulation of gas.

Xylazine administration decreases gastrointestinal motility and prolongs gastrointestinal transit time in several species. In dogs, it decreases gastrin secretion and gastrointestinal motility, and prolongs gastrointestinal transit time.[147–149] In sheep and cattle, cyclical contractions of the reticulum and rumen are inhibited by administration of xylazine and other α_2-agonists, and administration of α_2-antagonists (tolazoline or yohimbine) antagonizes these gastrointestinal effects.[150] In horses, motility of the cecum and colon are inhibited by administration of xylazine or xylazine-butorphanol, and normal bowel myoelectrical activity returns slowly after administration of xylazine-ketamine.[151,152] However, intestinal smooth muscle relaxation and analgesia me-

diated by activation of central and peripheral α_2 receptors also play an important role in the relief of visceral pain.[153] Indeed, xylazine is reportedly more effective than either opioids or nonsteroidal anti-inflammatory drugs in relieving visceral pain in ponies and horses.[119,154] In addition to increasing the visceral pain threshold, xylazine administration effectively sedates and calms painful horses and helps to prevent self-induced trauma. As expected, these desirable modifications in behavior are also accompanied by a decrease in intestinal motility and blood flow. This decrease in intestinal blood flow is disproportionate to the total decrease in cardiac output, which suggests that α_2 receptors mediate vasoconstriction within the intestinal vasculature.[155] Additionally, administration of an α_2-antagonist (yohimbine) attenuates ileus and hypoperfusion associated with endoxemia in horses, which provides further evidence of the important role of α_2 receptors in the regulation of gastrointestinal function.[156]

Urine output increases after xylazine administration in cattle, horses, ponies, and cats.[157–160] Urine specific gravity and osmolality also decrease in horses and ponies.[158,159] Although urethral closure pressure decreases in both male and female dogs given xylazine, normal micturition reflexes are maintained.[161] Decreases in urethral closure pressure are coupled to a reduction in electromyographic activity of the urethral sphincter, but xylazine administration does not appear to alter the detrusor reflex in dogs.[162,163]

Transient hypoinsulinemia and hyperglycemia have been reported in several species sedated with xylazine or that are anesthetized using a regimen that incorporates xylazine.[164–169] Hyperglycemia results from α_2-receptor–mediated inhibition of insulin release from pancreatic beta cells, and the magnitude and duration of these actions appear to be dose dependent.[167] Other hormonal changes induced by xylazine include transient alterations in growth hormone, testosterone, prolactin, antidiuretic hormone, and follicle-stimulating hormone levels.

Myometrial tone and intrauterine pressure increase after xylazine administration in cattle.[170] In pregnant sheep, myometrial activity doubled for 1 h after xylazine administration, whereas fetal diaphragmatic activity is reduced.[171] In horses, administration of equipotent doses of xylazine, detomidine, or romifidine produces comparable increases in intrauterine pressure.[172] Clinically, α_2-agonists have been administered during all stages of pregnancy in several domestic species but have not been definitively associated with an increased incidence of reproductive complications.[63] α_2-Agonists also reduce cardiac output and could impair fetal oxygen delivery. Although administration of xylazine and other α_2-agonists has not been linked definitively to abortion and premature labor, the indiscriminate use of these drugs in pregnant animals during the last trimester is not advised.

Xylazine administration causes mydriasis, which may be due to either central inhibition of parasympathetic input to the iris, direct activation of α_2 receptors located in the iris, or both.[173,174] Xylazine administration also lowers intraocular pressure in rabbits, cats, and monkeys by reducing sympathetic tone and decreasing aqueous flow.[175] More importantly, administration of xylazine to dogs and cats can cause vomiting, which increases intraocular pressure dramatically.

Xylazine can also be administered epidurally to horses and cattle. In addition to an analgesic effect mediated by activation of spinal α_2 receptors (heteroceptors), xylazine has a significant membrane-stabilizing or local anesthetic effect when applied to neurons or nerve fibers. This effect is characterized by a reduction in conduction velocity and blockade of action potentials.[176] Iontophoretic application of xylazine to rat cortical neurons suppresses spontaneous firing rates, and this effect is not blocked by an α_2-antagonist.[177] The results of these studies suggest that the action of locally applied xylazine is caused in part by a local anesthetic effect.

In horses, xylazine can be administered epidurally alone or in combination with a local anesthetic. When comparing xylazine and lidocaine at equal doses and volumes in ponies, xylazine induces more profound and longer-lasting analgesia after epidural administration.[178] Analgesia induced by epidural administration of xylazine does not cause the same degree of motor nerve paralysis as that caused by administration of local anesthetics.[179] In horses, the duration of epidural analgesia can be significantly prolonged by coadministration of lidocaine and xylazine, and is not associated with enhanced neurotoxicity or dramatic changes in cardiopulmonary function.[180]

In cattle, epidural administration of xylazine produces longer-lasting analgesia than does epidurally administered lidocaine or IM administered xylazine.[181] Cardiopulmonary and GI effects of epidural administration of xylazine (0.05 mg/kg) include decreases in heart rate, respiratory rate, and rumen motility.[182] Intravenous administration of tolazoline (0.3 mg/kg) rapidly antagonizes these effects but does not alter sedative and regional analgesic effects.[182] In sheep, intrathecal administration of xylazine or clonidine produces dose-dependent analgesia of the forelimbs, and analgesia is abolished by intrathecal administration of an α_2-antagonist (idazoxan).[183] These results indicate that xylazine produces part of its analgesic effect through activation of spinal α_2 receptors. This mechanism of analgesic action is further substantiated by the prolongation of analgesia observed after coadministration of morphine and a selective α_2-agonist (medetomidine) epidurally.[184]

Clinical Uses The clinical uses of xylazine are usually restricted to healthy animals. There is considerable variation among species in the dose of xylazine required to produce an equivalent sedative effect (Table 9.6). Generally, the lowest dose that will provide the required degree of sedation is administered to limit cardiovascular side effects. Xylazine is currently approved for use as a sedative in cats, dogs, horses, deer, and elk in the United States, and for cats, dogs, horses, and cattle in Canada. Xylazine—especially the 10% (100 mg/mL) solution—should be handled carefully to avoid accidental self-administration. If the drug is absorbed through mucous membranes or administered IM, profound sedation and bradycardia can occur. Medical treatment should be sought immediately, and the package insert should be given to the attending physician.

In dogs and cats, xylazine is used alone or in combination with opioids to provide sedation and analgesia for diagnostic and minor surgical procedures. The drug is also used in combination

Table 9.6. Xylazine doses for several domesticated species

Species	Dose
Cats	0.25–0.5 mg/kg IV
	0.5–1.0 mg/kg IM
Dogs	0.25–0.5 mg/kg IV
	0.5–1.0 mg/kg IM
Horses	0.5–1.0 mg/kg IV
	1.0–2.0 mg/kg IM
Cattle	0.05–0.1 mg/kg IV
	0.1–0.2 mg/kg IM
Sheep	0.05–0.1 mg/kg IV
	0.1–0.2 mg/kg IM
Goats	0.05–0.1 mg/kg IV
	0.1–0.2 mg/kg IM
Llama	0.1–0.2 mg/kg IV
	0.2–0.4 mg/kg IM

IM, intramuscularly; IV, intravenously.

with ketamine, ketamine-diazepam, or tiletamine-zolazepam to provide anesthesia for brief surgical procedures. As a preanesthetic, xylazine is used alone or in combination with opioids to facilitate placement of IV catheters and to decrease requirements for injectable and inhalational anesthetics. Anticholinergics (atropine and glycopyrrolate) can be administered with xylazine to prevent development of severe bradyarrhythmias perioperatively. Small doses of xylazine (0.1 mg/kg) can be administered postoperatively to smooth recovery and to potentiate the effects of other analgesic drugs (opioids), provided that patients are hemodynamically stable. Xylazine can be given IV or IM, but the IM route is preferred because cardiovascular side effects are reduced. Intramuscular doses for healthy dogs and cats range from 0.5 to 1.0 mg/kg.

In horses and cattle, xylazine is used alone or in combination with butorphanol to provide sedation and analgesia for diagnostic and surgical procedures. Xylazine can also be used as a preanesthetic before induction of anesthesia with ketamine, ketamine-diazepam, ketamine-guaifenesin, or thiopental-guaifenesin. In horses anesthetized with halothane, isoflurane, or sevoflurane, small doses of xylazine (0.1 to 0.2 mg/kg) can be given IV during the maintenance and recovery phases to reduce anesthetic requirements and smooth recovery, respectively. Xylazine can be also be used in combination with ketamine and guaifenesin for total IV anesthesia. After induction of anesthesia with xylazine and ketamine, anesthesia can be maintained with a combination of xylazine, ketamine, and guaifenesin ("triple drip") for approximately 1 h.

As a general rule, cattle usually require one-tenth of the dose of xylazine that horses require to produce an equivalent level of sedation. For sedation and analgesia alone or in combination with butorphanol, IV doses for horses range from 0.2 to 0.8 mg/kg, and those for cattle range from 0.02 to 0.08 mg/kg. As a preanesthetic before induction with an injectable anesthetic and maintenance with an inhalational anesthetic, IV doses for horses range from

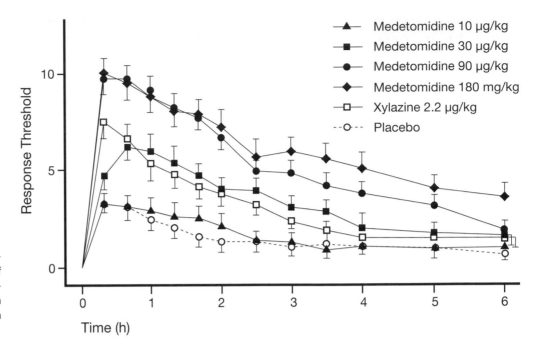

Fig. 9.9. Analgesic effects of intramuscular administration of medetomidine in dogs. Higher response threshold equates with improved analgesic action. With permission from Vainio et al.[115]

0.4 to 0.8 mg/kg, and those for cattle range from 0.04 to 0.08 mg/kg. As a preanesthetic before induction of anesthesia with ketamine or ketamine-diazepam, an IV dose of 1.0 mg/kg is typically administered to horses and a dose of 0.1 mg/kg is given to cattle. Xylazine can be administered to healthy foals and calves over 1 month of age but is not usually given to neonates. Doses of xylazine should be decreased in very large animals (draft horses and bulls) and in breeds with increased sensitivity to the drug (Brahman and Brahman crosses).[63] Xylazine doses should also be decreased in sick or debilitated animals but may need to be increased in excited animals. In horses or cattle that are fractious and difficult to restrain, xylazine can be administered IM at a dose of 1.0 to 2.0 mg/kg or 0.1 to 0.2 mg/kg, respectively.

Sudden death has been reported in horses after xylazine administration.[77] Excitement, violent seizures, and collapse can occur after accidental intracarotid injection or after IV administration of an overdose. Seizure activity that occurs immediately after intracarotid administration of xylazine is probably mediated by the activation of central α_1 receptors.[74,75] After intracarotid injection, pharmacodynamic effects extend beyond the "window of sedation" typically achieved when recommended doses of xylazine are administered IV or IM. Seizures caused by accidental intracarotid injection of xylazine can usually be controlled by IV administration of thiopental or thiopental-guaifenesin to effect. Once seizures are controlled, the horse should be intubated and supplemental oxygen administered.[63]

Medetomidine

This is the most widely used α_2-agonist in small animals. The chemical name for the drug is (±)-4-(1-[2,3-dimethylphenyl]ethyl)-1H-imidazole monohydrochloride (Fig. 9.6). It is more potent than xylazine and is dosed on a microgram-per-kilogram basis rather than a milligram-per-kilogram basis. In North America, medetomidine is approved for use in dogs as a sedative-

analgesic. Studies on the sedative, analgesic, and cardiopulmonary effects of medetomidine in cats have also been reported.[185–187]

Pharmacokinetics Medetomidine is a highly selective α_2-agonist that is supplied as a racemic mixture of two optical enantiomers. Dexmedetomidine is the active enantiomer, and levomedetomidine has no apparent pharmacological activity.[188–192] Shortly after medetomidine was approved for use in dogs as a sedative-analgesic in North America, dexmedetomidine was approved for use in people as a postoperative sedative in the United States. As expected, dexmedetomidine is approximately twice as potent as the racemic mixture that is available for use in animals. In dogs and cats, medetomidine has a rapid onset of action and can be administered IV or IM. After IM administration, the drug is rapidly absorbed, and peak plasma concentrations are reached within 30 min. The elimination half-life of medetomidine (80 µg/kg) after IV and IM administration in dogs and after IM administration in cats is 0.97, 1.28, and 1.35 h, respectively.[193] At this dose, the apparent volume of distribution after IV and IM administration in dogs and after IM administration in cats is 2.8, 3.0, and 3.5 L/kg, respectively.[193] Therapeutic effects of medetomidine are terminated by removal from target tissues, which parallels clearance of the drug from plasma. Elimination occurs mainly by biotransformation in the liver, and inactive metabolites are excreted in the urine.

Pharmacodynamics Onset of sedation, analgesia, and muscle relaxation is rapid after IM administration of medetomidine to dogs and cats, and the intensity and duration of these effects depend on dose. When medetomidine is given IM to dogs at a dose of 30 µg/kg, significant sedation is apparent within 5 min and persists for 1 to 2 h.[115] Similarly, when medetomidine is given to cats at a dose of 50 µg/kg, significant sedation is apparent within 15 min and persists for 1 to 2 h.[186] At these doses, analgesia peaks within 30 min and persists for 1 to 2 h (Fig. 9.9).[115,186] In dogs, sedation induced by IM administration of medetomidine at a dose of 30 µg/kg is comparable in intensity to that induced by IM administration of xylazine at a dose of 2.2 mg/kg but lasts longer.[115] Medetomidine has also been used as a sedative-analgesic and as a preanesthetic in horses, but, even at low doses (5 to 10 µg/kg IV), ataxia is a significant problem.[117,194,195] Sedation following IV administration of a 10-µg/kg dose of medetomidine in horses is comparable to that induced by a 1-mg/kg IV dose of xylazine.[194]

Medetomidine administration decreases injectable and inhalational anesthetic requirements dramatically in several species. Premedication with medetomidine decreases induction doses of thiopental and propofol by over 50% in dogs. Administration of medetomidine IM at doses of 10, 20, and 40 µg/kg decreases the amount of thiopental required for intubation to 7.0, 4.5, and 2.4 mg/kg, respectively.[85,196] Similarly, administration of medetomidine IM at a dose of 20 µg/kg decreases the amount of propofol required for intubation to 1.8 mg/kg.[122] Administration of medetomidine IM also appears to reduce the dose of ketamine required to induce anesthesia in dogs and cats.[197–199] Premedication with medetomidine also reduces halothane and isoflurane requirements. Administration of medetomidine IV at a dose of 10 µg/kg is reported to decrease the MAC of halothane by 90%.[200] In contrast, administration of medetomidine IV at a dose of 30 µg/kg decreased the MAC of isoflurane by only 47%.[87] Additionally, administration of medetomidine IM at a dose of 8 µg/kg consistently reduced the bispectral index value (an index of anesthetic depth) in dogs anesthetized with isoflurane (1.0, 1.5, and 2.0 MAC).[201]

As with other α_2-agonists, medetomidine administration produces dose-dependent changes in cardiovascular function.[202] Cardiovascular effects are best described in two phases: an initial peripheral phase characterized by vasoconstriction, increased blood pressure, and reflex bradycardia; and a subsequent central phase characterized by decreased sympathetic tone, heart rate, and blood pressure. Occasionally, AV blockade occurs secondary to the initial increase in blood pressure, and reflex (baroreceptors) increase in vagal tone. In conscious dogs, mean arterial pressure increases transiently, and heart rate and cardiac index decrease by approximately 60% after IV administration of medetomidine at doses ranging from 5 to 20 µg/kg.[202] At these doses, changes in mean arterial pressure, central venous pressure, and vascular resistance are dose dependent, whereas changes in heart rate and cardiac index are not. In conscious cats, mean arterial pressure does not appear to change, and heart rate and cardiac index decrease by approximately 50% after IM administration of medetomidine at a dose of 20 µg/kg (Fig. 9.10).[187] In conscious horses, IV administration of a low dose of medetomidine (4 µg/kg) produces less dramatic changes in arterial pressure, heart rate, and cardiac output.[117] In cats anesthetized with isoflurane (2%), mean arterial pressure increases from 77 to 122 mm Hg, heart rate decreases from 150 to 125 beats/min, and mean arterial flow decreases from 578 to 325 mL/min, 20 min after the IM administration of medetomidine at a dose of 10 µg/kg.[203] As with xylazine, cardiovascular responses to medetomidine administration appear to be attenuated in animals anesthetized with isoflurane.[89,90] Cerebral vasodilation is attenuated

by the IV administration of low doses of dexmedetomidine (0.5, 1.0, and 2.0 µg/kg) in dogs anesthetized with isoflurane or sevoflurane (0.5, 1.0, and 1.5 MAC).[204] In dogs anesthetized with isoflurane for ovariohysterectomy, heart rate is lower but blood pressure better maintained with medetomidine premedication (20 µg/kg IM) when compared with acepromazine premedication (0.05 mg/kg IM) (Fig. 9.11).[205] In conscious animals, the decrease in cardiac output is caused primarily by the decrease in heart rate and increase in vascular resistance, and not by a direct depression of myocardial contractility.[206,207] Peripheral cardiovascular effects are most pronounced when α_2-agonists are administered IV at high doses, and these effects can be reduced by administering α_2-agonists IM at low doses.[126,208] Although cardiac output decreases after medetomidine or dexmedetomidine administration, blood flow to the heart, brain, and kidneys is maintained by redistribution of flow from less vital organs and tissues.[209]

Medetomidine administration has little effect on pulmonary function. Respiratory rate and minute ventilation decrease after medetomidine administration, but this decrease in minute ventilation appears to coincide with a decrease in carbon dioxide production, and arterial blood-gas values do not change. In conscious dogs, IV administration of medetomidine (5 to 10 µg/kg) decreases the neurorespiratory response (ventilatory drive) to increases in inspired carbon dioxide.[210] In another study in conscious dogs and cats, IM administration of medetomidine at doses of 40 and 20 µg/kg, respectively, does not alter arterial pH, PCO_2, and PO_2.[187,211] Similarly, IV administration of medetomidine (4 µg/kg) does not alter arterial pH, PCO_2, and PO_2 in conscious horses.[117] The IV administration of medetomidine (20 µg/kg) or dexmedetomidine (3 µg/kg) does not alter arterial blood-gas values and produces less depression of ventilatory drive than does isoflurane (1 MAC) in dogs.[212,213] Parenteral administration of a low dose of dexmedetomidine (0.5 µg/kg) also appears to protect against bronchoconstriction induced by nebulization of histamine in dogs anesthetized with thiopental.[214]

Medetomidine administration has significant effects on gastrointestinal function in animals. Vomiting occurs in 10% of dogs and over 50% of cats administered medetomidine IM at mean doses of 40 and 80 µg/kg, respectively.[185] Normally, this is not a problem and can be advantageous if owners or hospital staff fail to withhold food from patients before induction of anesthesia. However, the potential for development of aspiration pneumonia exists if a properly inflated, cuffed endotracheal tube is not in place. Vomiting also dramatically increases intraocular pressure, which is a potential problem for some patients with ocular injury or disease. Medetomidine administration decreases gastrin release and intestinal and colonic motility in dogs.[149,215] These effects are mediated by activation of visceral α_2 receptors and inhibition of acetylcholine release.

Medetomidine administration has significant effects on renal and urogenital function in animals. In dogs, administration of medetomidine (10 to 20 µg/kg IV) decreases urine specific gravity and increases urine production for approximately 4 h.[216] Apparently, α_2-agonists interfere with the action of antidiuretic hormone on the renal tubules and collecting ducts, which increases the production of dilute urine.[217,218] Activation of α_1 re-

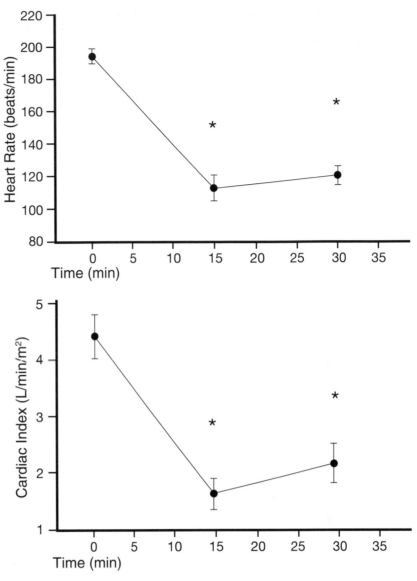

Fig. 9.10. Hemodynamic effects of intramuscular administration of medetomidine (20 μg/kg) in conscious cats. With permission from Lamont et al.[187]

*Significantly (P<0.05) different from baseline

ceptors increases myometrial contractility, and activation of α_2 receptors has limited effects on uterine tone in most species. In dogs, IV administration of medetomidine at a dose of 20 μg/kg decreases electrical activity of the myometrium, and a dose of 40 μg/kg increases electrical activity in dogs during the last trimester of pregnancy.[219] Medetomidine administration also produces significant cardiovascular effects, and use of the drug in animals during the last trimester of pregnancy should be avoided.

Medetomidine administration has dramatic effects on endocrine function in animals. In dogs, IM administration of medetomidine (10 to 80 μg/kg) decreases plasma norepinephrine, epinephrine, and nonesterified fatty acid concentrations for up to 4 h, whereas cortisol and glucagon concentrations do not change.[76] Preoperative administration of α_2-agonists also attenuates the stress response associated with surgical trauma. In dogs undergoing ovariohysterectomy, preoperative administration of medetomidine reduces catecholamine and cortisol concentrations post-

operatively.[220,221] Similarly, preoperative administration of medetomidine (20 μg/kg IM) attenuates perioperative increases in norepinephrine, epinephrine, and cortisol concentrations to a greater degree than does acepromazine (Fig. 9.12).[205] Administration of xylazine or medetomidine activates α_2 receptors on pancreatic beta cells and inhibits release of insulin for approximately 2 h.[76,168,222] Although both drugs produce a comparable inhibition of insulin release, medetomidine produces a less dramatic change in plasma glucose concentrations.[76,222] This difference may be due to a difference in selectivity for the α_2 receptor compared with the α_1 receptor. Xylazine, a less selective agonist, appears to increase plasma glucose concentrations directly by activating α_1 receptors and stimulating hepatic glucose production. Changes in catecholamine, nonesterified fatty acids, insulin, and glucose concentrations induced by administration of α_2-agonists (xylazine or medetomidine) are reversed by administration of α_2-antagonists (yohimbine or atipamezole).[223]

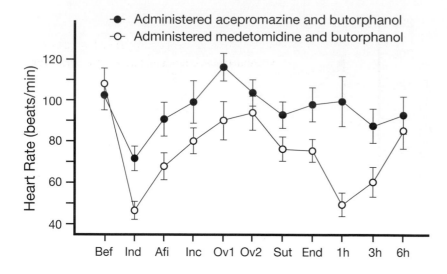

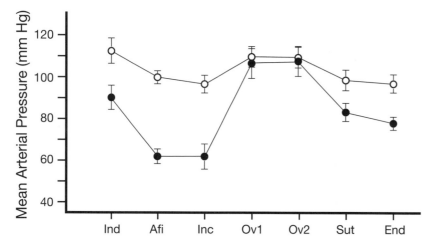

Fig. 9.11. Effects of preoperative intramuscular administration of medetomidine (20 µg/kg) or acepromazine (0.05 mg/kg) on heart rate and mean arterial pressure in dogs anesthetized with isoflurane for ovariohysterectomy. Bef, before surgery; Ind, induction; Afi, after induction; Inc, abdominal incision; OV1, removal of ovary; OV2, removal of second ovary; Sut, abdominal suturing; End, end of surgery; and 1h, 3h, and 6h mean 1 h, 3 h, and 6 h after surgery. With permission from Vaisanen et al.[205]

Medetomidine administration has significant effects on pupillary diameter and intraocular pressure. Topical administration of medetomidine readily induces mydriasis and decreases intraocular pressure in rabbits and cats.[224,225] In contrast, the IV administration of medetomidine to dogs reportedly induces miosis and does not alter intraocular pressure.[226] Administration of medetomidine to dogs and cats can cause vomiting, which increases intraocular pressure dramatically.

Medetomidine administration also has significant effects on cerebral blood flow, intracranial pressure, and thermoregulation. In one study performed in spontaneously breathing dogs anesthetized with isoflurane (0.5 and 1.5 MAC), the administration of dexmedetomidine (10 µg/kg IV) decreased cerebral blood flow but did not alter cerebral metabolic rate.[227] In another study in mechanically ventilated dogs anesthetized with isoflurane (1.0 MAC), the administration of medetomidine (30 µg/kg IV) increased cerebral perfusion pressure but did not change intracranial pressure.[90] Again, administration of medetomidine to dogs and cats can cause vomiting, which increases intracranial pressure dramatically. Decreases in body temperature are attributed to depression of the thermoregulatory center, muscle relaxation, and reduced shivering. In conscious dogs, only slight reductions

in body temperature (1°C over 1 h) are observed after IV administration of medetomidine at doses ranging from 1 to 20 µg/kg.[202]

Clinical Uses   As an adjunct to general anesthetics, medetomidine has a favorable pharmacodynamic profile in dogs and cats. In addition to providing sedation, analgesia, and muscle relaxation, the preoperative administration of medetomidine substantially reduces the amount of injectable and inhalational anesthetic required to induce and maintain anesthesia. Medetomidine administration also attenuates the stress response to surgical trauma by reducing catecholamine and cortisol levels postoperatively.[220,221] The initial increase in vascular resistance and blood pressure and subsequent bradycardia are potential problems, but these side effects are well tolerated by healthy dogs and cats. Vomiting is also a potential problem for some patients. As a general rule, medetomidine should not be administered to pediatric or geriatric animals, or to animals with significant neurological, cardiovascular, respiratory, hepatic, or renal disease. Once preanesthetic and anesthetic drugs are administered, patients should be monitored carefully throughout the perioperative period, with special attention being paid to heart rate and rhythm.

α_2-Agonists and acepromazine are the only reliable sedatives

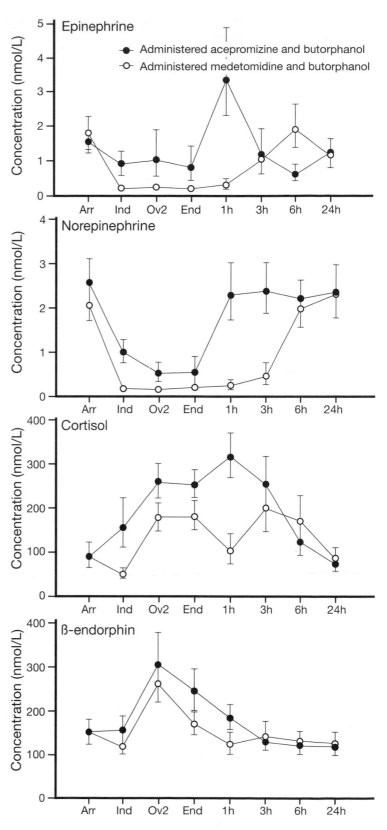

Fig. 9.12. Effects of preoperative intramuscular administration of medetomidine (20 µg/kg) or acepromazine (0.05 mg/kg) on norepinephrine, epinephrine, cortisol, and ß-endorphin concentrations in dogs undergoing ovariohysterectomy. Arr, arrival; Ind, induction; OV2, removal of second ovary; End, end of surgery; and 1h, 3h, 6h, and 24h mean 1 h, 3 h, 6 h, and 24 h after surgery. With permission from Vaisanen et al.[205]

currently available for use in dogs and cats. Acepromazine is routinely used preoperatively to provide sedation for catheter placement and induction of anesthesia, and is often given in combination with opioids to provide both sedation and analgesia. However, acepromazine is not suitable for every patient (e.g.,

brachycephalics, epileptics, and boxers) and can cause significant hypotension in animals anesthetized with isoflurane.[41] Medetomidine can be administered preoperatively at low doses to healthy dogs and cats, alone or in combination with opioids (Table 9.7).[67] Compared with acepromazine, low doses of

Table 9.7. Medetomidine doses for preoperative sedation and analgesia in healthy dogs and cats

Drugs	Canine Doses[a]	Feline Doses[b]
Medetomidine	10–20 µg/kg IM	20–40 µg/kg IM
with or without		
Atropine	0.04 mg/kg IM	0.04 mg/kg IM
Medetomidine	5–10 µg/kg IM	10–20 µg/kg IM
Butorphanol	0.2–0.4 mg/kg IM	0.2–0.4 mg/kg IM
with or without		
Atropine	0.04 mg/kg IM	0.04 mg/kg IM
Medetomidine	5–10 µg/kg IM	10–20 µg/kg IM
Morphine	0.2–0.4 mg/kg IM	0.2–0.4 mg/kg IM
with or without		
Atropine	0.04 mg/kg IM	0.04 mg/kg IM
Medetomidine	5–10 µg/kg IM	10–20 µg/kg IM
Hydromorphone	0.04–0.08 mg/kg IM	0.04–0.08 mg/kg IM
with or without		
Atropine	0.05 mg/kg IM	0.04 mg/kg IM
Medetomidine	5–10 µg/kg IM	10–20 µg/kg IM
Oxymorphone	0.04–0.08 mg/kg IM	0.04–0.08 mg/kg IM

IM, intramuscularly.
[a]Medetomidine should not be given to dogs with significant neurological, cardiac, respiratory, hepatic, or renal disease. Some of these drugs are not approved for use in dogs in Canada or the United States.
[b]Medetomidine should not be given to cats with significant neurological, cardiac, respiratory, hepatic, or renal disease. Some of these drugs are not approved for use in cats in Canada or the United States.

Table 9.8. Medetomidine and opioid doses for postoperative sedation and analgesia in healthy dogs and cats

Drugs	Canine Doses[a]	Feline Doses[b]
Medetomidine	2–4 µg/kg IM	4–8 µg/kg IM
Medetomidine	1–2 µg/kg IM	2–4 µg/kg IM
Butorphanol	0.1–0.2 mg/kg IM	0.1–0.2 mg/kg IM
Medetomidine	1–2 µg/kg IM	2–4 µg/kg IM
Morphine	0.1–0.2 mg/kg IM	0.1–0.2 mg/kg IM
Medetomidine	1–2 µg/kg IM	2–4 µg/kg IM
Hydromorphone	0.02–0.04 mg/kg IM	0.02–0.04 mg/kg IM
Medetomidine	1–2 µg/kg IM	2–4 µg/kg IM
Oxymorphone	0.02–0.04 mg/kg IM	0.02–0.04 mg/kg IM

IM, intramuscularly.
[a]Medetomidine should not be given to dogs with significant neurological, cardiac, respiratory, hepatic, or renal disease. Some of these drugs are not approved for use in dogs in Canada or the United States.
[b]Medetomidine should not be given to cats with significant neurological, cardiac, respiratory, hepatic, or renal disease. Some of these drugs are not approved for use in cats in Canada or the United States.

medetomidine produce better analgesia for catheter placement and greater reductions in anesthetic requirements, and are less likely to cause hypotension in animals anesthetized with isoflurane. In patients with good cardiopulmonary reserve, the concurrent administration of an anticholinergic agent will prevent bradyarrhythmias while slightly improving cardiac output at the expense of a rather large increase in myocardial work and oxygen consumption. Thus, the use of an anticholinergic preoperatively with α2-agonists to prevent bradycardia and AV blockade continues to be somewhat controversial.[208,211,228,229] The use of an anticholinergic has been recommended for the following reasons: Firstly, even at low preanesthetic doses, significant bradycardia can occur if an anticholinergic is not administered concurrently. Secondly, the potential for severe vagotonic responses and profound bradycardia, secondary to surgical manipulation and administration of other anesthetic drugs (opioids), is higher during the perioperative period. Thirdly, while the concurrent administration of anticholinergics with high doses of medetomidine can cause dramatic increases in vascular resistance and myocardial work, these increases can be minimized and are generally well tolerated by healthy patients given low doses of medetomidine prior to inhalant (vasodilatory) anesthesia.

Bradycardia and AV blockade are more consistently prevented when anticholinergics are given 10 to 20 min before medetomidine administration, although this is not always practical.[97,211,230] Atropine has a more rapid onset of action than does glycopyrrolate and can be given at the same time as low doses of medetomidine (5 to 20 µg/kg). However, anticholinergic administration increases vagal tone transiently, which can increase the incidence of bradyarrhythmias induced by administration of any α2-agonist. For example, if atropine or glycopyrrolate is administered at the same time as, or after, high doses of medetomidine (30 to 60 µg/kg), bradycardia and AV blockade are not consistently prevented and ventricular arrhythmias may develop.[228] Therefore, when high doses of medetomidine are administered, the use of anticholinergics should be avoided, heart rate and rhythm should be monitored closely, and atipamezole should be administered to correct severe bradyarrhythmias. Concurrent administration of anticholinergics with α2-agonist–ketamine combinations should also be avoided, because a prolonged high heart rate can occur.[231]

Very low doses of medetomidine have been given postoperatively to dogs and cats, alone or in combination with opioids (Table 9.8).[67] Administration of selective α2-agonists in very low doses may enhance and prolong the analgesic effects of opioids, with limited effects on cardiovascular function. Lower doses of opioids may also be used, which reduces the frequency of postoperative respiratory depression. α2-Agonists also can be used to manage anxiety and dysphoria postoperatively. Because the duration of action of medetomidine is significantly less than that of acepromazine, sedation can be more readily controlled.

Detomidine

This agent is used primarily for sedation and analgesia in horses. The chemical name for the drug is 1H-imidazole, 4-([2,3-

dimethylphenyl]methyl)-hydrochloride (Fig. 9.6). Detomidine is more potent than xylazine and is dosed on a microgram-per-kilogram basis rather than a milligram-per-kilogram basis. The drug produces sedation, analgesia, and muscle relaxation that are comparable to those produced by xylazine in intensity but last longer. In North America and Europe, the drug is sold as detomidine hydrochloride and is approved for use in horses as a sedative-analgesic.

Pharmacokinetics Pharmacokinetic parameters have been determined in calves and horses after IV administration of detomidine at a dose of 50 μg/kg.[232] In calves, the drug is 86% protein bound, and the elimination half-life, clearance, and volume of distribution are 20.0 h, 24.9 mL/min · kg, and 29.4 L/kg, respectively. In horses, the drug is 84% protein bound, and the elimination half-life, clearance, and volume of distribution are 9.7 h, 8.1 mL/min · kg, and 6.8 L/kg, respectively. In calves, detomidine is eliminated primarily by metabolism, and most of the metabolites are excreted in the urine. Tissue liver residues are less than 1 μg/kg at 80 h.

Pharmacodynamics Onset of sedation, analgesia, and muscle relaxation is rapid after IV or IM administration of detomidine. When detomidine is administered IV to horses at a dose of 20 μg/kg, peak sedation and analgesia are achieved within 15 min and persist for approximately 1 h.[116,233] When the same dose is administered IM, depth of sedation and intensity of analgesia are reduced, and peak effects are achieved within 30 min and persist for approximately 1 h.[233] Sedative and analgesic effects are comparable in duration when electrical stimulation is used to evaluate somatic analgesia. Administration of detomidine at a dose of 20 μg/kg induces sedation and analgesia comparable in intensity to, but longer than, those induced by administration of xylazine at a dose of 1.1 mg/kg.[116,233] At these doses, detomidine and xylazine also induce comparable levels of muscle relaxation and ataxia.[116] In a colic model (ponies with cecal balloons), IV administration of detomidine at a dose of 20 μg/kg provides analgesia for 45 min, whereas IV administration of xylazine at a dose of 1.1 mg/kg provides analgesia for approximately 20 min.[234] Sedation lasted longer than analgesia when a cecal balloon was used to evaluate visceral analgesia. In a 2003 placebo-controlled study using electrical stimulation to evaluate somatic analgesia, IV administration of detomidine at a dose of 20 μg/kg provided analgesia for approximately 30 min, whereas administration of xylazine at a dose of 1.1 mg/kg provided analgesia for approximately 15 min (Fig. 9.13).[82] Detomidine administration also reduces catecholamine and cortisol concentrations in horses.[235]

Detomidine administration produces dose-dependent changes in cardiovascular function. In conscious ponies, arterial pressure increases and heart rate decreases by over 50% immediately (1 min) after IV administration of detomidine at doses ranging from 10 to 60 μg/kg.[236] In conscious horses, heart rate decreases by 30% to 35% and cardiac output decreases by 40% to 45% after IV administration at doses of 10 to 20 μg/kg.[237] At these doses, 30% of horses develop AV block within 5 min, heart rate

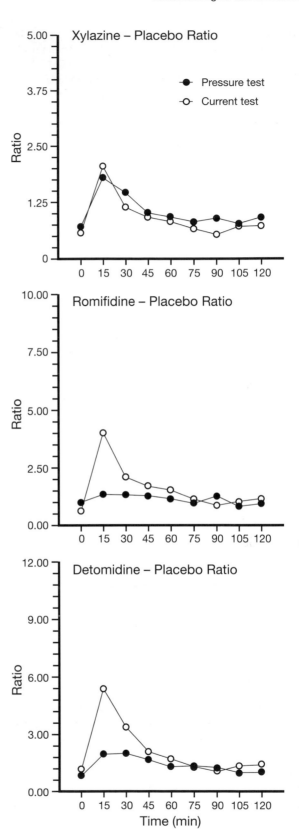

Fig. 9.13. Antinociceptive effects of intravenous administration of xylazine (1.1 mg/kg), detomidine (20 μg/kg), or romifidine (80 μg/kg) in horses. With permission from Moens et al.[82]

and cardiac output are reduced for 45 min to 1 h, and mean arterial pressure is reduced for 90 min to 2 h. After IM administration of detomidine at a dose of 40 µg/kg, heart rate and cardiac output decrease by 27% and 39%, respectively.[237] Intravenous infusion of detomidine at a constant rate produces decreases in heart rate and cardiac output that are comparable to bolus administration, but mean arterial pressure remains elevated for the duration of the infusion.[238] Hematocrit and total protein decrease after parenteral administration of detomidine.[237,238] These changes are probably produced by fluid shifts and sequestration of erythrocytes in the spleen that occur as sympathetic tone decreases.

Detomidine administration has little effect on pulmonary function. Respiratory rate decreases after detomidine administration, but the apparent decrease in minute ventilation appears to coincide with a decrease in carbon dioxide production, and arterial blood-gas values do not change appreciably. In horses administered detomidine IV at doses of 10 to 20 µg/kg, respiratory rate decreases by approximately 50% for 2 h after drug administration.[237] At these doses, arterial pH and PCO_2 do not change, and PO_2 decreases transiently but returns to normal values within 15 to 30 min. The decrease in arterial PO_2 coincides with the dramatic drop in heart rate and cardiac output that occurs immediately after administration of detomidine. Intravenous infusion of detomidine at a constant rate alters respiratory rate and arterial blood-gas values that are comparable to bolus administration.[238]

Detomidine administration has significant effects on esophageal transit time and gastrointestinal motility. In horses, IV administration of detomidine (10 to 20 µg/kg) produces dose-dependent increases in esophageal transit time and retrograde peristalsis, and a decrease in duodenal motility.[239,240] Detomidine administration also reduces cecal and colonic motility in ponies.[153] Detomidine is a very effective visceral analgesic, and its use in horses with colic should not be abandoned because of unwarranted concerns about gastrointestinal side effects. After all, increases in sympathetic tone associated with uncontrolled abdominal pain also reduce gastrointestinal motility.

Detomidine produces sedation and analgesia in horses when administered epidurally at the first intercoccygeal space. Its administration at doses of 30 to 60 µg/kg diluted in 10 mL of sterile water produces perineal analgesia with variable bilateral analgesia up to the 14th thoracic dermatome.[241,242] Analgesia begins in 10 to 15 min and lasts for 2 to 3 h. Doses under 30 µg/kg do not produce reliable analgesia, and those over 60 µg/kg may cause recumbency. The drug is lipophilic and is rapidly absorbed into the systemic circulation from the epidural space. Systemic effects include marked sedation and ataxia, a decrease in heart rate and 2° AV blockade, an increase followed by a decrease in mean arterial pressure, decreases in respiratory rate and arterial PO_2, and diuresis.[241,242] Caudal epidural administration of xylazine (0.25 mg/kg) produces longer-lasting perineal analgesia with fewer systemic side effects than does caudal epidural administration of detomidine.[243] Detomidine has also been administered epidurally in combination with morphine to horses with experimentally induced hind-limb lameness and to horses undergoing bilateral stifle arthroscopy.[244–246]

Clinical Uses Detomidine administration produces reliable sedation, analgesia, and muscle relaxation in horses. The drug is used alone and in combination with butorphanol to produce standing sedation for diagnostic and surgical procedures, and as an analgesic for horses with abdominal pain. Detomidine is usually given IV at doses ranging from 5 to 20 µg/kg, but it can be given IM at doses ranging from 10 to 40 µg/kg. Sedation is more reliable and horses are less responsive to external stimuli when detomidine is given with butorphanol or another opioid.[247] As with other α₂-agonists, excited or fractious animals may require higher doses of detomidine. Ataxia can be a problem in healthy horses, and the drug should be used with discretion in animals with neurological disease. Detomidine administration also produces marked cardiovascular side effects, and it should be used with caution in horses with significant cardiovascular disease and in those with endotoxic or traumatic shock.

Romifidine

This selective α₂-agonist derived from clonidine is used primarily to produce sedation and analgesia in horses. The chemical name for the drug is 2-([2-bromo-6-flourophenyl]imino)-imidazolidine hydrochloride. Romifidine administration produces sedation and analgesia that are comparable in duration to those produced by detomidine administration.[82,116] Muscle relaxation is comparable but with less ataxia than seen with equivalent sedative doses of xylazine or detomidine.[116] Romifidine is approved or licensed for use in horses in North America and Europe. Although not approved for use in small animals, the sedative and cardiovascular effects of romifidine have been reported in both dogs and cats.[248–251]

Pharmacokinetics and Pharmacodynamics Onset of sedation and analgesia is rapid after parenteral administration of romifidine. When romifidine is administered IV to horses at doses of 40 to 80 µg/kg, sedation begins within 2 min, peak effects are reached within 10 min, and sedation lasts for 40 to 80 min.[116] Similar results were reported after IV administration of romifidine at a dose of 80 µg/kg (Fig. 9.13).[82] In small animals, romifidine has a longer duration of action than xylazine or medetomidine. In dogs, the IM administration of romifidine at doses of 10 to 40 µg/kg produces mild to moderate sedation within 10 min and lasts for 1 to 2 h.[248] Sedation produced by IM administration of romifidine at a dose of 40 µg/kg is comparable in intensity to that produced by xylazine at a dose of 1 mg/kg but lasts longer.[248] The onset of action is faster after IV administration of romifidine at doses ranging from 20 to 120 µg/kg, but the incidence of neuromuscular, respiratory, and cardiovascular side effects increases.[249,250] In cats, IM administration of romifidine (40 µg/kg) in combination with butorphanol produces moderate sedation.[251]

Romifidine can also be used preoperatively to facilitate induction of anesthesia with ketamine and postoperatively to facilitate recovery from inhalational anesthesia. In horses, administration of romifidine before induction of anesthesia with diazepam and ketamine produces short-term anesthesia that is comparable to that produced by preanesthetic administration of xylazine.[252] Romifidine has also been used as a preanesthetic before induction and maintenance of anesthesia with ketamine and halothane, respectively.[253] Small doses of romifidine have also been administered postoperatively to facilitate recovery from isoflurane anesthesia.[254] Like other α_2-agonists, preanesthetic administration of romifidine (20 to 40 µg/kg IV) to dogs reduces the amount of thiopental or propofol required to induce anesthesia by 40% to 60% and the amount of halothane required to maintain anesthesia by 20%.[255,256]

At doses that produce equivalent degrees of sedation, romifidine produces changes in cardiovascular function that are comparable to those produced by other α_2-agonists. In conscious horses, IV administration of romifidine (80 µg/kg) induces a 20% increase in mean arterial pressure and a 30% to 60% decrease in heart rate within 5 min.[257] During the next 30 min, bradycardia persists, AV blockade is common, and cardiac output decreases by 30% to 40%.[257,258] As with other α_2-agonists, respiratory rate decreases, but arterial pH, PCO_2, and PO_2 do not change, and gastrointestinal motility decreases after romifidine administration.[257–259] In dogs, IV administration of romifidine at doses ranging from 5 to 50 µg/kg induces a dose-dependent increase in mean arterial pressure and decreases in heart rate and cardiac output.[260] After IM administration of romifidine (20 to 40 µg/kg), bradycardia lasts for up to 2 h, respiratory rate decreases, and arterial pH, PCO_2, and PO_2 do not change.[18] Administration of glycopyrrolate 15 min before administration of romifidine (20 to 40 µg/kg IM) reduces the incidence and severity of bradycardia but is associated with a dose-dependent increase in mean arterial pressure.[18]

Clinical Uses Romifidine administration produces reliable sedation and analgesia in horses. The drug is used alone and in combination with butorphanol to produce standing sedation for diagnostic and surgical procedures, and can also be used as an analgesic. Romifidine is usually administered IV to horses at doses ranging from 40 to 80 µg/kg and produces less ataxia than equivalent sedative doses of xylazine or detomidine.[116] Sedation is more reliable and horses are less responsive to external stimuli when romifidine is administered in combination with butorphanol.[257,261] Romifidine (100 µg/kg IV) has also been given as a preanesthetic before induction of anesthesia with diazepam and ketamine.[252] As with other α_2-agonists, fractious or excited animals may require higher doses of romifidine. Romifidine also produces marked cardiovascular side effects and should be used with caution in horses with significant cardiovascular disease and in those with endotoxic or traumatic shock. Romifidine is not labeled for use in dogs and cats, and its use in small animals is not recommended until further studies are completed.

α_2-Antagonists

α_2-Antagonists are used to reverse the sedative and cardiovascular effects of α_2-agonists. Currently, three antagonists (tolazoline, yohimbine, and atipamezole) are available for use in animals. Tolazoline is a relatively nonselective α-receptor antagonist, and receptor binding or selectivity ratios (α_2/α_1) for yohimbine and atipamezole are 40:1 and 8526:1, respectively.[262] Tolazoline and yohimbine are used primarily to reverse the effects

of xylazine in dogs, cats, ruminants, and several exotic species.[63,263] Atipamezole is used primarily to reverse the effects of medetomidine is dogs, cats, and several exotic species.[69,264–266]

In addition to reversing the sedative and cardiovascular effects of α_2-agonists, α_2-antagonists can produce significant side effects. If a relative overdose of an antagonist is administered, neurological (excitement and muscle tremors), cardiovascular (hypotension and tachycardia), and gastrointestinal (salivation and diarrhea) side effects can occur. Death has also been reported after rapid IV administration of tolazoline or yohimbine to sheep sedated with xylazine.[267] Therefore, the dose of antagonist should be calculated carefully, and these calculations should be based on the amount of agonist administered initially and the time that has elapsed since the agonist was administered. Generally, calculations are based on an agonist/antagonist ratio, not a simple milligram-per-kilogram calculation. When in doubt, it is usually better to underdose than to overdose the antagonist. α_2-Mediated analgesia is also reversed, and antagonists should be used with discretion postoperatively.

Tolazoline

This agent is a nonselective α-receptor antagonist used primarily to reverse the sedative and cardiovascular effects of xylazine in ruminants.[63,263] The drug is a synthetic imidazoline derivative (2-benzyl-2-imidazoline) that produces histaminergic and cholinergic effects in addition to producing nonspecific blockade of α receptors (Fig. 9.14). Tolazoline is approved for use in horses in Canada but not the United States.

Pharmacokinetics and Pharmacodynamics Tolazoline is effective in reversing the sedative cardiovascular and gastrointestinal effects of xylazine in ruminants. Administration of tolazoline (2 mg/kg IV) reverses the sedative and cardiovascular effects of xylazine (0.3 to 0.4 mg/kg IV) in sheep, 5- to 7-month old calves, and adult cattle equally well.[142,267–270] In steers and lactating dairy cattle given tolazoline IV at a relatively high dose (4 mg/kg), tolazoline concentrations were below 10 µg/kg by 4 days in tissue samples and by 2 days in milk samples.[113]

Clinical Uses Tolazoline is used primarily to reverse the sedative and cardiovascular effects of xylazine in ruminants. Dose calculations are made based on an agonist/antagonist ratio of approximately 1:10. Therefore, if the initial xylazine dose is 0.1 to 0.2 mg/kg, then tolazoline would be administered IV at a dose of 1 to 2 mg/kg. The time that has elapsed since the agonist was administered should be considered, as well. Tolazoline should be administered slowly when given IV to avoid neurological (excitement) and cardiovascular (hypotension and tachycardia) side effects.

Yohimbine

This agent is used as a selective α_2-receptor antagonist of the sedative and cardiovascular effects of xylazine in dogs, cats, and several exotic species.[63,263] This drug is an indolealkylamine alkaloid (17-hydroxyyohimban-16-carboxylic acid methyl ester) that is related structurally to reserpine (Fig. 9.14). At high con-

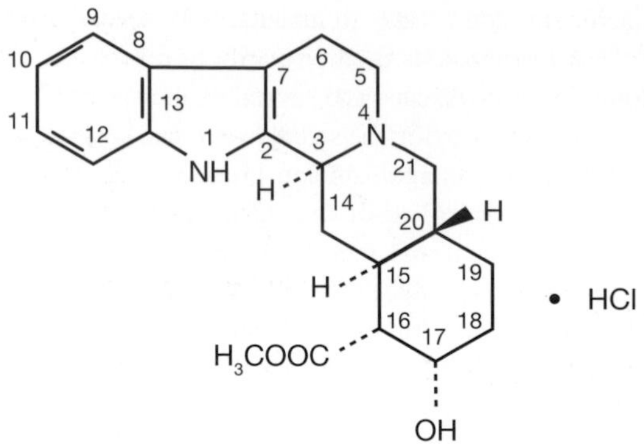

Fig. 9.14. Chemical structures of α_2-receptor antagonists. With permission from Gross.[325]

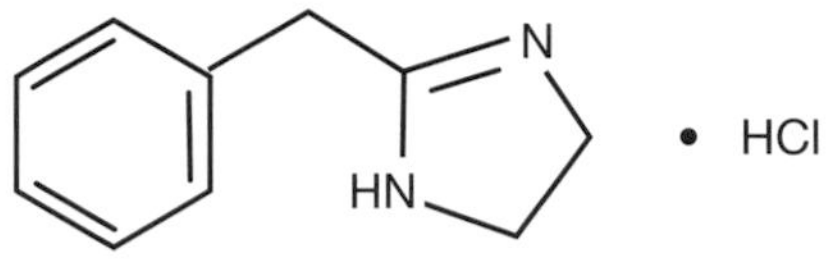

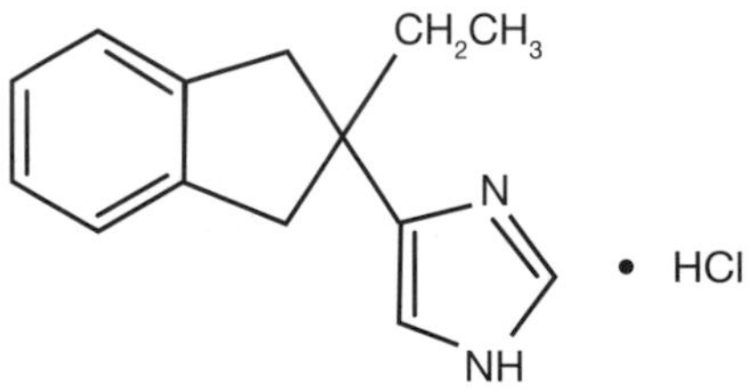

centrations, yohimbine may interact with dopaminergic and serotonergic receptors, and, at very high concentrations, it may have a nonspecific local anesthetic effect.[271] Yohimbine is approved for use in dogs in Canada and in dogs and deer in the United States.

Pharmacokinetics and Pharmacodynamics The pharmacokinetics of yohimbine have been reported for dogs, horses, and cattle.[272]

In dogs given yohimbine (0.4 mg/kg IV), the volume of distribution, total body clearance, and elimination half-life were 4.5 L/kg, 30 mL/min · kg, and 104 min, respectively. In horses given yohimbine (0.15 mg/kg IV), the volume of distribution, total body clearance, and elimination half-life were 4.6 L/kg, 40 mL/min · kg, and 76 min, respectively. In cattle given yohimbine (0.25 mg/kg IV), the volume of distribution, total body clearance, and elimination half-life were 4.9 L/kg, 70 mL/min · kg, and 47 min, respectively.

Many reports on a variety of species have documented yohimbine's efficacy in antagonizing the various actions of xylazine. Examples include use in dogs where yohimbine (0.1 mg/kg IV) reverses the sedative and cardiovascular effects of xylazine (1 mg/kg) when administered IV or IM[263,273–275] and in cats where

yohimbine (0.5 mg/kg IV) reverses the sedative and cardiovascular effects of xylazine (1 mg/kg IM).[263] In white-tailed deer, yohimbine (0.3 mg/kg IV) reportedly reverses the sedative and cardiovascular effects of a high dose of xylazine (3 mg/kg IM),[263,276] whereas, in calves, it (0.25 mg/kg IV) rapidly reverses the cardiovascular and gastrointestinal effects of xylazine (0.05 mg/kg IV), with minimum effect on sedation.[277]

Clinical Uses Dose calculations are made based on agonist/antagonist ratios of approximately 10:1, 2:1, and 10:1, for dogs, cats, and deer, respectively. Therefore, if the initial dose of xylazine is 0.5 mg/kg for a dog, then yohimbine would be given IV at a dose of 0.05 mg/kg. The time that has elapsed since the agonist was administered should be considered, as well. Like tolazoline, yohimbine is usually administered slowly IV to avoid neurological (excitement) and cardiovascular (hypotension and tachycardia) side effects.

Atipamezole
This highly selective α_2-receptor antagonist is used to reverse the sedative and cardiovascular effects of medetomidine in dogs, cats, and several other species.[69,264–266,278] The chemical name of the drug is (4-2-ethyl-2,3-dihydro-1H-inden-2-yl)-1H-imidazole (Fig. 9.14). Atipamezole is 200 to 300 times more selective for the α_2 receptor than is yohimbine and has no effect at β-adrenergic, dopaminergic, serotonergic, histaminergic, muscarinic, opiate, γ-aminobutyric acid (GABA), or benzodiazepine receptors.[262] Atipamezole is approved for use in dogs in North America and Europe.

Pharmacokinetics and Pharmacodynamics The pharmacokinetics of atipamezole (250 µg/kg IM), alone and 30 min after administration of medetomidine (50 µg/kg IV), have been reported for dogs.[279] When atipamezole is given alone, peak plasma concentrations are reached within 15 min, and the volume of distribution, total body clearance, and elimination half-life are 2.3 L/kg, 27 mL/min · kg, and 56 min, respectively. When atipamezole is given after medetomidine, peak plasma concentrations are reached within 25 min, and the volume of distribution, total body clearance, and elimination half-life are 2.5 L/kg, 24 mL/min · kg, and 72 min, respectively. Apparently, prior administration of medetomidine reduces cardiac output and hepatic blood flow, which delays absorption and metabolism of atipamezole.

Atipamezole is used primarily to reverse the sedative and cardiovascular effects of medetomidine in dogs.[264,265] Animals given atipamezole (200 µg/kg IM), 15 to 30 min after administration of medetomidine (40 µg/kg IM), show increases in heart rate and initial signs of arousal within 5 min and are walking within 10 min. Occasionally, tachycardia and excitation occur shortly after atipamezole administration, and resedation can occur 30 to 60 min after administration of the antagonist. Atipamezole has also been used to reverse the sedative and cardiovascular effects of medetomidine in cats.[266] Cats administered atipamezole (200 to 400 µg/kg IM), 15 to 30 min after administration of medetomidine (100 µg/kg IM), show increases in heart rate and initial signs of arousal within 5 min and are walking within 10 min. Occasionally,

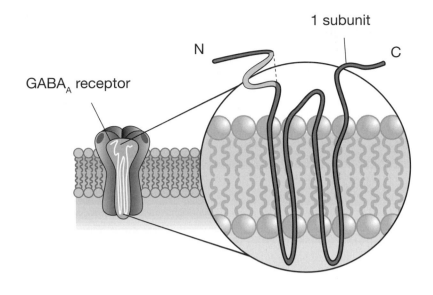

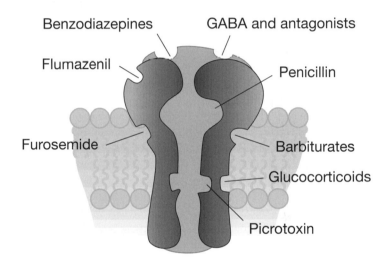

Fig. 9.15. The structure and major binding sites of the GABA$_A$-receptor complex. GABA, γ-aminobutyric acid. With permission from Chou.[326]

tachycardia and excitation occur shortly after atipamezole administration. Atipamezole has also been used to reverse the sedative effects of medetomidine in cattle[278] and several exotic species.[69] Medetomidine/atipamezole ratios for nondomestic carnivores and ruminants are 1:2–3 and 1:4–5, respectively. Atipamezole has been used to reverse the sedative and cardiovascular effects of xylazine in several species.[69,280–283] The xylazine/atipamezole ratio for reversal of most mammals is approximately 10:1.

Clinical Uses   Atipamezole is usually administered to reverse the effects of medetomidine after nonpainful diagnostic or therapeutic procedures, and it is not usually administered perioperatively. Complete reversal of the sedative, analgesic, and cardiovascular effects of medetomidine is achieved when atipamezole is administered IM to dogs and cats at four to six times and two to four times the dose of medetomidine, respectively.[265,266] Therefore, if the initial dose of medetomidine is 20 µg/kg for a dog, then atipamezole would be given IM at a dose of 100 µg/kg. Similarly, if the initial dose of medetomidine is 40 µg/kg for a cat, then atipamezole would be given IM at a dose of 120 µg/kg.

In both of these examples, the dose of atipamezole should be reduced if more than 30 min has elapsed since medetomidine administration. Because of the potential for excitation and cardiovascular side effects (hypotension and tachycardia), atipamezole is not labeled for IV use. However, it can be given IV to reverse the cardiovascular effects of medetomidine in emergency situations. Atipamezole and anticholinergics can both cause dramatic increases in heart rate, and the concurrent use of these drugs should be avoided.

Benzodiazepine Agonists

Benzodiazepines produce most of their pharmacological effects by modulating GABA-mediated neurotransmission.[284] GABA is the primary inhibitory neurotransmitter in the mammalian nervous system and cell membranes of most CNS neurons express GABA receptors. These receptors are also found outside the CNS in autonomic ganglia. Two main types of GABA receptors are involved in neuronal transmission: The GABA$_A$ receptor complex is a ligand-gated chloride channel that consists of a central pore surrounded by five glycoprotein subunits (Fig. 9.15).

Activation requires binding of GABA molecules to both α subunits of the receptor. The $GABA_B$ receptor is a metabotropic receptor that consists of a single glycoprotein subunit that is closely associated with a G protein. These G proteins are coupled directly to potassium or calcium channels or to a second-messenger system (adenylate cyclase or phospholipase C). Activation of ionotropic $GABA_A$ receptors increases chloride conductance rapidly and generates fast inhibitory postsynaptic potentials. Activation of metabotropic $GABA_B$ increases potassium conductance slowly and generates slow inhibitory postsynaptic potentials. Presynaptic $GABA_B$ autoreceptors are coupled to calcium channels and regulate neurotransmitter release.

The benzodiazepine-binding site, as well as the binding sites for other injectable anesthetics (barbiturates, propofol, and etomidate), is located on the $GABA_A$ receptor complex (Fig. 9.15). Benzodiazepines enhance binding between GABA and the $GABA_A$ receptor, and increase the frequency of channel opening. In contrast, barbiturates enhance intrinsic activity and increase the duration of channel opening. Both mechanisms increase chloride conductance and hyperpolarize the cell membrane, which reduces neuronal excitability. Benzodiazepines have no intrinsic agonist activity and cannot alter chloride conductance in the absence of GABA. This lack of intrinsic activity limits CNS depression and provides benzodiazepines with a much wider margin of safety than barbiturates.

Modulation of GABA-mediated neurotransmission also plays a role in nociception.[285] At the supraspinal level, activation of $GABA_A$ receptors inhibits descending antinociceptive pathways and enhances sensitivity to noxious stimuli. In fact, systemic administration of benzodiazepines and barbiturates antagonizes the analgesic effect of opioids.[286,287] However, at the spinal level, activation of $GABA_A$ and $GABA_B$ receptors produces an antinociceptive effect, and antagonism of spinal $GABA_B$ receptors may contribute to the development of allodynia.

Ligands that bind to benzodiazepine receptors are classified as agonists, inverse agonists, and antagonists. *Agonists* bind to benzodiazepine receptors and produce sedative, anxiolytic, muscle relaxant, and anticonvulsant effects in most animals. *Inverse agonists* bind to the same receptor and produce the opposite effects. *Antagonists* have high affinity for the benzodiazepine receptor and have little or no intrinsic activity. These ligands block or reverse the effects of both agonists and inverse agonists. Diazepam, midazolam, and zolazepam are the benzodiazepine agonists used most commonly in animals. Diazepam and midazolam are used primarily as sedatives, muscle relaxants, and anticonvulsants. Zolazepam is available in combination with a dissociative anesthetic (tiletamine), which is approved for use as an anesthetic in dogs and cats in the United States.

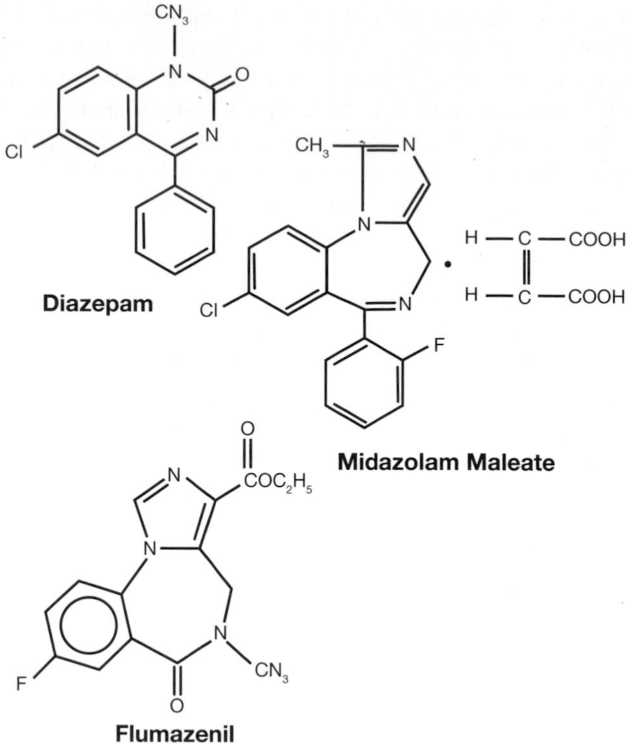

Diazepam

This is the most widely used benzodiazepine in both small and large animals. The chemical name for the drug is 7-chloro-1,3-dihydro-1-methyl-5-phenyl-2H-1,4-benzodiazepin-2-one (Fig. 9.16). Diazepam is not soluble in water, and parenteral formulations contain 40% propylene glycol and 10% ethanol. Because of this insolubility, diazepam should not be mixed with diluents or

Fig. 9.16. Chemical structures of benzodiazepine receptor agonists and antagonists. With permission from Gross.[325]

other drugs. Further, the drug should not be administered IM because it is very irritating and is poorly absorbed. The parenteral formulation of diazepam is administered by slow IV injection to avoid pain, thrombophlebitis, and cardiotoxicity. The drug is also sensitive to light and adheres to plastic, so therefore should not be stored in plastic syringes for extended periods.[288] Diazepam is used primarily as a muscle relaxant and as an anticonvulsant for dogs, cats, and horses. The drug is not approved for use in animals in Canada or the United States.

Pharmacokinetics Diazepam is highly lipid soluble and is rapidly distributed throughout the body. Approximately 90% of the drug is protein bound, and diazepam is metabolized by demethylation and hydroxylation to *N*-desmethyldiazepam (nordiazepam), 3-hydroxydiazepam, and oxazepam.[289] Nordiazepam and oxazepam produce significant pharmacological effects at clinically relevant concentrations. The pharmacokinetics of diazepam have been determined in dogs, cats, and horses. In dogs, the elimination half-life of diazepam after administration of a relatively high dose (2 mg/kg IV) is 3.2 h.[290] Nordiazepam appears rapidly in plasma and quickly exceeds concentrations of diazepam, whereas oxazepam concentrations peak within 2 h. The elimination half-lives of nordiazepam and oxazepam are 3.6 and 5.7 h, respectively. In cats, the mean elimination half-life of diazepam after administration of relatively high doses (5, 10, and 20 mg/kg IV) is 5.5 h.[291] Approximately 50% of the diazepam dose is converted to nordiazepam, and the mean elimination half-life of the metabolite is 21 h—which is approximately four times longer than the half-life of diazepam. In horses, the elimination half-life ranges from 7 to 22 h after IV administration of diazepam at a dose 0.2 mg/kg.[292] Metabolites are not detectable in plasma, but glucuronide conjugates are detectable in the urine. In contrast to dogs and cats, conjugation and elimination of the nordiazepam and oxazepam is rapid in the horse.

Pharmacodynamics Diazepam does not sedate dogs and horses reliably, and can cause excitement, dysphoria, and ataxia. In dogs, IV administration of diazepam (0.5 mg/kg) produces arousal and excitement.[293] Diazepam administration can produce dysphoria and aggressive behavior in cats, and the drug should be used with caution in this species.[120] In horses, IV administration of diazepam at doses greater than 0.2 mg/kg produces mild sedation but also marked muscle relaxation, ataxia, and recumbency.[292] Because of these behavioral effects, diazepam alone has limited value as a sedative for dogs, cats, and horses. In dogs and horses, it is used primarily as a muscle relaxant before induction of anesthesia with ketamine. Diazepam administration (0.3 to 0.5 mg/kg IV) immediately before ketamine administration improves muscle relaxation and facilitates intubation in dogs.[293,294] In horses premedicated with xylazine, diazepam administration (0.05 to 0.1 mg/kg IV) immediately before ketamine administration improves muscle relaxation and induction quality.[295] In cats premedicated with diazepam and then administered either ketamine or thiopental, dysphoria and aggressive behavior can occur during the recovery period.[120,296] This type of aberrant behavior limits the utility of diazepam as an anesthetic adjunct in cats.

Diazepam administered preoperatively reduces injectable and inhalational anesthetic requirements. Preoperative administration of diazepam (0.1 to 0.2 mg/kg IV) reduces the dose of thiamylal required to induce anesthesia, whereas the intraoperative administration reduces the amount of inhalant required to maintain anesthesia.[297] Diazepam reduces isoflurane requirements by 20% in dogs anesthetized with isoflurane and fentanyl.[298] Similarly, in horses, diazepam administration (0.04 mg/kg) reduces halothane requirement by 29%.[299] Not surprisingly, diazepam administration (0.2 mg/kg IV) decreases the absolute power of the electroencephalogram in all frequencies in dogs anesthetized with isoflurane.[300]

Diazepam produces limited effects on cardiovascular and pulmonary function in animals. In dogs, heart rate, myocardial contractility, cardiac output, and arterial blood pressure do not change appreciably after the IV administration of diazepam at doses of 0.5, 1.0, and 2.5 mg/kg.[301] The IV administration of diazepam at a dose of 0.5 mg/kg followed by the IV administration of ketamine (10 mg/kg) increases heart rate, as well cardiac output, with little change in blood pressure.[293] Respiratory rate decreases, but tidal volume is unchanged after ketamine administration. In horses, IV administration of diazepam over a wide range of doses (0.05 to 0.4 mg/kg) does not produce significant changes in heart rate, cardiac output, arterial blood pressure, respiratory rate, or arterial blood-gas values.[292]

Clinical Uses Diazepam is not a reliable sedative, but is a good muscle relaxant and anticonvulsant in most species. In dogs, diazepam is commonly administered IV at a dose of 0.3 to 0.5 mg/kg immediately before induction of anesthesia with ketamine.[293,302] Diazepam also can be administered prior to induction of anesthesia with thiopental, propofol, etomidate, or an opioid. Diazepam appears to be a more reliable sedative in older dogs and can be administered alone or in combination with an opioid to produce sedation in this subpopulation. In horses premedicated with xylazine or romifidine, diazepam is routinely administered IV at a dose of 0.05 to 0.1 mg/kg immediately before induction of anesthesia with ketamine.[295,303] Diazepam is also a reliable sedative in foals under 1 month of age and can be administered IV at a dose of 0.1 to 0.2 mg/kg. Higher doses are often administered when diazepam is used as an anticonvulsant. In small animals, diazepam in administered IV at a dose of 0.5 to 1.0 mg/kg to control seizures, and, in large animals, a dose of 0.1 to 0.2 mg/kg is usually effective. Again, the parenteral formulation of diazepam is very irritating and potentially cardiotoxic, and should always be administered by slow IV injection.

Midazolam

This is probably the most underutilized sedative in veterinary medicine. Although the drug is not a reliable sedative in dogs and cats, it produces excellent sedation and muscle relaxation in many small mammals (ferrets and rabbits), some large mammals (swine), and many birds. Midazolam is a benzodiazepine with a fused imidazole ring that accounts for the water solubility of the drug at pH values below 4.0. The chemical name of midazolam is 8-chloro-6-(2-fluorophenyl)-1-methyl-4H-imidazo(1,5-α)(1,4)-benzodiazepine (Fig. 9.16). The pH of the parenteral formulation is 3.5, and the drug is light sensitive like diazepam. After injection, midazolam changes its chemical configuration and becomes lipid soluble at physiological pH. Unlike diazepam, the drug is nonirritating and well absorbed after IM administration. Midazolam is used primarily as a perioperative sedative and muscle relaxant in ferrets, rabbits, swine, and birds. In dogs, it can be used as a sedative in older or debilitated animals, and in combination with ketamine to induce anesthesia. Midazolam is not approved for use in animals in Canada or the United States.

Pharmacokinetics In dogs, midazolam is almost completely (>90%) absorbed after IM injection, and peak plasma concentrations are reached within 15 min.[304] The drug is also highly protein bound (>95%) and rapidly crosses the blood-brain barrier. Midazolam is hydroxylated in the liver, and glucuronide conjugates are excreted in the urine.[305] After IV administration of midazolam (0.5 mg/kg), the volume of distribution, elimination half-life, and clearance are 3.0 L/kg, 77 min, and 27 mL/kg · min, respectively.[304] In dogs given midazolam (0.5 mg/kg IV) and ketamine (10 mg/kg IV) as a bolus, the elimination half-life of midazolam is 28 min.[306] In dogs anesthetized with enflurane, the volume of distribution, elimination half-life, and clearance of midazolam when given IV as a bolus are 3.9 L/kg, 98 min, and 29 mL/kg · min, respectively.[307] In piglets given midazolam (0.4 mg/kg) IV or intranasally, the elimination half-lives were 138 and 158 min, respectively.[308] Bioavailability is 64% and maximum plasma concentrations are reached within 5 min after intranasal administration.

Pharmacodynamics Midazolam is more lipophilic than diazepam and has twice the affinity for the benzodiazepine receptor. It also appears to have a greater sedative effect than diazepam in most species. Onset of sedation and muscle relaxation is rapid after IV or IM administration in most species. In most dogs administered midazolam (0.5 mg/kg) IV or IM, muscle relaxation, ataxia, transient agitation, or mild sedation are quickly observed.[304] In cats administered midazolam IV or IM over a wide range of doses (0.05 to 5.0 mg/kg), muscle relaxation becomes evident but so does arousal and excitement in many cats.[309–311] Some cats are difficult to approach and restrain after midazolam administration. Likewise, many cats administered midazolam and ketamine exhibit abnormal behavior (excitation or vocalization) during recovery. In contrast to its effect on cats, midazolam reliably sedates many other small mammals. In ferrets and rabbits, IM administration of midazolam at a dose of 0.5 to 1.0 mg/kg produces excellent sedation and muscle relaxation. It can also be administered intranasally to rabbits at dose of 2.0 mg/kg.[312] In piglets and adult swine, midazolam is an effective sedative when administered either IM or intranasally at a dose of 0.1 to 0.2 mg/kg.[308,313] In parrots and raptors, IM administration of midazolam at dose of 0.5 to 1.0 mg/kg produces mild to moderate sedation and muscle relaxation. It is also effective as a sedative in quail and geese when administered IM at doses ranging from 2 to 4 mg/kg.[314,315]

Midazolam is commonly given to enhance muscle relaxation and facilitate intubation in dogs and cats coadministered ketamine.[294,311] Preanesthetic administration (0.1–0.2 mg/kg IV) reduces the induction dose of barbiturates and propofol and the concentration of isoflurane required to maintain anesthesia during surgery.[316–318] Like diazepam, midazolam (0.2 mg/kg IV) decreases the absolute power of the electroencephalogram in dogs anesthetized with isoflurane.[319]

Midazolam administration produces minimal effects on cardiopulmonary function in mammals and birds. In dogs, heart rate and cardiac output increase by 10% to 20% after IV administration of midazolam at doses of 0.25 and 1.0 mg/kg.[301] In swine, even though heart rate decreases by 20% and respiratory rate decreases by 50%, cardiac output and blood-gas values do not change after IM midazolam injection (0.1 mg/kg).[313] The IV coadministration of midazolam with ketamine induces changes in cardiopulmonary function comparable to those induced by diazepam and ketamine in dogs.[294]

Clinical Uses Midazolam can be used alone and in combination with opioids to sedate older dogs, small mammals, swine, and birds. It is also administered in combination with injectable anesthetics to improve muscle relaxation and to reduce the dose of anesthetic required to induce anesthesia. Because midazolam has limited effects on cardiopulmonary function, the drug is an ideal sedative for many older or compromised animals. In dogs, midazolam is typically administered alone at doses of 0.2 to 0.4

mg/kg IM or in combination with opioids (butorphanol, hydromorphone, or oxymorphone) to induce sedative-analgesic effects. It can be administered IV at doses of 0.1 to 0.2 mg/kg before induction of anesthesia with ketamine, thiopental, propofol, or etomidate. In ferrets and rabbits, midazolam is administered IM at doses of 0.5 to 1.0 mg/kg, either alone or in combination with opioids (butorphanol or hydromorphone), prior to induction of anesthesia with ketamine. A 0.5- to 1.0-mg/kg dose given IM alone or in combination with butorphanol before induction of anesthesia with isoflurane or sevoflurane has proven quite effective in calming parrots and raptors. Midazolam is also an excellent sedative for most birds undergoing routine diagnostic procedures. In swine, midazolam is typically given IM at doses of 0.1 to 0.2 mg/kg, alone or in combination with opioids, prior to induction with ketamine. Midazolam can also be combined with ketamine to immobilize swine for diagnostic procedures and to facilitate placement of IV catheters. Anticonvulsant doses of midazolam are comparable to those for diazepam in most species. Midazolam is not approved for use in animals in Canada or the United States.

Benzodiazepine Antagonists

These bind to the $GABA_A$ receptor complex and block the effects of both agonists and inverse agonists. Antagonists have a strong affinity for the benzodiazepine receptor but have no intrinsic activity and are relatively free of side effects. Additionally, benzodiazepine antagonists cannot reverse the effects of anesthetic drugs (barbiturates) that bind to other sites on the $GABA_A$ receptor complex. Flumazenil is the only benzodiazepine antagonist currently available for clinical use. In animals, it is used primarily to reverse the sedative and muscle-relaxant effects of diazepam and other benzodiazepines.

Flumazenil

This is a highly selective, competitive benzodiazepine receptor antagonist. The chemical name of the drug is ethyl-8-fluro-5,6-dihydro-5-methyl-6-oxo-4H-imidazolo-(1,5-α)benzodiazepine-3-carboxylate (Fig. 9.16). Flumazenil has a strong affinity for the benzodiazepine receptor and has minimal intrinsic activity. The drug is used to reverse the unwanted behavioral and muscle relaxing effects of diazepam and midazolam in mammals and birds. Flumazenil is not approved for use in animals in Canada or the United States.

Pharmacokinetics and Pharmacodynamics Limited pharmacokinetic data are available for animals. An elimination half-life of 0.4 to 1.3 h has been reported for dogs.[320] In people, midazolam and flumazenil have similar pharmacokinetic profiles, which makes flumazenil a suitable antagonist for midazolam.[321] After IV administration, flumazenil is widely distributed and has an elimination half-life of approximately 1 h. The drug is not highly protein bound (<40%) and has a relatively high hepatic extraction ratio (0.6). Flumazenil undergoes hepatic metabolism and the primary metabolite is inactive.

Flumazenil rapidly reverses the sedative and muscle relaxant effects of benzodiazepine agonists in animals. In dogs, flumazenil administration completely reverses the behavioral and muscle-relaxant effects of an overdose of diazepam (2 mg/kg IV) or midazolam (1 mg/kg IV) within 5 min.[320] In addition, flumazenil may reverse the anticonvulsant effects of benzodiazepine agonists. Although flumazenil has minimal intrinsic activity, administration of the antagonist could facilitate development of seizures in predisposed animals. Flumazenil also appears to have minimal effects on cardiopulmonary function in animals.

Clinical Uses   Currently, flumazenil is the only benzodiazepine antagonist used in veterinary medicine. In dogs, an overdose of diazepam (2.0 mg/kg IV) or midazolam (1.0 mg/kg IV) can be effectively antagonized with flumazenil at a dose of 0.08 mg/kg.[320] These doses correspond to agonist/antagonist ratios of 26:1 and 13:1 for diazepam/flumazenil and midazolam/flumazenil, respectively. Flumazenil can be used in combination with opioid antagonists to reverse diazepam-oxymorphone sedation in dogs or alone to improve recoveries in cats given benzodiazepine-ketamine combinations.[322,323] In birds, flumazenil (0.1 mg/kg IM) has been used to reverse sedation and muscle relaxation induced by high doses of midazolam (2 to 6 mg/kg IM).[314] Following tiletamine-zolazepam (Telazol) administration in pigs, flumazenil can be used to reverse rear-limb muscle paralysis during recovery.

References

1. Hendrix PK, Robinson EP. Effects of a selective and a nonselective muscarinic cholinergic antagonist on heart rate and intestinal motility in dogs. J Vet Pharmacol Ther 1997;20:387–395.
2. Teixeira Neto FJ, McDonell WN, Black WD, et al. Effects of a muscarinic type-2 antagonist on cardiorespiratory function and intestinal transit in horses anesthetized with halothane and xylazine. Am J Vet Res 2004;65:464–472.
3. van der Linde-Sipman JS, Hellebrekers LJ, Lagerwey E. Myocardial damage in cats that died after anaesthesia. Vet Q 1992;14:91–94.
4. Roush JK, Keene BW, Eicker SW, et al. Effects of atropine and glycopyrrolate on esophageal, gastric, and tracheal pH in anesthetized dogs. Vet Surg 1990;19:88–92.
5. Galatos AD, Raptopoulos D. Gastro-oesophageal reflux during anaesthesia in the dog: The effect of preoperative fasting and premedication. Vet Rec 1995;137:479–483.
6. Ducharme NG, Fubini SL. Gastrointestinal complications associated with the use of atropine in horses. J Am Vet Med Assoc 1983;182:229–231.
7. Stormont C, Suzuki Y. Atropinesterase and cocainesterase of rabbit serum: Localization of the enzyme activity in isozymes. Science 1970;167:200–202.
8. Ludders JW, Heavner JE. Effect of atropine on tear formation in anesthetized dogs. J Am Vet Med Assoc 1979;175:585–586.
9. Arnett BD, Brightman AH, Musselman EE. Effect of atropine sulfate on tear production in the cat when used with ketamine hydrochloride and acetylpromazine maleate. J Am Vet Med Assoc 1984;185:214–215.
10. Vestre WA, Brightman AH, Helper LC, et al. Decreased tear production associated with general anesthesia in the dog. J Am Vet Med Assoc 1979;174:1006–1007.
11. Kantelip JP, Alatienne M, Gueorguiev G, et al. Chronotropic and dromotropic effects of atropine and hyoscine methobromide in unanaesthetized dogs. Br J Anaesth 1985;57:214–219.
12. Richards DL, Clutton RE, Boyd C. Electrocardiographic findings following intravenous glycopyrrolate to sedated dogs: A comparison with atropine. J Assoc Vet Anaesth 1989;16:46–50.
13. Muir WW. Effects of atropine on cardiac rate and rhythm in dogs. J Am Vet Med Assoc 1978;172:917–921.
14. Wellstein A, Pitschner HF. Complex dose-response curves of atropine in man explained by different functions of M1- and M2-cholinoceptors. Naunyn Schmiedebergs Arch Pharmacol 1988;338:19–27.
15. Weil AB, Keegan RD, Greene SA. Effect of low-dose atropine administration on dobutamine dose requirement in horses anesthetized with detomidine and halothane. Am J Vet Res 1997;58:1436–1439.
16. Paret G, Mazkereth R, Sella R, et al. Atropine pharmacokinetics and pharmacodynamics following endotracheal versus endobronchial administration in dogs. Resuscitation 1999;41:57–62.
17. Proakis AG, Harris GB. Comparative penetration of glycopyrrolate and atropine across the blood-brain and placental barriers in anesthetized dogs. Anesthesiology 1978;48:339–344.
18. Lemke KA. Electrocardiographic and cardiopulmonary effects of intramuscular administration of glycopyrrolate and romifidine in conscious beagle dogs. Vet Anaesth Analg 2001;28:75–86.
19. Frischmeyer KJ, Miller PE, Bellay Y, et al. Parenteral anticholinergics in dogs with normal and elevated intraocular pressure. Vet Surg 1993;22:230–234.
20. Singh S, McDonell WN, Young SS, et al. The effect of glycopyrrolate on heart rate and intestinal motility in conscious horses. J Vet Anaesth 1997;24:14–19.
21. Short CE, Paddleford RR, Cloyd GD. Glycopyrrolate for prevention of pulmonary complications during anesthesia. Mod Vet Pract 1974;55:194–196.
22. Dyson DH, James-Davies R. Dose effect and benefits of glycopyrrolate in the treatment of bradycardia in anesthetized dogs. Can Vet J 1999;40:327–331.
23. Dyson DH, Pascoe PJ, McDonell WN. Effects of intravenously administered glycopyrrolate in anesthetized horses. Can Vet J 1999;40:29–32.
24. Teixeira Neto FJ, McDonell WN, Black WD, et al. Effects of glycopyrrolate on cardiorespiratory function in horses anesthetized with halothane and xylazine. Am J Vet Res 2004;65:456–463.
25. McGrath CJ, Rempel WE, Addis PB, et al. Acepromazine and droperidol inhibition of halothane-induced malignant hyperthermia (porcine stress syndrome) in swine. Am J Vet Res 1981;42:195–198.
26. Redman HC, Wilson GL, Hogan JE. Effect of chlorpromazine combined with intermittent light stimulation on the electroencephalogram and clinical response of the Beagle dog. Am J Vet Res 1973;34:929–936.
27. Cornick JL, Hartsfield SM. Cardiopulmonary and behavioral effects of combinations of acepromazine/butorphanol and acepromazine/oxymorphone in dogs. J Am Vet Med Assoc 1992;200:1952–1956.
28. Smith LJ, Yu JK, Bjorling DE, et al. Effects of hydromorphone or oxymorphone, with or without acepromazine, on preanesthetic sedation, physiologic values, and histamine release in dogs. J Am Vet Med Assoc 2001;218:1101–1105.
29. Ballard S, Shults T, Kownacki AA, et al. The pharmacokinetics, pharmacological responses and behavioral effects of acepromazine in the horse. J Vet Pharmacol Ther 1982;5:21–31.

30. Marroum PJ, Webb AI, Aeschbacher G, et al. Pharmacokinetics and pharmacodynamics of acepromazine in horses. Am J Vet Res 1994;55:1428–1433.

31. Dewey EA, Maylin GA, Ebel JG, et al. The metabolism of promazine and acetylpromazine in the horse. Drug Metab Dispos 1981;9:30–36.

32. Heard DJ, Webb AI, Daniels RT. Effect of acepromazine on the anesthetic requirement of halothane in the dog. Am J Vet Res 1986;47:2113–2115.

33. Webb AI, O'Brien JM. The effect of acepromazine maleate on the anesthetic potency of halothane and isoflurane. J Am Anim Hosp Assoc 1988;24:609–613.

34. Doherty TJ, Geiser DR, Rohrbach BW. Effect of acepromazine and butorphanol on halothane minimum alveolar concentration in ponies. Equine Vet J 1997;29:374–376.

35. Doherty TJ, Rohrbach BW, Geiser DR. Effect of acepromazine and butorphanol on isoflurane minimum alveolar concentration in goats. J Vet Pharmacol Ther 2002;25:65–67.

36. Gaynor JS, Dunlop CI, Wagner AE, et al. Complications and mortality associated with anesthesia in dogs and cats. J Am Anim Hosp Assoc 1999;35:13–17.

37. Coulter DB, Whelan SC, Wilson RC, et al. Determination of blood pressure by indirect methods in dogs given acetylpromazine maleate. Cornell Vet 1981;71:75–84.

38. Stepien RL, Bonagura JD, Bednarski RM, et al. Cardiorespiratory effects of acepromazine maleate and buprenorphine hydrochloride in clinically normal dogs. Am J Vet Res 1995;56:78–84.

39. Colby ED, Sanford TD. Blood pressure and heart and respiratory rates of cats under ketamine/xylazine, ketamine/acepromazine anesthesia. Feline Pract 1981;11:19–24.

40. Ludders JW, Reitan JA, Martucci R, et al. Blood pressure response to phenylephrine infusion in halothane-anesthetized dogs given acetylpromazine maleate. Am J Vet Res 1983;44:996–999.

41. Bostrom I, Nyman G, Kampa N, et al. Effects of acepromazine on renal function in anesthetized dogs. Am J Vet Res 2003;64:590–598.

42. Muir WW, Skarda RT, Sheehan W. Hemodynamic and respiratory effects of a xylazine-acetylpromazine drug combination in horses. Am J Vet Res 1979;40:1518–1522.

43. Steffey EP, Kelly AB, Farver TB, et al. Cardiovascular and respiratory effects of acetylpromazine and xylazine on halothane-anesthetized horses. J Vet Pharmacol Ther 1985;8:290–302.

44. Popovic NA, Mullane JF, Yhap EO. Effects of acetylpromazine maleate on certain cardiorespiratory responses in dogs. Am J Vet Res 1972;33:1819–1824.

45. Boyd CJ, McDonell WN, Valliant A. Comparative hemodynamic effects of halothane and halothane-acepromazine at equipotent doses in dogs. Can J Vet Res 1991;55:107–112.

46. Muir WW, Werner LL, Hamlin RL. Effects of xylazine and acetylpromazine upon induced ventricular fibrillation in dogs anesthetized with thiamylal and halothane. Am J Vet Res 1975;36:1299–1303.

47. Dyson D, Pettifer G. Evaluation of the arrhythmogenicity of a low dose of acepromazine: Comparison with xylazine. Can J Vet Res 1997;61:241–245.

48. Lemke KA, Tranquilli WJ. Anesthetics, arrhythmias, and myocardial sensitization to epinephrine. J Am Vet Med Assoc 1994;205:1679–1684.

49. Valverde A, Cantwell S, Hernandez J, et al. Effects of acepromazine on the incidence of vomiting associated with opioid administration in dogs. Vet Anaesth Analg 2004;31:40–45.

50. Strombeck DR, Harrold D. Effects of atropine, acepromazine, meperidine, and xylazine on gastroesophageal sphincter pressure in the dog. Am J Vet Res 1985;46:963–965.

51. Hall JA, Magne ML, Twedt DC. Effect of acepromazine, diazepam, fentanyl-droperidol, and oxymorphone on gastroesophageal sphincter pressure in healthy dogs. Am J Vet Res 1987;48:556–557.

52. Scrivani PV, Bednarski RM, Myer CW. Effects of acepromazine and butorphanol on positive-contrast upper gastrointestinal tract examination in dogs. Am J Vet Res 1998;59:1227–1233.

53. Davies JV, Gerring EL. Effect of spasmolytic analgesic drugs on the motility patterns of the equine small intestine. Res Vet Sci 1983;34:334–339.

54. Doherty TJ, Andrews FM, Provenza MK, et al. The effect of sedation on gastric emptying of a liquid marker in ponies. Vet Surg 1999;28:375–379.

55. Marks SL, Straeter-Knowlen IM, Moore M, et al. Effects of acepromazine maleate and phenoxybenzamine on urethral pressure profiles of anesthetized, healthy, sexually intact male cats. Am J Vet Res 1996;57:1497–1500.

56. Lang SM, Eglen RM, Henry AC. Acetylpromazine administration: Its effect on canine haematology. Vet Rec 1979;105:397–398.

57. Barr SC, Ludders JW, Looney AL, et al. Platelet aggregation in dogs after sedation with acepromazine and atropine and during subsequent general anesthesia and surgery. Am J Vet Res 1992;53:2067–2070.

58. Pearson H, Weaver BM. Priapism after sedation, neuroleptanalgesia and anaesthesia in the horse. Equine Vet J 1978;10:85–90.

59. Dodman NH, Waterman AE. Paradoxical excitement following the intravenous administration of azaperone in the horse. Equine Vet J 1979;11:33–35.

60. Porter DB, Slusser CA. Azaperone: A review of a new neuroleptic agent for swine. Vet Med 1985;3:88–92.

61. Clarke KW. Effect of azaperone on the blood pressure and pulmonary ventilation in pigs. Vet Rec 1969;85:649–651.

62. Marsboom R, Symoens J. Azaperone (R1929) as a sedative for pigs. Neth J Vet Sci 1968;1:124–131.

63. Greene SA, Thurmon JC. Xylazine: A review of its pharmacology and use in veterinary medicine. J Vet Pharmacol Ther 1988;11:295–313.

64. England GC, Clarke KW. Alpha 2 adrenoceptor agonists in the horse: A review. Br Vet J 1996;152:641–657.

65. Cullen LK. Medetomidine sedation in dogs and cats: A review of its pharmacology, antagonism and dose. Br Vet J 1996;152:519–535.

66. Sinclair MD. A review of the physiological effects of alpha2-agonists related to the clinical use of medetomidine in small animal practice. Can Vet J 2003;44:885–897.

67. Lemke KA. Perioperative use of selective alpha-2 agonists and antagonists in small animals. Can Vet J 2004;45:475–480.

68. Klein LV, Klide AM. Central alpha2 adrenergic and benzodiazepine agonists and their antagonists. J Zoo Wildl Med 1989;20:138–153.

69. Jalanka HH, Roeken BO. The use of medetomidine and medetomidine-ketamine combinations, and atipamezole in nondomestic mammals: A review. J Zoo Wildl Med 1990;21:259–282.

70. Lemke KA. Understanding the pathophysiology of perioperative pain. Can Vet J 2004;45:405–413.

71. Maze M, Tranquilli W. Alpha-2 adrenoceptor agonists: Defining the role in clinical anesthesia. Anesthesiology 1991;74:581–605.

72. Maze M, Fujinaga M. Alpha2 adrenoceptors in pain modulation: Which subtype should be targeted to produce analgesia? Anesthesiology 2000;92:934–936.

73. Guimaraes S, Moura D. Vascular adrenoceptors: An update. Pharmacol Rev 2001;53:319–356.

74. Monti JM. Catecholamines and the sleep-wake cycle. I. EEG and behavioral arousal. Life Sci 1982;30:1145–1157.

75. Puumala T, Riekkinen P Sr, Sirvio J. Modulation of vigilance and behavioral activation by alpha-1 adrenoceptors in the rat. Pharmacol Biochem Behav 1997;56:705–712.

76. Ambrisko TD, Hikasa Y. Neurohormonal and metabolic effects of medetomidine compared with xylazine in beagle dogs. Can J Vet Res 2002;66:42–49.

77. Fuentes VO. Sudden death in a stallion after xylazine medication. Vet Rec 1978;102:106.

78. Doze V, Chen BX, Li Z, et al. Pharmacologic characterization of the receptor mediating the hypnotic action of dexmedetomidine. Acta Vet Scand Suppl 1989;85:61–64.

79. Guo TZ, Tinklenberg J, Oliker R, et al. Central alpha 1-adrenoceptor stimulation functionally antagonizes the hypnotic response to dexmedetomidine, an alpha 2-adrenoceptor agonist. Anesthesiology 1991;75:252–256.

80. Ansah OB, Raekallio M, Vainio O. Correlation between serum concentrations following continuous intravenous infusion of dexmedetomidine or medetomidine in cats and their sedative and analgesic effects. J Vet Pharmacol Ther 2000;23:1–8.

81. Virtanen R. Pharmacological profiles of medetomidine and its antagonist, atipamezole. Acta Vet Scand Suppl 1989;85:29–37.

82. Moens Y, Lanz F, Doherr MG, et al. A comparison of the antinociceptive effects of xylazine, detomidine and romifidine on experimental pain in horses. Vet Anaesth Analg 2003;30:183–190.

83. Tranquilli WJ, Benson GJ. Advantages and guidelines for using alpha-2 agonists as anesthetic adjuvants. Vet Clin North Am Small Anim Pract 1992;22:289–293.

84. Klide AM. Precautions when using alpha-2 agonists as anesthetics or anesthetic adjuvants. Vet Clin North Am Small Anim Pract 1992;22:294–296.

85. Bergstrom K. Cardiovascular and pulmonary effects of a new sedative/analgesic (medetomidine) as a preanesthetic drug in the dog. Acta Vet Scand 1988;29:109–116.

86. Cullen LK, Reynoldson JA. Xylazine or medetomidine premedication before propofol anesthesia. Vet Rec 1993;132:378–383.

87. Ewing KK, Mohammed HO, Scarlett JM, et al. Reduction of isoflurane anesthetic requirement by medetomidine and its restoration by atipamezole in dogs. Am J Vet Res 1993;54:294–299.

88. Steffey EP, Howland D Jr. Isoflurane potency in the dog and cat. Am J Vet Res 1977;38:1833–1836.

89. Lemke KA, Tranquilli WJ, Thurmon JC, et al. Hemodynamic effects of atropine and glycopyrrolate in isoflurane-xylazine–anesthetized dogs. Vet Surg 1993;22:163–169.

90. Keegan RD, Greene SA, Bagley RS, et al. Effects of medetomidine administration on intracranial pressure and cardiovascular variables of isoflurane-anesthetized dogs. Am J Vet Res 1995;56:193–198.

91. Tranquilli WJ, Thurmon JC, Benson GJ. Alterations in epinephrine-induced arrhythmogenesis after xylazine and subsequent yohimbine administration in isoflurane-anesthetized dogs. Am J Vet Res 1988;49:1072–1075.

92. Lemke KA, Tranquilli WJ, Thurmon JC, et al. Alterations in the arrhythmogenic dose of epinephrine after xylazine or medetomidine administration in isoflurane-anesthetized dogs. Am J Vet Res 1993;54:2139–2144.

93. Lemke KA, Tranquilli WJ, Thurmon JC, et al. Alterations in the arrhythmogenic dose of epinephrine after xylazine or medetomidine administration in halothane-anesthetized dogs. Am J Vet Res 1993;54:2132–2138.

94. Pettifer GR, Dyson DH, McDonell WN. An evaluation of the influence of medetomidine hydrochloride and atipamezole hydrochloride on the arrhythmogenic dose of epinephrine in dogs during halothane anesthesia. Can J Vet Res 1996;60:1–6.

95. Hayashi Y, Sumikawa K, Maze M, et al. Dexmedetomidine prevents epinephrine-induced arrhythmias through stimulation of central alpha-2 adrenoceptors in halothane-anesthetized dogs. Anesthesiology 1991;75:113–117.

96. Dyson DH, Maxie MG, Schnurr D. Morbidity and mortality associated with anesthetic management in small animal veterinary practice in Ontario. J Am Anim Hosp Assoc 1998;34:325–335.

97. Muir WW III, Ford JL, Karpa GE, et al. Effects of intramuscular administration of low doses of medetomidine and medetomidine-butorphanol in middle-aged and old dogs. J Am Vet Med Assoc 1999;215:1116–1120.

98. Grimm JB, Delormier LT, Grimm KA. Medetomidine-butorphanol-glycopyrrolate sedation for radiation therapy: An 8 year study [Abstract]. In: Proceedings of the Second Annual Veterinary Midwest Anesthesia and Analgesia Conference (VMAAC), Indianapolis, Indiana. Columbus: Ohio State University, 2004:18.

99. Clarke KW, Hall LW. "Xylazine": A new sedative for horses and cattle. Vet Rec 1969;85:512–517.

100. Burns SJ, McMullen WC. Clinical application of Bay Va 1470 in the horse. Vet Med 1971;67:77–79.

101. Garner HE, Amend JF, Rosborough JP. Effects of Bay Va 1470 on cardiovascular parameters in ponies. Vet Med 1971;66:1016–1021.

102. DeMoor A, Desmit P. Effect of Rompun on acid-base equilibrium and arterial oxygen pressure in cattle. Vet Med Rev 1971;2–3:163–169.

103. Kerr DD, Jones EW, Huggins K, et al. Sedative and other effects of xylazine given intravenously to horses. Am J Vet Res 1972;33:525–532.

104. Kerr DD, Jones EW, Holbert D, et al. Comparison of the effects of xylazine and acetylpromazine maleate in the horse. Am J Vet Res 1972;33:777–784.

105. Amend JF, Klavano PA, Stone EC. Premedication with xylazine to eliminate muscular hypertonicity in cats during ketamine anesthesia. Vet Med Small Anim Clin 1972;67:1305–1307.

106. Moye RJ, Pailet A, Smith MW Jr. Clinical use of xylazine in dogs and cats. Vet Med Small Anim Clin 1973;68:236–241.

107. Yates WD. Clinical uses of xylazine: A new drug for old problems. Vet Med Small Anim Clin 1973;68:483–486.

108. Hoffman PE. Clinical evaluation of xylazine as a chemical restraining agent, sedative, and analgesic in horses. J Am Vet Med Assoc 1974;164:42–45.

109. McCashin FB, Gabel AA. Evaluation of xylazine as a sedative and preanesthetic agent in horses. Am J Vet Res 1975;36:1421–1429.

110. Hsu WH. Xylazine-induced depression and its antagonism by alpha adrenergic blocking agents. J Pharmacol Exp Ther 1981;218:188–192.

111. Clough DP, Hatton R. Hypotensive and sedative effects of alpha-adrenoceptor agonists: Relationship to alpha 1- and alpha 2-adrenoceptor potency. Br J Pharmacol 1981;73:595–604.

112. Garcia-Villar R, Toutain PL, Alvinerie M, et al. The pharmacokinetics of xylazine hydrochloride: An interspecies study. J Vet Pharmacol Ther 1981;4:87–92.

113. Delehant TM, Denhart JW, Lloyd WE, et al. Pharmacokinetics of xylazine, 2,6-dimethylaniline, and tolazoline in tissues from yearling cattle and milk from mature dairy cows after sedation with xylazine hydrochloride and reversal with tolazoline hydrochloride. Vet Ther 2003;4:128–134.

114. Chamberlain PL, Brynes SD. The regulatory status of xylazine for use in food-producing animals in the United States. J Vet Pharmacol Ther 1998;21:322–329.

115. Vainio O, Vaha-Vahe T, Palmu L. Sedative and analgesic effects of medetomidine in dogs. J Vet Pharmacol Ther 1989;12:225–231.

116. England GC, Clarke KW, Goossens L. A comparison of the sedative effects of three alpha 2-adrenoceptor agonists (romifidine, detomidine and xylazine) in the horse. J Vet Pharmacol Ther 1992;15:194–201.

117. Bueno AC, Cornick-Seahorn J, Seahorn TL, et al. Cardiopulmonary and sedative effects of intravenous administration of low doses of medetomidine and xylazine to adult horses. Am J Vet Res 1999;60:1371–1376.

118. Pippi NL, Lumb WV. Objective tests of analgesic drugs in ponies. Am J Vet Res 1979;40:1082–1086.

119. Kalpravidh M, Lumb WV, Wright M, et al. Effects of butorphanol, flunixin, levorphanol, morphine, and xylazine in ponies. Am J Vet Res 1984;45:217–223.

120. Hatch RC, Kitzman JV, Zahner JM, et al. Comparison of five preanesthetic medicaments in thiopental-anesthetized cats: Antagonism by selected compounds. Am J Vet Res 1984;45:2322–2327.

121. Hatch RC, Wilson RC, Jernigan AD, et al. Reversal of thiopental-induced anesthesia by 4-aminopyridine, yohimbine, and doxapram in dogs pretreated with xylazine or acepromazine. Am J Vet Res 1985;46:1473–1478.

122. Redondo JI, Gomez-Villamandos RJ, Santisteban JM, et al. Romifidine, medetomidine or xylazine before propofol-halothane-N$_2$O anesthesia in dogs. Can J Vet Res 1999;63:31–36.

123. Tranquilli WJ, Thurmon JC, Corbin JE, et al. Halothane-sparing effect of xylazine in dogs and subsequent reversal with tolazoline. J Vet Pharmacol Ther 1984;7:23–28.

124. Bennett RC, Steffey EP, Kollias-Baker C, et al. Influence of morphine sulfate on the halothane sparing effect of xylazine hydrochloride in horses. Am J Vet Res 2004;65:519–526.

125. Steffey EP, Pascoe PJ, Woliner MJ, et al. Effects of xylazine hydrochloride during isoflurane-induced anesthesia in horses. Am J Vet Res 2000;61:1225–1231.

126. Klide AM, Calderwood HW, Soma LR. Cardiopulmonary effects of xylazine in dogs. Am J Vet Res 1975;36:931–935.

127. Haskins SC, Patz JD, Farver TB. Xylazine and xylazine-ketamine in dogs. Am J Vet Res 1986;47:636–641.

128. Tranquilli WJ, Thurmon JC, Paul AJ, et al. Influence of nifedipine on xylazine-induced acute pressor response in halothane-anesthetized dogs. Am J Vet Res 1985;46:1892–1895.

129. Hubbell JA, Muir WW. Effect of xylazine hydrochloride on canine splenic weight: An index of vascular capacity. Am J Vet Res 1982;43:2188–2192.

130. Antonaccio MJ, Robson RD, Kerwin L. Evidence for increased vagal tone and enhancement of baroreceptor reflex activity after xylazine (2-(2,6-dimethylphenylamino)-4-H-5,6-dihydro-1,3-thiazine) in anesthetized dogs. Eur J Pharmacol 1973;23:311–316.

131. Campbell KB, Klavano PA, Richardson P, et al. Hemodynamic effects of xylazine in the calf. Am J Vet Res 1979;40:1777–1780.

132. Kolata RJ, Rawlings CA. Cardiopulmonary effects of intravenous xylazine, ketamine, and atropine in the dog. Am J Vet Res 1982;43:2196–2198.

133. Reutlinger RA, Karl AA, Vinal SI, et al. Effects of ketamine HCl–xylazine HCl combination on cardiovascular and pulmonary values of the rhesus macaque (*Macaca mulatta*). Am J Vet Res 1980;41:1453–1457.

134. Wright M, Heath RB, Wingfield WE. Effects of xylazine and ketamine on epinephrine-induced arrhythmia in the dog. Vet Surg 1987;16:398–403.

135. Haskins SC, Peiffer RL Jr, Stowe CM. A clinical comparison of CT1341, ketamine, and xylazine in cats. Am J Vet Res 1975;36:1537–1543.

136. Lavoie JP, Pascoe JR, Kurpershoek CJ. Effects of xylazine on ventilation in horses. Am J Vet Res 1992;53:916–920.

137. Broadstone RV, Gray PR, Robinson NE, et al. Effects of xylazine on airway function in ponies with recurrent airway obstruction. Am J Vet Res 1992;53:1813–1817.

138. Gustin P, Dhem AR, Lekeux P, et al. Regulation of bronchomotor tone in conscious calves. J Vet Pharmacol Ther 1989;12:58–64.

139. Nolan A, Livingston A, Waterman A. The effects of alpha 2 adrenoceptor agonists on airway pressure in anesthetized sheep. J Vet Pharmacol Ther 1986;9:157–163.

140. Waterman AE, Nolan A, Livingston A. Influence of idazoxan on the respiratory blood gas changes induced by alpha 2-adrenoceptor agonist drugs in conscious sheep. Vet Rec 1987;121:105–107.

141. Doherty TJ, Pascoe PJ, McDonell WN, et al. Cardiopulmonary effects of xylazine and yohimbine in laterally recumbent sheep. Can J Vet Res 1986;50:517–521.

142. Hsu WH, Hanson CE, Hembrough FB, et al. Effects of idazoxan, tolazoline, and yohimbine on xylazine-induced respiratory changes and central nervous system depression in ewes. Am J Vet Res 1989;50:1570–1573.

143. Celly CS, McDonell WN, Black WD. Cardiopulmonary effects of the alpha2-adrenoceptor agonists medetomidine and ST-91 in anesthetized sheep. J Pharmacol Exp Ther 1999;289:712–720.

144. Celly CS, Atwal OS, McDonell WN, et al. Histopathologic alterations induced in the lungs of sheep by use of alpha2-adrenergic receptor agonists. Am J Vet Res 1999;60:154–161.

145. Hikasa Y, Ogasawara S, Takase K. Alpha adrenoceptor subtypes involved in the emetic action in dogs. J Pharmacol Exp Ther 1992;261:746–754.

146. Haskins SC. Abdominal distension associated with xylazine use. Mod Vet Pract 1979;60:433–438.

147. Hsu WH, McNeel SV. Effect of yohimbine on xylazine-induced prolongation of gastrointestinal transit in dogs. J Am Vet Med Assoc 1983;183:297–300.

148. McNeel SV, Hsu WH. Xylazine-induced prolongation of gastrointestinal transit in dogs: Reversal by yohimbine and potentiation by doxapram. J Am Vet Med Assoc 1984;185:878–881.

149. Nakamura K, Hara S, Tomizawa N. The effects of medetomidine and xylazine on gastrointestinal motility and gastrin release in the dog. J Vet Pharmacol Ther 1997;20:290–295.

150. Ruckebusch Y, Allal C. Depression of reticulo-ruminal motor functions through the stimulation of alpha 2-adrenoceptors. J Vet Pharmacol Ther 1987;10:1–10.

151. Rutkowski JA, Ross MW, Cullen K. Effects of xylazine and/or butorphanol or neostigmine on myoelectric activity of the cecum and right ventral colon in female ponies. Am J Vet Res 1989;50:1096–1101.

152. Lester GD, Bolton JR, Cullen LK, et al. Effects of general anesthesia on myoelectric activity of the intestine in horses. Am J Vet Res 1992;53:1553–1557.

153. Roger T, Ruckebusch Y. Colonic alpha 2-adrenoceptor–mediated responses in the pony. J Vet Pharmacol Ther 1987;10:310–318.

154. Muir WW, Robertson JT. Visceral analgesia: Effects of xylazine, butorphanol, meperidine, and pentazocine in horses. Am J Vet Res 1985;46:2081–2084.

155. Rutkowski JA, Eades SC, Moore JN. Effects of xylazine butorphanol on cecal arterial blood flow, cecal mechanical activity, and systemic hemodynamics in horses. Am J Vet Res 1991;52: 1153–1158.

156. Eades SC, Moore JN. Blockade of endotoxin-induced cecal hypoperfusion and ileus with an alpha 2 antagonist in horses. Am J Vet Res 1993;54:586–590.

157. Thurmon JC, Nelson DR, Hartsfield SM, et al. Effects of xylazine hydrochloride on urine in cattle. Aust Vet J 1978;54:178–180.

158. Thurmon JC, Steffey EP, Zinkl JG, et al. Xylazine causes transient dose-related hyperglycemia and increased urine volumes in mares. Am J Vet Res 1984;45:224–227.

159. Trim CM, Hanson RR. Effects of xylazine on renal function and plasma glucose in ponies. Vet Rec 1986;118:65–67.

160. Hartsfield SM. The effects of acetylpromazine, xylazine, and ketamine on urine production in cats [Abstract]. Presented at the American College of Veterinary Anesthesiologists Annual Scientific Meeting, 1980.

161. Moreau PM, Lees GE, Gross DR. Simultaneous cystometry and uroflowmetry (micturition study) for evaluation of the caudal part of the urinary tract in dogs: Reference values for healthy animals sedated with xylazine. Am J Vet Res 1983;44:1774–1781.

162. Richter KP, Ling GV. Effects of xylazine on the urethral pressure profile of healthy dogs. Am J Vet Res 1985;46:1881–1886.

163. Johnson CA, Beemsterboer JM, Gray PR, et al. Effects of various sedatives on air cystometry in dogs. Am J Vet Res 1988;49: 1525–1528.

164. Thurmon JC, Neff-Davis C, Davis LE, et al. Xylazine hydrochloride–induced hyperglycemia and hypoinsulinemia in thoroughbred horses. J Vet Pharmacol Ther 1982;5:241–245.

165. Tranquilli WJ, Thurmon JC, Neff-Davis CA, et al. Hyperglycemia and hypoinsulinemia during xylazine-ketamine anesthesia in Thoroughbred horses. Am J Vet Res 1984;45:11–14.

166. Symonds HW, Mallinson CB. The effect of xylazine and xylazine followed by insulin on blood glucose and insulin in the dairy cow. Vet Rec 1978;102:27–29.

167. Hsu WH, Hummel SK. Xylazine-induced hyperglycemia in cattle: A possible involvement of alpha 2-adrenergic receptors regulating insulin release. Endocrinology 1981;109:825–829.

168. Benson GJ, Thurmon JC, Neff-Davis CA. Effect of xylazine hydrochloride upon plasma glucose and serum insulin concentrations in adult pointer dogs. J Am Anim Hosp Assoc 1984;20:791–794.

169. Eichner RD, Prior RL, Kvasnicka WG. Xylazine-induced hyperglycemia in beef cattle. Am J Vet Res 1979;40:127–129.

170. LeBlanc MM, Hubbell JA, Smith HC. The effects of xylazine hydrochloride on intrauterine pressure in the cow. Theriogenology 1984;21:681–690.

171. Jansen CA, Lowe KC, Nathanielsz PW. The effects of xylazine on uterine activity, fetal and maternal oxygenation, cardiovascular function, and fetal breathing. Am J Obstet Gynecol 1984;148: 386–390.

172. Schatzmann U, Jossfck H, Stauffer JL, et al. Effects of alpha 2-agonists on intrauterine pressure and sedation in horses: Comparison between detomidine, romifidine and xylazine. Zentralbl Veterinarmed [A] 1994;41:523–529.

173. Hsu WH, Betts DM, Lee P. Xylazine-induced mydriasis: Possible involvement of a central postsynaptic regulation of parasympathetic tone. J Vet Pharmacol Ther 1981;4:209–214.

174. Hsu WH, Lee P, Betts DM. Xylazine-induced mydriasis in rats and its antagonism by alpha-adrenergic blocking agents. J Vet Pharmacol Ther 1981;4:97–101.

175. Burke JA, Potter DE. The ocular effects of xylazine in rabbits, cats, and monkeys. J Ocul Pharmacol 1986;2:9–21.

176. Aziz MA, Martin RJ. Alpha agonist and local anesthetic properties of xylazine. Zentralbl Veterinarmed [A] 1978;25:181–188.

177. O'Regan MH. Xylazine-evoked depression of rat cerebral cortical neurons: A pharmacological study. Gen Pharmacol 1989;20: 469–474.

178. Fikes LW, Lin HC, Thurmon JC. A preliminary comparison of lidocaine and xylazine as epidural analgesics in ponies. Vet Surg 1989;18:85–86.

179. LeBlanc PH, Caron JP, Patterson JS, et al. Epidural injection of xylazine for perineal analgesia in horses. J Am Vet Med Assoc 1988;193:1405–1408.

180. LeBlanc PH, Eberhart SW. Cardiopulmonary effects of epidurally administered xylazine in the horse. Equine Vet J 1990;22: 389–391.

181. Caron JP, LeBlanc PH. Caudal epidural analgesia in cattle using xylazine. Can J Vet Res 1989;53:486–489.

182. Skarda RT, Jean GS, Muir WW III. Influence of tolazoline on caudal epidural administration of xylazine in cattle. Am J Vet Res 1990;51:556–560.

183. Waterman A, Livingston A, Bouchenafa O. Analgesic effects of intrathecally-applied alpha 2-adrenoceptor agonists in conscious, unrestrained sheep. Neuropharmacology 1988;27:213–216.

184. Branson KR, Ko JC, Tranquilli WJ, et al. Duration of analgesia induced by epidurally administered morphine and medetomidine in dogs. J Vet Pharmacol Ther 1993;16:369–372.

185. Vaha-Vahe T. Clinical evaluation of medetomidine, a novel sedative and analgesic drug for dogs and cats. Acta Vet Scand 1989;30: 267–273.

186. Ansah OB, Raekallio M, Vainio O. Comparison of three doses of dexmedetomidine with medetomidine in cats following intramuscular administration. J Vet Pharmacol Ther 1998;21:380–387.

187. Lamont LA, Bulmer BJ, Grimm KA, et al. Cardiopulmonary evaluation of the use of medetomidine hydrochloride in cats. Am J Vet Res 2001;62:1745–1749.

188. Vickery RG, Sheridan BC, Segal IS, et al. Anesthetic and hemodynamic effects of the stereoisomers of medetomidine, an alpha 2-adrenergic agonist, in halothane-anesthetized dogs. Anesth Analg 1988;67:611–615.

189. Segal IS, Vickery RG, Maze M. Dexmedetomidine decreases halothane anesthetic requirements in rats. Acta Vet Scand Suppl 1989;85:55–59.

190. MacDonald E, Scheinin M, Scheinin H, et al. Comparison of the behavioral and neurochemical effects of the two optical enantiomers of medetomidine, a selective alpha-2-adrenoceptor agonist. J Pharmacol Exp Ther 1991;259:848–854.

191. Savola JM, Virtanen R. Central alpha 2-adrenoceptors are highly stereoselective for dexmedetomidine, the dextro enantiomer of medetomidine. Eur J Pharmacol 1991;195:193–199.

192. Kuusela E, Raekallio M, Anttila M, et al. Clinical effects and pharmacokinetics of medetomidine and its enantiomers in dogs. J Vet Pharmacol Ther 2000;23:15–20.

193. Salonen JS. Pharmacokinetics of medetomidine. Acta Vet Scand Suppl 1989;85:49–54.

194. Bryant CE, England GC, Clarke KW. Comparison of the sedative effects of medetomidine and xylazine in horses. Vet Rec 1991;129: 421–423.

195. Yamashita K, Muir WW III, Tsubakishita S, et al. Clinical comparison of xylazine and medetomidine for premedication of horses. J Am Vet Med Assoc 2002;221:1144–1149.

196. Young LE, Brearley JC, Richards DL, et al. Medetomidine as a premedicant in dogs and its reversal by atipamezole. J Small Anim Pract 1990;31:554–559.

197. Moens Y, Fargetton X. A comparative study of medetomidine/ketamine and xylazine/ketamine anesthesia in dogs. Vet Rec 1990;127:567–571.

198. Verstegen J, Fargetton X, Ectors F. Medetomidine/ketamine anesthesia in cats. Acta Vet Scand Suppl 1989;85:117–123.

199. Verstegen J, Fargetton X, Donnay I, et al. Comparison of the clinical utility of medetomidine/ketamine and xylazine/ketamine combinations for the ovariectomy of cats. Vet Rec 1990;127:424–426.

200. Vickery RG, Maze M. Action of the stereoisomers of medetomidine, in halothane-anesthetized dogs. Acta Vet Scand Suppl 1989;85:71–76.

201. Greene SA, Tranquilli WJ, Benson GJ, et al. Effect of medetomidine administration on bispectral index measurements in dogs during anesthesia with isoflurane. Am J Vet Res 2003;64:316–320.

202. Pypendop BH, Verstegen JP. Hemodynamic effects of medetomidine in the dog: A dose titration study. Vet Surg 1998;27:612–622.

203. Golden AL, Bright JM, Daniel GB, et al. Cardiovascular effects of the alpha2-adrenergic receptor agonist medetomidine in clinically normal cats anesthetized with isoflurane. Am J Vet Res 1998;59:509–513.

204. Ohata H, Iida H, Dohi S, et al. Intravenous dexmedetomidine inhibits cerebrovascular dilation induced by isoflurane and sevoflurane in dogs. Anesth Analg 1999;89:370–377.

205. Vaisanen M, Raekallio M, Kuusela E, et al. Evaluation of the perioperative stress response in dogs administered medetomidine or acepromazine as part of the preanesthetic medication. Am J Vet Res 2002;63:969–975.

206. Schmeling WT, Kampine JP, Roerig DL, et al. The effects of the stereoisomers of the alpha-2 adrenergic agonist medetomidine on systemic and coronary hemodynamics in conscious dogs. Anesthesiology 1991;75:499–511.

207. de Morais HS, Muir WW III. The effects of medetomidine on cardiac contractility in autonomically blocked dogs. Vet Surg 1995;24:356–364.

208. Vainio O, Palmu L. Cardiovascular and respiratory effects of medetomidine in dogs and influence of anticholinergics. Acta Vet Scand 1989;30:401–408.

209. Lawrence CJ, Prinzen FW, de Lange S. The effect of dexmedetomidine on nutrient organ blood flow. Anesth Analg 1996;83:1160–1165.

210. Lerche P, Muir WW III. Effect of medetomidine on breathing and inspiratory neuromuscular drive in conscious dogs. Am J Vet Res 2004;65:720–724.

211. Alibhai HI, Clarke KW, Lee YH, et al. Cardiopulmonary effects of combinations of medetomidine hydrochloride and atropine sulfate in dogs. Vet Rec 1996;138:11–13.

212. Bloor BC, Abdul-Rasool I, Temp J, et al. The effects of medetomidine, an alpha 2-adrenergic agonist, on ventilatory drive in the dog. Acta Vet Scand Suppl 1989;85:65–70.

213. Nguyen D, Abdul-Rasool I, Ward D, et al. Ventilatory effects of dexmedetomidine, atipamezole, and isoflurane in dogs. Anesthesiology 1992;76:573–579.

214. Groeben H, Mitzner W, Brown RH. Effects of the alpha2-adrenoceptor agonist dexmedetomidine on bronchoconstriction in dogs. Anesthesiology 2004;100:359–363.

215. Maugeri S, Ferre JP, Intorre L, et al. Effects of medetomidine on intestinal and colonic motility in the dog. J Vet Pharmacol Ther 1994;17:148–154.

216. Burton S, Lemke KA, Ihle SL, et al. Effects of medetomidine on serum osmolality; urine volume, osmolality and pH; free water clearance; and fractional clearance of sodium, chloride, potassium, and glucose in dogs. Am J Vet Res 1998;59:756–761.

217. Gellai M, Edwards RM. Mechanism of alpha 2-adrenoceptor agonist–induced diuresis. Am J Physiol 1988;255(2 Pt 2):F317–F323.

218. Rouch AJ, Kudo LH, Hebert C. Dexmedetomidine inhibits osmotic water permeability in the rat cortical collecting duct. J Pharmacol Exp Ther 1997;281:62–69.

219. Jedruch J, Gajewski Z, Ratajska-Michalczak K. Uterine motor responses to an alpha 2-adrenergic agonist medetomidine hydrochloride in the bitches during the end of gestation and the post-partum period. Acta Vet Scand Suppl 1989;85:129–134.

220. Benson GJ, Grubb TL, Neff-Davis C, et al. Perioperative stress response in the dog: Effect of pre-emptive administration of medetomidine. Vet Surg 2000;29:85–91.

221. Ko JC, Mandsager RE, Lange DN, et al. Cardiorespiratory responses and plasma cortisol concentrations in dogs treated with medetomidine before undergoing ovariohysterectomy. J Am Vet Med Assoc 2000;217:509–514.

222. Burton SA, Lemke KA, Ihle SL, et al. Effects of medetomidine on serum insulin and plasma glucose concentrations in clinically normal dogs. Am J Vet Res 1997;58:1440–1442.

223. Ambrisko TD, Hikasa Y. The antagonistic effects of atipamezole and yohimbine on stress-related neurohormonal and metabolic responses induced by medetomidine in dogs. Can J Vet Res 2003;67:64–67.

224. Jin Y, Wilson S, Elko EE, et al. Ocular hypotensive effects of medetomidine and its analogs. J Ocul Pharmacol 1991;7:285–296.

225. Potter DE, Ogidigben MJ. Medetomidine-induced alterations of intraocular pressure and contraction of the nictitating membrane. Invest Ophthalmol Vis Sci 1991;32:2799–2805.

226. Verbruggen AM, Akkerdaas LC, Hellebrekers LJ, et al. The effect of intravenous medetomidine on pupil size and intraocular pressure in normotensive dogs. Vet Q 2000;22:179–180.

227. Zornow MH, Fleischer JE, Scheller MS, et al. Dexmedetomidine, an alpha 2-adrenergic agonist, decreases cerebral blood flow in the isoflurane-anesthetized dog. Anesth Analg 1990;70:624–630.

228. Short CE. Effects of anticholinergic treatment on the cardiac and respiratory systems in dogs sedated with medetomidine. Vet Rec 1991;129:310–313.

229. Ko JC, Fox SM, Mandsager RE. Effects of preemptive atropine administration on incidence of medetomidine-induced bradycardia in dogs. J Am Vet Med Assoc 2001;218:52–58.

230. Ansah OB, Vainio O, Hellsten C, et al. Postoperative pain control in cats: Clinical trials with medetomidine and butorphanol. Vet Surg 2002;31:99–103.

231. Magoon KE, Hsu WH, Hembrough FB. The influence of atropine on the cardiopulmonary effects of a xylazine-ketamine combination in dogs. Arch Int Pharmacodyn Ther 1988;293:143–153.

232. Salonen JS. Pharmacokinetics of detomidine. Acta Vet Scand Suppl 1986;82:59–66.

233. Jochle W, Hamm D. Sedation and analgesia with Domosedan (detomidine hydrochloride) in horses: Dose response studies on efficacy and its duration. Acta Vet Scand Suppl 1986;82:69–84.

234. Lowe JE, Hilfiger J. Analgesic and sedative effects of detomidine compared to xylazine in a colic model using i.v. and i.m. routes of administration. Acta Vet Scand Suppl 1986;82:85–95.

235. Raekallio M, Leino A, Vainio O, et al. Sympatho-adrenal activity and the clinical sedative effect of detomidine in horses. Equine Vet J Suppl 1992;11:66–68.

236. Sarazan RD, Starke WA, Krause GF, et al. Cardiovascular effects of detomidine, a new alpha 2-adrenoceptor agonist, in the conscious pony. J Vet Pharmacol Ther 1989;12:378–388.

237. Wagner AE, Muir WW III, Hinchcliff KW. Cardiovascular effects of xylazine and detomidine in horses. Am J Vet Res 1991;52:651–657.

238. Daunt DA, Dunlop CI, Chapman PL, et al. Cardiopulmonary and behavioral responses to computer-driven infusion of detomidine in standing horses. Am J Vet Res 1993;54:2075–2082.

239. Watson TD, Sullivan M. Effects of detomidine on equine oesophageal function as studied by contrast radiography. Vet Rec 1991;129:67–69.

240. Merritt AM, Burrow JA, Hartless CS. Effect of xylazine, detomidine, and a combination of xylazine and butorphanol on equine duodenal motility. Am J Vet Res 1998;59:619–623.

241. Skarda RT, Muir WW. Physiologic responses after caudal epidural administration of detomidine in horses and xylazine in cattle. In: Short CE, Poznak AV, eds. Animal Pain. New York: Churchill Livingstone, 1992:292–315.

242. Skarda RT, Muir WW III. Caudal analgesia induced by epidural or subarachnoid administration of detomidine hydrochloride solution in mares. Am J Vet Res 1994;55:670–680.

243. Skarda RT, Muir WW III. Comparison of antinociceptive, cardiovascular, and respiratory effects, head ptosis, and position of pelvic limbs in mares after caudal epidural administration of xylazine and detomidine hydrochloride solution. Am J Vet Res 1996;57:1338–1345.

244. Sysel AM, Pleasant RS, Jacobson JD, et al. Efficacy of an epidural combination of morphine and detomidine in alleviating experimentally induced hind limb lameness in horses. Vet Surg 1996;25:511–518.

245. Sysel AM, Pleasant RS, Jacobson JD, et al. Systemic and local effects associated with long-term epidural catheterization and morphine-detomidine administration in horses. Vet Surg 1997;26:141–149.

246. Goodrich LR, Nixon AJ, Fubini SL, et al. Epidural morphine and detomidine decreases postoperative hind limb lameness in horses after bilateral stifle arthroscopy. Vet Surg 2002;31:232–239.

247. Clarke KW, Paton BS. Combined use of detomidine with opiates in the horse. Equine Vet J 1988;20:331–334.

248. Lemke KA. Sedative effects of intramuscular administration of a low dose of romifidine in dogs. Am J Vet Res 1999;60:162–168.

249. England GC, Flack TE, Hollingworth E, et al. Sedative effects of romifidine in the dog. J Small Anim Pract 1996;37:19–25.

250. Sinclair MD, McDonell WN, O'Grady MR, et al. The cardiopulmonary effect of romifidine in dogs with or without prior or concurrent administration of glycopyrrolate. Vet Anesth Analg 2002;29:1–13.

251. Selmi AL, Barbudo-Selmi GR, Moreira CF, et al. Evaluation of sedative and cardiorespiratory effects of romifidine and romifidine-butorphanol in cats. J Am Vet Med Assoc 2002;221:506–510.

252. Kerr CL, McDonell WN, Young SS. A comparison of romifidine and xylazine when used with diazepam/ketamine for short duration anesthesia in the horse. Can Vet J 1996;37:601–609.

253. Diamond MJ, Young LE, Bartram DH, et al. Clinical evaluation of romifidine/ketamine/halothane anesthesia in horses. Vet Rec 1993;132:572–575.

254. Santos M, Fuente M, Garcia-Iturralde R, et al. Effects of alpha-2 adrenoceptor agonists during recovery from isoflurane anesthesia in horses. Equine Vet J 2003;35:170–175.

255. England GC, Andrews F, Hammond RA. Romifidine as a premedicant to propofol induction and infusion anesthesia in the dog. J Small Anim Pract 1996;37:79–83.

256. England GC, Hammond R. Dose-sparing effects of romifidine premedication for thiopentone and halothane anesthesia in the dog. J Small Anim Pract 1997;38:141–146.

257. Clarke KW, England GC, Goossens L. Sedative and cardiovascular effects of romifidine, alone and in combination with butorphanol, in the horse. J Vet Anaesth 1991;18:25–29.

258. Freeman SL, Bowen IM, Bettschart-Wolfensberger R, et al. Cardiovascular effects of romifidine in the standing horse. Res Vet Sci 2002;72:123–129.

259. Freeman SL, England GC. Effect of romifidine on gastrointestinal motility, assessed by transrectal ultrasonography. Equine Vet J 2001;33:570–576.

260. Pypendop BH, Verstegen JP. Cardiovascular effects of romifidine in dogs. Am J Vet Res 2001;62:490–495.

261. Browning AP, Collins JA. Sedation of horses with romifidine and butorphanol. Vet Rec 1994;134:90–91.

262. Virtanen R, Savola JM, Saano V. Highly selective and specific antagonism of central and peripheral alpha 2-adrenoceptors by atipamezole. Arch Int Pharmacodyn Ther 1989;297:190–204.

263. Gross ME, Tranquilli WJ. Use of alpha 2-adrenergic receptor antagonists. J Am Vet Med Assoc 1989;195:378–381.

264. Vainio O, Vaha-Vahe T. Reversal of medetomidine sedation by atipamezole in dogs. J Vet Pharmacol Ther 1990;13:15–22.

265. Vaha-Vahe AT. The clinical effectiveness of atipamezole as a medetomidine antagonist in the dog. J Vet Pharmacol Ther 1990;13:198–205.

266. Vaha-Vahe AT. Clinical effectiveness of atipamezole as a medetomidine antagonist in cats. J Small Anim Pract 1990;1:193–197.

267. Hsu WH, Schaffer DD, Hanson CE. Effects of tolazoline and yohimbine on xylazine-induced central nervous system depression, bradycardia, and tachypnea in sheep. J Am Vet Med Assoc 1987;190:423–426.

268. Roming LG. Tolazoline as a xylazine antagonist in cattle [in German]. Dtsch Tierarztl Wochenschr 1984;91:154–157.

269. Takase K, Hikasa Y, Ogasawara S. Tolazoline as an antagonist of xylazine in cattle. Nippon Juigaku Zasshi 1986;48:859–862.

270. Powell JD, Denhart JW, Lloyd WE. Effectiveness of tolazoline in reversing xylazine-induced sedation in calves. J Am Vet Med Assoc 1998;212:90–92.

271. Goldberg MR, Robertson D. Yohimbine: A pharmacological probe for study of the alpha 2-adrenoreceptor. Pharmacol Rev 1983;35:143–180.

272. Jernigan AD, Wilson RC, Booth NH, et al. Comparative pharmacokinetics of yohimbine in steers, horses and dogs. Can J Vet Res 1988;52:172–176.

273. Hatch RC, Booth NH, Clark JD, et al. Antagonism of xylazine sedation in dogs by 4-aminopyridine and yohimbine. Am J Vet Res 1982;43:1009–1014.

274. Hsu WH. Effect of yohimbine on xylazine-induced central nervous system depression in dogs. J Am Vet Med Assoc 1983;182:698–699.

275. Hsu WH, Lu ZX, Hembrough FB. Effect of xylazine on heart rate and arterial blood pressure in conscious dogs, as influenced by atropine, 4-aminopyridine, doxapram, and yohimbine. J Am Vet Med Assoc 1985;186:153–156.

276. Hsu WH, Shulaw WP. Effect of yohimbine on xylazine-induced immobilization in white-tailed deer. J Am Vet Med Assoc 1984;185:1301–1303.

277. Guard CL, Schwark WS. Influence of yohimbine on xylazine-induced depression of central nervous, gastrointestinal and cardiovascular function in the calf. Cornell Vet 1984;74:312–321.

278. Ranheim B, Arnemo JM, Ryeng KA, et al. A pharmacokinetic study including some relevant clinical effect of medetomidine and atipamezole in lactating dairy cows. J Vet Pharmacol Ther 1999;22:368–373.

279. Salonen S, Vuorilehto L, Vainio O, et al. Atipamezole increases medetomidine clearance in the dog: An agonist-antagonist interaction. J Vet Pharmacol Ther 1995;18:328–332.

280. Jarvis N, England GC. Reversal of xylazine sedation in dogs. Vet Rec 1991;128:323–325.

281. Thompson JR, Kersting KW, Hsu WH. Antagonistic effect of atipamezole on xylazine-induced sedation, bradycardia, and ruminal atony in calves. Am J Vet Res 1991;52:1265–1268.

282. Arnemo JM, Moe SR, Soli NE. Xylazine-induced sedation in axis deer (Axis axis) and its reversal by atipamezole. Vet Res Commun 1993;17:123–128.

283. Tendillo FJ, Mascias A, Santos M, et al. Cardiopulmonary and analgesic effects of xylazine, detomidine, medetomidine, and the antagonist atipamezole in isoflurane-anesthetized swine. Lab Anim Sci 1996;46:215–219.

284. Tanelian DL, Kosek P, Mody I, et al. The role of the GABA$_A$ receptor/chloride channel complex in anesthesia. Anesthesiology 1993;78:757–776.

285. Hammond DL, Graham BA. GABAergic drugs and the clinical management of pain. In: Yaksh TL, Lynch C, Zapol WM, eds. Anesthesia: Biologic Foundations. Philadelphia: Lippincott-Raven, 1997:969–975.

286. Kissin I, Brown PT, Bradley EL Jr. Morphine and fentanyl anesthetic interactions with diazepam: Relative antagonism in rats. Anesth Analg 1990;71:236–241.

287. Kitahata LM, Saberski L. Are barbiturates hyperalgesic? Anesthesiology 1992;77:1059–1061.

288. Winsnes M, Jeppsson R, Sjoberg B. Diazepam adsorption to infusion sets and plastic syringes. Acta Anaesthesiol Scand 1981;25:93–96.

289. van der Klejin E, van Rossum JM, Muskens ET, et al. Pharmacokinetics of diazepam in dogs, mice and humans. Acta Pharmacol Toxicol 1971;29(Suppl 3):109–127.

290. Loscher W, Frey HH. Pharmacokinetics of diazepam in the dog. Arch Int Pharmacodyn Ther 1981;254:180–195.

291. Cotler S, Gustafson JH, Colburn WA. Pharmacokinetics of diazepam and nordiazepam in the cat. J Pharm Sci 1984;73:348–351.

292. Muir WW, Sams RA, Huffman RH, et al. Pharmacodynamic and pharmacokinetic properties of diazepam in horses. Am J Vet Res 1982;43:1756–1762.

293. Haskins SC, Farver TB, Patz JD. Cardiovascular changes in dogs given diazepam and diazepam-ketamine. Am J Vet Res 1986;47:795–798.

294. Hellyer PW, Freeman LC, Hubbell JA. Induction of anesthesia with diazepam-ketamine and midazolam-ketamine in greyhounds. Vet Surg 1991;20:143–147.

295. Brock N, Hildebrand SV. A comparison of xylazine-diazepam-ketamine and xylazine-guaifenesin-ketamine in equine anesthesia. Vet Surg 1990;19:468–474.

296. Reid JS, Frank RJ. Prevention of undesirable side reactions of ketamine anesthesia in cats. J Am Anim Hosp Assoc 1972;8:115–119.

297. Muir WW III, Bednarski L, Bednarski R. Thiamylal- and halothane-sparing effect of diazepam in dogs. J Vet Pharmacol Ther 1991;14:46–50.

298. Hellyer PW, Mama KR, Shafford HL, et al. Effects of diazepam and flumazenil on minimum alveolar concentrations for dogs anesthetized with isoflurane or a combination of isoflurane and fentanyl. Am J Vet Res 2001;62:555–560.

299. Matthews NS, Dollar NS, Shawley RV. Halothane-sparing effect of benzodiazepines in ponies. Cornell Vet 1990;80:259–265.

300. Greene SA, Moore MP, Keegan RD, et al. Quantitative electroencephalography for measurement of central nervous system responses to diazepam and the benzodiazepine antagonist, flumazenil, in isoflurane-anesthetized dogs. J Vet Pharmacol Ther 1992;15:259–266.

301. Jones DJ, Stehling LC, Zauder HL. Cardiovascular responses to diazepam and midazolam maleate in the dog. Anesthesiology 1979;51:430–434.

302. Wright M. Pharmacologic effects of ketamine and its use in veterinary medicine. J Am Vet Med Assoc 1982;180:1462–1471.

303. Kerr CL, McDonell WN, Young SS. A comparison of romifidine and xylazine when used with diazepam/ketamine for short duration anesthesia in the horse. Can Vet J 1996;37:601–609.

304. Court MH, Greenblatt DJ. Pharmacokinetics and preliminary observations of behavioral changes following administration of midazolam to dogs. J Vet Pharmacol Ther 1992;15:343–350.

305. Vree TB, Baars AM, Booij LH, et al. Simultaneous determination and pharmacokinetics of midazolam and its hydroxymetabolites in plasma and urine of man and dog by means of high-performance liquid chromatography. Arzneimittelforschung 1981;31: 2215–2219.

306. Brown SA, Jacobson JD, Hartsfield SM. Pharmacokinetics of midazolam administered concurrently with ketamine after intravenous bolus or infusion in dogs. J Vet Pharmacol Ther 1993;16: 419–425.

307. Hall RI, Szlam F, Hug CC Jr. Pharmacokinetics and pharmacodynamics of midazolam in the enflurane-anesthetized dog. J Pharmacokinet Biopharm 1988;16:251–262.

308. Lacoste L, Bouquet S, Ingrand P, et al. Intranasal midazolam in piglets: Pharmacodynamics (0.2 vs 0.4 mg/kg) and pharmacokinetics (0.4 mg/kg) with bioavailability determination. Lab Anim 2000;34:29–35.

309. Ilkiw JE, Suter CM, Farver TB, et al. The behaviour of healthy awake cats following intravenous and intramuscular administration of midazolam. J Vet Pharmacol Ther 1996;19:205–216.

310. Ilkiw JE, Suter CM, McNeal D, et al. The effect of intravenous administration of variable-dose midazolam after fixed-dose ketamine in healthy awake cats. J Vet Pharmacol Ther 1996;19:217–224.

311. Ilkiw JE, Suter C, McNeal D, et al. The optimal intravenous dose of midazolam after intravenous ketamine in healthy awake cats. J Vet Pharmacol Ther 1998;21:54–61.

312. Robertson SA, Eberhart S. Efficacy of the intranasal route for administration of anesthetic agents to adult rabbits. Lab Anim Sci 1994;44:159–165.

313. Smith AC, Zellner JL, Spinale FG, et al. Sedative and cardiovascular effects of midazolam in swine. Lab Anim Sci 1991;41:157–161.

314. Day TK, Roge CK. Evaluation of sedation in quail induced by use of midazolam and reversed by use of flumazenil. J Am Vet Med Assoc 1996;209:969–971.

315. Valverde A, Honeyman VL, Dyson DH, et al. Determination of a sedative dose and influence of midazolam on cardiopulmonary function in Canada geese. Am J Vet Res 1990;51:1071–1074.

316. Tranquilli WJ, Graning LM, Thurmon JC, et al. Effect of midazolam preanesthetic administration on thiamylal induction requirement in dogs. Am J Vet Res 1991;52:662–664.

317. Greene SA, Benson GJ, Hartsfield SM. Thiamylal-sparing effect of midazolam for canine endotracheal intubation: A clinical study of 118 dogs. Vet Surg 1993;22:69–72.

318. Stegmann GF, Bester L. Some clinical effects of midazolam premedication in propofol-induced and isoflurane-maintained anesthesia in dogs during ovariohysterectomy. J S Afr Vet Assoc 2001;72:214–216.

319. Keegan RD, Greene SA, Moore MP, et al. Antagonism by flumazenil of midazolam-induced changes in quantitative electroencephalographic data from isoflurane-anesthetized dogs. Am J Vet Res 1993;54:761–765.

320. Tranquilli WJ, Lemke KA, Williams LL, et al. Flumazenil efficacy in reversing diazepam or midazolam overdose in dogs. J Vet Anaesth 1992;19:65–68.

321. Amrein R, Hetzel W. Pharmacology of Dormicum (midazolam) and Anexate (flumazenil). Acta Anaesthesiol Scand Suppl 1990;92:6–15.

322. Lemke KA, Tranquilli WJ, Thurmon JC, et al. Ability of flumazenil, butorphanol, and naloxone to reverse the anesthetic effects of oxymorphone-diazepam in dogs. J Am Vet Med Assoc 1996;209:776–779.

323. Ilkiw JE, Farver TB, Suter C, et al. The effect of intravenous administration of variable-dose flumazenil after fixed-dose ketamine and midazolam in healthy cats. J Vet Pharmacol Ther 2002;25:181–188.

324. Stoelting RK. Anticholinergic drugs. In: Pharmacology and Physiology in Anesthetic Practice, 2nd ed. Philadelphia: JB Lippincott, 1987:232–239.

325. Gross ME. Tranquilizers, α_2-adrenergic agonists, and related agents. In: Adams HR. Veterinary Pharmacology and Therapeutics, 8th ed. Ames: Iowa State University Press, 2001:299–342.

326. Chou J. Pharmacology of excitatory and inhibitory neurotransmission. In: Golan DE, Tashjian AH Jr, Armstrong EJ, et al., eds. Principles of Pharmacology: The Pathophysiologic Basis of Drug Therapy. Philadelphia: Lippincott Williams and Wilkins, 2004:139–160.

Chapter 10

Opioids, Nonsteroidal Anti-inflammatories, and Analgesic Adjuvants

Leigh A. Lamont and Karol A. Mathews

Introduction

There are three major classes of analgesic agents employed in veterinary medicine for the management of pain: opioids, nonsteroidal anti-inflammatory drugs (NSAIDs), and local anesthetics. In addition to these three traditional drug classes, another diverse group of agents used to manage pain is known collectively as analgesic adjuvants. This chapter reviews the pharmacology of the opioids, NSAIDs, and analgesic adjuvants. For a complete discussion of the local anesthetics, the reader is referred to Chapter 14.

Opioids

All opioid analgesics are chemically related to a group of compounds that have been purified from the juice of a particular species of poppy: *Papaverum somniferum*. The unrefined extract from the poppy is called *opium* and contains approximately 20 naturally occurring pharmacologically active compounds, including familiar ones like morphine and codeine. This group of purified natural agents is specifically referred to as *opiates*. In addition, numerous semisynthetic and synthetic analogs of the opiates have been developed for clinical use. The word *opioid* is used broadly to cover all drugs that are chemical derivatives of the compounds purified from opium and is the term that is used throughout this chapter.

The opioids continue to be the cornerstone of effective pain treatment in veterinary medicine. They are a versatile group of drugs with extensive applications in the management of pain in patients with acute trauma, in patients undergoing surgical procedures, in patients with painful medical conditions or disease processes, and in patients suffering from chronic pain that require long-term therapy. In order for today's practitioner to be in a position to exploit this class of drugs to their fullest potential, a discussion encompassing the current state of knowledge of opioid pharmacology is appropriate.

Receptors

It is well known that exogenously administered opioids such as morphine or heroin exert their effects by interacting with specific opioid receptors and mimicking naturally occurring molecules known as *endogenous opioid peptides*. Based on work carried out over the past 20 years, it is now accepted that there are three well-defined types of opioid receptors, most commonly known by their Greek letter designations as μ (mu), δ (delta), and κ (kappa).[1–4] This classic system of nomenclature has been under reconsideration for a number of years and, during this time, several alternative naming systems have been proposed, leading to considerable confusion. In addition, a fourth type of opioid receptor, the nociceptin receptor (also known as the orphanin FQ receptor) has been characterized.[5,6] According to the most recent recommendations of the International Union of Pharmacology Subcommittee on Nomenclature, variations based on the Greek letters remain acceptable. Thus, mu, μ, or MOP (for *mu opioid peptide*); delta, δ, or DOP (for *delta opioid peptide*); kappa, κ, or KOP (for *kappa opioid peptide*); and NOP (for *nociceptin opioid peptide*) are considered interchangeable abbreviations. Distinct complementary DNA (cDNA) sequences have been cloned for all four opioid receptor types, and each type appears to have a unique distribution in the brain, spinal cord, and periphery.[7]

The diversity of opioid receptors is further extended by the existence of several subtypes of μ, δ, and κ receptors. Based on pharmacological studies, there are thought to be at least three μ-receptor subtypes, μ_1, μ_2, and μ_3; two δ-receptor subtypes, δ_1

and δ_2; and perhaps as many as four κ-receptor subtypes, κ_{1a}, κ_{1b}, κ_2, and κ_3.[7] The discovery of opioid receptor subtypes generated great enthusiasm among researchers and introduced the possibility of developing subtype-specific therapeutic agents with favorable side-effect profiles. At this point, however, the functional significance of these receptor subtypes remains unclear, and distinct cDNA sequences corresponding to these subtypes have not yet been identified.[7]

In general, it appears that the μ receptor mediates most of the clinically relevant analgesic effects, as well as most of the adverse side effects associated with opioid administration.[2] Drugs acting at the δ receptor tend to be poor analgesics, but may modify μ receptor–mediated antinociception under certain circumstances and mediate opioid receptor "crosstalk." The κ receptor mediates analgesia in several specific locations in the central nervous system (CNS) and the periphery, but distinguishing μ- and κ-mediated analgesic effects has proven to be difficult.[2,7] In contrast to the classic opioid receptors, the nociceptin receptor does not mediate typical opioid analgesia,[3,6] but instead produces antiopioid (pronociceptive) effects.[5,6] Because of the considerable structural homology among the three classically described opioid receptors, it is likely that there are significant interactions among these receptors in different tissues, and the loosely defined physiological roles ascribed to each receptor type still require further clarification.

Endogenous Receptor Ligands

The aforementioned opioid receptors discussed are part of an extensive opioid system that includes a large number of endogenous opioid peptide ligands. *Endogenous opioid peptides* are small molecules that are naturally produced in the CNS and in various glands throughout the body, such as the pituitary and the adrenal.[3] Three distinct families of endogenous opioid peptides have been identified: the enkephalins, the dynorphins, and β-endorphin. Each of these is derived from a distinct precursor polypeptide: proenkephalin, prodynorphin, and proopiomelanocortin, respectively.[3] These endogenous opioid peptides are expressed throughout the CNS, and their presence has been confirmed in peripheral tissues, as well.[3] There are considerable structural similarities among these three groups of peptides, and each family demonstrates variable affinities for μ, δ, and κ receptors. None of them bind exclusively to a single opioid receptor, and none of them have any significant affinity for the nociceptin receptor. The physiological roles of these peptides are not completely understood at this time. They appear to function as neurotransmitters, neuromodulators and, in some cases, as neurohormones. They mediate some forms of stress-induced analgesia and also play a role in analgesia induced by electrical stimulation of discrete regions in the brain, such as the periaqueductal gray area of the mesencephalon.[4]

Nociceptin (also known as orphanin FQ) is the endogenous ligand for the more recently discovered nociceptin receptor. Nociceptin is derived from pronociceptin, and its amino acid sequence is closely related to that of the aforementioned endogenous opioid peptides.[3,5] Despite this homology, nociceptin binding is specific for the nociceptin receptor, and the peptide does not appear to interact with μ, δ, or κ receptors. Furthermore, the physiological effects of nociceptin are in direct contrast to the actions of the classical endogenous opioid peptides, with nociceptin producing a distinctly pronociceptive effect.[3,5,6] The functional significance of nociceptin and its receptor remains to be elucidated, but additional insight into this novel opioid peptide may have substantial implications in future therapeutic drug development.

In addition to the enkephalins, dynorphins, β-endorphin, and nociceptin, there are now two other recently discovered endogenous opioid peptides called endomorphin 1 and endomorphin 2.[8] These peptides are putative products of an, as yet, unidentified precursor and have been proposed to be the highly selective endogenous ligands for the μ receptor.[3,8] The endomorphins are small tetrapeptides that are structurally unrelated to the endogenous opioid peptides.[8] Their identification has heralded a new era in research of the μ opioid system, which may contribute to our understanding of the neurobiology of opioids and provide new avenues for therapeutic interventions.

Signaling and Mechanisms of Analgesia

Binding of an opioid agonist to a neuronal opioid receptor, regardless of whether the agonist is endogenous or exogenous, typically leads to several events that serve to inhibit the activation of the neuron. Opioid receptors are part of a large superfamily of membrane-bound receptors that are coupled to G proteins.[7] As such, they are structurally and functionally related to receptors for many other neurotransmitters and neuropeptides that act to modulate the activity of nerve cells. Opioid receptor binding, via activation of various types of G proteins, may inhibit adenylyl cyclase (cyclic adenosine monophosphate) activity, activate receptor-operated phosphate ion (K^+) currents, and suppress voltage-gated calcium ion (Ca^{2+}) currents.[4]

At the presynaptic level, decreased Ca^{2+} influx will reduce release of transmitter substances, such as substance P, from primary afferent fibers in the spinal cord dorsal horn thereby inhibiting synaptic transmission of nociceptive input.[4] Postsynaptically, enhanced K^+ efflux causes neuronal hyperpolarization of spinal cord projection neurons and inhibits ascending nociceptive pathways. A third potential mode of opioid action involves upregulation of supraspinal descending antinociceptive pathways in the periaqueductal gray matter. It is now known that this system is subject to tonic inhibition mediated by GABAergic neurons, and opioid receptor activation has been shown to suppress this inhibitory influence and augment descending antinociceptive transmission.[4,9] The proposed cellular basis for this involves μ receptors that activate voltage-dependent K ions present on presynaptic GABAergic nerve terminals that inhibit γ-aminobutyric acid (GABA) release into the synaptic cleft.[9] It is important to note that although our collective understanding of opioid receptor–mediated signaling has increased dramatically in recent years, the relationship of such subcellular events to clinical analgesia at the level of the organism continues to require further clarification.

Distribution and Therapeutic Implications

Although cellular and molecular studies of opioid receptors and ligands are invaluable in understanding their function, it is critical to place opioid receptors in their anatomical and physiological context to fully appreciate the opioid system and its relevance to pain management. It has long been a principle tenet of opioid analgesia that these agents are centrally acting, and this understanding has shaped the way we use opioid analgesics clinically. It has been well established that the analgesic effects of opioids arise from their ability to directly inhibit the ascending transmission of nociceptive information from the spinal cord dorsal horn, and to activate pain-control circuits that descend from the midbrain via the rostral ventromedial medulla to the spinal cord. Within the CNS, evidence of μ, δ, and κ opioid receptor messenger RNA and/or opioid peptide binding has been demonstrated in supraspinal sites, including the mesencephalic periaqueductal gray matter, the mesencephalic reticular formation, various nuclei of the rostral ventromedial medulla, and forebrain regions including the nucleus accumbens, as well as spinally within the dorsal horn.[10,11] The interactions between groups of opioid receptors at various spinal and supraspinal locations, as well as interactions among different receptor types within a given location are complex and incompletely understood at this time.

Systemic administration of opioid analgesics via intravenous, intramuscular, or subcutaneous injection will induce a relatively rapid onset of action via interaction with these CNS receptors. Oral, transdermal, rectal, or buccal mucosal administration of opioids will result in variable systemic absorption, depending on the characteristics of the particular agent, with analgesic effects being mediated largely by the same receptors within the CNS. In addition, neuraxial administration, either into the subarachnoid or epidural space, is a particularly efficacious route of administration. Small doses of opioids introduced via these routes readily penetrate the spinal cord and interact with spinal and/or supraspinal opioid receptors to produce profound and potentially long-lasting analgesia, the characteristics of which will depend on the particular drug used.

Even though opioids have long been considered the prototype of centrally acting analgesics, a body of evidence has emerged that clearly indicates that opioids can produce potent and clinically measurable analgesia by activation of opioid receptors in the peripheral nervous system.[12] Opioid receptors of all three major types have been identified on the processes of sensory neurons,[13,14] and these receptors respond to peripherally applied opioids and locally released endogenous opioid peptides when upregulated during inflammatory-pain states.[12,15,16] Furthermore, although sympathetic neurons and immune cells have also been shown to express opioid receptors, their functional role remains unclear.[14] Although the binding characteristics of peripheral and central opioid receptors are similar, the molecular mass of peripheral and central μ opioid receptors appears to be different, suggesting that selective ligands for these peripheral receptors could be developed that would produce opioid analgesia without the potential to induce centrally mediated adverse side effects.[12,14,17–19]

Side Effects

Although opioids are used clinically primarily for their pain-relieving properties, they also produce a host of other effects on a variety of body systems. This is not surprising in light of the wide distribution of endogenous opioid peptides and their receptors in supraspinal, spinal, and peripheral locations. Some of these side effects, such as sedation, may be classified as either desirable or undesirable depending on the clinical circumstances. The following is a brief summary of these major side effects as they relate to opioids as a class of drugs.

Central Nervous System

Arousal   There are considerable species differences in the CNS response to opioid analgesics that cannot be attributed to pharmacokinetic variations alone. CNS depression (i.e., sedation) is typically seen in dogs, monkeys, and people, whereas CNS stimulation (i.e., excitement and/or spontaneous locomotor activity) may be elicited in cats, horses, goats, sheep, pigs, and cows after systemic administration of various opioids, most notably morphine.[20] Reasons for these different responses are not entirely clear at this time, but are presumably related to differing concentrations and distributions of μ, δ, and κ receptors in various regions of the brain in these species.[21] Despite these fundamental differences, it must be remembered that there are numerous factors that may affect the CNS response to opioids within a given species, including the temperament or condition of the patient; the presence or absence of pain; the dose, route, and timing of drug administration; and the specific opioid administered.

Thermoregulatory Center   The hypothalamic thermoregulatory system is also affected by opioid administration. Hypothermia tends to be the most common response, particularly when opioids are used during the perioperative period in the presence of other CNS-depressant drugs.[10,20] Under some clinical circumstances, however, opioid administration causes hyperthermia in cats, horses, swine, and ruminants. Part of this increase in body temperature may be attributed to an increase in muscle activity associated with CNS excitation in these species; however, a specific central hypothalamic mechanism has also been implicated, but remains poorly understood.[20] Panting is seen commonly after opioid administration, most often in dogs, but this effect tends to decrease with the onset of hypothermia.

Emetic Center   Nausea and vomiting associated with opioid administration are caused by direct stimulation of the chemoreceptor trigger zone for emesis located in the area postrema of the medulla.[10,22] As with the other centrally mediated side effects, species plays a role in determining an individual's tendency to vomit after an opioid is administered. Horses, rabbits, ruminants, and swine do not vomit with opioid administration. Cats may vomit, but usually at doses that are greater than those which stimulate vomiting in dogs. Dogs will commonly vomit after opioid administration, especially with morphine. Emesis is rarely seen when opioids are administered in the immediate postoperative period or in any patient that may be experiencing some degree of pain.

Cough Center   Opioids have variable efficacy in depressing the cough reflex, at least in part by a direct effect on a cough center located in the medulla.[10] Certain opioids are more effective anti-tussives than others, and drugs like codeine, hydrocodone, and butorphanol are occasionally prescribed specifically for this indication.

Pupillary Diameter   As a general rule, opioids tend to produce mydriasis in those species that exhibit CNS excitation, and miosis in those that become sedated after opioid administration.[20,23–25] Miosis is produced by an excitatory action of opioids on neuronal firing in the oculomotor nucleus.[22,24,25] In cats, and presumably in other species that exhibit mydriasis, this increase in activity in the oculomotor nuclear complex still occurs, but the miotic effect is masked by increased release of catecholamines, which produces mydriasis.[25]

Respiratory System

Opioids produce dose-dependent depression of ventilation, primarily mediated by μ_2 receptors, leading to a direct depressant effect on brain-stem respiratory centers.[10,22] This effect is characterized by decreased responsiveness of these centers to carbon dioxide and is reflected in an increased resting arterial carbon dioxide partial pressure and displacement of the carbon dioxide response curve to the right. This effect is compounded by the coadministration of sedative and/or anesthetic agents, meaning that significant respiratory depression and hypercapnia are much more likely to occur in anesthetized patients that receive opioids compared with those that are conscious. It should be noted that, in general, humans tend to be more sensitive to the respiratory-depressant effects of opioids when compared with most veterinary species, and the risk of hypoventilation would rarely constitute a legitimate reason for withholding opioid treatment in clinical practice.

Cardiovascular System

Most opioids have minimal effects on cardiac output, cardiac rhythm, and arterial blood pressure when clinically relevant analgesic doses are administered. Bradycardia may be caused by opioid-induced medullary vagal stimulation and will respond readily to anticholinergic treatment if warranted. Particular opioids (morphine and meperidine) can cause histamine release, especially after rapid intravenous administration, which may lead to vasodilation and hypotension.[20,26] Because of their relatively benign effects on cardiovascular function, opioids commonly form the basis of anesthetic protocols for patients with preexisting cardiovascular disease.

Gastrointestinal System

The gastrointestinal effects of the opioids are mediated by μ and δ receptors located in the myenteric plexus of the gastrointestinal tract.[10,20] Opioid administration will often stimulate dogs and, less frequently, cats to defecate. After this initial response, spasm of gastrointestinal smooth muscle predisposes patients to ileus and constipation. Horses and ruminants in particular may be predisposed to gastrointestinal complications associated with opioid administration, such as colic and ruminal tympany, respectively. These side effects tend to be most significant with prolonged ad-

ministration of opioids in dogs and cats experiencing chronic pain, and such patients may require dietary modifications and stool-softening medications to manage these adverse effects.

In human patients, opioids (most notably fentanyl and morphine) have been shown to increase bile duct pressure through constriction of the sphincter of Oddi.[27] The incidence of this side effect in people is, however, quite low.[28] Despite anatomical differences, this observation has led to concerns about opioid administration to dogs and cats with pancreatitis and/or cholangitis. A study reviewing the body of human literature found that, despite widespread clinical practice, there was no evidence to indicate that morphine is contraindicated for use in acute pancreatitis.[29] As there are no studies that specifically evaluate the effects of opioids in dogs and cats with pancreatitis, it does not at this time seem appropriate to withhold this class of drugs from this subset of severely painful patients.

Genitourinary System

Opioids, particularly when administered neuraxially, may cause urinary retention through dose-dependent suppression of detrusor contractility and decreased sensation of urge.[30,31] Manual expression of the urinary bladder or catheterization may be required in certain individuals until urodynamic function returns to normal.

Urine volume may also be affected by opioids, and the mechanism of this effect appears to be multifactorial. μ-Agonists tend to produce oliguria in the clinical setting, and this is in part a due to increased antidiuretic hormone release leading to altered renal tubular function.[22,32] Elevations in circulating plasma atrial natriuretic peptide may also play a role in morphine-induced antidiuresis.[32] Conversely, κ-agonists tend to produce a diuretic effect, possibly through inhibition of antidiuretic hormone secretion.[22,32] Other peripheral mechanisms involving stimulation of renal α_2-adrenergic receptors may also contribute to this κ-agonist effect.[32]

Agonists

Almost all clinically useful opioids exert their analgesic effects by acting as agonists at μ receptors. Although a few opioids act as κ-agonists, these drugs also tend to have antagonist or partial agonist effects at μ and/or δ receptors and are thus not classified as *pure* agonists. Pure or full opioid agonists can elicit maximal activation of the receptor when they bind it, and the subsequent downstream processes produce a maximal analgesic effect (Fig. 10.1). Clinically, the full μ-agonists are superior analgesics and are the drugs of choice for pain of moderate to severe intensity in many veterinary species (see Table 10.1 for recommended dosages). The following section contains brief descriptions of full μ-agonists that are in current clinical use.

Morphine (Morphine Sulfate)

Morphine is the prototypical opioid analgesic and acts as a full agonist not only at μ receptors, but also at δ and κ receptors.[10] Despite the development of numerous synthetic opioids, many of which are more potent than morphine and may have other characteristics that make them desirable alternatives to morphine in certain circumstances, no other drug has been shown to be more

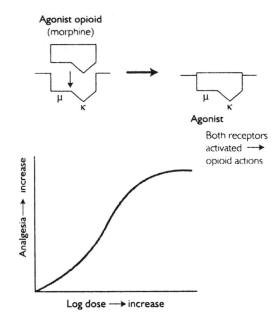

Agonist opioid
(morphine)

Agonist

Both receptors
activated →
opioid actions

Fig. 10.1. A lock-and-key analogy is used to illustrate full agonist drug interactions at opioid receptors, with a relative dose-response curve for analgesic efficacy shown below. A full opioid agonist (in this case, morphine) stimulates both μ- and κ-receptor types, which produces increased analgesic effect with increased dose. Modified from Nicholson and Christie,[270] p. 273, with permission from Elsevier.

Table 10.1. Dosage ranges (mg/kg) for opioid agonists in several domestic species

Opioid	Dogs	Cats	Horses	Cattle	Swine
Morphine	0.3–2.0 IM, SC 0.1–0.5 IV 0.1–0.3/h IV CRI 0.1–0.2 epidural[a] 1.5–3 PO[b]	0.05–0.2 IM, SC 0.1–0.2 epidural[a]	0.1–0.3 IM, SC 0.1–0.2 epidural[a]	?	0.5–2.0? IM, SC
Oxymorphone	0.05–2.0 IV, IM, SC	0.05–0.1 IV, IM, SC	0.01–0.03 IV, IM, SC	NR	0.05–0.2? IM, SC
Hydromorphone	0.05–2.0 IV, IM, SC	0.05–0.1 IV, IM, SC	0.01–0.03 IV, IM, SC	NR	0.05–0.2? IM, SC
Meperidine	3–5 IM, SC	3–5 IM, SC	1–3 IM, SC 0.2–1.0 IV	3–4? IM, SC	1–2? IM, SC
Fentanyl	0.002–0.01 IV 0.002–0.03c/h IV CRI 0.001–0.005/h epidural[a] CRI 0.002–0.005/h transdermal[d]	0.001–0.005 IV 0.002–0.03c/h IV CRI 0.001–0.005/h epidural[a] CRI 0.002–0.005/h transdermal[d]	0.001–0.002/h transdermal[d]	0.001–0.002/h transdermal[d]	NR
Alfentanil	?	?	NR	NR	?
Sufentanil	0.001–0.005 IV loading dose 0.001–0.01c/h IV CRI	?	NR	NR	?
Remifentanil	0.004–0.01 IV loading dose 0.004–0.06c/h IV CRI	?	NR	NR	?
Methadone	0.05–0.2 PO, IM, SC	0.05–0.2 PO, IM, SC	NR	NR	NR
Codeine	1–2 PO	0.1–1.0 PO	NR	NR	NR
Oxycodone	0.1–0.3? PO	?	NR	NR	NR
Hydrocodone	?	?	NR	NR	NR

CRI, continuous-rate infusion; IM, intramuscular(ly); IV, intravenous(ly); NR, not recommended for administration in this species; PO, per os (orally); SC, subcutaneous(ly); ?, reliable doses have not been established for this species.
[a]Preservative-free formulations are recommended for epidural administration.
[b]Doses are for sustained-release product (MS Contin), which should be dosed q 12 h.
[c]Lower IV infusion rates are suitable for management of most types of pain, whereas higher rates will produce profound analgesia suitable for surgery.
[d]Fentanyl transdermal patches are available in 0.025-, 0.05-, 0.075-, or 0.1-mg/h sizes.

efficacious than morphine at relieving pain. Compared with the synthetic opioid agonists, morphine is relatively hydrophilic and crosses the blood-brain barrier more slowly than fentanyl or oxymorphone, thereby delaying the peak effect somewhat even after intravenous administration.[10,22] Clinically, this lag is not likely to be significant under most circumstances, with the onset of analgesia occurring reasonably promptly after a single dose of morphine and typically lasting 3 to 4 h.[33,34] Morphine's poor lipid solubility means that it can produce long-lasting analgesia when administered into the epidural or subarachnoid space, with effects persisting for 12 to 24 h. The first-pass effect is significant after oral administration, and the bioavailability of oral morphine preparations is only in the range of 25%. If dose adjustments are made, adequate pain relief can be achieved with oral morphine administration, and the duration of action tends to be somewhat longer with this route.

In most species, the primary metabolic pathway for morphine involves conjugation with glucuronic acid leading to the formation of two major metabolites: morphine 6-glucuronide and morphine 3-glucuronide.[10,35] Despite the low levels of glucuronyl transferase in cats, the pharmacokinetics of morphine in this species seem to be broadly comparable to those in dogs and people, though clearance rates may be marginally slower.[33–35] This suggests that morphine must undergo a different type of conjugation reaction in this species. Morphine 6-glucuronide has pharmacological activities that are indistinguishable from those of morphine in animal models and in people, whereas morphine 3-glucuronide appears to have little affinity for opioid receptors, but may contribute to the excitatory effects of morphine in some situations.[10,36] With chronic morphine administration, it is likely that the active metabolite, morphine 6-glucuronide, contributes significantly to clinical analgesia.

Very little morphine is excreted unchanged in the urine. The major metabolites—morphine 3-glucuronide and, to a lesser extent, morphine 6-glucuronide—are eliminated almost entirely via glomerular filtration. In human patients, renal failure may lead to accumulation of morphine 6-glucuronide and persistent clinical effects, whereas liver dysfunction seems to have minimal impact on morphine clearance.[10,22]

The side effects associated with morphine administration are typical of most opioid agonists and have been discussed previously in this chapter. In particular, the increased incidence of vomiting after morphine administration, as well as its potential to cause histamine release after intravenous administration, helps to distinguish morphine from other full opioid agonists.

Clinically, morphine is a useful analgesic in dogs, cats, horses, and rats. It is often administered to dogs and cats at fixed dosing intervals via the intramuscular, subcutaneous or, less commonly, intravenous routes to manage pain associated with a variety of traumatic injuries and disease processes. Morphine has also been used extensively throughout the perioperative period in these species to manage pain associated with surgical procedures. In dogs and cats, the sparing effect of morphine on both injectable and inhalant anesthetic requirements can be significant.[37,38] Morphine is particularly effective in dogs when administered intravenously as a continuous infusion, which facilitates more pre-cise dose titration to achieve optimal analgesic effects.[38,39] Subcutaneous infusions of morphine and other opioids are being employed in human patients experiencing cancer pain,[40–43] and, as subcutaneous infusion devices are developed that are applicable to dogs and cats, this route of administration may be accessed by veterinarians in the future. Administration of the drug into the epidural or, less commonly, subarachnoid space is a common analgesic technique employed in both dogs and cats in a variety of clinical situations.[44,45] More recently, the discovery of peripheral μ opioid receptors has led to the clinical practice of instilling morphine locally into inflamed joints[46,47] and even topically onto damaged corneas[48] to supplement analgesia in canine patients.

The analgesic benefits of morphine use in horses are less clear-cut than in dogs and cats. Low doses of morphine can be administered systemically without adverse side effects and may relieve pain in conscious horses, though the analgesic response has been difficult to demonstrate in numerous clinical studies.[49] A 2003 study showed that morphine, in the absence of other drugs, actually increased the minimum alveolar concentration (MAC) of isoflurane in horses anesthetized in an experimental setting.[50] While this finding would appear to discourage routine use of morphine in the perioperative period, another retrospective study failed to demonstrate any adverse effects associated with perioperative morphine administration in a typical clinical setting in the presence of other drugs, such as α_2-agonists and ketamine.[51] Thus, the routine systemic administration of morphine to horses, especially those undergoing surgery, remains controversial.

Regional administration of morphine to horses, however, is becoming increasingly common, and a growing body of evidence seems to support this practice. Morphine produces significant analgesia with few adverse side effects when administered epidurally or intra-articularly and is often combined with other analgesic agents, such as α_2-agonists and local anesthetics, when administered via these routes.[49,52,53]

Morphine is used infrequently in ruminants and swine in the clinical setting, and its effects have not been well studied in these species. It is likely that regional and perhaps even systemic administration of morphine may play a role in pain management of these species in the future.

Oxymorphone (Oxymorphone Hydrochloride [Numorphan])

Oxymorphone is a synthetic opioid that acts as a full agonist at μ receptors and is comparable to morphine in its analgesic efficacy and duration of action. It is a more lipid soluble drug than morphine and is readily absorbed after intramuscular or subcutaneous administration. Oxymorphone is not available as an oral formulation.

When compared with morphine, oxymorphone is less likely to cause dogs and cats to vomit, and tends to produce more sedation when administered to these species. Its respiratory-depressant effects are similar to those induced by morphine, but oxymorphone seems more likely to cause dogs to pant. It does not produce histamine release, even when administered intravenously.[26] Oxymorphone's other side effects are typical of other full μ-agonist opioids and have been discussed previously.

Oxymorphone has been used extensively in dogs and cats, and is most often administered at fixed dosing intervals, either intramuscularly, subcutaneously, or intravenously, to manage pain in a variety of clinical settings. It is also commonly used in the preanesthetic, intraoperative, and postoperative periods in surgical patients. Oxymorphone has been administered epidurally in dogs, but its relative lipid solubility means that its analgesic action is briefer when administered by this route compared with the action of morphine.[54]

Oxymorphone is not commonly administered to horses, ruminants, or swine, and little data exist in these species to make any therapeutic recommendations.

Hydromorphone (Hydromorphone Hydrochloride [Dilaudid])

Hydromorphone is a synthetic opioid that acts as a full agonist at μ receptors and is used in both human and veterinary medicine. Clinically, hydromorphone and oxymorphone have similar efficacy, potency, duration of analgesic action, and side-effect profiles, but hydromorphone remains significantly less expensive. Like oxymorphone, hydromorphone is not associated with histamine release, so bolus intravenous administration is considered safe.[26]

In dogs and cats, hydromorphone can be used in any clinical situation where oxymorphone is used. Evidence from the human literature suggests that hydromorphone may be suitable for administration via a continuous infusion, either intravenously, subcutaneously, or epidurally,[42,55,56] and these routes of administration may further expand the use of hydromorphone in veterinary patients in the future. There is little published on the use of hydromorphone in large animal species at this time.

Meperidine (Meperidine Hydrochloride or Pethidine [Demerol])

Meperidine is a synthetic opioid that exerts its analgesic effects through agonism at μ receptors. Interestingly, it also appears able to bind other types of receptors, which may contribute to some of its clinical effects other than analgesia. Meperidine can block sodium channels and inhibit activity in dorsal horn neurons in a manner analogous to local anesthetics.[57,58] Meperidine also exerts agonist activity at α_2 receptors, specifically the α_{2B} subtype, suggesting that it may possess some α_2-agonist-like properties.[59,60]

Meperidine has a shorter analgesic action compared with morphine, oxymorphone, or hydromorphone, typically not extending beyond 1 h.[20] Metabolic pathways vary among different species, but, in general, most of the drug is demethylated to normeperidine in the liver and then undergoes further hydrolysis and ultimately renal excretion.[20,34,61] Normeperidine is an active metabolite and has approximately one-half the analgesic efficacy of meperidine.[10,20] Normeperidine has produced toxic neurological side effects in human patients receiving meperidine for prolonged periods, especially in the presence of impaired renal function.[22,62]

Unlike most of the other opioids in clinical use, meperidine has been shown to produce significant negative inotropic effects when administered alone to conscious dogs.[63] Because of its modest atropine-like effects, meperidine tends to increase heart rate rather than predispose patients to bradycardia, as is often seen with other opioids.[20,22] The clinical significance of these cardiovascular effects in the perianesthetic period has never been clearly ascertained. Like morphine, meperidine also causes histamine release when administered intravenously.[20]

A rare, but life-threatening, drug interaction that may have relevance in veterinary medicine has been reported in human patients receiving meperidine. The combination of meperidine (and perhaps other opioids) with a monoamine oxidase inhibitor may lead to *serotonin syndrome*, which is characterized by a constellation of symptoms, including confusion, fever, shivering, diaphoresis, ataxia, hyperreflexia, myoclonus, and diarrhea.[64–67] A monoamine oxidase inhibitor, selegiline (Deprenyl), has been used in canine patients to treat pituitary-dependent hyperadrenocorticism or to modify behavior in patients with canine cognitive dysfunction. Though there have not, to date, been any scientific studies of adverse meperidine-selegiline interactions in dogs, veterinarians must be aware of the potential for complications if analgesia is required in patients receiving monoamine oxidase inhibitors. A recent study that evaluated the effects of other opioids (oxymorphone and butorphanol) in selegiline-treated dogs did not identify any specific adverse drug interactions in these animals.[68]

Clinically, meperidine has been used primarily in dogs and cats during the preanesthetic period, often in combination with sedatives or tranquilizers. In patients undergoing surgery, administration of another full μ-agonist opioid with a longer duration of action is recommended for use postoperatively. Meperidine appears to offer few, if any, advantages over other opioids, such as oxymorphone or hydromorphone, in these species during the perioperative period.

Meperidine is not commonly used in large animals, but may, like morphine, produce useful analgesic effects when administered into the epidural space in these species.[69] Because of its local anesthetic-like effects, caudal epidural meperidine may offer advantages over other epidural opioids when perineal analgesia is specifically indicated.

Fentanyl (Fentanyl Citrate [Sublimaze])

Fentanyl is a highly lipid soluble, short-acting synthetic μ opioid agonist. A single dose of fentanyl administered intravenously has a more rapid onset and a much briefer action than morphine. Peak analgesic effects occur in about 5 min and last approximately 30 min.[10,22] Rapid redistribution of the drug to inactive tissue sites, such as fat and skeletal muscle, leads to a decrease in plasma concentration and is responsible for the prompt termination of clinical effects. In most veterinary species, the elimination half-life after a single bolus or a brief infusion is in the range of 2 to 3 h.[70–72] Administration of very large doses or prolonged infusions may cause saturation of inactive tissues, with termination of clinical effects becoming dependent on hepatic metabolism and renal excretion.[10,22] Thus, the context-sensitive half-life of fentanyl increases significantly with the duration of the infusion, and clinical effects may persist for an extended period following termination of a long-term intravenous infusion.

Side effects associated with fentanyl administration are similar to those of the other full μ-agonist opioids. In general, cardiovascular stability is excellent with fentanyl, and intravenous administration is not associated with histamine release.[10,22] Bradycardia may be significant with bolus doses, but readily responds to anticholinergics if treatment is warranted.[10,20] In human patients, muscle rigidity, especially of the chest wall, has been noted after administration of fentanyl or one of its congeners.[65,73,74] The potential significance of this adverse effect in animal patients is not clear at this time, and the risk is considered minimal if large, rapid bolus administrations are avoided.

Clinically, fentanyl is used most frequently in dogs and cats, but is also a potentially useful analgesic in other species, including horses, cows, sheep, goats, and pigs. Historically, fentanyl was available in combination with the butyrophenone tranquilizer, droperidol, in a product called Innovar-Vet, which was typically administered in the preanesthetic period to provide sedation and analgesia. This product is no longer available, and systemic administration of fentanyl today is usually via the intravenous route.

Because of its shorter action, fentanyl is typically administered as a continuous infusion to provide analgesia. Intravenous fentanyl can be infused at relatively low doses to supplement analgesia intraoperatively and/or postoperatively in dogs and cats. It is also useful for management of nonsurgical pain, such as that associated with pancreatitis. Alternatively, larger doses can be administered, often in combination with a benzodiazepine like midazolam, to induce general anesthesia in canine patients with cardiovascular or hemodynamic instability. Similarly, higher infusion rates of fentanyl can be used as the primary anesthetic agent for surgical maintenance in patients who will not tolerate significant concentrations of volatile inhalant anesthetics.[75–77] In the clinical setting, there are few reports of intravenous fentanyl administration in large animal species, though fentanyl infusions have been employed in a variety of surgical animal research models involving calves, sheep, and pigs.[78,79]

In addition to intravenous administration, fentanyl may be deposited into the epidural space to produce analgesia. Because of its high lipid solubility, epidural fentanyl, unlike morphine, is rapidly absorbed into the systemic circulation. Consequently, the clinical effects associated with a single bolus of epidural fentanyl resemble those of an intravenous injection. However, the benefits of neuraxial administration can be achieved by administering epidural fentanyl as a continuous infusion through an indwelling epidural catheter, often in combination with other analgesic agents. This technique is typically used in canine patients for management of severe acute pain, but it may have additional applications for the management of chronic pain as well.

The development of novel, less invasive, routes of opioid administration for use in human patients led to the marketing of transdermal fentanyl patches (Duragesic). The patches are designed to release a constant amount of fentanyl per hour that is then absorbed across the skin and taken up systemically. Fentanyl patches are designed for human skin and human body temperature, but their use has been evaluated in a number of veterinary species.[70,72,80–86] Though transdermal fentanyl appears to be an effective means of providing analgesia in a number of clinical settings, substantial variations in plasma drug concentrations have been documented, and significant lag times after patch placement are common prior to onset of analgesia.[70,71,83,84] Furthermore, changes in body temperature have been shown to affect fentanyl absorption significantly in anesthetized cats,[87] and it is likely that other factors associated with skin preparation and patch placement have the potential to alter plasma fentanyl levels and analgesic efficacy substantially. Two recent studies evaluating the efficacy of pluronic lecithin organogel (PLO gel) delivery of fentanyl through skin in dogs and cats concluded that this method of administration did not result in measurable plasma concentrations and thus could not be justified as an effective means of systemic administration.[88,89]

Alfentanil, Sufentanil, and Remifentanil (Alfenta, Sufenta, and Ultiva)

Alfentanil, sufentanil, and remifentanil are all structural analogs of fentanyl that were developed for use in human patients in an effort to create analgesics with a more rapid onset of action and predictable termination of opioid effects. All three are similar with regard to onset, and all have context-sensitive half-lives that are shorter than that of fentanyl after prolonged infusions.[22] Remifentanil is unique among opioids because it is metabolized by nonspecific plasma esterases to inactive metabolites.[90,91] Thus, hepatic or renal dysfunction will have little impact on drug clearance, and this, in combination with the robust nature of the esterase metabolic system, contributes to the predictability associated with remifentanil infusion.[10,22]

All three of these drugs are used during general anesthesia for procedures requiring intense analgesia and/or blunting of the sympathetic nervous system response to noxious stimulation. As yet, they have limited applications for postoperative or chronic pain management. Like fentanyl, they can be administered at relatively low infusion rates as adjuncts to general anesthetic protocols based on volatile inhalant or other injectable agents, or they can be administered at higher rates as primary agents for total intravenous anesthesia. The minimum alveolar-sparing properties of these agents have been demonstrated in both dogs[91,92] and cats.[77,93,94] In horses, systemic infusions of alfentanil did not have significant effects on MACs of inhalant anesthetics and, when administered to conscious horses, were associated with increases in locomotor activity.[95–97] There is little evidence to suggest that any of the fentanyl analogs offer advantages over morphine when administered into the epidural space for analgesia.[52]

Methadone (Methadone Hydrochloride [Dolorphine])

Methadone is a synthetic μ opioid agonist with pharmacological properties qualitatively similar to those of morphine, but possessing additional affinity for N-methyl-D-aspartate (NMDA) receptors.[98,99] Methadone's unique clinical characteristics include excellent absorption after oral administration, no known active metabolites, high potency, and an extended duration of action.[10,20,99] In human patients, the drug has been used primarily in the treatment of opioid-abstinence syndromes, but is being used increasingly for the management of chronic pain. Though there are reports of intramuscular or intravenous administration of methadone in the perioperative period in dogs, cats, and horses,[100–102] the drug is not commonly used in this setting in North America at this time. Additional studies may identify a role for oral methadone in the management of chronic pain syndromes in veterinary patients.

Codeine (Codeine Phosphate)

Codeine is the result of substitution of a methyl group onto morphine, which acts to limit first-pass hepatic metabolism and accounts for codeine's high oral bioavailability.[10,22] Codeine is well known for its excellent antitussive properties and is often combined in an oral formulation with a nonopioid analgesic, such as acetaminophen, for the management of mild to moderate pain in human patients. Codeine, alone or in combination with acetaminophen (Tylenol 3), has been used in dogs for the management of mild pain on an outpatient basis.

Oxycodone and Hydrocodone (Oxycodone Hydrochloride and Hydrocodone Bitartrate)

Oxycodone and hydrocodone are opioids that are typically administered orally for the treatment of pain in human patients. Though oxycodone is available as a single-drug continuous-release formulation (Oxycontin), these drugs are most often prepared in combination with nonopioid analgesics, such as aspirin and acetaminophen (e.g., Percocet, Percodan, Lorcet, and Vicodan). Little has been published regarding the use of these opioids in veterinary patients, and thus specific recommendations regarding their use cannot be made at this time.

Etorphine and Carfentanil (M-99 and Wildnil)

These two opioids are discussed together because they are both used exclusively for the restraint and capture of wild animals rather than as analgesic agents. They are extremely potent opioids, and the immediate availability of a suitable antagonist is mandatory before these drugs are to be used, not only to reverse drug effects in animal patients, but also as a safety precaution in the event of accidental human injection. Though etorphine and carfentanil are most often injected intramuscularly (usually using a remote drug-delivery technique), studies suggest that carfentanil is useful when administered orally in a variety of species.[103–106] A number of different drugs have been used in combination with etorphine or carfentanil to enhance muscle relaxation, including acepromazine, xylazine, and medetomidine.[107–110] For more detailed information on the use of these agents for immobilization of free-ranging wildlife, readers are referred to Chapters 12, 31, and 32 in this text.

Agonist-Antagonists and Partial Agonists

This group includes drugs that have varying opioid receptor–binding profiles, but that have one thing in common: They all occupy μ opioid receptors, but do not initiate a maximal clinical response. Drugs such as butorphanol and nalbuphine are classified as agonist-antagonists. They are competitive μ-receptor antagonists, but exert their analgesic actions by acting as agonists at κ receptors (Fig. 10.2). Buprenorphine, on the other hand, is

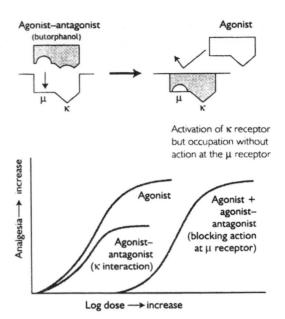

Fig. 10.2. A lock-and-key analogy is used to illustrate agonist-antagonist drug interactions at opioid receptors, with a relative dose-response curve for analgesic efficacy shown below. An agonist-antagonist opioid (in this case, butorphanol) has agonist activity at κ receptors and antagonist activity at μ receptors. In the presence of a full μ-agonist, these opioids tend to have antagonistic effects and will increase the dose of full agonist required to achieve maximal analgesic effect. Modified from Nicholson and Christie,[270] p. 273, with permission from Elsevier.

classified as a partial agonist and binds μ receptors, but produces only a limited clinical effect (Fig. 10.3). These mixed agonist-antagonist drugs were developed for the human market in an attempt to create analgesics with less respiratory depression and addictive potential. Because of their opioid receptor–binding affinities, the side effects associated with these drugs demonstrate a so-called ceiling effect, whereby increasing doses do not produce additional adverse responses. Unfortunately, the benefits of this ceiling effect on ventilatory depression come at the expense of limited analgesic efficacy and only a modest ability to decrease anesthetic requirements.

The coadministration of opioids with differing receptor-binding profiles is currently an active area of research that deserves further attention. The interactions in this setting are complex, and opioid coadministration appears to have the potential to produce additive, synergistic, or antagonistic analgesic effects, depending on the particular species, dosage, drugs, and pain model being evaluated. The following section contains brief descriptions of opioid agonist-antagonists and partial agonists that are currently in clinical use (see Table 10.2 for recommended dosages).

Butorphanol (Butorphanol Tartrate [Torbugesic])

Butorphanol is a synthetic agonist-antagonist opioid and has been used extensively in a wide variety of veterinary species. The drug was originally labeled as an antitussive agent in dogs and,

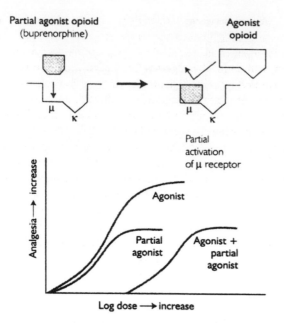

Fig. 10.3. A lock-and-key analogy is used to illustrate partial agonist drug interactions at opioid receptors, with a relative dose-response curve for analgesic efficacy shown below. A partial opioid agonist (in this case, buprenorphine) weakly stimulates μ receptors, which produces a reduced maximal analgesic effect compared with a full agonist. A large dose of partial agonist will block the receptor actions of a full agonist, moving its dose-response curve to the right and depressing its maximal analgesic effect. Modified from Nicholson and Christie,[270] p. 273, with permission from Elsevier.

even now, is approved as an analgesic in cats and horses only.[20] Butorphanol exerts its relevant clinical effects through its interactions at κ receptors and acts as an antagonist at μ receptors. The duration of butorphanol's analgesic effects remains somewhat debatable and likely varies with species, type and intensity of pain, dosage, and route of administration.[111–113] In general, its effects are shorter-lived than those of morphine and are probably in the range of 1 to 3 h. Butorphanol is typically administered via

the intramuscular, subcutaneous, or intravenous route, though an oral formulation is available and is occasionally prescribed for outpatient analgesia in dogs.

Butorphanol does not induce histamine release when administered intravenously and has minimal effects on cardiopulmonary function. There is conflicting evidence regarding the effects of butorphanol on inhalant anesthetic requirements in the dogs, cats, and horses. Earlier studies failed to demonstrate a significant sparing effect on MAC when butorphanol was coadministered with halothane in dogs and ponies.[114–116] More recently, isoflurane MAC reductions have been documented after administration of clinically relevant doses of butorphanol in both dogs and cats.[37,117] Reasons for these discrepancies are probably related to differences in study techniques, and, in dogs and cats specifically, it seems that butorphanol can induce at least modest reductions in inhalant anesthetic requirements.

When administered alone to healthy dogs and cats, butorphanol produces minimal sedation only. However, the drug is commonly used in combination with a variety of sedatives and tranquilizers, such as acepromazine, medetomidine, or midazolam, to produce sedation and analgesia for minimally invasive procedures.[118] It is also used during the preanesthetic and postoperative periods to provide analgesia for surgical procedures associated with mild to moderate pain.[85,119,120] Butorphanol does not appear to be an effective monoanalgesic for moderate to severe pain in these species, especially when pain is orthopedic in origin.[121–123]

Butorphanol, which is the opioid most commonly used in horses, is almost always coadministered with an α2-agonist or, occasionally, acepromazine. It is administered intravenously for a variety of standing procedures or prior to induction of general anesthesia. Butorphanol has been shown to be an effective, though short-lived, analgesic for visceral pain in this species, but the α2-agonists still seem to be superior for treatment of this type of pain in horses.[124,125] One study has documented the safety and apparent efficacy of a continuous intravenous infusion of butorphanol that maintained therapeutic plasma levels of drug while minimizing the potential for adverse gastrointestinal and behavioral effects.[113] Butorphanol has not been shown to be particu-

Table 10.2. Dosage ranges (mg/kg) for opioid agonist-antagonists and partial agonists in several domestic species

Opioid	Dogs	Cats	Horses	Cattle	Swine
Butorphanol	0.1–0.4 IV, IM, SC 0.5–2.0 PO[a]	0.1–0.8 IV, IM, SC 0.5–1.0 PO[a]	0.02–0.04 IV, IM, SC 0.02–0.04/h IV CRI 0.04 epidural	0.01–0.04 IV, IM, SC	0.1–0.5 IV, IM, SC
Nalbuphine	0.3–0.5 IM, SC 0.1–0.3 IV	0.2–0.4 IM, SC 0.1–0.2 IV	?	?	?
Pentazocine	1–3 IV, IM, SC	1–3 IV, IM, SC	0.1–1.0 IV, IM, SC	?	?
Buprenorphine	0.005–0.02 IV, IM, SC	0.005–0.02 IV, IM, SC 0.01–0.02 PO[b]	0.005–0.01 IV, IM, SC	0.005–0.01 IV, IM, SC	0.01–0.1 IV, IM, SC

CRI, continuous-rate infusion; IM, intramuscularly; IV, intravenously; PO, per os (orally); SC, subcutaneously; ?, reliable doses have not been established for this species.

[a]Butorphanol's oral bioavailability remains uncertain.

[b]Buprenorphine injectable solution has been shown to be effective when administered to the buccal mucosa in cats.

larly effective when administered into the caudal epidural space in horses, and other opioids, such as morphine, produce superior analgesia when given by this route.[52,126]

Butorphanol is occasionally administered to cattle, sheep, goats, and pigs to provide analgesia, but there is limited information in the literature on its analgesic efficacy in these species. The combination of butorphanol with xylazine or detomidine appears to enhance and prolong the sedation induced by the α_2-agonist. Additional studies evaluating the analgesic potential of butorphanol and other opioids in these species are certainly warranted.

Traditionally, it was thought that the simultaneous or sequential administration of butorphanol with a pure μ opioid agonist such as morphine or hydromorphone would be counterproductive from an analgesic standpoint because butorphanol's ability to antagonize μ receptors could inhibit or even reverse the effects of the agonist drug. Certainly, it has been clearly demonstrated that excessive sedation associated with a pure μ-agonist can be partially reversed by the administration of low doses of butorphanol, and it was presumed that butorphanol would similarly reverse the μ-mediated analgesic effects, as well. It would now appear that the potential interactions between butorphanol and full μ opioid agonists are more complex than originally believed. One study demonstrated that coadministration of butorphanol and oxymorphone to cats subjected to a visceral noxious stimulus enhanced analgesic effects.[127] A more recent feline study, however, which evaluated the combination of butorphanol and hydromorphone in a thermal threshold-pain model, failed to demonstrate enhanced analgesia and suggested that butorphanol actually did inhibit hydromorphone's analgesic effects.[128]

These contradictory findings illustrate that we still have much to learn about coadministration of opioid agents with differing receptor-binding profiles, and the clinical effects produced by such coadministration likely depend on many factors, including species, type of pain, dose, and the specific drugs involved.

Nalbuphine and Pentazocine (Nalbuphine Hydrochloride [Nubain] and Pentazocine Hydrochloride [Talwin])

Nalbuphine and pentazocine are classified as agonist-antagonist opioids and are clinically similar to butorphanol. They induce mild analgesia accompanied by minimal sedation, respiratory depression, or adverse cardiovascular effects. In human patients, nalbuphine is used more commonly than butorphanol, whereas, in veterinary medicine, butorphanol is used far more frequently. In the past, pentazocine was used in equine patients for management of colic pain, but it has largely been replaced by the α_2-agonists (xylazine and detomidine), nonsteroidal anti-inflammatories (flunixin meglumine), and butorphanol. Like butorphanol, nalbuphine is occasionally used to partially reverse the effects of a full μ-agonist opioid while maintaining some residual analgesia.

Buprenorphine (Buprenex [Temgesic])

Buprenorphine is a semisynthetic, highly lipophilic opioid derived from thebaine. Unlike other opioids in this category, buprenorphine is considered to be a partial agonist at μ opioid receptors. The drug binds avidly to, and dissociates slowly from, μ receptors, but cannot elicit a maximal clinical response. Because of its receptor-binding characteristics, buprenorphine has a delayed onset of action and takes at least 1 h to attain peak effect after intramuscular administration. It also has a relatively long action, with clinical analgesic effects persisting for 6 to 12 h in most species. Also, its high affinity for the μ receptor means that it may be difficult to antagonize its effects with a drug such as naloxone. Buprenorphine has most often been administered intravenously or intramuscularly; however, because of the long lag time before clinical effects are achieved after intramuscular administration, the intravenous route is preferred. A recent study has documented comparable plasma drug levels and analgesic efficacy with oral transmucosal administration in cats.[129] This route seems to be well tolerated by feline patients and is becoming increasingly popular in clinical practice. A transdermal buprenorphine patch (Transtec) is now commercially available and currently being evaluated in cats.

In dogs and cats, buprenorphine is used most often in the postoperative period to manage pain of mild to moderate intensity.[130-132] As with the other opioids in this category, buprenorphine may not be adequate for management of severe pain such as that associated with thoracotomies or invasive orthopedic procedures.[133] The drug is a popular analgesic in laboratory-animal species because it can be formulated with a variety of foodstuffs and given orally to rodents.

In horses, buprenorphine is occasionally administered in combination with an α_2-agonist to enhance and prolong sedation and analgesia.[134] There is little information published on the use of buprenorphine in cattle, and, though the drug is commonly used as an analgesic agent in research laboratories in sheep and swine, few reports actually evaluate its analgesic efficacy in these species.

Antagonists

These drugs have high affinities for the opioid receptors and can displace opioid agonists from μ and κ receptors. After this displacement, the pure antagonists bind to and occupy opioid receptors, but do not activate them (Fig. 10.4). Under ordinary circumstances, in patients that have not received exogenous agonist opioids, the opioid antagonists have few clinical effects when administered at clinically relevant dosages.[10] It is important to recognize that these drugs will rapidly reverse all opioid-induced clinical effects, including analgesia (see Table 10.3 for recommended dosages). Therefore, use of pure opioid antagonists should be reserved for emergency situations such as opioid overdose or profound respiratory depression. Their routine use for reversal of excessive sedation in patients experiencing prolonged anesthetic recoveries or in patients that develop bradycardia secondary to opioid administration is inappropriate and may cause the development of intense acute pain and activation of the sympathetic nervous system.

Naloxone (Naloxone Hydrochloride [Narcan])

The use of this pure opioid antagonist can reverse all opioid agonist effects, producing increased alertness, responsiveness, coordination and, potentially, increased perception of pain. Naloxone's effects are shorter than that of many of the opioid agonists, with recommended intravenous doses lasting between 30

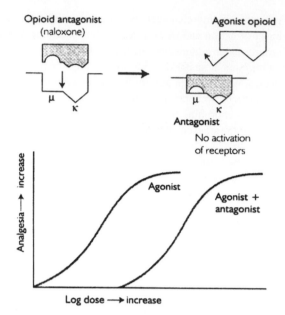

Fig. 10.4. A lock-and-key analogy is used to illustrate pure antagonist drug interactions at opioid receptors, with a relative dose-response curve for analgesic efficacy shown below. A pure opioid antagonist (in this case, naloxone) blocks both μ- and κ-receptor types, but has no intrinsic activity at these receptors. Receptor binding is competitive, so more agonist is required in the presence of antagonist to produce a maximal analgesic effect. Modified from Nicholson and Christie,[270] p. 273, with permission from Elsevier.

and 60 min. Consequently, animals need to be closely monitored for renarcotization after a dose of naloxone. Occasionally, excitement or anxiety may be seen after naloxone reversal of an opioid agonist. Premature ventricular contractions have also been documented after reversal, but are not common and seem to be more likely if there are high levels of circulating catecholamines. This drug is sometimes administered sublingually to neonatal patients exhibiting respiratory depression that have been delivered by cesarean section after maternal administration of an opioid agonist.

Naloxone has also been shown in animal models and human patients to produce a dose-related improvement in myocardial contractility and mean arterial blood pressure during shock.[135–137] Further studies are needed to clarify the role of the endogenous opioid system in the pathophysiology of various forms of shock.

Nalmefene and Naltrexone (Revex and Trexonil)
Both of these drugs are pure opioid antagonists with clinical effects that last approximately twice as long as those of naloxone.[138] Though little is published about the use of these drugs in veterinary patients, they may be advantageous in preventing renarcotization when used to antagonize the effects of a long-acting opioid.

Nonsteroidal Anti-inflammatories

The nonsteroidal anti-inflammatory drugs (NSAIDs) relieve mild to moderately severe pain, with efficacy dependent on the particular NSAID administered. This class of analgesics dates back thousands of years, with the salicylates being among the oldest and still most commonly used analgesics.[139] *Salicylate* is a naturally occurring substance found in willow bark and, prior to production of the synthetic compound, was used for centuries to manage pain associated with rheumatism. In 1878, Felix Hoffman, working at Bayer in Germany, made the acetylated form of salicylic acid that has come to be known as aspirin.[139] Although aspirin (acetylsalicylic acid or ASA) has been found to be effective in the management of acute and chronic mild discomfort, the newer injectable NSAIDs appear to have comparable efficacy to the pure μ-agonist opioids in controlling moderate to severe soft tissue and orthopedic pain. The NSAIDs appear to confer synergism when used in combination with opioids and may demonstrate an opioid-sparing effect should lower dosages of opioid be required. Their extended duration of action, in addition to their analgesic efficacy, make the NSAIDs ideal for treating acute and chronic pain in veterinary patients. Careful patient and drug selection is critical, however, because of their potential for harmful side effects.

Cyclooxygenases and Prostaglandin Synthesis

In 1971, Vane discovered the mechanism by which aspirin exerts its anti-inflammatory, analgesic, and antipyretic actions. He proved that aspirin and other NSAIDs inhibited the activity of a cyclooxygenase (COX) enzyme that produced prostaglandins (PGs) involved in the pathogenesis of inflammation, swelling, pain, and fever.[140] Twenty years later, a second COX enzyme was discovered and, more recently, a newly identified COX-3 has been identified.[141–143] *Cyclooxygenase* (previously termed *prostaglandin synthase*) oxidizes arachidonic acid (previously termed *eicosatetraenoic acid*) to various eicosanoids (including PGs and other related compounds) (Fig. 10.5).[144] Oxidation of arachidonic

Table 10.3. Dosage ranges (mg/kg) for opioid antagonists in several domestic species

Opioid	Dogs	Cats	Horses	Cattle	Swine
Naloxone	0.002–0.02 IV	0.002–0.02 IV	0.002–0.02 IV	a	a
Nalmefene	0.025–0.03? IV	0.025–0.03? IV	?	?	?
Naltrexone	0.0025–0.003? IV	0.0025–0.003? IV	?	?	?

IV, intravenously; ?, reliable doses have not been established for this species.
[a]Doses have not been specifically reported for these species; however, 0.01 mg/kg IV is probably appropriate

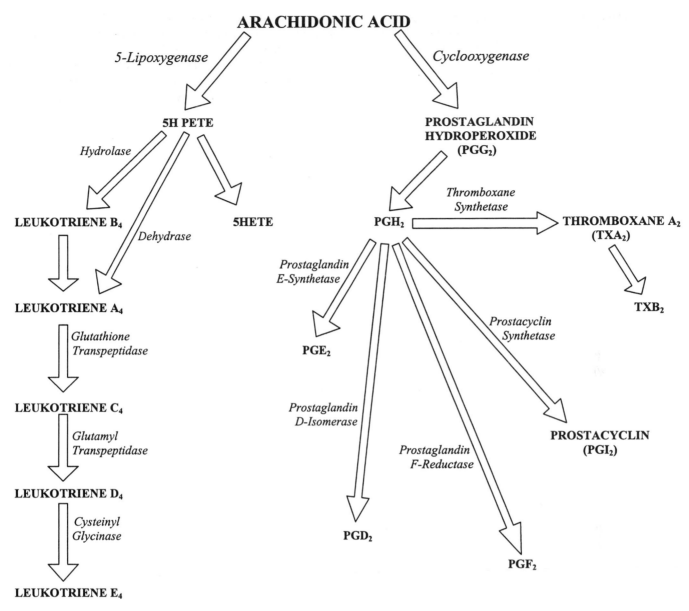

Fig. 10.5. The arachidonic acid cascade: eicosanoid synthesis. 5-HETE, 5-hydroxy-6,8,11,14-eicosatetraenoic acid; and 5-HPETE, 5-hydroperoxy-6,8,11,14-eicosatetraenoic acid.

acid by 5-lipoxygenase (5-LOX), the most biologically important of the mammalian oxygenases, produces the series of eicosanoids termed *leukotrienes* (Fig. 10.5). The release of arachidonic acid from membrane phospholipid is catalyzed by the enzyme phospholipase A_2 and is the rate-limiting step in PG and leukotriene synthesis. Prostaglandin G_2 is the initial prostenoid formed, followed by prostaglandin H_2, which serves as a substrate for prostaglandin E synthetase, prostaglandin D isomerase, prostaglandin F reductase, prostacyclin synthetase, and thromboxane synthetase for conversion to a variety of other prostenoids ubiquitous throughout cells and tissues in the body.[144] These include the PGs PGE_2, PGD_2, PGF_2, and PGI_2 (prostacyclin), and the thromboxanes TXA_2 and TXB_2, all with diverse functions.[145] The PGs are not stored, but are synthesized at a constant rate. They have

short half-lives of 4 to 6 min at 37°C and act locally at the site of production.

The PGs produced by both COX-1 and COX-2 are ubiquitous throughout the body and serve to facilitate many physiological functions during both health and illness. Consequently, the clinical use of NSAIDs has the potential to disrupt these functions, with the possibility of significant organ dysfunction. Thus, in addition to their role as analgesics, the effects of NSAIDs on the constitutive functions of the PGs must always be considered. There are several key points to note: (a) COX-1 generates PGs that are responsible for *mucosal defense* (i.e., secretion of bicarbonate and mucus, mucosal blood vessel attenuation of constriction, and mucosal epithelial regeneration), as well as TXA_2, which is necessary for platelet function; (b) COX-2 produces

PGs that function in the prevention and promotion of healing of mucosal erosions, and exert anti-inflammatory effects by inhibiting leukocyte adherence, as well as play a role in renal protection and maturation;[145] and (c) COX-3 produces PGs that exert a protective function by initiating fever.[143]

Thus, depending on the NSAID selected, primary plug formation of platelets, modulation of vascular tone in the kidney and gastric mucosa, cytoprotective functions within the gastric mucosa, smooth muscle contraction, and regulation of body temperature will all be affected.[145] In this regard, however, not all NSAIDs are created equal. As already noted, the COX-1, COX-2, and COX-3 enzymes make variable contributions to these functions, and individual NSAIDs inhibit each of these enzymes differently. Some NSAIDs inhibit both COX-1 and COX-2 (i.e., aspirin, phenylbutazone, ketoprofen [Anafen], ketorolac [Toradol], and flunixin meglumine [Banamine]); other NSAIDs preferentially inhibit COX-2 with only weak inhibition of COX-1 (i.e., meloxicam [Metacam], carprofen [Rimadyl], etodolac [Etogesic], vedaprofen [Quadrisol-5], and tolfenamic acid [Tolfedine]); and others inhibit COX-2 exclusively (i.e., deracoxib [Deramaxx] and firocoxib [Previcox]); whereas still another drug, acetaminophen, only weakly inhibits both COX-1 and COX-2 while inhibiting COX-3 activity preferentially.[141]

Several in vitro studies investigating NSAID selective inhibition of the COX-1 and COX-2 isoenzymes have been published, but their findings are very difficult to interpret because of inconsistencies in the assays used.[146] Clinically, this information is confusing because it does not consider the pharmacokinetics of particular drugs and their concentrations in various tissues.[147] Most NSAIDs that inhibit COX have been shown to result in diversion of arachidonate to the 5-LOX pathway. The 5-LOX is principally found in polymorphonuclear cells, mast cells, monocytes, basophils, and B lymphocytes that are recruited during inflammatory and immune reactions.[147] This enzyme catalyzes the initial step in leukotriene biosynthesis, which subsequently produces various eicosanoids, with leukotriene B_4 (LTB_4) being the most notable potent mediator of inflammation. The excessive production of leukotrienes has been implicated in the creation of NSAID-induced ulcers.[148,149] As always, however, the biological system is not clear-cut. Although the LOX pathway is proinflammatory, there is also an anti-inflammatory pathway,[150] which is discussed in more detail later.

The contribution of the leukotrienes to the inflammatory process would seem to suggest that inhibition of both the COX and 5-LOX pathways by a therapeutic agent would enhance the safety profile and may confer even greater analgesic efficacy because of broader anti-inflammatory and antinociceptive effects.[151] Data available show that dual acting compounds are effective in arthritic models, where they also retain antithrombotic activity, produce little or no gastrointestinal damage, and do not adversely affect the asthmatic state.[147] A dual COX–5-LOX inhibitor (tepoxalin [Zubrin]) has undergone clinical trials and is now approved for veterinary use.[151,152] Tepoxalin has demonstrated gastrointestinal anti-inflammatory activity in mice,[153] which supports the theory that 5-LOX inhibition can play a vital role in preventing NSAID-induced gastric inflammation.

Mechanisms of Analgesia

Prostaglandins, notably PGE_2 and prostacyclin, are potent mediators of inflammation and pain. These molecules exert hyperalgesic effects and enhance nociception produced by other mediators, such as bradykinin. The NSAIDs' analgesic mechanism of action is through inhibition of COX-1, COX-2, and COX-3 activity, with subsequent prevention of PG synthesis.

The antinociceptive effects of the NSAIDs are exerted both peripherally and centrally.[154] The NSAIDS penetrate inflamed tissues, where they have a local effect, which makes them excellent analgesic choices for treatment of injuries with associated inflammation, as well as conditions such as synovitis, arthritis, cystitis, and dermatitis.[154] The central action is at both the spinal and the supraspinal levels, with contributions from both COX-1 and COX-2.[154–158] This central effect may account for the overall well-being and improved appetite that are often observed in patients receiving parenterally administered NSAIDs for relief of acute pain.

The rational use of NSAIDs as analgesics should be based on an understanding of pain physiology and pathophysiology. Nociceptive pathways may involve either the COX-1 or COX-2 gene, and these genes are expressed in different locations and under different circumstances. The COX-2 isoenzyme, which is known as the inducible isoform because it is upregulated in inflammatory states, is known to play a key role in nociception. Although the COX-1 gene has traditionally been thought of as being expressed constitutively, this isoenzyme also plays an integral role in the pain experience.[142] The COX-1-selective NSAIDs are superior to COX-2-selective NSAIDs at inhibiting visceronociception caused by chemical pain stimulators in a mouse peritoneal model.[159] This has been confirmed by visceronociception being greatly reduced in COX-1, but not COX-2, knockout mice.[160] These studies concluded that peripheral COX-1 mediates nociception in slowly developing pain in mice, such as in visceral pain, and that central COX-1 may be involved in rapidly transmitted, nonvisceral pain, such as that caused by thermal stimulation.[160] Visceral pain may be mediated, at least in part, by stimulation of intraperitoneal receptors located on sensory fibers by COX-1-produced prostacyclin.[143] There may even be gender differences as in Ballou's mouse model, which demonstrated that spinal COX-2 did in fact contribute to visceral nociception, but only in female mice.[160] The analgesic potency of a range of NSAIDs in relieving tooth-extraction pain in human patients correlates closely with increasing selectivity toward COX-1 rather than COX-2. These findings highlight the importance of both COX-1 and COX-2 contributions to pain and the selective efficacy of the NSAIDs in treating various painful conditions and syndromes.

The COX-2 or inducible isoenzyme can increase by 20-fold over baseline in the presence of tissue injury and inflammation.[155] Proinflammatory cytokines and mitogens, such as interleukin 1β (IL-1β), interferon γ, and tumor necrosis factor α (TNF-α), induce COX-2 expression in macrophages, as can platelet-activating factor and PGE_2.[147] These events may also occur in chondrocytes, osteoblasts, and synovial microvessel endothelial cells. Higher COX levels increase prostenoid production where these compounds serve as amplifiers of nociceptive input and transmission in both the peripheral and central nervous systems.[155] The COX-2-selective NSAIDs have been shown to be clinically useful in managing inflammatory pain in human and animal patients. This has been a focus of the pharmaceutical industry as a more selective COX-2 inhibitor might show efficacy in alleviating pain and hyperalgesia while sparing COX-1-constitutive activity and potential adverse effects traditionally associated with NSAID administration. Unfortunately, this biological system is not as simple as first envisioned. Although COX-2 is induced during inflammation, it has also been shown to be induced during resolution of the inflammatory response where the anti-inflammatory PGs (PGD_2 and $PGF_{2\alpha}$), but not proinflammatory PGE_2, are produced. Potentially, inhibition of COX-2 during this phase may actually prolong inflammation.[147] As is the case for COX-1, it now appears that the COX-2 isoenzyme also has important constitutive functions. Studies indicate there may be a protective role for COX-2 in maintenance of gastrointestinal integrity,[161] in ulcer healing,[162] and in experimental colitis in rats.[163] In addition, the COX-2 isoenzyme appears to have constitutive functions associated with nerve, brain, ovarian and uterine function, and bone metabolism.[161] Therefore, the potential for NSAID-associated side effects with these systems is of concern. Of major importance are the COX-2-constitutive functions within the kidney, which differ from those of COX-1 in hypotensive and hypovolemic states.[164] Also, COX-2 appears to be important in nephron maturation.[165] The canine kidney is not fully mature until 3 weeks after birth,[166] and administration of a NSAID during this time, or to the bitch prior to birth, may cause a permanent nephropathy. In fact, in COX-2 null mice, which lack the gene for COX-2, all animals die of renal failure before 8 weeks of age.[167] Renal failure does not occur in COX-1-null–developing mice, and they do not develop gastric pathology.[167]

When considering the COX selectivity of a particular NSAID, the concentration (i.e., dose) of the NSAID may also influence its actions. A drug may function as a competitive, nonpreferential, or selective COX inhibitor (COX-1 or COX-2) at higher concentrations, and as a COX-2-selective inhibitor at lower concentrations.[168] The significance of this is the potential for inhibition of COX-1 with administration of an allegedly COX-2-selective NSAID. The COX selectivity may be present in vitro; however, at the dosing required to achieve analgesia, such selectivity may be lost. Cloning studies comparing canine COX isoenzymes with human COX isoenzymes found that they are highly homologous.[169] Canine COX-1 and COX-2 had a 96% and 93% DNA-sequence homology, respectively, with their human counterparts. This suggests that they would be similarly affected by pharmaceuticals such as NSAIDs designed to inhibit their function. However, the distribution of the COX enzymes may differ among species. When reviewing the adverse effects of NSAIDs (e.g., gastrointestinal ulceration, renal perturbations, and hemorrhage), hemorrhage is the only pathology that appears to be clinically diminished by the use of the more COX-2-selective NSAIDs.

COX 2 is reduced after administration of glucocorticoids, which may partially explain the anti-inflammatory and analgesic effects of this class of medications. Of interest, in addition to the

COX-2 role in inflammation, aberrantly upregulated COX-2 expression is increasingly implicated in the pathogenesis of a number of epithelial cell carcinomas, including colon, esophagus, breast, and skin, and in Alzheimer's disease and other neurological conditions.[170–172] For this reason, the COX-2 inhibitors are being researched as potential anticarcinogenic agents.[173]

Dissecting out the details of the derivation and specific actions of COX-1 and COX-2 continues to provide important insight into the management of pain with NSAIDs. The picture, however, remains incomplete because some NSAIDS do not significantly inhibit these enzymes. This finding stimulated the search for a potential COX-3 isoenzyme. Based on studies using canine cortex, a COX-3 isoenzyme was discovered that was derived from the same gene as COX-1.[142] The COX-3 isoenzyme is also present in human brain and heart tissues. It is distinct from COX-1 and COX-2 as demonstrated in studies using common analgesic-antipyretic NSAIDS in suppressing COX production. Acetaminophen inhibited COX-3 activity, but not COX-1 and COX-2, as does dipyrone.[142] Both of these agents are frequently used to reduce fever in animals. Other analgesic-antipyretic NSAIDs found to be effective COX-3 inhibitors are diclofenac (the most potent) and aspirin and ibuprofen (which preferentially inhibit COX-3 over COX-1 and COX-2). The overall conclusion of this particular study was that COX-3 possesses COX activity that differs pharmacologically from both COX-1 and COX-2, but is more similar to COX-1.[142] These findings indicate that the COX-3 isoenzyme is more susceptible to inhibition by drugs that are analgesic and antipyretic, but that lack anti-inflammatory activity. This observation again emphasizes the potential utility of administering NSAIDs with different COX selectivities for managing pain of different etiologies. As the COX-3 isoenzyme genetic profile is derived from the COX-1 gene, it appears that the COX-1 gene plays an integral role in pain and/or fever, depending on the physiological context.[142] This has been confirmed by the aforementioned studies.[143,159,160] The COX-1-selective NSAIDs with poor CNS penetration (i.e., ketoprofen and ketorolac) that are used in veterinary and human patients may, in fact, reach sufficient concentrations in the brain to inhibit COX-3.[174] It is also recognized that the analgesic effects of these NSAIDs frequently occur at lower dosages than those required to inhibit inflammation.

Fever Inhibition

Just as the relationship between pain and the various activities of the COX system is complex, so too is the association between fever and the COX isoenzymes. The mechanisms leading to the generation of fever vary depending on the inciting factor, which may be peripheral (i.e., endotoxin) or central (i.e., endogenous pyrogens, such as interleukin 1). Interspecies variation is also substantial, and the definitive role of the COXs in pyresis remains to be clearly elucidated. Evidence suggests that COX-2 plays a role in endotoxin pyrexia, whereas, based on the antipyretic effects of acetaminophen and aspirin, COX-1 and COX-3 appear to function in endogenous pyrexia.[141–143] Both of these drugs are effective in reducing fever in dogs. As an alternative in feline patients, ketoprofen[175] and meloxicam[176] have been shown to be effective antipyretic agents. Ketoprofen appears to be a good antipyretic in both cats and dogs, and this action can often be achieved at a relatively low dose.

Endogenous Anti-inflammatory Mechanisms

Endogenously generated small chemical mediators, or *autacoids*, play a key role in controlling inflammation by inhibiting polymorphonuclear cell recruitment and enhancing monocyte activity in a nonphlogistic manner.[149] Arachidonic acid–derived lipoxins, particularly lipoxin A_4, have been identified as anti-inflammatory mediators, indicating that the LOX pathway has a dual proinflammatory and anti-inflammatory function.

The NSAIDs may amplify or decrease this endogenous anti-inflammatory system. Aspirin is more COX-1 selective and can impair many components of mucosal defense and enhance leukocyte adherence within the gastric and mesenteric microcirculation.[177] However, with chronic use of aspirin, an adaptation of the gastric mucosa is associated with a marked upregulation of COX-2 expression and lipoxin production. This lipoxin is specifically termed *aspirin-triggered lipoxin* (ATL). Aspirin is unique among current therapies because it acetylates COX-2, thereby enabling the biosynthesis of 15(R)-hydroxyeicosatetraenoic acid from arachidonic acid, which is subsequently converted to ATL by 5-LOX. Inhibition of either the COX-2 or 5-LOX enzymes causes blockade of ATL synthesis.[177] Lipoxin A_4 and ATL (a carbon-15 epimer of lipoxin) attenuate aspirin-induced leukocyte adherence, whereas administration of selective COX-2 inhibitors blocks ATL synthesis and has been shown to augment aspirin-induced damage and leukocyte adherence to the endothelium of mesenteric venules in rats.[177]

In addition to the lipoxins, aspirin-induced COX-2 acetylation generates numerous other endogenous autacoids derived from dietary omega-3 fatty acids.[178] Some of these local autacoids are potent inhibitors of neutrophil recruitment, thereby limiting the role of these cells during the resolution phase of inflammation, and thus are referred to as *resolvins*.[178] The identification of both the lipoxins and the resolvins has introduced new potential therapeutic avenues for the treatment of inflammation, cardiovascular disease, and cancer.

Pharmacological Considerations

The NSAIDs are effective analgesics as indicated by the human consumption of 120 billion aspirin tablets per year in addition to the many other NSAIDs currently on the market. Despite this, the safety profile of these analgesics remains a concern. A search for the NSAID without adverse gastrointestinal effects is still ongoing. Incorporation of a nitric oxide–generating moiety into the molecule of several NSAIDs has shown attenuation of the ulcerogenic effects of these drugs. However, nitric oxide has also been implicated in the pathogenesis of arthritis and subsequent tissue destruction.[147]

Because of their high protein binding, NSAIDs can displace other drugs from their plasma protein-binding sites and potentially increase their plasma concentration. This is rarely a concern unless NSAIDs are administered to patients with organ dys-

function or in those receiving other highly protein-bound medications with a narrow therapeutic index. Interference with the metabolism and excretion of certain coadministered drugs may occur; therefore, verifying the safety of combination therapy is always mandatory.

Some NSAIDs may induce the syndrome of inappropriate secretion of antidiuretic hormone (ADH). Renal water reabsorption depends on the action of ADH mediated by cyclic adenosine monophosphate (cAMP). As PGs exert a controlled negative-feedback action on cAMP production, inhibition of PG synthesis produces above-normal levels of cAMP with potential for enhanced ADH activity. In addition, the administration of a COX-2-selective NSAID may enhance sodium and water reabsorption. Clinically, both mechanisms may result in high-specific-gravity urine with dilutional hyponatremia. Urine volume may be decreased through this mechanism, but without renal injury.[179,180]

NSAID-induced renal insufficiency is usually temporary and reversible with drug withdrawal and administration of intravenous fluids. Accidental ingestion of NSAIDs should be managed with gastric lavage (if within 1 h) followed by administration of activated charcoal and gastric protectants. If evidence of gastric ulcers exist, aggressive sucralfate therapy is necessary. Intravenous fluid therapy should continue for at least 1 day. Therapy beyond this period will depend on the renal and gastric status of the individual patient.

Patient Selection and Therapeutic Considerations

The general health of a patient greatly influences the decision to use NSAIDs. Cats and dogs are more susceptible than people to the adverse effects of this class of drugs. Thus, the reported safety of any one NSAID in human patients should not be assumed to be so in veterinary patients. Most NSAIDs have a narrow safety margin, so accurate dosing is absolutely necessary.

The administration of NSAIDs for perioperative pain management should be restricted to animals older than 6 weeks that are well hydrated and normotensive. Patients should have normal hemostatic function, no evidence or concern for gastric ulceration, and normal renal and hepatic function. Although these are general guidelines, future studies may indicate that short-term management of acute pain by using COX-1-sparing and, to some degree, COX-2-sparing NSAIDs may prove safe in animals with minimally compromised liver or renal function. Patients should not receive corticosteroids and NSAIDs concurrently,[181] nor should different NSAIDs be administered concurrently.

The preemptive use of NSAIDs is controversial because of their potential for harm. An earlier study assessing the effects on the kidney of preoperative administration of ketorolac, ketoprofen, or carprofen resulted in variable alterations in parameters measured. The conclusions of the study were that, in clinically normal dogs undergoing elective surgery, the use of these NSAIDs was not contraindicated, although renal function was not measured and two dogs in each of the ketoprofen and ketorolac groups were azotemic.[182] Another study assessing effects of preoperative administration of ketoprofen on whole blood platelet aggregation, buccal mucosal bleeding time, and hematologic indices in dogs undergoing elective ovariohysterectomy showed a decrease in platelet aggregation for at least 1 day after surgery. Mucosal bleeding time and hematologic indices did not change.[183] Other studies, specifically assessing efficacy and safety of NSAIDs given preoperatively in a variety of surgical procedures where intraoperative fluid therapy was administered and patient monitoring was conducted, noted adverse reactions with some of the NSAIDs.[123,184,185] A study conducted at the Ontario Veterinary College demonstrated no adverse effects with the administration of meloxicam or carprofen prior to orthopedic or soft tissue surgery in both cats (meloxicam) and dogs (meloxicam or carprofen) (unpublished data). In these studies, the preoperative administration of a NSAID provided very good to excellent analgesia. A laboratory study investigating potential adverse effects on glomerular filtration rate in dogs receiving meloxicam, carprofen, or saline prior to anesthesia and a painful stimulus failed to demonstrate a reduced glomerular filtration rate, and intravenous fluids were not administered in this study.[186] The benefit of preoperative administration of NSAIDs is the potential for a preemptive effect and the presence of analgesia upon recovery. When NSAIDs are administered postoperatively, opioids are often given concurrently, as 45 min is required to obtain a therapeutic effect with a NSAID, regardless of route. Another potential approach could be to administer the NSAID parenterally prior to completing the surgical procedure at least 45 min prior to extubation. Often it is difficult to distinguish the difference in the analgesic effects produced by preoperative versus intraoperative NSAID administration. For prolonged operative procedures, the benefit of a longer postoperative effect may be seen with administration of the NSAID upon completion, rather than at the start, of the procedure.

Effective plasma levels of NSAIDs are reached within 1 h after oral administration.[187–189] When NSAIDs are administered per os, they must be given with food to protect the gastric mucosa. If food is not present in the stomach, the contact area of the tablet on the mucosa results in a high localized concentration of the drug, increasing the potential for localized ulcer formation. It is important to remember that the potential for ulceration exists with all NSAIDs regardless of the route of administration.

Pain Management

The indications proposed here assume there are no contraindications to their use.

Postoperative Pain

The NSAIDs are extremely valuable in selected orthopedic[123,182,190,191] and soft tissue surgical procedures,[184,192–197] especially where extensive inflammation or soft tissue trauma is present. Opioid administration is preferred immediately after any surgical procedure, because the sedative-analgesic effects of this class of drugs help to ensure a smooth recovery. Injectable NSAIDs (carprofen, ketoprofen, meloxicam, or tolfenamic acid) can be coadministered initially with an opioid and subsequently used alone following orthopedic and selected soft tissue surgery; however, this depends on the degree of pain an animal is experiencing. Oral NSAIDs may be administered when an animal is able to eat. The initial dose of NSAID depends on the expected severity of pain. For example, a difficult fracture repair would require the recommended loading dose, but a laparotomy without complications could be successfully treated with half this dose. A sliding-scale approach similar to that used with the opioids for managing varying degrees of anticipated pain is also recommended for the NSAIDs; however, the upper dosing limit must not be exceeded.

Inflammatory Conditions

For relief of pain caused by meningitis, bone tumors (especially after biopsy), soft tissue swelling (mastitis), polyarthritis, cystitis, otitis, or severe inflammatory dermatologic diseases or injury (e.g., degloving and animal bites), the NSAIDs may be more efficacious than opioids. However, as many of these patients may be more prone to NSAID toxicity, careful patient selection and management are advised. The combination of an opioid with a low dose of NSAID is also effective in these conditions. An exception is necrotizing fasciitis, where NSAIDs may actually increase morbidity and mortality.[198]

Osteoarthritis

Few long-term studies evaluating the adverse effects of NSAIDs have been completed. A short-term study (12 days) assessing the effect of carprofen on platelet aggregation and activated partial thromboplastin time in Labrador retrievers showed, after 5 days of treatment, a reduction in platelet aggregation that persisted after treatment was discontinued for 7 days. The activated partial thromboplastin time was similarly affected as times were prolonged over baseline during this period, although they remained within normal range. The conclusions of this study, however, were that these alterations were minor and not clinically important.[199] The major adverse effects associated with long-term use of carprofen,[200] meloxicam,[201] or etodolac[202] for osteoarthritis are predominantly associated with the gastrointestinal tract. Gastroduodenal pathology associated with buffered aspirin, carprofen, etodolac, and placebo has been evaluated in healthy dogs after a 4-week course of administration. Two independent studies concluded that the administration of carprofen, etodolac, or placebo produced significantly fewer gastroduodenal lesions in dogs than did buffered aspirin.[203,204] Similar studies comparing ketoprofen with aspirin and placebo,[205] and comparing carprofen, meloxicam, and ketoprofen to aspirin and placebo,[206] noted that these NSAIDs produced mild to moderate gastrointestinal lesions that were similar to placebo, but significantly less severe than those produced by aspirin. A sliding-scale approach of NSAID administration for chronic use is highly recommended. As many patients with osteoarthritis are geriatric, a rapid reduction of the dose to affect a comfortable state is advised to reduce potential toxicity. For example, alternating to every-third-day therapy of meloxicam with half the recommended label dose proved efficacious in some dogs during a 1-year period.[201] If an individual patient requires persistent high doses of a particular NSAID to manage pain, prescribing a different NSAID may be more effective because of individual variation in response and effect, as previously discussed. When the adverse effects of a NSAID are a concern, reducing the dose and adding an analgesic of a different class (e.g., tramadol) may be equally effective for the treatment of chronic severe pain. However, for many geriatric animals with renal insufficiency, NSAIDs may be the only effective class of analgesic. For these animals, quality of life is a major issue. In this situation, meloxicam (in both cats and dogs) or carprofen (in dogs only) titrated down to the lowest effective dose has been used in patients with renal insufficiency with minimal or no worsening of renal function over time (personal communication).

During NSAID therapy, all patients should be monitored for hematochezia or melena, vomiting, increased water consumption, and nonspecific changes in demeanor. If any of these occur, the owner should be instructed to stop the medication and consult a veterinarian. Intermittent monitoring of creatinine and alanine aminotransferase (ALT) is recommended when the use of NSAIDs is prescribed on a chronic basis. Another important consideration for chronic use is the potential effect of NSAID therapy on joint and cartilage metabolism. Studies investigating the effects of carprofen[207,208] and meloxicam[209] at therapeutic doses found no toxicological or pharmacological actions on cartilage proteoglycan metabolism. In addition, meloxicam may have the potential for controlling cellular inflammatory reactions at inflamed sites in the joints of patients with osteoarthritis.[209]

Miscellaneous Conditions

Other indications for the use of NSAIDs are panosteitis, hypertrophic osteodystrophy (HOD), cancer pain (especially of bone), and dental pain. The NSAIDs with selective COX-1 inhibition should be used with caution after dental extractions where bleeding is, or may be, of concern. Meloxicam and carprofen have minimal, if any, antithromboxane activity and should, therefore, not interfere with platelet adhesion. For severe panosteitis and HOD, the full loading dose of a NSAID is required to obtain a suitable effect. The HOD of Weimaraners is poorly responsive to NSAID therapy and is better treated with high-dose, short-term corticosteroids, provided infectious disease has been ruled out and clinical signs are consistent with HOD alone.[210]

Contraindications

NSAIDs should not be administered to patients with acute renal insufficiency, hepatic insufficiency, dehydration, hypotension, or conditions associated with low *effective circulating volume* (e.g., congestive heart failure or ascites), coagulopathies (e.g., factor deficiencies, thrombocytopenia, or von Willebrand's disease), or evidence of gastric ulceration (i.e., vomiting with or without the presence of "coffee ground material" or melena). Administration of NSAIDs following gastrointestinal surgery must be determined by the overall health of the gut at the time of surgery. As the COX-2 isoenzyme is important for healing, intuitively NSAIDs producing potent COX-2 enzyme inhibition would be contraindicated where compromised bowel is noted. Concurrent use of other NSAIDs (e.g., aspirin) or corticosteroids is not recommended. The use of COX-1-preferential NSAIDs is contraindicated in patients with spinal injury (including herniated in-

tervertebral disc) because of the potential for hemorrhage and neurological deterioration, and because of excessive bleeding at the surgical site should surgical treatment be pursued. The NSAIDs should never be administered to patients in shock, trauma patients upon presentation, or patients with evidence of hemorrhage (e.g., epistaxis, hemangiosarcoma, or head trauma). The condition of patients with severe or poorly controlled asthma, such as feline asthma, or other types of moderate to severe pulmonary disease, may deteriorate with NSAID administration. Aspirin administration has been documented to exacerbate asthma in human patients, but the administration of COX-2-specific NSAIDs did not worsen clinical signs.[211] It is unknown whether animals may be affected in this way. Although administration of NSAIDs in head trauma, pulmonary diseases, or thrombocytopenia is generally contraindicated, the use of COX-2-preferential NSAIDs (i.e., meloxicam, etodolac, carprofen, tolfenamic acid, firocoxib, or deracoxib) may prove to be safe with further study. Because of inhibition of PG activity, the NSAIDs may be detrimental to reproductive function. Indomethacin may block prostaglandin activity in pregnant women, causing cessation of labor, premature closure of the ductus arteriosus in the fetus, and disruption of fetal circulation.[161] These effects may also occur in animals, so NSAIDs should not be administered during pregnancy. As COX-2 induction is necessary for ovulation and subsequent implantation of the embryo,[161] the use of NSAIDs should also be avoided in breeding females during this stage of the reproductive cycle. As previously mentioned, the COX-2 isoenzyme is required for maturation of the embryological kidney, so COX-2 administration to lactating mothers should be avoided.

Topical NSAIDs do not appear to be associated with the same adverse gastrointestinal effects noted when these same drugs are taken orally,[212] and topical administration has proven to be significantly more effective than placebo in many human clinical trials involving acute and chronic painful conditions.[213] A liposomal topical cream formulation of 1% diclofenac sodium (Surpass) has recently been approved by the U.S. Food and Drug Administration as a topical anti-inflammatory cream for the control of joint pain and inflammation associated with osteoarthritis in horses. The results of clinical field trials indicate that the product is safe, easy to use, and effective in reducing lameness caused by degenerative joint disease in this species. When applied topically (a 5-inch strip of cream) for 10 consecutive days to a single fetlock, diclofenac was present in all serum samples up to 2 days after the final application.[214] The term *locally enhanced topical delivery* (LETD) has been used to describe the local accumulation of drug to the target tissues. This effect has been documented in horses when using the 1% diclofenac liposomal formulation.[215] Consistent with its prolonged effect at the target tissue, diclofenac was slowly absorbed and eliminated following its application. When compared with other conventional topical creams and ointments, liposomal preparations provide better penetration and a more sustained release of agent. There are no well controlled published studies investigating the clinical use of topical formulations of NSAIDs in dogs and cats at the date of this writing.

Specific NSAIDs

Recommended dosages are listed in Tables 10.4 through 10.6.

Meloxicam (Oral Liquid and Parenteral Formulations)

Meloxicam is a COX-2-preferential NSAID approved for oral use in dogs in Australasia, Europe, and North America. The parenteral formulation is approved for cats in Australasia and the United States. Its use in cats in Canada is under investigation at the time of this writing, with completed studies indicating safety and efficacy. Its use in horses is also under investigation, with pharmacokinetic studies indicating that the half-life is shorter and clearance greater than in dogs, which suggests that dosing more than once a day may be necessary.[216]

Studies indicate no renal or hepatic abnormalities with acute administration[184] and minimal to no antithromboxane activity,[217] suggesting that hemostasis in normal animals may not be a problem. Very few adverse reactions have been documented, and most involve the gastrointestinal tract. A 2003 study showed no difference in gastric erosions over saline placebo when meloxicam was administered at 0.1 mg/kg for 3 days after electrical stimulation (i.e., surgical simulation) under anesthesia. However, the administration of corticosteroids plus meloxicam caused significant gastric erosions.[181] A case report of the administration of a combination of aspirin and meloxicam in a dog detected duodenal perforation.[218] This case illustrates the importance of COX-2 in intestinal protection when aspirin is coadministered, and rein-

Table 10.4. Dosage ranges (mg/kg unless otherwise indicated) for NSAIDs in dogs and cats

NSAID[a]	Indication	Species/Dose/Route	Frequency
Ketoprofen	Surgical pain	Dogs, ≤ 2.0 IV, SC, IM, PO	Once
		Cats, ≤ 2.0 SC	Once
		then dogs and cats, ≤ 1.0 IV, SC, IM, PO	q 24 h
		Dogs and cats, ≤ 2.0 PO	
	Chronic pain	then ≤ 1.0	Once
Meloxicam	Surgical pain	Dogs, ≤ 0.2 IV, SC	Once
		then ≤ 0.1 IV, SC, PO	q 24 h
	Chronic pain	Dogs, ≤ 0.2 PO	Once
		then ≤ 0.1 PO	q 24 h
	Surgical pain	Cats, ≤ 0.2 SC, PO	Once
		then ≤ 0.1 SC, PO lean weight	q 24 h for 2–3 days
	Chronic pain	Cats, ≤ 0.2 SC, PO	Once
		then ≤ 0.1 PO lean weight	q 24 h for 2–3 days
		then 0.025 PO or (0.1 mg/CAT max) lean weight	3–5 × weekly
Carprofen	Surgical pain	Dogs, ≤ 4.0 IV, SC, IM	Once at induction
		then ≤ 2.2 PO	Repeat q 12–24 h
		Cats, ≤ 4.0 SC lean weight	Once at induction only
	Chronic pain	Dogs, ≤ 2.2 PO	q 12–24 h
Etodolac	Chronic pain	Dogs, ≤ 10–15 PO	q 24 h
Tolfenamic acid	Acute, chronic pain	Dogs and cats, ≤ 4 SC, PO	q 24 h for 3 days, 4 days off, then repeat cycle
Firocoxib	Chronic pain	Dogs, 5.0 PO	q 24 h
Flunixin meglumine	Surgical pain	Dogs, ≤ 1.0 IV, SC, IM	Once
		Cats, 0.25 SC	q 12–24 h PRN × 1 or 2 doses
	Pyrexia	Dogs and cats, 0.25 SC	q 12–24 h PRN × 1 or 2 doses
	Ophthalmologic procedures	Dogs, 0.25–1.0 SC, IM	q 12–24 h PRN × 1 or 2 doses
Ketorolac	Surgical pain	Dogs, 0.3–0.5 IV, IM	q 8–12 h × 1 or 2 doses
		Cats, 0.25 IM	q 12 h × 1 or 2 doses
	Panosteitis	Dogs, 10-mg total dose in dogs ≥ 30 kg PO	q 24 h for 2–3 days
		5-mg total dose in dogs > 20 kg < 30 kg PO	
Deracoxib	Surgical pain	Dogs, ≤ 3–4 PO	q 24 h for 3–7 days
	Chronic pain	Dogs, ≤ 1–2 PO	q 24 h
Tepoxalin	Chronic pain	Dogs, 10 PO	q 24 h
Piroxicam	Inflammation of the lower urinary tract	Dogs, 0.3 PO	q 24 h × 2 doses then q 48 h
Acetaminophen	Acute, chronic pain	Dogs, 15 PO (contraindicated in cats)	q 8 h
Aspirin	Acute, chronic pain	Dogs, 10 PO	q 12 h

CAT max, maximal dose in cats; IM, intramuscularly; IV, intravenously; NSAID, nonsteroidal anti-inflammatory drug; PO, per os (orally); PRN, as necessary; SC, subcutaneously.

[a]See the text for details on contraindications for use.

Table 10.5. Dosage ranges (mg/kg) of NSAIDs in horses

NSAID[a]	Dose	Route	Frequency	Notes
Phenylbutazone	2–4	PO, IV	q 12 h	Reduce to 2 mg/kg on day 2
Flunixin meglumine	1	PO, IV, IM	q 12–24 h	
Ketoprofen	2–3	IV	q 24 h	
Carprofen	0.7	IV	q 24 h	
Eltenac	0.5	IV	q 24 h	
Diclofenac	5-inch ribbon of cream	Transdermal	q 12 h	Apply liposomal cream over 1 joint only twice daily
Vedaprofen	1	IV	q 24 h	
Meloxicam	0.6	IV	q 12 h	

IM, intramuscularly; IV, intravenously; NSAID, nonsteroidal anti-inflammatory drug; PO, per os (orally).
[a]See text for details on contraindications for use.

Table 10.6. Dosage ranges (mg/kg) of NSAIDs in ruminants

NSAID[a]	Dose	Route	Frequency	Notes
Phenylbutazone	2–6	PO, IV	q 24 h	Prohibited in dairy cattle >20 months of age
Flunixin meglumine	1	PO, IV, IM	q 12 or 24 h	
Ketoprofen	3	IV, PO	q 24 h	
Carprofen	0.7	IV	q 24–48 h	Sheep
Aspirin	100	PO	q 12 h	

IM, intramuscularly; IV, intravenously; NSAID, nonsteroidal anti-inflammatory drug; PO, per os (orally).
[a]See text for details on contraindications for use.

forces the concept that different NSAIDs should not be administered concurrently. Analgesia is excellent when meloxicam is combined with an opioid. Meloxicam has proven to be beneficial in the treatment of sodium urate–induced synovitis[219] and panosteitis[220] in dogs, and radiation-induced stomatitis in cats.[221]

Carprofen (Tablet and Parenteral Formulations)

Although classified as a NSAID, carprofen administration to beagles did not inhibit PGE_2, 12-hydroxyeicosatetraenoic acid, or TXB_2 synthesis in an experimental study using subcutaneous tissue cage fluids.[222] It was concluded that the principle mode of action of carprofen must be by mechanisms other than COX or 12-lipoxygenase inhibition. However, more recent studies indicate that it is a COX-2-preferential NSAID.[146,223] Carprofen is approved for perioperative and chronic pain management in dogs in Australasia, Europe, and North America. Carprofen is approved for single-dose, perioperative use in cats in Europe and is licensed for use in horses in the United Kingdom. In sheep, carprofen (0.7 mg/kg intravenously) produced plasma concentrations of 1.5 μg/mL, similar to those required to confer analgesia in horses, for up to 48 h.[224] However, analgesia was not assessed in this sheep study.[224] Antithromboxane activity is minimal,[217,225] suggesting that induced coagulopathy may not be a problem in patients with intact hemostatic mechanisms.

According to the European literature, potential adverse effects of NSAIDs, such as nephrotoxicity, hepatotoxicity, gastrointestinal bleeding, or hemostatic deficiencies have not been reported with carprofen use.[198] Acute hepatotoxicity and death after carprofen administration have been reported among dogs with previously reported normal liver function (with Labrador retrievers highly represented).[226] Carprofen provides good analgesia from 12 h[182,192] to 18 h after a variety of orthopedic procedures. In cats undergoing ovariohysterectomy, carprofen administration provided profound analgesia between 4 and 20 h postoperatively.[193]

Ketoprofen (Tablet and Parenteral Formulations)

Ketoprofen is approved for treatment of postoperative and chronic pain in both dogs and cats in Europe and Canada. It is also approved for use in horses and ruminants. As ketoprofen is an inhibitor of both COX-1 and COX-2, adverse effects are a potential problem requiring careful patient selection. Although several studies using ketoprofen preoperatively indicate its effectiveness in controlling postoperative pain,[182,184,190] a general consensus among practitioners has restricted its use primarily to the postoperative period to reduce the potential for hemorrhage. Ketoprofen should not be administered to patients with risk factors for hemorrhage. It is often administered to animals immediately after orthopedic procedures (e.g., fracture repair, cruciate repair, or onychectomy); however, it is advised to restrict administration after laparotomy or thoracotomy until such time that hemorrhage is not a concern and when intracavitary drainage tubes have been removed.

In a study investigating the efficacy of NSAIDs in controlling postoperative pain, ketoprofen conferred a very good to excellent analgesic state for up to 24 h when compared with butorphanol.[184] Ketoprofen administration has also been suggested for management of pain associated with hypertrophic osteodystrophy and panosteitis in dogs. Gastroprotectants should be coadministered. Occasional vomiting may be seen when ketoprofen is administered chronically. It has also been recommended in horses.[227] In foals less than 1 day old, the volume of distribution is larger and the clearance is reduced, which indicate that this drug has a longer elimination half-life in foals.[228] In ponies, synovial concentrations of ketoprofen are achieved after intravenous injection and will last for up to 4 h.[229] After oral administration, ketoprofen was an effective analgesic in 4- to 8-week-old calves undergoing dehorning,[230] and in 8- to 16-week-old calves when administered intravenously in conjunction with lidocaine injection of the testicles for castration.[231]

Etodolac (Tablet Formulation)

Etodolac is a COX-2-preferential NSAID approved in the United States for use in dogs for the management of pain and inflammation associated with osteoarthritis,[202,232] but is also useful in other painful conditions. The adverse effects appear to be primarily restricted to the gastrointestinal tract.

Deracoxib and Firocoxib (Tablet Formulations)

Deracoxib is a coxib-type COX-2-specific inhibitor approved in the United States and Canada for control of postoperative pain and inflammation associated with orthopedic surgery and chronic osteoarthritic pain in dogs. Firocoxib is the most COX-2 selective NSAID available in veterinary medicine and the most recently approved NSAID for the control of osteoarthritic pain in dogs in the United States. The incidence of vomiting and diarrhea were similar in dogs receiving deracoxib and those receiving placebo in a perioperative field trial, and overall the drug was well tolerated and effective.[233] It was also shown to be effective in attenuating lameness in dogs with urate crystal–induced synovitis after prophylactic and therapeutic administration.[234,235] The coxib group of NSAIDs were originally marketed as being more gastroprotective in human patients when compared with the less COX-1-sparing NSAIDs such as aspirin.[236] However, more recent findings and large-scale usage in human patients have indicated that coxib NSAIDs do not necessarily guarantee gastroprotection with chronic use. In a more recent canine study comparing the gastrointestinal safety profile of licofelone (a dual COX-LOX inhibitor) with rofecoxib (a similar coxib-type COX-2 inhibitor to deracoxib and firocoxib), rofecoxib was found to induce significant gastric and gastroduodenal lesions.[237] It has been recommended by some investigators that coxib-type NSAIDs not be administered for a period of 1 week after a previously administered NSAID or steroid has been discontinued.

Tepoxalin (Dissolvable Wafer)

Tepoxalin is a COX-1, COX-2, and LOX inhibitor of varying degrees with efficacy comparable to meloxicam or carprofen and safety comparable to placebo.[238] Tepoxalin has been approved for management of osteoarthritic pain in dogs. The safety profile of tepoxalin showed no difference from that of placebo when administered prior to a 30-min anesthesia period and a minor surgical procedure in dogs.[239]

Tolfenamic Acid (Tablet and Parenteral Formulations)

Tolfenamic acid is approved for use in cats and dogs in Europe and Canada for controlling acute postoperative and chronic pain. The dosing schedule is 3 days on and 4 days off, which must be strictly adhered to. Reported adverse effects are diarrhea and occasional vomiting. Tolfenamic acid has significant anti-inflammatory and antithromboxane activity,[240] so posttraumatic and surgical hemostasis may be compromised during active bleeding after administration of this NSAID.

Flunixin Meglumine (Parenteral Formulation)

Flunixin meglumine, which is a COX-1 and COX-2 inhibitor, is approved for use in dogs in Europe, but not in North America. It is also approved for use in ruminants and horses. Flunixin is commonly used to treat colic pain in horses. In foals less than 1 day old, pharmacokinetic data suggest increasing the dose by as much as 1.5 times the adult dose to achieve comparable therapeutic concentrations; however, longer dosing intervals are necessary to avoid toxicity.[241] Dosages for cattle are similar to those in horses. In dogs, it is reported to be an effective analgesic for surgical pain;[123,195] however, the potential for side effects such as increased ALT,[123] nephrotoxicity,[123,185,242] and gastric ulceration[243] is a major concern. Flunixin is also used as an anti-inflammatory in selected ophthalmologic surgical procedures, but safer NSAIDs appear to be as effective in this setting.

Phenylbutazone (Powder and Parenteral Formulations)

Phenylbutazone is approved for use in horses, cattle, and dogs in North America. Since safer NSAIDs are approved for dogs, phenylbutazone is not recommended for this species. In horses, there is high risk of gastric ulceration and nephrotoxicity,[244] where signs of toxicity may progress from inappetence and depression to colic, gastrointestinal ulceration, and weight loss.[245,246] In horses recovering from arthroscopic surgery, phenylbutazone administered prior to surgery and for 21/2 days afterward improved analgesic outcome when compared with a placebo group.[247] Phenylbutazone has a prolonged elimination half-life in cattle, ranging from 30 to 82 h.[248,249] Phenylbutazone administration to dairy cattle 20 months of age or older is prohibited by the U.S. Food and Drug Administration to avoid the presence of residues that are toxic to people.

Eltenac (Parenteral Formulation and Topical Gel)

In horses, eltenac induced minimal side effects when 0.5 mg/kg was used during an investigative study.[250] When used in an endotoxemic horse model, eltenac improved outcome parameters when compared with placebo, and it was proposed that this NSAID may provide clinical benefit in horses with naturally occurring endotoxemia.[251]

Vedaprofen (Oral and Parenteral Formulations)

The oral form is approved for use in dogs in Europe and Canada. The parenteral form is approved for use in horses in Europe and North America and has very similar pharmacokinetic and pharmacodynamic properties to those of ketoprofen.[252,253]

Ketorolac (Parenteral Formulation)

Ketorolac, which is a COX-1 and COX-2 inhibitor, is not approved for use in veterinary patients, but is included for the benefit of those working in the research setting where the availability of ketorolac is more likely than other NSAIDs. Ketorolac is comparable to oxymorphone in efficacy and to ketoprofen in duration and efficacy in managing postlaparotomy and orthopedic pain in dogs.[123] Only one to two doses should be administered to dogs or cats. Ketorolac has been used successfully for treatment of severe panosteitis in dogs where all other therapies had failed. It is recommended that ketorolac be administered with food or gastroprotectants to decrease the incidence of gastric irritation.

Piroxicam (Capsule Formulation)

Piroxicam is not approved for use in veterinary patients, but has proven valuable for its anti-inflammatory effects on the lower urinary tract in dogs with transitional cell carcinoma or cystitis and urethritis. The administration of gastroprotectants is recommended.[254]

Acetaminophen (Tablet and Oral Suspension Formulations)

Acetaminophen is a COX-3 inhibitor with minimal COX-1 and COX-2 effects. It is not approved for use in veterinary patients. It should not be administered to cats because of deficient glucuronidation of acetaminophen in this species.[255] It may be administered to dogs as an antipyretic and analgesic for mild pain and can be used in combination with opioids for a synergistic analgesic effect or opioid-sparing effect.[141,142] It can be prescribed as an individual drug that can be coadministered with an opioid (this approach allows more flexibility in dosing of the opioid), or in a proprietary combined formulation with an opioid (e.g., codeine plus acetaminophen, or oxycodone plus acetaminophen).

Aspirin (Tablet Formulation)

Aspirin, which is primarily a COX-1 inhibitor, is most commonly used as an analgesic for osteoarthritic pain in dogs. It is also available in proprietary combinations with various opioids (aspirin plus codeine, or aspirin plus oxycodone) to achieve a synergistic effect for the treatment of moderate pain. It is also used as an antipyretic and anticoagulant in dogs and cats. Aspirin has also been evaluated as an analgesic in cattle.[256]

Dipyrone (Tablet and Parenteral Formulations)

Dipyrone, which is a COX-3 inhibitor, is approved for use in cats and dogs in Europe and Canada. It should be given intravenously to avoid the irritation experienced when given intramuscularly. The analgesia produced is not usually adequate for moderate to severe postoperative pain, and dipyrone is reserved for use as an antipyretic in cases where other NSAIDs are contraindicated. Nephrotoxicity or gastric ulceration is not a major concern in the short term even in critically ill patients. Dipyrone administration induces blood dyscrasias in human patients, but this has not been reported in animals.

Diclofenac (Topical Liposomal Cream Formulation)

Diclofenac is a phenylacetic acid NSAID that is a nonselective cyclooxygenase inhibitor commonly used in human patients. There is no oral or parenteral formulation available in veterinary medicine, but a topical cream has recently been approved by the Food and Drug Administration for use in horses. This liposomal cream formulation of 1% diclofenac provides a novel therapeutic modality for the local application of NSAID-type anti-inflammatory drugs. Dosing is achieved by applying a 5-inch ribbon of topical cream to only one affected joint twice daily for no more than 10 consecutive days. Rubber gloves should be worn when applying and rubbing the cream into the skin covering the painful joint. The cream is stored at room temperature and should not be frozen. Simultaneous multiple-joint application can result in excessive absorption and high serum concentrations with an increased potential for severe NSAID-type adverse reactions.

Analgesic Adjuvants

Analgesic adjuvants are defined as drugs that have primary indications other than pain, but that possess analgesic actions in certain painful conditions. This definition encompasses a very diverse group of drugs and distinguishes the analgesic adjuvants from the so-called traditional analgesics, which include the opioids, the NSAIDs, and the local anesthetics. It is only recently that analgesic adjuvants have begun to be used in veterinary medicine, and most therapeutic recommendations have been extrapolated from experience with human patients and subsequently applied to companion animals.

As the name implies, these agents are typically coadministered with the traditional analgesics. They have been used most often in the management of chronic pain states; however, their use in acute pain settings is increasing, and certain adjuvant agents have become common analgesic supplements during the perioperative period. In the chronic pain setting, the adjuvant analgesics are administered (a) to manage pain that is refractory to traditional analgesics, (b) to enable the dose of traditional analgesics to be reduced in order to lessen side effects, and (c) concurrently to treat a symptom other than pain. In some clinical settings, such as chronic neuropathic pain syndromes, adjuvant analgesics have become so well accepted that they are administered as the first-line therapy in human patients.

When contemplating administration of an adjuvant analgesic, veterinarians must be aware of the drug's clinical pharmacology and its particular use in patients with pain. The following information about the drug is necessary: (a) approved indications, (b) unapproved indications (e.g., for analgesia) that are widely accepted in veterinary medical practice, (c) common side effects and uncommon but potentially severe adverse effects, (d) important pharmacokinetic features, and (e) specific dosing guidelines for pain.

Table 10.7. Potential analgesic adjuvants in veterinary clinical practice

α₂-Agonists	NMDA receptor antagonists
Medetomidine	Ketamine
Detomidine	Amantadine
Romifidine	Methadone
Antidepressants	Memantine
Amitriptyline	Anticonvulsants
Imipramine	Gabapentin
Paroxetine	Carbamazepine
Oral local anesthetics	Clonazepam
Mexiletine	Miscellaneous analgesics
Tocainide	Tramadol
Flecainide	
Others	
Capsaicin	
Calcitonin	
Magnesium	
Bisphosphonates	
Radiopharmaceuticals	

NMDA, *N*-methyl-D-aspartate.

Table 10.8. Dosage ranges (mg/kg) for analgesic adjuvants in selected domestic species

Analgesic Adjuvant	Dogs	Cats
Ketamine	0.5 IV loading dose 0.1–0.5/h IV CRI	0.5 IV loading dose 0.1–0.5/h IV CRI
Medetomidine	0.002–0.015 IV, IM	0.005–0.02 IV, IM
Gabapentin	2–10 PO q 8–12 h	2–10 PO q 8–12 h
Amantadine	3–5 PO q 24 h	3–5 PO q 24 h
Tramadol	2–10 PO q 12–24 h	?

CRI, continuous-rate infusion; IM, intramuscular(ly); IV, intravenous(ly); PO, per os (orally); ?, reliable doses have not been established for this species.

Numerous drugs may be considered as analgesic adjuvants in veterinary medicine today (Table 10.7). Some of these, such as ketamine and the α₂-agonists, are familiar to practitioners, whereas others have not been used historically in veterinary medicine. Much of the evidence substantiating the use of these agents comes from laboratory-animal research, clinical trials in humans, or anecdotal reports in human or animal patients. The following section briefly reviews the current state of knowledge regarding selected analgesic adjuvants in veterinary medicine (see Table 10.8 for recommended dosages).

Ketamine

Ketamine is a dissociative anesthetic and has been used for decades in veterinary medicine. More recently, it has been recognized as an NMDA receptor antagonist and, at very low doses, can contribute substantially to analgesia by minimizing CNS sensitization.

α₂-Agonists

Xylazine and, more recently, medetomidine, detomidine, and romifidine have been used extensively to provide sedation in a variety of veterinary species. Medetomidine and detomidine in particular have considerable analgesic potential, even in microdoses, and can be administered via a number of novel routes and techniques to supplement analgesia and enhance the analgesic actions of other agents in various painful conditions.

Gabapentin

Gabapentin is a human anticonvulsant drug that has been approved by the U.S. Food and Drug Administration since 1993.[10] Several years later, reports of its antihyperalgesic effects in rodent experimental pain models, as well as case reports and un-

controlled clinical trials involving human patients suffering from neuropathic pain, began to appear in the literature. Gabapentin's mechanism of analgesic action is unknown, but there is evidence to suggest that it may increase central inhibition or reduce the synthesis of glutamate, even though it does not appear to interact directly with NMDA receptors.[99]

Despite the lack of controlled data available at this time, gabapentin administration has been advocated for the management of a variety of human neuropathic pain syndromes[99,257] and more recently for management of incisional pain and arthritis.[258–261] In human clinical trials, side effects occur in approximately 25% of patients, are usually mild and self-limiting, and include drowsiness, fatigue, and weight gain with chronic administration. There are only anecdotal reports of its use in veterinary patients. Dosing guidelines in dogs and cats have been extrapolated from human dosing recommendations. Dosage modifications are often based on the clinical efficacy achieved in individual veterinary patients. Though it is not possible to make specific scientific recommendations of dosage and indication in specific species, with owner consent, both gabapentin and pregabalin have been increasingly used by veterinary practitioners striving to better manage chronic neuropathic pain of both malignant and nonmalignant origins in companion animals.

Amantadine

Amantadine is an antiviral agent developed to inhibit the replication of influenza A in human patients.[10] It has also been shown to have efficacy in the treatment of drug-induced extrapyramidal effects and in the treatment Parkinson's disease. More recently, amantadine administration has been advocated for the treatment of various types of pain. The drug appears to exert its analgesic effects through antagonism of NMDA receptors in a manner analogous to ketamine. Though controlled clinical human trials are lacking, amantadine seems most efficacious in the management of chronic neuropathic types of pain characterized by hyperalgesia and allodynia.[262,263] Patients suffering from opioid tolerance may also respond favorably to amantadine therapy, and some studies suggest that the drug may even find a place in perioperative pain management.[264] There are, at this writing, no well-controlled published studies evaluating the analgesic effects of amantadine in veterinary patients, and dosing recommendations are based largely on anecdotal reports. As the management of chronic pain in companion animals continues to receive much attention in veterinary medicine, the use of amantadine and other drugs with a similar mechanism of action is likely to become more prevalent.

Tramadol

Tramadol is a synthetic codeine analog that is a weak μ-receptor agonist.[10] In addition to its opioid activity, tramadol also inhibits neuronal reuptake of norepinephrine and 5-hydroxytryptamine (serotonin), and may actually facilitate 5-hydroxytryptamine release.[22] It is thought that these effects on central catecholaminergic pathways contribute significantly to the drug's analgesic efficacy.[265] Tramadol is recommended for the management of acute and chronic pain of moderate to moderately severe intensity associated with a variety of conditions, including osteoarthritis, fibromyalgia, diabetic neuropathy, neuropathic pain, and even perioperative pain in human patients.[266–268]

A study published in 2003 compared the effects of intravenous tramadol and morphine administered prior to ovariohysterectomy in dogs.[269] In this particular study, tramadol was comparable to morphine in its analgesic efficacy for this type of surgical pain. Clearly, additional studies are necessary before definitive therapeutic recommendations can be made for the management of perioperative pain in a variety of species. There are also anecdotal reports of singular oral tramadol administration for the management of chronic pain in dogs and cats when NSAID usage is contraindicated because of advanced renal disease. Because of its inhibitory effect on 5-hydroxytryptamine uptake, tramadol should not be used in patients that may have received monoamineoxidase inhibitors (MAOIs) such as selegiline (see also the section on meperidine) or in those patients with a recent history of seizure activity.

References

1. Harrison LM, Kastin AJ, Zadina JE. Opiate tolerance and dependence: Receptors, G-proteins, and antiopiates—Further evidence for heterogeneity. Peptides 1998;19:1603–1630.
2. Kieffer BL. Opioids: First lessons from knockout mice. Trends Pharmacol Sci 1999;20:19–26.
3. Janecka A, Fichna J, Janecki T. Opioid receptors and their ligands. Curr Top Med Chem 2004;4:1–17.
4. Inturrisi CE. Clinical pharmacology of opioids for pain. Clin J Pain 2002;18(Suppl):S3–S13.
5. Moran TD, Abdulla FA, Smith PA. Cellular neurophysiological actions of nociceptin/orphanin FQ. Peptides 2000;21:969–976.
6. Smith PA, Moran TD. The nociceptin receptor as a potential target in drug design. Drug News Perspect 2001;14:335–345.
7. Smith AP, Lee NM. Opioid receptor interactions: Local and nonlocal, symmetric and asymmetric, physical and functional. Life Sci 2003;73:1873–1893.
8. Zadina JE, Martin-Schild S, Gerall AA, et al. Endomorphins: Novel endogenous mu-opiate receptor agonists in regions of high mu-opiate receptor density. Ann NY Acad Sci 1999;897:136–144.
9. Christie MJ, Connor M, Vaughan CW, Ingram SL, Bagley EE. Cellular actions of opioids and other analgesics: Implications for synergism in pain relief. Clin Exp Pharmacol Physiol 2000;27:520–523.
10. Gutstein HB, Akil H. Opioid analgesics. In: Harman JG, Limbird LE, Goodman Gilman A, eds. Goodman and Gilman's The Pharmacological Basis of Therapeutics, 10th ed. New York: McGraw-Hill, 2001:569–619.
11. Yaksh TL. Pharmacology and mechanisms of opioid analgesic activity. In: Yaksh TL, Lynch C III, Zapol WM, Maze M, Biebuyck JF, Saidman LJ, eds. Anesthesia: Biologic Foundations. Philadelphia: Lippincott-Raven, 1998:921–934.
12. Stein C, Machelska H, Schafer M. Peripheral analgesic and antiinflammatory effects of opioids. Z Rheumatol 2001;60:416–424.
13. Fields HL, Emson PC, Leigh BK, Gilbert RF, Iversen LL. Multiple opiate receptor sites on primary afferent fibres. Nature 1980;284:351–353.
14. Stein C, Schafer M, Machelska H. Attacking pain at its source: New perspectives on opioids. Nat Med 2003;9:1003–1008.
15. Stein C, Hassan AH, Lehrberger K, Giefing J, Yassouridis A. Local analgesic effect of endogenous opioid peptides. Lancet 1993;342:321–324.
16. Stein C. Peripheral mechanisms of opioid analgesia. Anesth Analg 1993;76:182–191.
17. Stein C, Yassouridis A. Peripheral morphine analgesia. Pain 1997;71:119–121.
18. Stein C. The control of pain in peripheral tissue by opioids. N Engl J Med 1995;332:1685–1690.
19. Stein C, Pfluger M, Yassouridis A, et al. No tolerance to peripheral morphine analgesia in presence of opioid expression in inflamed synovia. J Clin Invest 1996;98:793–799.
20. Branson KR, Gross ME, Booth NH. Opioid agonists and antagonists. In: Adams HR, ed. Veterinary Pharmacology and Therapeutics. Ames: Iowa State Press, 2001:274–310.
21. Hellyer PW, Bai L, Supon J, et al. Comparison of opioid and alpha-2 adrenergic receptor binding in horse and dog brain using radioligand autoradiography. Vet Anaesth Analg 2003;30:172–182.
22. Stoelting RK. Opioid agonists and antagonists. In: Stoelting RK, ed. Pharmacology and Physiology in Anesthetic Practice. Philadelphia: Lippincott Williams & Wilkins, 1999:77–112.
23. Stephan DD, Vestre WA, Stiles J, Krohne S. Changes in intraocular pressure and pupil size following intramuscular administration of hydromorphone hydrochloride and acepromazine in clinically normal dogs. Vet Ophthalmol 2003;6:73–76.
24. Lee HK, Wang SC. Mechanism of morphine-induced miosis in the dog. J Pharmacol Exp Ther 1975;192:415–431.
25. Wallenstein MC, Wang SC. Mechanism of morphine-induced mydriasis in the cat. Am J Physiol 1979;236:R292–R296.
26. Smith LJ, Yu JKA, Bjorling DE, Waller K. Effects of hydromorphone or oxymorphone, with or without acepromazine, on preanesthetic sedation, physiologic values, and histamine release in dogs. J Am Vet Med Assoc 2001;218:1101–1105.
27. Radnay PA, Duncalf D, Novakovic M, Lesser ML. Common bile duct pressure changes after fentanyl, morphine, meperidine, butorphanol, and naloxone. Anesth Analg 1984;63:441–444.
28. Jones RM, Detmer M, Hill AB, Bjoraker DG, Pandit U. Incidence of choledochoduodenal sphincter spasm during fentanyl-supplemented anesthesia. Anesth Analg 1981;60:638–640.
29. Thompson DR. Narcotic analgesic effects on the sphincter of Oddi: A review of the data and therapeutic implications in treating pancreatitis. Am J Gastroenterol 2001;96:1266–1272.

30. Kuipers PW, Kamphuis ET, van Venrooij GE, et al. Intrathecal opioids and lower urinary tract function: A urodynamic evaluation. Anesthesiology 2004;100:1497–1503.

31. El Bindary EM, Abu el-Nasr LM. Urodynamic changes following intrathecal administration of morphine and fentanyl to dogs. East Mediterr Health J 2001;7:189–196.

32. Mercadante S, Arcuri E. Opioids and renal function. J Pain 2004; 5:2–19.

33. Barnhart MD, Hubbell JAE, Muir WW, Sams RA, Bednarski RM. Pharmacokinetics, pharmacodynamics, and analgesic effects of morphine after rectal, intramuscular, and intravenous administration in dogs. Am J Vet Res 2000;61:24–28.

34. Taylor PM, Robertson SA, Dixon MJ, et al. Morphine, pethidine and buprenorphine disposition in the cat. J Vet Pharmacol Ther 2001;24:391–398.

35. Faura CC, Collins SL, Moore RA, McQuay HJ. Systematic review of factors affecting the ratios of morphine and its major metabolites. Pain 1998;74:43–53.

36. Smith MT. Neuroexcitatory effects of morphine and hydromorphone: Evidence implicating the 3-glucuronide metabolites. Clin Exp Pharmacol Physiol 2000;27:524–528.

37. Ilkiw JE, Pascoe PJ, Tripp LD. Effects of morphine, butorphanol, buprenorphine, and U50488H on the minimum alveolar concentration of isoflurane in cats. Am J Vet Res 2002;63: 1198–1202.

38. Muir WW, Wiese AJ, March PA. Effects of morphine, lidocaine, ketamine, and morphine-lidocaine-ketamine drug combination on minimum alveolar concentration in dogs anesthetized with isoflurane. Am J Vet Res 2003;64:1155–1160.

39. Lucas AN, Firth AM, Anderson GA, Vine JH, Edwards GA. Comparison of the effects of morphine administered by constant-rate intravenous infusion or intermittent intramuscular injection in dogs. J Am Vet Med Assoc 2001;218:884–891.

40. Mikkelsen Lynch P, Butler J, Huerta D, Tsals I, Davidson D, Hamm S. A pharmacokinetic and tolerability evaluation of two continuous subcutaneous infusion systems compared to an oral controlled-release morphine. J Pain Symptom Manage 2000;19:348–356.

41. Devulder JE. Subcutaneous morphine is superior to intrathecal morphine for pain control in a patient with hypernephroma. J Clin Anesth 1998;10:163–165.

42. Fudin J, Smith HS, Toledo-Binette CS, Kenney E, Yu AB, Boutin R. Use of continuous ambulatory infusions of concentrated subcutaneous (s.q.) hydromorphone versus intravenous (i.v.) morphine: Cost implications for palliative care. Am J Hosp Palliat Care 2000;17:347–353.

43. Nelson KA, Glare PA, Walsh D, Groh ES. A prospective, within-patient, crossover study of continuous intravenous and subcutaneous morphine for chronic cancer pain. J Pain Symptom Manage 1997;13:262–267.

44. Troncy E. Results of preemptive epidural administration of morphine with or without bupivacaine in dogs and cats undergoing surgery: 265 cases (1997–1999). J Am Vet Med Assoc 2002;221: 666–672. Erratum in J Am Vet Med Assoc 2002;221:1149.

45. Pacharinsak C, Greene SA, Keegan RD, Kalivas PW. Postoperative analgesia in dogs receiving epidural morphine plus medetomidine. J Vet Pharmacol Ther 2003;26:71–77.

46. Day TK, Pepper WT, Tobias TA, Flynn MF, Clarke KM. Comparison of intra-articular and epidural morphine for analgesia following stifle arthrotomy in dogs. Vet Surg 1995;24:522–530.

47. Sammarco JL, Conzemius MG, Perkowski SZ, Weinstein MJ, Gregor TP, Smith GK. Postoperative analgesia for stifle surgery: A comparison of intra-articular bupivacaine, morphine, or saline. Vet Surg 1996;25:59–69.

48. Stiles J, Honda CN, Krohne SG, Kazacos EA. Effect of topical administration of 1% morphine sulfate solution on signs of pain and corneal wound healing in dogs. Am J Vet Res 2003;64:813–818.

49. Bennett RC, Steffey EP. Use of opioids for pain and anesthetic management in horses. Vet Clin North Am Equine Pract 2002; 18:47–60.

50. Steffey EP, Eisele JH, Baggot JD. Interactions of morphine and isoflurane in horses. Am J Vet Res 2003;64:166–175.

51. Mircica E, Clutton RE, Kyles KW, Blissitt KJ. Problems associated with perioperative morphine in horses: A retrospective case analysis. Vet Anaesth Analg 2003;30:147–155.

52. Natalini CC, Robinson EP. Evaluation of the analgesic effects of epidurally administered morphine, alfentanil, butorphanol, tramadol, and U50488H in horses. Am J Vet Res 2000;61:1579–1586.

53. Goodrich LR, Nixon AJ, Fubini SL, et al. Epidural morphine and detomidine decreases postoperative hindlimb lameness in horses after bilateral stifle arthroscopy. Vet Surg 2002;31:232–239.

54. Vesal N, Cribb PH, Frketic M. Postoperative analgesic and cardiopulmonary effects in dogs of oxymorphone administered epidurally and intramuscularly, and medetomidine administered epidurally: A comparative clinical study. Vet Surg 1996;25:361–369.

55. Chaplan SR, Duncan SR, Brodsky JB, Brose WG. Morphine and hydromorphone epidural analgesia: A prospective, randomized comparison. Anesthesiology 1992;77:1090–1094.

56. Sinatra RS, Eige S, Chung JH, et al. Continuous epidural infusion of 0.05% bupivacaine plus hydromorphone for labor analgesia: An observational assessment in 1830 parturients. Anesth Analg 2002; 94:1310–1311, table.

57. Wagner LE, Eaton M, Sabnis SS, Gingrich KJ. Meperidine and lidocaine block of recombinant voltage-dependent Na+ channels: Evidence that meperidine is a local anesthetic. Anesthesiology 1999;91:1481–1490.

58. Wolff M, Olschewski A, Vogel W, Hempelmann G. Meperidine suppresses the excitability of spinal dorsal horn neurons. Anesthesiology 2004;100:947–955.

59. Takada K, Tonner PH, Maze M. Meperidine functions as an alpha(2B) adrenoceptor agonist. Anesthesiology 1999;91:A363.

60. Takada K, Clark DJ, Davies MF, et al. Meperidine exerts agonist activity at the alpha(2B)-adrenoceptor subtype. Anesthesiology 2002;96:1420–1426.

61. Yeh SY, Krebs HA, Changchit A. Urinary excretion of meperidine and its metabolites. J Pharm Sci 1981;70:867–870.

62. Stone PA, Macintyre PE, Jarvis DA. Norpethidine toxicity and patient controlled analgesia. Br J Anaesth 1993;71:738–740.

63. Priano LL, Vatner SF. Generalized cardiovascular and regional hemodynamic effects of meperidine in conscious dogs. Anesth Analg 1981;60:649–654.

64. Sporer KA. The serotonin syndrome: Implicated drugs, pathophysiology and management. Drug Saf 1995;13:94–104.

65. Bowdle TA. Adverse effects of opioid agonists and agonist-antagonists in anaesthesia. Drug Saf 1998;19:173–189.

66. Heinonen EH, Myllyla V. Safety of selegiline (Deprenyl) in the treatment of Parkinson's disease. Drug Saf 1998;19:11–22.

67. Tissot TA. Probable meperidine-induced serotonin syndrome in a patient with a history of fluoxetine use. Anesthesiology 2003;98: 1511–1512.

68. Dodam JR, Cohn LA, Durham HE, Szladovits B. Cardiopulmonary effects of medetomidine, oxymorphone, or butorphanol in selegiline-treated dogs. Vet Anaesth Analg 2004;31:129–137.

69. Skarda RT, Muir WW III. Analgesic, hemodynamic, and respiratory effects induced by caudal epidural administration of meperidine hydrochloride in mares. Am J Vet Res 2001;62:1001–1007.

70. Carroll GL, Hooper RN, Boothe DM, Hartsfield SM, Randoll LA. Pharmacokinetics of fentanyl after intravenous and transdermal administration in goats. Am J Vet Res 1999;60:986–991.

71. Lee DD, Papich MG, Hardie EM. Comparison of pharmacokinetics of fentanyl after intravenous and transdermal administration in cats. Am J Vet Res 2000;61:672–677.

72. Maxwell LK, Thomasy SM, Slovis N, Kollias-Baker C. Pharmacokinetics of fentanyl following intravenous and transdermal administration in horses. Equine Vet J 2003;35:484–490.

73. Fahnenstich H, Steffan J, Kau N, Bartmann P. Fentanyl-induced chest wall rigidity and laryngospasm in preterm and term infants. Crit Care Med 2000;28:836–839.

74. Muller P, Vogtmann C. Three cases with different presentation of fentanyl-induced muscle rigidity: A rare problem in intensive care of neonates. Am J Perinatol 2000;17:23–26.

75. Hellyer PW, Mama KR, Shafford HL, Wagner AE, Kollias-Baker C. Effects of diazepam and flumazenil on minimum alveolar concentrations for dogs anesthetized with isoflurane or a combination of isoflurane and fentanyl. Am J Vet Res 2001;62:555–560.

76. Martin MF, Lima JR, Ezquerra LJ, Carrasco MS, Uson-Gargallo J. Prolonged anesthesia with desflurane and fentanyl in dogs during conventional and laparoscopic surgery. J Am Vet Med Assoc 2001;219:941–945.

77. Mendes GM, Selmi AL. Use of a combination of propofol and fentanyl, alfentanil, or sufentanil for total intravenous anesthesia in cats. J Am Vet Med Assoc 2003;223:1608–1613.

78. Wilson DV, Kantrowitz A, Pacholewicz J, et al. Perioperative management of calves undergoing implantation of a left ventricular assist device. Vet Surg 2000;29:106–118.

79. Kurita T, Morita K, Kazama T, Sato S. Comparison of isoflurane and propofol-fentanyl anaesthesia in a swine model of asphyxia. Br J Anaesth 2003;91:871–877.

80. Gilberto DB, Motzel SL, Das SR. Postoperative pain management using fentanyl patches in dogs. Contemp Top Lab Anim Sci 2003;42:21–26.

81. Franks JN, Boothe HW, Taylor L, et al. Evaluation of transdermal fentanyl patches for analgesia in cats undergoing onychectomy. J Am Vet Med Assoc 2000;217:1013–1020.

82. Wilkinson AC, Thomas ML, Morse BC. Evaluation of a transdermal fentanyl system in yucatan [sic] miniature pigs. Contemp Topi Lab Anim Sci 2001;40:12–16.

83. Egger CM, Duke T, Archer J, Cribb PH. Comparison of plasma fentanyl concentrations by using three transdermal fentanyl patch sizes in dogs. Vet Surg 1998;27:159–166.

84. Egger CM, Glerum LE, Allen SW, Haag M. Plasma fentanyl concentrations in awake cats and cats undergoing anesthesia and ovariohysterectomy using transdermal administration. Vet Anaesth Analg 2003;30:229–236.

85. Gellasch KL, Kruse-Elliott KT, Osmond CS, Shih AN, Bjorling DE. Comparison of transdermal administration of fentanyl versus intramuscular administration of butorphanol for analgesia after onychectomy in cats. J Am Vet Med Assoc 2002;220:1020–1024.

86. Robinson TM, Kruse-Elliott KT, Markel MD, Pluhar GE, Massa K, Bjorling DE. A comparison of transdermal fentanyl versus epidural morphine for analgesia in dogs undergoing major orthopedic surgery. J Am Anim Hosp Assoc 1999;35:95–100.

87. Pettifer GR, Hosgood G. The effect of rectal temperature on perianesthetic serum concentrations of transdermally administered fen-

tanyl in cats anesthetized with isoflurane. Am J Vet Res 2003;64:1557–1561.

88. Krotscheck U, Boothe DM, Boothe HW. Evaluation of transdermal morphine and fentanyl pluronic lecithin organogel administration in dogs. Vet Ther 2004;5:202–211.

89. Robertson SA, Taylor PM, Sear JW, Keuhnel G. Relationship between plasma concentrations and analgesia after intravenous fentanyl and disposition after other routes of administration in cats. J Vet Pharmacol Ther 2005;28:87–93.

90. Chism JP, Rickert DE. The pharmacokinetics and extra-hepatic clearance of remifentanil, a short acting opioid agonist, in male beagle dogs during constant rate infusions. Drug Metab Dispos 1996;24:34–40.

91. Hoke JF, Cunningham F, James MK, Muir KT, Hoffman WE. Comparative pharmacokinetics and pharmacodynamics of remifentanil, its principle metabolite (GR90291) and alfentanil in dogs. J Pharmacol Exp Ther 1997;281:226–232.

92. Michelsen LG, Salmenpera M, Hug CC Jr, Szlam F, VanderMeer D. Anesthetic potency of remifentanil in dogs. Anesthesiology 1996;84:865–872.

93. Ilkiw JE, Pascoe PJ, Fisher LD. Effect of alfentanil on the minimum alveolar concentration of isoflurane in cats. Am J Vet Res 1997;58:1274–1279.

94. Pascoe PJ, Ilkiw JE, Fisher LD. Cardiovascular effects of equipotent isoflurane and alfentanil/isoflurane minimum alveolar concentration multiple in cats. Am J Vet Res 1997;58:1267–1273.

95. Pascoe PJ, Taylor PM. Effects of dopamine antagonists on alfentanil-induced locomotor activity in horses. Vet Anaesth Analg 2003;30:165–171.

96. Pascoe PJ, Steffey EP, Black WD, Claxton JM, Jacobs JR, Woliner MJ. Evaluation of the effect of alfentanil on the minimum alveolar concentration of halothane in horses. Am J Vet Res 1993;54:1327–1332.

97. Pascoe PJ, Black WD, Claxton JM, Sansom RE. The pharmacokinetics and locomotor activity of alfentanil in the horse. J Vet Pharmacol Ther 1991;14:317–325.

98. Gorman AL, Elliott KJ, Inturrisi CE. The d- and l-isomers of methadone bind to the non-competitive site on the N-methyl-D-aspartate (NMDA) receptor in rat forebrain and spinal cord. Neurosci Lett 1997;223:5–8.

99. Ripamonti C, Dickerson ED. Strategies for the treatment of cancer pain in the new millennium. Drugs 2001;61:955–977.

100. Kramer S, Nolte I, Jochle W. Clinical comparison of medetomidine with xylazine/l-methadone in dogs. Vet Rec 1996;138:128–133.

101. Dobromylskyj P. Cardiovascular changes associated with anaesthesia induced by medetomidine combined with ketamine in cats. J Small Anim Pract 1996;37:169–172.

102. Fisher RJ. A field trial of ketamine anaesthesia in the horse. Equine Vet J 1984;16:176–179.

103. Mortenson J, Bechert U. Carfentanil citrate used as an oral anesthetic agent for brown bears (Ursus arctos). J Zoo Wildl Med 2001;32:217–221.

104. Pollock CG, Ramsay EC. Serial immobilization of a Brazilian tapir (Tapirus terrestrus) with oral detomidine and oral carfentanil. J Zoo Wildl Med 2003;34:408–410.

105. Kearns KS, Swenson B, Ramsay EC. Oral induction of anesthesia with droperidol and transmucosal carfentanil citrate in chimpanzees (Pan troglodytes). J Zoo Wildl Med 2000;31:185–189.

106. Mama KR, Steffey EP, Withrow SJ. Use of orally administered carfentanil prior to isoflurane-induced anesthesia in a Kodiak brown bear. J Am Vet Med Assoc 2000;217:546–549.

107. Caulkett NA, Cribb PH, Haigh JC. Comparative cardiopulmonary effects of carfentanil-xylazine and medetomidine-ketamine used for immobilization of mule deer and mule deer/white-tailed deer hybrids. Can J Vet Res 2000;64:64–68.

108. Miller BF, Muller LI, Storms TN, et al. A comparison of carfentanil/xylazine and Telazol/xylazine for immobilization of white-tailed deer. J Wildl Dis 2003;39:851–858.

109. Ramdohr S, Bornemann H, Plotz J, Bester MN. Immobilization of free-ranging adult male southern elephant seals with Immobilon™ (etorphine/acepromacine) and ketamine. S Afr J Wildl Res 2001;31:135–140.

110. Roffe TJ, Coffin K, Berger J. Survival and immobilizing moose with carfentanil and xylazine. Wildl Soc Bull 2001;29:1140–1146.

111. Sawyer DC, Rech RH, Durham RA, Adams T, Richter MA, Striler EL. Dose response to butorphanol administered subcutaneously to increase visceral nociceptive threshold in dogs. Am J Vet Res 1991;52:1826–1830.

112. Robertson SA, Taylor PM, Lascelles BDX, Dixon MJ. Changes in thermal threshold response in eight cats after administration of buprenorphine, butorphanol and morphine. Vet Rec 2003;153:462–465.

113. Sellon DC, Monroe VL, Roberts MC, Papich MG. Pharmacokinetics and adverse effects of butorphanol administered by single intravenous injection or continuous intravenous infusion in horses. Am J Vet Res 2001;62:183–189.

114. Quandt JE, Raffe MR, Robinson EP. Butorphanol does not reduce the minimum alveolar concentration of halothane in dogs. Vet Surg 1994;23:156–159.

115. Doherty TJ, Geiser DR, Rohrbach BW. Effect of acepromazine and butorphanol on halothane minimum alveolar concentration in ponies. Equine Vet J 1997;29:374–376.

116. Matthews NS, Lindsay SL. Effect of low-dose butorphanol on halothane minimum alveolar concentration in ponies. Equine Vet J 1990;22:325–327.

117. Ko JCH, Lange DN, Mandsager RE, et al. Effects of butorphanol and carprofen on the minimal alveolar concentration of isoflurane in dogs. J Am Vet Med Assoc 2000;217:1025–1028.

118. Grimm KA, Tranquilli WJ, Thurmon JC, Benson GJ. Duration of nonresponse to noxious stimulation after intramuscular administration of butorphanol, medetomidine, or a butorphanol-medetomidine combination during isoflurane administration in dogs. Am J Vet Res 2000;61:42–47.

119. Ansah OB, Vainio O, Hellsten C, Raekallio M. Postoperative pain control in cats: Clinical trials with medetomidine and butorphanol. Vet Surg 2002;31:99–103.

120. Carroll GL, Howe LB, Slater MR, et al. Evaluation of analgesia provided by postoperative administration of butorphanol to cats undergoing onychectomy. J Am Vet Med Assoc 1998;213:246–250.

121. Borer LR, Peel JE, Seewald W, Schawalder P, Spreng DE. Effect of carprofen, etodolac, meloxicam, or butorphanol in dogs with induced acute synovitis. Am J Vet Res 2003;64:1429–1437.

122. Mathews KA, Pettifer G, Foster R, McDonell W. Safety and efficacy of preoperative administration of meloxicam, compared with that of ketoprofen and butorphanol in dogs undergoing abdominal surgery. Am J Vet Res 2001;62:882–888.

123. Mathews KA, Paley DM, Foster RA, Valliant AE, Young SS. A comparison of ketorolac with flunixin, butorphanol, and oxymorphone in controlling postoperative pain in dogs. Can Vet J 1996;37:557–567.

124. Kalpravidh M, Lumb WV, Wright M, Heath RB. Effects of butorphanol, flunixin, levorphanol, morphine, and xylazine in ponies. Am J Vet Res 1984;45:217–223.

125. Muir WW, Robertson JT. Visceral analgesia: Effects of xylazine, butorphanol, meperidine, and pentazocine in horses. Am J Vet Res 1985;46:2081–2084.

126. Doherty TJ, Geiser DR, Rohrbach BW. Effect of high volume epidural morphine, ketamine and butorphanol on halothane minimum alveolar concentration in ponies. Equine Vet J 1997;29:370–373.

127. Briggs SL, Sneed K, Sawyer DC. Antinociceptive effects of oxymorphone-butorphanol-acepromazine combination in cats. Vet Surg 1998;27:466–472.

128. Lascelles BD, Robertson SA. Antinociceptive effects of hydromorphone, butorphanol, or the combination in cats. J Vet Intern Med 2004;18:190–195.

129. Robertson SA, Taylor PM, Sear JW. Systemic uptake of buprenorphine by cats after oral mucosal administration. Vet Rec 2003;152:675–678.

130. Stanway GW, Taylor PM, Brodbelt DC. A preliminary investigation comparing pre-operative morphine and buprenorphine for postoperative analgesia and sedation in cats. Vet Anaesth Analg 2002;29:29–35.

131. Dobbins S, Brown NO, Shofer FS. Comparison of the effects of buprenorphine, oxymorphone hydrochloride, and ketoprofen for postoperative analgesia after onychectomy or onychectomy and sterilization in cats. J Am Anim Hosp Assoc 2002;38:507–514.

132. Brodbelt DC, Taylor PM, Stanway GW. A comparison of preoperative morphine and buprenorphine for postoperative analgesia for arthrotomy in dogs. J Vet Pharmacol Ther 1997;20:284–289.

133. Kramer S, Nolte I, Albrecht J, et al. Pain relief in dogs and cats: Clinical experience with buprenorphine (Temgesic®). Berl Munch Tierarztl Wochenschr 1998;111:285–290.

134. van Dijk P, Lankveld DPK, Rijkenhuizen ABM, Jonker FH. Hormonal, metabolic and physiological effects of laparoscopic surgery using a detomidine-buprenorphine combination in standing horses. Vet Anaesth Analg 2003;30:72–80.

135. Boeuf B, Gauvin F, Guerguerian AM, Farrell CA, Lacroix J, Jenicek M. Therapy of shock with naloxone: A meta-analysis. Crit Care Med 1998;26:1910–1916.

136. Boeuf B, Poirier V, Gauvin F, et al. Naloxone for shock. Cochrane Database Syst Rev 2003, Issue 3 Art. no.: CD004443. DOI: 10.1002/14651858.CD004443.

137. Murray MJ, Offord KP, Yaksh TL. Physiologic and plasma hormone correlates of survival in endotoxic dogs: Effects of opiate antagonists. Crit Care Med 1989;17:39–47.

138. Veng-Pedersen P, Wilhelm JA, Zakszewski TB, Osifchin F, Waters SJ. Duration of opioid antagonism by nalmefene and naloxone in the dog: An integrated pharmacokinetic/pharmacodynamic comparison. J Pharm Sci 1995;84:1101–1106.

139. Vane JR, Botting RM. The mechanism of action of aspirin. Thromb Res 2003;110:255–258.

140. Vane JR. Inhibition of prostaglandin synthesis as a mechanism of action for aspirin-like drugs. Nat New Biol 1971;231:232–235.

141. Botting RM. Mechanism of action of acetaminophen: Is there a cyclooxygenase 3? Clin Infect Dis 2000;31(Suppl 5):S202–S210.

142. Chandrasekharan NV, Dai H, Roos KL, et al. COX-3, a cyclooxygenase-1 variant inhibited by acetaminophen and other analgesic/antipyretic drugs: Cloning, structure, and expression. Proc Natl Acad Sci USA 2002;99:13926–13931.

143. Botting R. COX-1 and COX-3 inhibitors. Thromb Res 2003;110:269–272.

144. Livingston A. Mechanism of action of nonsteroidal anti-inflammatory drugs. Vet Clin North Am Small Anim Pract 2000;30:773–781.

145. Vane JR, Botting RM. New insights into the mode of action of anti-inflammatory drugs. Inflamm Res 1995;44:1–10.

146. Kay-Mugford P, Benn SJ, LaMarre J, Conlon P. In vitro effects of nonsteroidal anti-inflammatory drugs on cyclooxygenase activity in dogs. Am J Vet Res 2000;61:802–810.

147. Bertolini A, Ottani A, Sandrini M. Dual acting anti-inflammatory drugs: A reappraisal. Pharmacol Res 2001;44:437–450.

148. Hudson N, Balsitis M, Everitt S, Hawkey CJ. Enhanced gastric mucosal leukotriene B4 synthesis in patients taking non-steroidal anti-inflammatory drugs. Gut 1993;34:742–747.

149. Rainsford KD. Mechanisms of NSAID-induced ulcerogenesis: Structural properties of drugs, focus on the microvascular factors, and novel approaches for gastro-intestinal protection. Acta Physiol Hung 1992;80:23–38.

150. Serhan CN, Chiang N. Novel endogenous small molecules as the checkpoint controllers in inflammation and resolution: Entree for resoleomics. Rheum Dis Clin North Am 2004;30:69–95.

151. Kirchner T, Argentieri DC, Barbone AG, et al. Evaluation of the antiinflammatory activity of a dual cyclooxygenase-2 selective/5-lipoxygenase inhibitor, RWJ 63556, in a canine model of inflammation. J Pharmacol Exp Ther 1997;282:1094–1101.

152. Argentieri DC, Ritchie DM, Ferro MP, et al. Tepoxalin: A dual cyclooxygenase/5-lipoxygenase inhibitor of arachidonic acid metabolism with potent anti-inflammatory activity and a favorable gastrointestinal profile. J Pharmacol Exp Ther 1994;271:1399–1408.

153. Kirchner T, Aparicio B, Argentieri DC, Lau CY, Ritchie DM. Effects of tepoxalin, a dual inhibitor of cyclooxygenase/5-lipoxygenase, on events associated with NSAID-induced gastrointestinal inflammation. Prostaglandins Leukotrienes Essent Fatty Acids 1997;56:417–423.

154. Chopra B, Giblett S, Little JG, et al. Cyclooxygenase-1 is a marker for a subpopulation of putative nociceptive neurons in rat dorsal root ganglia. Eur J Neurosci 2000;12:911–920.

155. Malmberg AB, Yaksh TL. Antinociceptive actions of spinal nonsteroidal anti-inflammatory agents on the formalin test in the rat. J Pharmacol Exp Ther 1992;263:136–146.

156. McCormack K. Non-steroidal anti-inflammatory drugs and spinal nociceptive processing. Pain 1994;59:9–43.

157. McCormack K. The spinal actions of nonsteroidal anti-inflammatory drugs and the dissociation between their anti-inflammatory and analgesic effects. Drugs 1994;47(Suppl 5):28–45.

158. Yaksh TL, Dirig DM, Malmberg AB. Mechanism of action of nonsteroidal anti-inflammatory drugs. Cancer Invest 1998;16:509–527.

159. Ochi T, Motoyama Y, Goto T. The analgesic effect profile of FR122047, a selective cyclooxygenase-1 inhibitor, in chemical nociceptive models. Eur J Pharmacol 2000;391:49–54.

160. Ballou LR, Botting RM, Goorha S, Zhang J, Vane JR. Nociception in cyclooxygenase isozyme-deficient mice. Proc Natl Acad Sci USA 2000;97:10272–10276.

161. DuBois RN, Abramson SB, Crofford L, et al. Cyclooxygenase in biology and disease. FASEB J 1998;12:1063–1073.

162. Schmassmann A, Peskar BM, Stettler C, et al. Effects of inhibition of prostaglandin endoperoxide synthase-2 in chronic gastrointestinal ulcer models in rats. Br J Pharmacol 1998;123:795–804.

163. Reuter BK, Asfaha S, Buret A, Sharkey KA, Wallace JL. Exacerbation of inflammation-associated colonic injury in rat through inhibition of cyclooxygenase-2. J Clin Invest 1996;98:2076–2085.

164. Imig JD. Eicosanoid regulation of the renal vasculature. Am J Physiol Renal Physiol 2000;279:F965–F981.

165. Harris RC. Cyclooxygenase-2 in the kidney. J Am Soc Nephrol 2000;11:2387–2394.

166. Horster M, Kemler BJ, Valtin H. Intracortical distribution of number and volume of glomeruli during postnatal maturation in the dog. J Clin Invest 1971;50:796–800.

167. Morham SG, Langenbach R, Loftin CD, et al. Prostaglandin synthase 2 gene disruption causes severe renal pathology in the mouse. Cell 1995;83:473–482.

168. Lipsky PE, Brooks P, Crofford LJ, et al. Unresolved issues in the role of cyclooxygenase-2 in normal physiologic processes and disease. Arch Intern Med 2000;160:913–920.

169. Gierse JK, Staten NR, Casperson GF, et al. Cloning, expression, and selective inhibition of canine cyclooxygenase-1 and cyclooxygenase-2. Vet Ther 2002;3:270–280.

170. Fosslien E. Molecular pathology of cyclooxygenase-2 in neoplasia. Ann Clin Lab Sci 2000;30:3–21.

171. Lipsky PE. Specific COX-2 inhibitors in arthritis, oncology, and beyond: Where is the science headed? J Rheumatol 1999;26(Suppl 56):25–30.

172. Smalley WE, DuBois RN. Colorectal cancer and nonsteroidal anti-inflammatory drugs. Adv Pharmacol 1997;39:1–20.

173. FitzGerald GA, Patrono C. The coxibs, selective inhibitors of cyclooxygenase-2. N Engl J Med 2001;345:433–442.

174. Warner TD, Giuliano F, Vojnovic I, Bukasa A, Mitchell JA, Vane JR. Nonsteroid drug selectivities for cyclo-oxygenase-1 rather than cyclo-oxygenase-2 are associated with human gastrointestinal toxicity: A full in vitro analysis. Proc Natl Acad Sci USA 1999;96:7563–7568.

175. Glew A, Aviad AD, Keister DM, Meo NJ. Use of ketoprofen as an antipyretic in cats. Can Vet J 1996;37:222–225.

176. Justus C, Quirke JF. Dose-response relationship for the antipyretic effect of meloxicam in an endotoxin model in cats. Vet Res Commun 1995;19:321–330.

177. Wallace JL, Fiorucci S. A magic bullet for mucosal protection ... and aspirin is the trigger! Trends Pharmacol Sci 2003;24:323–326.

178. Serhan CN, Hong S, Gronert K, et al. Resolvins: A family of bioactive products of omega-3 fatty acid transformation circuits initiated by aspirin treatment that counter proinflammation signals. J Exp Med 2002;196:1025–1037.

179. Petersson I, Nilsson G, Hansson BG, Hedner T. Water intoxication associated with non-steroidal anti-inflammatory drug therapy. Acta Med Scand 1987;221:221–223.

180. Dunn AM, Buckley BM. Non-steroidal anti-inflammatory drugs and the kidney. Br Med J 1986;293:202–203.

181. Boston SE, Moens NM, Kruth SA, Southorn EP. Endoscopic evaluation of the gastroduodenal mucosa to determine the safety of short-term concurrent administration of meloxicam and dexamethasone in healthy dogs. Am J Vet Res 2003;64:1369–1375.

182. Lobetti RG, Joubert KE. Effect of administration of nonsteroidal anti-inflammatory drugs before surgery on renal function in clinically normal dogs. Am J Vet Res 2000;61:1501–1507.

183. Lemke KA, Runyon CL, Horney BS. Effects of preoperative administration of ketoprofen on whole blood platelet aggregation, buccal mucosal bleeding time, and hematologic indices in dogs undergoing elective ovariohysterectomy. J Am Vet Med Assoc 2002;220:1818–1822.

184. Mathews KA, Pettifer G, Foster RF. A comparison of the safety and efficacy of meloxicam to ketoprofen and butorphanol for control of post-operative pain associated with soft tissue surgery in dogs. In: Proceedings of the Symposium on Recent Advances in Nonsteroidal Anti-inflammatory Therapy in Small Animals, Paris, 1999:67.

185. Mathews KA, Doherty T, Dyson D. Nephrotoxicity in dogs associated with methoxyflurane anesthesia and flunixin meglumine analgesia. Can Vet J 1990;31:766–771.

186. Crandell DE, Mathews KA, Dyson D. The effect of meloxicam and carprofen on renal function when administered to healthy dogs prior to anesthesia and painful stimulation. Am J Vet Res 2004;65:1384–1390.

187. Cayen MN, Kraml M, Ferdinandi ES, Greselin E, Dvornik D. The metabolic disposition of etodolac in rats, dogs, and man. Drug Metab Rev 1981;12:339–362.

188. Pasloske K, Burger J, Conlon P. Plasma prostaglandin E2 concentrations after single dose administration of ketorolac tromethamine (Toradol) in dogs. Can J Vet Res 1998;62:237–240.

189. Schleimer RP, Benjamini E. Effects of prostaglandin synthesis inhibition on the immune response. Immunopharmacology 1981;3:205–219.

190. Pibarot P, Dupuis J, Grisneaux E, et al. Comparison of ketoprofen, oxymorphone hydrochloride, and butorphanol in the treatment of postoperative pain in dogs. J Am Vet Med Assoc 1997;211:438–444.

191. Grisneaux E, Pibarot P, Dupuis J, Blais D. Comparison of ketoprofen and carprofen administered prior to orthopedic surgery for control of postoperative pain in dogs. J Am Vet Med Assoc 1999;215:1105–1110.

192. Lascelles BD, Butterworth SJ, Waterman AE. Postoperative analgesic and sedative effects of carprofen and pethidine in dogs. Vet Rec 1994;134:187–191.

193. Lascelles BD, Cripps P, Mirchandani S, Waterman AE. Carprofen as an analgesic for postoperative pain in cats: Dose titration and assessment of efficacy in comparison to pethidine hydrochloride. J Small Anim Pract 1995;36:535–541.

194. Lascelles BD, Cripps PJ, Jones A, Waterman-Pearson AE. Efficacy and kinetics of carprofen, administered preoperatively or postoperatively, for the prevention of pain in dogs undergoing ovariohysterectomy. Vet Surg 1998;27:568–582.

195. Nolan A, Reid J. Comparison of the postoperative analgesic and sedative effects of carprofen and papaveretum in the dog. Vet Rec 1993;133:240–242.

196. Slingsby LS, Waterman-Pearson AE. Comparison of pethidine, buprenorphine and ketoprofen for postoperative analgesia after ovariohysterectomy in the cat. Vet Rec 1998;143:185–189.

197. Taylor PM. Newer analgesics: Nonsteroid anti-inflammatory drugs, opioids, and combinations. Vet Clin North Am Small Anim Pract 1999;29:719–735.

198. Prescott JF, Miller CW, Mathews KA, Yager JA, DeWinter L. Update on canine streptococcal toxic shock syndrome and necrotizing fasciitis. Can Vet J 1997;38:241–242.

199. Hickford FH, Barr SC, Erb HN. Effect of carprofen on hemostatic variables in dogs. Am J Vet Res 2001;62:1642–1646.

200. Holtsinger RH, Parker RB, Beale BS. The therapeutic efficacy of carprofen (Rimadyl-V) in 209 clinical cases of canine degenerative joint. J Vet Comp Orthop Trauma 1992;5:140–144.

201. Doig PA, Purbrick KA, Hare JE, McKeown DB. Clinical efficacy and tolerance of meloxicam in dogs with chronic osteoarthritis. Can Vet J 2000;41:296–300.

202. Budsberg SC, Johnston SA, Schwarz PD, DeCamp CE, Claxton R. Efficacy of etodolac for the treatment of osteoarthritis of the hip joints in dogs. J Am Vet Med Assoc 1999;214:206–210.

203. Allyn M, Johnston SA, Schwartz PD. The gastroduodenal effects of buffered aspirin, carprofen and etodolac in the dog. In: Proceedings of the 16th Annual American College of Veterinary Internal Medicine, San Diego. Vet Med Forum 1998:731.

204. Reimer ME, Johnston SA, Leib MS, et al. The gastroduodenal effects of buffered aspirin, carprofen, and etodolac in healthy dogs. J Vet Intern Med 1999;13:472–477.

205. Forsyth SF, Guilford WG, Lowoko CRO. Endoscopic evaluation of the gastroduodenal mucosa following non-steroidal anti-inflammatory drug administration in the dog. NZ Vet J 1996;44:179–181.

206. Forsyth SF, Guilford WG, Haslett SJ, Godfrey J. Endoscopy of the gastroduodenal mucosa after carprofen, meloxicam and ketoprofen administration in dogs. J Small Anim Pract 1998;39:421–424.

207. Benton HP, Vasseur PB, Broderick-Villa GA, Koolpe M. Effect of carprofen on sulfated glycosaminoglycan metabolism, protein synthesis, and prostaglandin release by cultured osteoarthritic canine chondrocytes. Am J Vet Res 1997;58:286–292.

208. Budsberg SC, Schneider TA, Reynolds L. Plasma and synovial concentrations of carprofen in dogs with chronic unilateral stifle osteoarthritis. In: Proceedings of the Veterinary Orthopedic Society 26th Annual Conference, Sun Valley, ID, 1999:44.

209. Rainsford KD, Skerry TM, Chindemi P, Delaney K. Effects of the NSAIDs meloxicam and indomethacin on cartilage proteoglycan synthesis and joint responses to calcium pyrophosphate crystals in dogs. Vet Res Commun 1999;23:101–113.

210. Abeles V, Harrus S, Angles JM, et al. Hypertrophic osteodystrophy in six weimarancr [sic] puppies associated with systemic signs. Vet Rec 1999;145:130–134.

211. West PM, Fernandez C. Safety of COX-2 inhibitors in asthma patients with aspirin hypersensitivity. Ann Pharmacother 2003;37:1497–1501.

212. Evans JM, McMahon AD, McGilchrist MM, et al. Topical non-steroidal anti-inflammatory drugs and admission to hospital for upper gastrointestinal bleeding and perforation: A record linkage case-control study. Br Med J 1995;311:22–26.

213. McQuay H, McMahon A, McGilchrist M. Topically applied non-steroidal anti-inflammatory drugs. In: McQuay H, Moore A, eds. An Evidence-Based Resource for Pain Relief. New York: Oxford University Press, 1998:102–107.

214. Anderson D, Kollias-Baker C, Colahan P, Keene R, Lynn R, Helper D. Urinary and serum concentrations of diclofenac after topical application to horses. Vet Ther 2005;6:57–66.

215. Caldwell FJ, Mueller PO, Lynn RC, Budsberg SC. Effect of topical application of diclofenac liposomal suspension on experimentally induced subcutaneous inflammation in horses. Am J Vet Res 2004;3:271–276.

216. Sinclair M, Mealey KL, Mathews NS, Peck KE. The pharmacokinetics of meloxicam in horses. In: Proceedings of the Eighth World Congress of Veterinary Anesthesia, Knoxville, TN, 2003:112.

217. Poulsen Nautrep B, Justus, C. Effects of some veterinary NSAIDs on ex vivo thromboxane production and in vivo urine output in the dog. In: Proceedings of the Symposium on Recent Advances in Non-steroidal Anti-inflammatory Therapy in Small Animals, Paris, 1999:25.

218. Reed S. Nonsteroidal anti-inflammatory drug-induced duodenal ulceration and perforation in a mature rottweiler. Can Vet J 2002;43:971–972.

219. Cross AR, Budsberg SC, Keefe TJ. Kinetic gait analysis assessment of meloxicam efficacy in a sodium urate–induced synovitis model in dogs. Am J Vet Res 1997;58:626–631.

220. Edgar PC. Seven cases of panosteitis in the German shepherd dog. Vet Times 1998;11:22–23.

221. Lascelles BD, Waterman A. Analgesia in cats. In Pract 1997;19:203–213.

222. McKellar QA, Delatour P, Lees P. Stereospecific pharmacodynamics and pharmacokinetics of carprofen in the dog. J Vet Pharmacol Ther 1994;17:447–454.

223. Ricketts AP, Lundy KM, Seibel SB. Evaluation of selective inhibition of canine cyclooxygenase 1 and 2 by carprofen and other nonsteroidal anti-inflammatory drugs. Am J Vet Res 1998;59:1441–1446.

224. Welsh EM, Baxter P, Nolan AM. Pharmacokinetics of carprofen administered intravenously to sheep. Res Vet Sci 1992;53:264–266.

225. McKellar QA, Pearson T, Bogan JA. Pharmacokinetics, tolerance and serum thromboxane inhibition of carprofen in the dog. J Small Anim Pract 1990;31:443–448.

226. MacPhail CM, Lappin MR, Meyer DJ, Smith SG, Webster CR, Armstrong PJ. Hepatocellular toxicosis associated with administration of carprofen in 21 dogs. J Am Vet Med Assoc 1998;212:1895–1901.

227. Owens JG, Kamerling SG, Barker SA. Pharmacokinetics of ketoprofen in healthy horses and horses with acute synovitis. J Vet Pharmacol Ther 1995;18:187–195.

228. Wilcke JR, Crisman MV, Scarratt WK, Sams RA. Pharmacokinetics of ketoprofen in healthy foals less than twenty-four hours old. Am J Vet Res 1998;59:290–292.

229. Verde CR, Simpson MI, Frigoli A, Landoni MF. Enantiospecific pharmacokinetics of ketoprofen in plasma and synovial fluid of horses with acute synovitis. J Vet Pharmacol Ther 2001;24:179–185.

230. Faulkner PM, Weary DM. Reducing pain after dehorning in dairy calves. J Dairy Sci 2000;83:2037–2041.

231. Stafford KJ, Mellor DJ, Todd SE, Bruce RA, Ward RN. Effects of local anaesthesia or local anaesthesia plus a non-steroidal anti-inflammatory drug on the acute cortisol response of calves to five different methods of castration. Res Vet Sci 2002;73:61–70.

232. Glaser K, Sung ML, O'Neill K, et al. Etodolac selectively inhibits human prostaglandin G/H synthase 2 (PGHS-2) versus human PGHS-1. Eur J Pharmacol 1995;281:107–111.

233. Deracoxib Information Sheet from Novartis, 2004.

234. McCann ME, Andersen DR, Zhang D, et al. In vitro effects and in vivo efficacy of a novel cyclooxygenase-2 inhibitor in dogs with experimentally induced synovitis. Am J Vet Res 2004;65:503–512.

235. Millis DL, Weigel JP, Moyers T, Buonomo FC. Effect of deracoxib, a new COX-2 inhibitor, on the prevention of lameness induced by chemical synovitis in dogs. Vet Ther 2002;3:453–464.

236. Silverstein FE, Faich G, Goldstein JL, et al. Gastrointestinal toxicity with celecoxib vs nonsteroidal anti-inflammatory drugs for osteoarthritis and rheumatoid arthritis: The CLASS study—A randomized controlled trial. Celecoxib Long-Term Arthritis Safety Study. J Am Med Assoc 2000;284:1247–1255.

237. Moreau M, Daminet S, Martel-Pelletier J, Fernandes J, Pelletier JP. Superiority of the gastroduodenal safety profile of licofelone over rofecoxib, a COX-2 selective inhibitor, in dogs. J Vet Pharmacol Ther 2005;28:81–86.

238. Zubrin (Tepoxalin) Freedom of Information Summary. Rockville, MD: Center for Veterinary Medicine, Food and Drug Administration, 2004.

239. Kay-Mugford PA, Grimm KA, Weingarten AJ, Brianceau P, Lockwood P, Cao J. Effect of preoperative administration of tepoxalin on hemostasis and hepatic and renal function in dogs. Vet Ther 2004;5:120–127.

240. McKellar QA, Lees P, Gettinby G. Pharmacodynamics of tolfenamic acid in dogs: Evaluation of dose response relationships. Eur J Pharmacol 1994;253:191–200.

241. Crisman MV, Wilcke JR, Sams RA. Pharmacokinetics of flunixin meglumine in healthy foals less than twenty-four hours old. Am J Vet Res 1996;57:1759–1761.

242. McNeil PE. Acute tubulo-interstitial nephritis in a dog after halothane anaesthesia and administration of flunixin meglumine and trimethoprim-sulphadiazine. Vet Rec 1992;131:148–151.

243. Vonderhaar MA, Salisbury SK. Gastroduodenal ulceration associated with flunixin meglumine administration in three dogs. J Am Vet Med Assoc 1993;203:92–95.

244. MacAllister CG, Morgan SJ, Borne AT, Pollet RA. Comparison of adverse effects of phenylbutazone, flunixin meglumine, and ketoprofen in horses. J Am Vet Med Assoc 1993;202:71–77.

245. Collins LG, Tyler DE. Phenylbutazone toxicosis in the horse: A clinical study. J Am Vet Med Assoc 1984;184:699–703.

246. Snow DH, Douglas TA, Thompson H, Parkins JJ, Holmes PH. Phenylbutazone toxicosis in equidae: A biochemical and pathophysiological study. Am J Vet Res 1981;42:1754–1759.

247. Raekallio M, Taylor PM, Bennett RC. Preliminary investigations of pain and analgesia assessment in horses administered phenylbutazone or placebo after arthroscopic surgery. Vet Surg 1997;26:150–155.

248. DeBacker P, Braeckman R, Belpaire F. Bioavailability and pharmacokinetics of phenylbutazone in the cow. J Vet Pharmacol Ther 1980;3:29–33.

249. Arifah AK, Lees P. Pharmacodynamics and pharmacokinetics of phenylbutazone in calves. J Vet Pharmacol Ther 2002;25:299–309.

250. Goodrich LR, Furr MO, Robertson JL, Warnick LD. A toxicity study of eltenac, a nonsteroidal anti-inflammatory drug, in horses. J Vet Pharmacol Ther 1998;21:24–33.

251. MacKay RJ, Daniels CA, Bleyaert HF, et al. Effect of eltenac in horses with induced endotoxaemia. Equine Vet J Suppl 2000;26–31.

252. Lees P, May SA, Hoeijmakers M, Coert A, Rens PV. A pharmacodynamic and pharmacokinetic study with vedaprofen in an equine model of acute nonimmune inflammation. J Vet Pharmacol Ther 1999;22:96–106.

253. Bergman JG, Laar P. Field trial with vedaprofen, a new nonsteroidal anti-inflammatory drug. Vet Q 1996;18:S20.

254. Knapp DW, Richardson RC, Chan TC, et al. Piroxicam therapy in 34 dogs with transitional cell carcinoma of the urinary bladder. J Vet Intern Med 1994;8:273–278.

255. Court MH, Greenblatt DJ. Molecular basis for deficient acetaminophen glucuronidation in cats: An interspecies comparison of enzyme kinetics in liver microsomes. Biochem Pharmacol 1997;53:1041–1047.

256. Gingerich DA, Baggot JD, Yeary RA. Pharmacokinetics and dosage of aspirin in cattle. J Am Vet Med Assoc 1975;167:945–948.

257. Bennett MI, Simpson KH. Gabapentin in the treatment of neuropathic pain. Palliat Med 2004;18:5–11.

258. Turan A, Karamanlioglu B, Memis D, Usar P, Pamukcu Z, Ture M. The analgesic effects of gabapentin after total abdominal hysterectomy. Anesth Analg 2004;98:1370–1373, table of contents.

259. Turan A, Karamanlioglu B, Memis D, et al. Analgesic effects of gabapentin after spinal surgery. Anesthesiology 2004;100:935–938.

260. Whiteside GT, Harrison J, Boulet J, et al. Pharmacological characterisation of a rat model of incisional pain. Br J Pharmacol 2004;141:85–91.

261. Mao J, Chen LL. Gabapentin in pain management. Anesth Analg 2000;91:680–687.

262. Amin P, Sturrock ND. A pilot study of the beneficial effects of amantadine in the treatment of painful diabetic peripheral neuropathy. Diabet Med 2003;20:114–118.

263. Fukui S, Komoda Y, Nosaka S. Clinical application of amantadine, an NMDA antagonist, for neuropathic pain. J Anesth 2001;15:179–181.

264. Snijdelaar DG, Koren G, Katz J. Effects of perioperative oral aman-tadine on postoperative pain and morphine consumption in patients after radical prostatectomy: Results of a preliminary study. Anesthesiology 2004;100:134–141.

265. Desmeules JA, Piguet V, Collart L, Dayer P. Contribution of monoaminergic modulation to the analgesic effect of tramadol. Br J Clin Pharmacol 1996;41:7–12.

266. Shipton EA. Tramadol: Present and future. Anaesth Intensive Care 2000;28:363–374.

267. Scott LJ, Perry CM. Tramadol: A review of its use in perioperative pain. Drugs 2000;60:139–176.

268. Desmeules JA. The tramadol option. Eur J Pain 2000;4(Suppl A):15–21.

269. Mastrocinque S, Fantoni DT. A comparison of preoperative tra-madol and morphine for the control of early postoperative pain in canine ovariohysterectomy. Vet Anaesth Analg 2003;30:220–228.

270. Nicholson A, Christie M. Opioid analgesics. In: Maddison J, Page S, Church DB, eds. Small Animal Clinical Pharmacology. Philadelphia: WB Saunders, 2002:271–292.

Chapter 11
Injectable and Alternative Anesthetic Techniques

Keith R. Branson

Introduction

No injectable anesthetic produces all of the components of general anesthesia without depressing some vital organ function. Because the available drugs have rather selective actions within the central nervous system (CNS), combinations of drugs are necessary to provide surgical anesthesia without depressing vital functions. Other than ketamine, intravenous anesthetics generally provide only the mental depression of the anesthetic state. Additional analgesics, inhaled anesthetics, and/or muscle relaxants are required to provide and maintain all of the components of general anesthesia. Thus, drugs discussed in this chapter have been variously described as sedatives, hypnotics, anxiolytics, and incomplete anesthetics. The terms *sleep*, *hypnosis*, and *unconsciousness* have often been used interchangeably in describing the drug-induced sleep produced by these drugs. Characteristics of the ideal injectable anesthetic are listed in Table 11.1.

Injectable drugs are used to induce an unconscious state or are administered by repeated injection and infusion to maintain the mental depression necessary for anesthesia. In recent years, more specific and controllable compounds that provide hypnosis, analgesia, and muscle relaxation have been developed (e.g., propofol). Total intravenous anesthesia refers to the production of general anesthesia with injectable drugs only. The advantage of total intravenous anesthesia is its facility to provide each component of anesthesia with a dose of a specific drug. In contrast, inhalation anesthetics increase or decrease the intensity of all components of anesthesia (CNS depression, analgesia, and muscle relaxation) simultaneously, including their unwanted side effects. The search for new drugs and combinations with appropriate pharmacokinetic-pharmacodynamic profiles for use in domestic and wild animals is ongoing. In animals, unlike in people, a state approaching general anesthesia is not achievable with the use of opioids alone. Consequently, in veterinary anesthesia, opioids have been primarily used as analgesics perioperatively and as anesthetic adjuncts to induce a state of neuroleptanesthesia and are not employed alone as intravenous anesthetics. Because the dissociatives have such a widespread use in domestic, feral, and wild species, and are commonly combined with a variety of other drugs, they are discussed in Chapter 12.

Structure-Activity Relationships

Structure-activity relationships are descriptions of the way modifications of chemical structure affect pharmacological activity. The addition, modification, or removal of functional groups on the fundamental structure of a drug lends it physiochemical properties that alter its ability to access its site of action (receptor) and determines the effect it has on the receptor and cellular function (intrinsic activity). The structure-activity relationships of anesthetic induction drugs have been reasonably described.

Modification of the structure of barbituric acid converts the inactive compound into a hypnotic. The addition of aliphatic side chains in position 5 and 5′ produces hypnotic activity. The length of the side chains influences the duration of action, as well as potency. Replacement of the oxygen atom in position 2 of an active barbiturate with a sulfur atom produces a drug with a faster onset and a shorter action (e.g., thiopental or thiamylal). An active barbiturate methylated in position 1 produces a drug with a rapid onset and short action at the expense of excitatory side effects (e.g., methohexital). Generally, any modification that increases

Table 11.1. Characteristics of an ideal injectable anesthetic.

I. Physiochemical and pharmacokinetic
  a. Water soluble
  b. Long shelf life
  c. Stable when exposed to light
  d. Small volume required for induction of anesthesia
II. Pharmacodynamics
  a. Minimal individual variation
  b. Safe therapeutic ratio
  c. Onset, one vein to brain circulation time
  d. Short duration of action
  e. Inactivated to nontoxic metabolites
  f. Smooth emergence
  g. Absence of anaphylaxis
  h. Absence of histamine release
III. Side effects
  a. Absence of local toxicity
  b. No effect on vital organ function, except anesthetically desirable effects on the central nervous system

lipophilicity will increase a drug's potency and rate of onset and shorten its action.

Several imidazoles have hypnotic activity. This activity in such a molecule requires an alkyl branched carbon atom between the aryl moiety and the imidazole nitrogen and an ester moiety. Etomidate is the most widely used imidazole anesthetic derivative. Propofol is a diortho-substituted phenol with strong hypnotic actions. Sleep time increases with side-chain length. Potency increases with the length of the side chain up to a total of seven to eight carbon atoms. Longer chains decrease potency, while induction and recovery times are prolonged. The arylcycloalkylamines, of which ketamine is a derivative, derive their anesthetic activity from a cyclohexanone ring geminally substituted with an aromatic ring and a basic nitrogen. The potency of these compounds is influenced by substitution on the nitrogen, but their pharmacological activity is unaffected.

An often-overlooked aspect of structure-activity relationships is the role of stereoisomerism to biological activity. Except for the asymmetrical centers, the stereoisomers of a given molecule are physically and chemically identical. Nevertheless, activity is predicated on the active stereoisomer of a given neurotransmitter, hormone, or drug interfacing with the chiral active center of a receptor or enzyme. Because side effects are often caused by nonspecific action of drugs, the inactive stereoisomer can contribute to side effects of racemic mixtures. Some isomers may have the opposite effect on a receptor or enzyme than that of the active isomer. Several barbiturates have asymmetrical carbon atoms with isomers of varying potency. Nevertheless, all barbiturates are marketed as racemic mixtures. The (+) isomer of etomidate has hypnotic activity and is the only anesthetic to be marketed as a single active isomer. The stereoisomers of ketamine vary in their hypnotic and analgesic potency, with the (+) isomer being threefold more potent than the (−) isomer. The (−) isomer produces more untoward emergence reactions. Nevertheless, keta-

mine is marketed as a racemic mixture. Neither propofol nor the benzodiazepines have asymmetrical carbon atoms.[1]

Mechanisms of Action

The complexity of the CNS has contributed to the lack of a full understanding of the mechanisms of action of injectable anesthetic drugs. No drug has a single action. Some theories suggest that anesthetics alter cell membranes. Other theories emphasize interaction with neurotransmitter-receptor-ionophore systems. Considerable evidence suggests that most injectable anesthetics alter γ-aminobutyric acid (GABA)–mediated neurotransmission. GABA is an inhibitory neurotransmitter that activates postsynaptic receptors that, in turn, increase chloride conductance, thus hyperpolarizing and inhibiting the neuron. The specific mechanism of action of each injectable anesthetic will be described subsequently in this chapter.

Barbiturate Drugs

Barbituric acid was first prepared by Conrad and Gutzeit in 1882. In 1903, Fischer and von Mering introduced a derivative, diethyl barbituric acid (veronal or barbital), for use as a hypnotic. Fischer is believed to have named the drug veronal from the Latin *vera*, because he thought it to be the "true" hypnotic.

Chemical Structure

The barbiturates all contain a pyrimidine nucleus produced by the condensation of malonic acid and urea (Fig. 11.1). Barbituric acid itself has no hypnotic activity. Substituting alkyl or aryl groups on the R_1 or R_2 positions (Fig. 11.2) produces various compounds with hypnotic activity. Replacement of the oxygen atom in position X by a sulfur atom produces the ultra-short-acting thiobarbiturates.

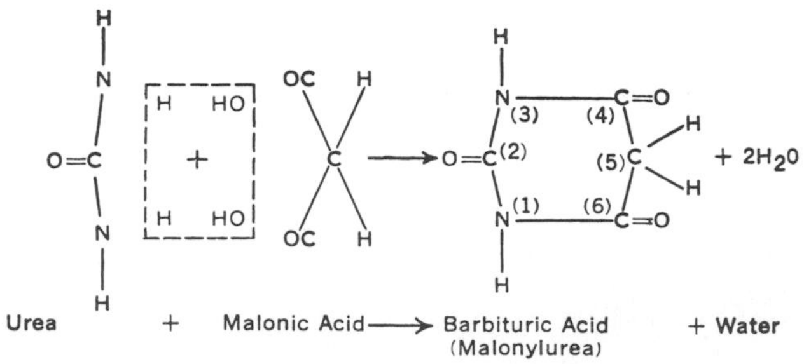

Fig. 11.1. Formation of barbituric acid from urea and malonic acid.

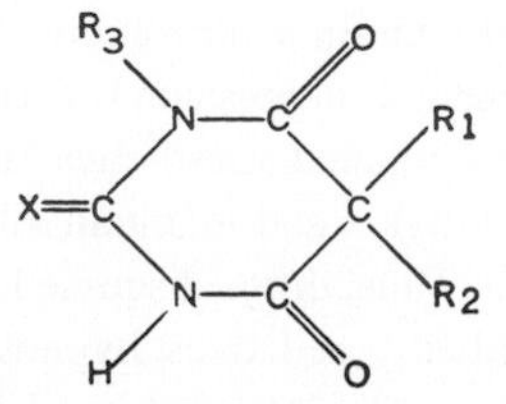

Fig. 11.2. General formula of the barbiturates.

Table 11.2. Names, status, chemical structures, duration of action, and excretion of the barbiturates

Barbiturate	Status	Commercial Names or Synonyms	R_1	R_2	R_3	X	Duration of Action	Organ of Degradation and/or Excretion
Allylbarbituric acid	NF	Sandoptal	allyl	isobutyl	H	O	Intermediate	III
Amobarbital	USP	Amytal	ethyl	isoamyl	H	O	Intermediate	III
Aprobarbital	NF	Alurate	allyl	isopropyl	H	O	Intermediate	II
Barbital	NF	Veronal Barbitone	ethyl	ethyl	H	O	Long	I
Butabarbital[a]	NNR	Butisol	ethyl	sec-butyl	H	O	Intermediate	—
Butallylonal[a]	NF	Pernoston	2-bromallyl	sec-butyl	H	O	Intermediate	II
Butethal	NF	Neonal	ethyl	n-butyl	H	O	Intermediate	II
Cyclobarbital	NF	Phanodorn	ethyl	cyclohexenyl	H	O	Short	II
Cyclopal	—	—	allyl	cyclopentenyl	H	O	Short	II
Diallylbarbituric acid	NF	Dial	allyl	allyl	H	O	Long	II
Hexethal[a]	NNR	Ortal	ethyl	n-hexyl	H	O	Intermediate	III
Hexobarbital[b]	NF	Evipal Hexobarbitone	methyl	cyclohexenyl	CH_3	O	Ultrashort	IV
Kemithal[b]	—	—	allyl	cyclohexenyl	H	S	Ultrashort	IV
Mephobarbital	NF	Mebaral	ethyl	phenyl	CH_3	O	Long	II
Pentobarbital	USP	Nembutal	ethyl	1-methylbutyl	H	O	Short	III
Phenobarbital	USP	Luminal Phenobarbitone	ethyl	phenyl	H	O	Long	I
Probarbital[a]	NF	Ipral	ethyl	isopropyl	H	O	Intermediate	III
Propallylonal	—	Nostal	isopropyl	2-bromallyl	H	O	Intermediate	III
Secobarbital[a]	USP	Seconal	allyl	1-methylbutyl	H	O	Short	III
Thiamylal[b]	NNR	Surital	allyl	1-methylbutyl	H	S	Ultrashort	IV
Thiopental[b]	USP	Pentothal	ethyl	1-methylbutyl	H	S	Ultrashort	IV
Vinbarbital[a]	NF	Delvinal	ethyl	1-methyl-1-butenyl	H	O	Intermediate	II

[a]Employed principally as the sodium salt.
[b]Used for intravenous anesthesia, as sodium salt.
I Mainly excreted by kidney.
II Degraded by liver and excreted by kidney.
III Degraded by liver.
IV Absorbed by body fat, degraded by liver, and excreted by kidney.
Adapted from Goodman and Gilman.[134]

Substituted R_1-R_2 derivatives of barbituric acid behave as weak acids and unite with fixed alkalies to form soluble salts. These salts hydrolyze in water to varying degrees and form alkaline solutions. Those commonly employed in veterinary medicine have a pH of 10 or above, and for this reason may cause severe tissue damage and slough if injected perivascularly in any appreciable quantity.

Classification

The barbiturates have been classified into four groups according to duration of action (Fig. 11.3 and Tables 11.2 and 11.3): long, intermediate, short, and ultrashort. All of those used for clinical anesthesia fall in the short or ultrashort classification, whereas those used for sedation or control of convulsions are of long or intermediate action.

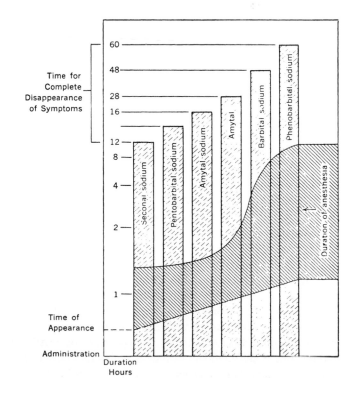

Fig. 11.3. Time of appearance, duration of anesthesia, and time needed for complete disappearance of symptoms after oral administration of equivalent single anesthetic doses in animals. From Jones et al.[139]

Table 11.3. Historical and clinical data of the oxybarbiturates and thiobarbiturates.

| Agent Generic Name | Oxybarbiturates | | |
	Pentobarbital	Secobarbital	Hexobarbital
Trade name	Nembutal Sodium Registered by Abbott Laboratories	Seconal Sodium Registered by Eli Lilly	Evipal Sodium Registered by Parke, Davis
Chemical name	Sodium 5-ethyl-5(1-methylbutyl)-barbiturate	Sodium 5-allyl-5-(1-methylbutyl)-barbiturate	Sodium 1,5-dimethyl-5-(1-cyclohexenyl)-barbiturate
Formula	$C_{11}H_{17}N_2O_3$ Na	$C_{12}H_{17}N_2O_3$ Na	$C_{12}H_{15}N_2O_5$ Na
Discovery of compound	1930 by Volwiler	1930 by Shonle	1932 by Krepp and Taub
Discovery of anesthetic or relaxant properties	1930 by Volwiler and Tabern	1931 by Swanson	1932 by Weese and Scharpff
Type of compound	5-Substituted barbiturate	5-Substituted barbiturate	N-substituted barbiturate
Molecular weight	248.26	260.27	258.25
Buffer employed	None	None	None
Preservative or stabilizing agent used	None	Phenol, 0.25%, and poly-ethylene glycol 200, 50%	None
Thermostability	Precipitates on heating	Precipitates on heating	Free acid melts at 146°C
Chemostability	Solution stable indefinitely	Solution stable up to 18 months in sealed container; decomposes on exposure to air	Solution stable for 48 h if tightly stoppered
Onset of action	30–60 s	30–60 s	30–60 s
Duration of action	1–2 h	1–2 h	15–30 min
Route and/or organ of detoxification or elimination	Detoxified by the liver	Detoxified by the liver	Detoxified by the liver
Usual mode of administration	Intravenous, intrathoracic, intraperitoneal	Intravenous	Intravenous
Specific pharmacological antagonist	Yohimbine plus 4-aminopyridine will partially antagonize pentobarbital and probably other barbiturates. Oxygen administration and artificial respiration are recommended in respiratory arrest.		
Solution pH	6% mixture (10.0–10.3)	5% mixture (9.8–10.1)	2.5% mixture (8.5–10.5)

Adapted from data compiled by Dr. W. H. L. Dornette and published by the Ohio Chemical and Surgical Equipment Company.

General Pharmacology

Racemic mixtures of the barbiturates are used both as hypnotics and as general anesthetics. The principal effect of a barbiturate is depression of the CNS by interference with passage of impulses to the cerebral cortex. Barbiturates act directly on CNS neurons in a manner similar to that of the inhibitory transmitter GABA. At clinical drug concentrations, barbiturates have two mechanisms of action at $GABA_A$ receptors. At lower concentrations, barbiturates exert a GABA-mimetic effect by decreasing the rate of dissociation of GABA from the $GABA_A$ receptor.[2,3] At increasing drug concentrations, barbiturates directly activate the chloride-ion channel associated with the $GABA_A$ receptor.[4,5] The GABA-mimetic effects of barbiturates are thought to produce their sedative hypnotic effects, whereas the direct chloride-ion channel activation produces their anesthetic effects. Barbiturates also inhibit the synaptic actions of some excitatory neurotransmitters such as glutamate and acetylcholine.[6–8] The role of this action in the production of the anesthetic state remains uncertain.

Ganglionic transmission is approximately 20 times more sensitive to pentobarbital than is axonal conduction.[9] The fast excitatory postsynaptic potential (EPSP) is approximately 10 times more sensitive to pentobarbital than are the slow potentials (slow EPSP and slow inhibitory PSP). Phenobarbital also exerts some degree of selectivity toward the fast EPSP. Anesthetic concentra-

Oxybarbiturates (cont.)	Thiobarbiturates		
Methohexital	**Thiamylal**	**Thiopental**	**Thialbarbitone**
Brevital Registered by Eli Lilly	Surital Sodium Registered by Parke, Davis	Pentothal Sodium Registered by Abbott Laboratories	Kemithal Sodium Registered by Fort Dodge Laboratories
Sodium a-dl-1-methyl-5-allyl-5- (1-methyl-2-pentynyl)- barbiturate	Sodium 5-allyl-5-(1-methylbutyl)- 2-thiobarbiturate	Sodium 5-ethyl-5-(1-methylbutyl)- 2-thiobarbiturate	Sodium 5-allyl-5-(2-cyclohexenyl)- 2-thiobarbiturate
$C_{14}H_{17}N_2O_3$ Na	$C_{12}H_{17}N_2O_2$ SNa	$C_{11}H_{17}N_2O_2$ SNa	$C_{13}H_{15}N_2O_2$ SNa
1955 by Doran	1929 by Dox	1929 by Taburn and Volwiler	1938 by Carrington
1955 by Gibson	1933 by Gruhzit	1933 by Tatum	1946 by Carrington and Raventos
N-5-substituted barbiturate	5-Substituted thiobarbiturate	5-Substituted thiobarbiturate	5-Substituted thiobarbiturate
284.0	276.33	264.23	286.3
Sodium carbonate	6% Sodium carbonate	6% Sodium carbonate	None
None	None	None	None
Deteriorates when boiled	Precipitates when boiled	Precipitates when boiled	Thermolabile
Solution stable at room temperature for 6 months	Solution stable for 48–72 h if tightly stoppered	Solution stable for 48–72 h if tightly stoppered	Solution stable 7 days; indefinitely, if frozen
10–30 s	20–30 s	20–30 s	20–30 s
5–15 min	10–15 min	10–15 min	15–45 min
Detoxified by the liver	Absorbed by fat and detoxified by the liver	Absorbed by fat and detoxified by the liver	Absorbed by fat and detoxified by the liver
Intravenous	Intravenous	Intravenous	Intravenous, intrathoracic, intraperitoneal
Yohimbine plus 4-aminopyridine will partially antagonize pentobarbital and probably other barbiturates. Oxygen administration and artificial respiration are recommended in respiratory arrest.			
5% mixture (10.4–11.4)	2.5% mixture (10.5–11.0)	2.5% mixture (10.5–11.0)	10% mixture (10.6)

tions of pentobarbital selectively block the fast EPSP. A selective postsynaptic block of the nicotinic action of acetylcholine also occurs and may account for the anesthetic-depressant effects of pentobarbital on ganglionic transmission. This selective depression on the nicotinic action of acetylcholine could occur by various molecular mechanisms, for example, by altering the binding of acetylcholine.

In hypnotic doses, the barbiturates have little effect on respiration, whereas, in anesthetic doses, respiration is depressed. Overdosage produces respiratory paralysis and death. With anesthetic doses, there is cardiovascular depression, both centrally and peripherally, with a fall in blood pressure. In hypnotic doses,

barbiturates have little effect on the basal metabolic rate. With anesthetic doses, basal metabolism is depressed, resulting in lowered body temperature.

Following barbiturate administration, leukocyte counts decrease in normal and splenectomized dogs.[10] Packed cell volume also decreases in nonsplenectomized dogs, presumably owing to splenic sequestration of red blood cells. There is no significant change in the differential counts (Tables 11.4 and 11.5).

The oxidation of pentobarbital, hexobarbital, and amobarbital is noncompetitively inhibited by halothane, methoxyflurane, and diethyl ether.[11] Saturation of the enzyme system by the anesthetic appears responsible. Chloramphenicol, a microsomal in-

Table 11.4. Leukocyte counts and packed cell volumes (PCVs) in 12 dogs after barbiturate anesthesia.

Time in minutes	Pentobarbital		Thiopental		Thiamylal		Methohexital	
	Leukocytes × 10³	PCV, %	Leukocytes × 10³	PCV, %	Leukocytes × 10³	PCV, %	Leukocytes × 10³	PCV, %
−30	13.7 ± 1.5[a]	50 ± 1.2	12.4 ± 1.0	49 ± 1.2	12.5 ± 1.1	48.5 ± 1.5	13.4 ± 1.4	50 ± 1.4
Anesthesia begins	13.6 ± 1.5	48 ± 1.5	12.2 ± 0.9	47 ± 1.0	12.7 ± 1.0	48 ± 1.2	13.5 ± 1.4	49 ± 1.1
+30	10.8 ± 1.3	40 ± 1.2	10.8 ± 1.0	40 ± 1.4	10.8 ± 1.0	41 ± 1.2	10.9 ± 1.2	42 ± 0.7
+60	10.9 ± 1.3	40 ± 1.5	10.7 ± 0.9	40 ± 1.6	10.1 ± 1.0	41 ± 1.4	11.0 ± 1.4	42 ± 1.0
+120	10.7 ± 1.4	40 ± 1.4	10.9 ± 1.1	42 ± 1.6	10.3 ± 1.1	43 ± 1.2	11.1 ± 1.2	44 ± 1.0
+180	10.8 ± 1.3	41 ± 1.0	11.3 ± 1.2	42 ± 1.3	10.7 ± 1.1	43 ± 1.2	10.9 ± 1.4	44 ± 1.1

[a]Mean ± standard deviation.
From Usenik and Cronkite.[10]

Table 11.5. Leukocyte counts and packed cell volumes (PCVs) in six splenectomized dogs (two trials per dog) after pentobarbital anesthesia.

Time in Minutes	Leukocytes × 10³	PCV, %
−30	14.2 ± 1.0[a]	46.5 ± 1.6
Anesthesia begins	13.9 ± 1.0	46 ± 1.9
+30	11.6 ± 1.1	45 ± 1.8
+60	11.2 ± 1.0	45 ± 1.8
+120	11.0 ± 1.1	45 ± 1.8
+180	11.0 ± 1.0	45 ± 1.9

[a]Mean ± standard deviation.
From Usenik and Cronkite.[10]

pK_a = dissociation constant
or
pH at which equal amount of drug is in ionized and unionized forms.

$$HA \rightleftharpoons H^+ + A^-$$

Barbiturate	pK_a
Thiopental	7.4
Secobarbital	7.9
Pentobarbital	8.0

Fig. 11.4. Dissociation of barbiturates.

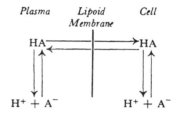

Fig. 11.5. Barbiturate dissociation. Cell membrane is permeable only to undissociated (nonionized) barbiturate.

hibitor, can markedly prolong recovery from pentobarbital anesthesia.

Barbiturates administered during the prenatal period can produce permanent alterations in sexual maturity of hamsters and rats,[12,13] and perhaps an increased incidence of congenital malformations in humans.[14,15]

Distribution

Barbiturates diffuse throughout the body, penetrating cell walls and crossing the placenta. The extent of ionization, lipid solubility (partition coefficient), and protein binding are the three most important factors in distribution and elimination of barbiturates.

Barbiturates are sodium salts of barbituric acid derivatives. When dissolved in water, they ionize. The degree of ionization is determined by the pH of the solution and the dissociation constant (pKa) of the agent. This dissociation constant is the pH at which the compound exists in equal quantities in the dissociated (ionized or polar) and undissociated (nonionized or nonpolar) forms (Fig. 11.4). For a barbiturate to penetrate the lipoid layer of cell membranes, it must be in the undissociated or nonpolar form (Fig. 11.5). The more acidic the solution is containing the drug, the more undissociated form that exists and the greater the amount that can penetrate cell membranes to produce deeper anesthesia.

The reverse is also true: The more alkaline the solution is, the greater the dissociation and the lesser the cell penetration.

At a blood pH of 7.4, a barbiturate assumes a "normal" distribution within the cells of the CNS and produces the desired degree of anesthesia. A change in blood pH, however, may lead to a change in the depth of anesthesia. An increase in acidity, such as commonly occurs with respiratory or metabolic acidosis, increases the depth. An increase in alkalinity, caused by hyperventilation or administration of alkalinizing agents, increases dissociation, and barbiturate migrates outward from the cells to the plasma, and anesthesia will lighten.[16] Alkalinization of the urine also decreases tubular reabsorption.

The undissociated form has a high affinity for nonpolar solvents. This varies between compounds, as shown in Table 11.6.

Table 11.6. Barbiturates: relation between physicochemical factors, distribution, and fate.

Barbiturate	Partition Coefficient[a]	Plasma Protein Binding[b]	Brain Protein Binding[c]	Delay in Onset of Activity[d]	Excreted by Kidney[e]	Degradation by Liver Slices[f]	pKa[g]
Barbital	1	0.05	0.06	22	65–90	—	7.8
Phenobarbital	3	0.20	0.19	12	30	—	7.3
Pentobarbital	39	0.35	0.29	0.1	—	0.21	8.0
Secobarbital	52	0.44	0.39	0.1	—	0.28	7.9
Thiopental	580	0.65	0.50	—	—	0.38	7.4

[a](Concentration in methylene chloride): (concentration in aqueous phase) of the nonionized form at approximately 25°C.
[b]Binding of 0.001 M barbituric acid by 1% bovine serum albumin in M/15 phosphate buffer at pH 7.4; fraction bound.
[c]Fraction of barbiturate bound by rabbit brain homogenates.
[d]Minutes until anesthesia after intravenous injection in mice.
[e]Approximate percentage of total dose excreted unchanged in urine of humans.
[f]Fraction degraded in vitro by liver slices in 3 h.
[g]Ionization exponent at 25°C.
From Goodman and Gilman.[135]

Table 11.7. Rates of passage of drugs from bloodstream into the cerebrospinal fluid of dogs and degrees of ionization of drugs at pH 7.4.

Drug	% Nonionized at pH 7.4	Permeability Coefficient[a]	Heptane-Water Partition Coefficient of Unionized Form of Drug
Barbital	55.7	0.026	0.002
Thiopental	61.3	0.50	3.3
Pentobarbital	83.4	0.17	0.05

[a]The higher the permeability coefficient, the more rapid is the rate of entry into the CSF.
From Shanker.[136]

Table 11.8. Influence of carbon dioxide on penetration of brain by drugs.

Area	Concentration in the Brain		
	Hypercapnic Acidosis	Hypocapnic Alkalosis	Relative Penetration
Urea (1 h)			
Gray	0.40	0.16	2.50
White	0.12	0.05	2.40
Phenobarbital (1/2 h)			
Gray	1.20	0.72	1.67
White	1.08	0.40	2.70
Salicylic Acid (1 h)			
Gray	0.44	0.11	4.00
White	0.38	0.04	9.50

Concentration in brain is expressed as a fraction of levels in plasma (relative penetration is brain fractions under conditions of hypercapnia to brain fraction under conditions of hypocapnia). Note the disproportionate increase in penetration of white matter by salicylic acid under conditions of hypercapnia. Gray, cerebral cortex; white, cerebral white matter.
From Roth and Barlow.[137] Copyright 1961 by the American Association for Advancement of Science.

The highly lipid-soluble agents have a rapid onset and are short-acting. They are rapidly metabolized and also easily reabsorbed by the kidney tubules.

A reversible bond develops to plasma proteins, chiefly albumin, the degree of which agrees roughly with the partition coefficient. Because cerebrospinal fluid is practically protein free, it contains less barbiturate than does plasma (Table 11.7). Organ tissues contain a slightly higher level of barbiturate, whereas fat contains very high concentrations. Highly lipid-soluble compounds penetrate brain tissue quite rapidly, reaching equilibrium with two or three circulations of blood. Gray matter of the brain is penetrated rapidly, with white matter being slower to reach equilibrium (Table 11.8).

Barbiturate anesthesia is terminated by physical redistribution, metabolic degradation, and renal excretion. Again, the solubility coefficient dictates the chief route of elimination. Short-acting agents with a high solubility coefficient are largely reabsorbed from the kidney tubules. Their action ceases when they are metabolically transformed into inactive substances, principally in the liver. Long-acting agents with low lipid solubility are chiefly excreted through the kidneys. As much as 85% of barbital and phenobarbital may be recovered from the urine over several days following administration.[17] The short-acting barbiturates (pentobarbital, amobarbital, and secobarbital) are destroyed principally by the liver. Their rapid destruction in the body accounts for their shorter action. With anesthetic-inducing doses ultra-short-acting barbiturates are quickly redistributed, accounting for their short action. Thiobarbiturates are not metabolized more rapidly than the oxybarbiturates.

The "Glucose Effect"?

A unique reanesthetizing action, termed the *glucose effect*, has been observed in animals recovering from barbiturate anesthesia that were subsequently given glucose. A species variation in susceptibility to this effect has been demonstrated: Guinea pigs, chickens, pigeons, rabbits, and hamsters are susceptible; dogs are intermediate; and mice, rats, goldfish, and tadpoles are refractory or negative. Intermediates in the glycolysis of glucose and in the Krebs cycle have been shown to have the same effect. The glucose effect presumably occurs with most barbiturates and thiobarbiturates, but not with inhalation or other anesthetics. Glucose causes a decrease in activity of the components of the microsomal electron chain, resulting in decreased microsomal metabolism.[18] A study on the glucose effect on respiration and electroencephalogram in dogs following pentobarbital administration found no evidence of significant deepening of anesthesia as judged by cortical depression, decreasing rate or depth of respiration, or a decrease in minute volume.[19]

Epinephrine given intravenously (IV) to dogs or mice also causes a return of sleep on awakening from hexobarbital or chloral hydrate anesthesia. Norepinephrine is less effective in producing this effect.[20] This phenomenon presumably is caused by increased glucose levels in the blood and should be remembered when the use of epinephrine is considered in barbiturate-anesthetized dogs. The effect of glucose, sodium lactate, and epinephrine on thiopental anesthesia in dogs has also been studied (Table 11.9). The glucose effect does not appear to be of practical concern as long as these drugs are used in therapeutic doses.[21]

Therapeutic Uses

Barbiturates are used to induce sedation and hypnosis, as anticonvulsants, and as anesthetics. Their use as sedatives and hypnotics in low doses has been supplanted, in most instances, by tranquilizers. The ability of barbiturates to depress the motor cortex has been used to treat convulsions associated with poisoning, particularly strychnine, "running fits," distemper encephalitis, and overdosage of local anesthetics. In modern veterinary medicine, the thiobarbiturates are primarily used as induction agents or short-acting anesthetics, whereas pentobarbital is now used sparingly because of its propensity to cause prolonged, rough recoveries when administered in anesthetic doses.

Addiction

Although barbiturate addiction can be produced in animals, it is by its very nature self-limiting; however, in humans, repeated oral use of barbiturates as soporifics or sedatives may become habit forming. For this reason, legislation in many countries prohibits use of these drugs without a prescription. Veterinarians should be acquainted with applicable laws regarding the use and sale of barbiturates to avoid infraction and to prevent liability.

Oxybarbiturates

Phenobarbital Sodium

Phenobarbital was synthesized in 1912 in Germany and marketed under the trade name Luminal. It is a long-acting barbiturate, and advantage has been taken of its prolonged action in treating various convulsive disorders (Fig. 11.3). In control of convulsions caused by distemper encephalitis, it appears to be as effective as any of the newer drugs and considerably cheaper. Because it is excreted slowly in the urine, it tends to be cumulative. An oral loading dose should be administered first, followed by a daily maintenance dose. In average dogs (10 kg), this would be 60 mg initially, followed by 15 mg three times a day. Overdosage causes loss of motor coordination; when this occurs, the dose should be reduced. Serial assays on serum, saliva, and cerebrospinal fluid have shown considerable daily fluctuation in phenobarbital levels, even after several weeks of therapy. The phenobarbital concentration increases gradually in the three fluids up to doses of 9.0 mg/kg. Serum or saliva assays can accurately indicate the phenobarbital concentration in cerebrospinal fluid.[22]

In animals suffering from strychnine poisoning, phenobarbital solution may be given IV to effect in the same manner as one would administer pentobarbital sodium. Phenobarbital is a hepatic microsomal enzyme inducer. Concomitant administration of phenobarbital and digoxin can shorten the biological half-life of the latter by approximately 30%.[23]

Pentobarbital Sodium

This drug came into general use as an anesthetic agent for dogs and cats in the early 1930s and slowly supplanted ether administered by open-mask methods as the anesthetic of choice. By 1940, its use was widespread. Today, it has largely been replaced by inhalation and balanced anesthetic techniques.

Commercial preparations of pentobarbital are racemic mixtures. Administration of subanesthetic doses is often associated with CNS stimulation and preanesthetic excitation. The R-isomer of pentobarbital causes a transient period of hyperexcitability before depressing the CNS, whereas the S-isomer produces relatively smooth and progressively deeper hypnosis.[24] Evidence suggests the S-isomer is more potent, possibly because of increased uptake by the brain.[25,26]

Table 11.9. Relative ability of glucose, sodium lactate, and epinephrine to cause anesthetic rebound[a] in dogs recovering from thiopental anesthesia.

Drug and Dosage	Dogs Given Injections (No.)	Dogs Rebounded (No.)	Dogs Rebounded %	Average Increase in Sleep Time (%)
Glucose, 600.0 mg/kg	18	2	11.1	47.9
Sodium lactate, 60.0 mg/kg	18	7	38.9	48.9
Epinephrine, 0.1 mg/kg	13	11	84.6	38.8
Saline solution, 1.0 mL/kg	12	0	0	0

[a]Apparent reanesthetization as indicated by loss of voluntary and involuntary movements and possible loss of pedal reflexes.
From Hatch.[21]

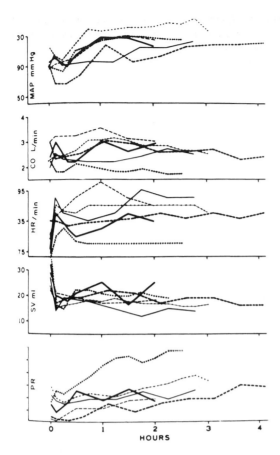

Fig. 11.6. Long-term changes from pentobarbital in six dogs. Note the large and abrupt increase in heart rate and decrease in stroke volume at the onset of the experiments. CO, cardiac output; HR, heart rate; MAP, mean arterial pressure; PR, peripheral resistance; and SV, stroke volume. From Olmsted and Page.[140].

Pentobarbital sodium occurs as a white powder or crystalline granules. It is freely soluble in water or alcohol. It forms a clear, colorless solution that is marketed under several trade names. Aqueous solutions have an alkaline pH and may precipitate on standing, but the drug can be redissolved by addition of an alkali such as sodium hydroxide. The calculated dose for dogs and cats is 30 mg/kg of body weight; however, it should be emphasized that pentobarbital is given *to effect*. Following a single intravenous dose of pentobarbital, arterial blood pressure decreases. The heart rate increases for 10 to 20 min and then stabilizes or decreases. Cardiac output is variable, whereas peripheral vascular resistance increases (Fig. 11.6).

The cardiovascular effects of prolonged pentobarbital (2.5 h) anesthesia in dogs have been assessed. Systolic blood pressure, initial ventricular impulse, stroke volume, pulse pressure, central venous pressure, arterial oxygen partial pressure, pH, and body temperature all decrease after anesthetic doses of pentobarbital. Heart rate, arterial carbon dioxide partial pressure, and peripheral resistance increased after 1.5 h. Cardiac output eventually decreases. Mean arterial pressure significantly decreases during induction, but usually returns to awake values in approximately 30

min (Table 11.10).[27] Intravenous pentobarbital administration alters myocardial function and distribution of blood flow. In dogs, it was found that intravenous pentobarbital decreases contractile force by 17.4%, arterial blood pressure by 4.8%, and renal blood flow by 8.4%, while increasing cardiac output by 4.8% and superior mesenteric artery flow by 14.1%. The decreased arterial blood pressure was believed to be caused by vasodilation of major vascular beds, and the increased cardiac output to be caused by increased venous return.[28] Respiration is initially depressed and gradually increases during recovery.[29]

Light pentobarbital anesthesia has little influence on renal hemodynamics. Deep anesthesia depresses renal function, both blood and urine flow, by circulatory depression and also by reflex vasoconstriction. Pentobarbital inhibits water diuresis by stimulating release of antidiuretic hormone.[30]

Leukopenia is found in dogs anesthetized with pentobarbital.[31] Leukocyte counts drop to 20% of control values (Fig. 11.7). Although the absolute differential white cell count decreases, there is a relative lymphocytosis that reaches its peak at 90 min and then returns to normal. Red cell numbers decrease also. Hemoglobin and hematocrit values show corresponding changes. Pentobarbital, amobarbital, and thiopental administration dilates the spleen, which presumably accounts for the decrease in erythrocytes via the sequestration of red blood cells.[32] Maximum dilation usually occurs 20 to 30 min after injection of the anesthetic. Sedimentation rate and coagulation time are both increased, whereas prothrombin time is decreased. Oral administration of pentobarbital sodium in sedative doses does not affect the blood constituents in the same fashion.

In some animals, the effect produced by high doses of pentobarbital is difficult to differentiate from shock. The size of the dose and method of its administration are the major factors in variation of response to pentobarbital. Individual variations undoubtedly exist. Roughly one of four animals given a dose of 30 mg/kg develops side effects that mimic some phase of shock.[33]

On intraperitoneal administration, the peak concentration in the blood is reached more slowly than with intravenous injection, and the portion of drug absorbed into the portal system is subjected to early destruction in the liver. When a 2.5% aqueous solution is given intraperitoneally in a dose of 30 mg/kg of body weight, anesthesia is not accompanied by impaired renal function, and arterial blood pressure increases.[34] When given radiolabeled pentobarbital orally, dogs excrete about 60% of the total dose in the urine during the first 24 h.[35] Over 92% is excreted as metabolic products derived from the drug, and only 3% is in the form of pentobarbital. Pentobarbital elimination from the blood of both intact and bilaterally nephrectomized dogs is similar because elimination is totally dependent on biotransformation of pentobarbital by the liver.[36] The absence of renal function per se does not seem to alter the pharmacokinetics of pentobarbital; however, the sensitivity of a patient to the action of barbiturates may be increased by uremia. This phenomenon is probably caused by the decreased capacity of plasma protein to bind acidic drugs.

Pentobarbital freely crosses the placental barrier and enters the fetus. For this reason, its use as a monoanesthetic (high dose) for

Table 11.10. Cardiovascular responses to pentobarbital anesthesia in 12 dogs.

Parameters	Control	Time After Pentobarbital Administration					
		0 h[a]	0.5 h	1 h	1.5 h	2 h	2.5 h
Systolic blood pressure	142 ± 3	116 ± 5[c]	123 ± 4[c]	121 ± 3[c]	122 ± 3[c]	124 ± 3[c]	130 ± 3[c]
(mm Hg)	100%[b]	82 ± 3	87 ± 3	86 ± 3	86 ± 2	88 ± 2	92 ± 2
Mean blood pressure	108 ± 4	95 ± 4[c]	104 ± 4	106 ± 3	108 ± 2	111 ± 3	117 ± 3
(mm Hg)	100%	89 ± 4	97 ± 4	99 ± 4	101 ± 3	104 ± 4	109 ± 4
Diastolic blood pressure	83 ± 3	80 ± 4	89 ± 4	93 ± 3[c]	95 ± 2[c]	90 ± 3[c]	105 ± 3[c]
(mm Hg)	100%	98 ± 5	109 ± 5	115 ± 6	117 ± 5	122 ± 6	127 ± 6
Pulse pressure (mm Hg)	59 ± 2.6	36 ± 2.4[c]	34 ± 1.9[c]	28 ± 2.2[c]	27 ± 1.9[c]	26 ± 1.3[c]	25 ± 1.4[c]
Central venous pressure	+1.44 ± 0.7	+0.14 ± 0.4[c]	−0.4 ± 0.4[c]	−1.00 ± 0.5[c]	−1.25 ± 0.5[c]	−1.08 ± 0.5[c]	−1.55 ± 0.6[c]
(mm Hg)							
Heart rate (beats/min)	96 ± 5	157 ± 5[c]	153 ± 7[c]	157 ± 8[c]	141 ± 7[c]	135 ± 7[c]	146 ± 10[c]
	100%	167 ± 9	165 ± 11	168 ± 9	155 ± 10	146 ± 11	157 ± 12
Initial ventricular	7 ± 0.4	9 ± 0.4[c]	9.8 ± 0.5[c]	10.1 ± 1[c]	12.5 ± 0.9[c]	13.8 ± 1[c]	14.7 ± 0.9[c]
impulse (angle in °)	100%	130 ± 6	142 ± 8	147 ± 15	180 ± 11	193 ± 11	212 ± 11
Cardiac output (L/min)	1.734 ± 0.15	1.834 ± 0.14	1.811 ± 0.09	1.502 ± 0.11[c]	1.324 ± 0.12[c]	1.195 ± 0.10[c]	1.172 ± 0.09[c]
	100%	111 ± 8	111 ± 8	90 ± 5	79 ± 6	71 ± 5	70 ± 5
Stroke volume	18.6 ± 2	11.8 ± 1[c]	12.3 ± 1[c]	10.1 ± 1[c]	9.5 ± 1[c]	9.4 ± 1[c]	8.9 ± 1[c]
(mL/beat)	100%	66 ± 4	68 ± 3	54 ± 2	51 ± 1	50 ± 3	47 ± 4
Total peripheral resistance	5287 ± 558	4574 ± 385	4819 ± 419	6200 ± 551	7370 ± 696[c]	8535 ± 942[c]	8864 ± 1928[c]
(dynes-s/cm^5)	100%	91 ± 7	95 ± 6	124 ± 11	142 ± 8	163 ± 10	168 ± 8
PaO$_2$ (mm Hg)	93.5 ± 3	60 ± 5[c]	70 ± 3[c]	73.5 ± 6[c]	70 ± 6[c]	77 ± 4[c]	75 ± 5[c]
	100%	61 ± 5	72 ± 4	75 ± 7	80 ± 6	79 ± 5	76 ± 6
PaCO$_2$ (mm Hg)	30.9 ± 0.8	40.9 ± 3[c]	44 ± 2[c]	41 ± 3[c]	38 ± 3[c]	38 ± 3[c]	38 ± 3[c]
	100%	132 ± 9	141 ± 5	133 ± 8	121 ± 7	123 ± 9	123 ± 7
pH arterial	7.38 ± 0.01	7.27 ± 0.03[c]	7.27 ± 0.03[c]	7.29 ± 0.03[c]	7.30 ± 0.02[c]	7.30 ± 0.03[c]	7.32 ± 0.03[c]
Temperature (°C)	38.8 ± 0.2	38.7 ± 0.2[c]	38.5 ± 0.2[c]	38.1 ± 0.2[c]	37.9 ± 0.2[c]	37.6 ± 0.2[c]	37.4 ± 0.2[c]

[a]0, time values taken 3 to 5 min after intravenous pentobarbital.

[b]Each value indicates mean ± standard error with percent of control ± standard error below.

[c]Denotes statistically significant changes with $P < 0.05$.

From Priano et al.[27]

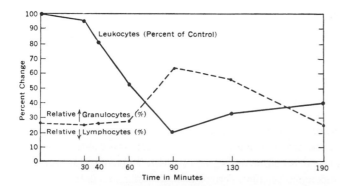

Fig. 11.7. The relative percentage change in white cell counts with intravenous pentobarbital sodium anesthesia in 12 dogs as compared with control levels in unanesthetized dogs. The relative percentage distribution of lymphocytes and granulocytes is shown on the same scale. From Graca and Garst.[31]

cesarean section causes high mortality among newborns. Neonates can be viable at birth, but usually do not recover from anesthesia and cannot nurse.

The duration of surgical analgesia with anesthetizing doses of pentobarbital varies widely with individual animals, averaging about 30 min. Complete recovery usually occurs in 6 to 18 h. Occasionally, animals, particularly cats, may not rouse for as long as 24 to 72 h.

Pentobarbital is no longer used in North America to produce anesthesia in most small companion animals, cattle, and horses, owing to the prolonged recovery period and marked respiratory depression. It has been administered by slow intravenous injection (15 to 30 mg/kg) in foals and young cattle. Because of prolonged recovery, pentobarbital should not be administered to animals younger than 1 month of age. In adult cattle, anesthesia has been induced with 14 mg/kg IV; half of the dose is injected rapidly, the animal is positioned on its sternum, and the remainder is injected slowly to effect.[37] Pentobarbital has also been administered with chloral hydrate or thiopental sodium to induce anesthesia in adult horses[38] and in goats before administration of inhalant anesthetics.[39]

The intravenous anesthetic dose in adult goats is 30 mg/kg, which maintains anesthesia for approximately 20 min. Anesthesia can be maintained by doses of 6 to 36 mg · kg^{-1} · h^{-1} of pentobarbital. The induction and intubation dose ranges from 10 to 42 mg/kg. A similar technique for intravenous pentobarbital in

Table 11.11. Effect of methohexital sodium on the horse after premedication with morphine, meperidine, or promazine (using four horses per treatment).

Premedication	Induction Time (s)		Duration (min)		Time to Stand (min)		Number of Horses and Type of Recovery[a]
	Mean	Range	Mean	Range	Mean	Range	
None	26	23–32	4	3–5.5	21	15–29	4 +++
Meperidine[b]	18	10–25	6	3–16	18	11–30	2 +++ 2 ++
Morphine[b]	16	10–20	5	2–9	19	10–27	2 +++ 1 ++ 1 +
Meperidine Morphine	20	20–21	5	2–7	17	10–34	2 +++ 1 ++ 1 +
Promazine[b]	32	25–35	9	7–10	12	9–16	4 +++
Promazine Meperidine	21	13–30	10	7–13	18	9–26	1 ++ 3 +
Promazine Morphine	24	20–30	7	4–9	27	22–30	1 ++ 3 +
Promazine Meperidine Morphine	27	21–35	8	6–11	17	5–30	1 ++ 3 +

[a]+, Hyperesthesia; ++, mild paddling; +++, severe paddling.
[b]The dose rates used in this trial were meperidine, 1 mg/lb body weight subcutaneously; morphine sulfate, 20 mg/100 lb body weight; promazine, 0.25 mg/lb body weight; methohexital sodium, 1 g/300 to 400 lb body weight.
From Grono.[42]

sheep has been described.[40] Like goats, sheep rapidly metabolize pentobarbital, and additional doses are required to maintain anesthesia for periods longer than 20 to 30 min. The anesthetic dose of pentobarbital sodium is approximately 25 mg/kg in adult sheep. In all ruminants, immediate intubation to prevent aspiration of regurgitated rumen contents is essential.

In swine, a 10- to 30-mg/kg dose of pentobarbital given IV provides anesthesia for 15 to 45 min. If anesthesia is induced until reflex response to surgical stimulation is abolished, respiratory depression is often severe, and apnea may occur.

Animals awakening from pentobarbital anesthesia tend to exhibit the same signs as when they are anesthetized, except in reverse order. These include crying, shivering, involuntary running movements, thrashing, increased respiratory movements followed by recovery of the righting reflex, and, later, ability to stand with a staggering gait. Because recovery is slow, without preanesthetic medication these actions may become so exaggerated that the animal injures itself through contact with the cage or stall or causes wound disruption. Greyhounds are notable for this effect. Show animals have been known to break teeth, much to the embarrassment of the veterinarian. Administration of a narcotic or a tranquilizer is indicated in cases of emergence excitement. Yohimbine plus 4-aminopyridine will incompletely antagonize pentobarbital-induced CNS depression in dogs preanesthetized with atropine-xylazine or atropine–acepromazine.[41]

Methohexital Sodium

This is an ultra-short-acting barbiturate that is unique in that it contains no sulfur atom. Its short duration owes more to redistribution than to rapid metabolism. Blood concentrations necessary to produce anesthesia are approximately one-half of those required with thiopental or thiamylal. According to the manufacturer, a double dose rapidly administered IV causes temporary apnea. The lethal dose is said to be approximately 2.5 times greater than the median anesthetic dose. Animals die of respiratory failure. Methohexital sodium is supplied as 500 mg of dry powder in glass vials. It is diluted with water or normal saline to form a 2.5% solution for injection. Solutions are said to be stable for as long as 6 months at room temperature. The dose for dogs or cats is 6 to 10 mg/kg of body weight. Half of the estimated dose is injected IV at a rapid rate, following which administration is continued to effect. Surgical anesthesia for 5 to 15 min is obtained by an initial injection. More prolonged anesthesia can be maintained by intermittent administration or continuous drip. Recovery is quick and may be accompanied by muscular tremors and violent excitement, which detract from the usefulness of the drug. Dogs are usually ambulatory 30 min after administration ceases.

Methohexital has been used alone and with several preanesthetics in horses (Table 11.11). Even with preanesthetic sedation, the recovery period is characterized by muscle tremors and struggling.[42] For this reason, the anesthesia produced is undesirable except when followed by administration of an inhalant anesthetic. Under these circumstances, it proves to be a good drug for induction, because its effects are short-lasting. One injection provides just sufficient time for intubation and administration of the inhalant before its effect ceases, leaving horses anesthetized with only the inhalant. The induction dose in horses is approximately 6 mg/kg. It must be given rapidly or anesthesia will not be achieved.

Methohexital has been used to induce anesthesia in calves at the rate of 3 to 5 mg/kg. A smooth, rapid induction enabling endotracheal intubation is produced.[43] In adult cattle, the dose for induction is 6 mg/kg.[44]

A high percentage of the metabolites of methohexital is excreted in the bile of dogs and rats. Following administration of [14C]methohexital to dogs and rats, 30.1% and 82.7% of the radioactivity is found in the feces, respectively. Dogs excrete 21.7% in bile and urine in the first hour and 52.4% in 8 h.[45]

Thiobarbiturates
Thiopental Sodium

Thiopental was the first thiobarbiturate to gain popularity as an anesthetic agent for animals. It is the thio analog of pentobarbital sodium, and differs only in that the number 2 carbon has a sulfur atom instead of an oxygen atom attached to it. Thiopental sodium is a yellow crystalline powder that is unstable in aqueous solution or when it is exposed to atmospheric air. For this reason, it is dispensed in sealed containers as a powder buffered with sodium carbonate. It is usually mixed with sterile water or saline to form 2.5%, 5.0%, or 10% solutions. Thiopental solutions should be stored in a refrigerator at 5° to 6°C (41° to 42°F) to retard deterioration. As solutions age, they become turbid and crystals precipitate, which results in progressive loss of activity, but does not increase its toxicity. Because the potency is decreased, larger quantities of solution must be used to produce the desired effect.[46]

The metabolism of thiopental is exceedingly complex. Following injection with thiopental containing radioactive sulfur (^{35}S), monkeys produce at least 12 different metabolic products that are excreted in the urine. About 86% is found in the urine within 4 days after intravenous injection; small amounts are also found in the tissues and feces.[47]

The initial toxic effect produced by thiopental is a marked depression of the respiratory centers. Both rate and amplitude are affected. By 5 min after administration of thiopental, heart rate, aortic pressure, peripheral vascular resistance, and left ventricular systolic and end-diastolic pressures increase.[48] Bigeminy is common. Cardiac arrhythmias associated with thiobarbiturate anesthesia can be accentuated by xylazine, halothane, methoxyflurane, and epinephrine.[49–52] Observed arrhythmias include sinus tachycardia, bigeminy, extrasystoles, ventricular tachycardia, multifocal ventricular tachycardia, and ventricular fibrillation. Administration of a lidocaine bolus concurrently with thiopental (11 mg/kg) reduces the cardiopulmonary depressive effects of the latter and has been advocated for anesthetic induction of patients predisposed to cardiac arrhythmias.[48]

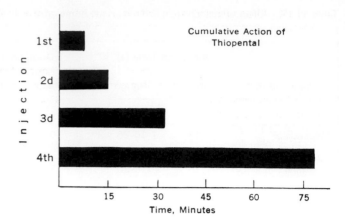

Fig. 11.8. The average duration of anesthesia after successive hourly intravenous injections of equal doses of thiopental to dogs. From Wyngaarden et al.[141]

During prolonged thiopental anesthesia, there is a pronounced hyperglycemia, increased lactic acid and amino acids in blood, and decreased liver glycogen.[53] Insulin either prevents a decrease or favors increased storage of liver glycogen. Repeated doses of thiopental have a cumulative effect, as shown in Figure 11.8. Prolonged periods of anesthesia may result from this effect if numerous doses are administered.

Thiopental has an ultrashort action because it is rapidly redistributed (e.g., into muscle tissue) and becomes localized in body fat.[54] As concentrations in the plasma, muscle, and viscera fall, the thiopental concentration in fat continues to rise. On the other hand, an appreciable amount is metabolized by the liver, and this contributes to the early rapid reduction of arterial thiopental concentration.[55] The same effect occurs after a fatty meal. A high chylomicron level in the blood reduces sleeping time significantly because thiopental is in more intimate contact with chylomicrons and a smaller diffusion distance is present. Blood fat is more potent than depot fat in decreasing thiopental sleeping time.[56] Leukopenia, hyperglycemia, elevated arterial partial pressure of carbon dioxide, and decreased arterial partial pressure of oxygen have been observed in thiopental-anesthetized horses (Table 11.12) and are comparable to changes observed with the use of other barbiturates and in other species.

For small animals, 1.25%, 2.5%, and 5.0% solutions of thiopental are used, depending on the animal's size. Whenever convenient, the more dilute solutions should be used, because overdosing is less likely and irritation is less in the event of accidental perivascular injection. As in other species, thiopental may be used in dogs and cats as the sole anesthetic or for induction prior to inhalation anesthesia. For rapid induction of anesthesia of short duration, the dose is 10 to 12 mg/kg. Should 10 to 20 min of surgical anesthesia be required, the dose range is 20 to 30 mg/kg. One-third of the estimated dose is injected rapidly within 15 s, and the remainder is administered slowly to effect. Additional doses may be administered to prolong anesthesia when required. Following large-dose administration, recovery (to standing) usually requires 1 to 1.5 h. Large doses will saturate the

Table 11.12. Mean values of the parameters listed below after a single intravenous anesthetic dosage of thiopental sodium in 8 horses[a].

	Preanesthetic Value	Minutes After Administering Anesthesia			Statistical Differences
		5	15	25	
Leukocyte count cell/mm^3	9700	7800	7500	6100	I
Packed-cell volume (vol %)	32	31	30.5	31	
Blood glucose (mg %)	82.1	85.0	91.2	103.1	I
Heart rate[b] (per min)	61	85	95	81	I
Blood pressure[c] (mm Hg)					
Systolic/diastolic	158/117	188/153	173/141	176/140	I
Respiratory rate[c] (per min)	29	8	14	21	I
Oxygen content of arterial blood (vol %)	19.2	19.0	18.2	18.4	II
Oxygen content of venous blood (vol %)	14.3	13.5	13.0	12.8	II
Carbon dioxide content of arterial blood (PaCO$_2$)	43.3	44.2	49.9	49.2	I
Arterial blood (pH)	7.39	7.31	7.21	7.22	I
Plasma level of thiopental sodium (mg/L)	—	49.3	37.1	35.8	I

[a]To produce surgical anesthesia, 9 to 17 mg/kg were required.
[b]Mean values in six horses because of equipment failure.
[c]Mean values in five horses because of equipment failure.
I Statistically significant difference at the 1% level before and after administration of thiopental sodium.
II Statistically significant difference at the 5% level before and after administration of thiopental sodium.
From Tyagi et al.[138]

tissues and cause a prolonged emergence. When induction is preceded by preanesthetic sedation, a dose range of 8 to 15 mg/kg is used. As in other species, too large a dose prior to inhalation anesthesia depresses respiration and impairs the uptake of inhaled gases. The use of thiopental is contraindicated in neonates and in feline porphyria.

Thiopental was commonly used for rapid induction of anesthesia in horses during the 1950s and early 1960s. After preanesthetic sedation with a suitable tranquilizer (e.g., xylazine or acepromazine), 6 to 10 mg/kg of thiopental are injected IV. If injected as rapidly as possible, 6 to 9 mg/kg are adequate. The smaller dose is used prior to the use of inhalant anesthetics, whereas the larger dose is used when a short period of surgical anesthesia is required. Thiopental is more commonly mixed with 5% guaifenesin when used for equine anesthesia. Two or three grams of thiopental are added to 1 L of 5% guaifenesin and administered rapidly IV to effect. It is often preceded by tranquilization with xylazine, detomidine, or acetylpromazine. The time of induction can be decreased by administering an additional 1 g of thiopental as an adult horse (400 to 500 kg) begins to relax. Once the horse is recumbent, the anesthesia can be maintained by continuing the infusion of thiopental and guaifenesin at a slower rate or by intubating and administering an inhalant anesthetic. The induction dose alone will produce anesthesia lasting 10 to 20 min. Total anesthesia time should be limited to less than 1 h when the combination of thiopental and guaifenesin is used as the maintenance anesthetic or recovery can be very prolonged and of poor quality. To minimize the recovery time when thiopental and guaifenesin are used for anesthetic maintenance, the amount of thiopental should be decreased by 50% in subsequent liters of the mixture.

Similar doses of thiopental alone (4 to 6 mg/kg) or with 5% guaifenesin in 5% dextrose in water may be given to induce anesthesia in cows. Once anesthesia is induced in cattle, endotracheal intubation is essential to prevent possible aspiration of rumen contents. The possibility of this is reduced by positioning animals so that the anterior thoracic and caudal cervical region is higher than any other part of the body. As in newborn foals, use of thiopental is contraindicated in the neonatal calves. Thiopental is also used in doses of 8 to 15 mg/kg in small ruminants. Rapid intravenous induction can be achieved with 8 to 12 mg/kg, whereas larger doses are given by slow intravenous injection to effect. The latter technique provides 10 to 20 min of surgical anesthesia.

The dose of thiopental required to induce anesthesia in swine is variable. The minimal dose required ranges from 4.0 to 8.0 mg/kg. Half the dose is injected rapidly, and the remainder more slowly over the next several minutes. Even during light anesthesia, respiratory depression, irregular breathing, and apnea commonly occur in swine.

Thiamylal Sodium

This is the thio analog of the barbiturate secobarbital sodium. It differs from thiopental sodium in that the ethyl radical of the latter (on R$_1$) is replaced by an allyl radical.[57] In dogs, the anesthetic potency of thiamylal is about 1.5 times that of thiopental.[58]

Administration

Barbiturates are administered by several routes, depending on the patient and the desired effect. For anesthesia, the intravenous route is preferable because the anesthetic can be given to effect. Because of wide variation in patient response, this type of dose control is desirable. Intraperitoneal administration and intramuscular administration are not widely employed. The oral route is slow and unpredictable, and therefore is used chiefly when sedation is sought.

Care should be taken in selection of needles and syringes for administration. In large species of animals, 12- to 18-gauge 1.5- to 2.0-inch needles are used, depending on the quantity of anesthetic that must be injected rapidly to carry the patient through the excitement stage. When large quantities are to be injected, a vascular catheter is preferred. In smaller animals, 20- to 24-gauge needles aid in venipuncture and help slow the rate of injection. There is a careless tendency to use large syringes on very small animals. This is dangerous because the dose cannot be accurately controlled. A syringe size commensurate with the dose should always be employed; use of large syringes with small doses is an invitation to disaster.

In many practices, an indwelling venous catheter is inserted prior to anesthetic administration. This is used for anesthetic injection and subsequent fluid administration during surgery. It also helps ensure that inadvertent perivascular injection does not occur when animals are transported. In small animals (weighing less than 5 kg), it is advisable to dilute the anesthetic with sterile water. By making a 100% dilution, more accurate dose control is achieved.

When intravenous injection is to be made, hair over the vein may be removed with clippers and the skin prepared by swabbing with a suitable antiseptic. The latter procedure, in addition to cleaning the area, tends to distend the vein. For intravenous anesthesia, the cephalic vein on the anterior aspect of the forelimb is most commonly used in small animals. In dogs, the second choice is generally the saphenous vein on the lateral surface of the hind limb just proximal to the hock. In cats, the saphenous or femoral vein on the inner surface of the thigh is a good second choice. Other veins less frequently used are the jugular and the marginal vein of the ear. In large dogs already anesthetized, the lingual veins on the ventral surface of the tongue are easily accessible. These veins tend to bleed rather profusely, however. In horses, cattle, and sheep, the jugular vein is used almost exclusively. In swine, the marginal vein of the ear or the anterior vena cava is most commonly employed.

In dogs, if injection is to be made into the cephalic vein of the right foreleg, the assistant stands by the animal's left side with the left arm circling the dog's neck and the right arm extended over its back. The right hand grasps the right foreleg just below the elbow. The right index finger is extended over the dorsal surface of the limb, the thumb is held around the ventral surface of the leg, and, by compressing thumb and forefinger, the vein is occluded, causing it to distend with blood. The assistant turns his or her wrist slightly so that the skin covering the dorsal aspect of the foreleg and the cephalic vein is rotated outward. The veterinarian grasps the paw of the right foot with the left hand and, if the vein is not easily seen, by rapidly squeezing the paw several times, pumps blood from the paw to distend the vein. If the carpus is flexed acutely, the vein is stretched tightly over the underlying muscles and rolling is prevented. Good technique demands that the needle used for injection be threaded into the vein so that the hub is at the site of venipuncture. The leg and syringe are both held in the veterinarian's left hand during injection so they will move as a unit if the animal moves. This prevents accidental retraction of the needle from the vein.

Persons experienced with administration of barbiturates to dogs and cats usually estimate the weight of the animal and draw an excess of solution into a syringe. The first one-third to one-half of the dose is rapidly injected while watching the animal's facial expression closely. As injection is made, the animal often licks its lips as though tasting the drug. Frequently, dogs move the head from side to side as the anesthetic effect begins. These movements are seen early in the administration and indicate more drug must be given. The eyes begin to lose their alert expression, and the animal then relaxes. As injection is continued, the veterinarian can, with thumb and forefinger placed behind the canine teeth, open the animal's jaw. If in a light state of anesthesia, the patient will further open the jaw, curl the tongue, and simulate a yawn. At this point, the cornea and pedal reflexes are still present, and the animal is not in a state of surgical anesthesia. Administration of anesthetic should be continued cautiously and in small amounts, with careful attention paid to respiration and reflexes. Surgical anesthesia is reached when the pedal reflex is abolished. At this point, further administration of drug is not necessary.

Intraperitoneal Injection

This has been employed extensively in the past, but has the disadvantage that the dose cannot be as accurately controlled as it can by intravenous administration. Usually with this method, the animal is restrained in a vertical position against the assistant's body with the animal's abdomen facing outward. An area just lateral to the umbilicus is clipped and a suitable antiseptic applied. The needle is passed through the abdominal wall and the injection made. The dose for intraperitoneal administration is calculated in the same manner as the intravenous dose. The peak concentration in the blood is reached more slowly, and drug absorbed into the portal system is subject to early metabolism.[34] This technique is not recommended in the clinical practice of veterinary anesthesia and may be quite painful to the animal.

Intramuscular and Intrathoracic Injection

Under unusual circumstances, such as when wild animals are anesthetized, intramuscular or subcutaneous injection of barbiturates may be indicated. Because of their high alkalinity, there is a tendency for tissue necrosis to develop following this procedure. For moderate anesthesia, 30 mg/kg, and for surgical anesthesia of 1 to 2 h, 40 mg/kg of pentobarbital can be administered. Induction requires about 15 min, and anesthesia reaches its peak effect about 30 min after injection.

Although pentobarbital has been given intrathoracically using the same dose as for intravenous anesthesia, veterinarians should strongly oppose intrathoracic administration of anesthetic because there is risk of puncture to the heart, pericardium, and lung, and barbiturates irritate the serosal surfaces. The latter fact can be confirmed on necropsy of animals destroyed with intrathoracic barbiturates. Pleural thickening, bronchitis, and coagulative necrosis of the lung have been observed on examination of experimentally injected cats.

In general, thiobarbiturates produce more respiratory depression on induction than do oxybarbiturates: Often one-third of the calculated dose causes the patient to collapse and respiration to stop. This transient apnea is alarming to those not aware of this reaction. When it occurs, injection of anesthetic should be suspended until spontaneous rhythmic respirations resume. This usually occurs as soon as the blood carbon dioxide level rises to stimulate respiration and rapid redistribution decreases CNS concentration.

Barbiturate Slough

Occasionally, animals may struggle during induction of barbiturate anesthesia, and some of the drug may be administered perivascularly. This should be avoided if at all possible because a tissue slough may develop. Experienced anesthetists prevent barbiturate slough by threading the needle into the vein. This procedure makes it unlikely that the needle will come out of the vein if the syringe is jarred or the animal moves. Sloughs caused by anesthesia require 2 to 4 weeks to heal and leave an unsightly scar. Nothing can infuriate owners more than development of a slough in their animal.

If it is suspected that barbiturate solution has been injected perivascularly, the area should be infiltrated with 1 or 2 mL of 2% procaine solution.[59] Lidocaine can also be used for this purpose. Local anesthetics are effective for two reasons. First, they are vasodilators and prevent vasospasm in the area, and thus aid in dilution and absorption of the barbiturate. Second, they are broken down in an alkaline medium, and this reaction neutralizes the alkali (barbiturate). The use of hot packs or hydrotherapy may be beneficial, as is infiltration of the area with saline to dilute the barbiturate further. Additionally, systemic antiinflammatory drugs may be of benefit.

Barbiturate Euthanasia

All of the euthanasia solutions that are commercially available in the United States contain pentobarbital as their active ingredient. Some include other drugs, but the additional ingredients do not make the product a more effective euthanasia agent. The combination products are schedule III controlled substances compared with the schedule II products that contain only pentobarbital. The usual dose of pentobarbital for euthanasia of dogs and cats is 120 mg/kg for the first 4.5 kg of body weight and 60 mg/kg for each additional 4.5 kg. Large animals usually require 10 to 15 mL per 45 kg of body weight. Pentobarbital should not be used for euthanasia of animals intended for consumption by people or other animals, and carcasses should be disposed of in a manner that prevents consumption by domestic or wild animals. Pentobarbital can be administered orally as a sedative prior to euthanasia. The dose is approximately 60 mg/kg, and the time to lateral recumbency is approximately 60 min.

Nonbarbiturate Drugs

Although the barbiturates have been the most commonly used short-acting anesthetics, many other injectable drugs have been used to induce and maintain unconsciousness. Chloral hydrate alone and in combination with magnesium sulfate and pentobarbital sodium has been used for induction and maintenance of anesthesia in large domestic animals (i.e., horses and cows). Many drugs used to depress the CNS and immobilize laboratory animals do not find application in routine small animal clinical use. Among them are chloral hydrate, chloralose, urethan, metomidate, and magnesium sulfate. Newer drugs, such as etomidate and propofol, have been developed to provide short periods of unconsciousness from which recovery is rapid. These hypnotic drugs are most effective when given in combination with preanesthetics and analgesics to achieve anesthesia and analgesia. Several of these combinations have recently been developed and assessed for use in animal anesthesia.

Neurosteroids

This class of drugs was first evaluated as a combination of two steroids: alphaxalone and alphadolone acetate (Althesin or Saffan). The solubility of alphaxalone (9 mg/mL) is increased by alphadolone acetate (3 mg/mL) and by 20% wt/vol polyoxyethylated castor oil (Cremophor EL). The combination of the two steroids has an exceptionally high therapeutic index (30.6). It has little cumulative effect (Fig. 11.9), and the duration of anesthesia varies with species (Fig. 11.10). Administration of the combination before or after barbiturates is not advised, although adverse effects when used with other anesthetic drugs have not been reported. Evidence suggests the neurosteroid anesthetics work by enhancing GABA-mediated neurodepression.[60,61] In addition, the activation of centrally located inhibitory glycine receptors may be involved.[61]

A new neurosteroid product has been developed that is a 10-mg/mL solution of alphaxalone in 2-hydroxypropyl-ß-cyclodextrin (Alfaxan-CD; Jurox, Rutherford, Australia). This preparation does not appear to cause histamine release, which has been associated with the vehicle used in earlier neurosteroid preparations.[62]

In cats, the dose of Althesin is 9 mg/kg for intravenous administration and 12 to 18 mg/kg for intramuscular administration. Intravenous injection produces relaxation in approximately 9 s and surgical anesthesia in about 25 s. Intramuscular administration produces variable results, but may be useful in fractious animals. The onset occurs in 6 to 12 min and lasts for approximately 15 min. A quiet area for induction is desirable. In fractious cats, when drugs must be administered intramuscularly, ketamine is the drug of choice because Althesin is less reliable by this route.[63]

Althesin has a neutral pH and does not produce pain or inflammation when injected perivascularly or intramuscularly. Additional doses can be given to prolong anesthesia without cumulative effects, and recovery is rapid. In contrast to ketamine, Althesin produces good muscular relaxation. Althesin has a slightly protective effect against epinephrine-induced arrhythmias in cats.[64] Urination, defecation, muscle tremors, paddling, salivation, and hyperesthesia have been reported as side effects. Edema of the feet, ears, and muzzle occurs in approximately 25% of cats injected, but is usually transient and disappears within 2

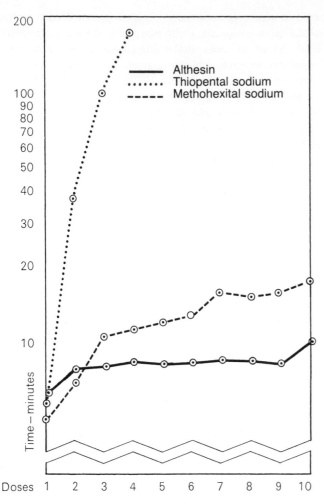

Fig. 11.9. Duration of loss of righting reflex in mice given repeated intravenous doses of Althesin and other anesthetics (five mice per group). Second and subsequent doses were given 30 s after return of the righting reflex. After Child et al.[65]

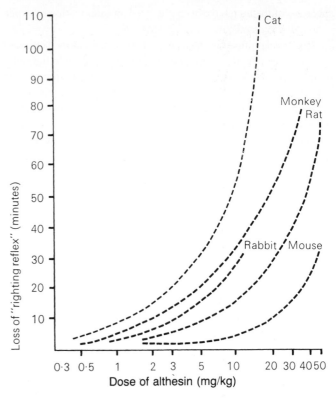

Fig. 11.10. Anesthetic activity of Althesin in different species. After Child et al.[65]

h. This condition apparently occurs in females more often than in males. Antihistamine administration reduces this occurrence.

In dogs and some other canidae, the use of polyoxyethylene derivatives of hexitol anhydride partial fatty acid esters produces an allergic response.[65] This response is manifested by a prolonged fall in blood pressure and a positive skin wheal if the drug is injected intradermally. Urticaria and erythema are believed to be caused by the release of histamine or histamine-like substances. Cremophor EL, a nonionic polyoxyethylated emulsifying agent used as the vehicle in Althesin, elicits the same response. Apparently, allergic reactions can be caused by the vehicle (polyoxyethylated castor oil). The reaction can be of the true-hypersensitivity type, which requires previous exposure to the drug, or of the complement-activation type, which requires no previous sensitization.[66]

Horses anesthetized with Althesin can develop violent paddling and galloping movements during recovery, which can be prevented by prior administration of xylazine (1 mg/kg).[67] The minimum dose of Althesin for induction of anesthesia is approx-

imately 1.2 to 1.34 mg/kg in non-premedicated horses. Although xylazine administration lengthens the recovery time, its administration would appear prudent.

The dose of Althesin for sheep is approximately 2.2 mg/kg IV. This produces light surgical anesthesia for 8 to 15 min. The average maintenance dose to produce surgical anesthesia for a 3-h period is 0.23 mg · kg^{-1} · min^{-1}. Sheep given Althesin develop bradycardia, with a decrease in systolic and diastolic pressures of 20% to 35% of preinjection levels. Left ventricular end-diastolic pressure elevates, and cardiac output decreases. These parameters return to normal within 6 to 8 min of injection. Myocardial depression measured as a decrease in maximum dp/dt is produced.[67] Althesin has also been used to induce anesthesia prior to the administration of inhalants to maintain anesthesia in ruminants (goats, sheep, and young calves).[68] The dose of Althesin for pigs is approximately 6 mg/kg to produce 10 to 15 min of anesthesia. In pigs known to develop malignant hyperthermia under anesthesia, Althesin does not induce this reaction, and it has been used safely in animals known to be susceptible to this condition.[67]

Althesin decreases cerebral blood flow accompanied by a fall in intracranial pressure in baboons.[69] Neither of the two steroids is extensively protein bound by the serum of rats, cats, horses, or people. Approximately 60% to 70% of a radioactive dose of alphaxalone or alphadolone acetate is excreted as metabolic products in the feces during the 5 days following intravenous injection; the other 20% to 30% appears in the urine within the same period.[70]

Chloral Hydrate

Liebrich, who introduced chloral hydrate as a hypnotic in 1869, thought that, because it released chloroform in vitro, it would do the same in vivo. This has subsequently been proved a misconception. Chloral hydrate occurs as colorless translucent crystals that volatilize with an aromatic, penetrating odor on exposure to air. It has a bitter, caustic taste. One gram of the crystals dissolves in 0.25 mL of water. It may be administered orally, or solutions may be injected IV or intraperitoneally. It irritates the gastric mucosa and may cause vomiting if not diluted in water, but is readily absorbed from the gastrointestinal tract. A small amount of chloral hydrate is excreted unchanged in the urine. The greater portion is reduced to trichloroethyl alcohol, a less potent hypnotic, and this in turn is conjugated with glucuronic acid to form urochloralic (trichloroethylglucuronic) acid, which has no hypnotic property. The latter is excreted in the urine. In animals with liver damage, chloral hydrate may be found in larger quantities and urochloralic acid in smaller quantities in the urine.

Chloral hydrate depresses the cerebrum, with loss of reflex excitability. In subanesthetic doses, motor and sensory nerves are not affected. Chloral hydrate is a good hypnotic but a poor anesthetic; the amount needed to produce anesthesia approaches the minimal lethal dose, and it produces deep sleep that lasts for several hours. It has weak analgesic action. In hypnotic doses, the medullary centers are not affected. Anesthetic doses of chloral hydrate depress the vasomotor center severely, causing a fall in blood pressure. Hypnotic doses depress respiration, and anesthetic doses markedly depress the respiratory center. Death from chloral hydrate administration is caused by progressive depression of the respiratory center. The margin of safety is such that it is not a satisfactory surgical anesthetic.

Chloral hydrate is not used for small animal anesthesia and has lost most of its popularity as a general anesthetic in large animals. Its continued use in large animals depends on the simplicity of administration and on the duration of effect of the induction dose—an interval adequate for many routine procedures. It is relatively inexpensive and may be combined with barbiturates. It is an irritant when inadvertently injected outside the vein. Use of a vascular catheter obviates this hazard. The concentration of the chloral hydrate solution should not be too high: 7% to 12% wt/vol aqueous solutions are generally used.

Doses reported for intravenous chloral hydrate vary extensively, probably owing to the rate of administration and to varying interpretations of the depth of resulting anesthesia. The recommended intravenous dose for chloral hydrate in horses varies from 2 to 3 g/45 kg as a sedative and up to 10 g/45 kg when used alone for general anesthesia. When the drug is used to enhance xylazine or xylazine-butorphanol sedation, a dose of 0.6 to 1.2 g/45 kg is usually effective. A dose of 1.8 g/45 kg may be necessary. This mixture of drugs can be used to provide effective standing restraint during low epidural analgesia achieved with a local anesthetic in horses undergoing surgical correction of a rectovaginal fistula.

Chloral hydrate solution was once commonly administered at 15 to 30 g/min and was given until the horse was about to fall, at which time the intravenous tubing was disconnected and the ani-

mal restrained until recumbent. If necessary, additional solution was administered slowly until the desired degree of sedation or anesthesia was achieved. Because of conversion to trichloroethanol and slow passage across the blood-brain barrier, anesthetic depression increases for several minutes after initial induction. Therefore, additional doses should not be administered immediately. The chief disadvantage with chloral hydrate is that the dose required to induce general anesthesia prolongs recovery. For this reason, in modern practice, chloral hydrate is primarily used to induce a degree of narcosis or sedation, and analgesia is produced by means of local or regional anesthesia. Premedication with tranquilizers reduces the amount of chloral hydrate required, facilitates induction, and minimizes struggling during recovery.[71]

The time required for horses to stand after cessation of administration of anesthetic doses varies from 1 to 4 h and is similar in duration to that observed after chloral hydrate and magnesium sulfate administration. If anesthesia is maintained for a long period, recovery may also be prolonged. The nature of the recovery period can vary; if left undisturbed, horses often pass quietly into a hypnotic state, remaining thus until they are ready to stand. Excitement and struggling during recovery are not uncommon and can be minimized by use of tranquilizers.

Chloral hydrate is also occasionally used to induce narcosis or anesthesia in cattle and swine. In the former, it has been largely replaced by xylazine. The chloral hydrate dose required is similar to that for horses. In cattle, premedication with atropine sulfate and early intubation are indicated. Chloral hydrate may also be administered to horses and cattle by stomach tube to induce varying degrees of sedation or narcosis (3 to 6 g/45 kg of body weight).

Chloral hydrate has been combined with magnesium sulfate or with magnesium sulfate and pentobarbital sodium for anesthesia in horses and cattle (Fig. 11.11). Investigators claimed that these drug combinations produced a more rapid and excitement-free induction, an increased anesthetic depth, a smoother emergence, a wider margin of safety, and less irritation than does anesthesia achieved with chloral hydrate alone. Nevertheless, with the advent of rapid-onset, short-acting, and safer drugs, there seems to be little merit in the use of chloral hydrate alone or in combination with other drugs to induce and maintain anesthesia in any species.

Chloralose

This is prepared by heating anhydrous glucose and trichloroacetaldehyde (anhydrous chloral) in a water bath. Both α-chloralose and ß-chloralose are formed, with the α form being active. Chloralose has been advocated for use in cardiovascular studies because it produces minimal depression and maintains more active reflexes than other anesthetics.[72]

Chloralose is usually prepared as a 1.0% aqueous solution. Heat is necessary to dissolve the drug, but solutions should not be boiled. The intravenous anesthetic dose of α-chloralose is approximately 110 mg/kg in dogs and 80 mg/kg in adult cats.[73] α-Chloralose appears to depress neuronal function of the cortex and routes of afferent input less than pentobarbital. Many investigators still consider chloralose a valuable drug for maintenance of unconsciousness for long, nonsurvival, surgical experiments.[74]

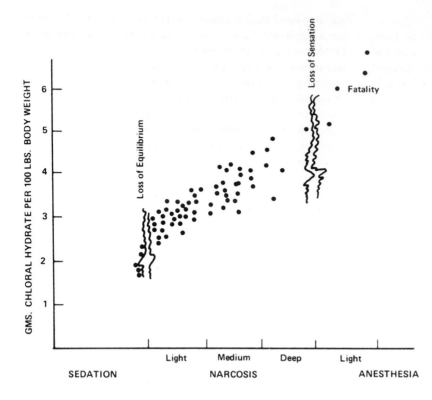

Fig. 11.11. Chloral hydrate and magnesium sulfate anesthesia (2:1) in horses: dose of chloral hydrate used and degree of anesthesia obtained in clinical cases.

Urethan

This is prepared by heating urea with alcohol under pressure or by warming urea nitrate with alcohol and sodium nitrite. The drug is marketed in the crystalline state. One gram dissolves in 0.5 mL of water, the aqueous solution being neutral. It is most often used as an anesthetic in laboratory animals and fish. The lethal intravenous dose for rabbits is 2.0 g/kg. The dose for dogs and cats is 0.6 to 2.0 g/kg. Up to 0.5 g/kg may be used as a hypnotic dose.

Urethan is mutagenic, carcinostatic, and carcinogenic.[75] Mice given urethan develop an exceptionally high incidence of lung tumors, regardless of the route of administration. Tumors also develop in treated rats and rabbits. Concern over the health of individuals in prolonged contact with urethan or its solutions is justified.[76] For this reason, urethan is no longer commonly used in any species.

Magnesium Sulfate

A saturated solution of magnesium sulfate has been used for euthanasia. However, it should be administered only after animals have been rendered unconscious with a barbiturate or another rapid-acting anesthetic. In small animals, anesthesia has been achieved with dilute solutions of magnesium sulfate; however, the CNS is globally depressed and respiratory arrest often occurs at anesthetic doses. Animals will become excited just prior to collapse. Respiratory arrest likely is caused by complete neuromuscular block and paralysis of the muscles of respiration rather than being a consequence of CNS depression. Therefore, one cannot be assured that magnesium sulfate administered alone is

a humane method for achieving anesthesia or euthanasia. Magnesium sulfate is better thought of as a muscle relaxant and CNS depressant than as a stand-alone anesthetic and is not recommended as such.

Metomidate

Metomidate hydrochloride is a hypnotic with muscle relaxant properties. Its hypnotic effect is exerted on mammals, birds, reptiles, and fish. Given alone, it induces sleep without analgesia. General anesthesia can be produced by combining it with neuroleptics or analgesics. It is available in powdered form, which dissolves readily in water to make 1% or 5% solutions. These solutions have a pH of 2.9 and 2.4, respectively. Combined with the butyrophenone tranquilizer azaperone, metomidate produces anesthesia in swine for approximately 2 h. Respiration slows and deepens. With rapid intravenous injection, apnea may occur. The cardiovascular system remains stable. It is often used as a sedative-anesthetic for fish.

Etomidate

This is an imidazole derivative that was synthesized in 1965 and first used for induction of anesthesia in people in 1975. It is a congener of metomidate and contains 2 mg/mL of the drug in 35% propylene glycol. Etomidate appears to work in a fashion similar to that of propofol and the barbiturates in that it enhances the action of the inhibitory neurotransmitter GABA.[77,78] Single injections produce relatively brief hypnosis. In dogs, doses of 1.5 and 3.0 mg/kg last 8 ± 5 and 21 ± 9 min, respectively.[79] The duration of hypnosis is dose related. Etomidate is rapidly hydrolyzed in the liver and excreted in the urine. The pharmacokinetics of a 3-mg/kg intravenous dose of etomidate in cats are best described as a three-compartment open model similar to those determined in people and rats. Induction and recovery are rapid, with a brief period of myoclonus early in the recovery period.[80]

Etomidate in powder and injectable forms has been used as an anesthetic for exotic species of animals. It was introduced in the United States as an induction agent for poor-risk human patients because it does not depress the cardiovascular and respiratory systems or release histamine. When used alone in dogs, it produces no change in heart rate, blood pressure, or myocardial performance.[79] Neonates born to mothers anesthetized with etomidate have minimal respiratory depression. Etomidate does not trigger malignant hyperthermia in susceptible swine.[81] Etomidate qualifies as a good induction drug for neurosurgical procedures. It decreases cerebral metabolic rate of oxygen consumption ($CMRO_2$) and has anticonvulsant properties. It may have brain-protective properties following episodes of global ischemia associated with cardiac arrest.

Etomidate inhibits adrenal steroidogenesis in dogs, suppressing the usual increase in plasma cortisol observed during surgery. A single induction dose of etomidate may depress adrenal function for up to 3 h. However, the lack of a stress response to surgery does not have deleterious effects, and it has been argued that attenuation of metabolic and endocrine responses to surgery actually reduces morbidity and may make this unique action of etomidate beneficial to overall patient outcome. Attention has been given to the development of Addisonian crisis produced by etomidate-induced blockade of corticosteroid production during prolonged infusion to maintain sedation in intensive care patients. Consequently, long-term infusion is not recommended.[82,83] Etomidate (2 mg/kg) can cause acute hemolysis. The mechanism of hemolysis appears to be propylene glycol, which causes a rapid osmolality increase that causes red cell rupture.[84]

Etomidate is compatible with other common preanesthetic agents. Venous pain is common on injection in humans, and myoclonia may occur if premedication is not administered. Nausea and vomiting are troublesome, especially after the use of multiple doses, and can occur at recovery, as well as induction. For the most part, these side effects can be prevented by adequate preanesthetic sedation. In summary, etomidate may be one of the better induction drugs in traumatized patients and those with severe myocardial disease, cardiovascular instability, cirrhosis, or intracranial lesions, or in patients requiring cesarean section surgery.[81]

Propofol

Propofol (2,6-diisopropylphenol) is unrelated to barbiturates, euganols, or steroid anesthetics. It is only slightly soluble in water and is marketed as an aqueous emulsion containing 10 mg of propofol, 100 mg of soybean oil, 22.5 mg of glycerol, and 12 mg of egg lecithin/mL. Sodium hydroxide is added to adjust the pH. It is available in sterile glass ampules and contains no preservatives. Propofol emulsion can support microbial growth and endotoxin production.[85] Because of the potential for iatrogenic sepsis, unused propofol remaining in an open ampule should be discarded and not be kept overnight for use the next day. Some formulations contain bacterial growth inhibitors to slow the growth rate of contaminants after a vial is opened, but these additives will not completely inhibit bacterial growth, so any unused propofol should still be discarded 6 h after a vial or ampule is opened. The growth inhibitors used are 0.005% disodium edentate or 0.025% sodium metabisulfite.

The pharmacokinetics of propofol in dogs fit a two-compartment open model. Rapid onset of action is caused by rapid uptake into the CNS. The short action and rapid smooth emergence result from rapid redistribution from the brain to other tissues and efficient elimination from plasma by metabolism.[86] Propofol has a large volume of distribution, as would be expected from its lipophilic nature. It is metabolized primarily by conjugation, but propofol's rapid disappearance from plasma is greater than hepatic blood flow, suggesting extra hepatic sites of metabolism.[87] The pharmacokinetics of propofol have not been reported in cats, but its anesthetic action is similar to that in dogs.[88] In general, after a single bolus injection, propofol induces a rapid, smooth induction followed by a short period of unconsciousness.[89] In people, recovery is rapid and free of emergence excitement after constant infusion or repeated bolus administration. In dogs, especially greyhounds, recoveries may be prolonged after continuous infusion of propofol exceeding 30 min.[90]

Propofol is usually injected as a single bolus for induction of general anesthesia in dogs and cats to enable intubation and initiation of inhalation anesthesia.[89] It should be remembered that propofol is a sedative-hypnotic and has only minimal analgesic action at a subanesthetic dose. As with other hypnotics, even when an animal is rendered unconscious with propofol, it will respond to painful stimuli unless analgesic drugs such as the opioids or α_2-agonists are administered concurrently. If administration is preceded by a preanesthetic such as morphine or medetomidine, the induction dose of propofol can be decreased substantially. The dose for induction of anesthesia in non-premedicated dogs ranges from 6 to 8 mg/kg IV, whereas the dose in sedated animals may be as low as 2 to 4 mg/kg IV.[85,86] Following a single dose of 6 mg/kg IV, recovery in dogs is complete in approximately 20 min. A similar dose given to cats provides about 30 min of anesthesia to complete recovery. The incidence of postanesthetic side effects, such as vomiting, sneezing, or pawing, is about 15%, but can be decreased with acepromazine or α_2-agonist premedication. When a patient is premedicated with 0.02 to 0.04 mg/kg of acepromazine, the induction dose of propofol is decreased by approximately 30% to 40%. Propofol can be used for maintenance of anesthesia in dogs either by intermittent bolus or continual infusion.[91,92] The rate of administration depends on the adjunctive drugs administered and the degree of surgical stimulation.[92] The continuous infusion rate ranges from 0.15 to 0.4 mg · kg^{-1} · min^{-1}. When using an intermittent-bolus technique, doses of 0.5 to 2 mg/kg are administered as needed. If the bolus dose used is kept constant, the interval between bolus administrations will stabilize and remain constant after 1 to 2 boluses are administered.

Propofol induces depression by enhancing the effects of the inhibitory neurotransmitter GABA and decreasing the brain's metabolic activity.[93] Propofol decreases intracranial and cerebral perfusion pressures. It transiently depresses arterial pressure and myocardial contractility similar to the ultra-short-acting thiobarbiturates. Hypotension is primarily the result of arterial and venous vasodilation.[94] Propofol enhances the arrhythmogenic effects of epinephrine, but is not inherently arrhythmogenic.[95]

Propofol is a phenolic compound and, as such, can induce oxidative injury to feline red blood cells when administered repeatedly over several days. This toxicity is likely the result of the cat's reduced ability to conjugate phenol. Heinz bodies form, and clinical signs of anorexia, diarrhea, and malaise can result.[96] Brief apnea may occur after induction with propofol. Animals breathing spontaneously may experience hypercapnia for a short period after rapid bolus injection.[97] Propofol is primarily metabolized in the liver by conjugation pathways to form inactive metabolites, which are then excreted in the urine and, to a much lesser extent, in bile.[98] Evidence suggests a variability in the capacity of the hepatic cytochrome P-450 enzyme system involved in propofol metabolism among dog breeds.[99] This may explain some of the breed variability in recovery times seen after propofol administration (e.g., the slower recoveries seen in greyhounds). Propofol has been used for cesarean section surgery with generally good results.[89,100] Because puppies have good conjugation enzyme activity, there is minimal fetal depression among neonates delivered from mothers anesthetized with propofol.

Complaints of pain by people injected with propofol IV are common. Pain likely occurs in small animals, but the prevalence appears to be much less. Pain can be minimized by premedication with an opioid or α_2-agonist and/or injection into larger vessels. Propofol, unlike barbiturates, does not damage tissue when injected perivascularly or intra-arterially. When combined with an opioid, acepromazine, or an α_2-agonist, propofol provides dependable short anesthesia for procedures such as castrations, ear flushes, exploration for foxtails, ultrasound examinations, biopsies, and suturing of small lacerations. Additionally, the advantage of rapid smooth recovery is beneficial in patients with chronic respiratory disease or those undergoing bronchoscopy or transtracheal aspiration procedures. Light propofol anesthesia has been advocated for patients undergoing upper-airway examination.[101]

Propofol is a satisfactory drug for immobilization of neonatal foals when given in combination with 0.5 mg/kg of xylazine IV. Immobilization is induced with 2 mg/kg propofol IV and maintained with 0.33 mg · kg^{-1} · min^{-1} IV. Cardiovascular changes are characterized by decreased pressure and cardiac output, and a decrease in respiration rate.

Propofol anesthesia has been used in full-sized horses, as well. It is usually employed in conjunction with an α_2-agonist such as detomidine or xylazine and can be used to maintain, as well as induce, general anesthesia. The induction dose of propofol is 2 to 4 mg/kg administered IV to premedicated horses.[102–104] Limited data on maintenance of propofol anesthesia suggest an infusion rate of approximately 0.2 mg/kg/min is acceptable.[104] The quality of the induction and recovery seen with the use of propofol in horses is acceptable.[102–105]

Alternative Methods of Anesthesia and Analgesia

Hypothermia

As the body temperature of warm-blooded animals falls, their metabolism is reduced, and therefore the need for oxygen is diminished. Oxygen uptake in dogs is reduced by approximately 50% at 30°C and 65% at 25°C.[106] The metabolic rate of isolated slices of rat heart is reduced 90% by lowering the temperature to 10°C.[107] The potassium-arrested heart at 37°C used four times as much glycogen and produced three times as much lactic acid as the heart at 17°C.[108] Thus, the heart, brain, liver, or other vital organs can survive at a low temperature for a considerably increased period when deprived of all or a portion of their blood supply. Hypothermia may be artificially produced in the entire body or in only a portion, such as the heart or head. It has found its greatest usefulness in surgery of the heart and CNS.[109]

The colder an animal becomes, the less oxygen is required by a given organ. It has been shown, however, that the reduction of oxygen consumption varies for different organs. For example, the work done by the heart at 26° to 27°C is a little less than that at normal temperature, and while the general oxygen uptake by the body at this temperature is reduced to 40% of normal, that of the heart is still 50%. In monkeys, little change in cerebral oxygen uptake occurs until a temperature of 31°C is reached.[110] At this point, it falls sharply, and through the next 4°C there is a drop of about 25%. Below 27°C, oxygen consumption continues to fall, but at a much slower rate. The relationship of cerebral oxygen consumption to temperature is sigmoid rather than linear (Fig. 11.12).

Several species of warm-blooded animals have been subjected to drastic hypothermia. Small laboratory animals can be cooled to 0°C, and even lower, and still recover. Between 80% and 100% of rats recovered after being cooled to temperatures just above the freezing point with cardiac and respiratory arrest for 1 h.[111] Golden hamsters have been kept on ice with circulatory arrest for up to 7 h. These animals even survived supercooling to −5° or −6°C.[112] When the circulation is maintained with a pump-oxygenator, dogs have survived cooling to 1.5°C.[113]

To induce the hypothermic state as quickly as possible, shivering must be controlled, because it is an important mechanism in protection against cold. Shivering is induced by an increased temperature gradient between cold receptors in the skin and centers in the hypothalamus.[114] Even without visible shivering, there is general hypertonicity of the skeletal muscles, which results in increased metabolic, heart, and respiratory rates. Shivering can be prevented by deep anesthesia or by light anesthesia with curarization or tranquilization with a phenothiazine. The latter drugs exert their effect through a peripheral action on muscle fibers and on the hypothalamic temperature control center.

Moderate hypothermia produces a rectilinear decrease in anesthetic requirements (minimum alveolar concentration [MAC]) for cyclopropane, diethyl ether, fluroxene, halothane, and methoxyflurane (Fig. 11.13).[115] Moderate hypothermia also reduces the concentration of anesthetic required to produce apnea. There is little difference between halothane, pentobarbital, and

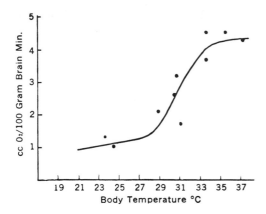

Fig. 11.12. Relation of oxygen uptake by the brain to temperature. From Bering et al.[110]

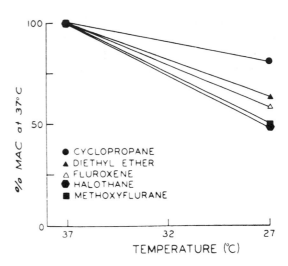

Fig. 11.13. The percentage decline between 37° and 27°C of the minimum alveolar concentration (MAC) required for anesthesia. Cyclopropane, the least oil-soluble agent, declines least, and halothane and methoxyflurane, the most oil-soluble agents, decline most. From Regan and Eger.[115]

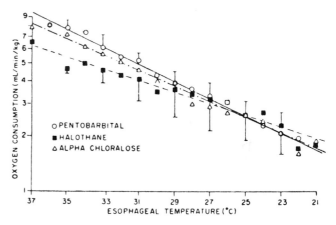

Fig. 11.14. Whole-body oxygen consumption compared with esophageal temperature during surface cooling in dogs. The least-squares best-fit lines are shown for three anesthetics: pentobarbital, halothane, and α-chloralose. Each point represents the mean, and each bar 1 SD. From Westenskow et al.[116]

chloralose in their effects on whole-body oxygen consumption during surface cooling in dogs (Fig. 11.14).[116]

Three methods of whole-body cooling have been used: surface, body cavity, and extracorporeal. *Surface cooling* is usually accomplished by directly immersing the unprotected body in ice water or by placing the body on a mattress through which ice water is circulated. Hyperventilation is maintained throughout the procedure to keep the blood pH on the alkaline side of normal. This has been shown to reduce cardiac arrhythmias and fibrillation. Below 28°C (82.4°F), no anesthetic is needed, and the patient is maintained on artificial ventilation alone. Active cooling is stopped when approximately two-thirds of the desired temperature fall has been accomplished. Otherwise, the temperature continues to drop once the desired degree of hypothermia has been reached.

Body cavity cooling is accomplished by pouring cold saline solution into the open thoracic cavity.[117] This method has the disadvantage of being slow and requiring large volumes of saline solution.

Extracorporeal cooling can be accomplished by running blood from a cannulated artery through a heat exchanger using cold tap water as the cooling medium. A pump is required to force the blood through the system. Thrombosis is prevented by administration of heparin. Extracorporeal cooling has been used to lower the brain temperature below that of the general body temperature, but carries with it the dangers of hemolysis, interference with the blood coagulation mechanism, and thrombosis. The most obvious advantage is that it provides the best control over body temperature, and rewarming can be performed quickly and efficiently by running warm water through the heat exchanger. Warming also may be accomplished by covering the patient with electric blankets or by using warm-water baths. Microwave rewarming has been used experimentally.[116]

Since hypothermia is a form of general anesthesia, it carries the risks of profound depression of the CNS and vital organs. In addition, it has its own hazards for the circulatory system, skin and internal organs, and metabolism. Blood pressure falls during hypothermia, owing to decreased cardiac output, whereas periph-

eral vascular resistance increases. Occasionally, blood pressure may drop severely. The fall in heart rate seen with hypothermia is caused by depression of the sinoatrial node and the bundle of His. These conduction changes are manifested by a prolonging of the PR interval, spreading of the QRS complex, and lengthening of the ST interval. In dogs, a cardiac crisis occurs between 23° and 15°C. This is characterized by cessation of sinus rhythm, intense bradycardia, ventricular extrasystoles, and ventricular fibrillation or standstill. As expected, atropine does not relieve the bradycardia. Ventricular fibrillation has been shown to occur most often when the temperature of the heart muscle is below

28°C and when the heart is manipulated. Fibrillation rapidly depletes cardiac muscle energy stores. It occurs less frequently in young animals than in adults. Hypercapnia with acidemia, hyperkalemia, and myocardial hypoxia also appears to cause fibrillation. The incidence of spontaneous ventricular fibrillation has been shown to vary with the anesthetic used to initiate hypothermia. For example, administration of pentobarbital produces a higher incidence than does use of thiopental or ether.[118]

Several cardioplegic solutions have been used to stop the heart and to prevent fibrillation. Hypothermia plus cardioplegia is more protective of cardiac tissue than is hypothermia alone.[119,120] Combined with deep hypothermia, cardioplegia solutions have provided 30 min of cardiac arrest without heart-lung bypass.

During hypothermia, clotting time is prolonged. In addition, the platelet count decreases, hemoconcentration occurs with sludging, and eosinophil and leukocyte counts decrease, accompanied by a fall in the mean corpuscular hemoglobin concentration.

Prolonged periods of hypothermia have detrimental effects on patients.[121–123] In dogs held at 29°C for 24 h, cardiac output and whole-body oxygen consumption decreased progressively to 7% and 28% of control, respectively. Cerebral blood flow and cerebral oxygen consumption responded similarly. On rewarming, cardiovascular collapse with severe tissue hypoxia and metabolic acidosis occurs. Cerebral blood flow becomes grossly inadequate, with depletion of brain energy stores. Hypothermia severely damages the liver, kidneys, and adrenal glands in dogs when temperatures of around 25°C are maintained for several hours.[124] Short periods (1 to 2 h) of cooling, however, do not appear to cause demonstrable damage.

Hypothermia has been used for surgery of the heart and great vessels, brain, and spinal cord, and in some other surgical procedures. It also has been advocated in treatment of shock, stroke, and cerebral and spinal contusion, and in prevention of brain damage following a severe hypoxic episode. The chief factor limiting its use alone in heart surgery is the danger of hypoxic brain damage. For this reason, older patients and those with cardiac defects requiring extensive repair should be managed with heart-lung bypass. Hypothermia has also been used in dogs to remove heartworms and to repair cardiac anomalies, but its use is not widespread. This is probably because many veterinarians are unaware of the simplicity of the technique and do not appreciate its potential.

Induction

To produce hypothermia in dogs, a phenothiazine tranquilizer may be given IV as a preanesthetic agent. A thiobarbiturate is injected for general anesthesia, following which an endotracheal catheter is inserted and an inhalant anesthetic is used for maintenance. A slow intravenous drip of Ringer's lactate solution or 5% dextrose is started, and a muscle relaxant is given in the drip tubing to abolish respirations. Controlled ventilation is then initiated. Unless a cooling mattress is available, the animal is positioned in a sink, bathtub, or other container, with its head above water. Electronic thermometer probes are placed in the esophagus at heart level and in the rectum, and electrodes of an electrocardiograph are attached to the feet. From this point, constant monitoring of the electrocardiogram on an oscilloscope is desirable, because cardiac fibrillation may occur at any time during the cooling period and requires immediate corrective measures.

Ice water is used for rapid cooling. It should be constantly agitated by hand or with a pump. The dog should be removed from the bath before the desired body temperature is reached, because temperature will continue to decline even after the dog's removal from the water.

After removal, the dog should be dried with towels and placed on an inactive heating pad during the operative period. Rewarming can then be started as soon as closure of the surgical wound is begun. As anesthesia is discontinued and shivering commences, the body temperature quickly begins to rise. If the operation is short, rewarming in a water bath may be necessary, along with administration of atropine and neostigmine to reverse the effects of the muscle relaxant.

Electronarcosis and Immobilization

Electric stimulation of the brain can activate either opioid or nonopioid pain-control pathways or both.[125] Passage of electricity through the brain to produce anesthesia has been investigated for many years. In the veterinary field, clinical trials were conducted by Sir Frederic Hobday in England as early as 1932. Despite extensive research, much remains to be learned about this technique. Early work documented the occurrence of respiratory depression, hyperthermia, convulsions, and fatalities. Electronarcosis may be of greatest use in situations where prolonged anesthesia is required for experimental purposes.

Most instruments deliver the current through needle electrodes applied to the head. Direct, pulsating direct, and alternating current have been used to produce electronarcosis. Alternating current of 700 cycles, 35 to 50 mA, and approximately 40 V has been employed.[126] Others have used combined direct and alternating current, modified to produce a rectangular wave for 1.0 to 1.4 ms, with a frequency of 100 waves/s.[127] Continuous electrode contact is important to maintain electronarcosis anesthesia. Individual variation among animals requires that the current be adjusted for each according to the response observed.

Electronarcosis is characterized by convulsions on induction unless a muscle relaxant is first administered. An exception to this is the method employing direct current for induction and then both direct and alternating current.[127] Profuse salivation develops on induction and continues throughout. This can be counteracted by using atropine. Endotracheal intubation should always be performed. Hyperthermia, probably caused by disturbance of the thermoregulatory center in the hypothalamus, is commonly seen. The electroencephalogram immediately following anesthesia is decreased in amplitude and increased in frequency, but returns to normal within 30 min. Brain lesions have been found following electronarcosis,[128] and skin burns from the electrodes have been reported.[129]

Electronarcosis appears to produce severe stress, as evidenced by an increased plasma level of hydroxycorticoids, epinephrine, and norepinephrine (Fig. 11.15). The blood pressure rises sharply and then gradually falls to near normal levels (Fig. 11.16). The clotting time, sedimentation rate, hemoglobin, hematocrit, and

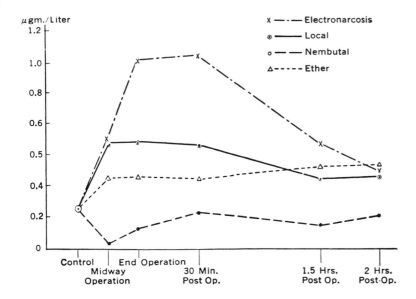

Fig. 11.15. Epinephrine secretion in response to a standard laparotomy: a comparison of different agents for anesthesia. The points on each curve represent the average values from seven dogs. Electronarcosis and laparotomy produced the greatest rise in epinephrine secretion, with response to procaine and to ether next in order, respectively. Nembutal (pentobarbital) depressed the epinephrine level of plasma despite the associated surgery. From Hardy et al.[142]

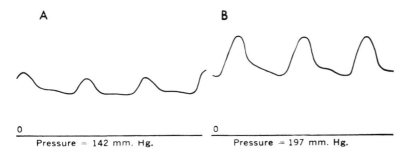

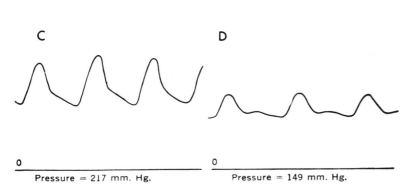

Fig. 11.16. Mean femoral artery blood pressure in a dog under electronarcosis: preinduction **(A)**, induction **(B)**, beginning surgical anesthesia **(C)**, and 15 min after onset of surgical anesthesia **(D)**. Courtesy of Dr. R.A. Herin, Colorado State University, Fort Collins, Colorado.

total and differential white blood cell counts do not differ from preinduction values.[130] There is little effect on arterial oxygen partial pressure; carbon dioxide content and pH decrease, whereas blood glucose rises. It was originally thought that electronarcosis, which produces an uninhibited response of the adrenal medullary and cortical systems, may be more desirable than drug-induced anesthesia, which usually depresses this response.[131] This is in contrast to the modern concept of anesthesia, which endeavors to minimize sympathetic nervous system response associated with the production of general anesthesia. Consequently, there has been a loss of interest in electronarcosis and immobilization as humane alternatives for producing general anesthesia.

In addition to questionable humaneness, it is difficult to assess the depth of unconsciousness achieved by electronarcosis. Muscle relaxation varies from adequate to poor. Pain induced by surgery may cause body movements in animals that appear unconscious. The photomotor reflex is probably the best means of determining the depth of anesthesia if a large dose of atropine has not been used. Early investigators indicated that analgesia persists for several minutes after removal of the current and the animal often appears hypnotized. A slight stimulus may then cause complete arousal, and the patient resumes all normal activities.

In the mid-1980s, electroimmobilization was advocated and

used by sheep and cattle producers and some veterinarians for restraint and processing of food animals. This technique was recommended for minor surgery, although strong evidence exists that electroimmobilization is aversive and does not eliminate pain. Amnesia and unconsciousness are not achieved with the manufacturer's recommended electrode placement and electric current application, and this technique may induce pain and dysphoria. Consequently, electroimmobilization is no longer widely used, nor can it be recommended as a humane method of animal restraint.[132]

Acupuncture

This technique has been advocated for providing analgesia during the operative and postoperative periods, to treat chronic pain, and even to treat selected disease states. Charts for people and farm animals (horses, cattle, and pigs) can be commonly found in the Oriental literature. Acupuncture points can be stimulated in many different ways, including needling, injection of saline, electric stimulation, and metal implantation. It has been shown that electroacupuncture minimally decreases halothane MAC in dogs. Although the mechanism of action of acupuncture has been suggested to be the activation of the endogenous opioid neurotransmitter system, the administration of opioid antagonists does not reverse acupuncture-induced decreases in halothane MAC. Some investigators have indicated that acupuncture induces surgical analgesia. However, there appear to be three reasons why acupuncture should not be solely relied upon for surgical anesthesia: lack of restraint, inadequate analgesia, and lack of adequate information on acupuncture points to be used for specific surgical sites. These factors—along with the disadvantages of unfamiliarity, time-consuming methods of application, and inconsistent effects—have made acupuncture an unreliable and nonviable method of producing general anesthesia. Acupuncture may be best used for treatment of chronic pain in animals. Treatment of laminitis and chronic back pain in horses has reportedly been effective.[133] See Chapter 24 for further discussion.

Physiological Hypnosis

Certain species of animals are highly susceptible to hypnosis (immobility reflex). These include arthropods, amphibians, reptiles, birds, guinea pigs, and rabbits. This modality is seldom used in animal anesthesia because of a lack of analgesia associated with the state of physiological hypnosis. Hypnosis should be viewed as a legitimate method of producing immobilization, not anesthesia.

References

1. Fragen RJ, Avram MJ. Nonopioid intravenous anesthetics. In: Barash PG, Cullen BF, Stoelting RK, eds. Clinical Anesthesia. Philadelphia: JB Lippincott, 1989:227.
2. Dunwiddie TV, Worth TS, Olsen RW. Facilitation of recurrent inhibition in rat hippocampus by barbiturate and related nonbarbiturate depressant drugs. J Pharmacol Exp Ther 238:564, 1986.
3. Tanelian DL, Kosek P, Mody I, MacIver MB. The role of the GABAA receptor/chloride channel complex in anesthesia [Review with 200 references]. Anesthesiology 78:757, 1993.
4. Schwartz RD, Jackson JA, Weigert D, Skolnick P, Paul SM. Characterization of barbiturate-stimulated chloride efflux from rat brain synaptoneurosomes. J Neurosci 5:2963, 1985.
5. Huidobro-Toro JP, Bleck V, Allan AM, Harris RA. Neurochemical actions of anesthetic drugs on the gamma-aminobutyric acid receptor–chloride channel complex. J Pharmacol Exp Ther 242:963, 1987.
6. Collins GG, Anson J. Effects of barbiturates on responses evoked by excitatory amino acids in slices of rat olfactory cortex. Neuropharmacology 26:167, 1987.
7. Downie DL, Franks NP, Lieb WR. Effects of thiopental and its optical isomers on nicotinic acetylcholine receptors. Anesthesiology 93:774, 2000.
8. Sloan T. Anesthetics and the brain. Anesthesiol Clin North Am 20:265, 2002.
9. Nicoll RA, Iwamoto ET. Action of pentobarbital on sympathetic ganglion cells. J Neurophysiol 41:977, 1978.
10. Usenik EA, Cronkite EP. Effects of barbiturate anesthetics on leukocytes in normal and splenectomized dogs. Anesth Analg 44:167, 1965.
11. Brown BR, Vandam LD. A review of current advances in metabolism of inhalation anesthetics. Ann NY Acad Sci 179:235, 1971.
12. Clemens LG, Popham RV, Ruppert PH. Neonatal treatment of hamsters with barbiturate alters adult sexual behavior. Dev Psychobiol 12:49, 1979.
13. Gupta C, Sonawane BR, Yaffe SJ. Phenobarbital exposure in utero: Alterations in female reproductive function in rats. Science 208:508, 1980.
14. Aase JM. Anticonvulsant drugs and congenital abnormalities. Am J Dis Child 127:758, 1974.
15. Barr M Jr, Poznanski AK, Schmikel RD. Digital hypoplasia and anticonvulsants during gestation: A teratogenic syndrome? J Pediatr 84:254, 1974.
16. Waddell WJ, Butler TC. The distribution and excretion of phenobarbital. J Clin Invest 36:1217, 1957.
17. Maynert EW, Van Dyke HB. The absence of localization of barbital in divisions of the central nervous system. J Pharmacol Exp Ther 98:184, 1950.
18. Peters M, Strother A. A study of some possible mechanisms by which glucose inhibits drug metabolism in vivo and in vitro. J Pharmacol Exp Ther 180:151, 1972.
19. Hamlin RL, Redding RW, Rieger JE, Smith RC, Prynn B. Insignificance of the "glucose effect" in dogs anesthetized with pentobarbital. J Am Vet Med Assoc 146:238, 1965.
20. Lamson PD, Greig ME, Williams L. Potentiation by epinephrine of the anesthetic effect in chloral and barbiturate anesthesia. J Pharmacol Exp Ther 106:219, 1952.
21. Hatch RC. The effect of glucose, sodium lactate, and epinephrine on thiopental anesthesia in dogs. J Am Vet Med Assoc 148:135, 1966.
22. Skinner SF, Robertson LT, Artero M, Gerding RK. Longitudinal study of phenobarbital in serum, cerebrospinal fluid, and saliva in the dog. Am J Vet Res 41:600, 1980.
23. Breznock EM. Effects of phenobarbital on digitoxin and digoxin elimination in the dog. Am J Vet Res 364:371, 1975.
24. Huang LYM, Barker JL. Pentobarbital: Stereospecific actions of (+) and (−) isomers revealed on cultured mammalian neurons. Science 207:195, 1980.
25. Tomlin SL, Jenkins A, Lieb WR, Franks NP. Preparation of barbiturate optical isomers and their effects on GABA(A) receptors. Anesthesiology 90:1714, 2004.

26. Mather LE, Edwards SR, Duke CC. Electroencephalographic effects of thiopentone and its enantiomers in the rat: Correlation with drug tissue distribution. Br J Pharmacol 128:83, 1999.

27. Priano LL, Traber DL, Wilson RD. Barbiturate anesthesia: An abnormal physiologic situation. J Pharmacol Exp Ther 165:126, 1969.

28. MacCannell KL. The effect of barbiturates on regional blood flows. Can Anaesth Soc J 16:1, 1969.

29. Hamlin RL, Smith CR. Characteristics of respiration in healthy dogs anesthetized with sodium pentobarbital. Am J Vet Res 28:173, 1967.

30. Blake WD. Some effects of pentobarbital and anesthesia on renal hemodynamics: Water and electrolyte excretion in the dog. Am J Physiol 191:393, 1957.

31. Graca JG, Garst EL. Early blood changes in dogs following intravenous pentobarbital anesthesia. Anesthesiology 18:461, 1957.

32. Hausner E, Essex HE, Mann FC. Roentgenologic observations of the spleen of the dog under ether, sodium amytal, pentobarbital sodium and pentothal sodium anesthesia. Am J Physiol 121:387, 1938.

33. Mylon E, Winternitz MC, De Suto-Nagy GJ. Studies on therapy in traumatic shock. Am J Physiol 139:313, 1943.

34. Corcoran AC, Page IH. Effects of anesthetic dosage of pentobarbital sodium on renal function and blood pressure in dogs. Am J Physiol 140:234, 1943.

35. Van Dyke HB, Scudi JV, Tabern DL. The excretion of N^{15} in the urine of dogs after the administration of labeled pentobarbital. J Pharmacol Exp Ther 90:364, 1947.

36. Davis LE, Baggot JD, Davis CAN, Powers TE. Elimination kinetics of pentobarbital in nephrectomized dogs. Am J Vet Res 34:231, 1973.

37. Toosey MB. The uses of concentrated pentobarbitone sodium solution in bovine practice. Vet Rec 71:24, 1959.

38. Jones EW, Johnson L, Heinze CD. Thiopental sodium anesthesia in the horse: A rapid induction technique. J Am Vet Med Assoc 137:119, 1960.

39. Linzell JL. Some observations on general and regional anesthesia in goats. In: Graham-Jones O, ed. Small Animal Anaesthesia, 2nd ed. London: Pergamon, 1964.

40. Harrison FA. The anaesthesia of sheep using pentobarbitone sodium and cyclopropane. In: Small Animal Anaesthesia, 2nd ed. London: Pergamon, 1964.

41. Hatch RC, Clark JD, Booth NH, Kitzman JV. Comparison of five preanesthetic medicaments in pentobarbital-anesthetized dogs: Antagonism by 4-aminopyridine, yohimbine, and naloxone. Am J Vet Res 44:2312, 1983.

42. Grono LR. Methohexital sodium anaesthesia in the horse. Aust Vet J 42:398, 1966.

43. Robertshaw D. Methohexital sodium anaesthesia in calves. Vet Rec 76:357, 1964.

44. Monahan CM. The use of methohexitone for induction of anaesthesia in large animals. Vet Rec 76:1333, 1964.

45. Welles JS, McMahon RE, Doran WJ. The metabolism and excretion of methohexital in the rat and dog. J Pharmacol Exp Ther 139:166, 1963.

46. Robinson MH. Deterioration of solutions of pentothal sodium. Anesthesiology 8:166, 1947.

47. Taylor JD, Richards RK, Tabern DL. Metabolism of S35 thiopental (pentothal): Chemical and paper chromatographic studies of S35 excretion by the rat and monkey. J Pharmacol Exp Ther 104:93, 1952.

48. Rawlings CA, Kolata RJ. Cardiopulmonary effects of thiopental/lidocaine combination during anesthetic induction in the dog. Am J Vet Res 44:144, 1983.

49. Muir WW. Electrocardiographic interpretation of thiobarbiturate-induced dysrhythmias in dogs. J Am Vet Med Assoc 170:1419, 1977.

50. Wiersig DO, Davis RH, Szabuniewicz M. Prevention of induced ventricular fibrillation in dogs anesthetized with ultrashort acting barbiturates and halothane. J Am Vet Med Assoc 165:341, 1974.

51. Szabuniewicz M, Davis RH, Wiersig DO. Prevention of methoxyflurane and thiobarbiturate cardiac sensitization to catecholamines in dogs. Pract Vet 47:12, 1975.

52. Muir WW, Werner LL, Hamlin RL. Effect of xylazine and acetylpromazine upon induced ventricular fibrillation in dogs anesthetized with thiamylal and halothane. Am J Vet Res 36:1299, 1975.

53. Booker WM, Maloney AH, Tureman JR, Ratliff C. Some metabolic factors influencing the course of thiopental anesthesia in dogs. Am J Physiol 170:168, 1952.

54. Brodie BB, Bernstein E, Mark LC. The role of body fat in limiting the duration of action of thiopental. J Pharmacol Exp Ther 105:424, 1952.

55. Saidman LJ, Eger EI. The effect of thiopental metabolism on duration of anesthesia. Anesthesiology 27:118, 1966.

56. Anderson EG, Magee DF. A study of the mechanism of the effect of dietary fat in decreasing thiopental sleeping time. J Pharmacol Exp Ther 117:281, 1956.

57. Swanson EE. Sodium 5-allyl-5-(1-methylbutyl)-2-thiobarbiturate, a short acting anaesthetic. J Pharm Pharmacol 3:112, 1951.

58. Wyngaarden JB, Woods LA, Seevers MH. The cumulative action of certain thiobarbiturates in dogs. Fed Proc 6:38, 1947.

59. Elder CK, Harrison EM. Pentothal sodium slough: Prevention by procaine hydrochloride. J Am Med Assoc 125:116, 1944.

60. Nadeson R, Goodchild CS. Antinociceptive properties of neurosteroids. III. Experiments with alphadolone given intravenously, intraperitoneally, and intragastrically. Br J Anaesth 86:704, 2001.

61. Weir CJ, Ling AT, Belelli D, Wildsmith JA, Peters JA, Lambert JJ. The interaction of anaesthetic steroids with recombinant glycine and GABAA receptors. Br J Anaesth 92:704, 2002.

62. Best P, Pearson M. Report on the Safety of an Alphaxalone-CD Anaesthetic Compound. Rutherford, Australia: Jurox, 1997.

63. Jones RS. Injectable anaesthetic agents in the cat: A review. J Small Anim Pract 20:345, 1979.

64. Dodds MG, Twissell DJ. Effect of Althesin (CT 1341) on circulatory responses to adrenaline and on halothane-adrenaline cardiac dysrhythmias in the cat. Postgrad Med J 48(Suppl 2):17, 1972.

65. Child KJ, Currie JP, Davis B, Dodds MG, Pearce DR, Twissell DJ. The pharmacological properties in animals of CT 1341: A new steroid anaesthetic agent. Br J Anaesth 43:2, 1971.

66. Watkins J, Clark RSJ. Report of a symposium: Adverse responses to intravenous agents. Br J Anaesth 50:1159, 1978.

67. Hall LW. Althesin in the larger animal. Postgrad Med J 48(Suppl 2):55, 1972.

68. Camburn MA. Use of alphaxalone-alphadolone in ruminants. Vet Rec 111:166, 1982.

69. Pickerodt V, McDowall DG, Coroneos NJ, Keaney NP. Effect of Althesin on carotid blood flow and intracranial pressure in the anaesthetized baboon: Preliminary communication. Postgrad Med J 48(Suppl 2):58, 1972.

70. Child KJ, Harnby G, Gibson W, Hart JW. Metabolism and excretion of Althesin (CT 1341) in the rat. Postgrad Med J 48(Suppl 2):37, 1972.

71. Stopiglia AV. Contribuicao para o estudo da anestesia genal de equideos [Abstract]. Sao Paulo: Faculty of Veterinary Medicine, University of Sao Paulo, 1962.

72. Brown RV, Hilton JG. The effectiveness of the baroreceptor reflexes under different anesthetics. J Pharmacol Exp Ther 118:198, 1956.

73. King EE, Unna KR. The action of mephenesin and other interneuron depressants on the brain stem. J Pharmacol Exp Ther 111:293, 1954.

74. Harding GW, Stogsdill RM, Towe AL. Relative effects of pentobarbital and chloralose on the responsiveness of neurons in sensorimotor cerebral cortex of the domestic cat. Neuroscience 4:369, 1979.

75. Auerbach C. The chemical production of mutations. Science 158:1141, 1967.

76. Wood EM. Urethane as a carcinogen. Prog Fish Cult 18:135, 1956.

77. Lingamaneni R, Hemmings HCJ. Differential interaction of anaesthetics and antiepileptic drugs with neuronal Na$^+$ channels, Ca^{++} channels, and GABA(A) receptors. Br J Anaesth 90:199, 2003.

78. Blednov YA, Jung S, Alva H, et al. Deletion of the alpha1 or beta2 subunit of GABAA receptors reduces actions of alcohol and other drugs. J Pharmacol Exp Ther 304:30, 2003.

79. Nagel ML, Muir WW, Nguyen K. Comparison of the cardiopulmonary effects of etomidate and thiamylal in dogs. Am J Vet Res 40:193, 1979.

80. Wertz EM, Benson GJ, Thurmon JC, Tranquilli WJ. Pharmacokinetics of etomidate in cats. Am J Vet Res 51:281, 1990.

81. Robertson S. Advantages of etomidate use as an anesthetic agent. Vet Clin North Am Small Anim Pract 22:277, 1992.

82. Kruse-Elliott KT, Swanson CR, Aucion DP. Effects of etomidate function on canine surgical patients. Am J Vet Res 48:1098, 1987.

83. Muir WW, Mason DE. Side effects of etomidate in dogs. J Am Vet Med Assoc 194:1430, 1989.

84. Ko JCH, Thurmon JC, Benson GJ, Tranquilli WJ, Hoffmann WE. Acute hemolysis associated with etomidate–propylene glycol infusion in dogs. J Vet Anesth 20:92, 1993.

85. Arduino MJ, Bland LA, McAllister SK, et al. Microbial growth and endotoxin production in the intravenous anesthetic propofol. Infect Control Hosp Epidemiol 12:535, 1991.

86. Zoran DL, Riedesel DH, Dyer DC. Pharmacokinetics of propofol in mixed breed dogs and greyhounds. Am J Vet Res 54:755, 1993.

87. Langley MS, Heel RC. Propofol: A review of its pharmacodynamic and pharmacokinetic properties and use as an intravenous anaesthetic. Drugs 35:334, 1988.

88. Weaver BM, Raptopoulos D. Induction of anaesthesia in dogs and cats with propofol. Vet Rec 126:617, 1990.

89. Morgan DWT, Legge K. Clinical evaluation of propofol as an intravenous anaesthetic agent in cats and dogs. Vet Rec 124:31, 1989.

90. Robertson SA, Johnston S, Beemsterboer J. Cardiopulmonary, anesthetic, and postanesthetic effects of intravenous infusions of propofol in greyhounds and non-greyhounds. Am J Vet Res 53:1027, 1992.

91. Thurmon JC, Ko JCH, Benson GJ, Tranquilli WJ, Olson WA. Hemodynamic and analgesic effects of propofol infusion in medetomidine-premedicated dogs. Am J Vet Res 55:363, 1994.

92. Smith JA, Gaynor JS, Bednarski RM, Muir WW. Adverse effects of administration of propofol with various preanesthetic regimens in dogs. J Am Vet Med Assoc 202:1111, 1993.

93. Concas A, Santoro G, Serra M, Sanna E, Biggio G. Neurochemical action of the general anaesthetic propofol on the chloride ion channel coupled with GABA receptors. Brain Res 542:225, 1991.

94. Ilkiw JE, Pascow PJ, Haskins SC, Patz JD. Cardiovascular and respiratory effects of propofol administration in hypovolemic dogs. Am J Vet Res 53:2323, 1992.

95. Branson KE, Gross ME. Propofol in veterinary medicine. J Am Vet Med Assoc 204:1888, 1994.

96. Day TK, Andress DG, Day DG. Effects of consecutive day propofol anesthesia on feline red blood cells [Abstract]. In: Proceedings of the Annual Meeting of the American College of Veterinary Anesthesiologists, Washington, DC, 1993:15.

97. Smith I, White PF, Nathanson M, Gouldson R. Propofol, an update on its clinical use. Anesthesiology 81:1005, 1994.

98. Simons PJ, Cockshott ID, Douglas EJ, Gordon EA, Knott S, Ruane RJ. Species differences in blood profiles, metabolism and excretion of ^{14}C-propofol after intravenous dosing to rat, dog and rabbit. Xenobiotica 21:1243, 1991.

99. Hay Kraus BL, Greenblatt DJ, Venkatakrishman K, Court MH. Evidence for propofol hydroxylation by cytochrome P4502B11 in canine liver microsomes: Breed and gender differences. Xenobiotica 30:575, 2004.

100. Dailland P, Cockshott ID, Litzin JD, et al. Intravenous propofol during cesarean section: Placental transfer, concentrations in breast milk, and neonatal effects—A preliminary study. Anesthesiology 71:827, 1989.

101. Ilkiw JE. Other potentially useful new injectable anesthetic agents. Vet Clin North Am Small Anim Pract 22:281, 1992.

102. Oku K, Yamanaka T, Ashihara N, Kawasaki K, Mizuno Y, Fujinaga T. Clinical observations during induction and recovery of xylazine-midazolam-propofol anesthesia in horses. J Vet Med Sci 65:805, 2003.

103. Frias AF, Marsico F, Gomez de Segura IA, et al. Evaluation of different doses of propofol in xylazine pre-medicated horses. Vet Anaesth Analg 30:193, 2003.

104. Matthews NS, Hartsfield SM, Hague B, Carroll GL, Short CE. Detomidine-propofol anesthesia for abdominal surgery in horses. Vet Surg 28:196, 1999.

105. Mama KR, Pascoe PJ, Steffey EP, Kollias-Baker C. Comparison of two techniques for total intravenous anesthesia in horses. Am J Vet Res 59:1292, 2004.

106. Bigelow WG, Lindsay WK, Harrison RC, Gordon RA, Greenwood WF. Oxygen transport and utilization in dogs at low body temperatures. Am J Physiol 160:125, 1950.

107. Fuhrman GJ, Fuhrman FA, Field J. Metabolism of rat heart slices, with special reference to effects of temperature and anoxia. Am J Physiol 163:642, 1950.

108. Gott VL, Bartlett M, Long DM, Lillehei CW, Johnson JA. Myocardial energy substances in the dog heart during potassium and hypothermic arrest. J Appl Physiol 17:815, 1962.

109. Swan H, Zeavin I, Holmes JH, Montgomery V. Cessation of circulation in general hypothermia. Ann Surg 138:360, 1953.

110. Bering EA Jr, Taren JA, McMurray JD, Bernhard WF. Studies on hypothermia in monkeys. II. The effect of hypothermia on the general physiology and cerebral metabolism of monkeys in the hypothermic state. Surg Gynecol Obstet 102:134, 1956.

111. Andjus RK, Lovelock JE. Reanimation of rats from body temperatures between 0 and 1°C by microwave diathermy. J Physiol 128:541, 1955.

112. Smith AU. Resuscitation of hypothermic, supercooled and frozen mammals. Proc R Soc Med 49:357, 1956.

113. Gollan F, Tysinger DS Jr, Grace JT, Kory RC, Meneely GR. Hypothermia of 1.5 degree C in dogs followed by survival. Am J Physiol 181:297, 1955.

114. Davis TRA, Mayer J. Nature of the physiological stimulus for shivering. Am J Physiol 181:669, 1955.

115. Regan MJ, Eger EI. Effect of hypothermia in dogs on anesthetizing and apneic doses of inhalation agents. Anesthesiology 23:689, 1967.

116. Westenskow DR, Wong KC, Johnson CC, Wilde CS. Physiologic effects of deep hypothermia and microwave rewarming: Possible

application for neonatal cardiac surgery. Anesth Analg 58:397, 1979.

117. Blades B, Pierpont HC. A simple method for inducing hypothermia. Ann Surg 140:557, 1954.

118. Covino BG, Charleson DA, D'Amato HE. Ventricular fibrillation in the hypothermic dog. Am J Physiol 178:148, 1954.

119. Hess ML, Krause SM, Greenfield LJ. Assessment of hypothermic, cardioplegic protection of the global ischemic canine myocardium. J Thorac Cardiovasc Surg 80:293, 1980.

120. Rosenfeldt FL, Hearse DJ, Cankovic-Darracott S, Braimbridge MV. The additive protective effects of hypothermia and chemical cardioplegia during ischemic cardiac arrest in the dog. J Thorac Cardiovasc Surg 79:29, 1980.

121. Michenfelder JD, Milde JH. Failure of prolonged hypocapnia, hypothermia or hypertension to favorably alter stroke in primates. Stroke 8:87, 1977.

122. Steen PA, Soule EH, Michenfelder JD. The detrimental effect of prolonged hypothermia in cats and monkeys with and without regional cerebral ischemia. Stroke 10:522, 1979.

123. Steen PA, Milde JH, Michenfelder JD. The detrimental effects of prolonged hypothermia and rewarming in the dog. Anesthesiology 52:224, 1980.

124. Knocker P. Effects of experimental hypothermia on vital organs. Lancet 2:837, 1955.

125. Watkins LR, Mayer DJ. Organization of endogenous opiate and nonopiate pain control systems. Science 216:1185, 1982.

126. Hardy JD, Turner MD, McNeil CD. Electrical anesthesia. III. Development of a method and laboratory observations. J Surg Res 1:152, 1961.

127. Smith RH, Goodwin C, Fowler E, Smith GW, Volpitto PP. Electronarcosis produced by a combination of direct and alternating current: A preliminary study. Anesthesiology 22:163, 1961.

128. Herin RA. Electroanesthesia: A review of the literature (1819–1965). Act Nerv Super (Praha) 10:439, 1968.

129. Smith RH, Gramling ZW, Smith GW, Volpitto PP. Electronarcosis by combination of direct and alternating current. 2. Effects on dog brain as shown by EEG and microscopic study. Anesthesiology 22:970, 1961.

130. Herin RA. Electrical anesthesia in the dog. J Am Vet Med Assoc 142:865, 1963.

131. McNeil CD, Hardy JD. Electrical anesthesia: Some metabolic observations and comparisons. Surg Forum 9:394, 1959.

132. Thurmon JC. Injectable anesthetic agents and techniques in ruminants and swine. Vet Clin North Am Food Anim Pract 2:567, 1986.

133. Klide AM. Acupuncture analgesia. Vet Clin North Am Small Anim Pract 374, 1992.

134. Goodman LS, Gilman A. The Pharmacological Basis of Therapeutics, 2nd ed. New York: Macmillan, 1958.

135. Goodman LS, Gilman A, eds. The Pharmacological Basis of Therapeutics, 4th ed. New York: Macmillan, 1970.

136. Shanker LS. Penetration of drugs into the central nervous system. In: Papper EM, Kitz RJ, eds. Uptake and Distribution of Anesthetic Agents. New York: McGraw-Hill, 1963.

137. Roth LJ, Barlow CF. Drugs in the brain. Science 134:22, 1961.

138. Tyagi RPS, Arnold JP, Usenik EA, Fletchers TP. Effects of thiopental sodium (Pentothal Sodium) anesthesia on the horse. Cornell Vet 54:584, 1964.

139. Jones LM, Booth N, McDonald L, eds. Veterinary Pharmacology and Therapeutics, 4th ed. Ames: Iowa State University Press, 1977.

140. Olmsted F, Page IH. Hemodynamic changes in dogs caused by sodium pentobarbital anesthesia. Am J Physiol 210:817, 1966.

141. Wyngaarden JN, Woods LA, Ridley R, Seevers MH. Anesthetic properties of sodium-5-allyl-5-(1-methylbutyl)-2-thiobarbiturate (Surital) and certain other thiobarbiturates in dogs. J Pharmacol Exp Ther 95:322, 1949.

142. Hardy JD, Carter T, Turner MD. Catechol amine metabolism. Ann Surg 150:669, 1959.

Chapter 12
Dissociative Anesthetics

Hui-Chu Lin

Introduction

The term *dissociative anesthesia* is used to describe an anesthetic state induced by drugs that interrupt ascending transmission from the parts of the brain responsible for unconscious and conscious functions, rather than by generalized depression of all brain centers as seen with most other general anesthetics.[1] Dissociative anesthesia is characterized by a cataleptoid state in which the eyes remain open with a slow nystagmic gaze.[2] Varying degrees of hypertonus and purposeful or reflexive skeletal muscle movements often occur unrelated to surgical stimulation. Although somatic analgesia may be intense, it is relatively brief.

Phencyclidine, ketamine, and tiletamine are dissociative anesthetics that have been used clinically for immobilization and anesthesia.[3,4] Phencyclidine was the first dissociative used in veterinary anesthesia, but it is no longer available for clinical use. Tiletamine is available for use only in combination with the benzodiazepine zolazepam. In a 1:1 ratio, this drug combination is marketed as Telazol in the United States and as Zoletil in Europe. In most respects, the pharmacodynamics of tiletamine are similar to those of ketamine (the most commonly used dissociative anesthetic), but tiletamine's potency and duration of action are intermediate between those of phencyclidine, the most potent, and ketamine, the least potent.

Pharmacology
Effects on the Nervous System

Dissociative anesthetics produce dose-related unconsciousness and analgesia. Because of their low molecular weight, a pK_a near physiological pH, and high lipid solubility, dissociative anesthetics have a rapid onset of action. Classically, the mechanism of action has been described as selective depression of neuronal function of the neocorticothalamic axis and the central nucleus of the thalamus with concurrent stimulation of selected parts of the limbic system, including the hippocampus.[5,6] More recently, antagonism of the *N*-methyl-D-aspartate (NMDA) receptor has been proposed as the most likely molecular mechanism responsible for most of the anesthetic, analgesic, psychotomimetic, and neuroprotective effects of the drug.[7] Alternatively, effects could be mediated in part by one or more of the following: (a) action on voltage-dependent sodium, potassium, and calcium channels; (b) depression of acetylcholine receptors; (c) enhancement and prolongation of γ-aminobutyric acid (GABA) receptors that link to chloride channels (GABA$_A$ receptors); and (d) depression of nociceptive cells in the medial medullary reticular formation and activity of cells in laminae I and V of the dorsal horn.[8–10]

Dissociative anesthetic administration to people with a history of seizures does not promote seizure activity despite the presence of thalamic and limbic epileptiform electroencephalogram patterns.[11,12] In fact, low doses of ketamine may have anticonvulsant properties through antagonism of NMDA receptors.[13–16] Nevertheless, ketamine-associated seizures have been reported in some animals, and use of ketamine, or any other dissociative anesthetic, in animals with a history of epilepsy or other seizure disorders should be avoided, if possible.[17–20]

Analgesia produced by dissociative anesthetics occurs at subanesthetic doses. Elevated pain thresholds correlate with plasma ketamine concentrations of 0.1 μg/mL or greater.[21] The degree of analgesia appears to be greater for somatic pain than for visceral pain.[22] In cats, visceral analgesia induced by ketamine (2, 4, and 8 mg/kg intravenously [IV]) is similar to that produced by butorphanol (0.1 mg/kg IV). With increasing doses of ketamine, or when ketamine and butorphanol are administered simultaneously, visceral analgesia is not increased.[23] At a high dose of ketamine (8 mg/kg), cats appear anesthetized but still respond to colonic nociceptor stimulation, suggesting limited visceral analgesia in cats and probably other species. Dissociative anesthetics appear to be more useful for anesthesia and postoperative analgesia related to integumentary and superficial musculoskeletal surgery.[23,24] Furthermore, NMDA receptors appear to be involved in hyperalgesic responses after peripheral tissue injury and inflammation, suggesting that ketamine (and possibly other dissociatives) would be effective at reducing hyperalgesia following tissue trauma.[25–29]

Local infiltration of ketamine may produce a brief period of local anesthetic effect.[30,31] When administered simultaneously with bupivacaine, ketamine doubles the duration of analgesic and local anesthetic effects of bupivacaine.[32] This peripheral analgesic effect of ketamine may be attributed to one or all of the following mechanisms: (a) blockade of sodium and potassium currents in peripheral nerves, (b) blockade of NMDA, α-amino-hydroxy-5-methyl-4-isoxazoleproprionic acid (AMPA), and kainite receptors on unmyelinated axons, and (c) blockade of glutamate effects on C-fiber free-nerve endings.[33–37]

Similar to systemic administration, epidural ketamine appears to produce profound somatic but poor visceral analgesia. Epidural administration produces a dose-dependent analgesic action.[38,39] In rats, a dose of 6 mg/kg induces motor blockade lasting 5 to 15 min, whereas sensory blockade alone occurs with lower doses (4 mg/kg).[40] In horses, the caudal epidural injection of lower doses of ketamine (0.5, 1.0, or 2.0 mg/kg) prevents nociceptive responses initiated by surgical incision and is associated with dose-dependent perineal analgesia.[41,42] In halothane-anesthetized ponies, epidural ketamine reduces the minimum alveolar concentration (MAC) of halothane between 14% (at a dose of 0.8 mg/kg) and 12% (at a dose of 1.2 mg/kg), which is similar to the reduction in MAC achieved with epidural morphine administration (14%).[43] When combined with epidural xylazine (0.5 mg/kg), ketamine (1 mg/kg) induces perineal analgesia lasting 20 min or longer. In some horses, analgesia is extended to the thigh and flank regions.[44] In another study, the subarachnoid administration of ketamine (1 to 2 mg/kg) at the L1-L2 intervertebral space of dogs produced analgesia of the hind limbs.[45]

Tissue trauma produces continuous nociceptive stimulation of C fibers that activates NMDA receptors in the central nervous system (CNS). This activation of NMDA receptors decreases the threshold to glutamate, making them more responsive to stimuli. As a result, *windup* may develop, which is clinically manifested as an exaggerated response to subthreshold noxious stimuli following a primary injury and amplification of postoperative pain.[46,47] These results have led to the concept of preemptively treating central sensitization as an important part of pain management. Consequently, the administration of ketamine at subanesthetic doses as a continuous-rate infusion in combination with other analgesics (e.g., opioids) has gained popularity in preventing or minimizing pain following surgery in both people and animals.[48–53]

Dissociative anesthetics induce significant increases in cerebral blood flow (CBF), intracranial pressure (ICP), and cerebrospinal fluid pressure as a result of cerebral vasodilation and elevated systemic blood pressure.[54–60] The mechanism of ketamine-induced elevated ICP remains controversial. Ketamine increases CBF and ICP in awake goats when arterial carbon dioxide partial pressure ($PaCO_2$) is allowed to rise but has no effect on CBF and ICP when $PaCO_2$ is maintained at a preketamine level, suggesting an indirect mechanism.[61–63] In piglets with preexisting intracranial hypertension, ketamine induced further increases in ICP, paralleling a rise in $PaCO_2$. When ventilation was controlled, no increase in ICP was observed in piglets with normal or elevated ICP.[62] These studies suggest that initiating controlled ventilation is prudent when dissociative anesthetics must be administered to patients with intracranial disease. Increased skeletal, thoracic, and abdominal muscle tone can also impede venous return from the head, increasing intracranial blood volume and pressure.[62,63]

Dissociative anesthetics may not be contraindicated in all patients at risk for intracranial hypertension, particularly when administered in the presence of another anesthetic and/or when controlled ventilation is instituted. It has been hypothesized that when ketamine is administered in the presence of another anesthetic, the second anesthetic may suppress ketamine's excitatory effect on the CNS. Nevertheless, administration of ketamine should be avoided in spontaneously breathing patients with suspected intracranial hypertension or disease until scientific evidence to the contrary emerges.

Abnormal behavior, which may progress to delirium, may occur during emergence from dissociative anesthesia. Depression of the inferior colliculus and medial geniculate nucleus leading to misperception of auditory and visual stimuli may be responsible for this reaction.[64] Emergence reactions are characterized by ataxia, increased motor activity, hyperreflexia, sensitivity to touch, and sometimes violent recovery.[16,65,66] These reactions usually disappear within several hours without recurrence. Premedication with or concurrent administration of α₂-adrenergic agonists, acetylpromazine, or a benzodiazepine (e.g., diazepam, midazolam, or zolazepam),decreases the incidence and/or severity of emergence reactions.[67–72]

Effects on the Cardiovascular System

The cardiovascular effects of dissociative anesthetics are characterized by indirect cardiovascular stimulation. Various effects on target organs include sympathomimetic effects mediated from within the CNS, inhibition of neuronal uptake of catecholamines by sympathetic nerve endings, direct vasodilation of vascular smooth muscle, and an inotropic effect on the myocardium.[73–76] Heart rate and arterial blood pressure usually increase as a result of increased sympathetic efferent activity.[77] Plasma concentrations of epinephrine and norepinephrine can increase within 2 min of intravenous administration of ketamine and return to control levels 15 min later.[78] In dogs and cats anesthetized with ketamine, mean arterial pressure, heart rate, and cardiac output increase while peripheral vascular resistance remains mostly unchanged.[22,79–84] Myocardial stimulation is associated with increased cardiac work and myocardial oxygen consumption. In healthy animals, increases in myocardial oxygen supply usually result from increased cardiac output and a decrease in coronary vascular resistance such that increases in coronary blood flow parallel the increase in oxygen consumption.[85,86] However, some studies indicate that ketamine-induced increases in coronary blood flow may be insufficient to meet myocardial oxygen demand, especially if cardiovascular disease is present.[87,88] The cardiovascular stimulating effects induced by dissociative anesthetics are blunted or prevented by prior administration of a benzodiazepine, droperidol, acetylpromazine, or α₂-adrenergic agonists, or the concomitant administration of inhalation anesthetics, including nitrous oxide.[89–93]

The direct effect of ketamine on the myocardium remains incompletely characterized. Positive inotropic effects have been demonstrated in patients whose heart rates were kept constant by atrial pacing and in isolated mammalian papillary muscle.[76,94-97] However, in denervated hearts, ketamine (and presumably other dissociative anesthetics) induces direct myocardial depression in vivo and in vitro.[97-102] Cook et al.[97] suggested that the predominant inotropic mechanism of ketamine is inhibition of catecholamine reuptake at the neuroeffector junction, leading to stimulation of β-adrenoceptors. The importance of an intact and normally functioning nervous system in stimulating cardiovascular function is underscored when ketamine is administered in the presence of other anesthetics. For example, when administered to dogs anesthetized with pentobarbital, ketamine induces a biphasic response in blood pressure, whereas in conscious dogs it induces only a pressor response.[79,100]

A direct dose-dependent negative inotropic effect of ketamine on failing and nonfailing human myocardium has been demonstrated. The negative inotropic effect of ketamine cannot be attributed primarily to the absence of sympathetic tone but rather to other direct negative inotropic mechanisms. Therefore, ketamine administration for induction of anesthesia may induce an unanticipated decrease in myocardial contractility in patients with end-stage heart disease.[103]

The survival rate of animals in shock is reportedly greater when they are anesthetized with ketamine versus halothane.[104] Ketamine has been shown to suppress activation of endotoxin-induced neuronal nuclear factor κB, which regulates the production of proinflammatory cytokines, including tumor necrosis factor α in human glioma cells in vitro and intact mouse brain cells in vivo. Therefore, in theory, ketamine may offer some neuroprotective effects during endotoxemia.[105] Furthermore, intravenous administration of ketamine (10 mg/kg/h) prior to injection of endotoxin to rats completely inhibits the hemodynamic effects (profound hypotension), metabolic acidosis, and the release of cytokines associated with endotoxin shock. However, the hemodynamic effect and the release of cytokine are only modestly suppressed when ketamine is administered after exposure to endotoxin. Thus, ketamine may have protective effect in patients with endotoxemia, but only when given preemptively.[106] Critically ill patients occasionally respond to ketamine with an unexpected decrease in blood pressure and cardiac output.[94] This likely results from depletion of catecholamine stores and an uncovering of ketamine's direct myocardial depressant effects.[107]

Effects on the Respiratory System

Dissociative anesthetics, when given alone, differ from most other anesthetics in that they do not depress ventilatory responses to hypoxia.[108] In dogs anesthetized with ketamine, respiratory rate and minute volume decrease initially, but both return to baseline values within 15 min.[109] In cats and sheep, ketamine induces a dose-dependent transient decrease in arterial oxygen partial pressure (PaO_2) in the presence of decreased or increased respiratory rate.[22,110-114] At higher doses, respiration is characterized by an apneustic, shallow, and irregular pattern.[3,19,84] Severe res-

piratory depression or arrest with an overdose of dissociative anesthetic has been reported in human patients and cats.[84,115-117]

Dissociatives often cause increased salivation and respiratory-tract secretions, which can be partially controlled by administration of an antimuscarinic (e.g., atropine). Laryngeal and pharyngeal reflexes usually are partially or fully maintained during dissociative anesthesia. Nevertheless, swallowing reflexes may be somewhat obtunded because most species can be intubated when anesthetized with ketamine. Careful airway management and/or endotracheal intubation should always be performed to prevent aspiration.

Effects on the Hepatic and Renal Systems

Hepatic dysfunction following clinical use of ketamine, and other dissociatives, is not evident in either people or dogs.[1,118] A significant increase in serum concentrations of liver enzymes has been observed in people anesthetized with a ketamine infusion and dogs given higher intramuscular doses (40 mg/kg daily for 6 weeks).[1,118] In rats, ketamine induces hepatic microsomal enzymes but to a lesser extent than that seen with phenobarbital.[119] The effect of ketamine-associated liver microsomal enzyme induction on drug interactions during anesthesia is largely uncharacterized.

Dissociative anesthetics generally undergo extensive hepatic biotransformation in dogs, horses, and people. Some hepatic metabolism occurs in cats, but normally the majority of drug is excreted via the kidney.[113,120] Rapid recovery following intravenous bolus ketamine administration is by rapid redistribution of ketamine from the CNS to other tissues, primarily fat, lung, liver, and kidney.[121] Clinically, animals with significant hepatic dysfunction do not metabolize ketamine as rapidly as do healthy animals. Animals with renal dysfunction or obstruction to urine flow also have prolonged sleep times when larger doses of ketamine are given.[112] Generally speaking, dissociative anesthetics should be given cautiously to animals that have significant hepatic or renal dysfunction.

Effects on Intraocular Pressure

In people, a slight increase in intraocular pressure (IOP) independent of changes in blood pressure has been observed during ketamine anesthesia.[122,123] However, conflicting results have been reported. Intravenous or intramuscular administration of ketamine alone (2 to 8 mg/kg) reportedly did not affect IOP significantly.[124,125] IOP increases during xylazine and ketamine anesthesia in dogs, whereas it tends to decrease in horses.[126,127] Increases in extraocular muscle tone induced by ketamine may be responsible for the IOP increase.[128] With this in mind, ketamine should be used with caution in patients with corneal injuries where increased IOP may result in expulsion of intraocular contents.

Clinical Use

Dogs

Dissociatives can increase muscle tone and can induce spontaneous movement and rough recoveries, and occasionally convulsions, in dogs (Tables 12.1 and 12.2).[66,109] To reduce these undesirable effects, dissociatives are often used in combination with adjunctive drugs. Benzodiazepines induce a central muscle relaxant effect that decreases the muscle hypertonus associated with ketamine.[129] In a comparative study, both midazolam-ketamine and diazepam-ketamine combinations induced minimal cardiovascular and respiratory effects. Time to intubation was significantly shorter with midazolam-ketamine, but recovery seemed to be smoother with diazepam-ketamine.[130] Zolazepam is combined with tiletamine in a fixed ratio in the proprietary mixture Telazol. This combination reduces the adverse effects of tileta-

mine when given alone, although the metabolism of zolazepam can vary among species and may result in a longer or shorter effect relative to tiletamine. Intravenous administration of acepromazine (0.11 mg/kg) and ketamine (11 mg/kg) induces anesthesia for 10 to 35 min, with good muscle relaxation and smooth recovery.[66]

Xylazine (1.1 mg/kg intramuscularly [IM]) or medetomidine (10 to 30 µg/kg [IM]) is often used with ketamine (5 to 10 mg/kg IM) for short-term anesthesia of 25 to 40 min. The ketamine dose can be adjusted, depending on the desired duration of surgery.[109,131] In high-strung small-breed dogs, small ketamine

Table 12.1. Use of ketamine alone or ketamine combinations in dogs.

Drug(s)	Dose(mg/kg) and Route	Duration (min)	Comment
Ketamine alone	10, IV	15±8	↑ Muscle tone Short duration Anesthesia inadequate for surgery
	1 or 2, intrathecally	—	Analgesia of the hind limbs
	10 µg/kg/min, CRI	—	↓ Isoflurane MAC by 25%
Ketamine Lidocaine Morphine	K 10 µg/kg/min; L 50 µg/kg/min; M 3.3 µg/kg/min, IV Simultaneously for CRI	—	↓ Isoflurane MAC by 45%
Acepromazine Ketamine Thiamylal	0.55, IM 11–22, IM To effect, IV	20–90	Occasional seizures
Acepromazine Ketamine	A 0.5, IV; K 10 IM	—	Good restraint
	A 0.2, IV; K 10 IV	39±8	Clinical anesthesia, less muscle rigidity
	A 0.22, IM; K 11–18 IM	—	Restraint, spastic movements, and prolonged recovery
Xylazine and Ketamine	X 0.55–1.1, IM; K 22, IV, to effect	—	Surgical anesthesia, muscle relaxation, and analgesia for abdominal surgery
	X 2.2, IM; K 11 IM	—	Occasional seizures
	X 2.2 IM; K 5.5 IM	—	Occasional seizures
	X 0.22, IM; K 10, IM	28–36	—
	X 1, IV; K 10, IM	32±6	Better muscle relaxation than ketamine alone
	X 1, IM; K15, IM	24.0±5.5	—
Xylazine Ketamine Thiamylal	1.1, IM 11–22, IM To effect, IV	25–60	Occasional seizures
Atropine Xylazine Ketamine	A 0.04, IV; X 1.1, IV; K 11, IV	—	—
	A 0.044, IM; X 1.1 IM; K 22 IM	17–35	↑ Risk in dogs with cardiopulmonary disease
Guaifenesin Xylazine Ketamine	G 50 mg/mL; X 0.25 mg/mL; K 1 mg/mL Induction, 0.55 mL/kg, IV Maintenance, 2.2 mL/kg/h, IV	120	Stable anesthesia
Medetomidine Ketamine	M 0.04, IM; K 2.5, IM	7.0±0.9	—
	M 0.04, IM; K 5, IM	30.0±4.9	Longer duration of muscle relaxation, and recovery than xylazine-ketamine, and prolonged recovery
	M 0.04, IM; K 7.5, IM	51±8	—
	M 0.04, IM; K 5, IM	>75	Significant cardiovascular changes
Diazepam Ketamine	D 0.28, IV; K 5.5, IV	—	Suitable induction for greyhound
Midazolam	M 0.5, IV; K 10, IV	13.3±3.1	↑ Heart rate, mild respiratory depression, and better muscle relaxation
Ketamine	M 0.28, IV; K 5.5, IV	—	More myoclonic movements, shorter time to intubation, and suitable induction for greyhound

CRI, continuous-rate infusion; IM, intramuscularly; IV, intravenously; MAC, minimum alveolar concentration.

Table 12.2. Use of Telazol alone or Telazol combinations in dogs.

Drug(s)	Dose and Route (mg/kg)	Duration (min)	Comment
Telazol alone	9.9, IM	21.0±10.9	Unsatisfactory recovery in two dogs
	9.9, IV	20.1±6.38	—
Telazol alone	6.6, IV	17.5±11.7	Smooth recovery
	13.2, IV	37.0±18.1	Rougher recovery
	19.8, IV	50.8±27.27	Rougher recovery
Telazol alone	6.6–9.9, IM	30	Diagnostic examinations
			Restraint
	2–4, IV	15–20	Diagnostic examinations
			Restraint
	9.9–13.2 IM	30–90	Minor surgical procedures (mild to moderate analgesia)
	4.0–9.9 IV	20–80	—
Telazol alone	2, IV	11.9±6.6	Minor procedures require no intubation
			Easy intubation
	4, IV	22.7±7.3	—
Telazol alone	15.4, IM	40	Anesthesia
	6.6, IV or IM	20–25	Light surgical anesthesia
Telazol alone	5.7, IM (4.0–8.6)	41.5 (15–77)	Satisfactory anesthesia
	9.7, IM (8.8–13.0)	56.6 (33–106)	Satisfactory anesthesia
	17.8, IM (13–22)	79.7 (37–124)	Satisfactory anesthesia
Telazol alone	4, IV	—	Satisfactory restraint for intradermal skin testing
Telazol alone	5, IV	38.5±23.0	Injection of flumazenil shortens recovery
Telazol alone	6–12, IM	—	—
Telazol alone	4–100, IM	—	—
Telazol	8.8, IM	100	Anesthesia
Xylazine	1.1, IM		Good muscle relaxation
Butorphanol	0.22, IM		Good analgesia
Telazol alone	19.7±3.3, IM	—	Unsatisfactory sedation in vicious dogs
Butorphanol	0.7, IM	—	Unsatisfactory sedation in vicious dogs
Telazol	10.6±1.3, IM		
Acepromazine	1.8±1.2, IM	—	Adequate sedation in vicious dogs
Telazol	19.3±1.8, IM		

IM, intramuscularly; IV, intravenously.

doses produce insufficient anesthesia and have a greater tendency to cause seizure. Dogs might salivate excessively during ketamine anesthesia, but this can be controlled with atropine or glycopyrrolate. α_2-Adrenergic agonist–induced bradycardia and second-degree atrioventricular block may be minimized by ketamine's sympathomimetic effect. However, atropine should be given if cardiac slowing is pronounced. An advantage of α_2-adrenergic agonist–ketamine combinations is the reversibility of CNS and cardiopulmonary depression. Antagonism should not be initiated for at least 20 min after ketamine administration unless required to treat severe adverse effects. Earlier antagonism may cause ketamine-induced hyperexcitability and seizures.[132]

In dogs, intravenous continuous-rate infusion of a low dose of ketamine (10 µg/kg/min) reduces the isoflurane MAC by 25%, whereas the continuous-rate infusion of a combination of morphine (3.3 µg/kg/min), lidocaine (50 µg/kg/min), and ketamine (10 µg/kg/min) has reduced the isoflurane requirement as much as 45%.[133] Concurrent administration of either morphine-lidocaine or morphine-ketamine combinations reportedly reduces CNS hypersensitivity in people suffering inflammatory or neuropathic pain.[134–137] Tables 12.1 and 12.2 further summarize the use of ketamine and Telazol either alone or in combination with various other classes of drugs when employed as anesthetics in dogs.

Cats

In cats, dissociatives have been used as primary anesthetic agents. Diazepam (0.3 mg/kg) is commonly mixed in the same syringe with ketamine (5.5 mg/kg) and given slowly IV for short-term anesthesia. This has proven to be a safe combination in cats with compromised cardiovascular function. Diazepam (0.22 mg/kg IV or 0.44 mg/kg IM) followed by ketamine (1 to 5 mg/kg IM) has also been used successfully in geriatric cats.[138] Administration of butorphanol prior to diazepam-ketamine may increase analgesia and enable diagnostic or surgical procedures to be performed when endotracheal intubation and delivery of an inhalant anesthetic are not feasible.[132] When various doses of midazolam (0.05, 0.5, 1.0, 2.0, or 5.0 mg/kg IV) are combined with ketamine (3 mg/kg IV), the duration of anesthesia increases slightly. However, increasing the intravenous midazolam dose (5 mg/kg) will often prolong objectionable behavioral signs (restlessness, vocalization, and changes in ability to approach and restrain).[139] Telazol has been used alone or in combination in cats. Zolazepam appears to be metabolized at a slower rate than tiletamine in this species, resulting in residual muscle relaxation and sedation, which often prolongs complete recovery. Xylazine and ketamine have been combined with Telazol to alter the dissociative anesthetic–benzodiazepine ratio, improving recovery characteristics, as well as facilitating possible antagonism with an α_2-adrenergic antagonist. This combination, which has been called *TKX* (Telazol-ketamine-xylazine), is made by reconstituting 500 mg of Telazol powder with 100 mg (1 mL of 100 mg/mL) of xylazine and 400 mg (4 mL) of ketamine. The resulting solution is very potent and, by using an insulin syringe, is more accurately dosed at 0.1 mL/5 kg of body weight.

Phenothiazine tranquilizers such as acepromazine have been combined with ketamine for better muscle relaxation and a smoother recovery. However, phenothiazine derivatives are α-adrenoceptor antagonists, and hypotension, prolonged recovery, and hypothermia may occur if they are used in higher doses.

α_2-Adrenergic agonist–ketamine combinations have often been used in cats. Xylazine (0.5 to 1.1 mg/kg IM), with or without atropine, is administered 20 min before ketamine (11 to 22 mg/kg IM).[68,140] Emesis is a common side effect of xylazine in cats, and it has been suggested that this should be allowed to occur prior to ketamine administration so as to prevent aspiration of stomach contents.[66] When compared with acepromazine (0.11 mg/kg IM)-ketamine (4.6 mg/kg IM), the simultaneous administration of xylazine (0.23 mg/kg IM)-ketamine (4.6 mg/kg IM) produces a longer anesthetic action. However, xylazine-ketamine anesthesia is also accompanied by longer-lasting cardiopulmonary depression.[141]

Medetomidine (10 to 80 μg/kg IM) has been combined with several different doses of ketamine (2.5, 5, 7.5, and 10 mg/kg IM) in cats undergoing ovariohysterectomy. The dose of ketamine is usually reduced as the medetomidine dose increases. Apnea may occur when the ketamine dose approaches 10 mg/kg. Good muscle relaxation and profound analgesia are comparable to that achieved with xylazine (1 mg/kg IM)-ketamine (10 mg/kg IM), and anesthesia lasts longer than it typically does with the acepromazine (1 mg/kg IM)-ketamine (10 mg/kg IM) combination.[142,143] Specific α_2-adrenergic antagonists such as atipamezole have been used to reverse medetomidine-ketamine anesthesia. Atipamezole dosed at two- to threefold the medetomidine dose is effective in antagonizing most of the anesthetic and analgesic effects of the medetomidine-ketamine combination.[144,145] Recovery to sternal recumbency usually occurs within 10 to 12 min after injection.[146] Bradycardia, vomiting, and excessive salivation, not unlike those seen with xylazine-ketamine, are the most common side effects following (2 to 5 min) medetomidine-ketamine administration.[147]

The use of oxymorphone, morphine, meperidine, and butorphanol has been assessed in combination with ketamine in cats.[148,149] When administered at oxymorphone's peak effect, the ketamine requirement is decreased by 2.5% to 10%.[148] Apparently, the administration of morphine or meperidine neither improves nor reduces the anesthetic effects of ketamine.[149] Adding butorphanol (0.1 mg/kg IV) to ketamine (8 mg/kg IV) appears to increase the intensity and duration of analgesia for a variety of procedures. The most effective dose of butorphanol ranges from 0.05 to 0.2 mg/kg IV. Some clinicians' experiences suggest that doses below and above this range provide less analgesia. It is important to realize that butorphanol is an opioid agonist-antagonist that has a *ceiling effect* on analgesia as well as undesirable opioid actions (e.g., respiratory depression). Doses above 0.2 mg/kg may cause CNS stimulation that is unaccompanied by an increased analgesic action. Tables 12.3 and 12.4 further summarize the use of ketamine and Telazol either alone or in combination with other drugs for use as anesthetics in cats.

Horses

Dissociatives should not be used as a monoanesthetics in horses because of the potential for dangerous and uncontrollable behavior and muscle incoordination. Preanesthetic sedation and tranquilization must be present before ketamine is administered. α_2-Adrenergic agonists (xylazine, detomidine, or romifidine) are most commonly used for this purpose. Xylazine (1.1 mg/kg IV), followed in 5 to 10 min by ketamine (2.2 to 3.0 mg/kg IV), induces a short period of anesthesia in horses. Higher doses of ketamine (2.75 to 3.0 mg/kg IV) are usually required for ponies, young "high-strung" Arabians, Hackneys, and thoroughbreds.[150] Ketamine should not be administered if xylazine fails to produce adequate sedation, and an alternative anesthetic technique (e.g., guaifenesin-thiobarbiturate mixture) should be considered.[150] It is not uncommon for heart and respiratory rates to decrease by one-third after xylazine administration.[151] After ketamine injection, heart rate may remain decreased while respiratory rate returns to prexylazine values.[151] Cardiac output and systemic arterial, pulmonary, and central venous pressures remain within normal ranges during xylazine-ketamine anesthesia.[151] Duration of anesthesia (15 to 20 min) is related to redistribution of ketamine to other body tissues and hepatic metabolism. In horses, approximately 60% of ketamine is metabolized by the liver, with the remainder excreted unchanged in the urine.[152] Anesthesia can be extended by administering one-third to one-half of the original dose of each drug.

In horses, the addition of butorphanol (0.01 or 0.02 mg/kg) enhances muscle relaxation and analgesia when using a xylazine-ketamine combination.[153] Behavioral changes caused by butorphanol may be breed dependent. CNS stimulation characterized by hyperresponsiveness and spasmodic lip movements has been reported in high-strung individuals after butorphanol intravenous administration, whereas deep sedation and ataxia were observed at the same dose when given to a Belgian stallion.[154] For extremely painful procedures, methadone with and without acepromazine has been administered to enhance analgesia during xylazine-ketamine anesthesia.[155,156]

Ketamine (1.5 to 2.0 mg/mL) can be added directly to a 5% solution of guaifenesin and the mixture administered as a rapid infusion, or ketamine can be administered as a bolus (1.5 to 2.2 mg/kg IV) after administration of enough guaifenesin to produce limb weakness (e.g., 1 to 2 mL/kg of a 5% solution). Less cardiovascular depression occurs with this combination, as compared

Table 12.3. Use of ketamine alone or ketamine combinations in cats.

Drug(s)	Dose and Route (mg/kg)	Duration (min)	Comment
Ketamine alone	2, 4, or 8, IV	105–115	Visceral analgesia
	4–30, IM	20–45	Incomplete immobilization and chemical restraint
		(11–40, IM)	Little analgesia, better muscle relaxation, and minor surgical procedures
	22–44, IM	—	Chemical restraint, cataleptoid anesthesia, and lack of muscle relaxation
	22, IM		Castration, onychectomy, and restraint
	33, IM	77	Ovariohysterectomy, cesarean section, laparotomy, orthopedic procedures; little analgesia, respiratory depression, and occasional apnea
Oxymorphone Triflupromazine Ketamine	0.16, SC, IM, IV 1.1, SC, IM, IV 1.1–2.2, SC, IM, IV	10–20	Light anesthesia
Xylazine Ketamine	X 1.1, IM; K 15.4–22, IM	25–40	Vomiting
	X 2.2, IM; K 11, IM	118	Vomiting
	X 0.23, IM; K 4.6, IM	85–135	Vomiting, and longer duration of anesthesia than acepromazine-ketamine
	X 2.2–4.4, IM; K 6.6, IM	60–100	—
	X 1, IM; K 10, IM	46.0±22.6	Satisfactory anesthesia, and depression of cardiovascular system
Atropine Xylazine Ketamine	0.3, IM 1.1, IM 22, IM	20	Satisfactory anesthesia
Guaifenesin Xylazine Ketamine	G 10 mg/mL; X 0.05 mg/mL; K 0.2 mg/mL Induction, 1.32±0.33 mL/kg, IV Maintenance, 10 mL/kg/h, IV	360	Easy administration, stable anesthesia, rapid recovery, and reversible with yohimbine or tolazoline
Acepromazine Ketamine	A 0.11, IM; K 4.6, IM	35–45	Better maintained heart rate than xylazine-ketamine
	A 1, IM; K 10, IM	20.0±14.8	Poor muscle relaxation and analgesia
	A 0.1, IV; K 2, IV	65	Visceral analgesia
	A 0.1, IV; K 4, IV	80	Visceral analgesia
	A 0.1, IV; K 8, IV	125±22	Visceral analgesia
Butorphanol Ketamine	B 0.1, IV; K 2, IV	280	Visceral analgesia
	B 0.1, IV; K 4, IV	325	Visceral analgesia
	B 0.1, IV; K 8, IV	360	Visceral analgesia
Medetomidine Ketamine	M 0.08, IM; K 2.5, IM	36.2±11.5	Better muscle relaxation and satisfactory anesthesia
	M 0.08, IM; K 5, IM	59.0±6.4	Better muscle relaxation and satisfactory anesthesia
	M 0.08, IM; K 7.5, IM	65.6±22.9	Better muscle relaxation and satisfactory anesthesia
	M 0.08, IM; K 10, IM	99.7±26.7	Better muscle relaxation, satisfactory anesthesia, and occasional apnea
	M 0.08, IM; K 7, IM	46±15	Vomiting, surgical anesthesia, and good muscle relaxation
	M 0.08, IM; K 5, IM	50.2	—
Detomidine Ketamine	D 0.5; K 10, oral	—	Greater sedation than oral xylazine-ketamine or medetomidine-ketamine
Diazepam Ketamine	D 0.2, IV; K 2, IV	20	Visceral analgesia
	D 0.2, IV; K 4, IV	60	Visceral analgesia
	D 0.2, IV; K 8, IV	100	Visceral analgesia
Midazolam Ketamine	M 0.5, IV; K 3, IV	—	↓ Muscle tone, dose-related behavioral signs, and suitable for clinical use
	M 0.5, IV; K 3, IV	5.0±1.1	Muscle relaxation and suitable for clinical use
	M 1, IV; K 3, IV	—	Suitable for clinical use
	M 2, IV; K 3, IV	—	—
	M 5, IV; K 5, IV	6.2±1.62	Prominent and long-lasting behavioral signs
Ketamine Propofol	K 23 or 46 µg/kg/min; P 0.025 mg/kg/min, IV Simultaneously	—	↓ Propofol dose requirement

IM, intramuscularly; IV, intravenously; SC, subcutaneously.

Table 12.4. Use of Telazol alone or Telazol combinations in cats.

Drug(s)	Dose and Route (mg/kg)	Duration (min)	Comment
Telazol alone	6–40, IM	—	—
Telazol alone	6–12, IM	—	Anesthesia
Telazol alone	12.8, IM	52.6±22.0	Salivation
			Apneustic breathing
	12.8, IV	52.8±17.3	Salivation
			Apneustic breathing
Telazol alone	7.5, IM	49.9±12.7	Surgical anesthesia
			Mild muscle relaxation
			Rough recovery
Telazol alone	9.7–11.9, IM	30	Diagnostic examinations
			Dentistry
	9.9, IV	25	Diagnostic examinations
			Dentistry
	10.6–12.5, IM	60	Minor procedure (mild to moderate analgesia)
	4.5, IM	30–60	Ovariohysterectomy
	4.5, IM	—	Onychectomy
	14.3–15.8, IM	60–135	—
Telazol alone	10.4, IM (6–16)	64.6 (32–135)	Satisfactory surgical anesthesia
			Salivation
Telazol alone	9.7, IV	60	—
	15.8, IV	>90	Respiratory depression
	23.7, IV	>90	Respiratory depression
Telazol alone	3.1±0.99, IM	—	Inadequate analgesia for castration
Acepromazine	A 0.1, IM; T, 3.4±1.09, IM or	—	Adequate anesthesia for castration
Telazol	2.7±0.97, IV		
Telazol alone	4.5±0.9, IM	—	Adequate anesthesia for castration
	4.5±0.9, IV	—	—
Telazol alone	5, IV	20.2±10.3	Injection of doxapram and flumazenil speed recovery
Telazol[a]	3.3, IM	43.4±9.1	Smooth induction and recovery
Ketamine	2.64, IM		Excellent muscle relaxation
Xylazine	0.66, IM		Good analgesia

IM, intramuscularly; IV, intravenously.
[a]Reconstitute with 4 mL of ketamine and 1 mL of 10% xylazine.

with thiopental-guaifenesin or thiamylal-guaifenesin anesthetic induction.[150,157] Bolus administration of ketamine plus guaifenesin in foals rapidly induces anesthesia with good muscle relaxation and analgesia followed by a smooth recovery.[158]

Continuous infusion of a guaifenesin-ketamine-xylazine combination is safe and effective for extending anesthesia in adult horses after xylazine (1.1 mg/kg IV) and ketamine (2.2 to 3.0 mg/kg IV) induction. This drug combination is prepared by adding 500 mg of xylazine and 2000 mg of ketamine to 1 L of 5% guaifenesin.[159–161] In ponies anesthetized for 2 h with this mixture, arterial blood pressure and left ventricular stroke work index were transiently decreased for the first 15 to 30 min after induction.[160] Cardiac index and arterial pH were also decreased for 15 min after induction. Hypoventilation with mild hypercapnia was noted throughout the study. These changes are transient and comparable to those reported for other injectable anesthetic drugs or drug combinations. In ponies and foals, anesthesia can be induced with a rapid intravenous injection of 1.1 mL/kg of the guaifenesin-ketamine-xylazine mixture. Anesthesia may be maintained by continuous intravenous infusion of 2 to 4 mL · kg^{-1} ·

h^{-1}, depending on anesthetic requirement. Standing recovery usually occurs within 25 to 45 min of discontinuation of the mixture.[150–162] An α_2-adrenergic antagonist such as tolazoline (2 to 4 mg/kg) can be administered IV to hasten recovery. When diazepam (0.1 mg/kg) is combined with xylazine (0.3 mg/kg) and ketamine (2 mg/kg), muscle relaxation is improved when compared with the administration of xylazine-ketamine alone. Diazepam provides practical advantages over guaifenesin in commercial preparation, small volume, and ease of administration.[163]

Detomidine is approved for use in horses in the United States as a sedative-analgesic for colic. Short-term anesthesia in horses can be achieved with detomidine (20 µg/kg IV) sedation followed in 6 to 8 min by ketamine (2.2 mg/kg IV). Mean arterial blood pressure increases after detomidine-ketamine injection.[164,165] When compared with xylazine, detomidine may induce better muscle relaxation when combined with ketamine. Recovery can be somewhat unpredictable. Occasionally, horses and ponies experience a rough recovery.[166] This may result from the longer sedation and muscle relaxation achieved with detomidine in some animals.[164–166]

Romifidine (100 µg/kg IV) has also been used in combination with ketamine (2.0 to 2.2 mg/kg IV) for short-term anesthesia or for induction prior to inhalation anesthesia in horses. The anesthesia duration produced by this combination is 10 to 25 min, similar to that of xylazine-ketamine.[167–169] Tables 12.5 and 12.6 further summarize ketamine and Telazol combination anesthesia in horses.

Ruminants

Xylazine (0.1 to 0.2 mg/kg IV) is commonly administered prior to, or concomitantly with, ketamine (2.2 to 3.0 mg/kg IV) for short-term anesthesia of ruminants. Tracheal intubation is easily achieved in cattle anesthetized with this combination.[170,171] Anesthesia may be safely prolonged by administering ketamine (1 to 2 mg/kg) slowly to effect. Alternatively, anesthesia can be

Table 12.5. Use of ketamine alone or ketamine combinations in horses.

Drug(s)	Dose and Route (mg/kg)	Duration (min)	Comment
Xylazine Ketamine	X 1.1, IV, wait 3–5 min; K 2.2, IV	16.1±7.3	Excellent analgesia and light anesthesia
	X 1.1, IV; K 2.2, IV Simultaneously	—	Excitement following induction
	X 1.1, IV, wait 3–5 min; K 6.6, IV	12.1±3.2	Muscle twitching, rapid nystagmus, and prolonged and rough recovery
	X 1.1, IV; K 2.2, IV	24	Inadequate muscle relaxation
	X 1.1, IV; K 2.2, IV	12–35	Smooth induction and recovery
Xylazine Butorphanol Ketamine	X 1.1, IV; B 0.1 or 0.2, IV; K 2.2, IV	Arabian, 18.25 Belgian, 52.5 Appaloosa: 56.5	Behavioral changes and enhanced muscle relaxation and analgesia
	X 1.1, IV; B 0.044, IV; K 2.2, IV	37	Adequate muscle relaxation and good analgesia
Xylazine Ketamine Methadone	X 1.1, IV; K 2.2, IV; M 0.1, IV	—	Satisfactory anesthesia
Methadone Acepromazine Xylazine Ketamine	M 0.1, IV; A 0.15, IV; X 1.1, IV; K 2.2, IV	—	Inadequate anesthesia
Acepromazine Methadone Ketamine	A 0.1, IV; M 0.1, IV; K 2.2, IV	—	—
	A 0.04, IV; M 0.04, IV; K 2.0–2.5, IV	10.2 (3–18)	Muscle tremor lasted < 1 min after induction
Guaifenesin Xylazine Ketamine	G 50 mg/mL; X 0.5 mg/mL; K 1 mg/mL Induction, 1.1 mL/kg, IV Maintenance, 2.75 mL/kg/h, IV	120	↓ Blood pressure initially and hypoventilation
	G 50 mg/mL; X 0.5 mg/mL; K 1 mg/mL Induction, 1.1 mL/kg, IV Maintenance, 4.5 mL/kg/h, IV	49±3	Surgical anesthesia
	G 50 mg/mL; X 0.5 mg/mL; K 2 mg/mL Induction, 1.1 mL/kg, IV Maintenance, 4.3 mL/kg/h, IV	44±2	Better muscle relaxation, analgesia, and surgical anesthesia
	G 100 mg/mL; X 1 mg/mL; K 2 mg/mL Maintenance, 1.1 mL/kg/h, IV	51–95	Presence of swallowing reflex, not suitable for laryngeal surgery, surgical anesthesia, and smooth recovery
	X 1.1, IV; G 100, IV; K 2, IV	—	Supplemental ketamine 200–1000 mg, maintain with halothane, and good muscle relaxation
Guaifenesin Ketamine	G 50 mg/mL; K 2 mg/mL at 1.5– 2.2 mg/kg K, IV	—	Less cardiovascular depression than thiamylal-guaifenesin or thiopental-guaifenesin
	K 6 mg/mL in 150 mg/mL G; IV infusion of 7.8 µg/kg/min initially	—	↓ Halothane MAC by 50%
Xylazine Diazepam Ketamine	X 0.3, IV; D 0.05, IV; K 2, IV	—	Supplemental ketamine 200–500 mg, maintain with halothane
	X 1.1, IV; D 0.1, IV; K 2, IV	—	Supplemental ketamine 200–750 mg, maintain with halothane, good muscle relaxation

(continued)

Table 12.5. Use of ketamine alone or ketamine combinations in horses (*continued*).

Drug(s)	Dose and Route (mg/kg)	Duration (min)	Comment
Xylazine Temazepam Ketamine	X 1.1, IV; T 0.044, IV; K 2.2, IV	—	Longer recumbency
Romifidine Ketamine	R 0.1, IV; K 2.0–2.2, IV	10–25	Initial limb rigidity and mild muscle tremor
Romifidine Midazolam Ketamine	R 0.08, IV; M 0.06, IV; K 2.2, IV R 20 mg, M 15 mg, K 500 mg in 50 mL 0.9% NaCl; maintenance, 0.24 mL/kg/h, IV; one-third of induction MK, IV if spontaneous movements occur	25–40	May require additional dose of MK Smooth recovery
Ketamine alone	5–6 mg/100 kg in subarachnoid space	—	Effective spinal block
	10–12 mg/100 kg in subarachnoid space	—	Blockade of T13 to L3 Effective surgical analgesia
	0.5, 1, 2 mg/100 kg in caudal epidural space	10–15	Dose-dependent perineal analgesia
	5 mL of 1, 2, or 3% solution, infiltration at the base of the proximal sesamoid		↓ Halothane MAC by 14% and 12%, respectively Abaxial sesamoid nerve block
Xylazine Ketamine	X 0.5 mg/100 kg; K 1 mg/100 kg; simultaneously in caudal epidural space	>20	Perineal analgesia may extend to the thigh and flank region
Methotrimeprazine Midazolam Guaifenesin Ketamine	Me 0.5, IV; Mi 0.1, IV; G 100, IV; K 1.6, IV	—	Induction of anesthesia, smooth recovery
Detomidine Ketamine	D 0.02, IV; K 2.2, IV	—	Second dose of ketamine (1.4 mg/kg) given 15 min after first dose; improve anesthesia
	D 0.02, IV; K 2.2, IV	10–43	Required more time than xylazine-ketamine to assume recumbency, occasional poor recovery, and longer-lasting hypertension
	D 0.02 IV; K 2.2, IV	26.8 (14–42)	Smooth induction and occasional rough recovery
Guaifenesin Detomidine Ketamine	G 50 mg/mL; D 5 µg/mL; K 2 mg/mL Induction, 0.67–1.1 mL/kg, IV Maintenance, 2.2 mL/kg/h, IV	—	Good muscle relaxation and analgesia, and minimal cardiovascular effects
	G 100 mg/mL; D 0.04 mg/mL; K 4 mg/mL Maintenance, 0.67±0.17 mL/kg/h, IV	140	Surgical anesthesia but may require additional ketamine during surgery Good recovery
Detomidine Butorphanol Ketamine	0.02, IV 0.04, IV 2.2, IV	36.2 (18–67)	Smooth induction Smoother recovery Muscle relaxation

IM, intramuscularly; IV, intravenously; MAC, minimum alveolar concentration.

maintained in adult cattle with a continuous infusion of ketamine in saline or 5% dextrose solution (2 mg/mL) at a rate of 10 mL/min.[172] Clinical experience shows that guaifenesin-ketamine-xylazine mixture is an effective anesthetic combination in ruminants. The concentration of each drug in the mixture is 50 mg/mL, 2 mg/mL, and 0.1 mg/mL for guaifenesin, ketamine, and xylazine, respectively. Anesthesia can be induced with 0.55 to 1.1 mL/kg initially and maintained with adjustment for surgical stimulation with 2.2 mL · kg^{-1} · h^{-1} in adult cattle and 1.65 mL · kg^{-1} · h^{-1} in calves, kids, and lambs. Anesthesia onset is gradual but smooth. Muscle relaxation is excellent, easily enabling tracheal intubation. Supplementation with oxygen (5 to 10 L/min) during procedures may help prevent hypoxemia. Mild hypoventilation is induced by the anesthetic mixture. Surgical procedures that can be performed in cattle anesthetized with guaifenesin-ketamine-xylazine include femoral fracture plating and pinning, penile surgery, umbilical hernia repair, cesarean section, and celiotomy.[172] Tables 12.7 and 12.8 further summa-

Table 12.6. Use of Telazol alone or Telazol combinations in equids.

Species	Drug(s)	Dose and Route (mg/kg)	Duration (min)	Comment
Horses	Xylazine Telazol	1.1, IV 1.65, IV	—	Anesthesia Smooth recovery
		1.1, IV 0.5, IV	26.25	Adequate anesthesia Easy intubation Hyperresponsiveness during recovery
		1.1, IV 0.75, IV	29.25	Adequate anesthesia Easy intubation Hyperresponsiveness during recovery
		1.1, IV 2.2, IV	34.33	Adequate anesthesia Easy intubation Smooth recovery
		1.1, IV 1.65, IV	32.8±2.8	Good muscle relaxation Smooth recovery[b]
	Detomidine Telazol	0.02, IV 2, IV	38.5±9.0	Balanced anesthesia Smooth recovery[b]
		0.04, IV 2, IV	66.5±10.3	Balanced anesthesia Excellent recovery[a]
		0.06, IV 3, IV	91.5±18.0	Balanced anesthesia Prolonged duration Rough recovery[c]
		0.015, IV 2, IV	25.5±3.0	Satisfactory induction and recovery
	Xylazine Telazol	1.1, IV 1.1, IV	30.7 (24–35)	Good muscle relaxation Smooth recovery[b]
	Xylazine Butorphanol Telazol	1.1, IV 0.04, IV 1.1, IV	41.3 (33–66)	Good muscle relaxation Prolonged analgesia Smooth recovery[b]
	Detomidine Telazol	0.02, IV 1.1, IV	26±4	Good muscle relaxation Prolonged analgesia Hypoxemia
		0.04, IV 1.4, IV	39±11	Good muscle relaxation Prolonged analgesia Hypoxemia
	Detomidine Ketamine Telazol	0.013, IV 0.53, IV 0.67, IV	—	Poor recovery
	Telazol alone	0.5 and 1.0 in caudal epidural space	60–90	Perineal analgesia One horse had muscle fasciculation and central nervous system excitation after high dose Ataxia
Mules	Xylazine Telazol	1.1, IV 1.1, IV	21.1	Smooth recovery[b]
Donkeys	Xylazine Telazol	1.1, IV 1.1, IV	46	Satisfactory anesthesia Good muscle relaxation Smooth recovery[b]
Miniature donkeys	Xylazine Butorphanol Telazol	1.1, IV 0.044, IV 1.1, IV	33.8±6.3	Satisfactory anesthesia Good recovery IM, intramuscularly; IV, intravenously.

IM, intramuscularly; IV, intravenously.
[a]Animals stood at first attempt.
[b]Animals stood requiring less than three attempts.
[c]Animals stood requiring greater than five attempts.

Table 12.7. Use of ketamine alone or ketamine combinations in ruminants.

Species	Drug(s)	Dose and Route (mg/kg)	Duration (min)	Comment
Cattle	Ketamine alone Xylazine Ketamine	2 mg/mL in saline, given at 10 mL/min, IV 0.1, IV 2, IV Suppl,[a] 2% ketamine in saline	— —	— Recovery in 45 min
	Ketamine alone	1.5–4.6, IV	—	—
	Xylazine Ketamine	0.22, IM, IV 1.8–4.6, IV	—	Muscle relaxation adequate for tracheal intubation
	Xylazine Ketamine	0.22, IM 11, IM	40–55	Good muscle relaxation Surgical anesthesia
	Ketamine alone	11, IV	—	Dose repeated every 30 min for a duration of 3–4 h
	Xylazine Ketamine	0.14, IM 2.8, IV	—	Better muscle relaxation
	Xylazine Ketamine	0.2, IM 5, IV Given separately	20	Rapid onset of action Easy tracheal intubation Transient respiratory depression
	Xylazine Ketamine	0.2, IM 10, IM Given separately	23.5±1.8	Rapid breathing Easy tracheal intubation Good muscle relaxation
	Xylazine Ketamine	0.2, IM 10, IM Simultaneously	37.0±3.4	Good muscle relaxation Good analgesia
	Xylazine Ketamine	0.088, IM 4.4, IM	55.7±10.4	Good muscle relaxation Good analgesia
	Medetomidine Ketamine	0.02, IV 2.2, IV	94±25	Sternal recumbency
	Diazepam Guaifenesin Ketamine	1.16±0.05, IV 115.23±5.13, IV 5.49±0.6, IV	22.2±3.2	Surgical anesthesia
	Diazepam Ketamine	1.18±0.04, IV 10.63±0.56, IV	36.0±3.67	Smooth induction and recovery
Sheep	Ketamine alone	22, IV	23.0±12.05	Marked muscle rigidity Mild salivation
	Xylazine Ketamine	0.2, IM 22, IV	67.0±21.6	Salivation Regurgitation ↓ Muscle rigidity Prolonged anesthesia
	Atropine Xylazine Ketamine	0.2, IM 0.2, IM 22, IV	34.0±5.5	↓ Salivation Urination Regurgitation Tachycardia
	Diazepam Ketamine	0.375, IV 7.5, IV	15	↓ Cardiac output ↑ Systemic vascular resistance
	Xylazine Ketamine	0.1, IV 7.5, IV	25	↓ Cardiac output, systemic vascular resistance and mean arterial pressure Avoid in compromised heart function
	Medetomidine Ketamine	0.025, IM 1, IM	—	Good muscle relaxation Tachypnea

(continued)

Table 12.7. Use of ketamine alone or ketamine combinations in ruminants (*continued*).

Species	Drug(s)	Dose and Route (mg/kg)	Duration (min)	Comment
Sheep	Diazepam Ketamine	0.375, IV 7.5, IV Maintenance, D 0.188, IV; K 3.75, IV; every 15 min	120	Satisfactory anesthesia Hypotension Respiratory acidosis ↑ Systemic and pulmonary vascular resistance
	Guaifenesin Xylazine Ketamine	50 mg/mL 0.1 mg/mL 1 mg/mL Induction, 0.67–1.1 mL/kg, IV Maintenance, 2.2 mL/kg, IV	60	Surgical anesthesia ↑ Respiratory rate, ↓ PaO$_2$[b] Supplemental 100% oxygen
Goats	Atropine Xylazine Ketamine	0.44, IM 0.22, IM 11, IM	40–45	Good muscle relaxation
	Ketamine alone	3, IV	—	Adequate for tracheal intubation
	Ketamine alone	22, IM	10.3	Apneustic breathing
	Atropine Ketamine	0.44, IM 22, IM	10.2	↓ Salivation
	Atropine Acepromazine Ketamine	0.44, IM 0.88, IM 22, IM	22.2	↑ Duration and degree of analgesia and muscle relaxation
	Atropine Diazepam Ketamine	0.44, IM 0.88, IM 22, IM	22.4	↑ Duration and degree of analgesia and muscle relaxation
	Atropine Xylazine Ketamine	0.44, IM 0.22, IM 11, IM	45.2	↑ Duration and degree of analgesia and muscle relaxation
	Midazolam Ketamine	0.4, IM 4, IM	16–39	Surgical anesthesia
	Ketamine alone	3 in subarachnoid space	48.8±3.5	Analgesia up to L1 Sedation, ataxia, and sternal recumbency
Llamas	Xylazine Ketamine	0.35, IM or 0.25, IV 5–8, IM or 3–5, IV	30–60	Restraint Anesthesia
	Xylazine Ketamine	0.4, IM or 0.8, IM 4, IM or 8, IM	— 73±18	Low doses of XK induced sternal recumbency High doses of XK induced analgesia Hypoxemia
	Guaifenesin Ketamine	80, IV 1.6, IV	15–20	Good muscle relaxation Little analgesia
	Diazepam Ketamine	0.2–0.3, IM or 0.1–0.2, IV 5–8, IM or 3–5, IV	—	Anesthesia

IM, intramuscularly; IV, intravenously; SC, subcutaneously.
[a]Suppl, supplemental dose.
[b]PaO$_2$, arterial oxygen partial pressure.

Table 12.8. Use of Telazol alone or Telazol combinations in ruminants.

Species	Drug(s)	Dose and Route (mg/kg)	Duration (min)	Comment
Calves	Telazol alone	4, IV	50–60	Anesthesia
	Xylazine Telazol	0.1, IV 4, IV	66	Anesthesia
Cattle	Telazol alone	2–6	—	—
Sheep	Telazol Butorphanol	12, IV 0.5, IV	31 (25–45)	Adequate anesthesia
	Telazol alone	11.9±2.7, IV (8.1–16.8) Suppl,ᵃ 5.7, IV	150 (48–222) 210 (48–318)	Cataleptoid anesthesia Excellent muscle relaxation Muscle relaxation not as good as single dose
	Telazol alone	14.4, IV (12–22)	41.5 (25–65)	Satisfactory anesthesia for neurosurgical procedures
	Telazol alone	2.2–4.4, IM	—	Immobilization
	Telazol alone	8–22	—	—
	Telazol alone	12, IV	39±5	Smooth induction Gradual but unremarkable recovery Apneustic breathing
	Telazol alone	24, IV	40±14	Smooth induction Gradual but unremarkable recovery Apneustic breathing
	No atropine Telazol Telazol Telazol	9, IM 12, IM 15, IM	14 35 51	Variable anesthetic response Surgical anesthesia Prolonged anesthetic duration
	With atropine Telazol Telazol Telazol	0.04, IM 9, IM 12, IM 15, IM	13 28 42	— — —
	Atropine Telazol	0.03, IM 13.2, IV	41.6±15.0	—
	Xylazine Telazol	0.01, IM 13.2, IV	101.7±26.0	Better muscle relaxation Longer anesthetic duration Apnea
Llamas	Telazol alone	4.4, IM	25–50	Chemical restraint

IM, intramuscularly; IV, intravenously.
ᵃSuppl, supplemental dose.

rize the use of ketamine combinations and Telazol for anesthesia in ruminants.

In llamas, xylazine (0.25 mg/kg IM) followed in 15 min by ketamine (5 mg/kg IM) induces 30 to 60 min of anesthesia and restraint sufficient for minor procedures such as suturing lacerations, abscess drainage, or cast application.[173] If tracheal intubation is desired, xylazine (0.25 mg/kg IV) with ketamine (2.5 mg/kg IV) can be used. Changes in heart rate and blood pressure are similar to those observed in other species. A recent study compared the anesthetic effects of two combinations of xy-

lazine (0.4 and 0.8 mg/kg IM) and ketamine (4 and 8 mg/IM) in llamas. The low-dose combination induced sternal recumbency, but analgesia-anesthesia was observed in only two llamas. The high-dose combination produced longer recumbency (87 vs. 19 min) and analgesia (73 vs. 18 min). Severe hypoxemia was observed in llamas receiving the high-dose combination, as evidenced by low saturation of peripheral oxygen measured by pulse oximeter and low PaO_2 measured from arterial blood gas. Hypoxemia can be treated effectively with nasal insufflation of 100% oxygen.[174]

Swine

Ketamine has been used extensively in pigs premedicated with atropine (0.04 mg/kg IM) for minor surgical and diagnostic procedures. At intramuscular doses of 11 to 20 mg/kg, muscle relaxation is poor and analgesia is brief. Green et al.[175] reported that pigs react violently to intramuscular injections of ketamine and then exhibit muscle tremor, extensor rigidity, panting respiration, and erythema. These responses can be minimized by combining diazepam (1 mg/kg IM) or xylazine (2 mg/kg IM) with ketamine (10 to 20 mg/kg IM). Deep sedation and good muscle relaxation occur with these drug combinations, but pigs may still respond to noxious stimuli such as incision of the abdominal wall.[175,176] Alternatively, a combination of oxymorphone (0.075 mg/kg), xylazine (2 mg/kg), and ketamine (2 mg/kg) mixed in the same syringe and given IV induces surgical anesthesia. When given IM, satisfactory anesthesia can be achieved by doubling the dose of each drug.[171,177]

Short-term anesthesia in pigs can also be achieved with at-ropine (0.025 mg/kg IM)-butorphanol (0.2 mg/kg IM)-xylazine (2 mg/kg IM)-ketamine (10 mg/kg IM) (ABXK) or with atropine (0.025 mg/kg IM)-butorphanol (0.2 mg/kg IM)-medetomidine (80 µg/kg IM)-ketamine (10 mg/kg IM) (ABMK). Anesthesia is induced rapidly with both combinations, but ABMK appears to induce more effective anesthesia for major surgery, which is characterized by good muscle relaxation enabling endotracheal intubation for over 1.5 h. Atipamezole (240 µg/kg IV or IM) can be administered to shorten the anesthesia.[178] Medetomidine-ketamine appears to produce longer periods of muscle relaxation (43.6 vs. 12.7 min vs. 21.0 vs. 14 min) and anesthesia (49.4 vs. 13.5 min vs. 34.6 vs. 17.2 min) than does xylazine-ketamine in pigs. Slight cardiovascular stimulation with minimal respiratory effect occurs during medetomidine-ketamine anesthesia.[179] Tables 12.9 and 12.10 further summarize the use of ketamine combinations and the use of Telazol for anesthesia in swine.

Table 12.9. Use of ketamine alone or ketamine combinations in swine.

Drug(s)	Dose and Route (mg/kg)	Duration (min)	Comment
Atropine Ketamine	0.044, IM 20, IM	10–30	Poor muscle relaxation and analgesia
Xylazine Ketamine	2, IM 20, IM	—	Required supplemental dose for intubation
Innovar-Vet Ketamine	1 mL/13.6 kg, IM 11, IM	41.75	Good muscle relaxation
Acepromazine Ketamine	0.5, IM 15, IM	18.25	Strong, sharp muscle activity
Xylazine Ketamine	0.2, IM 11, IM	24.5	Strong, sharp muscle activity
Ketamine alone	10–20, IM	—	Violent reaction, muscle tremor, extensor rigidity, ↑ heart rate and respiratory rate, panting respiration, and erythema
Diazepam Ketamine	1, IM 10, IM	40	Deep sedation and response to incision Good muscle relaxation
Xylazine Ketamine	2, IM 15, IM	40	Deep sedation Good analgesia Excellent muscle relaxation
Xylazine Ketamine Oxymorphone	2, IV 2, IV 0.075, IV	20–30	Good analgesia and muscle relaxation Smooth recovery, which can be shortened by naloxone
Xylazine Ketamine	1, IV 10, IV	25	Good analgesia
Guaifenesin Xylazine Ketamine	50 mg/mL 1 mg/mL 1 mg/mL Induction, 0.67–1.1 mL/kg, IV Maintenance, 2.2 mL/kg/h, IV	120	Good muscle relaxation and analgesia Minimal cardiovascular changes
Atropine Butorphanol Xylazine Ketamine	0.025, IM 0.2, IM 2, IM 10, IM	—	Rapid induction of anesthesia

(continued)

Table 12.9. Use of ketamine alone or ketamine combinations in swine (*continued*).

Drug(s)	Dose and Route (mg/kg)	Duration (min)	Comment
Atropine Butorphanol Medetomidine Ketamine	0.025, IM 0.2, IM 0.08, IM 10, IM	—	Rapid induction of anesthesia Good muscle relaxation
Meperidine Azaperone Ketamine Morphine	2.2, IM 2.2, IM 22, IM 1.7, IM	60.6±18.6	Surgical anesthesia Rapid and smooth recovery Anesthesia can be prolonged by supplemental ketamine and morphine
Miniature Pigs Xylazine Ketamine Butorphanol	2, IM 5, IM 0.1–0.22, IM	—	Light anesthesia
Xylazine Ketamine	2.2, IM 11.0–17.6, IM	—	Induction of anesthesia Short procedures
Diazepam Ketamine	1.1, IM 11.0–17.6, IM	—	—
Diazepam Ketamine	0.05–0.1, IM 10–30, IM	20–30	Deep sedation
Midazolam Ketamine	0.2–0.4, IM 10–30, IM	20–30	Deep sedation
Xylazine Ketamine	4, IM 5–10, IM	20–30	Deep sedation
Innovar-Vet Ketamine	1 mL/20 kg, IM 10–20, IM	20–30	Deep sedation
Atropine Xylazine Ketamine	0.04, IM 2.2, IM 12–20, IM	—	Anesthesia can be prolonged with supplemental ketamine 2–4 mg/kg IV
Diazepam Ketamine	1–2, IM 12–20, IM	—	—
Butorphanol Xylazine Ketamine	0.22, IM 2, IM 11, IM	—	Enhanced analgesia Satisfactory anesthesia for abdominal surgery

IM, intramuscularly; IV, intravenously.

Table 12.10. Use of Telazol alone or Telazol combinations in swine.

Drug(s)	Dose and Route (mg/kg)	Duration (min)	Comment
Xylazine Telazol	1.1, IM 6, IM	47±11	Satisfactory anesthesia Easy administration
Xylazine Telazol	2.2, IM 6, IM	67.5±9.0	Longer duration of analgesia
Telazol alone	10, IM	33.7±15.0	Good muscle relaxation Poor analgesia Excited recovery
	2–4, IM	—	Immobilization
	4.0–8.8, IM		Anesthesia
Telazol[a] Ketamine Xylazine	0.006–0.013 mL/kg, IM or 0.02–0.026 mL/kg, IM	35–40 25–35	Sedation and immobilization Surgical anesthesia

IM, intramuscularly.

[a]Reconstitute Telazol with 2.5 mL of ketamine and 2.5 mL of 10% xylazine.

Table 12.11. Use of ketamine alone or ketamine combinations in exotic and wildlife animals.

Common Names (Genus and Species)	Drug(s)	Dose and Route (mg/kg)	Duration (min)	Comment	Reference
Order Artiodactyla, family Bovidae					
Buffalo calf (*Bubalus bubalis*)	Ketamine alone	2, IV	4.45±0.34 (3.0–5.5)	—	187
	Ketamine Chlorpromazine	2, IV 2, IM	11.17±0.77 (6–14)	Prolongs analgesia, recovery time, and degree of muscle relaxation	
	Ketamine alone	Induction, 2, IV Maintenance, 0.2% infusion	60	Abdominal muscle relaxation	188
Alpine goat (*Capra hircus*)	Xylazine Ketamine	0.35, IM (0.1–0.62) 2.92, IM (1.65–6.2)	—	—	189
Goat (*Capra hircus*)	Ketamine alone	10–20, IM	—	—	190
Bighorn sheep (*Ovis canadensis*)	Xylazine Ketamine	Male: 70–300 mg, IM Female: 70–250 mg, IM Lambs: 80–90 mg, IM; 200 mg, IM	—	—	191
Alpine ibex (*Capra ibex*)	Medetomidine Ketamine	0.08–0.1, IM 1.5–2.0, IM	—	Complete immobilization	192
Barbary sheep (*Ammotragus lervia*)	Medetomidine Ketamine	0.08–0.1, IM 1.5–2.0, IM	—	Satisfactory immobilization Supplemental IV medetomidine (20%–25% of first dose) induced complete immobilization	193
Markhor (*Capra falconerii megaceros*)	Medetomidine Ketamine	0.069, IM 1.6, IM	—	Immobilization Good muscle relaxation	193
Mouflon sheep (*Ovis musimon*)	Medetomidine Ketamine	0.125, IM 2.5, IM	—	Complete immobilization	192
Zebu (*Bos indicus*)	Ketamine alone	5–20, IM	—	—	190
Order Artiodactyla, family Cervidae					
Chital deer (*Axis axis*)	Xylazine-ketamine mix (1:1) Xylazine, 100 mg/mL Ketamine, 100 mg/mL	Stags (90–100 kg), 1.5–2.0 mL, IM total dose	—	—	194
Fallow deer (*Dama dama*)	Xylazine-ketamine mix (1:1) Xylazine, 125 mg/mL Ketamine, 100 mg/mL	Yearlings (30–50 kg), 1 mL[a] Young buck (50–75 kg), 1.5 mL[a] Adult (35–45 kg), 1.5 mL[a] Large buck (>75 kg), 2 mL[a] Large buck (>90 kg), 2.5 mL[a] All doses are IM	—	— — — — — —	194
	Xylazine Ketamine	4, IM 3, IM	—	—	195

(continued)

317

Table 12.11. Use of ketamine alone or ketamine combinations in exotic and wildlife animals (*continued*).

Common Names (Genus and Species)	Drug(s)	Dose and Route (mg/kg)	Duration (min)	Comment	Reference
Fallow deer (*Dama dama*)	Medetomidine Ketamine	0.08–0.12, IM 1–2, IM	—	Complete immobilization	192
Red deer (*Cervus elaphus*)	Xylazine-ketamine mix (1:1) Xylazine, 125 mg/mL Ketamine, 100 mg/mL	Mature stags, 2 mL, IM[a] Yearlings, 1.5 mL, IM[a]	— —	— —	194
	Xylazine Ketamine	1.2, IM 1, IM	—	—	195
Domestic reindeer	Medetomidine Ketamine	0.025, IM 0.5, IM	—	Complete immobilization	192
Forest reindeer (*Rangifer tarandus fennicus*)	Medetomidine Ketamine	0.059±0.013, IM (0.037–0.084 range) 0.9±0.3, IM (0.4–1.9 range)	—	Immobilization	196
	Medetomidine Ketamine	0.0487, IM 1.1, IM	—	Complete immobilization	193
White-tailed deer (*Odocoileus virginianus*)	Xylazine Ketamine	0.54–1.99, IM 3.78–14.77, IM	—	Immobilization	197
	Xylazine Ketamine	100 mg total, IM 300 mg total, IM	—	—	198
	Xylazine Ketamine	0.35, IM (0.1–0.62) 2.92, IM (1.65–6.2)	—	—	189
	Medetomidine Ketamine	0.06, IM 1.7, IM	—	Complete immobilization	192
	Medetomidine Ketamine	0.0593, IM 1.7, IM	—	Complete immobilization	193
Formosan sika deer (*Cervus nippon taiouanus*)	Medetomidine Ketamine	0.233±0.061, IM (0.169–0.363) 2.33±0.61, IM (1.69–3.63)	—	Immobilization	192
Elk (*Cervus canadensis*)	Xylazine Ketamine	600 mg total, IM 1200 mg, total, IM	—	Immobilization	199
Order Carnivora, family Canidae					
Coyote (*Canis latrans*)	Ketamine alone	12.3, IM	52	Immobilization Extensive salivation Rigidity	200
	Xylazine Ketamine	1.8–2.9, IM 9.2–14.7, IM	—	Chemical restraint	(continued)

Table 12.11. Use of ketamine alone or ketamine combinations in exotic and wildlife animals (continued).

Common Names (Genus and Species)	Drug(s)	Dose and Route (mg/kg)	Duration (min)	Comment	Reference
Coyote (Canis latrans)	Xylazine Ketamine	2, IM 4, IM	—	—	201
Cape hunting dogs (Lycaon pictus)	Medetomidine Ketamine	0.043–0.121, IM 2.6–3.0, IM	—	Partial or complete immobilization Bradycardia ↓ Respiration rate	202
Arctic fox (Alopex lagopus)	Medetomidine Ketamine	0.05, IM 2.5, IM	—	Complete immobilization	192
Blue fox (Alopex lagopus)	Medetomidine Ketamine	0.05–2.5, IM 2.5, IM	—	Immobilization	203
Gray fox (Urocyon cinereoargenteus)	Xylazine Ketamine	6.6–11.0, IM 11.0–17.6, IM	—	Chemical restraint	200
Kit fox (Vulpes macrotis)	Xylazine Ketamine	6.6–11.0, IM 11.0–17.6, IM	—	Chemical restraint	200
Red fox (Vulpes fulva)	Xylazine Ketamine	6.6–11.0, IM 22–33, IM	—	Chemical restraint	200
Gray wolf (Canis lupus)	Xylazine Ketamine	2.2, IM 6.6, IM	—	Significant bradycardia	204
Wolf (Canis lupus L.)	Xylazine Ketamine	30 mg total, IM 400 mg total, IM	148.0±52.7	—	205
	Xylazine Ketamine	2–3, IM 5–6, IM	35–40	—	206
Order Carnivora, family Felidae					
Bobcat (Lynx rufus)	Acepromazine Ketamine	0.66–1.1, IM 17.6, IM (11.9–34.9)	—	Immobilization	200
	Ketamine alone	33.4, IM (22.4–60.3)	—	—	200
California bobcat (Felis rufus californieus)	Ketamine alone	5.5–17.0, IM	—	—	207
Fishing cat (Felis viverrina)	Ketamine alone	19–25, IM	—	—	208
Flat-headed cat (Felis planiceps)	Ketamine alone	8, IM	—	—	208
Jungle cat (Felis chaus)	Medetomidine Ketamine	0.1, IM 2.5, IM	—	Immobilization	192

(continued)

Table 12.11. Use of ketamine alone or ketamine combinations in exotic and wildlife animals (continued).

Common Names (Genus and Species)	Drug(s)	Dose and Route (mg/kg)	Duration (min)	Comment	Reference
Leopard cat (Felis bengalensis)	Ketamine alone	8–25, IM	—	—	209
Cheetah (Acinonyx jubatus)	Ketamine alone	8–12, IM	—	—	209
	Ketamine alone	10	—	—	208
	Medetomidine Ketamine	0.06–0.07, IM 2.5–3.0, IM	—	Immobilization	292
Jaguar (Panthera onca)	Ketamine alone	13–18, IM	—	—	209
	Medetomidine Ketamine	0.05, IM 1.5–2.0, IM	—	Immobilization	192
Leopard (Panthera pardus)	Medetomidine Ketamine	0.07–0.08,IM 2.5–3.0, IM	—	Immobilization	192
Black leopard (Panthera pardus)	Ketamine alone	15, IM	—	Occasional convulsion Inadequate muscle relaxation	209
	Ketamine alone	11 (5.5–17.0 range), IM	—	—	207
	Ketamine alone	7.5, IM	—	—	210
Chinese leopard (Panthera pardus japonensis)	Ketamine alone	15, IM	—	Occasional convulsion Inadequate muscle relaxation	209
Clouded leopard (Neofelis nebulosa)	Ketamine alone	8.6, IM	—	Occasional convulsion Inadequate muscle relaxation	209
		7, IM	—	—	208
Snow leopard (Panthera uncia)	Ketamine alone	10, IM	—	—	208
	Medetomidine Ketamine	0.06–0.08, IM 2.5–3.0, IM	—	Complete immobilization	192
	Medetomidine Ketamine	0.067±0.016, IM (0.038–0.107 range) 2.7±0.8, IM (1.3–5.7 range)	45	Complete immobilization Allowed tracheal intubation	193
	Xylazine Ketamine	2.2±0.2, IM (1.9–2.6 range) 10.9±1.0, IM (9.6–12.8 range)	30–45	Immobilization Moderate to good muscle relaxation	211

(continued)

Table 12.11. Use of ketamine alone or ketamine combinations in exotic and wildlife animals (*continued*).

Common Names (Genus and Species)	Drug(s)	Dose and Route (mg/kg)	Duration (min)	Comment	Reference
Snow leopard (*Panthera uncia*)	Medetomidine	0.067±0.014, IM (0.038–0.109 range)	30–60	Immobilization Shorter recovery compared with xylazine-ketamine	211
	Ketamine	2.9±0.8, IM (1.6–5.7 range)		Good to excellent muscle relaxation	
Lion (*Panthera leo*)	Medetomidine	0.03, IM	—	Immobilization	192
	Ketamine	1.0–1.5, IM			
	Ketamine alone	10–20, IM	—	Rapid immobilization	209
		5–7, IM	—	—	212
		5.0–7.5, IM	—	—	210
	Xylazine	110 total, IM	240	Immobilization	190
	Ketamine	450 total, IM			
	Xylazine	3.2, IM	—	—	213
	Ketamine	8, IM			
Mountain lion, puma (*Felis concolor*)	Xylazine	0.88–0.99, IM	—	Immobilization	200
	Ketamine	7.3–7.7, IM Suppl,[b] 4.4–8.8, IM			
	Ketamine alone	11–25, IM	—	—	209
	Xylazine	1.8, IM	—	—	214
	Ketamine	11, IM			
Margay (*Felis wiedii*)	Ketamine alone	15, IM	—	Occasional convulsion Inadequate muscle relaxation	209
Tiger (*Panthera tigris*)	Ketamine alone	7–14, IM	—	—	209
	Medetomidine	0.03, IM	—	Immobilization	192
	Ketamine	1.0–1.5, IM			
Order Carnivora, family Mustelidae					
Badger (*Taxidea taxus*)	Ketamine alone	11–33, IM	—	Immobilization	200
Beaver (*Castor canadensis*)	Ketamine alone	22, IM	—	Immobilization	215
	Aceceromazine	0.22, IM	—	Immobilization	200
	Ketamine	11, IM			
	Diazepam	0.1, IM	—	Smooth induction	216
	Ketamine	25, IM			

(continued)

321

Table 12.11. Use of ketamine alone or ketamine combinations in exotic and wildlife animals (*continued*).

Common Names (Genus and Species)	Drug(s)	Dose and Route (mg/kg)	Duration (min)	Comment	Reference
Ferret (*Mustela putorius furo*)	Ketamine alone	20–25, IM	—	—	217
	Xylazine Ketamine	2, IM 25, IM	80.0±11.4	—	218
	Ketamine alone	60, IM	—	Muscle rigidity Incomplete analgesia	219
	Diazepam Ketamine	3, IM 35, IM	—	Muscle rigidity Incomplete analgesia	219
	Xylazine Ketamine	2, IM 25, IM	—	Acceptable analgesia Muscle relaxation	219
	Ketamine alone	25, IM	—	Excessive salivation Muscle tremor Paddling motions	220
	Xylazine Ketamine	2, IM 25, IM	—	Good muscle relaxation	220
Fisher (*Martes pennati*)	Ketamine or with acepromazine	7.5, IM (11.0–24.2) 1.1, IM	—	Immobilization	200
Mink	Ketamine alone	5–20, IM	—	—	217
(*Mustela vision*)		10–15, IM	—	Suitable for electroejaculation Surgical anesthesia	217
		100, IM	—	Immobilization	217
		15.4–22.0, IM	—		217
Pine marten (*Marten americana*)	Ketamine alone	11–22, IM	—	Immobilization	200
European otter (*Lutra lutra*)	Diazepam Ketamine	0.5, IM 18, IM	—	Good muscle relaxation Smooth recovery	221
Asian small-clawed otter (*Aonyx cinerea*)	Medetomidine Ketamine	0.1–0.12, IM 4–5, IM	—	Good muscle relaxation Immobilization	222
River otter (*Lutra canadensis*)	Ketamine alone	22, IM	—	—	200
Sea otter (*Enhydra lutris*)	Ketamine alone	1, IM	—	Immobilization	200

(continued)

322

Table 12.11. Use of ketamine alone or ketamine combinations in exotic and wildlife animals (continued).

Common Names (Genus and Species)	Drug(s)	Dose and Route (mg/kg)	Duration (min)	Comment	Reference
Australian skink and bobtail skink (Tiliqua rugosa)	Ketamine alone	170–230 mg total, IM	—	Good muscle relaxation	223
King's skink (Egernia kingii)	Ketamine alone	170–230 mg total, IM	—	Good muscle relaxation	223
Common skunk (Mephitis mephitis nigra)	Ketamine alone	10–20, IM	—	—	224
Spotted skunk (Spilogale gracilis)	Ketamine alone	30.1, IM	—	Immobilization	200
Striped skunk (Mephitis mephitis)	Ketamine alone	4.5–60.0, IM	—	Immobilization	225
		26.8, IM	44	Immobilization	200
Weasel (Mustela frenata)	Ketamine alone	15.4–22.0, IM	—	Immobilization	200
Order Carnivora, family Ursidae					
American black bear (Ursus americana)	Medetomidine	0.03–0.04, IM	—	Immobilization	192
	Ketamine	1.0–1.5, IM			
	Xylazine	2.0–4.5, IM	—	Good chemical restraint	180
	Ketamine	5–9, IM			
		1.9–9.25, IM	45–100	—	181
		1.9–9.25, IM			
		3.6–10.5, IM	—	Immobilization	226
		3.6–10.5, IM			
Brown bear (Ursus arctos horribilis)	Medetomidine	Zoo: 0.02–0.03, IM Wild: 0.06–0.08, IM UK: 0.03–0.04, IM	—	Immobilization	192
	Ketamine	Zoo: 0.5–1.0, IM Wild: 1.0–1.6, IM UK: 1.0–1.5, IM			
Grizzly bear (Ursus arctos)	Xylazine	11.1, IM (6.3–14.0 range)	—	—	226
	Ketamine	11.1, IM (6.3–14.0 range)			
Himalayan bear (Selnarctos thibetanus)	Medetomidine	0.03–0.04, IM	—	—	192
	Ketamine	1.0–1.5, IM			
Polar bear (Ursus maritimus)	Medetomidine	0.03, IM	—	Immobilization	192
	Ketamine	1.0–1.5, IM			

(continued)

323

Table 12.11. Use of ketamine alone or ketamine combinations in exotic and wildlife animals *(continued)*.

Common Names (Genus and Species)	Drug(s)	Dose and Route (mg/kg)	Duration (min)	Comment	Reference
Polar bear (*Ursus maritimus*)	Xylazine Ketamine	6.8, IM 6.8, IM	—	Immobilization Good muscle relaxation	182
Sloth bear (*Melursus ursinus*)	Xylazine Ketamine	1.4–2.44, IM 5.8–9.75, IM	—	Immobilization	227
Other species					
Camel (*Camelus bactrianus*)	Xylazine Ketamine	0.25, IM 5.5, IM	—	Good muscle relaxation Good analgesia	228
		0.15, IM 2.5, IM	—	Good muscle relaxation Good analgesia	228
African elephant (*Loxodonta africana*)	1st dose Xylazine Ketamine 2nd dose Xylazine Ketamine or Ketamine	1st dose 0.14±0.03, IM 1.14±0.21, IM 2nd dose 0.08±0.03, IM 0.61±0.19, IM 0.47, IV	11.6±6.9 (7–31) 27.0±8.9 (13–50)	Deep sedation to immobilization	229
	Xylazine Ketamine	0.2, IM 1.0–1.5, IM	—	—	230
		0.1±0.04, IM 0.6±0.13, IM	—	Chemical restraint only	231
Spotted hyena (*Crocuta crocuta*)	Xylazine Ketamine	6.3, IM 13.2, IM	100	Immobilization	232
Collared peccaries (*Tayassu tajacu*)	Ketamine alone	14.71–24.61, IM	71.7	Smooth recovery	233
Rabbit (*Sylvilagus floridanus*)	Xylazine Ketamine	5, IM 70, IM	—	—	234
	Ketamine EMTU[c]	35, IM 25.0–45.5, IV	18.75 (15–60)	Lack of consistency in induction of surgical anesthesia	235
	Xylazine Acepromazine Ketamine	5, SC 0.75, IM 35, IM	95.25 (58–177)	Respiratory depression Hypothermia Surgical anesthesia	235
	Ketamine Chloral hydrate	20, IM 250, IV	15 (0–30)	Lack of consistency in induction of surgical anesthesia	235
	Xylazine Ketamine	5, IM 35, IM	46.5 (15–83)	Lack of consistency in induction of surgical anesthesia	235

(continued)

324

Table 12.11. Use of ketamine alone or ketamine combinations in exotic and wildlife animals (*continued*).

Common Names (Genus and Species)	Drug(s)	Dose and Route (mg/kg)	Duration (min)	Comment	Reference
Rabbit (*Sylviiagus floridanus*)	Xylazine Ketamine	5, IM 35, IM	—	—	236
	Xylazine Butorphanol Ketamine	5, IM 0.1, IM 35, IM	68±2	—	236
New Zealand white rabbit (*Oryctolagus cuniculus*)	Xylazine Ketamine	5, IM 35, IM	35±6	Surgical anesthesia	237
	Xylazine	5, IV 25, IV	—	—	238
		5, IM 35, IM	77±5	—	239
	Xylazine Acepromazine Ketamine	5, IM 0.75, IM 35, IM	99±20	—	239
	Guaifenesin Ketamine	200, IV 50, IM	30	Surgical anesthesia	240
Raccoon (*Procyon lotor*)	Ketamine alone	10–14, IM	—	Inadequate jaw muscle relaxation	241
		20–29, IM	180 (150–270 range)	Adequate jaw relaxation (30–100 min) Immobilization	241
	Ketamine alone	16.7, IM	—	Chemical restraint	200
	Xylazine Ketamine	2.2–3.3, IM 11.0–16.5, IM	—	Incomplete restraint with lower dose of ketamine	200
	Acepromazine Ketamine	1.25, IM 13.6, IM	—	—	200
Feral pig (*Sus scrofa*)	Xylazine Ketamine	9.8–19.6, IM 9.8–19.6, IM	47.9±12.7	Immobilization	242
Ringtail (*Bassariscus astutus*)	Ketamine alone	15, IM	—	Immobilization	200
Gopher snake (*Pituophis melanoleucus catenifer*)	Ketamine alone	75, IM	43.6±8.1 (11–63)	Sedation to surgical anesthesia	243

(continued)

Table 12.11. Use of ketamine alone or ketamine combinations in exotic and wildlife animals (continued).

Common Names (Genus and Species)	Drug(s)	Dose and Route (mg/kg)	Duration (min)	Comment	Reference
Richardson's ground squirrel (*Spermophilus richardsonii*)	Xylazine Ketamine	10.6±0.5, IM 85.5±3.4, IM or 10.7±0.7, SC 85.6±4.0, SC	16±3 19±9	Surgical anesthesia —	244 244
	Ketamine alone	86±7, IM	12±10	Did not induce surgical anesthesia	244
Bennett wallaby (*Protemnodon rufogrisea*)	Xylazine Ketamine	187.5, IM 150, IM	— —	Rapid immobilization Rapid immobilization	245 245
		80, IM 160, IM			
Marine animals					
Crabeater seal (*Lobodon carcinophagus*)	Diazepam Ketamine	0.2, IM 6, IM	20–40	—	246
Northern elephant seal (*Mirounga angustirostris*)	Ketamine alone	1.4–6.9, IM	—	Immobilization	247
Fur seal (*Arctocephalus galapagoensis*)	Xylazine Ketamine	0–1.16 3.1–18.7	—	Satisfactory immobilization	248
Gray seal (*Halischoerus grypus*)	Xylazine Ketamine	5.15, IM 4.96, IM	—	—	249
	Diazepam Ketamine	0.3, IM 6, IM	—	Immobilization	250
	Diazepam Ketamine	0.03–0.1, IM 1–3, IM	—	—	251
Harbor seal (*Phoca vitulina*)	Ketamine alone	3.0–3.2, IM	—	—	251
	Diazepam Ketamine	0.04–0.06, IM 1.4–1.9, IM	—	—	252
		0.05, IM, IV 1.5, IM, IV	45	Immobilization	252
	Ketamine alone	4.5, IM	<70	Smooth induction and recovery	252
Ringed seal (*Pusa hispida*)	Ketamine alone	4.5–11.0, IM	—	Sedation to surgical anesthesia	252
Southern elephant seal (*Miroubga leonina*)	Diazepam Ketamine	0.3, IM 6, IM	—	Immobilization	250
					(continued)

326

Table 12.11. Use of ketamine alone or ketamine combinations in exotic and wildlife animals (*continued*).

Common Names (Genus and Species)	Drug(s)	Dose and Route (mg/kg)	Duration (min)	Comment	Reference
Weddell seal (*Leptonychotes weddellii*)	Diazepam Ketamine	0.05±0.01, IM 7.99±1.99, IM	12.7±20.7	Immobilization	253
California sea lion (*Zalophus californianus*)	Ketamine	4.5–5, IM	<65	Avoid use in ill patients	252
Galapagos sea lion (*Zalophus californianus wollebaeki*)	Xylazine Ketamine	0.3–1.43, IM 2.1–7.1, IM	—	—	248

IM, intramuscularly; IV, intravenously; SC, subcutaneously.
[a]Total dose.
[b]Suppl, supplemental dose.
[c]EMTU, ethyl-(1-methyl-propyl)malonyl-thio-urea.

Table 12.12. Use of ketamine alone or ketamine combinations in birds.

Common Names (Genus and Species)	Drug(s)	Dose and Route (mg/kg)	Duration (min)	Comment	Reference
Accipiters	Diazepam Ketamine	1, IM 30, IM	—	—	254
Bald eagle (*Haliaeetus leucocephalus*)	Diazepam Ketamine	1, IM 10–30, IM	—	—	254
Budgerigar (*Melopsittacus undulatus*)	Xylazine Ketamine	10, IM 40, IM	—	—	255
Double-wattled cassowary (*Casuarius casuarius*)	Etorphine Ketamine	10–12 total, IM 200–300 total, IM	—	Immobilization suitable for minor procedures	256
Chicken (*Gallus gallus*)	Ketamine alone	1–160, IM 14, IV	15	Muscle tremor LD_{50},[b] 67.5 mg/kg	257
Columbiformes and corvids	Diazepam Ketamine	2–5, IM 20–40, IM	—	—	254
Ducks and geese	Diazepam Ketamine	2–4 20–60	—	—	254
Pekin duck (*Anas platyrhyncos*)	Ketamine alone	20, IV	—	—	258
	Xylazine Ketamine	1, IV 20, IV	—	Respiratory depression	258
Emu (*Dromiceius novaehollandiae*)	Ketamine alone	25, IM initially 5–8, IV additionally	—	Anesthesia	259
		25 initially, IM 5, suppl[a] IV	—	Short-term immobilization	259
Leghorn (*Gallus domesticus*)	Xylazine Ketamine	2, IM 2, IM	—	—	260
Red-tailed hawk (*Buteo jamaicensis*)	Xylazine Ketamine	2.2, IV 4.4, IV	—	—	261
Herons	Diazepam Ketamine	1–2, IM 20, IM	—	—	254
Ostrich (*Struthio camelus*)	Diazepam Ketamine	0.22, IV 4.4, IV	—	Good induction and recovery	262
	Xylazine	0.33, IV 6.6, IV	—	Poor induction Good recovery	262
	Xylazine Diazepam Ketamine	0.44, IM 0.15, IV 2.8, IV	—	Poor induction Good recovery	262
	Xylazine	0.9, IM	—	Fair induction	262

Table 12.12. Use of ketamine alone or ketamine combinations in birds (*continued*).

Common Names (Genus and Species)	Drug(s)	Dose and Route (mg/kg)	Duration (min)	Comment	Reference
Ostrich (*Struthio camelus*)	Xylazine Ketamine	0.03, IV 4.8, IV		Poor recovery	262
Blue-necked ostrich (*Struthio camelus austrealis*)	Etorphine Ketamine	10–12 total, IM 200–300 total, IM	—	Immobilization suitable for minor procedure	256
Barred, long-eared, and short-eared owls	Diazepam Ketamine	1, IM 10, IM	—	—	254
Great horned (*Bubo virginianus*) and screech owls (*Otus asio*)	Diazepam Ketamine	1, IM 25, IM	—	—	254
Parakeets	Ketamine alone	1 total, IM 2 total, IM 3 total, IM	— — —	Sedation Surgical anesthesia Surgical anesthesia	263
Pigeon (*Columbia livia*)	Ketamine alone	1 total, IM 2 total, IM 3 total, IM	— — —	Respiratory depression — —	263
Cape vulture (*Gyps coprotheres*)	Ketamine	7.5–28.8, IM	—	Immobilization	264
Turkey vulture (*Cathartes aura*)	Xylazine Ketamine	1, IM 10, IM	19.8±25.4	Good muscle relaxation Consistent level of anesthesia	265

IM, intramuscularly; IV, intravenously.
[a]Suppl, supplemental dose.
[b]LD$_{50}$, median lethal dose.

329

Table 12.13. Use of Telazol alone or Telazol combinations in exotic and wildlife animals.

Common Names (Genus and Species)	Drug(s)	Dose and Route (mg/kg)	Duration (min)	Comment	Reference
Order Artiodactyla, family Bovidae					
Aoudad (*Ammotagus lervia*)	Telazol	3.5–8.6, IM	—	Immobilization	183
Bison (*Bison bison*)	Telazol	2.2–4.4, IM	—	Good immobilization	184
White-tailed gnu (*Connochaeters gnou*)	Telazol	37, IM	—	Immobilization	184
African pygmy goat (*Capre hircus*)	Telazol	2.2, IM	—	Immobilization	184
		4.4–27.6, IM	—	—	183
Mexican goat *Capra* species	Telazol	5.5–9.5, IM	—	Immobilization	184
Mouflon sheep (*Ovis musimon*)	Telazol	5.5–7.5, IM	—	Immobilization	184
Rocky Mountain bighorn sheep (*Ovis canadensis*)	Telazol	4.4–5.5, IM	—	Immobilization	184
Tahr (*Hemitragus jemlahicus*)	Telazol	3.3–4.4, IM	—	Immobilization	184
Order Artiodactyla, family Cervidae					
Pronghorn antelope (*Antilocapra americana*)	Telazol	4.6, IM	—	Good chemical restraint	184
Sable antelope (*Hippotragus niger*)	Telazol	22.0–23.8,IM	—	—	183
Sitatunga antelope (*Tragelaphus spekii*)	Telazol	8.3–20.7, IM	—	—	183
		1.7–4.25, IM	—	—	165
Suni antelope (*Neotragus moschatus*)	Telazol	6.6–30.0, IM	—	—	183
Blesbuck (*Damaliscus dorcus*)	Telazol	3.09–11.0, IM	—	—	183
Bushbuck (*Tragelaphus scriptus*)	Telazol	8.5–12.7, IM	—	—	183
Black-tailed deer (*Odocoileus hemionus*)	Telazol	2.5–20.0, IM	—	—	194

(continued)

330

Table 12.13. Use of Telazol alone or Telazol combinations in exotic and wildlife animals (*continued*).

Common Names (Genus and Species)	Drug(s)	Dose and Route (mg/kg)	Duration (min)	Comment	Reference
White-tailed deer (*Odocoileus virginianus*)	Telazol	4.4, IM (1.1–8.8)	30–60 (3–186)	—	184
		5, IM	21	Good immobilization	266
		8.9, IM	—	Immobilization	267
		1.5–10.0, IM	—	—	194
Fallow deer (*Dama dama*)	Telazol	33, IM	—	Immobilization	184
Luzon sambar deer (*Cervus meriannus meriannus*)	Telazol	6.6, IM	—	Immobilization	184
Mule deer (*Odocoileus hemionus*)	Telazol	14.6–22.0, IM	—	Immobilization	184
		14–20, IM	—	—	194
Sika deer (*Cervus nippon pseudaxis*)	Telazol	4.4, IM	—	Immobilization	184
Crowned duiker (*Sylvicapra grimmia coronata*)	Telazol	4.4–11.0, IM	—	—	183
Maxwell duiker (*Cephalophus maxwelli*)	Telazol	2.2–13.2, IM	—	—	183
Common eland Cape eland (*Taurotragus oryx*)	Telazol	11.5, IM	—	—	183
Dorcas gazelle (*Gazella dorcas*)	Telazol	2.6–16.5, IM	—	Supplemented with inhalation anesthesia Good restraint for minor surgery	184
		4.4–22.0, IM	—	—	184
Grant's gazelle (*Gazella granti*)	Telazol	4.8–13.2, IM	—	Immobilization	184
		7.3–15.4, IM	—	—	183
Persian gazelle (*Gazella subgutturosa*)	Telazol	6.6, IM	—	Immobilization	184
Slender-horned gazelle (*Gazella leptoceros*)	Telazol	6.6–11.4, IM	—	Immobilization	184
		4.8–15.4, IM	—	—	183
Soemmering's gazelle (*Gazella soemmeringi*)	Telazol	11, IM	—	—	183
Thomson's gazelle (*Gazella thomsoni*)	Telazol Acepromazine	8.8, IM 5 mg total dose, IM	—	Immobilization	184
	Telazol	4.4–14.1, IM	—	—	183

(continued)

Table 12.13. Use of Telazol alone or Telazol combinations in exotic and wildlife animals (*continued*).

Common Names (Genus and Species)	Drug(s)	Dose and Route (mg/kg)	Duration (min)	Comment	Reference
Gemsbok (*Oryx gazella*)	Telazol	31, IM	—	Immobilization	184
		5.5, IM	—	—	183
Blue-bearded gnu (*Connochaetes taurinus taurinus*)	Telazol	6.6, IM	—	—	183
Brindled gnu (*Connochaettes taurinus*)	Telazol	4.4, IM	—	—	183
Impala (*Aepyceros melampus*)	Telazol	4.85, IM	—	—	183
Greater kudu (*Tragelaphus strepsiceros*)	Telazol	6.1, IM	—	—	183
Alaskan moose (*Alces alces gigas*)	Telazol	4.4–7.9, IM	—	Chemical restraint Lower dose produces ataxia	184
		2.4–5.3, IM	0–103	Unpredictable response Prolonged ataxia during recovery	268
Nyala (*Tragelaphus angasi*)	Telazol	6.6–11.0, IM	—	—	183
Siberian reindeer (*Rangifer tarandus*)	Telazol	4.4–5.3, IM	—	Immobilization	184
Springbok (*Antidorcas marsupialis*)	Telazol	10.6, IM	—	—	183
Wapiti (*Cervus canadensis*)	Telazol	9.2, IM	—	Immobilization	184
Zebu (*Bos indicus*)	Telazol	3.6, IM	—	—	183
Order Carnivora, family Canidae					
Cacomistle (*Bassariscus astutus*)	Telazol	3.3–16.5, IM	—	Desirable immobilization	184
Coyote (*Canis latrans*)	Telazol	11, IM	—	Desirable immobilization	184
Cape hunting dog (*Lycaon pictus*)	Telazol	8.8–10.0, IM	—	Desirable immobilization	184
Racoon dog (*Nyctereutes procyonoides*)	Telazol	6.6, IM	—	Desirable immobilization	184
Red fox (*Vulpes vulpes*)	Telazol	10, IM	25.1±2.5	Good cardiovascular and respiratory support Desirable immobilization	269

(continued)

Table 12.13. Use of Telazol alone or Telazol combinations in exotic and wildlife animals (*continued*).

Common Names (Genus and Species)	Drug(s)	Dose and Route (mg/kg)	Duration (min)	Comment	Reference
Red fox (*Vulpes vulpes*)		8.8, IM	—	Excellent immobilization	184
		4, IM	34		185
Fennec fox (*Fennecus zerda*)	Telazol	13, IM (12–16 range)	53 (32–65 range)	Excellent immobilization	185
Gray wolf (*Urocyon cinereoargenteus*)	Telazol	5.3, IM (2.6–14.1 range)	63 (12–135 range)	Surgical anesthesia	185
		8.8, IM	—	Desirable immobilization	184
Iranian wolf	Telazol	3.6, IM (2.1–5.5 range)	(15–78 range)	Excellent immobilization	185
Timber wolf (*Canis iupis*)	Telazol	2.2–6.6, IM	—	Needed physical restraint	184
Order Carnivora, family Felidae					
Caracal (*Felis caracal*)	Telazol	3.3–5.5, IM	—	Needed some restraint	184
		6.6–7.3, IM	—	—	183
African wildcat (*Felis libyca* Forster)	Telazol	4.4, IM	—	Desirable immobilization	184
Bobcat (*Lynx rufus*)	Telazol	13.3, IM	99	Additional dose for maintenance	185
Dusky jungle cat (*Felis chaus*)	Telazol	1.1–5.5, IM	—	Desirable immobilization	184
Geoffrey cat (*Felis geoffreyi*)	Telazol	4, IM	—	Desirable immobilization	184
Golden cat (*Felis temnincki*)	Telazol	4, IM (4.0–4.1 range)	31 (26–37 range)	Excellent immobilization	185
		2.0–4.4	—	Desirable immobilization	184
Fishing cat (*Felis viverrina*)	Telazol	2.2–4.4, IM	—	Desirable immobilization	184
Jungle cat (*Felis chaus*)	Telazol	4.2, IM	58	Surgical anesthesia	185
		1.1–5.5, IM	—	—	184
Leopard (*Felis begalensis*)	Telazol	7, IM (5–10 range)	61 (25–87 range)	Excellent immobilization	185
		2.2–6.6, IM	—	Desirable immobilization	184
Pampas cat (*Felis manul*)	Telazol	2.2–5.5, IM	—	Desirable immobilization	184
					(*continued*)

Table 12.13. Use of Telazol alone or Telazol combinations in exotic and wildlife animals (*continued*).

Common Names (Genus and Species)	Drug(s)	Dose and Route (mg/kg)	Duration (min)	Comment	Reference
Cheetah (*Acinonyx jubatus*)	Telazol	1.6–3.5, IM	60–90	Light anesthesia Moderate muscle relaxation Muscle rigidity and voluntary movement with low dose	270
		4.6, IM (2.9–9.2 range)	117 (39–395 range)	Surgical anesthesia Salivation	185
		2.2–2.75, IM	—	Desirable immobilization	184
		2.2–8.8, IM	—	—	183
Jaguar (*Panthera onca*)	Telazol	4.2, IM (3.5–4.4 range)	60 (40–115 range)	Excellent immobilization	185
		2–4, IM	—	Desirable immobilization	184
Jaguarondi (*Felis jaguarondi*)	Telazol	6.6, IM	—	Desirable immobilization	184
Black leopard	Telazol	5.0–6.25, IM	<180	Desirable immobilization	271
(African spotted leopard) (*Panthera pardus*)		6.6, IM (1.4–11.5 range)	141 (23–228 range)	Surgical anesthesia at higher dose Lowest dose did not produce immobilization	185
		3.4–11.0, IM	—	—	183
		3.6–6.0, IM	—	—	272
		4–5, IM	—	—	184
Clouded leopard (*Panthera nebulosa*)	Telazol	4.7, IM (1.5–8.3 range)	121 (23–293 range)	Excellent immobilization	185
Snow leopard (*Panthera unicia*)	Telazol	4, IM (3.9–4.0 range)	65 (56–75 range)	Good immobilization	185
Lion (*Panthera leo*)	Telazol	3.76±0.48, IM	—	Rapid induction time Good muscle relaxation No convulsions	273
		1.6–2.9, IM	—	Sufficient muscle relaxation Licking movement	184
		2.2–3.0, IM	—	Desirable immobilization	183
		2.2–8.4, IM	—	—	183
		5, IM (3.2–8.9 range)	69 (21–139 range)	Good immobilization	185
		<2.2, IM	—	Some immobilization	184

(*continued*)

Table 12.13. Use of Telazol alone or Telazol combinations in exotic and wildlife animals (*continued*).

Common Names (Genus and Species)	Drug(s)	Dose and Route (mg/kg)	Duration (min)	Comment	Reference
Mountain lion, puma (*Felis concolor*)	Telazol	8.2, IM (2.7–16 range)	96 (20–280 range)	Poor muscle relaxation at lower dose Repeated doses for root canal and tooth capping	185
		2.2–3.3, IM	—	Needed a little physical restraint	184
Ocelot (*Felis pardalis*)	Telazol	8.3, IM (4.5–12.2 range)	42 (30–55 range)	Surgical anesthesia	185
		4.4, IM	—	—	183
Serval (*Felis serval*)	Telazol	4.4–5.5, IM	—	Desirable immobilization	184
		2.2–12.2, IM	—	—	183
Tiger (*Panthera tigris*)	Telazol	2.0–2.8, IM	—	Slight physical restraint needed	184
		4, IM	—	Anesthesia	184
		3.5–4.0, IM	180–300	Desirable immobilization	271
		2.3–11.7, IM	—	Minimum dose of 4.6 mg/kg for female and 4 mg/kg for male	274
		4.4–19.3, IM	—	—	183
Order Carnivora, family Ursidae					
American black bear (*Ursus americana*)	Telazol	4.7±0.8, IM	—	—	275
		0.6–0.73, IV 3.3–7.0, IM	—	—	183
Asiatic bear (*Selenarctos thibetanus*)	Telazol	2.8–4.4, IM	—	—	183
Brown bear (*Ursus arctos syriacus*)	Telazol	3.5±1.8, IM	—	—	275
Grizzly bear (*Ursus arctos horribilis*)	Telazol	7–9, IM	45–75	Rapid induction Predictable recovery Wide safety margin Few adverse side effects	276
		2.4–6.3, IM	—	—	183
Kamchacka bear (*Ursus arctos beringianus*)	Telazol	4.3, IM (3.1–5.2 range)	41 (26–75 range)	Surgical anesthesia Additional half dose can be given for prolonged procedures	185
Kodiak bear (*Ursus arctos middendorffi*)	Telazol	5.5, IM	20	Good anesthesia	184
					(*continued*)

Table 12.13. Use of Telazol alone or Telazol combinations in exotic and wildlife animals (continued).

Common Names (Genus and Species)	Drug(s)	Dose and Route (mg/kg)	Duration (min)	Comment	Reference
Polar bear (*Ursus maritimus*)	Telazol	4.9, IM (3.5–7.0 range)	83 (15–230 range)	Surgical anesthesia Additional IM or IV dose may be necessary to maintain anesthesia	185
		5, IM	—	Immobilization Inadequate analgesia	277
		8–9,IM	—	Immobilization Satisfactory analgesia Fast recovery	278
		3.5–7.0, IM	—	—	185
Sloth bear (*Melursus ursinus*)	Telazol	5.5–6.6, IM	—	—	183
Spectacled bear (*Tremartos ornatus*)	Telazol	5.7, IM (3.2–11.1 range)	35 (23–45 range)	Excellent immobilization	185
		2.8±0.5, IM	—	—	275
Sun bear (*Helarctos malaynus*)	Telazol	4.0–5.5, IM	—	—	185
		2.8–4.7, IM Suppl,[a] 29%–75% of original dose	15–180	Adequate immobilization Rapid induction Smooth recovery Free of convulsions	275
		4.8, IM (4.0–5.5 range)	35 (30–45 range)	Surgical anesthesia	185
Order Carnivora, family Viverridae					
Binturong (*Arctictis binturong*)	Telazol	1.1, IM	—	A litter but able to handle	184
African palm civet (*Nandinia binotata*)	Telazol	5.5–8.8, IM	—	Needed higher dose	184
Banded palm civet (*Hemigalus derbyanus*)	Telazol	6.6, IM	—	Desirable immobilization	184
Formosan masked civet (*Paguma larvata*)	Telazol	<2–4, IM	—	Manual restraint needed	184
Palm civet (*Paradoxurus hermaphroditus*)	Telazol	2.2–4.9, IM	—	Needed some restraint	184
Lesser oriental civet (*Viverricula indica*)	Telazol	4.4, IM	—	Desirable immobilization	184

(continued)

Table 12.13. Use of Telazol alone or Telazol combinations in exotic and wildlife animals (continued).

Common Names (Genus and Species)	Drug(s)	Dose and Route (mg/kg)	Duration (min)	Comment	Reference
Fanaloka (Cryptoprocta fosse)	Telazol	2–8, IM	—	Needed some physical restraint	184
Genet (Genetta tigrina)	Telazol	2.2, IM	—	Desirable immobilization	184
Linsand (Prionodon linsang)	Telazol	4.4, IM	—	Desirable immobilization	184
African water mongoose (Atilax paludinosus)	Telazol	5.5, IM	—	Desirable immobilization	184
Ring-tail mongoose (Gallidia elegans)	Telazol	4.4, IM	—	Desirable immobilization	184
Black-footed mongoose Bdeogale species	Telazol	4.4, IM	—	Desirable immobilization	184
Ratel (Melivora capnsis)	Telazol	2.2, IM	—	Awakened fast	184
Other species					
Acouchi (Myoprocta pratti)	Telazol	4.4–6.6, IM	—	—	184
Badger (Taxidea taxus)	Telazol	4.4, IM	—	Surgical anesthesia	185
Chimpanzee (Pan troglodytes)	Telazol	16, orally Suppl,[a] 2.5, IM	40	Immobilization Analgesia <40	279
Chinchilla (Chinchilla villidera laniger)	Telazol	11–44, IM	115–431	Surgical anesthesia	280
		4.4, IM	—	—	183
		5.5–44, IM	—	—	184
African elephant (Loxodonta africana)	Telazol	3, IM	—	—	184
Ferret (Mustela putorius)	Telazol	12, IM	31 (15–51 range)	Poor analgesia Immobilization	281
		22, IM	73 (45–165 range)	Immobilization Good muscle relaxation Adequate analgesia	281
		19.8, IM	—	—	183
		5.8, IM (1.5–10.0 range)	32 (17–58 range)	Excellent immobilization Halothane can be used for prolonged anesthesia	185

(continued)

337

Table 12.13. Use of Telazol alone or Telazol combinations in exotic and wildlife animals (*continued*).

Common Names (Genus and Species)	Drug(s)	Dose and Route (mg/kg)	Duration (min)	Comment	Reference
Gerbil (*Meriones unguiculatus*)	Telazol	60, IM	Male, 5.7±0.37 Female, 4.3±1.18 1.58–4.03	Surgical anesthesia	282
		20–40, IM		Immobilization	282
Guinea pig (*Cavia porcellus*)	Telazol	52, IM	122 (70–163 range)	Unsatisfactory anesthesia Useful for procedures requiring prolonged recumbency without manipulation	283
Hamster Outbred Syrian	Telazol	20–80, IP	7–27	Immobilization Inadequate analgesia	284
		60–80, IM	19–32	Immobilization Inadequate analgesia	
European hedgehog (*Erinaceus europaeus*)	Telazol	0.75–10.0, IM	—	—	183
Feral horse (*Equus equus*)	Telazol Butorphanol Xylazine	3.5, IM 0.07, IM 3, IM	88 (16–210 range)	Immobilization	285
Hutia (*Plagiodontia aedium*)	Telazol	6.6, IM	—	—	185
Spotted hyena (*Crocuta crocuta*)	Telazol	1.8, IM	—	Desirable immobilization	185
Long-nose rat kangaroo (*Potorous tridactylus*)	Telazol	14.7, IM	—	—	286
Red kangaroo (*Mactropus rufus*)	Telazol	4.1, IM (2.8–6.9 range)	107 (30–217 range)	Desirable anesthesia Salivation	287
		<4, IM	—	Poor muscle relaxation	287
		>4, IM	—	Good muscle relaxation	
		6–8, IM	20–30	Prolonged procedures	287
		1.8–6.2, IM Suppl.[a] 25%–60% of original IM dose	60–120	Sufficient anesthesia	286
Tree kangaroo (*Dendrolagus matschiei*)	Telazol	1.6–4.9, IM	20	Minor muscle rigidity Adequate immobilization	286
Kinkajou (*Potos flavus*)	Telazol	0.7–7.7, IM	—	Desirable immobilization Higher dose may be necessary for surgery	185

(*continued*)

Table 12.13. Use of Telazol alone or Telazol combinations in exotic and wildlife animals (*continued*).

Common Names (Genus and Species)	Drug(s)	Dose and Route (mg/kg)	Duration (min)	Comment	Reference
Koala (*Phascolarctos cinereus*)	Telazol	7, IM (5.0–7.7 range) Suppl,[a] 2.5	30–45	Anesthesia Mild salivation	288
		6.9, IM	90	Surgical anesthesia	289
Mice Outbred or inbred	Telazol	100–160, IP or IM	86.3±1.1 (80–98 range)	Respiratory depression	284
			4–119		
Mink (*Mustela vison*)	Telazol	30, IM	27	Surgical anesthesia	185
		1.2–2.6, IM	—	Good immobilization	184
		3.6–7.5, IM	5–35	Surgical anesthesia	
		12–16, IM	36–57	Surgical anesthesia	
Monkeys	Telazol	5–10, IM	30–55	Excellent muscle relaxation Absence of ocular movement Gradual emergence	290
Red howler monkey (*Alouatta seniculus*)	Telazol	23.3, IM (13.0–37.5)	45	Good muscle relaxation Immobilization	291
River otter (*Lutra canadensis*)	Telazol	5.4, IM (4.1–6.7 range)	38 (20–57)	Surgical anesthesia	185
		2.2, IM	10	Chemical restraint	184
		4.1–6.7, IM	—	—	185
		0.66–11.0, IM	—	—	183
Sea otter (*Enhydra lutris*)	Telazol	1.2, IM	40	Unable to resist handling	292
		1.4–2.9, IM	25–45	Surgical anesthesia	292
		9.3, IM	360	Surgical anesthesia but with apnea	292
		1–2, IM	—	Immobilization	200
Pacarana (*Dinomys branickii*)	Telazol	4.4, IM	—	—	184
Lesser panda (*Ailurus fulgens*)	Telazol	4.1, IM (1.8–6.3)	25–40	Moderate muscle relaxation Mild salivation Increased salivation Muscle tremors	255

(*continued*)

339

Table 12.13. Use of Telazol alone or Telazol combinations in exotic and wildlife animals (*continued*).

Common Names (Genus and Species)	Drug(s)	Dose and Route (mg/kg)	Duration (min)	Comment	Reference
Collared peccary (*Tayassu tajacu sonoriensis*)	Telazol	4.6–32.3, IM >19, IM	— —	Good immobilization Surgical anesthesia	184
Phalanger (*Trichosurus vulpecula*)	Telazol	7.7–11.5, IM	—	—	286
Nonhuman primates	Telazol	0.6–10.0, IM 2–22, IM	—	Chemical immobilization Surgical anesthesia	293
Rabbits (*Sylvigalus floridanus*)	Telazol Xylazine	15, IM 5, IM	72±8	Surgical anesthesia Profound visceral analgesia	237
	Telazol	23.6, IM (13–40 range)	68 (20–120 range)	Unsatisfactory surgical anesthesia Immobilization	283
	Telazol	8.8–23.4, IM	—	—	183
Raccoon (*Procyon lotor*)	Telazol	11.8, IM (4.3–225.0 range)	45 (17–65 range)	Surgical anesthesia with higher dose Poor muscle relaxation with lower dose Desirable immobilization	185
		5.9–13.7, IM	—	Lower dose given IV	184
		0.8–7.0, IM	—	—	184
		6.6–14.8, IM	—	—	183
Rat					
Sprague-Dawley	Telazol	20–30, IP	68 (41–110 range)	Satisfactory anesthesia Good muscle relaxation	283
Outbred or inbred	Telazol	20–40, IP or IM	6 to >300	Satisfactory anesthesia	284
Rhesus monkey (*Macaca mulatta*)	Telazol	3–5, IM	—	—	294
Hoffman's sloth (*Choloepus hoffmanni*)	Telazol	2.2–4.4, IM	—	—	184
Striped skunk (*Mephitis mephitis*)	Telazol	9.3, IM (3–14 range)	42 (10–102 range)	Surgical anesthesia	185
		5.5–11.0, IM	—	Desirable immobilization	184
		17.6–54.2, IM	—	—	183
Gray squirrel (*Scirus carolinensis*)	Telazol	4.4–6.6, IM	—	—	183
Formosan tree squirrel (*Callosciurus erythraeus*)	Telazol	8.3–17.0, IM	—	—	184
					(*continued*)

Table 12.13. Use of Telazol alone or Telazol combinations in exotic and wildlife animals (*continued*).

Common Names (Genus and Species)	Drug(s)	Dose and Route (mg/kg)	Duration (min)	Comment	Reference
Tayra (*Eira barbara*)	Telazol	3.3, IM	—	—	184
Mainland wombat (*Phascolomis hirsutus*)	Telazol	2.0–2.2, IM	—	—	286
Gray seal (*Halischoerus grypus*)	Telazol	1, IM	—	—	295
Elephant seal (*Mirounga anqustirostris*)	Telazol	0.7–1.6, IM	—	Lower dose not sufficient for good restraint	184
		1–2, IM	—	Satisfactory immobilization	184
Southern elephant seal (*Miroubna leonina*)	Telazol	1, IM	—	—	285
Tasmanian devil (*Sarcophilus harrisii*)	Telazol	2.8–5.5, IM	—	Higher dose may be necessary	184
Northern sea lion (*Eumetopias jubatus*)	Telazol	1.8–2.5, IM	—	Smooth recovery	296
Tapir (*Tapirus terrestris*)	Telazol	2.8, IM	—	Immobilization	184

IM, intramuscularly; IP, intraperitoneally; IV, intravenously.
aSuppl, supplemental dose.

Table 12.14. Use of Telazol alone or Telazol combinations in reptiles.

Common Names (Genus and Species)	Drug(s)	Dose and Route (mg/kg)	Duration (min)	Comment	Reference
Alligator (Alligator Mississippiensis)	Telazol	15, IM	183.8±33.8	Long induction time Painful on injection Incomplete loss of response	297
Boa constrictor (Boa constrictor)	Telazol	15–29, IM	—	Adequate for minor procedures	184
Crocodile (Crocodylus noloticus)	Telazol Acepromazine	5–10, IM 1, IM	—	Sedation	298
Common iguana (Iguana iguana)	Telazol	10, IM	—	Desirable immobilization	184
		26.5, IM	—	—	183
Indian python (Python molurus)	Telazol	15.4, IM	—	—	183
Rattlesnake (Crotalus atrox)	Telazol	35–210, IM	—	Long duration of sedation	184
Timber rattlesnake (Crotalus horridus)	Telazol	75, IM	—	Prolonged recovery	184
Tortoise Testudo species	Telazol	1.1–22.0, IM	—	—	183

Table 12.15. Use of Telazol alone or Telazol combinations in birds.

Common Names (Genus and Species)	Drug(s)	Dose and Route (mg/kg)	Duration (min)	Comment	Reference
Mynah bird (*Acridotheres tristis*)	Telazol	26.5, IM	—	—	183
Sulfur-crested cockatoo (*Cacatua galerita*)	Telazol	2.64–25.2, IM	—	—	183
Ring-necked dove (*Streptopelia risoria*)	Telazol	50–75, IM	—	—	184
Rock dove (*Columba livia*)	Telazol	10–70, IM	—	—	283
Muscovy duck (*Cairina moschate*)	Telazol	5.9–15.6, IM	—	5.9 and 8.4 mg/kg did not produce sufficient analgesia	184
	Telazol	13.2–22.0, IM	—	—	183
Bald eagle (*Haliaetus leucocephalus*)	Telazol	13.2–22.0, IM	—	—	183
Emu (*Dromaius novaehollandiae*)	Telazol	15, IM / 22, IM	— / —	Needed some physical restraint / —	183
Flamingo *Phoenicopteri* species	Telazol	22, IM	—	—	183
Chilean flamingo (*Phoenicopterus ruber chilensis*)	Telazol	6.6, IM	—	Desirable immobilization	184
Egyptian goose (*Alopochen aegyptiacus*)	Telazol	22.0–24.5, IM	—	—	183
Lesser Magellan goose (*Choephaga picta*)	Telazol	6.6–8.8, IM	—	Desirable immobilization	184
White-fronted goose (*Anser aibiforms frontalis*)	Telazol	2.7, IM	—	Desirable immobilization	184
Roadside hawk (*Buteo magnirostris*)	Telazol	16–33, IM	—	Desirable immobilization	184
Pea hen (*Pavo cristatus*)	Telazol	11.3, IM	—	—	183
Green heron (*Butorides virescens*)	Telazol	75, IM	—	Excellent anesthesia	184
Rhinoceros hornbill (*Buceros rhinoceros*)	Telazol	28.7, IM	—	—	183
Blue-gold macaw (*Ara ararauna*)	Telazol	12.1–22.0, IM	—	—	183

(continued)

343

Table 12.15. Use of Telazol alone or Telazol combinations in birds. (*continued*)

Common Names (Genus and Species)	Drug(s)	Dose and Route (mg/kg)	Duration (min)	Comment	Reference
Scarlet macaw (*Ara macao*)	Telazol	4.4–11.0, IM	—	—	184
		5.5–19.8, IM	—	—	183
Mallard (*Anas platyrhynchos*)	Telazol	44.1–55.1, IM	—	—	183
Osprey (*Pardion haliaetus*)	Telazol	9.26–17.6, IM	—	—	183
Ostrich	Telazol	4–5, IM	—	Desirable immobilization	184
(*Sruthio camelus*)		3.7, IV	—	Good induction Poor recovery	262
Barn owl (*Tyto alba*)	Telazol	8.8–30.2, IM	—	—	183
African ring-neck parakeet (*Psittacula krameri*)	Telazol	26, IM	—	Desirable immobilization	184
Parakeet (*Melopsittacus undulatus*)	Telazol	20–22, IM	—	—	183
Patagonian parrot (*Cyrsolophus patagonus*)	Telazol	11, IM	—	Excellent immobilization	184
Crested green wood partridge (*Rollulus roulroul*)	Telazol	10, IM	—	Good immobilization	184
Pigeon (*Columbia livia*)	Telazol	30.6, IM (20–48 range)	41.4 (25–70 range)	Immobilization Poor relaxation	283
		40–60, IM	—	Good anesthesia	184
Plover *Charadriidae* species	Telazol	17.6, IM	—	—	183
Rhea (*Rhea americana*)	Telazol	2–5, IM	—	Tranquilized, resisted handling	184
Greater rhea (*Rhea americana*)	Telazol	2–22, IM	—	—	184
		35.8	—	—	183
Yellow-bellied sapsucker (*Sphyrapicus varius*)	Telazol	33–100, IM	—	Good immobilization	184
Black swan (*Cygnus atratus*)	Telazol	6.6, IM	—	—	184
Black-neck swan (*Cygnus malanocoryphus*)	Telazol	4.4–6.6, IM	—	Some physical restraint needed	184

(*continued*)

Table 12.15. Use of Telazol alone or Telazol combinations in birds. (*continued*)

Common Names (Genus and Species)	Drug(s)	Dose and Route (mg/kg)	Duration (min)	Comment	Reference
Wood stork (*Mycteria americana*)	Telazol	11, IM	—	—	183
Blue-wing teal (*Anas discors*)	Telazol	22–35, IM	—	Prolonged recovery with higher dose	184
Green-wing teal (*Anas crecca carolinensis*)	Telazol	35, IM	—	Prolonged recovery with higher dose	184
Woodcock (*Philohela minor*)	Telazol	44, IM	—	Desirable immobilization	184

IM, intramuscularly; IV, intravenously.

Nondomestic Animals

Ketamine and Telazol have both been used extensively in various combinations for the immobilization of captured and wild animals. Ketamine usage has been somewhat limited because of its relatively low concentration, requiring a large volume be delivered to many larger species. Ketamine can be lypholized and reconstituted to a smaller volume to create a higher concentration when a larger dose is required via a remote delivery device (e.g., darts).[180–182] In contrast, Telazol has the advantage of being reconstituted to a small volume with potent sedatives or adjunctive analgesic drugs to increase overall potency. Both anesthetics have been used alone or in combination in many wild and exotic species.[183–186] Tables 12.11 through 12.15 further summarize the use of ketamine and Telazol, alone and in combination with other drugs, in nondomesticated species.

References

1. Corssen G, Miyasaka M, Domino EF. Changing concepts in pain control during surgery: Dissociative anesthesia with CI-581—A progress report. Anesth Analg 47:746, 1968.
2. Winters WD, Ferrer-Allado T, Guzman-Flores C. The cataleptic state induced by ketamine: A review of the neuropharmacology of anesthesia. Neuropharmacology 11:303, 1972.
3. Thurmon JC, Nelson DR, Christie GJ. Ketamine anesthesia in swine. J Am Vet Med Assoc 160:1325, 1972.
4. Chen G, Ensor C. 2-(Ethylamino)-2-(2-thienyl) cyclohexanone–HCl (CI-634): A taming, incapacitating, and anesthetic agent for the cat. Am J Vet Res 29:863, 1968.
5. Miyasaka M, Domino EF. Neuronal mechanisms of ketamine-induced anesthesia. Int J Neuropharmacol 7:557, 1968.
6. Massopust LC, Wolin LR, Albin MS. The effects of a new phencyclidine derivative and diazepinone derivative on the electroencephalographic and behavioral responses in the cat. TIT J Life Sci 3:1, 1973.
7. Kohrs R, Durieux ME. Ketamine: Teaching an old drug new tricks. Anesth Analg 87:1186, 1998.
8. Brockmeyer DM, Kendig JJ. Selective effects of ketamine on amino acid-mediated pathways in neonatal rat spinal cord. Br J Anaesth 74:79, 1995.
9. Ohtani M, Kikuchi H, Kitahata LM, Taub A, Toyooka H, Hannaoka K, Dohi S. Effects of ketamine on nociceptive cells in the medial medullary reticular formation of the cat. Anesthesiology 51:414, 1979.
10. Kitahata LM, Taub A, Kosaka Y. Lamina-specific suppression of dorsal-horn unit activity by ketamine hydrochloride. Anesthesiology 38:4, 1973.
11. Corssen G, Little SG, Tavakoli M. Ketamine and epilepsy. Anesth Analg 53:319, 1974.
12. Ferrer-Allado T, Brechner VL, Dymond A, Cozen H, Crandall P. Ketamine-induced electroconvulsive phenomena in the human limbic and thalamic regions. Anesthesiology 38:333, 1973.
13. Reder BS, Trapp LD, Troutman KG. Ketamine suppression of chemically induced convulsions in the two-day-old white leghorn cockerel. Anesth Analg 59:406, 1980.
14. Church J. The anticonvulsant activity of ketamine and other phencyclidine receptor ligands, with particular reference to N-methyl-D-aspartate receptor mediated events. In: Domino EF, ed. Status of Ketamine in Anesthesiology. Ann Arbor, MI: NPP, 1990:521.
15. Anis NA, Bery SC, Burton NR, Lodge D. The dissociative anesthetics, ketamine and phencyclidine, selectively reduce excitation of central mammalian neurons by N-methyl-D-aspartate. Br J Pharmacol 79:565, 1983.
16. Velisek L, Mares P. Anticonvulsant action of ketamine in laboratory animals. In: Domino EF, ed. Status of Ketamine in Anesthesiology. Ann Arbor, MI: NPP, 1990:541.
17. Kaplan B. Ketamine HCl anesthesia in dogs: Observation of 3 cases. Vet Med Small Anim Clin 67:631, 1972.
18. Humphrey WJ. Ketamine HCl as a general anesthetic in dogs. Mod Vet Pract 52:38, 1971.
19. Evans AT, Krahwinkel DJ, Sawyer DC. Dissociative anesthesia in the cat. J Am Vet Med Assoc 8:371, 1972.
20. Beck CC. Evaluation of Vetalar (ketamine HCl): A unique feline anesthetic. Vet Med Small Anim Clin 66:993, 1971.
21. Nimmo WS, Clements JA. Ketamine. In: Prys-Roberts C, Hug CC, eds. Pharmacokinetics of Anesthesia. Boston: Blackwell Scientific, 1984:235.
22. Haskins SC, Peiffer RL, Stowe CM. A clinical comparison of CT-1341, ketamine, and xylazine in cats. Am J Vet Res 36:1537, 1975.
23. Sawyer DC, Rech RH, Durham RA. Effects of ketamine and combination with acetylpromazine, diazepam, or butorphanol on visceral nociception in the cat. In: Domino EF, ed. Status of Ketamine in Anesthesiology. Ann Arbor, MI: NPP, 1990:247.
24. Sawyer DC, Rech RH, Durham RA. Does ketamine provide adequate visceral analgesia when used alone or in combination with acepromazine, diazepam, or butorphanol in cats? J Am Anim Hosp Assoc 29:257, 1993.
25. Castroman PJ, Ness TN. Ketamine, an N-methyl-D-aspartate receptor antagonist, inhibits the reflex responses to distension of the rat urinary bladder. Anesthesiology 96:1401, 2002.
26. Castroman PJ, Ness TN. Ketamine, an N-methyl-D-aspartate receptor antagonist, inhibits the spinal neuronal responses to distension of the rat urinary bladder. Anesthesiology 96:1410, 2002.
27. Olivar T, Laird JM. Differential effects of N-methyl-D-aspartate receptor blockade on nociceptive somatic and visceral reflexes. Pain 79:67, 1999.
28. Alams S, Saito Y, Kosaka Y. Antinociceptive effects of epidural and intravenous ketamine to somatic and visceral stimuli in rats. Can J Anaesth 43:408, 1996.
29. Iwasaki H, Collins JG, Namiki A, Yamasawa Y, Omote K, Omote T. Effects of ketamine on behavioral responses to somatic and visceral stimuli in rats. Masui 40:1691, 1991.
30. Pederson JL, Galle TS, Kehlet H. Peripheral analgesic effects of ketamine in acute inflammatory pain. Anesthesiology 89:58, 1998.
31. Warncke T, Jørum E, Stubhaug A. Local treatment with the N-methyl-D-aspartate receptor antagonist, ketamine, inhibits development of secondary hyperalgesia in man by a peripheral action. Neurosci Lett 227:1, 1997.
32. Tverskoy M, Oren M, Vaskovich M, Dashkovsky I, Kissin I. Ketamine enhances local anesthetic and analgesic effects of bupivacaine by peripheral mechanism: A study in postoperative patients. Neurosci Lett 215:5, 1996.
33. Brau ME, Sander F, Vogel W, Hemelmann G. Blocking mechanisms of ketamine and its enantiomers in enzymatically demyelinated peripheral nerves as revealed by single-channel experiments. Anesthesiology 86:394, 1997.
34. Orser BA, Pennefather PS, MacDonald JF. Multiple mechanisms of ketamine blockade of N-methyl-D-aspartate receptors. Anesthesiology 86:903, 1997.

35. Carlton SM, Hargett GL, Coggeshall RE. Localization and activation of glutamate receptors in unmyelinated axons of rats' glabrous skin. Neurosci Lett 197:25, 1995.

36. MacIver MB, Tanelian DL. Structural and functional specialization of A delta and C fiber free nerve endings innervating rabbit corneal epithelium. J Neurosci 13:4511, 1993.

37. Lopez-Sanrom FJ, Cruz JM, Santos M, Mazzini RA, Tabanera A, Tendillo FJ. Evaluation of the local analgesic effect of ketamine in the palmar digital nerve block at the base of the proximal sesamoid (abaxial sesamoid block) in horses. Am J Vet Res 64:475, 2003.

38. El-Khateeb OE, Ragab A, Metwalli M, Hassan HA. Assessment of epidural ketamine for relief of pain following vaginal and lower abdominal surgery. In: Domino EF, ed. Status of Ketamine in Anesthesiology. Ann Arbor, MI: NPP, 1990:403.

39. El-Khateeb OE. Caudal ketamine for relief of pain following anorectal surgery. In: Domino EF, ed. Status of Ketamine in Anesthesiology. Ann Arbor, MI: NPP, 1990:411.

40. Guinto-Enriquez G, Enriquez RY, Reyes de Castro L. Epidural injection of ketamine hydrochloride: An experimental study in rats. In: Domino EF, ed. Status of Ketamine in Anesthesiology. Ann Arbor, MI: NPP, 1990:381.

41. Réduo MA, Valvadão CAA, Duque JC, Balestrero LT. The preemptive effect of epidural ketamine on wound sensitivity in horses tested by using von Frey filaments. Vet Anaesth Analg 29:200, 2002.

42. Gomez de Segura IA, De Rossi R, Santos M, San-Roman JL, Tendillo FJ. Epidural injection of ketamine for perineal analgesia in the horse. Vet Surg 217:384, 1998.

43. Doherty JJ, Geiser DR, Rohrbach BW. Effects of high-volume epidural morphine, butorphanol, and ketamine on halothane MAC in the horse. J Vet Anaesth 22:37, 1995.

44. Kariman A, Nowrouzian I, Bkhtiari J. Caudal epidural injection of a combination of ketamine and xylazine for perineal analgesia in horses. Vet Anaesth Analg 27:115, 2000.

45. Baha F, Malbert CH. Effect of ketamine given by the intrathecal route in dogs. Rev Med Vet 142:283, 1991.

46. Woolfe CJ, Thompson SWN. The induction and maintenance of central sensitization is dependent on N-methyl-D-aspartate receptor activation: Implication for the treatment of post-injury pain hypersensitivity state. Pain 44:293, 1991.

47. Stubburg A, Breivik H, Eide PK, Kreunen M, Foss A. Mapping of punctuate hyperalgesia around a surgical incision demonstrates that ketamine is a powerful suppressor of central sensitization to pain following surgery. Acta Anaesthesiol Scand 41:1124, 1997.

48. Fu ES, Miguel R, Scharf JE. Preemptive ketamine decreases postoperative narcotic requirements in patients undergoing abdominal surgery. Anesth Analg 84:1086, 1997.

49. Warwick D, Kee N, Khaw KS, Ma ML, Mainlans P-A, Gin T. Postoperative analgesic requirement after cesarean section: A comparison of anesthetic induction with ketamine or thiopental. Anesth Analg 85:1294, 1997.

50. Guillou N, Tanguy M, Seguin P, Branger B, Campion J-P, Malledant Y. The effects of small-dose ketamine on morphine consumption in surgical intensive care unit patients after major abdominal surgery. Anesth Analg 97:843, 2003.

51. Kwok RFK, Lim J, Chan MTV, Gin T, Chiu WKY. Preoperative ketamine improves postoperative analgesia after gynecologic laparoscopic surgery. Anesth Analg 98:1044, 2004.

52. Lucas AN, Firth AM, Anderson GA, Vine JH, Edwards GA. Comparison of the effects of morphine administered by constant-rate infusion or intermittent intramuscular injection in dogs. J Am Vet Med Assoc 218:884, 2001.

53. Wagner AE, Walton JA, Hellyer PW, Gaynor JS, Mama KR. Use of low doses of ketamine administered by constant rate infusion as an adjunct for postoperative analgesia in dogs. J Am Vet Med Assoc 221:72, 2002.

54. Evans J, Rosen M, Weeks RD, Wise C. Ketamine in neurosurgical procedures. Lancet 1:40, 1971.

55. Gardner AE, Olson BE, Lichtiger M. Cerebrospinal fluid pressure during associative anesthesia with ketamine. Anesthesiology 35:226, 1971.

56. Shapiro HM, Wyte SR, Harris AB. Ketamine anesthesia in patients with intracranial pathology. Br J Anaesth 44:1200, 1972.

57. Takeshita H, Okuda Y, Sari A. The effects of ketamine on cerebral circulation and metabolism in man. Anesthesiology 36:69, 1972.

58. List WF, Crumrine RS, Cascorbi HF, Weiss MH. Increased cerebrospinal fluid pressure after ketamine. Anesthesiology 36:98, 1972.

59. Wyte SR, Shapiro HM, Turner P, Harris AB. Ketamine-induced intracranial hypertension. Anesthesiology 36:174, 1972.

60. Schulte am Esch J, Pfeifer G, Thiemig I, Entzian W. The influence of intravenous anaesthetic agents on primarily increased intracranial pressure. Acta Neurochir (Wien) 51:560, 1979.

61. Schwedler M, Miletich DJ, Albrecht RF. Cerebral blood flow and metabolism following ketamine administration. Can Anaesth Soc J 29:222, 1982.

62. Pfenninger E, Reith A. Ketamine and intracranial pressure. In: Domino EF, ed. Status of Ketamine in Anesthesiology. Ann Arbor, MI: NPP, 1990:109.

63. Lassen NA. Cerebral and spinal cord blood flow. In: Cottrell JE, Turndoff H, eds. Anesthesia and Neurosurgery. St Louis: CV Mosby, 1986:1.

64. White PF, Way WL, Trevor AJ. Ketamine: Its pharmacology and therapeutic uses. Anesthesiology 56:119, 1982.

65. Beck CC. Vetalar (ketamine hydrochloride): A unique cataleptoid anesthetic agent for multispecies usage. J Zoo Anim Med 7:11, 1976.

66. Wright M. Pharmacologic effects of ketamine and its use in veterinary medicine. J Am Vet Med Assoc 180:1462, 1982.

67. Faulk RH. Xylazine and ketamine synergism for ultrashort anesthesia in cats. Feline Pract 8:15, 1978.

68. Amend JF, Klavano PA, Stone EC. Premedication with xylazine to eliminate muscular hypertonicity in cats during ketamine anesthesia. Vet Med Small Anim Clin 67:1305, 1972.

69. Manziano CF, Manziano JR. The combination of ketamine HCl and acepromazine maleate as a general anesthetic in dogs. Vet Med Small Anim Clin 73:727, 1978.

70. Kothary SP, Zsigmond EK. A double-blind study of the effective antihallucinatory doses of diazepam prior to ketamine anesthesia. Clin Pharmacol Ther 21:108, 1977.

71. Cartwright PD, Pingel SM. Midazolam and diazepam in ketamine anesthesia. Anaesthesia 59:439, 1984.

72. Toft P, Romer U. Comparison of midazolam and diazepam to supplement total intravenous anesthesia with ketamine for endoscopy. Can J Anaesth 34:466, 1987.

73. Ivankovitch AD, Miletich DJ, Reinmann C, Albrecht RF, Zahed B. Cardiovascular effects of centrally administered ketamine in goats. Anesth Analg 53:924, 1974.

74. Salt PJ, Barnes PK, Beswick FJ. Inhibition of neuronal and extraneuronal uptake of noradrenaline by ketamine in the isolated perfused rat heart. Br J Anaesth 51:835, 1979.

75. Altura BM, Altura BT, Carella A. Effects of ketamine on vascular smooth muscle function. Br J Pharmacol 70:257, 1980.

76. Tweed WA, Minuck M, Nymin D. Circulatory responses to ketamine anesthesia. Anesthesiology 37:613, 1972.

77. Wong DHW, Jenkins LC. An experimental study of the mechanism of action of ketamine on the central nervous system. Can Anaesth Soc J 21:57, 1974.

78. Baraka A, Harrison T, Kachachi T. Catecholamine levels after ketamine anesthesia in man. Anesth Analg 52:198, 1973.

79. Traber DL, Wilson RD, Priano LL. A detailed study of the cardiopulmonary response to ketamine and its blockade by atropine. South Med J 63:1077, 1970.

80. McCarthy DA, Chen G, Kaump DH, Ensor C. General anesthetic and other pharmacological properties of 2-(O-chlorophenyl)-2-methylamino cyclohexanone HCl (CI-581). J New Drugs 5:21, 1965.

81. Traber DL, Wilson RD, Priano LL. Blockade of the hypertensive response to ketamine. Anesth Analg 49:420, 1970.

82. Traber DL, Wilson RD, Priano LL. The effect of alpha-adrenergic blockade on the cardiopulmonary response to ketamine. Anesth Analg 50:737, 1971.

83. Nakajima T, Azumi T, Yatabe Y. Mechanism of positive chronotropic response of the canine SA node to selective administration of ketamine. Arch Int Pharmacodyn Ther 234:247, 1978.

84. Child KJ, Davis B, Dodds MG, Twissell DJ. Anaesthetic, cardiovascular and respiratory effects of a new steroidal agent CT 1341: A comparison with other intravenous anaesthetic drugs in the unrestrained cat. Br J Pharmacol 46:189, 1972.

85. Sonntag H, Heiss HW, Knoll D, Regensburger D, Schenk HD, Bretschneider HJ. Myocardial perfusion and myocardial oxygen consumption in patients during induction of anesthesia using dehydrobenzperidol-fentanyl or ketamine [in German]. Z Kreislaufforsch 61:1092, 1972.

86. Smith G, Thorburn J, Vance JP, Brown DM. The effect of ketamine on the canine coronary circulation. Anaesthesia 34:555, 1979.

87. Folts JD, Afonso S, Rowe GG. Systemic and coronary hemodynamic effects of ketamine in intact anaesthetized and unanaesthetized dogs. Br J Anaesth 47:686, 1975.

88. Kaukinen S. The combined effects of antihypertensive drugs and anaesthetics (halothane and ketamine) on the isolated heart. Acta Anaesthesiol Scand 22:649, 1978.

89. Zsigmond EK, Kothary SP, Matsuki A, Kelsch RC, Martinez O. Diazepam for prevention of the rise in plasma catecholamines caused by ketamine. Clin Pharmacol Ther 15:223, 1974.

90. Jackson APF, Dhadphale PR, Callaghan ML. Haemodynamic studies during induction of anaesthesia for open-heart surgery using diazepam and ketamine. Br J Anaesth 50:375, 1978.

91. Båfors E, Haggmark S, Nyhman H, Rydvall A, Reiz S. Droperidol inhibits the effects of intravenous ketamine on central hemodynamics and myocardial O₂ consumption in patients with generalized atherosclerotic disease. Anesth Analg 62:193, 1983.

92. Bidwai AV, Stanley TH, Graves CL, Sentker CR. The effects of ketamine on cardiovascular dynamics during halothane and enflurane anesthesia. Anesth Analg 54:588, 1975.

93. Reich DL, Silvay G. Ketamine: An update on the first twenty-five years of clinical experience. Can J Anaesth 36:186, 1989.

94. Barrigin S, De Miguel B, Tamargo J, Tejerina T. The mechanism of the positive inotropic effect of ketamine on isolated atria of the rat. Br J Pharmacol 76:85, 1982.

95. Riou B, Lecarpentier Y, Viars P. Inotropic effect of ketamine on rat cardiac papillary muscle. Anesthesiology 71:116, 1989.

96. Riou B, Viars P, Lecarpentier Y. Effects of ketamine on the cardiac papillary muscle of normal hamsters and those with cardiomyopathy. Anesthesiology 73:910, 1990.

97. Cook DJ, Carton EG, Housemans PR. Mechanism of the positive inotropic effect of ketamine in isolated ferret ventricular papillary muscle. Anesthesiology 74:880, 1991.

98. Schwartz DA, Horwitz LD. Effects of ketamine on left ventricular performance. J Pharmacol Exp Ther 194:410, 1975.

99. Waxman K, Shoemaker WC, Lippmann M. Cardiovascular effects of anesthetic induction with ketamine. Anesth Analg 59:355, 1980.

100. Dowdy EG, Kaya K. Studies of the mechanism of cardiovascular responses to CI-581. Anesthesiology 29:931, 1968.

101. Urthaler F, Walker AA, James TN. Comparison of the inotropic action of morphine and ketamine studied in canine cardiac muscle. J Thorac Cardiovasc Surg 72:142, 1976.

102. Rusy BF, Amuzu JK, Bosscher HA, Redon D, Komai H. Negative inotropic effect of ketamine in rabbit ventricular muscle. Anesth Analg 71:275, 1990.

103. Sprung J, Schuetz SM, Stewart RW, Moravec CS. Effects of ketamine on the contractility of failing and nonfailing human heart muscles in vitro. Anesthesiology 88:1202, 1998.

104. Longnecker DE, Sturgill BC. Influence of anesthetic agents on survival following hemorrhage. Anesthesiology 45:516, 1976.

105. Sakai T, Ichiyama T, Whitten CW, Gieseeke AH, Lipton JM. Ketamine suppresses endotoxin-induced NF-kappaB expression. Can J Anesth 47:1019, 2000.

106. Taniguchi T, Shibata K, Yamamoto K. Ketamine inhibits endotoxin-induced shock in rats. Anesthesiology 95:928, 2001.

107. Stoelting RK. Nonbarbiturate induction drugs. In: Pharmacology and Physiology in Anesthetic Practice. Philadelphia: JB Lippincott, 1991:134.

108. Booth NH. Intravenous and other parenteral anesthetics. In: Booth NH, McDonald LE, eds. Veterinary Pharmacology and Therapeutics. Ames, IA: Iowa State University Press, 1988:212.

109. Haskins SC, Farver TB, Patz JD. Ketamine in dogs. Am J Vet Res 46:1855, 1985.

110. Hatch RC. Prevention of ketamine catalepsy and enhancement of ketamine anesthesia in cats pretreated with methiothepin. Pharmacol Res Commun 5:311, 1973.

111. Hatch RC, Ruch T. Experiments on antagonism of ketamine anesthesia in cats given adrenergic, serotonergic, and cholinergic stimulants alone and in combination. Am J Vet Res 35:35, 1974.

112. Short CE. Dissociative anesthesia. In: Short CE, ed. Principles and Practice of Veterinary Anesthesia. Baltimore: Williams and Wilkins, 1987:158.

113. Waterman A, Livingston A. Some physiological effects of ketamine in sheep. Res Vet Sci 25:225, 1978.

114. Thurmon JC, Kumar A, Link RP. Evaluation of ketamine hydrochloride as an anesthetic in sheep. J Am Vet Med Assoc 162:293, 1973.

115. Sears BE. Complications of ketamine. Anesthesiology 35:231, 1971.

116. Lofty AO. Anesthesia with ketamine: Indications, advantages, and shortcomings. Anesth Analg 49:969, 1970.

117. Szappanyas G, Gemperle M, Isard A. Utilization of ketamine (Ketalar) as an anesthetic in veterinary surgery. Bull Soc Sci Vet Med Comp 72:149, 1970.

118. Dundee JW, Fee JPH, Moore J, McIlroy PD, Wilson DB. Liver function studies after ketamine infusions. Br J Clin Pharmacol 6:450, 1978.

119. Marietta MP, Vore ME, Way WL, Trevor AJ. Characterization of ketamine induction of hepatic microsomal drug metabolism. Biochem Pharmacol 26:2451, 1977.

120. Paddleford RR. General anesthesia. In: Paddleford RR, ed. Manual of Small Animal Anesthesia. New York: Churchill Livingstone, 1988:31.

121. Lanning CF, Harmel MH. Ketamine anesthesia. Annu Rev Med 26:137, 1975.

122. Yoshikawa K, Murai Y. Effect of ketamine on intraocular pressure in children. Anesth Analg 50:199, 1971.

123. Corssen G, Hoy JE. A new parenteral anesthetic CI 581: Its effect on intraocular pressure. J Pediatr Ophthalmol 4:20, 1967.

124. Peuler M, Glass DD, Arens JF. Ketamine and intraocular pressure. Anesthesiology 43:575, 1975.

125. Ausinsch B, Rayburn RL, Munson ES, Levy NS. Ketamine and intraocular pressure in children. Anesth Analg 55:773, 1976.

126. Gelatt KN, Peiffer RL, Gum GG, Gwin RM, Erickson JL. Evaluation of applanation tonometers for the dog eye. Invest Ophthalmol Vis Sci 16:963, 1977.

127. Trim CM, Colbern GT, Martin CL. Effect of xylazine and ketamine on intraocular pressure in horses. Vet Rec 117:442, 1985.

128. Wilson RP. Complications associated with local and general ophthalmic anesthesia. In: Smolin G, Friedlaender MH, eds. Complications of Ocular Surgery. Int Ophthalmol Clin 32:1, 1992.

129. Rucker MC. Panel report on combining anesthesia in dogs. Mod Vet Pract 57:319, 1976.

130. Hellyer PW, Freeman L, Hubbell JAE. Induction of anesthesia with diazepam-ketamine and midazolam-ketamine in greyhounds. Vet Surg 20:143, 1991.

131. Kirkpatrick RM. Use of xylazine and ketamine as a combination anesthetic. Canine Pract 5:53, 1978.

132. Hartsfield SM. Advantages and guidelines for using ketamine for induction of anesthesia. Vet Clin North Am Small Pract 22:266, 1992.

133. Muir WW, Wiese AJ, March PA. Effects of morphine, lidocaine, ketamine, and morphine-lidocaine-ketamine drug combination on minimum alveolar concentration in dogs anesthetized with isoflurane. Am J Vet Res 64:1155, 2003.

134. Bossard AE, Guirimand F, Fletcher D, Gaude-Joindreau V, Chauvin M, Bouhassira D. Interaction of a combination of morphine and ketamine on the nociceptive flexion reflex in human volunteers. Pain 98:47, 2002.

135. Cherry DA, Plummer JL, Gourlay GK, Coates KR, Odgers CL. Ketamine as an adjunct to morphine in the treatment of pain. Pain 94:119, 2001.

136. Reeves M, Lindholm DE, Myles PS, Fletcher H, Hunt JO. Adding ketamine to morphine for patient-controlled analgesia after major abdominal surgery: A double-blinded, randomized controlled trial. Anesth Analg 93:116, 2001.

137. Wu CL, Tella P, Staats PS, Vaslav R, Kazim DA, Wesselmann U, Raja SN. Analgesic effects of intravenous lidocaine and morphine on postamputation pain. Anesthesiology 96:841, 2002.

138. Hartsfield SM. Injectable drugs and drug combinations for feline premedication, sedation, anesthesia and analgesia [Abstract]. In: Proceedings of the 54th Annual Meeting (Feline medicine) of the American Animal Hospital Association, Phoenix, AZ, 1987:277.

139. Ilkiw JE, Suter C, McNeal D, Steffey EP. Effect of intravenous administration of variable-dose midazolam following fixed-dose ketamine in healthy awake cats. In: Proceedings of the Annual Meeting of the American College of Veterinary Anesthesiologists, Las Vegas, NV, 1990:18.

140. Cullen LK, Jones RS. Clinical observations on xylazine/ketamine anesthesia in the cat. Vet Rec 101:115, 1977.

141. Colby ED, Sanford TD. Feline anesthesia with mixed solutions of ketamine/xylazine and ketamine/acepromazine. Feline Pract 12:14, 1982.

142. Verstegen J, Fargetton X, Ectors F. Medetomidine/ketamine anesthesia in cats. Acta Vet Scand 85:117, 1989.

143. Verstegen J, Fargetton X, Donnay I, Ectors F. An evaluation of medetomidine/ketamine and other drug combinations for anaesthesia in cats. Vet Rec 128:32, 1991.

144. Young LE, Jones RS. Clinical observations on medetomidine/ketamine anesthesia and its antagonism by atipamezole in the cat. J Small Anim Pract 31:221, 1990.

145. Verstegen J, Fargetton X, Zanker S, Donnay I, Ectors F. Antagonistic activities of atipamezole 4-aminopyridine and yohimbine against medetomidine/ketamine-induced anesthesia in cats. Vet Rec 128:57, 1991.

146. Dobromylskyj P. Cardiovascular changes associated with anaesthesia induced by medetomidine combined with ketamine in cats. J Small Anim Pract 37:169, 1996.

147. Grove DM, Ramsey EC. Sedative and physiologic effects of orally administered alpha 2-adrenoceptor agonists and ketamine in cats. J Am Vet Med Assoc 216:1929, 2000.

148. Reid JS, Frank RJ. Prevention of undesirable side reactions of ketamine anesthesia in cats. J Am Anim Hosp Assoc 8:115, 1972.

149. Hatch RC. Effects of ketamine when used in conjunction with pethidine or morphine in cats. J Am Vet Med Assoc 162:964, 1973.

150. Benson GJ, Thurmon JC. Intravenous anesthesia. In: Riebold TW, ed. Principles and Techniques of Equine Anesthesia. Vet Clin North Am 6:513, 1990.

151. Muir WW, Skarda RT, Milne DW. Evaluation of xylazine and ketamine hydrochloride for anesthesia in horses. Am J Vet Res 38:195, 1977.

152. Heath RB, Hubbell JAE, Muir WW. Intravenous anesthesia. In: Mansmann RA, McAllister ES, Pratt PW. Equine Medicine and Surgery, 3rd ed. Santa Barbara, CA: American Veterinary, 1982:257.

153. Matthews NS, Taylor TS, Sullivan JA. A comparison of three combinations of injectable anesthetics in miniature donkeys. Vet Anaesth Analg 29:36, 2002.

154. Tranquilli WJ, Thurmon JC, Turner TA, Benson GJ, Lock TF. Butorphanol tartrate as an adjunct to xylazine-ketamine anesthesia in the horse. Equine Pract 5:26, 1983.

155. Fisher RJ. A field trial of ketamine anaesthesia in the horse. Equine Vet J 16:176, 1984.

156. Parsons LE, Walmsley JP. Field use of an acetylpromazine/methadone/ketamine combination for anaesthesia in the horse and donkey. Vet Rec 111:395, 1982.

157. Muir WW. Intravenous anesthetics and anesthetic techniques in horses. In: Muir WW, Hubbell JAE, eds. Equine Anesthesia: Monitoring and Emergency Therapy. St Louis: Mosby Year Book, 1991:281.

158. Hikasa Y, Takase K, Kakuta T, Ogasawara S. Clinical application of 0.2% ketamine micro-drip infusion anesthesia in foals. Bull Equine Res Inst Jpn 26:31, 1989.

159. Spadavecchia C, Stucki F, Moens Y, Schatzmann U. Anaesthesia in horses using halothane and intravenous ketamine-guaiphenesin: A clinical study. Vet Anaesth Analg 29:20, 2002.

160. Greene SA, Thurmon JC, Tranquilli WJ, Benson GJ. Cardiopulmonary effects of continuous intravenous infusion of guaifenesin, ketamine, and xylazine in ponies. Am J Vet Res 47:2364, 1986.

161. Lin HC, Thurmon JC, Benson GJ, Tranquilli WJ, Olson WA. Guaifenesin-ketamine-xylazine anesthesia for castration in ponies: A comparative study with two different doses of ketamine. J Equine Vet Sci 13:29, 1993.

162. Young LE, Bartram DH, Diamond MJ, Gregg AS, Jones RS. Clinical evaluation of an infusion of xylazine, guaifenesin and ketamine for maintenance of anaesthesia in horses. Equine Vet J 25:115, 1993.

163. Brock N, Hildebrand SV. Xylazine–diazepam–ketamine compared with xylazine–guaifenesin-ketamine in equine anesthesia [Abstract]. Vet Surg 19:468, 1990.

164. Clarke KW, Taylor PM, Watkins SB. Detomidine/ketamine anesthesia in the horse. Acta Vet Scand 82:167, 1986.

165. Matthews NS, Hartsfield SM, Cornick JL, Williams JD, Beasley A. A comparison of injectable anesthetic combinations in horses. Vet Surg 20:268, 1991.

166. Thurmon JC, Ko JCH, Benson GJ, Tranquilli WJ, Olson WA. Guaifenesin-ketamine-detomidine anesthesia for castration of ponies: A preliminary report. In: Fourth International Congress of Veterinary Anesthesia, Utrecht, The Netherlands, 1991:48.

167. Taylor PM, Clarke KW. Intravenous anesthesia. In: Handbook of Equine Anaesthesia. London: WB Saunders, 1999:33.

168. Diamond MJ, Young LE, Bartram DH, Gregg AS, Clutton RE, Long KJ, Jones RS. Clinical evaluation of romifidine/ketamine/halothane anesthesia in horses. Vet Rec 132:572, 1993.

169. Bouts T, Gasthuys F, Vlaminck L, Van Branteghem L. Comparison of romifidine-ketamine-midazolam and romifidine-tiletamine-zolazepam total intravenous anaesthesia (TIVA) for clinical anesthesia in horses. Vet Anaesth Analg 29:90, 2002.

170. Fuentes VO, Tellez E. Ketamine dissociative analgesia in cattle. Vet Rec 94:482, 1974.

171. Thurmon JC, Benson GJ. Anesthesia in ruminants and swine. In: Howard JL, ed. Current Veterinary Therapy: Food Animal Practice. Philadelphia: WB Saunders, 1993:58.

172. Thurmon JC. Injectable anesthetic agents and techniques in ruminants and swine. Vet Clin North Am Food Anim Pract 2:567, 1986.

173. Gavier D, Kittleson MA, Fowler ME, Johnson LE, Hall G, Nearenberg D. Evaluation of a combination of xylazine, ketamine, and halothane for anesthesia in llamas. Am J Vet Res 49:2047, 1988.

174. DuBois WR, Prado TM, Ko JCH, Mandsager RE. A comparison of two intramuscular doses of xylazine-ketamine combination and tolazoline reversal in llamas. Vet Anaesth Analg 31:90, 2004.

175. Green CJ, Knight J, Precious S, Simpkin S. Ketamine alone and combined with diazepam or xylazine in laboratory animals: A 10 year experience. Lab Anim 15:163, 1981.

176. Kyle OC, Novak S, Bolooki H. General anesthesia in pigs. Lab Anim Sci 29:123, 1979.

177. Breese CE, Dodman NH. Xylazine-ketamine-oxymorphone: An injectable anesthetic combination in swine. J Am Vet Med Assoc 184:182, 1984.

178. Sakaguchi M, Nishimura R, Sasaki N, Ishiguro T, Tamura H, Takeuchi A. Anesthesia induced in pigs by use of a combination of medetomidine, butorphanol, and ketamine and its reversal by administration of atipamezole. Am J Vet Res 57:529, 1996.

179. Sakaguchi M, Nishimura R, Sasaki N, Ishiguro T, Tamura H, Takeuchi A. Chemical restraint by medetomidine-ketamine and its cardiopulmonary effects in pigs. Zentrabl Veterinarmed [A] 42:293, 1995.

180. Addison EM, Kolensky GB. Use of ketamine hydrochloride, and xylazine hydrochloride to immobilize black bears (Ursus americanus). J Wildl Dis 15:253, 1977.

181. Haigh JC. Freeze-dried ketamine and Rompun for use in exotic species. Proc Am Assoc Zoo Vet 1978:21.

182. Lee J, Schweinsburg R, Kernan F, Haigh J. Immobilization of polar bears (Ursus maritimus, Phipps) with ketamine hydrochloride and xylazine hydrochloride. J Wildl Dis 17:331, 1981.

183. Schobert E. Telazol use in wild and exotic animals. Vet Med 82:1080, 1987.

184. Gray CW, Bush M, Beck CC. Clinical experience using CI-744 in chemical restraint and anesthesia of exotic specimens. J Zoo Anim Med 5:12, 1974.

185. Boever WJ, Holden J, Kane KK. Use of Telazol (CI-744) for chemical restraint and anesthesia in wild and exotic carnivores. Vet Med Small Anim Clin 72:1722, 1977.

186. King JM, Bertram BCR, Hamilton PH. Tiletamine and zolazepam for immobilization of wild lions and leopards. J Am Vet Med Assoc 171:894, 1977.

187. Pathak SC, Nigam JM, Peshin PK, Singh AP. Anesthetic and hemodynamic effects of ketamine hydrochloride in buffalo calves (Bubalus bubalis). Am J Vet Res 43:875, 1982.

188. Ramakrishna O, Murphy DK, Nigam JM. Ketamine anesthesia in buffalo calves. Indian Vet J 58:503, 1981.

189. Dew TL. Use of tolazoline hydrochloride to reverse multiple anesthetic episodes induced with xylazine hydrochloride and ketamine hydrochloride in white-tailed deer and goats. J Zoo Anim Med 19:8, 1988.

190. Langrehr D, Muller R. Significance of CI-581 for anesthesiology in veterinary medicine with special attention to zoo animals. In: Proceedings of the Ninth International Symposium on Disease in Zoo Animals. Berlin: Akademie, 1967.

191. Festa-Bianchet M, Jorgenson JT. Use of xylazine-ketamine to immobilize bighorn sheep in Alberta. J Wildl Dis 49:162, 1985.

192. Barnett JEF, Lewis JCM. Medetomidine and ketamine anesthesia in zoo animals and its reversal with atipamezole: A review and update with specific reference to work in British zoos. In: Proceedings of the American Zoo Veterinarians, South Padre Island, TX, 1990:207.

193. Jalanka H. The use of medetomidine, medetomidine-ketamine combinations and atipamezole at Helsinki Zoo: A review of 240 cases. Acta Vet Scand 85:193, 1989.

194. English AW. Chemical restraint of deer. Proc Deer Refresher Course Vet Univ Sydney 72:325, 1984.

195. Keep JM. The sedation and immobilization of deer. Proc Deer Refresher Course Vet Univ Sydney 49:21, 1984.

196. Jalanka HH. Medetomidine- and ketamine-induced immobilization in forest reindeer (Rangifer tarandus fennicus) and its reversal by atipamezole. In: Proceedings of the American Zoo Veterinarians, Greensboro, NC, 1989:1.

197. Mech LD, Giudice GDD, Karns PD, Seal US. Yohimbine hydrochloride as an antagonist to xylazine hydrochloride immobilization of white-tailed deer. J Wildl Dis 21:405, 1985.

198. Kreeger TJ, Giudice GDD, Seal US, Karns PD. Immobilization of white-tailed deer with xylazine hydrochloride and ketamine hydrochloride and antagonism by tolazoline hydrochloride. J Wildl Dis 22:407, 1986.

199. Golightly RT, Hofstra TD. Immobilization of elk with a ketamine-xylazine mix and rapid reversal with yohimbine hydrochloride. Wildl Soc Bull 17:53, 1989.

200. Jessup DA. Restraint and chemical immobilization of carnivores and furbearers. In: Nielsen L, Haigh JC, Fowler ME, eds. Chemical Immobilization of North American Wildlife. Milwaukee, WI: Wisconsin Humane Society, 1982:227.

201. Kreeger TJ, Seal US. Immobilization of coyotes with xylazine hydrochloride–ketamine hydrochloride and antagonism by yohimbine hydrochloride. J Wildl Dis 22:604, 1986.

202. Heerden JV, Swan GE, Dauth J, Burroughs REJ, Dreyer MJ. Sedation and immobilization of wild dogs (Lycaon pictus) using medetomidine or a medetomidine-ketamine combination. S Afr J Wildl Res 21:88, 1991.

203. Jalanka HH. Medetomidine- and medetomidine-ketamine–induced immobilization in blue foxes (*Alopex lagopus*) and its reversal by atipamezole. Acta Vet Scand 31:63, 1990.

204. Kreeger TJ, Faggella AM, Seal US, Mech LD, Callahan M, Hall B. Cardiovascular and behavioral responses of gray wolves to ketamine-xylazine immobilization and antagonism by yohimbine. J Wildl Dis 23:463, 1987.

205. Kreeger TJ, Seal US, Faggella AM. Xylazine hydrochloride–ketamine hydrochloride immobilization of wolves and its antagonism by tolazoline hydrochloride. J Wildl Dis 22:397, 1986.

206. Fuller TK, Kuehn DW. Immobilization of wolves using ketamine in combination with xylazine or promazine. J Wildl Dis 19:69, 1983.

207. Mathews M. The use of ketamine to immobilize a black leopard. J Zoo Anim Med 2:25, 1971.

208. Dolensek EP. Reports to Parke-Davis, Detroit, MI, 1971.

209. Hime JM. Use of ketamine hydrochloride in non-domesticated cats. Vet Rec 95:193, 1974.

210. Parke-Davis. Reports on file, Detroit, MI, 1965-1971.

211. Jalanka HH. Evaluation and comparison of two ketamine-based immobilization techniques in snow leopards (*Panthera uncia*). J Zoo Wildl Med 20:163, 1989.

212. Herbst LH, Packer C, Seal US. Immobilization of free-ranging African lions (*Panthera leo*) with a combination of xylazine hydrochloride and ketamine hydrochloride. J Wildl Dis 21:401, 1985.

213. Wyk TCV, Berry HH. Tolazoline as an antagonist in free-ranging lions immobilized with a ketamine-xylazine combination. J S Afr Vet Assoc 57:221, 1986.

214. Logan KA, Thorne ET, Irwin LL, Skinner R. Immobilizing wild mountain lions (*Felis concolor*) with ketamine hydrochloride and xylazine hydrochloride. J Wildl Dis 22:97, 1986.

215. Melquist WE, Hornocker MG. Methods and techniques for studying and censusing river otter populations. For Wildl Range Exp Stn Univ Idaho 1979:no. 54.

216. Greene SA, Keegan RD, Gallagher LV, Alexander JE, Harari J. Cardiovascular effects of halothane anesthesia after diazepam and ketamine administration in beavers (*Castor canadensis*) during spontaneous or controlled ventilation. Am J Vet Res 52:665, 1991.

217. Aulerich RJ. Reports to Parke-Davis, Detroit, MI, 1971.

218. Sylvina TJ, Berman NG, Fox JG. Effects of yohimbine on bradycardia and duration of recumbency in ketamine/xylazine anesthetized ferrets. Lab Anim Sci 40:178, 1990.

219. Moreland AF, Glaser C. Evaluation of ketamine, ketamine-xylazine and ketamine-diazepam anesthesia in the ferret. Lab Anim Sci 35:287, 1985.

220. Bone L, Battles AH, Goldfarb RD, Lombard CW, Moreland AF. Electrocardiographic values from clinically normal, anesthetized ferrets (*Mustela putorius furo*). Am J Vet Res 49:1884, 1988.

221. Kuiken T. Anesthesia in the European otter (*Lutra lutra*). Vet Rec 123:59, 1988.

222. Lewis JCM. Reversible immobilization of Asian small-clawed otters with medetomidine and ketamine. Vet Rec 128:86, 1991.

223. Arena PC, Richardson KC, Cullen LK. Anaesthesia in two species of large Australian skunk. Vet Rec 123:155, 1988.

224. Beck CC. Chemical restraint of exotic species. J Zoo Anim Med 3:3, 1972.

225. Rosatte RC, Hobson DP. Ketamine hydrochloride as an immobilizing agent for striped skunk. Can Vet J 24:134, 1983.

226. Lynch GM, Hall W, Pelchat B, Hanson JA. Chemical immobilization of black bear with special reference to the use of ketamine-xylazine. In: Nielsen L, Haigh JC, Fowler ME, eds. Chemical Immobilization of North American Wildlife. Milwaukee, WI: Wisconsin Humane Society, 1982:245.

227. Page CD. Sloth bear immobilization with a ketamine-xylazine combination: Reversal with yohimbine. J Am Vet Med Assoc 189:1050, 1986.

228. White RJ, Bali S, Bark H. Xylazine and ketamine anaesthesia in the dromedary camel under field conditions. Vet Rec 120:110, 1987.

229. Jacobson ER, Allen J, Martin H, Kollins GV. Effects of yohimbine on combined xylazine-ketamine–induced sedation and immobilization in juvenile African elephants. J Am Vet Med Assoc 187:1195, 1985.

230. Allen JL. Use of tolazoline as an antagonist to xylazine-ketamine–induced immobilization in African elephants. Am J Vet Res 47:781, 1986.

231. Heard DJ, Kollias GV, Webb AI, Jacobson ER, Brock KA. Use of halothane to maintain anesthesia induced with etorphine in juvenile African elephants. J Am Vet Med Assoc 193:254, 1988.

232. Stander PE, Gasaway WC. Spotted hyenas immobilized with ketamine/xylazine and antagonized with tolazoline. Afr J Ecol 29:168, 1991.

233. Gallagher JF, Lochmiller RL, Grant WE. Immobilization of collared peccaries with ketamine hydrochloride. J Wildl Manag 49:356, 1985.

234. Mills TM, Copland JA. Effects of ketamine-xylazine anesthesia on blood levels of luteinizing hormone and follicle stimulating hormone in rabbits. Lab Anim Sci 32:619, 1982.

235. Hobbs BA, Ralhall TG, Sprenkel TL, Anthony KL. Comparison of several combinations for anesthesia in rabbits. Am J Vet Res 52:669, 1991.

236. Marini RP, Avison DL, Corning BF, Lipman NS. Ketamine/xylazine/butorphanol: A new anesthetic combination for rabbits. Lab Anim Sci 42:57, 1992.

237. Popilskis SJ, Oz MC, Gorman P, Florestal A, Kohn DF. Comparison of xylazine with tiletamine-zolazepam (Telazol) and xylazine-ketamine anesthesia in rabbits. Lab Anim Sci 41:51, 1991.

238. Borkowski GL, Danneman PJ, Russell GB, Lang CM. An evaluation of three intravenous anesthetic regimens in New Zealand rabbits. Lab Anim Sci 40:270, 1990.

239. Lipman NS, Marini RP, Erdman SE. A comparison of ketamine/xylazine and ketamine/xylazine/acepromazine anesthesia in the rabbit. Lab Anim Sci 40:395, 1990.

240. Olson ME, McCabe K, Walker RL. Guaifenesin alone or in combination with ketamine or sodium pentobarbital as an anesthetic in rabbits. Can J Vet Res 51:383, 1987.

241. Gregg DA, Olson LD. The use of ketamine hydrochloride as an anesthetic for raccoons. J Wildl Dis 11:335, 1975.

242. Baber DW, Coblentz BE. Immobilization of feral pigs with a combination of ketamine and xylazine. J Wildl Manag 46:557, 1982.

243. Custer RS, Bush M. Physiologic and acid-base measures of gopher snakes during ketamine or halothane–nitrous oxide anesthesia. J Am Vet Med Assoc 177:870, 1980.

244. Olson ME, McCabe K. Anesthesia in the Richardson's ground squirrel: Comparison of ketamine, ketamine and xylazine, droperidol and fentanyl, and sodium pentobarbital. J Am Vet Med Assoc 189:1035, 1986.

245. England GCW, Kock RA. The use of two mixtures of ketamine and xylazine to immobilise free ranging Bennett wallabies. Vet Rec 122:11, 1988.

246. Shaughnessy PD. Immobilization of crabeater seals, *Lobodon carcinophagus*, with ketamine and diazepam. Wildl Res 18:165, 1991.

247. Briggs GD, Henrickson RV, Boeuf JL. Ketamine immobilization of northern elephant seals. J Am Vet Med Assoc 167:546, 1975.

248. Trillmich F. Ketamine/xylazine combination for the immobilization of Galapagos sea lions and fur seals. Vet Rec 112:279, 1983.

249. Baker JR, Gatesman TJ. Use of carfentanil and a ketamine-xylazine mixture to immobilise wild grey seals (*Halichoerus grypus*). Vet Rec 116:208, 1985.

250. Baker JR, Anderson SS, Fedak MA. The use of ketamine-diazepam mixture to immobilise wild grey seals (*Halichoerus grypus*) and southern elephant seals (*Mirounga leonina*). Vet Rec 123:287, 1988.

251. Geraci JR, Skirnisson K, St Aubin DJ. A safe method for repeatedly immobilizing seals. J Am Vet Med Assoc 179:1192, 1981.

252. Geraci JR. An appraisal of ketamine as an immobilizing agent in wild and captive pinnipeds. J Am Vet Med Assoc 163:574, 1973.

253. Gales NJ, Burton HR. Use of emetics and anaesthesia for dietary assessment of Weddell seals. Aust Wildl Res 15:423, 1988.

254. Evans RH. Anesthesia for orthopedics. Vet Tech 6:44, 1985.

255. Heaton JT, Brauth SE. Effects of yohimbine as a reversing agent for ketamine-xylazine anesthesia in budgerigars. Lab Anim Sci 42:54, 1992.

256. Stoskopf MJ, Beall FB, Ensley PK, Neely E. Immobilization of large ratites: Blue necked ostrich (*Struthio Camelus austrealis*) and double wattled cassowary (*Casuarius casuarius*) with hematologic and serum chemistry data. J Zoo Anim Med 13:160, 1982.

257. McGrath CJ, Lee TC, Campbell VL. Dose-response anesthetic effects of ketamine in the chicken. Am J Vet Res 45:531, 1984.

258. Ludders JW, Rode J, Mitchell GS, Nordheim EV. Effects of ketamine, xylazine, and a combination of ketamine and xylazine in Pekin ducks. Am J Vet Res 50:245, 1989.

259. Grubb B. Use of ketamine to restrain and anesthetize emus. Vet Med Small Anim Clin 78:247, 1983.

260. Harvey RB, Kubena LF, Lovering SL, Phillips TD. Ketamine/xylazine anesthesia for chickens. Avian/Exotic Pract 2:6, 1985.

261. Degernes LA, Kreeger TJ, Mandsager R, Redig PT. Ketamine-xylazine anesthesia in red-tailed hawks with antagonism by yohimbine. J Wildl Dis 24:322, 1988.

262. Cornick JL, Jensen J. Anesthetic management of ostriches. J Am Vet Med Assoc 200:1661, 1992.

263. Stunkard JA, Miller JC. An outline guide to general anesthesia in exotic species. Vet Med Small Anim Clin 69:1181, 1974.

264. Heerden JV, Komen J, Myer E. The use of ketamine hydrochloride in the immobilization of the cape vulture (*Gyps coprotheres*). J S Afr Vet Assoc 58:143, 1987.

265. Allen JL, Oosterhuis JE. Effect of tolazoline on xylazine-ketamine–induced anesthesia in turkey vultures. J Am Vet Med Assoc 189:1011, 1986.

266. Lindzey J, Griel LC. Laboratory Study of CI-744 as an Anesthetic Agent in Deer. State College: Pennsylvania State University, August 1972.

267. Mautz WW, Seal US, Boardman CB. Blood serum analyses of chemically and physically restrained white-tailed deer. J Wildl Manag 44:343, 1980.

268. Franzmann AW, Arneson PD. Immobilization of Alaskan moose. J Zoo Anim Med 5:26, 1974.

269. Kreeger TJ, Seal US, Tester JR. Chemical Immobilization of red foxes (*Vulpes vulpes*). J Wildl Dis 26:95, 1990.

270. Smeller J, Bush M. A physiological study of immobilized cheetahs (*Acinonyx jubatus*). J Zoo Anim Med 7:5, 1976.

271. Seidensticker J, Tamang KM, Gray CW. The use of CI-744 to immobilize free-ranging tigers and leopards. J Zoo Anim Med 5:22, 1974.

272. Bertram BCR, King JM. Lion and leopard immobilization using CI-744. East Afr Wildl J 14:237, 1976.

273. Bush M, Custer R, Smeller J, Bush LM, Seal US, Barton R. The acide-base status of lions, *Panthera leo*, immobilized with four drug combinations. J Wildl Dis 14:102, 1978.

274. Smith JLD, Sunquist ME, Tamang KM, Rai PB. A technique for capturing and immobilizing tigers. J Wildl Manag 47:255, 1983.

275. Bush M, Custer RS, Smith EE. Use of dissociative anesthesia for the immobilization of captive bear: Blood gas, hematology and biochemistry values. J Wildl Dis 16:481, 1980.

276. Taylor WP, Reynolds HV, Ballard WB. Immobilization of grizzly bears with tiletamine hydrochloride and zolazepam hydrochloride. J Wildl Manag 53:978, 1989.

277. Haigh JC, Stirling I, Broughton E. Clinical experiences with Telazol for polar bear (*Ursus maritimus*, Phipps) immobilization. Am Assoc Zoo Vet 130:1984.

278. Stirling I, Spencer C, Andriashek D. Immobilization of polar bears (*Ursus maritimus*) with Telazol in the Canadian Arctic. J Wildl Dis 25:159, 1989.

279. Knottenbelt MK, Knottenbelt DC. Use of oral sedative for immobilization of a chimpanzee (*Pan troglodytes*). Vet Rec 126:404, 1990.

280. Schultz TA, Fowler ME. The clinical effects of CI-744 in chinchillas, *Chinchilla villidera* (Laniger). Lab Anim Sci 24:810, 1974.

281. Payton AJ, Pick JR. Evaluation of a combination of tiletamine and zolazepam as an anesthetic for ferrets. Lab Anim Sci 39:243, 1989.

282. Hrapkiewicz KL, Stein S, Smiler KL. A new anesthetic agent for use in the gerbil. Lab Anim Sci 39:338, 1989.

283. Ward GS, Johnson DO, Roberts CR. The use of CI-744 as an anesthetic for laboratory animals. Lab Anim Sci 24:737, 1974.

284. Silverman J, Huhndorf M, Balk M, Slater G. Evaluation of a combination of tiletamine and zolazepam as an anesthetic for laboratory rodents. Lab Anim Sci 33:457, 1983.

285. Matthews NS, Myers MM. The use of tiletamine-zolazepam for darting feral horses. J Equine Vet Sci 13:264, 1993.

286. Smeller JM, Bush M, Custer RW. The immobilization of marsupials. J Zoo Anim Med 8:16, 1977.

287. Boever WJ, Stuppy D, Kane KK. Clinical experience with Telazol (CI-744) as a new agent for chemical restraint and anesthesia in the red kangaroo (*Macropus rufus*). J Zoo Anim Med 8:14, 1977.

288. Bush M, Graves J, O'Brian SJ, Wildt DE. Dissociative anesthesia in free-ranging male koalas and selected marsupials in captivity. Aust Vet J 67:449, 1990.

289. Wildt DE, O'Brian SJ, Graves JAE, Murray ND, Hurlbut S, Bush M. Anesthesia and reproductive characteristics of free-ranging male koalas (*Phascolarctos cinereus*). Am Assoc Zoo Vet 109, 1988.

290. Kaufman L, Hahnenberger R. CI-744 anesthesia for ophthalmological examination and surgery in monkeys. Invest Ophthalmol 14:788, 1975.

291. Crissey SD, Edwards MS. Telazol immobilization of red howlers (*Alouatta seniculus*) under free-ranging conditions [Abstract]. In: Proceedings of the American Association of Zoo Veterinarians, 1989:207.

292. Williams TD, Kocher FH. Comparison of anesthetic agents in the sea otter. J Am Vet Med Assoc 173:1127, 1978.

293. Eads FE. Telazol (CI-744): A new agent for chemical restraint and anesthesia in nonhuman primates. Vet Med Small Anim Clin 71:648, 1976.

294. Bree MM. Dissociative anesthesia in *Macaca mulatta*: Clinical evaluation of CI 744. J Med Primatol 1:256, 1972.

295. Baker JR, Fedak MA, Anderson SS, Arnbom T, Baker R. Use of tiletamine-zolazepam mixture to immobilize wild grey seals and southern elephant seals. Vet Rec 126:75, 1990.

296. Loughlin TR, Spraker T. Use of Telazol to immobilize female northern sea lions (*Eumetopias jubatus*) in Alaska. J Wildl Dis 25:353, 1989.

297. Clyde VL, Cardeilhac P, Jacobson E. Chemical restraint of American alligator (*Alligator Mississippiensis*) with atracurium and tiletamine-zolazepam. In: Proceedings of the American Zoo Veterinarians, South Padre Island, TX, 1990:288.

298. Bonath KH, Haller RD, Bonath I, Amelang D. Tiletamine-zolazepam-acepromazine sedation in *Crocodylus niloticus* with regard to respiratory and cardiovascular system [Abstract]. In: Proceedings of the Fourth International Congress of Veterinary Anaesthesia, 1991:78.

Chapter 13
Inhalation Anesthetics

Eugene P. Steffey and Khursheed R. Mama

Introduction

Inhalation anesthetics are used widely for the anesthetic management of animals. They are unique among the anesthetic drugs because they are administered, and in large part removed from the body, via the lungs. Their popularity arises in part because their pharmacokinetic characteristics favor predictable and rapid adjustment of anesthetic depth. In addition, a special apparatus is usually used to deliver the inhaled agents. This apparatus includes a source of oxygen (O_2) and a patient breathing circuit that in turn usually includes an endotracheal tube or face mask, a means of eliminating carbon dioxide (CO_2), and a compliant gas reservoir. These components help minimize patient morbidity or mortality because they facilitate lung ventilation and improved arterial oxygenation. In addition, inhalation anesthetics in gas samples can now be readily and affordably measured almost instantaneously. Measurement of inhalation anesthetic concentration enhances the precision and safety of anesthetic management beyond the extent commonly possible with injectable anesthetic agents.

Over the nearly 150 years that inhalation anesthesia has been used in clinical practice, fewer than 20 agents have actually been introduced and approved for general use with patients (Fig. 13.1).[1] Fewer than ten of these have had any history of widespread clinical use in veterinary medicine, and only 5 are of current clinical veterinary importance in North America. It is this group of anesthetics that are the focus of this chapter. Isoflurane is generally considered the most widely used inhalation anesthetic in veterinary medicine, having replaced halothane in this regard. The gaseous agent nitrous oxide (N_2O) and the newest volatile agent sevoflurane, along with halothane, enjoy varying degrees of popularity and are grouped in an intermediary category. It is important to note that, at the time of updating this chapter, suppliers are considering no longer making and distributing halothane, at least in North America. However, because the decision at this time is not final, for purposes of this chapter, the author will continue to include information on halothane. The other newer volatile anesthetic, desflurane, is presently only of limited use in veterinary medicine but is grouped among the five contemporary agents. Two additional volatile agents receive brief attention for different reasons. Methoxyflurane, an agent popular during the period of about 1960 to 1990, is no longer commercially available in North America. However, because of some of its physical-chemical characteristics, mention here has value to the reader in comparing agents of more current interest. Enflurane, introduced for use in human patients in 1972 and still commercially available, has little or no use in veterinary practice in the United States but remains in limited use elsewhere for management of small companion animal patients or laboratory animals. Although of investigational interest, a review of xenon is not included in this clinically focused chapter.

In this edition, information on agents of largely historical interest has not been included. Readers interested in aspects of these formally used agents are referred to the earlier editions of this and other textbooks.[2–6] Such agents include diethyl ether, chloroform, and others noted in Fig. 13.1.

Physiochemical Characteristics

The chemical structure of inhalation anesthetics and their physical properties determine their actions and safety of administration. An in-depth analysis of the impact of agent chemical structure and physical properties is beyond the scope of this chapter. However, brief discussion of aspects of Fig. 13.2 and Table 13.1 is appropriate because the physiochemical characteristics summarized determine and/or influence practical considerations of

Inhalation Anesthetics in Clinical Practice

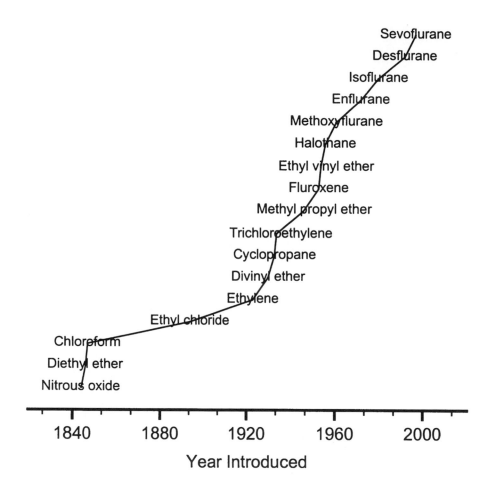

Fig. 13.1. Inhalation anesthetics introduced for widespread clinical use. Adapted from Eger[1] and Karzai et al.[323]

their clinical use. For example, they determine the form in which the agents are supplied by the manufacturer (i.e., as a gas or liquid) and account for the resistance of the anesthetic molecule to degradation by physical factors (e.g., heat and light) and substances it contacts during use (e.g., metal components of the anesthetic-delivery apparatus and the CO_2 absorbents such as soda lime). The equipment necessary to deliver the agent safely to patients (e.g., vaporizer and breathing circuit) is influenced by some of these properties, as are the agent's uptake, distribution within, and elimination (including potential for metabolic breakdown) from the patient. In summary, a knowledge and understanding of fundamental properties enable more intelligent use of contemporary anesthetics.

Chemical Characteristics

All contemporary inhalation anesthetics are organic compounds except N_2O (Fig. 13.2) (cyclopropane and xenon are other no-

table inorganic anesthetics). Agents of current interest are further classified as either aliphatic (i.e., straight or branch chained) hydrocarbons or ethers (i.e., two organic radicals attached to an atom of O_2; the general structure is ROR). In the continued search for a less reactive, more potent, nonflammable inhalation anesthetic, focus on halogenation (i.e., addition of fluorine, chlorine, or bromine; iodine is least useful) of these compounds has predominated. Chlorine and bromine especially convert many compounds of low anesthetic potency into more potent drugs. Historically, interest in fluorinated derivatives was delayed until the 1940s because of difficulties in synthesis, and thus quantities available for study were limited. Methods of synthesis, although difficult, have improved considerably and facilitated new agent discovery (Fig. 13.2). It is interesting that organic fluorinated compounds are a group of extreme contrasts—some are toxic, others are not; some are extremely inert, others are highly reactive. In some anesthetics, fluorine is substituted for chlorine or

Table 13.1. Some physical and chemical properties of inhalation anesthetics in current clinical use for animals

Property	Desflurane	Enflurane	Halothane	Isoflurane	Methoxyflurane[a]	N₂O	Sevoflurane
Molecular weight (g)	168	185	197	185	165	44	200
Liquid specific gravity (20°C) (g/mL)	1.47	1.52	1.86	1.49	1.42	1.42	1.52
Boiling point (°C)	23.5	57	50	49	105	−89	59
Vapor pressure (mm Hg)							
20°C	700[325]	172	243	240	23	—	160
24°C	804	207	288	286	28	—	183
mL vapor/mL liquid at 20°C	209.7	197.5	227	194.7	206.9	—	182.7
Preservative	None	None	Yes	None	Not available	None	Yes
Stability in							
Soda lime	Yes	Yes	No	Yes	No	Yes	No
Ultraviolet light	Yes	Yes	No	Yes	No	Yes	?

Excepting for new citations where noted, references appear in the immediate past edition of this text and chapter. N₂O, nitrous oxide.
[a]Methoxyflurane is no longer available.

bromine to improve stability but at the expense of reduced anesthetic potency and solubility.

Halothane (Fig. 13.2) is a halogenated, aliphatic saturated hydrocarbon (ethane). Predictions that halogenated structure would provide nonflammability and molecular stability encouraged the development of halothane in the early 1950s. However, soon after clinical introduction it was observed that the concurrent presence of halothane and catecholamines increased the incidence of cardiac arrhythmias, especially in human patients. An ether linkage in the molecule favors a reduced incidence of cardiac arrhythmias. Consequently, this chemical structure is a predominant characteristic of all agents developed or proposed for clinical use since the introduction of halothane (Fig. 13.2).

Despite many favorable characteristics and improvements over earlier anesthetics (Fig. 13.1) that included improved chemical stability, halothane is susceptible to decomposition. Accordingly, halothane is stored in dark bottles, and a very small amount of a preservative, thymol, is added to it to retard breakdown. Thymol is much less volatile than halothane and over time collects within the devices used to control delivery of the volatile anesthetic (i.e., vaporizers) and causes them to malfunction. To accomplish greater molecular stability, fluorine is substituted for chlorine or bromine in the anesthetic molecule. This chemical manipulation added shelf life to the substance and negated the need for additives such as thymol. Unfortunately, the fluorine ion is also toxic to some tissues (e.g., kidneys), which is of clinical concern if the parent compound (e.g., sevoflurane and, historically, most notably methoxyflurane) is not resistant to metabolism (Fig. 13.2).

Physical Characteristics

There is a constant interchange of respiratory gases (O₂ and CO₂) between cells and the external environment via blood. Inhalation anesthesia involves additional considerations whereby an anesthetic must be transferred under control from a container to sites of action in the central nervous system (CNS). Early in this process the agent is diluted to an appropriate amount (concentration) and supplied to the respiratory system in a gas mixture that contains enough O₂ to support life. The chain of events that en-

sues is influenced by many physical and chemical characteristics that can be quantitatively described (Tables 13.1 to 13.4). The practical clinical applications of these quantitative descriptions are reviewed here. Limited space does not permit in-depth review of all underlying principles, and readers interested in further background information are referred elsewhere.[7,8]

The physical characteristics of importance to our understanding of the action of inhalation anesthetics can be conveniently divided into two general categories: those that determine the means by which the agents are administered and those that help determine their kinetics in the body. This information is applied in the clinical manipulation of anesthetic induction and recovery and in facilitating changes in anesthetic-induced CNS depression in a timely fashion.

Properties Determining Methods of Administration

A variety of physical and chemical properties determine the means by which inhalation anesthetics are administered. These include characteristics such as molecular weight, boiling point, liquid density (specific gravity), and vapor pressure.

General Principles: A Brief Review Molecules are in a constant state of motion and exhibit a force of mutual attraction. The degree of attraction is evident by the state in which the substance exists (i.e., solid, liquid, or gas). Molecular motion increases as energy (e.g., in the form of heat) is added to the molecular aggregate and decreases as energy is removed. With increased motion the intermolecular forces are reduced; if conditions are extreme enough, a change in physical state may ensue. All substances exist naturally in a particular state but can be made to exist (at least in theory) in any or all phases by altering conditions. Water, as an example, exists as ice (mutual molecular attraction is great), liquid water, or water vapor (attraction considerably reduced), depending on conditions.

Gas versus Vapor Inhalation anesthetics are either gases or vapors. In relation to inhalation anesthetics the term *gas* refers to an agent, such as N₂O, that exists in its gaseous form at room tem-

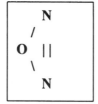

Enflurane
(Ethrane®)

```
      Cl  F       F
      |   |       |
  H – C – C – O – C – H
      |   |       |
      F   F       F
```

Desflurane
(Suprane®, 1653)

```
      F   H       F
      |   |       |
  F – C – C – O – C – H
      |   |       |
      F   F       F
```

Halothane
(Fluothane®)

```
      Br  F
      |   |
  H – C – C – F
      |   |
      Cl  F
```

Isoflurane
(Forane®, Aerrane®)

```
      F   Cl      F
      |   |       |
  F – C – C – O – C – H
      |   |       |
      F   H       F
```

Nitrous oxide

```
       N
      /
  O   ||
      \
       N
```

Sevoflurane
(Ultane®, Sevoflo®)

```
                  F
                  |
      H     F – C – F
      |         |
  F – C – O – C – H
      |         |
      H     F – C – F
                  |
                  F
```

Fig. 13.2. Chemical structure of inhalation anesthetics in current use for animals. Trade names are in parentheses.

perature and sea level pressure. The term *vapor* indicates the gaseous state of a substance that at ambient temperature and pressure is a liquid. With the exception of N_2O, all the contemporary anesthetics fall into this category. Desflurane (Table 13.1) is one of the new volatile liquids that comes close to the transition stage and offers some unique (among the inhalation anesthetics) considerations to be discussed later in this chapter.

Whether inhalation agents are supplied as a gas or volatile liquid under ambient conditions, the same physical principles apply to each agent when it is in the gaseous state. Molecules move about haphazardly at high speeds and collide with each other (more frequently in liquid than in gas) or the walls of the containing vessel. The force of the bombardment is measurable and referred to as pressure. In the case of gases, if the space or volume in which the gas is enclosed is increased, the number of bombardments decreases (i.e., a smaller number of molecular collisions per unit time) and then the pressure decreases. The behavior of gases is predictably described by various gas laws. Relationships such as those described by Boyle's law (volume vs. pressure), Charles's law (volume vs. temperature), Gay-Lussac's law (temperature vs. pressure), and Dalton's Law of Partial Pressure (the total pressure of a mixture of gases is equal to the sum of the partial pressures of all of the gaseous substances present), among others, are important to our overall understanding of aspects of respiratory and anesthetic gases and vapors. However, in-depth descriptions of these principles are beyond the scope of this chapter, and readers are referred elsewhere for this information.[8]

Methods of Description Quantities of inhalation anesthetic agent are usually characterized by one of three methods: pressure (i.e., in millimeters of mercury [mm Hg]), concentration (in volume percent [vol%]) or mass (in milligrams [mg] or grams [g]). The form most familiar to clinicians is that of concentration (e.g., *X*% of agent A in relation to the whole gas mixture). Modern monitoring equipment samples inspired and expired gases and provides concentration readings for inhalation anesthetics. Precision vaporizers used to control delivery of inhalation anesthetics are calibrated in percentage of agent, and effective doses are almost always reported in percentages.

Pressure is also an important way of describing inhalation anesthetics and is further discussed as a measure of anesthetic potency. A mixture of gases in a closed container will exert a pressure on the walls of the container. The individual pressure of each gas in a mixture of gases is referred to as its *partial pressure*. As noted earlier, this expression of the behavior of a mixture of gases is known as Dalton's law, and its use in understanding inhalation anesthesia is inescapable. Use of the concept of partial pressure is important in understanding inhalation anesthetic action in a multiphase biological system because, unlike concentration, the partial pressure of an agent is the same in different compartments that are in equilibrium with each other. That is, in contradistinction to concentration or volume percent, an expression of the relative ratio of gas molecules in a mixture, partial pressure is an expression of the absolute value.

Molecular weight and agent density are used in many calculations to convert from liquid to vapor volumes and mass. Briefly

Table 13.2. Partition coefficients (solvent and gas) of inhalation anesthetics at 37°C

Solvent	Desflurane	Enflurane	Halothane	Isoflurane	Methoxyflurane	N₂O	Sevoflurane
Water	—	0.78	0.82	0.62	4.50	0.47	0.60
Blood	0.42	2.00	2.54	1.46	15.00	0.47	0.68
Olive oil	18.70	96.00	224.00	91.00	970.00	1.40	47.00
Brain	1.30	2.70	1.90	1.60	20.00	0.50	1.70
Liver	1.30	3.70	2.10	1.80	29.00	0.38	1.80
Kidney	1.00	1.90	1.00	1.20	11.00	0.40	1.20
Muscle	2.00	2.20	3.40	2.90	16.00	0.54	3.10
Fat	27.00	83.00	51.00	45.00	902.00	1.08	48.00

Tissue samples are derived from human sources. Data are from sources referenced in the immediate past edition of this text and chapter. N₂O, nitrous oxide.

Table 13.3. Solvent-gas partition coefficients for halothane at 37°C in a variety of species[327]

Solvent	Dog	Horse	Ox	Rabbit
Blood	3.51	1.77	2.40	4.02
Brain	6.03	5.42	4.80	6.22
Liver	6.64	8.51	5.10	9.17
Kidney	4.95	3.21	3.80	6.96
Muscle	5.45	3.55	5.40	3.67

Table 13.4. Rubber or plastic-gas partition coefficients at room temperature

Solvent	Desflurane	Enflurane	Halothane	Isoflurane	Methoxyflurane	N₂O	Sevoflurane	Reference
Rubber	—	74	120	62	630	1.2	—	Eger[1]
	19	—	190	49	—	—	29	Targ et al.[328]
Polyvinyl chloride	—	120	190	110	—	—	—	Eger[1]
	35	—	233	114	—	—	69	Targ et al.[328]
Polyethylene	—	~2	26	~2	118	—	—	Eger[1]
	16	—	128	58	—	—	31	Targ et al.[328]

These data are summarized from multiple sources as reported in Eger,[1] with some differences in methods of determination. The data from Targ et al.[328] indicate more recently derived data that, unlike earlier data, were recorded following complete equilibration with these materials. Where there is overlap, the ranking of partition coefficients is consistent with halothane > isoflurane > sevoflurane > desflurane. Combining both groupings yields methoxyflurane > halothane > enflurane > isoflurane > sevoflurane > desflurane > nitrous oxide.

(and in simplified fashion), Avogadro's principle is that equal volumes of all gases under the same conditions of temperature and pressure contain the same number of molecules (6.0226×10^{23} [Avogadro's number] per gram molecular weight). Furthermore, under standard conditions the number of gas molecules in a gram molecular weight of a substance occupies 22.4 L. To compare properties of different substances of similar state, it is necessary to do so under comparable conditions; with respect to gases and liquids this usually means with reference to pressure and temperature. Physical scientists have arbitrarily selected *standard conditions* as being 0°C (273 K in absolute scale) and 760 mm Hg pressure (1 atmosphere at sea level). If conditions differ, appropriate temperature and/or pressure corrections must be applied to resultant data.

The weight of a given volume of liquid, gas, or vapor may be expressed in terms of its density or specific gravity. The density is an absolute value of mass (usually grams) per unit volume (for liquids, volume = 1 mL; for gases, 1 L at standard conditions). The specific gravity is a relative value; that is, the ratio of the weight of a unit volume of one substance to a similar volume of water in the case of liquids or air in the case of gases (or vapors) under similar conditions. The value of both air and water is 1. At least for clinical purposes, the value for density and specific gravity for an inhalation anesthetic is the same. Thus, for example, we can determine the volume of isoflurane gas (vapor) at 20°C from a mL of isoflurane liquid according to the scheme given in Fig. 13.3. This type of calculation has practical applications. For example, to determine the savings in isoflurane liquid afforded by reducing the fresh gas (e.g., O₂) inflow rate, a series of calculations as presented in Fig. 13.4 can be made.

a. Isoflurane specific gravity = 1.49 g/mL, therefore:
   1 mL liquid isoflurane = 1 mL x 1.49 g/mL = 1.49 g

b. Since molecular weight of isoflurane = 185 g (from Table 13-1, then:
   1.49 g ÷ 185 g = 0.0081 mol of liquid

c. Since 1 mol of gas = 22.4 L, then:
   0.0081 mol x 22,400 mL/mol = 181.4 mL of isoflurane vapor at 0C, 1 atm

d. But vapor is at 20C not 0C (i.e., 273 K),
   So, 181.4 x 293/273 = 194.7 mL vapor/mL liquid isoflurane at 20C and at sea level pressure

   For substantial variation in ambient pressure, the final figure noted above would have to be further "corrected" by a factor of: 760/ambient barometric pressure

Fig. 13.3. Example of calculations to determine the volume of isoflurane vapor at 20°C from 1 mL of isoflurane liquid.

a. Total isoflurane vapor delivered over 2 hours (120 min) estimated at:

   3%/100 x 6 LPM = 0.18 LPM x 120 min = 21.60 L/120 min = 21,600 mL/120 min

   vs

   3%/100 x 4 LPM = 0.12 LPM x 120 min = 14.4 L/120 min = 14,400 mL/120 min

b. Total vapor volume saved:

   21,600 mL/120 min – 14,400 mL/120 min = 7,200 mL vapor/120 min saved

c. Total liquid isoflurane volume saved/2 hours

   7,200 mL vapor ÷ 194.7 mL vapor/mL liquid = 36.98 mL of isoflurane liquid

   (194.7 mL vapor/mL liquid can be calculated as in Fig. 13.4 or taken from Table 13-1)

   The economic value of reducing isoflurane consumption can then be determined by calculating the product of the liquid volume saved and the purchase cost/mL of isoflurane liquid

Fig. 13.4. Problem: Determine the savings in isoflurane liquid afforded by reducing the fresh gas (e.g., O_2) inflow rate from 6 Lpm (L/min) to 4 Lpm, given that the average delivered (vaporizer setting) concentration for 2 h is 3%.

Vapor Pressure Molecules of liquids are in constant random motion. Some of those in the surface layer gain sufficient velocity to overcome the attractive forces of neighboring molecules and in escaping from the surface enter the vapor phase. The change in state from a liquid to a gas phase is known as *vaporization* or *evaporation*. This process is dynamic and in a closed container that is kept at a constant temperature eventually reaches an equilibrium whereby there is no further net loss of

Vapor Pressure - Temperature Relationship

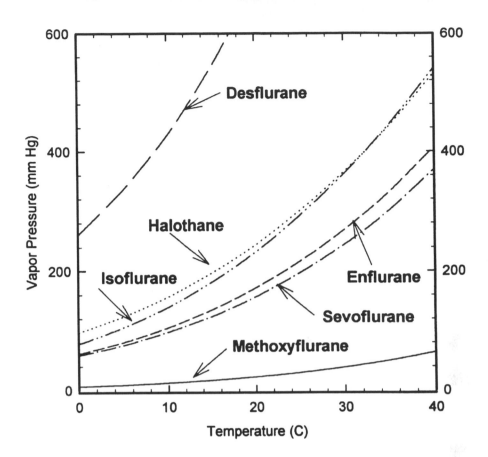

Fig. 13.5. Vapor pressure as a function of temperature for six volatile anesthetics. Curves are generated from Antoine equations.[324,325]

molecules to the gas phase (i.e., the numbers of molecules leaving and returning to the liquid phase are equal). The gas phase at this point is saturated.

Molecules of a vapor exert a force per unit area or pressure in exactly the same manner as do molecules of a gas. The pressure (mm Hg) that the vapor molecules exert when the liquid and vapor phases are in equilibrium is known as the *vapor pressure.* Thus, the vapor pressure of an anesthetic is a measure of its ability to evaporate; that is, it is a measure of the tendency for molecules in the liquid state to enter the gaseous (vapor) phase. The vapor pressure of a volatile anesthetic must be at least sufficient to provide enough molecules of anesthetic in the vapor state to produce anesthesia at ambient conditions. The *saturated vapor pressure* represents a maximum concentration of molecules in the vapor state that exists for a given liquid at each temperature. Herein lies a practical difference between substances classified as a gas or vapor: A gas can be administered over a range of concentrations from 0 to 100%, whereas the vapor has a ceiling that is dictated by its vapor pressure. The saturated vapor concentration can be easily determined by relating the vapor pressure to the ambient pressure. For example, in the case of halothane (Table 13.1), a maximal concentration of 32% halothane is possible under usual conditions (i.e., [244/760] × 100 = 32%, where 760 mm Hg is the barometric pressure at sea level). With other variables considered constant, the greater the vapor pressure, the

greater is the concentration of the drug deliverable to a patient. Therefore, again from Table 13.1, halothane, for example, is more volatile than methoxyflurane under similar conditions. The barometric pressure also influences the final concentration of an agent. For example, in locations such as Denver, Colorado, where the altitude is about 5000 feet above sea level and the barometric pressure is only about 635 mm Hg, the saturated vapor concentration of halothane at 20°C is now (243/635) × 100 = 38.3%.

It is important to recognize that the saturated vapor pressure at 1 atmosphere is unique for each volatile anesthetic agent and depends only on its temperature. In this case, the effect of barometric pressure can be neglected over ranges normally encountered in the practice of anesthesia. Thus, for a given agent, the graph of the saturated vapor pressure versus temperature is a curve as shown in Fig. 13.5. From this graph it can be seen that if the temperature of the liquid is increased, more molecules escape the liquid phase and enter the gaseous phase. The greater number of molecules in the vapor phase produces a greater vapor pressure and vapor concentration. Conversely, if the liquid is cooled, the reverse occurs and vapor concentration decreases. Liquid cooling may occur not only because of changing ambient conditions but also as a natural consequence of the vaporization process. For example, during vaporization the "fastest" molecules at the surface escape first. With depletion of these "high energy" molecules, the average kinetic energy of those left behind is reduced, and there is a tendency for the temperature of the remaining liquid to fall if this process is not compensated for externally. As the temperature decreases, the vapor pressure, and thus the vapor concentration, also decreases.

Boiling Point   The *boiling point* of a liquid is defined as the temperature at which the vapor pressure of the liquid is equal to the atmospheric pressure. Customarily, the boiling temperature is stated at the standard atmospheric pressure of 760 mm Hg. The boiling point decreases with increasing altitude because the vapor pressure does not change, but the barometric pressure decreases. The boiling point of N_2O is $-89°C$ (Table 13.1) at 1 atmosphere pressure at sea level. It is thus a gas under operating-room conditions. Because of this, it is distributed for clinical purposes in steel tanks compressed to the liquid state at about 750 psi (pounds per square inch; 750 psi/14.9 psi [1 atmosphere] = 50 atmospheres). As the N_2O gas is drawn from the tanks, liquid N_2O is vaporized, and the overriding gas pressure remains constant until no further liquid remains in the tank. At that point, only N_2O gas remains, and the gas pressure decreases from this point as remaining gas is vented from the tank. Consequently, the weight of the N_2O minus the weight of the tank, rather than the gas pressure within the tank, is a more accurate guide to the remaining amount of N_2O in the tank.[9]

Desflurane, the newest clinically available volatile anesthetic, also possesses an interesting consideration because its boiling point (Table 13.1) is near room temperature. This characteristic accounted for an interesting engineering challenge in developing an administration device (i.e., a vaporizer) for routine use in the relatively constant environment of the operating room and limits further consideration of its use in all but a narrow range of circumstances commonly encountered in veterinary medical applications. For example, because of its low boiling point, even evaporative cooling has large influences on vapor pressure and thus the vapor concentration of gas mixtures delivered to patients.

Calculation of Anesthetic Concentration Delivered by a Vaporizer
The saturated vapor pressure of most volatile anesthetics is of such magnitude that the maximal concentration of anesthetic attainable at usual operating-room conditions is above the range of concentrations that are commonly necessary for safe clinical anesthetic management. Therefore, some control of the delivered concentration is necessary and usually provided by a device known as a *vaporizer*. The purpose of the vaporizer is to dilute the vapor generated from the liquid anesthetic with O_2 (or an O_2 and N_2O mixture) to produce a more satisfactory inspired-anesthetic concentration. This anesthetic dilution is usually accomplished as indicated in the Fig. 13.6 model by diverting the gas entering the vaporizer into two streams, one that enters the vaporizing chamber (anesthetic chamber volume: V_{anes}) and the other that bypasses the vaporizing chamber (dilution volume or $V_{dilution}$). If the vaporizer is efficient, the carrier gas passing through the vaporizing chamber becomes completely saturated to an anesthetic concentration (%) reflected by (anesthetic-agent vapor pressure/atmospheric pressure) $\times$ 100, at the vaporizer chamber temperature. The resultant anesthetic concentration then

is decreased (diluted) downstream by the second gas stream to a "working" concentration. In modern, precision, agent-specific vaporizers no mental effort is required—just set the dial; the manufacturers have precalibrated the vaporizer for accurate delivery of the dialed concentration. Nevertheless, it is helpful to our overall understanding to know the principles underlying this convenience and how to apply these principles in the use of older noncompensated measured-flow vaporizers.

To calculate the anesthetic concentration from the vaporizer, one must know the vapor pressure of the agent (at the temperature of use), the atmospheric pressure, the fresh gas flow entering the vaporizing chamber, and the diluent gas flow. Then,

% anesthetic = flow of anesthetic from the vaporizing chamber/total gas flow

More detail for interested readers is presented in Fig. 13.6.

Properties Influencing Drug Kinetics: Solubility
Anesthetic gases and vapors dissolve in liquids and solids. The solubility of an anesthetic is a major characteristic of the agent and has important clinical ramifications. For example, anesthetic solubility in blood and body tissues is a primary factor in the rate of uptake and its distribution within the body. It is therefore a primary determinant of the speed of anesthetic induction and recovery. Solubility in lipid bears a strong relationship to anesthetic potency, and its tendency to dissolve in anesthetic-delivery components such as rubber goods influences equipment selection and other aspects of anesthetic management.

Solubility of Gases   As previously mentioned, molecules of a gas that overlie a liquid surface are in random motion, and some penetrate the liquid surface. After entering the liquid they intermingle with the molecules of the liquid (i.e., the gas dissolves in the liquid). There is a net movement of the gas into the liquid until equilibrium is established between the dissolved gas in the liquid and the undissolved portion above the liquid. At this time there is no further net gain of gas molecules by the liquid, and the number of gas molecules entering the liquid equals the number leaving. The gas molecules within the liquid exert the same pressure or tension that they exert in the gas phase. If the pressure (i.e., the number of gas molecules overlying the liquid) is increased, more molecules pass into the liquid, and the pressure within the liquid is increased. This net inward movement of gas molecules continues until a new equilibrium is established between the pressure of the gas in the liquid and that overlying the liquid. Alternatively, if the pressure of gas overlying the liquid is somehow decreased below that in the liquid, gas molecules escape from the liquid. This net outward movement of gas molecules from the liquid phase continues until equilibrium between the two phases is reestablished.

The amount, that is, the total number of molecules of a given gas dissolving in a solvent depends on the chemical nature of the gas itself, the partial pressure of the gas, the nature of the solvent, and the temperature. This relationship is described by Henry's law,

$$V = S \times P$$

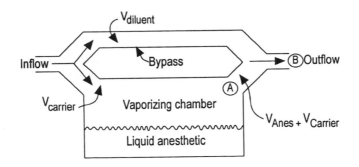

Steps:

1. The saturated *concentration* of anesthetic in the anesthetic vaporizing chamber and leaving it (ideally at A above) is calculated knowing the saturated vapor pressure (P_{VP}) (from Table 2) and barometric pressure (P_B).

For example:

$$\text{Halothane\%} = \frac{243}{760} \times 100 = 32.0\% \tag{a}$$

2. The *volume* of anesthetic leaving the vaporizing chamber is the original volume of the carrier gas (O_2) entering the anesthetic vaporizing chamber ($V_{carrier}$) and the volume of anesthetic (V_{halo}) added to it.

$$\text{Halothane\%} - \frac{V_{halo}}{V_{carrier} + V_{halo}} \times 100 \tag{b}$$

Halothane% is known from (a) above and $V_{carrier}$ is known from control of a flowmeter (e.g., a measured flow vaporizer) or via the design characteristics of a commercial, agent-specific, vaporizer that automatically "splits" the fresh gas flow from a single flow meter. In the first case, two gas flow controls are necessary, one for $V_{carrier}$ and one for a larger gas dilution flow ($V_{dilution}$). In either the case of manual or automatic fresh gas flow alteration, the equation is then solved for V_{halo} (expressed in ml of halothane vapor).

For example, if $V_{carrier} = 100$ mL O_2, then

$$32\% = \frac{V_{halo}}{100 + V_{halo}} \times 100$$

$$3200 + 32V_{halo} = 100V_{halo}$$

$$3200 = 68V_{halo}$$

$$V_{halo} = 47.1 \text{ mL halothane vapor}$$

3. V_{halo} is then contained in a total gas volume at B of

$$V_{total\ gas} = V_{halo} + V_{carrier} + V_{diluent} \tag{c}$$

Where $V_{diluent}$ is set by the anesthetist using a second gas control (i.e., flowmeter; units here of mL/min) or by the vaporizer design and dial setting.

Then in our example for a $V_{diluent}$ of 1000 mL (in 1 minute)

$$V_{total} = 47.1 + 100 + 1000$$
$$= 1147 \text{ ml (rounded off)}$$

4. So the final halothane vapor concentration is determined by

$$\text{halothane \%} = \frac{V_{halo}}{V_{Total}} \times 100$$

Again, in our example,

$$\text{halothane \%} = \frac{47.1}{1147} = 4.1\%$$

Alternatively, with some basic algebraic work with equations given above, the same numbers can be applied to the resultant formula given below to arrive at the anesthetic concentration. The condensed formula is:

$$\text{Anesthetic concentration (\%)} = \frac{V_{carrier} \cdot P_{VP} \cdot 100}{V_{diluent} \cdot (P_B - P_{VP}) + (V_{carrier} \cdot P_B)}$$

Fig. 13.6. An anesthetic vaporizer model to assist in illustrating the principles associated with the calculation of the vapor concentration of an inhalation anesthetic emerging from a vaporizer. Conditions associated with halothane delivery in San Francisco (i.e., at sea level; barometric pressure = 760 mm Hg) at 20°C are used as an example of general principles.

where V is the volume of gas, P is the partial pressure of the gas, and S is the solubility coefficient for the gas in the solvent at a given temperature. Henry's law applies to gases that do not combine chemically with the solvent to form compounds.

Before leaving this basic information, a brief focus on a number of variations may be helpful. First, it is important to recognize that if the atmosphere that overlies the solvent is made up of a mixture of gases, then each gas dissolves in the solvent in proportion to the partial pressure of the individual gases. The total pressure exerted by the molecules of all gases within the solvent equals the total gas pressure lying above the solvent.

Within the body there is a partition of anesthetic gases between blood and body tissues in accordance with Henry's law. This process can be perhaps better understood by visualizing a system composed of three compartments (e.g., gas, water, and oil) contained in a closed container (Fig. 13.7). In such a system the gas overlies the oil, which in turn overlies the water. Because

there is a passive gradient from the gas phase to the oil, gas molecules move into the oil compartment. This movement in turn develops a gradient for the gas molecules in oil relative to water. If gas is continually added above the oil, there will be a continual net movement of the gas molecules from the gas phase into both the oil and, in turn, the water. At a given temperature, when no more gas dissolves in the solvent, the solvent is said to be *fully saturated*. At this point the pressure of the gas molecules within the three compartments will be equal, but the amount (i.e., the number of molecules or volume of gas) partitioned between the two liquids will vary with the nature of the liquid and gas. Finally, it is important to understand that the amount of gas that goes into solution depends on the temperature of the solvent. Less gas dissolves in a solvent as temperature increases, and more gas is taken up as solvent temperature decreases. For example, as water is heated, air bubbles appear inside the container as a result of the decreasing solubility of the air in water.

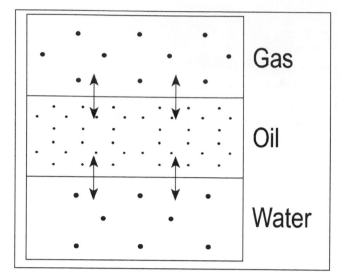

Fig. 13.7. Diagrammatic representation of an anesthetic gas distributing itself among three compartments (gas, oil, and water). At equilibrium, the number of anesthetic molecules in the three compartments differs, but the pressure exerted by the anesthetic molecules is the same in each compartment.

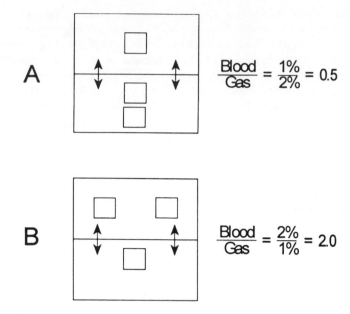

Fig. 13.8. Blood-gas partition coefficient illustration. Adapted from Eger.[10]

Conversely, as blood is cooled from a normal body temperature (e.g., hypothermia), gases become more soluble in blood.

The extent to which a gas will dissolve in a given solvent is usually expressed in terms of its solubility coefficient (Table 13.2). With inhalation anesthetics, solubility is most commonly measured and expressed as a *partition coefficient* (PC). Other measurements of solubility include the Bunsen and Ostwald solubility coefficients.[8,10]

The PC is the concentration ratio of an anesthetic in the solvent and gas phases (e.g., blood and gas) (Fig. 13.8) or between two tissue solvents (e.g., brain and blood) (Table 13.2). It thus describes the capacity of a given solvent to dissolve the anesthetic gas; that is, how the anesthetic will *partition* itself between the gas and the liquid solvent phases after equilibrium has been reached. Remember, anesthetic gas movement occurs because of a partial pressure difference in the gas and liquid solvent phases, so when there is no longer any anesthetic partial pressure difference there is no longer any net movement of anesthetic, and equilibrium has been achieved. Solvent-gas PCs are summarized in Table 13.2. The values noted in this table are for human tissues because these values are most widely available in the anesthesia literature. Comparative data for halothane with some species of clinical interest in veterinary medicine is listed in Table 13.3. Regardless of the species, it is important to emphasize that many factors can alter anesthetic-agent solubility.[10–13] Perhaps the most notable after the nature of the solvent is temperature.

Of all the PCs that have been described or are of interest, two are of particular importance in the practical understanding of anesthetic action. They are the blood-gas and the oil-gas solubility coefficients.

Blood-Gas Partition Coefficient Blood-gas solubility coefficients (Tables 13.2 and 13.3) provide a means for predicting the speed of anesthetic induction, recovery, and change of anesthetic depth. Assume, for example, that anesthetic A has a blood-gas PC value of 15. This means that the concentration of the anesthetic in blood will be 15 times greater at equilibrium than that in alveolar gas. Expressed differently, the same volume of blood, say 1 mL, will hold 15 times more of anesthetic A than 1 mL of alveolar gas despite an equal partial pressure. Alternatively, consider anesthetic B with a PC of 1.4. This PC indicates that, at equilibrium, the amount of anesthetic B is only 1.4 times greater in blood than it is in alveolar air. Comparing the PC of anesthetic A with that of anesthetic B indicates that anesthetic A is much more soluble in blood than B (nearly 11 times more soluble: 15/1.4). From this, and assuming other conditions are equal, anesthetic A will require a longer time of administration to attain a partial pressure in the body for a particular end point (say, anesthetic induction) than will anesthetic B. Also, since there is more of anesthetic A contained in blood and other body tissues under similar conditions, elimination (and therefore anesthetic recovery) will be prolonged when compared with anesthetic B.

Oil-Gas Partition Coefficient The oil-gas PC is another solubility characteristic of clinical importance (Table 13.2). This PC describes the ratio of the concentration of an anesthetic in oil (olive oil is the standard) and gas phases at equilibrium. The oil-gas PC correlates directly with anesthetic potency (see the section Anesthetic Dose: The Minimum Alveolar Concentration) and describes the capacity of lipids for anesthetic.

Other Partition Coefficients Solubility characteristics for various tissues (Tables 13.2 and 13.3) and other media, such as rubber and plastic (Table 13.4), are also important. For example, the solubility of a tissue determines in part the quantity of anesthetic removed from the blood to which it is exposed. The higher the tissue solubility, the longer it will take to saturate the tissue with anesthetic agent. Thus, other things considered equal, anesthetics that are very soluble in tissues will require a longer period for induction and recovery. If the amount of rubber goods in the apparatus used to deliver the anesthetic to a patient is substantial, and the anesthetic-agent solubility in rubber is large, the amount of uptake of anesthetic agent by the rubber may be of clinical significance.

Pharmacokinetics: Uptake and Elimination of Inhalation Anesthetics

The aim in administering an inhalation anesthetic to a patient is to achieve an adequate partial pressure or tension of anesthetic (P_{anes}) in the CNS (e.g., brain; for purposes of this discussion, considerations of anesthetic delivery to spinal cord sites of action are considered similar to those of the brain) to cause a desired level of CNS depression commensurate with the definition of general anesthesia. Anesthetic depth varies directly with P_{anes} in brain tissue. The rate of change of anesthetic depth is of obvious clinical importance and depends directly on the rate of change in anesthetic tensions in the various media in which it is contained before reaching the brain. Thus, knowledge of the factors that govern these relationships is of fundamental importance to skillful control of general inhalation anesthesia.

Inhalation anesthetics are unique among the classes of drugs that are used to produce general anesthesia because they are administered via the lungs. The pharmacokinetics of the inhaled anesthetics describe the rate of their uptake by blood from the lungs, distribution in the body, and eventual elimination by the lungs and other routes. Readers seeking more in-depth coverage are directed to reviews by Eger,[10,14] Eger et al.,[15] and Mapleson.[16]

Inhalation anesthetics, similar to the gases of respiration (i.e., O_2 and CO_2), move down a series of partial pressure gradients from regions of higher tension to those of lower tension until equilibrium (i.e., equal pressure throughout the apparatus and body tissues) is established. Thus on induction, the P_{anes} at its source in a vaporizer is high, as is dictated by the vapor pressure, and progressively decreases as anesthetic travels from vaporizer to patient breathing circuit, from circuit to lungs, from lungs to arterial blood, and, finally, from arterial blood to body tissues (e.g., the brain) (Fig. 13.9). Of these the alveolar partial pressure (P_A) of anesthetic is pivotal. The brain has a rich blood supply, and the anesthetic in arterial blood (P_aAnes) rapidly equilibrates with brain tissue ($P_{brain}Anes$). Usually gas exchange at the alveolar level is sufficiently efficient that the P_aAnes is close to P_AAnes. Thus, the $P_{brain}Anes$ closely follows P_AAnes, and by controlling the P_AAnes there is a reliable indirect way for controlling $P_{brain}Anes$ and anesthetic depth.

At this point it may be also helpful to recall that although the partial pressure of anesthetic is of primary importance, we frequently define clinical dose of an inhaled anesthetic in terms of concentration (C; i.e., vol%). As previously noted this is because it is common practice for clinicians to regulate and/or measure

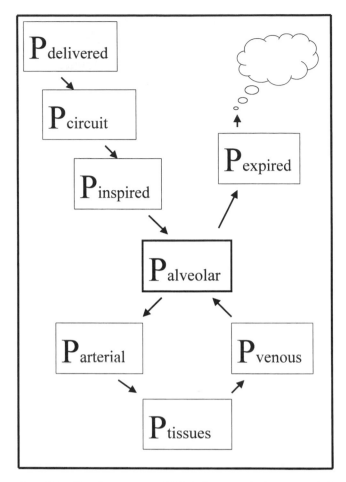

Fig. 13.9. The flow pattern of inhalation anesthetic agents during anesthetic induction and recovery. Inhalation anesthesia may be viewed as the development of a series of partial pressure (tension) gradients. During induction there is a high anesthetic tension in the vaporizer that decreases progressively as the flow of anesthetic gas moves from its source to the brain. Some of these gradients are easily manipulated by the anesthetist; others are not or are done so with difficulty.

respiratory and anesthetic gases in volume percent. In addition, in the gaseous phase, the relationship between the P_{anes} and the C_{anes} is a simple one:

$$P_{anes} = \text{fractional anesthetic concentration} \times \text{total ambient pressure}$$

The fractional anesthetic concentration is of course $C_{anes}/100$. However, as reviewed in the preceding section, in blood or tissues the actual *quantity* of anesthetic depends on both the P_{anes} and the anesthetic solubility (as measured by PC) within the solvent (e.g., blood or oil). Consequently, at equilibrium, the *partial pressure* of the gas in the alveoli and among tissue compartments will be equal although *concentrations* will vary within these tissues.

Anesthetic Uptake

The P_A of anesthetic is a balance between anesthetic input (i.e., delivery to the alveoli) and loss (uptake by blood and body tissues) from the lungs. A rapid rise in the P_A of anesthetic is asso-

A. Increased alveolar delivery
  1. Increased inspired anesthetic concentration
    a. Increased vaporization of agent
    b. Increased vaporizer dial setting
    c. Increased fresh gas inflow
    d. Decreased gas volume of patient breathing circuit
  2. Increased alveolar ventilation
    a. Increased minute ventilation
    b. Decreased dead space ventilation
B. Decreased removal from the alveoli
  1. Decreased blood solubility of anesthetic
  2. Decreased cardiac output
  3. Decreased alveolar-venous anesthetic gradient

Fig. 13.10. Factors related to a change in alveolar anesthetic tension (P_A, alveolar partial pressure).

ciated with a rapid anesthetic induction or change in anesthetic depth. Factors that contribute to a rapid change in the P_A of anesthetic are summarized in Fig. 13.10.

Delivery to the Alveoli

Delivery of anesthetic to the alveoli and therefore the rate of rise of the alveolar concentration or fraction (F_A) toward the inspired concentration or fraction (F_I) depends on the inspired-anesthetic concentration itself and the magnitude of alveolar ventilation. Increasing either one of these or both increases the rate of rise of the P_A of anesthetic; that is, with other things considered equal there is an increase in speed of anesthetic induction or change in anesthetic level.

Inspired Concentration   The inspired concentration has a number of variables controlling it. First of all, the upper limit of inspired concentration is dictated by the agent vapor pressure, which in turn depends on temperature. This may be especially important considering the breadth of veterinary medical application of inhaled anesthesia and methods of vaporizing volatile

anesthetics under widely diverse conditions (some environmental conditions are quite hostile).

Characteristics of the patient breathing system can also be a major factor in generating a suitable inspired concentration under usual operating-room conditions. Characteristics of special importance include the volume of the system, the amount of rubber or plastic components of the system, the position of the vaporizer relative to the breathing circuit (i.e., within or outside of the circuit), and the fresh gas inflow to the patient breathing circuit. The patient breathing circuit contains a gas volume that must be replaced with gas containing the desired anesthetic concentration. Thus, the volume of the breathing circuit serves as a buffer to delay the rise of anesthetic concentration. In the management of small animals (i.e., animals weighing less than 10 kg) a nonrebreathing patient circuit and/or a relatively high fresh gas inflow into the patient breathing circuit is usually used, so there should *not* be a clinically important difference between the delivered (e.g., vaporizer dial setting) and the inspired concentrations. That is, when the vaporizer dial setting is adjusted to the desired concentration setting, the fresh gas plus anesthetic flowing from the vaporizer almost immediately contains the dialed anesthetic vapor concentration. In addition, the total gas flow is high relative to the volume of the delivery circuit, so the anesthetic concentration in the inspired breath is rapidly increased. However, with animals weighing more than 10 kg, a circle, CO_2 absorber (i.e., rebreathing), patient breathing circuit is most commonly used for inhalation anesthesia. The volume of this breathing circuit may be very large compared with fresh gas inflow. This volume markedly delays the rate of rise of inspired-anesthetic concentration because the residual gas volume must be "washed out" and replaced by anesthetic containing fresh gas in order for the inspired concentration to increase to that delivered from the vaporizer (Fig. 13.11). In addition, exhaled gas (minus CO_2) is rebreathed to varying degrees with these circuits. The inspired gas is composed of exhaled and fresh gases. Because the expired gas contains less anesthetic than does the fresh gas, the inspired-anesthetic gas concentration

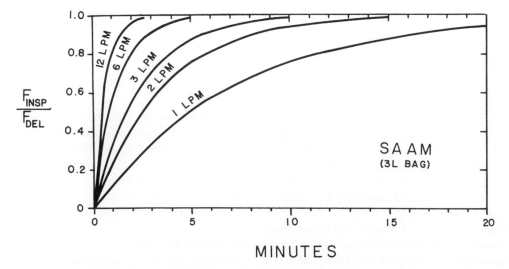

MINUTES

Fig. 13.11. A comparison of the rate of increase of inspired-halothane concentration toward a constant-delivered concentration F_{insp}/F_{del} in a 7-L small animal anesthetic breathing circuit (SAAM) at fresh gas flow rates of 1, 3, 6, and 12 L/min (LPM).[17]

Table 13.5. Vaporizer positioning within or outside of a circle patient rebreathing circuit influences inspired anesthetic concentration

Factor	Vaporizer Positioning	
	Out of Circuit	In Circuit
Increase ventilation	Decrease	Increase
Increase fresh gas (O_2) inflow to circuit	Increase	Decrease

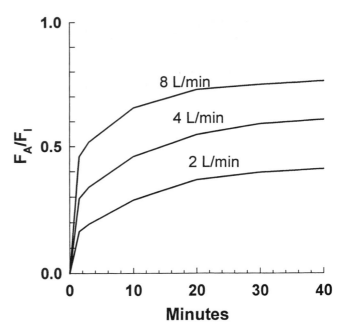

Fig. 13.12. The effect of ventilation on the rise of the alveolar concentration (F_A) of halothane toward the inspired (F_I) concentration. As noted, the F_A/F_I ratio increases more rapidly as ventilation is increased from 2 to 8 L/min. Redrawn from Eger,[10] with permission.

will be less than that of the fresh gas leaving the vaporizer.

In veterinary applications, the delaying influence of the circle circuit is most notable with anesthetic management of very large animals such as horses[17] and cattle and/or when using a closed-circuit fresh gas flow rate (i.e., where O_2 is the fresh gas, and its inflow [plus anesthetic] to the circuit just meets the metabolic needs of the patient). With closed-circuit delivery, the fresh gas inflow is very low relative to the circuit volume.[7,10,17]

The high solubility of some older anesthetics (e.g., methoxyflurane) (Table 13.4) in rubber and plastic also delays development of an appropriate inspired-anesthetic concentration. The loss of anesthetic to these equipment "sinks" serves to increase the apparent volume of the anesthetic circuitry and may, in some cases, be clinically important (e.g., the use of rubber hoses and a large rubber rebreathing bag on circuits designed for anesthetic management of horses). With the newest inhalation anesthetics and more modern anesthetic-delivery equipment this issue is of minor or no clinical importance.

Positioning the vaporizer in relation to the patient breathing circuit will influence inspired-anesthetic concentration.[16,18] For example, with the vaporizer positioned within a circle rebreathing circuit, a decrease in inspired concentration will follow an increase in fresh gas inflow to the circuit, whereas an increase in inspired concentration will result if the vaporizer is positioned outside the circuit (Table 13.5). With the loss of methoxyflurane to clinical practice most vaporizers in use, at least in North America, are agent-specific, precision vaporizers. This style of vaporizer is always placed upstream and outside of the patient breathing circuit.

Alveolar Ventilation An increase in alveolar ventilation increases the rate of delivery of inhalation anesthetic to the alveolus (Fig. 13.12). If unopposed by blood and tissue uptake of anesthetic, alveolar ventilation would rapidly increase the alveolar concentration of anesthetic so that within minutes the alveolar concentration would equal the inspired concentration. However, in reality the input created by alveolar ventilation is countered by absorption of anesthetic into blood. Predictably, hypoventilation decreases the rate at which the alveolar concentration increases over time compared with the inspired concentration (i.e., anesthetic induction is slowed). Alveolar ventilation is altered by changes in anesthetic depth (increased depth usually means de-

creased ventilation), mechanical ventilation (usually increased ventilation), and dead-space ventilation (i.e., for any constant minute ventilation, a decrease in dead-space ventilation results in an increase in alveolar ventilation).

Alveolar ventilation and thus the alveolar anesthetic concentration can also be influenced by administering a potent inhalation anesthetic like halothane in conjunction with N_2O. Very early in the administration of N_2O (during the period of large volume uptake; the first 5 to 10 min of delivery) the rate of rise of the alveolar concentration of the concurrently administered inhalation anesthetic is increased. This is commonly referred to as the *second gas effect*, and this phenomenon can be applied clinically to speed anesthetic induction.[10,14,19]

Removal from Alveoli: Uptake by Blood
As noted by Eger,[10] anesthetic uptake is the product of three factors: solubility (S, the blood-gas solubility [Table 13.4]), cardiac output (CO), and the difference in the anesthetic partial pressure between the alveolus and venous blood returning to the lungs (P_A − P_I), expressed in mm Hg:

$$uptake = S \times CO(P_A - P_I/P_{bar})$$

where P_{bar} = barometric pressure in mm Hg. Note that if any of these three factors equals zero there is no further uptake of anesthetic by blood.

Solubility As previously discussed the solubility of an inhalation anesthetic in blood and tissues is characterized by its PC (Tables 13.2 and 13.3). Remember that a PC describes how an in-

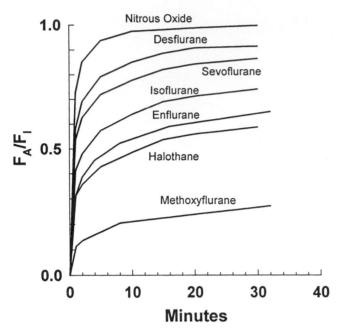

Fig. 13.13. The rise in the alveolar anesthetic concentration (F_A) toward the inspired concentration (F_I). Note that the rise is most rapid with the least soluble anesthetic, nitrous oxide, and slowest with the most soluble anesthetic, methoxyflurane. All data are from studies in people. The curves are redrawn from Eger.[1,326]

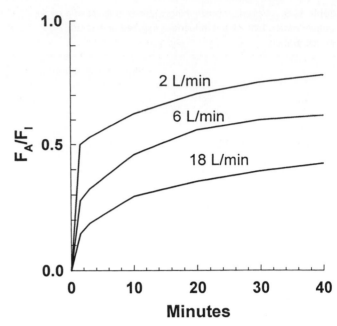

Fig. 13.14. The effect of cardiac output on the rise of the alveolar concentration (F_A) of halothane toward the inspired concentration (F_I). As noted, the F_A/F_I ratio increases more rapidly as cardiac output is decreased from 18 to 2 L/min. Redrawn from Eger.[10]

halation anesthetic distributes itself between two phases or two solvents (e.g., the quantity of agent in blood and alveoli [gas] or blood and muscle, respectively) once equilibrium is established (i.e., when the anesthetic partial pressure is equal). Based on blood-gas PCs, inhalation anesthetics range from highly soluble (methoxyflurane) to poorly soluble (N_2O, desflurane, and sevoflurane). Agents such as halothane and isoflurane are intermediary.

Compared with an anesthetic with high blood solubility (PC), an agent with low blood solubility is associated with a more rapid equilibration because a smaller amount of anesthetic must be dissolved in the blood before equilibrium is reached with the gas phase. In the case of the agent with a high blood-gas PC the blood acts like a large "sink" into which the anesthetic is poured, and accordingly blood is "reluctant" to give up the agent to other tissues (such as the brain). The blood serves as a conduit for drug delivery to the brain and as such can be visualized as a pharmacologically inactive reservoir that is interposed between the lungs and the agent's site of desired pharmacological activity (i.e., brain). Therefore, an anesthetic agent with a low blood-gas PC is usually more desirable than a highly soluble agent, because it is associated with (a) a more rapid anesthetic induction (i.e., more rapid rate of rise in alveolar concentration during induction [Fig. 13.13]); (b) a more precise control of anesthetic depth (i.e., alveolar concentration during the anesthetic maintenance); and (c) a more rapid elimination of anesthetic and recovery (i.e., a rapid decrease in alveolar concentration during recovery).

Cardiac Output The amount of blood flowing through the lungs and into body tissues also influences anesthetic uptake from the lungs. The greater the CO, the more blood is passing through the lungs carrying away anesthetic from the alveoli. Thus, a large CO, like increased anesthetic-agent blood solubility, delays the alveolar rise of P_{anes} (Fig. 13.14). Patient excitement is an example in which a relatively large CO is anticipated. Conversely, a reduced CO should be anticipated with a patient in shock. Such a situation would be associated with an increase in the rate of the P_A increase of the anesthetic, and this, along with other factors, make the anesthetic induction more rapid and risky.

Alveolar to Venous Anesthetic Partial Pressure Difference The magnitude of difference in anesthetic partial pressure between the alveoli and mixed venous blood is related to the amount of uptake of anesthetic by tissues. It is not surprising that the largest gradient occurs during induction. Once the tissues no longer absorb anesthetic (i.e., equilibrium is reached), there is no longer any uptake of anesthetic from the lungs because $P_I = P_A$ (i.e., the mixed venous blood returning to the lungs contains as much anesthetic as when it left the lungs). The changes in gradient between the initiation of induction and equilibration result in part from the relative distribution of CO. In this regard it is important to recognize that roughly 70% to 80% of the CO is normally directed to only a small volume of body tissues in a lean individual.[20,21] Tissues such as the brain, heart, hepatoportal system, and kidneys represent only about 10% of the body mass but normally receive about 75% of the total blood flow each minute. As a result these highly perfused tissues equilibrate rapidly with arterial anesthetic partial pressure when compared with other body

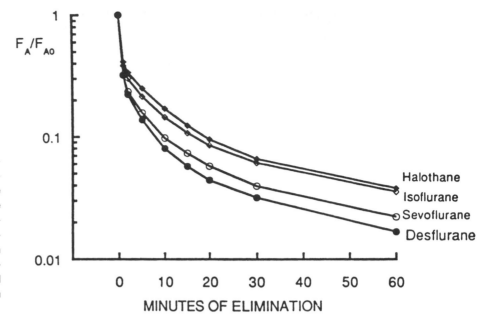

Fig. 13.15. The fall in alveolar concentration (F_A) relative to the alveolar concentration at the end of anesthesia (F_{AO}). Note that the newest, most insoluble volatile anesthetic, desflurane, is eliminated in humans more rapidly than are the other contemporary potent anesthetics. Not shown is information for methoxyflurane. If present, the curve for methoxyflurane would appear above that for halothane. From Eger,[326] with permission.

tissues (actual timing is influenced by agent solubility). Since the venous anesthetic pressure or tension equals that in the tissue within 10 or 15 min, about 75% of the blood returning to the lungs is the same as the alveolar tension. This presumes there has been no change in arterial anesthetic partial pressure during this time and thus uptake is reduced. Skin and muscle comprise the major bulk of the body (about 50% in humans) but at rest receive only about 15% to 20% of the CO, so saturation of these tissues requires several hours. Fat is a variable component of body bulk and receives only a small proportion of blood flow. Consequently, anesthetic saturation of this tissue is very slow because all anesthetics are considerably more soluble in fat than in other tissue groups (Table 13.2).

Other factors can influence the magnitude of the alveolar to arterial anesthetic partial pressure gradient. For example, abnormalities of ventilation-perfusion cause an alveolar-arterial gradient proportional to the degree of abnormality.[10,22,23] Others include loss of anesthetic via the skin[24–26] and into closed gas spaces[10,14,19] and metabolism.[10,14]

Overview

The rate with which the alveolar anesthetic concentration increases relative to the inspired concentration (i.e., the rate of change in anesthetic level) is often summarized as a plot of the ratio of F_A/F_I versus time. The position of individual curves representing different anesthetics on a plot is related to the solubility characteristics of the anesthetics (Fig. 13.13). The shape of the graph of F_A/F_I versus time is similar for all anesthetics (Fig. 13.13). A rapid initial rise results from the effect of alveolar ventilation bringing anesthetic into the lung. The rate of rise of the curve then decreases as uptake by the blood occurs. With time the highly perfused tissues of the body equilibrate with incoming blood so that eventually about three-quarters of the total blood flow returning to the heart has the same anesthetic partial pres-

sure as it had when it left the lungs. Thus, further uptake from the lung is decreased, and the rate of approach of the F_A to F_I over time is further decreased.

Anesthetic Elimination

Recovery from inhalation anesthesia results from the elimination of anesthetic from the CNS. This requires a decrease in alveolar anesthetic partial pressure (concentration), which in turn fosters a decrease in arterial and then CNS anesthetic partial pressure (Fig. 13.9). Prominent factors accounting for recovery are the same as those for anesthetic induction. Therefore, factors such as alveolar ventilation, CO, and especially agent solubility greatly influence recovery from inhalation anesthesia. Indeed, the graphic curves representing the washout of anesthetic from alveoli versus time (Fig. 13.15) are essentially inverses of the wash-in curves. That is, the washout of the less soluble anesthetics is high at first (i.e., rapid washout by ventilation of the lung functional residual capacity) and then rapidly declines to a lower output level that continues to decrease but at a slower rate. The washout of more soluble agents is also high at first, but the magnitude of decrease in alveolar anesthetic concentration is less and decreases more gradually with time (Fig. 13.15).

An important factor during the washout period is the duration of anesthesia. This effect and a comparison of this effect between three agents spanning a range of blood solubilities is summarized in Fig. 13.16.[27] If a patient rebreathing anesthetic circuit (e.g., circle system) is in use and the patient is not disconnected from the circuit at the end of anesthesia, the circuit itself may also reduce the rate of recovery, just as the circuit was shown to decrease the rate of rise of anesthetic during induction. This influence of rebreathing circuits can be reduced by directing high flow rates of anesthetic-free O_2 into the anesthetic circuit (i.e., applying principles of a non-rebreathing circuit).

Other factors that are important to varying degrees to inhala-

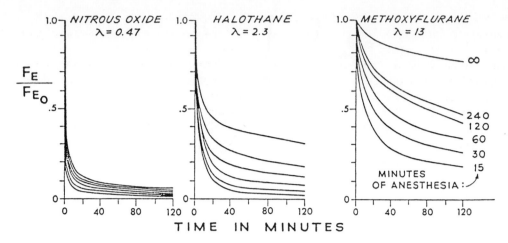

Fig. 13.16. The decrease in the alveolar anesthetic concentration (F_E) from the concentration at the time of breathing circuit disconnect (i.e., the beginning of recovery from anesthesia; F_{EO}) is influenced by both the solubility (λ) of anesthetic and the duration of anesthesia. From Stoelting and Eger,[27] with permission.

tion anesthetic elimination from the body include percutaneous loss, intertissue diffusion of agents, and metabolism. Transcutaneous movement of inhalation agent occurs, but the amount under consideration is small.[24–26,28] Intertissue diffusion is of theoretical interest, but its clinical importance is limited.[29–31] Metabolism may also play a small role with some inhalation anesthetics (e.g., methoxyflurane and perhaps even halothane), especially when associated with prolonged anesthesia.[29,32–34]

A special consideration associated with recovery after use of N_2O also deserves comment. *Diffusion hypoxia* is a possibility at the end of N_2O administration when the patient breathes air immediately rather than O_2 for at least a brief transition period (i.e., 5 to 10 min).[35–37] In this case a large volume of N_2O enters the lung from the blood. This early rapid inflow of N_2O to the lung displaces other gases within the lung. If at this time the patient is breathing air (only about 21% O_2) rather than 100% O_2, N_2O dilutes alveolar O_2, further reducing O_2 tension from levels found in ambient air. This action may cause life-threatening reductions in arterial oxygenation. Since the major effect is in the first few minutes after discontinuing N_2O, the condition can be prevented by administering pure O_2 at the conclusion of N_2O administration rather than allowing the patient to breathe ambient air immediately.

Biotransformation

Inhalation anesthetics are not chemically inert.[38] They undergo varying degrees of metabolism primarily in the liver but also to lesser degrees in the lung, kidney, and intestinal tract.[32,39–42] The importance of this is twofold. First, in a very limited way with older anesthetics, metabolism may facilitate anesthetic recovery. Second and more important is the potential for acute and chronic toxicities by intermediary or end metabolites of inhalation agents, especially on kidneys, liver, and reproductive organs.[32,42]

The magnitude of metabolism of inhalation anesthetic agents is determined by a variety of factors, including the chemical structure, hepatic enzyme activity (cytochrome P-450 enzymes located in the endoplasmic reticulum of the hepatocyte), the blood concentration of the anesthetic,[43] disease states, and ge-

Table 13.6. Biotransformation of inhalation anesthetics in humans

Anesthetic	% Anesthetic Metabolized	References
Methoxyflurane	50–75	34, 41
Halothane	20–46	34, 40, 329
Sevoflurane	2–5	53, 330
Enflurane	2–8	34, 331
Isoflurane	0.2	332
Desflurane	0.02	56
Nitrous oxide	0.004	293, 294

netic factors (i.e., some species and individuals are more active metabolizers of these drugs than are others, e.g., humans compared with rats).

An indication of the extent of biotransformation of contemporary inhalation anesthetics is presented in Table 13.6. Sevoflurane degrades in vivo to about the same extent as isoflurane and as indicated by transient postanesthetic increases in blood and urinary fluoride levels in rats,[44–48] dogs,[47] horses,[49–51] swine,[52] and people.[53] The peak serum fluoride concentrations observed in people during and after sevoflurane anesthesia are low, and nephrotoxicity is not expected.[53,54] Desflurane resists degradation in vivo.[52,55,56] The increase in serum inorganic fluoride is much smaller than that found with isoflurane.[52,55,56]

For further information on the biotransformation of inhalation anesthetics in general and for specific details regarding individual anesthetic agents, readers are referred to reviews by Baden and Rice[32] and Mazze and Fujinaga.[42]

Anesthetic Dose: The Minimum Alveolar Concentration

In 1963 Merkel and Eger described what has become the standard index of anesthetic potency for inhalation anesthetics: the *minimum alveolar concentration* (MAC).[57] The *MAC* is defined as the minimum alveolar concentration of an anesthetic at 1 atmosphere that produces immobility in 50% of subjects exposed to a supramaximal noxious stimulus. Thus, the MAC corresponds to the median effective dose (ED_{50}): Half of the subjects are anesthetized and half have not yet reached that "level." The dose that corresponds to the ED_{95} (95% of the individuals are anesthetized), at least in people, is 20% to 40% greater than the MAC.[58] Anesthetic potency of an inhaled anesthetic is inversely related to the MAC (i.e., potency = 1/MAC). From information presented earlier, it also follows that the MAC is inversely related to the oil-gas PC. Thus, a very potent anesthetic like the formally available agent methoxyflurane, which has a high oil-gas PC, has a lower MAC, whereas an agent with a low oil-gas PC has a higher MAC.

A number of characteristics of the MAC deserve emphasis.[10] First, the A in MAC represents *alveolar* concentration, not inspired or delivered (e.g., as from a vaporizer). This is important because the alveolar concentration is easily monitored with contemporary technology. Also, as we reviewed earlier, after sufficient time for equilibration (minutes), alveolar partial pressure will more closely approximate arterial and brain anesthetic partial pressures.

Second, the MAC is defined in terms of volume percent of 1 atmosphere and therefore represents an anesthetic partial pressure (P) at the anesthetic site of action; that is, remember, $P_x = (C/100) \cdot P_{bar}$, where P_x stands for the partial pressure of the anesthetic in the gas mixture, C is the anesthetic concentration in volume percent, and P_{bar} is the barometric or total pressure of the gas mixture. Thus, although the concentration at the MAC for a given agent may vary depending on ambient pressure conditions (e.g., sea level vs. high altitude), the anesthetic partial pressure always remains the same. For example, the MAC for isoflurane in healthy dogs is reported as 1.63 vol%. The study reporting this value was conducted at near sea level conditions at Davis, California (i.e., $P_{bar} = 760$ mm Hg). Based on the foregoing discussion, a MAC of 1.63 vol% represents an alveolar isoflurane partial pressure (P_{iso}) of 11.6 mm Hg. In comparison, for the same dog at Mexico City (elevation, 2240 m above sea level; $P_{bar} = 584$ mm Hg) the alveolar P_{iso} at the MAC is expected to be the same as determined at Davis (i.e., 11.6 mm Hg), whereas the MAC (i.e., the alveolar concentration) would be about 2.17 vol%.

Finally, it is important to note that the MAC is determined in healthy animals under laboratory conditions in the *absence* of other drugs and circumstances common to clinical use that may modify the requirements for anesthesia. General techniques for determining the MAC in animals are given elsewhere.[10,59–62] In determining the MAC in people the initial surgical skin incision has been the standard noxious stimulus used.[10] For the determination of the MAC in smaller animals (mice to dogs and pigs)[10,63,64] the standard stimulus has been application of a forceps or other surgical clamp to the base of the tail or the base of the dewclaw of the limb (e.g., pigs[62]), whereas electrical stimulus applied beneath the oral mucous membranes is most commonly used in larger species such as horses.[60]

The MAC values for contemporary inhalation anesthetics for a variety of animals commonly encountered in veterinary medicine are summarized in Table 13.7a and b. Values for humans are also listed for comparison. For values of agents of historical interest such as methoxyflurane, enflurane, or diethyl ether, readers are referred to the review in an earlier edition of this book or elsewhere.[10,64]

Since its original introduction, the MAC concept has been extended to other stimulus end points in an effort to better define and understand the anesthetic state. For example, Stoelting and coworkers[65] determined the value for the MAC of an anesthetic at which people opened their eyes on verbal command during emergence from anesthesia; this has been termed *MAC-awake*. The verbal stimulus is of course less intense than the surgical incision in people and thus the response occurs at a lower concentration of anesthetic than movement following incision. The end-tidal concentration preventing movement in response to tracheal intubation (the MAC for intubation) is more stimulating to people than is surgical incision and was described by Yakaitis and colleagues.[66,67] Roizen and colleagues[68] reported an even greater alveolar concentration necessary to prevent adrenergic response (rise in endogenous catecholamines) to skin incision (also in human patients) compared with the concentration necessary to just prevent movement; this is known as *MAC-BAR*. Thus, a group of response curves is possible and depends on the chosen strength of the stimulus applied.

In a single species the variability in the MAC (response to a noxious stimulus) is generally small and not substantially influenced by gender, duration of anesthesia, variation in arterial CO_2 partial pressure ($PaCO_2$) (from 10 to 90 mm Hg), metabolic alkalosis or acidosis, variation in arterial oxygen partial pressure (PaO_2) (from 40 to 500 mm Hg), moderate anemia, or moderate hypotension[10,64,69] (Table 13.8). Even between species the variability in the MAC for a given agent is usually not large. However, there is at least one notable exception (Table 13.7a). In humans, the MAC for N_2O is 104%, making it the least potent of the inhalation anesthetics currently used in this species. Its potency in other species is less than half that in humans (i.e., around 200%). Because the N_2O MAC is above 100% it cannot be used by itself at 1 atmosphere pressure in any species and still provide adequate amounts of O_2. Consequently, and assuming that the MAC values for combinations of inhaled anesthetics are additive, N_2O is usually administered with another more potent inhalant agent to thereby reduce the concentration of the second agent necessary for anesthesia (Fig. 13.17). However, because of the potency difference between animals and people, the amount of reduction differs in an important way. For example, administration of 60% N_2O with halothane reduces the amount of halothane needed to produce the MAC by about 55% in healthy people (Fig. 13.17) but reduces it only by about 20% to 30% in dogs. As noted in Fig. 13.17, the response of other animals most closely resembles that of dogs. Some physiological factors and drugs that influence the MAC are listed in Table 13.8.

Equipotent doses (i.e., equivalent concentrations of different anesthetics at the MAC) are useful for comparing effects of inhalation anesthetics on vital organs. In this regard anesthetic dose is commonly defined in terms of multiples of the MAC (i.e., 1.5

Table 13.7a. Minimum alveolar concentration values (%) for a variety of mammals at sea level or near sea level conditions

	Desflurane	Halothane	Isoflurane	Sevoflurane	N₂O
Cat	9.79[333] 10.27[334]	0.99[335,336] 1.14[337] 1.19[338]	1.28[339] 1.50[336] 1.61[338] 1.63[165] 1.90[334] 2.21[340]	2.58[341] 3.07[336] 3.41[334]	255[337]
Cow		0.76[342](calf)	1.14[343]		223[342] (calf)
Dog	7.2[344] 7.68–8.19[345] 10.3[346]	0.86[347] 0.87[337,348,349] 0.89[164,350] 0.92[351] 0.93[352]	1.28[165] 1.30[140] 1.31[353] 1.39[165] 1.39–1.50[354]	2.10[86] 2.36[350]	188[348] 222[337] 297[355]
Ferret		1.01[356]	1.52[356] 1.74[357]		267[356]
Goat		1.29[358] 1.3[359]	1.2[71] 1.23[360] 1.29[358] 1.31[361] 1.43[362] 1.5[359]	2.33[358]	
Horse	7.02[363] 8.06[151]	0.88[60] 0.95[364] 1.02[365] 1.05[142]	1.31[60] 1.43[141] 1.44[366] 1.64[367]	2.31[368] 2.84[369]	205[213]
Monkey		0.89[337] 1.15[370]	1.28[370] 1.46[140]		200[337]
Mouse	6.6–9.1[a,371]	0.95[372] 1.00[373] 1.19–1.37[a,371] 1.59[374]	1.31–1.77[a,371] 1.35[372] 1.41[373]	2.7[375]	150[376] 275[373]
Pig	10.00[62]	0.90[377] 0.91[378] 1.25[379]	1.45[380] 1.48[377] 1.51[140] 1.55[381] 1.75[382] 2.04[62]	1.97[383] 2.12[377] 2.53[384] 2.66[92]	162[381] 195[382] 277[379]
Rabbit	8.90[344]	0.80[385] 0.82[386] 1.05[387] 1.39[388] 1.42[389] 1.44[390] 1.56[391]	2.05[388] 2.07[389] 2.12[390]	3.70[392]	

or 2.0 times the MAC or simply 1.5 MAC or 2.0 MAC). From the preceding discussion, therefore, the ED_{50} equals the MAC or 1.0 MAC and represents a light level of anesthesia (clearly inadequate in 50% of otherwise unmedicated, healthy animals). The ED_{95} is 1.2 to 1.4 MAC, and 2.0 MAC represents a deep level of anesthesia, in some cases even an anesthetic overdose. The concept of MAC multiples can be used to compare drug effects and contrast pharmacodynamics of multiple doses of a specific drug.

Pharmacodynamics: Actions and Toxicity of the Volatile Anesthetics

All contemporary inhalation anesthetic agents in one way or another influence vital organ function. Some actions are inevitable and accompany the use of all agents, whereas other actions are a special or prominent feature of one or a number of the agents. In addition, dose-response relationships of inhalation anesthetics are not necessarily parallel. Differences in action, and especially

Table 13.7a. Minimum alveolar concentration values (%) for a variety of mammals at sea level or near sea level conditions (*continued*)

	Desflurane	Halothane	Isoflurane	Sevoflurane	N$_2$O
Rat	5.72[393]	0.81[397]	1.17[397]	2.99[399]	136[407]
	6.48[394]	0.95[398]	1.28[405]	2.40[400]	155[408]
	6.85[395]	1.02[399]	1.30[406]	2.50[44]	204[172]
	7.10[396]	1.03[372]	1.38[401]		221[409]
		1.10[400]	1.46[372]		235[409]
		1.11[401]	1.46[395]		
		1.13[402,403]	1.58[357,398]		
		1.17[404]			
		1.23[395]			
Sheep		0.97[410]	1.58[410]		
Human (30–60 years)	6.00[411]	0.73[412]	1.15[416]	1.58[417]	104[423]
		0.74[413,414]		1.71[418]	
		0.77[415]		1.83[419]	
				1.84[420]	
				1.85[421]	
				1.9[422]	
				2.05[392]	

N$_2$O, nitrous oxide. Superscript numbers are reference numbers.
[a]Absolute value related to strain.

Table 13.7b. ED$_{50}$ values for a variety of nonmammals[a]

	Desflurane	Halothane	Isoflurane	Sevoflurane	N$_2$O
Birds					
Chicken		0.85[61]			
Cockatoo			1.44[424]		
Crane			1.34[425]		
Duck		1.04[426]	1.30[427]		
Hawk			1.45[428]		220[428]
Parrot					
Amazon			1.47[424]		
African gray			1.91[424]		
Pigeon			1.51[428]		154[428]
Other					
Goldfish		0.76[429]			
Toad		0.67[430]			82.2[430]

ED$_{50}$, median effective dose; N$_2$O, nitrous oxide. Superscript numbers are reference numbers.
[a]Sea level or near sea level conditions.

undesirable action, of specific anesthetic agents form the basis for selecting one agent over another for a particular patient and/or procedure. Undesirable actions also provide primary impetus for development of new agents and/or anesthetic techniques.

Data from healthy animals exposed to equipotent alveolar concentrations of these drugs under controlled circumstances provide foundation information for this review. In other cases, results of studies of human volunteers form the basis of our understanding of some drug actions. Because animals are com-

monly allowed to breathe spontaneously during clinical management of general anesthesia (versus controlled mechanical ventilation) investigational results obtained from spontaneously breathing test animals are often considered baseline by veterinarians. In the broader anesthesiology and pharmacology literature, however, results of studies from human volunteers or animals administered precise amounts of inhalation anesthetics during controlled ventilation (and normocapnia) most commonly form the basis of comparison of pharmacodynamic differences. It is important to stress that many variables other than mode of ventila-

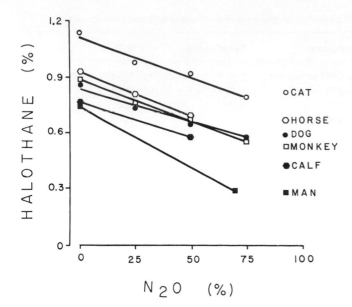

Fig. 13.17. When nitrous oxide (N_2O) is combined with halothane the alveolar concentration of halothane at minimum alveolar concentration is decreased. However, the halothane sparing imposed by nitrous oxide (N_2O) is less in animals compared with humans. From Steffey and Eger,[216] with permission.

tion commonly accompany anesthetic management of animals in both clinical and laboratory settings. These variables influence drug pharmacodynamics and may cause individuals to respond differently than test subjects that were studied under standardized conditions. Such confounding variables include species, duration of anesthesia, noxious (painful) stimulation, coexisting disease, concurrent medications, variation in body temperature, and extremes of age as examples.

Central Nervous System

Inhalation anesthetics affect the CNS in many ways. Mostly these agents are selected because they induce a reversible, dose-related state of CNS (somatic and motor), but also hemodynamic and endocrine, unresponsiveness to noxious stimulation: that is, a state of *general anesthesia*. Interestingly, although clinical anesthesia was introduced more than 150 years ago, the sites and mechanisms by which general anesthetics (including the inhalation anesthetics) cause unresponsiveness to surgical or other forms of noxious stimulation remain unknown. Traditionally, this summary state we refer to as general anesthesia was assumed to result from a focus in the brain. However, mounting evidence is causing a shift in thinking such that this state we know as general anesthesia is likely the collection of a number of end points that are distinct and site specific, and include supraspinal and spinal events. For example, actions focused in the brain (especially the cerebral cortex and thalamus) mediate such centrally recognized components of general anesthesia as amnesia (at least in humans) and hypnosis (sleep), whereas the spinal cord appears to be a critical site of anesthetic action that suppresses noxious-evoked movement.[70–72] In-depth review of known neural effects and theories of mechanism of action of inhalation anesthetics is beyond

the scope of this clinically focused review. Accordingly, readers with further interest in these subjects are referred to recent reviews by investigators currently active in this work.[73,74]

Inhalation anesthetics influence electrical activity of the brain, cerebral metabolism, cerebral perfusion, intracranial pressure, and analgesia—issues of critical importance to anesthetic management of animals.

Electroencephalographic Effects

The electroencephalograph (EEG) is used to help identify pathological brain disorders and to predict the outcome of brain insults. Studies have also shown that general anesthesia alters EEG parameters, and we apply this knowledge to better understand anesthetic circumstances. The EEG signal (wave) contains two basic parameters within a time frame (i.e., continues or an epoch): amplitude and frequency. *Amplitude* is the electrical height of the waves in volts, and *frequency* is the number of times per second the wave crosses the zero voltage reference point. The signal from an alert, attentive brain is usually low amplitude and high frequency. When events that lead the brain to produce higher frequencies occur, the EEG is described as *activated*, and it is considered *depressed* when slower frequencies are noted. General characteristics of the normal EEG are that it is symmetrical, the patterns are predictable, and spike waveforms are not present. All anesthetics do not produce exactly the same changes in EEG pattern as dose (anesthetic depth) increases, so the generic correlation of the raw EEG pattern with anesthetic dose is not precise. Indeed, despite some weak correlations and its usefulness as an indication of changing anesthetic depth, no parameter has had sensitivity and specificity sufficient to justify use of the EEG alone as a reliable index of anesthetic depth.[75] With technological advances of recent years, research has focused on use of processed EEG parameters (e.g., the bispectral index) as improved descriptions of anesthetic states. However, this subject is beyond the scope of this chapter and therefore is explored elsewhere (see Chapter 38).

In general, as the depth of anesthesia increases from awake states, the electrical activity of the cerebral cortex becomes desynchronized. Using isoflurane as an example of the general EEG response to volatile anesthetics,[1] the frequency of the EEG activity (alveolar concentrations of <0.4 MAC) initially increases. With further increases in anesthetic concentration, a decrease in frequency and increased amplitude of the EEG waves occur. The wave amplitude increases to a peak (about 1 MAC), and then, with further dose increase, the amplitude progressively declines (burst suppression occurs at about 1.5 MAC; i.e., bursts of slow high-voltage activity separated by electrical silence) and eventually becomes flatline (predominance of electrical silence). With isoflurane, an isoelectric pattern occurs at about 2.0 MAC, whereas, on the other extreme, it is not seen with halothane until >3.5 MAC. Electrical silence does not occur with enflurane. The two newest volatile anesthetics—sevoflurane and desflurane—cause dose-related changes similar to those of isoflurane.[76–78]

Several anesthetics in contemporary use have epileptogenic potential, especially in individuals predisposed to seizures. Enflurane is most prominent in this regard among the inhalation

Table 13.8. Some factors that influence the value of the minimum alveolar concentration (anesthetic requirement)

No Change	Increase	Decrease
Arterial blood pressure >50 mm Hg[431]	Drugs causing CNS stimulation	Drugs causing CNS depression[a]
Atropine, glycopyrrolate, and scopolamine[335]	Amphetamine	Other inhaled anesthetic
Duration of anesthesia	Ephedrine	Nitrous oxide[19]
Gender	Morphine (horse[141])	Injectable anesthetics
Hyperkalemia and hypokalemia	Laudanosine[391]	Ketamine[243]
Metabolic acid-base change	Physostigmine[432]	Lidocaine[340,352]
$PaO_2 > 40$ mm Hg	Hyperthermia (to 42°C)	Thiopental[433]
$PaCO_2 = 15–95$ mm Hg		Preanesthetic medication
		Acepromazine[434–436]
		Diazepam[437–439]
		Detomidine[366]
		Fentanyl[440]
		Medetomidine[441,442]
		Meperidine[241]
		Midazolam[443]
		Morphine[444]
		Xylazine[367]
		Other
		Adenosine
		Central anticholinergic[432]
		5-HT antagonist[445]
		Arterial blood pressure < 50 mm Hg
		Hyponatremia
		Hypothermia
		Increasing adult age
		$PaO_2 < 40$ mm Hg
		$PaCO_2 > 95$ mm Hg
		Pregnancy

5-HT, 5-hydroxytryptophan; CNS, central nervous system; PaO_2, arterial oxygen partial pressure; $PaCO_2$, arterial carbon dioxide partial pressure. Superscript numbers are reference numbers.

[a]List of example drugs are intended to be representative, not exhaustive. The list is summarized from previous reviews[10,59,64] except where indicated by superscript reference numbers.

anesthetics. Seizure activity is of concern because neuronal injury may result if demands for substrate (especially O_2) for maintaining neuronal function are greater than supply. A second concern is trauma to patients experiencing tonic-clonic muscle twitching, especially among horses. People assisting in the anesthetic and surgical management of these large patients may become injured. Finally, there is concern that seizures may persist into the postanesthetic period, especially unpredictably and when they occur in less well-controlled circumstances.

Systematic studies of EEG activity in people[79] and dogs[80] showed that enflurane was associated with spontaneous or noise-initiated intensified seizures. In addition, enflurane induces seizure activity that is associated with substantial increases in cerebral blood flow and cerebral metabolic use of O_2. In the studies by Joas et al.,[80] halothane, methoxyflurane, and isoflurane did not cause the frank epileptoid activity in dogs that was induced by enflurane. Indeed, both halothane and isoflurane have the capacity to produce an isoelectric EEG, with isoflurane doing so at a lower dose.[1] Present wide-spread opinion is that epileptogenesis is not a clinical concern with either agent.

The EEG responses to the two newest anesthetics—desflurane and sevoflurane—are reportedly similar to those of isoflurane,[76–78] and all three can suppress drug-induced convulsive behavior.[81–85] However, there are reports of seizure activity in animals[86,87] and human patients[88,89] during sevoflurane anesthesia. Because of the EEG-activating property of enflurane and perhaps sevoflurane it seems prudent to avoid their use in situations when events might predispose patients to seizures and when reasonable anesthetic alternatives exist.

Cerebral Metabolism
All volatile anesthetics decrease cerebral metabolic rate (CMR; cerebral O_2 consumption). The magnitude of decrease is least with halothane but similar with isoflurane, sevoflurane, and desflurane.[76,81,86,90,91]

Cerebral Blood Flow
The volatile anesthetics cause no change or often an increase in cerebral blood flow (CBF).[76,81,86,91,92] The effect on CBF is likely the sum of a tendency both to decrease as a result of anes-

thesia reducing cerebral O_2 consumption and increase due to vasodilation caused by direct anesthetic action on vascular smooth muscle.[93] This can be summarized by saying the ratio of CBF relative to CMR is increased by the potent inhalation anesthetics. The effect is anesthetic dose related and influenced by agent. The rank order of CBF increase is generally regarded as halothane > enflurane, isoflurane, desflurane, and sevoflurane (all four being similar).[69] Effects on CBF have been shown to be time dependent in animals[94–96] but not in humans.[97]

Intracranial Pressure

The inhalation anesthetics increase intracranial pressure (ICP), and this change parallels the CBF increase that similarly accompanies these agents.[76,98] In larger animals such as horses, body and head position further impacts the heart-to-brain hydrostatic gradient, which in turn can further impact ICP. Consequently, body position necessitates even greater consideration in anesthetized horses than is commonly considered in smaller species so as to minimize risks of inadequate CBF and cerebral ischemia.[99] It is generally regarded across species lines that ICP increases can be decreased by hyperventilation and decreasing $PaCO_2$.[100] Accordingly, use of hyperventilation is a common strategy in clinical situations in which even small elevations in ICP are of special concern. Mechanical ventilation and accompanying reduced $PaCO_2$ also reduce ICP in horses.[101] However, because of the commonly associated, often large decrease in systemic blood pressure in this species, cerebral perfusion pressure may decrease out of proportion and further reduce CBF.

Analgesia

A clinically desirable general anesthetic includes both hypnotic and analgesic actions. However, studies to differentiate hypnotic potency from analgesic potency within the anesthetic-concentration range is, at the least, difficult to interpret. Studies of subanesthetic concentrations of inhalation anesthetics have been preformed but with conflicting results. Some inhalation anesthetics have been reported to increase the response threshold to noxious stimulation compared with like, but unmedicated, conditions (e.g., diethyl ether), whereas others (e.g., isoflurane and sevoflurane) do not change the threshold,[102,103] and still others, like halothane,[104] may decrease the threshold for response and contribute a heightened awareness to noxious stimulation (i.e., antianalgesia). More recent work even suggests that inhalation anesthetics (including diethyl ether and N_2O) can be antianalgesic.[105] An antianalgesic effect may enhance perception of noxious stimulation (pain) for varying periods during, for example, recovery from anesthesia when low-level alveolar concentrations are reached.

Respiratory System

Inhalation anesthetics depress respiratory system function. The volatile agents, in particular, decrease ventilation in a drug-specific and species-specific manner. Depending on conditions, including species of interest, some of the most commonly considered measures of breathing effectiveness—that is, breathing rate and depth (tidal volume)—may not be revealing or may even

Table 13.9. Apneic index (AI) in various species

	Desflurane		Halothane		Isoflurane	
	MAC	AI	MAC	AI	MAC	AI
Cat					1.63	2.4[165]
Dog	7.2	2.4[119]	0.87	2.9[349]	1.28	2.5[165]
Horse			0.88	2.6[60]	1.31	2.3[60]
Pig	9.8	1.6[119,446]				
Rat			1.11	2.3[173]	1.38	3.1[172]
Human	7.25	1.8[121]	0.77	2.3[121]	1.15	1.7[121]

Minimum alveolar concentration (MAC) is given in volume percent, and the AI is a ratio of the end-tidal anesthetic concentration at apnea and MAC. Similar data are not currently available for sevoflurane.

be misleading. In general, spontaneous ventilation progressively decreases as inhalation anesthetic dose is increased, because at low-dose tidal volume decreases more than frequency increases. As anesthetic dose is further increased, respiratory frequency also decreases. In otherwise unmedicated animals (as well as people) anesthetized with volatile agents, respiratory arrest occurs at 1.5 to 3.0 MAC (Table 13.9). The overall decrease in minute ventilation and the likely variable increase in dead-space ventilation (causing an increase in the dead space to tidal volume ratio, V_D/V_t, from a normal of about 0.3 to 0.5 or more) reduce alveolar ventilation. Decreases in alveolar ventilation are out of proportion to decreases in CO_2 production (O_2 use is decreased by general anesthesia), such that $PaCO_2$ increases (Fig. 13.18). In addition, the normal stimulation to ventilation caused by increased $PaCO_2$ (or decreased PaO_2) is depressed by the inhalation anesthetics, presumably via the action of these agents directly on the medullary and peripheral (aortic and carotid body) chemoreceptors.[106–109] Changes in perianesthetic PaO_2 other than what might be related to the magnitude of alveolar ventilation are not notably different among the various inhalation anesthetics in a given species.

Bronchospasm is associated with some diseases and other patient conditions and contributes to increased airway resistance. A variety of early studies indicated that, among anesthetics available at the time, halothane was the most effective bronchodilator.[110,111] The effect is believed to result at least partially by decreasing cholinergic neurotransmission.[112,113] For years, therefore, it has been the anesthetic agent of choice for patients at risk of bronchospasm. The work of Hirshman and colleagues[114,115] suggests that isoflurane and perhaps enflurane were as effective in decreasing experimentally produced airway resistance and therefore were good alternatives to halothane. More recent work with isoflurane, sevoflurane, and desflurane indicates that relaxation of constricted bronchial muscles by these agents is at least equal to or exceeds that caused by halothane.[113,116,117]

Avoidance of airway irritation by inspiring inhalation anes-

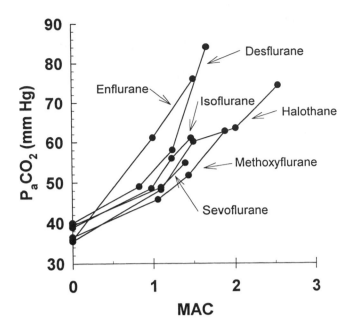

Fig. 13.18. Respiratory response to an increase in the alveolar concentration (expressed in as a multiple of the minimum alveolar concentration [MAC]) of inhalation anesthetics in humans. PaCO2, arterial carbon dioxide partial pressure. Data are taken from multiple sources.[107,121–125]

thetics is important especially during induction of anesthesia because the irritation may cause breath holding, coughing, and laryngospasm (particularly in some species such as primates [human and nonhuman]) that, in turn, result in arterial oxyhemoglobin desaturation. At least in humans, none of the potent inhalation anesthetics seem to have irritant properties at subanesthetic concentrations. However, patient objection and airway irritation is evident with desflurane (and to a lesser degree with isoflurane[118]) at concentrations of 7% or greater,[119,120] and as a result desflurane is not commonly used for anesthetic induction in human patients. Airway irritation has not been a generally recognized problem associated with induction of anesthesia in animals commonly anesthetized by veterinarians.

Arterial Carbon Dioxide Tension
The PaCO2 is the most frequently used index of respiratory system response to general anesthetics. All contemporary inhalation anesthetics depress alveolar ventilation and, as a consequence, increase PaCO2 in dose-related fashion. Figure 13.18 summarizes the effects of inhalation anesthetics in humans, the species for which data are most complete.[107,121–125] Actual rank order of the magnitude of hypoventilation imposed by the four contemporary volatile anesthetics at a common alveolar dose differs slightly depending on the species.

Factors Influencing Respiratory Effects
Mode of Ventilation Ventilation is often assisted or controlled during inhalation anesthesia to compensate for the anesthetic-induced respiratory depression. Controlled mechanical ventilation (i.e., the anesthetist controls both respiratory frequency and tidal volume) is used to predictably maintain a normal, or some other specific, PaCO2 during anesthesia. Assisted ventilation (i.e., the anesthetist augments tidal volume, but the animal determines its own breathing frequency) is used to attempt to improve the efficiency of oxygenating arterial blood and reduce the work of breathing but is usually not effective in substantially lowering PaCO2 compared with circumstances associated with spontaneous ventilation (i.e., the animal controls both the rate and depth of breathing).[126,127]

Duration of Anesthesia Respiratory function, including PaCO2, is little changed for as long as up to 10 h of constant, low-dose halothane (or methoxyflurane) in dogs.[128,129] This is also supported by work in humans[130] anesthetized with constant low-dose halothane. However, in horses anesthetized for 5 h with a constant dose of 1.2 MAC isoflurane a substantial temporal increase in PaCO2 was noted.[131] A similar, but more modest, trend was noted in horses when halothane was used for anesthesia.[132,133] At least in some species, if alveolar dose of halothane is increased above about 1.0 to 1.3 MAC and maintained constant at a heightened level, the magnitude of change in hypoventilation also worsens with time.[129] Conversely, there is evidence for recovery from the ventilatory depressant effects of volatile anesthetics in humans.[125]

Surgery and Other Noxious Stimulation Noxious stimulation may cause sufficient central nervous stimulation to lessen the ventilatory depression of the inhalation anesthetic.[134–137] This effect is of course diminished with increasing anesthetic depth.

Concurrent Drug Administration In humans the substitution of N2O for an equivalent amount of a concurrently administered, more potent volatile agent such as isoflurane lowers PaCO2 more (prevents hypoventilation) than does the volatile agent alone.[19] In dogs and monkeys anesthetized with halothane, ventilation was at least as, and sometimes more, depressed when N2O was substituted for a portion of the halothane requirement.[138,139] The addition of opioid drugs like morphine may increase the respiratory depression produced by an inhalation anesthetic.[136,140–142]

Cardiovascular System
All of the volatile inhalation anesthetics cause dose-dependent and drug-specific changes in cardiovascular performance. The magnitude and sometimes direction of change may be influenced by other variables that often accompany general anesthesia (Table 13.10). The mechanisms of cardiovascular effects are diverse but often include direct myocardial depression and a decrease in sympathoadrenal activity.

Cardiac Output
All of the volatile anesthetics decrease CO. The magnitude of change is dose related and depends on agent. In general, among the contemporary agents in use with animals, halothane depresses CO the most.[1,143–145] Desflurane in many ways is similar in cardiovascular action to isoflurane, whereas sevoflurane has

Table 13.10. Factors that influence cardiovascular effects of inhalation anesthetics

Anesthetic dose
Duration of anesthesia
Concurrent drug therapy
Intravenous fluid therapy
Magnitude of PaCO$_2$
Mechanical ventilation
Noxious stimulation

PaCO$_2$, arterial carbon dioxide partial pressure.

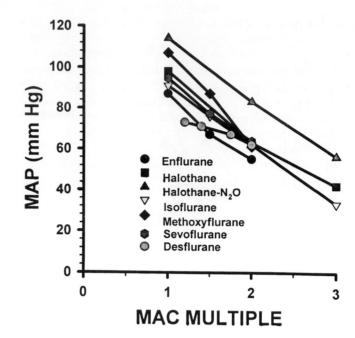

Fig. 13.19. Inhalation anesthetics cause a dose (expressed as multiples of the minimum alveolar concentration [MAC])-dependent decrease in mean arterial blood pressure (MAP) in dogs whose ventilation is mechanically controlled to produce eucapnia. N$_2$O, nitrous oxide. Data are from many sources and referenced in the text.

characteristics resembling both halothane and isoflurane. All three of the newer volatile anesthetics tend to preserve CO at clinically useful concentrations.[51,119,146–154] The decrease in CO is largely due to a decrease in stroke volume as a result of dose-related depression in myocardial contractility.[1,119,150,155–157]

The effect of inhalation anesthetics on heart rate (HR) is variable and depends on agent and species. For example, in humans, HR is not substantially altered with halothane anesthesia but is usually increased by isoflurane, desflurane, and sevoflurane.[153,158,159] Compared with conditions in awake, calm dogs, HR is increased with the use of any of the four anesthetics listed.[149,154] There is evidence to suggest that differences between agents in the degree of increase in HR in dogs are explained by differences in the vagolytic activity of the agents.[152] In dogs the HR usually remains constant over a range of clinically useful alveolar concentrations in the absence of other modifying factors (e.g., noxious stimulation).[143,144,149,154,160,161] The distribution of blood flow to organs is altered during inhalation anesthesia. Readers with special interest in these changes are referred elsewhere for further information.[162,163]

Arterial Blood Pressure

Volatile anesthetics cause a dose-dependent decrease in arterial blood pressure (Fig. 13.19).[15,51,143,147,151,154,164–168] In general the dose-related decrease in arterial blood pressure is similar regardless of the species studied.[60,143,145,148,164–166,168–170] In animals the dose-related decrease in blood pressure with all four of the contemporary agents is usually related mostly to a decrease in stroke volume. In some cases (agent and/or species) a decrease in peripheral vascular resistance may also play an important, but lesser, role. This common scenario in animals differs from results generally reported from studies with people anesthetized at least with isoflurane, sevoflurane, and desflurane, whereby pressure decreases primarily from a decrease in systemic vascular resistance.[15,171] Indices of anesthetic influence on cardiovascular collapse are listed in Table 13.11.[143,172,173]

Cardiac Rhythm and Catecholamines

Inhalation anesthetics may increase the automaticity of the myocardium and the likelihood of propagated impulses from ectopic sites, especially from within the ventricle.[174] Although spontaneously derived dysrhythmias were most notable with earlier inhalation anesthetics (e.g., halothane), none of the three most re-

Table 13.11. Anesthetic-induced cardiovascular depression as expressed by cardiovascular anesthetic indices

	Desflurane	Halothane	Isoflurane
Dog[a]		2.84	2.69
Pig[b]		2.45	3.02
Rat[c]		3.0	5.7

[a]The anesthetic concentration causing death in ventilated dogs related to the minimum alveolar concentration (MAC).[119]
[b]Mean fatal dose related to the MAC.[446]
[c]Heart concentration of anesthetic at cardiovascular failure related to heart concentration of anesthetic at establishment of anesthesia.[172,173]

cently introduced ether-derivative agents appear to predispose the heart to generated extrasystoles. However, any such effect can be exaggerated by adrenergic agonists.[175] The association of cardiac dysrhythmias with adrenergic drugs and anesthetic agents has received extensive study.

Inhalation anesthetics may sensitize the heart to arrhythmogenic effects of catecholamines. Halothane is most notable in this regard, as it markedly reduces the amount of epinephrine necessary to cause ventricular premature contractions.[176] There is some evidence that deeper levels of halothane decrease this incidence,[177–179] but this is not a consistent finding.[180] Enflurane and methoxyflurane are less potent in regard to their ability to sensitize the heart to arrhythmogenic effects of epinephrine, and isoflurane, desflurane, and sevoflurane are least arrhythmogenic.[1,179,181–186] The potential for dysrhythmias follows administration of most catecholamine-type drugs, although the magnitude of such potential varies with the drug coadministered[186–191] and other associated conditions.[192] Such considerations are important in the design of anesthetic plans for patients in which it is desirable or necessary to administer catecholamines, for example, local application to minimize blood oozing from highly vascular surgical sites, to minimize blood pressure, or for CO support, or in patients in which high blood levels of endogenous catecholamines are anticipated.

Factors Influencing Circulatory Effects

A variety of circumstances occasionally associated with the anesthetic management of veterinary patients may add to or negate the primary effects of the anesthetic. In most cases the most profound modifications of drug action are on cardiovascular function. Some factors influencing cardiovascular performance include mechanical ventilation and alterations in $PaCO_2$, noxious (surgical) stimulation, duration of anesthesia, and coexisting drugs.

Mode of Ventilation and $PaCO_2$ There may be considerable difference in the cardiovascular effects of inhalation anesthetics in animals breathing spontaneously compared with when their breathing is mechanically controlled (e.g., intermittent positive-pressure ventilation [IPPV]) to produce and maintain a normal $PaCO_2$. In general, and considering a broad range of circumstances, cardiovascular function is usually depressed during IPPV relative to actions during spontaneous ventilation. Such action results from either the direct mechanical actions (e.g., intermittent elevation of intrathoracic pressure and resultant decrease in venous return to the heart) or lessening of the indirect pharmacological action of $PaCO_2$[193] or both. Carbon dioxide has pharmacological actions important for these considerations. For example, an increased $PaCO_2$ has direct depressant actions on the heart and smooth muscle of the peripheral blood vessels (i.e., vessel dilation) but indirect (via sympathetic nervous system) stimulation of circulatory function.

In generally healthy, sympathetically intact animals (light anesthesia) the stimulatory actions of hypercapnia usually predominate, so increased CO and arterial blood pressure usually accompany an increase in $PaCO_2$, becoming lower when $PaCO_2$ is normalized.[51,126,145,151,164,168,169,194–197]

Noxious Stimulation   Noxious stimulation during anesthesia modifies the circulatory effect of inhalation anesthetics via stimulation of the sympathetic nervous system. An increase in arterial blood pressure and HR (CO) commonly accompanies noxious stimulation.[68,136,137,198,199] The response is anesthetic dose related. For example, Roizen et al.[68] and Yasuda et al.[198] showed that deeper levels of halothane and enflurane decreased or prevented surgically induced increases in serum norepinephrine levels in human patients.[68] Anesthetic doses that block the response are in the range of 1.5 to 2.0 MAC.

Duration of Anesthesia   Some cardiovascular effects of inhalation anesthetics may change with duration of anesthesia. For example, in humans, halothane anesthesia lasting 5 to 6 h is associated with an increase in values of some measures of cardiovascular function, such as CO and HR.[195,200] Similarly, varying degrees of time-related changes have been reported with the use of enflurane,[125] desflurane,[159,201,202] and others.[158,201–205]

Temporal changes in cardiovascular function have also been reported in a variety of animals with the use of halothane,[129,132,206,207] isoflurane,[131,206,208] and sevoflurane.[208] Dose of anesthetic[129,158,209] and body posture during anesthesia[133,210] apparently also play a temporal role in some species.

The causes of these changes remain unclear. In vitro, depression of the cat papillary muscle exposed to a constant concentration of halothane does not vary over a 3-h period.[211] This observation suggests that temporal effects associated with inhalation anesthetics are not the result of improved intrinsic cardiac function. Studies on human volunteers have shown that temporal responses to halothane can be prevented if the subjects are given propranolol before anesthesia, which suggests that the mechanism is related to increasing sympathetic nervous system activity.[212]

Usually the temporal changes associated with inhalation anesthetics are of only minor or no concern to clinicians. However, such changes must be considered when interpreting results of laboratory studies in which these agents are used for anesthetic management.

Concurrent Drug Administration   Drugs administered immediately before or in conjunction with inhalation anesthetics (preanesthetic medication, injectable anesthetic induction drugs, vasoactive and cardiotonic drugs, etc.) may influence cardiovascular function by altering the anesthetic requirement (i.e., the MAC and thereby increase or decrease anesthetic level) or by their own direct action on cardiovascular performance.

For example, N_2O is used on occasion as a substitute for a portion of a more potent inhalation anesthetic. Because of its own anesthetic potency (albeit small; remember, the MAC for N_2O in animals is in the range of 2 atmospheres [Table 13.7]) its use may facilitate delivery of a reduced amount of the potent volatile agent and thereby contribute to some cardiovascular sparing. Nitrous oxide may depress the myocardium directly, but this effect is usually counterbalanced by its sympathomimetic effect, often resulting in a net improvement in cardiovascular function compared with conditions without N_2O. In animal patients the magnitude of N_2O effect is clinically limited and species dependent.[138,139,166,213,214] More complete summaries of its cardiovascular actions have been published elsewhere.[215,216]

Injectable drugs, such as acepromazine, α_2-agonists, thiobarbiturates, and dissociatives (e.g., ketamine), are frequently administered to animals as part of their anesthetic management. These drugs confound the primary effects of the inhalation anesthetics and may accentuate cardiovascular depression. On the other hand, sympathomimetic drugs, such as ephedrine,[217] dopamine, and dobutamine,[218,219] are frequently given to counteract unwanted cardiovascular depression of the anesthetic.

Effects on the Kidneys

It is generally regarded that present-day volatile inhalation anesthetics produce similar mild, reversible, dose-related decreases in renal blood flow and glomerular filtration rate and that such changes largely reflect an anesthetic-induced decrease in CO.[171] However, some studies show little or no change in these kidney-related parameters.[44,163,220,221]

As a consequence of the anesthetic-induced decrease in glomerular filtration, healthy anesthetized animals commonly produce a smaller volume of concentrated urine compared with when awake. An increase in serum urea nitrogen, creatinine, and inorganic phosphate may accompany especially prolonged anesthesia.[222-225] The reduction in renal function is highly influenced by an animal's state of hydration and hemodynamics during anesthesia.[226] Accordingly, attendant intravenous fluid therapy and prevention of a marked reduction in renal blood flow will lessen or counteract the tendency for reduced renal function. In most cases, effects of inhalation anesthesia on renal function are rapidly reversed after anesthesia.

Among the inhalation anesthetics, methoxyflurane is the most nephrotoxic. Although it is no longer available for use in human or animal patients, its actions are of pathophysiological interest and therefore is briefly reviewed here. Particularly in humans and some strains of rats, the use of methoxyflurane caused renal failure that was characterized not by oliguria but by a large urine volume unresponsive to vasopressin.[32] This was caused by the biotransformation of methoxyflurane and the large release of free fluoride ion that, in turn, directly damaged the renal tubules. Although renal injury in animals is rare, renal injury has been reported in dogs when methoxyflurane was used in combination with tetracycline antibiotics[227] and flunixin.[227]

With the possible exception of enflurane and sevoflurane, the breakdown of other inhalation anesthetics does not pose a risk of fluoride-induced nephrotoxicity. Biotransformation of enflurane and sevoflurane by humans following a moderate duration of anesthesia causes serum inorganic fluoride concentrations to increase even beyond the 50-μmol/L level, which is normally considered the nephrotoxic threshold in humans.[32,171,228,229] However, clinical, histological, or biochemical evidence of injury related to increases in fluoride has only rarely been reported in human patients. The overriding consensus is that sevoflurane has little potential for nephrotoxicity caused by defluorination.[32,171] Two factors may explain the general lack of injury despite the body's ability to degrade sevoflurane. In 1977, Mazze et al.[230] proposed that the area under the serum fluoride concentration-versus-time curve may be a more important determinant of nephrotoxicity than is peak serum fluoride concentration. Because sevoflurane is poorly soluble and is rapidly eliminated via the lungs the duration of its availability for biotransformation is notably limited. More recently, Kharasch and coworkers[231] proposed another consideration: Sevoflurane is primarily metabolized by the liver, whereas hepatic and renal sites are important for methoxyflurane breakdown. The relative lack of intrarenal anesthetic defluorination may markedly reduce its nephrotoxic potential. Studies have confirmed the increase in serum fluoride in horses anesthetized with sevoflurane.[49-51] In these reports the magnitude and time course of fluoride increase were similar to that reported for humans. In addition, as with humans, no evidence has been reported of untoward renal effects associated with the increase in fluoride in horses.

Sevoflurane is degraded by CO_2 absorbents such as soda lime and Baralyme.[45,53] A nephrotoxic breakdown product—compound A—is produced.[45,232] Compound A can cause renal injury and death in rats,[233] and the concentration threshold for nephrotoxicity in rats[234-236] is within the range of concentrations that may be found associated with the anesthetic management of human patients.[237] Not surprisingly, compound A is formed in the breathing circuits used for animals in veterinary medical practice.[238] The ultimate importance of in vitro sevoflurane degradation to the well-being of veterinary patients like dogs, cats, and horses[50] remains to be established. Until such time that additional data appear, it seems prudent to avoid sevoflurane for prolonged anesthesia especially with concurrent low fresh gas inflow to the breathing circuit (which promotes the concentration of compound A) and in patients with known or marginal kidney disease.

Effects on the Liver

Depression of hepatic function and hepatocellular damage may be caused by the action of volatile anesthetics. Effects may be mild and transient or permanent, and injury may be by direct or indirect action. Studies by Reilly et al.[239] suggested that at least halothane (but likely also other potent inhalation anesthetics) substantially inhibits the drug-metabolizing capacity of the liver. A reduction in intrinsic hepatic clearance of drugs along with anesthetic-induced alteration of other pharmacokinetically important variables (e.g., reduced hepatic blood flow) fosters a delayed drug removal or an increase in plasma drug concentration during anesthesia. Examples of such circumstances have been reported.[239-243] Prolonged or increased (relative to conditions in the unanesthetized animal) plasma concentrations of some drugs have important toxic implications, especially in physiologically comprised patients.

All of the potent inhalation anesthetics can cause hepatocellular injury by reducing liver blood flow and oxygen delivery. However, available data suggest that, of the four contemporary volatile anesthetics, isoflurane is most likely to better maintain tissue O_2 supply and thereby is the agent least likely to produce liver injury even when administered for prolonged periods. The effects of the two newest agents sevoflurane and desflurane are nearly similar to isoflurane, whereas halothane produces the most striking adverse changes.[32,147,163,167,244-250] Results of investigations indicate that ancillary influences, including the use of N_2O,[251] concurrent hypoxia,[249,252-254] prior induction of hepatic drug-metabolizing enzymes,[255,256] mode of ventilation,[257] and positive end-expired pressure,[258] may worsen conditions and increase the likelihood of hepatocellular damage.

It now appears that especially halothane produces two types of hepatotoxicity in susceptible individuals. One is a mild, self-limiting postanesthetic form of hepatocellular destruction and associated increase in serum concentrations of liver enzymes. Signs of hepatotoxicity occur shortly after anesthetic exposure. The other is a rare, severe, often fatal hepatotoxicity with delayed onset and largely clinically limited to human patients (i.e., halothane hepatitis) and thought to be an immune-mediated toxicity.[259,260] The mechanism of halothane hepatitis may also be family related.[261] The increased incidence of hepatic injury associated with halothane was the principal factor leading to the decrease in the use of halothane for human patients nearly three decades ago.

Effects on Skeletal Muscle: Malignant Hyperthermia

Malignant hyperthermia (MH) is a potentially life-threatening pharmacogenetic myopathy that is most commonly reported in susceptible human patients[262,263] and swine[264] (e.g., Landrace, Pietrain, or Poland China strains). However, reports of its occurrence in other species are available.[265–271] Its clinicopathological, histopathological, and genetic basis has recently been further described for horses.[272,273] All of the four contemporary volatile anesthetics can initiate MH, but halothane is the most potent triggering agent relative to other inhalation anesthetics.[263] The syndrome is characterized by a rapid rise in body temperature that, if not treated quickly, causes death. Monitoring of temperature and CO_2 production is warranted in susceptible or suspected patients. Patients known to be susceptible to MH can be anesthetized safely. Avoiding the use of triggering agents and administering prophylactic dantrolene before anesthesia are effective in preventing the onset of MH.[263]

Further discussions on the clinical pharmacology and use of volatile inhalant anesthetics in various species and disease conditions, and for special procedures and patients, can be found in other sections of this book that emphasize individual anesthetic patient management.

The Gaseous Anesthetic: Nitrous Oxide

Nitrous oxide was introduced into clinical practice more than 150 years ago. Since then, its use has formed the basis for the use of more general anesthetic techniques in human patients than any other single inhalation agent.[19] Its use became widespread because of its many desirable properties, including low blood solubility (Table 13.2), limited cardiovascular and respiratory system depression, and minimal toxicity.[19] Its use in the anesthetic management of animals became a natural extension of its use in people.

Dose

Nitrous oxide is not the ideal anesthetic for people or animals. As discussed earlier in this chapter, N_2O is not a potent anesthetic (Table 13.7a and b) and will not anesthetize a fit, healthy individual. To derive the important benefits from the use of N_2O, it is usually administered in high inspired concentrations. However, as the concentration of N_2O is increased, there is a change in the proportion and partial pressure of the various other constituents of the inspired breath, notably O_2. Consequently, to avoid hypoxemia, 75% of the inspired breath is the highest concentration that can be administered safely under conditions at sea level. Use of N_2O at locations above sea level requires a lower N_2O concentration to ensure an adequate partial pressure of inspiratory O_2

(PiO_2). Nitrous oxide has less value in the anesthetic management of animals than in that of human patients because the anesthetic potency of N_2O in animals is only about half that found for humans (e.g., the MAC for dogs is about 200% vs. about 100% for people [Table 13.7a]).[10,216] Thus, the value of N_2O in veterinary clinical practice is primarily as an anesthetic adjuvant, that is, accompanying other inhaled or injectable drugs. Since the effects of N_2O on vital organ function (including cardiovascular and respiratory) in the absence of hypoxemia are small in most veterinary patients, benefit is afforded by enabling a certain reduction in the amount of the primary, more potent, inhaled or injectable anesthetic agent.

Kinetics

Nitrous oxide's low blood solubility (Table 13.2) is responsible for a rapid onset of action. Although it does not have the potency to produce anesthesia, it may be used to speed induction of inhalation anesthesia as a result of its own (albeit limited) CNS effects and, as mentioned earlier, also by augmenting the uptake of a concurrently administered more potent volatile anesthetic such as halothane: the second gas effect.[10,19,274,275] When a high concentration of N_2O is administered concurrently in a mixture with an inhalation agent (e.g., N_2O plus halothane), the alveolar concentration of the simultaneously administered anesthetic (halothane) increases more rapidly than when the "second" gas has been administered without N_2O. The second gas effect is the result of an increased inspiratory volume secondary to the large volume of N_2O taken up (remember, N_2O is used at high concentrations)[274] and a concentrating effect on the second gas in a smaller volume (and thus increased gradient for transfer to blood) as a result of the uptake of the large volume of N_2O.[10,275] Results of a more recent study with desflurane confirms previous findings for the second gas effect.[276]

Pharmacodynamics

As noted previously, N_2O's effects on cardiovascular and respiratory function (other than reducing the inspired O_2 concentration) are small compared with other inhalation anesthetics. It does depress myocardial function directly, but its sympathetic stimulation properties counteract some of the direct depression (its own as well as that from accompanying volatile anesthetics).[216] As a result of its sympathetic nervous system activation it may contribute to an increased incidence of cardiac arrhythmias.[277,278] There is evidence to suggest that its use contributes to myocardial ischemia in some circumstances.[279–282] Overall, a conservative outlook regarding N_2O use relative to respiration and circulation is that significant concern is warranted only in patients with initially compromised function.[283,284] As with any agent, its advantages and disadvantages should be weighed on an individual patient basis.

Nitrous oxide has little or no effect on liver and kidney function.[285–287] Although there is evidence of N_2O-induced interference with the production of red and white blood cells by bone marrow, the risk of adverse outcomes to a patient exposed under most clinical veterinary circumstances is little or none.[286,288] However, prolonged exposure to N_2O causes megaloblastic hematopoiesis and polyneuropathy. Seriously ill patients may have increased sensitivity to these toxicities. Problems result from N_2O-induced inactivation of the vitamin B_{12}–dependent enzyme methionine synthase, an enzyme that controls interrelations between vitamin B_{12} and folic acid metabolism.[289] Although an occasional patient may develop signs suggestive of vitamin B_{12} and folic acid deficiency after an anesthetic technique that includes the use of N_2O, this is a rare event in human and animal patients.[286,290] Prolonged occupational or abusive exposure to N_2O may be equally harmful, and this potential harm should be considered in management plans of veterinary practices.[32,286,291,292] Nitrous oxide is rapidly and mainly eliminated in the exhaled breath. The extent of biotransformation (to molecular nitrogen [N_2]) is very small and mainly by intestinal flora[32,293,294] (Table 13.6).

Transfer of Nitrous Oxide to Closed Gas Spaces

Gas spaces exist or may exist in the body under a variety of conditions and to varying degrees. For example, gas is normally found in the stomach and intestines. The gut is a dynamic reservoir; the gas it contains is freely movable into and out of it according to the laws of diffusion. The gas in the gut originates from air swallowing, normal production of bacterial behavior, chemical reactions, and diffusion from the blood. There is marked variability in both composition and volume of stomach and bowel gas (e.g., herbivore vs. carnivore). There are other natural air cavities, such as the air sinuses and the middle ear, and then there are circumstances in which air may be electively or inadvertently introduced as part of diagnostic or therapeutic actions (e.g., pneumoencephalogram, pneumocystogram, endoscopy, and vascular air emboli).

Potential problems associated with gas spaces arise when an animal breathing air is given a gas mixture containing N_2O.[10,19] Nitrogen is the major component of air (80%) and of most gas spaces (methane, CO_2, and hydrogen are also found in variable quantities in the gut). When N_2O is introduced into the inspired breath, a reequilibration of gases in the gas space begins with N_2O quickly entering and N_2 slowly leaving. That is, because of its greater blood solubility, the volume of N_2O that can be transported to a closed gas space is many times the volume of N_2 that can be carried away.[10] For example, the blood-gas PC for N_2O is 0.47 (Table 13.2), whereas that for N_2 is about 0.015.[295] Thus, N_2O is more than 30 times more soluble in blood than is N_2 (0.47/0.015). The result of the net transfer of gas to the gas space can be manifested as an increase in volume, as with the gut,[296,297] pneumothorax,[297] or blood embolus;[298,299] an increase in pressure (e.g., middle ear[300,301] or pneumoencephalogram[302]); or both (as the distending limits of the compliant space are reached). Usually air is used to inflate the cuff of an endotracheal tube. This cuff is another relatively compliant, enclosed air space. Nitrous oxide will similarly expand this gas space and may increase the pressure exerted on the tracheal wall.[303–305]

Diffusion Hypoxia

A further issue requiring consideration for the differential movement of N_2O and N_2 is at the end of anesthesia when N_2O is dis-

continued. Because of the large volume of N_2O stored in the body during anesthesia and the unequal change of N_2O for N_2, a deficiency in blood oxygenation may occur at the end of anesthesia if air is abruptly substituted for N_2O. As discussed earlier in this chapter, this condition is referred to as *diffusion hypoxia*.[35,36] The rapid outpouring of N_2O from the blood into the lung causes a transient but marked decrease in alveolar PO_2, with a resultant decrease in PaO_2.

Interaction with Respiratory Gas Monitoring

Routine monitoring of expired CO_2 is increasingly important and possible in the operating room of veterinary hospitals. Nitrous oxide interferes with the accurate recording of CO_2 with some monitoring devices. This interaction must be considered in decisions regarding the purchasing of equipment and overall anesthetic management plan. A more complete summary of the advantages and disadvantages of N_2O use is available elsewhere.[19] Brief summaries of practical considerations of N_2O use in veterinary practice have also been published.[306,307]

Occupational Exposure: Trace Concentrations of Inhalation Anesthetics

Operating-room personnel are often exposed to low concentrations of inhalation anesthetics. Ambient air is contaminated via vaporizer filling, known and unknown leaks in the patient breathing circuit, and careless spillage of liquid agent. Measurable amounts of anesthetic gases and vapors are present in operating-room air under a variety of conditions.[308–315] Personnel inhale and, as shown by studies, retain these agents for some time.[316,317] The slow rate of elimination of some vapors (especially the more blood-soluble agents like halothane) enables retained trace anesthetic quantities to accumulate from one day to the next.

Concern is raised because epidemiological studies of humans and laboratory studies of animals have suggested that chronic exposure to trace levels of anesthetics may constitute a health hazard. The possibility that chronic exposure to low levels of anesthetic agents constitutes a hazard to health science personnel has attracted and maintained worldwide interest since the early 1970s. Of particular concern are reports that inhaled anesthetics possess mutagenic, carcinogenic, or teratogenic potential. Depending on the point in life at which exposure occurs, there is concern that these underlying mechanisms in turn may be responsible for an increased incidence of fetal death, spontaneous abortion, birth defects, or cancer in exposed workers.[318–320] However, to date, no genotoxic effect of long-term or short-term exposure to inhaled anesthetics has been demonstrated in humans, and "the conclusion from both animal and human studies is that there is no carcinogenic risk either from exposure to the currently used inhaled anesthetics."[32]

Although the data to date, especially regarding effects on human reproduction, remain equivocal, a firm cause-and-effect relationship between chronic exposure to trace levels of anesthetics and human health problems does not exist. Although the risk

Table 13.12. Methods to reduce occupational exposure to inhalation anesthetics in the operating room

1. Use waste gas *scavenger* to collect gas from the pressure-relief (pop-off) valve of the patient breathing circuit and ventilator
2. Conduct *regular inspection* and *maintenance* to detect and repair leaks in anesthetic machines and patient breathing circuits, piped gas supplies (nitrous oxide), etc.
3. *Alter work practices* (e.g., minimize leaks around the face mask and turn off the vaporizer and fresh gas flow when the patient breathing circuit is not attached to the patient)
4. Ventilate operating rooms adequately
5. Monitor room trace anesthetic gas levels
6. Educate personnel

of long-term exposure to trace concentrations of anesthetics for those in operating-room conditions appears minimal, current evidence is suggestive enough to cause concern and to encourage practices to reduce the contamination by anesthetics of operating-room personnel. Indeed, exposure levels have been recommended by the government: 2.0 parts per million (ppm) for volatile agents and 25 ppm for N_2O.[318] In this regard, inexpensive methods to reduce and control anesthetic exposure by operating-room personnel are available and should be used (Table 13.12).

Frequent monitoring of actual levels of anesthetic gas or vapor is of obvious value and is encouraged in specialized circumstances and/or environments where there is high use. Likely the greatest impact results from educating personnel about the potential problem of waste anesthetic gases and methods for controlling exposure levels.[318–321] For further information on this subject, readers are directed to a more complete report of current knowledge and conclusions from available data that have been developed by the American Society of Anesthesiologists (ASA) Task Force on Trace Anesthetic Gases of the ASA Committee on Occupational Health of Operating Room Personnel.[322]

References

1. Eger EI II. Isoflurane (Forane): A Compendium and Reference. Madison, WI: Anaquest, 1985:79–90.
2. Soma LR. Textbook of Veterinary Anesthesia. Baltimore: Williams and Wilkins, 1971.
3. Hall LW. Wright's Veterinary Anaesthesia and Analgesia. London: Bailliere Tindall, 1971.
4. Lumb WV, Jones EW. Veterinary Anesthesia. Philadelphia: Lea and Febiger, 1973.
5. Short CE. Inhalant anesthetics. In: Short CE, ed. Principles & Practice of Veterinary Anesthesia. Baltimore: Williams and Wilkins, 1987:70–90.
6. Steffey EP. Inhalation anesthetics In: Thurmon JC, Tranquilli W, Benson GJ, eds. Lumb & Jones' Veterinary Anesthesia, 3rd ed. Philadelphia: Lea and Febiger, 1996:297–329.
7. Lowe HJ, Ernst EA. The Quantitative Practice of Anesthesia: Use of Closed Circuit. Baltimore: Williams and Wilkins, 1981.
8. Hill DW. Physics Applied to Anaesthesia, 4th ed. London: Butterworths, 1980.
9. Haskins S, Sansome AL. A time-table for exhaustion of nitrous oxide cylinders using cylinder pressure. Vet Anesth 1979;6:6–8.
10. Eger EI II. Anesthetic Uptake and Action. Baltimore: Williams and Wilkins, 1974.
11. Mapleson WW, Allott PR, Steward A. The variability of partition coefficients for halothane in the rabbit. Br J Anaesth 1972;44:656–681.
12. Eger RR, Eger EI II. Effect of temperature and age on the solubility of enflurane, halothane, isoflurane, and methoxyflurane in human blood. Anesth Analg 1985;64:640–642.
13. Lerman J, Schmitt-Bantel BI, Gregory GA, et al. Effect of age on the solubility of volatile anesthetics in human tissues. Anesthesiology 1986;65:307–312.
14. Eger EI II. Uptake and distribution. In: Miller RD, ed. Anesthesia, 5th ed. Philadelphia: Churchill Livingstone, 2000:74–95.
15. Eger EI II, Eisenkraft JB, Weiskopf RB. The Pharmacology of Inhaled Anesthetics. San Francisco: Dannemiller Memorial Educational Foundation, 2003.
16. Mapleson WW. Pharmacokinetics of inhalational anaesthetics. In: Nunn JF, Utting JE, Brown BR Jr, eds. General Anaesthesia, 5th ed. London: Butterworths, 1989:44–59.
17. Steffey EP, Howland DJ. Rate of change of halothane concentration in a large animal circle anesthetic system. Am J Vet Res 1977;38:1993–1996.
18. Mapleson WW. The concentration of anaesthetics in closed circuits, with special reference to halothane. I. Theoretical studies. Br J Anaesth 1960;32:298–309.
19. Eger EI II. Nitrous Oxide/N2O. New York: Elsevier, 1985.
20. Webb AI. The effect of species differences in the uptake and distribution of inhalant anesthetic agents. In: Grandy J, Hildebrand S, McDonell W, et al., eds. Proceedings of the Second International Congress of Veterinary Anesthesia. Santa Barbara, CA: Veterinary Practice, 1985:27–32.
21. Staddon GE, Weaver BMQ, Webb AI. Distribution of cardiac output in anaesthetized horse. Res Vet Sci 1979;27:38–45.
22. Eger EI II, Severinghaus JW. Effect of uneven pulmonary distribution of blood and gas on induction with inhalation anesthetics. Anesthesiology 1964;25:620–626.
23. Stoelting RK. The effect of right to left shunt on the rate of increase of arterial anesthetic concentration. Anesthesiology 1972;36:352–356.
24. Stoelting RK, Eger EI II. Percutaneous loss of nitrous oxide, cyclopropane, ether and halothane in man. Anesthesiology 1969;30:278–283.
25. Fassoulaki A, Lockhart SH, Freire BA, et al. Percutaneous loss of desflurane, isoflurane, and halothane in humans. Anesthesiology 1991;74:479–483.
26. Lockhart SH, Yasuda N, Peterson N, et al. Comparison of percutaneous losses of sevoflurane and isoflurane in humans. Anesth Analg 1991;72:212–215.
27. Stoelting RK, Eger EI II. The effects of ventilation and anesthetic solubility on recovery from anesthesia: An in vivo and analog analysis before and after equilibration. Anesthesiology 1969;30:290–296.
28. Cullen BF, Eger EI II. Diffusion of nitrous oxide, cyclopropane, and halothane through human skin and amniotic membrane. Anesthesiology 1972;36:168–173.
29. Carpenter RL, Eger EI II, Johnson BH, et al. Does the duration of anesthetic administration affect the pharmacokinetics or metabolism of inhaled anesthetics in humans? Anesth Analg 1987;66:1–8.
30. Bunemann L, Jensen K, Thomsen L, et al. Central blood flow and metabolism during controlled hypotension with sodium-

nitroprusside and general anaesthesia for total hip replacement a.m. Charnley. Acta Anaesthesiol Scand 1987;31:487–491.

31. Laster MJ, Taheri S, Eger EI II, et al. Visceral losses of desflurane, isoflurane, and halothane in swine. Anesth Analg 1991;73: 209–212.

32. Baden JM, Rice SA. Metabolism and toxicity of inhaled anesthetics. In: Miller RD, ed. Anesthesia, 5th ed. New York: Churchill Livingstone, 2000:147–173.

33. Cahalan MK, Johnson BH, Eger EI II. Relationship of concentrations of halothane and enflurane to their metabolism and elimination in man. Anesthesiology 1981;54:3–8.

34. Carpenter RL, Eger EI II, Johnson BH, et al. The extent of metabolism of inhaled anesthetics in humans. Anesthesiology 1986;65: 201–206.

35. Fink BR. Diffusion anoxia. Anesthesiology 1955;16:511–519.

36. Rackow H, Salanitre E, Frumin MH. Dilution of alveolar gases during nitrous oxide excretion in man. J Appl Physiol 1961;16:723–728.

37. Sheffer L, Steffenson JL, Birch AA. Nitrous oxide–induced diffusion hypoxia in patients breathing spontaneously. Anesthesiology 1972;37:436–439.

38. Van Dyke RA, Chenoweth MB, Van Poznak A. Metabolism of volatile anesthetics. I. conversion in vivo of several anesthetics to $^{14}CO_2$ and chloride. Biochem Pharmacol 1964;13:1239–1247.

39. Stier A, Alter H, Hessler O, et al. Urinary excretion of bromide in halothane anesthesia. Anesth Analg 1964;43:723–728.

40. Rehder K, Forbes J, Alter H, et al. Halothane biotransformation in man: A quantitative study. Anesthesiology 1967;28:711–715.

41. Holaday DA, Rudofsky S, Treuhaft PS. The metabolic degradation of methoxyflurane in man. Anesthesiology 1970;33:579–593.

42. Mazze RI, Fujinaga M. Biotransformation of inhalational anaesthetics. In: Nunn JF, Utting JE, Brown BR, eds. General Anaesthesia, 5th ed. London: Butterworths, 1989:73–85.

43. Sawyer DC, Eger EI II, Bahlman SH, et al. Concentration dependence of hepatic halothane metabolism. Anesthesiology 1971;34: 230–235.

44. Cook TL, Beppu WJ, Hitt BA, et al. Renal effects and metabolism of sevoflurane in Fischer 344 rats: An in-vivo and in-vitro comparison with methoxyflurane. Anesthesiology 1975;43:70–77.

45. Wallin RF, Regan BM, Napoli MD, et al. Sevoflurane: A new inhalational anesthetic agent. Anesth Analg 1975;54:758–766.

46. Cook TL, Beppu WJ, Hitt BA, et al. A comparison of renal effects and metabolism of sevoflurane and methoxyflurane in enzyme-induced rats. Anesth Analg 1975;54:829–835.

47. Martis L, Lynch S, Napoli MD, et al. Biotransformation of sevoflurane in dogs and rats. Anesth Analg 1981;60:186–191.

48. Rice SA, Dooley JR, Mazze RI. Metabolism by rat hepatic microsomes of fluorinated ether anesthetics following ethanol consumption. Anesthesiology 1983;58:237–241.

49. Aida H, Mizuno Y, Hobo S, et al. Cardiovascular and pulmonary effects of sevoflurane anesthesia in horses. Vet Surg 1996;25:164–170.

50. Driessen B, Zarucco L, Steffey EP, et al. Serum fluoride concentrations, biochemical and histopathological changes associated with prolonged sevoflurane anaesthesia in horses. J Vet Med [A] 2002; 49:337–347.

51. Steffey EP, Woliner MJ, Mama KR, et al. Effects of sevoflurane in horses. Am J Vet Res 2005;20 (in press).

52. Koblin DD, Weiskopf RB, Holmes MA, et al. Metabolism of I-653 and isoflurane in swine. Anesth Analg 1989;68:147–149.

53. Holaday DA, Smith FR. Clinical characteristics and biotransformation of sevoflurane in healthy human volunteers. Anesthesiology 1981;54:100–106.

54. Frink EJ Jr, Malan TP Jr, Brown EA, et al. Plasma inorganic fluoride levels with sevoflurane anesthesia in morbidly obese and nonobese patients. Anesth Analg 1993;76:1333–1337.

55. Koblin DD, Eger EI II, Johnson BH, et al. I-653 resists degradation in rats. Anesth Analg 1988;67:534–539.

56. Sutton TS, Koblin DD, Gruenke LD, et al. Fluoride metabolites after prolonged exposure of volunteers and patients to desflurane. Anesth Analg 1991;73:180–185.

57. Merkel G, Eger EI II. A comparative study of halothane and halopropane anesthesia including method for determining equipotency. Anesthesiology 1963;24:346–357.

58. de Jong RH, Eger EI II. MAC expanded: AD_{50} and AD_{95} values of common inhalation anesthetics in man. Anesthesiology 1975;42: 408–419.

59. Stanski DR. Monitoring depth of anesthesia. In: Miller RD, ed. Anesthesia, 5th ed. Philadelphia: Churchill Livingstone, 2000: 1087–1116.

60. Steffey EP, Howland DJ, Giri S, et al. Enflurane, halothane and isoflurane potency in horses. Am J Vet Res 1977;38:1037–1039.

61. Ludders JW, Mitchell GS, Schaefer SI. Minimum anesthetic dose and cardiopulmonary response for halothane in chickens. Am J Vet Res 1988;49:929–933.

62. Eger EI II, Johnson BH, Weiskopf RB, et al. Minimum alveolar concentration of I-653 and isoflurane in pigs: Definition of a supramaximal stimulus. Anesth Analg 1988;67:1174–1177.

63. Eger EI II, Saidman LJ, Brandstater B. Minimal alveolar anesthetic concentration: A standard of anesthetic potency. Anesthesiology 1965;26:756–763.

64. Quasha AL, Eger EI II, Tinker JH. Determination and applications of MAC. Anesthesiology 1980;53:315–334.

65. Stoelting RK, Longnecker DE, Eger EI II. Minimum alveolar concentrations in man on awakening from methoxyflurane, halothane, ether and fluroxene anesthesia: MAC awake. Anesthesiology 1970;33:5–9.

66. Yakaitis RW, Blitt CD, Angiulo JP. End-tidal halothane concentration for endotracheal intubation. Anesthesiology 1977;47:386–388.

67. Yakaitis RW, Blitt CD, Angiulo JP. End-tidal enflurane concentration for endotracheal intubation. Anesthesiology 1979;50:59–61.

68. Roizen MF, Horrigan RW, Frazer BM. Anesthetic doses blocking adrenergic (stress) and cardiovascular responses to incision: MAC BAR. Anesthesiology 1981;54:390–398.

69. Drummond JC, Patel PM. Cerebral physiology and the effects of anesthetics and techniques. In: Miller RD, ed. Anesthesia, 5th ed. Philadelphia: Churchill Livingstone, 2000:695–733.

70. Rampil IJ, Mason P, Singh H. Anesthetic potency (MAC) is independent of forebrain structures in the rat. Anesthesiology 1993;78: 707–712.

71. Antognini JF, Schwartz K. Exaggerated anesthetic requirements in the preferentially anesthetized brain. Anesthesiology 1993;79: 1244–1249.

72. Rampil IJ. Anesthetic potency is not altered after hypothermic spinal cord transection in rats. Anesthesiology 1994;80:606–610.

73. Antognini JF, Carstens E, Raines DE. Neural Mechanisms of Anesthesia. Totowa, NJ: Humana, 2003.

74. Koblin DD. Mechanisms of action. In: Miller RD, ed. Anesthesia, 5th ed. New York: Churchill Livingstone, 2000:48–73.

75. Dwyer RC, Rampil IJ, Eger EI II, et al. The electroencephalogram does not predict depth of isoflurane anesthesia. Anesthesiology 1994;81:403–409.

76. Scheller MS, Tateishi A, Drummond JC, et al. The effects of sevoflurane on cerebral blood flow, cerebral metabolic rate for oxy-

gen, intracranial pressure, and the electroencephalogram are similar to those of isoflurane in the rabbit. Anesthesiology 1988;68: 548–552.

77. Rampil IJ, Weiskopf RB, Brown JG, et al. I-653 and isoflurane produce similar dose-related changes in the electroencephalogram of pigs. Anesthesiology 1988;69:298–302.

78. Rampil IJ, Lockhart SH, Eger EI II, et al. The electroencephalographic effects of desflurane in humans. Anesthesiology 1991;74: 434–439.

79. Neigh JL, Garman JK, Harp JR. The electroencephalographic pattern during anesthesia with Ethrane: Effects of depth of anesthesia, PaCO$_2$ and nitrous oxide. Anesthesiology 1971;35:482–487.

80. Joas TA, Stevens WC, Eger EI II. Electroencephalographic seizure activity in dogs during anaesthesia: Studies with Ethrane, fluroxene, halothane, chloroform, divinyl ether, diethyl ether, methoxyflurane, cyclopropane and Forane. Br J Anaesth 1971;43:739–745.

81. Todd MM, Drummond JC. A comparison of the cerebrovascular and metabolic effects of halothane and isoflurane in the cat. Anesthesiology 1984;60:276–282.

82. Karasawa F. The effects of sevoflurane on lidocaine-induced convulsions. J Anesth 1991;5:60–67.

83. Fukuda H, Hirabayashi Y, Shimizu R, et al. Sevoflurane is equivalent to isoflurane for attenuating bupivacaine-induced arrhythmias and seizures in rats. Anesth Analg 1996;83:570–573.

84. Murao K, Shingu K, Tsushima K, et al. The anticonvulsant effects of volatile anesthetics on penicillin-induced status epilepticus in cats. Anesth Analg 2000;90:142–147.

85. Murao K, Shingu I, Tsushima K, et al. The anticonvulsant effects of volatile anesthetics on lidocaine-induced seizures in cats. Anesth Analg 2000;90:148–155.

86. Scheller MS, Nakakimura K, Fleischer JE, et al. Cerebral effects of sevoflurane in the dog: Comparison with isoflurane and enflurane. Br J Anaesth 1990;65:388–392.

87. Osawa M, Shingu K, Murakawa M, et al. Effect of sevoflurane on central nervous system electrical activity in cats. Anesth Analg 1994;79:52–57.

88. Woodforth IJ, Hicks RG, Crawford MR, et al. Electroencephalographic evidence of seizure activity under deep sevoflurane anesthesia in a nonepileptic patient. Anesthesiology 1997;87:1579–1582.

89. Komatsu H, Tale S, Endo S, et al. Electrical seizures during sevoflurane anesthesia in two pediatric patients with epilepsy. Anesthesiology 1994;81:1535–1537.

90. Cucchiara RF, Theye RA, Michenfelder JD. The effects of isoflurane on canine cerebral metabolism and blood flow. Anesthesiology 1974;40:571–574.

91. Lutz LJ, Milde JH, Milde LN. The cerebral functional, metabolic, and hemodynamic effects of desflurane in dogs. Anesthesiology 1990;73:125–131.

92. Manohar M, Parks CM. Porcine systemic and regional organ blood flow during 1.0 and 1.5 minimum alveolar concentrations of sevoflurane anesthesia without and with 50% nitrous oxide. J Pharmacol Exp Ther 1984;231:640–648.

93. Drummond JC, Todd MM, Scheller MS, et al. A comparison of the direct cerebral vasodilating potencies of halothane and isoflurane in the New Zealand white rabbit. Anesthesiology 1986;65:462–468.

94. Albrecht RF, Miletich DJ, Madala LR. Normalization of cerebral blood flow during prolonged halothane anesthesia. Anesthesiology 1983;58:26–31.

95. Boarini DJ, Kassell NF, Coester HC, et al. Comparison of systemic and cerebrovascular effects of isoflurane and halothane. Neurosurgery 1984;15:400–409.

96. Warner DS, Boarini DJ, Kassell NF. Cerebrovascular adaptation to prolonged halothane anesthesia is not related to cerebrospinal fluid pH. Anesthesiology 1985;63:243–248.

97. Kuroda Y, Murakami M, Tsuruta J, et al. Blood flow velocity of middle cerebral artery during prolonged anesthesia with halothane, isoflurane, and sevoflurane in humans. Anesthesiology 1997;87: 527–532.

98. Artru AA. Relationship between cerebral blood volume and CSF pressure during anesthesia with halothane or enflurane in dogs. Anesthesiology 1983;58:533–539.

99. Brosnan RJ, Steffey EP, LeCouteur RA, et al. Effects of body position on intracranial and cerebral perfusion pressures in isoflurane-anesthetized horses. J Appl Physiol 2002;92:2542–2546.

100. Adams RW, Cucchiara RF, Gronert GA, et al. Isoflurane and cerebrospinal fluid pressure in neurosurgical patients. Anesthesiology 1981;54:97–99.

101. Brosnan RJ, Steffey EP, LeCouteur RA, et al. Effects of ventilation and isoflurane end-tidal concentration on intracranial and cerebral perfusion pressures in horses. Am J Vet Res 2003;64:21–25.

102. Tomi K, Mashimo T, Tashiro C, et al. Alterations in pain threshold and psychomotor response associated with subanaesthetic concentrations of inhalation anaesthetics in humans. Br J Anaesth 1993; 70:684–686.

103. Petersen-Felix S, Arendt-Nielsen L, Bak P, et al. Analgesic effects in humans of subanaesthetic isoflurane concentrations evaluated by experimentally induced pain. Br J Anaesth 1995;75:55–60.

104. Dundee JW, Moore J. Alterations in response to somatic pain associated with anaesthesia. IV. The effect of sub-anaesthetic concentrations of inhalation agents. Br J Anaesth 1960;32: 453–459.

105. Zhang Y, Eger EI, Dutton RC, et al. Inhaled anesthetics have hyperalgesic effects at 0.1 minimum alveolar anesthetic concentration. Anesth Analg 2000;91:462–466.

106. Knill RL, Kieraszewicz HT, Dodgson BG, et al. Chemical regulation of ventilation during isoflurane sedation and anaesthesia in humans. Br J Anaesth 1983;49:957–963.

107. Fourcade HE, Stevens WC, Larson CP Jr, et al. The ventilatory effects of Forane, a new inhaled anesthetic. Anesthesiology 1971;35:26–31.

108. Hirshman CA, McCullough KE, Cohen PJ, et al. Depression of hypoxic ventilatory response by halothane, enflurane and isoflurane in dogs. Br J Anaesth 1977;49:947–962.

109. Knill RL, Manninen PH, Clement JL. Ventilation and chemoreflexes during enflurane sedation and anaesthesia in man. Can Anaesth Soc J 1979;26:353–360.

110. Coon RL, Kampine JP. Hypocapnic bronchoconstriction and inhalation anesthetics. Anesthesiology 1975;43:635–641.

111. Klide AM, Aviado DM. Mechanism for the reduction in pulmonary resistance induced by halothane. J Pharmacol Exp Ther 1967;158: 28–35.

112. Tobias JD, Hirshman CA. Attenuation of histamine-induced airway constriction by albuterol during halothane anesthesia. Anesthesiology 1990;72:105–110.

113. Habre W, Petak F, Sly PD, et al. Protective effects of volatile agents against methacholine-induced bronchoconstriction in rats. Anesthesiology 2001;94:348–353.

114. Hirshman CA, Bergman NA. Halothane and enflurane protect against bronchospasm in an asthma dog model. Anesth Analg 1978; 57:629–633.

115. Hirshman CA, Edelstein H, Peetz S, et al. Mechanism of action of inhalational anesthesia on airways. Anesthesiology 1982;56:107–111.

116. Mazzeo AJ, Cheng EY, Bosnjak ZJ, et al. Differential effects of desflurane and halothane on peripheral airway smooth muscle. Br J Anaesth 1996;76:841–846.

117. Wiklund CU, Lim S, Lindsten U, et al. Relaxation by sevoflurane, desflurane and halothane in the isolated guinea-pig trachea via inhibition of cholinergic neurotransmission. Br J Anaesth 1999;83:422–429.

118. Doi M, Ikeda K. Airway irritation produced by volatile anaesthetics during brief inhalation: Comparison of halothane, enflurane, isoflurane and sevoflurane. Can J Anaesth 1993;40:122–126.

119. Eger EI II. Desflurane (Suprane): A Compendium and Reference. Rutherford, NJ: Healthpress, 1993.

120. TerRiet MF, DeSouza GJA, Jacobs JS, et al. Which is most pungent: Isoflurane, sevoflurane or desflurane? Br J Anaesth 2000;85:305–307.

121. Lockhart SH, Rampil IJ, Yasuda N, et al. Depression of ventilation by desflurane in humans. Anesthesiology 1991;74:484–488.

122. Munson ES, Larson CP Jr, Babad AA, et al. The effects of halothane, fluroxene and cyclopropane on ventilation: A comparative study in man. Anesthesiology 1966;27:716–728.

123. Larson CP Jr, Eger EI II, Muallem M, et al. The effects of diethyl ether and methoxyflurane on ventilation. II. A comparative study in man. Anesthesiology 1969;30:174–184.

124. Doi M, Ikeda K. Respiratory effects of sevoflurane. Anesth Analg 1987;66:241–244.

125. Calverley RK, Smith NT, Jones CW, et al. Ventilatory and cardiovascular effects of enflurane anesthesia during spontaneous ventilation in man. Anesth Analg 1978;51:610–618.

126. Hodgson DS, Steffey EP, Grandy JL, et al. Effects of spontaneous, assisted, and controlled ventilation in halothane-anesthetized geldings. Am J Vet Res 1986;47:992–996.

127. Steffey EP, Wheat JD, Meagher DM, et al. Body position and mode of ventilation influences arterial pH, oxygen and carbon dioxide tensions in halothane-anesthetized horses. Am J Vet Res 1977;38:379–382.

128. Brandstater B, Eger EI II, Edelist G. Constant-depth halothane anesthesia in respiratory studies. J Appl Physiol 1965;20:171–174.

129. Steffey EP, Farver TB, Woliner MJ. Cardiopulmonary function during 7 h of constant-dose halothane and methoxyflurane. J Appl Physiol 1987;63:1351–1359.

130. Fourcade HE, Larson CP Jr, Hickey RF, et al. Effects of time on ventilation during halothane and cyclopropane anesthesia. Anesthesiology 1972;36:83–88.

131. Steffey EP, Hodgson DS, Dunlop CI, et al. Cardiopulmonary function during 5 hours of constant-dose isoflurane in laterally recumbent, spontaneously breathing horses. J Vet Pharmacol Ther 1987;10:290–297.

132. Steffey EP, Kelly AB, Woliner MJ. Time-related responses of spontaneously breathing, laterally recumbent horses to prolonged anesthesia with halothane. Am J Vet Res 1987;48:952–957.

133. Steffey EP, Kelly AB, Hodgson DS, et al. Effect of body posture on cardiopulmonary function in horses during five hours of constant-dose halothane anesthesia. Am J Vet Res 1990;51:11–16.

134. France CJ, Plumer HM, Eger EI II, et al. Ventilatory effects of isoflurane (Forane) or halothane when combined with morphine, nitrous oxide and surgery. Br J Anaesth 1974;46:117–120.

135. Eger EI II, Dolan WM, Stevens WC, et al. Surgical stimulation antagonizes the respiratory depression produced by Forane. Anesthesiology 1972;36:544–549.

136. Steffey EP, Eisele JH, Baggot JD, et al. Influence of inhaled anesthetics on the pharmacokinetics and pharmacodynamics of morphine. Anesth Analg 1993;77:346–351.

137. Steffey EP, Pascoe PJ. Xylazine blunts the cardiovascular but not the respiratory response induced by noxious stimulation in isoflurane anesthetized horses [Abstract]. In: Proceedings of the Seventh International Congress of Veterinary Anaesthesia, 2000:55.

138. Steffey EP, Gillespie RJ, Berry JD, et al. Circulatory effects of halothane and halothane–nitrous oxide anesthesia in the dog: Spontaneous ventilation. Am J Vet Res 1975;36:197–200.

139. Steffey EP, Gillespie JR, Berry JD, et al. Cardiovascular effects with the addition of N$_2$O to halothane in stump-tailed macaques during spontaneous and controlled ventilation. J Am Vet Med Assoc 1974;165:834–837.

140. Steffey EP, Baggot JD, Eisele JH, et al. Morphine-isoflurane interaction in dogs, swine and rhesus monkeys. J Vet Pharmacol Ther 1994;17:202–210.

141. Steffey EP, Eisele JH, Baggot JD. Interactions of morphine and isoflurane in horses. Am J Vet Res 2003;64:166–175.

142. Bennett RC, Steffey EP, Kollias-Baker C, et al. Influence of morphine sulfate on the halothane sparing effect of xylazine hydrochloride in horses. Am J Vet Res 2004;65:519–526.

143. Steffey EP, Howland D Jr. Potency of enflurane in dogs: Comparison with halothane and isoflurane. Am J Vet Res 1978;39:673–677.

144. Klide AM. Cardiovascular effects of enflurane and isoflurane in the dog. Am J Vet Res 1976;37:127–131.

145. Steffey EP, Howland D Jr. Comparison of circulatory and respiratory effects of isoflurane and halothane anesthesia in horses. Am J Vet Res 1980;41:821–825.

146. Eger EI II. New inhaled anesthetics. Anesthesiology 1994;80:906–922.

147. Merin RG, Bernard JM, Doursout MF, et al. Comparison of the effects of isoflurane and desflurane on cardiovascular dynamics and regional blood flow in the chronically instrumented dog. Anesthesiology 1991;74:568–574.

148. Weiskopf RB, Holmes MA, Eger EI II, et al. Cardiovascular effects of I-653 in swine. Anesthesiology 1988;69:303–309.

149. Pagel PS, Kampine JP, Schmeling WT, et al. Comparison of the systemic and coronary hemodynamic actions of desflurane, isoflurane, halothane, and enflurane in the chronically instrumented dog. Anesthesiology 1991;74:539–551.

150. Warltier DC, Pagel PS. Cardiovascular and respiratory actions of desflurane: Is desflurane different from isoflurane? Anesth Analg 1992;75:S17–S31.

151. Steffey EP, Woliner MJ, Puschner B, et al. Effects of desflurane in the horse. Am J Vet Res 2005;66:669–677.

152. Picker O, Scheeren TWL, Arndt JO. Inhalation anaesthetics increase heart rate by decreasing cardiac vagal activity in dogs. Br J Anaesth 1988;87:748–754.

153. Malan TP, DiNardo JA, Isner J, et al. Cardiovascular effects of sevoflurane compared with those of isoflurane in volunteers. Anesthesiology 1995;83:918–928.

154. Mutoh T, Nishimura R, Kim H, et al. Cardiopulmonary effects of sevoflurane, compared with halothane, enflurane, and isoflurane, in dogs. Am J Vet Res 1997;58:885–890.

155. Pagel PS, Kampine JP, Schmeling WT, et al. Influence of volatile anesthetics on myocardial contractility in vivo: Desflurane versus isoflurane. Anesthesiology 1991;74:900–907.

156. Pagel PS, Kampine JP, Schmeling WT, et al. Evaluation of myocardial contractility in the chronically instrumented dog with intact autonomic nervous system function: Effects of desflurane and isoflurane. Acta Anaesthesiol Scand 1993;37:203–210.

157. Boban M, Stowe DF, Buljubasic N, et al. Direct comparative effects of isoflurane and desflurane in isolated guinea pig hearts. Anesthesiology 1992;76:775–780.

158. Stevens WC, Cromwell TH, Halsey MJ, et al. The cardiovascular effects of a new inhalation anesthetic, Forane, in human volunteers at constant arterial carbon dioxide tension. Anesthesiology 1971;35:8–16.

159. Weiskopf RB, Cahalan MK, Eger EI II, et al. Cardiovascular actions of desflurane in normocarbic volunteers. Anesth Analg 1991;73:143–156.

160. Bernard J-M, Wouters PF, Doursout M-F, et al. Effects of sevoflurane and isoflurane on cardiac and coronary dynamics in chronically instrumented dogs. Anesthesiology 1990;72:659–662.

161. Clarke KW, Alibhai HIK, Lee Y-HL, et al. Cardiopulmonary effects of desflurane in the dog during spontaneous and artificial ventilation. Res Vet Sci 1996;61:82–86.

162. Seyde WC, Longnecker DE. Anesthetic influences on regional hemodynamics in normal and hemorrhaged rats. Anesthesiology 1984;61:686–698.

163. Bernard J-M, Doursout MF, Wouters P, et al. Effects of enflurane and isoflurane on hepatic and renal circulations in chronically instrumented dogs. Anesthesiology 1991;74:298–302.

164. Steffey EP, Farver TB, Woliner MJ. Circulatory and respiratory effects of methoxyflurane in dogs: Comparison of halothane. Am J Vet Res 1984;45:2574–2579.

165. Steffey EP, Howland D Jr. Isoflurane potency in the dog and cat. Am J Vet Res 1977;38:1833–1836.

166. Steffey EP, Gillespie JR, Berry JD, et al. Circulatory effects of halothane and halothane–nitrous oxide anesthesia in the dog: Controlled ventilation. Am J Vet Res 1974;35:1289–1293.

167. Frink EJ Jr, Morgan SE, Coetzee A, et al. The effects of sevoflurane, halothane, enflurane, and isoflurane on hepatic blood flow and oxygenation in chronically instrumented greyhound dogs. Anesthesiology 1992;76:85–90.

168. Steffey EP, Howland DJ. Cardiovascular effects of halothane in the horse. Am J Vet Res 1978;39:611–615.

169. Steffey EP, Gillespie JR, Berry JD, et al. Cardiovascular effect of halothane in the stump-tailed macaque during spontaneous and controlled ventilation. Am J Vet Res 1974;35:1315–1319.

170. Pypendop BH, Ilkiw JE. Hemodynamic effects of sevoflurane in cats. Am J Vet Res 2004;65:20–25.

171. Stoelting RK. Inhaled anesthetics. In: Pharmacology and Physiology in Anesthetic Practice, 3rd ed. Philadelphia: Lippincott-Raven, 1999:36–76.

172. Wolfson B, Hebrick WD, Lake CL, et al. Anesthetic indices: Further data. Anesthesiology 1978;48:187–190.

173. Wolfson B, Kielar CM, Lake C, et al. Anesthetic index: A new approach. Anesthesiology 1973;38:583–586.

174. Price HL. The significance of catecholamine release during anesthesia. Br J Anaesth 1966;38:705–711.

175. Katz RL, Epstein RA. The interaction of anesthetic agents and adrenergic drugs to produce cardiac arrhythmias. Anesthesiology 1968;29:763–784.

176. Raventos J. The action of fluothane: A new volatile anaesthetic. Br J Pharmacol 1956;11:394–409.

177. Muir BJ, Hall LW, Littlewort MCG. Cardiac irregularities in cats under halothane anaesthesia. Br J Anaesth 1959;31:488–489.

178. Ueda I, Hirakawa M, Arakawa K, et al. Do anesthetics fluidize membranes? Anesthesiology 1986;64:67–72.

179. Joas TA, Stevens WC. Comparison of the arrhythmic doses of epinephrine during Forane, halothane, and fluroxene anesthesia in dogs. Anesthesiology 1971;35:48–53.

180. Muir WW III, Hubbell JAE, Flaherty S. Increasing halothane concentration abolishes anesthesia-associated arrhythmias in cats and dogs. J Am Vet Med Assoc 1988;192:1730–1735.

181. Moore MA, Weiskopf RB, Eger EI II, et al. Arrhythmogenic doses of epinephrine are similar during desflurane or isoflurane anesthesia in humans. Anesthesiology 1993;79:943–947.

182. Munson ES, Tucker WK. Doses of epinephrine causing arrhythmia during enflurane, methoxyflurane and halothane anesthesia in dogs. Can Anaesth Soc J 1975;22:495–501.

183. Navarro R, Weiskopf RB, Moore MA, et al. Humans anesthetized with sevoflurane or isoflurane have similar arrhythmic response to epinephrine. Anesthesiology 1994;80:545–549.

184. Weiskopf RB, Eger EI II, Holmes MA, et al. Epinephrine-induced premature ventricular contractions and changes in arterial blood pressure and heart rate during I-653, isoflurane, and halothane anesthesia in swine. Anesthesiology 1989;70:293–298.

185. Johnston RR, Eger EI II, Wilson C. A comparative interaction of epinephrine with enflurane, isoflurane and halothane in man. Anesth Analg 1976;55:709–712.

186. Hikasa Y, Okabe C, Takase K, et al. Ventricular arrhythmogenic dose of adrenaline during sevoflurane, isoflurane, and halothane anaesthesia either with or without ketamine or thiopentone in cats. Res Vet Sci 1996;60:134–137.

187. Tucker WK, Rackstein AD, Munson ES. Comparison of arrhythmic doses of adrenaline, metaraminol, ephedrine, and phenylephrine during isoflurane and halothane anesthesia in dogs. Br J Anaesth 1974;46:392–396.

188. Maze M, Smith CM. Identification of receptor mechanisms mediating epinephrine-induced arrhythmias during halothane anesthesia in the dog. Anesthesiology 1983;59:322–326.

189. Light GS, Hellyer PW, Swanson CR. Parasympathetic influence on the arrhythmogenicity of graded dobutamine infusions in halothane-anesthetized horses. Am J Vet Res 1992;53:1154–1160.

190. Lemke KA, Tranquilli WJ, Thurmon JC, et al. Alterations in the arrhythmogenic dose of epinephrine after xylazine or medetomidine administration in halothane-anesthetized dogs. Am J Vet Res 1993;54:2132–2138.

191. Lemke KA, Tranquilli WJ, Thurmon JC, et al. Alterations in the arrhythmogenic dose of epinephrine after xylazine or medetomidine administration in isoflurane-anesthetized dogs. Am J Vet Res 1993;54:2139–2144.

192. Robertson BJ, Clement JL, Knill RL. Enhancement of the arrhythmogenic effect of hypercarbia by surgical stimulation during halothane anaesthesia in man. Can Anaesth Soc J 1981;28:342–349.

193. Cullen DJ, Eger EI II. Cardiovascular effects of carbon dioxide in man. Anesthesiology 1974;41:345–349.

194. Grandy JL, Hodgson DS, Dunlop CI, et al. Cardiopulmonary effects of halothane anesthesia in cats. Am J Vet Res 1989;50:1729–1732.

195. Bahlman SH, Eger EI II, Halsey MJ, et al. The cardiovascular effects of halothane in man during spontaneous ventilation. Anesthesiology 1972;36:494–502.

196. Cromwell TH, Stevens WC, Eger EI II, et al. The cardiovascular effects of compound 469 (Forane) during spontaneous ventilation and CO_2 challenge in man. Anesthesiology 1971;35:17–25.

197. Cullen LK, Steffey EP, Bailey CS, et al. Effect of high $PaCO_2$ and time on cerebrospinal fluid and intraocular pressure in halothane-anesthetized horses. Am J Vet Res 1990;51:300–304.

198. Yasuda N, Weiskopf RB, Cahalan MK, et al. Does desflurane modify circulatory responses to stimulation in humans? Anesth Analg 1991;73:175–179.

199. Zbinden AM, Petersenfelix S, Thomson DA. Anesthetic depth defined using multiple noxious stimuli during isoflurane/oxygen anesthesia. II. Hemodynamic responses. Anesthesiology 1994;80:261–267.

200. Eger EI II, Smith NT, Stoelting RK, et al. Cardiovascular effects of halothane in man. Anesthesiology 1970;32:396–409.

201. Eger EI II, Bowland T, Ionescu P, et al. Recovery and kinetic characteristics of desflurane and sevoflurane in volunteers after 8-h exposure, including kinetics of degradation products. Anesthesiology 1997;87:517–526.

202. Tayefeh F, Larson MD, Sessler DI, et al. Time-dependent changes in heart rate and pupil size during desflurane or sevoflurane anesthesia. Anesth Analg 1997;85:1362–1366.

203. Cullen BF, Eger EI II, Smith NT, et al. Cardiovascular effects of fluroxene in man. Anesthesiology 1970;32:218–230.

204. Libonati M, Cooperman LH, Price HL. Time-dependent circulatory effects of methoxyflurane in man. Anesthesiology 1971;34:439–444.

205. Gregory GA, Eger EI II, Smith NT. The cardiovascular effects of diethyl ether in man. Anesthesiology 1971;34:19–24.

206. Dunlop CI, Steffey EP, Miller MF, et al. Temporal effects of halothane and isoflurane in laterally recumbent ventilated male horses. Am J Vet Res 1987;48:1250–1255.

207. Steffey EP, Dunlop CI, Cullen LK, et al. Circulatory and respiratory responses of spontaneously breathing, laterally recumbent horses to 12 hours of halothane anesthesia. Am J Vet Res 1993;54:929–936.

208. Yamanaka T, Oku K, Koyama H, et al. Time-related changes of the cardiovascular system during maintenance anesthesia with sevoflurane and isoflurane in horses. J Vet Med Sci 2001;63:527–532.

209. Whitehair KJ, Steffey EP, Willits NH, et al. Recovery of horses from inhalation anesthesia. Am J Vet Res 1993;54:1693–1702.

210. Steffey EP, Woliner MJ, Dunlop C. Effects of five hours of constant 1.2 MAC halothane in sternally recumbent, spontaneously breathing horses. Equine Vet J 1990;22:433–436.

211. Shimosato S, Yasuda I. Cardiac performance during prolonged halothane anaesthesia in the cat. Br J Anaesth 1978;50:215–219.

212. Price HL, Skovsted P, Pauca AL, et al. Evidence for β-receptor activation produced by halothane in man. Anesthesiology 1970;32:389–395.

213. Steffey EP, Howland D Jr. Potency of halothane-N₂O in the horse. Am J Vet Res 1978;39:1141–1146.

214. Bahlman SH, Eger EI II, Smith NT, et al. The cardiovascular effects of nitrous oxide–halothane anesthesia in man. Anesthesiology 1971;35:274–255.

215. Eisele JH Jr. Cardiovascular effects of nitrous oxide. In: Eger EI II, ed. Nitrous Oxide/N₂O. New York: Elsevier, 1985;125–156.

216. Steffey EP, Eger EI II. Nitrous oxide in veterinary practice and animal research. In: Eger EI II, ed. Nitrous Oxide/N₂O. New York: Elsevier, 1984:305–312.

217. Grandy JL, Hodgson DS, Dunlop CI, et al. Cardiopulmonary effects of ephedrine in halothane-anesthetized horses. J Vet Pharmacol Ther 1989;12:389–396.

218. Dyson DH, Pascoe PJ. Influence of preinduction methoxamine, lactated Ringer solution, or hypertonic saline solution infusion or postinduction dobutamine infusion on anesthetic-induced hypotension in horses. Am J Vet Res 1990;51:17–21.

219. Swanson CR, Muir WW III, Bednarski RM, et al. Hemodynamic responses in halothane-anesthetized horses given infusions of dopamine or dobutamine. Am J Vet Res 1985;46:365–371.

220. Priano LL, Marrone B. Effect of halothane on renal hemodynamics during normovolemia and acute hemorrhagic hypovolemia. Anesthesiology 1985;63:357–364.

221. Gelman S, Fowler KC, Smith LR. Regional blood flow during isoflurane and halothane anesthesia. Anesth Analg 1984;63:557–566.

222. Steffey EP, Zinkl J, Howland DJ. Minimal changes in blood cell counts and biochemical values associated with prolonged isoflurane anesthesia of horses. Am J Vet Res 1979;40:1646–1648.

223. Steffey EP, Farver T, Zinkl J, et al. Alterations in horse blood cell count and biochemical values after halothane anesthesia. Am J Vet Res 1980;41:934–939.

224. Stover SM, Steffey EP, Dybdal NO, et al. Hematologic and biochemical values associated with multiple halothane anesthesias and minor surgical trauma of horses. Am J Vet Res 1988;49:236–241.

225. Steffey EP, Giri SN, Dunlop CI, et al. Biochemical and haematological changes following prolonged halothane anaesthesia in horses. Res Vet Sci 1993;55:338–345.

226. Nuñez E, Steffey EP, Ocampo L, et al. Effects of α₂-adrenergic receptor agonists on urine production in horses deprived of food and water. Am J Vet Res 2004;65:1342–1346.

227. Pedersoli WM. Blood serum inorganic ionic fluoride tetracycline and methoxyflurane anesthesia in dogs. J Am Anim Hosp Assoc 1977;13:242–246.

228. Mazze RI, Trudell JR, Cousins MJ. Methoxyflurane metabolism and renal dysfunction: Clinical correlation in man. Anesthesiology 1971;35:247–252.

229. Leiman BC, Katz J, Stanley TH, et al. Removal of tracheal secretions in anesthetized dogs: Balloon catheters versus suction. Anesth Analg 1987;66:529–533.

230. Mazze RI, Calverley RK, Smith NT. Inorganic fluoride nephrotoxicity: Prolonged enflurane and halothane anesthesia in volunteers. Anesthesiology 1977;46:265–271.

231. Kharasch ED, Hankins DC, Thummel KE. Human kidney methoxyflurane and sevoflurane metabolism: Intrarenal fluoride production as a possible mechanism of methoxyflurane nephrotoxicity. Anesthesiology 1995;82:689–699.

232. Newsome HH Jr, Turley GT, Kennerly M. Bioavailability of synthetic steroids for canine adrenal suppression. J Surg Res 1977;23:315–320.

233. Morio M, Fujii K, Satoh N, et al. Reaction of sevoflurane and its degradation products with soda lime. Anesthesiology 1992;77:1155–1164.

234. Gonsowski CT, Laster MJ, Eger EI II, et al. Toxicity of compound A in rats: Effect of a 3-hour administration. Anesthesiology 1994;80:556–565.

235. Gonsowski CT, Laster MJ, Eger EI II, et al. Toxicity of compound A in rats: Effect of increasing duration of administration. Anesthesiology 1994;80:566–573.

236. Kandel L, Laster MJ, Eger EI II, et al. Nephrotoxicity in rats undergoing a one-hour exposure to compound A. Anesth Analg 1995;81:559–563.

237. Frink EJ Jr, Malan TP Jr, Isner RJ, et al. Renal concentrating function with prolonged sevoflurane or enflurane anesthesia in volunteers. Anesthesiology 1994;80:1019–1025.

238. Muir WW III, Gadawski JE. Cardiorespiratory effects of low-flow and closed circuit inhalation anesthesia, using sevoflurane delivered with an in-circuit vaporizer and concentrations of compound A. Am J Vet Res 1998;59:603–608.

239. Reilly CS, Wood AJJ, Koshakji RP, et al. The effect of halothane on drug disposition: Contribution of changes in intrinsic drug metabolizing capacity and hepatic blood flow. Anesthesiology 1985;63:70–76.

240. Pearson GR, Bogan JA, Sanford J. An increase in the half-life of pentobarbitone with the administration of halothane in sheep. Br J Anaesth 1973;45:586–591.

241. Steffey EP, Martucci R, Howland D, et al. Meperidine-halothane interaction in dogs. Can Anaesth Soc J 1977;24:459–467.

242. Smith CM, Steffey EP, Baggot JD, et al. Effects of halothane anesthesia on the clearance of gentamicin sulfate in horses. Am J Vet Res 1988;49:19–22.

243. White PF, Johnston RR, Pudwill CR. Interaction of ketamine and halothane in rats. Anesthesiology 1975;42:179–186.

244. Subcommittee of the National Halothane Study of the Committee on Anesthesia NAS-NRC. Summary of the national halothane study: Possible association between halothane anesthesia and postoperative hepatic necrosis. J Am Med Assoc 1966;197:121–134.

245. Inman WHW, Mushin WW. Jaundice after repeated exposure to halothane: An analysis of reports to the Committee on Safety of Medicines. Br Med J 1974;1:5–10.

246. Gelman S, Fowler KC, Smith LR. Liver circulation and function during isoflurane and halothane anesthesia. Anesthesiology 1984;61:726–731.

247. Holmes MA, Weiskopf RB, Eger EI II, et al. Hepatocellular integrity in swine after prolonged desflurane (I-653) and isoflurane anesthesia: Evaluation of plasma alanine aminotransferase activity. Anesth Analg 1990;71:249–253.

248. Eger EI II, Johnson BH, Ferrell LD. Comparison of the toxicity of I-653 and isoflurane in rats: A test of the effect of repeated anesthesia and use of dry soda lime. Anesth Analg 1987;66:1230–1233.

249. Strum DP, Eger EI II, Johnson BH, et al. Toxicity of sevoflurane in rats. Anesth Analg 1987;66:769–773.

250. Eger EI II, Johnson BH, Strum DP, et al. Studies of the toxicity of I-653, halothane, and isoflurane in enzyme-induced, hypoxic rats. Anesth Analg 1987;66:1227–1230.

251. Ross JAS, Monk SJ, Duffy SW. Effect of nitrous oxide on halothane-induced hepatotoxicity in hypoxic, enzyme-induced rats. Br J Anaesth 1984;56:527–533.

252. Shingu K, Eger EI II, Johnson BH. Hypoxia per se can produce hepatic damage without death in rats. Anesth Analg 1982;61:820–823.

253. Shingu K, Eger EI II, Johnson BH. Hypoxia may be more important than reductive metabolism in halothane-induced hepatic injury. Anesth Analg 1982;61:824–827.

254. Whitehair KJ, Steffey EP, Woliner MJ, et al. Effects of inhalation anesthetic agents on response of horses to three hours of hypoxemia. Am J Vet Res 1996;57:351–360.

255. Reynolds ES, Moslen MT. Liver injury following halothane anesthesia in phenobarbital-pretreated rats. Biochem Pharmacol 1974;23:189–195.

256. Reynolds ES, Moslen MT. Halothane hepatotoxicity: Enhancement by polychlorinated biphenyl pretreatment. Anesthesiology 1977;47:19–27.

257. Cooperman LH, Warden JC, Price HL. Splanchnic circulation during nitrous oxide anesthesia and hypocarbia in normal man. Anesthesiology 1968;29:254–258.

258. Johnson EE, Hedley-Whyte J. Continuous positive-pressure ventilation and choledochoduodenal flow resistance. J Appl Physiol 1975;39:937–942.

259. Davis M, Eddleston ALWF, Neuberger JM, et al. Halothane hepatitis. N Engl J Med 1980;303:1123–1124.

260. Kitteringham NR, Kenna JG, Park BK. Detection of autoantibodies directed against human hepatic endoplasmic reticulum in sera from patients with halothane-associated hepatitis. Br J Clin Pharmacol 1995;40:379–386.

261. Farrell G, Prendergast D, Murray M. Halothane hepatitis: Detection of a constitutional susceptibility factor. N Engl J Med 1985;313:1310–1315.

262. Denborough MA, Forster JFP, Lovell RRH. Anaesthetic deaths in a family. Br J Anaesth 1962;34:395–396.

263. Gronert GA, Antognini JF, Pessah IN. Malignant hyperthermia. In: Miller RD, ed. Anesthesia, 5th ed. Philadelphia: Churchill Livingstone, 2000:1033–1052.

264. Hall LW, Woolf N, Bradley JWP, et al. Unusual reaction to suxamethonium chloride. Br Med J 1966;2:1305.

265. Kirmayer AH, Klide AM, Purvance JE. Malignant hyperthermia in a dog: Case report and review of the syndrome. J Am Vet Med Assoc 1984;185:978–983.

266. Deuster PA, Bockman EL, Muldoon SM. In vitro responses of cat skeletal muscle to halothane and caffeine. J Appl Physiol 1985;58:521–528.

267. Bagshaw RJ, Cox RH, Knight DH, et al. Malignant hyperthermia in a greyhound. J Am Vet Med Assoc 1978;172:61–62.

268. Rosenberg H, Waldron-Maese E. Malignant hyperpyrexia in horses: Anesthetic sensitivity proven by muscle biopsy. In: Abstracts of the Annual Meeting of the American Society of Anesthesiologists, 1977:333–334.

269. Hildebrand SV, Howitt GA. Succinylcholine infusion associated with hyperthermia in ponies anesthetized with halothane. Am J Vet Res 1983;44:2280–2284.

270. Short C, Paddleford RR. Malignant hyperthermia in the dog [Letter]. Anesthesiology 1973;39:462–463.

271. de Jong RH, Heavner JE, Amory DW. Malignant hyperpyrexia in the cat. Anesthesiology 1974;41:608–609.

272. Aleman M, Brosnan RJ, Williams DC, et al. Malignant hyperthermia in a horse anesthetized with halothane. J Vet Intern Med 2005;19:363–366.

273. Aleman M, Riehl J, Aldridge BM, et al. Association of a mutation in the ryanodine receptor 1 gene with equine malignant hyperthermia. Muscle Nerve 2004;30:356–365.

274. Epstein RM, Rackow H, Salanitre E, et al. Influence of the concentration effect on the uptake of anesthetic mixtures: The second gas effect. Anesthesiology 1964;25:364–371.

275. Stoelting RK, Eger EI II. An additional explanation for the second gas effect: A concentrating effect. Anesthesiology 1969;30:273–277.

276. Taheri S, Eger EI II. A demonstration of the concentration and second gas effects in humans anesthetized with nitrous oxide and desflurane. Anesth Analg 1999;89:774–780.

277. Liu WS, Wong KC, Port JD, et al. Epinephrine-induced arrhythmia during halothane anesthesia with the addition of nitrous oxide, nitrogen or helium in dogs. Anesth Analg 1982;61:414–417.

278. Lampe GH, Donegan JH, Rupp SM, et al. Nitrous oxide and epinephrine-induced arrhythmias. Anesth Analg 1990;71:602–605.

279. Philbin DM, Foex P, Drummond G, et al. Postsystolic shortening of canine left ventricle supplied by a stenotic coronary artery when nitrous oxide is added in the presence of narcotics. Anesthesiology 1985;62:166–174.

280. Leone BJ, Philbin DM, Lehot JJ, et al. Gradual or abrupt nitrous oxide administration in a canine model of critical coronary stenosis induces regional myocardial dysfunction that is worsened by halothane. Anesth Analg 1988;67:814–822.

281. Nathan HJ. Nitrous oxide worsens myocardial ischemia in isoflurane-anesthetized dogs. Anesthesiology 1988;68:407–416.

282. Diedericks J, Leone BJ, Foex P, et al. Nitrous oxide causes myocardial ischemia when added to propofol in the compromised canine myocardium. Anesth Analg 1993;76:1322–1326.

283. Saidman LJ, Hamilton WK. We should continue to use nitrous oxide. In: Eger EI II, ed. Nitrous Oxide/N$_2$O. New York: Elsevier, 1985:345–353.

284. Eger EI II, Lampe GH, Wauk LZ, et al. Clinical pharmacology of nitrous oxide: An argument for its continued use. Anesth Analg 1990;71:575–585.

285. Lampe GH, Wauk LZ, Whitendale P, et al. Nitrous oxide does not impair hepatic function in young or old surgical patients. Anesth Analg 1990;71:606–609.

286. Brodsky JB. Toxicity of nitrous oxide. In: Eger EI II, ed. Nitrous Oxide/N₂O. New York: Elsevier, 1985:259–279.

287. Lampe GH, Wauk LZ, Donegan JH, et al. Effect on outcome of prolonged exposure of patients to nitrous oxide. Anesth Analg 1990;71:586–590.

288. Waldman FM, Koblin DD, Lampe GH, et al. Hematologic effects of nitrous oxide in surgical patients. Anesth Analg 1990;71:618–624.

289. Nunn JF, Chanarin I. Nitrous oxide inactivates methionine synthetase. In: Eger EI II, ed. Nitrous Oxide/N₂O. New York: Elsevier, 1985:211–233.

290. Koblin DD, Tomerson BW, Waldman FM, et al. Effect of nitrous oxide on folate and vitamin B12 metabolism in patients. Anesth Analg 1990;71:610–617.

291. Layzer RB, Fishman RA, Schafer JA. Neuropathy following abuse of nitrous oxide. Neurology 1978;28:504–506.

292. Layzer RB. Myeloneuropathy after prolonged exposure to nitrous oxide. Lancet 1978;2:1227–1230.

293. Hong K, Trudell JR, O'Neil JR, et al. Biotransformation of nitrous oxide. Anesthesiology 1980;53:354–355.

294. Hong K, Trudell JR, O'Neil JR, et al. Metabolism of nitrous oxide by human and rat intestinal contents. Anesthesiology 1980;52:16–19.

295. Weathersby PK, Homer LD. Solubility of inert gases in biological fluids and tissues: A review. Undersea Biomed Res 1980;7:277–296.

296. Steffey EP, Johnson BH, Eger EI II, et al. Nitrous oxide increases the accumulation rate and decreases the uptake of bowel gases. Anesth Analg 1979;58:405–408.

297. Eger EI II, Saidman LJ. Hazards of nitrous oxide anesthesia in bowel obstruction and pneumothorax. Anesthesiology 1965;26:61–66.

298. Steffey EP, Gauger GE, Eger EI II. Cardiovascular effects of venous air embolism during air and oxygen breathing. Anesth Analg 1974;53:599–604.

299. Munson ES, Merrick HC. Effect of nitrous oxide on venous air embolism. Anesthesiology 1966;27:783–787.

300. Davis I, Moore JRM, Lahiri SK. Nitrous oxide and the middle ear. Anaesthesia 1979;34:147–151.

301. Perreault L, Normandin N, Plamondon L, et al. Middle ear pressure variations during nitrous oxide and oxygen anaesthesia. Can Anaesth Soc J 1982;29:428–434.

302. Saidman LJ, Eger EI II. Change in cerebrospinal fluid pressure during pneumoencephalography under nitrous oxide anesthesia. Anesthesiology 1965;26:67–72.

303. Stanley TH, Kawamura R, Graves C. Effects of N₂O on volume and pressure of endotracheal tube cuffs. Anesthesiology 1974;41:256–262.

304. Stanley TH. Effects of anesthetic gases on endotracheal tube cuff gas volumes. Anesth Analg 1974;53:480–482.

305. Stanley TH. Nitrous oxide and pressures and volumes of high- and low-pressure endotracheal-tube cuffs in intubated patients. Anesthesiology 1975;42:637–640.

306. Bednarski RM. Advantages and guidelines for using nitrous oxide. Vet Clin North Am Small Anim Pract 1992;22:313–314.

307. Klide AM, Haskins SC. Precautions when using nitrous oxide. Vet Clin North Am Small Anim Pract 1992;22:314–316.

308. Linde HW, Bruce DL. Occupational exposure of anesthetists to halothane, nitrous oxide and radiation. Anesthesiology 1969;30:363–368.

309. Whitcher CE, Cohen EN, Trudell JR. Chronic exposure to anesthetic gases in the operating room. Anesthesiology 1971;35:348–353.

310. Ward GS, Byland RR. Concentrations of methoxyflurane and nitrous oxide in veterinary operating rooms. Am J Vet Res 1982;43:360–362.

311. Ward GS, Byland RR. Concentrations of halothane in veterinary operating and treatment rooms. J Am Vet Med Assoc 1982;180:174–177.

312. Milligan JE, Sablan JL, Short CE. A survey of waste anesthetic gas concentrations in US Air Force veterinary surgeries. J Am Vet Med Assoc 1980;177:1021–1022.

313. Dreesen DW, Jones GL, Brown J, et al. Monitoring for trace anesthetic gases in a veterinary teaching hospital. J Am Vet Med Assoc 1981;179:797–799.

314. Manley SV, McDonell WF. Recommendations for reduction of anesthetic gas pollution. J Am Vet Med Assoc 1980;176:519–524.

315. Manley SV, Taloff P, Aberg N, et al. Occupational exposure to waste anesthetic gases in veterinary practice. Calif Vet 1982;36:14–19.

316. Pfaffli P, Nikki P, Ahlman K. Halothane and nitrous oxide in end-tidal air and venous blood of surgical personnel. Ann Clin Res 1972;4:273–277.

317. Corbett TH. Retention of anesthetic agents following occupational exposure. Anesth Analg 1973;52:614–618.

318. Ad Hoc Committee on Effects of Trace Anesthetic Agents on Health of Operating Room Personnel. Waste Anesthetic Gases in Operating Room Air: A Suggested Program to Reduce Personnel Exposure. Park Ridge, IL: American Society of Anesthesiologists, 1983:1–19.

319. Cohen EN, Bellville JW, Brown BW. Anesthesia, pregnancy, and miscarriage: A study of operating room nurses and anesthetists. Anesthesiology 1971;35:343–347.

320. Cohen EN, Brown BW Jr, Bruce DL, et al. A survey of anesthetic health hazards among dentists. J Am Dent Assoc 1975;90:1291–1296.

321. Lecky JH. Anesthetic pollution in the operating room: A notice to operating room personnel. Anesthesiology 1980;52:157–159.

322. Berry A, McGregor DG, Baden JM, et al. Waste Anesthetic Gases: Information for Management in Anesthetizing Areas and the Postanesthetic Care Unit (PACU). Park Ridge, IL: American Society of Anesthesiologists, 2005:1–45.

323. Karzai W, Haberstroh J, Muller W, et al. Rapid increase in inspired desflurane concentration does not elicit a hyperdynamic circulatory response in the pig. Lab Anim 1997;31:279–282.

324. Rodgers RC, Hill GE. Equations for vapour pressure versus temperature: Derivation and use of the Antoine equation on a hand-held programmable calculator. Br J Anaesth 1978;50:415–424.

325. Susay SR, Smith MA, Lockwood GG. The saturated vapor pressure of desflurane at various temperatures. Anesth Analg 1996;83:864–866.

326. Eger EI II. Desflurane animal and human pharmacology: Aspects of kinetics, safety, and MAC. Anesth Analg 1992;75:S3–S9.

327. Webb AI, Weaver BMQ. Solubility of halothane in equine tissues at 37°C. Br J Anaesth 1981;53:479–486.

328. Targ AG, Yasuda N, Eger EI II. Solubility of I–653, sevoflurane, isoflurane, and halothane in plastics and rubber composing a conventional anesthetic circuit. Anesth Analg 1989;69:218–225.

329. Cascorbi HF, Blake DA, Helrich M. Differences in the biotransformation of halothane in man. Anesthesiology 1970;32:119–123.

330. Shiraishi Y, Ikeda K. Uptake and biotransformation of sevoflurane in humans: A comparative study of sevoflurane with halothane, enflurane and isoflurane. J Clin Anesth 1990;2:377–380.

331. Chase RE, Holaday DA, Fiserova-Bergerova V, et al. The biotransformation of ethrane in man. Anesthesiology 1971;35:262–267.

332. Holaday DA, Fiserova-Bergerova V, Latto IP, et al. Resistance of isoflurane to biotransformation in man. Anesthesiology 1975; 43:325–332.

333. McMurphy RM, Hodgson DS. The minimum alveolar concentration of desflurane in cats. Vet Surg 1995;24:453–455.

334. Barter LS, Ilkiw JE, Steffey EP, et al. Animal dependence of inhaled anaesthetic requirements in cats. Br J Anaesth 2004;92:275–277.

335. Webb AI, McMurphy RM. Effect of anticholinergic preanesthetic medicaments on the requirements of halothane for anesthesia in the cat. Am J Vet Res 1987;48:1733–1736.

336. Ide T, Sakurai Y, Aono M, et al. Minimum alveolar anesthetic concentrations for airway occlusion in cats: A new concept of minimum alveolar anesthetic concentration airway occlusion response. Anesth Analg 1998;86:191–197.

337. Steffey EP, Gillespie JR, Berry JD, et al. Anesthetic potency (MAC) of nitrous oxide in the dog, cat and stumptail monkey. J Appl Physiol 1974;36:530–532.

338. Drummond JC, Todd MM, Shapiro HM. Minimal alveolar concentrations for halothane, enflurane, and isoflurane in the cat. J Am Vet Med Assoc 1983;182:1099–1101.

339. Ilkiw JE, Pascoe PJ, Fisher LD. Effect of alfentanil on the minimum alveolar concentration of isoflurane in cats. Am J Vet Res 1997;58:1274–1279.

340. Pypendop BH, Ilkiw JE. The effects of intravenous lidocaine administration on the minimum alveolar concentration of isoflurane in cats. Anesth Analg 2005;100:97–101.

341. Doi M, Yunoki H, Ikeda K. The minimum alveolar concentration of sevoflurane in cats. J Anesth 1988;2:113–114.

342. Steffey EP, Howland D Jr. Halothane anesthesia in calves. Am J Vet Res 1979;40:372–376.

343. Cantalapierdra AG, Villanueva B, Pereira JL. Anaesthetic potency of isoflurane in cattle: Determination of the minimum alveolar concentration. Vet Anaesth Analg 2000;27:22–26.

344. Doorley MB, Waters SJ, Terrell RC, et al. MAC of I-653 in beagle dogs and New Zealand white rabbits. Anesthesiology 1988;69:89–92.

345. Wang BG, Tang J, White PF, et al. The effect of GP683, an adenosine kinase inhibitor, on the desflurane anesthetic requirement in dogs. Anesth Analg 1997;85:675–680.

346. Hammond RA, Alibhai HIK, Walsh KP, et al. Desflurane in the dog: Minimum alveolar concentration (MAC) alone and in combination with nitrous oxide. J Vet Anaesth 1994;21:21–23.

347. Eger EI II, Saidman LJ, Brandstater B. Temperature dependence of halothane and cyclopropane anesthesia in dogs: Correlation with some theories of anesthetic action. Anesthesiology 1965;26:764–770.

348. Eger EI II, Brandstater B, Saidman LJ, et al. Equipotent alveolar concentrations of methoxyflurane, halothane, diethyl ether, fluroxene, cyclopropane, xenon, and nitrous oxide in the dog. Anesthesiology 1965;26:771–777.

349. Regan MJ, Eger EI II. Effect of hypothermia in dogs on anesthetizing and apneic doses of inhalation agents: Determination of the anesthetic index (apnea/MAC). Anesthesiology 1967;28:689–700.

350. Kazama T, Ikeda K. Comparison of MAC and the rate of rise of alveolar concentration of sevoflurane with halothane and isoflurane in the dog. Anesthesiology 1988;68:435–438.

351. Steffey EP, Eger EI II. Hyperthermia and halothane MAC in the dog. Anesthesiology 1974;41:392–396.

352. Himez RS Jr, DiFazio CA, Burmey RC. Effects of lidocaine on the anesthetic requirements of nitrous oxide and halothane. Anesthesiology 1977;47:437–440.

353. Schwieger IM, Szlam F, Hug CC. Absence of agonistic or antagonistic effect of flumazenil (Ro 15-1788) in dogs anesthetized with enflurane, isoflurane, or fentanyl-enflurane. Anesthesiology 1989; 70:477–481.

354. Schwartz AE, Maneksha FR, Kanchuger MS, et al. Flumazenil decreases the minimum alveolar concentration of isoflurane in dogs. Anesthesiology 1989;70:764–767.

355. DeYoung DJ, Sawyer DC. Anesthetic potency of nitrous oxide during halothane anesthesia in the dog. J Am Anim Hosp Assoc 1980;16:125–128.

356. Murat I, Housmans PR. Minimum alveolar concentrations of halothane, enflurane, and isoflurane in ferrets. Anesthesiology 1988;68:783–787.

357. Imai A, Steffey EP, Farver TB, et al. Assessment of isoflurane-induced anesthesia in ferrets and rats. Am J Vet Res 1999;60: 1577–1583.

358. Hikasa Y, Okuyama K, Kakuta T, et al. Anesthetic potency and cardiopulmonary effects of sevoflurane in goats: Comparison with isoflurane and halothane. Can J Vet Res 1998;62:299–306.

359. Antognini JF, Eisele PH. Anesthetic potency and cardiopulmonary effects of enflurane, halothane, and isoflurane in goats. Lab Anim Sci 1993;43:607–610.

360. Doherty TJ, Rohrbach BW, Geiser DR. Effect of acepromazine and butorphanol on isoflurane minimum alveolar concentration in goats. J Vet Pharmacol Ther 2002;25:65–67.

361. Doherty TJ, Rohrbach BW, Ross L, et al. The effect of tiletamine and zolazepam on isoflurane minimum alveolar concentration in goats. J Vet Pharmacol Ther 2002;25:233–235.

362. Doherty TJ, Will WA, Rohrbach BW, et al. Effect of morphine and flunixin meglumine on isoflurane minimum alveolar concentration in goats. Vet Anaesth Analg 2004;31:97–101.

363. Tendillo FJ, Mascias A, Santos M, et al. Anesthetic potency of desflurane in the horse: Determination of the minimum alveolar concentration. Vet Surg 1997;26:354–357.

364. Steffey EP, Willits N, Woliner M. Hemodynamic and respiratory responses to variable arterial partial pressure of oxygen in halothane-anesthetized horses during spontaneous and controlled ventilation. Am J Vet Res 1992;53:1850–1858.

365. Pascoe PJ, Steffey EP, Black WD, et al. Evaluation of the effect of alfentanil on the minimum alveolar concentration on halothane in horses. Am J Vet Res 1993;54:1327–1332.

366. Steffey EP, Pascoe PJ. Detomidine reduces isoflurane anesthetic requirement (MAC) in horses. Vet Anaesth Analg 2002;29: 223–227.

367. Steffey EP, Pascoe PJ, Woliner MJ, et al. Effects of xylazine hydrochloride during isoflurane-induced anesthesia in horses. Am J Vet Res 2000;61:1225–1231.

368. Aida H, Mizuno Y, Hobo S, et al. Determination of the minimum alveolar concentration (MAC) and physical response to sevoflurane inhalation in horses. J Vet Med Sci 1994;56:1161–1165.

369. Steffey EP, Mama KR, Galey F, et al. Effects of sevoflurane in horses. Am J Vet Res 2005;66:606–614.

370. Tinker JH, Sharbough FW, Michenfelder TD. Anterior shift of the dominant EEG rhythm during anesthesia in the Java monkey. Anesthesiology 1977;46:252–259.

371. Sonner JM, Gong D, Eger EI II. Naturally occurring variability in anesthetic potency among inbred mouse strains. Anesth Analg 2000;91:720–726.

372. Mazze RI, Rice SA, Baden JM. Halothane, isoflurane, and enflurane MAC in pregnant and nonpregnant female and male mice and rats. Anesthesiology 1985;62:339–342.

373. Deady JR, Koblin DD, Eger EI II, et al. Anesthetic potencies and the unitary theory of narcosis. Anesth Analg 1981;60:380–384.

374. Quinlan JJ, Homanics GE, Firestone LL. Anesthesia sensitivity in mice that lack the β3 subunit of the γ-aminobutyric acid type A receptor. Anesthesiology 1998;88:775–780.

375. Dahan A, Sarton E, Teppema L, et al. Anesthetic potency and influence of morphine and sevoflurane on respiration in mu-opioid receptor knockout mice. Anesthesiology 2001;94:824–832.

376. Miller KW, Paton WDM, Smith EB, et al. Physiochemical approaches to the mode of action of general anesthetics. Anesthesiology 1972;36:339–351.

377. Lerman J, Oyston JP, Gallagher TM, et al. The minimum alveolar concentration (MAC) and hemodynamic effects of halothane, isoflurane, and sevoflurane in newborn swine. Anesthesiology 1990;73:717–721.

378. Tranquilli WJ, Thurmon JC, Benson GJ, et al. Halothane potency in pigs (Sus scrofa). Am J Vet Res 1983;44:1106–1107.

379. Weiskopf R, Bogetz MS. Minimum alveolar concentrations (MAC) of halothane and nitrous oxide in swine. Anesth Analg 1984;63:529–532.

380. Lundeen G, Manohar M, Parks C. Systemic distribution of blood flow in swine while awake and during 1.0 and 1.5 MAC isoflurane anesthesia with or without 50% nitrous oxide. Anesth Analg 1983;62:499–512.

381. Eisele PH, Talken L, Eisele JH Jr. Potency of isoflurane and nitrous oxide in conventional swine. Lab Anim Sci 1985;35:76–78.

382. Tranquilli WJ, Thurmon JC, Benson GJ. Anesthetic potency of nitrous oxide in young swine (Sus scrofa). Am J Vet Res 1985;46:58–61.

383. Gallagher TM, Burrows FA, Miyasaka K, et al. Sevoflurane in newborn swine: Anesthetic requirements (MAC) and circulatory responses [Abstract]. Anesthesiology 1987;67:A503.

384. Hecker KE, Baumert JH, Horn N, et al. Minimum anesthetic concentration of sevoflurane with different xenon concentrations in swine. Anesth Analg 2003;97:1364–1369.

385. Wear R, Robinson S, Gregory GA. Effect of halothane on baroresponse of adult and baby rabbits. Anesthesiology 1982;56:188–191.

386. Davis NL, Nunnally RL, Malinin TI. Determination of the minimum alveolar concentration (MAC) of halothane in the white New Zealand rabbit. Br J Anaesth 1975;47:341–345.

387. Sobair ATH, Cottrell DF, Camburn MA. Focal heat stimulation for the determination of the minimum alveolar concentration of halothane in the rabbit. Vet Res Commun 1997;21:149–159.

388. Drummond JC. MAC for halothane, enflurane, and isoflurane in the New Zealand white rabbit: And a test for the validity of MAC determinations. Anesthesiology 1985;62:336–339.

389. Imai A, Steffey EP, Ilkiw JE, et al. Comparison of clinical signs and hemodynamic variables used to monitor rabbits during halothane- and isoflurane-induced anesthesia. Am J Vet Res 1999;60:1189–1195.

390. McLain GE, Sipes IG, Brown B, et al. The noncompetitive N-methyl-D-aspartate receptor antagonist, MK-810 profoundly reduces volatile anesthetic requirements. Neuropharmacology 1989;28:677–681.

391. Shi WZ, Fahey MR, Fisher DM, et al. Increase in minimum alveolar concentration (MAC) of halothane by laudanosine in rabbits [Abstract]. Anesth Analg 1985;64:282.

392. Scheller MS, Saidman LJ, Partridge BL. MAC of sevoflurane in humans and the New Zealand white rabbit. Can J Anaesth 1988;35:153–157.

393. Eger EI II, Johnson BH. MAC of I-653 in rats, including a test of the effect of body temperature and anesthetic duration. Anesth Analg 1987;66:974–977.

394. Yost CS, Hampson AJ, Leonoudakis D, et al. Oleamide potentiates benzodiazepine-sensitive γ-aminobutyric acid receptor activity but does not alter minimum alveolar anesthetic concentration. Anesth Analg 1998;86:1294–1300.

395. Laster MJ, Liu J, Eger EI II, et al. Electrical stimulation as a substitute for the tail clamp in the determination of minimum alveolar concentration. Anesth Analg 1993;76:1310–1312.

396. Taheri S, Halsey MJ, Liu J, et al. What solvent best represents the site of action of inhaled anesthetics in humans, rats, and dogs? Anesth Analg 1991;72:627–634.

397. Vitez TS, White PF, Eger EI II. Effects of hypothermia on halothane MAC and isoflurane MAC in the rat. Anesthesiology 1974;41:80–81.

398. Cole DJ, Kalichman MW, Shapiro HM, et al. The nonlinear potency of sub-MAC concentrations of nitrous oxide in decreasing the anesthetic requirement of enflurane, halothane, and isoflurane in rats. Anesthesiology 1990;73:93–99.

399. Steffey MA, Brosnan RJ, Steffey EP. Assessment of halothane and sevoflurane anesthesia in spontaneously breathing rats. Am J Vet Res 2003;64:470–474.

400. Crawford MW, Lerman J, Saldivia V, et al. Hemodynamic and organ blood flow responses to halothane and sevoflurane anesthesia during spontaneous ventilation. Anesth Analg 1992;75:1000–1006.

401. White PF, Johnston RR, Eger EI II. Determination of anesthetic requirement in rats. Anesthesiology 1974;40:52–57.

402. Strout CD, Nahrwold MC. Halothane requirement during pregnancy and lactation in rats. Anesthesiology 1981;55:322–323.

403. Roizen MF, White PF, Eger EI II, et al. Effects of ablation of serotonin or norepinephrine brain-stem areas on halothane and cyclopropane MACs in rats. Anesthesiology 1978;49:252–255.

404. Waizer PR, Baez S, Orkin LR. A method for determining minimum alveolar concentration of anesthetic in the rat. Anesthesiology 1973;39:394–397.

405. Russell GB, Graybeal JM. Differences in anesthetic potency between Sprague-Dawley and Long-Evans rats for isoflurane but not nitrous oxide. Pharmacology 1995;50:162–167.

406. Rampil IJ, Laster M. No correlation between quantitative electroencephalographic measures and movement response to noxious stimuli during isoflurane anesthesia in rats. Anesthesiology 1992;77:920–925.

407. DiFazio CA, Brown RE, Ball CG, et al. Additive effects of anesthetics and theories of anesthesia. Anesthesiology 1972;36:57–63.

408. Russell GB, Graybeal JM. Direct measurement of nitrous oxide MAC and neurologic monitoring in rats during anesthesia under hyperbaric conditions. Anesth Analg 1992;75:995–999.

409. Gonsowski CT, Eger EI II. Nitrous oxide minimum alveolar anesthetic concentration in rats is greater than previously reported. Anesth Analg 1994;79:710–712.

410. Palahniuk RJ, Shnider SM, Eger EI II. Pregnancy decreases the requirement for inhaled anesthetic agents. Anesthesiology 1974;41:82–83.

411. Rampil IJ, Lockhart SH, Zwass MS, et al. Clinical characteristics of desflurane in surgical patients: Minimum alveolar concentration. Anesthesiology 1991;74:429–433.

412. Miller RD, Wahrenbrock EA, Schroeder CF, et al. Ethylene-halothane anesthesia: Addition or synergism? Anesthesiology 1969;31:301–304.

413. Saidman LJ, Eger EI II. Effect of nitrous oxide and of narcotic premedication on the alveolar concentration of halothane required for anesthesia. Anesthesiology 1964;25:302–306.

414. Gibbons RT, Steffey EP, Eger EI II. The effect of spontaneous versus controlled ventilation on the rate of rise of alveolar halothane concentration in dogs. Anesth Analg 1977;56:32–34.

415. Saidman LJ, Eger EI II, Munson ES, et al. Minimum alveolar concentrations of methoxyflurane, halothane, ether and cyclopropane in man: Correlation with theories of anesthesia. Anesthesiology 1967;28:994–1002.

416. Stevens WC, Dolan WM, Gibbons RD, et al. Minimum alveolar concentrations (MAC) of isoflurane with and without nitrous oxide in patients of various ages. Anesthesiology 1975;42:197–200.

417. Kimura T, Watanabe S, Asakura N, et al. Determination of end-tidal sevoflurane concentration for tracheal intubation and minimum alveolar anesthetic concentration in adults. Anesth Analg 1994;79:378–381.

418. Katoh T, Ikeda K. The minimum alveolar concentration (MAC) of sevoflurane in humans. Anesthesiology 1987;66:301–304.

419. Katoh T, Ikeda K. The effect of clonidine on sevoflurane requirements for anaesthesia and hypnosis. Anaesthesia 2005;52:364–381.

420. Katoh T, Ikeda K. The effects of fentanyl on sevoflurane requirements for loss of consciousness and skin incision. Anesthesiology 1998;88:18–24.

421. Katoh T, Kobayashi S, Suzuki A, et al. The effect of fentanyl on sevoflurane requirements for somatic and sympathetic responses to surgical incision. Anesthesiology 1999;90:398–405.

422. Suzuki A, Katoh T, Ikeda K. The effect of adenosine triphosphate on sevoflurane requirements for minimum alveolar anesthetic concentration and minimum alveolar anesthetic concentration awake. Anesth Analg 1998;86:179–183.

423. Hornbein TF, Eger EI II, Winter PM, et al. The minimum alveolar concentration of nitrous oxide in man. Anesth Analg 1982;61:553–556.

424. Curro TG, Brunson DB, Paul-Murphy J. Determination of the ED50 of isoflurane and evaluation of the isoflurane-sparing effect of butorphanol in cockatoos (Cacatua spp.). Vet Surg 1994;23:429–433.

425. Ludders JW, Rode J, Mitchell GS. Isoflurane anesthesia in sandhill cranes (Grus canadensis): Minimal anesthetic concentration and cardiopulmonary dose-response during spontaneous and controlled breathing. Anesth Analg 1989;68:511–516.

426. Ludders JW. Minimal anesthetic concentration (MAC) and cardiopulmonary dose-response of halothane in Pekin ducks [Abstract]. J Vet Anaesth Suppl 1991:131.

427. Ludders JW, Mitchell GS, Rode J. Minimal anesthetic concentration and cardiopulmonary dose response of isoflurane in ducks. Vet Surg 1990;19:304–307.

428. Fitzgerald G, Blais D. Effect of nitrous oxide on the minimal anesthetic dose of isoflurane in pigeons and red-tailed hawks [Abstract]. In: Proceedings, Fourth International Congress of Veterinary Anaesthesia, Utrecht, The Netherlands, 1991:27.

429. Cherkin A, Catchpool JF. Temperature dependence of anesthesia in goldfish. Science 1964;144:1460–1462.

430. Shim CY, Andersen NB. The effects of oxygen on minimal anesthetic requirements in the toad. Anesthesiology 1971;34:333–337.

431. Wouters P, Doursout M-F, Merin RG, et al. Influence of hypertension on MAC of halothane in rats. Anesthesiology 1990;72:843–845.

432. Zucker J. Central cholinergic depression reduces MAC for isoflurane in rats. Anesth Analg 1991;72:790–795.

433. Stone DJ, Moscicki JC, DiFazio CA. Thiopental reduces halothane MAC in rats. Anesth Analg 1992;74:542–546.

434. Doherty TJ, Geiser DR, Rohrbach BW. Effect of acepromazine and butorphanol on halothane minimum alveolar concentration in ponies. Equine vet J 1997;29:374–376.

435. Heard DJ, Webb AI, Daniels RT. Effect of acepromazine on the anesthetic requirement of halothane in the dog. Am J Vet Res 1986;47:2113–2116.

436. Webb AI, O'Brien JM. The effect of acepromazine maleate on the anesthetic potency of halothane and isoflurane. J Am Anim Hosp Assoc 1988;24:609–615.

437. Matthews NS, Dollar NS, Shawley RV. Halothane-sparing effect of benzodiazepines in ponies. Cornell Vet 1990;80:259–265.

438. Hellyer PW, Mama KR, Shafford HL, et al. Effects of diazepam and flumazenil on minimum alveolar concentrations for dogs anesthetized with isoflurane or a combination of isoflurane and fentanyl. Am J Vet Res 2001;62:555–560.

439. Perisho JA, Buechel DR, Miller RD. The effect of diazepam on minimum alveolar anesthetic requirement (MAC) in man. [Abstract] Can Anaesth Soc J 1971;18:536.

440. Murphy MR, Hug CC Jr. The anesthetic potency of fentanyl in terms of its reduction of enflurane MAC. Anesthesiology 1982;57:485–488.

441. Ewing KK, Mohammed HO, Scarlett JM, et al. Reduction of isoflurane anesthetic requirement by medetomidine and its restoration by atipamezole in dogs. Am J Vet Res 1993;54:294–299.

442. Gross ME, Clifford CA, Hardy DA. Excitement in an elephant after intravenous administration of atropine. J Am Vet Med Assoc 1994;205:1437–1438.

443. Melvin MA, Johnson BH, Quasha AL, et al. Induction of anesthesia with midazolam decreases halothane MAC in humans. Anesthesiology 1982;57:238–241.

444. Lambert-Zechovsky N, Bingen E, Bourillon A, et al. Effects of antibiotics on the microbial intestinal ecosystem. Dev Pharmacol Ther 1984;7:150–157.

445. Doherty TJ, McDonell WN, Dyson DH, et al. The effect of a 5-hydroxytryptamine antagonist (R51703) on halothane MAC in the dog. J Vet Pharmacol Ther 1995;18:153–155.

446. Weiskopf RB, Holmes MA, Rampil IJ, et al. Cardiovascular safety and actions of high concentrations of I-653 and isoflurane in swine. Anesthesiology 1989;70:793–799.

Chapter 14
Local Anesthetics

Roman T. Skarda and William J. Tranquilli

Introduction

Local anesthetics are a group of chemically related compounds that reversibly bind sodium channels and block impulse conduction in nerve fibers.[1] The interruption of neural transmission in sensory afferent nerves or tracts by a local anesthetic drug after local tissue infiltration, regional nerve blocks, or epidural or intrathecal (subarachnoid) injection uniquely and most effectively prevents or reduces pain or nociceptive input during and after surgery. Analgesia in the desensitized area is not only complete by such techniques, but it also removes the immediate secondary (central) sensitization to pain and reduces the central facilitation of the nociceptive pathway. The use of a local anesthetic is essential if surgery is to be performed in a conscious patient and the pain associated with trauma and inflammation is to be relieved. The use of a local anesthetic technique before surgery may also benefit patients by avoiding general anesthesia or reducing the amount of required general anesthetics. Sustained analgesia into the recovery period is a great benefit to patients when a local anesthetic with a longer anesthetic effect is used. Knowledge of the clinical pharmacology of individual local anesthetics enables the achievement of effective and safe neural blockade. Each of the local anesthetic techniques discussed herein has its own particular rate of onset, duration, and risk of complication.

History

The 100-year history of local anesthetic use in humans has typically involved self-experimentation, followed by widespread application with little testing for electrophysiology and neurotoxicity in animals and humans. Desensitization of a body region dates from 1884, when Koller reported the first topical use of cocaine for rendering the eye temporarily insensible to pain at the Congress of the German Society for Ophthalmology.[2] However, cocaine was found to be extremely toxic and addictive. Einhorn synthesized procaine, the first nontoxic prototype of amino-ester local anesthetics, in 1904. Subsequently, other amino-ester local anesthetics, including tetracaine in 1932 and 2-chloroprocaine in 1955, were synthesized. The next milestone in local anesthetic synthesis was in 1943, when Lofgren developed lidocaine, the prototype for all subsequent amide-type local anesthetics. Within 60 years thereafter, additional amide local anesthetics were produced, including mepivacaine (1956), bupivacaine (1957), prilocaine (1959), etidocaine (1971), articaine (1974), and ropivacaine (1980s).[3,4] Levobupivacaine is the newest member of the

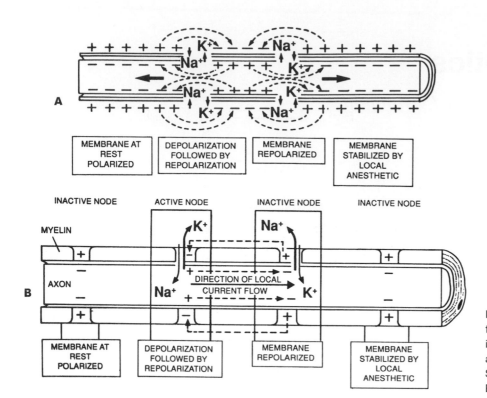

MEMBRANE AT REST POLARIZED | DEPOLARIZATION FOLLOWED BY REPOLARIZATION | MEMBRANE REPOLARIZED | MEMBRANE STABILIZED BY LOCAL ANESTHETIC

INACTIVE NODE   ACTIVE NODE   INACTIVE NODE   INACTIVE NODE

MYELIN

AXON

DIRECTION OF LOCAL CURRENT FLOW

MEMBRANE AT REST POLARIZED | DEPOLARIZATION FOLLOWED BY REPOLARIZATION | MEMBRANE REPOLARIZED | MEMBRANE STABILIZED BY LOCAL ANESTHETIC

Fig. 14.1. Sodium-ion and potassium-ion flux across the axolemma and propagation of impulse: an unmyelinated nerve fiber **(A)** and a myelinated nerve fiber **(B)**. Reprinted from Skarda,[224] p. 200, with permission from Elsevier.

amino-amide class of long-lasting local anesthetics approved by the Food and Drug Administration (FDA) in 1999.

Electrophysiological Effects

The conduction of impulses in excitable membranes requires a flow of sodium ions through selective sodium channels into the nerve in response to depolarization of the nerve membrane.[5] Mammalian voltage-gated sodium channels consist of one large alpha subunit that contains four homologous domains (D1 to D4), each with six putative α-helical transmembrane segments (S1 to S6) and one or two smaller auxiliary beta subunits.[6] Under resting conditions, sodium ions are at a higher concentration outside than inside the nerve, and a voltage difference across the axonal membrane, known as *resting potential*, of −70 mV exists. When the nerve is stimulated, the permeability of the membrane to sodium ions increases transiently, and sodium passes through the membrane by way of sodium-selective ionic channels that exist in various conformations (i.e., resting, open, or inactivated), depending on the transmembrane potential, depolarizing the plasma membrane. During the depolarization, the action potential moves in obligatory fashion along the axon, allowing for impulse propagation along the nerve membrane (Fig. 14.1). After a few milliseconds, the membrane repolarizes as a result of inactivation or "closing" of the sodium channels. During repolarization, the membrane is no longer permeable to sodium ions, but potassium channels open, and potassium ions flow down their electrochemical gradient out of the cell.[1]

Mechanisms of Action

The precise mode of action of local anesthetic drugs is unknown. A number of theories have been offered: (a) the surface-charge theory (benzene's lipophilic end binds to the membrane hydrophilic end in solution and increases the transmembrane potential), (b) the membrane-expansion theory (benzocaine expands the axonal membrane, compressing the ionic channels), (c) the specific-receptor theory (the biotoxins tetrodoxin and saxitoxin bind to receptors at the external surface at or near the sodium channels, producing a potent conduction block, and (d) the combination membrane-expansion and specific-receptor theory. In this theory, the quaternary ammonium compounds (amides) and ester local anesthetics first pass through the cell membrane as the uncharged base (B) to reach the intracellular site where the uncharged base is protonated and the charged cation (conjugated acid, BH^+) binds to the receptor and "plugs" the channel (Fig. 14.2).[1] Charged or hydrophilic drugs reach the receptor primarily through the open sodium channels and bind more strongly to the closed than open channel. Highly lipid-soluble molecules approach the receptor through the membrane. Perhaps best accepted is the idea that local anesthesia results when local anesthetics bind to sodium-selective ionic channels in nerves, inhibiting the sodium permeability that underlies action potential and depolarization of the cell membrane.[7] Electrical transmission through a myelinated axon stops when enough concentration of the anesthetic is applied to bathe at least three consecutive nodes of Ranvier.[8,9] More recently, local anesthetic binding has been mapped to homologue domains D4 to S6 and inactivation to D3

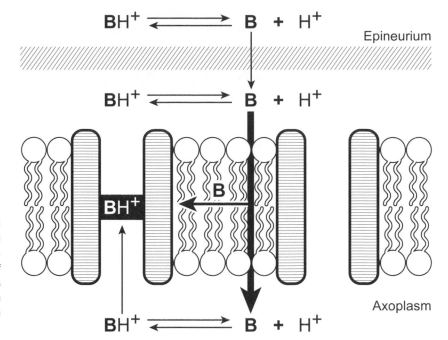

Fig. 14.2. Site of action of amino-ester and amino-amide local anesthetics. The uncharged base form diffuses most readily across the lipid barriers and interacts at the intermembrane portion of the sodium channel. The charged form (BH+) gains access to a specific receptor via the axoplasmic surface of the sodium channel pore. Modified from Carpenter and Mackey,[76] p. 414, with permission.

to S6 of α-helical transmembrane segments of membrane proteins in sodium channels.[6]

Frequency-Dependent Block

Local anesthetics may differ in their ability to bind to sodium channels, depending on the channel status.[10] Open ion-conducting and inactivated sodium channels have a greater local anesthetic affinity than resting, nonconducting sodium channels. If a frog sciatic nerve preparation is stimulated at low frequency (3 Hz) and exposed to a low concentration of a local anesthetic (1.5 mM lidocaine, 0.125 mM etidocaine, or 0.06 mM tetracaine), a minor decrease in impulse transmission develops. An increase in the stimulus frequency (100 Hz) increases the degree of block.[11] Repetitive stimulation of nerve fibers increases the binding affinity of the receptor site for local anesthetics and facilitates the development of neural blockade, a phenomenon called *use-dependent* or *frequency-dependent block*, or *phasic block*.

Other Mechanisms of Action

Local anesthetics will bind to many different sites that may contain a variety of different sodium channels. The sodium channels in the heart, brain, and axons are not identical.[12] However, if local anesthetics achieve a sufficient tissue concentration, they will affect all excitable membranes, including such as exist in the heart, brain, and neuromuscular junction. The molecular mechanisms by which local anesthetics produce epidural or spinal (subarachnoid) analgesia may include local anesthetic binding to sodium and potassium channels within the dorsal and ventral horns[13] and binding to neural calcium channels, which causes hyperpolarization of cell membranes.[14] Alterations in membrane calcium ion (Ca^{2+}) may be responsible for deformation or expansion of the cell membrane and thus the transmission or conduction of nerve impulses.[15] Local anesthetics may inhibit substance P binding and evoked increases in intracellular calcium (Ca^{2+}),[16] and potentiate γ-aminobutyric acid (GABA)–mediated chloride currents by inhibiting GABA uptake.[17] Spinal anesthesia may also be mediated via complex interactions at neural synapses and disruption of electrical information coding.[18]

Other chemicals, such as toxins, α_2-adrenergic agonists, ketamine, meperidine, calcium-channel blockers, antihistamines, anticholinergics, alcohol, anticonvulsants, barbiturates, and volatile general anesthetics also bind and inhibit sodium channels and often exhibit weak local anesthetic activity.[19–21] Xylazine,[22] ketamine,[23] and meperidine[24] have reportedly produced perineal anesthesia when applied to the caudal epidural space of horses.

Antimicrobial Activity

Additional and sometimes controversial benefits of local anesthetics, which are routinely administered before minor skin surgery and for postoperative pain relief, include both a potent antimicrobial effect[25–27] and improved wound healing.[28,29]

Administration of 1%, 2%, and 4% lidocaine demonstrates a dose-dependent inhibition of growth for all strains of bacteria tested (e.g., *Staphylococcus aureus*, *Escherichia coli*, *Pseudomonas aeruginosa*, and *Enterococcus faecalis*) and no change in the susceptibility of the bacteria to lidocaine by the addition of epinephrine.[26] Likewise, administration of 2% and 5% lidocaine and 1% prilocaine demonstrates a powerful antimicrobial effect on various bacteria, including *Escherichia coli*, *Staphyloccocus aureus*, *Pseudomonas aeruginosa*, and *Candida albicans*.[27] In contrast, 0.25% and 0.5% bupivacaine shows poor antimicrobial effectiveness, and ropivacaine has no antimicrobial effect on such microorganisms.

Investigation of the in vivo effects of lidocaine on leukocyte function in surgical wounds of rats demonstrates lower leukocyte cell counts in the wounds of lidocaine-treated versus placebo-treated rats 48 and 72 h after surgical implantation of hollow titanium implants.[28] At least one histopathological study indicates that local infiltration of 0.5% and 2.0% lidocaine and 0.5% bupivacaine does not substantially alter the healing of midline abdominal incisions in rabbits.[30]

Clinical Pharmacology

Chemical Structure

All local anesthetics contain an aromatic ring at one end of the molecule and an amine at the other, separated by a hydrocarbon chain (Table 14.1).[1,31,32] The aromatic end is derived from benzoic acid or aniline and is lipophilic. The amine end is derived from ethyl alcohol or acetic acid and is hydrophilic. Substitution of alkyl groups on the aromatic ring or amine end increases lipid solubility and potency.

Chirality

In general, local anesthetics are supplied commercially as racemic mixtures of both $R-(+)$ and $S-(-)$ optical stereoisomers. Differences in structure result in various pharmacodynamic and pharmacokinetic actions.

Ropivacaine is provided as the hydrochloride of the pure $S-(-)$ enantiomer.[33,34] It is associated with a reduced incidence of both cardiovascular and central nervous system (CNS) toxicity, a concern with use of racemic bupivacaine.[35] In addition, epidural ropivacaine is similar to bupivacaine in onset, depth, duration, and extent of sensory blockade, although motor block is less intense and briefer.[36]

More recently, levobupivacaine, the pure $S-(-)$ enantiomer of bupivacaine, has been produced. In common with ropivacaine, levobupivacaine is less toxic than bupivacaine, which is attributable to a lesser affinity for brain and myocardial tissue than either that of the $R-(+)$ enantiomer or racemic bupivacaine.[37]

Grouping of Local Anesthetics

The clinically useful local anesthetic drugs essentially segregate into amino esters and amino amides, based on the chemical link between the aromatic moiety and the hydrocarbon chain (Table 14.1). Amino esters have an ester link, and the amino amides have an amide link, respectively. The nature of linkage (ester versus amide) has a notable effect on the chemical stability and the route of metabolism. Ester-linked local anesthetics are cocaine, benzocaine, procaine, chloroprocaine, and tetracaine. Most esters are readily hydrolyzed by plasma cholinesterase and have short half-lives when stored in solution without preservatives. Amide-linked local anesthetics are lidocaine, prilocaine, dibucaine, etidocaine, mepivacaine, bupivacaine, levobupivacaine, ropivacaine, and articaine. The amide agents are very stable, cannot be hydrolyzed by cholinesterase, and rely on enzymatic degradation in the liver. The amide structure of articaine is similar to that of other local anesthetics but contains an additional ester group, which is quickly hydrolyzed by esterases, shortening its duration of action. Ropivacaine and levobupivacaine are synthesized as

single $S-(-)$ optical isomers. Other local anesthetics exist as racemates or have no asymmetrical carbons.

The clinical action of local anesthetics may be described by their inherent anesthetic potency, speed of onset of action, duration of action, and tendency for differential block (Table 14.2). These properties do not sort independently.

Local Anesthetic Potency

There tends to be an association between the lipid solubility (octane-water partition coefficient) of a local anesthetic and the local anesthetic potency in vitro.[38] The smaller the molecule and larger the lipophilic property of the local anesthetic, the more readily the anesthetic permeates the axonal nerve membranes, which are highly lipid in composition, and binds sodium channels with greater affinity. The addition of side chains to the lipophilic end of the basic chemical structure increases the lipid solubility and potency of the local anesthetics. The addition of a butyl group to the lipophilic end of procaine forms tetracaine, which is 80 times more lipid soluble and 8 times more potent than procaine. Similarly, replacement of the methyl group with a butyl group on the lipophilic end of mepivacaine yields bupivacaine, which is approximately 30 times more lipid soluble and 8 times more potent than procaine, making it also 15 times more lipid soluble and 4 times more potent than mepivacaine (Table 14.2).

Speed of Onset

The onset of local anesthetic effects in isolated nerves is most likely associated inversely with the lipid solubility and acid dissociation constant (pK_a) of the anesthetic. Most local anesthetics have pK_a values that range from 7.7 to 9.1 (Table 14.2). The percentage of local anesthetic molecules present in the uncharged, nonionized base form, which is primarily responsible for membrane permeability, decreases with increased pK_a at any given tissue pH.[39] When comparing mepivacaine (pK_a, 7.7) with bupivacaine (pK_a, 8.1), mepivacaine with its pK_a nearer to tissue pH 7.4 has a noticeable faster onset of action than bupivacaine (5 to 10 vs. 20 to 30 min). Etidocaine is highly lipid soluble (partition coefficient, 140) and has a low pK_a (7.74), so it penetrates diffusion barriers around A-α nerves relatively easily, producing good motor block within 5 to 10 min. Articaine has good lipid solubility (partition coefficient, 52) and low pK_a (7.8). Articaine (4% solution) produces successful (complete) local anesthesia for periodontal surgery or tooth extraction in 1 to 3 min that lasts for 50 to 60 min.[40] Although chloroprocaine has a higher pK_a than procaine (9.1 vs. 8.9), chloroprocaine is more potent and has a faster onset of action. The pK_a of ropivacaine is 8.07, approximately the same as bupivacaine (8.1) or mepivacaine (7.7). However, ropivacaine has an intermediate degree of lipid solubility (partition coefficient of 14 at pH 7.4) compared with bupivacaine (partition coefficient, 30) and mepivacaine (partition coefficient, 2).

Duration of Anesthetic Effect

The duration of clinical local anesthetic action correlates with the high lipid solubility, which also relates to increased potency, as previously described, and to increased protein binding within the axonal membrane and the vasoactivity of the local anesthetic

Table 14.1. Trade names, chemical structure, and main clinical uses of ester-linked and amide-linked local anesthetic agents

Trade Name	Chemical Structure	Main Clinical Use
Amides		
Lidocaine	Xylocaine / Lignocaine	Infiltration, nerve blocks, intra-articular, epidural
Prilocaine	Citanest	Infiltration, nerve blocks, epidural
Etidocaine	Duranest	Infiltration, nerve blocks, epidural
Mepivacaine	Carbocaine	Infiltration, nerve blocks, intra-articular, epidural
Bupivacaine	Marcaine	Infiltration, nerve blocks, epidural, subarachnoid
Levobupivacaine	Chirocaine	Infiltration, nerve blocks, epidural, subarachnoid
Ropivacaine	Naropin	Infiltration, nerve blocks, epidural, subarachnoid
Articaine	Ultracain / Carticain	Infiltration, nerve blocks, intravenous, regional anesthesia, epidural

(continued)

drug. Increasing the side chain of the local anesthetic molecule increases the protein binding and prolongs the duration of action. More lipid-soluble local anesthetics are relatively water insoluble and, therefore, highly protein bound (Table 14.2).

The duration of effect of local anesthetics at the site of action is inversely related to the rate of systemic absorption. The rate of vascular absorption varies directly with the vascularity of the injection site and the physicochemical and pharmacological prop-

Table 14.1. Trade names, chemical structure, and main clinical uses of ester-linked and amide-linked local anesthetic agents (*continued*)

Trade Name	Chemical Structure		Main Clinical Use

Esters

Cocaine			Topical
Benzocaine	Americaine	H_2N—⟨⟩—$\overset{O}{\overset{\|}{C}}OC_2H_5$	Topical
Procaine	Novocain	H_2N—⟨⟩—$COOCH_2CH_2N(CH_2CH_3)_2$	Infiltration, nerve blocks, epidural
Chloroprocaine	Nesacaine	H_2N—⟨⟩—$COOCH_2CH_2N(C_2H_5)_2 \cdot HCl$ (Cl)	Infiltration, nerve blocks, epidural
Tetracaine	Pontocaine Amethocaine	$CH_3(CH_2)_3NH$—⟨⟩—$COOCH_2CH_2N(CH_3)_2 \cdot HCl$	Topical, subarachnoid

Cocaine structure: CH_3, N, $COOCH_3$, $OOCC_6H_5$, H

erty and dose of the local anesthetic. Lidocaine is a better va-sodilator than prilocaine, so lidocaine is removed from the site of injection faster. This makes lidocaine a shorter-acting anesthetic than prilocaine (60 to 120 vs. 120 to 180 min), even though lido-caine is more protein bound (65% vs. 55%).

Articaine is better able to diffuse away through soft tissues and bone than are other local anesthetics, and it contains an ester group, which is quickly hydrolyzed by esterases, shortening its duration to approximately 30 to 45 min.[41] By using articaine in peribulbar anesthesia for cataract surgery, corneal sensation returns quickly, thereby reducing the likelihood of inadvertent damage to an anesthetized eye after discharge.[42]

Tonicaine is a lidocaine derivative compound that produces sciatic nerve blockade with a relatively fast onset (<10 min) and long duration (12 to 16 h). Tonicaine requires additional local and systemic toxicity studies before it can be safely used in animals and people.[43]

Bupivacaine, tetracaine, etidocaine, and ropivacaine are highly lipid-soluble local anesthetics that are only slowly "washed out" from isolated nerves in vitro, and they are not readily removed by the bloodstream from nerve membranes, making their duration of action long (180 to 480 min) (Table 14.2).

Mixtures of Local Anesthetics

Neural blockade produced by mixing of local anesthetics is un-predictable and controversial and may depend on a number of factors, which include not only the types of drugs but also the pH of the mixture. If lidocaine (with fast onset and intermediate du-ration) and bupivacaine (with long onset and duration of action)

are mixed, neural blockade may begin faster and last longer.[44] One study suggests that there is no clinical advantage, with re-spect to onset and duration of sensory blockade in humans, to using a 50:50 mixture of plain lidocaine (1%) and plain bupiva-caine (0.25%) in place of their independent use.[45] Prior adminis-tration of chloroprocaine (with fast onset and brief duration) to bupivacaine (with longer onset and duration) shortens the dura-tion of bupivacaine-induced nerve blockade, because the metabo-lites of chloroprocaine may inhibit the binding of bupivacaine to sodium-channel receptor sites.[46,47] Administration of bupiva-caine (2.4 μg/mL) and etidocaine (2.3 μg/mL) causes 38% and 21% inhibition, respectively, of the rate of chloroprocaine hy-drolysis by human serum.[48] A mixture of equal parts of 2% chloroprocaine and 0.5% bupivacaine produces a rat sciatic nerve blockade with the characteristics of a chloroprocaine block. Changing the pH of this mixture from 3.6 to 5.6 changes the characteristics to a blockade resembling that produced by bupi-vacaine.[49] For mixtures of lidocaine-bupivacaine and lidocaine-tetracaine, there is no evidence of a synergistic or antagonistic in-teraction in rats.[50]

Novel Local Anesthetic Delivery Systems

Vehicles for Sustained Release of Local Anesthetics

Various approaches have been tried to prolong neural blockade and postoperative analgesia for several hours or days after a sin-gle administration of a local anesthetic drug. Polyactic, polycar-

Table 14.2. Physical, chemical, and biological properties of currently available local anesthetic agents.

Drug	Lipid Solubility	Relative Anesthetic Potency[a]	pK_a	Plasma Protein Binding (%)	Onset of Action	Duration of Action (min)
Ester linked						
Low potency, short duration						
Procaine	1	1	8.9	6	Slow	45–60
Chloroprocaine	1	1	9.1	7	Fast	30–60
High potency, long duration						
Tetracaine	80	8	8.6	80	Slow	60–360
Amide linked						
Intermediate potency, short duration						
Articaine	52	4	7.8	65	Fast	30–45
Intermediate potency and duration						
Lidocaine	3.6	2	7.86	65	Fast	60–120
Mepivacaine	2	2	7.7	75	Fast	90–180
Prilocaine	1	2	7.7	55	Fast	120–180
Intermediate potency, long duration						
Ropivacaine	14	6	8.07	95	Intermediate	180–480
High potency, long duration						
Bupivacaine	30	8	8.1	95	Intermediate	180–480
Levobupivacaine	31.1	ND	8.09	>97	Intermediate	180–480
Etidocaine	140	6	7.74	95	Fast	180–480

[a]The potency given is relative to procaine. ND, not determined.

bonate, and polymer microspheres containing local anesthetics,[51–53] lecithin-coated methoxyflurane microdroplets,[54] local anesthetics from biodegradable polymer matrices,[55] lecithin-coated tetracaine microcrystals,[56] and liposome-encapsulated lidocaine[57] or bupivacaine[58] have been developed to serve as vehicles for sustained release of local anesthetic agents.

The large unilamellar vehicles (diameter, 300 nm) that exhibit a pH gradient (pH 7.4, outside; and pH 4.0, inside) and encapsulate 0.75% bupivacaine can subsequently provide a sustained-release system that increases the duration of neural blockade from 2 to 6.5 h.[58] In the guinea pig cutaneous wheal model, more than 85% of the liposomal carrier remains at the site of administration for 2 days.[58] The duration of intercostal nerve blockade in sheep increases from 4 to 13 days after using the controlled release of 8 to 80 mg of bupivacaine/kg of body weight and 0.05% dexamethasone from polymer microspheres (470 mg of microspheres containing 352 mg of bupivacaine per nerve).[53]

Continuous Peripheral Nerve Blockade

This can be accomplished by the use of a continuous-catheter insertion system and a disposable infusion pump.[59] Local anesthetic delivery has been applied at the end of surgery on 17 dogs submitted for forelimb amputation, total ear-canal ablation with lateral bulla osteotomy, or median and lateral thoracotomies. The continuous infusion of 2% lidocaine (2 mL/h) into the surgical sites was well tolerated by the patients, producing good postoperative analgesia for up to 50 h, with no acute local anesthetic toxicity, hemodynamic instability, or breakthrough pain.[60]

Differential Nerve Blockade

Controversy still surrounds the differential susceptibility of nerve fibers to local anesthetics and its relation to selective functional deficit. It is apparent that differential block of impulses in nerve fibers exists, varying among different anatomical features (different peripheral nerves, fiber diameter, presence or absence of myelination, and surrounding tissue), different local anesthetics, critical duration of drug exposure (absorption, distribution, and elimination of drug from the site of injection), and different animal species (e.g., frogs, rats, cats, and people).

Sensory and motor fibers have a characteristic neurophysiological profile, motor and sensory function, and conduction-block susceptibility (Table 14.3).

In Vitro Studies

One of the oldest observations about local anesthetic block with cocaine is that dogs and frogs lose sensation before motor function.[61] In vitro studies with desheathed rabbit vagus and sciatic nerve indicate that various local anesthetics (i.e., cocaine, procaine, chloroprocaine, tetracaine, lidocaine, bupivacaine, etidocaine, tetrodoxin, and saxitoxin) block C fibers before A-α fibers.[62] These findings have led to the belief that the susceptibility to local anesthetic depends inversely on fiber diameter. The "size principle" that smaller (slower) axons are always blocked first, however, is not always true. When equilibrium is achieved between the nerve and the local anesthetic solutions, the large A-α fibers are blocked at the lowest drug concentration, the inter-

Table 14.3. Classification of nerve fibers and order of blockade

	Fiber Type					
	A-α	A-β	A-γ	A-δ	B	C
Function	Somatic motor	Touch, pressure	Proprioception	Fast pain, temperature	Vasoconstriction, preganglionic sympathetic	Slow pain, postganglionic sympathetic polymodal nociceptors
Myelin	Heavy	Moderate	Moderate	Light	Light	None
Diameter (μM)	12–20	5–15	3–6	2–5	1–3	0.4–1.5
Priority of blockade	⟵ 5	⟵ 4	⟵ 3	⟵ 2	⟵ 1	⟶ 2
Signs of blockade	Loss of motor function	Loss of sensation to touch and pressure	Loss of proprioception	Pain relief, loss of temperature sensation	Increased skin temperature	Pain relief, loss of temperature sensation

mediate B fibers are blocked at a higher concentration, and the smallest, slowest-conducting C fibers require the highest drug concentration for conduction blockade.[63,64]

Similarly, earlier reports indicate that the larger A-β fibers in rabbit vagus nerve are more susceptible to the local anesthetic blockade than are the small, preganglionic, myelinated B fibers.[64–66] The larger A-δ fibers in the dorsal roots of saphenous nerve of cats are also reported to be more susceptible to procaine blockade than are the C fibers.[63]

In Situ Studies

Local anesthetics have been found to block pain fibers (small un-myelinated C fibers and myelinated A-δ fibers) more readily and before other sensory and motor fibers (large myelinated A-γ, A-β, and A-α fibers) (Table 14.3). Local anesthetics also will block small-diameter myelinated or unmyelinated fibers at a lower concentration than is required to block large fibers of the same type. This is probably attributable to the longer action potentials and the discharge at higher frequencies of smaller fibers.

A recent in vivo electrophysiological study with rats con-firmed such results.[67] If the minimal effective threshold concentration of lidocaine in rat sciatic nerve was measured that pro-duced 50% of tonic fiber blockade in large, myelinated A-α and A-β fibers, small myelinated A-δ fibers, and unmyelinated C fibers of sensory axons, and in large myelinated A-α fibers and small A-γ of motor axons, then the order was motor = proprio-ception (A-γ > A-δ = A-α > A-β fibers) > nociception (C fibers). At 1% lidocaine, all fibers were tonically blocked.

On the other hand, if compound action potentials of the saphe-nous nerve were recorded before and during blockade with low concentrations with either a low lipid-soluble local anesthetic (e.g., procaine or 2-chloroprocaine) or intermediate lipid-soluble anesthetic (e.g., lidocaine or bupivacaine), then priority of fiber blockade appeared to be C > A-δ > A-α fibers.[68] However, with very lipid-soluble etidocaine, A-δ fibers are blocked before C fibers. Of the local anesthetics tested, 2-chloroprocaine produced the greatest differential rate of block of peripheral nerve fibers, and etidocaine produced the least. Mepivacaine appears to block

sensory and motor fibers at the same rate, and bupivacaine and ropivacaine can produce selective sensory analgesia, with little or no motor blockade.[69–71]

Brachial Plexus Infiltration

Deposition of local anesthetics to the brachial plexus of humans has produced either equally fast anesthesia and paralysis by 1% lidocaine or a more rapid motor blockade than sensory blockade by 1% mepivacaine,[72] 0.5% bupivacaine, or 0.5% ropiva-caine.[73,74] Similarly, brachial plexus block in dogs produced more rapid onset of motor block when compared with sensory block after the administration of bupivacaine (0.375% with 5 Mg/mL epinephrine, 4 mg/kg) (9.7 vs. 26.2 min, mean values).[75] This phenomenon has been explained by some authors by the so-matotopical arrangement of nerve fibers such that the motor fibers would be located at the periphery of the nerve trunk (man-tle bundles) and the sensory fibers in the center (or core) (Fig. 14.3).[72,76] Consequently, if sufficient analgesic drug is applied to produce motor blockade, the diffusion of the analgesic or its transport into the nerve by the local blood supply will first affect the motor fibers. However, anatomical studies of the radial, me-dian, and ulnar nerves in humans do not support this concept, making the mechanism for the differential rate of brachial plexus blockade controversial.[77] Analgesia during brachial plexus block in dogs lasted 11 ± 0.5 h in one study, but the relative rates of re-covery of motor activity and sensation in dogs after brachial plexus blockade have not been investigated.[75]

Differential Epidural and Spinal Blockade

In general, progression of epidural and spinal anesthesia is re-lated to the diameter, myelination, and conduction velocity of af-fected nerve fibers. Exposure of mixed-nerve trunks within the spinal vertebral column to a sufficient concentration of an anal-gesic drug might cause a loss of sensation in this order: pain, heat and cold, touch, proprioception, and skeletal muscle tone. Re-covery of sensation is expected to be in the reverse order.[78]

Autonomic small unmyelinated C fibers and myelinated B fibers seem to be readily desensitized after epidural or spinal ad-

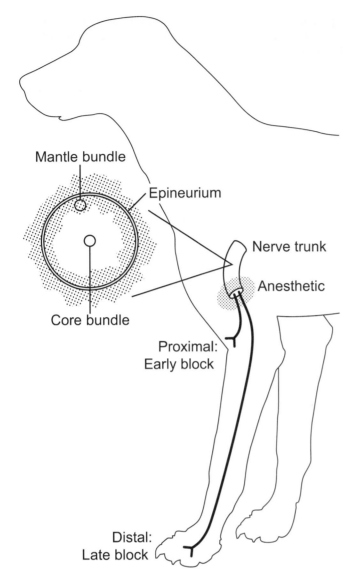

Fig. 14.3. Somatosensory arrangement of nerve fibers in the trunk of the brachial plexus of the dog. Nerve fibers in the mantle or peripheral bundles innervate primarily motor fibers of the proximal limb, whereas nerve fibers in the core or center bundles innervate for the most part the sensory fibers of the distal foot. The concentration gradient that develops during initial diffusion of local anesthetic into the nerve trunk causes onset of anesthesia to proceed from proximal to distal. Recovery from anesthesia also proceeds from proximal to distal because of absorption of local anesthetic into the circulation surrounding the nerve trunk.

ministration of local anesthetics. Spinal anesthesia is generally characterized by preganglionic sympathetic nerve blockade (B fibers) that extends further than sensory block (A-δ fibers), and sensory block extends further than somatic motor block (A-α fibers).[79]

The relative importance of blockade of each class of fiber (A-β, A-δ, and C) for surgical anesthesia has been assessed by measuring cutaneous perception thresholds in people. In this study, A-β, A-δ, and C fibers of the skin were stimulated at 2000, 250, and 5 Hz, and demonstrated differential block by the sequential return of sensation to touch (A-β function), then pinprick (A-δ function), and lastly cold (C-fiber function), respectively.[80]

Sensory anesthesia sufficient for surgery usually cannot be obtained without motor impairment. Adequate sensory analgesia with little or no motor blockade can be achieved with the epidural administration of low concentrations of bupivacaine or ropivacaine combined with opioids and/or α2-agonists. Epidural blockade may be able to differentiate between sympathetic, somatic, and central pain in patients with chronic pain.

Factors Influencing Anesthetic Activity

A variety of factors can influence the quality of regional anesthesia, including the local anesthetic dose, site of administration, additives such as epinephrine or hyaluronidase, pH adjustment and carbonation, baricity, temperature, mixtures of local anesthetics, and pregnancy.

Dose of Local Anesthetic Agent

A greater dose (volume and/or concentration) will facilitate overall efficacy, thereby decreasing the delay of onset of action and increasing both the likelihood of successful anesthesia and its duration. The potential of systemic toxicity by inadvertent intravenous injection of an anesthetic,[81] or neurotoxicity after inadvertent subarachnoid injection,[82] precludes the routine administration of larger doses of local anesthetic.

All local anesthetics can be neurotoxic, particularly in concentrations and doses larger than those used clinically. Large-scale surveys, using histopathological, electrophysiological, behavioral, and neuronal cell models, indicate that lidocaine and tetracaine seem to have a greater potential for neurotoxicity than does bupivacaine at clinically relevant concentrations administered intrathecally (spinal).[83]

Volume of Local Anesthetic
Generally, a larger volume of local anesthetic will produce a faster and denser block. An exception to this rule is articaine, which readily penetrates tissues and produces anesthesia in approximately 2 min, irrespective of the volume injected. The necessity of a larger injected volume of anesthetic solution for a high rate of complete sensory block can be minimized during axillary plexus blocks in people[84] and dogs[75] if an adequate concentration of a local anesthetic agent (e.g., 1% mepivacaine or 0.375% bupivacaine) is precisely administered at multiple injection sites covering all major nerves of the brachial plexus.

Administration of large volumes (0.22 to 0.33 mL/kg) of bupivacaine (0.75%), lidocaine (2%), or 2-chloroprocaine (3%) into the subarachnoid space of sheep and monkeys has produced neurological deficits and histological abnormalities of the spinal cord, but no one local anesthetic was considered more neurotoxic than another.[82]

Concentration of Local Anesthetic
A higher concentration of local anesthetic will also produce a faster and denser block. Increasing the concentration of lidocaine

and bupivacaine during phasic ("use dependent") inhibition of sodium currents increases the rate of binding but has no effect on unbinding sodium channels.[85] In general, the chance for successful desensitization and anesthesia decreases when the concentration is lowered. One study suggests that lumbar epidural anesthesia with 10 mL of 2% lidocaine in humans produces more intense blockade of large-diameter and small-diameter sensory nerve fibers than that with 20 mL of 1% lidocaine.[86] Similarly, administration of 0.75% ropivacaine into the lumbar epidural space of dogs produces a higher rate of complete anesthesia than does 0.5% ropivacaine of similar volume (0.22 mL/kg).[87]

Injection Site

In general, the fastest onset (within 3 to 5 min) and shortest duration (1 h) of anesthesia is usually produced after subcutaneous and intrathecal injections of 2% lidocaine or mepivacaine hydrochloride solution, followed in order of increasing onset time for minor nerve blocks (5 to 10 min), major nerve blocks, and epidural anesthesia (10 to 20 min).

Additives

Vasoconstrictors

As a general rule, the addition of a vasoconstrictor to a local anesthetic agent, such as epinephrine, allows for decreased local perfusion, delayed rate of vascular absorption of local anesthetic, and therefore increased intensity and prolonged anesthetic activity. Lumbar epidural anesthesia, using 10 mL of 1% lidocaine with epinephrine 1:200,000 produces a more intense block of both large-diameter and small-diameter sensory nerve fibers than that achieved with lidocaine alone.[88]

The usual concentration of epinephrine is 5 µg/mL or 1:200,000 (1 mg/200 mL of saline), which may be obtained by adding 0.1 mL of 1:1000 (0.1 mg) epinephrine to 20 mL of local anesthetic solution. Alternatively, 1:1000 epinephrine may be diluted with preservative-free normal saline. The maximum safe concentration of epinephrine is 1:50,000; concentrations less than 1:200,000 are less effective.

Market preparations of local anesthetics that contain epinephrine 1:200,000 have a lower pH (to retard oxidation) than do plain solutions; for example, 2% lidocaine without and with epinephrine 1:200,000 has a pH of 6.78 and 4.55; and 0.5% bupivacaine without and with epinephrine (1:200,000) has a pH of 6.04 and 3.73, respectively. The pH of solutions freshly prepared with epinephrine is higher than the pH of commercial preparations containing epinephrine; for example, the pH of 2% lidocaine and 0.5% bupivacaine with freshly added epinephrine 1:200,000 is 6.33 and 5.99, respectively. The low pH of the epinephrine preparations will potentially decrease the amount of free protonated anesthetic base available for diffusion through the axonal membrane, thereby slowing the onset of action.

Epinephrine effects depend on the injection site and the local anesthetic, but, in general, it reduces the potential toxicity of local anesthetics by causing vasoconstriction and thus preventing higher blood concentrations.[89] Epinephrine (1:200,000) reduces the average anesthetic blood concentration in dogs given an epidural injection of either 3 mL of 1% ropivacaine or 0.75%

bupivacaine at various time intervals, but not the time to achieve maximal blood levels, and it does not alter onset or duration of sensory or motor blockades produced by epidural ropivacaine 1% or bupivacaine 0.75% in dogs.[90]

Acidic epinephrine-containing local anesthetic solutions can decrease the pH at the site of injection, depending on the buffer demand of the injectate and the buffer capacity of the tissue. Epinephrine should not be added to local anesthetics intended for nerve blocks that have an erratic blood supply and for intravenous regional anesthesia with use of a tourniquet because it can cause nerve ischemia and prolonged blockade. Epinephrine often causes tissue necrosis along wound edges. Lidocaine, bupivacaine, and etidocaine equally protect against epinephrine (5 µg/kg/min)-induced arrhythmias in dogs anesthetized with a 1.4 minimum alveolar concentration of halothane.[91] Norepinephrine and phenylephrine appear to have no clinical advantage over epinephrine.

Hyaluronidase

This depolymerizes hyaluronic acid, the tissue cement or ground substance of the mesenchyme, aiding in the local anesthetic spread of an anesthetic agent.[92] The addition of hyaluronidase 3.75 IU/mL to 2% lidocaine, 0.75% bupivacaine, or a 1:1 mixture of 0.75% bupivacaine and 2% lidocaine is reported to improve the diffusion of local anesthetics, resulting in more effective retrobulbar-peribulbar anesthesia and extraocular muscle akinesia after retrobulbar injections.[93,94] Increasing the concentration of hyaluronidase to 7.5 IU/mL does not provide any further advantage over 3.75 IU/mL. The increased permeability of tissues may enhance systemic absorption (and toxicity) but shortens the duration of anesthetic effects because more drug is available in base form. The addition of 5 IU of hyaluronidase/mL of 1% lidocaine with 1:200,000 epinephrine solution in a standard dose and technique for ophthalmic surgery (2 mL as retrobulbar injection for intraocular anesthesia, 2 mL for upper-eyelid anesthesia, and 4 mL for extraorbital facial nerve blockade) reportedly does not increase the systemic absorption and cerebrospinal fluid (CSF) concentration of lidocaine in dogs.[95] However, administration of hyaluronidase does not seem to enhance the efficacy of newer local anesthetics with improved spreading power (e.g., articaine and ropivacaine). Administration of 2% articaine or 1% ropivacaine produces a faster onset of anesthesia and less pain on injection than does administration of 1% bupivacaine.[42,96] Hyaluronidase is a protein that cannot be heat sterilized.[97]

pH Adjustment and Carbonation

The pH of the local anesthetic solution affects the local distribution of the anesthetic. Extracellular increase of bicarbonate increases the cross-membrane pH gradient, the intracellular concentration of the ionized local anesthetic, and local anesthetic effects.

The addition of sodium bicarbonate to procaine, chloroprocaine, mepivacaine, or lidocaine will shorten the onset of nerve block, enhance the density of block, and prolong the duration of block in isolated nerve preparations.[98] This is likely because the amount of nonionized base increases, which enhances diffusion of the local anesthetic through axonal membranes and ion trapping due to the increased cross-membrane pH gradient.

The efficacy of alkalinization depends on the local anesthetic and regional block techniques. The addition of sodium bicarbonate for median nerve block in humans decreases the pain on injection and increases the rate of onset of motor block, but has no effect on duration of sensory anesthesia.[99] Similarly, adjusting the pH of 1% lidocaine or 0.25% bupivacaine with sodium bicarbonate to 7.4 has little effect on duration of anesthesia after injection into the infraorbital area or abdominal musculature.[100]

In humans, alkalinization produces the best results with 2% lidocaine and 0.5% bupivacaine for epidural block, with 2% lidocaine for axillary brachial plexus block, and with 2% mepivacaine for sciatic and femoral nerve blocks.[101] Bicarbonate has minimal effects when added to ropivacaine.

Increasing the pH of lidocaine or mepivacaine from 4.5 to 7.2 by adding 1 mEq of sodium bicarbonate/10 mL of local anesthetic before injection has been shown to accelerate the onset of epidural anesthesia in humans.[102,103] A pH increase of 2% 2-chloroprocaine from 7.1 to 7.7 with sodium bicarbonate accelerates epidural anesthesia in humans, but a pH increase from 7.1 to 7.7 with tromethamine does not, indicating that factors other than just pH are responsible for the more rapid onset of anesthesia.[104]

Local anesthetic solutions may deteriorate with time upon addition of bicarbonate. Solutions of lidocaine and 2-chloroprocaine readily alkalinize to near physiological pH without precipitation. Mepivacaine 1.5% precipitates above neutral pH within 20 min. Bupivacaine and etidocaine precipitate after the addition of small amounts of sodium bicarbonate and cannot be alkalinized to physiological pH.[105] The mixtures should be used within 20 min of their preparation.

The addition of carbon dioxide to lidocaine produces a more rapid onset and better quality of epidural anesthesia in humans.[106] Marketed solutions of carbonated lidocaine have an adjusted pH ranging from 6.35 to 6.9, and the PCO_2 is 700 mm Hg.[102] Opening the vial lets the carbon dioxide escape, thereby increasing the pH to above 7.0.

The use of carbonated lidocaine for epidural anesthesia in horses did not demonstrate the theoretical expectations of increased diffusion and faster onset of perineal anesthesia.[107]

Baricity

This is defined as the calculated ratio of the density of a solution to the density of CSF. One of the most important physical properties affecting the spread of local anesthetic solutions and level of analgesia achieved after intrathecal administration of a local anesthetic is its density relative to the density of CSF at 37°C.[108]

Density is the weight of a unit volume of solution (grams per milliliter) at a specific temperature, whereas the *specific gravity* (SG) is the calculated ratio of the density of a solution (x) to the known density of water (y), (SG = x/y). The density of a drug in solution cannot be determined from a simple formula because it depends on the physical state of that substance in solution.[109] The density of intrathecal agents is usually compared with the density of the CSF. At room temperature, most glucose-free drugs are isobaric with respect to CSF, but as drugs warm to body temperature they become relatively hypobaric. The densities of 2% lidocaine and 0.5% and 0.75% bupivacaine, for example, are slightly less than that of normal range of CSF in humans and therefore can be considered slightly hypobaric.[110] The density of 0.2% tetracaine is the same as water (0.993 g/mL). Continued dilution of 0.75% bupivacaine with water produces increasingly hypobaric solutions. The 0.075% bupivacaine (1:9 dilution) has a density comparable to that of water (0.993 g/mL).[111]

Hypobaric solutions have a baricity less than that of CSF and will migrate to nondependent areas during and immediately after the injection. Glucose-free 0.5% bupivacaine acts as a hypobaric solution, which produces a higher level of analgesia in the nondependent side compared with the dependent side in patients positioned laterally.[112] The unpredictability of extent of spinal block provided by spinal bupivacaine (0.5%) and tetracaine (0.5%) in humans may be related to individual variations in CSF densities.[113] Humans with higher CSF densities demonstrate a higher spinal block after administration of plain bupivacaine (0.5%, 3 mL).[114]

Dextrose and hypertonic saline–containing local anesthetic solutions (e.g., tetracaine in 10% glucose, and dibucaine in 5% hyperbaric saline) have a specific gravity greater than that of CSF. They will migrate from the site of injection to dependent areas.[115] Hyperbaric solutions are created by combining local anesthetics (e.g., 0.5% bupivacaine or 0.5% ropivacaine) with an equal volume of 10% dextrose, producing final drug and dextrose concentrations of 0.25% and 5%, respectively.[116] Lidocaine (1.5%) in 7.5% dextrose in water is clinically indistinguishable from 5% lidocaine in 7.5% dextrose in water as a spinal anesthetic for lower abdominal surgery in humans.[117]

Local anesthetic agents and solvent solutions often contain additives, which affect pH, osmolality, preservation, and vasoconstriction, that may in turn alter the density and specific gravity of the local anesthetic and, therefore, spread of spinal anesthesia.[118] CSF pH and the addition of vasopressors (0.2 mg of epinephrine or 2 mg of phenylephrine) minimally affect the onset of spinal anesthesia with 10 mg of tetracaine and 1 mL of 10% dextrose. However, the addition of epinephrine or phenylephrine at these doses prolonged spinal anesthesia by 53% and 72%, respectively.[119]

Temperature

The cooling of mammalian nerves in vitro slows the conduction velocity and increases the susceptibility to local anesthetic inhibition of transmission.[120] The potency of local anesthetics increases in vitro and in vivo with cooling in some instances but not in others. Inhibition of C fibers (as assessed by galvanic skin potentials) is marginally faster when ice-cold lidocaine (1%) is used compared with room-temperature lidocaine (1%) for median nerve blocks in volunteers.[121] Cooling of lidocaine increases its pK_a and the relative amount of the protonated (active) form within lipid, thereby potentiating the anesthetic effect.[122] On the other hand, a decrease in temperature from 37° to 20°C decreases the uptake of lidocaine in mammalian sciatic nerve by 45%. It is unlikely that cooling of local anesthetics (5°C) before injection of small volumes (5 mL) will be of any effect under clinical condi-

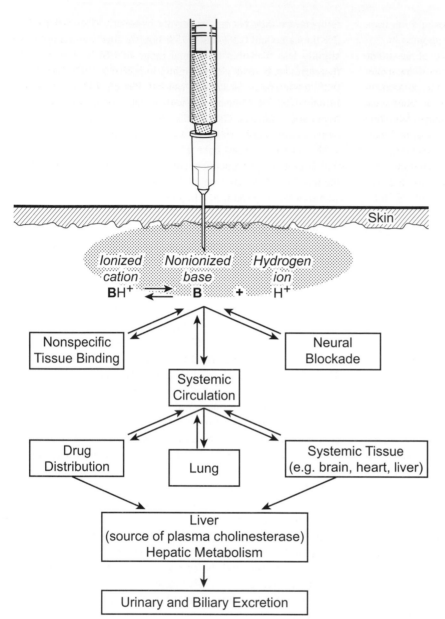

Fig. 14.4. Factors that determine the diffusion of local anesthetic near the site of injection and within the body. The nonionized base of the anesthetic (B) diffuses into the axon and nonspecific tissues. Nonspecific tissue binding and absorption into the bloodstream reduce the mass of drug available to diffuse into neural tissue. Further explanation is under the Drug Disposition section.

tions because of rapid warming of the local anesthetic by the surrounding tissue, preventing the nerve itself from growing cold.[123]

Pregnancy

This appears to increase the susceptibility of nerves to local anesthetics. Pregnant women with lidocaine (1%)-induced median nerve block at the wrist have a greater decrease in sensory nerve action potential than do nonpregnant women, indicating that pregnancy increases median nerve susceptibility to lidocaine desensitization.[121] Similarly, isolated vagus nerves removed from pregnant rabbits are more susceptible to bupivacaine-induced conduction block than are nerve fibers from nonpregnant animals.[124,125] Progesterone administration to nonpregnant rabbits replicates the increased local anesthetic susceptibility of pregnancy. Distention of the lumbar epidural venous plexus during pregnancy may displace the local anesthetic solution to more cra-

nial regions of the spinal canal. Therefore, to prevent excessive cranial spread of anesthesia, a reduced dose of epidural and spinal anesthetics during pregnancy is recommended.

Drug Disposition

Local anesthetics, as the name implies, are deposited at or near the desired site of action. In general, local anesthetics are injected near a nerve bundle. Intraneural injection is painful and may cause nerve damage. The factors that determine the distribution of local anesthetic near the injection site are illustrated in Fig. 14.4. Most clinically used local anesthetics are weak bases and are supplied as mildly acidic hydrochloride salts to improve solubility and stability. In solution, local anesthetics exist as nonionized base (B) and ionized cation (BH$^+$). The nonionized anesthetic (B) diffuses across the tissue barriers and into the axonal nerve membrane, where membrane stability and neural blockade occur.[1] Nonspecific binding of anesthetic in connective tissue, fat, and muscles and absorption of anesthetic into the vascular and lymph systems reduce the mass (volume × concentration) of the anesthetic available at the neural tissue. Once absorbed into the bloodstream, the local anesthetic is distributed to the lungs, where a significant part (20% to 30%) is absorbed, depending mainly on the physicochemical properties of the local anesthetic.[126,127] After back diffusion of the anesthetic from the lung into the blood, the anesthetic is distributed to systemic tissues (e.g., brain, heart, and liver) and is metabolized in the liver to compounds that are primarily excreted by the kidney and bile.

Absorption

Systemic absorption of local anesthetics is determined primarily by the drug dose (volume or concentration), duration of effect at the site of action, vascularity of the injection site, and use of a vasoconstrictor. Local anesthetic solutions generally are ineffective when applied to the intact skin.

Topical Application Products

Topical application of local anesthetics includes transdermal patches, creams, and iontophoretic delivery systems. Proparacaine is the topical local anesthetic most commonly used in veterinary medicine.

After application of a lidocaine patch (Lidoderm; Endo Laboratories, Chadds Ford, PA), a sufficient amount of 5% lidocaine penetrates the human intact skin to produce analgesia in patients with neuropathic pain associated with postherpetic neuralgia and in patients with postthoracotomy and postmastectomy pain, but less than the amount necessary to produce a complete sensory block.[128] A single patch (10 × 14-cm adhesive bandage) contains 700 mg of lidocaine, which is used in a 12-h-on and 12-h-off period to minimize systemic absorption.

The eutectic mixture of 2.5% lidocaine and 2.5% prilocaine (EMLA Cream; Astra Pharmaceuticals, Wilmington, DE) contains 25 mg of lidocaine and 25 mg of prilocaine per each gram or milliliter, which has a sufficiently high concentration of readily available anesthetic base and high water content to penetrate the intact skin and produce reliable cutaneous anesthesia for a wide range of applications in people (e.g., venipuncture in children, radial artery cannulation in adults, and laser treatment)[129,130] and for venipuncture in dogs, cats, rabbits, and rats.[131] In humans, the EMLA preparation is applied as a thick layer under an occlusive dressing, and maximum depth of analgesia of approximately 5 mm is achieved for 30 min after a 90-min application and for a 60-min period after a 120-min application of the cream.[129] In general, the depth of cutaneous analgesia in people ranges from 1 to 6 mm and is believed to be time dependent (1 to 4 h).[132]

Amethocaine cream 1 g (5% wt/wt) applied for 30 or 60 min on the dorsum of the hand produces good analgesia for venous cannulation similar to analgesia produced by 5% EMLA Cream (2.5 g) applied for 30 or 60 min.[133] In comparison to the gel preparation, a 30-min application of the amethocaine-patch system provides profound topical anesthesia of human skin that lasts longer than a 60-min application of EMLA (3 to 6 h vs. 20 min).[134]

ELA-Max Cream (Ferndale Laboratories, Ferndale, MI) is designed to produce analgesia of the skin to reduce venipuncture pain in 20 to 30 min in children without the use of an occlusive dressing. The preparation contains 4% lidocaine, which is liposome encapsulated to enable fast penetration into the stratum corneum. It remains in the epidermis after absorption and minimizes the rapid metabolism of lidocaine.[135] ELA-Max Cream lacks the active ingredient of prilocaine (EMLA Cream), which has been associated with methemoglobinemia in infants.[128,135] ELA-Max Cream may be more suitable for use in cats, which are susceptible to methemoglobin formation.[136]

Numby Stuff patches (Iomed; Salt Lake City, UT), which consist of 2% lidocaine and 1:100,000 epinephrine, are percutaneously administered through iontophoretic drug administration by using a battery generator to deliver small electrical current (4 mA) through two small electrodes.[137,138] Each application device delivers 1 mL of the anesthetic to a depth up to 10 mm in 10 min, giving a transient blanching and tingling of the skin.[138]

Transdermal local anesthesia by iontophoresis, but not EMLA, reduces the pain of intravenous injection of hyperosmolar saline, whereas venipuncture is painless with both methods.[139] The technique involves the use 0.5 mL of lidocaine (2% to 4%) with or without epinephrine 1:50,000 and a current intensity of 0.1 to 0.2 mA/cm^2 at the anode and placement of the cathode on the dorsal surface of the forearm for 10 min.

Although veterinary applications of Lidoderm patches, ELA-Max Cream, Numby Stuff patches, and transdermal local anesthesia by iontophoresis have been minimal, potential uses include local analgesia for small-wound repair, venipuncture, or catheter placement (intravenous and epidural).

Distribution

Local distribution of local anesthetic at the injection site depends on the volume of local anesthetic injected, inclusion of a vasoconstrictor or hyaluronidase in the local anesthetic solution, and the specific drug employed. The specific gravity (baricity) of the solution relative to the specific gravity of the CSF influences distribution within the CNS.

The distribution of amino-ester local anesthetics (e.g., procaine, chloroprocaine, and tetracaine) in body tissues is limited because of their rapid enzymatic hydrolysis by nonspecific plasma pseudocholinesterases. Amide-type local anesthetics (e.g., lidocaine, mepivacaine, prilocaine, bupivacaine, levobupivacaine, etidocaine, and ropivacaine) are widely distributed in the body after intravenous bolus injection or a fast rate of vascular absorption. Their pharmacokinetic properties are usually described by a two- or three-compartment model.[140,141]

Plasma Protein Binding

The *plasma protein binding* of local anesthetic drugs refers to the mode by which drugs are transported in the blood. It has a significant effect on numerous aspects of clinical pharmacokinetics and pharmacodynamics.[142] In blood, all amide-linked local anesthetics are partially protein bound, primarily to α_1-acid glycoprotein (AAG) and, to a lesser extent, to albumin[32,141,143] In general, the protein binding of local anesthetics is positively correlated with the degree of ionization in the physiological pH range and the drug's potency. Plasma protein binding of local anesthetics ranges from 6% for the least potent and short-acting procaine to 95% for the more potent and longer-persisting bupivacaine, etidocaine, and ropivacaine (Table 14.2). Plasma protein binding for articaine and its metabolite articainic acid is between 57% and 90% (average 65%), and the resultant half-lives of the substances are between 1 and 3.9 h.[41]

The free drug concentration in plasma, but not the protein-bound concentration of drug, governs tissue concentrations. The effect of serum protein binding on lidocaine distribution into the brain and CNS in dogs after intravenous lidocaine administration indicates that the free or unbound fraction of lidocaine is an important determinant of lidocaine entry into the brain and CSF.[144] Protein binding of lidocaine in dogs that receive a loading dose (2 mg/kg) and a maintenance infusion (50 µg/kg/h) of lidocaine is associated with increased protein binding and only slight increases of free plasma concentrations of lidocaine.[145]

In dogs, the concentration of lidocaine bound to AAG varies considerably, and it is higher in dogs with inflammatory disease than in healthy dogs.[146] Studies in normal subjects and patients with myocardial infarction, renal disease, hepatic failure, and in patients that are receiving antiepileptic drug therapy, demonstrate a good relationship between the AAG concentration and the binding ratio for lidocaine.[147]

Local anesthetic protein binding approaches saturation only at very high drug concentrations, primarily after prolonged infusion of a long-acting local anesthetic (e.g., ropivacaine or levobupivacaine) and local anesthetic-opioid combination to provide prolonged postoperative analgesia. The slow rise in total plasma concentration with increasing duration of infusion of ropivacaine and levobupivacaine appears to be the predominant reason for rare complications related to systemic toxicity produced by these drugs.[37]

Biotransformation and Excretion

The liver and lungs are major sites for plasma clearance of local anesthetics. Metabolism converts relatively lipid-soluble local anesthetics into smaller, more water-soluble agents.

For esters, the primary step is ester hydrolysis, catalyzed by nonspecific plasma cholinesterases. The rate of plasma hydrolysis is rapid, yielding half-lives measured in seconds, and is inversely related to toxicity (chloroprocaine [most rapid] > procaine > tetracaine [least rapid]).[32,143]

Procaine and benzocaine are metabolized to paraaminobenzoic acid (PABA),[148,149] a breakdown product responsible for allergic reactions and anaphylaxis in some human patients. The majority of the PABA is excreted unchanged or as conjugated product in the urine.[32] Chloroprocaine and tetracaine are metabolized similarly, but not to PABA.

Cocaine is an atypical ester in that it undergoes either ester hydrolysis or N-demethylation to norcocaine and then ester hydrolysis and significant hepatic metabolism and urinary excretion. Cocaine is rarely used in veterinary medicine, although it can be abused for stimulation of horses before a race. An intravenous dose of above 0.04 mg/kg increases spontaneous locomotor activity of horses,[150] whereas 200 mg of intravenous cocaine to adult horses undergoing an increased treadmill exercise increased the time to exhaustion by 92 s (15%).[151]

Ester metabolism can, theoretically, be slowed by reduced cholinesterase activity during pregnancy and long-term cholinesterase inhibition via poisons, thereby prolonging the clearance of ester anesthetics and increasing the potential for toxicity.

The amino-amide local anesthetics undergo nearly exclusive metabolism by the liver and hepatic degradation, which requires conjugation with glucuronic acid.[25] Cats glucuronidate drugs to a lesser extent than dogs, making cats more prone to develop toxic side effects when given amide local anesthetics.[25] Little (<5%) of these agents is excreted unchanged in urine.

The order of clearance of amides is prilocaine (most rapid) > etidocaine > lidocaine > mepivacaine or ropivacaine > bupivacaine (least rapid). Lidocaine undergoes oxidative N-dealkylation by cytochrome P450IIIA4.[32,143] Mepivacaine, etidocaine, bupivacaine, and ropivacaine also undergo N-dealkylation and hydroxylation. They are further conjugated with glucuronide before they are excreted from the body via the urine or bile. Prilocaine undergoes hydrolysis to o-toluidine, a compound that can oxidize hemoglobin to methemoglobin.[32,143]

Since all amide local anesthetics are metabolized by the liver, drug clearance is highly dependent on hepatic blood flow, hepatic extraction, and enzyme function. Clearance of amide local anesthetics can be reduced or prolonged by factors that decrease hepatic blood flow, such as β-adrenergic or H_2-receptor blockers, by hypotension during regional and general anesthesia, or by heart or liver failure.[32,143]

Local Anesthetic Toxicity

When careful technique and appropriate dose are used, local anesthetics are relatively free of harmful side effects. However, as with any pharmacological agents, local anesthetics may cause severe toxic reactions after unintentional intravenous administration,[35] vascular absorption of an excessive dose (large volume or high concentration) of the local anesthetic agent,[152] or ingestion of topical local anesthetic preparations.[153]

Doses of local anesthetics, especially those for cats and small dogs, should always be carefully calculated and reduced in sick animals. For example, in healthy dogs and cats, the dose of lidocaine should not exceed 12 and 6 mg/kg, respectively, to prevent toxicity. Repeated applications, the application of higher than the recommended doses, or impaired elimination may all contribute to increasing blood concentration of local anesthetics. Potential damage may also occur from chemical contamination of the local anesthetic solution, allergic reactions, or methemoglobinemia, or from neural ischemia produced by local pressure or hypotension. The systemic toxicity of local anesthetics involves primarily alterations in the CNS and the cardiovascular system.

Central Nervous System Toxicity

In general, toxic and lethal doses of local anesthetic drugs produce signs of CNS excitation leading ultimately to convulsive activity followed by CNS depression (unconsciousness and coma)

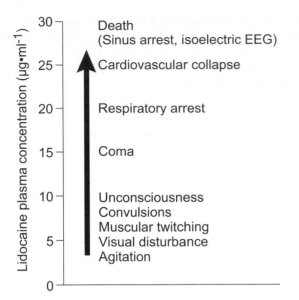

Fig. 14.5. Toxic effects produced by increasing lidocaine plasma concentrations. EEG, electroencephalogram.

with eventual respiratory arrest and cardiovascular collapse.[10] Acute CNS toxicity occurs at lower doses than those required to produce acute cardiovascular system toxicity.

As the plasma concentration of the drug increases, humans experience a predictable sequence of signs and symptoms, such as numbness of tongue, light-headedness, visual disturbance, muscle twitching, unconsciousness, and convulsions, which may progress to coma, respiratory arrest, cardiovascular depression, and death (Fig. 14.5). The seizure frequency and accompanying cardiovascular changes in patients undergoing various regional block techniques (e.g., brachial plexus block or epidural and caudal regional anesthesia) have been reviewed, indicating a rate of seizure development with caudal > brachial > epidural anesthetics and no adverse cardiovascular, pulmonary, or nervous system events occurring with seizures.[154]

In small animals, low concentrations of local anesthetics produce sedation, whereas higher concentrations produce seizures, probably because of selective depression of inhibitory fibers in the subcortical area (amygdala), with subsequent spread, leading to grand mal seizures. Muscle twitching and convulsions are usually the first signs of local anesthetic toxicity observed in dogs and cats. More potent local anesthetics consistently produce seizures at lower blood concentrations and lower doses than do the less potent local anesthetics.

In awake dogs, the mean cumulative dose of serially and rapidly administered intravenous local anesthetics to produce convulsions is 4.0 mg/kg tetracaine, 5.0 mg/kg bupivacaine, 8.0 mg/kg etidocaine, and 22 mg/kg lidocaine, indicating a relative CNS toxicity of tetracaine, bupivacaine, etidocaine, and lidocaine of about 1:1.2:2:4.[81]

In cats, procaine (the least potent CNS depressant, less lipid soluble and less protein bound) produces seizures at 35 mg/kg intravenously (IV), whereas bupivacaine (one of the most potent CNS depressants, highly lipid soluble and highly protein bound) induces convulsions at approximately 5 mg/kg IV.[155,156] Intravenously administered lidocaine at a dose of 11.7 ± 4.6 mg/kg causes seizures in cats.[157] Increased arterial PCO_2 (68 to 81 mm Hg) and decreased pH reportedly decrease the convulsive dose of procaine, lidocaine, and bupivacaine by approximately 50% in cats.[155]

Horses are reported to be more sensitive to the CNS toxicity of lidocaine than other species, although the mechanism of this increased sensitivity is not known. Seizures in horses may occur at plasma levels of 600 ng of procaine/mL[158] and 6.0 μg of lidocaine/mL,[159] respectively, and usually are brief because of rapid redistribution. Such concentrations are not readily achieved with careful local and regional anesthetic techniques; for example, the procaine plasma concentration can reach 400 ng/mL within 1 h after subcutaneous injection of 3.3 mg of procaine/kg of horse body weight, whereas the lidocaine plasma concentration approaches 3.5 μg/mL approximately 15 min after a flank "line block" using 10 mg of lidocaine/kg of body weight.

The toxic effects of local anesthetics within the CNS are enhanced by increased cerebral blood flow, by increased concentration of ionized drug in the brain, or by the direct excitatory effect on subcortical structures.

Cardiovascular Toxicity

Since an alarming editorial in 1979 about cardiac arrest in humans following regional anesthesia with etidocaine and bupivacaine,[160] ropivacaine and, recently, levobupivacaine were developed as alternative long-acting amide local anesthetics with less potential for cardiovascular toxicity.[161–166]

Local anesthetic cardiovascular toxicity may result from direct electrophysiological and mechanical effects on the heart or the peripheral circulation and from local anesthetic actions on the autonomic nervous system. The use of lower concentrations can result in CNS excitation, with increased heart rate, arterial blood pressure, pulmonary artery pressure, and cardiac output. With larger toxic blood concentrations, the systemic effects are characterized by decreased heart rate, arterial blood pressure, pulmonary artery pressure, and cardiac output.[167,168]

Results from animal studies demonstrate increased systemic toxicity associated with bupivacaine and etidocaine as compared with lidocaine, the most extreme of which include severe CNS and cardiovascular reactions, eventually leading to hemodynamic instability, cardiovascular collapse, and death. In intact, ventilated dogs anesthetized with pentobarbital, minimal changes in various cardiovascular functions are seen with lidocaine, mepivacaine, prilocaine, bupivacaine, and etidocaine at doses of 0.3 to 3 mg/kg. At 10 mg/kg, lidocaine, mepivacaine, and prilocaine produce moderate hypotension and increased pulmonary vascular resistance, and bupivacaine and etidocaine produce significant decreases in cardiac output and stroke volume.[81] Irreversible cardiovascular depression is not produced with lidocaine, bupivacaine, etidocaine, or tetracaine in ventilated dogs anesthetized with pentobarbital, until the blood concentration is at least 3.5 to 6.7 times the dose producing seizures.[81] However, in humans and animals, both bupivacaine and etidocaine administration have produced simultaneous CNS and cardiovascular toxicity manifested as severe cardiac dysrhythmia, fibrillation, and cardiac arrest.[32,160,168,169]

In another study of pentobarbital-anesthetized dogs, the intravenous administration of bupivacaine (4 mg/kg) or etidocaine (8 mg/kg) depressed electrophysiological and hemodynamic function; lidocaine (16 mg/kg) induced bradycardia and arterial hypotension, whereas mepivacaine (12 mg/kg) induced minimal cardiovascular changes.[170] The cumulative lethal dose varies from approximately 80 mg/kg for lidocaine and mepivacaine to 40 mg/kg for etidocaine and 20 mg/kg for bupivacaine in ventilated dogs anesthetized with pentobarbital.[171] Direct injection of equipotent doses of 2% lidocaine (8 mg) or 0.5% bupivacaine (2 mg) in a 4:1 ratio into a branch of the left coronary artery in morphine (2.5 mg/kg subcutaneously) + α-chloralose (10 mg/kg/h IV)–anesthetized and ventilated dogs produced a 50% reduction of systolic contraction that lasted 25% longer after bupivacaine than after lidocaine injection.[172]

When a comparable prolongation of the QRS interval (as a measure of electrophysiological toxicity) was recorded in pentobarbital-anesthetized pigs after injection of 2 mg of bupivacaine, 4.5 mg of ropivacaine, or 30 mg of lidocaine into the left anterior descending coronary artery, the electrophysiological toxicity ratio for bupivacaine-ropivacaine-lidocaine was 15:6.7:1.[173] Thus, ropivacaine appears to provide a much greater margin of safety than does bupivacaine.

In sheep, the mean fatal dose of intravenous lidocaine is 30.8 ± 5.8 mg/kg, that of bupivacaine is 3.7 ± 1.1 mg/kg, and that of ropivacaine is 7.3 ± 1.0 mg/kg; thus the ratio of fatal doses of lidocaine, bupivacaine, and ropivacaine is approximately 9:1:2.[174] Respiratory depression with bradycardia and hypotension without arrhythmias were the causes of death in lidocaine-treated sheep, whereas most bupivacaine-treated or ropivacaine-treated sheep died after sudden onset of ventricular tachycardia and fibrillation. Not surprisingly, the cardiotoxicity of lidocaine and bupivacaine in awake, unanesthetized sheep is enhanced by hypercarbia, acidosis, and hypoxia.[175]

Local anesthetics bind and inhibit cardiac sodium channels.[168,176] Bupivacaine binds more readily and for a longer duration to cardiac sodium channels than does lidocaine.[177] The bupivacaine $S-(-)$ isomer binds cardiac sodium channels less readily than does the $R-(+)$ isomer, forming the basis for the development of levobupivacaine and ropivacaine.[37] In vitro studies of guinea pig hearts (Langendorff model) indicate that $R-(+)$ bupivacaine, based on intracardiac distribution, prolongs atrioventricular (AV) conduction more and produces more second-degree AV conduction blocks than does $S-(-)$ or racemic bupivacaine.[178] Similarly, $S-(-)$ bupivacaine produces less QRS widening and fewer AV conduction blocks, less ventricular fibrillation, and less asystole in paced rabbit hearts than does $R-(+)$ or racemic bupivacaine.[179] Comparative effects of equal concentrations of bupivacaine, levobupivacaine, and ropivacaine in electrically paced rabbit hearts (210 beats/min) indicate that the free concentration of the three drugs necessary to double the basal QRS duration is 2.4, 7.2, and 14.4 μg/mL

for race-mic bupivacaine, levobupivacaine, and ropivacaine, respectively.[180]

Toxicosis After Ingestion or Application of Topical Preparations

Topical local anesthetic preparations containing lidocaine, benzocaine, tetracaine, and dibucaine, which are in many prescription and nonprescription products, such as ointments, teething gels, suppositories, and aerosols, can be hazardous to animals if ingested. Ingestion of topical benzocaine preparations or spray before endotracheal intubation has produced varying degrees of vomiting, cyanosis, dyspnea, respiratory depression, prolonged sedation, hypotension, cardiac arrhythmias, tremors, seizures, and death in dogs and cats. Likewise, digestion of ointments and creams containing 0.5% and 1.0% dibucaine hydrochloride, which may not be considered dangerous by pet owners, has produced salivation, vomiting, hypothermia, bradycardia, hypotension, weakness, seizures, dysrhythmia, and death in dogs and cats. Between 1995 and 1999 the National Animal Poison Control Center (NAPCC) recorded over 70 cases of toxicosis induced by either ingestion or the inappropriate use of lidocaine, benzocaine, or dibucaine in a variety of animals, including dogs, cats, and ferrets. The clinical signs in a variety of animal species, including dogs, cats, and ferrets, with lidocaine and dibucaine toxicosis included salivation, vomiting, hypothermia, depression, tremors, weakness, bradycardia, hypotension, and seizures.[153]

Local Toxicity

Neurotoxicity

When properly used, local anesthetics rarely produce neurotoxic effects or localized tissue damage. Neurotoxicity of local anesthetics can be demonstrated in vitro by the collapse of growth cones and neuritis in cultured neurons.[181] Comparison of seven local anesthetics in a study on growing neurons of the freshwater snail demonstrates neurotoxicity in this order: procaine = mepivacaine (least neurotoxic) < ropivacaine = bupivacaine < lidocaine < tetracaine < dibucaine (most neurotoxic). Similarly, mepivacaine also induced less growth cone collapse and neurite degeneration in the growing dorsal root ganglion neurons from chick embryos than did lidocaine, bupivacaine, or ropivacaine, indicating that mepivacaine is the safest among clinically used local anesthetics.[182]

During the 1980s, 2-chloroprocaine (Nesacaine) occasionally produced cauda equina syndrome in people when large doses (formulated with the antioxidant sodium metabisulfite at an acidic pH) were accidentally injected into the subarachnoid space.[32,183–185] Experiments with sheep and monkeys document that a large volume (10 mL) of subarachnoid administration of 2-chloroprocaine (3%), bupivacaine (0.75%), or the carrier solution of 2-chloroprocaine (Nesacaine) is neurotoxic and that no local anesthetic appears to be more toxic than another when injected in large volumes into the subarachnoid space of sheep and monkeys.[186] The large doses and volumes of local anesthetics simulate the clinical reality of accidental spinal anesthesia when epidural anesthesia is intended.

Several studies have been completed since then to evaluate the potential neurotoxicity of repeated injections or continuous infusions of local anesthetics in laboratory animals in situ and vitro. Experiments using surgically exposed vagus nerves in rabbits bathed in situ for up to 1 h in 1.5% 2-chloroprocaine, 2% lidocaine, or 0.75% bupivacaine indicate that 2-chloroprocaine is more neurotoxic than either lidocaine or bupivacaine.[187] Histological sections of nerves excised 10 to 12 days after drug exposure revealed epineurial cellular infiltration and fibrosis, perineurial fibrosis, and axonal degeneration following the administration of 2-chloroprocaine or a mixture of 2-chloroprocaine and bupivacaine, and only minor pathology following exposure to lidocaine or bupivacaine.

Controversy exists about whether lidocaine produces persisting sacral deficits and whether it may be associated with an excessive incidence of transient radicular irritation after spinal anesthesia in humans.[188] Solutions of 5% lidocaine and 0.5% tetracaine, unlike other spinal local anesthetic solutions (1.5% lidocaine with or without 7.5% dextrose, or 0.75% bupivacaine without dextrose), have been associated with clinical cases of cauda equina syndrome after continuous spinal anesthesia. These solutions cause irreversible conduction block in desheathed amphibian nerves 15 min after exposure to 5% lidocaine or 0.5% tetracaine.[189] Neurotoxic effects, including paralysis, have been produced after subarachnoid infusion of 100 μL/h of 1.5% lidocaine, 0.5% bupivacaine, or 2% 2-chloroprocaine in rats. The incidence of paralysis depended on the duration of exposure to the local anesthetic and was more intense in rats receiving lidocaine or 2-chloroprocaine than those infused with bupivacaine.[190]

Myotoxicity

All clinically used local anesthetics are myotoxic, with a drug-specific and dose-dependent rate of toxicity that worsens with serial or continuous administration.[191] Some reports indicate that single and repeated injections of clinical doses of mepivacaine (Carbocaine)[192] or bupivacaine (Marcaine)[193] produce skeletal muscle damage in rats. With 200 μL of local anesthetic (1% procaine, 0.2% tetracaine, 0.5% lidocaine, 0.75% bupivacaine, 2% chloroprocaine, 0.25% dibucaine, and 0.5% lidocaine with 1:200,000 epinephrine, and 2% piperocaine) injected into the tibialis anterior muscle of rats, the muscle fibers recovered from the initial damage in 30 days, with relatively few long-term residual effects.[194]

The administration of 20 mL of bupivacaine (5 mg/mL) or ropivacaine (7.5 mg/mL) via catheter to the femoral nerve of minipigs, and subsequent continuous infusion of bupivacaine (2.5 mg/mL) or ropivacaine (3.75 mg/mL) over 6 h, induced necrosis and apoptosis in muscle fibers with bupivacaine and less severe fiber injury with ropivacaine, without affecting vasculature, neural structures, and connective tissues.[195] The administration of bupivacaine and ropivacaine induces Ca^{2+} release of the sarcoplasmic reticulum and simultaneously inhibits Ca^{2+} reuptake into the sarcoplasmic reticulum, suggesting that these synergistic effects may be an important mechanism in bupivacaine and ropivacaine's observed myotoxicity.[195]

Although skeletal muscle damage from local anesthetics is not a major clinical problem, case reports have been published of local anesthetic-induced myotoxicity in humans after local and regional anesthesia, peripheral nerve blocks, retrobulbar injections, and trigger-point infiltration for treatment of myofascial pain.[191]

Methemoglobinemia

Methemoglobinemia (MHG) or increased concentration of methemoglobin (MHb) in the blood is defined as an altered state of hemoglobin whereby the ferrous form of iron (Fe^{2+}) is oxidized to the ferric state (Fe^{3+}), which increases oxygen affinity for hemoglobin (as seen with MHG) and reduces oxygen release at tissues.[196] In addition, oxidative denaturation of hemoglobin can cause Heinz-body formation, which can lead to erythrocyte lysis. MHG can cause hypoxia, cyanosis, or even death.

A number of local anesthetic agents, most notably benzocaine and prilocaine, and less often procaine and lidocaine, are implicated as causative agents. Benzocaine induces MHG in several species, whereas lidocaine may increase MHG in cats and people.[197] It appears that these agents do not directly produce MHG, but rather that one of their metabolites, i.e., o-toluidine, is responsible.

An intense chocolate brown–colored blood and central cyanosis unresponsive to the administration of 100% oxygen suggest the diagnosis of MHG. MHb concentrations of 15% or more cause a brown discoloration to the blood, which is visible on a white paper towel. Laboratory confirmation is by blood cooximetry, indicating an MHb concentration of greater than 15% (1% to 2% is normal). Spectrophotometry for quantitating the percentage of MHb may be available in a local human hospital laboratory. Blood smears can be useful in determining the presence and degree of Heinz-body formation.

The clinical consequences of MHG are related to the blood concentration of MHb. In humans, dyspnea, nausea, and tachycardia occur at an MHb concentration of > 30%, whereas lethargy, stupor, and deteriorating consciousness occur as the MHb concentration approaches 55%.[198] Acquired toxic MHG has been induced with benzocaine topical anesthetics (spray, cream, and ointment), which were used for bronchoscopic procedures,[199] transesophageal echocardiography,[200] fiberoptic orotracheal intubation, and skin application.[201] Peak MHb concentrations were directly related to the total dose of benzocaine or prilocaine administered and did not occur until 4 to 8 h after epidural administration of prilocaine.[202]

MHG has been induced by the nasal, oropharyngeal, and dermal applications of benzocaine in sheep,[203] dogs, and cats.[204–206] A 2-s spray of benzocaine (estimated dose, 56 mg) to the mucous membranes of the nasopharynx of dogs, cats, monkeys, rabbits, and miniature pigs produces MHb concentrations, ranging from 3.5% to 38%, 15 to 60 min after drug administration.[191] A 2-s benzocaine dose and a 10-s dose produce MHb up to 26.4 and 50.5%, respectively, in sheep.[197]

Benzocaine is combined with butamben and tetracaine in a topical anesthetic spray (Cetacaine) that has been commonly used to desensitize the larynx before intubation.[201] Cats are well recognized to be at an increased risk for developing MHG and Heinz-body anemia with benzocaine-containing products, including Cetacaine. Because of the susceptibility of cats, ferrets, or other exotic animals to MHG, the topical use of Cetacaine should be avoided in these species.

Allergic Reactions

Although allergic reactions to local anesthetics may occur, they are uncommon and often misdiagnosed after accidental intravenous injection of local anesthetics. True anaphylaxis or life-threatening allergic immune reaction is mediated by immunospecific antibodies (immunoglobulins E or G) that interact with mast cells, basophils, or the complement system to liberate vasoactive mediators and recruit other inflammatory cells. Such reactions have been documented with amino-ester local anesthetics (e.g., procaine), particularly those that are metabolized directly to PABA, which is a common allergen. Anaphylaxis to amide local anesthetics (e.g., lidocaine) is much less common.[207] Some reaction may result from hypersensitivity to a preservative (e.g., methylparaben, whose chemical structure is similar to that of PABA). Allergic reactions of dogs and cats treated with amide-linked local anesthetics are very rare, which is probably because of their different metabolism and breakdown products when compared with humans.

Adverse drug reactions may mimic anaphylaxis, characterized by bronchospasm, upper-airway edema, vasodilatation, increased capillary permeability, and cutaneous wheal and flare. Rapid cardiopulmonary intervention with airway maintenance, epinephrine administration, and volume expansion is essential to avoid a fatal outcome. Patients with local anesthetic allergy can have their skin tested to determine nonreactive agents.

Treatment of Adverse Reactions

Treatment of adverse reactions after administration of local anesthetics depends on an animal's presenting signs, and involves stabilizing, decontaminating, and supporting the patient.

When local anesthetic-induced convulsions occur, hypoxia, hypercarbia, and acidosis develop rapidly.[208] Because these metabolic changes greatly increase the toxicity of local anesthetics,[175,209,210] prompt therapy with oxygen administration by mask to a dyspneic patient and supporting ventilation (e.g., endotracheal intubation, oxygen supplementation, and positive-pressure ventilation) is indicated.[211]

The administration of oxygen by mask and intravenous fluids are often all that is necessary to treat mild signs of local anesthetic toxicity, including mild seizures.[212] Anticonvulsant drug therapy is indicated if seizure activity interferes with ventilation or is prolonged. Diazepam or midazolam can be given intravenously in dogs and cats at 0.5 to 1 mg/kg in increments of 5 to 10 mg to effect, with minimal side effects. Thiopental or propofol (1 to 2 mg/kg IV) acts more rapidly but may produce greater cardiorespiratory depression than that produced with benzodiazepine therapy.[213,214]

Acute hypotension may be treated with intravenous fluids (10 mL/kg/h) and vasopressors (phenylephrine, 0.5 to 5.0 μg/kg/min, or norepinephrine, 0.02 to 0.2 μg/kg/min). Hemoglobin-based oxygen carriers (HBOCs), such as HBOC 301 (Oxyglobin) or HBOC 201 (Hemopure and Biopure) (Biopure, Cambridge, MA), are polymerized bovine hemoglobin glutamers that provide a most effective colloid, similar to plasma, and oxygen-carrying effect.[215,216] Oxyglobin can be a good substitute for stored blood, which may not always be available. Severely hypotensive dogs and cats with obvious severe blood loss (>30 mL/kg in dogs, 15 mL/kg in cats) and those that continue to be dyspneic despite oxygen therapy may rapidly improve from an initial Oxyglobin bolus (4 to 6 mL/kg in dogs, and 2 to 3 mL/kg in cats) as a stop-gap measure to prevent cardiovascular collapse. A one-time intravenous dose of 30 mL/kg Oxyglobin at a rate of 10 mL/kg/h may be given to hypotensive dogs to increase arterial pressure and flow. Every 10 mL of Oxyglobin infused contains 1.3 g of HBOC. Caution must be exercised to avoid intravascular volume overload, which can produce pulmonary edema, pleural effusion, mucous membrane discoloration, pigmenturia, vomiting, and neurological abnormalities, particularly in small dogs and cats.[215]

An intravenous bolus of epinephrine (1 to 15 μg/kg) may be required in presence of myocardial failure. Guidelines for cardiopulmonary resuscitation should be followed when toxicity progresses to cardiac arrest. Animal studies suggest that lidocaine intoxication causes myocardial depression that can be successfully treated with continued advanced cardiac life support.[217] In contrast, cardiotoxic effects in anesthetized dogs associated with incremental overdosage of bupivacaine, levobupivacaine, or ropivacaine are not as easily treated by resuscitation efforts. The administration of epinephrine may lead to severe arrhythmias, including ventricular fibrillation, with a subsequent mortality rate from bupivacaine, levobupivacaine, ropivacaine, and lidocaine of approximately 50%, 30%, 10%, and 0%, respectively.[217]

Even though the risk of cardiovascular toxicity of ropivacaine has not been completely eliminated, ropivacaine may offer clear advantages over bupivacaine, in that ropivacaine accumulates less sodium-channel blockade at physiological heart rates, dissociates from sodium channels more rapidly, is less cardiotoxic, and is more susceptible to treatment than is bupivacaine.[218,219]

Ventricular dysrhythmias, including life-threatening ventricular tachycardia associated with local anesthetic toxicity in dogs, have been treated with bretylium tosylate (2 to 6 mg/kg IV).[220,221] Procainamide and quinidine may be effective treatments for ventricular antiarrhythmias in dogs and cats. Lidocaine is generally contraindicated in patients with amide local anesthetic toxicity.

MHG is easily treated and rapidly reduced to hemoglobin by slow (over several minutes) intravenous administration of a 1% solution of methylene blue (methylthioninium chloride, 4 mg/kg in dogs and 1 to 2 mg/kg in cats).[198] The dose can be repeated in dogs, but repeated administration of methylene blue in cats is controversial because of the risk of Heinz-body anemia and the aggravation of subsequent hemolysis without further lowering MHb content.[222]

Tachyphylaxis

Tachyphylaxis, or the acute tolerance to local anesthetic agents, is defined as decreases in intensity, segmental spread, or duration after repeated administration of equal doses of an anesthetic. Various ester-amide–type local anesthetics (e.g., cocaine, procaine, and tetracaine) and amide-type local anesthetics (e.g., lidocaine, lidocaine–carbon dioxide, mepivacaine, bupivacaine, etidocaine, and dibucaine) have been used at increasing doses to maintain a similar level of effect during surface anesthesia, nerve blocks, brachial plexus block, and epidural and subarachnoid anesthesia. The underlying mechanisms of tachyphylaxis are not well understood. Local alterations in disposition and absorption of local anesthetics—but not in structure (ester vs. amide) or the pharmacological properties of local anesthetics themselves (e.g., brief vs. long acting), technique, mode of administration (intermittent vs. continuous), and pharmacodynamic processes (interactions at receptor sites)—may all play a role in the development of tachyphylaxis.[223]

Choices of Local Anesthetics

The use of specific local anesthetics for local and regional anesthetic and analgesic techniques in animals is described in Chapters 20 (dogs), 21 (cats), 22 (horses), and 23 (cattle, sheep, goats, and pigs).

Local Anesthetics Approved for Veterinary Use by *Codified Federal Register* (*CFR*)

Lidocaine injection with epinephrine: cats, cattle, dogs, and horses (21 *CFR* 522.1244, p. 280, April 1, 1993, editions).

Mepivacaine hydrochloride injection: horses (21 *CFR* 522.1372, p. 281, April 1, 1993, editions).

Proparacaine hydrochloride ophthalmic solution: animal species not specified (21 *CFR* 524.1883, p. 338, April 1, 1993, editions).

The *CFR* also lists a number of combination products containing local anesthetics plus corticosteroid or antimicrobial agents for treatment of surface bacterial infections and/or allergy.

References

1. Butterworth JF IV, Strichartz GR. Molecular mechanisms of local anesthesia: A review. Anesthesiology 1990;72:711–734.
2. Liljestrand G. Carl Koller and the development of local anesthesia. Acta Physiol Scand Suppl 1967;299:1–30.
3. Liljestrand G. The historical development of local anesthesia. In: Lechart P, ed. International Encyclopedia of Pharmacology and Therapeutics, vol 1: Local Anesthetics, Sect 8. Oxford: Pergamon, 1971:1–38.
4. Vandam LD. Some aspects of the history of local anesthesia. In: Strichartz BR, ed. Local Anesthetics. Berlin: Springer-Verlag, 1987:1–19.
5. Hodgkin AL, Huxley AF. A quantitative description of membrane current and its application to conduction and excitation in nerve. J Physiol (Lond) 1952;117:500–544.
6. Wang S-Y, Nau C, Wang GK. Residues in Na^+ channel D3–S6 segment modulate both batrachotoxin and local anesthetic affinities. Biophys J 2000;79:1379–1387.
7. Heavner JE. Molecular action of local anesthetics. In: Raj PP, ed. Clinical Practice of Regional Anesthesia. New York: Churchill Livingstone, 1991:67–71.
8. Franz DN, Perry RS. Mechanisms for differential block among single myelinated and non-myelinated axons by procaine. J Physiol 1974;236:193–210.
9. Raymond SA, Steffenson SC, Gugino LD, Strichartz GR. The role of nerve exposed to local anesthetics in impulse blocking action. Anesth Analg 1989;68:563–570.
10. Covino BG, Vassallo HG. Local Anesthetics: Mechanisms of Action and Clinical Use. New York: Grune and Stratton, 1976.
11. Scurlock E, Meymaris E, Gregus J. The clinical character of local anesthetics: A function of frequency-dependent conduction block. Acta Anaesthesiol Scand 1978;22:601–608.
12. Cattrall WA. Structure and function of voltage-sensitive ion channels. Science 1988;242:50–61.
13. Olschewski A, Hempelmann G, Vogel W, Safronov BV. Blockade of Na^+ and K^+ currents by local anesthetics in the dorsal horn neurons of the spinal cord. Anesthesiology 1998;88:172–179.
14. Sugiyama K, Muteki T. Local anesthetics depress the calcium current of rat sensory neurons in culture. Anesthesiology 1994;80:1369–1378.
15. Ritchie JM, Greengard P. On the mode of action of local anesthetics. Annu Rev Pharmacol 1966;6:405–408.
16. Li YM, Wingrove DE, Too HP, et al. Local anesthetics inhibit substance P binding and evoked increases in intracellular Ca^{++}. Anesthesiology 1995;82:166–173.
17. Nordmark J, Rydquist B. Local anesthetics potentiate GABA-mediated Cl-currents by inhibiting GABA uptake. Neuroreport 1997;8:465–468.
18. Raymond SA. Subblocking concentrations of local anesthetics: Effects on impulse generation and conduction in single myelinated sciatic nerve axons in frogs. Anesth Analg 1992;75:906–921.
19. Staiman A, Seeman P. The impulse-blocking concentrations of anesthetics, alcohols, anticonvulsants, barbiturates, and narcotics on phrenic and sciatic nerves. Can J Physiol Pharmacol 1974;52:535–550.
20. Århem P, Rydqvist B. The mechanism of action of ketamine on the myelinated nerve membrane. Eur J Pharmacol 1968;126:245–251.
21. Bräu ME, Koch ED, Vogel W, Hempelmann G. Tonic blocking action of meperidine on Na^+ and K^+ channels in amphibian peripheral nerves. Anesthesiology 2000;92:147–155.
22. LeBlanc PH, Caron JP, Patterson JS, Brown M, Matta MA. Epidural injection of xylazine for perineal analgesia in horses. J Am Vet Med Assoc 1988;193:1405–1408.
23. Gómez de Segura IA, Rossi R-de, Santos M, San-Roman JL, Tendillo FJ. Epidural injection of ketamine for perineal analgesia in the horse. Vet Surg 1998;27:384–391.
24. Skarda RT, Muir WW III. Analgesic, hemodynamic, and respiratory effects induced by caudal epidural administration of meperidine hydrochloride in mares. Am J Vet Res 2001;62:1001–1007.
25. Steffey EP, Booth NH. Local anesthetics. In: Adams HR, ed. Veterinary Pharmacology and Therapeutics, 7th ed. Ames: Iowa State University Press, 1995:358–371.
26. Parr AM, Zoutman DE, Davidson JSD. Antimicrobial activity of lidocaine against bacteria associated with nosocomial wound infection. Ann Plast Surg 1999;43:239–245.

27. Aydin ON, Eyigor M, Aydin N. Antimicrobial activity of ropivacaine and other local anaesthetics. Eur J Anaesthesiol 2001;18:687–694.

28. Eriksson AS, Sinclair R, Cassuto J, Thomsen P. Influence of lidocaine on leukocyte function in the surgical wound. Anesthesiology 1992;77:74–78.

29. Drucker M, Cardenas E, Arizzi P, Valenzuela A, Gamboa A. Experimental studies on the effect of lidocaine on wound healing. World J Surg 1998;22:394–398; Discussion, 397–398.

30. Vasseur PB, Paul HA, Dybdal N, Crumley L. Effects of local anesthetics on healing of abdominal wounds of rabbits. Am J Vet Res 1984;45:2385–2388.

31. Courtney KR, Strichartz GR. Structural elements which determine local anesthetic activity. In: Strichartz GR, ed. Handbook of Experimental Pharmacology, vol 81: Local Anesthetics, Berlin: Springer-Verlag, 1987:53–94.

32. De Jong RH. Local Anesthetics, 2nd ed. Springfield, IL: Charles C Thomas, 1977.

33. De Jong RH. 1995 Gaston Labat Lecture. Ropivacaine: White knight or dark horse? Reg Anesth 1995;20:474–481.

34. Etches RC, Writer WDR, Ansley D, et al. Continuous epidural ropivacaine 2% for analgesia after lower abdominal surgery. Anesth Analg 1997;84:784–790.

35. Feldman HS, Arthur GR, Covino BG. Comparative systemic toxicity of convulsant and supraconvulsant doses of intravenous ropivacaine, bupivacaine, and lidocaine in the conscious dog. Anesth Analg 1989;69:794–801.

36. Zaric D, Nydahl PA, Philipson L, Samuelsson L, Heierson A, Axelsson K. The effect of continuous lumbar epidural infusion of ropivacaine (0.1%, 0.2%, and 0.3%) and 0.25% bupivacaine on sensory and motor block in volunteers: A double blind study. Reg Anesth 1996;21:14–25.

37. Thomas JM, Schug SA. Recent advances in the pharmacokinetics of local anesthetics: Long-acting amide enantiomers and continuous infusion. Clin Pharmacokinet 1999;36:67–83.

38. Sanchez V, Arthur GR, Strichartz GR. Fundamental properties of local anesthetics. I. The dependence of lidocaine's ionization and octane: Buffer partitioning on solvent and temperature. Anesth Analg 1987;66:159–165.

39. Levy RH. Local anesthetic structure, activity and mechanism of action. In: Eger EI II, ed. Anesthetic Uptake and Action. Baltimore: Williams and Wilkins, 1974:323–327.

40. Hofer H, Eberl R, Altmann H. Pharmakokinetische Untersuchung mit ^{35}S-markiertem Carticaine. Prakt Anaesth 1974;9:157–161.

41. Oertel R, Rahn R, Kirch W. Clinical pharmacokinetics of articaine. Clin Pharmacokinet 1997;33:417–425.

42. Allman KG, McFayden JG, Armstrong J, Sturrock GD, Wilson IH. Comparison of articaine and bupivacaine/lidocaine for single medial canthus peribulbar anaesthesia. Br J Anaesth 2001;87:584–587.

43. Wang GK, Quan C, Vladimirov M, Mok W-M, Thalhammer JG. Quaternary ammonium derivative of lidocaine as a long acting local anesthetic. Anesthesiology 1995;83:1293–1301.

44. De Jong RH, Bonin JD. Mixtures of local anesthetics are no more toxic than the parent drugs. Anesthesiology 1981;54:177–181.

45. Ribotsky BM, Berkowitz KD, Montague JR. Local anesthetics: Is there an advantage to mixing solutions? J Am Podiatr Med Assoc 1996;86:487–491.

46. Cohen SE, Thurlow A. Comparison of a chloroprocaine-bupivacaine mixture with chloroprocaine and bupivacaine used individually for obstetric epidural analgesia. Anesthesiology 1979;51:288–292.

47. Corke BC, Carlson CG, Dettbarn WD. The influence of 2-chloroprocaine on the subsequent analgesic potency of bupivacaine. Anesthesiology 1984;60:25–27.

48. Lalka D, Vicuna N, Burrow SR, et al. Bupivacaine and other amide local anesthetics inhibit the hydrolysis of chloroprocaine by human serum. Anesth Analg 1978;57:534–539.

49. Galindo A, Witcher T. Mixtures of local anesthetics: Bupivacaine-chloroprocaine. Anesth Analg 1980;59:683–685.

50. Spiegel DA, Dexter F, Warner DS, Baker MT, Todd MM. Central nervous system toxicity of local anesthetic mixtures in the rat. Anesth Analg 1992;75:922–928.

51. Wakiyama N, Juni K, Nakano M. Preparation and evaluation in vitro of polylactic microspheres containing local anesthetics. Chem Pharm Bull (Tokyo) 1982;30:3719–3727.

52. Kojima T, Nakano M, Juni K, Inoue S, Yoshida Y. Preparation and evaluation in vitro of polycarbonate microspheres containing local anesthetics. Chem Pharm Bull (Tokyo) 1984;32:2725–2802.

53. Dräger C, Benzinger D, Gao F, Berde B. Prolonged intercostal nerve blockade in sheep using controlled-release of bupivacaine and dexamethasone from polymer microspheres. Anesthesiology 1998;89:969–979.

54. Haynes DH, Kirkpatrick AF. Ultra-long-duration of local anesthesia produced by injection of lecithin-coated methoxyflurane microdroplets. Anesthesiology 1985;63:490–499.

55. Masters DB, Berde CB, Dutta SK, et al. Prolonged regional nerve blockade by controlled release of local anesthetic from a biodegradable polymer matrix. Anesthesiology 1993;79:340–346.

56. Boedecker BH, Lojeski EW, Kline MD, Haynes DH. Ultra-long duration of local anesthesia produced by injection of lecithin-coated tetracaine microcrystals. J Clin Pharmacol 1994;34:699–702.

57. Mashimo T, Uchida I, Pak M, et al. Prolongation of canine epidural anesthesia by liposome encapsulation of lidocaine. Anesth Analg 1992;74:827–834.

58. Mowat JJ, Mok MJ, MacLeod BA. Liposomal bupivacaine: Extended duration nerve blockade using large unilamellar vesicles that exhibit a proton gradient. Anesthesiology 1996;85:635–643.

59. Klein SM, Grant SA, Greengrass RA, et al. Interscalene brachial plexus block with continuous catheter insertion system and a disposable infusion pump. Anesth Analg 2000;91:1473–1478.

60. Wolfe TM, Muir WW. Local anesthetics: Pharmacology and novel applications. Compend Contin Educ Pract Vet 2003;25:916–927.

61. Gasser HS, Erlanger J. Role of fiber size in establishment of nerve block by pressure or cocaine. Am J Physiol 1929;88:581–591.

62. De Jong RH. Physiology and Pharmacology of Local Anesthesia. Springfield, IL: Charles C Thomas, 1970.

63. Franz DN, Perry RS. Mechanisms of differential block among single myelinated and non-myelinated axons of procaine. J Physiol (Lond) 1974;236:193–210.

64. Gissen AJ, Covino BG, Gregus J. Differential sensitivity of mammalian nerve fibers to local anesthetic agents. Anesthesiology 1980;53:467–474.

65. Heavner JE, de Jong RH. Lidocaine blocking concentrations for B- and C-nerve fibers. Anesthesiology 1974;40:228–233.

66. Fink BR, Cairns AM. Lack of size-related differential sensitivity to equilibrium conduction block among mammalian myelinated axons exposed to lidocaine. Anesth Analg 1987;66:948–953.

67. Gokin AP, Philip B, Strichartz GR. Preferential block of small myelinated sensory and motor fibers by lidocaine: In vivo electrophysiology in the rat sciatic nerve. Anesthesiology 2001;95:1441–1454.

68. Ford DJ, Raj PP, Pritam S, Regan KR, Ohlweiler D. Differential peripheral nerve block by local anesthetics in the cat. Anesthesiology 1984;60:28–33.

69. Wildsmith JA. Peripheral nerve and local anaesthetic drugs. Br J Anaesth 1986;58:692–700.

70. Feldman HS, Covino BG. Comparative motor-blocking effects of bupivacaine and ropivacaine, a new amino amide local anesthetic, in the rat and dog. Anesth Analg 1988;67:1047–1052.

71. Feldman HS, Dvoskin S, Arthur GR, Doucette AM. Antinociceptive and motor-blocking efficacy of ropivacaine and bupivacaine after epidural administration in the dog. Reg Anesth 1996; 21:318–326.

72. Winnie AP, La Vallee DA, Pe Sosa B, Masud KZ. Clinical pharmacokinetics of local anesthetics. Can Anaesth Soc J 1977;24:252–262.

73. Hickey R, Hoffman J, Ramamurthy J. A comparison of ropivacaine 0.5% and bupivacaine 0.5% for brachial plexus block. Anesthesiology 1991;74:599–602.

74. Hickey R, Rowley CL, Candido KD, Hoffman J, Ramamurthy S, Winnie AP. A comparative study of 0.25% ropivacaine and 0.25% bupivacaine for brachial plexus block. Anesth Analg 1992;75:602–606.

75. Futema F, Fantoni DT, Auler JOC Jr, Cortopassi SRG, Acaui A, Stopiglia AJ. A new brachial plexus block technique in dogs. Vet Anaesth Analg 2002;29:133–139.

76. Carpenter RL, Mackey DC. Local anesthetic. In: Barash PG, Cullen BF, Stoelting RK, eds. Clinical Anesthesia, 3rd ed. Philadelphia: Lippincott-Raven, 1997:413–439.

77. Sunderland S, Ray LJ. The interneural topography of the radial, median and ulnar nerves. Brain 1945;68:1243–1299.

78. Covino BG, Vassallo HG. Local Anesthetics: Mechanisms of Action and Clinical Use, 1st ed. New York: Grune and Stratton, 1976.

79. Green NM. Area of differential block in spinal anesthesia with hyperbaric tetracaine. Anesthesiology 1958;19:45–50.

80. Liu S, Kopacz DJ, Carpenter RL. Quantitative assessment of differential sensory nerve block after lidocaine spinal anesthesia. Anesthesiology 1995;82:60–63.

81. Liu PL, Feldman HS, Giasi R, Patterson MK, Covino BG. Comparative CNS toxicity of lidocaine, etidocaine, bupivacaine, and tetracaine in awake dogs following rapid intravenous administration. Anesth Analg 1983;62:375–379.

82. Rosen MA, Baysinger CL, Shnider SM, et al. Evaluation of neurotoxicity after subarachnoid injection of large volumes of local anesthetic solutions. Anesth Analg 1983;62:802–808.

83. Hodgson PS, Neal JM, Pollock JE, Liu SS. The neurotoxicity of drugs given intrathecally (spinal). Anesth Analg 1999;88:797–809.

84. Serradell A, Herrero R, Villanueva JA, Santos JA, Moncho JM, Masdeu J. Comparison of three different volumes of mepivacaine in axillary plexus block using multiple nerve stimulation. Br J Anaesth 2003;4:519–524.

85. Chernoff DM. Kinetic analysis of phase inhibition of neuronal sodium currents by lidocaine and bupivacaine. Biophys J 1990;58:53–68.

86. Sakura S, Sumi M, Kushizaki H, Saito Y, Kosaka Y. Concentration of lidocaine affects intensity of sensory block during lumbar epidural anesthesia. Anesth Analg 1999;88:123–127.

87. Duke T, Caulkett NA, Ball SD, Remedios AM. Comparative analgesic and cardiopulmonary effects of bupivacaine and ropivacaine in the epidural space of the conscious dog. Vet Anaesth Analg 2000;27:13–21.

88. Sakura S, Sumi M, Morimoto N, Saito Y. The addition of epinephrine increases intensity of sensory block during epidural anesthesia with lidocaine. Reg Anesth Pain Med 1999;24:541–546.

89. Burfoot MF, Bromage PR. The effects of epinephrine on mepivacaine absorption from the spinal epidural space. Anesthesiology 1971;35:488–492.

90. Hurley RJ, Feldman HS, Latka C, Arthur GR, Covino BG. The effects of epinephrine on the anesthetic and hemodynamic properties of ropivacaine and bupivacaine after epidural administration in the dog. Reg Anesth 1991;16:303–308.

91. Chapin JC, Kushins LG, Munson ES, Schick LM. Lidocaine, bupivacaine, etidocaine, and epinephrine-induced arrhythmias during halothane anesthesia in dogs. Anesthesiology 1980;52:23–26.

92. Vickers MD, Schnieden H, Wood-Smith FG. Drugs in Anaesthetic Practice, 6th ed. London: Butterworth's, 1984.

93. Nicoll JMV, Treuren B, Acharya PA, Ahlen K, James M. Retrobulbar anesthesia: The role of hyaluronidase. Anesth Analg 1986;65:1324–1328.

94. Kallio H, Paloheimo M, Maunuksela E-L. Hyaluronidase as an adjuvant in bupivacaine-lidocaine mixture for retrobulbar/peribulbar block. Anesth Analg 2000;91:934–937.

95. Cudmore I, O'Sullivan K, Casey P, Goggin M, Cunningham AJ. Retrobulbar block: Effect of hyaluronidase on lidocaine systemic absorption and CSF diffusion in dogs. Anesth Analg 1989; 68(Suppl):65.

96. Nociti JR, Serzedo PS, Zuccolotto EB, Cagnolati CA, Nues AM. Ropivacaine in peribulbar block: A comparative study with bupivacaine. Acta Anaesthesiol Scand 1999;43:799–802.

97. Moore DC. The use of hyaluronidase in local and nerve block analgesia other than spinal block: 1520 cases. Anesthesiology 1951;12:611–626.

98. Chernoff DM, Strichartz. Kinetics of local anesthetic inhibition of neural sodium currents, pH and hydrophobicity dependence. Biophys J 1990;58:69–81.

99. Ririe DG, Walker FO, James RL, Butterworth J. Effect of alkalinization of lidocaine on median nerve block. Br J Anaesth 2000;84:163–168.

100. Buckley FP, Neto GD, Fink BR. Acid and alkaline solutions of local anesthetics: Duration of nerve block and tissue pH. Anesth Analg 1985;64:477–482.

101. Capogna G, Celleno D, Laudano D, Giunta F. Alkalinization of local anesthetics. Which block, which local anesthetic? Reg Anesth 1995;20:369–377.

102. Di Fazio CA, Carron H, Grosslight KR, Moscicki JC, Bolding WR, Johns RA. Comparison of pH-adjusted lidocaine solutions for epidural anesthesia. Anesth Analg 1986;65:760–764.

103. McMorland GH, Douglas MJ, Jeffery WK, et al. Effect of pH-adjustment of bupivacaine on onset and duration of epidural analgesia in parturients. Can Anaesth Soc J 1986;33:537–541.

104. Ackerman WE, Juneja MM, Denson DD, et al. The effect of pH and PCO_2 on epidural analgesia with 2% 2-chloroprocaine. Anesth Analg 1989;68:593–598.

105. Peterfreund RA, Datta S, Ostheimer GW. pH adjustment of local anesthetic solutions with sodium bicarbonate: Laboratory evaluation of alkalinization and precipitation. Reg Anesth 1989;14:265–270.

106. Bromage PR, Burfoot MF, Crowell DE, Truant AP. Quality of epidural blockade. 3. Carbonated local anesthetic solutions. Br J Anaesth 1967;39:197–209.

107. Schelling CG, Klein LV. Comparison of carbonated lidocaine and lidocaine hydrochloride for caudal epidural anesthesia in horses. Am J Vet Res 1985;46:1375–1377.

108. Greene NM. Distribution of local anesthetic solutions within the subarachnoid space. Anesth Analg 1985;64:715–730.

109. Nicol ME, Holdcroft A. Density of intrathecal agents. Br J Anaesth 1992;68:60–63.

110. Thage B, Callesen T. Bupivacaine in spinal anesthesia: The spread of analgesia—Dependence on baricity, positioning, dosage, technique of injection and patient characteristics [in Danish]. Ugeskr Laeger 1993;39:104–108.

111. Horlocker TT, Wedel DJ. Density, specific gravity, and baricity of spinal anesthetic solutions at body temperature. Anesth Analg 1993;76:1015–1018.

112. Blomqvist H, Nilsson A. Is glucose-free bupivacaine isobaric or hypobaric? Reg Anesth 1989;14:195–198.

113. Masuda R, Yokoyama K. Density, specific gravity and baricity of various spinal anesthetics and those of normal human cerebrospinal fluid in Japanese [in Japanese]. Masui 1995;44:1527–1532.

114. Schiffer E, Van Gessel E, Fournier R, Weber A, Gamulin Z. Cerebrospinal fluid density influences extent of plain bupivacaine spinal anesthesia. Anesthesiology 2002;96:1325–1330.

115. Davis H, King WR. Densities of common spinal anesthetic solutions at body temperature. Anesthesiology 1952;13:184–188.

116. McDonald SB, Liu SS, Kopacz DJ, Stephenson CA. Hyperbaric spinal ropivacaine: A comparison to bupivacaine in volunteers. Anesthesiology 1999;90:971–977.

117. Markey JR, Montiague R, Winnie AP. A comparative efficacy study of hyperbaric 5% lidocaine and 1.5% lidocaine for spinal anesthesia. Anesth Analg 1997;85:1105–1107.

118. Masuda R, Yokoyama K, Inoue T. Spread of spinal anesthesia with 3 different hyperbaric solutions used in Japan [in Japanese]. Masui 1998;47:1444–1450.

119. Park WY, Balingit PE, Macnamara TE. Effects of patient age, pH of cerebrospinal fluid, and vasopressors on onset and duration of spinal anesthesia. Anesth Analg 1975;54:455–458.

120. Rosenberg PH, Heavner JE. Temperature-dependent nerve-blocking action of lidocaine and halothane. Acta Anaesthesiol Scand 1980;24:314–320.

121. Butterworth JF IV, Walker FO, Neal JM. Cooling potentiates lidocaine inhibition of median nerve sensory fibers. Anesth Analg 1990;70:507–511.

122. Sanchez V, Arthur R, Strichartz GR. Fundamental properties of local anesthetics. I. The dependence of lidocaine's ionization and octanol:buffer partitioning on solvent and temperature. Anesth Analg 1987;66:159–165.

123. Butterworth JF, Walker FO, Neal JM. Cooling lidocaine from room temperature to 5°C (neither hastens nor improves median nerve block). Anesth Analg 1989;68(Suppl):S45.

124. Datta S, Lambert DH, Gregus J, Gissen AJ, Covino BG. Differential sensitivities of mammalian nerve fibers during pregnancy. Anesth Analg 1983;62:1070–1072.

125. Flanagan HL, Datta S, Lambert DH, Gissen AJ, Covino BG. Effects of pregnancy on bupivacaine-induced conduction blockade in the isolated rabbit vagus nerve. Anesth Analg 1987;66:123–126.

126. Post C, Andersson RGG, Ryrfeldt Å, Nilsson E. Physico-chemical modification of lidocaine uptake in rat lung tissue. Acta Pharmacol Toxicol 1979;44:103–109.

127. Ohmura S, Sugano A, Kawada M, Yamamoto K. Pulmonary uptake of ropivacaine and levobupivacaine in rabbits. Anesth Analg 2003;97:893–897.

128. Devers A, Galer BS. Topical lidocaine patch relieves a variety of neuropathic pain conditions: An open-label study. Clin J Pain 2000;16:205–208.

129. Bjerring P, Arendt-Nielsen L. Depth and duration of skin analgesia to needle insertion after topical application of EMLA Cream. Br J Anaesth 1990;64:173–177.

130. Gajraj NM, Pennant JH, Watcha MF. Eutectic mixture of local anesthetics (EMLA®) cream. Anesth Analg 1994;78:574–583.

131. Flecknell PA, Liles JH, Williamson HA. The use of lignocaine-prilocaine local anaesthetic cream for pain-free venepuncture in laboratory animals. Lab Anim Sci 1990;24:142–146.

132. Wahlgren CF, Quiding H. Depth of cutaneous analgesia after application of a eutectic mixture of the local anesthetics lidocaine and prilocaine (EMLA Cream). J Am Acad Dermatol 2000;42:584–588.

133. Molodecka J, Stenhouse C, Jones JM, Tomlinson A. comparison of percutaneous anaesthesia for venous cannulation after topical application of either amethocaine or EMLA Cream. Br J Anaesth 1993;72:174–176.

134. McCafferty DF, Woolfson AD. New patch delivery system for percutaneous local anaesthesia. Br J Anaesth 1993;71:370–374.

135. Eichenfield LF, Funk A, Fallon-Friedlander S, Cunningham BB. A clinical study to evaluate the efficacy of ELA-Max (4% liposomal lidocaine) as compared with eutectic mixture of local anesthetics cream for pain reduction of venipuncture in children. Pediatrics 2002;109:1093–1099.

136. Fransson BA, Peck KE, Smith JK, Anthony JR, Mealey KL. Transdermal absorption of a liposome-encapsulated formulation of lidocaine following topical administration in cats. Am J Vet Res 2002;63:1309–1312.

137. Squire SJ, Kirchoff KT, Hissong K. Comparing two methods of topical anesthesia used before intravenous cannulation in pediatric patients. J Pediatr Health Care 2000;14:68–72.

138. Wallace MS, Ridgeway B, Jun E, Schulteis G, Rabussay D, Zhang L. Topical delivery of lidocaine in healthy volunteers by electroporation, electroincorporation, or iontophoresis: An evaluation of skin analgesia. Reg Anesth Pain Med 2001;26:229–238.

139. Irsfeld S, Klement W, Lipfert P. Dermal anaesthesia: Comparison of EMLA Cream with iontophoretic local anaesthesia. Br J Anaesth 1993;71:375–378.

140. Covino BG. Pharmacodynamic and pharmacokinetic aspects of local anesthetics. Ann Chir Gynaecol 1984;73:188–122.

141. Tucker G. Pharmacokinetics of local anesthetics. Br J Anaesth 1986;58:717–731.

142. Wright JD, Boudinot FD, Ujhelyi MR. Measurement and analysis of unbound drug concentrations. Clin Pharmacokinet 1996;30:445–462.

143. Strichartz GR, Ritchie JM. The action of local anesthetics on ionic channels of excitable tissues. In: Strichartz GR, ed. Local Anesthetics. Berlin: Springer-Verlag, 1987:21–52.

144. Marathe PH, Shen DD, Artru AA, Bowdle TA. Effect of serum protein binding on the entry of lidocaine into brain and CSF in dogs. Anesthesiology 1991;75:804–812.

145. De Rick AF, Belpaire FM, Dello C, Bogaert MG. Influence of enhanced alpha-1-acid glycoprotein concentration on protein binding, pharmacokinetics and antiarrhythmic effect of lidocaine in the dog. J Pharmacol Exp Ther 1987;241:289–293.

146. Belpaire FM, De Rick A, Dello C, Fraeyman N, Bogaert MG. Alpha 1-acid glycoprotein and serum binding of drugs in healthy and diseased dogs. J Vet Pharmacol Ther 1987;10:43–48.

147. Shand DG. alpha 1-Acid glycoprotein and plasma lidocaine binding. Clin Pharmacokinet 1984;9:27–31.

148. Brodie BB, Lief PA, Poet R. The fate of procaine in man following intravenous administration and methods for the estimation of pro-

caine and diethylaminoethanol. J Pharmacol Exp Ther 1948;94: 359–366.

149. O'Brien JE, Abbey V, Hinsvark O, Perel J, Finster M. Metabolism and measurement of chloroprocaine, an ester-type local anesthetic. J Pharm Sci 1979;68:75–78.

150. Queiroz-Neto A, Zamur G, Lacerda-Neto, Tobin T. Determination of the highest no-effect dose (HNED) and of the elimination pattern of cocaine in horses. J Appl Physiol 2002;22:117–121.

151. McKeever KH, Hinchcliff KW, Gerken DF, Sams RA. Effects of cocaine on incremental treadmill exercise in horses. J Appl Physiol 1993;75:2727–2733.

152. Lambert LA, Lambert DH, Strichartz GR. Irreversible conduction block in isolated nerve by high concentrations of local anesthetics. Anesthesiology 1994;80:1082–1093.

153. Welch SL. Local anesthetic toxicosis. Vet Med 2000;95:670–673.

154. Brown DL, Ransom DM, Hall JA, Leicht CH, Schroeder DR, Offord KP. Regional anesthesia and local anesthetic-induced systemic toxicity: Seizure frequency and accompanying cardiovascular changes. Anesth Analg 1996;82:669–670.

155. Englesson S. The influence of acid-base changes on central nervous system toxicity of local anaesthetic agents. I. An experimental study in cats. Acta Anaesthesiol Scand 1974;18:79–87.

156. Englesson S, Grevsten S. The influence of acid-base changes on central nervous system toxicity of local anaesthetic agents. Acta Anaesthesiol Scand 1974;18:88–103.

157. Chadwick HS. Toxicity and resuscitation in lidocaine- or bupivacaine-infused cats. Anesthesiology 1985;63:385–390.

158. Tobin T, Blake JW, Sturma L, Amett S, Truelove J. Pharmacology of procaine in the horse: Pharmacokinetics and behavioral effects. Am J Vet Res 1977;38:637–647.

159. Courtot D. Elimination of lignocaine in the horse. Irish Vet J 1979;33:205–215.

160. Albright GA. Cardiac arrest following regional anesthesia with etidocaine or bupivacaine. Anesthesiology 1979;51:285–287.

161. Rutten AJ, Nancarrow C, Mather LE, Ilsley AH, Runciman WB, Upton RN. Hemodynamic and central nervous system effects of intravenous bolus doses of lidocaine, bupivacaine, and ropivacaine in sheep. Anesth Analg 1989;69:291–299.

162. Nancarrow C, Rutten AJ, Runciman WB, Mathes LE, Carapetis RJ, McLean CF. Myocardial and cerebral drug concentrations and the mechanisms of death after fatal intravenous doses of lidocaine, bupivacaine, and ropivacaine in the sheep. Anesth Analg 1989;69: 276–283.

163. Scott DB, Lee A, Fagan D, Bowler GM, Bloomfield P, Lundh R. Acute toxicity of ropivacaine compared with that of bupivacaine. Anesth Analg 1989;69:563–569.

164. Huang YF, Pryor ME, Mather LE, Veering BT. Cardiovascular and central nervous system effects of intravenous levobupivacaine in sheep. Anesth Analg 1998;86:797–804.

165. Chang DH, Ladd LA, Wilson KA, Gelgor L, Mather LE. Tolerability of large-dose intravenous levobupivacaine in sheep. Anesth Analg 2000;91:671–679.

166. Ohmura S, Kawada M, Ohta T, Yamamoto K, Kobayashi T. Systemic toxicity and resuscitation in bupivacaine-, levobupivacaine-, or ropivacaine-infused rats. Anesth Analg 2001;93: 743–748.

167. Blair MR. Cardiovascular pharmacology of local anaesthetics. Br J Anaesth 1975;47(Suppl):247–252.

168. Strichartz GR, Berde CB. Local anesthetics. In: Miller RD, ed. Anesthesia, 4th ed. New York: Churchill Livingstone, 1994: 489–521.

169. Kotelko DM, Shnider SM, Dailey PA, et al. Bupivacaine-induced cardiac arrhythmias in sheep. Anesthesiology 1984;60:10–18.

170. Bruelle P, Lefrant J-Y, de La Coussaye JE, et al. Comparative electrophysiologic and hemodynamic effects of several amide local anesthetic drugs in anesthetized dogs. Anesth Analg 1996;82:648–656.

171. Liu P, Feldman HS, Covino BM, Giasi R, Covino BG. Acute cardiovascular toxicity of intravenous amide local anesthetics in anesthetized ventilated dogs. Anesth Analg 1992;61:317–322.

172. Buffington CW. The magnitude and duration of direct myocardial depression following intracoronary local anesthetics: A comparison of lidocaine and bupivacaine. Anesthesiology 1989;70:280–287.

173. Reiz S, Haggmark S, Johansson G, Nath S. Cardiotoxicity of ropivacaine: A new amide local anesthetic agent. Acta Anaesthesiol Scand 1989;33:93–98.

174. Nancarrow C, Rutten AJ, Runciman WB, et al. Myocardial and cerebral drug concentrations and the mechanisms of death after fatal intravenous doses of lidocaine, bupivacaine, and ropivacaine in the sheep. Anesth Analg 1989;69:276–283.

175. Rosen MA, Thigpen JW, Shnider SM, Foutz SE, Levinson G, Koike M. Bupivacaine-induced cardiotoxicity in hypoxic and acidotic sheep. Anesth Analg 1985;64:1089–1096.

176. Heavner JE. Cardiac toxicity of local anesthetics in the intact isolated heart model: A review. Reg Anesth Pain Med 2002;27: 545–555.

177. Chernoff DM. Kinetic analysis of phasic inhibition of neuronal sodium currents by lidocaine and bupivacaine. Biophys J 1990;58:53–68.

178. Graf BM, Martin E, Bosnjak ZJ, Stowe DF. Stereospecific effect of bupivacaine isomers on atrioventricular conduction in the isolated perfusion guinea pig heart. Anesthesiology 1997;86:410–419.

179. Mazoit JX, Boico O, Samii K. Myocardial update of bupivacaine. II. Pharmacokinetics and pharmacodynamics of bupivacaine enantiomers in the isolated perfused rabbit heart. Anesth Analg 1993; 77:477–482.

180. Mazoit JX, Decaux A, Bouaziz H, Edouard A. Comparative ventricular electrophysiologic effect of racemic bupivacaine, levobupivacaine and ropivacaine on the isolated rabbit heart. Anesthesiology 2000;93:784–792.

181. Kasaba T, Onizuka S, Takasaki M. Procaine and mepivacaine have less toxicity in vitro than other clinically used local anesthetics. Anesth Analg 2003;97:85–90.

182. Radwan IA, Saito S, Goto F. The neurotoxicity of local anesthetics on growing neurons: A comparative study of lidocaine, bupivacaine, mepivacaine, and ropivacaine. Anesth Analg 2002;94: 319–324.

183. Covino BG, Marx GF, Finster M, Zsigmond EK. Prolonged sensory/motor deficits following inadvertent spinal anesthesia. Anesth Analg 1980;59:399–400.

184. Ravindran RS, Turner MS, Muller J. Neurologic effects of subarachnoid administration of 2-chloroprocaine-CE, bupivacaine, and low pH normal saline in dogs. Anesth Analg 1982;61:279–283.

185. Tetzlaff J. Clinical Pharmacology of Local Anesthetics. Woburn, MA: Butterworth-Heinemann, 2000.

186. Rosen MA, Baysinger MD, Shnider SM, et al. Evaluation of neurotoxicity after subarachnoid injection of large volumes of local anesthetic solutions. Anesth Analg 1983;62:802–808.

187. Barsa J, Batra M, Fink BR, Sumi SM. A comparative in vivo study of local neurotoxicity of lidocaine, bupivacaine, 2-chloroprocaine, and a mixture of 2-chloroprocaine and bupivacaine. Anesth Analg 1982;61:961–967.

188. Hodgson PS, Neal JM, Pollock JE, Liu SS. The neurotoxicity of drugs given intrathecally (spinal). Anesth Analg 1999;88:797–809.

189. Lambert LA, Lambert DH, Strichartz GR. Irreversible conduction block in isolated nerve by high concentrations of local anesthetics. Anesthesiology 1994;80:1082–1093.

190. Li DF, Bahar M, Cole G, Rosen M. Neurological toxicity of the subarachnoid infusion of bupivacaine, lignocaine or 2-chloroprocaine in the rat. Br J Anaesth 1985;57:424–429.

191. Hogan Q, Dotson R, Erickson S, Kettler R, Hogan K. Local anesthetic myotoxicity: A case and review. Anesthesiology 1994;80:942–947.

192. Basson MD, Carlson BM. Myotoxicity of single and repeated injections of mepivacaine (Carbocaine) in the rat. Anesth Analg 1980;59:275–282.

193. Benoit PW, Belt WD. Destruction and regeneration of skeletal muscle after treatment with a local anesthetic, bupivacaine (Marcaine). J Anat 1970;107:547–556.

194. Foster AH, Carlson BM. Myotoxicity of local anesthetics and regeneration of the damaged muscle fibers. Anesth Analg 1980;59:727–736.

195. Zink W, Seif C, Bohl JRE, et al. The acute myotoxic effects of bupivacaine and ropivacaine after continuous peripheral nerve blockades. Anesth Analg 2003;97:1173–1179.

196. Hall AH, Kulig KW, Rumack BH. Drug- and chemical-induced methemoglobinemia: Clinical features and management. Med Toxicol 1986;1:253–260.

197. Guertler AT, Lagutchik MS, Martin DG. Topical anesthetic-induced methemoglobinemia in sheep: A comparison of benzocaine and lidocaine. Fundam Appl Toxicol 1992;18:294–298.

198. Coleman MD, Coleman NA. Drug-induced methemoglobinemia: Treatment issues. Drug Saf 1996;14:394–405.

199. Saleem MA, McClung JA, Peterson SJ. Hypoxemia sans hypoxemia. Heart Dis 2000;2:116–117.

200. Vidyarthi V, Manda R, Ahmed A, Khosla S, Lubell DL. Severe methemoglobinemia after transesophageal echocardiography. Am J Ther 2003;10:225–227.

201. Ferraro-Borgida MJ, Mulhern SA, DeMeo MO, Bayer MJ. Methemoglobinemia from perineal application of an anesthetic cream. Ann Emerg Med 1996;27:785–788.

202. Arens JF, Carrera AE. Methemoglobin levels following peridural anesthesia with prilocaine for vaginal deliveries. Anesth Analg 1970;49:219–222.

203. Lagutchik MS, Mundie TG, Martin DG. Methemoglobinemia induced by a benzocaine-based topically administered anesthetic in eight sheep. J Am Vet Med Assoc 1992;201:1407–1410.

204. Harvey JW, Sameck JH, Burgard FJ. Benzocaine-induced methemoglobinemia in dogs. J Am Vet Med Assoc 1979;175:1171–1175.

205. Wilkie DA, Kirby R. Methemoglobinemia associated with dermal application of benzocaine cream in a cat. J Am Med Vet Assoc 1988;192:85–86.

206. Davis JA, Greefield RE, Brewer TG. Benzocaine-induced methemoglobinemia attributed to topical application of the anesthetic in several laboratory animal species. Am J Vet Res 1993;54:1322–1326.

207. Levy JH. Allergic reactions during anesthesia. J Clin Anesth 1988;1:39–46.

208. Munson ES, Tucker WK, Ausinsch B, Malagodi MH. Etidocaine, bupivacaine, and lidocaine seizure thresholds in monkeys. Anesthesiology 1975;42:271–478.

209. Englesson S, Matousek M. Central nervous system effects of local anaesthetic agents. Br J Anaesth 1975;47:241–246.

210. Heavner JE, Dryden CF, Sanghani V, Huemer G, Bessire A, Badgwell JM. Severe hypoxia enhances central nervous system and cardiovascular toxicity of bupivacaine in lightly anesthetized pigs. Anesthesiology 1992;77:142–147.

211. Mallampati SR, Liu PL, Knapp RM. Convulsions and ventricular tachycardia from bupivacaine with epinephrine: Successful resuscitation. Anesth Analg 1984;63:856–859.

212. Moore DC, Brindenbaugh LD. Oxygen: The antidote for systemic reactions from local anesthetic drugs. J Am Med Assoc 1960;174:842–847.

213. Bernards CM, Carpenter RL, Rupp SM, et al. Effect of midazolam and diazepam premedication on central nervous system and cardiovascular toxicity of bupivacaine. Anesthesiology 1989;70:318–323.

214. Heavner JE, Arthur J, Zou J, McDaniel K, Tyman-Szram B, Rosenberg PH. Comparison of propofol with thiopentone for treatment of bupivacaine-induced seizures in rats. Br J Anaesth 1993;71:715–719.

215. Gibson GR, Callan MB, Hoffman V, Giger U. Use of hemoglobin-based oxygen-carrying solution in cats: 72 cases (1998–2000). J Am Vet Med Assoc 2002;221:96–102.

216. Muir WW, Wellman ML. Hemoglobin solutions and tissue oxygenation. J Vet Intern Med 2003;17:127–135.

217. Groban L, Deal DD, Vernon JC, James RL, Butterworth J. Cardiac resuscitation after incremental overdosage with lidocaine, bupivacaine, levobupivacaine, and ropivacaine in anesthetized dogs. Anesth Analg 2001;92:37–43.

218. Arlock P. Actions of three local anaesthetics: lidocaine, bupivacaine and ropivacaine on guinea pig papillary muscle sodium channels (V_{max}). Pharmacol Toxicol 1988;63:96–104.

219. Ohmura S, Kawada M, Ohta T, Yamamoto K, Kobayashi T. Systemic toxicity and resuscitation in bupivacaine-, levobupivacaine-, or ropivacaine-infused rats. Anesth Analg 2001;93:743–748.

220. Kittleson MD. Drugs used in treatment of cardiac arrhythmias. In: Duncan L, ed. Small Animal Cardiovascular Medicine. St Louis: CV Mosby, 1998:203–220.

221. Kasten GW, Martin ST. Bupivacaine cardiovascular toxicity: Comparison of treatment with beryllium and lidocaine. Anesth Analg 1985;64:911–916.

222. Harvey JW, Keitt AS. Studies of the efficacy and potential hazards of methylene blue therapy in aniline-induced methaemoglobinaemia. Br J Haematol 1983;54:29–41.

223. Lipfert P. Tachyphylaxie von Lokalanaesthetika: Der Anesthesist. Reg Anesth 1989;38:13–20.

224. Skarda RT. Local anesthetics and local anesthetic techniques in horses. In: Muir WW, Hubbell JAE, eds. Equine Anesthesia Monitoring and Emergency Therapy. St Louis: CV Mosby, 1991:199–246.

Chapter 15

Muscle Relaxants and Neuromuscular Blockade

Elizabeth A. Martinez and Robert D. Keegan

Introduction

Muscle relaxants are anesthetic adjuncts administered to improve relaxation of skeletal muscles during surgical or diagnostic procedures. The term *neuromuscular blocking agents* (NMBAs) is a cumbersome, but descriptive, name that refers to this class of drugs producing their effect by actions at the neuromuscular junction. The more general term *muscle relaxant* refers to any drug that has relaxant properties and would include centrally acting agents such as benzodiazepines, α_2-adrenoceptor agonists, and guaifenesin. Beneficial effects of NMBA administration during general anesthesia include facilitation of tracheal intubation, reduction of skeletal muscle tone at light planes of inhalant or injectable anesthesia, and prevention of patient movement during delicate ocular, neurological, or cardiac surgery. Although used frequently in human anesthesia and in some veterinary specialties such as ophthalmology, the use of NMBAs in general veterinary practice is limited. Inhalant anesthetics such as isoflurane are complete anesthetics in that they fulfill the *triad* of anesthesia: unconsciousness, analgesia, and muscle relaxation. All three of these properties are required in order to perform most invasive surgical procedures. Of the three properties of the triad, inhalant anesthetics are very good at producing loss of consciousness at comparatively light planes of anesthesia, whereas substantially deeper planes are required to obtund nociceptive processing and skeletal muscle contraction. Indeed, these last two properties are provided by potent inhalant anesthetics only by virtue of more profound depression of the central nervous system (CNS). Unfortunately, deeper planes of inhalant anesthetics are associated with a decrease in cardiovascular function; thus, the properties of muscle relaxation and analgesia are accompanied by reduced cardiovascular performance. In young, healthy animals having good cardiovascular reserve, this may be well tolerated; in patients having poor cardiovascular function, however, significant morbidity and mortality may result. Rather than using inhalant anesthetics to provide all three components of the triad, a safer approach may be one that uses lower concentrations of an inhalant to provide unconsciousness, an analgesic to inhibit nociceptive processing, and an NMBA to relax skeletal muscle. This approach has historically been termed *balanced anesthesia*. Balanced anesthetic techniques are frequently chosen because they provide optimal conditions for both the surgeon and the patient.

History of Muscle Relaxants

The introduction of NMBAs into anesthesiology in 1942 is a relatively recent event in medical practice. Indigenous South Americans had been using a paralyzing poison for centuries on the heads of their hunting arrows. This lethal compound was derived from the tropical plant *Chondodendron tomentosum* and caused paralysis and death to quarry that had been impaled by a coated arrow. Such a poison was an advantage because animals suffering a normally nonlethal wound would succumb and could be harvested by the hunter. The existence of this poison, known as curare, was recognized outside of South America, but its medical uses were not realized. The link was made when an explorer, Richard Gill, returned from the jungles of South America and was diagnosed with multiple sclerosis. The suggestion that the spastic paralysis might be relieved by administration of the arrow poison led Gill to overcome his disability and return to the South American jungle. He returned to the United States in the late 1930s having obtained a quantity of curare, which he sold to a pharmaceutical company that then purified the raw curare and marketed it under the trade name of Intocostrin. Initially, Intocostrin was used only in psychiatric medicine to control seizures that were associated with treatments of psychotic states. A physician in the company realized the potential the drug might have in the field of anesthesiology and convinced an anesthesiologist to undertake studies in humans. This was to be a monumental undertaking because the anesthesia community of the day was understandably not receptive to administration of a paralytic arrow poison to surgical patients. Indeed, the mere suggestion that one would administer a drug that would intentionally cause respiratory arrest was unthinkable to a generation of physicians who had grown up with the motto "Where there is breath, there is hope." Studies which suggested that d-tubocurarine, a quaternary alkaloid isolated from raw curare, was safe and useful for relaxing abdominal muscles during general anesthesia began to emerge, and use of the drug spread to Great Britain by 1945.[1] Another drug with paralytic properties similar to d-tubocurarine, but having the advantage of rapid onset and offset (succinylcholine), was introduced into human practice in the early 1950s.[2] Reports of the use of NMBA in dogs also began to appear in the early 1950s, and administration of succinylcholine to horses was described in the 1960s.[3,4] Both d-tubocurarine and succinylcholine have a number of undesirable cardiovascular effects. These agents can affect autonomic ganglia and cardiac muscarinic receptors, as well as induce histamine release. Although succinylcholine has the advantage of rapid onset and offset compared with d-tubocurarine, the additional disadvantages of hyperkalemia, arrhythmias, postanesthetic myalgia, and the changing nature of its block dictated that other NMBAs be developed.

Synthetic relaxants developed during the ensuing years included gallamine, decamethonium, alcuronium and, finally, steroid-based pancuronium. Most are now only of historical interest, although alcuronium is still frequently used in many parts of the world, and pancuronium serves as a parent molecule of several contemporary NMBAs. Atracurium and vecuronium, introduced in the 1980s, have the advantage of minimal to no cardiovascular effects, minimal histamine release, and a controllable and predictable duration of action. Both are widely used in human anesthesia practice. Mivicurium, an analogue of atracurium with a rapid onset and brief action, was developed to take advantage of rapid onset of action in facilitating tracheal intubation after induction of anesthesia. It is essentially devoid of the problems of hyperkalemia, arrhythmia, and myalgia. Recently developed NMBAs include doxacurium, pipecuronium, and rocuronium, which represent an effort to produce an NMBA that has a precise, predictable duration of action and minimal untoward cardiovascular side effects.

Physiology of the Neuromuscular Junction

All muscle relaxants exert their effects at the *neuromuscular junction*, which forms the interface between the large myelinated motor nerve and the muscle that is supplied by that nerve. The neuromuscular junction itself may be divided into the prejunctional motor nerve ending, the synaptic cleft, and the postjunctional membrane of the skeletal muscle fiber. Present on the prejunctional and postjunctional areas of the neuromuscular junction are nicotinic receptors, which bind and respond to acetylcholine (ACh) or another suitable ligand. The prejunctional receptor is thought to be important in the synthesis and mobilization of ACh stores, but not for its release.[5] There appear to be two types of postjunctional receptors: junctional and extrajunctional.[6] The *junctional receptors* are found on the motor end plates of normal adult animals and are responsible for interacting with the released ACh, initiating muscle contraction. Antagonism of ACh at the junctional receptors is responsible for the relaxant effect seen when an NMBA is administered. The *extrajunctional receptors* are not present in high numbers on the skeletal muscle membranes of adult mammals, but are important because they are synthesized by muscles that are receiving a less than normal degree of motor nerve stimulation.[7] Thus, their number may be increased following spinal cord injury or after a period of muscle disuse, such as when a limb is cast. They are also present in neonates. The location of extrajunctional receptors is not restricted to the motor end plate and they may be located over the entire muscle cell surface.[8,9] Extrajunctional receptors appear to be more responsive to depolarizing NMBAs such as succinylcholine and less responsive to nondepolarizing NMBAs such as atracurium.[10] If the degree of neuromuscular deficit is severe, extrajunctional receptors may be more numerous and widely distributed over the muscle membrane. Such patients may have a more intense response to the actions of a depolarizing NMBA and a more profound release of intracellular potassium ions (K^+) with its concomitant adverse cardiac effects.[11]

The prejunctional nerve endings synthesize and store a quantity of ACh in synaptic vesicles. During normal neuromuscular transmission, an action potential arrives at the prejunctional motor nerve ending, causing depolarization of the nerve terminal. The depolarization of the nerve membrane activates adenylate cyclase, which converts adenosine triphosphate to cyclic adenosine monophosphate. The resultant conversion results in calcium-

Neuromuscular Contraction

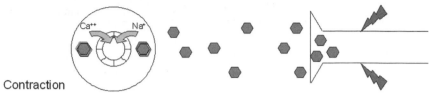

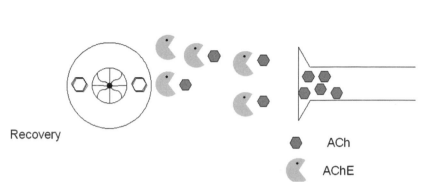

Contraction

Recovery

⬡ ACh

◖ AChE

Fig. 15.1. Top: Normal neuromuscular transmission. An action potential arriving at the motor end plate causes the release of acetylcholine (ACh) into the synaptic cleft. ACh binds to both postsynaptic receptors, which opens the ion channel and subsequent muscular contraction. **Bottom:** Recovery and repolarization occur when ACh is degraded by acetylcholinesterase (AChE), the receptor sites are cleared, and the ion channel closes. Ca+, calcium ions; and Na+, sodium ions.

ion (Ca^{2+}) entry into the nerve terminal and resultant release of ACh into the synaptic cleft. ACh can then diffuse to the postsynaptic membrane and interact with postjunctional nicotinic receptors, resulting in the development of an end-plate potential (a muscle cell action potential) and ultimately muscular contraction (Fig. 15.1). ACh is rapidly hydrolyzed into choline and acetate by acetylcholinesterase. Thus, the muscle cell is depolarized by the end-plate potential created by the binding of ACh to the receptor and then is repolarized as the ACh is removed from the receptor and hydrolyzed.

The postjunctional receptors are concentrated on the end plate immediately opposite the sites of ACh release.[12] Electron microscopy of these receptors shows them to have a central pit surrounded by a raised circular area; thus, they look similar to a spool of thread that is viewed end on.[13,14] The raised circular area is the mouth of a cylinder of protein that protrudes through the cell membrane, and it contains the binding sites for ACh and other ligands. The pit is the extracellular opening of an ion channel that runs throughout the cylinder's length. The receptor is composed of five subunits of four distinct subunit types designated alpha, beta, gamma, and delta. The two alpha subunits of each receptor and the others are arranged into a cylinder having a potential space, the ion channel, contained within.[15] The functional opening of the channel is controlled by the ACh-binding sites present in the two alpha subunits. When two molecules of ACh are bound to the two binding sites on each of the two alpha subunits, the protein rotates into a new conformation and, in so doing, opens the ion channel and permits ion flow.[16] The open channel enables flow of small cations (sodium ions [Na$^+$] and Ca^{2+} flow in and K$^+$ flows out) but not large cations or anions. Ion-current flow depolarizes the postjunctional membrane.[17] As the ACh molecules dissociate from the nicotinic receptors and are hydrolyzed by acetylcholinesterase, the ion channel closes, current flow stops, and the membrane is repolarized.

Binding of ligands to the nicotinic receptor at the neuromuscular junction is competitive and reversible. Since two molecules of ACh bound to each of the receptor alpha subunits are required for normal function, antagonists have a distinct advantage in that they need only bind to one of the subunits to prevent normal neuromuscular transmission and thus paralysis.[18] The interaction of ACh and NMBA at the postjunctional receptors is a dynamic process of binding and dissociation and, coupled with the sheer number of receptors present (10,000 to 20,000/μm^2), the success or failure of neuromuscular transmission in the presence of an NMBA is determined by the concentration of the NMBA versus the concentration of ACh. A high percentage of receptors binding ACh favors muscular contraction, whereas a high percentage of receptors binding NMBA favors paralysis. This suggests a method for reversing paralysis induced by an NMBA. Increasing the concentration of ACh compared with the concentration of NMBA will increase the probability that the receptor will bind ACh and normal neuromuscular transmission will again result. Clinically, ACh concentration is increased by administration of inhibitors of acetylcholinesterase, such as neostigmine. When acetylcholinesterase is inhibited, ACh is not degraded immediately after release from the receptor, its half-life within the synapse is longer, and more of it is available to interact with receptors. Increased ACh activity is also seen as the concentration of an NMBA declines due to degradation of the drug. As the concentration declines, the competitive balance favors ACh and more normal neuromuscular transmission returns.

Pharmacology

Ligand-Receptor Interactions

The classic mechanism of action of an NMBA such as d-tubocurarine or atracurium is the competitive binding of the drug to the receptor thus blocking transmission of the nerve action potential. There are at least two other less well understood mechanisms: desensitization and channel blockade.

Earlier it was stated that the cholinergic receptor is inactive with its potential ion channel collapsed when two molecules of ACh are not attached to the alpha subunits of the receptor. Binding of ACh to each of the two alpha subunits of the receptor causes the conformational change to the active state and enables the ion channel to open. However, the channel does not have to exist only in the open or collapsed state. A third possible conformation is the desensitized state, in which receptors bind ACh to the alpha subunits, but a conformational change and channel opening do not occur. A number of drugs, including agonists, antagonists, and inhalant anesthetics, appear to be able to switch the cholinergic receptor to the desensitized state. The desensitized-state hypothesis explains the synergistic action that inhalant anesthetics have with NMBAs because it is known clinically that much lower doses of NMBAs achieve an acceptable degree of relaxation when a patient is anesthetized with a volatile anesthetic. A large number of drugs may cause or promote desensitization, such as succinylcholine, thiopental, Ca^{2+}-channel blockers, local anesthetics, phenothiazines, cyclohexamines, inhalant anesthetics, and some antibiotics.[19–22]

Channel blockade occurs when a molecule becomes stuck within the channel, obstructing normal ion flux. This is possible because the mouth of the ion channel is much wider than the transmembrane portion, which enables molecules to enter the channel but not necessarily pass completely through it. Therefore, channel blockade blocks normal neuromuscular transmission not by competing for binding sites on the nicotinic receptor, but by interfering with the depolarization process in response to binding of an agonist.[23,24] This is an important distinction because the paralysis induced by channel blockade may not be antagonized by administration of an anticholinesterase. In fact, inhibition of cholinesterase enzyme may intensify the block because the opening of more ion channels in response to a greater concentration of ACh may provide a greater opportunity for the offending molecules to become trapped within the channel. It is known that many drugs can cause channel blockade, but the fact that NMBAs themselves can block the neuromuscular receptor channels may partially explain why administration of an anticholinesterase drug in an effort to antagonize neuromuscular blockade may sometimes intensify rather than lessen the paralysis.[25,26]

Depolarizing and Nondepolarizing Drugs

Depolarizing and nondepolarizing neuromuscular junction–blocking drugs both have an affinity for, and bind to, nicotinic ACh receptors at the neuromuscular junction; however, their intrinsic activity at the receptor is very different. Nondepolarizing drugs bind to the receptor but do not activate it (Fig. 15.2). Their onset of action is characterized by a progressive weakening of muscle contraction and, ultimately, flaccid paralysis. Depolarizing drugs also bind to the receptor and, similar to ACh, the receptor is stimulated, causing depolarization of the postjunctional membrane. Unlike ACh, succinylcholine and other depolarizing NMBAs are not susceptible to breakdown by acetylcholinesterase and thus the ion channel remains open and repo-

larization does not occur. The persistent state of depolarization associated with administration of depolarizing NMBAs causes inexcitability of the motor end plate and, as with nondepolarizing NMBA, a flaccid paralysis results. In addition to the differing mechanism of action of depolarizing drugs, several other differences are clinically apparent when comparing depolarizing and nondepolarizing NMBAs. Succinylcholine administration can cause muscle fasciculations immediately prior to the development of flaccid paralysis. Large doses, repeated administration, or administration of succinylcholine as an infusion causes the character of the block to change from the aforementioned classic depolarizing action (i.e., phase I block) to a phase II block which resembles that of nondepolarizing drugs such as d-tubocurarine. Despite years of investigation into the genesis of phase II block, its mechanism is still not clearly understood. Prolonged exposure of the cholinergic receptors to the agonist succinylcholine likely causes receptor desensitization, channel blockade, or a combination of both. Both receptor desensitization and channel blockade have properties that would mimic those of the nondepolarizing NMBAs and thus would change the mechanism and nature of the succinylcholine-induced block.

Individual Neuromuscular Blocking Drugs

The NMBAs are quaternary ammonium compounds that mimic the quaternary nitrogen atom of ACh. They are attracted to the nicotinic receptors at the motor end plate, as well as to nicotinic receptors located in autonomic ganglia. Most NMBAs are positively charged, water-soluble compounds that have a limited volume of distribution and, in many cases, limited hepatic biotransformation.[27] The water-soluble nature of these compounds suggests their pharmacokinetics differ markedly from those of most anesthetic drugs, such as thiopental and propofol. A hallmark of lipid-soluble anesthetic agents is their rapid onset of action and their rapid termination of effect after intravenous administration.

In contrast, the low lipid solubility exhibited by the NMBAs limits drug transfer across membrane structures, including the placenta and blood-brain barrier. Hepatic metabolism and redistribution to sites other than the skeletal muscles are not major mechanisms in the termination of NMBA effects. An exception is vecuronium, where biliary excretion is important in its elimination from the body.[28] Because of their water solubility, most NMBAs are excreted by glomerular filtration and are generally not reabsorbed by the renal tubules. The water-soluble nature of these drugs may also contribute to the observation that neonates may require relatively higher doses of NMBAs because neonates have a higher percentage of body water than do adults and typically higher apparent volumes of distribution for water-soluble drugs. Recommended doses of muscle relaxants used in common domesticated species are listed in Table 15.1.

Succinylcholine

This is currently the only depolarizing NMBA used in veterinary medicine. Structurally, the succinylcholine molecule is two ACh molecules joined end to end. This drug is rapidly hydrolyzed in

Neuromuscular Blockade

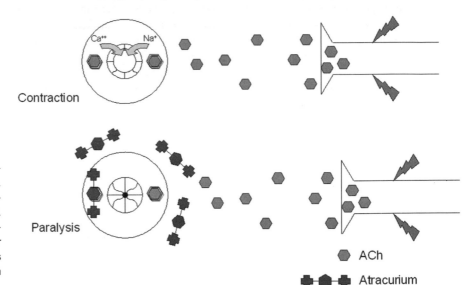

Fig. 15.2. **Top:** Normal neuromuscular transmission proceeds as described in Fig. 15.1. **Bottom:** Atracurium competes with acetylcholine (ACh) at the postsynaptic receptor. The occupation of at least one of the two receptor sites by atracurium prevents receptor activation, and the ion channel remains closed. Ca$^+$, calcium ions; and Na$^+$, sodium ions.

Table 15.1. Doses of commonly used neuromuscular blocking agents in some domestic species.

Drug (mg/kg)	Dog	Cat	Horse
Succinylcholine	0.3–0.4	0.2	0.12–0.15
Pancuronium	0.07	0.06	0.12
Atracurium	0.15–0.2	0.15–0.25	0.07–0.15
Vecuronium	0.1–0.2	0.025–0.05	0.1
Pipecuronium	0.05	0.003	

plasma by pseudocholinesterase (plasma cholinesterase), so only a small fraction of the injected dose survives degradation in plasma to reach the site of action at the neuromuscular junction. Very little pseudocholinesterase is present in the synaptic cleft, so succinylcholine-induced paralysis is terminated by diffusion of the drug away from the neuromuscular junction and into the extracellular fluid. Paradoxically, the rapid degradation of succinylcholine in the plasma is in some way responsible for the rapid onset of effect achieved by the drug. Because of the rapid degradation by plasma pseudocholinesterase, comparatively large doses of succinylcholine may be administered without worry of an increased duration of effect. The higher the succinylcholine dose, the more rapid the onset of paralysis will be. This strategy does not apply when using nondepolarizing NMBAs, where a significant increase in the duration of action will follow increased dosages. Because of its rapid onset of effect and brief action, succinylcholine is often the relaxant of choice to facilitate rapid human endotracheal intubation. Use of NMBAs to facilitate endotracheal tube placement is not common in veterinary practice because, with the arguable exception of cats and pigs, laryngeal contraction is rarely an impediment to tracheal intuba-

tion. Pseudocholinesterase is synthesized in the liver, and production is decreased by liver disease, chronic anemia, malnutrition, burns, pregnancy, cytotoxic drugs, metoclopramide, and cholinesterase-inhibitor drugs.[29-32] Additionally, species differences in pseudocholinesterase activity may exist. A reduction in plasma cholinesterase activity can be expected to prolong the action of succinylcholine. Administration of organophosphate insecticides, such as dichlorvos and trichlorfon, to horses has been shown to reduce pseudocholinesterase activity and prolong the duration of succinylcholine-induced neuromuscular blockade.[33] Conversely, cats wearing a dichlorvos flea collar had no increased duration of succinylcholine effect.[34]

Pancuronium

This was the first in a series of nondepolarizing NMBAs having a steroid nucleus. The drug has a dose-dependent onset of approximately 5 min and action ranging from 40 to 60 min in dogs. A large fraction of the drug is excreted by the kidney, and the remainder is metabolized by the liver. As may be expected, the action lasts longer in patients with renal insufficiency. In addition to having affinity for the nicotinic receptors at the neuromuscular junction, pancuronium can also inhibit cardiac muscarinic receptors, thus mildly to moderately increasing heart rate in some patients. This effect appears to vary among species. The muscarinic receptor–blocking effect and associated increase in heart rate appear to be caused by a second positive charge attached to the steroid ring. Removal of a single methyl group and, thus, of the positive charge, creates vecuronium, which is devoid of these cardiovascular effects.

Atracurium

This is a short-acting nondepolarizing NMBA having a benzylisoquinoline structure similar to that of d-tubocurarine. The drug has a dose-dependent onset of action of approximately 5 min, and its action lasts approximately 30 min in dogs. Repeated doses do not tend to be cumulative, so neuromuscular blockade is sometimes maintained via continuous intravenous infusion. Atracurium is unique in that almost half of it is degraded by Hofmann elimination and nonspecific ester hydrolysis. The remaining fraction is degraded by as yet undefined routes, although evidence exists that its action is not prolonged in people in hepatic or renal failure.[35,36] Hepatic metabolism and renal excretion are not necessary for termination of effect. Consequently, atracurium may be administered to patients with hepatic or renal insufficiency without significantly increasing its duration of action.

Hofmann elimination is a process of spontaneous molecular decomposition and appears to be pH and temperature dependent. It does not require enzymatic activity. Because Hofmann elimination may occur ex vivo, atracurium should be kept refrigerated and is supplied at a pH of 3.25 to 3.65. When injected intravenously, it spontaneously decomposes into laudanosine and a quaternary monoacrylate at physiological pH and temperature. The laudanosine metabolite is a known CNS stimulant and can induce seizures. Unlike atracurium, laudanosine is almost totally dependent on hepatic biotransformation for elimination; thus, laudanosine plasma concentrations may be elevated in patients who have hepatic insufficiency and are given atracurium for longer surgical procedures. Laudanosine-induced CNS stimulation and seizures are unlikely unless atracurium is administered for prolonged periods, as might occur in intensive care settings. Since Hofmann elimination is pH and temperature dependent, hypothermia may increase the duration of atracurium neuromuscular blockade and require a decrease in the infusion rate necessary to maintain neuromuscular blockade.[37] Ester hydrolysis of atracurium is accomplished by several plasma esterases unrelated to plasma cholinesterase. In contrast to succinylcholine metabolism, the duration of action of atracurium is not prolonged in the presence of cholinesterase inhibitors.

Many NMBAs having the benzylisoquinoline structure are associated with histamine release and a varying degree of hypotension. d-Tubocurarine, the prototypical benzylisoquinoline NMBA, is among the most potent at releasing histamine, but newer drugs having the benzylisoquinoline structure, such as atracurium and mivacurium, require several times the effective dose for neuromuscular blockade before appreciable amounts of histamine are released.[38,39] Although signs of histamine release, such as hypotension and tachycardia, are not usually observed when atracurium is administered, slow intravenous administration is always preferred.

Cisatracurium

Atracurium is a racemic mixture of ten optical isomers. The 1R-*cis*, 1R′-*cis* isomer, or cisatracurium, comprises approximately 15% of racemic atracurium, is approximately four times more potent, and has much less potential for histamine release. For example, in cats, plasma histamine concentrations were unchanged when up to 60 times the effective dose of cisatracurium was administered.[40] Cisatracurium has a similar onset time and duration

of action to atracurium. Hofmann elimination metabolizes more than half the administered dose of cisatracurium, but, unlike with the racemic compound, ester hydrolysis does not occur. As with atracurium, Hofmann elimination causes laudanosine production. Since cisatracurium is approximately fourfold as potent as atracurium, the administered dose is correspondingly less, as is production of laudanosine.[41]

Vecuronium

Introduced in the 1980s, this was one of the first NMBAs free of cardiovascular effects. The discovery that the vagolytic properties and associated tachycardia seen with pancuronium administration were caused by two positive charges within the steroid molecule led investigators to remove a single methyl group from the parent pancuronium molecule. Vecuronium, the resultant drug, has remarkable cardiovascular stability and does not induce tachycardia nor release histamine.[42] This drug has a dose-dependent onset of action of approximately 5 min and an intermediate duration of action similar to that of atracurium: 30 min. As with atracurium, a cumulative effect with subsequent doses is not a prominent feature of this drug. Vecuronium is unstable when prepared in solution and is supplied as a lyophilized powder that is reconstituted with sterile water prior to injection. The powder does not need refrigeration, and, once reconstituted, the solution is stable for 24 h. Slightly more than half of the drug is metabolized by hepatic microsomal enzymes and excreted in the bile while a significant fraction undergoes renal elimination.[43] In humans, the action of vecuronium is either slightly prolonged or unchanged in patients who exhibit renal insufficiency but not in patients who suffer hepatic failure unless increased doses are administered.[44]

Rocuronium

This is a derivative of vecuronium, having approximately one-eighth the potency of the parent compound. Since vecuronium and rocuronium have similar molecular weights and rocuronium has lower potency, a higher injected dose of rocuronium places a greater number of molecules near the neuromuscular junction translating into a more rapid onset of neuromuscular blockade. The rapid onset of effect of rocuronium makes the drug an attractive nondepolarizing alternative to succinylcholine for tracheal intubation. Its duration of action in dogs is similar to that of vecuronium and atracurium.[45] Similar to vecuronium, rocuronium seems to be without cardiovascular effects and does not release histamine.[46] The primary route of elimination is via the hepatic system while a small fraction is eliminated via the kidney.[42]

Doxacurium

This is a very potent benzylisoquinoline NMBA with a long duration of action.[47] Similar to other benzylisoquinoline NMBAs, such as atracurium, doxacurium does not have vagolytic properties or cause ganglion blockade. Similar to cisatracurium, administration of clinical doses does not cause appreciable histamine release. Doxacurium appears to be minimally metabolized and is excreted unchanged into the bile and urine.

Mivacurium

This drug is a rapid-acting, short-duration NMBA marketed for use in humans for facilitating tracheal intubation at anesthetic induction. Similar to atracurium, mivacurium can induce histamine release if high doses are administered. Mivacurium is rapidly biotransformed by plasma pseudocholinesterase, and metabolites do not have appreciable neuromuscular blocking activity. Its dose-dependent duration of action differs between species. The action of typical doses used in humans lasts approximately 25 min, about one-half to one-third less than that of atracurium. Mivacurium also shows marked differences in potency among species, being much more potent in dogs than in people. In dogs, one-third of the human dose is associated with blockade that is five times longer.[48] The differences in duration of action between species may in part reflect the reduced activity of pseudocholinesterase in dogs, because normal plasma cholinesterase concentrations for dogs are reportedly from 19% to 76% of human values.[49] Also, canine pseudocholinesterase enzyme might have differing affinity for the three primary isomers of mivacurium.[49] Clinical observations indicate that mivacurium has a much briefer action in cats than in dogs.

Nonneuromuscular Effects

The NMBAs primary action is at the nicotinic receptors at the motor nerve plate, but most drugs affect other cholinergic receptors, including the cardiac muscarinic receptors and nicotinic ganglionic receptors within the autonomic nervous system. Many undesirable effects can be caused by either the blocking of receptors or the mimicking actions of ACh.

Cardiovascular Effects

ACh is the primary neurotransmitter of preganglionic and postganglionic neurons within the parasympathetic nervous system, whereas the sympathetic nervous system employs ACh only as a preganglionic neurotransmitter in most tissues. The ubiquitous presence of ACh and the structural similarities between ACh and the NMBAs provides an opportunity to induce physiological effects other than paralytic actions. Agonist or antagonist action at cardiac muscarinic receptors or nicotinic receptors at sympathetic ganglia may decrease or increase heart rate and cause cardiac dysrhythmias. Succinylcholine can mimic the effect of ACh at cardiac muscarinic receptors, leading to sinus bradycardia, junctional rhythms, and even sinus arrest.[50,51] Alternatively, by virtue of its ACh-like effects at sympathetic ganglia, administration of succinylcholine may increase heart rate and blood pressure.[52] The net clinical effect observed in an individual animal is probably a function of the species, dose, and timing of administration.

Nondepolarizing drugs, particularly the older agents, may also influence a patient's cardiovascular status. The rapid intravenous injection of a paralyzing dose of d-tubocurarine can decrease blood pressure significantly. This may occur by blocking the action of ACh at sympathetic ganglia, which then decreases sympathetic efferent activity, leading to hypotension. Alternatively, histamine release associated with the rapid intravenous administration of d-tubocurarine could cause hypotension. This mechanism probably causes the majority of hypotension, because either slow intravenous administration, or prior administration of an antihistamine, usually attenuates the response.[53]

Rapid intravenous administration of clinically used doses of pancuronium may produce an increase in heart rate and corresponding increases in arterial pressure and cardiac output.[54,55] This response is caused by blockade of cardiac muscarinic receptors and resultant decreased parasympathetic nervous system effects on the heart.[56] In addition, there is evidence that pancuronium may stimulate the release of norepinephrine from sympathetic adrenergic nerves.[57] A modest increase in heart rate is not always disadvantageous, particularly when drugs having vagomimetic effects (e.g., opioids and α_2-adrenergic agonists) are concurrently administered to a patient. The ability of pancuronium to increase heart rate is inconsistent among species, however. In dogs, heart rate, blood pressure, and cardiac output typically increase.[55,56] Heart rate does not change in horses anesthetized with halothane and administered pancuronium, whereas both heart rate and blood pressure may increase in ponies.[58,59] Pancuronium administration does not change heart rate or blood pressure in anesthetized calves, but increases heart rate and blood pressure in pigs.[60,61] The newer, intermediate-duration agents, such as atracurium and vecuronium, are virtually devoid of these cardiovascular effects. Atracurium and mivacurium may release histamine, but blood pressure is rarely decreased when modest doses of these NMBAs are used.

The newest NMBAs—pipecuronium, doxacurium, and rocuronium—were designed with cardiovascular stability in mind and their administration is unlikely to be associated with profound changes in cardiovascular function. Rapacuronium induces histamine release, but this is minimized if rapid intravenous administration is avoided.[62]

Histamine Release

The quaternary ammonium structure inherent in the NMBAs is responsible for the propensity of many of these compounds to stimulate histamine release following intravenous injection. Release of histamine in animals causes vasodilation, a decrease in blood pressure, and possibly a compensatory increase in heart rate. Histamine release is usually associated with administration of the benzylisoquinoline class of NMBAs but has been reported with low-potency steroid relaxants.[63] Because d-tubocurarine is a potent inducer of histamine release at doses required to produce clinically useful neuromuscular block, vasodilation and increased heart rate are commonly encountered.[54] For newer NMBAs, the dose necessary to evoke clinically significant histamine release is much higher than the dose necessary to produce relaxation. For example, in people, approximately 2.5 times the effective dose of atracurium is required to stimulate histamine release.[64] Pretreatment of patients with H_1-receptor and H_2-receptor antagonists is effective in preventing the cardiovascular effects associated with NMBA-induced histamine release.[65] Worries about histamine release with newer NMBAs may be avoided simply by administering relaxants more slowly and refraining from administering higher doses.

Placental Transfer

All clinically used NMBAs are large, hydrophilic, polar molecules. As a consequence, their transfer across cell membranes, including the placenta, is limited. At clinical doses, placental transfer of relaxants is minimal and effects on the neonate are unlikely. There is widespread use of NMBAs during human cesarean operations, and atracurium and succinylcholine have been used clinically in small and large domestic animals without consequence to neonates. Administration of NMBAs—such as pancuronium, succinylcholine, gallamine, and d-tubocurarine—to pregnant ferrets and cats does not impair muscle-twitch strength in neonates.[66]

Central Nervous System Effects

Being large, polar, hydrophilic molecules, the NMBAs do not cross cell membranes readily, but evidence exists that most of these drugs do gain limited entrance into the cerebrospinal fluid and may be associated with CNS effects. Pancuronium administration reportedly reduced the minimum alveolar concentration of halothane in humans.[67] However, a subsequent study in humans found that pancuronium, atracurium, or vecuronium administration had no effect on the minimum alveolar concentration (MAC) of halothane.[68] Accidental administration of NMBAs into the cerebrospinal fluid has caused myotonia, autonomic effects, and seizures.[69,70] Laudanosine, a metabolite of atracurium, easily crosses the blood-brain barrier in dogs, and high concentrations may stimulate the CNS.[71] Clinically useful dosages of atracurium, however, are unlikely to result in the formation of a sufficient quantity of laudanosine to alter the CNS.

Protein Binding

All nondepolarizing NMBAs are protein bound, but the clinical significance of such binding is unclear. Presumably, only the unbound fraction of drug is available to interact at ACh receptors and induce paralysis. In studies of people who had hepatic cirrhosis with decreased plasma protein concentrations, the proportion of d-tubocurarine, pancuronium, and vecuronium bound to plasma protein was not different compared with healthy patients who had normal plasma protein concentrations.[72,73] Thus, despite the theoretical concerns of low plasma protein increasing the proportion of free, active drug, the amount of NMBA that is protein bound in hypoproteinemic patients appears to remain unchanged.

Nonneuromuscular Effects of Succinylcholine

Several, often undesirable, nonneuromuscular side effects are associated with the administration of succinylcholine. These sequelae include hyperkalemia; increased intraocular, intracranial, and intragastric pressure; and muscle soreness.

Hyperkalemia

Succinylcholine administration is associated with a transient increase in serum potassium levels. Succinylcholine activates the nicotinic motor end-plate receptors but, unlike ACh, is not immediately degraded by acetylcholinesterase. This produces depolarization characterized by open ion channels that enable potassium ions to egress from the muscle fiber into the extracellular space. As a result, serum potassium concentrations can rise transiently after drug administration. In healthy patients, this increase is usually without adverse effects, provided that cardiovascular disease is not present and preadministration serum potassium levels are normal. In patients with burns, severe muscle trauma, muscular denervation, nerve damage, or neuromuscular disease, extrajunctional ACh receptors proliferate over the surface of the muscle fiber. This increase in receptor density is accompanied by an increase in sensitivity to the depolarizing muscle relaxants and an increase in the amount of intracellular potassium released in response to succinylcholine administration. The increase in extrajunctional ACh receptor density begins to occur within 2 days after the injury and can persist for 2 to 3 months.[74]

Intraocular Pressure

Succinylcholine administration increases intraocular pressure. In humans, intraocular pressure usually peaks within 2 to 4 min and remains increased for at least 6 min after administration.[75] The mechanism responsible for the increase in intraocular pressure is presently unknown but likely involves altered circulation to the eye. The administration of the calcium-channel blocker nifedipine attenuates this increase.[76] Administration of succinylcholine to patients who have penetrating eye injuries should be avoided because it can cause ocular evisceration. Controversy exists as to whether administration of a nondepolarizing NMBA prior to succinylcholine prevents increases in intraocular pressure. It is important to realize that the use of any induction technique that might cause gagging or forceful coughing will raise intraocular and intracranial pressure and thus must be avoided in patients who have an open globe. Induction with a rapid-acting injectable anesthetic and being certain that adequate anesthetic depth has been achieved prior to attempting tracheal intubation are critical in preventing intraocular pressure increases.

Intragastric Pressure

Because succinylcholine administration causes muscle contraction that manifests clinically as fasciculations of the skeletal muscles, abdominal constriction and increases in intraabdominal and intragastric pressure can occur, increasing the potential for regurgitation.

Intracranial Pressure

Muscle fasciculations induced by succinylcholine may also increase intracranial pressure. In humans, prior administration of a nondepolarizing NMBA prevents the increase in intracranial pressure. Since most domestic animals can be easily intubated without use of an NMBA, it is recommended that succinylcholine be avoided in patients with intracranial hypertension. As with penetrating eye injuries, a rapid, smooth induction of anesthesia is a more desirable strategy in preventing unnecessary increases in intracranial pressure.

Muscle Responses

Succinylcholine administration is often associated with muscle soreness. Myalgia results from muscle fasciculations that occur during the initial depolarization of the motor end plate.[77] The intensity of the fasciculations and the intensity of muscle pain are correlated.[78] Although skeletal muscle enzymes such as creatine kinase increase after succinylcholine administration, whether animals experience muscle pain similar to that of humans is unknown, but likely.[79–81]

Muscle Relaxants in Anesthetized Animals

The use of muscle relaxants in veterinary practice is not as frequent as in human medicine. Human patients are frequently given muscle relaxants to facilitate endotracheal intubation and surgical access. Most animals can be intubated relatively easily without paralysis, and muscle relaxation caused by inhalant anesthetic agents is adequate for most procedures. Because of the need for familiarity with NMBA pharmacology and mechanical ventilation, the use of muscle relaxants in animals has been limited mostly to teaching hospitals and adequately equipped specialty practices and research institutions.

Indications

Muscle relaxants may be administered for numerous reasons. To facilitate intubation, muscle relaxants are typically given with hypnotic drugs to eliminate laryngeal spasm and provide rapid control of the airway. The need for a motionless, centrally positioned eye during intraocular or corneal surgery often requires the use of a muscle relaxant. Other indications include prevention of unconscious spontaneous movement, reduced resistance to controlled ventilation, and facilitation of surgical access during surgery.

Precautions

Because the muscles of respiration are paralyzed, ventilation must be controlled, either by a mechanical ventilator or by a staff member who can manually ventilate the patient until muscle strength is restored. Muscle relaxants have no sedative, anesthetic, or analgesic properties, so it is critical that the animal be adequately anesthetized to render it completely unconscious. Assessing the level of anesthesia in a paralyzed patient is more difficult than in a nonparalyzed patient because the usual indicators of depth (e.g., purposeful movement in response to a noxious stimulus, palpebral response, and jaw tone) are abolished. When including an NMBA in an anesthetic protocol, anesthetists must be certain they can reliably maintain an adequate plane of surgical anesthesia and level of ventilation.

Historically, muscle relaxants have been given alone to animals for capture or restraint, including use as the sole agent for brief surgical procedures (e.g., equine castration). At this time, the use of such inhumane practices is not justified because of the widespread availability of safe and effective anesthetics. The administration of an NMBA alone to an awake patient for immobilization purposes is also considered inhumane.

Selection

When choosing a muscle relaxant, one must consider many factors, including the species to be paralyzed, the reason for paraly-

sis, the duration of action required, the health status of the patient, and concurrent drug administration. Relaxants will differ in the onset of action, duration of action, recovery time, cardiovascular effects, and route of elimination. If a rapid onset and brief action are needed, the choice might be rocuronium or mivacurium, whereas doxacurium may be selected for longer action without significant cardiovascular effects. Atracurium is metabolized via Hofmann elimination and may be a good choice when hepatic or renal disease is present.[35,36]

Because many factors will affect the intensity and duration of muscle paralysis, monitoring of neuromuscular blockade is useful for titrating the dose needed for the desired effect. It is important to remember that individual muscle groups respond differently to muscle relaxants. The diaphragm is less sensitive to the effects of muscle relaxants compared with the muscles of the limbs.[82] Therefore, a higher dose may be required to abolish spontaneous ventilation compared with the dose for facilitation of fracture reduction. In horses, when a dose of muscle relaxant required to abolish the hoof twitch is administered, the facial twitch will often remain, though at reduced strength.[83,84] When not monitoring hoof-twitch tension, it should be appreciated that the facial twitch may be present even when adequate relaxation has been achieved in the limb for performing the surgical procedure.

Factors Affecting Neuromuscular Blockade

A number of factors can influence the duration of action, intensity, and recovery from neuromuscular blockade. Whenever a muscle relaxant is administered, neuromuscular function must be monitored during the anesthetic and recovery periods to avoid overdosing and residual paralysis.

Impaired Metabolism and Excretion

Hepatic failure may alter the initial effect of nondepolarizing muscle relaxants because of an increase in the volume of distribution. However, their effect may be increased from decreased metabolism, especially when drugs dependent on hepatic biotransformation (e.g., vecuronium) are administered.[85–87] Impaired liver function may also prolong or cause residual neuromuscular blockade.[88] In general, muscle relaxants are not highly protein bound to albumin, typically less than 50% bound.[89–92] Thus, the net effect of low albumin may not be clinically significant. Decreased esterase activity may slow the biotransformation of mivacurium and atracurium. Patients with biliary obstruction may have reduced hepatic clearance of muscle relaxants.[93] The clinical impact of hepatic failure depends on the specific NMBA and dose administered.

In patients with renal insufficiency, paralysis may be prolonged when muscle relaxants that rely predominantly on renal elimination (gallamine, pancuronium, or doxacurium) are given.[94–97] Recovery from mivacurium administration may also be prolonged, possibly because of decreased pseudocholinesterase activity.[98] Atracurium pharmacokinetics are generally unaffected, but if a constant-rate infusion is given to a patient with renal failure, laudanosine may accumulate.[99] It is best to avoid the use of high doses, repeated doses, or continuous infusions of muscle relaxants that primarily depend on renal elimination in patients with significant renal disease.

Anesthetic Drugs

Inhalant anesthetic agents cause a time and dose-dependent enhancement of the intensity and duration of block produced by muscle relaxants.[100] The explanation for this interaction is complex, with inhalational agents suppressing motor evoked potentials in response to spinal cord and transcranial stimulation. Muscle contractility is altered, and variation in regional muscle blood flow causes a greater fraction of the relaxant to reach the site of action.[101] The effects are greatest after administration of a long-acting relaxant or during a continuous infusion. The order of potency of some of the inhalational anesthetics in enhancing muscle relaxant effects is as follows: diethyl ether > enflurane > isoflurane > desflurane > halothane.[101] Also, antagonism of the block may be delayed, especially if inhalant anesthesia is continued after administration of the reversal agent. Monitoring of neuromuscular function helps to facilitate the appropriate dosing of muscle relaxants during inhalational anesthesia.

Most injectable anesthetic agents have only minor effects on the neuromuscular blocking properties of muscle relaxants. Induction agents, such as thiopental, ketamine and propofol, may minimally enhance neuromuscular blockade.[101]

Acid-Base Disturbances

Generally, respiratory acidosis increases the intensity of muscle blockade, whereas respiratory alkalosis decreases the effect.[102–105] Both metabolic acidosis and alkalosis may potentiate the effects of muscle relaxants and make it more difficult to antagonize relaxant-induced muscle paralysis.[102,103,105,106]

Electrolyte Disturbances

Alterations in serum concentration of potassium, magnesium, and calcium influence neuromuscular blockade. Decreases in extracellular potassium result in hyperpolarization of the end plate and resistance to ACh-induced depolarization.[107] A relative increase in extracellular potassium lowers the resting membrane potential, opposing the effect of the muscle relaxant.[107] Increased serum magnesium concentrations compete with ionized calcium, decreasing ACh release. Accordingly, in patients given magnesium sulfate, the duration of action of muscle relaxants may increase.[108] Hypocalcemia decreases ACh release, muscle action potential, and muscle contraction strength, thus increasing the effect of the neuromuscular block.[107,109] Typically, hypercalcemia decreases the effect of d-tubocurarine, pancuronium, and possibly other NMBAs, resulting in a higher dose requirement to achieve paralysis.[107]

Hypothermia

This generally slows drug elimination and decreases nerve conduction and muscle contraction. The overall clinical effect will vary with the degree of hypothermia. Care is required when administering muscle relaxants in cold environments. Doses may need to be reduced to prevent prolonged paralysis.

Age

Youth is associated with altered dose requirements of muscle relaxants. Receptor immaturity and decreased clearance appears to increase the potency of muscle relaxants in the young.[110–112] On the other hand, very young animals may require higher doses of muscle relaxants because of increased extracellular fluid and a larger volume of distribution when compared with adults. In addition, in younger animals, muscle relaxants usually have a faster onset of action while neuromuscular function recovers more quickly, so a lower dose of antagonist is usually required at the termination of the procedure.[113]

Although the data from published studies are not always clear-cut, old age may be associated with an increase in the effect of muscle relaxants, perhaps because of a lower volume of distribution and decreased rate of clearance. In elderly human patients, a delay in reversal and the need for higher doses of reversal agents are common, and likely attributable to slower spontaneous recovery.[114,115]

Neuromuscular Disorders

Animals with neuromuscular disorders may exhibit unpredictable responses to both depolarizing and nondepolarizing muscle relaxants. Care should be taken when administering muscle relaxants to patients with neuromuscular disorders or a history of muscle weakness or wasting.

Peripheral neuropathies may be classified as idiopathic, familial, metabolic, or immune mediated. In human patients, peripheral neuropathy may increase the effect of nondepolarizing muscle relaxants because of neural damage and the possibility of denervation-induced upregulation.[116] These patients may also be predisposed to succinylcholine-induced hyperkalemia.[117]

Diseases such as tick paralysis and botulism impair presynaptic release of ACh. Patients with presynaptic neuromuscular disorders show an increased sensitivity to nondepolarizing muscle relaxants. Myasthenia gravis is an autoimmune disease that causes generalized muscle weakness from a decrease in the number of ACh receptors on the motor end-plate muscle membrane. ACh is released normally, but its effect on the postsynaptic membrane is reduced. Patients with myasthenia gravis may be resistant to succinylcholine-induced paralysis, but are extremely sensitive to nondepolarizing relaxants and have an increased sensitivity toward succinylcholine-induced phase II block.[118,119] Patients with myasthenia gravis do not appear to be more sensitive to succinylcholine-induced hyperkalemia or malignant hyperthermia.[120] From published reports of dogs with myasthenia gravis, the initial dose recommendations of atracurium and vecuronium are 0.1 mg/kg and 0.02 mg/kg, respectively.[121,122]

Antimicrobial and Other Drug Interactions

The most notable effects on neuromuscular blockade occur with the administration of polymyxin and aminoglycoside antimicrobials, but can also occur with tetracycline, lincomycin, and clindamycin. Polymyxins may depress postsynaptic sensitivity to ACh and enhance channel block.[123,124] Antagonism with either neostigmine or calcium may be difficult and unreliable.[124] Aminoglycosides, such as gentamicin, kanamycin, neomycin, streptomycin, and tobramycin, have a presynaptic site of action, as evidenced by depressed ACh release. The ability to antagonize blockade with calcium supports this mechanism and site of action.[124] Studies in anesthetized cats and horses given atracurium have shown a significant decrease in twitch tension after administration of gentamicin (2 mg/kg intravenously [IV]), but recovery times were not significantly changed.[125,126] Cats given gentamicin (10 mg/kg IV) during neuromuscular blockade have shown a significant decrease in tibialis cranialis twitch response.[127] Furthermore, dogs given a single daily dose of gentamicin (6 mg/kg IV as a bolus) had significantly decreased twitch tension, while recovery time did not differ from that for controls.[128]

Tetracycline administration presumably depresses ACh release through calcium chelation. The enhanced blockade is usually reversible with calcium, but not neostigmine, administration.[124] The primary site of the inhibitory action of lincomycin may be directly on the muscle. It may also have slight presynaptic and postsynaptic activity. This effect is poorly reversed with neostigmine or calcium but partially reversed with 4-aminopyridine.[124] Clindamycin has a greater neuromuscular blocking effect than lincomycin: The mechanism is direct inhibition of the muscle, and reversal is difficult with either calcium or neostigmine administration.[124] Penicillins and cephalosporins appear to have a negligible effect on overall neuromuscular function.[124] Nevertheless, whenever an antibiotic is administered to a patient also given a muscle relaxant, the possibility of an enhanced block and/or residual paralysis should be considered. Close patient monitoring is recommended well into the recovery period.

Lithium administration may also increase or prolong neuromuscular blockade by competing with sodium and decreasing ACh release. The effects of muscle relaxants have been potentiated by numerous classes of drugs, including beta blockers, doxapram, anticonvulsants, steroids, and H_2-receptor antagonists.[101]

Monitoring Neuromuscular Blockade

Neuromuscular function should be monitored whenever a muscle relaxant is administered. Appropriate monitoring will facilitate proper dosing of both the muscle relaxant and its antagonist. To prevent residual paralysis and muscle weakness in the recovery period, it is critical that monitoring be continued until the function is fully restored. Evoked motor responses to peripheral nerve stimulation are used to evaluate the degree of neuromuscular blockade. Many handheld peripheral nerve stimulators are available (Fig. 15.3).

Sites of Stimulation

Sites for stimulation of peripheral motor nerves in dogs and cats include the peroneal and ulnar nerves (Figs. 15.4 and 15.5). In horses, the facial nerve and superficial peroneal nerve are most commonly used (Figs. 15.6 and 15.7). Contact electrodes are placed over the nerve to be stimulated, and the resultant motor response is compared with the prerelaxant response.

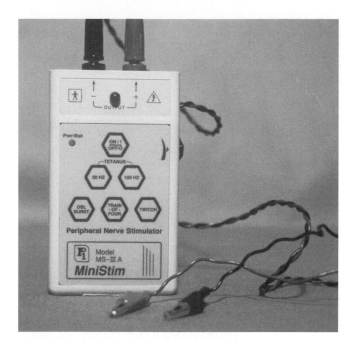

Fig. 15.3. Peripheral nerve stimulator.

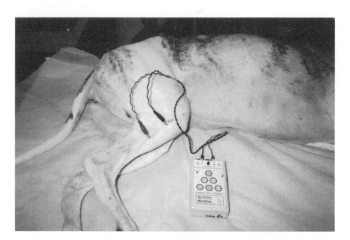

Fig. 15.4. Superficial peroneal nerve stimulation in a dog.

Electrical Stimulation Characteristics

When monitoring neuromuscular function in veterinary patients, there are standard methods for stimulating peripheral nerves. The output from the peripheral nerve stimulator should be a square-wave stimulus lasting 0.2 to 0.3 ms. Ideally, the output current of the nerve stimulator should be adjustable, enabling a *supramaximal impulse* (i.e., a current slightly greater than that required to elicit the maximum motor response) to be applied to the nerve. A supramaximal stimulus ensures that all fibers in the nerve bundle are depolarized. Since muscle fibers contract in an all-or-none fashion, any subsequent changes in the evoked motor response during supramaximal stimulation of the peripheral nerve are caused by changes at the neuromuscular junction or muscle level, not by loss of nerve fiber input.

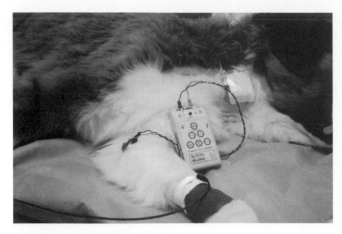

Fig. 15.5. Ulnar nerve stimulation in a dog.

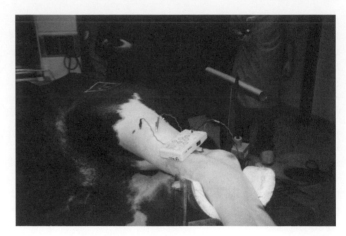

Fig. 15.7. Peroneal nerve stimulation in a horse.

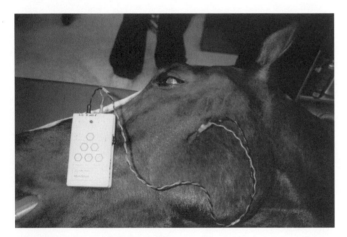

Fig. 15.6. Facial nerve stimulation in a horse.

Pattern of Stimulation

Ideally, the peripheral nerve stimulator should have a variable output and be capable of providing single-twitch, train-of-four, tetanic, and double-burst patterns of stimulation. Examples of the evoked muscle response to supramaximal stimulation before and after administration of a muscle relaxant are presented in Fig. 15.8. Partial neuromuscular block with depolarizing and nondepolarizing relaxants modifies the recorded responses to these stimulation patterns. These modified responses are summarized in Table 15.2.

Single Twitch

When using the single twitch, the simplest form of nerve stimulation, the degree of relaxation is assessed by dividing the elicited response by the prerelaxant response. The *prerelaxant response* is the twitch response measured immediately prior to the administration of the muscle relaxant. Since ACh release is decreased by the prejunctional effects of the relaxant, the frequency of single-twitch stimulation should be no greater than approximately one twitch every 7 to 10 s.[129] If the stimulus is applied too frequently, the resultant twitch response will be artificially low,

causing inaccuracy in determination of the degree of relaxation. Twitch response is not depressed until 75% to 80% of receptors are blocked and will be abolished when approximately 90% to 95% of receptors are blocked.[130]

Train of Four

The *train-of-four (TOF) pattern* of stimulation is the delivery of four supramaximal impulses over 2 s (2 Hz). The TOF can be repeated every 10 to 20 s without significant temporal effects. The relaxation level is determined by comparing the ratio of the intensity of the fourth twitch to the first twitch (T_4/T_1 ratio). Since the TOF serves as its own control, it is not necessary to determine baseline values prior to relaxant administration, although proper stimulator function should be verified before paralysis. In the absence of neuromuscular blockade, the T_4/T_1 ratio will be 1.0. After a nondepolarizing muscle relaxant is administered, when approximately 70% of receptors are occupied the twitches will fade, beginning with the fourth, followed by the third, second, and first twitches.[131] The dose of relaxant given will determine the degree of fade, the strength of any remaining twitches, and how long the twitches are absent. During recovery, the twitches will reappear in reverse order. A T_4/T_1 ratio of 0.7 or greater is associated with adequate clinical signs of recovery from the muscle relaxant.[132]

During the phase I block from a depolarizing relaxant, the TOF fade will be absent. However, repeat administration or continuous infusion of the depolarizing drug can cause a phase II block. When this occurs, fade will be seen following a TOF stimulus (Table 15.2).[133]

Tetanic Stimulation

Sustained muscle contraction is achieved by continuously delivering a high-frequency (50 Hz) supramaximal stimulus for 5 s.[133] Partial neuromuscular blockade from nondepolarizing relaxant administration will reduce tetanic height and cause fade.[134] Although this pattern of stimulation is helpful for detecting residual neuromuscular blockade during the anesthetic recovery period, it is important to remember that tetanic stimulation can be painful for lightly anesthetized or conscious patients.[135]

Table 15.2. Responses during partial neuromuscular block[a]

Criteria	Depolarizing Block	Nondepolarizing Block	Phase II Block
Fasciculation before onset of block	Yes	No	—
Time for onset	Short	Longer	—
Single twitch	Depressed	Depressed	Depressed
Tetanic height	Depressed	Depressed	Depressed
Tetanic fade	Minimal or absent	Present and marked	Present and marked
Train-of-four fade	Minimal or absent	Present and marked	Present and marked
Posttetanic facilitation	Minimal or absent	Present	Present
Response to anticholinesterases	Block is prolonged	Block is antagonized	Block is antagonized

[a]Distinguishing features of depolarizing, nondepolarizing, and succinylcholine–induced phase II block. The left column lists the different patterns of nerve stimulation or other characteristic, and the second, third, and fourth columns list the respective responses in the presence of partial neuromuscular block.

Posttetanic Facilitation

Posttetanic facilitation is an increase in an evoked response from a stimulus delivered shortly after tetanic stimulation. This is thought to be caused by increased ACh release from the nerve terminal, but other theories exist.[130] It is characterized by either an increase in twitch tension or a decrease in the degree of fade in response to either a single-twitch, TOF, or double-burst pattern of stimulation. Posttetanic facilitation is often the first clinical indicator of recovery from neuromuscular blockade.[136,137]

Double-Burst Stimulation

Double-burst stimulation (DBS) is the delivery of two minitetanic bursts, two to four impulses each, delivered at a rate of 50 Hz and 750 ms apart. When DBS is used, a ratio of the response to the second burst compared with the response to the first burst (D_2/D_1) is calculated. DBS may be superior to TOF because not only does DBS correlate highly to TOF when assessed via mechanomyography, but fade is more readily seen with DBS using both visual and tactile means.[130] An additional advantage

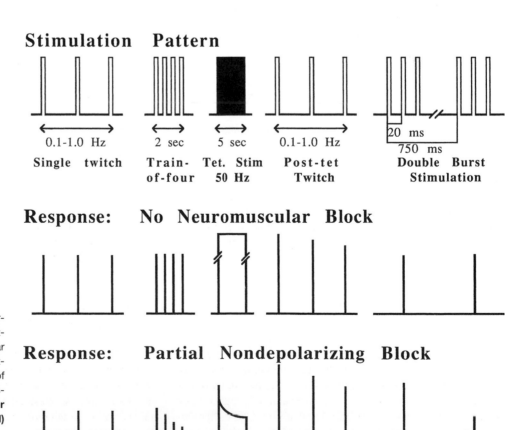

Fig. 15.8. Diagram showing different peripheral nerve stimulation patterns for monitoring neuromuscular function **(top panel)**. Under each pattern is shown the characteristics of the evoked muscle responses measured mechanically before **(center panel)** and during **(bottom panel)** partial block.

of DBS is that D_1 is detectable at a deeper level of neuromuscular blockade than is T_1.[138]

Quantifying Evoked Responses

Whenever a muscle relaxant is administered, neuromuscular function must be monitored until normal neuromuscular function is restored. Residual blockade during the recovery period can cause serious complications. Proper monitoring provides information about the degree and duration of neuromuscular blockade, and assures the observer that no residual blockade is present prior to recovery from anesthesia. In veterinary patients, the most common method used for assessing the degree of neuromuscular blockade is visual observation of the evoked response from peripheral nerve stimulation. With experienced observers, visual observation is adequate in most clinical situations. However, more accurate evaluation of the depth and duration of block is best achieved when the muscle response is recorded and measured. The two methods for accurately quantifying the evoked response are mechanically recorded, where the twitch tension by the muscle is measured using a force displacement transducer, and electromyographically recorded, where the muscle action potential is measured.

Mechanomyography

Mechanomyography (MMG) measures the evoked response of the stimulated muscle by force translation. The use of this method has been described in cats, dogs, horses, ponies, cows, and llamas.[45,125,126,139–141] With the limb immobilized, stimulating electrodes are placed over a peripheral nerve (peroneal or ulnar). The force transducer is attached to a paw or hoof at a right angle to the direction of muscle contraction. For maximum evoked muscle-twitch tension, a resting tension of 100 to 300 g should be applied. A supramaximal stimulus is applied to the nerve by using a single-twitch, TOF, or double-burst stimulation pattern. The resultant twitch tension can then be quantified. By using MMG, the depth and duration of neuromuscular blockade can be determined accurately. However, limitations make its use in many clinical situations impractical. To prevent changes in resting tension and twitch angle, the limb must be immobilized and no movement should occur during the recording period.[142]

Electromyography

Electromyography (EMG) measures the compound action potential of muscle fibers contracting during a supramaximal stimulus of a peripheral motor nerve. With the stimulating electrodes placed over a peripheral nerve, the recording electrode is placed over the innervation zone of the muscle, midway between its origin and insertion. Also required are a reference electrode, placed over the insertion site, and a ground electrode, placed between the other two electrodes. EMG has the advantage of requiring less or no limb immobilization and no resting tension, and there are more choices as to which muscles may be used.[142] In a study in dogs given atracurium, there was no statistical difference between MMG and EMG during TOF stimulation for either T_1 or T_4/T_1.[143] The disadvantage of EMG is that it may be difficult to obtain proper electrode placement for accurate results, particu-

larly in smaller patients. Until a standard method is developed and validated for various species and sites of monitoring, MMG will remain the gold standard for quantifying evoked responses.

Reversal of Neuromuscular Blockade

Nondepolarizing Blockade

As previously reviewed, acetylcholinesterase is present in high concentrations at the neuromuscular junction. It hydrolyzes ACh into choline and acetic acid, terminating the effects of ACh. The effects of nondepolarizing muscle relaxants are antagonized by administering an anticholinesterase (also known as an acetylcholinesterase inhibitor). This class of drugs inhibits the enzyme acetylcholinesterase, increasing the concentration of ACh molecules at the neuromuscular junction. Since nondepolarizing muscle relaxants and ACh compete for the same postsynaptic binding sites, the ACh increase can tip the balance of competition in favor of ACh, and neuromuscular transmission is restored.

The anticholinesterase drugs used to antagonize neuromuscular blockade include edrophonium, neostigmine, and pyridostigmine. They differ in how they inhibit acetylcholinesterase activity. Edrophonium produces a reversible inhibition by electrostatic attachment to the anionic site and by hydrogen bonding at the esteratic site on acetylcholinesterase. The action of edrophonium is relatively brief because a covalent bond is not formed and ACh can easily compete with edrophonium for access to the enzyme. Neostigmine and pyridostigmine inhibit acetylcholinesterase by forming a carbamyl-ester complex at the esteratic site of acetylcholinesterase. This bond lasts longer when compared with the bond of the enzyme with ACh, thereby preventing acetylcholinesterase from accessing ACh.

The reversal agents vary in their onset of action. In order from the shortest to the longest onset is edrophonium < neostigmine < pyridostigmine. In human patients, neostigmine is 4.4 times more potent than pyridostigmine and 5.7 times more potent than edrophonium for reversal of nondepolarizing neuromuscular blockade.[144] The duration of action is similar for both neostigmine and edrophonium, whereas that of pyridostigmine is approximately 40% longer.[144,145] In cats, neostigmine is 12 times more potent than edrophonium.[146]

Antiacetylcholinesterase agents are primarily metabolized by the liver, with hepatic biotransformation eliminating 50% of a neostigmine dose, 30% of an edrophonium dose, and 25% of a pyridostigmine dose. Renal excretion eliminates the remainder of the drug. Patients with renal failure will have prolonged elimination of an anticholinesterase drug.

The ACh accumulation following the administration of an anticholinesterase drug is not specific to the neuromuscular junction. While nicotinic effects occur at the neuromuscular junction and autonomic ganglia, muscarinic cholinergic effects occur because of inhibition of acetylcholinesterase at the sinus node, smooth muscle, and glands. Clinical effects of increased ACh concentrations at these sites include bradycardia, sinus arrest, bronchospasm, miosis, intestinal hyperperistalsis, and salivation. For this reason, it is advised that an anticholinergic drug, either atropine or glycopyrrolate, be administered immediately prior to reversal of neuromuscular blockade with an anticholinesterase. When choosing between atropine and glycopyrrolate, one must consider that atropine has a faster onset of action, which is more likely to cause an initial tachycardia, and will cross the blood-brain and blood-placental barriers. Compared with neostigmine and pyridostigmine, the muscarinic effects of edrophonium are mild, so it may be chosen for reversal when one wants to avoid the use of an anticholinergic. For example, edrophonium is frequently chosen in equine patients because anticholinergic drug administration has been associated with the development of ileus and colic.

Depolarizing Blockade

Recovery from succinylcholine (phase I block) is rapid and spontaneous because of succinylcholine hydrolysis by plasma cholinesterases. Recovery may be delayed in patients with decreases in plasma cholinesterase levels or activity. The administration of an anticholinesterase would actually prolong the depolarizing block.[147] On the other hand, a phase II block from succinylcholine can be antagonized similarly to the nondepolarizing muscle relaxants, emphasizing the need for determining the type (phase I or phase II) of block present when using succinylcholine (Table 15.2).[148,149]

Centrally Acting Muscle Relaxants

Guaifenesin is used routinely as a muscle relaxant in large animal species. Its mechanism of action is to disrupt nerve impulse transmission at the level of the internuncial neurons of the spinal cord, brain stem, and subcortical areas of the brain. At therapeutic doses, skeletal muscle relaxes, but there is little effect on the respiratory muscles or diaphragm. Guaifenesin does not provide analgesia or produce unconsciousness. Therefore, it should not be used alone for any painful surgical or diagnostic procedure. No antagonist is available to reverse the muscle relaxant effects of guaifenesin.

Guaifenesin is commercially available as either a powder, which is reconstituted to the desired concentration with sterile water, or as a ready-made solution. Concentrations of 5%, 10%, and 15% have been used, with a 5% solution in 5% dextrose being the most common. Guaifenesin administered intravenously in high concentrations (>10%) can cause hemolysis, hemoglobinuria, and venous thrombosis.[150] Tissue can be damaged if guaifenesin is inadvertently administered perivascularly.[150]

The cardiopulmonary effects of guaifenesin, alone or in combination with xylazine, ketamine, or thiobarbiturates, have been studied in horses. When guaifenesin is given alone, heart rate, respiratory rate, right atrial pressure, pulmonary arterial pressure, and cardiac output are unchanged. Systolic, diastolic, and mean arterial pressures are decreased. Xylazine (1.1 mg/kg IV), given prior to guaifenesin administration, reduced the dose necessary to achieve lateral recumbency (88 ± 10 mg/kg) compared with guaifenesin alone (134 ± 34 mg/kg). The addition of xylazine typically decreases heart rate, respiratory rate, cardiac output, and arterial oxygen partial pressure (PaO_2). Central venous pressure increases, whereas systolic, diastolic, and mean arterial blood pressures commonly decrease.[151,152]

Guaifenesin can be combined with thiopental for both induction and maintenance of anesthesia in horses. Following premedication with either xylazine or acepromazine, a combination of guaifenesin and thiopental (2 to 3 g of thiopental in 1 L of 5% guaifenesin) is given for induction or, alternatively, guaifenesin is given until the horse is wobbly and buckling at the knees, and then a bolus of thiopental (4 mg/kg) is administered. Short periods of anesthesia (<1 h) can be maintained by a continuous infusion of the guaifenesin-thiopental combination.

A significant amount of guaifenesin crosses the placental barrier in pregnant mares.[152] Stallions may have up to 1.5 times longer action compared with mares. The longer recovery time in male horses is attributed to slower drug elimination from the plasma.[153]

Guaifenesin has also been combined with thiobarbiturates or ketamine for use in cattle, small ruminants, and swine.[154,155] Although guaifenesin has been used in dogs, the large volume requirement makes it impractical for routine use in this species.[156] However, when combined with a thiobarbiturate or ketamine-xylazine, guaifenesin has proven an effective component when immobilizing dogs.[157]

Peripherally Acting Muscle Relaxants

Dantrolene is a hydantoin derivative that interferes with excitation-contraction coupling, thus relaxing skeletal muscle through a decrease in the amount of calcium released from the sarcoplasmic reticulum. Therapeutic doses do not adversely affect cardiac or smooth muscle and do not depress respiration.[158] Dantrolene is the drug of choice for the treatment of malignant hyperthermia. In swine, the recommended dose is 1 to 3 mg/kg IV when treating a malignant hyperthermia crisis and 5 mg/kg orally for prophylaxis.[159] Dantrolene is supplied in 20-mg vials in powder form with 3 g of mannitol to improve solubility. It is reconstituted using 60 mL of sterile water to achieve a concentration of 0.33 mg/mL. The oral preparation comes in 50-mg capsules.

The prophylactic use of dantrolene in animal patients prone to malignant hyperthermia is no longer routinely recommended. Pretreatment with dantrolene prior to anesthesia does not guarantee effective blood levels and, in equine patients, may produce unwanted skeletal muscle weakness during the recovery period. In susceptible patients, an anesthetic regimen using nontriggering anesthetics should be used, and dantrolene should be immediately available. However, the intravenous preparation of dantrolene may be cost prohibitive and not economically justifiable for many veterinary clinics to keep in stock. Most human hospital pharmacies have the intravenous formulation and may sell the needed amount to the veterinary clinic when required. Compounding the oral preparation for intravenous use has been described. The process is complex and time consuming, but dantrolene powder can be stored for rapid reconstitution during a malignant hyperthermia crisis.[160,161]

Metabolism of dantrolene is via the liver through oxidative and reductive pathways. Metabolites and the unchanged drug are excreted in the urine. Dantrolene can cause muscle weakness, nausea, and diarrhea. Fatal hepatitis has occurred in human patients after chronic treatment with dantrolene.[162] Severe myocardial depression has been reported when dantrolene is administered concurrently with verapamil or other calcium channel blockers.[163,164] Synergism, resulting in a delayed recovery of neuromuscular function, has been observed with dantrolene and vecuronium coadministration.[165]

References

1. Griffith HR, Johnson GE. The use of curare in general anaesthesia. Anesthesiology 1942;3:418–420.
2. Foldes FF, McNall PG, Borrego-Hinojosa JM. Succinylcholine: A new approach to muscular relaxation in anesthesiology. N Engl J Med 1952;247:596–600.
3. Pickett D. Curare in canine surgery. J Am Vet Med Assoc 1951; 119:346–353.
4. Miller RM. Psychological effects of succinylcholine chloride immobilization in the horse. Vet Med Small Anim Clin 1966;61:941–943.
5. Bowman WC. Prejunctional and postjunctional cholinoceptors at the neuromuscular junction. Anesth Analg 1980;59:935–943.
6. Edwards C. The effects of innervation on the properties of acetylcholine receptors in muscle. Neuroscience 1979;4:565–584.
7. Steinbach JH. Neuromuscular junctions and alpha-bungarotoxin-binding sites in denervated and contralateral cat skeletal muscles. J Physiol 1981;313:513–528.
8. Fambrough DM. Control of acetylcholine receptors in skeletal muscle. Physiol Rev 1979;59:165–227.
9. Stya M, Axelrod D. Mobility of extrajunctional acetylcholine receptors on denervated adult muscle fibers. J Neurosci 1984;4: 70–74.
10. Azar I. The response of patients with neuromuscular disorders to muscle relaxants: A review. Anesthesiology 1984;61:173–187.
11. Gronert GA, Theye RA. Pathophysiology of hyperkalemia induced by succinylcholine. Anesthesiology 1975;43:89–99.
12. Hirokawa N, Heuser JE. Internal and external differentiations of the postsynaptic membrane at the neuromuscular junction. J Neurocytol 1982;11:487–510.
13. Changeux JP, Bon F, Cartaud J, et al. Allosteric properties of the acetylcholine receptor protein from *Torpedo marmorata*. Cold Spring Harb Symp Quant Biol 1983;48(Pt 1):35–52.
14. Stroud RM, Finer-Moore J. Acetylcholine receptor structure, function, and evolution. Annu Rev Cell Biol 1982:1:317–351.
15. Fairclough RH, Finer-Moore J, Love RA, Kristofferson D, Desmeules PJ, Stroud RM. Subunit organization and structure of an acetylcholine receptor. Cold Spring Harb Symp Quant Biol 1983; 48(Pt 1):9–20.
16. Guy HR. A structural model of the acetylcholine receptor channel based on partition energy and helix packing calculations. Biophys J 1984;45:249–261.
17. Neubig RR, Boyd ND, Cohen JB. Conformations of *Torpedo* acetylcholine receptor associated with ion transport and desensitization. Biochemistry 1982;21:3460–3467.
18. Sheridan RE, Lester HA. Functional stoichiometry at the nicotinic receptor. J Gen Physiol 1982;80:499–515.
19. Brown RD, Taylor P. The influence of antibiotics on agonist occupation and functional states of the nicotinic acetylcholine receptor. Mol Pharmacol 1983;23:8–16.
20. Madsen BW, Albuquerque EX. The narcotic antagonist naltrexone has a biphasic effect on the nicotinic acetylcholine receptor. FEBS Lett 1985;182:20–24.
21. Albuquerque EX, Akiake A, Shaw DP, Rickett DL. The interaction of anticholinesterase agents with the acetylcholine receptor-ionic channel complex. Fundam Appl Toxicol 1984;4(2 Pt 2):S27–S33.
22. Cohen JB, Boyd ND, Shera NS. Interactions of anesthetics with nicotinic postsynaptic membranes isolated from *Torpedo* electric tissue. Prog Anesthesiol 1980;2:165–174.
23. Dreyer F. Acetylcholine receptor. Br J Anaesth 1982;54:115–130.
24. Lambert JJ, Durant NN, Henderson EG. Drug-induced modification of ionic conductance at the neuromuscular junction. Annu Rev Pharmacol Toxicol 1983;23:505–539.
25. Colquhoun D, Sheridan RE. The modes of action of gallamine. Proc R Soc Lond [B] 1981;211:181–203.
26. Ogden DC, Colquhoun D. Ion channel block by acetylcholine, carbachol, and suberyldicholine at the frog neuromuscular junction. Proc R Soc Lond [B] 1985;225:329–355.
27. Shanks CA. Pharmacokinetics of the nondepolarizing neuromuscular relaxants applied to calculation of bolus and infusion dosage regimens. Anesthesiology 1986;64:72–86.
28. Upton RA, Nguyen TL, Miller RD, Castagnoli N Jr. Renal and biliary elimination of vecuronium (ORG NC 45) and pancuronium in rats. Anesth Analg 1982;61:313–316.
29. Birch JH, Foldes FF, Rendell-Baker L. Causes and prevention of prolonged apnea with succinylcholine. Curr Res Anesth Analg 1956;35:609–633.
30. Pantuck EJ. Ecothiopate iodide eye drops and prolonged response to suxamethonium. Br J Anaesth 1966;38:406–407.
31. Kopman AF, Strachovsky G, Lichtenstein L. Prolonged response to succinylcholine following physostigmine. Anesthesiology 1978; 49:142–143.
32. Bentz EW, Stoelting RK. Prolonged response to succinylcholine following pancuronium reversal with pyridostigmine. Anesthesiology 1976;44:258–260.
33. Short CE, Cuneio J, Cupp D. Organophosphate-induced complications during anesthetic management in the horse. J Am Vet Med Assoc 1971;159:1319–1327.
34. Reynolds WT. Use of suxamethonium in cats fitted with dichlorvos flea collars. Aust Vet J 1985;62:106–107.
35. Fisher DM, Canfell PC, Fahey MR, et al. Elimination of atracurium in humans: Contribution of Hofmann elimination and ester hydrolysis versus organ-based elimination. Anesthesiology 1986;65: 6–12.
36. Fahey MR, Rupp SM, Fisher DM, et al. The pharmacokinetics and pharmacodynamics of atracurium in patients with and without renal failure. Anesthesiology 1984;61:699–702.
37. Playfor SD, Thomas DA, Choonara I. The effect of induced hypothermia on the duration of action of atracurium when given by infusion to critically ill children. Paediatr Anaesth 2000;10:83–88.
38. Scott RP, Savarese JJ, Basta SJ, et al. Clinical pharmacology of atracurium given in high dose. Br J Anaesth 1986;58:834–838.
39. Stoops CM, Curtis CA, Kovach DA, et al. Hemodynamic effects of mivacurium chloride administered to patients during oxygen-sufentanil anesthesia for coronary artery bypass grafting or valve replacement. Anesth Analg 1989;68:333–339.
40. Wastila WB, Maehr RB, Turner GL, Hill DA, Savarese JJ. Comparative pharmacology of cisatracurium (51W89), atracurium, and five isomers in cats. Anesthesiology 1996;85:169–177.
41. Sparr HJ, Beaufort TM, Fuchs-Buder T. Newer neuromuscular blocking agents: How do they compare with established agents? Drugs 2001;61:919–942.
42. Morris RB, Cahalan MK, Miller RD, Wilkinson PL, Quasha AL, Robinson SL. The cardiovascular effects of vecuronium (ORG

NC45) and pancuronium in patients undergoing coronary artery bypass grafting. Anesthesiology 1983;58:438–440.

43. Caldwell JE, Szenohradszky J, Segredo V, et al. The pharmacodynamics and pharmacokinetics of the metabolite 3-desacetylvecuronium (ORG 7268) and its parent compound, vecuronium, in human volunteers. J Pharmacol Exp Ther 1994;270:1216–1222.

44. Lebrault C, Berger JL, D'Hollander AA, Gomeni R, Henzel D, Duvaldestin P. Pharmacokinetics and pharmacodynamics of vecuronium (ORG NC 45) in patients with cirrhosis. Anesthesiology 1985;62:601–605.

45. Cason B, Baker DG, Hickey RF, Miller RD, Agoston S. Cardiovascular and neuromuscular effects of three steroidal neuromuscular blocking drugs in dogs (ORG 9616, ORG 9426, ORG 9991). Anesth Analg 1990;70:382–388.

46. Hudson ME, Rothfield KP, Tullock WC, Firestone LL. Haemodynamic effects of rocuronium bromide in adult cardiac surgical patients. Can J Anaesth 1998;45:139–143.

47. Martinez EA, Wooldridge AA, Hartsfield SM, Mealey KL. Neuromuscular effects of doxacurium chloride in isoflurane-anesthetized dogs. Vet Surg 1998;27:279–283.

48. Smith LJ, Moon PF, Lukasik VM, Erb HN. Duration of action and hemodynamic properties of mivacurium chloride in dogs anesthetized with halothane. Am J Vet Res 1999;60:1047–1050.

49. Smith LJ, Schwark WS, Cook DR, Moon PF, Looney AL. Pharmacokinetic variables of mivacurium chloride after intravenous administration in dogs. Am J Vet Res 1999;60:1051–1054.

50. Leigh MD, McCoy DD, Belton MK, Lewis GB Jr. Bradycardia following intravenous administration of succinylcholine chloride to infants and children. Anesthesiology 1957;18:698–702.

51. Schoenstadt DA, Whitcher CE. Observations on the mechanism of succinyldicholine-induced cardiac arrhythmias. Anesthesiology 1963;24:358–362.

52. Galindo AH, Davis TB. Succinylcholine and cardiac excitability. Anesthesiology 1962;23:32–40.

53. Moss J, Rosow CE, Savarese JJ, Philbin DM, Kniffen KJ. Role of histamine in the hypotensive action of d-tubocurarine in humans. Anesthesiology 1981;55:19–25.

54. Booij LH, Edwards RP, Sohn YJ, Miller RD. Cardiovascular and neuromuscular effects of Org NC 45, pancuronium, metocurine, and d-tubocurarine in dogs. Anesth Analg 1980;59:26–30.

55. Reitan JA, Warpinski MA. Cardiovascular effects of pancuronium bromide in mongrel dogs. Am J Vet Res 1975;36:1309–1311.

56. Durant NN, Marshall IG, Savage DS, Nelson DJ, Sleigh T, Carlyle IC. The neuromuscular and autonomic blocking activities of pancuronium, Org NC 45, and other pancuronium analogues, in the cat. J Pharm Pharmacol 1979;31:831–836.

57. Domenech JS, Garcia RC, Sastain JM, Loyola AQ, Oroz JS. Pancuronium bromide: An indirect sympathomimetic agent. Br J Anaesth 1976;48:1143–1148.

58. Klein L, Hopkins J, Beck E, Burton B. Cumulative dose responses to gallamine, pancuronium, and neostigmine in halothane-anesthetized horses: Neuromuscular and cardiovascular effects. Am J Vet Res 1983;44:786–792.

59. Manley SV, Steffey EP, Howitt GA, Woliner M. Cardiovascular and neuromuscular effects of pancuronium bromide in the pony. Am J Vet Res 1983;44:1349–1353.

60. Hildebrand SV, Howitt GA. Neuromuscular and cardiovascular effects of pancuronium bromide in calves anesthetized with halothane. Am J Vet Res 1984;45:1549–1552.

61. Muir AW, Marshall RJ. Comparative neuromuscular blocking effects of vecuronium, pancuronium, Org 6368 and suxametho-

nium in the anaesthetized domestic pig. Br J Anaesth 1987;59:622–629.

62. Levy JH, Pitts M, Thanopoulos A, Szlam F, Bastian R, Kim J. The effects of rapacuronium on histamine release and hemodynamics in adult patients undergoing general anesthesia. Anesth Analg 1999;89:290–295.

63. Savarese JJ, Caldwell JE, Lien CA, Miller RD. Pharmacology of muscle relaxants and their antagonists. In: Miller RD, ed. Anesthesia, 5th ed. Philadelphia: Churchill-Livingstone, 2000:412–490.

64. Basta SJ, Savarese JJ, Ali HH, Moss J, Gionfriddo M. Histamine-releasing potencies of atracurium, dimethyl tubocurarine and tubocurarine. Br J Anaesth 1983;55(Suppl 1):105S–106S.

65. Scott RP, Savarese JJ, Basta SJ, et al. Atracurium: Clinical strategies for preventing histamine release and attenuating the haemodynamic response. Br J Anaesth 1985;57:550–553.

66. Evans CA, Waud DR. Do maternally administered neuromuscular blocking agents interfere with fetal neuromuscular transmission? Anesth Analg 1973;52:548–552.

67. Forbes AR, Cohen NH, Eger EI II. Pancuronium reduces halothane requirement in man. Anesth Analg 1979;58:497–499.

68. Fahey MR, Sessler DI, Cannon JE, Brady K, Stoen R, Miller RD. Atracurium, vecuronium, and pancuronium do not alter the minimum alveolar concentration of halothane in humans. Anesthesiology 1989;71:53–56.

69. Peduto VA, Gungui P, Di Martino MR, Napoleone M. Accidental subarachnoid injection of pancuronium. Anesth Analg 1989;69:516–517.

70. Goonewardene TW, Sentheshanmuganathan S, Kamalanathan S, Kanagasunderam R. Accidental subarachnoid injection of gallamine: A case report. Br J Anaesth 1975;47:889–893.

71. Hennis PJ, Fahey MR, Canfell PC, Shi WZ, Miller RD. Pharmacology of laudanosine in dogs. Anesthesiology 1986;65:56–60.

72. Ghoneim MM, Kramer E, Bannow R, Pandya H, Routh JI. Binding of d-tubocurarine to plasma proteins in normal man and in patients with hepatic or renal disease. Anesthesiology 1973;39:410–415.

73. Duvaldestin P, Henzel D. Binding of tubocurarine, fazadinium, pancuronium and Org NC 45 to serum proteins in normal man and in patients with cirrhosis. Br J Anaesth 1982;54:513–516.

74. Carter JG, Sokoll MD, Gergis SD. Effect of spinal cord transection on neuromuscular function in the rat. Anesthesiology 1981;55:542–546.

75. Pandey K, Badola RP, Kumar S. Time course of intraocular hypertension produced by suxamethonium. Br J Anaesth 1972;44:191–196.

76. Indu B, Batra YK, Puri GD, Singh H. Nifedipine attenuates the intraocular pressure response to intubation following succinylcholine. Can J Anaesth 1989;36:269–272.

77. Waters DJ, Mapleson WW. Suxamethonium pains: Hypothesis and observation. Anaesthesia 1971;26:127–141.

78. Magee DA, Robinson RJ. Effect of stretch exercises on suxamethonium induced fasciculations and myalgia. Br J Anaesth 1987;59:596–601.

79. Maddineni VR, Mirakhur RK, Cooper AR. Myalgia and biochemical changes following suxamethonium after induction of anaesthesia with thiopentone or propofol. Anaesthesia 1993;48:626–628.

80. McLoughlin C, Leslie K, Caldwell JE. Influence of dose on suxamethonium-induced muscle damage. Br J Anaesth 1994;73:194–198.

81. Benson GJ, Hartsfield SM, Manning JP, Thurmon JC. Biochemical effects of succinylcholine chloride in mechanically ventilated horses anesthetized with halothane in oxygen. Am J Vet Res 1980;41:754–756.

82. Silverman DG, Brull SJ. Features of neurostimulation. In: Silverman DG, ed. Neuromuscular Block in Perioperative and Intensive Care. Philadelphia: JB Lippincott, 1994:23–36.

83. Klein LV. Neuromuscular blocking agents in equine anesthesia. Vet Clin North Am Large Anim Pract 1981;3:135–161.

84. Hildebrand SV, Holland M, Copland VS, Daunt D, Brock N. Clinical use of the neuromuscular blocking agents atracurium and pancuronium for equine anesthesia. J Am Vet Med Assoc 1989;195:212–219.

85. Duvaldstein P, Agoston S, Henzel D, Kersten UW, Desmonts JM. Pancuronium pharmacokinetics in patients with liver cirrhosis. Br J Anaesth 1978;50:1131–1136.

86. Duvaldstein P, Berger JL, Videcoq M, Desmonts JM. Pharmacokinetics and pharmacodynamics of Org NC 45 in patients with cirrhosis [Abstract]. Anesthesiology 1982;57:A238.

87. Bencine AF, Houwertjes MC, Agoston S. Effects of hepatic uptake of vecuronium bromide and its putative metabolites on their neuromuscular blocking actions in the cat. Br J Anaesth 1985;57:789–795.

88. Silverman DG, Mirakhur RK. Reversal of nondepolarizing block. In: Silverman DG, ed. Neuromuscular Block in Perioperative and Intensive Care. Philadelphia: JB Lippincott, 1994:217–238.

89. Wood M. Plasma binding and limitation of drug access to site of action. Anesthesiology 1991;75:721–723.

90. Wood M. Plasma drug binding: Implications for anesthesiologists. Anesth Analg 1986;65:786–804.

91. Wood M, Stone WJ, Wood AJ. Plasma binding of pancuronium: Effects of age, sex, and disease. Anesth Analg 1983;62:29–32.

92. Skivington MA. Protein binding of three titrated muscle relaxants. Br J Anaesth 1972;44:1030–1034.

93. Lebrault C, Duvaldestin P, Henzel D, Chauvin M, Guesnon P. Pharmacokinetics and pharmacodynamics of vecuronium in patients with cholestasis. Br J Anaesth 1986;58:983–987.

94. Agoston S, Vermeer GA, Kersten UW, Meijer DKF. The fate of pancuronium bromide in man. Acta Anaesthesiol Scand 1973;17:267–275.

95. Cook DR, Freeman JA, Lai AA, et al. Pharmacokinetics and pharmacodynamics of doxacurium in normal patients and in those with hepatic or renal failure. Anesth Analg 1991;72:145–150.

96. Miller RD, Stevens WC, Way WL. The effect of renal failure and hyperkalemia on the duration of pancuronium neuromuscular blockade in man. Anesth Analg 1972:52;661–666.

97. Cooper R, Maddineni VR, Mirakhur RK, Wierda JMKH, Brady M, Fitzpatrick KTJ. Time course of neuromuscular effect and pharmacokinetics of rocuronium bromide (ORG 9426) during isoflurane anesthesia in patients with and without renal failure. Br J Anaesth 1993;71:222–226.

98. Phillips BJ, Hunter JM. The use of mivacurium chloride by constant infusion in the anephric patient. Br J Anaesth 1992;68:492–498.

99. Ward S, Boheimer N, Weatherly BC, Simmonds RJ, Dopson TA. Pharmacokinetics of atracurium and its metabolites in patients with normal renal function, and in patients with renal failure. Br J Anaesth 1987;59:697–706.

100. Withington DE, Donati F, Bevan DR, Varin F. Potentiation of atracurium neuromuscular blockade by enflurane: Time-course of effect. Anesth Analg 1991;72:469–473.

101. Silverman DG, Mirakhur RK. Effect of other agents on nondepolarizing relaxants. In: Silverman DG, ed. Neuromuscular Block in Perioperative and Intensive Care. Philadelphia: JB Lippincott, 1994:104–122.

102. Crul-Sluijter EJ, Crul JF. Acidosis and neuromuscular blockade. Acta Anaesthesiol Scand 1974;18:224–236.

103. Funk DI, Crul JF, Pol FM. Effects of changes in acid-base balance on neuromuscular blockade produced by ORG-NC 45. Acta Anaesthesiol Scand 1980;24:119–124.

104. Gencarelli PJ, Swen J, Koot HWJ, Miller RD. The effects of hypercarbia and hypocarbia on pancuronium and vecuronium neuromuscular blockades in anesthetized humans. Anesthesiology 1983;59:376–380.

105. Hughes R, Chapple DJ. The pharmacology of atracurium: A new competitive neuromuscular blocking agent. Br J Anaesth 1981;53:31–44.

106. Miller RD, Roderick LL. The influence of acid-base changes on neostigmine antagonism of pancuronium neuromuscular blockade. Br J Anaesth 1978;50:317–324.

107. Waud BE, Waud DR. Interaction of calcium and potassium with neuromuscular blocking agents. Br J Anaesth 1980;52:863–866.

108. Ghoneim MM, Long JP. The interaction between magnesium and other neuromuscular blocking agents. Anesthesiology 1970;32:23–27.

109. Gramstad L, Hysing ES. Effect of ionized calcium on the neuromuscular blocking actions of atracurium and vecuronium in the cat. Br J Anaesth 1990;64:199–206.

110. Meakin G, Morton RH, Wareham AC. Age-dependent variations in response to tubocurarine in the isolated rat diaphragm. Br J Anaesth 1992;68:161–163.

111. Meretoja OA. Is vecuronium a long-acting neuromuscular blocking agent in neonates and infants? Br J Anaesth 1989;62:184–187.

112. Meakin G, Shaw EA, Baker RD, Morris P. Comparison of atracurium-induced neuromuscular blockade in neonates, infants, and children. Br J Anaesth 1988;60:171–175.

113. Debaene B, Meistelman C, d'Hollander A. Recovery from vecuronium neuromuscular blockade following neostigmine administration in infants, children, and adults during halothane anesthesia. Anesthesiology 1989;71:840–844.

114. Marsh RHK, Chjmielewski AT, Goat VA. Recovery from pancuronium: A comparison between old and young patients. Anaesthesia 1980;35:1193–1196.

115. Young WI, Matteo RS, Ornstein E. Duration of action of neostigmine and pyridostigmine in the elderly. Anesth Analg 1988;67:775–778.

116. Fikes LL, Dodman NH, Court MH. Anaesthesia for small animal patients with neuromuscular disease. Br Vet J 1990;146:487–499.

117. Fergusson RJ, Wright DJ, Willey RF, Crompton GK, Grant IWB. Suxamethonium is dangerous in polyneuropathy. Br Med J (Clin Res Ed) 1981;282:298–299.

118. Nilsson E, Meretoja OA. Vecuronium dose-response and maintenance requirements in patients with myasthenia gravis. Anesthesiology 1990;73:28–32.

119. Eisenkraft JB, Book WJ, Mann SM, Papatestas AE. Resistance to succinylcholine in myasthenia gravis: A dose-response study. Anesthesiology 1988;69:760–763.

120. Silverman DG. Myasthenia gravis and myasthenic syndrome. In: Silverman DG, ed. Neuromuscular Block in Perioperative and Intensive Care. Philadelphia: JB Lippincott, 1994:324–331.

121. Jones RS, Sharp NJH. Use of the muscle relaxant atracurium in a myasthenic dog. Vet Rec 1985;117:500–501.

122. Jones RS, Brown A, Watkins PE. Use of the muscle relaxant atracurium in a myasthenic dog. Vet Rec 1988;122:611.

123. Singh TN, Marshall IG, Harvey AC. Pre- and postjunctional blocking effects of aminoglycoside, polymyxin, tetracycline, and lincosamide antibiotics. Br J Anaesth 1982;54:1295–1305.

124. Sucoll MD, Gergis SD. Antibiotics and neuromuscular function. Anesthesiology 1981;55:148–159.

125. Hildebrand SV, Hill T. Interaction of gentamycin and atracurium in anaesthetized horses. Equine Vet J 1994;26:209–211.

126. Forsyth SF, Ilkiw JE, Hildebrand SV. Effect of gentamicin administration on the neuromuscular blockade induced by atracurium in cats. Am J Vet Res 1990;51:1675–1678.

127. Potter JM, Edeson RG, Campbell RJ, Forbes AM. Potentiation by gentamicin of non-depolarizing neuromuscular block in the cat. Anaesth Intensive Care 1980;8:20–25.

128. Martinez EA, Mealey KL, Wooldridge AA, et al. Pharmacokinetics, effects on renal function, and potentiation of atracurium-induced neuromuscular blockade after administration of a high dose of gentamicin in isoflurane-anesthetized dogs. Am J Vet Res 1996;57:1623–1626.

129. Ali HH, Savarese JJ. Stimulus frequency and dose-response curve to d-tubocurarine in man. Anesthesiology 1980;52:36–39.

130. Silverman DG, Brull SJ. Patterns of stimulation. In: Silverman DG, ed. Neuromuscular Block in Perioperative and Intensive Care. Philadelphia: JB Lippincott, 1994:37–50.

131. Waud BE, Waud DR. The relationship between the response to "train-of-four" stimulation and receptor occlusion during competitive neuromuscular block. Anesthesiology 1972;37:413–416.

132. Brand JB, Cullen DJ, Wilson NE, Ali HH. Spontaneous recovery from nondepolarizing neuromuscular blockade: Correlation between clinical and evoked response. Anesth Analg 1977;56:55–58.

133. Klein LV. Neuromuscular blocking agents. In: Short CE, ed. Principles and Practice of Veterinary Anesthesia. Baltimore: Williams and Wilkins, 1987:134–153.

134. Hildebrand SV. Neuromuscular blocking agents in equine anesthesia. Vet Clin North Am Equine Pract 1990;6:587–606.

135. Hildebrand SV. Neuromuscular blocking agents. Vet Clin North Am Small Anim Pract 1992;22:341–346.

136. Torda TA, Graham GG, Tsui D. Neuromuscular sensitivity to atracurium in humans. Anaesth Intensive Care 1990;18:62–68.

137. Viby-Morgenson J, Howardy-Hansen P, Chraemmer-Jorgensen B, Ording H, Engbaek J, Nielsen A. Posttetanic count (PTC): A new method of evaluating an intense nondepolarizing neuromuscular blockade. Anesthesiology 1981;55:458–461.

138. Braude N, Vyvyan HAL, Jordan MJ. Intraoperative assessment of atracurium-induced neuromuscular block using double burst stimulation. Br J Anaesth 1991;67:574–578.

139. Hildebrand SV, Howitt GA. Dosage requirement of pancuronium in halothane-anesthetized ponies: A comparison of cumulative and single-dose administration. Am J Vet Res 1984;45:2441–2444.

140. Bowen JM. Monitoring neuromuscular function in intact animals. Am J Vet Res 1969;30:857–859.

141. Hildebrand SV, Hill T. Neuromuscular blockade by atracurium in llamas. Vet Surg 1991;20:153–154.

142. Law SC, Cook DR. Monitoring the neuromuscular junction. In: Lake CL, ed. Clinical Monitoring. Philadelphia: WB Saunders, 1990:719–755.

143. Martinez EA, Hartsfield SM, Carroll GL. Comparison of two methods to assess neuromuscular blockade in anesthetized dogs [Abstract]. Vet Surg 1998;28:127.

144. Cronnelly R, Morris RB, Miller RD. Edrophonium: Duration of action and atropine requirement in humans during halothane anesthesia. Anesthesiology 1982;57:261–265.

145. Morris RB, Cronnelly R, Miller RD, Stanski DR, Fahey MR. Pharmacokinetics of edrophonium and neostigmine when antagonizing d-tubocurarine neuromuscular blockade in man. Anesthesiology 1981;54:399–402.

146. Baird WLM, Bowman WC, Kerr WJ. Some actions of NC 45 and of edrophonium in the anesthetized cat and man. Br J Anaesth 1982;54:375–385.

147. Jones RS, Heckmann R, Wuersch W. The effect of neostigmine on the duration of action of suxamethonium in the dog. Br Vet J 1980;136:71–73.

148. Lee C. Train-of-four fade and edrophonium antagonism of neuromuscular block by succinylcholine in man. Anesth Analg 1976;55:663–667.

149. Cullen LK, Jones RS. The effect of neostigmine on suxamethonium neuromuscular block in the dog. Res Vet Sci 1980;29:266–268.

150. Hall LW, Clarke KW, Trim CM. Veterinary Anaesthesia, 10th ed. London: WB Saunders, 2001:149–178.

151. Hubbell JAE, Muir WW, Sams RA. Guaifenesin: Cardiopulmonary effects and plasma concentrations in horses. Am J Vet Res 1980;41:1751–1755.

152. Greene Sa, Thurmon JC, Tranquilli WJ, Benson GJ. Cardiopulmonary effects of continuous intravenous infusion of guaifenesin, ketamine, and xylazine in ponies. Am J Vet Res 1986;47:2364–2367.

153. Davis LE, Wolff WA. Pharmacokinetics and metabolism of glyceryl guaiacolate in ponies. Am J Vet Res 1970;31:469–473.

154. Carroll GL, Hartsfield SM. General anesthetic techniques in ruminants. Vet Clin North Am Food Anim Pract 1996;12:627–661.

155. Moon PF, Smith LJ. General anesthetic techniques in swine. Vet Clin North Am Food Anim Pract 1996;12:663–691.

156. Tavernor WD, Jones EW. Observations on the cardiovascular and respiratory effects of guaiacol glycerol ether in conscious and anaesthetized dogs. J Small Anim Pract 1970;11:177–184.

157. Benson GJ, Thurmon JC, Tranquilli WJ, Smith CW. Cardiopulmonary effects of an intravenous infusion of guaifenesin, ketamine, and xylazine in dogs. Am J Vet Res 1985;46:1896–1898.

158. Pinder RM, Brogden RN, Speight TM, Avery GS. Dantrolene sodium: A review of its pharmacological properties and therapeutic efficacy in spasticity. Drugs 1977;13:3–23.

159. Gronert GA, Milde JH, Theye RA. Dantrolene in porcine malignant hyperthermia. Anesthesiology 1976;41:488–495.

160. Gronert GA, Mansfield E, Theye RA. Rapidly soluble dantrolene for intravenous use. In: Aldrete JA, Britt BA, eds. Malignant Hyperthermia. New York: Grune and Stratton, 1978:535–536.

161. O'Brien PJ, Forsyth GW. Preparation of injectable dantrolene for emergency treatment of malignant hyperthermia-like syndromes. Can Vet J 1983;24:200–204.

162. Stoelting RK. Pharmacology and Physiology in Anesthetic Practice, 2nd ed. Philadelphia: JB Lippincott, 1991:541–548.

163. Roewer N, Rumberger E, Bode H, Schulte Am Esch. Electrophysiological and mechanical interactions of verapamil and dantrolene on isolated heart muscle [Abstract]. Anesthesiology 1985;63:A274.

164. Bezer G. Dantrolene sodium intravenous: Verapamil. Anesth Intensive Care 1985;13:108–110.

165. Dreissen JJ, Wuis EW, Gieden JM. Prolonged vecuronium neuromuscular blockade in a patient receiving oral dantrolene. Anesthesiology 1985;62:523–524.

Chapter 16
Drug Interactions

Mark G. Papich

Introduction

When providing anesthesia and analgesia to animals, veterinarians often administer combinations of drugs without fully appreciating the possible interactions that may and do occur. Many interactions, both beneficial and harmful, are possible, considering the number of drugs that are coadministered. Although most veterinarians view drug interactions as undesirable, modern anesthesia and analgesic practice emphasizes the use of drug interactions for the benefit of the patient (multimodal anesthesia or analgesia).

A distinction should be made between drug interactions that occur in vitro (such as in a syringe or vial) from those that occur in vivo (in patients). Interactions and incompatibilities may occur as a consequence of mixing drugs in the same vial or syringe prior to administration, or when drugs interact in patients. Veterinarians frequently mix drugs together (compound) in syringes, vials, or fluids before administration to animals. In vitro reactions, also called *pharmaceutical interactions*, may form a drug precipitate or a toxic product or inactivate one of the drugs in the mixture. In vivo interactions are also possible, affecting the pharmacokinetics (absorption, distribution, or elimination) or the pharmacodynamics (mechanism of action) of the drugs and can result in enhanced or reduced pharmacological actions or increased incidence of adverse events.

Drug interactions usually result from administration of (a) two drugs in one formulation, as a fixed-dose mixture; (b) two drugs in separate formulations simultaneously; (c) a second drug during prolonged use of the first drug; and (d) two drugs at specific time intervals. Drug interactions can be classified as either pharmacokinetic or pharmacodynamic. *Pharmacokinetics* refers to what the body does to drugs, and *pharmacodynamics* refers to what drugs do to the body. Pharmacokinetic interactions produce changes in drug concentration at the receptor site by altering absorption, elimination, or distribution. Pharmacodynamic interactions occur when one drug alters the response to another.

In vitro Drug Interactions

Acid-Base Interactions

Mixing drugs or solutions that vary in pH or acid-base characteristics may result in an incompatible mixture because of opposition of charge (anion-cation) or interference with the stability of a solution because of acid-base interactions. For example, drugs formulated as hydrochloride salt (HCl) are done so to maintain a pH balance that will ensure that the drug is soluble in an aqueous solution. The HCl may also be critical for the solubility and stability of the compound. If the solution is alkalinized by adding bicarbonate or other bases, the compound may become unstable or precipitate.

The pH of common intravenous fluids is lower than many clinicians appreciate. For example, 0.9% sodium chloride and 5% dextrose solutions can have a pH as low as 3 (Table 16.1).[1] A drug added to a bag containing an acidic solution may lose activity or precipitate if alkalinity is needed for drug stability or solubility. The pH values of common intravenous solutions are listed in Table 16.1.

Chemical Incompatibilities

These reactions occur as a result of chemical interactions among active ingredients, inactive ingredients, vehicles, and preservatives. Veterinarians should not admix drug solutions without first consulting a pharmaceutical reference[2,3] or the drug manufacturer. The drugs listed in Table 16.2 have often been cited as being incompatible with other drugs or solutions. Interactions with injectable drugs can be found in Trissel's book of interactions or the *USP Drug Information*, volume 1.[2,3] Signs of interactions and incompatibilities can include haziness of the solutions, precipitation, bubble formation, or a color change. Some interactions cause drug hydrolysis and oxidation, for example, sympathomimetic catecholamines, such as dobutamine, dopamine, or epinephrine may oxidize to a slight pink without significant loss of potency. However, if the color changes to brownish, it should not be used because this is a sign of significant oxidation.

Solutions

These may be incompatible with other solutions because of ionic interactions. For example, sodium bicarbonate ($NaHCO_3$) reacts with calcium-containing solutions, forming calcium carbonate. Admixing tetracyclines with calcium-containing solutions results in precipitation. In general, hydrochloride salts (e.g., dobutamine HCl, dopamine HCl, and epinephrine HCl) should not be mixed with alkaline solutions. Vitamin B_1 (thiamine hydrochloride) is unstable in alkaline solutions and should not be mixed with alkalinizing solutions, carbonates, or citrates.

Table 16.1. Common fluid solutions and components.

Fluid	Na+	K+	Ca2+	Cl-	pH
0.9% Saline	154	0	0	154	4.5–5.7
0.45% Saline	77	0	0	77	4–7
Ringer's solution	147	4	4.5	156	5.0–7.5
Lactated Ringer's	130	4	3	109	6.0–7.5
5% Dextrose (D_5W)	0	0	0	0	3.2–6.5

D_5W, 5% dextrose solution.

Table 16.2. Anesthetic drug in vitro incompatibilities with other drugs and solutions.

Drug	Compatibility with Other Drugs	Compatibility with Fluid Solutions	Important Considerations
Bupivacaine HCl	pH 4.0–6.5. Avoid strongly acid or alkaline solutions. Sodium bicarbonate has been added to local anesthetics just prior to administration to decrease pain from injection. Raising the pH will accelerate the onset of anesthetic action.	Compatible with fluid solutions.	Do not use if solution becomes cloudy, yellow, or pink. If pH is adjusted (e.g., pH 6–7) with alkalinizing solutions, the drug is stable if used soon after mixing.
Buprenorphine		Infuse with sodium chloride.	
Butorphanol	Do not mix with sodium barbiturates.		Protect from light.
Calcium chloride	Will precipitate with sodium bicarbonate.		Do not mix with compounds known to chelate with calcium.
Dexamethasone sodium phosphate	pH 7.0–8.5. Do not mix with acidifying solutions.	Compatible with most IV solutions.	
Diazepam	pH 6.2–6.9. Hydrolysis will occur if combined with low pH solutions. Precipitation will occur with aqueous solutions.	Precipitation occurs when mixed with water-based (aqueous) solutions. Ringer's based solutions and dextrose will cause precipitation.	Protect from light. There is no loss if stored in hard plastic syringe. However, if stored in soft plastic (PVC) infusion bags or tubing, significant sorption will occur (e.g., 80%–90% in 24 h).
Dobutamine HCl	pH 2.5–5.5. Do not mix with alkalinizing drugs.	Do not mix with alkaline solutions. Compatible with most fluid solutions.	Slight pink tinge to solution can occur without loss of potency, but do not use if solution turns brown.
Dopamine HCl	pH 2.5–5.0. Do not mix with alkalinizing solutions.	Do not mix with alkaline fluids. Compatible with most fluid solutions.	Do not use if solution turns color.
Epinephrine HCl	pH of solution is acidic. It is destroyed by mixing with alkaline drugs.	Incompatible with alkaline solutions and oxidizing solutions.	Do not mix with bicarbonates, nitrates, citrates, and other salts. It is compatible with plastic in syringes. When solution becomes oxidized, it turns brown. Do not use if this color change is observed.

Table 16.2. Anesthetic drug in vitro incompatibilities with other drugs and solutions (*continued*).

Drug	Compatibility with Other Drugs	Compatibility with Fluid Solutions	Important Considerations
Fentanyl citrate		Compatible with most fluid solutions.	No loss measured when stored in plastic infusion sets.
Furosemide	pH of solution, 8.0–9.8. Stable with alkaline drugs, but do not mix with acidifying drug solutions with pH < 5.5	Do not mix with acidic solutions.	Compatible in plastic syringes and infusion sets.
Glycopyrrolate	Acidic pH (2–3). Do not mix with drugs that will alkalinize the solution.	Do not mix with alkaline solutions (pH > 6.0). Compatible with most other fluids.	
Heparin sodium	Heparin is acidic and will react with some basic compounds.	Infuse with dextrose solutions.	No loss occurs in various solutions. No sorption to plastic has been reported.
Hydromorphone HCl	Do not mix with diazepam or bicarbonate.	Stable in most fluid solutions.	
Isoproterenol HCl		Compatible with dextrose and saline solutions.	Degradation occurs at pH > 6.0.
Ketamine HCl	Acidic solution. Do not mix with alkaline solutions such as barbiturates. Avoid mixing ketamine and diazepam.	Compatible with saline and dextrose solutions.	Solution may turn slightly dark, which does not affect potency.
Lidocaine	pH of solution, 5–7. Compatible with most drugs. It can be alkalinized to pH 7.2 without loss of stability.	Stable in fluids, including dextrose solution.	Aqueous solution is stable in mildly acid and alkaline conditions. If pH is adjusted (e.g., pH 6–7) with alkalinizing solutions, the drug is stable if used soon after mixing. No sorption to plastic syringes has been reported.
Lorazepam		Compatible with fluid solutions such as dextrose and saline.	Dilute solution for IV use. There is significant sorption to PVC containers.
Meperidine HCl	Compatible with most drugs.	Compatible with most fluid solutions.	Compatible with plastic syringes.
Midazolam HCl	pH of solution, ca. 3.0. Increasing the pH to >7 will result in drug loss.	Compatible with fluid solutions.	No sorption with plastic or fluid containers is reported.
Morphine sulfate	pH of solution, 3.5–7.0. Stable at low pH, but degradation will occur at pH > 7.	Stable in most fluids (dextrose and saline solutions).	No sorption to plastic has been reported.
Nitroglycerin	pH of solution, 3.0–6.5. Do not mix with other drugs.	Compatible with most fluid solutions.	Sorption to containers, especially PVC plastic, is extensive and will result in significant loss.
Oxymorphone HCl	pH of solution, 2.7–4.5. Compatible with most drugs.	Compatible with most fluid solutions.	
Pentobarbital sodium	pH of solution is 9.0–10.5. It will precipitate if combined with most hydrochloride-based drugs or anything with low pH. Alkaline solution will affect other coadministered drugs.		Aqueous solutions are not stable. Will precipitate readily in solutions with low pH.

(continued)

441

Table 16.2. Anesthetic drug in vitro incompatibilities with other drugs and solutions (*continued*).

Drug	Compatibility with Other Drugs	Compatibility with Fluid Solutions	Important Considerations
Phenobarbital sodium	pH of solution, 9.2–10.2. It will precipitate if combined with most hydrochloride-based drugs or anything with low pH. Alkaline solution will affect other coadministered drugs.		Will precipitate readily in solutions with low pH.
Phenytoin sodium	pH of solution, 10.0–12.3. Do not mix with acidifying drugs.		Will precipitate readily in solutions with low pH.
Propofol	pH of solution, 7.0–8.5 and lower (depends on manufacturer).	Compatible with fluid solutions such as dextrose and saline.	Oil and water emulsion formulation that will encourage microbe growth. Do not freeze. More stable in glass than in plastic.
Sodium bicarbonate	Alkaline solution; pH 7.0–8.5. Do not mix with acid solutions.	Do not mix with solutions that contain calcium (e.g., Ringer's) or precipitation may occur.	
Sodium nitroprusside	pH of solution, 3.5–6.0.	Dextrose solution is recommended for infusion.	Very sensitive to light. Cover with foil during infusion.
Thiopental sodium	pH of solution, 10–11. If not kept at alkaline pH, precipitation will occur.		Reconstituted solution is stable for only 3 days at room temperature or 7 days refrigerated.

HCl, hydrochloride; IV, intravenous; and PVC, polyvinyl chloride.

Diazepam

Diazepam is notorious for its instability in solutions and its ability to adsorb to plastic containers. Diazepam is formulated in organic solvents (e.g., propylene glycol, ethanol, and benzyl alcohol) and is not soluble in aqueous solutions. If the diazepam solution is added to an aqueous solution, it will become hazy or precipitate unless the solution is very dilute (e.g., 1:50 to 1:100). In addition, diazepam is known to adsorb to soft plastic containers, such as those composed of polyvinyl chloride (e.g., PVC infusion bags and plastic tubing). Heparin, when used in flush solutions, is physically incompatible with diazepam.

Changes in pH That Affect Drug Stability or Solubility

According to the *USP-NF*,[3] improper pH ranks with exposure to elevated temperature as a factor most likely to cause a clinically significant loss of drug efficacy. A drug solution or suspension may be stable for days, weeks, or even years in its original formulation, but when mixed with another liquid that changes the pH, it can degrade in minutes, hours, or days. A pH change of 1 unit might decrease drug stability by a factor of 10 or greater. These types of interactions are more likely at the extremes of pH, for example outside the range of 4 to 8 (see Table 16.2 for pH values of commonly used anesthetic and adjunctive drugs). Some drugs undergo epimerization (steric rearrangement) when ex-

posed to a pH range higher than the optimum for the drug. Other drugs are oxidized, which is catalyzed by high pH, rendering the drug inactive. Oxidation is often visible through a color change.

Some drugs are alkaline when in solution and will raise the pH of other admixed drugs, resulting in instability or precipitation. Examples of drugs that will increase the pH of solution above 6 are sodium bicarbonate, barbiturates, alkaline-buffered antibiotics, and aminophylline. Barbiturates are notable because the alkalinity of their solutions. Sodium salts of barbiturates in solution (e.g., pentobarbital sodium, phenobarbital sodium, or sodium thiopental) have a pH of approximately 10. If mixed with any solution that lowers the pH, for example, a hydrochloride-based solution, precipitation will occur instantly.

In vivo Drug Interactions

These are reactions that occur in patients when more than one drug is administered. Studies in people have demonstrated that, as the number of drugs coadministered to a patient increases, the incidence of drug interactions also increases. The consequences of drug interactions are most severe for drugs that have a narrow therapeutic index (i.e., when the ratio of toxic dose to effective dose is small). In vivo drug interactions may change drug absorption, drug disposition, biotransformation, and excretion (pharmacokinetic interactions).

Pharmacokinetic Drug Interactions

These interactions include (a) alteration in absorption, (b) alteration in drug-biotransformation enzymes, (c) alteration in protein binding, (d) changes in renal or hepatic clearance, and (e) changes in drug distribution.

Absorption (Systemic Availability)

Most patients undergoing anesthesia are fasted; however, oral medications are occasionally administered in the immediate perioperative period (e.g., orally administered nonsteroidal anti-inflammatory drugs [NSAIDs]). Most anesthetic and anesthetic adjunctive drugs (e.g., opioids) slow gastrointestinal motility and can delay passage of drugs to the small intestine, where most oral drugs are absorbed. Some drugs require an acidic environment to dissolve before gastrointestinal absorption. Antacid compounds, proton-pump inhibitors (omeprazole), or H_2-receptor blockers (famotidine, ranitidine, and cimetidine) can suppress stomach acid production, which may decrease the absorption of other drugs. There are few documented examples where this type of interaction has affected analgesic or anesthetic drug efficacy, however. It is well documented that orally administered antifungal and antibiotic drugs are affected by stomach acidity. It should be noted that fasted animals have a higher stomach pH than normal and often in the same range as animals administered an H_2 blocker or proton-pump inhibitor.[4]

Divalent cations (Mg^{2+} and Ca^{2+}) in antacid drugs will bind to tetracyclines and prevent absorption from the gastrointestinal tract. Divalent and trivalent cations, especially Fe^{3+}, Ca^{2+}, Mg^{2+}, and Al^{3+}, can bind to and prevent absorption of fluoroquinolone antibiotics. Gastrointestinal protectants, such as sucralfate (which contains aluminum) and antacids (containing Mg^{2+} and/or Al^{3+}), will decrease absorption of fluoroquinolone antibiotics (e.g., enrofloxacin and ciprofloxacin) and tetracyclines.

Alteration in absorption as a desirable drug interaction is best demonstrated by the practice of adding epinephrine to local anesthetic solutions. Epinephrine prolongs the duration of local anesthetic action by reducing blood flow (secondary to epinephrine-induced vasoconstriction) and thus delaying systemic absorption of the local anesthetic. The second gas effect represents enhanced absorption from the alveoli of volatile anesthetics administered with nitrous oxide. Rapid absorption of nitrous oxide concentrates the other anesthetic in the alveoli, thereby enhancing absorption of the volatile agent.

EMLA cream (lidocaine 2.5% and prilocaine 2.5%) is an interesting example of a physical change that occurs when two drugs are mixed with a resulting favorable impact on absorption. The cream contains equal parts of the local anesthetics lidocaine and prilocaine that combine to produce a eutectic mixture. Neither local anesthetic is effective when applied to unbroken skin, but the eutectic mixture can penetrate skin.

Interactions Involving the Multidrug Resistance Efflux Pump

The multidrug resistance (MDR) efflux pump, also known as P glycoprotein (P-gp), is coded for by the MDR gene(s) and can be

Table 16.3. Substrates and inhibitors of P glycoprotein that may affect anesthetic drug actions.

P-glycoprotein substrates
  Opiates (loperamide, morphine)
  Digoxin
  Quinidine
  Ivermectin
  Verapamil
  Antihistamines
  Cyclosporine
  Doxorubicin
  Diltiazem
P-glycoprotein inhibitors
  Ketoconazole
  Erythromycin
  Cyclosporine
  Grapefruit juice
  Fluoxetine
  St. John's wort
  Paroxetine
  Verapamil
  Quinidine

involved in several important drug interactions.[5,6] The P-gp is located in membranes and is responsible for pumping drug compounds across a membrane and out of the cell. P-gp can be protective (e.g., removing ivermectin from the central nervous system [CNS]) or lead to decreased drug effectiveness (e.g., chemotherapeutic drug resistance in cancer cells).

P-gp is responsible for pharmacokinetic changes because it is located in the intestine, biliary tract, liver, placenta, and blood-brain barrier (BBB). The best-known pharmacokinetic effects are (a) the pumping of drugs into the intestinal lumen, thereby decreasing systemic absorption and increasing drug clearance from the body; and (b) the P-gp, located in the BBB, that affects the CNS uptake and elimination of certain compounds. P-gp is an integral part of the BBB and participates in neuroprotection of the brain by regulating drug entry.[7] Because P-gp is located also in the gastrointestinal tract, placenta, and kidneys, among other organs, inhibition of P-gp by ketoconazole, cyclosporine, calcium-channel blockers (diltiazem), and antiarrhythmics (lidocaine and quinidine) may have a variety of consequences.[8] In some cases, drugs such as cyclosporine can be both a substrate and an inhibitor of P-gp (see Table 16.3). Rifampin and corticosteroids can act as inducers (they increase the activity) of P-gp.

Ketoconazole can inhibit P-gp in the intestine and increase oral absorption of other drugs, including cyclosporine. Concurrent administration of ketoconazole has been known to decrease dose requirements for cyclosporine by one-third. Cyclosporine may inhibit P-gp in the BBB and increase the CNS concentration of some drugs, such as those within the avermectin group. There are anecdotal reports of dogs developing clinical signs consistent with avermectin toxicosis after having received both cyclosporine and avermectin-like drugs.

There have been no reports of anesthetic drugs affecting P-gp interactions. However, because inhibition of P-gp influences the BBB, clinicians should be aware of the potential for exaggerated CNS anesthetic effects when an animal has received a P-gp inhibitor. Some opiates are substrates for P-gp in the BBB, although this is less established in the veterinary species of interest. However, an exaggerated CNS response (e.g. sedation or respiratory depression) might result from administration of an opiate and an inhibitor of P-gp.

Interactions That Affect Hepatic Drug Clearance

Changes in hepatic clearance are usually a consequence of changes in hepatic blood flow, although other actions (e.g., effects on microsomal enzyme activity) can result from one drug influencing the metabolism of another. Blood-flow changes are most noted when the liver extracts a high fraction of drug from the blood presented to it. Drugs most affected are those known as *high clearance drugs*. Lidocaine, meperidine, and opiates (e.g., morphine, oxymorphone, and hydromorphone) are examples of analgesic drugs that have high hepatic extractions. Inhalational anesthetics, such as halothane, can reduce liver blood flow.

Many drugs must be biotransformed by microsomal enzymes in the liver to make them more water soluble for excretion into the bile or urine. Drugs metabolized by the liver can undergo phase I or phase II reactions. Phase I reactions metabolize the drug to a more water-soluble compound. These reactions often are oxidative, but other reactions, such as reduction, also occur. Phase II reactions occur via conjugation. The best-known example is that of conjugation with glucuronic acid, but other conjugation reactions with amino acids, acetyl groups, and sulfates are possible. Drugs that affect the liver's biotransformation enzymes can cause clinically significant drug interactions.

Cytochrome P-450 Family of Enzymes

The cytochrome P-450 (CYP) enzymes have been studied in great detail in humans, and a family of these enzymes have been identified that participate in the metabolism of drugs. The CYP-3A4 enzymes are probably the most important of this group because they have the largest number of substrates (about half the drugs currently prescribed clinically). However, CYP-2D6, CYP-1A2, CYP-2C9, and CYP-2C19 also can be important for drug metabolism. The presence and significance of these enzymes in domestic animals have not been documented nearly as well. Animals also have these families of enzymes, although the activity of each group is not the same.[9] Of the species compared (dogs, cats, and horses), none of them resemble the same pattern as humans.

Microsomal Enzyme Induction

Drugs and compounds can increase hepatic microsomal (cytochrome P-450) enzyme activity. Since some of these enzymes are found in intestine as well as the liver, enzyme induction can cause faster biotransformation, resulting in lower oral bioavailability and/or faster plasma clearance. The enzymes most commonly affected by induction are the mixed-function oxidases (phase I oxidation reactions). Enzyme induction causes an in-

Table 16.4. Cytochrome P-450 inducers.

Chlorinated hydrocarbons
Diazepam (Valium)
Diphenhydramine
Estrogens
Griseofulvin
Hyperthyroidism
Pentobarbital
Phenobarbital
Phenylbutazone
Phenytoin (Dilantin)
Progestogens
Rifampin

crease in activity as well as an increase in enzyme content within the endoplasmic reticulum.

Some drugs are specific in their inducing ability. For example, a drug may induce one group of enzymes without affecting another. The drugs that are most affected by enzyme inhibition are those that undergo metabolism by hepatic enzymes and are lipid soluble. Affected drugs usually have a low hepatic extraction ratio. The time for induction to occur is usually 2 to 3 weeks after initial exposure, and it may take weeks to months for enzyme activity to return to normal after the inducing drug is withdrawn. Potential enzyme inducers are listed in Table 16.4.

Microsomal Enzyme Inhibition

Hepatic microsomal enzymes responsible for drug biotransformation may be inhibited by certain drugs and compounds. Inhibition usually occurs via competitive binding to form an inactive drug-enzyme complex. Inhibition almost immediately follows drug exposure. In many cases, a metabolite of the drug is responsible for enzyme inhibition. Noncompetitive inhibition is also possible when a drug is not a substrate for the enzyme, but alters its function in some manner.

Examples of drugs that inhibit microsomal enzymes are listed in Table 16.5. Some of the microsomal enzyme inhibition–mediated drug interactions that have been described in veterinary patients include cimetidine inhibition of theophylline metabolism, chloramphenicol inhibition of barbiturate metabolism, ketoconazole inhibition (by as much as 85%) of cyclosporine metabolism, ketoconazole inhibition of prednisolone metabolism, and ethanol or 4-methyl-pyrazole inhibition of alcohol dehydrogenase, which converts ethylene glycol to toxic metabolites (this effect is used to treat toxicosis). One well-known example of enzyme inhibition that has clinical consequences in people is the inhibition of acetaminophen metabolism following alcohol consumption. This inhibition can lead to accumulation of hepatotoxic metabolites that form via other pathways.

During the anesthetic period, the nature of enzyme inhibition is important to patients that receive drugs requiring hepatic biotransformation to terminate their effect. For example, if there is concurrent enzyme inhibition, the risks of anesthesia may be altered. Veterinarians should be cognizant of the potential prob-

Table 16.5. Cytochrome P-450 enzyme inhibitors.

Chloramphenicol
Cimetidine
Cyclophosphamide
Erythromycin
Interferon (vaccines)
Ketoconazole
Morphine
Organophosphates
Quinidine
Tetracycline
Verapamil

lems that may occur if they administer or prescribe a drug that has enzyme-inhibiting effects when also administering anesthetics. Fortunately, clearance of inhalant anesthetics and drugs cleared via renal excretion are usually not directly affected.

Interactions That Involve Drug Protein Binding

Alterations in protein binding occur but are rarely of clinical significance. Drugs exist in unbound (free) and bound forms in the blood. The free form is generally immediately available to exert pharmacological effects, but the bound form is not. Drug displaced from protein distributes rapidly into tissue and is available for biotransformation and excretion. The net effect of a displacement interaction is usually small, transient, and frequently unrecognized.

Some drugs are known to compete for binding sites on albumin and other proteins, altering the unbound fraction of a second drug. For most drugs, the amount of protein (and protein-binding sites) in the plasma greatly exceeds the number of drug molecules in the plasma, and binding is rarely saturated. Interactions that involve displacement of protein-bound drugs are therefore rare unless there is severe hypoproteinemia or the drug is so highly protein bound that it occupies most of the binding sites. Only drugs that are highly protein bound (usually defined as approximately 80% to 85% or greater bound), exhibit high clearance rates, and have a low therapeutic index are likely to be involved in protein-binding interactions of clinical significance. Two recent reviews illustrate that drug protein-binding interactions have minimal consequences in most situations of multiple-drug administration.[10,11] Although changes in plasma protein binding may have an important influence on individual pharmacokinetic parameters, changes in plasma protein binding will usually not greatly influence the clinical exposure of a patient to a drug.[11]

Pharmacodynamic Drug Interactions

These interactions include drug interactions at the same receptor sites or at different sites. In anesthesiology, pharmacodynamic interactions are frequently used clinically, and pharmacokinetic interactions much less often. Pharmacodynamic interactions of marked clinical significance can affect the cardiovascular, respiratory, and central nervous systems, as well as the neuromuscular junction and metabolism.

It is also common to give drugs that interact to produce complementary effects, to reduce side effects, or to terminate an effect of a drug. Some examples of these types of desirable interaction are (a) the systemic administration of an opioid to reduce the concentration of inhalation agent required to prevent patient response to a noxious stimulus, (b) atropine administration to reduce or prevent the muscarinic effects (e.g., salivation or bradycardia) of anticholinesterases (e.g., neostigmine) when used to counter the action of nondepolarizing neuromuscular blocking agents, (c) administration of an opiate partial agonist or agonist/antagonist (e.g., buprenorphine or butorphanol) to blunt the effects of a pure opiate agonist, and (d) the use of anticholinesterase compounds to antagonize the action of nondepolarizing neuromuscular blocking agents by blocking the hydrolysis of endogenous acetylcholine.

Interactions are possible with the concomitant use of stimulants and sedatives and/or anesthetics. Among the commonly encountered stimulants are the sympathetic amines (phenylpropanolamine, ephedrine, and pseudoephedrine) and other drugs that exert their effects through dopaminergic mechanisms. Selegiline is a monoamine oxidase B (MAO-B) inhibitor at low doses (MAO-A *and* B inhibitor at high doses) that has been administered to animals for treatment of canine hyperadrenocorticism and cognitive disorder. In addition to its indirect dopaminergic effects, it is metabolized to *l*-amphetamine and *l*-methamphetamine in animals.[12] The amphetamine *l*-isomer is not as pharmacologically active as the d-isomer (e.g., dextroamphetamine), but high doses of selegiline (3 mg/kg) have caused excitement and restlessness in dogs, presumably via amphetamine effects.[13] MAO-B inhibitors are generally less likely than MAO-A inhibitors to cause severe anesthetic drug interactions, but they still may exacerbate CNS toxicity of other excitatory drugs. Of the interactions reported in humans, coadministration of selegiline with selective serotonin reuptake inhibitors (SSRIs) such as fluoxetine and paroxetine has caused CNS reactions and the potential for the *serotonin syndrome* characterized by muscle rigidity, tremors, restlessness, and altered mental status.[14] Other signs of serotonin syndrome may not involve the CNS and include dysfunction of the respiratory and cardiovascular system and hyperthermia. Such reactions associated with selegiline have not yet been documented in veterinary medicine. There does not appear to be a larger potential for severe interactions between selegiline and sympathomimetic amines (e.g., phenylpropanolamine and ephedrine) because selegiline does not inhibit MAO-A at clinically relevant doses. Nevertheless, when prescribing selegiline with sympathetic amines or MAO inhibitors such as amitraz (Mitaban), one should advise owners of the potential interaction and clinical manifestations. There have been reported serotonin-mediated reactions in humans when selegiline has been administered with the opiate meperidine, but documentation of the clinical occurrence of these reactions in veterinary patients is lacking. Because this reaction is caused by a metabolite of meperidine, other opiates are considered less likely to cause this reaction.

Nonsteroidal Anti-inflammatory Drug Interactions

NSAIDs such as carprofen, meloxicam, etodolac, tepoxalin, firocoxib, and deracoxib are used to treat pain and inflammation. In large animals, flunixin meglumine, ketoprofen, and phenylbutazone are often used. The mechanism of action of an NSAID is primarily via inhibition of cyclooxygenase (prostaglandin endoperoxide synthase) isoenzymes. Prostaglandin synthase 1 (cyclooxygenase 1 [COX-1]) is primarily a constitutive enzyme expressed in tissues. Prostaglandins, prostacyclin, and thromboxane synthesized by this enzyme are in part responsible for normal physiological functions. Prostaglandin synthase 2 (COX-2) is synthesized by macrophages and inflammatory cells and is inducible after stimulation by cytokines and other mediators of inflammation. Contrary to initial beliefs, though, COX-2 may be constitutive in some tissues. This has recently raised concerns about the ability of COX-2–selective drugs to spare physiological prostaglandin production in some tissues and their safety in certain situations. NSAID development in the 1990s and early 2000s focused on selective inhibition of COX-2, with the goal of producing analgesia and suppressing inflammation without inhibiting physiologically important prostanoids. However, more profound inhibition of COX-2 may not always be beneficial, because COX-2 products appear to be beneficial in some tissues and disease states. For example, COX-2 products have biological importance in angiogenesis, renal function, regulation of bone resorption, reproductive function, and healing of gastroduodenal ulcers.[15] Prolonged COX-2 inhibition has also been associated with a higher risk of cardiovascular complications (stroke and myocardial ischemia) in humans, because it unbalances the production of endogenous prostanoids by preserving COX-1 function, which may promote platelet aggregation and vasoconstriction.[16] Consequently, COX-2–selective drugs (valdecoxib, celecoxib, and rofecoxib) used in humans have received increased scrutiny by the medical community in recent years, and two have been voluntarily withdrawn from the U.S. market. Unbalanced COX-2 enzyme inhibition appears to increase risk of adverse events in some patient populations, and, because of this concern, future directions of NSAID development may need to be reexamined.[17]

The action of NSAIDs in animals raises questions about the potential for adverse interactions. Some theoretical interactions are worthy of consideration. NSAIDs might interfere with prostaglandin-mediated vasodilation that may be necessary for tissue perfusion during anesthesia. Prostaglandins may be important for the action of cardiovascular drugs such as angiotensin-converting enzyme (ACE) inhibitors (e.g., captopril, enalapril, benazepril, and lisinopril). Prostaglandins may also mediate some of the pharmacological effects of diuretics such as furosemide. Furosemide and ACE inhibitors stimulate prostaglandin synthesis to increase renal blood flow and produce vasodilation and natriuresis. Consequently, NSAID inhibition of prostaglandin synthesis may decrease the action of ACE inhibitors and furosemide.[18] NSAIDs may decrease the antihypertensive effect of ACE inhibitors. For aspirin, this action appears to be dose related.[19,20] This warning is listed in the United States Pharmacopeia-Drug Information (USP-DI 2004) and has been reported in people, but its clinical significance has been debated.[19,20] The administration of an ACE inhibitor with the NSAID tepoxalin is not associated with adverse renal effects.

Because NSAIDs are generally highly protein bound, interactions with other highly protein-bound drugs are possible, but as discussed previously, unlikely.[21] Manufacturers' labels on veterinary NSAIDs have warned veterinarians that coadministration of NSAIDs (many of which are over 90% protein bound) could increase free fractions of coadministered drugs such as phenobarbital and produce adverse effects. However, despite the frequently cited potential protein-binding interactions between NSAIDs and other drugs, there are very few documented cases where this has resulted in an adverse outcome, and the clinical significance of protein-binding interactions has likely been exaggerated.

One last possible NSAID interaction worthy of consideration is the combination of an NSAID with a fluoroquinolone antibiotic, causing CNS toxicity in people.[22] This type of interaction with currently available fluoroquinolones used in animals (enrofloxacin, marbofloxacin, orbifloxacin, and difloxacin) has not been reported, however.

Renal Interactions with NSAIDs and Anesthetics

In the kidney, prostaglandins play an important role in modulating the tone of blood vessels and regulating salt and water balance, especially during periods of renal stress. Renal injury caused by NSAID use has been described in people and horses. Reported cases of toxicity occur when high doses have been used or when there are other complicating factors (e.g., coadministration of methoxyflurane).[23] Renal injury probably occurs as a result of inhibition of renal prostaglandin synthesis and altered renal autoregulation during periods of renal stress or insult.[24] In animals that have decreased renal perfusion caused by dehydration, anesthesia, shock, or preexisting renal disease, this interference with prostaglandin synthesis can lead to renal ischemia.[25] Many cases of renal damage caused by anesthetic-NSAID interactions might be subclinical because of the reserve capacity of the kidney. Widespread nephron damage would be required (approximately 75%) before currently used laboratory benchmarks for renal function (blood urea nitrogen and creatinine) would significantly change.

Additional information is needed with regard to the safety of the effect of currently available COX-2 specific inhibitors on the kidney. Prostaglandins that play an important role in salt and water regulation and renal hemodynamics are synthesized by COX-2 enzymes.[26] Constitutive COX-2 is found in various sections of the kidney, and administration of drugs that selectively inhibit COX-2 may adversely affect overall renal function in some situations. Of the currently available NSAIDs, carprofen's effect on renal function has been the most extensively studied. Because carprofen is registered for use in perioperative situations in an injectable formulation, safety studies have been conducted to determine whether there is any evidence of an increased occurrence of renal toxicity with its use in the perioperative period, particularly during anesthesia. In one study, carprofen, ketorolac, and ketoprofen were examined in healthy dogs undergoing surgery, but without intravenous fluid administration. There were minor increases in renal tubular epithelial cells in urine sediment, but, overall, carprofen had no adverse effect on renal function.[27] In contrast, some ketorolac-treated and ketoprofen-treated dogs had transient azotemia. In two similar studies, carprofen administered to anesthetized healthy dogs had no adverse effect on renal function.[28,29] The renal effects of deracoxib administration have been reported by the manufacturer. At high doses, there is a dose-dependent effect on renal tubules. At up to 10 mg/kg for 6 months, it is well tolerated in most dogs, but there is a potential for a dose-dependent renal tubular degeneration/regeneration at doses of 6 mg/kg or higher with long-term usage. It should be remembered that the clinically approved dose of deracoxib for long-term treatment is only 1 to 2 mg/kg per day. Tepoxalin at a dose of 10 mg/kg (currently registered dose) has been evaluated in anesthetized, healthy, normotensive, normovolemic dogs. It has also been evaluated in dogs receiving ACE inhibitors. In both studies adverse effects on renal function were not detected.[30] Despite the apparent safety of perioperative NSAID administration documented by these studies, intravenous fluid administration and vigilant monitoring during prolonged anesthesia are clearly warranted to reduce the risk of either subclinical damage or overt renal complications.

Gastrointestinal Interactions with NSAIDs

In the gastrointestinal (GI) tract, prostaglandins play an important role in maintaining a healthy mucosa and cytoprotection and in regulation of acid and mucous secretion. Administration of NSAIDs typically alters GI physiology and may increase the risk of GI injury. GI effects range from mild gastritis and vomiting to severe GI ulceration and bleeding and even death. These effects have been documented for the past 3 decades in the veterinary literature. GI toxicity is caused by two main mechanisms: direct irritation of the GI mucosa and prostaglandin inhibition.[15] Direct irritation occurs because an acidic NSAID can become more lipophilic in the acid milieu of the stomach and cause injury by enhancing diffusion into the gastric mucosa. Secondly, prostaglandins have a cytoprotective effect on the GI mucosa, and inhibition of these compounds causes decreased cytoprotection, diminished blood flow, decreased synthesis of protective mucus, and inhibition of mucosal cell turnover and repair. In healthy dogs, COX-1 is the primary COX enzyme that produces prostaglandins (primarily prostaglandin E_2).[31] An examination of published reports of GI toxicity from the administration of an NSAID in animals indicates that the most serious problems are caused from doses that are higher than recommended, but toxicity has been observed also from relatively mild doses in susceptible individuals. Some factors may increase the risk of GI toxicosis, including concurrent corticosteroids and other GI diseases. Corticosteroids in particular are known to increase the risk of GI toxicity caused by NSAIDs.[25,32,33] Even meloxicam, which is relatively COX-1 sparing in the canine GI tract, has been associated with increased risk of GI mucosal injury when administered with a corticosteroid.[32] Other events that stress the gastric mucosa, such as decreased perfusion caused by shock, anesthesia, or

dehydration, increase risk of damage.[34] Clinical observations suggest that, although gastric ulceration can be significant with the administration of NSAIDs in some patients, catastrophic perforating ulceration can occur also in the proximal duodenum, especially in dogs.[34] Further investigation into the actions of NSAIDs on the duodenal mucosa are needed.

Opioid Interactions

Opioids are often administered with general anesthetics to provide analgesia and enhance their anesthetic action.[35] They are also commonly coadministered with sedative and tranquilizing agents to enhance sedation and analgesia. Clinical and research observations strongly support the concurrent use of opioids and anesthetic and anesthetic-adjunctive drugs; however, there is some evidence that this practice may actually decrease the magnitude and duration of opioid analgesic efficacy in some situations.[36,37]

As discussed previously in this chapter, there is a specific interaction between MAO inhibitors and meperidine described in people. The use of these drugs together has caused an unpredictable and sometimes fatal reaction, which includes excitation, sweating, rigidity, coma, and seizures. This reaction seems to be rather specific for meperidine because it is caused by one of its metabolites. If animals receive MAO inhibitors and another opiate, it is suggested first to administer a test dose of the opiate and observe the animal carefully. If there is no adverse reaction, subsequent doses can probably be administered safely. Although nonspecific MAO inhibitors are rarely used for treatment of depression in animals, other drugs with MAO-inhibiting properties are used in animals. For example, selegiline, a specific MAO type-B inhibitor, is used in dogs to treat canine hyperadrenocorticism and cognitive disorder. Amitraz, which is also an MAO inhibitor, is found in pet collars and dips to prevent and treat mite infestations. Although no adverse reactions in animals have been documented with amitraz or selegiline and opioid analgesic drugs, one should administer these drug combinations cautiously, at least for the first dose.

In recent years, tramadol has become increasingly popular as an oral analgesic medication for managing chronic pain, but its analgesic efficacy may be partially attributed to serotonin reuptake inhibition. The potential to induce CNS excitation and even seizures when tramadol is coadministered with known CNS stimulants, such as the tricyclic antidepressants, the SSRIs such as fluoxetine, and mood-altering herbal medication such as St. John's wort, should be appreciated by veterinarians. These combinations should be administered to animals with caution.

Interactions Among Opioid Drugs

In recent years, there has been some confusion as to whether the administration of opioid agonists with opioid agonist/antagonists will produce an interaction that diminishes the analgesic effect of the combination. In theory, drugs such as butorphanol and pentazocine have antagonistic properties on the μ receptor, so they should partially reverse some effects of μ-receptor agonists when administered together. The clinical significance of this antagonism has been debated, however. In dogs, for example, although butorphanol reverses some respiratory depression and sedation produced by pure agonists, the analgesic efficacy may be preserved.[38] Similarly, in dogs given butorphanol for postoperative pain associated with orthopedic surgery, there was no diminished efficacy with subsequent administration of oxymorphone.[39] However, in another study, dogs that had not responded to butorphanol after shoulder arthrotomy responded to subsequent administration of oxymorphone, but the oxymorphone dose required to produce an adequate effect was higher than what would be required if oxymorphone was used alone, suggesting that some antagonism of analgesia may have been present.[40] When butorphanol and oxymorphone have been administered together to cats, a greater efficacy has been reported than when either drug was used alone.[41,42] These clinical observations taken together suggest that antagonism may indeed occur in some clinical patients, but in other patients coadministration actually results in a synergistic analgesic effect. These divergent results from one individual to the next may be due to a variety of factors, including (a) differences in the pain syndrome being treated, (b) species variation in response to opioids, (c) dosage ratios of the specific opioids being administered and (d) variation in opioid efficacy between genders. For example, when looking at the first of these factors in humans, whether antagonism or synergism occurs with the coadministration of butorphanol and a pure opioid agonist appears to depend on whether somatic pain versus visceral pain is present. These types of studies have not been performed to date in common pet species.

Nomenclature

Commonly used terms to describe drug interactions are addition, antagonism, synergism, and potentiation.

In purely pharmacological terms that have underlying theoretical implications, *addition* refers to simple additivity of fractional doses of two or more drugs, the fraction being expressed relative to the dose of each drug required to produce the same magnitude of response; that is, response to X amount of drug A = response to Y amount of drug B = response to $1/2X_A + 1/2Y_B$, $1/4X_A + 3/4Y_B$, and so on. Additivity is strong support for the assumption that drug A and drug B act via the same mechanism (e.g., on the same receptors). Confirmatory data are provided by in vitro receptor-binding assays. Minimum alveolar concentration (MAC) fractions for inhalational anesthetics are additive.

Synergism refers to the situation where the response to fractional doses as described previously is greater than the response to the sum of the fractional doses (e.g., $1/2X_A + 1/2Y_B$ produces more than the response to X_A or Y_B).

Potentiation refers to the enhancement of action of one drug by a second drug that has no detectable action of its own.

Antagonism refers to the opposing action of one drug toward another. Antagonism may be competitive or noncompetitive. In competitive antagonism, the agonist and antagonist compete for the same receptor site. Noncompetitive antagonism occurs when the agonist and antagonist act via different receptors.

Experimental approaches to determine additivity etc. have included dose-response analysis (Fig. 16.1) and isobolographic analysis (Fig. 16.2).

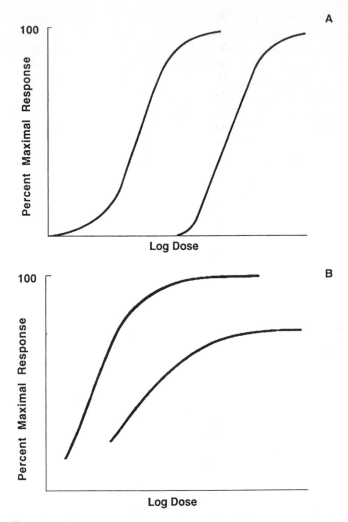

Fig. 16.1. Dose-response curve illustrating competitive antagonism **(A)** and noncompetitive antagonism **(B)**. In **A**, the dose-response curve is shifted to the right in the presence of an antagonist, but the shape of the curve is not changed. In **B**, the dose-response curve is shifted to the right in the presence of an antagonist, and the maximal response to the agonist is reduced.

Anesthetic Drug Interactions

The way anesthetic drugs are usually used raises special considerations with regard to drug interactions. For example, (a) drugs that act rapidly are usually used; (b) responses to administered drugs are measured, often very precisely; (c) drug antagonism is often relied upon; and (d) doses or concentrations of drugs are usually titrated to effect. Minor increases or decreases in responses are usually of little consequence and are dealt with routinely.

Commonly Used Anesthetic Drug Interactions

Two or more different kinds of injectable neuroactive agents are frequently used to induce anesthesia with the goal of achieving the highest quality of anesthesia with minimal side effects. The agents frequently have complementary effects on the brain, but

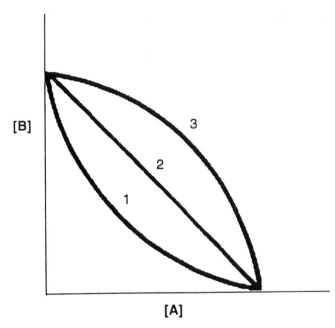

Fig. 16.2. Isobolograms for the response to mixtures of drugs. The sets of concentrations of drugs A and B, which as mixture produce an effect (e.g., 50% of a maximal response), are plotted. Strict additivity, which means [A] + [B] = a constant, results in a curve of slope −1 (2). If the curve is concave (3), some antagonism is present; if the curve is convex (1), synergism is present.

one agent may also antagonize an undesirable effect of the other. An example of such a combination is tiletamine and zolazepam (Telazol [tiletamine hydrochloride 50 mg/mL and zolazepam hydrochloride 50 mg/mL], an arylcycloalkylamine and a benzodiazepine).

Tiletamine produces sedation, immobility, amnesia, and marked analgesia, but may also produce muscle rigidity and grand mal seizures. Zolazepam produces sedation, reduces anxiety, and prevents muscle rigidity and seizures. Another arylcycloalkylamine-benzodiazepine combination commonly used is ketamine with either midazolam or diazepam. Ketamine is also frequently used in combination with xylazine, a potent sedative with central muscle relaxant and analgesic properties.

Acepromazine is often used as a preanesthetic agent. In addition to calming patients, acepromazine reduces the dose of anesthetic required to produce anesthesia and reduces the sensitivity of the myocardium to catecholamines, thereby reducing the risk of ventricular arrhythmias. On the other hand, acepromazine possesses α_1-adrenergic blocking activity such that the cardiovascular depressant effects of general anesthetics may interact to produce further vasodilation and hypotension.

Volatile anesthetics may potentiate cardiovascular depression in patients. Because nitrous oxide produces relatively less cardiovascular depression than does an equivalent dose of a volatile agent (it may even stimulate), at any given depth of anesthesia, the amount of cardiovascular depression is less with nitrous oxide plus a volatile agent than with the volatile agent alone at the same depth of anesthesia achieved.

To manage pain associated with surgical procedures better, it is becoming increasingly common to combine the use of regionally administered analgesics and light general anesthesia. An example of such an approach is to administer a local anesthetic alone or in combination with an opioid or an α_2-adrenergic agonist into the epidural space before or during general anesthesia. Benefits sought with this approach are reduction in the amount of general anesthetic required and the provision of preemptive analgesia. Reducing the amount of general anesthetic required reduces the magnitude of systemic side effects of the general anesthetic.

References

1. Papich MG. Incompatible critical care drug combinations. In: Bonagura JD, ed. Current Veterinary Therapy XII, 1995:194–198.
2. Trissel LA. Handbook on Injectable Drugs, 11th ed. Bethesda, MD: American Society of Health-System Pharmacists, 2001.
3. US Pharmacopeia. USP-DI, vol 1: Drug Information for the Health Care Professional. Rockville, MD: US Pharmacopeia, 2004.
4. Bersenas AME, Mathews KA, Allen DG, Conlon PD. Effects of ranitidine, famotidine, pantoprazole, and omeprazole on intragastric pH in dogs. Am J Vet Res 66:425–431, 2005.
5. Lin JH. Drug-drug interaction mediated by inhibition and induction of P-glycoprotein. Adv Drug Deliv Rev 55:53–81, 2003.
6. Mealey KL. Therapeutic implications of the MDR-1 gene. Vet Pharmacol Ther 27:257–264, 2004.
7. Lechardeur D, Phung-Ba V, Wils P, Scherman D. Detection of the multidrug resistance of P-glycoprotein in healthy tissues: The example of the blood-brain barrier. Ann Biol Clin (Paris) 54:31–36, 1996.
8. Preiss R. P-glycoprotein and related transporters. Int J Clin Pharmacol Ther 36:3–8, 1998.
9. Chauret N, Gauthier A, Martin J, Nicoll-Griffith DA. In vitro comparison of cytochrome P450-mediated metabolic activities in human, dog, cat, and horse. Drug Metab Dispos 25:1130–1136, 1997.
10. Toutain PL, Bousquet-Melou A. Free drug fraction vs free drug concentration: A matter of frequent confusion. J Vet Pharmacol Ther 25:460–463, 2002.
11. Benet LZ, Hoener B. Changes in plasma protein binding have little clinical relevance. Clin Pharmacol Ther 71:115–121, 2002.
12. Milgram NW, Ivy GO, Murphy MP, et al. Effects of chronic oral administration of L-deprenyl in the dog. Pharmacol Biochem Behav 51:421–428, 1995.
13. Head E, Milgram NW. Changes in spontaneous behavior in the dog following oral administration of L-deprenyl. Pharmacol Biochem Behav 43:749–757, 1992.
14. Mahmood I. Clinical pharmacokinetics and pharmacodynamics of selegiline. Clin Pharmacokinet 33:91–102, 1997.
15. Wolfe MM, Lichtenstein DR, Singh G. Gastrointestinal toxicity of nonsteroidal antiinflammatory drugs. N Engl J Med 340:1888–1899, 1999.
16. Mukherjee D, Nissen SE, Topol EJ. Risk of cardiovascular events associated with selective COX-2 inhibitors. J Am Med Assoc 286:954–959, 2001.
17. Topol EJ. Failing the public health: Rofecoxib, Merck and the FDA. N Engl J Med 351:1707–1709, 2004.
18. Wilson TW. Renal prostaglandin synthesis and angiotensin-converting enzyme inhibition. J Cardiovasc Pharmacol 19(Suppl 6):S39–S44, 1992.
19. Nawarskas JJ, Spinler SA. Does aspirin interfere with the therapeutic efficacy of angiotensin-converting enzyme inhibitors in hyperten-

sion or congestive heart failure? Pharmacotherapy 18:1041–1052, 1998.

20. Guazzi MD, Campodonico J, Celeste F, et al. Antihypertensive efficacy of angiotensin converting enzyme inhibition and aspirin counteraction. Clin Pharmacol Ther 63:79–86, 1998.

21. Verbeeck RK. Pathophysiologic factors affecting the pharmacokinetics of nonsteroidal anti-inflammatory drugs. J Rheumatol 15(Suppl 17):44–57, 1988.

22. Christ W, Lehnert T, Ulbrich B. Specific toxicologic aspects of the quinolones. Rev Infect Dis 10(Suppl 1):S141–S146, 1988.

23. Mathews KA, Doherty T, Dyson DH, Wilcock B, Valliant A. Nephrotoxicity in dogs associated with methoxyflurane anesthesia and flunixin meglumine analgesia. Can Vet J 31:766–771, 1990.

24. Brown SA. Renal effects of nonsteroidal anti-inflammatory drugs. In: Kirk RW, ed. Current Veterinary Therapy X. Philadelphia: WB Saunders, 1989:1158–1161.

25. Mathews KA. Nonsteroidal anti-inflammatory analgesics in pain management in dogs and cats. Can Vet J 37:539–545, 1996.

26. Rossat J, Maillard M, Nussberger JU, Brunner HR, Burnier M. Renal effects of selective cyclooxygenase-2 inhibition in normotensive salt-depleted subjects. Clin Pharmacol Ther 66:76–84, 1999.

27. Lobetti RG, Joubert KE. Effect of administration of nonsteroidal anti-inflammatory drugs before surgery on renal function in clinically normal dogs. Am J Vet Res 61:1501–1506, 2000.

28. Ko JCH, Miyabiyashi T, Mandsager RE, Heaton-Jones TG, Mauragis DF. Renal effects of carprofen administered to healthy dogs anesthetized with propofol and isoflurane. Am J Vet Med Assoc 217:346–349, 2000.

29. Boström IM, Nyman GC, Lord PF, Haggstrom J, Jones BE, Bohlin HP. Effects of carprofen on renal function and results of serum biochemical and hematologic analyses in anesthetized dogs that had low blood pressure during anesthesia. Am J Vet Res 63:712–721, 2002.

30. Fusellier M, Desfontis JC, Madec S, et al. Effect of tepoxalin on renal function in healthy dogs receiving an angiotensin-converting enzyme inhibitor. J Vet Pharmacol Ther 28:581–586, 2005.

31. Wilson JE, Chandrasekharan NV, Westover KD, Eager KB, Simmons DL. Determination of expression of cyclooxygenase-1 and -2 isozymes in canine tissues and their differential sensitivity to nonsteroidal anti-inflammatory drugs. Am J Vet Res 65:810–818, 2004.

32. Boston SE, Moens NMM, Kruth SA, Southorn EP. Endoscopic evaluation of the gastrointestinal mucosa to determine the safety of short-term concurrent administration of meloxicam and dexamethasone in healthy dogs. Am J Vet Res 63:1369–1375, 2003.

33. Dow SW, Rosychuk RA, McChesney AE, Curtis CR. Effects of flunixin and flunixin plus prednisone on the gastrointestinal tract of dogs. Am J Vet Res 51:1131–1138, 1990.

34. Vonderhaar MA, Salisbury SK. Gastroduodenal ulceration associated with flunixin meglumine administration in three dogs. J Am Vet Med Assoc 203:92–95, 1993.

35. Steffey EP, Baggot JD, Eisele JH, et al. Morphine-isoflurane interaction in dogs, swine, and Rhesus monkeys. J Vet Pharmacol Ther 17:202–210, 1994.

36. Haskins SC. Postoperative analgesia. Vet Clin N Am Small Anim Pract 22:353–356, 1992.

37. Sawyer DC, Rech RH, Stockdale AD, et al. Comparative effects of temazepam and diazepam on isoflurane MAC and oxymorphone analgesia in dogs. Vet Surg 19:314–321, 1990.

38. Lemke KA, Tranquilli WJ, Thurmon JC, Benson GJ, Olson WA. Ability of flumazenil, butorphanol, and naloxone to reverse the anesthetic effects of oxymorphone-diazepam in dogs. J Am Vet Med Assoc 209:776–779, 1996.

39. Pibarot P, Dupuis J, Grisneaux E, et al. Comparison of ketoprofen, oxymorphone hydrochloride, and butorphanol in the treatment of postoperative pain in dogs. J Am Vet Med Assoc 211:438–444, 1997.

40. Mathews KA, Paley DM, Foster RA, Valliant AE, Young SS. A comparison of ketorolac with flunixin, butorphanol, and oxymorphone in controlling postoperative pain in dogs. Can Vet J 37:557–567, 1996.

41. Briggs SL, Sneed K, Sawyer DC. Antinociceptive effects of oxymorphone-butorphanol-acepromazine combination in cats. Vet Surg 27:466–472, 1998.

42. Sawyer DC, Briggs S, Paul K. Antinociceptive effect of butorphanol-oxymorphone combination in cats. In: Scientific Abstracts of the Proceedings of the Fifth International Congress of Veterinary Anesthesia, Guelph, Ontario, August 21–25, 1994:161.

Section IV
EQUIPMENT AND MONITORING

Chapter 17
Anesthetic Machines and Breathing Systems

Sandee M. Hartsfield

Introduction

The halogenated hydrocarbon anesthetics are liquids that must be vaporized for administration. These volatile drugs are potent and should be delivered with accuracy. Nitrous oxide (N_2O) is a gas anesthetic, normally used in high concentrations. It should be administered with enough oxygen to assure an adequate inspired concentration of oxygen. Using contemporary methods, anesthesia machines and breathing systems are required for administration of inhalant anesthetics. Standards for performance and safety of anesthesia machines designed for use in human patients have been published.[1-4] Newer veterinary anesthesia machines meet some of these standards, but are not required to comply fully with the American Society for Testing and Materials (ASTM) guidelines.

Anesthesia Machines

Anesthesia machines have certain basic components, and are compatible with various breathing systems. An anesthesia machine prepares a precise, but variable, gas mixture (oxygen and anesthetic) for delivery to a breathing system.[2] The breathing system supplies oxygen and anesthetic to patients, eliminates carbon dioxide from exhaled gases, and provides a means for controlled ventilation. Sources for medical gases (e.g., cylinders for oxygen and N_2O), a regulator and a flowmeter for each gas, and a vaporizer for each volatile anesthetic are fundamental to the operation of an anesthesia machine.[5]

Pressures of gases vary at different locations in an anesthesia machine,[2,3] and knowledge of these pressures facilitates the evaluation and safe operation of these machines. There are low-, intermediate-, and high-pressure areas. The high-pressure area accepts gases at cylinder pressure and reduces and regulates the pressure; this area includes gas cylinders, hanger yokes, yoke blocks, high-pressure hoses, pressure gauges, and regulators, and the pressure may be as high as 2200 pounds per square inch (psi). The intermediate-pressure area accepts gases from the central pipeline or from the regulators on the anesthesia machine and conducts them to the flush valve and flowmeters; this area includes pipeline inlets, power outlets for ventilators, conduits from pipeline inlets to flowmeters, and conduits from regulators to flowmeters, the flowmeter assembly, and the oxygen-flush apparatus. The pressure usually ranges from 37 to 50 psi, although it may be lower on newer anesthesia machines. The low-pressure area consists of the conduits and components between the flowmeter and the common gas outlet; this area includes vaporizers located outside the breathing system, piping from the flowmeters to the vaporizer, conduit from the vaporizer to the common gas outlet, and conduit from the common gas outlet to the breathing system, and the pressure is only slightly above am-

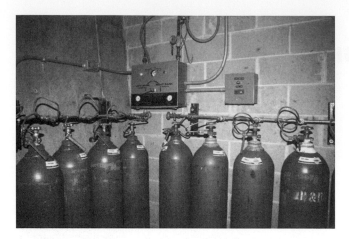

Fig. 17.1. Primary and reserve banks of large oxygen cylinders supplying the central medical gas pipeline system at a veterinary teaching hospital. The primary bank supplies oxygen to the pipeline system until the cylinders are depleted, at which time the system is automatically switched to the reserve bank.

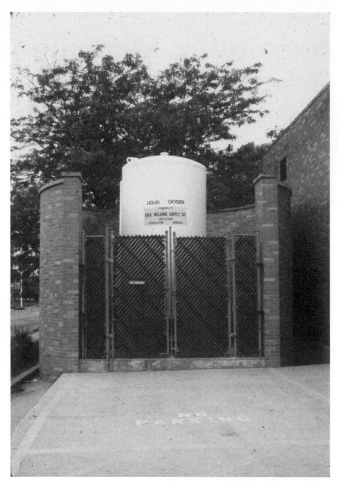

Fig. 17.2. An outside bulk container for liquid oxygen supplying the central medical gas pipeline system of a large hospital.

bient. Pressures in the breathing system itself vary, but usually range from 0 to 30 cm of water (cm H_2O) when used with normal, healthy patients.

Medical Gases

An anesthesia machine typically has two sources for each medical gas. First, small compressed-gas cylinders attach to the machine and the hanger yokes, and, second, the hospital's central gas supply enters the machine at pipeline inlets. Ideally, the hospital's pipeline should be the primary source of medical gases, and small cylinders should be reserved for emergencies or transport.[6] Generally, bulk sources of medical gases are more economic than small cylinders.

The pipeline source for N_2O originates from the bank of large (G or H) compressed-gas cylinders, and oxygen may be supplied similarly (Fig. 17.1). Alternately, the central source of oxygen may emanate from a bulk tank of liquid oxygen (Fig. 17.2) or possibly from an oxygen-concentrating system. The latter will not reliably deliver 100% oxygen. Pipeline systems (Fig. 17.3) convey gases from the central source to terminal units (station outlets) throughout the hospital. A noninterchangeable gas-specific connector at the station outlet accepts only its corresponding connector, which attaches to the pipeline inlet of an anesthetic machine through a flexible, high-pressure hose. The connector may be a threaded diameter index safety system (diss) or a proprietary (manufacturer specific) nonthreaded, noninterchangeable quick connector (Fig. 17.4).[3] The high-pressure hose connects to the anesthesia machine at a pipeline inlet, which is usually a diss male connector (Fig. 17.5).

Gases move to and from a cylinder through a brass valve (Fig. 17.6). The valve stem controls flow, and a safety relief device (e.g., a fusible plug with a low melting point) allows emergency escape of gas to prevent bursting of a cylinder during exposure to high temperatures.[2] The threaded outlets of the valve bodies on

large cylinders (G and H) are designed to prevent the accidental interchange of oxygen, N_2O, and other gases at regulators or manifolds. The valve bodies of small (E) cylinders of oxygen and N_2O attach directly to anesthesia machines at the hanger yokes, and they use the pin-index safety system (Fig. 17.7) to prevent interchange of oxygen and N_2O. Two pinholes and a port in the valve body correspond to two pins and a nipple on the hanger yoke. Spacing of the pins for each medical gas precludes the interchange of gases under ordinary conditions (Fig. 17.8).

Although the pin-index system is effective, the system has been defeated.[2] The pins can be removed (Fig. 17.9), bent, broken, or forced deeper into the yoke. The nipple can be stacked with enough washers to allow attachment of the wrong cylinder. Yoke blocks coupled to high-pressure hoses will accommodate alternate gas sources. Some of the older yoke blocks do not have pinholes, and some short blocks can be attached upside down (Fig. 17.9), allowing connection of the wrong gas. Older anesthesia machines should be inspected to assure the integrity of the pin-index system for oxygen and N_2O. Small cylinders should be aligned correctly to the hanger yoke to prevent the creation of a potential hazard. Directing the retaining screw into the safety re-

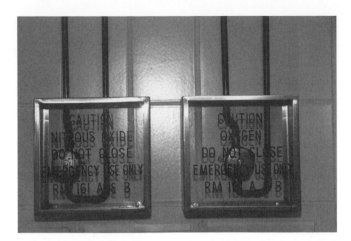

Fig. 17.3. A set of emergency shutoff valves for oxygen and nitrous oxide in a central pipeline system for medical gases in a veterinary teaching hospital. These valves should be placed strategically throughout the gas distribution system to control the flow of gases during emergencies or maintenance.

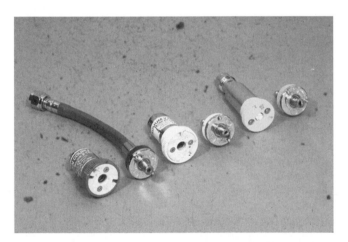

Fig. 17.4. A set of proprietary (Ohio or Ohmeda, Madison, WI) quick connects (quick couplers) for oxygen (male and female on the *left*), vacuum (male and female in the *center*), and air (male and female on the *right*). The female connectors are usually present at the site of use (station outlet) for attachment to the male counterparts from the anesthesia machine or other equipment via high-pressure flexible hose. Inadvertent interchange of the gases is prevented by variations in the spacing of corresponding components of the couplers.

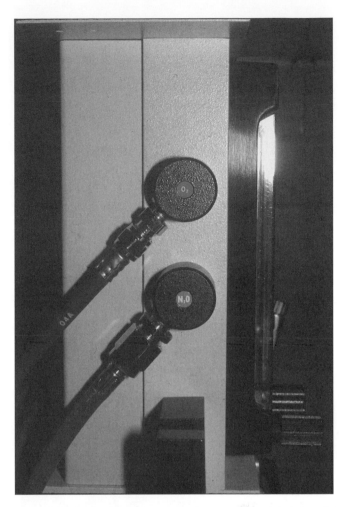

Fig. 17.5. Pipeline inlets for oxygen (*top* connector labeled as O_2) and nitrous oxide (*bottom* larger connector) on a Drager anesthesia machine (North American Drager, Telford, PA). The female diameter index safety system (diss) connectors from the high-pressure hoses couple to the male diss pipeline inlets on the anesthesia machine.

lief device instead of the conical depression has caused rapid decompression of a cylinder (Fig. 17.10).[7,8] If an anesthesia machine has multiple hanger yokes, each yoke should be fitted with a cylinder or a yoke plug (Fig. 17.11) when the machine is in operation.

An oxygen cylinder's service pressure is about 2200 psi. An E cylinder contains about 700 L of gaseous oxygen and an H cylinder about 7000 L (Table 17.1). The pressure is proportional to the contents, and an E cylinder with a pressure of 1100 psi contains about 350 L of oxygen. The pressure in a full N_2O cylinder is

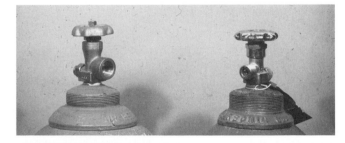

Fig. 17.6. Brass valves on large gas cylinders. The valve outlets on these two cylinders are designed to prevent an inadvertent connection to the wrong cylinder of gases. The valve on the *right* has external threads, whereas the one on the *left* has internal threads. The valve outlet for a large cylinder is distinguished by diameter, number of threads per inch, and type of threads (right hand or left hand and internal or external).

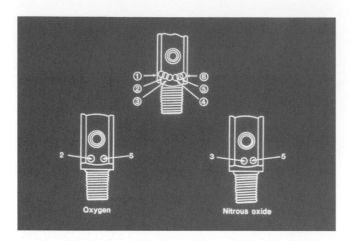

Fig. 17.7. Diagram of the pin-index safety system. The spacing between the valve outlet and the pinholes in the valve bodies for oxygen and nitrous oxide cylinders are illustrated. The pinholes and outlets correspond to the nipple and pins of hanger yokes on anesthesia machines and help to prevent the inadvertent incorrect use of medical gases. Note that pinholes 2 and 5 are used for oxygen, whereas pinholes 3 and 5 are used for nitrous oxide. From Hartsfield.[5]

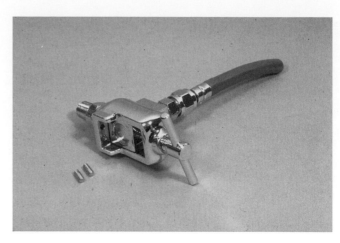

Fig. 17.9. An oxygen yoke showing a way in which the pin-index system for small gas cylinders can be defeated. The pins have been removed, and a short yoke block has been inserted upside down. Both will defeat the effectiveness of the pin-index system and allow connection to an inappropriate cylinder.

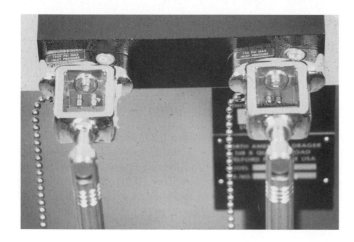

Fig. 17.8. Comparison of the yokes for small cylinders of oxygen (*left*) and nitrous oxide (*right*). The relationship of the pins and the nipple on each yoke show how the inadvertent interchange of oxygen and nitrous oxide cylinders is prevented. From Hartsfield.[5]

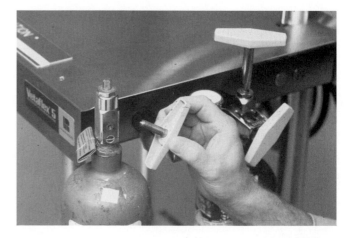

Fig. 17.10. The retaining screw of the yoke and a small (E) cylinder of oxygen next to a Vetaflex 5 veterinary anesthesia machine (Pitman-Moore, Washington Crossing, NJ). The retaining screw has been removed from the yoke to illustrate the pointed shape, which is intended to correspond to the conical depression of the cylinder valve and to secure the cylinder in the yoke. If the cylinder is positioned incorrectly in the yoke and the retaining screw is tightened into the fusible plug (the round, slotted device below the conical depression), the cylinder may decompress rapidly.

about 750 psi at normal room temperature, with N_2O in both liquid and gaseous phases. The vapor pressure of N_2O varies with temperature and determines the pressure in the cylinder. In a full cylinder, 95% of the volume is liquid,[9] and an E cylinder contains about 1600 L (Table 17.1). As liquid N_2O vaporizes, the cylinder cools, and frosting may occur. The contents of an N_2O cylinder is not directly proportional to the pressure. As pressure starts to decrease after all liquid N_2O has vaporized, about 25% of the original gas content remains. The remaining gas will then be depleted based on rate of flow.[10] Although the amount of N_2O is not directly related to pressure, the content of any cylinder can be de-

termined by weight regardless of the state of the material in the cylinder.[3]

In the United States, the Department of Transportation controls the construction and testing of gas cylinders. The service pressure, defined as the maximum filling pressure at 70°F (22°C),[2] is typically 1900 to 2200 psi for oxygen. Cylinders are designated alphabetically, size A being the smallest. Sizes E, G,

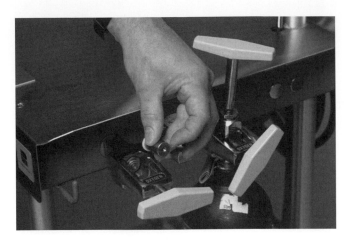

Fig. 17.11. Preparation for inserting a yoke plug into a yoke intended for a small (E) cylinder prior to use of the anesthesia machine. Since only one cylinder is present, the open yoke should be blocked with a yoke plug to prevent gas leaks, even if a check valve is present immediately upstream from the cylinder.

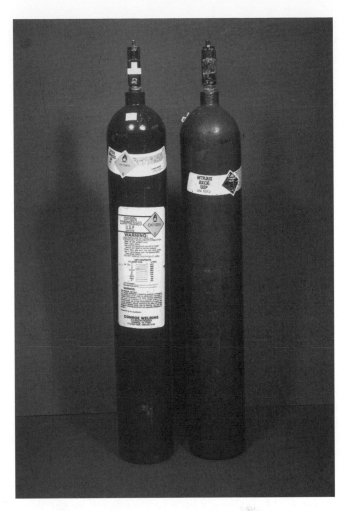

Fig. 17.12. Small (E) cylinders of oxygen and nitrous oxide, with labels and warnings. The diamond-shaped figure on each cylinder's label indicates the hazard class of the contents (yellow for oxygen, an oxidizer; and green for nitrous oxide, a nonflammable gas).

and H are common for medical oxygen and N_2O (Table 17.1). Permanent markings near the top of the cylinder indicate the Department of Transportation specification number, the type of material used in construction (e.g., steel or aluminum), service pressure in pounds per square inch, serial number, identification of the manufacturer, and testing dates. A five-point star after the last testing date qualifies the cylinder to be retested after 10 years.[3]

A color-coded label (green for oxygen and blue for N_2O) on the wall of the cylinder indicates the gas contents, warns of potential hazards (e.g., oxidizing agent), and names the manufacturer or distributor (Fig. 17.12). A single word appears on the label: *Danger* means an immediate threat to health or property if gas is released, *warning* indicates a less than immediate threat, and *caution* means no immediate hazard to health or property. A diamond-shaped area on the label indicates the hazard class of

Table 17.1. Characteristics of medical gas cylinders[3]

Size	Gas	Gas Symbol	Color Code (U.S.)	Capacity and Pressure (at 70°F)	Empty Cylinder Weight (pounds)
E	Oxygen	O_2	Green	660 L 1900 psi	14
E	Nitrous oxide	N_2O	Blue	1590 L 745 psi	14
G	Nitrous oxide	N_2O	Blue	13,800 L 745 psi	97
H	Oxygen	O_2	Green	6900 L 2200 psi	119
H	Nitrous oxide	N_2O	Blue	15,800 L 745 psi	119

psi, pounds per square inch.

the gas by words (oxidizer, nonflammable, or flammable) and color code (yellow, green, and red, respectively).[3] Distributors often attach a color-coded tag to the valve body, identifying a cylinder's contents. Tags incorporate sequential perforated tabs imprinted with the terms *full*, *in use*, and *empty* to track the use of the cylinder.

Extensive descriptions of the appropriate handling, storage, and use of compressed gas cylinders have been published.[2–4,8,11] Briefly, cylinders should not be stored near flammable materials and should be properly secured at all times, even during transport. Cylinders should be stored in a cool, dry, clean, well-ventilated room that is constructed of fire-resistant materials.[3] Before using a cylinder, the contents should be clearly identified from the label. The valve port should be pointed away from the operator, opened briefly to clear possible debris, and then closed before connection to a hanger yoke, regulator, or manifold. A sealing washer should be placed between a small cylinder valve and the hanger yoke. The valve should be opened slowly to pressurize the regulator and then opened fully.[2,3] Defective cylinders should not be used.

Pressure Gauges

Each compressed gas supplied to an anesthesia machine should have a corresponding pressure gauge (Fig. 17.13)[1–3] that is attached to the regulators for large cylinders and to manifolds for banks of cylinders. The gauge indicates pressure on the cylinder side of the regulator. Gauges are identified by the gas's chemical symbol or name and are usually color coded. The scale is graduated to indicate the units of measure in kilopascals (kPa) and pounds per square inch.[1] Bourdon tube-type gauges are typical for anesthesia machines.[12] Earlier standards for anesthesia machines required that the gauge's full-scale reading should be at least one-third greater than the maximum cylinder pressure, and that, on a given anesthesia machine, all gauges should displace a similar arc from the lowest to highest readings.[2] Pressure gauges are also incorporated into pipeline distribution systems at various locations. In addition, pressure gauges may be used on anesthesia machines to report pipeline pressure.[1,3] Pressure gauges do not accurately report the quantitative contents of a cylinder containing liquid gas.[1]

Regulators

An anesthesia machine should have a regulator for each medical gas supplied to the machine (Fig. 17.14).[1] The pressure in a gas cylinder varies with its content and temperature, and the pressure in a full cylinder is relatively high (e.g., 2000 psi in an oxygen cylinder). A regulator reduces the high and variable storage pressure to a lower and more constant pressure that is appropriate for the anesthesia machine.[6] By reducing and controlling pressure as gas exits a cylinder, a regulator maintains constant flow to the flowmeter, even though the pressure in the cylinder decreases as the contents are depleted.

Although regulators on newer anesthesia machines designed for human patients may be quite sophisticated, a simple regulator has a high-pressure chamber separated by a valve port from a low-pressure chamber (Fig. 17.15).[12] Movement of a flexible di-

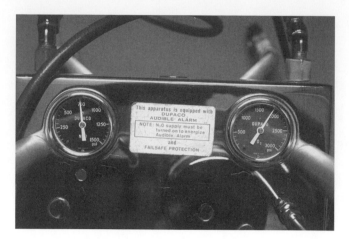

Fig. 17.13. Pressure gauges for oxygen (1900 psi) and nitrous oxide (750 psi) on a veterinary anesthesia machine.

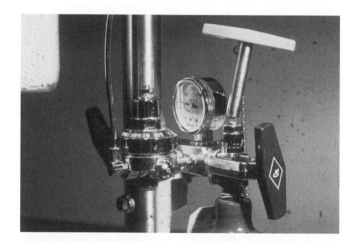

Fig. 17.14. Pressure regulator on a Pitman-Moore 970 veterinary anesthesia machine (Pitman-Moore, Washington Crossing, NJ). The triangular shaped regulator for oxygen is shown in-line between the yoke for the oxygen cylinder and the small-diameter oxygen line to the flowmeter. The pressure gauge indicates the pressure in the cylinder, and the pressure downstream from the regulator is reduced to 50 psi by the regulator.

aphragm opens or closes the valve, regulating a variable opening, and consequently the pressure in the low-pressure chamber. Increasing pressure on the low-pressure side tends to close the valve. The amount of pressure required to close the valve depends on a spring opposite the diaphragm. The exact construction varies among regulators, but the function is consistent. Regulators are designed for safety relief (at two to four times the pressure in the low-pressure chamber) in order to protect equipment and personnel.[3,12]

Regulators produce a safe operating pressure, prevent flowmeter fluctuations as cylinders empty, and decrease the sensitivity of the flowmeter indicator to slight movements of the control knob. The ASTM standard requires that regulators on anesthesia ma-

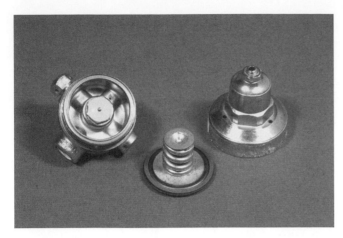

Fig. 17.15. A simple pressure regulator for oxygen that has been separated into its component parts. Shown are the body of the regulator with the entry port for high-pressure gas at 7 o'clock (*left*), the diaphragm and spring (*center*), and the cover (*right*) with holes for pressure relief through the diaphragm and the adjusting screw.

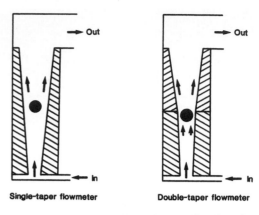

Fig. 17.16. Flowmeter diagram illustrating gas flow from bottom to top through flowmeters with single and double tapers. As the indicator (*black dot*) rises, flow increases because orifice size increases. The double taper tube allows increased accuracy at the lower end of the tube while accurately metering higher flow rates at the top. From Hartsfield.[5]

chines be set so that the pipeline gases are used preferentially.[1] Therefore, regulators may be set at about 45 psi (if a power outlet is present for a ventilator) or at 37 to 42 psi (without a power outlet), since pipeline pressure is usually 50 psi. Older anesthesia machines that have regulators set at 50 psi and open E cylinders located on the machine can allow E cylinder gas flow rather than pipeline gas flow when a pipeline check valve is not present, possibly depleting gases from the cylinder that should be saved for emergency situations (e.g., pipeline failure). Contemporary anesthesia machines designed for human patients have additional regulators (second stage) that deliver gases to the flowmeters at much lower pressures (e.g., 12 to 16 psi) to increase the constancy of the flowmeter.[3,6]

Flowmeters

Flowmeters for medical gases are positioned downstream from the regulators for each corresponding gas, and the portion of the flowmeter that is downstream from the flow-control valve is part of the low-pressure system of an anesthesia machine. A flowmeter measures and indicates the rate of flow of gas,[3] and enables precise control of oxygen or N_2O delivery to an out-of-system vaporizer and to the common gas outlet.

Gas moves through the flow-control valve to enter the bottom of the glass tube (i.e., Thorpe tube) of the flowmeter assembly. The gas then courses around a movable indicator (float) in the annular space between the indicator and the wall of the tube, and exits at the top of the tube (Fig. 17.16). The tube is larger at the top than at the bottom, and a greater volume of gas moves around the indicator as it rises.[2] The scale associated with the tube indicates rate of gas flow in milliliters per minute (mL/min) or in liters per minute (L/min). Some flowmeters, especially those on older anesthesia machines, have double tapers (Fig. 17.16). A slight taper in the lower part of the tube promotes accuracy at low flows (mL/min), and a greater taper at the top allows higher flow

rates (L/min). The current machine standard requires that the scale be on the glass tube itself or be located to the right of the tube (viewed from the front of the anesthesia machine).[1] The scale may be on the left in older anesthesia machines, and the operator should assure the proper adjustment of flowmeter control knobs when older equipment is used.[3]

Flowmeters are calibrated at 760 mm Hg and 20°C, and accuracy may change under other conditions.[3] Generally, the effects of temperature on flowmeter function are minimal, but changes in barometric pressure may be significant, producing a higher flow than indicated at lower barometric pressure (altitude) and a lower flow at high pressure (i.e., in a hyperbaric chamber).[3] Since a flowmeter (tube, indicator, and scale) is calibrated as a unit, parts from different flowmeters should not be interchanged. If a flowmeter fails, the glass tube, indicator, and scale should be replaced as a unit. The lowest mark on the scale is the first accurate setting, and extrapolation to lower flow rates is unreliable.[2] A flowmeter's indicator should be read at the top (Fig. 17.17), except for a ball-type float, which is read at the center (Fig. 17.18). The point of reference for reading the indicator should be shown on the flowmeter assembly.[1] Flowmeters should be used in the position on the machine as originally designed (e.g., vertical on newer machines or slanted in some older machines).

The flow-control knob for oxygen on contemporary anesthesia machines should be as large or larger than other flow-control knobs, it should have a fluted profile (Figs. 17.17 and 17.18) as dictated by the ASTM standard, and it should project beyond the control knobs for other gases.[1] This enables the operator to "feel" which gas is being adjusted ("touch coded").[2] A control knob is labeled with the gas symbol and is color coded (Figs. 17.17 and 17.18). Good flow controls have fine threads for accuracy and stops to prevent over tightening and damage to flow-control valves.

The size of the flowmeter's indicator in relation to the scale influences accuracy. Float indicators may be longer than 1 cm, and

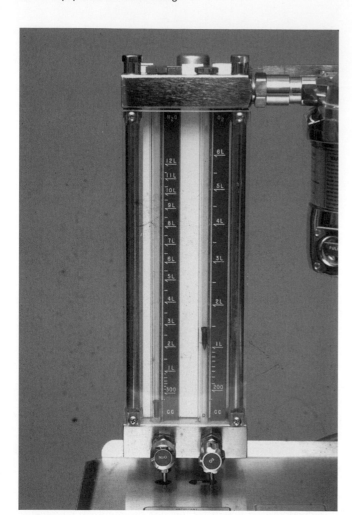

Fig. 17.17. Oxygen and nitrous oxide flowmeters on a Vetaflex 5 veterinary anesthesia machine (Pitman-Moore, Washington Crossing, NJ). The oxygen flowmeter is located to the right in the cluster, and the indicator should be read at its top (1.5 L/min). The indicator is relatively long compared with the calibrations on the scale. Erroneously reading the bottom of the indicator would result in a flow of oxygen that was 600 mL/min lower that intended. The O_2 flow-control knob is fluted and color coded.

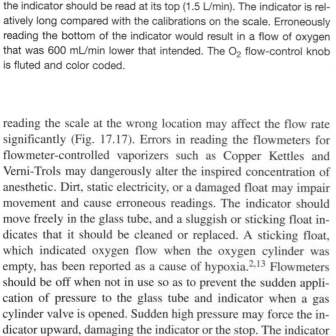

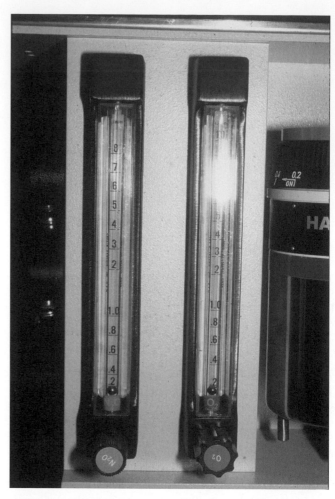

Fig. 17.18. Flowmeters for oxygen and nitrous oxide on a Drager anesthesia machine (North American Drager, Telford, PA). The oxygen flowmeter is located to the right of the nitrous oxide flowmeter, and the ball-type indicator should be read in the center (1 L/min). The flow-control knob for oxygen is fluted and color coded and is larger than the flowmeter for nitrous oxide.

reading the scale at the wrong location may affect the flow rate significantly (Fig. 17.17). Errors in reading the flowmeters for flowmeter-controlled vaporizers such as Copper Kettles and Verni-Trols may dangerously alter the inspired concentration of anesthetic. Dirt, static electricity, or a damaged float may impair movement and cause erroneous readings. The indicator should move freely in the glass tube, and a sluggish or sticking float indicates that it should be cleaned or replaced. A sticking float, which indicated oxygen flow when the oxygen cylinder was empty, has been reported as a cause of hypoxia.[2,13] Flowmeters should be off when not in use so as to prevent the sudden application of pressure to the glass tube and indicator when a gas cylinder valve is opened. Sudden high pressure may force the indicator upward, damaging the indicator or the stop. The indicator may jam at the top of the tube, where it may go unnoticed.[2]

The standard for modern anesthesia machines requires the presence of only one flow-adjustment control for each gas delivered to the common gas outlet.[1] Ideally, when there are two flowmeters for one gas, they should be connected in series and controlled by a single flow-control knob.[3] Some veterinary anesthesia machines (Fig. 17.19) and older machines for human and veterinary patients may have multiple flow controls for multiple flowmeters with different scales in a parallel arrangement, and the operator should assure proper settings with both control knobs. Similarly, the sequence of flowmeters is important with multiple gases on a single anesthesia machine. The machine standard requires that oxygen be delivered downstream of other gases when all gases use a common manifold.[1] If oxygen enters the manifold upstream from the other gases, the possibility exists for delivering hypoxic mixtures, which is a complication that has

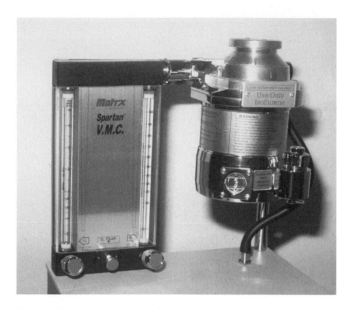

Fig. 17.19. Double oxygen flowmeters on a Matrx Spartan VMC veterinary anesthesia machine (Matrx, Orchard Park, NY). One flowmeter (*left*) is graduated from 0 to 1000 mL/min, whereas the other is graduated from 0.2 to 4.0 L/min. The intent is to increase accuracy at lower flow rates. Two flow-control knobs in parallel offer an opportunity for setting an incorrect flow of oxygen. With two flowmeters in parallel, the total flow is the sum of the flow rates set from each flowmeter.

been reported several times.[2] The U.S. and Canadian standard locates the oxygen flowmeter to the right in a cluster of flowmeters as viewed from the front of the anesthesia machine. If a specific flowmeter for a vaporizer is required, it should be to the right of the cluster, at least 10 cm from the oxygen flowmeter,[2] although flowmeter-controlled vaporizers are no longer covered in the ASTM standard.[1] For flowmeter-controlled vaporizers, this arrangement standardizes the location of control knobs and decreases the likelihood of adjusting the incorrect flowmeter. Standardization of location of the flowmeters for oxygen delivery and for vaporizers along with requiring touch-coded flow-control knobs for oxygen flowmeters are intended to reduce errors in oxygen flow rates. Locating the oxygen flowmeter to the right in a cluster of flowmeters is a North American standard, and the location may vary on older machines and in machines manufactured in other countries.[3] Other arrangements of flowmeters may exist in older anesthesia machines (e.g., oxygen flowmeter located to the left, to the right, or in the center in a cluster). The danger of delivering hypoxic mixtures by adjusting the wrong control knob when using both N_2O and oxygen must be guarded against.

The arrangement of flowmeters on older models of Drager anesthesia machines allowed delivery of hypoxic mixtures if both oxygen and N_2O were used and a leak developed at the base of the oxygen flowmeter (Fig. 17.20). This malfunction caused the death of a horse.[14] Similarly, cyanosis and light anesthesia were produced shortly after intubation and attachment of a dog

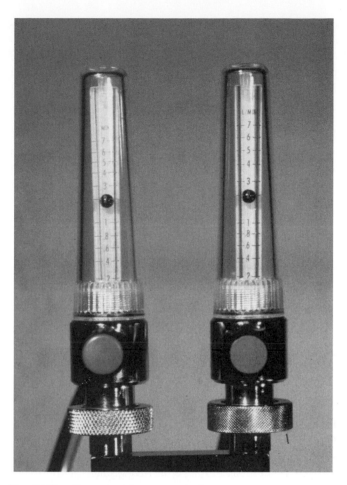

Fig. 17.20. Flowmeters for oxygen (*left*) and nitrous oxide (*right*) on a Drager Narkovet Stand Model anesthesia machine (North American Drager, Telford, PA) for small animals. A leak at the seal created by the nut below the flowmeter could result in delivery of a low or hypoxic concentration of oxygen to the breathing system.

to an anesthesia machine;[15] evaluation of the oxygen flowmeter revealed a leak at its base caused by a faulty seal with a folded washer. Because of this flowmeter's design, the indicator showed a correctly adjusted flow rate for oxygen, although total gas flow to the vaporizer and breathing system was very low. Leaks associated with flowmeters can occur at several locations, including cracks in the glass tube, as well as problems with O-rings and gaskets.[6] Leaks in the flowmeter should be detected by leak tests performed on the low-pressure area of an anesthesia machine.[16]

Flowmeters should be adjusted to assure an adequate total volume and an appropriate concentration of each medical gas. Flow rates should meet or exceed the patient's oxygen consumption and deliver an adequate inspired-oxygen concentration (usually a fraction of inspired oxygen [F_IO_2] ≥ 0.3). Delivery of an appropriate concentration of oxygen, as well as an adequate quantity of oxygen, is essential for saturating hemoglobin and for supplying the patient's metabolic needs. Accuracy becomes especially important with the administration of N_2O and with closed and low-flow breathing systems. The accuracy of flowmeters significantly decreases with flows lower than 1 L/min.[2] With low-flow systems, scrutiny of F_IO_2 becomes important; continuous monitoring of oxygen concentration on the inspiratory limb of the breathing system has been recommended. Indeed, to meet the ASTM standard, an oxygen analyzer is a required component of the anesthesia machine.[1,6]

Safety Devices for Oxygen Pressure and Flow

Anesthesia machines may be designed to alert the operator to a dangerously low pressure of oxygen flow.[3,4] When the oxygen pressure reaches a certain value, the machine may alert the user with an alarm, or the machine may be engineered to cut off the supply of all other gases (e.g., N_2O) to prevent the delivery of hypoxic mixtures. In addition, some anesthesia machines incorporate proportioning devices to assure that oxygen is flowing at some preset minimum portion of the total fresh gas flow. Dupaco anesthesia machines were once popular in veterinary anesthesia and incorporated an audible alarm if the pressure of oxygen became dangerously low. The Metomatic veterinary anesthesia machine reduces the flow of other gases (i.e., flow through the Verni-Trol) if oxygen flow is reduced. These safety mechanisms may malfunction, and continuously monitoring gases on the inspiratory limb of the breathing system is a more reliable way to assure the delivery of an adequate concentration of oxygen.

Flush Valves

Oxygen is supplied at approximately 50 psi to the flush valve of an anesthesia machine. The flush valve delivers a high, but unmetered, flow (35 to 75 L/min is the ASTM standard)[1] of oxygen to the common gas outlet or directly to the breathing system in some simple veterinary machines (e.g., Matrx small animal anesthesia machine). The contemporary machine standard does not allow piping of oxygen from the flush valve through the vaporizer. However, older anesthesia machines, especially those with precision vaporizers added after the machine was manufactured, may increase oxygen flow through the vaporizer, with the potential for increased output of anesthetic.[6]

At a flow rate of 50 L/min, oxygen from the flush valve can quickly fill the breathing system. In general, pediatric breathing systems (i.e., pediatric circles, Mapleson systems, or valved nonrebreathing systems) should not be filled via the flush valve because of the danger of overpressurizing a patient's respiratory system. Current machine standards require that the actuating device for the flush valve be recessed to prevent inadvertent activation and delivery of a high volume of gas to the breathing system (Fig. 17.21).[1] Other problems involving the flush valve include leaks in the flush-valve assembly and sticking of the flush valve in the on position.[3] A leak at the flush valve reportedly resulted in loss of anesthetic and oxygen at flow rates of less than 1 L/min, making it impossible to maintain surgical anesthesia with the typical fresh gas flow rates used with a semiclosed circle breathing system.[17]

Vaporizers

Except for N_2O, modern inhalant anesthetics are delivered with vaporizers. Concentration-calibrated, variable-bypass vaporizers,

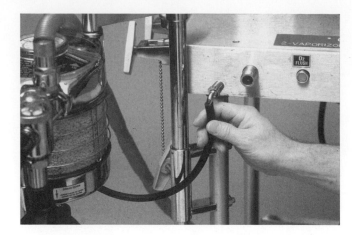

Fig. 17.21. Flush valve and common gas outlet on a veterinary anesthesia machine. The flush valve (labeled on the machine) is protected from inadvertent activation by a circular stainless-steel guard. The common gas outlet (open hole) received a connector to link the anesthesia machine through a rubber hose to the fresh gas inlet of the breathing system.

which are temperature, flow, and back-pressure compensated, are standard in human anesthesia and are recommended for delivery of volatile inhalant anesthetics to veterinary patients. However, nonprecision, uncompensated vaporizers (e.g., Stephens vaporizer) have also been marketed to veterinarians as a part of a complete anesthesia machine. In addition, an older vaporizer designed for less volatile inhalant anesthetics (Ohio #8 glass bottle), when modified by removal of the wick, has been evaluated for the delivery of halothane or isoflurane to veterinary patients.[18,19] Administering highly volatile, highly potent inhalant anesthetics with nonprecision, uncompensated vaporizers is associated with a high degree of risk unless instrumental monitoring (e.g., of inspired or expired anesthetic concentration) is available.

A vaporizer is designed to change a liquid anesthetic into its vapor and to add a specific amount of vapor to the gases being delivered to a patient.[2] Carrier gas, oxygen alone or with N_2O, passes through the vaporizer to acquire anesthetic vapor. Because the saturated vapor pressures of most inhalant anesthetics are significantly greater than the partial pressures required for clinical anesthesia (i.e., significantly greater than the minimum alveolar concentration [MAC]), a vaporizer should deliver a concentration that is close to the setting on the vaporizer control dial. Otherwise, the inspired concentration of anesthetic should be monitored. In general, the design of precision vaporizers allows dilution of a high concentration of anesthetic vapor from the vaporization chamber to a clinically usable and safe concentration.

Physics of Vaporizer Design and Function

Several principles of physics are involved in the function of a vaporizer for inhalant anesthetics.[2–4] Heat is required for vaporization of liquid anesthetics; the *latent heat of vaporization* is defined as the number of calories required to change 1 g of liquid into its vapor. This heat requirement causes liquid anesthetic to cool during vaporization. The vapor pressure of an anesthetic is the partial pressure of the aesthetic gas above the liquid at equilibrium, and vapor pressure varies directly with temperature. Thus, uncontrolled cooling limits a vaporizer's maximum output. A vaporizer made of a substance (e.g., copper) with a high *specific heat* (the quantity of heat required to raise the temperature of 1 g of the substance 1°C) supplies heat to the liquid anesthetic during vaporization, retarding the cooling process. If a vaporizer is constructed of a material with a high *thermal conductivity* (the rate at which heat flows through a substance), such as copper, heat flows from warmer ambient air into the vaporizer to impede cooling. Materials including copper and bronze are used in the construction of vaporizers because of favorable values of these metals for specific heat and thermal conductivity. More recently, stainless steel has been used in the construction of vaporizers.[4] The output of concentration-calibrated vaporizers is generally expressed as volume percent of anesthetic vapor in the gases exiting the vaporizer. This relative value changes with variation in barometric pressure.

Compensatory Mechanisms for Vaporizers

The conditions of use affect the performance of vaporizers and must be stated in the operation manual for a concentration-calibrated vaporizer to meet the ASTM standard.[1] The effects of changes in carrier-gas flow, temperature, ambient pressure, and back-pressure should be delineated. Vaporizers compensate in various ways for changes in flow, temperature, and pressure.[2–4]

Compensation for variations in temperature of the liquid anesthetic during vaporization can be accomplished by several mechanisms. As previously mentioned, copper and bronze materials with high specific heat and thermal conductivity values supply and conduct heat efficiently to the liquid anesthetic to promote a relatively constant temperature. This "heat sink" mechanism attenuates changes in temperature, producing a degree of thermostability. Bimetallic strip valves in Tec vaporizers, a gas-filled bellows linked to a valve in the bypass gas flow in Ohio calibrated vaporizers, and an expansion member (silicone cone) in Vapor/vaporizers that expand(s) and contract(s) with temperature changes, alter(s) carrier-gas flow through the vaporization chamber and controlling anesthetic output.[4] Manual adjustments in carrier-gas flow are required to compensate for temperature variations in measured-flow vaporizers (e.g., Verni-Trol vaporizer) and older Vapor vaporizers. Other vaporizers are electrically heated, and the mechanism for control of the temperature of the anesthetic is supplied heat (e.g., Verni-Trol vaporizer on the Ohio DM 5000 anesthesia machine). The Tec 6 vaporizer for desflurane is electrically heated and thermostatically controlled at 39°C.[16]

Differences in carrier-gas flow rates alter the output of uncompensated vaporizers. Modern flow-compensated vaporizers produce relatively accurate anesthetic concentrations over an approximate range of 250 mL/min to 15 L/min.[6] The *splitting ratio* (ratio of the bypass to the gas passing through the vaporization

chamber) determines the output of vapor,[4] and the resistance to flow through each of the two channels in the vaporizer allows the splitting ratio to be maintained at various rates of flow.[3] Below 250 mL/min and above 15 L/min, the output from most concentration-calibrated vaporizers is variable, and performance data outside that range may not be available. Output from older variable-bypass vaporizers (e.g., Fluotec Mark 2) may vary significantly from the setting on the control dial at flow rates less than 4 L/min. Measured-flow (flowmeter controlled) vaporizers (e.g., Copper Kettle) require adjustments in the flow of oxygen to the vaporization chamber when the total flow of gas is changed.

Vaporizer output may vary with the composition of the carrier gas; the output of anesthetic with oxygen as the carrier gas may differ from the output with a combination of oxygen and N_2O as the carrier gas.[2,4] The magnitude of effect is variable, depending on the specific vaporizer. With N_2O, newer vaporizers initially deliver concentrations that are less than the control-dial setting. With the Fluotec Mark 3, N_2O has little effect on output. However, N_2O as the carrier gas in the Fluotec Mark 2 increases the output of halothane.[2]

Back-pressure compensation is a design feature of modern vaporizers. Intermittent pressure transmitted to a vaporizer during activation of the flush valve and during application of positive-pressure ventilation may increase vaporizer output compared with output of anesthetic during free flow of gases through the vaporizer.[6] Newer vaporizers prevent or minimize this "pumping effect" by use of small vaporization chambers (e.g., Tecs), long spiral tubes at the inlet to the vaporization chamber (e.g., Vapor), pressure-check valves just downstream from the vaporizer, and relief valves at the vaporizer outlet.[2,3,6]

Effects of Barometric Pressure on Vaporizer Function

Variations in barometric pressure (e.g., high altitude or hyperbaric chambers) alter vaporizer output expressed in volume percent. A specific partial pressure of inhalant anesthetic (e.g., 1 MAC) represents the same anesthetic potency (partial pressure) at various barometric pressures.[20] However, anesthetic concentration is expressed as volume percent on most vaporizers, and MAC expressed as volume percent increases as barometric pressure decreases. Changing the barometric pressure also alters the viscosity and density of gases flowing through vaporizers and flowmeters and affects the output concentration.[20] The ASTM standard states that the effects of barometric pressure on the performance of a vaporizer must be described in catalogs and operation manuals.[1,3]

With decreasing barometric pressure, most concentration-calibrated vaporizers (e.g., Fluotec Mark 3) are considered "self-compensating" and deliver about the same partial pressure, but an increasing volume percent of anesthetic.[3,20] Basically, the vaporizer can be set normally in volume percent even though the volume-percent setting on the control dial is inaccurate.[20] In theory, a halothane vaporizer at an ambient pressure of 500 mm Hg should deliver twice the concentration on the control dial in volume percent and approximately 1.3 times the dialed concentration in terms of MAC or potency.[4] Since variations in resistance of flow through the vaporizer at differing ambient pressures cause small changes in concentration output,[3] the best approach is to measure partial pressure of anesthetic in inspired or expired gases when working at atypical barometric pressures.

With measured-flow vaporizers (e.g., Copper Kettle), changes in barometric pressure affect both partial pressure and volume percent of the delivered anesthetic.[20] If barometric pressure is low, the output expressed as volume percent and as partial pressure increases. When the barometric pressure is high, measured-flow vaporizers deliver a lower anesthetic concentration, expressed as either volume percent or partial pressure. Temperature, barometric pressure, and vapor pressure of the anesthetic all affect the final anesthetic concentration, but the greatest effects are on anesthetics with low boiling points and with vapor pressures that are near the barometric pressure.[3,20]

Changes in barometric pressure also affect the function of flowmeters. Actual flow increases, becoming higher than the indicator and scale of the flowmeter show, as barometric pressure decreases.[20] In, contrast, a flowmeter will deliver less flow than indicated when ambient pressure is higher than the barometric pressure at which the flowmeter was calibrated.[3]

Potential Problems with Vaporizers

The arrangement of vaporizers on anesthesia machines and how vaporizers are maintained affect their safety under clinical conditions. Filling errors, improper transport, using vaporizers in series, and improperly connecting a vaporizer to a machine may cause significant variations in output.

Veterinary practices often stock more than one inhalant anesthetic, and a vaporizer may be inadvertently filled with the wrong drug, especially if the vaporizer has a screw-cap filler port in contrast to a keyed filler port. Keyed filler systems are designed to prevent the introduction of the wrong anesthetic into a vaporizer (Fig. 17.22). However, they are more inconvenient, and screw-cap filler ports and a simple bottle adapter will decrease spillage (Fig. 17.23). Admittedly, there is an increased chance for incorrect filling of vaporizers (Fig 17.24). If an agent-specific vaporizer for a drug with a lower vapor pressure (e.g., methoxyflurane) is filled with a potent, highly volatile anesthetic, dangerously high concentrations may be produced. If this occurs, the vaporizer should be decontaminated before it is used for a patient. The best approach is to have the vaporizer serviced by a qualified vaporizer technician. For Ohio calibrated vaporizers, service is required because the paper wicks must be replaced. For a contaminated Tec vaporizer, an option is to drain the vaporizer, flush it with an oxygen flow of 5 L/min for 45 min or until no trace of a contaminant is present, allow it to stabilize thermally for about 2 h, and refill it with the appropriate anesthetic. Vaporizers contaminated with a nonvolatile contaminant (e.g., water or thymol) should be drained and serviced.[4]

Filler ports and sight glasses are designed to preclude overfilling of modern vaporizers, primarily to prevent liquid anesthetic from entering the fresh gas line of the vaporizer (Fig. 17.25). Recent designs for some vaporizers prevent liquid from entering the fresh gas line even during tipping or inversion. However, tip-

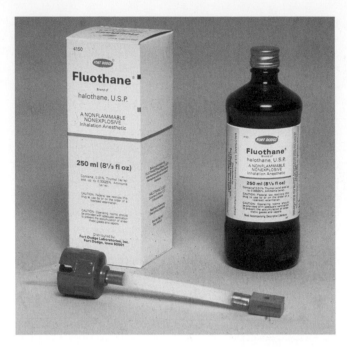

Fig. 17.22. Bottle adapter for halothane vaporizers with keyed filler systems. Such systems reduce the likelihood of introducing an inappropriate anesthetic into an agent-specific vaporizer. The larger end (*left*) of the device attaches to a bottle of halothane, and the opposite end corresponds to the vaporizer filler receptacle. A screw in the receptacle enables a tight seal to be created during the filling process. Bottles of inhalant liquid have a color-coded collar to accept only the correct bottle adapter (see Fig. 17.23).

ping of certain vaporizers may introduce liquid anesthetic into the bypass channel.[3] If this occurs, a high concentration of anesthetic vapor may be delivered: Tipping a vaporizer that was not securely attached to an anesthetic machine has reportedly caused a human patient's cardiac arrest.[21] Also, moving a vaporizer on a mobile anesthesia machine may alter vaporizer output if the machine is tipped or liquid anesthetic is sloshed as the machine is moved over doorway thresholds. Generally, vaporizers should be emptied before transport. Even portable anesthesia machines should be moved with care. If tipping occurs, a high flow of oxygen through the vaporizer for 20 min with the control dial at a low setting has been recommended, but servicing may be required.[2]

One anesthesia machine may be fitted with multiple vaporizers (Fig. 17.24). Modern anesthesia machines designed for use in human patients are equipped with interlocking mechanisms that do not allow two vaporizers to be on simultaneously.[6] Few veterinary practices have the luxury of owning anesthesia machines with interlocking vaporizers. In-line, noninterlocked vaporizers offer the possibility of operating two vaporizers concurrently, conceivably producing an excessive depth of anesthesia.[2] The simultaneous use of more than one vaporizer in series also increases the probability of contaminating a vaporizer with an inappropriate agent. If vaporizers are placed in series, the best order is methoxyflurane, sevoflurane, isoflurane, and halothane from upstream to downstream: This reduces the chance of contamination by taking into account both vapor pressure and po-

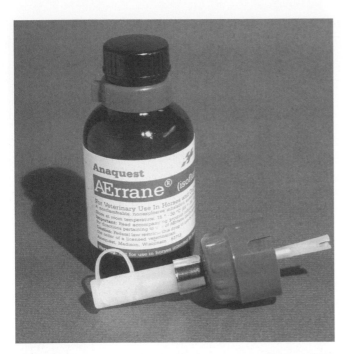

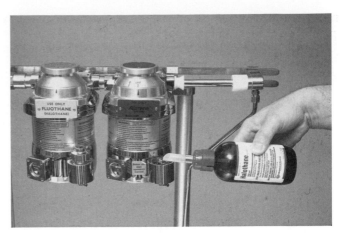

Fig. 17.24. Filling a vaporizer with a screw-cap filler port. Halothane is about to be poured into an isoflurane vaporizer, illustrating the possibility of filling a vaporizer with a screw-cap filler port with the wrong anesthetic. Tec 3 vaporizers for halothane (Fluotec Mark 3) and isoflurane (Isotec 3) are shown in series. The ideal order would be to reverse these vaporizers with the isoflurane immediately downstream from the flowmeters, followed by the halothane vaporizer (see the text for explanation).

Fig. 17.23. Bottle adapter (Southmedic, Beaumont, TX) for filling isoflurane vaporizers with screw-cap filler ports. The isoflurane bottle has a color-coded collar corresponding to the color on the bottle's label and the color of the bottle adapter. This type of bottle adapter is intended to reduce spillage during the filling of vaporizers with screw-cap filler ports.

tency.[3,4] Anesthesia machines with vaporizers in series should be used carefully if an interlocking mechanism is not in place.

Occasionally, veterinarians will use a freestanding, concentration-calibrated vaporizer that is periodically connected between the common gas outlet and the breathing system or between the outlet of another vaporizer and the breathing system. Also, freestanding vaporizers are commonly used with pump oxygenators for cardiopulmonary bypass procedure.[4] A freestanding vaporizer offers a greater opportunity for tipping. The flow through the vaporizer might be inadvertently reversed when vaporizer connections are changed periodically, and oxygen may be forced through the vaporizer with the flush valve if the vaporizer is located downstream from the flush valve. All of these situations lead to a significant increase in the output concentration.[6] Use of a freestanding vaporizer is not the safest approach for access to a second inhalant anesthetic.

In anesthesia machines designed for veterinary use, a concentration-calibrated vaporizer can be connected in reverse, even though the connections are labeled and different sizes. In this configuration, the vaporizer output can potentially be twice that indicated on the control dial.[6]

Classification of Vaporizers

Vaporizers have been classified according to several major characteristics:

1. Method of output regulation
2. Method of vaporization

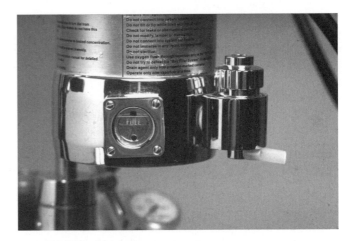

Fig. 17.25. Screw-cap filler system and sight glass for a Fluotec Mark 3 vaporizer. The location of the filler port prevents the operator from filling the vaporizer excessively because liquid will overflow if the maximum level on the sight glass is exceeded significantly. The plastic tubing on the bottom of the filler system facilitates drainage of the vaporizer.

3. Location
4. Mechanism of temperature compensation
5. Agent specificity
6. Resistance

Even though some authors have used only one feature in classifying vaporizers, such schemes are incomplete because of the variations among vaporizers.[3] As examples of classification

Table 17.2. Classification characteristics of some vaporizers used in veterinary anesthesia[2–4]

Vaporizer	Method of Output Regulation	Method of Vaporization	Location	Temperature Compensated	Resistance	Specificity
Ohio #8	VBP CC−	FO/wick	VIC	No	Low	No
Stephens	VBP CC−	FO/wick	VIC	No	Low	No
Tec 2	VBP CC+[a]	FO/wick	VOC	Yes	High	Yes
Tec 3	VBP CC+	FO/wick	VOC	Yes	High	Yes
Vapor	VBP CC+	FO/wick	VOC	Yes	High	Yes
Vapor 19.1	VBP CC+	FO/wick	VOC	Yes	High	Yes
Ohio Calibrated	VBP CC+	FO/wick	VOC	Yes	High	Yes
Siemens	NA CC+	Inject	VOC	No	High	Yes
Copper Kettle	MF CC−	Bubble-through	VOC	Yes	High	No
Verni-Trol	MF CC−	Bubble-through	VOC	Yes	High	No

CC+, concentration calibrated; CC−, not concentration calibrated; FO, flow-over; MF, measured flow through the vaporizer; NA, not applicable; VBP, variable bypass; VIC, vaporizer in circuit (i.e., in the breathing system); VOC, vaporizer out of circuit (i.e., out of the system).
[a]A Tec 2 vaporizer is concentration calibrated at higher flows of carrier gas, but output varies with low flows.

nomenclature, the characteristics of several vaporizers are summarized in Table 17.2.

1. Regulation of Output

Anesthetic output is regulated in volume percent by variable-bypass or measured-flow mechanisms.[3,4] With variable-bypass vaporizers, all fresh gas flows into the vaporizer, part being directed through and part bypassing the vaporization chamber. The gases rejoin before exiting the vaporizer, establishing the anesthetic concentration dialed with the control knob. The standard for these vaporizers is for the control dial to be turned on in a counterclockwise direction.[1] Concentration-calibrated variable-bypass vaporizers are quite accurate (e.g., Tecs), but uncalibrated variable-bypass vaporizers (e.g., Ohio #8) are inaccurate.

Measured-flow (flowmeter controlled) vaporizers are considered non–concentration-calibrated.[4] They route a small flow of carrier gas (i.e., oxygen) through the vaporizer, and this gas becomes fully saturated with anesthetic. A second source of gas (i.e., oxygen and possibly N_2O) that never enters the vaporizer dilutes the saturated gas to the desired concentration. Calculations are necessary to determine the concentration of anesthetic that is delivered to the common gas outlet and breathing system.

2. Method of Vaporization

The method of vaporization can be flow-over, bubble-through, or injection.[2–4] *Flow-over* vaporizers direct carrier gas over the surface of the liquid anesthetic. The surface area may be increased with wicks to improve the efficiency of vaporization (Figs. 17.26 and 17.27). The Stephens vaporizer can be used with or without a wick, depending on the anesthetic and the decision of the anesthetist.[22] The *bubble-through* method of vaporization delivers carrier gas below the surface of the liquid through a diffuser (a sintered bronze disk in the Copper Kettle) that disperses bubbles of carrier gas through the liquid anesthetic to increase the liquid-gas interface.[4] Efficiency of vaporization increases with smaller

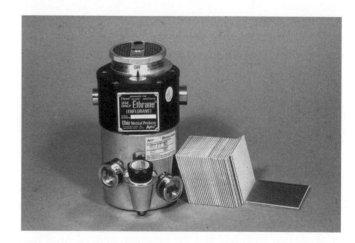

Fig. 17.26. Ohio calibrated vaporizer with paper wicks and copper spacers. The wicks function to increase the surface area for vaporization of inhalant anesthetic.

bubbles, deeper bubble dispersion, and slower carrier-gas flow.[2] *Injection* vaporizers deliver a known amount of liquid anesthetic or pure vapor into a known volume of gas to deliver an accurate concentration.[3]

3. Vaporizer Location

In relation to the breathing system, a vaporizer may be located either out of the system (vaporizer out of circuit [VOC]) (Fig. 17.28) or in the system (vaporizer in circuit [VIC]) (Fig. 17.29).[2] High-resistance vaporizers are used as VOC units, and low-resistance vaporizers are necessary for VIC use (because the patient must inspire through the vaporizer). Traditionally, highly potent, highly volatile anesthetics have been administered with VOC vaporizers. However, some VIC vaporizers have been used for delivery of isoflurane and halothane. VIC-type vaporizers have been characterized as being unpredictable in output.[3,23]

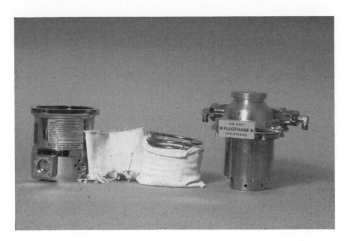

Fig. 17.27. Fluotec Mark 3 vaporizer with cloth wicks. The wicks function to increase the surface area for vaporization of inhalant anesthetic. From Hartsfield.[5]

4. Temperature Compensation

As discussed previously, heat is required to vaporize liquid anesthetics. To prevent or compensate for cooling that alters the rate of vaporization of the liquid anesthetic, heat must be supplied to maintain the temperature of the liquid anesthetic, or the flow of carrier gas through the vaporizer must be adjusted to account for the changing rate of vaporization. Heat may be supplied from the vaporizer itself if it is made of a material with high specific heat and high thermal conductivity (thermostability).[4] Electric heaters and warm-water jackets were used to supply heat for older vaporizers, and an electric heating device has been incorporated into newer vaporizers (e.g., the Tec 6) designed for desflurane.[16] In other vaporizers, alternative thermostatic mechanisms (e.g., a change in carrier gas flow through the vaporization chamber) have been used to counterbalance changes in temperature and vaporization. Manual adjustments of flow through the vaporization chamber are made to offset variations in temperature that occur with measured-flow vaporizers.

5. Agent Specificity

Vaporizers can be either *agent specific* (designed for a particular inhalant anesthetic) or *multipurpose* (used with any volatile liquid anesthetic).[2] A vaporizer that is designed and used for multiple agents should be clearly labeled with the name of the agent currently in the vaporizer. If the anesthetic is changed, the vaporizer should be cleared of the original anesthetic before another anesthetic is introduced into the vaporizer, and draining alone may not eliminate all of the original anesthetic.[3] The trend for vaporizer type has been toward agent-specific, concentration-calibrated vaporizers.

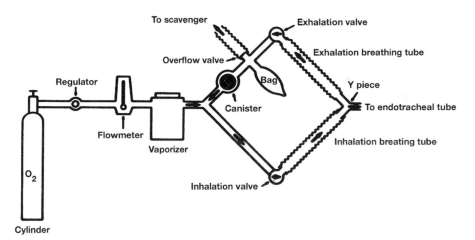

Fig. 17.28. Diagram of a vaporizer located outside the breathing system (vaporizer out of circuit [VOC]) and its relationship to the other basic components of the anesthesia machine and circle system. From Hartsfield.[5]

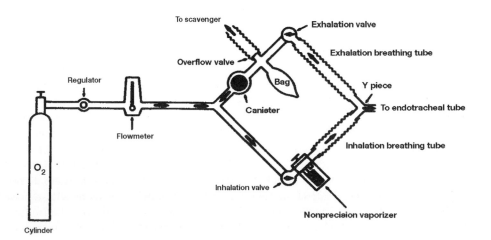

Fig. 17.29. Diagram of the vaporizer located inside the breathing system (vaporizer in circuit [VIC]) and its relationship to other basic components of the anesthesia machine and circle system. From Hartsfield.[5]

6. Resistance

Vaporizers have been classified according to resistance to flow.[3] Plenum-type vaporizers are high-resistance vaporizers designed for location outside of the breathing system, and high resistance is characteristic of contemporary concentration-calibrated, variable-bypass vaporizers. Low-resistance vaporizers are those designed for incorporation into the breathing system[3] and include the Ohio #8 and the Stephens vaporizers.

In-circuit Vaporizers (VICs)

Nonprecision, draw-over, VIC vaporizers were commonly used in veterinary anesthesia for many years. Until the introduction of halothane into veterinary anesthesia, perhaps the most widely used vaporizer for veterinary patients in the United States was the Ohio #8 glass bottle. Although it is no longer manufactured, it was the basic vaporizer on many veterinary anesthesia machines (Pitman-Moore models 960 and 970) sold in the 1970s for administration of methoxyflurane. In the 1990s, the Stephens vaporizer was also marketed for use in veterinary patients. Nevertheless, for safety reasons, VIC vaporizers have generally been recommended for use only with anesthetics of low potency (e.g., ether) or low vapor pressure (e.g., methoxyflurane). In human patients, the Ohio #8 glass bottle was used mostly for administration of diethyl ether and, to a lesser extent, methoxyflurane. The use of halothane and isoflurane in nonprecision vaporizers located within the circuit has been described specifically when used with low-flow or closed breathing systems.[24]

With VIC vaporizers, the inspired anesthetic concentration varies with a patient's respiratory minute volume, use of positive-pressure ventilation, changes in carrier-gas flow rate, and variations in temperature. At a given vaporizer setting, increased spontaneous ventilation, positive-pressure ventilation, and lower fresh gas flows increase the inspired anesthetic concentration. As has been stated specifically for the Ohio #8 vaporizer, "The delivered concentration is unknown and changes unpredictably with use."[23] Without instrumental monitoring of the inspired or expired anesthetic concentration, the anesthetist is completely dependent on the response of the patient to determine appropriate settings for the vaporizer. This is often referred to as *qualitative anesthesia* in contrast to *quantitative anesthesia*, where a known concentration of inhalant (with knowledge of its potency [i.e., MAC value]) is continually delivered to a patient.

Ohio #8 Glass-Bottle Vaporizer

The Ohio #8 vaporizer is classified as variable bypass, flow-over with wick, non–temperature-compensated, VIC, low resistance, and multipurpose.[2] It is designed very simply: The vaporization chamber is made of glass, and a cloth wick creates a large surface area for vaporization (Fig. 17.30). The vaporizer is not calibrated; thus, it is considered nonprecision. The vaporizer has no method of controlling the temperature of the liquid. Its low resistance allows it to be situated in the breathing system (VIC), usually on the inspiratory side of the circle. If positioned on the expiratory limb, the vaporization chamber may become contaminated with water condensing from expired gases. The control

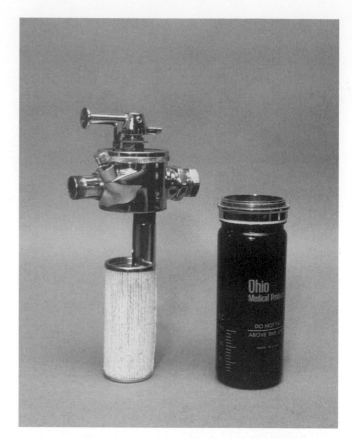

Fig. 17.30. Partially disassembled Ohio #8 glass bottle vaporizer. The cloth wick (*left*) functions to increase the surface area for vaporization of the anesthetic.

arm of the lever is adjustable from zero, corresponding to no gas flow through the vaporization chamber, to 10, corresponding to total inspiratory flow through the vaporization chamber (Fig. 17.31). The possibility of diverting all gas flow through the vaporization chamber makes the use of highly volatile anesthetics particularly dangerous, especially if the wick is in place. The concentration delivered is unknown and may change unpredictably. The function of this vaporizer is probably best summarized by the following statement: "Because of the variability associated with an in-system vaporizer, it is not possible to give performance data."[2] The Ohio #8 vaporizer is no longer being manufactured, and finding expertise and parts for repairing it may be difficult.

The Ohio #8 vaporizer, modified by the removal of the wick, has been proposed as an inexpensive alternative for administration of isoflurane[18] and halothane.[19] Use of an Ohio #8 vaporizer for administration of halothane or isoflurane with the wick in place is dangerous owing to the high concentration of anesthetic that may be delivered in the inspired gases, especially if all carrier gases are diverted through the vaporization chamber. Even with the wick removed, recommendations for using the Ohio #8 vaporizer for isoflurane include familiarity with guidelines for its use and understanding of its limitations.[18] The Ohio #8 vaporizer

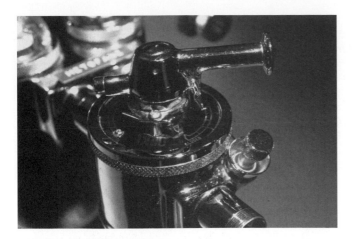

Fig. 17.31. Control lever for the Ohio #8 jar vaporizer set at position 2. The numbered positions (0 to 10) on the vaporizer correspond to increasing flow of carrier gas through the vaporization chamber. At the closed position (0), all gas entering the vaporizer should bypass the vaporization chamber, and, at full open (10), all gas entering the vaporizer should move through the vaporization chamber.

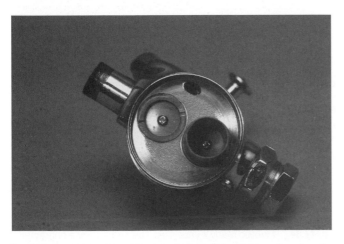

Fig. 17.32. Underside of the head of an Ohio #8 vaporizer showing valves and seats through which gases enter and leave the vaporization chamber. The integrity of these valves in the off position may be lost because of wear or corrosion leading to carrier-gas flow through the vaporization chamber, even when the control lever is in the zero or off position.

also has potential for leaking anesthetic into the breathing system when the control lever is off.[2] With age, the vaporizer's valves may not seat properly (Fig. 17.32), allowing continuous passage of fresh gases through the vaporization chamber and production of anesthetic-rich gases.

Stephens Vaporizer

The Stephens vaporizer is classified as variable bypass, flow-over, non–temperature-compensated, VIC, low resistance, and multipurpose. It is not a precision vaporizer. The vaporizer's low resistance allows it to be located within the breathing system on the inspiratory side. The vaporization chamber is made of glass

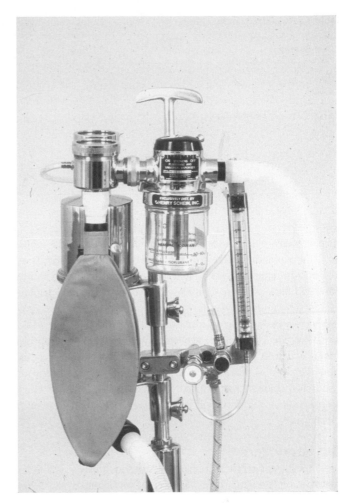

Fig. 17.33. Stephens anesthesia machine and vaporizer (Henry Schein, Port Washington, NY). The glass vaporizer can be set at the off and full-on positions with incremental settings marked in eighths. This vaporizer has been used with methoxyflurane (with a wick in place) and for halothane or isoflurane with the wick removed.

(Fig. 17.33), and a wick is provided for administration of methoxyflurane. The wick should not be used for administration of halothane or isoflurane.[22] The vaporizer is not calibrated and has no method for controlling the temperature of the liquid. The control knob is adjustable from the off position to the full-on position in increments of eighths. The off position indicates no flow through the vaporization chamber, and the on position corresponds to complete flow through the vaporization chamber. The Stephens vaporizer is intended for use in a low-flow circle breathing system.[22]

Out-of-circuit Vaporizers (VOCs)

Modern concentration-calibrated vaporizers located outside of the breathing circuit are considered precision vaporizers: Any volatile liquid anesthetic can be administered safely with a concentration-calibrated, agent-specific, VOC vaporizer. Several brands of VOC-type vaporizers are common in veterinary anes-

Table 17.3. Approximate output (vol%) from a Fluotec Mark 2 vaporizer at various flow rates and dial settings[15]

Dial Setting	1 L/min	2 L/min	3 L/min	4 L/min	6 L/min	8 L/min
0.5%	0	0	0	0.5	0.5	0.5
1.0%	0	0.5	1.0	1.0	1.0	1.0
1.5%	0.5	1.5	1.5	1.5	1.5	1.5
2.0%	1.8	2.0	2.0	2.0	2.0	2.0
2.5%	3.0	2.5	2.5	2.5	2.5	2.5
3.0%	4.0	3.1	3.0	3.0	3.0	3.0
3.5%	5.0	4.0	3.5	3.5	3.5	3.5
4.0%	6.5	5.0	4.1	4.0	4.0	4.0

thesia. Many older models of vaporizers, although no longer being manufactured, remain serviceable and may be purchased as used equipment. Newer VOC-type vaporizers are temperature, flow, and back-pressure compensated. The performance of older VOC-type vaporizers varies with changes in temperature, flow, and back-pressure, and performance data should be reviewed before using them. The concentration control dial and the vaporizer output generally are linear over a wide range of flow rates and temperatures in newer VOC-type vaporizers. The following discussion, though not exhaustive, includes information about several out-of-circuit vaporizers commonly used in veterinary anesthesia.

Tec Vaporizers

Tec vaporizers specifically designed for halothane or isoflurane vaporization, particularly the Fluotec Mark 3 and Isotec 3, are commonly used in veterinary anesthesia. They are considered reliable because they are temperature, flow, and back-pressure compensated under normal operating conditions. The Fluotec Mark 3's predecessor, the Fluotec Mark 2, is no longer being manufactured, but may still be available as used equipment. In some veterinary practices, Fluotec Mark 2 vaporizers remain in use. Tec 4, 5, and 6 vaporizers have superseded the Tec 3 vaporizers for use in contemporary human anesthesia machines.[6,16] Although these vaporizers have not been as commonly used in veterinary anesthesia, various publications and the specific operation manuals offer information about their use and performance.[3,4,6,16]

Fluotec Mark 2

This vaporizer (Fig. 17.34) is classified as variable bypass, flow-over with wick, VOC, temperature compensated, high resistance, and agent specific.[2] Temperature compensation is with a bimetallic strip valve at the outlet to the vaporization chamber.[3] Performance data show that the Mark 2 becomes imprecise at flow rates below 4 L/min, and inaccuracy increases distinctly below 2 L/min.[2] At flow rates and dial settings likely to be selected for small veterinary patients, the Mark 2's actual output tends to be lower than control-dial settings of less than 2% and higher than dial settings of 2% or greater (Table 17.3).

At the very low flow rates required for closed and low-flow maintenance techniques, the Mark 2's output may decrease to zero or increase to concentrations much higher than the dial set-

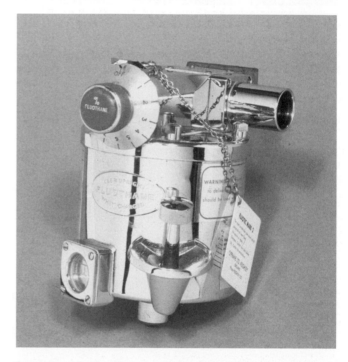

Fig. 17.34. Fluotec Mark 2 vaporizer. The performance characteristics for variations in carrier-gas flow are included on the plastic card attached to the vaporizer (see Fig. 17.35).

tings. Because of its unpredictable output characteristics, the Mark 2 has been categorized as unsuitable and unreliable for use with low fresh gas flow rates.[2,22,25] Back-pressure (e.g., positive-pressure ventilation) increases the output of the Mark 2 dramatically at flow rates less than 2 L/min.[2,26] A pressurizing valve was developed for the Mark 2 to minimize the effects of back-pressure,[2] but it may not be present on all Mark 2 vaporizers. The operator should fully understand the Mark 2's relatively poor performance characteristics before using the vaporizer clinically, and the output diagram for the Mark 2 should be available for consultation during clinical use (Fig. 17.35).

Tec Mark 3 Vaporizers

These vaporizers are classified as variable bypass, flow-over, temperature compensated, agent specific, high resistance, and

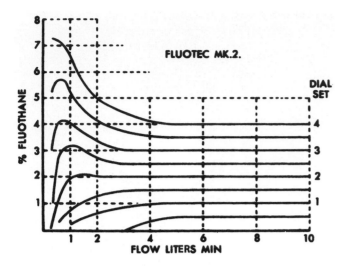

Fig. 17.35. Performance diagram for a Fluotec Mark 2 vaporizer. The diagram indicates expected output of halothane in volume percent for specific control-dial settings at specific carrier-gas flow rates.

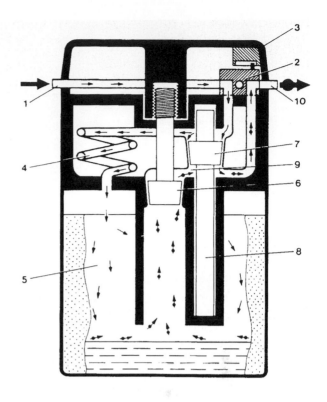

Fig. 17.36. Vapor 19.1 vaporizer (North American Drager, Telford, PA) for isoflurane and a cross-sectional diagram of the vaporizer: *1,* fresh gas inlet; *2,* on-and-off control (activated by concentration knob); *3,* concentration knob; *4,* pressure compensation; *5,* vaporizing chamber; *6,* control cone; *7,* vaporizing chamber-bypass cone; *8,* expansion member for temperature compensation; *9,* mixing chamber; and *10,* fresh gas inlet. From Lumb and Jones.[31]

VOC.[2,3] This model type includes the Fluotec Mark 3, the Pentec Mark 2, and the Isotec 3 vaporizers (Fig. 17.24). The Tec 3 vaporizer is temperature compensated with a bimetallic, temperature-sensitive element associated with the vaporization chamber. Output from the Tec 3 vaporizer is nearly linear over the range of concentrations and flow rates that would typically be selected for veterinary patients (250 mL/min to 6 L/min). Back-pressure compensation is accomplished in the internal design of the vaporizer with a long tube leading to the vaporization chamber, an expansion area in the tube, and exclusion of wicks from the area of the vaporization chamber near the inlet.[2]

Vapor Vaporizers: Vapor 19.1 and Vapor

The Vapor 19.1 vaporizer (Fig. 17.36) is classified as variable bypass, flow-over with wick, temperature compensated, high resistance, agent specific, and VOC.[2,3] Specific vaporizers are available for isoflurane and halothane administration. Temperature compensation is automatic with an "expansion member" that varies the flow of gas through the vaporization chamber with changes in temperature. Pressure compensation is accomplished by the presence of a long spiral inlet tube to the vaporization chamber.[4] This vaporizer is accurate from 0.3 to 15 L/min of fresh gas flow at the lower settings on the control dial, but complete saturation may not occur at higher settings with higher flows. The vaporizer is designed for operation (temperature compensation) in the range of 10° to 40°C.[2]

The Vapor vaporizer (Fig. 17.37) preceded the Vapor 19 and 19.1, and has been called "semiautomatic" because manual adjustments are required for complete temperature compensation (Fig. 17.38).[5] The unit is no longer being manufactured, but some vaporizers may still be in operation in veterinary practices. The vaporizer was available for both methoxyflurane and halothane administration. It is classified as variable bypass, flow-over with

wick, VOC, temperature compensated by manual flow alteration, high resistance, and agent specific, and is considered to be very accurate.[2] It was designed for thermostability and is constructed of a large mass of copper as a heat sink to prevent excessive cooling during vaporization.[2,27] The concentration dial must be manually adjusted to the temperature chamber within the vaporizer and the liquid between 16° and 28°C (Fig. 17.38).[28] The unit is flow compensated over a wide range (approximately 250 mL/min to 10 L/min), with some deviation at high concentrations at high flows. The mechanism for back-pressure compensation involves a long coiled tube at the inlet to the vaporization chamber.[2]

Other Vaporizers

Ohio Calibrated Vaporizer

This vaporizer (Fig. 17.26) has been available for veterinary use and was commonly employed on human anesthesia machines for many years. This vaporizer is classified as variable bypass, flow-

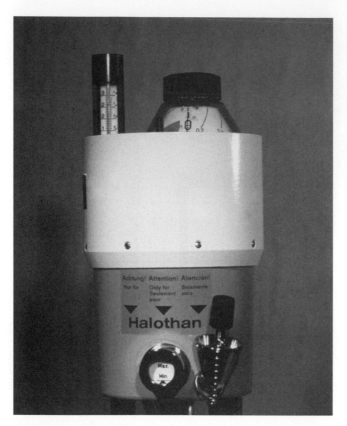

Fig. 17.37. A halothane Vapor vaporizer (North American Drager, Telford, PA).

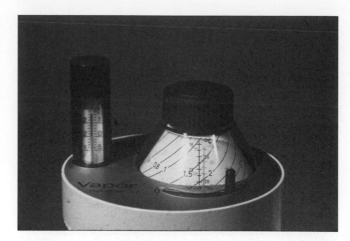

Fig. 17.38. Vapor vaporizer with a control-dial setting of 2% at 28°C. The thermometer (*left*) indicates the temperature within the vaporizer (liquid anesthetic). The control dial is used to manually align the curved line corresponding to the desired anesthetic concentration with the temperature of the liquid anesthetic (the vertical line with hash marks) within the vaporizing chamber. From Hartsfield.[5]

over with wick, automatically temperature compensated, agent specific, VOC, and high resistance.[2,3] Specific units are manufactured for isoflurane, halothane, and sevoflurane administration. These vaporizers were designed for accuracy at fresh gas flows between 0.3 to 10 L/min, and temperature compensation occurs between 16° and 32°C. Tilting these vaporizers up to 20° while in use or up to 45° when not in use does not cause problems. Greater tipping of the vaporizer may cause delivery of high concentrations. Between paper wicks, the vaporizer has plastic spacers that may react with enflurane or isoflurane to cause discoloration of the liquid anesthetic, apparently without significant consequences.[3]

Siemens Vaporizer

This vaporizer is a concentration-calibrated, injection-type, non-thermocompensated, agent-specific, and plenum (high resistance) unit.[3] It has not been used extensively in clinical veterinary anesthesia, except in laboratory-animal facilities associated with hospitals for human patients. The vaporizer was designed to couple with a specific Siemens ventilator. The function and evaluation of this vaporizer have been reviewed elsewhere.[3]

Measured-Flow Vaporizers

Verni-Trols and Copper Kettles (Fig. 17.39) are flowmeter-controlled vaporizers that formerly were popular for use in anesthesia of human patients.[2–4] Copper Kettles were the first devices

to enable precise vaporization of liquid anesthetics.[2] These flowmeter-controlled vaporizers are classified as measured flow, bubble-through, high resistance, VOC, temperature compensated (thermally stable with manual flow adjustments based on temperature of the liquid anesthetic), and multipurpose. They have been classified as saturation vaporizers. These vaporizers are constructed of copper (Copper Kettle) or silicon bronze (Verni-Trol) for thermostability. Back-pressure compensation mechanisms are present on more recent models and can be fitted on older models (e.g., check valves). These vaporizers are no longer being manufactured and are not covered by the ASTM standard of 1989.[6] However, they are available on used anesthesia machines and have been purchased for veterinary patient use. Since these vaporizers are multipurpose or universal, they can accurately vaporize halothane, isoflurane, sevoflurane, or methoxyflurane, and should be clearly labeled for the agent in use.

With measured-flow vaporizers, manual adjustments in flow rates are required to account for variations in total gas flow, day-to-day changes in temperature, and changes in liquid temperature during use, especially with high fresh gas flow rates. In most cases, a calculator (Fig. 17.40) is supplied with each vaporizer for determining proper flow rates. Anesthesia machines with measured-flow vaporizers have oxygen flowmeters for two purposes: One flowmeter routes all of its oxygen through the vaporization chamber, where it is fully saturated with anesthetic; the other flowmeter supplies oxygen that bypasses the vaporizer and supplies oxygen to meet the patient's requirements. Both gas sources combine at a mixing valve to achieve the proper anesthetic concentration before gases enter the breathing system.

Since the output of a measured-flow vaporizer is oxygen fully saturated with anesthetic, the concentration of halothane or isoflurane approaches 32%. Dangerously high concentrations of anesthetic can be delivered to the breathing system if flowmeters

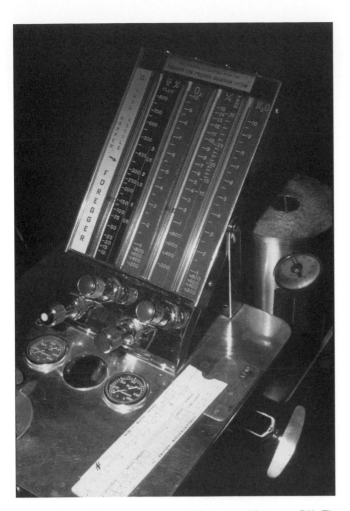

Fig. 17.39. Copper Kettle vaporizer (Foregger, Allentown, PA). The vaporization chamber (copper kettle) with its thermometer is behind the table top (*right rear*), and the vaporizer circuit control valve is attached to the left front corner of the tabletop. The flowmeter cluster from *left to right* includes the oxygen flowmeter to the vaporization chamber (black scale), two bypass oxygen flowmeters (green), and one nitrous oxide flowmeter (blue). This cluster does not meet recent standards for the arrangement of flowmeters. From Hartsfield.[5]

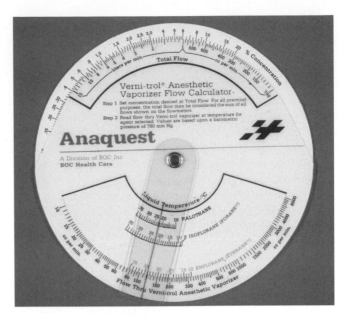

Fig. 17.40. A circular slide rule for calculation of oxygen flow rates for an anesthetic machine with a measured-flow vaporizer. The rule can be used for several different anesthetics at various total flow rates over a range of temperatures. This circular slide rule shows that 120 mL of oxygen must be supplied to the vaporizer to produce 3% halothane at a total gas flow rate of 2 L/min at a vaporizer temperature of 23°C.

are set carelessly or if the diluent flow is not turned on. It is also possible to misread the calculator and set incorrect flows.[2] Because such high concentrations can be achieved and because errors in adjustment of flowmeters are possible, the use of continuous monitoring of the inspired anesthetic agent concentration has been recommended.[4]

In addition to using a calculator, the output from measured-flow vaporizers can be calculated or estimated. Methods, including formulas, for calculating flow requirements for measured-flow vaporizers have been reviewed.[22] As previously stated, the vaporization chamber produces an anesthetic concentration equal to the anesthetic's saturated vapor pressure. Thus, if halothane's vapor pressure is 243 mm Hg at 20°C, approximately 32% halothane is delivered to the mixing valve. This concentration is diluted by bypass gases to an appropriate concentration for the patient.

If a patient is to be maintained with a total gas flow of 2 L/min and a halothane concentration of 1.5%, then 30 mL/min of halothane vapor ($1.5\% \times 2000$ m/L = 30 mL) must be delivered to the breathing system along with 1970 mL/min of oxygen. About 64 mL of oxygen must enter the vaporization chamber each minute to produce an output of 30 mL/min of halothane: 30 mL = $32\% \cdot X$, where X is the total gas flow exiting the vaporization chamber; thus, X = 94 mL, and 94 mL − 30 mL = 64 mL. The bypass oxygen flow must equal 2000 mL/min − 94 mL/min or 1906 mL/min. In all calculations, the total gas flow to the patient must be considered, including oxygen, N_2O, and vaporizer flows, for determination of anesthetic requirements.

Using similar computations for methoxyflurane administration at 20°C (vapor pressure = 23 mm Hg), a maximum vaporizer output of 3% can be predicted. Thus, with 2 L/min of total fresh gas flow to the breathing system and a desired concentration of 1%, 20 mL/min of methoxyflurane ($1\% \times 2000$ mL = 20 mL) must be delivered to the breathing system. About 647 mL of oxygen must enter the vaporization chamber to deliver 20 mL/min of methoxyflurane vapor to the breathing system: 20 mL = $3\% \cdot X$, where X is the total gas flow exiting the vaporization chamber; thus, X = 667 mL, and 667 mL − 20 mL = 647 mL. Therefore, 647 mL/min of oxygen must be delivered to the vaporization chamber to produce a total output of 667 mL/min, including 20 mL of methoxyflurane. The bypass flow must them be equal to 1333 mL/min, for a total flow of 2 L/min to the breathing system.

Most of the hazards associated with measured-flow vaporizers relate to incorrect use, including errors in calculation of the output of vapor, failure to turn on the vaporizer flowmeter or the vaporizer circuit control valve, and careless handling of the vaporizer during filling and transport. With tipping, liquid anesthetic may enter the discharge tube of the vaporizer, ultimately delivering very high concentrations of anesthetic to the breathing system. Overfilling is also possible in older models.[2] Older vaporizers may not be equipped for back-pressure compensation, and application of positive-pressure ventilation may significantly increase the concentration delivered.[2] An inflowing gas leak at a faulty O-ring on the base of a sidearm Verni-Trol has reportedly caused reduced oxygen concentration and hypoxia in human patients.[29] Later models of the same machine incorporated a check valve to prevent loss of fresh gas flow. Finally, flow rates below the lowest mark on the scale for the vaporizer's flowmeter should not be extrapolated.

Some measured-flow vaporizers, including the Verni-Trol on the Ohio DM 5000 anesthesia machine[2] and the vaporizer on the old Pitman-Moore 980 veterinary anesthesia machine (Fig. 17.41), designed specifically for methoxyflurane,[22,30] were calibrated for the vaporizer flowmeter to be measured in cubic centimeters (milliliters) per minute of anesthetic vapor rather than in milliliters per minute of oxygen flow to the vaporizer. Consequently, using the flow-rate calculation derived from calculators accompanying Copper Kettles or other Verni-Trol–type machines with these two machines will result in erroneously high delivered concentrations to the anesthetic circuit.[22,31] Volatile anesthetics other than methoxyflurane should not be used in the Pitman-Moore 980 machine's vaporizer.[22,30]

Maintenance of Vaporizers

Vaporizers should be conscientiously maintained. In general, the best policy is to follow the manufacturer's guidelines for care and servicing of vaporizers. Recommendations for maintenance vary. Returning a vaporizer to the manufacturer yearly for cleaning and calibration has been suggested.[32] One source recommends calibration and testing for leaks every 3 to 6 months.[3] Maintenance should be performed on a vaporizer if, based on the responses of patients, the dialed anesthetic concentration is suspected to be erroneous or if any of the components of the vaporizer function improperly (e.g., the control dial is difficult to adjust). Servicing, as recommended by the manufacturer, includes an evaluation of operation, cleaning, changing of filters, replacement of worn parts, and recalibration.[2] Halothane and methoxyflurane contain preservatives (thymol and butylated hydroxytoluene, respectively) that do not vaporize and thus collect in the vaporization chambers and on the wicks, potentially affecting anesthetic output. Vaporizers should be periodically drained to eliminate these preservatives. Vaporizers should not be overfilled or tipped when filled. Vaporizers should be emptied before removal from the anesthesia machine for service. In the past, flushing a vaporizer with ether to dissolve preservatives that collect in it has been recommended. Owing to the flammability and explosiveness of ether, extreme caution should be exercised. Flushing the vaporizer does not eliminate the need for regular service by a certified vaporizer technician.

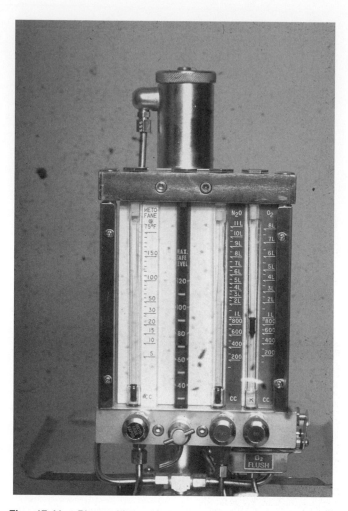

Fig. 17.41. Pitman-Moore 980 veterinary anesthesia machine (Pitman-Moore, Washington Crossing, NJ). This machine includes a Verni-Trol vaporizer with the oxygen flowmeter (*left*, white background) to the vaporization chamber calibrated in milliliters per minute of methoxyflurane vapor. From Hartsfield.[5]

Use of the Wrong Anesthetic in an Agent-Specific Vaporizer

Using an agent-specific vaporizer for an anesthetic for which the vaporizer is not calibrated is problematic, especially if the introduction of an anesthetic is unintentional (i.e., the operator does not realize the mistake). A low output of anesthetic is the expected result if an anesthetic with a lower vapor pressure is placed into a vaporizer designed for a drug with a higher vapor pressure. Conversely, a highly volatile anesthetic in an agent-specific vaporizer designed for a drug with a lower vapor pressure is likely to produce a high, potentially lethal concentration. The differential potencies of the drugs in question would be expected to affect the depth of anesthesia in either situation.

During the introduction of isoflurane into veterinary anesthesia, it was commonly administered with agent-specific, halothane vaporizers that were not recalibrated for isoflurane. Because the vapor pressures of halothane and isoflurane are similar, the out-

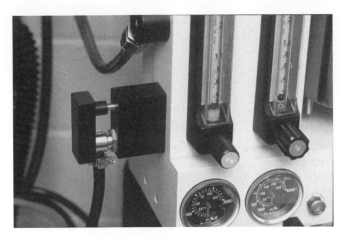

Fig. 17.42. Common gas outlet on a Drager anesthesia machine. The retaining device designed to prevent an accidental disconnection at the common gas outlet is in the closed down position.

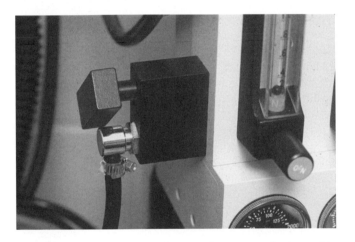

Fig. 17.43. Common gas outlet on a Drager anesthesia machine. The retaining device designed to prevent an accidental disconnection at the common gas outlet is in the open horizontal position.

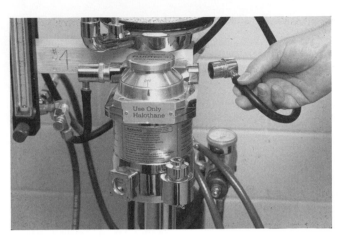

Fig. 17.44. The outlet hose on a Fluotec Mark 3 vaporizer mounted onto a small animal anesthesia machine. The vaporizer outlet connector is attached to a rubber hose that directs anesthetic and carrier gas to the circle system. Alternatively, the rubber hose could be attached to one of the Mapleson systems. A faulty connection to the vaporizer or disconnection of the rubber hose could be responsible for interfering with the delivery of oxygen and anesthetic to the breathing system.

Common Gas Outlet

This outlet is the site from which gases that have passed through the flowmeter, vaporizer (VOC), and flush valve exit the anesthesia machine on the way to the breathing system. Typically, there is a 15-mm internal diameter (ID) opening to which a fitting with rubber tubing attaches (Fig. 17.21). The other end of the tubing connects to the fresh gas inlet of the breathing circuit. In some simple veterinary anesthesia machines with VOC vaporizers, all gases flow directly from the vaporizer outlet to the fresh gas inlet of the breathing system.

Disconnections at the common gas outlet, the vaporizer outlet, or the fresh gas inlet can cause loss of gas flow to the breathing system. The ASTM standard requires that the common gas outlet incorporate a retaining device to prevent accidental disconnection (Figs. 17.42 and 17.43).[1] Disconnects should be detected during the checkout of the machine and breathing system before each case, but disconnects can occur during use of the machine if a retaining mechanism is not present.

A disconnection from the common gas outlet or from the outlet of the vaporizer (Fig. 17.44) during an anesthetic procedure may not be recognized immediately in a spontaneously breathing patient. With a circle system and a VOC, low inspired-oxygen fraction, increased respiratory efforts, and light anesthesia are likely. Some circle systems (Matrx VMS small animal circle) incorporate an air-intake valve (negative-pressure–relief valve [Fig. 17.45]) to entrain room air when the fresh gas flow is inadequate. With a non-rebreathing system and an outlet disconnect, exhaled carbon dioxide will be rebreathed, low F_IO_2 is probable, and the patient will appear lightly anesthetized with increased respiratory efforts. The use of an oxygen analyzer for continuous evaluation of inspired gases enables early detection of this problem.

put was not expected to differ greatly from the control-dial setting. Indeed, halothane vaporizers produce concentrations of isoflurane that are reasonably close to the dial setting for halothane.[33] Nevertheless, current manufacturer recommendations are against the use of isoflurane in halothane-specific vaporizers and vice versa.[3] Depending on the vaporizer and conditions of operation, isoflurane in a halothane vaporizer may produce 25% to 50% more vapor than expected, and halothane in an isoflurane-specific vaporizer usually delivers a concentration that is lower than expected.[3] If isoflurane is to be used in an agent-specific halothane vaporizer, the vaporizer should be serviced and completely recalibrated for isoflurane. Complete calibration implies that the vaporizer has been tested for accuracy with an anesthetic-gas analyzer at various carrier-gas flows and various temperatures to assure reliable function.

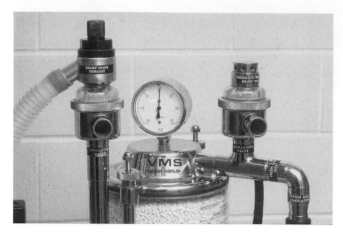

Fig. 17.45. Air-intake valve (negative pressure relief valve) on the dome of the inspiratory one-way valve of a circle system on a Fraser Harlake small animal anesthesia machine. The valve is designed to entrain room air if the supply of fresh gas to the circle breathing system is interrupted. In addition, the pop-off valve is attached to the expiratory one-way valve.

Breathing Systems

Anesthetic breathing systems deliver anesthetic gases and oxygen to the patient, remove carbon dioxide from exhaled gases, and usually provide a means to manually support ventilation. Spontaneously breathing patients inhale and exhale through the breathing system, and the breathing system should be able to supply enough gases to meet the peak inspiratory demands of the patient.

The breathing system adds resistance to the flow of gases, and the diameter of the breathing tubes and other conduits is a major factor in determining the amount of resistance. Doubling the radius decreases the resistance 16 times. Halving the length of the circuit halves the resistance. Changing the direction of gas flow or routing gases through restrictive orifices creates turbulent flow and increases resistance. Therefore, breathing systems should be as short as practical, with maximum diameters in the conduits and the fewest bends and restrictions in the path of gas flow.[2] Generally, the endotracheal tube has the smallest luminal diameter of the breathing apparatus, and the largest tube that is practical should be selected.

Classification of breathing systems has been called a favorite pastime among anesthesiology personnel.[3] Most systems of classification are confusing, not exclusive, and thus not helpful to veterinary students or personnel. When referring to a breathing system in the veterinary or medical literature, the system should be named and physically described, the fresh gas flow rates should be stated, and the patient's body weight and/or oxygen consumption should be listed.[5,34] This eliminates the need for cumbersome, obscure classification systems.

Systems Using Chemical Absorption of Carbon Dioxide

Circle and to-and-fro breathing systems use a chemical absorbent for exhaled carbon dioxide. They are termed *rebreathing* systems because part or all of the exhaled gases, after extraction of carbon dioxide, flow back to the patient. In contrast to *non-rebreathing* systems, rebreathing systems conserve anesthetic, oxygen, heat, and moisture, but impart more resistance to ventilation. Rebreathing systems are relatively expensive to purchase, but comparatively economic to operate.

Circle Systems

Pediatric, standard adult (small animal), and large animal circles differ primarily in their IDs and volumes. Arbitrarily, pediatric circles have been recommended for veterinary patients weighing less than 6.8 kg (15 lb), standard adult circles for patients between 6.8 kg and 135 kg (300 lb), and large animal circles for larger patients.[5] However, choosing the size of circle system for a veterinary patient may be influenced by the species, the practical availability of equipment, the type of ventilation used, and the veterinarian's preferences. In the anesthesia of human patients, a *pediatric circle* usually refers to a standard (adult) absorber assembly, short breathing tubes of small diameter (15 mm ID), and a small bag.[3]

All circle systems have the same basic components, arranged so that gases move in only one direction (Figs. 17.28 and 17.29). Exhaled gases enter the Y piece and flow through the expiratory breathing tube and the expiratory one-way valve. Gases may enter the reservoir bag before or after coursing through the carbon dioxide–absorbent canister. On inspiration, gases exit the reservoir bag and travel through the inspiratory one-way valve, the inspiratory breathing tube, and the Y piece to the patient.

Components of the Circle System

Y Piece This is usually constructed of plastic and unites the endotracheal tube connector and the inspiratory and expiratory breathing tubes. The Y piece contributes to the system's mechanical dead space, but a septum may be present in the Y piece to decrease dead space. It has been argued that the amount of dead space in a standard, adult (small animal) Y piece is not significantly greater than that in a non-rebreathing system.[35] A standard adult Y piece has a 15-mm female port for the endotracheal tube connector, and this port may have a 22-mm outer diameter (OD) to accept a mask. The two 22-mm male ports connect to the breathing tubes. Disposable systems may have the Y piece and breathing tubes permanently attached to each other. The dimensions of the Y piece in large animal circles vary among manufacturers, but approximate 50 mm (2 inches).

Breathing Tubes These tubes are usually made of rubber or plastic, and serve as flexible, low-resistance conduits between the Y piece and the one-way valves. Corrugations reduce the likelihood of obstructions if the tubes are bent. Breathing tubes add length and volume to the system, and increase resistance to ventilation; the tubes should have an ID larger than the ID of the patient's endotracheal tube. Standard adult breathing tubes have a 22-mm ID and have been recommended for small animals weighing more than 7 kg.[36] For smaller patients, 15-mm-ID tubes are available, whereas 50-mm-ID (2 inch) breathing tubes are used with large animal circle systems. Breathing tubes do not

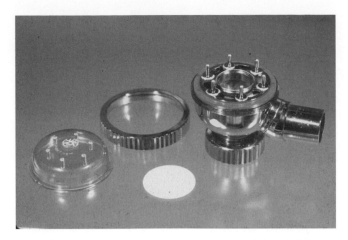

Fig. 17.46. Components of a unidirectional valve (North American Drager, Telford, PA) of a circle breathing system. From the *left*, the plastic dome, the retaining ring for the dome, the valve itself, and the valve housing are depicted. From Hartsfield.[5]

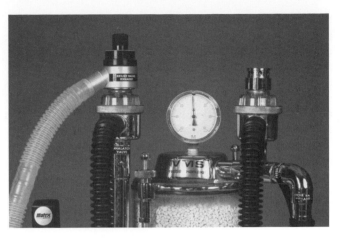

Fig. 17.47. Pop-off valve and manometer on a circle breathing system of a VMS anesthesia machine. The exhaust port (19-mm outer diameter) of the pop-off valve is attached to clear corrugated tubing, which directs waste gases to the scavenging system. The air-intake valve is mounted on the top of the dome for the inspiratory (*right*) one-way valve and functions to entrain room air if the fresh gas supply to the circle system fails.

contribute to mechanical dead space if the one-way valves are functional.

One-way (Unidirectional) Valves   These paired valves direct gas flow away from the patient on expiration and toward the patient on inspiration, preventing the rebreathing of exhaled gases before they pass through the absorbent canister. Gases enter a unidirectional valve from below, raise the disk, and pass under the dome (Fig. 17.46) to the reservoir bag, the absorbent canister, or the inspiratory breathing tube, depending on the location of the valve and the design of the circle. The one-way valves are usually attached to the canister on modern circle systems, but some older systems located the one-way valves within the Y piece, where they were more likely to become incompetent. Valves contribute to the resistance of breathing and should be inspected regularly to assure proper function.

Fresh Gas Inlet   This inlet is the location at which gases from the common gas outlet of the anesthesia machine or from the outlet of the vaporizer enter the circle system. The fresh gas inlet is located on the absorbent canister near the inspiratory one-way valve or on the inspiratory one-way valve. Entry of fresh gases on the inspiratory side of the circle minimizes dilution of fresh gases with exhaled gases with a VOC, prevents absorbent dust from being forced toward the patient, and reduces loss of fresh gases through the pop-off valve.

Pop-off Valve   This valve (adjustable pressure-limiting valve, relief valve, or overflow valve [Fig. 17.47]) vents gases to the scavenger system to prevent the buildup of excessive pressure within the circle, and it allows rapid elimination of anesthetic gases from the circle when 100% oxygen is indicated. The exhaust port of the pop-off valve through which overflow gases enter the scavenger system is designated to have a 10- or 30-mm male connector according to ASTM standards,[1,3] although older

overflow valve ports were sized at 22 mm OD. A pop-off valve should vent gases at pressures of 1 to 2 cm H_2O when it is fully opened. Several types of pop-off valves are available, but those with a spring-loaded disk are common. The pop-off valve is most convenient and relatively conservative with absorbent if it is located between the expiratory one-way valve and the absorbent canister. This location limits waste of fresh gases during exhalation. The pop-off valve is a major safety feature of a circle breathing system regardless of the mode of operation of the circle (e.g., closed, low-flow, or semiclosed fresh gas flow rates). The pop-off valve is designed to prevent the inadvertent buildup of pressure, and it should remain open except during the administration of positive-pressure ventilation.

Reservoir Bag   This bag is located on the absorber side of the circle, either upstream or downstream from the canister, depending on the manufacturer. The reservoir bag, which attaches to the bag port, has an outside diameter of 22 mm for small animal circles and 50 mm (2 inches) for large animal circle systems. Gas from an appropriately sized reservoir meets the patient's peak inspiratory flow demands and provides compliance in the system during exhalation.[3] The bag also provides a mechanism for assisted or controlled ventilation. Excursions of the bag during spontaneous ventilation enable the anesthetist to assess respiratory rate and to roughly estimate the tidal volume. In addition, if the pop-off valve is inadvertently left closed, the bag provides a compliant area of the system to prevent the immediate buildup of excessive pressure. Ideally, the bag should not allow pressures to exceed 60 cm H_2O.[3] The minimum size of the reservoir should be six times the patient's tidal volume, but as a matter of practicality, the bag's volume should exceed the patient's inspiratory capacity. Therefore, a spontaneous deep breath should not empty the bag.[4] For small animal circle systems, 1-, 2-, 3-, and 5-L bags are common, whereas 15-, 20-, or 30-L bags are used for large animals. An optimally sized bag enables the anesthetist to manually support ventilation comfortably and to observe ventilatory excursions. An unnecessarily large bag is cumbersome, impairs monitoring, and slows changes in the inspired anesthetic concentration when settings on an out-of-circuit vaporizer are increased or decreased.

Manometer   This device (Fig. 17.47) is a pressure gauge that is usually attached to the top of the absorber assembly. It is calibrated in centimeters of water (cm H_2O), although it may have a scale in kilopascals or in millimeters of mercury (mm Hg). Primarily, manometers are used to assess pressures during assisted or controlled ventilation.

Air-Intake Valve   This valve (negative-pressure–relief valve) is included on some veterinary anesthesia machines (Matrx VMS small animal) (Fig. 17.47). Located on the dome of the inspiratory one-way valve in these small circle systems, the valve will entrain room air in emergencies (i.e., absence of fresh gas inflow). If fresh gas flow is interrupted, the valve allows ambient air (21% oxygen) to enter the circle and prevents the patient from inspiring against a negative pressure and becoming hypoxic.

In-circuit Vaporizers   Vaporizers can be located within the breathing system (Fig. 17.29), the Ohio #8 glass bottle and the Stephens being the most likely vaporizers located in this position. The primary requirement is that the in-circuit vaporizer be of a low-resistance type, because patients must inspire through the vaporizer.

Absorber   This assembly, which contains the canister for the chemical absorbent for carbon dioxide, is located between the one-way valves, on the side of the circle opposite the patient (Fig. 17.48). The canister is usually one plastic container or two stacked plastic containers. For a specific patient, the canister should be large enough to contain an airspace between chemical granules that is equal to or greater than the patient's maximum tidal volume. The intergranular space is approximately 50% when a canister is filled with standard absorbent (4- to 8-mesh size).[4] Exhaled gases may enter the top or bottom of a canister, and baffles or annular rings (Fig. 17.49) in many absorbers move gases toward the center of the canister to compensate for lower resistance to gas flow near the canister wall. Without baffles or annular rings, channeling of gases and inefficient absorption of the carbon dioxide may occur. Internal tubes for gas return from an absorber may enhance the wall effect and gas channeling.[2] Some absorber units, especially those for large animals, have drain in the bottom to discharge water that condenses from exhaled gases.

The canister filled with absorbent, besides being a source of resistance during ventilation, is an important area for malfunctions in circle systems. The canister is removed regularly to change the absorbent, and failure to create a seal adequately when replacing the canister causes leaks. Normal wear and tear may damage the canister, the caustic effects of soda lime may

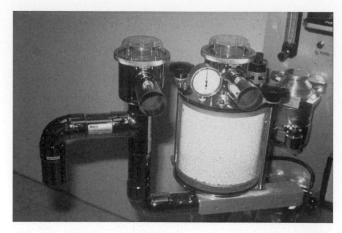

Fig. 17.48.   Absorber assembly for a Matrx (Orchard Park, NY) large animal circle breathing system. Attached to the absorber canister are the unidirectional valves, the manometer, the ports for the breathing hoses and reservoir bag, and the pop-off valve.

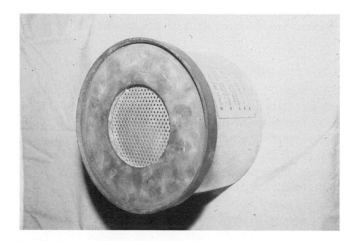

Fig. 17.49.   An absorber assembly with an annular ring. The ring diameter, being smaller than the canister diameter, promotes dispersion of gases throughout the canister and helps to prevent preferential flow of gases next to the walls of the canister leading to the development of dead space.

corrode metal parts, and aging causes gaskets to deteriorate. Simply leaving soda lime granules on the gaskets can make a tight seal impossible. One report described the bypass of soda lime with resultant hypercarbia because of the disconnection of the diffuser foot from the conduction tube in the canister on a veterinary anesthesia machine.[37] Newer circle systems are constructed with materials less vulnerable to the effects of soda lime.

Some circle systems were designed with a mechanism for purposely bypassing the absorbent canister (Fig. 17.50). The bypass was intended for use during the changing of soda lime and for intentionally elevating the inspired concentration of carbon dioxide.[2] If these obsolete systems are used in veterinary practices, the operator should understand the function of the bypass and its control apparatus and should not operate the circle in the bypass mode.

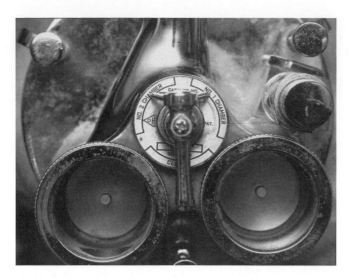

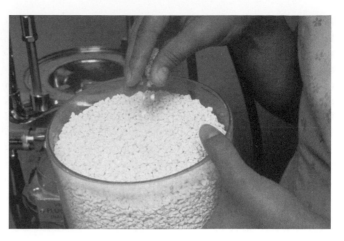

Fig. 17.50. The top of an absorber from an obsolete circle breathing system. The control on the absorber functions to direct exhaled gases through one or both chambers of the canister. With both indicators in the closed position, exhaled gases bypass the carbon dioxide absorbent completely.

Fig. 17.51. Evaluation of the consistency of soda lime granules. Functional granules are relatively soft and easily crushed, whereas expended granules are hard.

Chemical absorption of carbon dioxide is a fundamental function of circle and to-and-fro breathing systems. Depending on the fresh gas inflow, all or part of the exhaled carbon dioxide may be absorbed chemically. If the fresh gas flow approximates the patient's oxygen consumption, almost all exhaled carbon dioxide will be chemically neutralized. Chemical absorption of carbon dioxide allows lower fresh gas flows, reduces wastage of anesthetics and oxygen, and lowers the cost for anesthesia. With high fresh gas flows, much of the exhaled carbon dioxide escapes through the pop-off valve and into the scavenger system, and the dependence on chemical absorption of carbon dioxide is decreased.

Chemical Absorption of Carbon Dioxide

Calcium hydroxide is the primary component of soda lime and barium hydroxide lime, the two most common absorbents for carbon dioxide. Small amounts of sodium and potassium hydroxide in soda lime activate the reaction, and silica and kieselguhr are included to give hardness to the granules.[2,3] Barium hydroxide lime is inherently hard owing to bound water molecules and does not require silica.[2] For optimal absorption of carbon dioxide, 14% to 19% H_2O is required in soda lime. Water formed during granule reactions with carbon dioxide can be useful in humidifying dry gases from the fresh gas inlet, but does not participate in the reactions of chemical absorption of carbon dioxide. The overall chemical reaction of carbon dioxide with soda lime includes multiple steps (e.g., carbon dioxide first reacts with water to form carbonic acid), but can be summarized as follows:

$$2\,NaOH + 2\,H_2CO_3 + Ca(OH)_2 \rightarrow CaCO_3 + Na_2CO_3 + 4\,H_2O + heat$$

($CaCO_3$, calcium carbonate; $Ca[OH]_2$, calcium hydroxide; H_2CO_3, carbonic acid; Na_2CO_3, disodium carbonate; and $NaOH$, sodium hydroxide)

The granule size for chemical absorbents is typically 4 to 8 mesh and represents a compromise between absorptive activity and airflow resistance.[2] Small granules offer the most surface area for chemical reactions, but large granules impose less resistance to gas flow through the canister. Proper packing of a canister is necessary to prevent flow of gases over a single pathway in the canister, creating excessive dead space. Gentle shaking of the canister upon filling it with an absorbent will avoid loose packing and reduce channeling. Packing too tightly should be avoided to prevent formation of dust and increased resistance to ventilation.[4]

During evaluation of a rebreathing system, the anesthetist should confirm that the absorbent is functional. Fresh granules of calcium hydroxide are soft enough to be easily crushed, whereas expended granules have chemically changed to calcium carbonate and are hard (Fig. 17.51). Indicators of pH are added to absorbents to show color changes as chemical reactions proceed. Soda lime changes from white to violet as the granules are exhausted. The violet may revert to white during storage, but will reappear when the granules are exposed to carbon dioxide again. Newer CO_2 absorbents will maintain this color change and are less reactant producing less heat, carbon monoxide, and compound A. The absorption of carbon dioxide is an exothermic reaction, and a "heat line" should be detectable on the wall of the canister if carbon dioxide absorption is effective. Heat is particularly notable in canisters for large animals. The amount of carbon dioxide absorption is about 26 L/100 g,[4] but efficiency may vary, depending on the design of the canister and the method of packing. When using a circle system with a chemical absorbent, the inspired carbon dioxide should be near zero.[2] Measuring the concentration of carbon dioxide in inspired gases, with 0.1% to 1.0% being acceptable[38,39] is the most accurate way to determine whether the absorbent is functional.[2,3] Without such measurements, the absorbent should be exchanged when the color reaction is apparent in approximately two-thirds of the absorbent.[2,36]

Fresh Gas Flows for Circle Breathing Systems

Fresh gas flow–rate recommendations for circle systems are somewhat controversial. Semiclosed, low-flow, and closed circles are the options, and when all factors are considered, a veterinarian's personal preference usually determines the flow of fresh gas. Nevertheless, there are differing advantages to the various fresh gas flow rates discussed. The terms *closed, low-flow,* and *semiclosed* are often used in reference to circle breathing systems and refer to the fresh gas–inflow rate compared with the metabolic needs of the patient. The terms do not denote any structural differences among the breathing systems, and they do *not* relate any information about the state of the pop-off valve (open or closed).

Closed Circle System

Closed-system anesthesia occurs when there is a low flow of anesthetic gases and oxygen to the patient and system.[3] Thus, the oxygen flow into a closed circle approximates the patient's oxygen consumption, which varies with the patient's metabolic rate. Metabolic rate and oxygen consumption are influenced by the patient's body weight and body-surface area, its temperature, its state of consciousness, and the type of anesthetic. Table 17.4 lists values for oxygen consumption in dogs as reported in several publications. Table 17.5 includes published recommendations for fresh gas flows for closed circle systems in dogs, and all fall within the minimum and maximum rates of oxygen consumption reported for dogs as listed in Table 17.4. In practice, observation of the reservoir bag enables the anesthetist to adjust the fresh gas flow to approximate the patient's uptake of gases when using a closed system.

Although a patient's oxygen consumption is used to guide the rate of fresh gas flow into a closed system, the minimum flow of carrier gas for accurate function of the vaporizer should be considered. Concentration-calibrated, variable-bypass vaporizers (VOCs) require a certain minimum flow to assure proper performance, and flow below the minimum may cause erratic output of anesthetic. With a vaporizer, the lowest flow known to produce a reliable output should be the minimum acceptable flow for the breathing system. Strategies for using closed-system anesthesia with both in-circuit and out-of-circuit vaporizers have been reviewed.[24]

Generally, N_2O is not used in a closed breathing system because of the potential for developing hypoxic gas mixtures with low inflow of oxygen. If N_2O is administered in a closed system, continuous monitoring of F_IO_2 is imperative. With closed systems, denitrogenation of the system by emptying the reservoir bag through the pop-off valve and refilling the system with fresh gas should be done two to four times during the first 15 min of anesthesia and each 30 min thereafter to prevent exhaled nitrogen from diluting oxygen in the system.[31,40] A closed system is completely dependent on chemical carbon dioxide absorption, and the quality of the absorbent should be assured before each use. Ideally, the inspired concentration of carbon dioxide should be monitored to assure proper function of the absorbent. Closed systems are more economic, retain more heat and humidity, and are less likely to produce operating-room pollution than other systems.

Table 17.4. Values reported for consumption of oxygen in dogs

Oxygen Consumption ($mL \cdot kg^{-1} \cdot min^{-1}$)	Conditions	Reference
6 to 8 $mL \cdot kg^{-1} \cdot min^{-1}$	Anesthetized	Soma[46]
10 to 11 $mL \cdot kg^{-1} \cdot min^{-1}$	Anesthetized	Soma[46]
4 to 8 $mL \cdot kg^{-1} \cdot min^{-1}$	Awake, resting	Haskins[63]
9 to 14 $mL \cdot kg^{-1} \cdot min^{-1}$	Ketamine anesthesia	Haskins[63]
3 to 7 $mL \cdot kg^{-1} \cdot min^{-1}$	Barbiturate and inhalant anesthesia	Haskins[63]
4 to 7 $mL \cdot kg^{-1} \cdot min^{-1}$	Basal metabolic rate	Wagner and Bednarski[24]

Table 17.5. Recommendations for oxygen flow for closed circle systems in veterinary anesthesia

Oxygen Flow Rate	Reference
11 $mL \cdot kg^{-1} \cdot min^{-1}$	Hartsfield[5]
4.4 to 11 $mL \cdot kg^{-1} \cdot min^{-1}$	Muir and Hubbell[41]
4 to 7 $mL \cdot kg^{-1} \cdot min^{-1}$	Wagner and Bednarski[24]
4.4 to 6.6 $mL \cdot kg^{-1} \cdot min^{-1}$	Muir and Hubbell[32]

Low-Flow Circle System

Low-flow anesthesia for small animals has been defined as an oxygen flow rate greater than the patient's oxygen consumption (4 to 7 $mL \cdot kg^{-1} \cdot min^{-1}$) but less than 22 $mL \cdot kg^{-1} \cdot min^{-1}$.[24] In the definition, 22 $mL \cdot kg^{-1} \cdot min^{-1}$ was used because it is the lower limit of the traditional range of flow for a semiclosed circle system.[41] The advantages of a low-flow system are similar to those for a closed system, including economy, reduced waste gas, and some retention of heat and moisture.[42] The primary disadvantage of low-oxygen-flow techniques relates to the inadequate delivery of anesthetic from a concentration-calibrated, variable-bypass vaporizer during mask induction or during the transition from a short-acting injectable anesthetic induction to the maintenance of inhalant anesthesia. The suggested solution for this problem is the use of higher fresh gas flow rates for the first 15 to 30 min of anesthesia, followed by a change to low-flow technique after the uptake of inhalant anesthetic by the patient has decreased.[24] Similarly, changing depth of anesthesia is slower with low fresh gas flow rates. To increase anesthetic concentration in the system with a concentration-calibrated, out-of-circuit vaporizer, the fresh gas flow should be increased temporarily to speed the process. To lower the anesthetic concentration, the concentration setting on the vaporizer should be decreased and fresh gas inflow increased with either an out-of-circuit or in-circuit vaporizer location. For small animals, 10 to 15 $mL \cdot kg^{-1} \cdot min^{-1}$ has been suggested as an appropriate flow rate for a low-flow system.[24]

Semiclosed Circle System

This terminology describes a system in which the fresh gas inflow exceeds the uptake of oxygen and anesthetic by the patient.

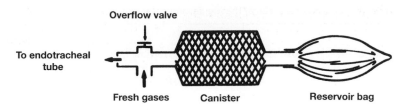

Fig. 17.52. Diagram of a to-and-fro rebreathing delivery system showing the component parts: patient connector, pop-off valve, fresh gas inlet, canister, and reservoir bag. From Hartsfield.[5]

Traditional flows for semiclosed circle systems range from 22 to 44 mL · kg^{-1} · min^{-1}.[24,41] A significant quantity of excess gas must be eliminated through the pop-off valve. The choice of flow rate for a semiclosed circle is based primarily on personal preference, but the patient's oxygen consumption times three has been a common guideline. For example, if a dog's oxygen consumption is 7 mL · kg^{-1} · min^{-1}, the fresh gas flow would be 21 mL · kg^{-1} · min^{-1}. Use of N$_2$O will increase total gas flow requirement. For a 50% N$_2$O mixture, oxygen flow would equal 21 mL · kg^{-1} · min^{-1}, and N$_2$O flow would equal 21 mL · kg^{-1} · min^{-1}, with a total fresh gas flow of 42 mL · kg^{-1} · min^{-1}. With a semiclosed circle, nitrogen accumulation within the system is not significant because gases are rapidly eliminated through the pop-off valve. N$_2$O can be used safely, the inspired anesthetic concentration can be changed rapidly, and dependency on the carbon dioxide absorbent is less because carbon dioxide is partly eliminated through the pop-off valve into the scavenging system. However, the retention of heat and humidity is lessened, and economy is less, compared with closed and low-flow systems.

Breathing systems that produce the least resistance to gas flow should be chosen for spontaneously breathing patients. Resistance to gas flow through a circle breathing system is influenced primarily by the pop-off valve, unidirectional valves, and carbon dioxide absorbent canister.[2] The total resistance in a circle system varies with the fresh gas flow rate and the type of ventilation. High fresh gas flow rates can increase flow through the pop-off valve and therefore may increase resistance to ventilation. The ventilation pattern affects the flow rate and therefore the resistance through the soda lime canister and the unidirectional valves.[2]

Resistance to breathing has been cited as a reason for not using adult circle systems for pediatric patients. However, Dorsch and Dorsch[2] suggest that the use of circle systems in spontaneously breathing pediatric patients may not be contraindicated solely on the basis of resistance. For veterinary patients, it has been recommended that circle breathing systems are appropriate for healthy animals weighing as little as 2.5 to 3.0 kg.[24,43,44]

Resistance to constant flow in large animal breathing circuits has been assessed.[45] Greater resistance occurs with higher flows through all of the breathing circuits. The Drager and Fraser Sweatman circuits were intermediate in total resistance when nine different circuits were compared, and each circuit had individual parts that contributed significantly to resistance in at least one of the circuit types. Since low resistance is considered an advantage, it has been suggested that most larger animal breathing circuits be redesigned to help minimize resistance.

To-and-Fro System

This type of rebreathing system (Fig. 17.52) is much less popular than the rebreathing circle and Mapleson systems. The to-and-fro system has a carbon dioxide–absorbent canister located between the endotracheal tube connector and a reservoir bag. A pop-off valve and the fresh gas inlet are positioned between the canister and the endotracheal tube connector. A to-and-fro system is suitable for both large and small animals if proper canisters are available.[28,46] With low flows approximating the patient's oxygen consumption, carbon dioxide removal depends on chemical absorption. With higher flows, part of the expired carbon dioxide is vented through the pop-off valve.

Portability, simplicity, and ease of disassembly for cleaning are advantages of the to-and-fro system. Disadvantages are related to the position of the system, including the canister, next to the patient. Heat produced during carbon dioxide absorption may be transferred to the patient during inspiration, there is greater potential for inhalation of alkaline dust from the absorbent than with a circle system, and the system is quite cumbersome. Over time, channeling of gases through the canister may create dead space in the absorbent, causing inefficient absorption of carbon dioxide. The horizontal position of the canister is probably less desirable than the vertical position used in most circle rebreathing systems.[4] As with circle systems, denitrogenation during the early phases of anesthesia is required to prevent hypoxia, especially with lower fresh gas flows.

Mapleson Systems

Breathing systems that use no chemical absorbent for carbon dioxide, but depend primarily on high fresh gas flow rates to flush exhaled carbon dioxide from the system, have been classified as Mapleson systems. They have been called *nonrebreathing systems* as a group, though this terminology is technically incorrect because some rebreathing of exhaled gases occurs in most of these systems, especially with lower recommended flow rates.[5]

The Mapleson systems are simple and easy to use, are easily cleaned and sterilized, are lightweight and compact, can be positioned conveniently, have few moving parts, are relatively inexpensive, impart little resistance to respiration, do not require carbon dioxide absorbents, add minimal mechanical dead space, and allow the inspired concentration of anesthetic to be changed rapidly. The main disadvantages of using Mapleson systems is the requirement for higher flow rates of fresh gas, which decreases temperature and increases cost. Higher flow rates promote hypothermia and drying of the respiratory tract. The Mapleson sys-

Table 17.6. Characteristics of the Mapleson breathing systems

Class	Fresh Gas Inlet	Overflow Location	Presence of a Reservoir	Corrugated Tubing	Example System
A	Near the reservoir	Near the patient	Yes	Yes	Magill
B	Near the patient	Near the patient	Yes	Yes	a
C	Near the patient	Near the patient	Yes	No	a
D	Near the patient	Away from the patient[b]	Yes	Yes	a
MD[c]	Near the patient	Away from the patient	Yes	Yes	Bain
E	Near the patient	Away from the patient	No	Yes	T-piece
F	Near the patient	Away from the patientb	Yes	Yes	Jackson-Rees

[a]No system in this classification is commonly used in veterinary anesthesia.
[b]The overflow may be located between the reservoir and the corrugated tubing of the system.
[c]MD, modified Mapleson D system.

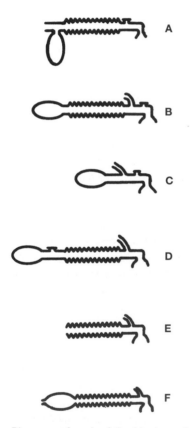

Fig. 17.53. Diagrams of each of the Mapleson breathing systems (*A–F*, Mapleson systems). From Rayburn.[64]

tems are diagramed in Fig. 17.53, and characteristics of the Mapleson systems are listed in Table 17.6.

Magill System
The Magill system (Fig. 17.54) is classified as a Mapleson A system and is characterized by a fresh gas inlet, an overflow valve near the patient, and a corrugated tube connecting the patient end of the system to a reservoir bag.[46] Fresh gas flows continuously

into the reservoir bag and into the corrugated tubing, moving carbon dioxide–rich gases through the overflow valve. The system is efficient during spontaneous ventilation, but, during controlled ventilation, some rebreathing of expired gases occurs. Fresh gas inflow should approximate the patient's minute volume,[9] with flows less than 0.7 of minute volume leading to some rebreathing.[2] The N_2O flow should be calculated as a part of the total fresh gas inflow. The volume of the corrugated tubing and the reservoir bag should be equal to or greater than the patient's tidal volume. Because of the location of the overflow valve, the system is relatively cumbersome during controlled ventilation.

Bain Coaxial System
This system (Fig. 17.55) is classified as a modified Mapleson D design. It is configured as a tube within a tube.[9] The internal tube (0.7 mm ID) supplies fresh gases to the patient end of the system (Fig. 17.56), minimizing mechanical dead space. The Bain system accepts an endotracheal connector (15 mm) or a mask (22 mm). The external corrugated tube conducts exhaled gases from the patient to a reservoir bag. The reservoir bag may attach directly to the corrugated tubing, in which case the pop-off valve is built into the bag, or the corrugated tubing may attach to a metal head with drilled channels and accommodations for the reservoir bag, the overflow valve, and optionally a manometer.[2,3]

Recommendations for total fresh gas flow into a Bain system are variable for both human and animal patients. Recommendations have been based on minute volume, body weight, and body surface area.[2] During spontaneous ventilation, 200 to 300 mL · kg^{-1} · min^{-1} has been recommended for anesthesia of human patients.[9] Fresh gas flows from 100 to 150 mL · kg^{-1} · min^{-1} have been recommended for veterinary patients.[36,47] Some investigators[48] have suggested a fresh gas flow rate of 200 mL · kg^{-1} min^{-1} for patients weighing less than 7 kg, whereas others have recommended a flow rate of 220 to 330 mL · kg^{-1} · min^{-1}.[32] The fresh gas flow that will eliminate rebreathing during spontaneous ventilation with a Bain system differs significantly from patient to patient. After reviewing numerous references, Dorsch and Dorsch[3] concluded that most studies recommended fresh gas flows of 1.5 to 3.0 times minute volume. Less than two to three

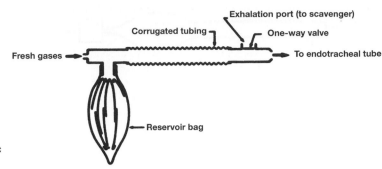

Fig. 17.54. Diagram of a Magill system illustrating the basic components and the entry of fresh gases. From Hartsfield.[5]

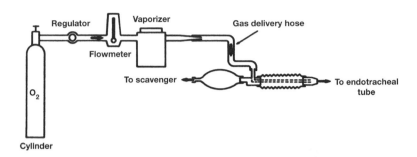

Fig. 17.55. Diagram of a Bain coaxial system attached to an anesthesia machine. Fresh gas flows from the outlet of the vaporizer or the common gas outlet of the anesthesia machine to enter the Bain system near the reservoir. Moving through the Bain's inner tube, fresh gas is delivered near the patient end of the system. Exhaled gases flow through the corrugated tubing to the reservoir and the overflow to the scavenging system.

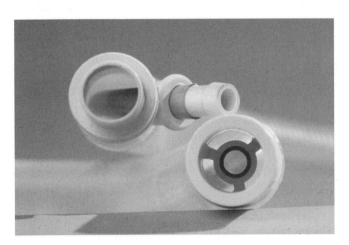

Fig. 17.56. The two ends of a Bain coaxial system showing the location for attachment of the reservoir bag (*top left*) and the endotracheal tube (*bottom right*). Fresh gases enter at the reservoir end (Y connection at the *top right*) and move through the small inner tube to the patient end of the system (triangular supports). From Hartsfield.[5]

times the minute volume will result in some rebreathing of carbon dioxide, but the end-tidal carbon dioxide concentration may remain normal even with some rebreathing of carbon dioxide.[3] For spontaneously breathing patients, 440 to 660 mL · kg^{-1} · min^{-1} may be used for maintenance of anesthesia with the Bain system to assure that rebreathing of exhaled gases does not contribute to increases in arterial carbon dioxide partial pressure. Without regular monitoring of carbon dioxide tensions or expired carbon dioxide values, the exact flow requirements are difficult

to define for an individual patient. Minute volumes for dogs and cats range from 170 to 350 mL · kg^{-1} · min^{-1} and 200 to 350 mL · kg^{-1} · min^{-1}, respectively.[49] Using these values for minute volume, an argument can be made for even higher flows than 660 mL · kg^{-1} · min^{-1}. In general, a total fresh gas flow of less than 500 mL/min or more than 3 L/min with a Bain system is not recommended for animals that weigh less than 6.8 kg. With controlled ventilation, 100 mL · kg^{-1} · min^{-1} is apparently an adequate flow for fresh gases.[50] For larger patients maintained with an adult Bain system, lower total fresh gas flow (e.g., 100 mL · kg^{-1} · min^{-1}) may be appropriate. Use of Bain systems has been effective in dogs weighing up to 35.5 kg.[47] Fresh gas flows higher than usually recommended are indicated in situations of increased carbon dioxide production, increased dead space, and decreased minute ventilation.[3] Flow rates of two to three times minute volume have been recommended for hypoventilating animals in which controlled ventilation was not corrective.[47]

During spontaneous ventilation, a Mapleson D system has been shown to function identically to a Mapleson F system.[2] The Bain's coaxial design has been shown to be effective in reducing loss of heat and humidity,[2] although the overall benefit is questionable in small veterinary patients maintained with relatively high fresh gas flow rates.

Ayre's T-Piece and Norman Mask Elbow Systems

Ayre's T-piece and Norman mask elbow systems (Fig. 17.57) equipped with an expiratory limb (corrugated tubing) and reservoir bag are classed as Mapleson F systems.[2] Without a reservoir bag, they are Mapleson E systems. The T piece itself is a T-shaped tube with a 1-cm ID. Fresh gas enters the tube from the side, perpendicular to the direction of gas glow during ventilation

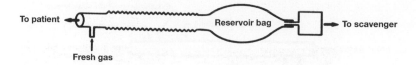

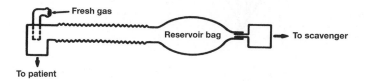

Fig. 17.57. Diagrams of Norman Mask Elbow system (*bottom*) and Ayre's T-piece system (*top*). From Hartsfield.[5]

(Fig. 17.57). One end of the tube attaches to the endotracheal tube connector, and the other end attaches to an expiratory arm (corrugated tubing equivalent to one-third of the patient's tidal volume) to which a reservoir bag may or may not be attached. The reservoir bag has an overflow valve. An Ayre's T piece with an expiratory tube and reservoir is a Rees modification of an Ayre's T piece or a Jackson-Rees system.[2]

During spontaneous ventilation, fresh gas flows to the patient during inspiration; during expiration and prior to the next inspiration, gas flows toward the reservoir. Gas flow follows the path of least resistance. Inspiratory flow requirements in excess of the fresh gas flow are obtained from the expiratory arm and reservoir. During expiration and before inspiration, high gas flow clears exhaled gases from the expiratory tube and washes out carbon dioxide. Such a system should have an ID of at least 1 cm to minimize resistance.

Generally, two to three times the patient's minute volume is recommended to prevent dilution of the inspired anesthetic concentration and rebreathing of carbon dioxide with Mapleson F systems. If N_2O is used, the desired concentration is calculated using N_2O as a portion of the total fresh gas flow. Variable recommendations for the most appropriate flow rates to use with these systems exist in the veterinary literature.

In a Norman mask elbow system, the direction of gas flow into the system is parallel to the flow of gases into the endotracheal tube during inspiration and expiration (Fig. 17.57). The fresh gas inlet is located in the center of the patient end of the system. This location probably reduces dead space slightly more than the Ayre's T-piece system. Also, the patient end of the elbow accepts a standard mask (22 mm). Recommendations for flow rates, tube sizes and volumes, and reservoir sizes and volumes are similar to those for the Ayre's T-piece system. Controlled ventilation can be used with either system by closing the overflow valve and compressing the reservoir bag. To prevent rebreathing during controlled ventilation, the expiratory tube's volume should be greater than the patient's tidal volume.

Resistance to ventilation in the Mapleson systems is minimal,[2] which may be advantageous for small patients. The advantages of modern "non-rebreathing" systems for very small patients include decreased resistance to ventilation, better gas exchange, greater control of the depth of anesthesia, and fewer mechanical

problems.[48] Hazards of non-rebreathing systems relate primarily to outflow occlusion, development of excessive airway pressure, and barotraumas to the lungs, including development of pneumothorax.

Care in positioning the Mapleson systems and judicious use of overflow valves during positive-pressure ventilation are important considerations. Activation of the flush valve when a non-rebreathing system is being used can overpressurize the respiratory system, causing volutrauma (rapid overexpansion of the lungs) and subsequent pneumothorax. Therefore, the machine's flush valve should not be used when one of the Mapleson systems is connected to a patient.

Systems with Non-rebreathing Valves

Numerous non-rebreathing valves (e.g., Stephens-Slater, Fink, and Digby-Leigh) have been designed for anesthesia breathing systems, but they are not commonly used today.[3] These breathing systems with one-way valves were cumbersome, and essentially have been replaced by the Mapleson and circle systems. Presently, non-rebreathing valves are used most in self-inflating bags for resuscitation or transport of patients requiring manual ventilation.

Stephens-Slater System

This system (Fig. 17.58) was in common use in veterinary anesthesia in the 1970s, but today is mainly of historical interest. The system was designed with two one-way valves, one directing gas from the reservoir to the patient and blocking exhaled gases from the reservoir and a second valve directing exhaled gases away from the system and preventing entry of ambient gases during inspiration. Fresh gases enter the system through the reservoir bag and move through the inspiratory valve to the patient. The recommended total fresh gas flow is equal to the patient's minute volume.[2,46] The flow of N_2O, if used, is calculated as a part of the total fresh gas flow. Since the valves are located near the patient, the system is cumbersome, especially with manual ventilation, during which the exhalation valve is held closed while the reservoir bag is compressed. The reservoir must be monitored closely to assure sufficient gas to meet inspiratory demands. This valved system added minimal dead space and resistance to respiration. However, the valve flaps could stick and obstruct ventilation. The

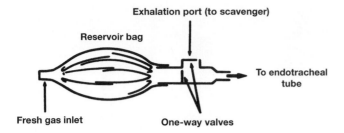

Fig. 17.58. Diagram of a Stephens-Slater system. From Hartsfield.[5]

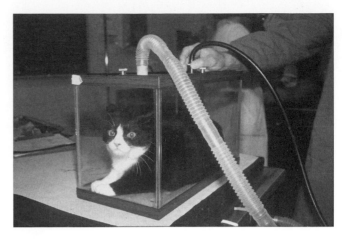

Fig. 17.59. Closed container for oxygenation and inhalant inductions in small patients. The container is clear so that the animal can be monitored during the induction process. The ports for the entrance of fresh gases and for attachment of a scavenging system are on the lid.

system was popular prior to the advent of scavenging, which presents some difficulty with the Stephens-Slater system.

Resuscitation Bags

These self-inflating bags incorporate non-rebreathing valves. As an example, an Ambu bag (a bag valve mask) facilitates resuscitation and transport of apneic or anesthetized patients. Oxygen can be delivered into the reservoir bag to increase F_IO_2. When the bag is compressed, the increase in pressure closes the exhalation port and gases enter the patient's respiratory system. When pressure on the bag is released, gas flows from the patient's respiratory system through the exhalation port. With spontaneous breathing, the Ambu valve allows the patient to inhale room air only. The Ambu E2 is a modification that allows the patient to inhale both from the reservoir and from the exhalation port, creating a mixture of fresh gas and air. During controlled ventilation, all gases originate from the reservoir.[2]

Closed Containers and Masks

Closed Containers

Closed containers are used for oxygenation and inhalant inductions in small veterinary patients. Inhalant inductions have decreased in popularity because of the difficulty associated with scavenging of waste gases, especially as an anesthetized patient is removed from the chamber. Perhaps, the only completely effective way to assure elimination of waste anesthetic gases with this system is the concurrent use of a fume hood. The primary advantage of induction in a closed container is the reduced requirement for physical restraint of the patient. Induction in a closed container is very effective for aggressive cats and for some laboratory and small wild or exotic species. Often, the container can be placed over the animal, eliminating the need for any physical contact and restraint.

Most containers for inhalant inductions are constructed of glass, Plexiglas, or other clear plastic materials (Fig. 17.59), allowing the patient to be observed during induction. Since the airway might become obstructed during a closed-container induction, ventilatory efforts should be monitored throughout the process. The chamber should be no larger than necessary, but the animal should be able to lie in lateral recumbency without having to flex its neck. A chamber that is too small for the patient promotes airway obstruction. Excessive chamber volume slows the rate of rise of anesthetic concentration and the onset of induc-

tion. When the patient is induced and is manageable, it should be removed from the chamber, and the induction should be completed by mask.

Relatively high flows of fresh gas facilitate inductions in closed containers. The outlet of the chamber should be attached to a scavenger system when anesthetic is being administered. Chamber inductions should be done in a well-ventilated area, ideally, under a fume hood that vents all waste gases from the working environment. Depending on the size of the chamber and the body weight of the patient, total flow of fresh gas into the chamber should be approximately 2 to 5 L/min.[51] Low flow rates of fresh gases slow induction and contribute to the development of excitement. Oxygen should be administered for about 5 min before the introduction of inhalant anesthetic. Then, the concentration of the inhalant should be increased at 0.5% increments every 10 s until 4% to 4.5% sevoflurane or isoflurane is being administered. Unless N_2O is contraindicated because of patient pathology, it can be used in concentrations of 60% to 70%.

Masks

Mask inductions (Fig. 17.60) are facilitated by anesthetic concentrations and fresh gas flows that are similar to those for closed containers. Mask inductions are smoothest in depressed, tranquilized, or sedated patients. Masks should fit snugly over the muzzle to minimize dead space, and the appropriate size for the patient should be used. A tight-fitting mask promotes a rapid induction and minimal contamination of the workplace with waste gases. A clear mask with a rubber diaphragm (Fig. 17.61) enables visualization of the nares and mouth during induction and creates a good seal around the animal's muzzle. The mask should be attached to a breathing system to provide a reservoir of gases to meet the patient's peak inspiratory flow demands, which may exceed the inflow of fresh gases. Most excess gases can be scavenged through the pop-off valve of the breathing system, but

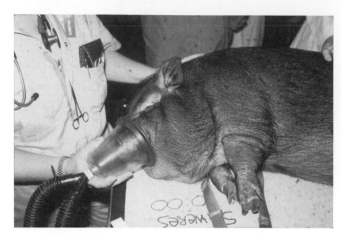

Fig. 17.60. Masking a tranquilized potbellied pig with isoflurane in oxygen administered with a transparent veterinary mask. The rubber diaphragm enables a good seal between the patient's snout and the mask, minimizing leakage.

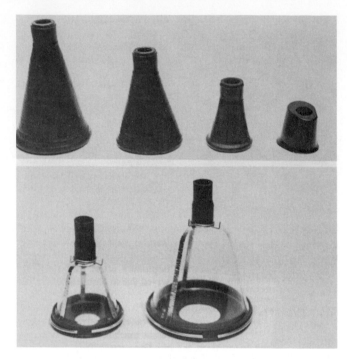

Fig. 17.61. Small animal masks of varying sizes. The clear masks with rubber diaphragms facilitate monitoring during the masking procedure, and they enable a good seal around the muzzle. A conical rubber mask of the correct size minimizes dead space under the mask. From Lumb and Jones.[31]

masking procedures should be done in a well-ventilated environment. High fresh gas flows (e.g., 3 to 5 L/min for most dogs and cats) during masking supply the oxygen demands of the patient, dilute and eliminate exhaled carbon dioxide, and provide inhalant anesthetic concentrations equivalent to the vaporizer setting (3% to 5% for isoflurane or 4% to 6% for sevoflurane) for a relatively rapid induction.

Scavenging Waste Anesthetic Gases

Over the last two decades, the exposure of medical and veterinary personnel to waste anesthetic gases has become a significant concern. A bulletin from the American Veterinary Medical Association's Liability Insurance Trust has stated the following: Numerous studies in the United States and abroad have found no conclusive evidence that waste gases or trace amounts of waste gas cause specific health problems. There is evidence, however, to suggest that removal of gases from veterinary facilities will likely improve the occupational health of the veterinary staff.[52]

At present, the Occupational Safety and Health Administration (OSHA) has no set limits for exposure to anesthetics, but OSHA can enforce recommendations of the National Institute for Occupational Safety and Health (NIOSH) under the general duty clause: The general duty of an employer is provision of a work environment that is free of recognized hazards that are likely to cause death or serious physical harm.[53,54] The recommended exposure limits from NIOSH vary from a maximum of 2 parts per million (ppm) for halogenated hydrocarbon anesthetics like halothane and isoflurane to an 8-h time-weighted average exposure to N_2O of 25 ppm. Used together, 0.5 ppm is the limit for the halogenated agent, with 25 ppm being the limit for N_2O.[55] The American Conference of Governmental Industrial Hygienists has recommended threshold-limit values of 50 ppm for halothane and N_2O as 8-h time-weighted averages.[56]

Recommendations for Controlling Waste Gases

Veterinary workers should be aware of potential risks so that they can take steps to minimize their exposure to the inhalant anesthetics. Women in the first trimester of pregnancy, individuals with hepatic or renal disease, and persons with a compromised immune system appear to be at greater risk.[57] The following considerations are important in regard to managing waste anesthetic gases:

1. All personnel should be educated about the potential health hazards associated with exposure to waste anesthetic gases.
2. Scavenger systems should be used with all anesthesia machines and breathing systems.
3. All rooms in which anesthetic gases are used should be well ventilated with an appropriate number of air exchanges (e.g., 15 air exchanges per hour).
4. Anesthetic machines and breathing systems should be maintained as leak free as possible, and the leakage tolerances should comply with established criteria (e.g., less than 300 mL/min at 30 cm H_2O for a circle breathing system with the pop-off valve closed).[3]
5. A log documenting the performance and maintenance procedures for anesthesia machines, vaporizers, and breathing systems should be maintained.

6. Personnel should minimize spillage when filling vaporizers, and keyed filling mechanisms should be considered.
7. Anesthetic concentrations in induction, operating, and recovery rooms should be periodically monitored to assure the efficacy of scavenging and other efforts to reduce contamination in the workplace.

Several ways of decreasing contamination of the occupational environment with anesthetic gases have been suggested. They include the following:

1. Avoid spills when filling vaporizers.
2. Start gas flows only after intubation of the patient.
3. Use endotracheal tubes with inflated cuffs.
4. Occlude the Y piece of the circle or the patient end of a Mapleson system if the system is disconnected from the patient.
5. Use a scavenging pop-off valve.
6. Discharge all gases through an effective scavenger system.
7. Flush breathing systems with oxygen before disconnecting the patient.
8. Use the minimum gas flow that promotes safe anesthesia.
9. Minimize the use of masks and closed containers. When using masks, be sure that they fit well, and use closed containers only in well-ventilated areas. Ideally, masks should be used under a fume hood.
10. Maintain proper ventilation in work areas and minimize exposure to exhaled gases during the initial phases of the recovery period whenever possible.

Having anesthetic machines and breathing systems properly outfitted and functional for administration of anesthetic gases is essential for assuring the minimum amount of environmental pollution. Each machine should be leak free, and each machine-breathing system combination should connect with a functional scavenger system. An efficient scavenging system is the most important factor in reducing trace anesthetic gases, because it will lower ambient concentrations by as much as 90%.[3]

Scavenging Systems

A scavenging system collects waste gases from the anesthetic breathing system and eliminates them from the workplace.[3,57] The scavenger system is composed of a gas-collecting assembly, an interface, and a disposal system (Figs. 17.62 and 17.63). Depending on the system, various types of tubing connects these parts.

The Gas-Collecting Assembly

This assembly gathers waste gases from the breathing system. At present, the exhaust outlet from the pop-off valve (Fig. 17.47) on a circle system must be either 19 mm or 30 mm in outside diameter. On older anesthesia machines, 22-mm connectors were used, which enabled the inadvertent interchange of scavenging hoses and breathing tubes. Depending on the location of the overflow in Mapleson systems (e.g., the Bain system), devices connecting the tail or the side of the reservoir bag serve as the gas-collecting assembly and attach to transfer tubing leading to the interface.

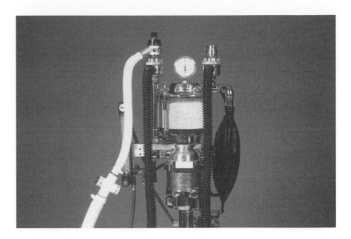

Fig. 17.62. A scavenging system (Vetroson; Summit Hill Laboratories, Navesink, NJ) on a veterinary anesthesia machine showing the pop-off valve of the circle breathing system attached to the corrugated tubing of the scavenging system that directs waste gases to the disposal system. The T-shaped component includes air-intake valves and is part of the interface that assists in the pressure regulation in the scavenging system.

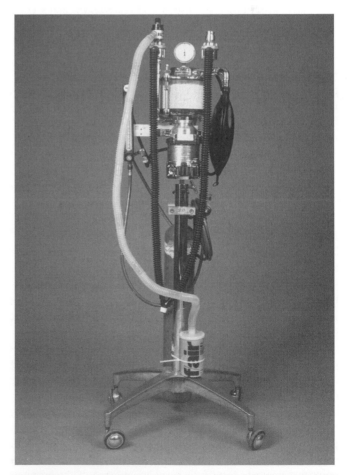

Fig. 17.63. A scavenging system including the pop-off valve, which is connected to a canister containing activated charcoal (F/air, Omnicon; Critical Care Products, Houston, TX). This system can be used for halogenated hydrocarbon anesthetics, but not for nitrous oxide.

The Interface

The interface is intended to prevent the transfer of pressure changes in the scavenging system to the breathing system. The inlet to the interface should be 19 or 30 mm OD, and the outlet can be of variable diameter (not 15 or 22 mm). Various interfaces are available (Fig. 17.62). An interface should provide positive-pressure relief to protect the patient from occlusions of the scavenging system, negative-pressure relief to limit the pressure effects of an active disposal system, and a reservoir for excess waste gas for use with active disposal systems. Interfaces may be opened or closed.[3]

The Disposal System

Disposal systems can be passive or active. Passive systems include non-recirculating ventilation systems, piping directly to the atmosphere, and absorption devices. Active systems include piped-vacuum and active duct systems. A non-recirculating ventilation system for the room allows the discharge of waste gases through an exhaust vent or grille. Discharging waste gases directly to the atmosphere is suitable for many veterinary hospitals because the distance from the gas-collecting assembly on the breathing system to the outside can be relatively short. Such systems can be affected by wind currents and should be designed so that water, wind, dust, and insects and other pests cannot enter the system from the outside.

Canisters containing activated charcoal (Fig. 17.63) will absorb halogenated hydrocarbon anesthetics with a varying degree of efficiency. The canisters are simple to use and portable. The effectiveness of absorption varies with different brands, styles of canisters, and rates of flow through the canisters. These devices must be changed regularly, making them rather expensive to use, and they do not absorb N_2O.[3] In general, other methods for scavenging waste gases are preferable, with absorption systems reserved for situations where more reliable methods are not accessible.

Central vacuum systems provide convenient anesthetic-gas disposal for hospitals with such systems already in place. The system should be able to create a flow of at least 30 L/min and functions best when the operator can manually adjust the flow.[3] The location for discharge of waste gases must be in an appropriate location and not situated where waste gases can reenter the ventilation system of the hospital. Ideally, a central vacuum system dedicated to scavenging, with another system to provide suction for other hospital needs (e.g., surgical suction), is most desirable.

An active duct system with a high volume of flow and a low negative pressure provides an excellent means of gas disposal (Fig. 17.64). Negative pressure is generated by a fan, pump, or other device in a large duct that is connected to smaller ducts that open into the room at the site of use. Such systems are effective, but regular maintenance is required to assure that the fan or pump is operational. This system is not affected by wind currents. With any disposal system, the ultimate elimination of gas must be at a point that prevents reentry of gases to any area of the hospital. The discharge site should be located away from any air-intake vents of the building, and the prevailing winds should not direct exhausted gases toward the air-intake vents of the building.

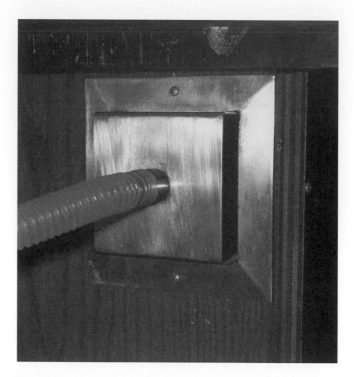

Fig. 17.64. Corrugated tubing from the pop-off valve of a circle breathing system attached to a high-volume, low-pressure scavenging system (an active duct system). Air is constantly entrained on each side of the stainless-steel plate, whereas waste gas from the breathing system enters the scavenging system through the corrugated tubing.

Anesthesia Apparatus: Checkout Recommendations

Evaluation of anesthesia machines and breathing systems is important to ensure safety for personnel and patients. For patients, delivery of appropriate concentrations and amounts of oxygen and anesthetics is essential. For personnel, the machine and breathing system should be maintained to prevent contamination of the workplace with anesthetics. The Food and Drug Administration has published "Anesthesia Apparatus Checkout Recommendations" for anesthesia-gas–delivery systems and recommends that this checkout or a reasonable equivalent be conducted before administering anesthesia. The intent is to improve patient safety.[58,59] Recommendations for checkout of veterinary machines have been published.[60]

The high-, intermediate-, and low-pressure areas of the anesthesia apparatus should be evaluated.[1–3] The high-pressure area includes gas cylinders, hanger yokes, yoke blocks, high-pressure hoses, pressure gauges, and regulators. These components are exposed to pressures up to 2200 psi for oxygen and up to 745 psi for N_2O. Testing should include inspection for loose connections and audible leakage, pressure checks (loss of pressure when cylinder valves are open and flowmeters are off), and use of soapy water solutions to "snoop" for leaks (creation of bubbles) especially at joints (Fig. 17.65). The intermediate-pressure area (approximately

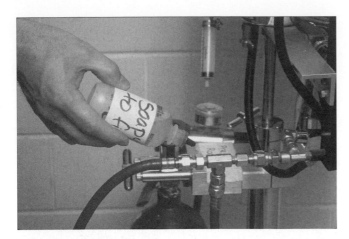

Fig. 17.65. Searching for leaks in the gas piping system of an anesthesia machine. With the cylinder valve on and pressure on the system, soapy water is applied to areas with potential for leaks. Bubbles will form if leaks are present.

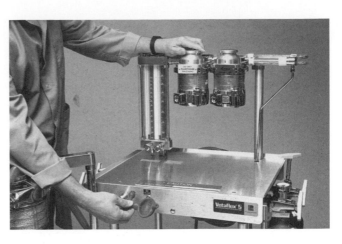

Fig. 17.66. Universal negative-pressure leak test. With all gases off and the vaporizer off, a compressed rubber bulb is attached to the common gas outlet of the anesthesia machine. The bulb should not reinflate in less than 10 s. The test should be repeated with the vaporizer control on. From Andrews.[16]

40 to 50 psi) includes pipeline inlets, conduits from pipeline inlets to flowmeters, and conduits from regulators to flowmeters, the flowmeter assembly, and the oxygen-flush apparatus. Tests include visual inspection, listening for leaks, and use of soapy water solutions. The low-pressure area includes the vaporizer(s), conduits from the flowmeters to the vaporizer, a conduit from the vaporizer to the common gas outlet, and a conduit from the common gas outlet to the breathing system. Pressures are slightly above atmospheric. Routing tests include visual inspection and pressure checks with the breathing system. In many anesthesia machines, pressure applied to the breathing system affects the low-pressure area of the machine. Some newer anesthesia machines have check valves near the common gas outlet.

A universal negative-pressure leak test has been proposed for contemporary anesthesia machines to evaluate the low-pressure area. The test requires a simple suction bulb.[16] The flowmeters and vaporizers are off during the test. The suction bulb is attached at the common gas outlet and squeezed until the bulb fully collapses, creating a vacuum in the low-pressure areas (Fig. 17.66). If the bulb reinflates in less than 10 s, a significant leak is present. The test is repeated with the control dial of the vaporizer on to detect any internal leaks that might not be found with the vaporizer off. This test differentiates between leaks in the low-pressure area of the machine (vaporizer) and the breathing system. The test can detect leaks as small as 30 mL/min and has been described as extremely reliable.

Anesthetic machines should be checked out each day before anesthetizing the first patient, and the breathing system should be evaluated before each patient. The operation manual for individual anesthesia machines gives specific guidelines for evaluation and checkout, and machines with special features require individualized attention. Ventilators on anesthesia machines and monitoring equipment should also be evaluated before beginning anesthesia. The following procedures are modified from the

"Anesthesia Apparatus Checkout Recommendations" from the FDA's Center for Devices and Radiological Health[1] and are appropriate for evaluation of anesthesia machines and breathing systems before the first case of the day:

1. Check central oxygen and N_2O supplies for adequate quantities of gases and pipeline pressures.

2. Inspect the flowmeters, vaporizers, gauges, and supply hoses. Assure correct mounting of cylinders in the hanger yokes; the presence of a wrench for cylinder valve; and a complete, undamaged breathing system with adequate absorbent for carbon dioxide.

3. Assure that the waste-scavenging system is connected to the pop-off valve and is working properly. Leak tests for the scavenger system have been recommended.[3] If a charcoal canister is being used, confirm that it is not exhausted.

4. Turn off the flow-control valves for the flowmeters.

5. Assure that the vaporizer is properly filled, with the filler cap sealed and the control dial off.

6. Check oxygen cylinders on the machine. With the pipeline supply disconnected, oxygen cylinder valve off, and pressure gauge at zero, slowly open the valve to check the pressure (500 psi) and determine the presence of leaks (a slow drop in pressure on the gauge) (Figs. 17.67 and 17.68). With multiple oxygen cylinders, each cylinder should be checked.

7. Check the N_2O supply (if present) as in step 6. If they are present, test the fail-safe devices to assure that N_2O cannot be delivered without an adequate amount of oxygen.

8. Test the flowmeters for each gas. With the flow-control valve off, the float should rest at the bottom of the glass tube. Adjust flow through the full range to assure proper function (no sticking or erratic movements).

9. Test the central pipeline supplies of oxygen and N_2O. With small (E) cylinders off and pipeline inlets connected to the cen-

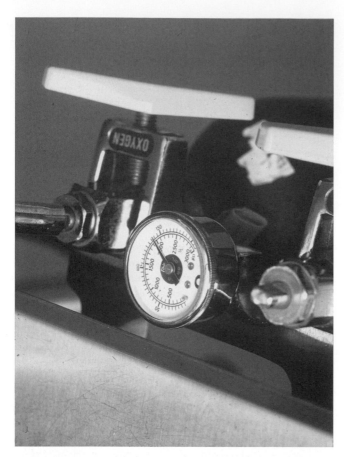

Fig. 17.67. Oxygen cylinder with the pressure gauge reading 2000 psi. An oxygen cylinder should have at least 500 psi before the cylinder and anesthesia machine are used with a patient. With oxygen flowmeters off, the cylinder valve should remain on to allow evaluation of the machine for slow leaks.

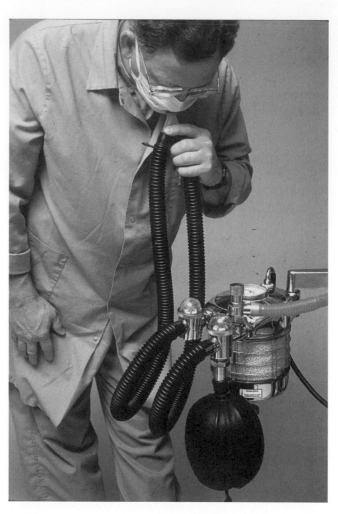

Fig. 17.69. Checking the function of the expiratory one-way valve of a circle system. Wearing a surgical mask, the evaluator exhales through the Y piece and observes the expiratory one-way valve to ensure that the valve disk moves appropriately. The reservoir bag should expand as air moves through the valve.

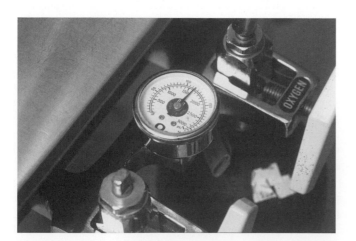

Fig. 17.68. Oxygen cylinder with the pressure gauge reading at 1700 psi after 15 min with the cylinder valve open. If the cylinder pressure was 2000 psi at the start of the test and the flowmeters were off, a significant leak is present and should be corrected before the anesthesia machine is used with a patient.

tral gas supply, adjust flows to a midrange and assure that supply pressures remain near 50 psi.

10. With the vaporizer off, no odor of anesthetic should be present when the oxygen flowmeter is on.

11. For a circle system, test the function of the unidirectional valves. Wearing a surgical mask (Fig. 17.69), exhale through the exhalation limb to check the exhalation valve, and compress the reservoir bag (pop-off valve closed and Y piece open) to check the inhalation valve (Fig. 17.70). Valve disks should be present and should rise and fall appropriately.

12. Test for leaks in the circle breathing system and the anesthesia machine. Close the pop-off valve, occlude the Y piece, fill the system with oxygen, and turn the oxygen flow to 5 L/min. As the pressure in the system reaches 20 cm H_2O, reduce the flow until the pressure in the system (manometer) no longer rises. The oxygen flow should be negligible; a high leakage rate is unacceptable. Squeeze the reservoir bag to create a relatively high pressure (40 to 50 cm H_2O) and assure a tight system. In check-

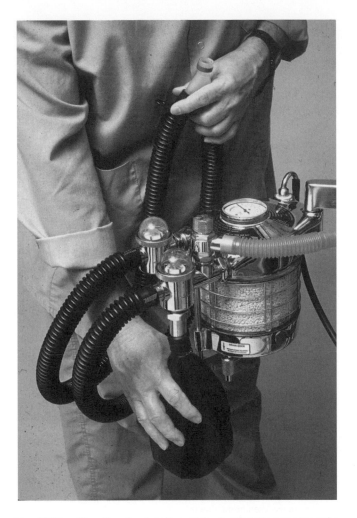

Fig. 17.70. Checking the function of the inspiratory one-way valve of a circle system. With the pop-off valve closed, the reservoir bag is compressed, and the valve disk of the inspiratory one-way valve should move appropriately.

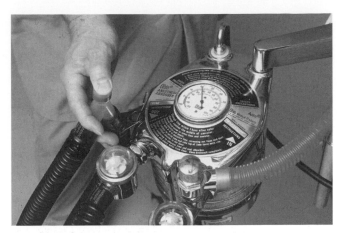

Fig. 17.71. Evaluation of the integrity of a circle breathing system. The pop-off valve is closed, the patient port is occluded, and the system is filled to a pressure of 30 cm H_2O for at least 10 s, or the leak as determined by use of the oxygen flowmeter should be less than 250 mL/min.

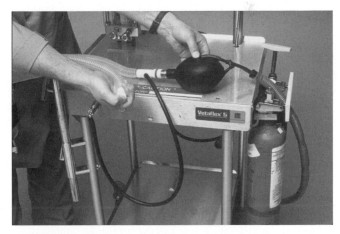

Fig. 17.72. Evaluation of a Bain breathing system (Kendall, Boston, MA) with a complete system check. With all gas flows off, the overflow valve is closed and the patient port is occluded. The bag is filled with the flush valve to a pressure of 30 cm H_2O, and a leak-free system should maintain this pressure for at least 10 s. If a leak is present, it can be quantified with the oxygen flowmeter and should not exceed 300 mL/min. From Dorsch and Dorsch.[3]

ing the circle system for leaks, one recommendation is to fill the circle (pop-off valve closed and Y piece occluded) to a pressure of 30 cm H_2O and assure that the leak rate is less than 250 mL/min[39] or that the pressure drop is less than 5 cm H_2O in 30 s or that the pressure remains at 30 cm H_2O for at least 10 s (Fig. 17.71).[3] Others have recommended similar testing procedures with slightly different values for testing pressures and acceptable leak rates.[61,62]

13. Open the pop-off valve slowly and observe the release of pressure. Occlude the Y piece and verify that only a negligible positive or negative pressure develops with an oxygen flow rate of zero or 5 L/min.

14. Assure that the pop-off valve provides relief of pressure when the flush valve is activated.

15. Similar to the circle system, non-rebreathing systems should be tested before use. For a complete system check of a Bain system, the patient port should be occluded, the relief valve closed, and the reservoir bag distended. The bag should remain

fully distended, and pressure within the system should not decrease (Fig. 17.72). The complete system check does not assure a leak-free inner tube of the coaxial system. Therefore, the inner tube is evaluated by temporarily occluding the inner tube at the patient end with oxygen flowing at approximately 1 to 2 L/min (Fig. 17.73). During a short period of occlusion with an instrument such as the plunger of a syringe, the float in the oxygen flowmeter should fall (Fig. 17.74).[2,3] The complete system check will usually suffice for other non-rebreathing systems (e.g., Norman mask elbow and Ayre's T-piece systems).

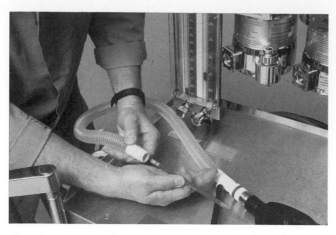

Fig. 17.73. Evaluation of the inner tube of a Bain breathing system. The first step is to turn on the oxygen flowmeter. In this example, the flow of oxygen was set at 1 L/min.

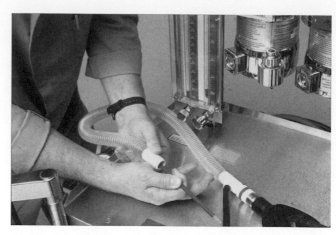

Fig. 17.74. Evaluation of the inner tube of a Bain breathing system. The second step is to occlude the patient end of the inner tube. If the inner tube is intact, the oxygen flowmeter's indicator (e.g., ball or bobbin) should fall (stop flow). From Dorsch and Dorsch.[3]

The tests mentioned here should be considered the minimum. The operation manual for a specific anesthesia machine usually provides appropriate per-use checkout procedures, and numerous other tests have been described to evaluate anesthesia apparatus.[3] Depending on the type of anesthesia machine, breathing system, ventilator (manual or mechanical), and monitoring equipment, other tests may be indicated. Veterinarians should familiarize themselves with the evaluation procedures that are most appropriate for their specific anesthesia apparatus.

References

1. American Society for Testing and Materials. Minimum Performance and Safety Requirements for Components and Systems of Anesthesia Gas Machines (ASTM F1161-99). Philadelphia: American Society for Testing and Materials, 1989.
2. Dorsch JA, Dorsch SE. Understanding Anesthesia Equipment: Construction, Care, and Complications, 2nd ed. Baltimore: Williams and Wilkins, 1984.
3. Dorsch JA, Dorsch SE. Understanding Anesthesia Equipment: Construction, Care, and Complications, 3rd ed. Baltimore: Williams and Wilkins, 1994.
4. Ehrenwerth J, Eisenkraft JB, eds. Anesthesia Equipment: Principles and Application. St Louis: CV Mosby, 1993.
5. Hartsfield SM. Machines and breathing systems for administration of inhalation anesthetics. In: Short CE, ed. Principles and Practice of Veterinary Anesthesia. Baltimore: Williams and Wilkins, 1987:395.
6. Andrews JJ. Inhaled anesthetic delivery systems. In: Miller RD, ed. Anesthesia, 3rd ed. New York: Churchill Livingstone, 1990:171.
7. Fox JWC, Fox EJ. An unusual occurrence with a cyclopropane cylinder. Anesth Analg 47:624, 1968.
8. Webb AI, Warren RG. Hazards and precautions associated with the use of compressed gases. J Am Vet Med Assoc 181:1491, 1982.
9. Stoelting RK, Miller RD. Basics of Anesthesia. New York: Churchill Livingstone, 1984.
10. Haskins SC, Sansome AL. A timetable for exhaustion of nitrous oxide cylinders using cylinder pressure. Vet Anesth 6:6, 1979.
11. Grant WJ. Medical Gases: Their Properties and Uses. Chicago: Year Book, 1978.
12. Schreiber P. Anesthesia Equipment: Performance, Classification and Safety. New York: Springer-Verlag, 1972.
13. Mazzia VDB. Oxygen and the anesthesia machine. NY State J Med 62:2845, 1962.
14. Gray PR. Anesthetic machine leak. J Am Vet Med Assoc 179:1348, 1981.
15. Hartsfield SM. Practical problems with veterinary anesthesia machines. In: Proceedings of the Fifth International Congress of Veterinary Anesthesia, Guelph, Ontario, 1994:21.
16. Andrews JJ. Understanding your anesthesia machine. In: Annual Refresher Course Lecture 163:1. Washington, DC: American Society of Anesthesiologists, 1993.
17. Hartsfield SM, Thurmon JC. Reduced anesthetic vapor concentration in a breathing circuit related to a leak in the oxygen flush apparatus. Vet Anesth 5:35, 1978.
18. Bednarski RM, Gaynor JS, Muir WW III. Vaporizer in circle for delivery of isoflurane to dogs. J Am Vet Med Assoc 202:943, 1993.
19. Gallagher LV, Klavano PA. Scavenging waste anesthetic gases from obsolescent anesthetic machines. J Am Vet Med Assoc 179:1393, 1981.
20. Schreiber PJ. Effects of barometric pressure on anesthetic equipment. Audio Digest (Anesthesiol) 17:14, 1975.
21. Munson WM. Cardiac arrest: Hazard of tipping a vaporizer. Anesthesiology 26:235, 1965.
22. Ludders JW. Vaporizers used in veterinary anesthesia. Semin Vet Med Small Anim 8:72, 1993.
23. Orkin FK. Anesthetic systems. In: Miller RD, ed. Anesthesia, 2nd ed. New York: Churchill Livingstone, 1986:117.
24. Wagner AE, Bednarski RM. Use of low-flow and closed-system anesthesia. J Am Vet Med Assoc 200:1005, 1992.
25. Lin C. Assessment of vaporizer performance in low-flow and closed-circuit anesthesia. Anesth Analg 59:359, 1980.
26. Hill DW, Lowe HJ. Comparison of concentration of halothane in closed and semiclosed circuits during controlled ventilation. Anesthesiology 23:291, 1962.

27. Hill DW. The design and calibration of vaporizers for volatile anesthetic agents. In: Scurr C, Feldman S, eds. Scientific Foundations of Anesthesia. Chicago: Year Book, 1974:71.

28. Thurmon JC, Benson GJ. Inhalation anesthetic delivery equipment and its maintenance. Vet Clin North Am Large Anim Pract 3:73, 1981

29. Mulroy M, Ham J, Eger EI II. Inflowing gas leak, potential source of hypoxia. Anesthesiology 45:102, 1976.

30. Operation and Maintenance Manual for the Metomatic Model 980 Veterinary Anesthesia Machine. Madison, WI: Ohio Medical Products.

31. Lumb WV, Jones EW. Veterinary Anesthesia, 2nd ed. Philadelphia: Lea and Febiger, 1984.

32. Muir WW III, Hubbell JAE. Handbook of Veterinary Anesthesia, 2nd ed. St Louis: Mosby, 1995.

33. Steffey EP, Woliner MJ, Howland D. Accuracy of isoflurane delivery by halothane-specific vaporizers. Am J Vet Res 44:1072, 1983.

34. Hamilton WK. Nomenclature of inhalation anesthetic systems. Anesthesiology 25:3, 1964.

35. Dunlop CI. The case for rebreathing circuits for very small animals. Vet Clin North Am Small Anim Pract 22:400, 1992.

36. Bednarski RM. Anesthetic breathing systems. Semin Vet Med Surg (Small Anim) 8:82, 1993.

37. Menhusen MJ. Anesthetic machine malfunctions resulting in soda lime bypass and hypercarbia. J Am Anim Hosp Assoc 15:507, 1979.

38. Jorgensen B, Jorgensen S. Carbon dioxide elimination from circle systems. Acta Anaesthesiol Scand Suppl 53:86, 1973.

39. Bednarski RM. Anesthetic equipment. In: Muir WW III, Hubbell JAE, eds. Equine Anesthesia, Monitoring and Emergency Therapy. St Louis: Mosby Year Book, 1991:325.

40. Tevik A, Nelson AW, Berkley WE, Lumb WV. Effect of nitrogen in a closed-circle system with low oxygen flows for equine anesthesia. J Am Vet Med Assoc 154:166, 1969.

41. Muir WW III, Hubbell JAE. Handbook of Veterinary Anesthesia. St Louis: CV Mosby, 1989.

42. Klide AM. The case for low gas flows. Vet Clin North Am Small Anim Pract 22:384, 1992.

43. Hartsfield SM, Sawyer DC. Cardiopulmonary effects of rebreathing and nonrebreathing systems during halothane anesthesia in the cat. Am J Vet Res 37:1461, 1976.

44. Suter CM, Pascoe PJ, McDonell WN, Wilson B. Resistance and work of breathing in the anesthetized cat: Comparison of a circle breathing circuit and a coaxial breathing system. In: Proceedings of the Annual Meeting of the American College of Veterinary Anesthesiologists, 1989.

45. Hodgson DS, McMurphy RM. Resistance to flow in large animal anesthetic machine breathing circuits. In: Proceedings of the Annual Meeting of the American College of Veterinary Anesthesiologists, Washington, DC, 1993.

46. Soma LR, ed. Textbook of Veterinary Anesthesiology. Baltimore: Williams and Wilkins, 1971.

47. Manley SV, McDonnell WN. Clinical evaluation of the Bain breathing circuit in small animal anesthesia. J Am Anim Hosp Assoc 15:67, 1979.

48. Hodgson DS. The case for nonrebreathing circuits for very small animals. Vet Clin North Am Small Anim Pract 22:397, 1992.

49. Haskins SC. Monitoring the anesthetized patient. In: Short CE, ed. Principles and Practice of Veterinary Anesthesia. Baltimore: Williams and Wilkins, 1987:455.

50. Manley SV, McDonnell WN. A new circuit for small animal anesthesia: The Bain coaxial circuit. J Am Anim Hosp Assoc 15:61, 1979.

51. Sawyer DC. The practice of small animal anesthesia. Philadelphia: WB Saunders, 1982.

52. Anesthetic gases. AVMA Professional Liability Insurance Trust Saf Bull 1(1):1, 1992.

53. Occupational Safety and Health Administration (OSHA). DVM Issues. Austin: Texas Veterinary Medical Association, May 1991.

54. Quick BA, Fountain BL. OSHA and the veterinary practice establishment. J Am Vet Med Assoc 195:302, 1989.

55. National Institute for Occupational Safety and Health (NIOSH). Criteria for a Recommended Standard Occupational Exposure to Waste Anesthetic Gases and Vapors. HEW Publ N105H. Washington, DC: US Government Printing Office, 1977.

56. Milligan JE. Anesthetic gas hazards. In: Heidelbaugh ND, Murnane TG, Rosser WW, eds. Health Hazards in Veterinary Practice, 2nd ed. Austin: Texas Department of Health, 1989:101.

57. Smith JA. Anesthetic pollution and waste anesthetic gas scavenging. Semin Vet Med Surg Small Anim 8:90, 1993.

58. Food and Drug Administration (FDA). Anesthesia apparatus checkout recommendations: Availability. Federal Register 52:5583, 1987.

59. March MG, Crowley JJ. An evaluation of anesthesiologists' present checkout methods and the validity of the FDA checklist. Anesthesiology 75:724, 1991.

60. Mason DE. Anesthesia machine checkout and troubleshooting. Semin Vet Med Surg Small Anim 8:104, 1993.

61. Paddleford RR. Exposure of veterinary personnel to waste anesthetic gases. Semin Vet Med Surg 1:249, 1986.

62. Manley SV, McDonell WN. Recommendations for reduction of anesthetic gas pollution. J Am Vet Med Assoc 176:519, 1980.

63. Haskins SC. Opinions in small animal anesthesia. Vet Clin North Am Small Anim Pract 22:245, 1992.

64. Rayburn RL. Pediatric anesthesia circuits. In: Annual Refresher Course Lecture 117. Washington, DC: American Society of Anesthesiologists, 1981.

Chapter 18
Airway Management and Ventilation

Sandee M. Hartsfield

Introduction

Safe anesthesia includes establishment of a patient airway with assurance of adequate ventilation and oxygenation. If spontaneous ventilation is insufficient, the anesthetist should provide supplemental oxygen during the preanesthetic, induction, maintenance, and recovery phases of anesthesia.

Endotracheal Intubation

Indications

Indications for endotracheal intubation include maintenance of a patent airway, protection of the airway from foreign material, application of positive-pressure ventilation, application of tracheal

or bronchial suction, administration of oxygen, and delivery of inhalant anesthetics. Placement of an endotracheal tube also reduces anatomical dead space if the tube is of the correct size and correctly positioned. For maintenance of inhalant anesthesia, an endotracheal tube should create a seal with the trachea to prevent leakage of anesthetic gases into the environment. An endotracheal tube is basic for endotracheal intubation, but ancillary equipment may be required in certain species. Intubation can be accomplished through the oral cavity, nasal passages, an external pharyngotomy, or tracheostomy.

Endotracheal Tubes

Murphy-type and Cole-type endotracheal tubes are commonly used in veterinary anesthesia. Uniquely, the Murphy tube has an opening, called a *Murphy eye* or *side hole*, in the wall opposite the bevel (Fig. 18.1); this hole allows gas flow, even if the end hole is occluded.[1] Characteristics of cuffed Murphy endotracheal tubes designed primarily for human patients are diagrammed in Fig. 18.2; such tubes are used in most veterinary patients for which appropriate sizes are available.

Cole tubes are uncuffed and are characterized by a shoulder near the distal end (Figs. 18.3 and 18.4); the diameter of the patient end of the Cole tube is smaller than the remainder of the tube.[1] Only the smaller portion of the tube should fit into the larynx and trachea. Although fitting the sloping shoulder of the Cole tube against the arytenoid cartilage creates a seal,[2] Dorsch and Dorsch indicate that, to avoid pressure against the laryngeal cartilages and to prevent laryngeal dilation, the shoulder should not contact the larynx.[1] The diameter of the tube should be such that the laryngotracheal part of the tube creates a seal, which guards against egress of gas and aspiration of foreign material. An effective seal can be established in veterinary patients of various sizes.[2,3]

Endotracheal tubes are made of polyvinyl chloride (PVC), rubber, silicone, and occasionally other plastic or rubberized materials. The most common tubes for human use are made of PVC,[1] many of which are used in small animals. Some endotracheal tubes, designed specifically for veterinary patients, are made of silicone rubber (Fig. 18.5). In general, endotracheal tubes should be clear so that they can be inspected for cleanliness or obstructions before each use. Red rubber tubes have been advertised for veterinary patients; such tubes are opaque, prone to cracking, and difficult to clean and disinfect.

Cuffed endotracheal tubes (Fig. 18.6) designed for human patients consist of a connector to fit the breathing system (15 mm

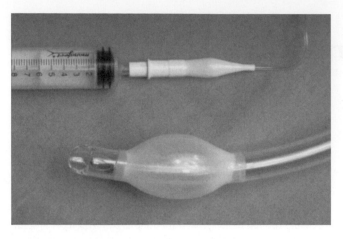

Fig. 18.1. A Murphy endotracheal tube characterized by a side hole (Murphy eye) opposite the bevel at the distal end of the tube. The inflatable cuff, pilot balloon, self-sealing inflation valve, and syringe for inflation of the cuff are shown. The parts and characteristics of a Murphy tube are diagramed and labeled in Fig. 18.2.

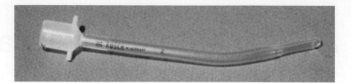

Fig. 18.3. A 10-French Cole endotracheal tube appropriate for small veterinary patients. Note the smaller diameter of the laryngotracheal portion of the tube (distal end of the tube, *right* side of the photograph).

OD [outer diameter]), the tube itself, and a cuff system (inflating valve, inflating tube, and pilot balloon). Labels on these tubes may include the manufacturer's name, internal and external diameters in millimeters, markings in centimeters indicating the length of the tube from the patient (distal) end, and IT, which indicates that the tube has been implantation tested. In addition, tubes labeled with either F29 or Z79 indicate that the tube material has been tested for tissue toxicity.[1,4] The terms *oral* and/or *nasal* may appear beside the tube's size for internal and external diameters, respectively. Some endotracheal tubes have the size in French units (French size = external diameter in millimeters times pi), which indicates the outside diameter of the tube. Radiopaque markers are embedded in some endotracheal tubes.

Inflation of the cuff of an endotracheal tube applies pressure to the tracheal mucosa. The perfusion pressure of the tracheal mucosa ranges from 25 to 35 mm Hg. A cuff pressure on the tracheal wall of 20 to 25 mm Hg will usually not interfere with tracheal mucosal blood flow.[5] Greater pressures in the cuff can lead to is-

Characteristics of Common Endotracheal Tubes

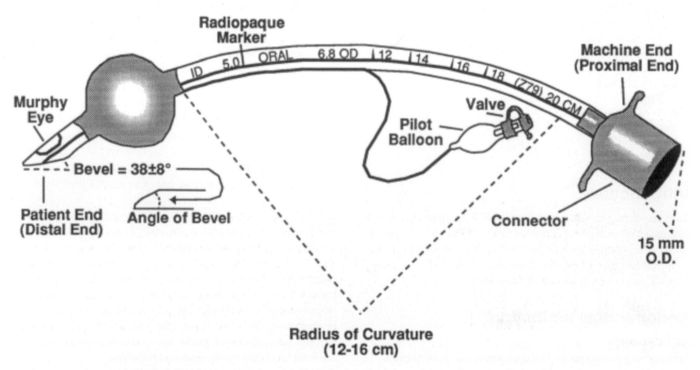

Fig. 18.2. Diagram illustrating the parts and desirable characteristics (e.g., radius of curvature and angle of the bevel) of a Murphy endotracheal tube. OD, outer diameter. From Dorsch and Dorsch.[1]

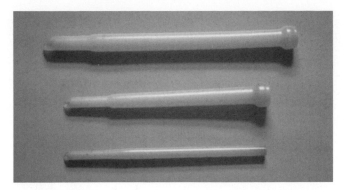

Fig. 18.4. Three sizes of Cole endotracheal tubes appropriate for large veterinary patients. Note the smaller diameter of the laryngotracheal portion of each tube (distal ends of the tubes, *left* side of the photograph). The proximal ends of the top two tubes are designed to fit the outside diameter of the Y piece of a circle breathing system for large animals.

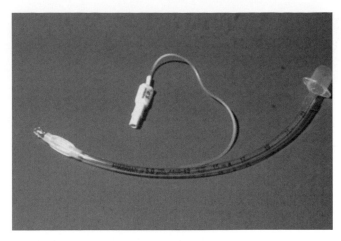

Fig. 18.6. A Murphy endotracheal tube designed for human patients, but commonly used for small animals. Numbers and markings indicate the internal (5.0 mm) and external (8.0 mm) diameters, the length (13, 15, 17, 19, 21, and 23 cm) of the tube from the patient end, the manufacturer (Sheridan), and tissue toxicity testing (Z79). The internal diameter (5.0 mm) and manufacturer are also shown on the pilot balloon.

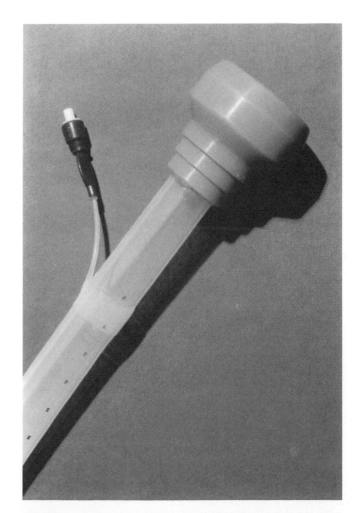

Fig. 18.5. Silicone rubber endotracheal tubes designed for veterinary use. The proximal end of the top tube has been fitted with a connector that will conform to the outside diameter of a Y piece of a circle breathing system for large animals.

chemic injury, mucosal damage, and ultimately tracheal strictures in serious cases. Therefore, the design of contemporary human endotracheal tubes includes a high-volume, low-pressure cuff that creates a good seal between the tracheal mucosa and the cuff wall when the cuff is properly inflated. The intent of the high-volume nonelastic cuff is to distribute the low-pressure seal over a relatively large area of the tracheal mucosa.[4] A cuff should be inflated with the smallest amount of air that will provide effective protection of the airway. A general recommendation is that pressure on the lateral wall of the trachea exerted by the cuff be maintained between 25 and 34 cm H_2O.[1] Generally, a leak should occur around the cuff when pressure equal to approximately 25 cm H_2O is applied to the airway.

Armored or reinforced endotracheal tubes (Fig. 18.7) are specially designed with helical wire or plastic implanted within the wall of the tube to prevent kinking of the tube and obstruction of the airway when the patient's head and neck are flexed. Such tubes are useful for ophthalmic surgery, cervical spinal taps, myelograms, oral surgery, and head and neck surgery. Armored tubes have thicker walls than standard tubes, causing them to have smaller internal diameters than standard tubes of equivalent external size.[4] Therefore, resistance to gas flow is increased, and reinforced tubes should not be used unnecessarily. Typically, these tubes are very flexible and more difficult to insert than standard PVC tubes. A stylet or guide tube will facilitate insertion of an armored tube into the larynx, but a stiff stylet should not extend past the distal end of the endotracheal tube.

Endotracheal intubation through a tracheostomy is sometimes necessary to provide a patent airway. Cuffed tracheostomy tubes with 15-mm-OD (outer diameter) connectors (Fig. 18.8) are available for use in human patients. However, standard endotracheal tubes for both large and small animals may be placed via

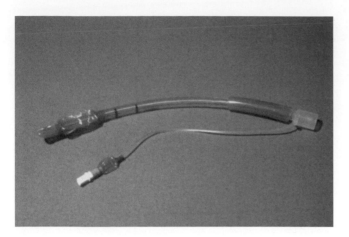

Fig. 18.7. An armored endotracheal tube with a spiral wire embedded in the wall of the tube: the endotracheal tube connector, bite guard near the proximal end of the tube, inflatable cuff, pilot balloon, inflation line, and self-sealing inflation valve.

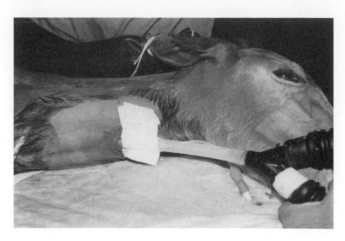

Fig. 18.9. A silicone rubber endotracheal tube placed through a tracheostomy site to facilitate inhalant anesthesia for oral and nasal surgery in a foal.

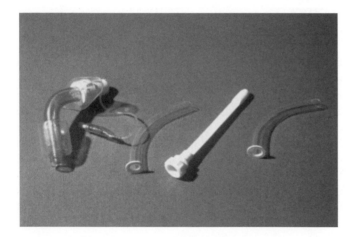

Fig. 18.8. A cuffed tracheostomy tube (*left*) designed for human patients, but applicable to veterinary patients. From *left to right* are the cuffed tracheostomy tube with inflation line and pilot balloon, a removable lumen for the tube, an obturator to facilitate insertion of the tube, and another removable lumen.

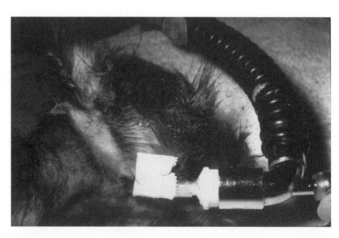

Fig. 18.10. An endotracheal tube placed by external pharyngotomy in a small dog to facilitate oropharyngeal surgery. From Hartsfield.[19]

tracheostomy to facilitate general anesthesia (Fig. 18.9). Endotracheal tubes are also recommended for intubation by external pharyngotomy (Fig. 18.10).[6]

Normally, endotracheal intubation is accomplished in anesthetized patients. Forced intubation in awake or lightly anesthetized patients should be avoided unless dictated by special circumstances. Traumatic intubation can produce laryngeal edema, laryngeal spasm, hemorrhage, and vagal stimulation leading to bradycardia and other arrhythmias. Direct application of a local anesthetic (e.g., lidocaine [Fig. 18.11]) to the larynx may prevent laryngeal spasms in susceptible animals (e.g., cats and swine). The local anesthetic can be sprayed into the larynx, applied with a cotton swab, or squirted from a syringe and hypodermic needle.

When using a syringe, the hypodermic needle must be firmly attached to prevent its dislodgment and entrance into the larynx. The total dose of local anesthetic should not approach a toxic dose, based on the patient's species and body weight. In very small patients, spraying local anesthetic onto the larynx can easily exceed a toxic dose.

Endotracheal and tracheostomy tubes should be cleaned thoroughly after use. The tubes should be gently scrubbed with a soft brush, rinsed, dried, and sterilized or disinfected. If ethylene oxide is not available, chemical disinfectants can be used; glutaraldehyde has been recommended.[7] After disinfection, tubes should be rinsed thoroughly, according to recommendations for use of the disinfectant, and dried. If tubes are inadequately

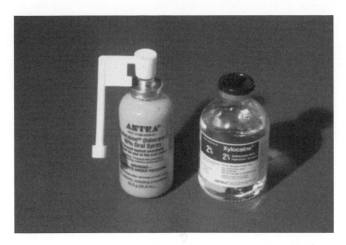

Fig. 18.11. Lidocaine as a spray (*left*) or as a liquid (applied with a cotton swab or delivered by squirting it with a syringe and needle) can be applied topically to the larynx to facilitate endotracheal intubation in various species. With either method of delivery, the anesthetist should keep the total dose of lidocaine less than the toxic dose for the patient and species involved.

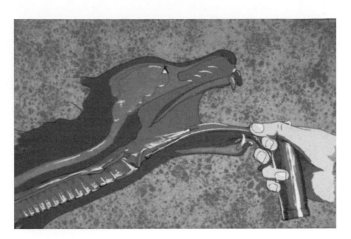

Fig. 18.12. Diagram of the correct positioning of a laryngoscope blade for maximum visualization of the larynx. Note that the dog's mouth is opened widely, its tongue is extended from its mouth maximally, and the tip of the laryngoscope blade is positioned at the base of the epiglottis.

rinsed, tissue reactions to the disinfectant can occur. Ethylene oxide sterilization should be performed according to the manufacturer's recommendations for the product and its sterilization equipment. Endotracheal tubes should be clean and dry before they are sterilized with ethylene oxide. Appropriate aeration time should be allowed between sterilizing a tube and its use in a patient: typically 2 days at 120°F (49°C) in an aeration chamber or 14 days if no aeration chamber is available. Failure to allow sufficient aeration time can cause serious respiratory complications.[8] Most endotracheal or tracheostomy tubes should not be autoclaved; however, silicone rubber tubes can be steam autoclaved.[7,9]

Laryngoscopy is required for endotracheal intubation of some species. Often, the laryngoscope's light source is the main benefit of laryngoscopy, but the blade can be used to manipulate the tongue, soft palate, and epiglottis to view the glottis (Fig. 18.12). Useful blades include the Miller, the McIntosh, and the Bizarri-Guiffrida (Figs. 18.13 and 18.14), and other blades are available. Different lengths of blades are needed for various species. As examples, very short blades designed for human infants are useful in rabbits, and blades up to 205 mm designed for human adults are appropriate for large dogs. Specially designed, very long (350 to 450 mm) blades can be purchased for veterinary use and may be needed in llamas, cattle, swine, and other species.

Techniques of Endotracheal Intubation
Dogs

For most dogs, an endotracheal tube and adequate lighting are the only necessities for intubation of the trachea. However, the use of a laryngoscope, a stylet to stiffen the endotracheal tube, a guide tube (Fig. 18.15), sterile water-soluble lubricant, a mouth speculum, and local anesthetic may be desirable and even necessary under certain circumstances.

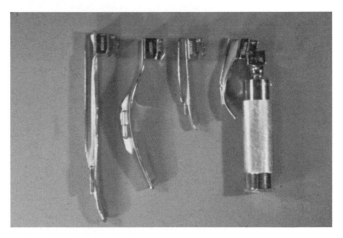

Fig. 18.13. From *left to right*, an adult Miller laryngoscope blade, an adult Bizarri-Guiffrida blade, a pediatric Miller blade, and a pediatric Bizarri-Guiffrida blade on a laryngoscope handle. The Bizarri-Guiffrida blades allow the maximum field of view without the interference of a flange.

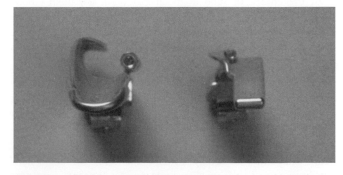

Fig. 18.14. End-on view of Miller (*left*) and Bizarri-Guiffrida (*right*) laryngoscope blades. The Bizarri-Guiffrida blade allows maximum space for passage of the endotracheal tube, and the Miller blade provides a flange to elevate redundant tissue (e.g., soft palate).

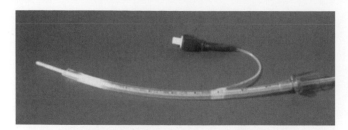

Fig. 18.15. Photograph of a silicone rubber endotracheal tube with a 10-French canine polyethylene urinary catheter preplaced for use as a guide tube. The guide tube will pass easily through the larynx and into the cranial part of the trachea to facilitate passage of the endotracheal tube.

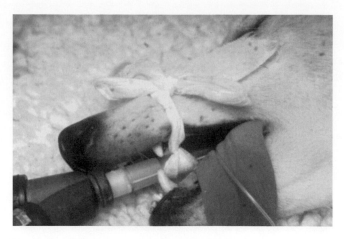

Fig. 18.17. An endotracheal tube secured to a dog's maxilla with a piece of rolled gauze. Note that the gauze is tied tightly around the tube without constricting the lumen, that the connector is at the level of the incisor teeth, and that the gauze is positioned immediately caudal to the maxillary canine teeth and tied in a bow.

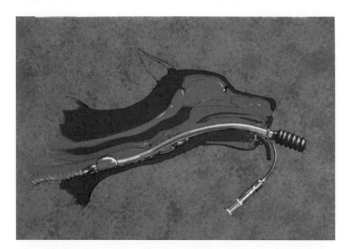

Fig. 18.16. Diagram of the correct placement of an endotracheal tube in a dog. Note that the connector is located near the incisor teeth to minimize mechanical dead space and that the cuffed end of the tube is in the cervical trachea near the thoracic inlet.

Sizes of endotracheal tubes for canine patients range from 1.5 mm to approximately 15 mm ID (internal diameter).[2] It is difficult, if not impossible, to find cuffed tubes smaller than 3.0 mm ID. There are breed differences that preclude generalizations about the choice of tube diameter based on a patient's body weight or some other arbitrary guide. For example, a 25-kg English bulldog usually accepts only about a 7.5-mm-ID endotracheal tube, but a 25-kg mixed-breed dog may easily accept a 10-mm tube. Most tubes designed for human patients are too long for dogs and should be cut at the proximal end to fit the patient; the connector should be positioned at the level of the dog's incisors, and the distal end should be located in the trachea near the thoracic inlet (Fig. 18.16).

After induction of anesthesia, the dog is positioned in sternal recumbency for intubation. An assistant holds the dog's head with one hand, placing the finger and thumb behind the maxillary canine teeth and pulling the dog's lips upward to create the best field of view. With the other hand, the assistant opens the dog's mouth widely and extends its tongue. The assistant should not put pressure under the dog's neck because the view of the larynx will be obstructed by the soft palate. With a good light source, most dogs can be intubated without a laryngoscope. If an assistant is unavailable, an oral speculum will keep the dog's mouth open during intubation. In small patients, dogs with oral or pharyngeal lesions, and brachycephalic dogs, a laryngoscope facilitates intubation and should always be available if difficulty should arise. The endotracheal tube should be secured to prevent its dislocation during anesthesia. Using a piece of rolled gauze, the tube can be tied to the maxilla (Fig. 18.17), the mandible, or behind the head, depending on the breed, the type of surgery, the presence and condition of the canine teeth, and the anesthetist's preference.

Extubation should be done when the dog's oral and pharyngeal reflexes have returned. The tube should be pulled directly between the upper and lower incisor teeth. If a tube is allowed to deviate laterally, the dog may shear the tube. This damages tubes and creates the potential for aspiration or ingestion of a part of the tube.

Cats

The primary equipment required for feline intubation are an endotracheal tube and a light source. However, a laryngoscope, a stylet to stiffen the endotracheal tube, a guide tube (canine polyethylene urinary catheter), sterile water-soluble lubricant, a mouth speculum, and local anesthetic may be useful. If a wire stylet is used to stiffen the tube, the stylet should not extend past the distal end of the tube to avoid injury to the trachea.[2] Inadequate depth of anesthesia is probably the most common reason for difficult intubation.

Sizes of endotracheal tubes for domestic cats range from 1.5 mm to approximately 5.5 mm ID; most adult cats readily accept 4.0- to 4.5-mm-ID tubes, a range that provides optimal internal diameter with minimal difficulty in intubation. It is difficult to

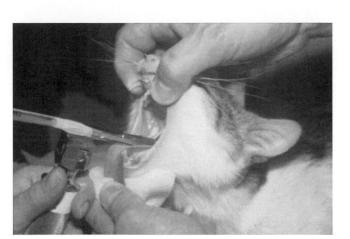

Fig. 18.18. Illustration of an excellent method of positioning a cat for endotracheal intubation. Note the secure grip on the maxilla with the index finger and thumb caudal to the canine teeth. The tongue is extended, maximizing the field of view.

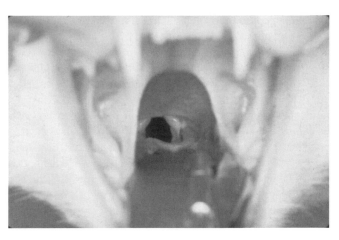

Fig. 18.19. View of a cat's glottis using the restraint and positioning depicted in Fig. 18.18. The laryngoscope blade is placed on the tongue with the tip just ventral to the epiglottis.

find cuffed tubes smaller than 3.0 mm ID, and such sizes may be needed for small kittens. One option is to use small Cole tubes. Since most endotracheal tubes designed for human patients are too long for cats, the tube should be cut at the proximal end to fit the patient. The proximal end of the tube should be positioned at the level of the cat's incisors, and the distal end should be located in the trachea near the thoracic inlet.

After induction of anesthesia, the cat should be positioned in sternal recumbency. Although not necessary in every case, local anesthetic (0.5% lidocaine) may be applied to the larynx to desensitize the arytenoid cartilage and epiglottis to help prevent laryngospasm during intubation. An assistant holds the head with one hand, placing a finger and thumb behind the cat's maxillary canine teeth and pulling the lips upward to create the best field of view (Figs. 18.18 and 18.19). With the other hand, the assistant extends the cat's tongue. If the tongue is not protruding from the mouth, the laryngoscope blade can be used to manipulate the tongue so that the assistant can grasp it. Neither the anesthetist nor the assistant should put their fingers into a lightly anesthetized cat's mouth. The assistant should not put pressure under the cat's neck because the view of the larynx may be obstructed by the soft palate. As in dogs, with a good light source, most cats can be intubated without the aid of a laryngoscope. However, a laryngoscope is often helpful. The blade should not touch the arytenoid cartilage or the epiglottis (Fig. 18.18) because such stimulation may cause active closure of the glottis. A laryngoscope should always be available for a difficult intubation (e.g., oral or pharyngeal lesions). If an assistant is unavailable, an oral speculum will keep the cat's mouth open while intubation is accomplished. The routine use of a guide tube (5- to 8-French canine urinary catheter) that extends past the cuffed end of the endotracheal tube (Fig. 18.18) for 2 or 3 cm often makes feline intubation easier. As the endotracheal tube is advanced toward the glottis, rotating it from 0° to 90° or greater will facilitate its passage. Rolled gauze can be used to secure the tube behind the

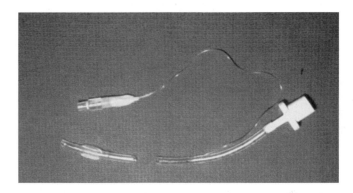

Fig. 18.20. A endotracheal tube (4-mm internal diameter) sheared during extubation of a cat at the time of recovery from anesthesia. Aspiration or ingestion of the smaller piece is possible.

cat's head with a simple bow knot. In cats, the tube should be tied for rapid removal at recovery.

Extubation should be done when the cat's oral and pharyngeal reflexes have returned. The tube should be pulled directly between the upper and lower incisor teeth. If a tube is allowed to move laterally, the cat may shear the tube (Fig. 18.20), which creates the potential for aspiration or ingestion of part of the tube.

Horses

Blind passage of the endotracheal tube in horses can be aided by a mouth speculum. For routine intubation, PVC connectors (10 cm long, variable diameters) for PVC pipe make economic, effective specula that can be placed between the horse's upper and lower incisors to protect the tube. The connectors can be wrapped with adhesive tape to increase friction between the teeth and the speculum.[7] Other supplies that may be useful for equine intubation under certain conditions include a guide tube (equine stomach tube), sterile water-soluble lubricant, local anesthetic, and a fiber-optic endoscope.

To assure an appropriate range of sizes of endotracheal tubes for equine patients (miniature horses to draft horses), tubes as small as 7 mm ID and as large as 30 mm ID should be available. Larger sizes (e.g., 35 mm ID) have been recommended for large thoroughbred and draft horses.[10] Tube size varies with the size of the patient and with the location of the tube (oral versus nasal intubation). Modern 26-mm-ID silicone rubber cuffed endotracheal tubes are appropriate for a high percentage of adult horses, with 30-mm tubes indicated for very large horses. In general, a tube that is passed nasally should be about two sizes smaller than a tube that is passed orally.[9]

In preparation for oropharyngeal intubation, the horse's mouth should be flushed with water to remove any debris that may be retained in the oropharynx, including the cheek pouches. Horses are positioned in lateral recumbency for intubation with a lubricated endotracheal tube. A sterile water-soluble lubricant should be used; lubricants containing local anesthetic are unnecessary and may irritate airway tissues.[7,11] The mouth speculum is placed between the upper and lower incisors, the head and neck are extended, and the endotracheal tube is advanced into the pharynx until the tip of the tube touches the larynx. In some patients, the tube enters the larynx without any interference. However, several attempts (a series of 10- to 15-cm advancements and retractions of the tube, with rotation of the tube from 0° to 90° or greater as it approaches the glottis) may be necessary for intubation, even in normal horses. Although the technique is somewhat of an art, intubation can be facilitated by maximally extending the horse's head and neck in a straight line with the its back (best done by an assistant), extending the tongue during intubation, and holding the endotracheal tube so that the proximal end is curved below the mandible during attempts at intubation. In general, an endotracheal tube of proper size can be passed into the larynx with little if any resistance once correct positioning and technique have been established.

For difficult intubation, an equine stomach tube (guide tube) may be passed into the larynx and trachea, over which the endotracheal tube can be manipulated through the larynx and into the trachea. In some instances (e.g., laryngeal or pharyngeal abnormalities), equine intubation may be successful only after visualizing the glottis with a fiber-optic endoscope; this allows adjustments in the position of the endotracheal tube or a guide tube as it approaches the glottis.

A properly positioned endotracheal tube is usually obvious to an experienced anesthetist because of the absence of resistance as the tube enters the larynx and trachea. Air flow into and out of the tube during spontaneous ventilation can be used to verify tube placement. Some veterinarians advocate compression of the thorax to create air flow from a properly placed tube, but this technique may not be foolproof. Finally, water may condense on the inner surface of the tube during exhalation if the tube is placed properly.

Swine

Endotracheal intubation of swine is relatively difficult for several reasons:[12] The distance from the tip of the snout to the larynx is

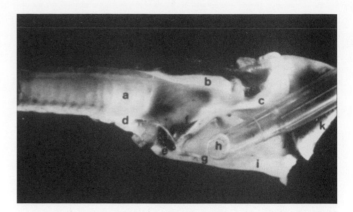

Fig. 18.21. Sagittal section of a pig's larynx. This illustrates the irregular course that an endotracheal tube must travel as it moves through the larynx and into the cranial trachea: *a*, tracheal opening; *b*, dorsal cricoid cartilage; *c*, arytenoids cartilage; *d*, ventral cricoid cartilage; *e* and *i*, thyroid cartilage; *f*, entrance to lateral laryngeal ventricle; *g*, posterior floor of the larynx; *h*, tip of endotracheal tube; *j*, middle laryngeal ventricle; and *k*, and epiglottis. Reproduced by permission of Dr. William Tranquilli.

comparatively long, the mouth does not open widely, the larynx is rather loosely attached, mobile, relatively small, and slopes ventrally, creating a sharp angle for passing an endotracheal tube (Fig. 18.21). In addition, laryngospasm is rather easily induced in lightly anesthetized pigs. An endotracheal tube, a laryngoscope, 2% lidocaine in a syringe, sterile water-soluble lubricant, and a guide tube should be available for intubation of swine.

Compared with other domestic species, swine have small laryngeal and tracheal diameters. Endotracheal tube sizes from 3 mm ID in piglets to 16 mm ID in larger swine may be needed. Mature sows and boars may accept even larger tubes. After induction of anesthesia, the pig is placed in sternal recumbency, an assistant holds the head with a small rope or piece of rolled gauze passed through the mouth, and the pig's tongue is extended. A mouth speculum can be employed, if necessary. Using the appropriate length of blade, the pig's larynx is visualized with the aid of a laryngoscope; this usually requires some manipulation to position the blade for a good view of the glottis, especially in large swine with a narrow pharynx and excessive tissue in the area of the soft palate. Lidocaine can be squirted onto the larynx for desensitization. The guide tube (usually two 10-French canine urinary catheters in tandem) is passed through the larynx and into the trachea; the guide tube should be manipulated through the larynx without excessive force, and best results are obtained by passing the guide tube along the dorsal aspect of the larynx to the midcervical trachea. Then, a well-lubricated endotracheal tube is directed over the guide tube, through the larynx, and into the trachea; firm, gentle advancement of the tube with a simultaneous twisting motion (0° to greater than 90°) is helpful. The tube should be positioned with the connector at the level of the tip of the snout, and the distal end should be near the thoracic inlet. The cuff should be inflated with the minimum amount of air that will create a seal. The tube can be secured to the snout with adhesive tape or behind the ears with rolled gauze.

Miniature pet pigs are intubated by using the same equipment (smaller sizes) and method just described, but gentle technique should be emphasized. Laryngospasm, laryngeal edema, and death have been associated with traumatic intubation in miniature pigs.[13]

Cattle

The primary implements for endotracheal intubation in adult cattle are endotracheal tube, a mouth speculum (e.g., Bayer dental wedge, Guenther mouth speculum, Weingart mouth speculum, or Drinkwater mouth gag), and an equine stomach tube (two to three times longer than the endotracheal tube) for use as a guide. For smaller cattle, a long laryngoscope blade (e.g., 14, 16, or 18 inches) may be necessary for passage of a guide tube. Sizes of endotracheal tubes ranging from 18 to 30 mm ID may be needed for adult cattle.

After induction of anesthesia, a mouth speculum is positioned to hold the mouth open; this helps to prevent damage to the endotracheal tube cuff and to the anesthetist's hand and arm during intubation. The cow's tongue is extended from the mouth as its head and neck are extended. The anesthetist passes one hand through the cow's mouth and palpates the epiglottis and glottis. The anesthetist passes the guide tube into the pharynx and then slides the tube through the glottis, assuring the tube's proper placement by palpation as it enters the larynx. The guide tube is advanced until its tip is in the midcervical trachea. After the anesthetist's arm is removed from the cow's mouth, the endotracheal tube is advanced over the guide tube and into the cow's larynx and trachea. Rotation of the tube from 0° to greater than 90° as the tube approaches the arytenoid cartilage will help to advance the endotracheal tube into the trachea. The cuff should be inflated immediately to decrease the likelihood of aspiration of regurgitated rumen contents. Should active or passive regurgitation of large quantities of ruminal content occur just before or simultaneously with endotracheal intubation, external pressure applied over the esophagus will halt the flow of ruminal contents. Alternatively, the endotracheal tube can be quickly passed into the esophagus and the cuff inflated, permitting the regurgitant to flow through the endotracheal tube beyond the pharynx and out of the mouth, preventing its aspiration into the lungs. A properly positioned endotracheal tube in a cow is shown in Fig. 18.22.

Bovine intubation can be accomplished without a guide tube. The endotracheal tube is passed beside or under the anesthetist's arm and palpated as it enters the cow's larynx.[12] Alternately, the anesthetists can take the tube into the cow's mouth, cupping the distal end of the tube in the hand.[14] The disadvantage of either method is that the size of the endotracheal tube that can be readily passed is limited, especially if the anesthetist has a large arm.

Small Ruminants

Equipment required for endotracheal intubation in small ruminants includes an endotracheal tube, a laryngoscope, and a guide tube. Endotracheal intubation in small ruminants (sheep, goats, calves, cattle weighing less than about 250 kg, deer, and exotic

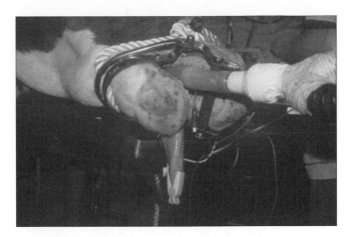

Fig. 18.22. A silicone rubber endotracheal tube (26-mm internal diameter) placed in a cow. The tube was passed with the Wiengart mouth speculum in place as shown.

ruminants) is best accomplished by direct visualization of the larynx with an illuminated laryngoscope. Sternal recumbency facilitates the procedure, but intubation can be achieved during lateral recumbency. After induction of anesthesia, an assistant holds the animal's head while the anesthetist extends its tongue. The anesthetist passes the laryngoscope blade over the base of the tongue to visualize the glottis, and then passes a guide tube (e.g., a small equine stomach tube in calves or a polyethylene catheter in sheep or goats) into the larynx and into the trachea to about the midcervical area. The laryngoscope is removed, and the endotracheal tube is passed over the guide tube and into the trachea. The cuff is inflated immediately to decrease the likelihood of aspiration of regurgitated rumen contents. The use of a metal rod has been advocated as a guide tube.[14] Excessive force with a metal guide tube increases the risk of damaging the larynx or trachea and is not recommended.

Nasotracheal Intubation

This is commonly used in foals for the administration of inhalant anesthetics during induction.[9] The technique can be also be used in calves and adult horses, and its use has been described in llamas.[15]

The characteristics of an ideal nasotracheal tube include a tube with minimal curvature and extra length (55 cm). The tube should be made of inert material (e.g., silicone rubber) and have relatively thin walls for maximum internal diameter. The tube should resist kinking. Low-volume, high-pressure cuffs may be less traumatic during placement, but high-volume, low-pressure cuffs may be best for longer periods of anesthesia. Tubes as small as 7 mm ID may be necessary for neonatal foals. In general, in any given patient a nasotracheal tube should be one to two sizes smaller than the appropriately sized orotracheal tube.[9] Once induction is completed using a nasotracheal tube, the nasotracheal tube can be removed and replaced with an appropriately sized orotracheal tube to decrease resistance to gas flow.

Nasotracheal intubation (Figs. 18.23 through 18.26) involves passage of a properly sized endotracheal tube through the nostril

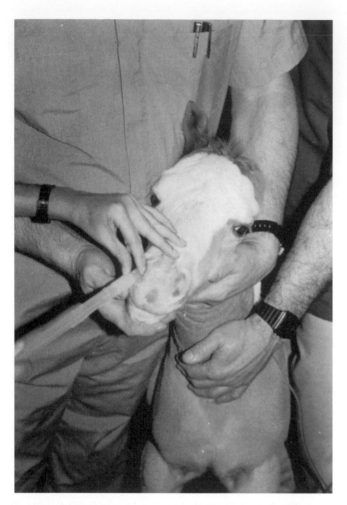

Fig. 18.23. Restraint of an nontranquilized foal for nasotracheal intubation. A lubricated tube is directed through the ventral meatus.

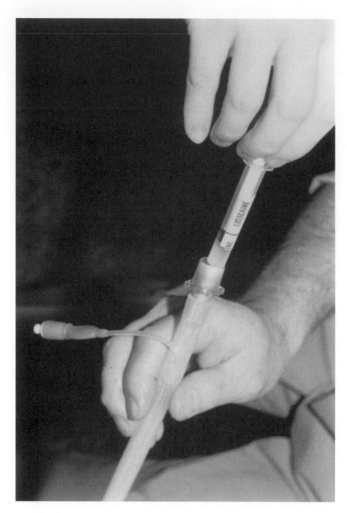

Fig. 18.24. Lidocaine (2%) being injected through the endotracheal tube, the distal end of which is near the foal's glottis. The lidocaine should desensitize the epiglottis and arytenoid cartilages to facilitate passage of the tube through the glottis.

(Fig. 18.23), ventral nasal meatus, and larynx and into the trachea. Lidocaine gel (10%) is a good lubricant for the tube and should be applied to the nostril and rostral portion of the nasal passage before advancing the tube in awake animals. A sterile water-soluble lubricant without lidocaine is appropriate for anesthetized patients. With the patient's head and neck extended, the tube is advanced into the pharynx and passed into the larynx on inspiration. Air moves freely through a correctly placed tube during spontaneous ventilation. Taping the tube to the muzzle is appropriate (Fig. 18.26).

For uncooperative foals and calves, sedation may facilitate nasotracheal intubation. Some awake patients cough and close the glottis in response to the tube contacting the larynx. With the nasotracheal tube positioned with the cuffed end near the larynx, 2% lidocaine solution can be flooded onto the larynx via the tube (Fig. 18.24). This desensitizes the larynx and eases intubation.

Extubation following nasotracheal intubation should be done carefully. After deflation of the cuff, the tube should be withdrawn slowly and deliberately, with the patient's head restrained to avoid any sudden, jerky motions. Rapid, rough extubation may cause unnecessary nasal hemorrhage.

Rabbits and Other Laboratory Animals

Intubation techniques for rabbits and other small laboratory animals have been described.[16] Most techniques for intubation of small laboratory animals include the use of a laryngoscope or a modified otoscope to expose the glottis, a catheter or stylet to serve as a guide tube, a small-diameter lubricated endotracheal tube, and lidocaine to desensitize the larynx before passing the endotracheal tube. In laboratory rabbits weighing about 3.0 kg, the use of 3.5-mm-ID, 14-cm-long endotracheal tubes are appropriate.[17]

The rabbit has been described as perhaps the most difficult animal to anesthetize.[18] Undoubtedly, problems with airway management influenced that opinion. However, the technique for endotracheal intubation in rabbits can be mastered with practice when using proper equipment. Guide-tube technique causes minimal trauma during intubation and allows selection of the largest suitable endotracheal tube. Endotracheal intubation in rabbits requires gentle manipulations. Rough technique invariably leads to

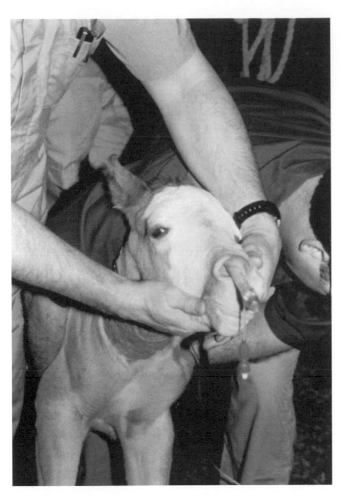

Fig. 18.25. A nasotracheal tube is positioned in the trachea and ready to be secured to the patient. The proximal end of the tube extends a few centimeters from the nostril to facilitate taping (see Fig. 18.26).

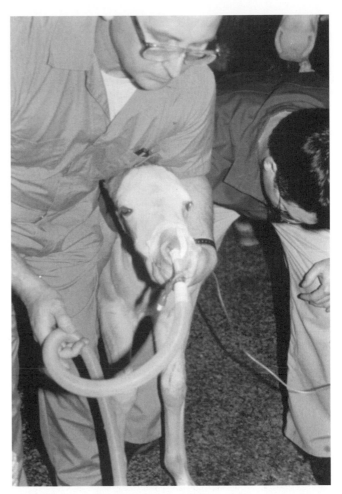

Fig. 18.26. A nasotracheal tube secured to a foal's muzzle. The cuff has been inflated, and an adult Bain breathing system has been connected to the endotracheal tube to facilitate induction of anesthesia with isoflurane in oxygen.

trauma to the tongue, pharynx, larynx, or trachea. Trauma with associated edema and hemorrhage can cause lethal complications.

Rabbits can be intubated when positioned in sternal recumbency with the head and neck extended and the fleshy tongue gently withdrawn from the mouth (Figs. 18.27 to 18.30). The rabbit's head can be held with a piece of rolled gauze placed caudal to the maxillary incisors. A size-0 Miller laryngoscope blade (75 mm long) is used to expose the glottis; the blade is carefully manipulated lateral to the maxillary incisors, into the mouth, and over the base of the tongue to expose the soft palate, epiglottis, and glottis. All are very fine, but distinct, anatomical structures. The epiglottis may be positioned behind the soft palate. The anesthetist should definitively identify the glottis before proceeding. Then, a guide tube (a 5- to 8-French canine urinary catheter) can be passed through the larynx and into the midcervical trachea, about 2 cm past the glottis (Fig. 18.27). The guide tube should not be forced because the trachea is easily torn, which can eventually lead to subcutaneous emphysema, pneumothorax, pneumomediastinum, pneumoabdomen, or death. The endotracheal tube is passed over the guide tube, through the larynx, and

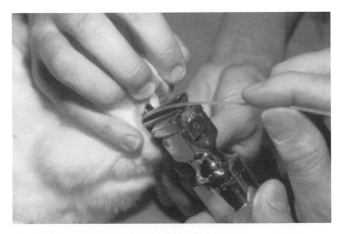

Fig. 18.27. Endotracheal intubation in a rabbit. The rabbit is positioned in sternal recumbency, the glottis has been exposed with a size-0 Miller blade, and the anesthetist is passing a 7-French canine urinary catheter to serve as a guide tube for intubation.

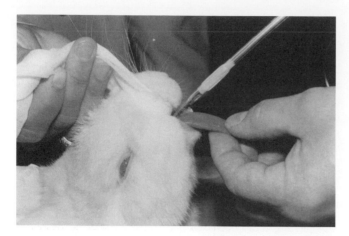

Fig. 18.28. Endotracheal intubation in a rabbit. The endotracheal tube is advanced over the guide tube and into the mouth (the distal end of the guide tube is located 2 cm caudal to the cricoid cartilage).

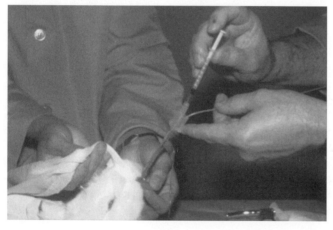

Fig. 18.29. Endotracheal intubation in a rabbit. The distal end of the endotracheal tube is located just rostral to the glottis, the tip of the guide tube is in the cervical trachea, and lidocaine is flushed through the lumen of the endotracheal tube to desensitize the larynx before advancement of the endotracheal tube.

into the trachea. If resistance to passing the endotracheal tube through the glottis is apparent, less than 0.5 mL of 2% lidocaine can be flushed through the endotracheal tube to the larynx. The lidocaine desensitizes the larynx, and intubation usually proceeds uneventfully. The cuff should be inflated minimally, the pilot balloon should remain soft, and a leak around the cuff should occur at an inspiratory pressure of about 15 cm H_2O. The tube should be secured with rolled gauze behind the rabbit's ears. Alternatively, in large rabbits, a blind approach to endotracheal intubation is often successful when the head and neck are maximally extended and the endotracheal tube is advanced into the remiglottis. Intubation of the trachea is expedited at this point by listening for air movement through the tube while gently advancing it beyond the larynx into the trachea.

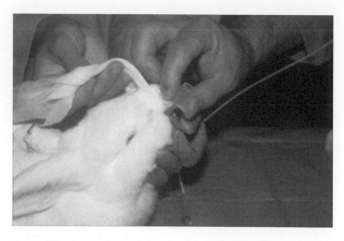

Fig. 18.30. Endotracheal intubation in a rabbit. The distal end of the endotracheal tube has been advanced through the larynx to its final position in the midcervical trachea. The anesthetist is preparing to extract the guide tube and secure the endotracheal tube behind the rabbit's ears.

Birds and Reptiles

Endotracheal intubation in birds and reptiles that are commonly presented for anesthesia is relatively easy. The glottis is usually located on the midline at the base of the tongue and is readily apparent when the patient's mouth is opened. Appropriately sized endotracheal tubes should be selected, and, to avoid damage to the tracheal rings if cuffed tubes are used, the cuff should not be overinflated. Owing to the small size of some birds and reptiles and the propensity for mucus to collect in the distal end of the tube, the anesthetist should be careful to assure a patent airway at all times. The use of lubricating jelly can also cause the obstruction of air flow through small endotracheal tubes.

Special Techniques for Endotracheal Intubation

The common techniques for endotracheal intubation may fail if oropharyngeal pathology is present (Fig. 18.31) or if movement of the temporomandibular joint is impaired. In such patients, "blind" intubation can be performed successfully on occasion. With the patient's head and neck extended, the larynx can be manipulated externally with one hand while the other hand maneuvers the tube through the larynx and into the trachea. However, if this technique is too traumatic or fails completely, other options for intubation are available.

Guide-Tube Technique

In some patients, a laryngoscope blade will allow exposure and illumination of the glottis by diverting the obstruction to one side, enabling direct placement of the endotracheal tube into the larynx. However, it may be easier to pass a small-diameter guide tube (e.g., a canine urinary catheter), rather than an endotracheal tube, through the glottis. Guide-tube technique has been previously described for various species, and it can be beneficial in dogs and cats with oropharyngeal pathology.[19] Once the tip of the guide

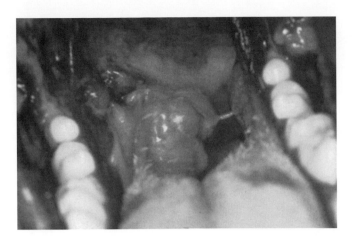

Fig. 18.31. In this dog, a pharyngeal tumor is obstructing the larynx and inhibiting passage of an endotracheal tube. Intubation was accomplished by using a laryngoscope blade to expose the glottis enough for a guide tube to enter the larynx, followed by passage of the endotracheal tube over the guide tube. From Hartsfield.[19]

tube is situated about half the distance from the cricoid cartilage to the thoracic inlet, the endotracheal tube can be passed into place (Fig. 18.32). Then, the guide tube is removed, and the endotracheal tube is secured as appropriate for the species involved.

Retrograde Intubation

If direct visualization of at least a portion of the glottis is impossible, other techniques of intubation have been advocated.[19,20] One method—use of a retrograde guide tube or wire—involves passing a hypodermic needle through the skin of the neck and into the trachea at the junction of the second and third tracheal rings. In human patients, the needle is passed through the crico-

thyroid membrane. A guidewire is then maneuvered through the needle cranially into the larynx, pharynx, and oral cavity until it can be used as a guide for passage of an endotracheal tube (Fig. 18.33). After the tip of the endotracheal tube is within the larynx, the needle and the guide tube are removed, and the endotracheal tube is manipulated into its final position with the cuffed end near the thoracic inlet. The cuff should be located caudal to the puncture site of the hypodermic needle to avoid forcing gases subcutaneously or into the mediastinum during positive-pressure ventilation. Subcutaneous emphysema and pneumothorax are possible complications with this technique.

Lateral Pharyngotomy

This technique has been described[6] and has been advocated for selected canine and feline patients requiring oropharyngeal surgery or orthopedic procedures involving the mandible or maxilla (Fig. 18.10). The major advantages are improved visualization within the operative field during oropharyngeal surgery and normal dental occlusion to aid in the proper reduction of mandibular or maxillary fractures.

The basics of tube placement involve passage of a correctly sized, cuffed endotracheal tube and a routine skin incision made near the angle of the mandible. Then, hemostats are bluntly passed through the skin incision into the caudal part of the pharynx. After the endotracheal tube adapter has been removed, the adapter end of the tube is grasped and pulled from the pharynx, through the subcutaneous tissue, and through the skin incision. The endotracheal tube adapter is replaced, and the tube is reconnected to the breathing system for maintenance. A correctly placed tube should be secured to the skin with tape and several sutures.

Using an Endoscope

Laryngoscopy with a flexible fiber-optic endoscope can be useful for intubation in patients with abnormal anatomy or disease

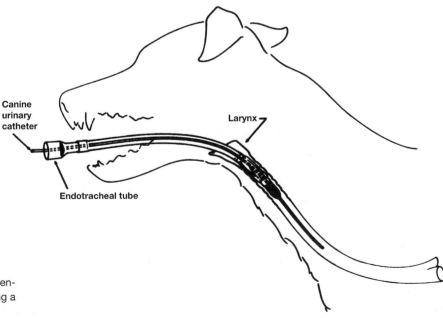

Fig. 18.32. Diagram illustrating passage of an endotracheal tube into the trachea of a dog by using a guide tube. From Hartsfield.[19]

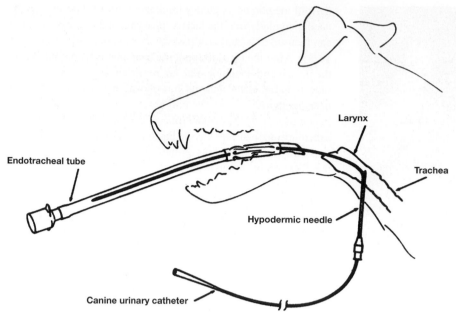

Larynx

Trachea

Endotracheal tube

Hypodermic needle

Canine urinary catheter

Fig. 18.33. Diagram illustrating the placement and use of a retrograde guide tube for passage of an endotracheal tube in a dog. This technique is reserved for patients that cannot be intubated by other methods. From Hartsfield.[19]

processes involving the pharynx or head and neck. Depending on the species and the specific conditions, the endoscope can be placed inside the endotracheal tube to directly guide intubation passed orally beside the endotracheal tube, or advanced through the nasal passage to view the endotracheal tube entering the glottis. The technique can be particularly advantageous in horses with abnormal oropharyngeal, laryngeal, and/or nasal anatomy, and can be helpful in small laboratory species that are difficult to intubate. The technique is applicable to any species that are difficult to intubate. The technique is applicable to any species in which intubation is impaired by anatomical abnormalities or disease. The technique is illustrated in a normal cat in Figs. 18.34 through 18.36.

Tracheostomy

A temporary tracheostomy can be chosen for airway management in lieu of the techniques suggested earlier for difficult cases. In some patients, the only reasonable option for intubation is tracheostomy, and some patients with airway disease arrive in the induction room with a tracheostomy tube in place. For anesthesia, intubation of the trachea through the tracheostomy site provides all of the advantages of oral intubation or intubation by pharyngotomy. However, tracheostomy has been associated with infection, granulomas, tracheal stricture, cartilage damage, hemorrhage, pneumothorax, tracheocutaneous or tracheo-esophageal fistula, aspiration, dysphagia, and tracheal malacia; thus, tracheostomy should not be considered an innocuous procedure.[21] Intubation via tracheostomy is generally reserved for patients requiring preoperative or postoperative tracheostomy for airway management. A tracheostomy tube with a replaceable lumen (Fig. 18.8) should be used, if available, but standard endotracheal tubes have been used satisfactorily (Fig. 18.9). Care of the tube is very important. Neglected tubes that are not cleaned regularly can be obstructed by mucus that dries within the lumen of the tube (Figs. 18.37 and 18.38).

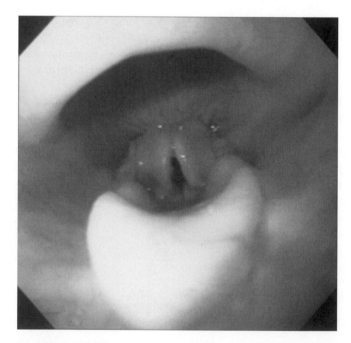

Fig. 18.34. Epiglottis, arytenoid cartilages, and glottis of a cat, as viewed through a fiber-optic endoscope.

Changing Endotracheal Tubes

Changing endotracheal tubes during a surgical or diagnostic procedure in an anesthetized animal is occasionally required due to a failing cuff or simply the need for a different size or length of tube. Patients positioned and draped for surgery are generally not ideally situated for intubation. Changing the tube with guide-tube technique is probably the easiest, most efficient way to accomplish the procedure.[19,22] Depending on the size of the patient and the endotracheal tube, two canine urinary catheters (8 to 10

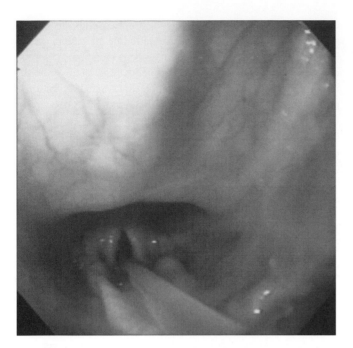

Fig. 18.35. A polyethylene guide tube (8-French) passing through the glottis and into the larynx and trachea of a cat as viewed through a fiber-optic endoscope. Although not generally necessary for intubation in cats, this technique is effective in other species.

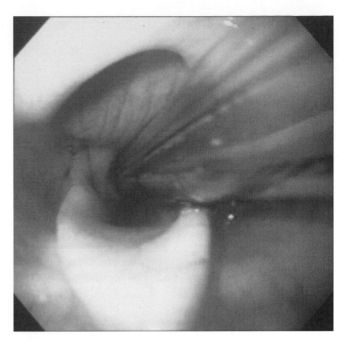

Fig. 18.36. An endotracheal tube passing into the larynx of a cat as viewed through a fiber-optic endoscope. Although not generally necessary for intubation in cats, this technique is effective in other species.

French) connected in tandem, or an equine stomach tube will make an excellent guide tube.

To change endotracheal tubes, the guide tube is inserted through the original endotracheal tube to the area of the midcervical trachea. Next, the endotracheal tube cuff is deflated, and the endotracheal tube is pulled over the guide tube without removing the guide tube from the trachea. Then, the new endotracheal tube is maneuvered through the larynx and into the trachea by using the guide tube to direct its passage. The cuff of the new tube is inflated to protect the airway, and the new tube is secured in the manner appropriate for the specific species.

Tracheal Extubation

Extubation is performed after patients regain the ability to swallow and protect their airways. When the cuff is deflated, the endotracheal tube is removed slowly and deliberately, with care taken to avoid damaging the patient's tissues with the endotracheal tube or damaging the cuff as the tube passes the teeth. After extubation, protection of the airway from foreign material and maintenance of a patent airway remain important. The type of surgical or diagnostic procedure, the species and breed, and pre-existing conditions all affect these considerations.

The anesthetist should be certain that no foreign material remains in the oropharynx before beginning extubation. In dogs and cats, the pharynx should be inspected visually, and any debris should be removed. Specifically, surgery of the mouth and pharynx, dental procedures, and endoscopy promote the accumu-

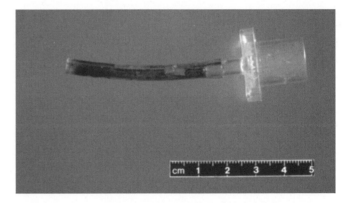

Fig. 18.37. An endotracheal tube that had been placed through a tracheostomy to maintain an airway in a cat during transport of the cat to a referral center. On presentation, the cat was dyspneic and cyanotic. The tube was filled with dried mucus, and the extent of the occlusion of the lumen is illustrated more dramatically in Fig. 18.38. The tube had not been changed or cleaned for several hours.

lation of blood, fluids, lubricants, tartar, or other materials. Animals anesthetized for gastrointestinal surgery are prone to passive movement of fluid into the pharynx; two examples are dogs with gastric dilation and volvulus (GDV) and horses with colic. Nasogastric or orogastric tubes commonly used in these procedures may promote flow of gastric contents into the pharynx during surgery or when the tube is removed. With either

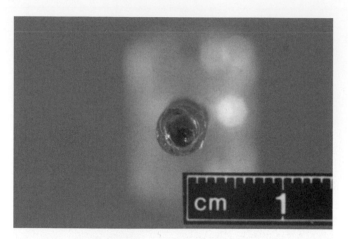

Fig. 18.38. End-on view of the endotracheal tube in Fig. 18.37 shows that the lumen was almost occluded. The cat was dyspneic prior to removal of the tube from the tracheostomy site.

species, the head should be positioned to allow drainage of fluid from the pharynx during surgery, and removing the endotracheal tube with the cuff inflated is advised.

Assuring a patent airway after extubation is essential, especially in patients with small-diameter upper airways (e.g., kittens, piglets, rabbits, and small brachycephalic dogs). A number of factors can be responsible for postextubation problems. Edema of the upper airway, including the larynx and nasal passages; laryngeal spasm; interference with the integrity of the airway by the soft palate; and laryngeal paralysis are all possible causes of obstructive problems. The anesthetist should be prepared to manage the airway at the time of extubation, knowing that these complications can impair ventilation and oxygenation. In some instances of postextubation airway obstruction, reanesthetizing the patient and reintubation may be the only feasible option.

Techniques of Oxygen Administration

Supplemental oxygen is used in anesthetized and critically ill patients to increase the partial pressure of oxygen in arterial blood (PaO_2) and to promote delivery of oxygen to the tissues. When a patient is breathing room air, values for PaO_2 that are less than 80 mm Hg indicate the potential for hypoxemia. If the PaO_2 decreases to less than 60 mm Hg, the need for supplemental oxygen is indicated.[23] Although ventilation is a factor in maintaining oxygenation, the fraction of oxygen in inspired gases (F_IO_2) plays a significant role in establishing the PaO_2. As a rule, the PaO_2 value is approximately five times the F_IO_2 value if there are no major abnormalities in the matching of pulmonary ventilation and perfusion. Supplemental oxygen may be the only effective way of correcting hypoxemia in animals with diffusion abnormalities and ventilation-perfusion mismatching. Supplemental oxygen may not significantly improve PaO_2 in patients with pulmonary or cardiac shunts.

Several techniques can be used to administer oxygen to anes-

thetized and critically ill patients. The effectiveness of oxygen supplementation is assessed by evaluation of the patient's clinical responses (e.g., improvement in mucous membrane color and character of ventilation), by measuring the F_IO_2, and by monitoring of PaO_2, arterial oxygen saturation (SaO_2), and saturation of peripheral oxygen (SpO_2). Although PaO_2 and SaO_2 data are reliable, they require periodic arterial blood sampling and the use of an acid-base, blood-gas analyzer. The SpO_2 can be conveniently measured by pulse oximetry. Pulse oximetry is a practical method for noninvasive, moment-to-moment estimation of the saturation of hemoglobin with oxygen in anesthetized, recovering, and critically ill patients.[24,25]

Mask Delivery

Masks for delivery of oxygen to veterinary patients are useful for preoxygenation immediately before induction of anesthesia and for emergency situations in awake patients. The use of masks for oxygenation requires constant attention, and some patients will not accept a mask unless they are sedated. Both factors limit the effectiveness of masks in awake patients. Indeed, some patients object to a mask so vigorously that the increase in oxygen consumption associated with restraint may nullify the benefits of a greater F_IO_2.

The flow rates generally recommended for increasing F_IO_2 when using masks are variable among species. For example, flow rates of 10 to 15 L/min of supplemental oxygen have been recommended to increase the inspired-oxygen concentration to approximately 35% to 60% in adult horses.[26] Flow rates for smaller patients, including dogs and cats, usually range from 3 to 5 L/min. With a tight-fitting mask, higher flow rates of oxygen will produce greater F_IO_2 values and less rebreathing of expired carbon dioxide.

A mask should be used with a breathing system with a reservoir that can meet the patient's tidal volume demands or with a valved system that allows room air to be entrained. As an example, a dog with a tidal volume of 300 mL and an inspiratory time of 1 s has a peak inspiratory gas flow of approximately 18 L/min, which exceeds the practical flow rate for oxygen during masking. High inspiratory flow rates can be provided if the mask is attached to a circle breathing system with a reservoir bag. In addition, a breathing system has an overflow (pop-off) valve that prevents the buildup of excessive pressure with a tight-fitting mask.

Nasal Insufflation

Insufflation involves delivery of oxygen into the patient's airway at relatively high flow rates (Fig. 18.39); the patient inspires both oxygen and room air, the relative proportions of each being determined primarily by the oxygen flow rate and the rate of gas flow during inspiration.

Insufflation can be accomplished by a variety of methods. For horses recovering from anesthesia, oxygen may be delivered from a flowmeter through a delivery tube and into an orotracheal, nasotracheal, or tracheostomy tube. For most awake patients, oxygen is insufflated through a nasal catheter, the tip of which is positioned in the nasopharynx. The catheter is usually made of soft rubber, and the tube should have several fenestrations to pre-

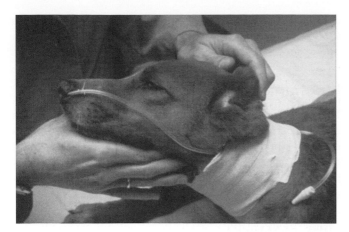

Fig. 18.39. A nasal catheter for administration of oxygen in a dogs. The tube is secured to the muzzle with a suture.

vent jetting lesions from developing in the nasopharyngeal mucosa.[27] For awake small animals, instilling 2% lidocaine into the nasal passage with the patient's head and neck extended and held upward may facilitate passage of the tube. Placement involves insertion of the rubber catheter into the nasal passage and the nasopharynx, the distance being approximately the same as from the tip of the nose to the medial canthus of the eye. The external portion of the catheter is secured to the patient's head with tissue adhesive, tape, and/or sutures. A flexible length of tubing supplies oxygen from a flowmeter and allows the patient some freedom for movement in a cage or stall. Changing the catheter to the opposite nasal passage every 1 to 2 days has been recommended to prevent pressure necrosis, jet lesions, and accumulation of mucus.[27]

The flow-rate requirements for oxygen during insufflation are quite variable, the patient's ventilation and the desired F_IO_2 being two important factors. Following anesthesia, adult horses require a minimum of 15 L/min of oxygen flow to improve the PaO_2 in arterial blood, and proportionally lower flows (e.g., 5 L/min) are suitable for smaller horses and foals.[26] In small animals, flow rates of 1 to 7 L/min are typically used for the administration of nasal oxygen. Approximate flow rates for dogs and cats to achieve rather specific ranges of F_IO_2 have been suggested.[27,28] In dogs, various flow rates of 100% oxygen administered intranasally were studied, and flow rates of 50, 100, 150, and 200 mL kg^{-1} min^{-1} produced inspired-oxygen concentrations measured at the tracheal bifurcation of 28%, 37%, 40%, and 47%, respectively.[29] To prevent mucosal drying with prolonged insufflation, oxygen should be flowed through a bubble-type humidifier.

Tracheal Insufflation

An intratracheal catheter placed percutaneously into the trachea through the cricothyroid membrane or between tracheal rings near the larynx can be used to insufflate oxygen to a compromised patient. Intratracheal administration of 100% oxygen has been evaluated in dogs, and flow rates of 10, 25, 50, 100, 150,

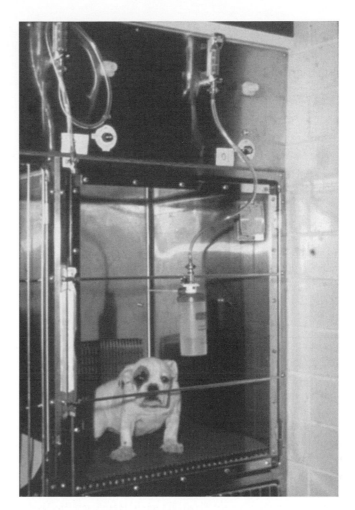

Fig. 18.40. A standard stainless-steel cage with a Plexiglas door facilitating administration of humidified oxygen to an English bulldog. Although concentrations of oxygen are unlikely to be very high, patients with respiratory distress often show clinical improvement.

200, and 250 mL kg^{-1} min^{-1} produced inspired-oxygen concentrations at the tracheal bifurcation of 25%, 32%, 47%, 67%, 70%, 78%, and 86%, respectively.[30] The technique for tracheal insufflation has been described for small animals.[27,30] The catheter should be placed aseptically, be of the over-the-needle type, relatively large bore, have several smooth fenestrations to prevent jet lesions, and ultimately positioned with the tip near the bronchial bifurcation. Oxygen should be humidified, and flow rates should approximate those used for nasal insufflation.

Oxygen Cages

Oxygen cages (Figs. 18.40 and 18.41) specifically designed for small animals are commercially available, but expensive. These cages regulate oxygen flow, control humidity and temperature, and eliminate carbon dioxide from exhaled gases. For small animals, flow rates of oxygen, cage temperature, and cage humidity have been recommended to be less than 10 L/min, approximately 22°C, and 40% to 50%, respectively.[27] With these flow rates,

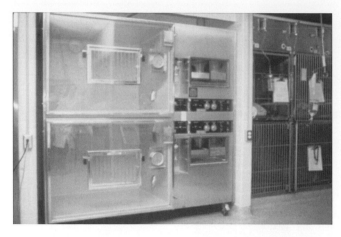

Fig. 18.41. Two commercial oxygen cages designed for small veterinary patients. The cages can control environmental temperature, deliver oxygen, and absorb carbon dioxide from expired gases.

most oxygen cages produce an environmental oxygen concentration of about 40% to 50%.[27] Oxygen concentrations of 30% to 40% generally are adequate for patients with moderate pulmonary disease.[23] Oxygen cages are not practical for large horses,[26] and, even in smaller animals, the effectiveness of an oxygen cage diminishes as body size increases. Because of this, nasal insufflation of oxygen has supplanted oxygen cages in many instances, even for smaller dogs and cats.

Smaller canine patients can be managed easily in oxygen cages, but temperature and humidity are more difficult to control with larger dogs. A major disadvantage of an oxygen cage is that the animal must be removed from the cage for examination and treatment, requiring the patient to breathe room air or oxygen by mask during this period. Clinically, some dogs and cats with serious ventilatory compromise respond very well to an oxygen-enriched environment as initial therapy; the increase in F_IO_2 is associated with decreased ventilatory effort, and the patient stabilizes and becomes more manageable prior to further examination and treatment.

Oxygen Toxicity

Oxygen toxicity develops with prolonged exposure to high oxygen concentrations.[31,32] Oxygen toxicity leads to the deterioration of pulmonary function, pulmonary edema, and death. The length of time that a patient's PaO_2 is elevated may be more predictive of oxygen toxicity than the duration of exposure to a high F_IO_2.[32] There is significant species and individual variability in susceptibility to oxygen toxicity.[27,32] In human patients, the guideline is that 100% oxygen should not be administered for more than 12 h of exposure.[27] In general, a patient should not be deprived of a high concentration of oxygen if a high F_IO_2 is required to maintain an adequate PaO_2; it has been stated that the brain softens (due to hypoxemia) before the lungs harden (owing to changes induced by prolonged exposure to high oxygen tensions).[33] As a guideline for prolonged administration of oxygen, 40% to 50% oxygen is generally safe, but higher inspired concentrations should be used if necessary to maintain a patient's PaO_2 at approximately 90 to 100 mm Hg and ensure hemoglobin saturation with oxygen.

Mechanical Ventilation

Essentially, all anesthetized patients hypoventilate; they do not maintain arterial carbon dioxide partial pressure ($PaCO_2$) values near 40 mm Hg because of abnormal alveolar ventilation. Although controlled ventilation is not necessary for all anesthetized patients, various circumstances may compel an anesthetist to employ intermittent positive-pressure ventilation (IPPV). The absolute indication for mechanical ventilation is apnea.[34] However, IPPV should be instituted if hypoventilation becomes significant, if neuromuscular blocking drugs are employed, or if intrathoracic surgery is performed.[35] General anesthesia for longer than 11/2 h may constitute a reason for IPPV.[36] In addition, IPPV may be needed to facilitate inhalant anesthesia. Hypoventilating animals may not absorb enough anesthetic to maintain surgical anesthesia. IPPV will enhance alveolar ventilation and increase the uptake of the inhalants. This may help in eliminating the oscillations between deep and light anesthesia associated with depression of spontaneous ventilation.

Maintaining relatively normal carbon dioxide tensions in arterial blood is the primary goal of mechanical ventilation in anesthetized patients. Normal values for $PaCO_2$ are generally in the range of 35 to 45 mm Hg for most species. However, controversy exists about the routine use of IPPV in anesthetized patients, particularly anesthetized horses, simply to keep $PaCO_2$ near 40 mm Hg. Because IPPV is associated with reduced cardiovascular function and moderate increases in $PaCO_2$ are associated with improvement in some cardiovascular variables, IPPV for every anesthetized patient is neither universally accepted nor universally practiced. The definition of an acceptable degree of hypercapnia in an anesthetized animal is not without debate. For spontaneously breathing horses, a range of 60 to 70 mm Hg of $PaCO_2$ has been suggested as perhaps safer than controlled ventilation with its potentially adverse effects on cardiovascular function and tissue perfusion.[36] Others have recommended IPPV for horses only when $PaCO_2$ values exceed 60 mm Hg[37] or even 70 mm Hg.[26,37] Employing IPPV in large anesthetized animals, including horses and other species, to maintain $PaCO_2$ values between 35 and 50 mm Hg remains common practice. For a more definitive answer to this debate, large-scale clinical trials with various sized horses and anesthetic-surgical conditions need to be completed.

The direct cardiovascular effects of carbon dioxide include dilation of peripheral arterioles and myocardial depression. Indirectly, carbon dioxide evokes sympathoadrenal responses, which cause blood pressure elevation, tachycardia, and increased myocardial contractility.[38] Moderate (60 to 70 mm Hg) to high (75 to 85 mm Hg) increases in $PaCO_2$ in spontaneously breathing and mechanically ventilated, lightly anesthetized horses were associated with augmented cardiovascular function compared with horses with normal carbon dioxide tensions; these hemodynamic effects were accompanied by increases in circulating catecholamines.[39] If more normal (35 to 45 mm Hg) arterial carbon

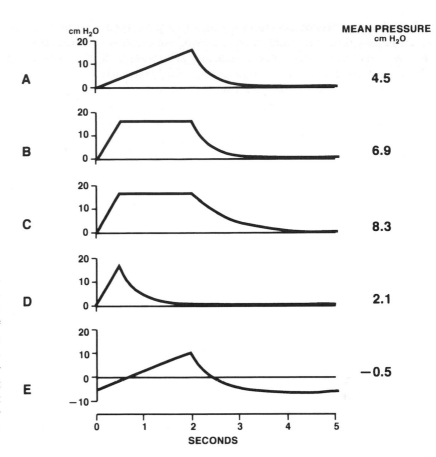

MEAN PRESSURE
cm H_2O

A   4.5

B   6.9

C   8.3

D   2.1

E   —0.5

Fig. 18.42. Diagrams illustrating the mean pressure in the lungs in relation to positive-pressure ventilation: the effects of a long inspiratory time **(A)**, an inspiratory plateau or holding pressure at the end of inspiration **(B)**, an inspiratory plateau with retarded expiration **(C)**, a rapid inspiration **(D)**, and a slow inspiration with a negative expiratory phase **(E)**. Lower mean pressure is most desirable from the standpoint of cardiovascular function, and **D** illustrates the most desirable type of ventilation, although the inspiratory time depicted is shorter than normally used clinically. From Mushin et al.,[71] in Lumb and Jones.[72]

dioxide tensions correlate with lower values for blood pressure, myocardial contractility, and cardiac output in anesthetized animals, the argument can be made that spontaneously breathing (slightly hypercapnic) anesthetized animals may maintain cardiovascular function better than animals whose ventilation is controlled with IPPV. The use of inotropic drugs may be necessary to maintain cardiovascular function during surgical anesthesia in mechanically ventilated horses. Nevertheless, there are good reasons to maintain $PaCO_2$ values within reasonable limits in anesthetized animals.

Inhalant anesthetics (e.g., halothane) and epidural or spinal anesthesia reduce the circulatory responses to carbon dioxide.[38,40] In addition, hypercapnia has been associated with increases in vagal tone and slowing of heart rate.[41] Indeed, hypercapnia has long been related to enhanced vagal responsiveness, bradycardia, and even cardiac arrest. It used to be said that "hypercarbia does not stimulate vagal activity directly, but it 'sets the stage' for cardiac arrest if such a stimulus is present."[42] It is known that carbon dioxide produces narcosis in dogs, the degree of which depends on the $PaCO_2$ value; narcosis progressively increases with $PaCO_2$ values above 95 mm Hg and induces complete anesthesia at 245 mm Hg.[43] Hypercapnia and the associated increases in circulating catecholamines have been linked to the development of cardiac arrhythmias, especially when the heart has been sensitized by halogenated inhalant anesthetics.[44] In human pediatric patients whose airways were managed by masks, hypercapnia was associated with an increased incidence

of arrhythmias.[45] The authors noted that light anesthesia or a combination of factors such as hypercapnia and halothane might have been as important as hypercapnia alone in the production of arrhythmias in these children. Thus, there is a negative side to uncontrolled hypercapnia that should be considered for anesthetized patients, and the veterinarian or anesthesiologist should weigh the advantages against the disadvantages in the anesthetic management of each patient.

Mechanical ventilation does negatively affect cardiovascular function (Fig. 18.42). The depression of cardiovascular function may be significant. When ventilation is controlled and negative pressures are not generated during inspiration, venous return is not enhanced. Indeed, IPPV may physically impede venous return to the right side of the heart, leading to decreases in stroke volume, cardiac output, and arterial blood pressure. In anesthetized, mechanically ventilated horses, a reduction in blood pressure and damping of the pressure waveform is not uncommon, especially in critically ill patients with a marginal blood volume. The negative effects of mechanical ventilation on cardiovascular function can be exacerbated by prolonging inspiratory time, holding positive pressure in the lungs at the end of inspiration, retarding exhalation, applying positive pressure during the expiratory phase, and employing an excessively rapid respiratory rate. Some of these effects are illustrated in Fig. 18.42. Fortunately, these negative effects can be overcome in many cases by the appropriate expansion of extracellular fluid volume and, if necessary, the administration of inotropic drugs.

Guidelines for mechanical ventilation usually include values for inspiratory time, respiratory rate, inspiratory to expiratory time ratio, and tidal volume. Some variations exist because of differences in body size, species, physical condition of the lungs and thorax, and existing disease processes.

Normal tidal volume is generally considered to range between 10 and 20 mL/kg of body weight.[46] A good working guideline for tidal volume in the domestic species is approximately 10 mL/kg.[47] For IPPV, the tidal volume set on a mechanical ventilator is usually increased above the normal spontaneous tidal volume to compensate for pressure-mediated increases in the volume of the breathing system and airway. Increasing the tidal volume (bellows volume) by 2.2 to 4.4 mL/kg has been recommended.[35] Settings for tidal volume—15 mL/kg in large animals and 20 mL/kg in small animals—have been suggested.[47] Use of small tidal volumes may cause atelectasis, which may only be recognized grossly during thoracotomy or with blood-gas analysis, because atelectasis contributes to mismatching of pulmonary ventilation and perfusion leading to decreased PaO_2. The tidal volume should be delivered to the patient over a relatively short period to avoid maintaining positive intrathoracic pressure. Inspiratory time should be approximately 1 to 1.5 s in small animals and 1.5 to 3 s in large animals.

The inspiratory time compared with time during the entire expiratory phase is termed the *I-E ratio*. That fraction should be 1:2 (I-E) or less for mechanical ventilation in all patients. Ratios that approach 1:1 produce a long duration of positive intrathoracic pressure, which interferes more with cardiovascular function. If a patient's respiratory rate is 10 breaths/min and the inspiratory time is 1.5 s, the I-E ratio will be 1:3. In general, the exact value of the I-E ratio is not important as long as the ratio is less than 1:2. With some ventilators that incorporate specific, unchangeable I-E ratios, the options for controlling respiratory rate may be limited.

Tidal volume and inspiratory time affect the development of peak inspiratory pressure. In general, 15 to 30 cm H_2O will expand the lung,[47] and 15 to 20 cm H_2O and 20 to 30 cm H_2O have been recommended as peak inspiratory pressures for mechanical ventilation of small animal species with normal lungs and large animal species with normal lungs, respectively.[35] Excessive or sustained pressure during IPPV can cause excessive expansion and volutrauma, leading to disruption of the alveolar membrane, to the development of interstitial air, and ultimately to the transfer of air into the mediastinum, pleural space, or abdomen.[48] A good guideline for peak inspiratory pressure is not to exceed 30 cm H_2O. Special attention to peak pressure is important for animals that have experienced lung trauma (e.g., diaphragmatic hernia).[49]

The appropriate respiratory rate for mechanical ventilation varies with the species and the tidal volume selected. The following recommendations have been published: dogs, 8 to 14 breaths/min; cats, 10 to 14 breaths/min; horses and cows, 6 to 10 breaths/min; and small ruminants and pigs, 8 to 12 breaths/min.[47] In patients requiring smaller than usual tidal volumes, to avoid excessive inspiratory pressures (e.g., lung trauma, diaphragmatic hernia, or gastrointestinal distension, including GDV), respiratory rates can be increased to maintain the appropriate minute ventilation.

When controlled ventilation is discontinued at the end of anesthesia, the return of spontaneous ventilation may be impaired. If $PaCO_2$ is low, spontaneous ventilation may not resume. Part of the management of controlled ventilation should be maintenance of relatively normal carbon dioxide tensions, and hypocarbia should be avoided. The residual effects of opioids, anesthetics, and adjunctive drugs (e.g., neuromuscular blocking drugs) at the end of anesthesia may contribute to a delayed return to spontaneous ventilation. Complicating factors associated with general anesthesia or surgery (e.g., hypothermia or hypovolemia) may slow an animal's return to consciousness and thus spontaneous ventilation. In general, the arterial tension of carbon dioxide must increase to stimulate the animal to breathe spontaneously, or the patient must regain a level of consciousness that promotes spontaneous ventilation. Before attempting to discontinue controlled ventilation, the anesthetist should ascertain that depth of anesthesia is decreasing, that the effects of muscle-relaxing drugs have subsided or have been antagonized, and that cardiovascular function is relatively normal. Then, the animal can be weaned from controlled ventilation.

The patient should continue to receive supplemental oxygen until spontaneous ventilation is relatively normal. Reducing the rate of controlled ventilation usually increases $PaCO_2$ enough to stimulate spontaneous breathing when an animal is regaining consciousness. Generally, the patient is mechanically or manually ventilated at a rate of one to four breaths per minute until spontaneous ventilation resumes. In many cases, animals begin to breathe spontaneously after the vaporizer has been turned off and most of the inhalant anesthetic has been eliminated, even though controlled ventilation has not been stopped. Some patients require some type of external stimulus to begin breathing (e.g., pinching the skin between a dog's toes). After the animal begins to breathe spontaneously, assisted ventilation and supplemental oxygen should be provided until the respiratory rate and tidal volume begin to normalize.

Anesthesia Ventilators

Anesthesia ventilators provide for mechanical ventilation of patients being maintained with inhalant anesthetics. Simply, an anesthesia ventilator is a reservoir bag (a bellows or concertina bag) in a closed container (bellows housing) that can substitute for the reservoir bag of an anesthesia breathing system. Within limits, the ventilator can drive its bellows to produce a specific tidal volume or a specific inspiratory pressure at a preselected rate. The anesthesia ventilator performs the same job as the anesthetist who periodically squeezes the circle system's reservoir bag to ventilate the patient. Some anesthesia ventilators are stand-alone units that are attached to an anesthesia machine when needed, whereas other ventilators are manufactured as an integral part of the anesthesia machine. Most anesthesia ventilators designed for human patients are appropriate for veterinary patients weighing less than approximately 140 kg. Ventilators specifically designed for large animals are needed for pa-

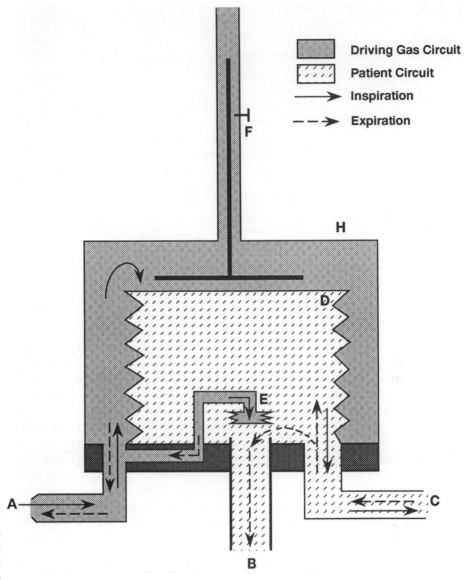

Fig. 18.43. Diagram of a generic, double-circuit ventilator. Driving gas enters at *A*, leading to compression of the bellows and forcing gas in the patient circuit toward the breathing system and the patient's respiratory system (*C*). Overflow gas from the patient circuit exits through the pop-off valve (*E*) and flows into the scavenger system (*B*). *F*, tidal volume adjustment; *D*, bellows; and *H*, bellows housing.

Double-Circuit Ventilator

tients weighing more than 140 kg. Admittedly, these guidelines for body weight and selection of a ventilator are somewhat arbitrary.

Classification

The power source, drive mechanism, cycling mechanism, and type of bellows have been used to classify anesthesia ventilators.[50] The power source may be electricity, compressed gas, or both. The drive mechanism is commonly compressed gas, even when electric controls are used. Anesthesia ventilators are usually double-circuit units (Fig. 18.43). *Double circuit* refers to two gas sources: (a) the driving-gas circuit (outside of the bellows), which compresses the bellows, and (b) the patient gas circuit (inside the bellows), which originates at the anesthesia machine and provides oxygen and anesthetic to the breathing system and pa-

tient. Specific ventilators for veterinary applications are classified in Table 18.1.

Anesthesia ventilators are typically, though not always, time cycled.[50] Fluidic timing devices were common in the late 1970s, and fluid-controlled ventilators remain in use. Newer electronic ventilators incorporate solid-state timing circuitry and are classified as time cycled and electronically controlled. A pressure-cycling mechanism may be present in some ventilators, and some have been described as volume cycled. In most cases, a timing mechanism plays a major role in a ventilator's function, and volume or pressure limits may affect the change in the respiratory cycle from inspiration to expiration.

The direction that the bellows moves during expiration, either ascending or descending, also helps to characterize anesthesia ventilators. Newer anesthesia ventilators usually have ascending

Table 18.1. Classification and characteristics of some anesthesia ventilators

Ventilator	Power Source	Drive Mechanism	Cycling Mechanism	Bellows[a]	Type of Ventilation
Drager SAV (SA)	Pneumatic	Pneumatic	Time-fluidic	Ascend	Control
Hallowell EMC 2000 (SA)	Pneumatic and electronic	Pneumatic	Time-electronic	Ascend	Control
Mallard 2400 V (SA)	Pneumatic and electronic	Pneumatic	Time-electronic	Ascend	Control
Metomatic (Ohio)-SA	Pneumatic	Pneumatic	Time-fluidic	Descend	Assist/control
Ohmeda 7000 (SA)	Pneumatic	Pneumatic	Time-electronic	Ascend	Control
ADS 1000 (SA)	Pneumatic and electronic	Pneumatic	Time-electronic	None	Control
SAV 75 (SA)	Pneumatic	Pneumatic	Time-pressure	Ascend	Assist/control
Drager AV (LA)	Pneumatic and electronic	Pneumatic	Time-fluidic	Descend	Control
Narkovet Electronic LA Control Center	Pneumatic and electronic	Pneumatic	Time-electronic	Descend	Control
LAVC 2000 (LA)	Pneumatic	Pneumatic	Time-pressure	Descend	Assist/control
Mallard 2800 (LA)	Pneumatic and electronic	Pneumatic	Time-electronic	Ascend	Control

LA (large animal) and SA (small animal) indicate the primary use of the ventilator.
[a]Bellows is described in reference to the direction of movement during expiration.

bellows. The ascending bellows is considered safer because it will not fill if a disconnection occurs in the breathing circuit.[50] The ascending bellows falls to the bottom of the bellows housing during a disconnection, giving an immediate visual indication of ventilator failure. Ascending bellows are incorporated into modern electronic ventilators. Ventilators with descending bellows may continue to cycle even with a complete disconnection of the ventilator from the breathing system.

The terms *tidal volume preset*, *volume preset*, and *volume constant* have been used to describe anesthesia ventilators; these terms have been included in operation manuals and other descriptive literature authored both by manufacturers and by medical personnel. The implication is that the ventilator delivers exactly the tidal volume selected despite the total inspiratory time or the amount of inspiratory pressure that develops. However, the tidal volume that actually reaches a patient's lungs may vary from the setting on the ventilator. Variations are related to the compliance of the breathing system, leaks in the system, and the entry of fresh gases into the breathing system. Although the terms *tidal volume preset*, *volume preset*, and *volume constant* may be practical, the user should understand the unknown influences on the quantity of gas actually delivered to the patient.

In addition, ventilators may be called *pressure preset*, indicating that inspiration continues until a selected pressure is reached, no matter what tidal volume is necessary to achieve the pressure. The amount of gas delivered to a patient depends on a number of factors, including the resistance and compliance of the breathing system and the patient's respiratory system. Although inspiratory pressure may not vary over time, the tidal volume may change as compliance of the respiratory system changes.

Even though ventilators have been classified as *volume limited* and *pressure limited*, and *pressure cycled*, *time cycled*, and *volume cycled*, these terms may be somewhat misleading or confusing because the mechanism that actually causes the change from expiration to inspiration is most often a timing mechanism.

Indeed, the change from one phase of ventilation to the other may involve more than one mechanism, including volume, pressure, and/or time. Some ventilators may use different cycling mechanisms depending on the mode of operation.[50] A pressure-limited ventilator is one that delivers gas to a patient during inspiration until a preset pressure develops in the bellows, at which point the expiratory phase begins. The disadvantage of pressure-limited ventilation is that the tidal volume delivered to a patient may decrease if respiratory compliance decreases during ventilation. A volume-limited ventilator delivers a present tidal volume (within the limits discussed earlier) without regard for the maximum inspiratory pressure (up to the preset maximum pressure for the ventilator). Inspiratory pressure may increase if compliance decreases during mechanical ventilation. Most anesthesia ventilators have a maximum pressure limit during inspiration for the safety of the patient, and that pressure limit varies with the model of the ventilator. Ventilators that are used as volume-limited units may truly be limited by time rather than by volume, and that fact becomes apparent if the inspiratory flow rate is too slow.

Terminology of Mechanical Ventilation

Several abbreviations are used in the medical literature to describe various types of ventilation. Common abbreviations are included and discussed in the following subsections.

IPPV (Intermittent Positive-Pressure Ventilation)

With IPPV, airway pressure is maintained above ambient pressure during inspiration, and airway pressure falls to ambient pressure to allow passive expiration.[48] *Conventional positive-pressure ventilation* (CPPV), also called *control-mode ventilation* (CMV), is a form of IPPV in which a ventilator delivers a preset tidal volume at a preset frequency.[51] *Assist-control-mode ventilation* (AMV) provides a preset tidal volume from the ventilator in response to patient-initiated attempts to inspire; a preset frequency of ventilation is delivered by the ventilator if the patient fails to initiate breathing.[51] The term *intermittent positive-pressure breathing* (IPPB) is synonymous with IPPV.

PEEP (Positive End-Expiratory Pressure)

With PEEP, airway pressure at end expiration is maintained above ambient pressure. The term *PEEP* is applied when positive pressure is maintained between inspirations that are delivered by a ventilator.[51] The term *ZEEP*, or *zero end-expiratory pressure*, has been used in studies comparing the effects of PEEP with the effects of ZEEP.[52] In addition, some ventilators can create negative pressure to assist expiration or to speed the egress of gases during the expiratory phase. This has been termed *NEEP* or *negative end-expiratory pressure*.

CPAP (Continuous Positive Airway Pressure)

When airway pressure is maintained above ambient pressure during spontaneous breathing, the term *CPAP* is applied instead of PEEP.[51]

IMV (Intermittent Mandatory Ventilation)

This method of ventilation is used for ventilatory support and for weaning of patients from ventilators. The technique allows patients to breathe spontaneously, but it inserts mechanical breaths at a preset tidal volume and frequency.[51,52] Most veterinary anesthesia ventilators are not designed for delivering this form of ventilation, and IMV is provided by critical care ventilators for human patients. The periodic sigh that anesthetists provide manually during spontaneous ventilation to expand the lung and decrease collapsed alveoli in anesthetized animals may be considered IMV.[26]

The terms *assisted ventilation* and *controlled ventilation* are common in the veterinary literature. Assisted ventilation can be performed manually by anesthetists, who synchronizes their compression of the breathing bag with a patient's spontaneous breathing to augment the tidal volume.[53] With a mechanical ventilator, assisted ventilation is basically patient-initiated ventilation, with the ventilator delivering the preselected tidal volume. Since the patient determines the frequency of ventilation, it also determines minute volume.[54] Some veterinary ventilators can provide assisted ventilation, delivering a tidal volume from the bellows when a patient creates negative pressure at the initiation of a breath.[55]

During *controlled ventilation* as defined earlier for CMV, inspiration is initiated by the ventilator and a preset respiratory rate is maintained. The ventilator sets frequency, tidal volume, and minute volume. Controlled ventilation is necessary in any situation that renders a patient unable to initiate an adequate number of breaths. Essentially all anesthesia ventilators will operate in this mode, and some operate only in this mode. Controlled ventilation can be provided manually by an anesthetist using the reservoir bag of the breathing system to establish both rate and tidal volume, and thus minute volume, for the patient.[53]

The term *assisted-controlled ventilation* has been defined as assisted ventilation (patient-controlled rate with ventilator-controlled tidal volume) with a preset minimum acceptable respiratory rate; if the patient-initiated rate falls below the preset rate, the ventilator will cycle at the minimum preset rate. This mode is similar to AMV as defined earlier. The use of assisted-controlled ventilation has been suggested for the transition period between spontaneous and controlled ventilation.

Guidelines for Use

The controls on most anesthesia ventilators include settings for tidal volume, inspiratory time, inspiratory pressure, respiratory rate, and I-E ratio (either adjustable or preset). Other controls may be present, but the four listed are basic. The following guidelines have already been discussed, but will again be briefly reviewed. The setting for tidal volume is usually between 10 and 20 mL/kg, and the inspiratory pressure is normally between 12 and 30 cm H_2O. In small patients, the respiratory rate should be set between 8 and 12 breaths/min, whereas the respiratory rate for large animals should be set between 6 and 10 breaths/min. In setting the ventilator, inspiratory time should be short in comparison to expiratory time so that positive interpleural pressure will minimally interfere with venous return and cardiac output. Inspiratory time should be 1 to 1.5 s in small animals and preferably less than 3 s in large animals. Therefore, the I-E ratio should be 1:2 or less (e.g., 1:3 or 1:4), depending on the respiratory rate.

Examples of Ventilators for Small Animals

Although not all-inclusive, the following discussion describes ventilators that are appropriate for small animal patients. Some of these ventilators were designed specifically to support anesthetized veterinary patients, whereas others were designed for human use, but are applicable to veterinary patients. The classification, principles of operation, and other points about the general function of each ventilator are included. Before operating a ventilator, the user should consult the operation manuals and follow all preuse evaluation procedures recommended by the manufacturer.

Drager Small Animal Ventilator (SAV)

This ventilator (Fig. 18.44) was marketed as an optional component for the Drager Narkovet 2 Anesthesia Machine, but was available on a mobile stand (universal pole) specifically designed for the ventilator.[56] Presently, the ventilator is not being manufactured, but these ventilators remain in use for veterinary anesthesia. The SAV is classified as double circuit, tidal volume preset, and time cycled, with an ascending bellows; it is pneumatically powered and has fluidic circuitry. The pressure of the driving gas should be between 40 to 60 pounds per square inch (psi). The controls include a power ("on-off") switch, a tidal volume adjustment rod to set the attached plate within the bellows housing to the selected tidal volume (200 to 1600 mL), a frequency control knob (10 to 30 breaths/min), and an inspiratory flow knob to control the rate of flow into the bellows housing to drive the bellows. The inspiratory flow knob should be set so that the bellows is fully compressed at the end of the inspiratory phase; however, the bellows should not be deformed at the end of inspiration. Deformation of the bellows at the end of inspiration my indicate an increase in tidal volume by as much as 100 mL. The inspiratory flow control setting affects the peak pressure that

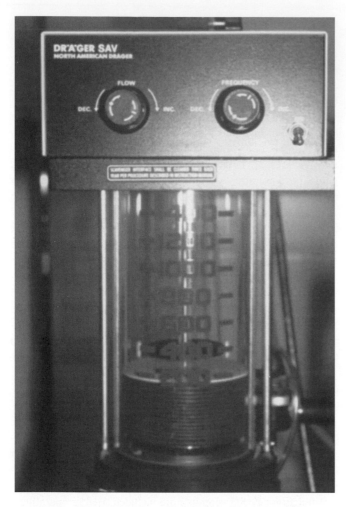

Fig. 18.44. Drager SAV (small animal ventilator; front view). The ascending bellows and the bellows housing with the tidal volume marked in milliliters are shown in the *bottom* of the photograph, and the inspiratory-flow control knob (*left*), the frequency control knob (*center right*), and the power switch (*far right*) are shown in the *top* of the photograph.

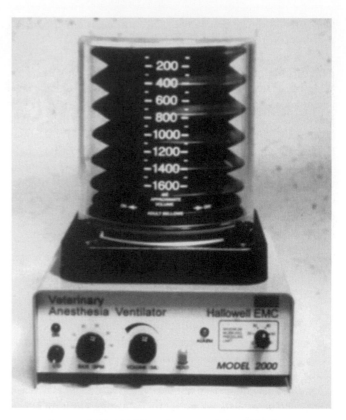

Fig. 18.45. Hallowell EMC Model 2000 Small Animal Veterinary Anesthesia Ventilator (front view). The bellows shown is the medium sized for tidal volumes between 300 and 1600 mL, and the basic control knobs and alarm indicator light are on the front panel. Photograph courtesy of W. Stetson Hallowell.

is achieved on inspiration and the inspiratory time. Higher inspiratory flows produce shorter inspiratory times and tend to produce higher peak inspiratory pressures. The ratio of inspiratory to expiratory time phase is preset to 1:2. This ventilator provides only controlled ventilation. The ventilator relief valve behind the bellows chamber compensates for the continuous entry of fresh gases into the breathing system. Because the ventilator uses an ascending bellows, the effect of gravity on the bellows maintains a PEEP of approximately 2 cm H_2O.

Before using the ventilator, the proper connections to the gas-supply and scavenger system should be made, and the appropriate preuse checkout procedures should be done for all equipment. Assuming that the anesthesia machine, breathing system, and ventilator are functional, the following is a reasonable step-by-step approach to the operation of this ventilator with a circle breathing system:

1. The tidal volume adjustment rod is set appropriately for the patient.
2. Corrugated tubing from the ventilator's breathing-hose terminal is connected to the circle system's reservoir-bag mount.
3. The circle system's APL valve (adjustable pressure-limiting or pop-off valve) is closed.
4. The ventilator's power switch is turned on.
5. The frequency of ventilation is adjusted to approximately the desired number of breaths per minute.
6. The inspiratory flow control knob is adjusted to produce the desired inspiratory time to deliver the preset tidal volume.
7. Frequency of ventilation and inspiratory flow may need to be readjusted to achieve the desired rate of breathing and inspiratory time.

Hallowell EMC Model 2000 Small Animal Veterinary Anesthesia Ventilator

This ventilator (Fig. 18.45) is designed for use with standard small animal anesthesia machines and breathing systems, and the connections to the breathing system, scavenger, and driving gas are shown in Fig. 18.46.[57] This ventilator is classified as double circuit and time cycled with an ascending bellows; it is pneumatically and electrically powered. The ventilator is essentially vol-

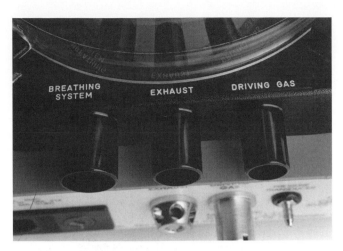

Fig. 18.46. Hallowell EMC Model 2000 Small Animal Veterinary Anesthesia Ventilator (rear view). Note the connectors on the bellows housing for the breathing system, scavenger system (exhaust), and driving gas. Photograph courtesy of W. Stetson Hallowell.

ume constant within the practical limits described earlier. The ventilator is pneumatically driven and electronically controlled by an electrically activated solenoid valve that allows gas pressure to be supplied to the volume control during the inspiratory phase of the ventilatory cycle. The ventilator's power switch is incorporated into the respiratory-rate control. Therefore, the ventilator is on when the rate selector is turned from the off position to the desired frequency of respiration (6 to 40 breaths/min). The pressure of the driving-gas supply (either oxygen, nitrogen, or clean dry air) should be regulated between 30 to 60 psi. This high flow is necessary only for larger patients.

The control module of the ventilator has the following adjustable components: the on-off and respiratory-rate control knob, a volume control knob, an inspiratory hold pushbutton, and a maximum working pressure limit (MWPL) selector. The ratio of inspiratory to expiratory time phase is preset at 1:2. However, this ventilator is available with an optional adjustable I-E ratio in the range of 1:1.5 to 1:4, enabling users to minimize the inspiratory time when ventilating at a lower frequency of ventilation. The volume control is a variable orifice-metering valve that regulates the driving-gas flow, which compresses the bellows. Basically, the volume control is used to set minute volume. It regulates the inspiratory flow rate directly, and a higher inspiratory flow rate at any given respiratory rate will produce a greater tidal volume. The inspiratory hold pushbutton interrupts the ventilatory cycle and prevents discharge of gas from the bellows housing until the button is released or the MWPL is reached. The MWPL can be set between 10 and 60 cm H_2O. If the MWPL is reached at any time, the inspiratory phase of ventilation is terminated and exhalation is allowed. Low breathing-system pressure will be detected if pressure at the end of inspiration is less than 5 cm H_2O, and a red warning light will illuminate and an alarm will sound indicating the possibility of a disconnection of the patient circuit from the ventilator. This

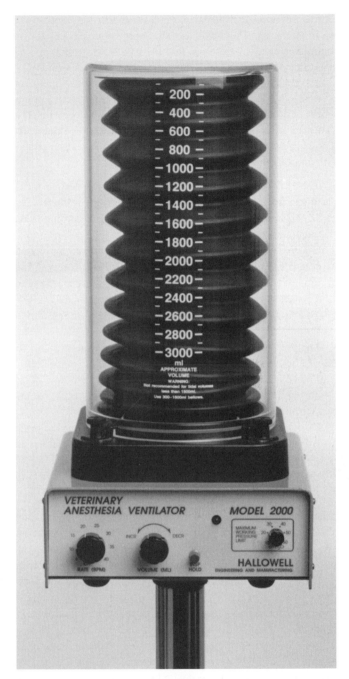

Fig. 18.47. Hallowell EMC Model 2000 Small Animal Veterinary Anesthesia Ventilator (front view). The bellows shown is the largest one for tidal volumes between 0 and 3000 mL. The basic control knobs and alarm indicator light are on the front panel. Photograph courtesy of W. Stetson Hallowell.

ventilator provides for controlled ventilation; assisted ventilation is not an option.

Three sizes of interchangeable bellows and bellows housings are available to enable various sizes of patients to be ventilated effectively (Fig. 18.47). With the proper bellows, the manufacturer indicates that tidal volumes as small as 20 mL and as large as 3 L can be delivered and that the patient can effectively breathe spontaneously from the bellows when the ventilator is not in operation. The ventilator relief valve compensates for the continuous entry of fresh gas into the breathing system, and the resistance of the relief valve creates a PEEP of 2 to 3 cm H_2O.

Before using the ventilator, connections to the gas-supply and scavenger system should be made, and the appropriate preuse checkout procedures should be done. Assuming proper function of the anesthesia machine, breathing system, and ventilator, the following is a reasonable operational approach for this ventilator with a circle breathing system:

1. The MWPL selector (Fig. 18.45) is set to the desired maximum pressure (safety limit), and the pressure transducer (Fig. 18.46) is connected to the breathing system according to the manufacturer's recommendations.
2. Corrugated tubing from the ventilator's breathing system connector is attached to the circle system's reservoir-bag mount, and the ventilator is attached to the scavenger system.
3. The circle system's pop-off (APL) valve is closed.
4. The ventilator's volume control is adjusted to the minimum setting.
5. The ventilator's power-rate switch is turned on, and the desired frequency of ventilation is set.
6. The volume control knob is adjusted to produce a flow of gas during inspiration that produces the desired tidal volume and/or peak inspiratory pressure.
7. During maintenance, the minute volume is adjusted with the volume control, and the rate control can be used to adjust the size of each tidal volume.

Mallard Medical Model 2400V Anesthesia Ventilator

This ventilator[58] (Fig. 18.48) was originally designed to allow continuous mechanical ventilation of anesthetized pediatric and adult human patients. It is sold to veterinarians as a stand-alone unit for use with breathing system and anesthesia machine. Classified as a double-circuit ventilator, it has electric and pneumatic power sources. The ventilator is controlled by a microprocessor, and the manufacturer describes the ventilator as electronically time cycled and volume limited. The tidal volume is selected by limiting the upward expansion of the bellows. Tidal volume is adjusted by moving a cylinder within the bellows housing to coincide with the desired setting in milliliters, and the cylinder within the bellows housing is secured by a control knob (nut) located on the top center of the housing. This ventilator employs an ascending bellows. The bellows is pneumatically driven, and the ventilator operates at a pressure of 50 ± 10 psi.

The controls are positioned on a console, which is located below the bellows housing. A master on/standby/off switch is present in the right lower corner of the console's front panel; the standby mode allows preselection of respiratory rate and inspiratory time, and the I-E ratio is computed and displayed digitally on light-emitting diode (LED) displays before mechanical ventilation is initiated. Respiratory rate and inspiratory time are controlled by ten-turn potentiometers to allow selection of 2 to 80 breaths/min (respiratory rate) and 0.1 to 3.0 s (inspiratory time), respectively. The I-E ratio display shows the relationship of in-

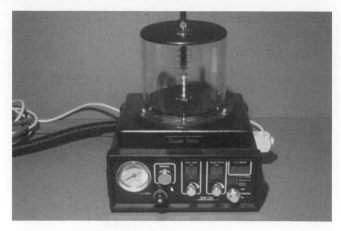

Fig. 18.48. Mallard 2400V Small Animal Anesthesia Ventilator. The bellows is collapsed on the floor of the bellows housing. The tidal volume control is set at approximately 1600 mL. The control knobs on the console are described in the text.

spiratory time to expiratory time, giving inspiratory time a value of 1. A black control knob located in the lower left portion of the front panel allows adjustment of inspiratory flow rate (10 to 100 L/min), and a display gauge near the control knob indicates whether the flow being used is low, medium, or high. A green pushbutton is located in the front center portion of the control console; this button activates inspiration as long as the button is pushed in. This button can be used to maintain mechanical ventilation in the event of a power failure and can be used to sigh the patient.

Two sizes of bellows are available. The adult bellows provides tidal volumes ranging from 200 to 2200 mL; the pediatric bellows produces volumes ranging from 50 to 300 mL. An exhalation valve assembly is located on the back of the control console. This valve is closed pneumatically during the inspiratory phase of ventilation, and it opens automatically during the expiratory phase. Excess gas from the patient circuit exits through this valve to prevent the buildup of excessive pressure. The post (19 mm) of this valve should be attached to a scavenger system for elimination of waste gases from the working environment. With an ascending bellows, PEEP (usually 2 or 3 cm H_2O) will be present. In addition, PEEP of up to 20 cm H_2O can be added to the system with the control knob of the optional PEEP valve. Also, an adjustable overpressure relief valve within the console is preset to 80 cm H_2O, and this limits the maximum pressure that can be developed in the patient breathing circuit. Externally, this pressure can be adjusted from 20 to 100 cm H_2O. This ventilator has audible alarms if the ventilator fails to cycle or if an electric power failure occurs. In addition, the LED displays will indicate selection of an inverse I-E ratio, failure of the ventilator to cycle, and low supply-gas pressure (<30 psi).

Before using the ventilator, the proper connections to the gas-supply and scavenger system should be made, and the appropriate preuse checkout procedures should be done for all equipment. Assuming proper function of the anesthesia machine, breathing

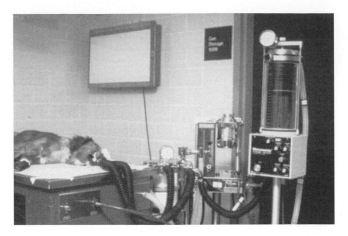

Fig. 18.49. Metomatic Veterinary Ventilator. The ventilator's bellows is connected by a corrugated breathing tube to the reservoir-bag port of the circle breathing system to enable controlled ventilation. Anesthesia was maintained with halothane in oxygen in this dog.

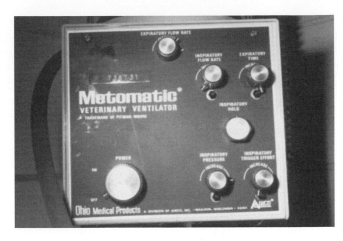

Fig. 18.50. Control panel of a Metomatic Veterinary Ventilator. The function of the various controls of this ventilator are discussed in the text.

system, and ventilator, the following is a reasonable operational approach for this ventilator with a circle breathing system:

1. Prior to clinical applications, refer to the operation manual for instructions and conduct performance verification procedures.
2. Select the appropriate control settings for the tidal volume by limiting the upward expansion of the bellows.
3. Place the master switch in the *standby* mode and dial the desired settings for the respiratory rate and the inspiratory time, based on the patient's needs.
4. Set the inspiratory flow control to the desired rate of flow—low, medium, or high—depending on the needs of the patient.
5. Connect the corrugated tubing from the ventilator's bellows to the circle system's reservoir-bag mount and attach the ventilator to the scavenger system.
6. Close the circle system's pop-off (APL) valve.
7. Set the master switch to the *on* position.
8. The ventilator should cycle according to the selected settings, and only minor adjustments should be necessary (i.e., slight alterations in inspiratory time).

Metomatic Veterinary Ventilator
This ventilator is shown in Figs. 18.49 and 18.50. This unit was designed to ventilate anesthetized small animals being maintained with circle breathing systems. The ventilator is no longer being manufactured, but many units are still in operation in veterinary hospitals.

This ventilator is classified as double circuit and time cycled, with fluidic circuitry and a descending bellows. Within the limits of the definitions, it can be used as a volume-preset ventilator or as a pressure-limited ventilator. The ventilator is powered pneumatically and will function properly with an oxygen-supply pressure to 45 to 55 psi.

Controls (Fig. 18.50) for this ventilator are as follows:[59,60] power (on-off) switch, tidal volume control, inspiratory flow-rate

control, expiratory time control, expiratory flow-rate control, inspiratory hold pushbutton, and inspiratory trigger-effort control. The power switch controls a valve that supplies pneumatic power (oxygen at 50 psi) to the ventilator. The tidal volume control adjusts the bellows from 0 to 1400 mL. The inspiratory flow-rate control regulates the rate of delivery of gas from the bellows to the patient during inspiration and is adjustable from 20 to 70 L/min. The inspiratory pressure control sets the maximum pressure that can be delivered to the patient circuit during inspiration, up to 40 cm H_2O; pressure is adjustable from 10 to 40 cm H_2O. The expiratory time control adjusts the time between the end of one inspiratory phase of respiration and the beginning of the next and can be varied from less than 1 to at least 12 s; essentially, it is a setting for respiratory rate although rate is influenced to some degree by other controls. The expiratory flow-rate control allows variation in the rate at which the bellows descends to the fully extended position and is adjustable from 15 to 100 L/min. The inspiratory hold pushbutton allows the initiation of inspiration at any point during the respiratory cycle by depressing and immediately releasing the button. If the pushbutton is depressed and held, inspiration will be initiated, and the bellows will remain at the end-inspiratory position until the button is released. The inspiratory trigger-effort control sets the sensitivity of the ventilator to the negative pressure produced by the patient's inspiratory effort. The setting can be low, which would require only a slight negative pressure to initiate a cycle, or high, which prevents the patient from triggering inspiration; the setting is adjustable from −0.5 to −5.0 cm H_2O. Many of these ventilators were equipped with a patient circuit pressure gauge (manometer) mounted on top of the bellows housing. This ventilator can be set to provide controlled or assisted ventilation.

The ventilator provides a relief valve (pop-off valve) to allow the escape of excess gases that are delivered to the patient circuit. Generally, the pressure in the patient circuit returns to zero at end expiration, since a descending bellows is employed.

Four modes of ventilation can be employed with this ventilator:

1. *Controller, volume controlled and pressure limited.* The rate and pattern of respiration are controlled by the ventilator. The selected tidal volume is delivered as long as inspiratory pressure does not exceed 40 cm H_2O. If the pressure limit is reached before the entire tidal volume is delivered, inspiration will cease.

2. *Controller, pressure controlled and volume limited.* The rate of ventilation is controlled by the ventilator. The ventilator delivers gas to the patient until the preset pressure limit is reached or until the contents of the bellows are fully discharged. Since tidal volume is affected by pressure, changes in airway resistance and compliance of the lungs can alter tidal volume.

3. *Assistor-controller, volume controlled and pressure limited.* The respiratory cycle is initiated by any spontaneous inspiratory effort on the part of the patient. The minimum frequency of ventilation is set by the ventilator, and if the patient fails to initiate the preset number of breaths, the ventilator will cycle at the minimum frequency. The preset tidal volume is delivered unless the inspiratory pressure reaches 40 cm H_2O, at which point inspiration will cease.

4. *Assistor-controller, pressure controlled and volume limited.* The respiratory cycle is initiated by spontaneous inspiratory efforts, and the minimum frequency is set by the ventilator. The patient may initiate a faster rate of respiration. The ventilator delivers gas to the patient until a preset pressure is reached or until the bellows is fully discharged. The tidal volume will be affected significantly by changes in compliance of the lung and airway resistance.

When using the Metomatic ventilator, the first mode (controller, volume controlled and pressure limited) is most frequently used. Before using the ventilator, the proper connections to the gas-supply and scavenger system should be made, and the appropriate preuse checkout procedures should be done. Assuming that the anesthesia machine, breathing system, and ventilator are functional, the following is a step-by-step approach to the operation of the ventilator with a circle breathing system:

1. Select the desired tidal volume.
2. Set the inspiratory trigger-effort control to a high setting, but not to the maximum.
3. Turn the inspiratory pressure control to a high setting (the maximum setting or high enough to assure that the bellows will deliver a complete tidal volume).
4. Set the inspiratory flow-rate control to a midrange setting. After the ventilator is in use, this control will be reset to deliver the tidal volume in approximately 1 to 1.5 s.
5. Set the expiratory flow rate to a midrange setting. This setting can be refined after the ventilator is in use; a setting is usually employed that will not impede ventilation.
6. Set the expiratory time control to a midrange setting. This control should be reset to allow the appropriate frequency of ventilation after the ventilator is in use.
7. Connect the corrugated tube from the ventilator's bellows to the circle system's reservoir-bag port.
8. Close the pop-off (APL) valve of the circle.
9. Turn the power switch on.

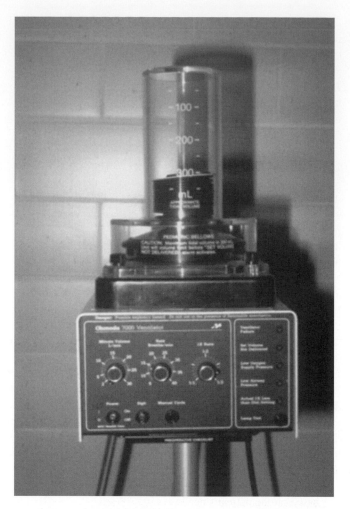

Fig. 18.51. Ohmeda 7000 Ventilator. The control module is shown with six controls on the *left* two-thirds of the panel and six warning indicators on the *right* two-thirds of the panel. This ventilator is equipped with a pediatric bellows assembly (0 to 300 mL for tidal volume).

10. Observe the character and rate of ventilation, and refine the adjustments of the various controls. Usually, inspiratory flow rate is adjusted first, followed by frequency or expiratory time, and expiratory flow rate.

Ohmeda 7000 Electronic Anesthesia Ventilator

The Ohmeda 7000 (Fig. 18.51) is a double-circuit ventilator with a pneumatically driven ascending bellows. The ventilator is electronically controlled with a preset minute volume. It is specifically designed as an anesthesia ventilator and can be fitted with either an adult or a pediatric bellows, and its application in human anesthesia has been described.[50,54,61] This ventilator and upgraded models are available for use in human patients[54] and are readily applicable to small animal anesthesia. The control module (Fig. 18.51) has six controls, including the minute volume dial (2 to 30 L/min with the adult bellows and 2 to 12 L/min with the pediatric bellows), the respiratory-rate dial (6 to 40 breaths/min), the I-E ratio dial (1:1, 1:2, and 1:3), power (on-off) switch, the sigh switch (to provide a "sigh" equal to 150% of the tidal volume once every 64 breaths), and a manual cycle button (used to manually initiate a ventilatory cycle only during the expiratory phase). The scale on the bellows housing ranges from 100 to 1600 mL on the adult bellows and from 0 to 300 mL on the pediatric bellows. The bellows assembly exhaust port is 19 mm OD, the connection to the anesthesia machine is 22 mm, and there is a high-pressure (50 psi) diameter index safety system (DISS) fitting for an oxygen line for the driving-gas circuit. The control module of the ventilator computes tidal volume, inspiratory time, expiratory time, and inspiratory flow based on the settings of the various control dials. The bellows should be fully distended (starts at the zero mark on the bellows housing scale) before inspiration begins.

The driving-gas supply is oxygen at 50 psi, which is reduced to 38 psi by a precision regulator within the ventilator; the gas line with the reduced pressure connects to a manifold of five solenoids. Electronic controls regulate the solenoid valves to deliver flows in 2-L/min increments from 4 to 60 L/min. Based on control settings, a precise volume of gas (equal to the tidal volume) is delivered to the bellows chamber to drive the bellows during the inspiratory phase, which forces gas from the bellows into the patient circuit. Flow stops when the full tidal volume has been delivered. A high-pressure relief valve opens at a pressure of 65 cm H_2O if such pressures should occur. During the expiratory phase, gas from the patient circuit (flow from the anesthesia machine) enters the bellows. The ventilator relief opens when the bellows is fully distended and a pressure of 2.5 cm H_2O has been exceeded; excess gas from the patient circuit is vented into the scavenger system.

The manufacturer recommends a bellows assembly-leak test. With the ventilator attached to a circle breathing system with the breathing system's pop-off valve closed, the Y piece occluded, all fresh gas flow off, and the bellows filled from the anesthesia machine's oxygen-flush valve, the bellows should drop no more than 100 mL/min. If a significant leak is present, the ventilator should not be used until the leak is sealed. If the anesthesia machine, breathing system, and ventilator are all in proper working order as indicated by preuse checkout procedures, the following guidelines are appropriate for use of the ventilator:

1. Properly connect the electric and pneumatic power sources for the ventilator.
2. Using the control dials, set the desired values for minute volume, respiratory rate (frequency), and I-E ratio.
3. Make the appropriate connections from the ventilator bellows to the circle system's reservoir-bag port and to the scavenger system.
4. Close the pop-off (APL) valve of the circle system.
5. Be sure that the bellows is completely filled with oxygen-anesthetic mixture.
6. Switch the power control to *on*.
7. Make final adjustments in minute volume and respiratory rate to meet the needs of the patient.

The next generation of ventilators from Ohmeda is the 7800 series of ventilators. The 7800 is available as a stand-alone unit and potentially could be applied to small animal patients. The ventilator is classified as electronically controlled, pneumatically driven, and tidal volume preset, and can accurately deliver tidal volumes of 50 to 1500 mL. A major difference between the 7000 and 7800 series is that tidal volume, rather than minute ventilation, is selected by the operator, which appears to be a significant advantage.[61]

Vet-Tec Small Animal Ventilator (SAV-75)

This ventilator is designed for use in small animal anesthesia.[62] The bellows is designed to ascend on expiration and is pneumatically driven by a Bird ventilator. Used without a bellows, Bird ventilators are classified as single-circuit ventilators, but the SAV-75 performs as a double-circuit unit. This ventilator can be used for ventilation in assist, control, or assist-control modes. When the system is operating, the Bird ventilator supplies gas to pressurize the space between the bellows and the bellows housing (canister) to force the bellows downward, which delivers gases from the bellows through the interface hose (corrugated breathing tube) to the breathing system. The controls on the Bird ventilator include inspiratory pressure, inspiratory flow rate, expiratory time (apnea control), and inspiratory sensitivity. In addition, a manometer, a hand timer (push-pull mechanism), and a DISS connector for the source of pneumatic power are prominent features of the ventilator. Inspiratory pressure can be varied to a maximum of 60 cm H_2O, inspiratory sensitivity from -0.5 to -5.0 cm H_2O, expiratory time to produce 4 to 60 controlled breaths/min, and inspiratory flow to a maximum of 70 L/min. Safety relief occurs on inspiration if a pressure of 65 cm H_2O develops. The pneumatic power source should be delivered to the ventilator inlet at 50 psi. The bellows can deliver a tidal volume of up to 2000 mL. Inspiration can be started or stopped by use of the hand timer. The Bird ventilator is time cycled unless the push-pull manual cycling rod is pulled out, causing the ventilator to be pressure cycled.[55] Figure 18.52 shows a Bird ventilator.

Before using the SAV-75 ventilator for controlling ventilation during anesthesia, the power-supply and scavenger system should be connected, and the appropriate preuse checkout procedures should be done for all equipment. Assuming proper function of the anesthesia machine, breathing system, and ventilator, the following is a reasonable operational approach for the ventilator with a circle breathing system in the control mode:

1. Set the inspiratory sensitivity control to a high setting to eliminate the possibility of patient-initiated ventilation.
2. Set the inspiratory pressure control to the range of 15 to 20 cm H_2O and readjust the setting to achieve the desired tidal volume after steps 5 and 6 have been completed.
3. Connect the corrugated hose (interface hose) from the ventilator's bellows to the reservoir-bag port of the circle system.
4. Close the pop-off (APL) valve of the circle system. At this point, the bellows may need to be filled by increasing the flow of oxygen to the patient circuit (oxygen flowmeter of the anesthesia machine).
5. Turn the inspiratory flow control on to start the ventilator and set the flow control to deliver a tidal volume in approximately 1 to 1.5 s.

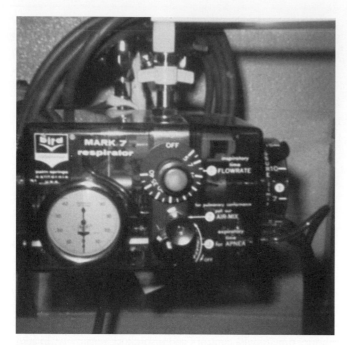

Fig. 18.52. A Bird Mark 7 Ventilator. The inspiratory-sensitivity control is on the *left* end of the ventilator, the inspiratory-pressure limit is on the *right* end, the driving gas inlet is on the *top*, and the manometer, inspiratory-flow control, air-mix selector, and expiratory-time control are on the *front* panel of the ventilator. From Lumb and Jones.[72]

6. Set the expiratory time control to establish a respiratory rate appropriate for the patient, often 8 to 12 breaths/min.
7. For final settings, the operator should understand that there are interactions between the controls on a Bird ventilator (e.g., changing inspiratory flow may affect respiratory rate).

ADS 1000 Veterinary Anesthesia Delivery System and Critical Care Ventilator

This microprocessor-controlled ventilator is marketed either for use with a vaporizer or for patients not requiring an anesthetic (e.g., critical care patients).[63] The ventilator-anesthesia system (Fig. 18.53) functions as a nonbreathing circuit, does not incorporate a bellows assembly, and does not include a canister for chemical absorbent to eliminate carbon dioxide. It is not intended for connection to another breathing system. Based on the patient's body weight, the microprocessor determines the values for the various ventilatory parameters to be provided by the ventilator.

This ventilator fits into the single-circuit class and is powered electrically and pneumatically. According to the operation manual, the ventilator must be supplied with oxygen at a pressure of 50 psi for the display to report the minute volume per kilogram of body weight accurately for the patient. Little published information other than testimonials is available about the clinical effectiveness of this ventilator system, but in vitro performance with a test lung has been studied.[64] The performance of the ventilator system in vitro changed across the range of body weights (1 to 20 kg) included in the study. Overventilation occurred at

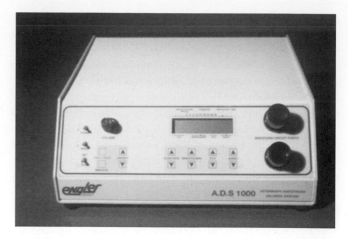

Fig. 18.53. ADS 1000 Veterinary Anesthesia Delivery System and Critical Care Ventilator. The ports for the breathing hoses are located on the *right* side of the ventilator, and the controls for the ventilator are located on the *front* panel of the console.

body weights less than 4 kg, and underventilation was evident at body weights greater than 8 kg. The authors concluded that the ventilator could support ventilation, but the displayed parameters did not always accurately reflect the actual performance of the ventilator.

The front panel of the ventilator has the following controls and components (Fig. 18.53): power switch, mask-mode switch, set-run switch, weight-selection buttons, fill-hold button, breathe button, display for various ventilatory parameters with adjustments for these parameters below the display, and two ports for attachment of corrugated breathing tubes. Before attempting to use the ventilator, the operator should read the manual supplied by the manufacturer. The following is a summary of the manufacturer's guidelines for operating the ventilator, but is not intended to replace or supplant the manual supplied for the ventilator:

1. Connect the green oxygen hose on the back of the ventilator to an oxygen source (50 psi).
2. Attach the breathing tubes to the breathing-circuit ports on the front of the ventilator.
3. Connect the scavenger *out* port on the back of the ventilator to the hospital scavenger system.
4. Connect the electric cord to the 120-VAC–1.5-amp port on the back of the ventilator to an electric outlet.
5. Attach the vaporizer connectors to the appropriate ports on the back of the ventilator.
6. Allow the ventilator to complete the self-diagnostic test described in the operator's manual. The test will help to determine failure of the safety pop-off valve, inadequate oxygen supply, and the presence of leaks.
7. After diagnostics are complete, the mask function should be off and the set-run switch should be in the *set* position. The display will then show settings for a 20-kg patient (minute volume of 24 L/min, 9 breaths/min, peak inspiratory pressure of 15 cm H_2O, and the assist mode in the *off* position).

8. Using the weight-up or weight-down button, enter the correct weight of the patient in kilograms into the display, and the ventilator will automatically set the ventilatory parameters based on the patient's weight. Ventilation will be completely controlled (the default setting for *assist* is off).

Once these steps are completed, the patient should be anesthetized and intubated with a cuffed endotracheal tube. The Y piece connecting the breathing tubes should be attached to the endotracheal tube connector, and the vaporizer should be set appropriately. The ventilator's set-run switch should be set to *run*. Controlled ventilation should begin.

Examples of Ventilators for Large Animals

Although not all-inclusive, the following discussion includes descriptions of ventilators that are appropriate for use during anesthesia in large animal patients. Classification, principles of operation, and function are discussed.

Drager Large Animal Anesthesia Ventilator

This ventilator (Fig. 18.54) is included as a part of the Narkovet-E Large Animal Anesthesia Machine; the entire system is called the Narkovet-E Large Animal Anesthesia Control Center. The ventilator was not marketed as a stand-alone unit for large animal anesthesia. Although they are no longer being manufactured, some of these ventilator-anesthesia machine combinations remain in use in veterinary hospitals. The ventilator is powered pneumatically, generally at a pressure of 50 psi.[65] It is classed as double circuit, tidal volume preset, time cycled, and pneumatically driven with a descending bellows, and it uses fluidic circuitry. The controls include an on-off switch, a tidal volume control with a scale of 4 to 15 L on the bellows housing, a frequency control (6 to 18 breaths/min), and a flow control knob that determines inspiratory flow (a combination of flow and maximum pressure being delivered to the bellows compartment); the manufacturer recommends that the flow setting be adjusted so that the bellows always reaches the upper stop. The inspiratory to expiratory time ratio of 1:2 is preset.

Before using the ventilator, the proper connections to the gas-supply and scavenger system should be made, and the appropriate preuse checkout procedures should be done. The instruction manual for ventilators includes a standard preuse check for the ventilator.[65] The following is a logical approach to the operation of the ventilator with a circle breathing system:

1. Connect the compressed-air-supply hose to the ventilator.
2. Adjust the tidal volume control to the appropriate setting for the patient and ensure that the self-locking mechanism is engaged to prevent inadvertent movement of the bellows stop plate during use.
3. Attach the corrugated breathing hose from the bellows to the reservoir-bag port of the circle system.
4. Close the pop-off (APL) valve on the circle system.
5. Turn the power switch on.
6. Adjust the frequency control knob to the desired respiratory rate.

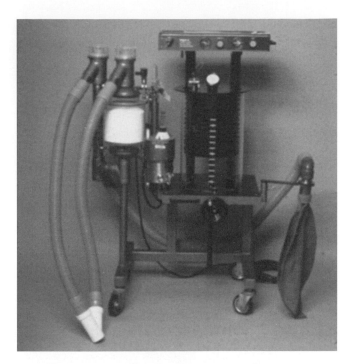

Fig. 18.54. Narkovet-E Large Animal Anesthesia Control Center: the ventilator's bellows and the bellows housing with tidal volume marking (4 to 15 L), with the large animal circle system on the *left* and the reservoir bag for the circle breathing system on the *right*. The controls for the ventilator are on the panel above the bellows housing at the *top* of the unit.

7. Adjust the flow control knob so that the bellows reaches the upper stop at end inspiration. If the bellows does not return to its original position during expiration (usually indicative of a leak in the patient circuit), the bellows can be filled by using a higher flow from the oxygen flowmeter, and the leak should be corrected.

Narkovet-E Electronic Large Animal Control Center

This is a combination of Drager's Narkovet E-2 Large Animal Anesthesia System (anesthesia machine and circle breathing system) with a Drager AV-E ventilator (Figs. 18.55 through 18.57). The ventilator is not available as a stand-alone unit for large animals and is no longer being manufactured, but machines are still in use. The ventilator is classified as double circuit, tidal volume preset, and time cycled, with a descending bellows. The ventilator is electronically controlled and pneumatically driven. It is powered electrically (120 VAC) and pneumatically (40 to 60 psi with oxygen, but air is an option).[66] The controls (Figs. 18.55 and 18.57) include an on-off switch, a self-locking knob located below the bellows assembly to control the tidal volume (4 to 15 L), a thumbwheel controller-indicator switch to adjust the respiratory rate (frequency control from 1 to 30 breaths/min), a flow control setting to determine the inspiratory flow rate, and the inspiratory-expiratory phase time ratio control (a thumbwheel indicator-controller to adjust the I-E ratio in increments of 0.5 from 1:1 to 1:4.5). The manufacturer recommends that the flow

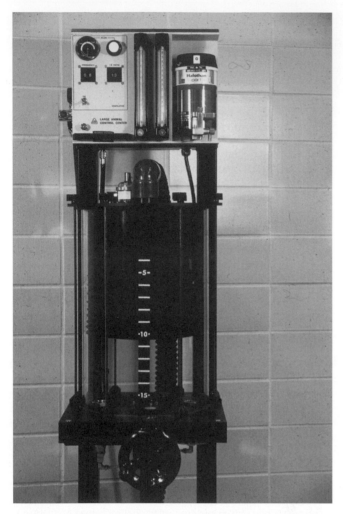

Fig. 18.55. Narkovet-E Electronic Large Animal Control Center: the bellows and bellows housing with markings for tidal volume (4 to 15 L), the corrugated breathing hose from the bellows to the circle system (behind the bellows housing), and the self-locking knob or wheel (*bottom center*) for selection of tidal volume. In addition, the controls for the ventilator and anesthesia machine (*top* of the photograph) are included and are shown in detail in Fig. 18.56.

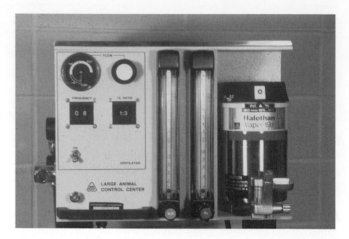

Fig. 18.56. Narkovet-E Electronic Large Animal Control Center: the control panel for the ventilator is on the *left* of the photograph. The power switch in the off position is directly under the thumbwheel controller-indicator switch for frequency (respiratory rate) selection on the *left* of the panel. The thumbwheel controller-indicator switch for inspiratory-expiratory ratio selection is on the *right* of the panel, with the inspiratory flow control directly above it. Some of the basic parts of the anesthesia machine, including the flowmeters (*center* of the photograph) for oxygen and nitrous oxide, the halothane vaporizer, and the flush valve (*bottom left*), are present.

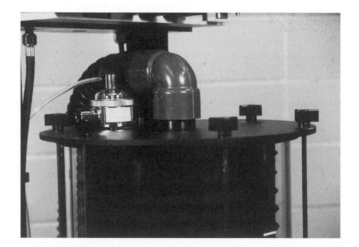

Fig. 18.57. Narkovet-E Electronic Large Animal Control Center: the top of the bellows and the bellows housing, with an elbow connecting the bellows to the corrugated breathing tube, which attaches to the reservoir port of the circle breathing system. To the *left* of the elbow is the overflow valve from the bellows, which is connected to the scavenger system from the ventilator when the ventilator is in use. The clear, small-diameter tubing attached to the pop-off valve is part of the mechanism for closing the pop-off valve during the inspiratory phase of controlled ventilation.

control knob be adjusted so that the bellows always reaches the upper stop of inspiration. The ventilator provides for controlled ventilation; assisted ventilation is not an option.

Before using the ventilator, the proper connections to the gas-supply and scavenger system should be made, and the appropriate preuse checkout procedures should be done. The instruction manual for the ventilator includes a standard preuse checklist. The following is a step-by-step approach to the operation of the ventilator with a circle breathing system:

1. Connect the gas supply (oxygen hose) to the anesthesia machine and ventilator.
2. Adjust the tidal volume control to the appropriate setting for the patient and ensure that the self-locking mechanism is engaged to prevent inadvertent movement of the bellows stop plate.
3. Select the desired frequency of ventilation.
4. Select the desired I-E ratio.
5. Attach the corrugated breathing hose from the bellows to the reservoir-bag port of the circle system.

6. Close the pop-off (APL) valve on the circle system.

7. Turn the power supply switch on.

8. Adjust the flow control knob so that the bellows reaches the upper stop at end inspiration. If the bellows does not return to its original location during expiration, it can be filled by increasing the flow from the oxygen flowmeter.

Mallard Medical Rachel Model 2800 Anesthesia Ventilator

This ventilator (Fig. 18.58) is a microprocessor-based, electronic control system that facilitates controlled ventilation in large animals being maintained on circle breathing systems (R. Pearson, personal communication, Mallard Medical, Irvine, CA).[58] The ventilator is designed to interface with currently available large animal circle systems. The stand for the ventilator and the bellows is designed for the attachment of a circle breathing system and at least two vaporizers for inhalant anesthetics, and it has shelves to accommodate physiological monitoring devices.

Most of the functional considerations for the Model 2800 are similar to those for the Model 2400V. The control console for the 2800 is located above the bellows housing instead of below the housing as it is in the 2400V, and LED displays are employed as they are in the 2400V. The ventilator is controlled by a microprocessor, but the pneumatics have been modified for generation of greater inspiratory flows, which are adjustable from 10 to 600 L/min. The bellows is inverted and ascends during expiration, and two sizes of bellows are available (3 and 21 L), allowing the selection of appropriate tidal volumes for patients with a wide range of body weights. Like other ventilators with inverted bellows, the Model 2800 produces PEEP because of the effect of gravity on the bellows. However, the amount of PEEP is controlled by a pneumatic vacuum pump on the 2800: the pump creates negative pressure between the bellows and the bellows housing during the expiratory phase of ventilation and functions to reduce the level of PEEP according to the adjustments made by the operator. An ambient end-expiratory pressure may be achieved.

Before using the ventilator, the proper connections to the gas

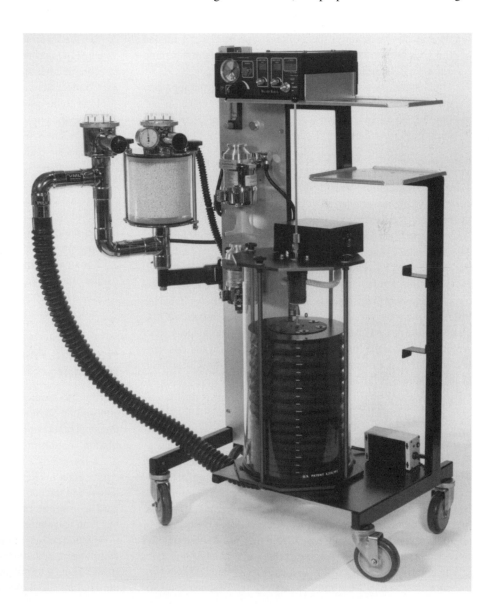

Fig. 18.58. Mallard Medical Rachel Model 2800 Large Animal Anesthesia Ventilator: the ventilator with a Matrx circle system attached (*left* side). The corrugated breathing hose that exits the bellows below the bellows housing is attached to the reservoir-bag port of the circle system. The control console for the ventilator is located at the *top* of the photograph. The controls for the 2800 are similar to those shown in Fig. 18.48 for the Model 2400V.

and electric power supplies and the scavenger system should be made, and the appropriate preuse checkout procedures should be done for all equipment. The following is a reasonable operational approach for the Model 2800 ventilator with a circle breathing system:

1. Place the master switch in the standby mode and dial the desired settings for respiratory rate and inspiratory time, according to the patient's needs.
2. Set the inspiratory flow control to the desired rate of flow—low, medium, or high—depending on the patient's needs (typically in the high range for large animals).
3. Connect the corrugated tubing from the ventilator's bellows to the circle system's reservoir-bag mount and the ventilator exhalation port to the scavenger system.
4. Close the circle system's pop-off (APL) valve and release the ventilator's bellows. Ensure that the bellows is fully inflated and positioned at zero.
5. Turn the master switch on, and inspiration should begin.
6. If the bellows does not return to zero during the expiratory phase, the bellows can be filled with flow from the oxygen flowmeter. Alternately, the bellows can be filled with the flush valve, but the anesthetic concentration in the breathing circuit will be reduced any time this is done.
7. The inspiratory time can be adjusted to produce the appropriate tidal volume for the patient.
8. Finally, the PEEP control is adjusted to set the desired end-expiratory pressure.

Vet-Tec Model 3000 Large Animal Anesthesia Ventilator
This is a large animal anesthesia ventilator designed for use in equine and bovine practices.[67] A similar ventilator in combination with a large animal anesthesia machine (Model 2000 Large Animal Anesthesia Machine and Ventilator) is also available.[67] The ventilator system has been described as a "bag-in-a-barrel" powered by a Bird ventilator.[35] The LAVC-2000 and the LAVC-3000 systems can be converted to a 5-L system for use in foals by adding a 5000-mL bellows and a canister (bellows housing) insert. Numerous variations of these ventilator-anesthesia machine combinations were possible, because the manufacturer would customize the unit upon request. The bellows in this ventilator system is driven by a modified Bird Mark 7 ventilator. Used without a bellows, the Bird Mark 7 is classed as a single-circuit ventilator, but the LAVC ventilator system is double circuit and has been classified as a pressure-preset ventilator.[35] The ventilator has been produced with a descending bellows, but literature from the manufacturer indicates the availability of an inverted bellows. The Bird ventilator is pneumatically powered. This ventilator system can be used for ventilation in assist, control, or assist-control modes. When the system is operating, the Bird ventilator supplies gas to pressurize the space between the bellows and the bellows housing (canister) to force the bellows in an upward motion delivering gases from the bellows, through the interface hose, to the breathing system.

The controls on a Bird Mark 7 (Fig. 18.52) include inspiratory pressure, inspiratory flow rate, expiratory time (apnea control),

and inspiratory sensitivity. In addition, a manometer, a hand timer (push-pull mechanism), and a DISS connector for the source of pneumatic power are prominent features of the ventilator. With the modified Bird Mark 7, inspiratory pressure can be varied from 5 to 65 cm H_2O, inspiratory sensitivity from -0.5 to -5 cm H_2O, expiratory time from 5 to 15 s, and inspiratory flow from 0 to over 450 L/min. The pneumatic power source should be delivered to the inlet of the ventilator at 50 psi. The bellows can deliver a tidal volume of up to 20 L. Inspiration can be started or stopped by use of a hand timer. The Bird Mark 7 is a time-cycled ventilator unless the push-pull manual cycling rod is pulled out, which causes the ventilator to be pressure cycled.[55]

Before using the Model LAV-3000 ventilator for controlling ventilation during anesthesia, the power-supply and scavenger system should be connected, and the appropriate preuse checkout procedures should be done for all equipment. The following is a reasonable operational approach for the ventilator with a circle breathing system in the control mode:

1. Set the inspiratory sensitivity control to a high setting to eliminate the possibility of patient-initiated ventilation.
2. Set the inspiratory pressure control to the range of 20 to 30 cm H_2O and readjust the setting to achieve the desired tidal volume after steps 5 and 6 have been completed.
3. Connect the corrugated hose (interface hose) from the bellows to the reservoir-bag port of the circle system.
4. Close the pop-off (APL) valve of the circle system. Then, the bellows may need to be filled by increasing the flow of oxygen to the patient circuit (oxygen flowmeter on the anesthesia machine).
5. Turn the inspiratory flow control on to start the ventilator and set the flow control to deliver a tidal volume in approximately 1.5 to 3.0 s.
6. Set the expiratory time control to establish a respiratory rate appropriate for the patient, often 7 to 10 breaths/min.
7. For final settings, the operator should understand that there are interactions between the controls on a Bird ventilator (e.g., changing inspiratory flow may affect respiratory rate and vice versa).

Hazards Associated with the Use of Ventilators

During anesthesia, the use of a ventilator allows the anesthetist to concentrate on monitoring and supportive procedures. If an anesthetist is preoccupied with manually controlling or assisting ventilation, monitoring and support may be neglected. A good example is the use of a mechanical ventilator in anesthesia for equine colic surgery. There is some loss of contact between the anesthetist and the patient when a ventilator is used, especially in regard to respiratory function. Without a "hand on the reservoir bag," an anesthetist may miss such developments as disconnections in the patient circuit, variations in respiratory resistance and compliance, and changes in the rate of spontaneous ventilation. In addition, a ventilator, because of its sounds and regularity, may lull an anesthetist into believing that ventilation is adequate when, in fact, it is not.[61] Ventilators are mechanical and may malfunction, and many veterinary ventilators are not equipped with the alarm systems that are now required for human ventilators. Finally, ventilators add a source of possible contamination to the breathing system.[61]

The hazards of mechanical ventilation are usually associated with malfunctions and failure of the equipment or inappropriate or inadvertently altered control settings. The operator should select a ventilator capable of meeting the respiratory requirements for the patient. Ventilators designed specifically for small animals or human patients are not necessarily appropriate for larger animals. A ventilator must be able to generate an adequate inspiratory flow rate and tidal volume if it is to be safe for use in larger animals. General hazards associated with ventilators include hypoventilation, hyperventilation, excessive airway pressure, negative pressure during expiration, and failure of alarms, if the ventilator is so equipped. Hypoventilation can be associated with power failure, dysfunction of the ventilator, cycling failure, inadequate design for the patient, leak of driving gas, loss of breathing-system gas, incorrect settings, and obstruction of flow.[61]

Respiratory Assist Devices

Several types and brands of respiratory assist devices are available. Some are completely manual in operation (resuscitation bags with one-way valves), and some use compressed gas (oxygen) to assist ventilation (demand valves). The mechanics of these devices have been reviewed.[61]

Manual Resuscitators

A manual resuscitator is appropriate for application of IPPV to small veterinary patients. Several brands of resuscitators are available. The basic components of a manual resuscitator are a compressible self-reexpanding bag, a bag-refill valve, and a non-rebreathing valve.[68] Some resuscitators can be attached to a source of oxygen to enrich the oxygen content of inspired gases (Fig. 18.59). Manual resuscitators can be fitted with a reservoir to serve as a source of oxygen when the oxygen flow to the resuscitator does not meet the filling demands of the resuscitator. The addition of such a reservoir makes the resuscitator more cumbersome to use.[68]

Demand Valves

A demand valve can be used to deliver intermittent positive pressure ventilation. The demand valve is set to deliver oxygen when the patient begins to inspire (creating a negative inspiratory pressure) until exhalation starts or until a certain preset pressure is reached.[68] Expiration is passive through the valve outlet. The outlet may be restrictive to expiration in large patients. The device can be disconnected from the endotracheal tube after inspiration to decrease the resistance to exhalation if the demand valve must be used for an extended time.[26] A demand valve can be triggered manually to deliver oxygen to the patient as long as the activation button is held down or until the preset pressure limit is reached. Alternately compressing and releasing the control button allows application of IPPV. A demand valve with the capacity for a high inspiratory flow rate is most desirable for use in large animals; demand valves generating low inspiratory flows will cause an excessively long inspiratory time in patients requiring a large tidal volume.

Demand valves are available from various manufacturers. The Hudson Demand Valve (Fig. 18.60) has been described for use in horses.[69] It delivers approximately 200 L/min if the oxygen-supply pressure is 50 psi and greater than 275 L/min if the supply pressure is 80 psi. This valve will accept a standard connector for an endotracheal tube (15 mm), and an adapter will allow attachment of the demand valve to a large animal endotracheal tube connector. The equine demand valve sold by J.D. Medical (Phoenix, AZ) functions at an inlet pressure of 50 to 75 psi. This

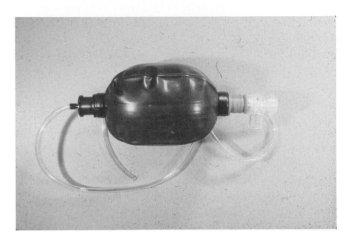

Fig. 18.59. A manual resuscitation bag. Plastic tubing, which may be connected to an oxygen flowmeter, is attached to the bag refill valve to facilitate the addition of oxygen to inspired gases. The components of the resuscitation bag include the clear elbow (*right*), which is a non-rebreathing valve, the black self-inflating bag, and a refill valve (the black apparatus on the *left* end of the bag). The non-rebreathing valve may be connected to a mask or to an endotracheal tube.

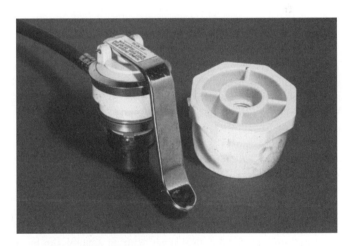

Fig. 18.60. The Hudson Demand Valve (*left*) with an adapter for attachment to a large animal endotracheal tube connector.

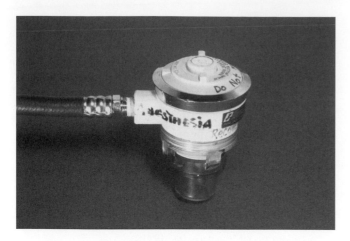

Fig. 18.61. The Elder CPR/Demand Valve. The oxygen inlet is shown with high-pressure oxygen hose connected. The clear plastic connector at the *bottom* of the photograph will fit endotracheal tube connectors, and the button in the *top center* of the demand valve activates and controls the flow of oxygen.

demand valve is available with various lengths of supply-gas hose and several sizes of adapters for endotracheal tubes. The Elder CPR/Demand Valve (Fig. 18.61) is intended to provide 100% oxygen to breathing or apneic patients.[70] The unit operates on a regulated inlet supply of oxygen at pressures between 40 and 80 psi. There is a variable pressure limit of 60 cm H_2O. Variable pressure (0 to 60 cm $H_2O \pm$ 5 cm H_2O) can be delivered to the patient, depending on the amount of pressure that is placed on the manual control button. Two models of this demand valve allow the choice of two set flow rates: 40 L/min at 40 psi and 160 L/min at 40 psi. The inlet for the valve is a DISS male oxygen fitting, and the outlet is 15 mm ID for attachment to an endotracheal tube connector and 22 mm OD for accepting a standard adult mask. This demand valve is easily adapted to fit both large and small animal endotracheal tubes with an adapter similar to the one shown in Fig. 18.60.

References

1. Dorsch JA, Dorsch SE. Tracheal tubes. In: Dorsch JA, Dorsch SE, eds. Understanding Anesthesia Equipment, 3rd ed. Baltimore: Williams and Wilkins, 1994:439.
2. Sawyer DC. Canine and feline endotracheal intubation and laryngoscopy. Compend Contin Educ Pract Vet 11:973, 1984.
3. Heath RB. Complications associated with general anesthesia of the horse. Vet Clin North Am Large Anim Pract 3:45, 1981.
4. Smith TC. Anesthesia breathing systems. In: Ehrenworth J, Eisenkraft JB, eds. Anesthesia Equipment, Principles and Applications. St Louis: CV Mosby, 1993:89.
5. Guyton DC. Endotracheal and tracheotomy tube cuff design: Influence on tracheal damage. Crit Care Update 1:1, 1990.
6. Hartsfield SM, Gendreau CL, Smith CW, Rouse GP, Thurmon JC. Endotracheal intubation by pharyngotomy. J Am Anim Hosp Assoc 12:71, 1977.
7. Shawley RV, Bednarski RM. Endotracheal intubation in the horse. In: Muir WW III, Hubbell JAE, eds. Equine Anesthesia. St Louis: CV Mosby, 1991:210.
8. Trim CM, Simpson ST. Complications following ethylene oxide sterilization. J Am Anim Hosp Assoc 18:507, 1982.
9. Webb AI. Nasal intubation in the foal. J Am Vet Med Assoc 185:48, 1984.
10. Soma LR. Intubation of the trachea. In: Textbook of Veterinary Anesthesia. Baltimore: Williams and Wilkins, 1971:229.
11. Loeser EA, Kaminsky A, Diaz A, Stanley TH, Pace NL. The influence of endotracheal tube cuff design and cuff lubrication on postoperative sore throat. Anesthesiology 58:376, 1983.
12. Thurmon JC, Benson GJ. Anesthesia in ruminants and swine. In: Howard JL, ed. Current Veterinary Therapy, Food Animal Practice 2. Philadelphia: WB Saunders, 1986:51.
13. Ko JCH, Thurmon JC, Tranquilli WA, Benson GJ, Olson WA. Problems encountered when anesthetizing potbellied pigs. Vet Med 88:435, 1993.
14. Hubbell JAE, Hill BL, Muir III WW. Perianesthetic considerations in cattle. Compend Contin Educ Pract Vet 8:F92, 1986.
15. Riebold TW, Engel HN, Grubb TL, Adams JG, Huber MJ, Schmotzer WB. Orotracheal and nasotracheal intubation in llamas. J Am Vet Med Assoc 204:779, 1994.
16. Sedgewick C, Jahn S. Techniques for endotracheal intubation and inhalation anesthesia for laboratory animals. Calif Vet 34:27, 1980.
17. Boothe HW, Hartsfield SM. Use of the laboratory rabbit in the small animal student surgery laboratory. J Vet Med Educ 17:16, 1990.
18. Hughes HC. Anesthesia of laboratory animals. Lab Anim 10:40, 1981.
19. Hartsfield SM. Alternate methods of endotracheal intubation in small animals with emphasis on patients with oropharyngeal pathology. Tex Vet Med J 47:25, 1985.
20. Borland LM, Swan DM, Leff S. Difficult pediatric endotracheal intubation: A new approach to the retrograde technique. Anesthesiology 55:557, 1981.
21. Hedlund CS. Tracheostomy. Probl Vet Med 3:198, 1991.
22. Millen JE, Glauser FL. A rapid, simple technique for changing endotracheal tubes. Anesth Analg 57:735, 1978.
23. Haskins SC. Standards and techniques of equipment utilization. In: Sattler FP, Knowles R, Whittick WG, eds. Veterinary Critical Care. Philadelphia: Lea and Febiger, 1981:60.
24. Fairman NB. Evaluation of pulse oximetry as a continuous monitoring technique in critically ill dogs in the small animal intensive care unit. J Vet Emerg Crit Care 2:50, 1992.
25. White GA, Matthews NS, Hartsfield SM, Walker MA, Slater MR. Pulse oximetry for estimation of oxygenation in dogs with experimental pneumothorax. J Vet Emerg Crit Care 4:69, 1994.
26. Hubbell JAE. Oxygen supplementation and ventilatory assist devices. In: Muir WW III, Hubbell JAE, eds. Equine Anesthesia, Monitoring and Emergency Therapy. St Louis: CV Mosby, 1991: 401.
27. Court MH. Respiratory support of the critically ill small animal patient. In: Murtaugh RJ, Kaplan PM, eds. Veterinary Emergency and Critical Care Medicine. St Louis: CV Mosby, 1992:575.
28. Mann FA, Wagner-Mann C, Albert JA, Smith J. Comparison of intranasal and intratracheal oxygen administration in healthy awake dogs. Am J Vet Res 53:856, 1992.
29. Fitxpatrick RK, Crowe DT. Nasal oxygen administration in dogs and cats: Experimental and clinical investigations. J Am Anim Hosp Assoc 22:293, 1986.
30. Haskins SC. Physical therapeutics for respiratory disease. Semin Vet Med Surg Small Animal 1:276, 1986.

31. Benumof JL. Respiratory physiology and respiratory function during anesthesia. In: Miller RD, ed. Anesthesia, 2nd ed. New York: Churchill Livingstone, 1986:1115.

32. Nunn JF. Hyperoxia and oxygen toxicity. In: Nunn JF, ed. Applied Respiratory Physiology, 3rd ed. London: Butterworth, 1987:478.

33. Winter PM. Pulmonary oxygen toxicity. In: Refresher Courses in Anesthesiology. American Society of Anesthesiologists. Philadelphia: JB Lippincott, 1974:163.

34. Steffey EP. Mechanical ventilation of the anesthetized horse. Vet Clin North Am Large Anim Pract 3:97, 1981.

35. Muir WW III, Hubbell JAE, Skarda RT, Bednarski RM. Ventilation and mechanical assist devices. In: Handbook of Veterinary Anesthesia, 2nd ed. St Louis: CV Mosby, 1995:209.

36. Thurmon JC. General clinical considerations for anesthesia of the horse. Vet Clin North Am Equine Pract 6:485, 1990.

37. Hodgson DS, Dunlop CE. General anesthesia for horses with specific problems. Vet Clin North Am Equine Pract 6:625, 1990.

38. Cullen DJ, Eger EI II. Cardiovascular effects of carbon dioxide in man. Anesthesiology 41:345, 1974.

39. Wagner AE, Bednarski RM, Muir WW III. Hemodynamic effects of carbon dioxide during intermittent positive-pressure ventilation in horses. Am J Vet Res 12:1922, 1990.

40. Shibata K, Futagami A, Take Y, Kobayashi T. Epidural anesthesia modifies the cardiovascular response to marked hypercapnia in dogs. Anesthesiology 81:1454, 1994.

41. Horwitz LD, Bishop BS, Stone HL. Effects of hypercapnia on the cardiovascular system of conscious dogs. J Appl Physiol 25:346, 1968.

42. Price HL. Effects of carbon dioxide on the cardiovascular system. Anesthesiology 21:652, 1960.

43. Eisele JH, Eger EI II, Muallem M. Narcotic properties of carbon dioxide in the dog. Anesthesiology 28:856, 1967.

44. Smith TC, Gross JB, Willman H. The therapeutic gases, oxygen, carbon dioxide, helium, and water vapor. In: Gilman AG, Goodman LS, Rail TW, Murad F, eds. Goodman and Gilman's the Pharmacological Basis of Therapeutics, 6th ed. New York: Macmillan, 1985:322.

45. Rold N, Cote CJ. Persistent cardiac arrhythmias in pediatric patients: Effects of age, expired carbon dioxide values, depth of anesthesia, and airway management. Anesth Analg 73:720, 1991.

46. Haskins SC. Monitoring the anesthetized patient. In: Short CE, ed. Principles and Practice of Veterinary Anesthesia. Baltimore: Williams and Wilkins, 1987:455.

47. Shawley RV. Controlled ventilation and pulmonary function. In: Short CE, ed. Principles and Practice of Veterinary Anesthesia. Baltimore: Williams and Wilkins, 1987:419.

48. Nunn JF. Artificial ventilation. In: Applied Respiratory Physiology, 3rd ed. London: Butterworth, 1987:392.

49. Bednarski RM. Diaphragmatic hernia: Anesthetic considerations. Semin Vet Med Surg Small Animal 1:256, 1986.

50. Andrews JJ. Inhaled anesthetic delivery systems. In: Miller RD, ed. Anesthesia, 3rd ed. New York: Churchill Livingstone, 1991:171.

51. Sassoon CSH, Mahutte CK, Light RW. Ventilator modes: Old and new. Crit Care Clin 6:605, 1990.

52. Wilson RS. Techniques of ventilatory control: Indications and complications. In: Refresher Courses in Anesthesiology. American Society of Anesthesiologists, 13:221, 1985.

53. Soma LR. Anesthetic management. In: Soma LR, ed. Textbook of Veterinary Anesthesia. Baltimore: Williams and Wilkins, 1971:287.

54. Grogono AW, Travis JT. Anesthesia ventilators. In: Ehrenworth J, Eisenkraft JB, eds. Anesthesia Equipment, Principles and Application. St Louis: CV Mosby, 1993:140.

55. Mushin WW, Rendel-Baker L, Thompson PW, Mapleson WW. The Bird ventilators. In: Mushin WW, ed. Automatic Ventilation of the Lungs, 3rd ed. Oxford: Blackwell Scientific Publications. 1980:373.

56. Operator's Instruction Manual, Narkovet 2 Small Animal Anesthesia Machine. Telford, PA: North American Drager, 1988:6.

57. Hallowell EMC Model 2000 Small Animal Veterinary Anesthesia Ventilator-Functional Description. Pittsfield, MA: Hallowell Engineering and Manufacturing, 1993:1.

58. Operator's Manual and Service Instructions, Mallard Medical Model 2400V Anesthesia Ventilator. Irvine, CA: Mallard Medical, 1991.

59. Soma LR. Controlled Ventilation of the Veterinary Patient. Washington Crossing, NJ: Pitmann-Moore, 1973.

60. Operation Maintenance, Metomatic Veterinary Ventilator. Madison, WI: Ohio Medical Products, 1978.

61. Dorsch JA, Dorsch SE. Anesthesia ventilators. In: Understanding Anesthesia Equipment, 3rd ed. Baltimore: Williams and Wilkins, 1994:255.

62. Vet-Tec SAV-75 Small Animal Anesthesia Ventilator. Phoenix, AZ: JD Medical Distributing, 1990.

63. ADS 1000 Veterinary Anesthesia Delivery System and Critical Care Ventilator Operation Manual. Hialeah, FL: Engler Engineering, 1994.

64. Faudskar L, Raffee M, Randall D. In vitro performance evaluation of the ADS 1000 veterinary ventilator [Abstract]. J Vet Emerg Crit Care 4:107, 1994.

65. Instruction Manual, Drager AV Anesthesia Ventilator. Telford, PA: North America Drager, 1982.

66. Instruction Manual, Drager AV-E Anesthesia Ventilator. Telford, PA: North American Drager, 1981.

67. Vet-Tec LAVC-2000 Large Animal Anesthesia Machine and Ventilator-Product Information Brochure. Phoenix, AZ: JD Medical Distributing, 1990.

68. Dorsch JA, Dorsch SE. Manual resuscitators. In: Understanding Anesthesia Equipment, 3rd ed. Baltimore: Williams and Wilkins, 1994:225.

69. Riebold TQ, Goble DO, Geiser DR. Clinical techniques for equine anesthesia. In: Riebold TO, ed. Large Animal Anesthesia. Ames: Iowa State University Press, 1982:41-33.

70. Elder CPR/Demand Valve Product Information Brochure. Irvine, CA: Life Support Products, 1990.

71. Mushin WW, Rendell-Baker L, Thompson PW, Mapleson WW. Automatic Ventilation of the Lungs, 2nd ed. Philadelphia: FA Davis, 1969.

72. Lumb WV, Jones EW. Oxygen administration and artificial respiration. In: Lumb WV, Jones EW, eds. Veterinary Anesthesia, 1st ed. Philadelphia: Lea and Febiger, 1973:141.

Chapter 19
Monitoring Anesthetized Patients

Steve C. Haskins

Introduction

The purpose of anesthesia is to provide reversible unconsciousness, amnesia, analgesia, and immobility for invasive procedures. The administration of anesthetic drugs and the unconscious, recumbent, and immobile state, however, compromise patient homeostasis. Anesthetic crises are unpredictable, and tend to be rapid in onset and devastating in nature. The purpose of monitoring is to achieve the goals while maximizing the safety of the anesthetic experience.

The purpose of preoperative monitoring is to determine the existence and magnitude of abnormal processes that might compromise a patient's response to anesthesia and the operative procedure, and to guide the development of the anesthetic plan. The preoperative assessment provides the basis for tailoring drug selection and the intraoperative and postoperative monitoring and support to the specific needs of the patient. Intraoperative monitoring, the subject of this chapter, focuses on insuring an optimum anesthetic depth with minimal physiological impairment. The purpose of postoperative monitoring is to warrant a full and complete recovery from the anesthetic state and to provide adequate analgesia.

Anesthetic Mortality

Anesthetic issues and problems are common, but mortality from them is rare. The difference is in the monitoring, which can lead to the early recognition and correction of the problem. Such events, when they are easily rectified, are seldom even defined as problems. An adverse event that threatens the life or causes the death of a patient is universally defined as a problem. Perioperative cardiac arrest, as opposed to the problem(s) that could potentially cause it, is objective and not likely to be underrecognized. Such mortality analyses may help define when and what should be monitored during anesthesia.

Earlier studies reported a perioperative mortality rate of 20 to 189 per 10,000 patients administered anesthetics.[1-4] Anesthesia contributed to 2.5 to 9.2 deaths per 10,000 patients administered anesthetics. Mortality rates were higher among patients with poorer preoperative physical status and greater age where biological reserves are limited, and among patients undergoing emergency procedures where preoperative planning and preparation are limited, but were still of notable frequency in young, healthy patients undergoing planned procedures. Of the deaths, 1% occurred at induction, 10% to 30% intraoperatively, 10% early postoperatively, and the remainder over the ensuing days.[3,4] Intraoperative causes of death included the primary disease process; aspiration; hypovolemia and hypotension; hypoxia secondary to airway or endotracheal tube problems, or pneumothorax; misdosing of drugs; and hypothermia. Postoperative causes of death included the primary disease process, arrest during endotracheal tube suctioning, aspiration, pneumonia, and heart failure.

Perioperative mortality was reported to be 8.8/10,000 patients administered anesthetics in a recent study of human patients.[5] Deaths attributed entirely to anesthesia were quite uncommon (0.1/10,000), but anesthetic-contributed mortality (anesthesia in combination with surgery and augmented by the underlying disease) was 1.4/10,000. In addition, there was a 0.5/10,000 incidence of postoperative coma 1 day after anesthesia. Of anesthesia-related deaths, 17% occurred in American Society of Anesthesiologist (ASA) classification 1 or 2, 45% in ASA class 3, and 38% in ASA class 4 or 5 patients. Of the deaths, 29% occurred intraoperatively, 6% in recovery, and the remainder postoperatively. No deaths were recorded at the time of induction, which is a notoriously dangerous point in the anesthetic experience. Many problems were noted during induction, but no deaths resulted from them. Of the anesthesia-related deaths, 52% involved cardiovascular problems (hypovolemia and inadequate volume replacement, hypotension and hypertension, ventricular arrhythmias, or heart failure), and 10% involved respiratory problems (inadequate oxygenation, airway problems, aspiration, or ventilatory failure). Metabolic problems were a distant third category.[6] Inadequate preoperative preparation was thought to occur in 25%, and inadequate monitoring in 10%, of the anesthesia-related deaths.

In a survey study reported in 1990, cardiac arrests, 55% of which were fatal, occurred in 2.6 per 10,000 patients administered anesthetics.[7] Anesthesia was thought to play a role in 45% of these cardiac arrests. Of anesthesia-related deaths, 23% occurred in ASA classification 1 or 2, 17% in ASA class 3, and 61% in ASA class 4 or 5 patients. Of the cardiac arrests, 47% were thought to be due to preventable causes, the most common of which were errors in drug administration and hypoxia.

A veterinary study in 1998 cited a complication rate of 2.1% in 8087 dogs and 1.3% in 8702 cats, and an overall mortality rate of 0.1% (10/10,000 anesthetics).[8]

Life-threatening perioperative problems, and therefore the thrust of monitoring, seem to focus on the cardiopulmonary system, although other organ systems and metabolic issues cannot be ignored. Certain patient groups appear to represent greater risk, although anesthesia and operation represent great risk to any patient. Critically ill patients are somewhat advantaged because we know in advance to pay special attention. Healthy patients undergoing routine procedures are perhaps disadvantaged if we let our guard down because we are not expecting a problem. Monitoring encompasses (a) assuring an appropriate anesthetic level and (b) guarding against excessive physiological impairment.

Monitoring Anesthetic Level

The purpose of assuring an appropriate level of anesthesia is to minimize the detrimental effects of excessively light levels of anesthesia (awareness, recall, pain, and movement), as well as those of excessively deep levels of anesthesia (hypoventilation and hypoxemia; reduced cardiac output, hypotension, and inadequate tissue perfusion; hypothermia; and prolonged recovery). The term *anesthetic depth* is somewhat of an anachronism because it is based on the concept that anesthetic agents cause pro-

gressive depression of central nervous system (CNS) function. It is clear that anesthetic agents have different mechanisms of action on the CNS, most of which are depressant, but some of which are stimulant.[9] Consciousness might better be represented as a sphere, as opposed to a line. When cortical function is pushed outside the boundaries of this sphere (in any direction) (as opposed to below a line), unconsciousness occurs. Consciousness might be viewed as a state of organized CNS function, and anesthesia as a state of disorganized CNS function produced by facilitated or impaired neurotransmitter release or receptor receptivity. The terms *level of anesthesia* and *anesthetic depth*, however, are familiar and are used in this chapter, but refer to the relationship between anesthetic-induced CNS function and the center of the *sphere of consciousness*.

The state of *general anesthesia* is defined as the lack of awareness of all aspects of one's environment (including pain). Anesthetic drugs, administered in small dosages, may cause sedation, but not anesthesia. There are, of course, degrees of sedation or obtundation between fully awake and anesthetized, but there is no consensus as to what to call them. An animal that is visibly lethargic, sluggish, and depressed, but is spontaneously aware of its environment, might be described as being mildly sedated or obtunded. An animal that is "sleeping" and does not appear to be aware of (or care about) its environment when unstimulated, but that is readily awakened with verbal or light tactile stimulation, might be described as being moderately sedated or obtunded. An animal that awakens only with strong tactile or noxious stimulation might be described as being more sedate or obtunded, whereas anesthetized or comatose patients cannot be awakened even by strong, painful stimulation. Some sedative drugs (e.g., opioids), even in high dosages, do not induce anesthesia reliably. Some sedative drugs administered in small dosages do not even induce sedation, but can decrease a patient's apprehension or anxiety: This is *tranquilization*. Tranquilizers (phenothiazines and benzodiazepines) can never be anesthetics, but they can potentiate the anesthetic effects of anesthetics. Anesthetic drugs, if dosed judiciously, can act as tranquilizers, sedatives, or true anesthetics. Opioids can induce an anesthesia-like state in high dosages, but, if used alone, spontaneous movement in animals and awareness in people are not uncommon.

Analgesia is the lack of awareness of nociceptive stimuli. Some agents (e.g., opioids and nitrous oxide) are good analgesics, but are not particularly good at inducing loss of awareness (anesthesia). Some anesthetic drugs (barbiturates, propofol, etomidate, halothane, and sevoflurane) are good anesthetics but have no analgesic qualities (in subanesthetic dosages). These agents can be used for surgical procedures, however, because, once anesthetized, animals lose their ability to perceive pain. The eminent problems with these agents are the variation in anesthetic depth associated with nociceptive stimulation during the operative procedure and the lack of postoperative analgesia. Some agents (ketamine and isoflurane) are good anesthetics, as well as good analgesics.

There are also levels of anesthesia. In Guedel's classic description of anesthetic depth,[10] loss of consciousness defines the border between stages I and II, and the cessation of spontaneous muscle movement the border between stages II and III (the surgical stage of anesthesia). In the lighter plane of stage III, a hemodynamic response and muscular movement in response to noxious stimuli might still be present, but stage II provided a comfortable margin between these responses and awareness of the noxious stimulus. A hemodynamic response or reflex muscular movement in response to a noxious stimulus proved a light level of surgical anesthesia and yet the patient was far removed from being aware of the noxious stimulus: the ideal anesthetic level. This is an important concept either to accept or to reject because it bears directly upon the philosophy of much of the recent research that equates a hemodynamic response, an electroencephalographic (EEG) response, or a muscular movement response to a noxious stimulus with the conscious awareness of pain.

One of the major goals of anesthesia is that the patient should lack awareness during the procedure. Amnesia is often listed as one of the goals of anesthesia, but it is somewhat of an oxymoron. If the first goal is met, then there is nothing to forget. It would hardly be philosophically acceptable to allow awareness of pain during the operative procedure, as long as the patient forgot about it afterward. It turns out that the first goal (lack of awareness) is not always met, but that awareness, and discomfort and pain, are also not synonymous. There is also a naturally high incidence of amnesia afterward. Awareness probably occurs considerably more frequently than people remember it.[11] In one study, 20 patients were deliberately awoken intraoperatively from propofol anesthesia and asked to perform cognitive tasks, and then were reanesthetized for completion of the surgical procedure.[12] Only 35% of these patients could remember the experience. Awareness, it turns out, is a very difficult thing to study because it can be studied only by asking patients whether they remember anything. There is also the difference between spontaneous, explicit recall of specific events and implicit, nonspecific recall that can be obtained only with extensive questioning or hypnosis. Explicit recall is often better 1 week after surgery than it is after 1 day, so the study results depend on when the question is asked. The incidence of explicit awareness in people is cited to be about 0.2%.[13] Intraoperative awareness is also not always associated with intraoperative pain nor posttraumatic suffering, but when it is, it is a serious problem.[13] Many reports of awareness in people are associated with insufficient dosages of anesthetic; for example, in cesarean section when fetal depression is a concern, and in cardiac and trauma patients where anesthetic-induced cardiovascular depression is a concern.[13] The easiest way to prevent intraoperative awareness is to provide adequate amounts of anesthetic. Preventing movement, hemodynamic, and EEG response to surgical stimulation, although not necessary in most patients, would seem to be the best means of minimizing intraoperative awareness in all patients.

In general, patients lose recall at the lightest levels of anesthesia first, awareness second, movement in response to a nociceptive stimulus third, and a hemodynamic or EEG response to a nociceptive stimulus fourth, with increasing anesthetic depth. For halothane, MAC_{awake} (minimum alveolar concentration [MAC] to prevent response to verbal command in 50% of patients: awareness) is about 0.4%; $MAC_{incision}$ (MAC to prevent muscu-

lar movement in response to a strong surgical stimulus) is about 0.9%; and MAC_{BAR} (MAC to block the autonomic response to skin incision) is about 1.1%.[14] The MAC_{awake} and the $MAC_{incision}$ were reported to be 0.39 and 1.3 for isoflurane and 0.61 and 2.0 for sevoflurane, respectively.[15] Patients maintained at an end-tidal anesthetic concentration that is sufficient to prevent movement in response to surgical stimulation, let alone sufficient to prevent a hemodynamic response, have a $2^{1}/_{2}$- to 3-fold anesthetic margin between them and awareness. The *bispectral index* (BIS) is a processed electroencephalogram that quantifies the degree of anesthetic-induced cortical electrical depression. A value below 60 is associated with loss of recall, below 50 with the loss of awareness, below 40 with the loss of muscular movement in response to a noxious stimulus, and below 20 with burst suppression (deep anesthesia). MAC_{BAR} and MAC_{BIS} (the MAC associated with an increase in BIS to 60 in response to nociceptive stimulation) were reported to be about the same in cats.[16] BIS has been used to help ensure that patients are well anesthetized, pain free, and unaware.[13,17]

A hemodynamic or EEG response or movement in response to a nociceptive stimulus does not mean that an animal is consciously aware of the stimulus; the evidence seems to be quite contrary to this assumption. These reactions might represent the ideal anesthetic level (light, but not too light). However, in the clinical practice of anesthesia, since a 100% lack of awareness is the goal, maintaining a depth of anesthesia that is free of hemodynamic, EEG, and movement response to surgical stimuli, as long as the cardiovascular system can handle it, would seem to maximize the likelihood of achieving the lack-of-awareness goal. Spontaneous movement during anesthesia is, however, a characteristic of some anesthetic agents (opioids, etomidate, and propofol) and is not synonymous with inadequate anesthetic depth.

Anesthetic level represents the balance between the amount of drug(s) administered, the amount of surgical stimulation (which tends to awaken patients), and the severity of illness (which tends to synergize the anesthetic). Anesthetic requirements change over time (with an overall decreasing trend) within a single anesthetic experience, because of variations in the magnitude of surgical stimulation, the gradual filling of redistribution sites, and variations in body temperature. It would not be appropriate to maintain initial vaporizer settings or drug infusion rates for the duration of the operative procedure, because animals would invariably be excessively anesthetized by the end of the procedure. Anesthetists should repeatedly try to decrease the amount of anesthetic administered during the course of an anesthetic. Since the dosage of anesthetic required for a patient cannot be predicted, however, the administration of each anesthetic should be considered a clinical experiment. If the signs of anesthetic depth suggest that an animal's anesthesia level is getting too light, then perhaps the anesthetic dose should be returned to its previous setting; unless, of course, one is at the end of the operative procedure: then light is right. The challenge is to keep the animal in a light to medium level of anesthesia; that is, deep enough to abate conscious perception and to provide adequate muscle relaxation, yet light enough that the signs of anesthesia clearly indicated that the animal is not too deeply anesthetized.

Single, point-in-time measurements are meaningful when they are severely abnormal; an animal that is prematurely leaving the operating table of its own will is a problem at the moment, and it does not matter what depth was assessed 5 min earlier. For the most part, though, measurements and evaluations are interpretable only in the context of previous measurements (the palpebral reflex at the moment, compared with what it was 15 min earlier) and with reference to other related parameters. (If an animal is scrambling to leave the table, who cares whether it has a palpebral reflex?) Given the mechanistic differences between anesthetic drugs and interindividual differences in response to them, monitoring of anesthetic level is, at best, very uncertain. It is nevertheless the explicit responsibility of anesthetists to ensure that these drugs are administered in the safest possible way by monitoring the animal's response to them.

Physical Signs of Anesthetic Depth

These depend, for the most part, on the evaluation of muscular tone and muscular reflexes. The signs of anesthetic depth vary from moment to moment, from individual to individual, and between species and anesthetic drugs. No one sign alone defines anesthetic depth. Assess as many signs as possible. They invariably suggest different levels of anesthesia, one sign suggesting a light level, one medium, and one deep, and the anesthetist is left to sort it all out. Observers should prioritize the signs (some are more reliable than others) and then average their findings (medium in the aforementioned example). The presence of a sign is much more meaningful than the absence of it. For instance, in most species and with most anesthetics, the presence of a palpebral reflex is a reliable sign of a light level of anesthesia. The absence of a palpebral reflex suggests that the level is not light. In some individuals, though, the sign is unreliable, and the level is light despite the absence of the reflex. When the signs of anesthetic depth are unclear or contradictory, anesthetic drug administration should be decreased until the animal is clearly at a light to medium level of anesthesia. Lastly, know that there is no obligatory correlation between level of anesthesia and physiological consequence of anesthesia; a light level does not preclude severe hypotension or hypoxemia. These are some points to remember:

1. The recent history of anesthetic dosing is an important component of the evaluation of the depth of anesthesia: Large dosages should be associated with a deep level of anesthesia and vice versa. The vaporizer setting or the drug infusion rate helps define the amount of anesthetic being delivered to a patient. End-tidal anesthetic concentrations and plasma drug concentrations define the amount of anesthetic in a patient. Usual vaporizer settings, drug administration rates, and end-tidal and plasma concentrations that are appropriate for induction (loading) and then maintenance for the various common anesthetics are discussed elsewhere in this text (Chapters 8 through 16). The issue here is that the anesthetic drug dosing is just the beginning of the evaluation of the depth of anesthesia, not the definition of it. "Usual" dosages may cause excessive anesthesia in animals with serious underlying disease and hypothermia. Normal anesthetic drug dosages do not guarantee that an animal will not be overanesthetized. Equally important is that vaporizers and infusion pumps do not always work properly, and normal settings may actually overshoot or undershoot the mark. Knowledge of anesthetic drug dosing and knowledge of the amount of drug "on board a patient" define only what they measure and are not the definition of anesthetic depth in an individual patient. You are going to need more information.

2. Spontaneous movement is a reliable sign of a light level of anesthesia with most anesthetics. Focal muscle twitching has been associated with etomidate and propofol administration and should not be interpreted, per se, to indicate a light level. Spontaneous muscular movement is common with opioid-based anesthetic protocols and also should not be interpreted to indicate a light level. Muscle hypertonus can be a feature of ketamine-based protocols and should not be interpreted to indicate a light level.

3. Reflex movement in response to surgical stimulation is a reliable sign of a light level of anesthesia. It does not, however, mean that an animal is experiencing pain from a nociceptive stimulus.

4. An abrupt increase in heart rate, blood pressure, or breathing rate, specifically in response to surgical stimulation, is generally considered to be a reliable sign of a light level of anesthesia. In general, physiological parameters such as heart rate, arterial blood pressure, breathing rate, and minute ventilation should trend upward as an animal becomes more lightly anesthetized and downward when an animal becomes deeply anesthetized. These are not, however, reliable *premonitory* indicators of anesthetic depth; they are often observed to be quite stable until after an animal abruptly awakes or suffers cardiovascular collapse. There are also many abnormalities that affect these parameters (in either direction) that have nothing to do with anesthetic level. Anesthetic level is only one of the differentials that should be considered when an animal develops a decreased or increased heart or breathing rate.

5. Mandibular muscle tone should be *lots*, *some*, and *none* in light, medium, and deep levels of anesthesia, respectively, in dogs and cats. The descriptors lots, some, and none must be indexed to the species and breed of an animal; one would never expect a cat to have the same muscle tone as a mastiff. Mandibular muscle tone is assessed by the resistance encountered when trying to just open the mandible. Puppies never have any mandibular muscle tone, and this parameter cannot be used to evaluate their depth of anesthesia. Large animals always have much muscle tone and this parameter cannot be used to evaluate their depth of anesthesia. Ruminants and swine exhibit a chewing reflex when they are lightly anesthetized.[18]

6. A change to an abdominal (diaphragm)-first breathing pattern signals a deeper level of anesthesia, as does bradypnea and hypoventilation.

7. The presence of a palpebral reflex is a reliable indicator of a light level of anesthesia. The absence of it suggests a medium or deep level. The goal would be an anesthetic depth where the palpebral reflex is either just barely present or just barely absent. Some individuals fail to exhibit a palpebral reflex even though their anesthesia level is actually light. With keta-

mine use, the palpebral reflex is always present and the eyelids remain open as opposed to the effect of most other anesthetics on this parameter.

8. The presence of a *pupillary light reflex* (pupillary constriction in response to a bright light shined upon the retina) and the presence of a *dazzle reflex* (a blink in response to a bright light) are reliable indicators of a light to light to medium level of anesthesia. The pupillary light reflex may be minimized or eliminated by parasympatholytics.

9. In small animals, with traditional anesthetics, eyeball position is central (and the pupil size is medium) when the animal's anesthesia level is light, is rotated ventromedially when the level is medium, and is central again (and the pupil is dilated) when the level is deep. The eyeball does not rotate when ketamine is used. In horses, the eyeball can rotate, though not reliably so, but spontaneous nystagmus does occur. A very slow, "roving" eyeball ("one minute it's here; the next it's over there") might represent a medium level of anesthesia, whereas a fast nystagmus represents a very light level in this species. Nystagmus may occur in light levels of anesthesia in ruminants and swine, but disappears at deeper levels. In these species, the eyeball rotates ventrally with deeper levels of anesthesia. Nystagmus does not normally occur in anesthetized small animals.

10. The lack of tear production as noted by a dry-appearing cornea is a sign of a deep level of anesthesia with traditional anesthetics. Lacrimation or "tearing" is seen in horses and is a sign of a light level.

11. The gag and swallow reflexes are reliable indicators of a light level of anesthesia in nearly all species.

EEG: Monitoring of Anesthetic Depth

Typically, the EEG pattern changes from a low-wave, high-frequency pattern during the awake state to high-wave, low-frequency with anesthesia to burst suppression (intermittent periods of electrical silence) and finally persistent electrical silence with deep levels of anesthesia. The raw EEG signals, however, require a considerable volume of recording and considerable specialized training and expertise to interpret subtle changes. Computerized analysis of raw EEG signals facilitates interpretation of those signals. EEG voltage changes (power) as a function of time (time domain) generate such indices as total EEG power, median power frequency, or burst suppression. Interpretational algorithms (by fast Fourier transformation) might also examine signal activity as a function of frequency (frequency domain) and generate such indices as spectral edge frequency (SEF_{95}) (the frequency below which 95% of the total EEG power resides), median frequency (the median EEG power frequency), and the relative power of the delta (0.5 to 3.5 Hz), theta (3.5 to 7.0 Hz), alpha (7 to 13 Hz), and beta (13 to 30 Hz) frequency ranges compared with total EEG power.[19] Such indices have been used to characterize anesthetic depth in people[6,20–22] and animals.[23–26] Other indices[27] and combinations of indices,[28] BIS and Narcotrend (Monitor Technik, Bad Bramstedt, Germany), may represent a more integrated approach to EEG analysis compared with the classic indices[19,22] and may be more user-friendly.

BIS analysis (Aspect Medical Systems, Newton, MA) repre-

sents a variably weighted value derived from four subparameters: (a) burst suppression ratio (time domain); (b) a quasi value (time domain); (c) β_2 power ratio in the 30- to 47-Hz range compared with that in the 11- to 20-Hz range (frequency domain); and (d) the bispectral biocoherence ratio of peaks in the 0.5- to 47-Hz range compared with the 40- to 47-Hz range (frequency domain).[17] BIS has been extensively studied in humans primarily as an index of sedation[29,30] or depth of anesthesia.[16,22,26,31–34] It has also been used as an index of brain function in neurological patients.[35,36] The BIS monitor does not require calibration and displays a bar graph denoting signal quality and amount of electromyographic interference. Excessive muscle movement can be a problem.[37] The monitor displays a number between 0 and 100: Values above 90 are compatible with awake and alert, 80 to 90 with anxiolysis, 60 to 80 with hypnotic or moderate obtundation, below 60 with loss of recall, below 50 with unresponsiveness to verbal stimuli, below 20 with burst suppression, and 0 with isoelectric stimuli (Aspect Medical Systems). Not all anesthetics affect BIS in the same way: Propofol, midazolam, and thiopental strongly depress it, inhalational anesthetics have an intermediate effect, opioids have little effect, and nitrous oxide and ketamine tend to increase the BIS value.[17]

Narcotrend analyzes the raw EEG data and then categorizes the levels of sedation as awake (A0), subvigilant (A1 and A2), sedation (B0, B1, and B2), anesthesia (C0, C1, and C2), moderate anesthesia (D0, D1, and D2), deep anesthesia or burst suppression (E), and coma/electrical silence (F).[38]

Auditory evoked EEG responses have been used primarily to assess neurological function in CNS disease, but have also been used to assess anesthetic depth and awareness or recall.[39] Many studies have used sensory (to a noxious stimulus)-evoked EEG or BIS, hemodynamic responses, and movement responses to evaluate nociception.

All EEG indices are subject to large individual and anesthetic drug variation. Depending on the magnitude of the stimulation and the depth of anesthesia, stimulus-induced EEG changes could represent either an arousal pattern or a pattern that suggests a deeper level of anesthesia (the *paradoxical* response).[23,40] The EEG changes do not reflect analgesic properties of an anesthetic drug, per se, but only its hypnotic properties. No EEG index has yet replaced physical evaluation of patients and common sense, although several indices clearly aide the evaluation of anesthetic depth, reduction of anesthetic drug dosages, and shortened recovery times.[38]

Monitoring Perioperative Pain and Analgesia

Nociception is the neural response to a noxious stimulus. *Pain* is the conscious interpretation that the nociceptive stimulus is sufficiently unpleasant to motivate its owner to do something about it. The evaluation of pain is more simple in communicative people (you ask them) than in neonates and animals. The existence of pain in an animal and the need for analgesic therapy depend on the observation of behavioral changes or abnormalities that can reasonably be attributed to pain. Unfortunately, none of the "pain signs" are specific to pain; many nonpainful situations cause them, as well.

Physical Signs of Pain

It might be helpful to divide pain into levels of magnitude: mild, moderate, and severe. *Severe pain* might be defined as that which is intolerable; the kind of pain where the animal throws itself about its cage in a mindless frenzy because the pain is so severe that it simply cannot deal with it in any other way. Unprovoked vocalizing (crying or whimpering) by an animal that does not have CNS disease and is not recovering from anesthesia, but does have a disease that might be painful, is taken as evidence of severe pain. *Mild pain* might be equated with that amount which one would consider to be a nuisance and not necessarily of such magnitude that its owner would seek out pain-relief medications. Such an animal can tolerate it well and can usually go about its normal daily activity. Since the pain does not interfere with behavior in any fashion, it defies recognition by an outside observer.

Moderate pain may be described as that which starts to interfere with normal behavior, appetite, or activity of an animal that has a disease or that has undergone a surgical procedure or experienced a trauma that is reported to be painful in people. The animal may exhibit an anxious expression and may not rest comfortably, and may be unable to sleep. The animal is less concerned with happenings in its environment. Appetite may be decreased or absent and the animal may lose weight, energy, or productivity. The animal's activity may be decreased (if the animal is trying to minimize pain associated with movement). It may just lie in one spot for extended periods with its eyes open, staring into space without focusing on anything in particular. The animal's activity may become increased (if the animal is trying to find a position wherein the pain is diminished), and the animal may assume abnormal positions. The animal may move, but infrequently, and stiffly, as though to guard and protect the painful area. The attitude may also change to that of an animal that is less tolerant to being handled than normal. The attitude may become more fearful or more aggressive.

The pain may be classified as moderate if an animal develops an anxious expression or tenses when the area in question is about to be touched, or if it cries out or responds aggressively when the area is touched (assuming that these represent inappropriate responses for this particular individual or species to an otherwise innocuous stimulus). Secondary physiological changes that may result from pain are tachycardia, tachypnea, hypertension, arrhythmias, dilated pupils, salivation, and/or hyperglycemia.

EEG: Monitoring of Analgesia

The EEG indices measure brain electrical activity that changes in an approximately consistent pattern with anesthetic depth in such a way that one can predict with some accuracy when a patient loses awareness, recall, and response to a noxious stimulus. EEG changes observed in response to nociceptive stimulation generally reflect a lighter level of anesthesia, although a "paradoxical arousal" response, reflective of a deeper level, is common.[23,40]

These EEG indices are not a measure of pain, per se, but of a cortical response to the nociceptive stimulus, in the same way that movement or a change in heart rate may occur in response to a nociceptive stimulus. These responses do not prove that an animal is experiencing pain, but only suggest a cortical electrical response to the nociceptive stimulus; the animal may or may not be experiencing pain.

Most studies use the EEG indices to measure the ability of various drugs to diminish a response to a specifically timed, induced surgical stimulus (such as an incision).[40-43] Although the administration of nitrous oxide did not affect 95% spectral edge frequency or BIS in the absence of surgical stimulation,[44] it was associated with a dose-dependent decrease in these parameters when administered during major lumbar surgery.[45] Although the administration of fentanyl did not affect 95% spectral edge frequency or BIS, per se, it prevented the decrease in these indices (paradoxical response) associated with skin incision.[43] Both results were attributed to the analgesic properties of the drugs. In a novel approach to studying preemptive analgesia, when the spectral edge frequency was maintained within the target range of 8 to 12 Hz, postoperative pain scores and morphine requirements were reduced.[46] There are no analgesia monitors per se, but only monitors of the cortical electrical response to nociceptive stimuli. When a drug diminishes the EEG response to a nociceptive stimulus, it is often presumed to be because of its analgesic qualities (unless, of course, it is because of its hypnotic qualities).

Analgesia assessment in the postoperative period is a different challenge from that of a specific, timed, nociceptive stimulus in the intraoperative period. Postoperatively, pain is pretty much ongoing. The objective might be to return the EEG index and the patient to a state that is relaxed, sedate, and pain free (that is clearly not an arousal nor a paradoxical arousal state) and to maintain them in that state. In EEG terms, this might be an SEF_{95} of 8 to 12 Hz or a BIS value below 60. In physical examination terms, this is represented by behavior which suggests that the animal is comfortable and reasonably pain free. The EEG indices are not likely to be particularly helpful in weaning an animal off of analgesic drugs; that is, in determining when it is okay to withdraw them and allow an animal to return to a normal, aroused, drug-free, pain-free state.

Important Concepts in the Provision of Analgesia

The administration of analgesic drugs prior to the nociceptive stimulus (preemptive analgesia) is thought to reduce the *ramping up* process (amplification of the nociceptive signal) by the modulatory interneurons within the spinal cord. Preemptive analgesia reduces the magnitude of postoperative pain as well as the dosages of analgesics administered.

Animals cannot truly be evaluated for pain during the recovery phase (the reflex phase) of anesthesia. Nevertheless, excessive vocalizing and activity during this time should be subdued with a sedative; they can cause the animal's owner considerable angst. Ensure that the source of the discomfort is not a full urinary bladder (animals typically receive a large volume of fluids during surgery and often do not urinate).

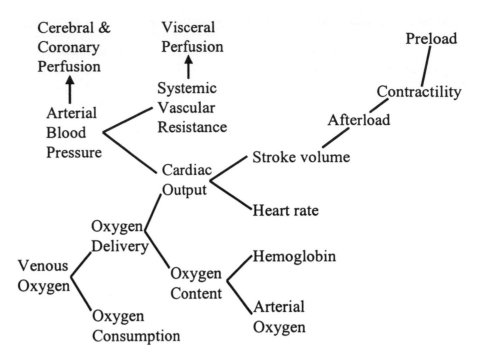

Fig. 19.1. Integration of cardiopulmonary performance.

In the postoperative period, after the evaluation of pain signs, because they are not specific, one is invariably left with doubt as to whether an animal is experiencing pain. In the end, the decision is subjective. Animals should subjectively appear to be comfortable, respond to human interaction normally, sleep, eat and drink, and move about with ease. If they do not present a comfortable picture, something should be done. Analgesic drugs are not without potential adverse effects, and there is sometimes great hesitancy to administer them to treat a problem that one is not sure exists. The relative risks, however, are low and by far outweighed by the potential harm associated with unremitting pain. When it is unclear whether an animal is experiencing undue pain and when it is unclear whether analgesics should be administered, it is appropriate to administer a full dose of an analgesic.

Free nerve endings transduce pressure, heat, or chemical nociceptive stimuli into an electrical signal (transduction) that is then transmitted to the spinal cord, brain stem, and thalamus (transmission). In the dorsal horn of the spinal cord, nociceptive signals can be diminished or augmented by ascending or descending interneuronal pathways (modulation). The somatosensory cortex then integrates, interprets, and quantifies the nociceptive stimulus (perception). Different analgesic drugs affect nociception at different levels of the process, and this justifies the use of drugs with multilevel effects and the use of multiple drugs to take advantage of their differential foci of effect. Transduction can be inhibited by local anesthetics, opioids, and antiprostaglandins; transmission by local anesthetics and α_2-agonists; spinal modulation by local anesthetics, opioids, α_2-agonists, N-methyl-D-aspartate antagonists (ketamine), antiprostaglandins, and anticonvulsants; and perception by general anesthetics, opioids, α_2-agonists, and tranquilizers (phenothiazines).[47]

When one or two dosages of an analgesic fail to alleviate the "pain signs," chances are that pain was not the problem in the first case. The use of anxiolytics may be indicated. Acepromazine (0.01 mg/kg) has been remarkably effective; diazepam (0.2 mg/kg) may or may not be effective.

Physiological Consequences of the Anesthetic State

Although the pharmacodynamic effects of the various anesthetic drugs vary, the mechanisms by which they cause morbidity and mortality are the same: excessive bradycardia, arrhythmias, myocardial depression, vasodilation, hypotension, hypoventilation, hypoxemia, or hypothermia. These common problems should be the focus of intraoperative monitoring of organ function. Ongoing, automatic, audible monitors of organ function are the mainstays of intraoperative monitoring and crisis prevention. Single, point-in-time measurements are meaningful when their results are severely abnormal: A heart rate of zero is a problem at the moment, and it does not matter what it was 15 min earlier. For the most part, though, measurements and evaluations are only interpretable in the context of previous measurements (trends) and with reference to related parameters (Fig. 19.1). A dog's heart rate of 50 beats/min may not be a problem if blood pressure and cardiac output are adequate to meet the tissue perfusion needs of the patient, or may even be an appropriate compensation if the arterial blood pressure is high. Some expected cardiopulmonary changes associated with the administration of various anesthetic agents are listed in Tables 19.1 (dogs) and 19.2 (horses).

Cardiovascular Monitoring
Heart Rate and Rhythm
Heart rate and stroke volume are important to cardiac output. Slower heart rates are usually associated with larger end-diastolic

Table 19.1. Cardiopulmonary effects of general anesthesia in dogs.

	Awake[a]	Ketamine[b]	Oxymorphone[c]	Halothane[d]	Pentobarbital[e]
HR	90 ± 21	166 ± 44	72 ± 14	97 ± 13	107 ± 20
CI	4.65 ± 1.09	6.55 ± 2.23	4.13 ± 1.13	3.22 ± 0.62	4.26 ± 0.51
CVP	3 ± 4	2 ± 4	12 ± 4	2 ± 1	NR
PAOP	5 ± 2	NR	15 ± 2	5 ± 2	NR
ABPm	104 ± 12	139 ± 13	112 ± 10	64 ± 9	118 ± 18
PAPm	15 ± 4	17 ± 6	21 ± 4	10 ± 2	17 ± 3
SVRI	(1787)	(1696)	(2166)	(1588)	(2215)
PaO_2	100 ± 6	96 ± 7	81 ± 6	540 ± 46	90 ± 7
PvO_2	50 ± 5	50 ± 5	49 ± 5	81 ± 8	51 ± 3
$PaCO_2$	40 ± 3	41 ± 6	50 ± 2	45 ± 8	43 ± 5
$A\text{-}aPO_2$	10 ± 5	6 ± 3	(14)	(120)	12 ± 5
Ven admix	4 ± 3	3 ± 3	13 ± 6	6 ± 1	7 ± 3
Hb	13.1 ± 1.7	14.9 ± 1.9	16.3 ± 1.8	14.0 ± 2.2	14.0 ± 1.0
DO_2	(801)	(1273)	(854)	(656)	(771)
VO_2	(149)	(230)	(153)	(84)	(126)
O_2 extr	(0.19)	(0.18)	(0.18)	(0.13)	(0.16)

HR, heart rate (beats/min); CI, cardiac index (L/min/m²); CVP, central venous pressure (cm H_2O); PAOP, pulmonary artery occlusion pressure (mm Hg); ABPm, mean arterial blood pressure (mm Hg); PAPm, mean pulmonary arterial blood pressure (mm Hg); SVRI, systemic vascular resistance index (dynes · s · cm^{-5}); PaO_2, arterial partial pressure of oxygen (mm Hg); PvO_2, venous partial pressure of oxygen; $PaCO_2$, arterial partial pressure of carbon dioxide (mm Hg); $A\text{-}aPO_2$, alveolar-arterial PO_2 gradient (mm Hg); Ven admix, venous admixture (%); Hb, hemoglobin (g/dL); DO_2, oxygen delivery (mL/min/m²); VO_2, oxygen consumption (mL/min/m²); O_2 extr, oxygen extraction (%).
Data expressed as mean ± 1 SD. Numbers in parentheses were recalculated from the available data.
[a]In unsedated, calm, recumbent dogs breathing room air
[b]15 min after ketamine (10 mg/kg) administered intravenously.
[c]75 min after 0.4 mg/kg oxymorphone, administered intravenously, followed by 0.2 mg/kg at 20, 40, and 60 min.
[d]30 min after mask induction and intubation with halothane.
[e]40 min after pentobarbital induction.

Table 19.2. Cardiopulmonary effects of general anesthesia in horses[58,59].

	Awake	Isoflurane (1.2 MAC)/ Halothane (1.0 MAC)
HR	37 ± 2	43 ± 5/39 ± 2
CI	69 ± 3	59 ± 8/35 ± 3
ABPm	133 ± 12	92 ± 5/98 ± 9
PAPm	29 ± 2	25 ± 2/26 ± 1
SVRI	333 ± 18	285 ± 28/579 ± 56
PaO_2	507 ± 14	318 ± 46/360 ± 28
PvO_2	52 ± 6	57 ± 4/ND
$PaCO_2$	45 ± 1	73 ± 4/65 ± 2

HR, heart rate (beats/min); CI, cardiac index (L/min/kg); ABPm, mean arterial blood pressure (mm Hg); PAPm, mean pulmonary arterial blood pressure (mm Hg); SVRI, systemic vascular resistance index (dynes · s · cm^{-5}); PaO_2, arterial oxygen partial pressure (mm Hg); PvO_2, venous partial pressure of oxygen; $PaCO_2$, arterial carbon dioxide partial pressure (mm Hg).
Data expressed as mean ± 1 SD.
MAC, minimum alveolar concentration; ND, not done.

ventricular volumes and larger stroke volumes; up to a point, cardiac output is preserved by the larger stroke volumes.[48] Heart rate is too slow when it is associated with low cardiac output, hypotension, or poor tissue perfusion. In lieu of this kind of evidence or a reasonable cause for the bradycardia, values of 60 beats/min for dogs, 90 for cats, and low 20s for horses are common triggers for treatment. Common causes and treatment for bradycardia are listed in Table 19.3. Verify that the problem is truly bradycardia as opposed to a slow pulse rate, which could be caused by ventricular arrhythmias. Excessive vagal tone can be caused by pharyngeal, laryngeal, or tracheal stimulation; by pressure on the eyeball or rectus muscles; or by visceral inflammation, distension, or traction.

Sinus tachycardia is primarily a sign of an underlying problem (Table 19.4). It becomes a problem for patients only when there is not enough time for diastolic filling: Cardiac output decreases. In people, because of coronary artery disease, sinus tachycardia is feared because the increased myocardial oxygen consumption may exceed oxygen-delivery capabilities. In lieu of cardiac output information, the trigger level for specific treatment of sinus tachycardia may be somewhere in the low 200s for dogs, the high 200s for cats, and 80 for horses.

Ventricular arrhythmias, in an animal that did not have them prior to anesthesia, are primarily a sign of an anesthetic-induced complication (Table 19.5). Make sure that the electrocardiographic abnormality is truly of ventricular origin as opposed to a right bundle branch block, which appears similar to a ventricular rhythm except that it is preceded by a P wave. Ventricular arrhythmias may also be caused by intrinsic myocardial disease or arrhythmogenic factors released from various debilitated abdom-

Table 19.3. Causes of perioperative bradycardia.

Cause	Treatment
Anesthetic overdosage	Lighten the level of anesthesia
Opioids	Administer a parasympatholytic
α_2-Agonists	No treatment
Excessive vagal tone caused by visceral stimulation	Less stimulation; parasympatholytic
Hypothermia	Rewarm
Hyperkalemia	Calcium or insulin-glucose therapy
Sick sinus syndrome	Administer a parasympatholytic or sympathomimetic
Atrioventricular conduction block	Administer a parasympatholytic or sympathomimetic
End-stage metabolic failure	Administer a parasympatholytic or sympathomimetic
Hypoxia	Administer oxygen
Parasympathomimetics (e.g., acetylcholine-sterase inhibitors)	Administer a parasympatholytic
Organophosphates	Administer a parasympatholytic
Digitalis	Administer a sympathomimetric

Table 19.4. Causes and treatment of tachycardia.

Cause	Treatment
Too light a level of anesthesia	Deepen the level of anesthesia
Ketamine	No treatment
Parasympatholytics (e.g., atropine)	Give less or by the subcutaneous or intramuscular route the next time; glycopyrrolate
Sympathomimetics	Decrease the infusion rate
Hypovolemia	Restore blood volume
Hyperthermia	Cool
Hypoxemia	Administer oxygen
Hypercapnia	Improve ventilation or eliminate rebreathing
Individual variation	No treatment
Paroxysmal supraventricular rhythm	Administer verapamil or diltiazem
Recovery phase	No treatment
Postoperative pain	Administer analgesics
Pheochromocytoma	Sypatholytic

Table 19.5. Causes of ventricular ectopic pacemaker activity.

Endogenous release of catecholamines or sympathomimetic therapy
Hypoxia or hypercapnia
Hypovolemia or hypotension
Myocardial inflammation, disease, or stimulation (intracardiac catheters or pleural tubes)
Thoracic and nonthoracic trauma
Certain anesthetics lower the threshold to endogenous or exogenous catecholamines (halothane, xylazine, thiamylal, or thiopental)
Hypokalemia (potentiated by respiratory or metabolic alkalosis, or glucose-insulin therapy)
Hyperkalemia (potentiated by acidosis, hypocalcemia, succinyl-choline, or may be iatrogenic)
Visceral organ disease (gastric volvulus and/or torsion)
Intracranial disorders (increased pressure or hypoxia)
Digitalis toxicity (potentiated by hypokalemia and hypercalcemia)

mic drugs have deleterious cardiovascular and neurological effects. A simple decrease in the rate or severity of the arrhythmia may be a suitable end point to the titration of antiarrhythmic drugs (Table 19.6).

Ventricular arrhythmias can be caused by several mechanisms that are not readily apparent from the electrocardiographic appearance of the arrhythmia: (a) abnormal automaticity characterized by rapid, spontaneous, phase 4 depolarization; (b) reentry of depolarization wave fronts because of unidirectional conduction blocks; (c) early after-depolarizations caused by diminished repolarizing potassium currents prolonging action potentials; and (d) delayed after-depolarizations caused by abnormal oscillations of cytosolic calcium concentrations after myocardial or Purkinje cell repolarization. A given antiarrhythmic may be effective in one mechanism and be ineffective, or even worsen the arrhythmia, in another. Antiarrhythmic therapy is always a bit of a clinical trial. Lidocaine is a first-choice antiarrhythmic because it selectively affects abnormal cells without affecting automaticity or conduction in normal cells.

Vasomotor Tone

Peripheral and visceral perfusion is primarily regulated by vasomotor tone. Vasodilation improves peripheral perfusion, whereas vasoconstriction impairs it. Vasodilation is a potent cause of hypotension, whereas vasoconstriction increases blood pressure. Vasomotor tone is assessed by mucous membrane color (pale = vasoconstriction, whereas red = vasodilation), capillary refill time (<1 s = vasoconstriction, whereas >2 s = vasodilation), toeweb to core temperature gradient (>4°C = vasoconstriction, whereas <2°C = vasodilation). Vasoconstriction may be caused by hypovolemia, heart failure, hypothermia, or the administration of vasoconstrictor drugs. Vasodilation may be caused by the systemic inflammatory response, hyperthermia or the administration of vasodilator drugs. Treatment should be directed to the underlying cause; vasocorrective therapy is only utilized as a last resort (Table 19.7).

inal organs. Ventricular arrhythmias become a problem for a patient when they interfere with cardiac output, arterial blood pressure, and tissue perfusion, or when they threaten to convert to ventricular fibrillation. Ventricular arrhythmias should be treated when (a) the minute-rate equivalent approaches the trigger point for treating sinus tachycardia, (b) they are multiform, or (c) the ectopic beat overrides the T wave of the preceding depolarization. Total elimination of the ventricular arrhythmia is not necessarily the goal of therapy, because large dosages of antiarrhyth-

Table 19.6. Antiarrhythmic drugs.

Drug	Mechanism	Indication	Intravenous Dosage
Lidocaine	Sodium-channel blocker	VPCs	1–4 mg/kg; 2–6 mg/kg/h
Procainamide	Sodium-channel blocker	VPCs; APCs	1–4 mg/kg; 2–6 mg/kg/h
Quinidine	Sodium-channel blocker	VPCs; APCs	5–15 mg/kg
Amiodarone	Sodium-channel blocker and other effects	VPCs	5 mg/kg over 20 min
Atenolol	ß Blocker	APCs; VPCs	0.2–1 mg/kg
Esmolol	ß Blocker	APCs; VPCs	0.2–0.5 mg/kg; 0.5–10 mg/kg/h
Propanolol	ß Blocker	APCs; VPCs	0.01–0.3 mg/kg
Diltiazem	Calcium-channel blocker	APCs	0.05–0.25 mg/kg; 0.05–0.3 mg/kg/h
Verapamil	Calcium-channel blocker	APCs	0.05–0.25 mg/kg

APCs (atrial premature contractions), supraventricular arrhythmia; VPCs (ventricular premature contractions), ventricular arrhythmia.

Table 19.7. Cardiovascular drugs.

Drug	Indication				Intravenous Dosage
	Contractility	Heart Rate	Vasomotor Tone		
			Art	Ven	
Dobutamine	↑↑↑	↑↑	↓		5–15 µg/kg/min
Dopamine	↑↑↑	↑↑	↑↑		5–15 µg/kg/min
Epinephrine	↑↑↑	↑↑↑	↑↑↑		0.1–1.0 µg/kg/min
Norepinephrine	0	nc	↑↑↑		0.2–2.0 µg/kg/min
Phenylephrine	0	↓	↑↑↑		1–5 µg/kg/min
Vasopressin	0	↓	↑↑		0.5 units/kg
Hydralazine	0	↑↑	↓↓	0	0.5–1.0 mg/kg
Nitroprusside	0	↑↑	↓↓↓	↓↓↓	1–5 µg/kg/min
Acepromazine	0	↑	↓	↓	0.01 mg/kg
Morphine	0	↓	↓	↓↓	0.1–0.5 mg/kg
Diltiazem	↓↓	↓	↓	↓	0.05–0.25 mg/kg; 0.05–0.3 mg/kg/h
Enalaprilat	0	nc	↓	↓	0.01–0.02 mg/kg

Art, arterial; Ven, venous; nc, no change.

Central Venous Pressure

Central venous pressure (CVP) is the luminal pressure of the intrathoracic vena cava. Peripheral venous pressure is variably higher than CVP, is subject to unpredictable extraneous influences, and is not a reliable indicator of CVP. CVP is the relationship between central blood volume and central blood volume capacity. Central blood volume is determined by venous return and cardiac output. Verification of a well-placed, unobstructed catheter can be ascertained by observing small fluctuations in the fluid meniscus within the manometer synchronous with the heartbeat, and larger excursions synchronous with ventilation. Large fluctuations synchronous with each heartbeat may indicate that the end of the catheter is positioned within the right ventricle. Direct observation of the CVP waveform may help identify the proper location of the catheter tip (Fig. 19.2). Measurements should be made during the expiratory pause phase (during either spontaneous or positive-pressure ventilation) because changes in pleural pressure affect the luminal pressure within the anterior vena cava.

The normal CVP in small animals is 0 to 10 cm H_2O. It is 15 to 30 cm H_2O in laterally recumbent horses, and 5 to 10 cm H_2O in dorsally recumbent horses.[49] Low-range or below-range values indicate hypovolemia and suggest that a rapid bolus of fluids should be administered. Above-range values indicate relative hypervolemia and that fluid therapy should be stopped. CVP is a measure of the relative ability of the heart to pump the venous return and should be measured whenever heart failure is a concern. CVP is also a measure of the relationship between blood volume and blood volume capacity and could be measured to help determine the end point for large fluid volume resuscitation. CVP measurements are used to determine whether there is "room" for additional fluid therapy in the management of hypotension.

CVP is not a measure of preload (only of preload pressure) and is a poor predictor of stroke volume or cardiac output.[50] Preload is end-diastolic muscle stretch that, in vivo, is mostly related to end-diastolic volume, which, clinically, is reflected in the measure of end-diastolic diameter. CVP is a filling pressure, not a vol-

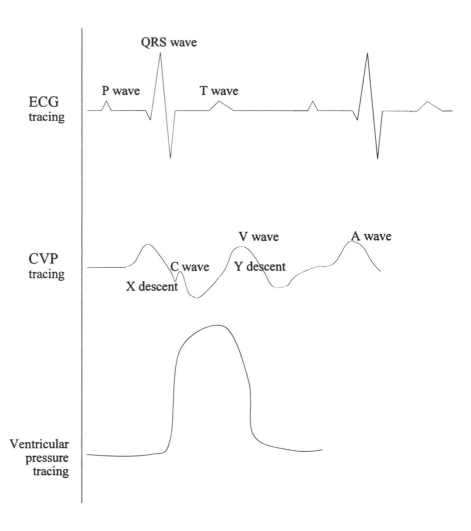

Fig. 19.2. Central venous and ventricular pressure waveforms. CVP, central venous pressure; and ECG, electrocardiogram.

ume, and will not be representative of preload in diseases associated with decreased ventricular compliance (i.e., hypertrophy, tamponade, and fibrosis). Diastolic performance (relaxation) is also adversely affected by some anesthetics.[51]

Arterial Blood Pressure

Arterial blood pressure is a consequence of the relationship between blood volume and blood volume capacity. Arterial blood volume is determined by cardiac output and systemic vascular resistance. Arterial blood pressure is a primary determinant of cerebral and coronary perfusion. Systolic blood pressure is primarily determined by stroke volume and arterial compliance. Diastolic blood pressure is primarily determined by systemic vascular resistance and heart rate. Mean blood pressure is the average pressure: one-half of the area of the pulse-pressure waveform. If the pulse-pressure waveform were a perfect triangle, mean pressure would be one-third of the difference between diastolic pressure and systolic pressure. To the extent that the pulse-pressure contour is not a perfect triangle—a tall, narrow pulse-pressure waveform is common—the mean pressure will be closer to diastolic. The mean arterial blood pressure is physiologically the most important because it represents the mean driving pressure for organ perfusion. Many clinical instruments, however, measure only

systolic blood pressure. The relationship between systolic blood pressure and mean arterial blood pressure is variable, depending on the shape of the pulse-pressure waveform; systolic blood pressure should always be assessed with this in mind.

Assessment of pulse quality by digital palpation is an evaluation of both the height and width of the pulse-pressure waveform compared with normal. Tall, wide pulse-pressure waveforms are seen in sepsis, whereas tall, narrow waveforms occur with a patent ductus and during cardiopulmonary resuscitation. Small, narrow pulse-pressure waveforms are seen with small stroke volumes and vasoconstriction. A small stroke volume can be seen with hypovolemia, poor heart function from any cause, tachycardia, and ventricular arrhythmias. The pulse-pressure waveform is largely a reflection of stroke volume and vessel size. It is not a measure of arterial blood pressure per se, although, in a species-dependent and very general way, vessels with low pressure are easier to collapse and vice versa. The weak, thready pulse that occurs with hypovolemia is caused by small stroke volumes and vessel constriction; patients with this symptom may be normotensive. Peripheral pulse quality (such as the dorsal metatarsal in dogs) decreases and disappears earlier than it does in larger, more central arteries (such as the femoral) with progressive hypovolemia. The relative pulse quality of more peripheral versus more central arteries may provide a rough index to the magnitude of the problem.

Arterial blood pressure can be measured indirectly by sphygmomanometry or directly via an arterial catheter attached to a transducer system. *Sphygmomanometry* involves the application of an occlusion cuff over an artery in a cylindrical appendage. The width of the occlusion cuff should be about 40% of the circumference of the leg to which it is applied. The occlusion cuff should be placed snugly around the leg. If it is applied too tightly, the pressure measurements will be erroneously low because the cuff itself, acting as a tourniquet, will partially occlude the underlying artery. If the cuff is too loose, the pressure measurements will be erroneously high because excessive cuff pressure will be required to occlude the underlying artery. Inflation of the cuff applies pressure to the underlying tissues and will totally occlude blood flow when the cuff pressure exceeds systolic blood pressure. As the cuff pressure is gradually decreased, blood will begin to flow intermittently when the cuff pressure falls below systolic pressure. When this occurs, (a) the manometer pressure at which needle oscillations begin to occur on the manometer during cuff deflation (caused by the pulse wave hitting the cuff) corresponds approximately to systolic blood pressure, and (b) the manometer pressure at which one can digitally palpate a pulse distal to the cuff corresponds approximately to diastolic blood pressure. *Doppler ultrasound* involves the application of a small piezoelectric ultrasound crystal over an artery. Some Doppler instruments measure blood flow and are used to measure systolic blood pressure, whereas other instruments generate signals from the movement of the arterial wall and can be used to measure both systolic and diastolic blood pressures. *Oscillometry* analyzes the fluctuation of pressure in the cuff as it is slowly deflated and provides a digital display of systolic, diastolic, and mean blood pressures, and heart rate. Most of these instruments can be set to recycle at discrete time intervals. Small vessel size and motion can interfere with measurements.

All external techniques are least accurate when vessels are small, when the blood pressure is low, and when the vessels are constricted. Direct measurement of arterial blood pressure is more accurate and continuous compared with indirect methods, but requires the introduction of a catheter into an artery by a percutaneous or cut-down procedure. The dorsal metatarsal and ear arteries in dogs and cats, and the facial and metatarsal arteries in horses and cows, are commonly used. The subcutaneous tissues around these arteries are relatively tight, and hematoma formation at the time of catheter removal is rarely a problem. Once the catheter is placed, it is connected to a monitoring device. The catheter must be flushed with heparinized saline at frequent intervals (hourly) or continuously to prevent blood clot occlusion. The measuring device could be a long fluid administration set suspended from the ceiling. Fluid is instilled into the tubing via a three-way stopcock to a very high level and then allowed to gravitate into the artery until the hydrostatic pressure of the column of water is equalized with the mean arterial blood pressure of the patient. Since blood pressure oscillates, leaving the system open between measurements is not advised because that will let blood enter the catheter and clot and occlude it. Alternatively, the measuring device could be an aneroid manometer (Fig. 19.3). Water or blood must not be allowed to enter the manometer.

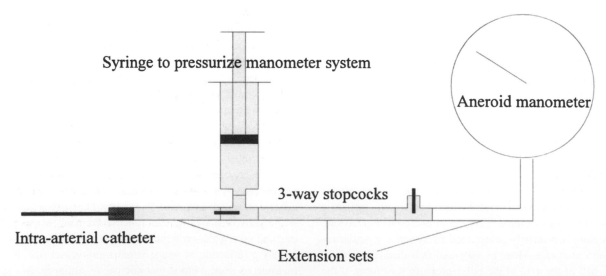

Fig. 19.3. Aneroid manometer system for measuring arterial blood pressure. The intra-arterial catheter is attached to a sterile length of extension tubing (since the system measures only mean pressure, the tubing does not have to be high-pressure, low-compliant tubing); a three-way stopcock; another extension tubing; another stopcock; and a third extension tubing, which is attached to the aneroid manometer. A saline-filled syringe is attached to the first stopcock, which is closed to the patient. Saline is injected into the tubing toward the manometer until the pressure registers at least 150 mm Hg (it needs to be only slightly higher than mean arterial blood pressure). The first stopcock is then closed to the syringe (opened between the pressurized manometer system and the arterial catheter), and the equilibrated pressure equals mean arterial blood pressure. Since blood pressure varies, do not leave the system open between measurements; blood will flow into the catheter and clot. This is an intermittent pressure-measuring device. The second stopcock enables the removal of excess saline from the tubing so that fluid does not get into the aneroid manometer.

Sterile saline is injected into the tubing toward the manometer via a three-way stopcock until the compressed air increases the registered pressure to a level above that of mean blood pressure. The pressurized manometer system is then allowed to equilibrate with the mean blood pressure of the patient. Arterial catheters can also be attached to a commercial transducer and recording system. The extension tubing between the catheter and the transducer should not be excessively long and should be constructed of nonexpansible plastic to avoid damped signals. The transducer should be "zeroed" periodically and calibrated with a mercury manometer to verify accurate blood pressure measurements. The stopcock that is opened to room air for the zeroing process must be at the level of the heart. With modern patient monitors, the transducer can be placed anywhere with reference to the patient (the monitor will compensate internally with an *offset pressure* for any vertical differences between the patient and the transducer). If the relative vertical position between the patient and the transducer changes, the transducer must be rezeroed. With older patient monitors without this offset feature, the transducer and the zeroing stopcock must be placed at the level of the heart.

The fidelity of the reproduction of the pulse-pressure waveform by a fluid-filled measurement system is the result of a rather complex interaction between the frequency response of the measurement system (resonant frequency and damping) and patient factors such as heart rate and systolic vigor. Generally, the intraarterial catheter should be large; the transducer should be placed close to the patient, with high-pressure tubing connecting the catheter to the transducer; and the measuring system should be free of blood clots or air bubbles (Table 19.8). *Underdamping* occurs when the frequency response of the measuring system is identical to one of the harmonics of the pulse-pressure waveform. The recorded waveform will be exaggerated—the systolic pressure will be erroneously high and the diastolic pressure will be erroneously low; pressure oscillations may override the recorded waveform (Fig. 19.4). *Overdamping* occurs also when the frequency response is less than all of the harmonics of the pulse-pressure waveform. The recorded waveform will be blunted—the systolic pressure will be erroneously low and the diastolic pressure will be erroneously high; the dicrotic notch is diminished or absent (Fig. 19.4).

The frequency response of the measurement system can be assessed by the dynamic pressure response test (Fig. 19.5). This involves the sudden release of pressure on the measurement system, such as is done by flushing the catheter with the continuous-flush device. During the flush procedure, the regis-

Table 19.8. Key features of a high-frequency response measuring system.

Large-inside-diameter catheter
Short (as opposed to long) catheter
Large, more central artery (as opposed to a small, peripheral artery)
Short-catheter-transducer connecting tubing
Noncompliant tubing
No loose, leaky connections
As few stopcocks as possible
No kinks in the tubing
Hyperflexed appendages avoided when the catheter is in a peripheral artery
No air bubbles in the measuring system
No blood clots in the catheter or measuring system (use a continuous-flush device)

tered pressure equals that of the pressure bag (>300 mm Hg). When the flushing procedure is abruptly terminated, the pressure should return to baseline after about one to two negative and one to two positive oscillations.[52] Ideally, the measuring system would have a high resonant frequency and low damping. The resonant frequency is calculated as 1 s divided by the length of time of one complete oscillation (peak to peak) (Fig. 19.5). Typical values are 10 to 50 Hz.[52] Damping is calculated as the amplitude reduction ratio: the height of one-half of a complete cycle (peak to trough or vice versa) divided by the height of the previous one-half cycle (Fig. 19.5). Typical values are 0.35 to 0.7.[52] The appropriateness of the frequency response of the measuring system for a particular patient is determined by a combination of the resonant frequency and the damping. Underdamping is caused by the combination of a low resonant frequency and minimal damping. Overdamping is caused by the combination of a low resonant frequency and excessive damping.

If overdamping or underdamping is noted, check for (and remove) blood clots or air bubbles from the measurement system, exchange low-compliant tubes with rigid tubes, shorten the length of tubing between the catheter and transducer, make sure there are no leaks, and eliminate kinks in the tubing or appendage (if a peripheral artery has been catheterized). If the underdamping problem continues, add a damping device (longer tubing, less rigid tubing, and a small air bubble at the transducer).

Normal systolic, diastolic, and mean blood pressures are ap-

Fig. 19.4. Underdamping and overdamping caused by a frequency response of the measuring system that is the same as one of the harmonics of the original pressure waveform or too low, respectively. **a:** Ideal pressure waveform. **b:** Underdamped pressure waveform. **c:** Overdamped pressure waveform.

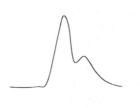

4a. Normal

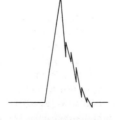

4b. Underdamped

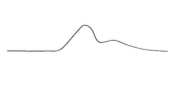

4c. Overdamped

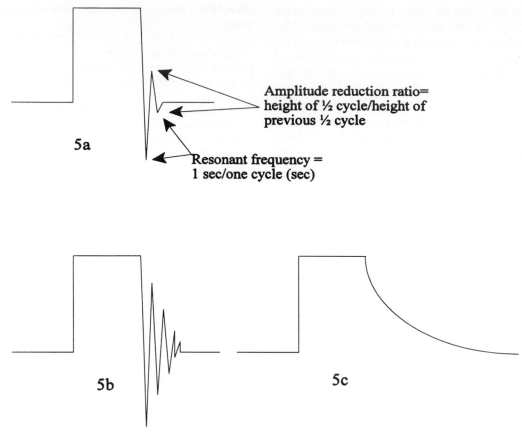

Amplitude reduction ratio=
height of ½ cycle/height of
previous ½ cycle

Resonant frequency =
1 sec/one cycle (sec)

5a

5b

5c

Fig. 19.5. Dynamic pressure response test to determine natural frequency response of a measuring system. The pressure is suddenly released and the fluctuations in pressure recorded. **a:** Optimal: The waveform should oscillate 1 to 1.5 full cycles before returning to baseline. The resonant frequency is calculated as 1 s divided by the duration of one complete cycle (peak to peak or trough to trough). The damping is calculated as the amplitude reduction ratio of the height of one-half cycle (peak to trough or trough to peak) divided by the previous one-half cycle. **b:** Underdamped: The waveform oscillates more than two full cycles. **c:** Overdamped: The waveform oscillates less than 0.5 full cycle.

proximately 100 to 140, 60 to 100, and 80 to 120 mm Hg, respectively. In general, one should be concerned when the systolic arterial blood pressure (ABPs) falls below 100 or when the mean arterial blood pressure (ABPm) falls below 80 mm Hg. In general, one should be very concerned when the ABPs falls below 80 or the ABPm falls below 60 mm Hg. Hypotension may be caused by hypovolemia, poor cardiac output, or vasodilation (Table 19.9). Hypertension (high ABPm) is generally attributed to vasoconstriction. High ABPs, not associated with a high ABPm, is generally attributed to an inappropriate frequency response of the measuring system (for that patient and that time). Hypertension can cause increased hemorrhage, retinal detachment, increased intracranial pressure, and high afterload to the heart, and should be treated when ABPm exceeds 140 mm Hg (Table 19.7). High ABPm may be produced by a light level of anesthesia, hyperthermia, sympathomimetic drugs, hyperthyroidism (thyroxine-catecholamine synergy), renal failure (renin-angiotensin), pheochromocytoma (epinephrine), or increased intracranial pressure. In the latter case, the hypertension is most likely caused by the Cushing's response, to maintain an adequate cerebral perfusion pressure, and should not be treated.

Cardiac Output

Poor cardiac output is implied when preload parameters (CVP, pulmonary artery occlusion pressure, jugular vein distension, postcava distension on chest radiograph, and end-diastolic diameter on cardiac ultrasound image) are high and the afterload parameters (cardiac output, arterial blood pressure, and physical and laboratory measures of tissue perfusion) are low or abnormal. Pulse-quality assessment provides an indirect measure of stroke volume. Cardiac output is a flow parameter and can be low even when arterial blood pressure is normal. Cardiac output in humans is most often measured by thermodilution techniques via the balloon-tipped pulmonary artery catheter. Lithium administration is another indicator-dilution technique that has been used.[53–56] It requires its own detector and computer; cardiac output can be measured only a finite number of times (because of lithium accumulation); the detector probes are fairly expensive; and, of course, pulmonary artery pressure and pulmonary artery occlusion pressure are not measured. Cardiac output can also be measured by esophageal Doppler ultrasonography, thoracic electrical bioimpedance, and pulse analysis.[53,56,57] Cardiac output in normal, awake dogs is 4.42 ± 1.24 L/min/m^2 (165 ± 43

Table 19.9. Causes of hypotension.

Low venous return
Hypovolemia
Preexisting dehydration
Blood loss, plasma exudation, or crystalloid transudation at operative site
Positive-pressure ventilation
Gastric distension
Iatrogenic inflow occlusion
Poor diastolic function
Hypertrophic cardiomyopathy
Pericardial tamponade
Tachycardia
Fibrosis
Poor systolic function (contractility)
Dilative cardiomyopathy
Negative inotropic effect of anesthetic drugs, β_1 blockers, or calcium-channel blockers
Ventricular arrhythmias
Impaired systolic efficiency
Atrioventricular valve insufficiency
Outflow-tract obstruction
Bradycardia
Low systemic vascular resistance
Vasodilating effect of anesthetic or other drugs
Patent ductus arteriosus

Table 19.10. Causes of tachypnea.

Too lightly anesthetized
Too deeply anesthetized
Agonal "gasps"
Hypoxemia
Hypercapnia
Hyperthermia
Hypotension
Sepsis
Atelectasis
Postoperative recovery phase
Postoperative pain
Drug-induced (opioids)
Individual variation

mL/min/kg) and is generally decreased by general anesthetics, except ketamine (Table 19.1). Cardiac output in awake horses is 70 to 90 mL/min/kg and is decreased to 35 to 60 mL/min/kg with general anesthesia.[58–60]

Cardiac output may be reduced by poor venous return and end-diastolic ventricular filling (hypovolemia, positive-pressure ventilation, or inflow occlusion); by ventricular restrictive disease (hypertrophic or restrictive cardiomyopathy, pericardial tamponade, or pericardial fibrosis); by decreased contractility; by excessive bradycardia, tachycardia, or arrhythmias; by regurgitant atrioventricular valves; or by outflow-tract obstruction. Poor cardiac output should be improved by correcting the underlying problem when possible. Preload should be optimized. When poor contractility is thought to be the problem, anesthetic dosage levels should be decreased to the least amount that will enable the completion of the surgical procedure. Sympathomimetic therapy (Table 19.7) is indicated when poor contractility is thought to be the problem, and fluid therapy and anesthetic drug reduction have failed to restore acceptable forward-flow parameters.

Oxygen Delivery

Oxygen delivery (DO_2) is the product of cardiac output and blood oxygen content (Fig. 19.1). Some myocardial depression is expected with general anesthesia, and this could be associated with a decrease in cardiac output and DO_2. In fact, DO_2 may be increased or decreased by anesthetic drugs (Table 19.1). A decrease in DO_2 during general anesthesia may not be a problem if oxygen consumption (VO_2) is also reduced by muscular inactivity

and hypothermia.[61,62] Oxygen consumption, however, like DO_2, is variably affected by anesthetic drugs[61,62] (Table 19.1). Critical DO_2, the DO_2 below which VO_2 decreases linearly, has been reported to be between 160 and 280 mL/min/m² (6 to 11 mL/min/kg) in dogs.[63–66] In critically ill human patients, a minimum oxygen delivery of 550 to 600 mL/min/m² has been recommended.[67,68] From our own experiments ($n = 97$), DO_2 in normal dogs is 790 ± 259 mL/min/m² (29.5 ± 8.8 mL/min/kg). Optimal DO_2 was thought to be associated with a minimum DO_2 of 600 mL/min/kg because, when DO_2 decreased below this level, oxygen extraction, arteriovenous oxygen content gradient and arteriovenous partial pressure of carbon dioxide (PCO_2) gradient increased, and central venous partial pressure of oxygen (PO_2) decreased. Alternatively, when cardiac output measurements are unavailable, oxygen extraction above 30%, arteriovenous oxygen content gradient above 5 mL/dL, arteriovenous PCO_2 gradient above 5 mm Hg, or central venous PO_2 (PvO_2) below 40 mm Hg may indicate a less than optimal DO_2. Most anesthetics (inhalationals, opioids, and barbiturates, but not ketamine) impair oxygen extraction and increase the critical DO_2 compared with baseline.[69]

Pulmonary Monitoring

Breathing Rate, Rhythm, Nature, and Effort

The breathing rate can vary widely, and except for extreme values is of limited value as a respiratory monitor. A change in breathing rate, however, is a sensitive indicator of an underlying change in the status of a patient. Bradypnea may be a sign of deep anesthesia or hypothermia. There are many causes of tachypnea, and it is important not to default to the conclusion that its occurrence represents too light a level of anesthesia (Table 19.10). Arrhythmic breathing patterns are indicative of a problem with the central pattern generator in the medulla. A *Cheyne-Stokes breathing pattern* (cycling between hyperventilation and hypoventilation) may be seen in otherwise healthy anesthetized horses and an apneustic breathing pattern (inspiratory hold) may be seen in otherwise healthy dogs and cats anesthetized with ketamine.

Ventilometry

Ventilation volume can be estimated by visual observation of the chest or rebreathing bag or measured by ventilometry. Normal tidal volume ranges between about 8 and 20 mL/kg. A small tidal volume may be acceptable if the breathing rate is fast enough to accomplish normal alveolar minute ventilation. Normal total minute ventilation ranges between 150 and 250 mL/kg/min for dogs. Dead-space ventilation is about 30% to 40% of tidal volume and minute ventilation in a normal patient breathing a normal tidal volume, but may be much higher with shallow breathing, upper-airway dead space, or pulmonary thromboembolism. Arterial PCO_2 ($PaCO_2$) is usually considered to be the definition of alveolar minute ventilation, and the measured minute ventilation should be appropriate. A large minute ventilation in combination with a normal (or high) $PaCO_2$ is indicative of a large dead-space ventilation.

Compliance is calculated as expired tidal volume divided by the change in pressure that it took to generate the tidal volume. A change in airway pressure is easy to measure during positive-pressure ventilation, but to measure the change in transpulmonary pressure during spontaneous ventilation requires the measurement of pleural pressure (which is usually done via the lower esophagus). If, for instance, 10 cm H_2O of pressure was required in order to generate a tidal volume of 10 mL/kg, the compliance would be calculated to be 1 mL/kg/cm H_2O. If the measurements are made during the cyclic breathing process, the value is termed *dynamic compliance*. If the measurements are made after an inspiratory pause, the value is termed *static compliance*. The manner in which these measurements would usually be obtained during general anesthesia would include a component of anesthetic-circuit gas compression and breathing-circuit expansion. Since anesthetic circuits and technique vary, you will need to establish expected values by using your particular equipment and technique. Compliance is decreased by restrictive pulmonary, pleural, or thoracic wall disease.

Partial Pressure of Carbon Dioxide

The $PaCO_2$ is a measure of the ventilatory status of a patient and normally ranges between 35 and 45 mm Hg. $PaCO_2$ values may be slightly higher in anesthetized small animals and is considerably higher (60 to 80 mm Hg) in anesthetized horses[49] (Table 19.2) and cattle.[18] A $PaCO_2$ in excess of 60 mm Hg may be associated with excessive respiratory acidosis and is usually considered to represent sufficient hypoventilation to warrant positive-pressure ventilation in small animals. $PaCO_2$ values below 20 mm Hg are associated with respiratory alkalosis and a decreased cerebral blood flow that may impair cerebral oxygenation.

Venous PCO_2 ($PvCO_2$) is usually 3 to 6 mm Hg higher than $PaCO_2$ in stable states and can generally be used as an approximation of $PaCO_2$. The venous partial pressure of carbon dioxide is variably higher in transition states and during hypovolemia or anemia. $PaCO_2$ may also be estimated by measuring the carbon dioxide in a sample of gas taken at the end of an exhalation (Fig. 19.6). End-tidal PCO_2 is usually 2 to 4 mm Hg lower than $PaCO_2$ in dogs and 10 to 15 mm Hg lower in horses.[70] Capnography en-

Table 19.11. Information derived from the capnogram[71-73].

Observed Problem	Possible Cause(s)
No waveform	Apnea; obstructed aspirating tubing
Increased baseline	Rebreathing malfunction or contaminated sample cell
Increased plateau	Hypoventilation or increased rate of carbon dioxide production
Decreased plateau To a new, stable level	Hyperventilation, hypothermia, airway leaks, tachypnea, pulmonary thromboembolism, or capnograph calibration error
Abruptly to zero	Airway obstruction, airway disconnect, apnea, or cardiac arrest
Flattened upsweep (line A in Fig. 19.6)	Small airway narrowing and increase in disparity of alveolar time constants
Flattened downsweep (line C in Fig. 19.6)	Rebreathing
Unstable, fluctuating plateau	Spontaneous breathing during mechanical ventilation

ables anesthetists to evaluate adequacy of ventilation, and many other problems, as well (Table 19.11).[71-73]

An increased arteriovenous PCO_2 gradient suggests decreased tissue perfusion. A note of caution: Do not contaminate the blood sample with sodium bicarbonate, because that will increase PCO_2 dramatically. The causes of hypercapnia and hypocapnia are listed in Table 19.12.

Partial Pressure of Oxygen

The PaO_2 measures the tension of oxygen dissolved in the plasma, irrespective of the hemoglobin concentration. The PaO_2 is a measure of the oxygenating efficiency of the lungs. The normal PaO_2 is considered to range between 80 and 110 mm Hg when an animal is breathing room air at sea level. When room air is being breathed, the PaO_2 would normally decrease during general anesthesia, because of anesthetic-induced hypoventilation, increased ventilation-perfusion mismatching, and atelectasis. Usually, however, anesthetized animals are attached to an anesthetic machine and breath 100% oxygen. The PaO_2 is usually above 500 mm Hg in small animals and above 200 mm Hg in horses.[49,58,60] Hypoxemia is usually defined as a PaO_2 below 80 mm Hg. Hypoxemia could be caused by low inspired oxygen, hypoventilation while breathing 21% oxygen, and venous admixture (Table 19.13). A PaO_2 below 60 mm Hg is a commonly selected trigger for symptomatic therapy.

PvO_2 reflects tissue PO_2 and bears no correlation to PaO_2. Mixed or central PvO_2 ranges between 40 and 50 mm Hg. Values below 30 mm Hg may be caused by anything that decreases the delivery of oxygen to the tissues (hypoxemia, anemia, low cardiac output, or vasoconstriction) (Fig. 19.1); values above 60 mm Hg suggest reduced tissue uptake of oxygen (shunting, septic shock, or metabolic poisons). Venous blood for such evaluations must be taken from a central vein such as the jugular, anterior

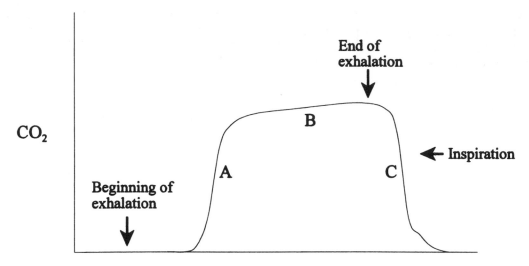

Fig. 19.6. Capnogram. The end-tidal carbon dioxide (CO_2) at the end of exhalation should be only a few mm Hg below arterial CO_2 partial pressure. *Line A* reflects the transition between CO_2-free anatomical and alveolar dead-space gases and functional alveolar gases. The slope of line A reflects variable emptying of fast and slow alveoli (airway disease flattens the slope of line A). *Line B*, the plateau of the capnogram, reflects alveolar gas; the slight upward slope to line B represents an increasing alveolar CO_2 during exhalation. *Line C* represents inspiration; the slope of line C is less steep with rebreathing.

Table 19.12. Causes of hypercapnia and hypocapnia.

Hypercapnia	Hypocapnia
Hypoventilation	Hyperventilation
Neuromuscular: excessive anesthetic depth; intracranial, cervical, neuromuscular	Light level of anesthesia
	Hypoxemia
	Hyperthermia
Airway obstruction: endotracheal tube; large or small airways	Hypotension
	Sepsis
Thoracic or abdominal restrictive disease	Postoperative recovery phase
Pleural space–filling disorder: air, fluid, or abdominal viscera	Postoperative pain
Pulmonary parenchymal disease	Inappropriate ventilator settings
Inappropriate ventilator settings	
Malfunctioning/exhausted soda lime	
Malfunctioning anesthetic machine: dead-space rebreathing	

Table 19.13. Causes of hypoxemia.

Low inspired oxygen
Depleted oxygen supply
Maladjusted flowmeter
Insufficient flow in a Bain's circuit
Anesthetic machine malfunction: dead-space rebreathing
Hypoventilation (when breathing room air)
Venous admixture
Low ventilation/perfusion regions: mild to moderate pulmonary parenchymal disease
Small airway and alveolar collapse (no ventilation but perfused regions): moderated to severe pulmonary parenchymal disease
Diffusion impairment: inhalation injury, oxygen toxicity, or inflammatory lung disease
Anatomic right-to-left shunts

vena cava, or pulmonary artery; peripheral PvO_2 values are highly variable and difficult to interpret.

Blood gases are measured at the temperature of the blood-gas analyzer water bath (usually 37°C). Ideally, the animal's body temperature would be identical to that of the water bath, but this seldom occurs. When the animal's body temperature differs from that of the water bath, there will be changes in the measured pH and blood gases associated with the in vitro change in temperature. There is some debate about whether to correct for these temperature changes. If one wants to know what is actually happening in a patient and wants to compare the current measurement with previous measurements, even though there has been a sub-

stantial change in body temperature, the temperature-corrected values should be used. If a clinician is contemplating therapy to "fix" an abnormality by using normothermic reference points, then the uncorrected values should be used.[74] "Normal values" for hypothermic or hyperthermic patients are different than those for normothermic patients, but these reference values have not been established for each level of hypothermia or hyperthermia that occurs.

Hemoglobin Saturation with Oxygen

When red to infrared light is transmitted through a blood sample, a certain proportion of it will be absorbed by the various hemoglobins present in the blood sample: oxyhemoglobin, methemoglobin, carboxyhemoglobin, and reduced hemoglobin. A bench-

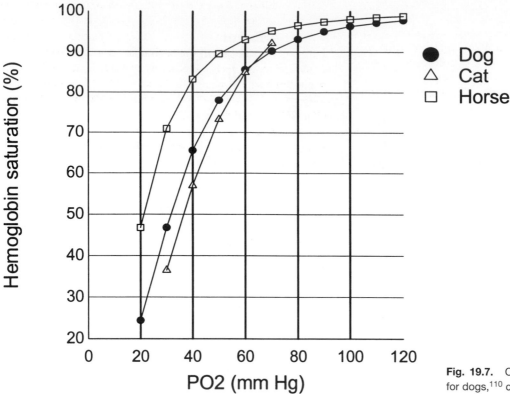

Fig. 19.7. Oxyhemoglobin dissociation curves for dogs,[110] cats,[111] and horses.[112]

top co-oximeter measures and displays values for the first three. The displayed oxyhemoglobin is functional; that is, it is expressed as a percentage of the amount of hemoglobin available for oxygen binding (total hemoglobin minus methemoglobin and carboxyhemoglobin) as opposed to fractional oxyhemoglobin, which is expressed as a percentage of total hemoglobin irrespective of methemoglobin or carboxyhemoglobin. Normal methemoglobin and carboxyhemoglobin levels are normally less than 1% each, and so, usually, functional and fractional oxyhemoglobin levels are quite similar. To the extent that either methemoglobin or carboxyhemoglobin are present in large concentrations, fractional oxyhemoglobin levels will be variably lower than functional oxyhemoglobin levels.

Hemoglobin-oxygen saturation (SO_2) measures the percent oxygen saturation of the hemoglobin and is related to PO_2 by a sigmoid curve. The clinical information derived from the measurement of arterial SO_2 (SaO_2) is similar to that obtained from a PaO_2 measurement in that they both are a measure of the ability of the lung to deliver oxygen to the blood. In this matter, functional oxyhemoglobin is the more meaningful number. The "numbers of concern" are, however, different. In general, a PO_2 of 100 mm Hg is equivalent to an SO_2 of 98%; a PO_2 of 80 mm Hg to an SO_2 of 95%; a PO_2 of 60 mm Hg to an SO_2 of 90%; and a PO_2 of 40 mm Hg to an SO_2 of 75%. Exact quantitative correlation depends on the hemoglobin affinity for oxygen. The P_{50} is the PO_2 at which the hemoglobin is 50% saturated and is commonly used to define hemoglobin affinity. The P_{50} for human hemoglobin is 26 to 28 mm Hg; it is slightly higher for dogs and goats; much higher for sheep, cats, and cattle; and lower for

horses. Figure 19.7 and Table 19.14 illustrate representative oxyhemoglobin dissociation curves for horses, dogs, and cats.

Pulse oximeters attach to a patient externally (e.g., tongue, lips, tail, or toenail). For most clinical purposes, most pulse-oximeter readings are sufficiently accurate approximations of oxyhemoglobin saturation, though accuracy should be verified by an in vitro standard if possible. There are substantial bias and precision variations and response times between different commercial products at different levels of saturation.[75] Tissue, venous and capillary blood, nonpulsatile arterial blood, and skin pigment also absorb infrared light. There is a fairly narrow spectrum of wavelengths that passes through skin and yet is absorbed by hemoglobin. A pulse oximeter must differentiate this background absorption from that of pulsatile arterial blood. It does this by measuring light absorbance during a pulse and subtracting from that the light absorbance occurring between the pulses. If the pulse oximeter cannot detect a pulse, it will not measure the oxyhemoglobin level.

The accuracy of a pulse oximeter is greatest within the range of 80% and 95%, and is determined by the accuracy of the empirical formula that is programmed into the instrument.[76] Differences in tissue absorption or scatter of light, different thicknesses of tissue, smaller pulsatile flow patterns and small signal-to-noise ratios, and incompletely compensated light-emitting diodes may account for some inaccuracies. Inaccuracies may also generate from baseline-read errors (motion), differences in sensor location, and electrical or optical interference. When a measurement is obtained, it may either be accurate or inaccurate. When inaccurate, it is usually inaccurately low. When a

Table 19.14. Oxyhemoglobin dissociation curve for dogs[110] and horses[112].

PO2	Dogs	Horses	PO2	Dogs	Horses
20	24.4	46.8	72	91.0	95.6
22	28.7	52.9	74	91.7	95.9
24	33.2	58.4	76	92.2	96.1
26	37.8	63.2	78	92.8	96.4
28	42.3	67.4	80	93.2	96.6
30	46.8	71.0	82	93.7	96.8
32	51.0	74.2	84	94.1	97.0
34	55.0	77.0	86	94.5	97.2
36	58.8	79.4	88	94.8	97.3
38	62.3	81.5	90	95.1	97.5
40	65.6	83.3	92	95.4	97.6
42	68.5	84.9	94	95.7	97.8
44	71.3	86.3	96	95.9	97.9
46	73.7	87.6	98	96.2	98.0
48	76.0	88.7	100	96.4	98.1
50	78.0	89.6	102	96.6	98.2
52	79.9	90.5	104	96.8	98.3
54	81.6	91.3	106	96.9	98.4
56	83.1	92.0	108	97.1	98.5
58	84.4	92.6	110	97.2	98.6
60	85.7	93.1	115	97.6	98.7
62	86.8	93.7	120	97.9	98.9
64	87.8	94.1	130	98.3	99.1
66	88.7	94.5	150	98.9	99.5
68	89.6	94.9	200	99.5	99.9
70	90.3	95.3	300	99.9	100.0

PO2, partial pressure of oxygen.

low measurement is obtained, particularly when it seems incongruous for the patient's condition at the time, it might be wise to retry the measurement in several different locations and then either take the average or the highest reading. If methemoglobin or carboxyhemoglobin were present in high concentrations, they would absorb light and would impact the measurement made by a two-wavelength pulse oximeter designed to measure only oxyhemoglobin. Because of the biphasic absorption of methemoglobin at both the 660- and 940-nm wavelengths, abnormal accumulations tend to push the oximeter reading toward 85% (underestimating measurements when SaO_2 is above 85%, and overestimating it when SaO_2 is below 85%).[77] Carboxyhemoglobin absorbs light like oxyhemoglobin at 660 nm, but hardly at all at 940 nm, and this would increase the apparent oxyhemoglobin measurement.[78] Fetal hemoglobin produces very little effect on measured hemoglobin saturation.[76] Indocyanine green dye and methylene blue dye absorb light and will generate falsely low saturation measurements.[76]

A pulse oximeter is an ideal perioperative monitor in that it is an automatic, continuous, audible monitor of mechanical cardiopulmonary function. It specifically measures pulse rate and hemoglobin saturation, and it requires a reasonable peripheral pulse quality in order to achieve a measurement. One of the common reasons for poor instrument performance is peripheral vasoconstriction. Its value as an ongoing monitor in detecting hypoxemia has been established.[75,76] The pulse oximeter is not discriminating for high PaO_2 values where the oxyhemoglobin curve is flat. The difference between a PaO_2 of 500 and 100 mm Hg in an animal breathing 100% oxygen is very important as an index of lung function; the corresponding decrease in SaO_2, from 99% to 98%, would hardly be noticed.

Venous Admixture

Pulmonary dysfunction interferes with the ability of the lungs to transfer oxygen efficiently from the alveoli to the blood, resulting in a lower-than-expected PaO_2. *Venous admixture* is the collective term for all of the ways in which blood can pass from the right side of the circulation to the left side of the circulation without being properly oxygenated (Table 19.13). Several methods are used to quantitate lung-oxygenating efficiency (Table 19.15).

Oxygen Content

This parameter can be measured, but is usually calculated: (hemoglobin concentration × 1.34 [oxygen content of fully saturated hemoglobin] × percent saturation) + (0.003 × PO_2).

Table 19.15. Formulas for quantifying lung-oxygenating efficiency (venous admixture).

Parameter	Formula
Alveolar PO_2 (P_AO_2)	([Barometric pressure − 50] × fractional inspired oxygen) − ($PaCO_2$ × 1.1), where 50 = saturated water-vapor pressure at 38.5°C, and 1.1 = 1/RQ when RQ = 0.9
Alveolar-arterial PO_2 gradient (for any F_IO_2)	Calculated P_AO_2 × measured PaO_2
PaO_2 + $PaCO_2$ (for F_IO_2 = 0.21 at sea level)	Measured PaO_2 + measured $PaCO_2$
PaO_2/F_IO_2 (PF) ratio (for $F_IO_2 > 0.4$)	PaO_2/F_IO_2, where F_IO_2 is expressed as a decimal fraction between 0.21 and 1.0
Arterial, mixed-venous, and pulmonary capillary oxygen content	(1.34 × Hb × SO_2) + (0.003 × PO_2), where 1.34 is 100% saturated hemoglobin (Hb) oxygen content, SO_2 is hemoglobin saturation, and PO_2 is partial pressure of oxygen in arterial, mixed-venous, or capillary blood
Venous admixture (for any F_IO_2)	(Capillary O_2 content × arterial O_2 content)/(capillary O_2 content × venous O_2 content)

F_IO_2, fraction of inspired oxygen; $PaCO_2$, arterial carbon dioxide partial pressure; PaO_2, arterial oxygen partial pressure; PO_2, partial pressure of oxygen; RQ, respiratory quotient.

Table 19.16. The relationship between partial pressure of oxygen (PO_2), hemoglobin saturation (SO_2), and oxygen content under different clinical circumstances.

	PO_2 (mm Hg)	SO_2 (%)	Hb (g/dL)	O_2 content (mL/dL)
Normal	100	96.4	15	19.7
Anemia	100	96.4	5	6.8
Methemoglobinemia (50%)	100	96.4	15	10.0
Hypoxemia	40	65.6	15	13.3
Hyperoxemia	500	100	15	21.6

The canine oxyhemoglobin relationship was used for determining SO_2. Hb, hemoglobin concentration. Oxygen content was calculated as $(1.34 \times Hb \times SO_2) + (0.003 \times PO_2)$.

Hemoglobin is by far the most important contributor to oxygen content. The PO_2, SO_2, and oxygen content are related, but each measure provides a distinctly different perspective of blood oxygenation, and the difference can be important (Table 19.16). An increased arteriovenous oxygen-content difference (>5 g/dL) suggests increased oxygen extraction, which is usually attributable to decreased oxygen delivery.

Renal Monitoring

Urine flow is used as an indirect measure of renal blood flow, and renal blood flow is used as an indirect measure of visceral blood flow. Urine output can be assessed by serial palpation of the urinary bladder or by actual measurement after the aseptic placement of a urinary catheter. Normal urine output should be about 1 to 2 mL/kg/h. Maintaining visceral blood flow is, of course, an important aspect of any anesthetic plan and is generally achieved by optimizing the circulating blood volume (sufficient, but not excessive, fluid therapy), monitoring and maintaining forward-flow cardiovascular parameters, and monitoring of laboratory indices of tissue perfusion (standard base excess, lactate concentration, and central PvO_2). Oliguria or anuria, per se, can be treated, after ensuring that renal perfusion is adequate, with furosemide (0.5- to 5-mg/kg bolus ± 0.1 to 0.5 mg/kg/h) or mannitol (0.5-g/kg bolus ± 0.1 g/kg/h). Statistically, diuretic therapy does not prevent acute renal failure, but it does facilitate the medical management of the case.

Temperature Monitoring

Hypothermia

Hypothermia during anesthesia may be associated with anesthetic drug depression of muscular activity, metabolism, and hypothalamic thermostatic mechanisms. Heat loss may be augmented by evaporation of surgical scrub solutions from the skin surface, by the infusion of room-temperature fluids, by contact with cold, noninsulated surfaces, and by evaporation of surface fluid from an exposed body cavity. Core temperature can be measured with either esophageal or rectal thermistors attached to a continuously displayed thermometer.

Core body temperatures down to 36°C (96°F) are not detrimental to patients.[79,80] Nonshivering thermogenesis will increase, and there may be some shivering thermogenesis during recovery. Recovery should not be prolonged in any noticeable way. Body temperatures of 32° to 34°C (90° to 94°F) are associated with reduced anesthetic requirements; recovery should be noticeably prolonged. Animals will shiver if they can, but some will not shiver and will have to be artificially rewarmed. Body temperatures of 28° to 30°C (82° to 86°F) have a marked CNS-depressant effect, and usually no anesthetic agent is required. Shivering thermogenesis will not occur, and the animal will have to be rewarmed artificially, at least initially. Atrial arrhythmias may occur. Oxygen consumption is reduced to about 50% of normal, heart rate and cardiac output to about 35% to 40% of normal, and arterial blood pressure to about 60% of normal.[79] Cerebral metabolism is about 25% of normal. These decreases in hemodynamic parameters are secondary to cold-induced hypometabolism. Measurements must be interpreted in this context rather than in comparison with normothermic values. Body temperatures of 25° to 26°C (77° to 80°F) are associated with prolongation of the PR interval and widened QRS complexes, increased myocardial automaticity, and decreased tissue oxygen delivery out of proportion to decreases in oxygen requirement, resulting in anaerobic metabolism, lactic acidosis, and rewarming acidemia. Blood viscosity is about 200% of normal. Body temperatures of 22° to 23°C (72° to 74°F) are usually associated with ventricular fibrillation and death.

Intraoperative hypothermia is usually mild to moderate and, as long as appropriate safeguards are exercised, is seldom detrimental to patients. The largest problem with intraoperative hypothermia is the nonrecognition of it. The continued administration of normothermic amounts of anesthetic to a hypothermic patient can produce a relative anesthetic overdose.

Passive rewarming (minimizing further heat loss and enabling patients to warm themselves metabolically) is usually effective in treating mild hypothermia (temperature above 34°C [94°F]) when a patient is capable of metabolic or shivering thermogenesis. Intraoperative heat loss can be minimized by warm room temperatures, insulating barriers between the patient and table surfaces, and administering warmed fluids. Active rewarming can be achieved by using circulating warm water or warm-air blankets, infrared heat lamps (optimal distance, 75 cm[81]) or radiant-heat warmers; by placing hot-water bottles under the drapes (avoid contact with skin if the water temperature exceeds 42°C); by flushing the abdominal cavity or colon with warm, sterile, isotonic, polyionic fluids; or by extracorporeal techniques.

Aggressive surface rewarming should be avoided in very cold patients[82–84] because peripheral vasodilation may induce excessive hypotension in the face of a cold-depressed heart. Ischemic peripheral tissues may have accumulated various metabolites, which may have deleterious cardiovascular effects when large quantities are washed into the central circulation. The rewarming rate should be limited to about 1°C/h.[80]

Hyperthermia

Fever is a reset thermostat and is caused by the release of endogenous pyrogens (interleukin 1) from monocytes[85] in response to infections, tissue damage, or antigen-antibody reactions. Interleukin 1 stimulates prostaglandin synthesis in the hypothalamic thermoregulatory center. Hyperthermia, without a reset thermostat, is pathological. It not uncommonly occurs in large dogs that are cocooned within many layers of drapes on an operating table. Hyperthermia may be potentiated by surface vasoconstriction, light levels of anesthesia, and ketamine administration.

Mild degrees of hyperthermia are not, per se, harmful to patients and may represent an appropriate response to an underlying disease (fever or infection). Mild hyperthermia (below 40°C [104°F]) does not normally require treatment, per se. Cell damage starts at body temperatures above 42°C (108°F), when oxygen delivery can no longer keep pace with the racing metabolic activity and increased oxygen consumption. Severe hyperthermia causes multiple organ dysfunction and failure: renal, hepatic, and gastrointestinal failure; myocardial and skeletal muscle damage; cerebral edema; disseminated intravascular coagulation; hypoxemia; metabolic acidosis; and hyperkalemia.[86]

Malignant hyperthermia—a rapidly, relentlessly, progressive increase in body temperature—is associated with the metabolic heat production of disturbed intracellular calcium recycling at the sarcoplasmic reticulum.[87,88] Muscle hypertonicity may or may not occur, depending on the calcium concentration in the sarcoplasm. The defect has been identified in families of people and pigs, and a malignant hyperthermia-like syndrome has been reported in dogs,[89,90] cats,[91,92] and horses.[93,94] Aggressive cooling of the animal, by any and all means possible, is indicated. Dantrolene administration (2.5 to 10.0 mg/kg intravenously) is the specific and often effective treatment for this syndrome.

Surface-cooling techniques are most effective with room-temperature fluids. The evaporation of the water from the skin surface causes the cooling. Ice water causes vasoconstriction that impedes heat loss from the core until skin temperature is below 10°C, at which time vessel paralysis and vasodilation occur, and core temperatures decrease precipitously.[95] Convective heat loss can be enhanced with fans. Conductive heat loss can be enhanced with ice packs. The administration of large volumes of cold crystalloid fluids intravenously into the colon or stomach or into a body cavity is an effective internal cooling technique. The administration of antipyretic drugs (antiprostaglandins, dipyrone, or aminopyrine) is generally an effective treatment for fever, but is ineffective for pathological hyperthermia.

Laboratory Monitoring

Hemoglobin

Whether or not animals are anemic prior to the operative procedure, hemoglobin concentrations will be decreased intraoperatively by anesthetic-induced vasodilation and splenic dilation, non-hemoglobin-containing fluid administration, and blood loss. Historically, in humans, the trigger for a hemoglobin transfusion has been a hemoglobin concentration of 10 g/dL (a packed cell volume [PCV] of 30%).[96] Recent studies in humans have suggested that a more relaxed trigger of 7 g/dL (PCV = 21%) is associated with at least as good, and perhaps better, morbidity and mortality statistics.[96] In veterinary medicine, in animals with immune-mediated hemolytic anemia, it is well accepted to withhold blood transfusions until the hemoglobin concentration is below 5 g/dL (PCV = 15%). In human medicine, in Jehovah Witness patients, mortality rate does not increase significantly until the hemoglobin concentration is 5 g/dL (PCV = 15%).[96] There are many examples of human and veterinary patients surviving much greater levels of anemia.

It may not actually be possible to define a minimum hemoglobin concentration, given the complexities of cardiac output and oxygen-extraction compensatory mechanisms. An animal can tolerate greater degrees of anemia if it has the wherewithal to increase cardiac output. If cardiac output were routinely measured, DO_2 could be calculated, which would eliminate some of the guesswork, but cardiac output is seldom measured. Anesthetic agents commonly decrease myocardial contractility and cardiac output (Tables 19.1 and 19.2), and oxygen extraction is often impaired during general anesthesia,[69] so it would be predicted that anesthetized patients require a hemoglobin concentration higher than the bare minimum. Metabolic markers of poor tissue oxygenation, such as a low PvO_2, a high arteriovenous oxygen-content gradient, or a high arteriovenous PCO_2 gradient, may help guide the need for hemoglobin transfusions. Lactic acidosis is a late, after-the-fact (but usually before-the-death) index of inadequate tissue perfusion.

Blood may need to be administered in volumes of 10 to 30 mL/kg, depending on the magnitude of anemia. Cats have a small blood volume (50 to 55 mL/kg) compared with most other species, and bolus dosages of all fluids should be approximately 50% of canine recommendations. The amount of blood to administer can also be calculated: (desired PCV − current PCV) × body weight (kg) × 2 mL whole blood (or 1 mL packed red blood cells).

Oncotic Pressure

Plasma oncotic pressure is an important vascular fluid–retention force. When depleted, there is an increased risk of interstitial edema, but, because of an offsetting decrease in perimicrovascular oncotic pressure, it is not as edemagenic as might be expected. An increased capillary hydrostatic pressure or vascular permeability are, in contrast, potent causes of edema. Colloidal osmotic pressure (COP) can be measured: Values in normal animals are 20 to 25 mm Hg. Values of 15 to 20 mm Hg are common in anesthetized and critically ill patients, but are not thought to be of important concern. Values in the low teens should trigger therapy, and values in the single digits should cause great concern. COP can be qualitatively approximated from an albumin measurement (albumin normally accounts for about 70% of the COP). Albumin values in normal dogs, cats, and horses are 2.9 to 4.2, 1.9 to 3.9, and 2.3 to 3.6, respectively. A 50% decrease in albumin is associated with about a 50% reduction in COP and so on. COP can also be approximated by calculation from albumin and globulin measurements:[97] dogs, −7.748 + (5.201 × albumin) + (4.857 × globulin); cats, −4.857 + (5.903 × albumin) +

$(3.378 \times$ globulin); and horses, $-4.3845 + (5.501 \times$ albumin) + $(2.475 \times$ globulin).

The cheapest way to augment COP is to administer an artificial colloid such as dextran 70 or hetastarch in bolus dosages (if volume augmentation is also desirable) of 10 to 30 mL/kg or in continuous infusions of 1 to 2 mL/kg/h. Plasma may be indicated if there are concurrent coagulation issues, and whole blood may be indicated if there are concurrent hemoglobin issues.

Bear in mind a note of caution regarding patients with portocaval shunts, which are often presented with single-digit colloid osmotic pressures. Aggressive colloid administration to "get the COP out of the basement" should be avoided because it upsets the COP–capillary hydrostatic pressure balance and causes edema.

Coagulation

Animals bleed perioperatively either because of a cut large vessel or coagulopathy. The latter can be caused by coagulation or platelet problems. Coagulation is assessed by in vitro tests such as partial thromboplastin time (PTT; normal values are laboratory dependent: 9 to 18 s), activated clotting time (ACT; <120 s at 37°C), and whole blood clotting time (<4 min at 37°C; 8 min at room temperature). The PIVKA test assesses for proteins induced by vitamin K antagonists (normal, 15 to 18 s). Elevated fibrin degradation products represent activation of the clotting and fibrinolytic cascades, and an elevated d-dimer level represents fibrinolysis. The results of these tests are usually normal to slightly abnormal in normal animals.[98–100] Decreased antithrombin (normal: dogs, 80% to 140%; and horses, 130% to 220%[100]) may be indicative of a protein-losing "-opathy" and a prothrombotic state or may represent consumption and disseminated intravascular coagulation (DIC). Platelet numbers can be assessed with a platelet count or a platelet screen on a blood smear (normal, 12 to 25 platelets per oil-emersion field, in a good blood smear without platelet clumping; the platelet count is estimated as $15,000 \times$ the number of platelets per oil-emersion field). Platelet function can be assessed by examining for petechia or a buccal mucosal bleeding time (normal, <4 min). Thromboelastography, which provides an integrated assessment of clot formation, can be used to assess for hyper- or hypocoagulopathy.[101,102]

Coagulopathies may or may not need to be treated. If bleeding is minor and not into a vital organ, and blood can easily be replaced by transfusion, specific therapy may not be necessary. Specific treatment with fresh plasma is necessary if platelets are required; fresh-frozen plasma is used if platelets are not required, but labile factors such as von Willebrand's factor, factor 8, or antithrombin are required. For vitamin K antagonist poisoning, any kind of plasma will suffice. The goal of plasma therapy is to stop the bleeding, not to return the abnormal laboratory test to normal. The latter would be very expensive and would probably not even be possible because of concerns about hypervolemia.

Glucose

An adequate level of blood glucose is important for cerebral metabolism. Hypoglycemia might occur during general anesthesia, but is most common as a nonspecific hormonal response to the stress of anesthesia and operation. A blood glucose concentration below 60 mg/dL should be treated with a 2.5% to 5.0% glucose infusion. Severe hypoglycemia should be treated, in addition, with a bolus of glucose (0.1 to 0.25 g/kg). There is growing evidence that persistent moderate hyperglycemia (>200 mg/dL; >11 mM/L) in the intensive care setting is associated with significantly poorer outcomes.[103–105] In this setting, it has been recommended to enforce glycemic control with insulin in quantities sufficient to maintain the blood glucose concentration below 150 to 200 mg/dL (8 to 11 mM/L).[104,105] Whether short-term hyperglycemia, as would occur with a typical anesthetic-surgical experience, is detrimental has not been investigated.

Metabolic Acid-Base Status

Metabolic and lactic acidosis result from inadequate tissue oxygenation. The marker for metabolic acidosis is a decreased bicarbonate concentration (normal: 20 to 24 mEq/L in dogs, 18 to 22 mEq/L in cats, and 24 to 28 mEq/L in horses), a decrease in total carbon dioxide concentration (a value 1 to 2 mEq/L higher than bicarbonate), or an increase in the base deficit (normal: 0 to -4 mEq/L in dogs, -3 to -7 in cats, and 4 to 0 in horses). Lactate is the marker for lactic acidosis (normal, <2 mM/L), which is usually presumed to represent inadequate tissue oxygenation.[106,107] However, the lactate level can also be elevated as a result of catecholamine-stimulated Na-K-ATPase activity.[108] A word of caution: Do not contaminate the blood sample with lactated Ringer's solution because that will cause a proportionate increase in the measured lactate concentration.

Mild to moderate metabolic acidosis does not need to be treated specifically; correction of the underlying problem should suffice. Severe metabolic acidosis (pH < 7.20) may benefit from therapy with sodium bicarbonate: desired base deficit $-$ measured base deficit $\times$ body weight (kg) $\times$ 0.3. These dosages of bicarbonate should be administered over a period of at least 20 min, and preferably longer.

Sodium

Sodium concentration is important to transcellular fluid flux, and it is important in fluid therapy not to change it too much, too rapidly. Abrupt changes of sodium concentrations of more than about 15 to 17 mEq/L (in either direction) should be avoided because they may be associated with untoward transcellular water shifts and irreversible brain damage.[109] Baseline sodium concentrations below 130 or above 165 mEq/L in dogs must especially be changed slowly (1 mEq/L/h when treating hypernatremia and 0.5 mEq/h when treating hyponatremia). Decreasing the sodium concentration too fast causes immediate intracellular edema (within hours), whereas increasing it too fast causes hemorrhage and central myelinolysis in 3 to 5 days.

Potassium

Hypokalemia is by far the most common electrolyte problem in critically ill animals, but hyperkalemia can also occur. Both are usually preexisting problems. Severe hypokalemia causes hyperpolarization of electrically excitable cells and, eventually, paralysis. Hypokalemia is potentiated by sodium bicarbonate therapy, respiratory alkalosis, and β_2-agonist therapy. Severe hypokalemia should be treated with a potassium infusion (up to 0.5 mEq/kg/h). Severe hyperkalemia causes hypopolarization of electrically excitable cells and myocardial arrhythmias and fibrillation, decreased conduction and contractility, and asystole. Severe hyperkalemia can be treated with either calcium gluconate (0.5 mL of 10% solution per kilogram) or 0.1 to 0.25 units of regular insulin per kilogram, followed by the infusion of 0.5 to 1.5 g/kg of glucose over the next 2 h.

Calcium

Hypocalcemia (ionized) could be a preexisting problem or could result from the administration of citrated blood products. Hypocalcemia can be potentiated by sodium bicarbonate therapy and, for unknown reasons, is commonly observed with hypothermia. Hypocalcemia can decrease myocardial contractility and cause vasodilation. There is no broad agreement as to when hypocalcemia should be treated, but, as a general guideline, ionized concentrations below 0.75 mM/L should perhaps be treated. Calcium gluconate can be administered as a bolus (0.5 mL of the 10% solution [9.3 mg/mL or 0.47 mEq/mL] per kilogram) or as an infusion of 0.5 to 1.5 mL of the 10% solution/kg/h.

Magnesium

Hypomagnesemia is usually a preexisting problem associated with malnutrition or refeeding, diuretic therapy, or diabetic ketoacidosis. It can also result from the administration of citrated blood products. Hypomagnesemia is generally associated with widespread cellular dysfunction manifested by neuromuscular excitability (muscle twitching, fasciculations, and tetany) and eventually paralysis. Hypomagnesemia may also be associated with ventricular arrhythmias and refractory hypokalemia, hypophosphatemia, hyponatremia, and hypocalcemia.

Hypomagnesemia should be treated if the ionized portion is less than 0.2 mM/L (0.45 mg/dL). A dose of magnesium sulfate (0.1 to 0.2 mEq/kg) can be administered slowly intravenously. Magnesium sulfate can then be administered at a daily dosage of 0.25 to 1.0 mEq/kg/day (3 to 12 mg/kg/day) as a continuous-rate infusion.

References

1. Vacanti CJ, VanHouten RJ, Hill RC. A statistical analysis of the relationship of physical status to postoperative morbidity in 68,388 cases. Anesth Analg 40:564–566, 1970.
2. Goldstein A, Keats AS. The risk of anesthesia. Anesthesiology 33:130–143, 1970.
3. Marx GF, Mateo CV, Orkin LR. Computer analysis of postanesthetic deaths. Anesthesiology 39:54–58, 1973.
4. Bodlander FMS. Deaths associated with anaesthesia. Br J Anaesth 47:36–40, 1975.
5. Arbous MS, Grobbee DE, van Kleef JW, et al. Mortality associated with anaesthesia: Quantitative analysis to identify risk factors. Anaesthesia 56:1141–1155, 2001.
6. Mi WD, Sakai T, Singh H, Kudo T, Kudo M, Matsuki A. Hypnotic endpoints vs the bispectral index, 95% spectral edge frequency and median frequency during propofol infusion with or without fentanyl. Eur J Anaesthesiol 16:47–54, 1999.
7. Chopra V, Bovill JG, Spierdijk J. Accidents, near accidents and complications during anaesthesia. Anaesthesia 45:3–6, 1990.
8. Dyson DH, Maxie MG, Schnurr D. Morbidity and mortality associated with anesthetic management in small animal veterinary practice in Ontario. J Am Anim Hosp Assoc 34:325–335, 1998.
9. Winters WD, Ferrar-Allado T. The cataleptic state induced by ketamine: A review of the neuropharmacology of anesthesia. Neuropharmacology 11:303–315, 1972.
10. Guedel AE. Inhalational Anesthesia: A Fundamental Guide. New York: Macmillan, 1937.
11. Kerssens C, Klein J, Bonke B. Awareness: Monitoring versus remembering what happened. Anesthesiology 99:570–575, 2003.
12. Nordstrom O, Sandin R. Recall during intermittent propofol anaesthesia. Br J Anaesth 76:699–701, 1996.
13. Sandin RH. Awareness 1960–2002, explicit recall of events during general anaesthesia. In: Vuyk J, Schraag S, eds. Advances in Modelling and Clinical Applications of Intravenous Anaesthesia. New York: Kluwer Academic/Plenum, 2003:135–147.
14. Stanski DR. Monitoring depth of anesthesia. In: Miller RD, ed. Anesthesia. New York: Churchill-Livingstone, 1990:1001–1029.
15. Katoh T, Suguro Y, Nakajima R, Kazama T, Ikeda K. Blood concentration of sevoflurane and isoflurane on recovery from anaesthesia. Br J Anaesth 69:259–262, 1992.
16. March PA, Muir WW. Minimum alveolar concentration measures of central nervous system activation in cats anesthetized with isoflurane. Am J Vet Res 64:1528–1533, 2003.
17. Vuyk J, Mertens M. Bispectral index scale (BIS) monitoring and intravenous anaesthesia. In: Vuyk J, Schraag S, eds. Advances in Modelling and Clinical Applications of Intravenous Anaesthesia. New York: Kluwer Academic/Plenum, 2003:95–104.
18. Tranquilli WJ. Techniques of inhalation anesthesia in ruminants and swine. Vet Clin North Am Food Anim Pract 2:593–619, 1986.
19. Rampil IJ. A primer for EEG signal processing in anesthesia. Anesthesiology 89:980–1002, 1998.
20. Schwender D, Daunderer M, Mulzer S, Klasing S, Finsterer U, Peter K. Spectral edge frequency of the electroencephalogram to monitor "depth" of anaesthesia with isoflurane or propofol. Br J Anaesth 77:179–184, 1996.
21. Drummond JC, Brann CA, Perkins DE, Wolfe DE. A comparison of median frequency, spectral edge frequency, a frequency band power ratio, total power, and dominance shift in the determination of depth of anesthesia. Acta Anaesthesiol Scand 35:693–699, 1991.
22. Schmidt GN, Bischoff P, Standl T, Lankenau L, Hilbert GD, Esch JS. Comparative evaluation of Narcotrend, Bispectral Index, and classical electroencephalographic variables during induction, maintenance, and emergence of a propofol/remifentanil anesthesia. Anesth Analg 98:1346–1353, 2004.
23. Otto KA, Mally P. Noxious stimulation during orthopaedic surgery results in EEG "arousal" or "paradoxical arousal" reaction in isoflurane-anaesthetised sheep. Res Vet Sci 75:103–112, 2003.
24. Otto KA, Short CE. Electroencephalographic power spectrum analysis as a monitor of anesthetic depth in horses. Vet Surg 20:362–371, 2004.
25. Miller SM, Short CE, Ekstrom PM. Quantitative electroencephalographic evaluation to determine the quality of analgesia during anesthesia of horses for arthroscopic surgery. Am J Vet Res 56:374–379, 2004.
26. Martin-Cancho MF, Lima JR, Luis L, et al. Bispectral index, spectral edge frequency 95%, and median frequency recorded for vari-

ous concentrations of isoflurane and sevoflurane in pigs. Am J Vet Res 64:866–873, 2003.

27. Muncaster ARG, Sleigh JW, Williams M. Changes in consciousness, conceptual memory, and quantitative electroencephalographical measures during recovery from sevoflurane- and remifentanil-based anesthesia. Anesth Analg 96:720–725, 2003.

28. Ortolani O, Conti A, Di Filippo A, et al. EEG signal processing in anaesthesia: Use of a neural network technique for monitoring depth of anaesthesia. Br J Anaesth 88:644–648, 2002.

29. Simmons LE, Riker RR, Prato BS, Fraser GL. Assessing sedation during intensive care unit mechanical ventilation with the Bispectral Index and the Sedation-Agitation Scale. Crit Care Med 27:1499–1504, 1999.

30. DeDeyne C, Struys M, Decruyenaere J, Hoste E, Colardyn F. Use of continuous bispectral EEG monitoring to assess depth of sedation in ICU patients. Intensive Care Med 24:1294–1298, 1998.

31. Greene SA, Benson GJ, Tranquilli WJ, Grimm KA. Relationship of canine bispectral index to multiples of sevoflurane minimal alveolar concentration, using patch or subdermal electrodes. Comp Med 52:424–428, 2002.

32. Muthuswamy J, Sharma A. A study of electroencephalographic descriptors and end-tidal concentration in estimating depth of anesthesia. J Clin Monit 12:353–364, 1996.

33. March PA, Muir WW. Use of the bispectral index as a monitor of anesthetic depth in cats anesthetized with isoflurane. Am J Vet Res 64:1534–1541, 2003.

34. Rosow C, Manberg PJ. Bispectral index monitoring. Anesthesiol Clin North Am 19:947–966, 2001.

35. Gilbert TT, Wagner MR, Halukurike V, Paz HL, Garland A. Use of bispectral electroencephalogram monitoring to assess neurologic status in unsedated, critically ill patients. Crit Care Med 29:1996–2000, 2001.

36. Fabregas N, Gambus PL, Valero R, et al. Can bispectral index monitoring predict recovery of consciousness in patients with severe brain injury? Anesthesiology 101:43–51, 2004.

37. Nasraway SA, Wu EC, Kelleher RM, Yasuda CM, Donnelly AM. How reliable is the Bispectral Index in critically ill patients? A prospective, comparative, single-blinded observer study. Crit Care Med 30:1483–1487, 2002.

38. Bauerle K, Greim CA, Schroth M, Geisselbrecht M, Kobler A, Roewer N. Prediction of depth of sedation and anaesthesia by the Narcotrend™ EEG monitor. Br J Anaesth 92:841–845, 2004.

39. Schraag S, Kenny GNC. Auditory evoked potentials: A clinical or a research tool? In: Vuyk J, Schraag S, eds. Advances in Modelling and Clinical Applications of Intravenous Anaesthesia. New York: Kluwer Academic/Plenum, 2003:105–113.

40. Kiyama S, Tsuzaki K. Processed electroencephalogram during combined extradural and general anaesthesia. Br J Anaesth 78:751–753, 1997.

41. Kiyama S, Takeda J. Effect of extradural analgesia on the paradoxical arousal response of the electroencephalogram. Br J Anaesth 79:750–753, 1997.

42. Singh H, Sakai T, Matsuki A. Movement response to skin incision: Analgesia vs bispectral index and 95% spectral edge frequency. Eur J Anaesthiol 16:610–614, 1999.

43. Hagihira S, Takashina M, Takahiko M, Ueyama H, Mashimo T. Electroencephalographic bicoherence is sensitive to noxious stimuli during isoflurane or sevoflurane anesthesia. Anesthesiology 100:818–825, 2004.

44. Barr G, Jakobsson JG, Lenhardt R, Negishi C, Sessler DI. Nitrous oxide does not alter bispectral index: Study with nitrous oxide as sole agent and as an adjunct to i.v. anaesthesia. Br J Anaesth 82:827–830, 1999.

45. Hans P, Bonhomme V, Benmansour H, Dewandre PY, Brichant JF, Lamy M. Effect of nitrous oxide on the bispectral index and the 95% spectral edge frequency of the electroencephalogram during surgery. Anaesthesia 56:999–1004, 2001.

46. Gurman GM, Popescu M, Weksler N, Steiner O, Avinoah E, Porath E. Influence of the cortical electrical activity level during general anaesthesia on the severity of immediate postoperative pain in the morbidly obese. Acta Anaesthesiol Scand 47:804–808, 2003.

47. Tranquilli WJ, Grimm KA, Lamont LA. Pain Management for the Small Animal Practitioner. Jackson, WY: Teton NewMedia, 2004.

48. Copland VS, Haskins SC, Patz JD. Atropine reversal of oxymorphone induced bradycardia. Vet Surg 21:414–417, 1992.

49. Riebold TW. Monitoring equine anesthesia. Vet Clin North Am Equine Pract 6:607–624, 1990.

50. Kumar A, Anel R, Bunnel E, et al. Pulmonary artery occlusion pressure and central venous pressure fail to predict ventricular filling volume, cardiac performance, or the response to volume infusion in normal subjects. Crit Care Med 32:691–699, 2004.

51. Pagel PS, Kampine JP, Schmeling WT, Warltier DC. Alteration of left ventricular diastolic function by desflurane, isoflurane, and halothane in the chronically instrumented dog with autonomic nervous system blockade. Anesthesiology 74:1103–1114, 1991.

52. Gardner RM. Direct blood pressure measurement: Dynamic response requirements. Anesthesiology 54:227–236, 1981.

53. Hett DA, Jonas MM. Noninvasive cardiac output monitoring. Intensive Crit Care Nurs 20:103–108, 2004.

54. Corley KT, Donaldson LL, Furr MO. Comparison of lithium dilution and thermodilution cardiac output measurements in anaesthetized neonatal foals. Equine Vet J 34:598–601, 2002.

55. Mason DJ, O'Grady M, McDonell W. Comparison of a central and a peripheral (cephalic vein) injection site for the measurement of cardiac output using the lithium-dilution cardiac output technique in anesthetized dogs. Can J Vet Res 66:207–210, 2002.

56. Linton RA, Young LE, Marlin DJ, et al. Cardiac output measured by lithium dilution, thermodilution, and transesophageal Doppler echocardiography in anesthetized horses. Am J Vet Res 61:731–737, 2000.

57. Corley KTT, Donaldson LL, Durando MM, Birks EK. Cardiac output technologies with special reference to the horse. J Vet Intern Med 17:262–272, 2003.

58. Steffey EP, Dunlop CI, Farver TB, Woliner MJ, Schultz LJ. Cardiovascular and respiratory measurements in awake and isoflurane-anesthetized horses. Am J Vet Res 48:7–12, 1987.

59. Steffey EP, Howland D. Cardiovascular effects of halothane in the horse. Am J Vet Res 69:611–615, 1978.

60. Hillidge CJ, Lees P. Cardiac output in the conscious and anaesthetised horse. Equine Vet J 7:16–21, 1975.

61. Mikat M, Peters J, Zindler M, Arndt JO. Whole body oxygen consumption in awake, sleeping, and anesthetized dogs. Anesthesiology 60:220–227, 1984.

62. Rock P, Beattie C, Kimball AW, et al. Halothane alters the oxygen consumption–oxygen delivery relationship compared with the conscious state. Anesthesiology 73:1186–1197, 1990.

63. Guzman JA, Lacoma FJ, Kuz JA. Relationship between systemic oxygen supply dependency and gastric intramucosal PCO_2 during progressive hemorrhage. J Trauma 44:696–700, 1998.

64. Cilley RE, Scharenberg AM, Bongiorno PF, Guire KE, Bartlett RH. Low oxygen delivery produced by anemia, hypoxia, and low cardiac output. J Surg Res 51:425–433, 1991.

65. Cilley RE, Polley TZ, Zwischenberger JB, Toomasian JM, Bartlett RH. Independent measurement of oxygen consumption and oxygen delivery. J Surg Res 47:242–247, 1989.

66. Van Der Linden P, Schmartz D, De Groote F, Willaert P, Rausin I, Vincent JL. Critical haemoglobin concentration in anaesthetized dogs: Comparison of two plasma substitutes. Br J Anaesth 81:556–562, 1998.

67. Shoemaker WC, Appel PL, Kram HB, Waxman K, Lee TS. Prospective trial of supranormal values of survivors as therapeutic goals in high-risk surgical patients. Chest 94:1176–1186, 1988.

68. Yu M, Levy MM, Smith P, Takiguchi SA, Miyasaki A, Myers SA. Effect of maximizing oxygen delivery on morbidity and mortality rates in critically ill patients: A prospective randomized, controlled study. Crit Care Med 21:830–838, 1993.

69. Van Der Linden P, Gilbart E, Engelman D, Schmartz D, Vincent JL. Effects of anesthetic agents on systemic critical O_2 delivery. J Appl Physiol 71:83–93, 1991.

70. Hubbell JAE. Monitoring. In: Muir WW, Hubbell JAE, eds. Equine Anesthesia Monitoring and Emergency Therapy. St Louis: Mosby Year Book, 1991:153–178.

71. Swedlow DB. Capnometry and capnography: The anesthesia disaster early warning system. Semin Anesth 5:194–205, 1986.

72. Gravenstein JS, Paulus DA, Hayes TJ. Capnography in Clinical Practice. London: Butterworth, 1989.

73. Schmitz BD, Shapiro BA. Capnography. Respir Care Clin North Am 1:107–117, 1995.

74. Shapiro BA, Peruzzi WT, Templin R. Clinical Application of Blood Gases. Chicago: Mosby Year Book, 1994.

75. Weingarten M. Respiratory monitoring of carbon dioxide and oxygen. J Clin Monit 6:217–225, 1990.

76. Tremper KK, Barker SJ. Pulse oximetry. Anesthesiology 79:98–108, 1989.

77. Barker SJ, Tremper KK, Hyatt J, Zaccari J. Effects of methemoglobinemia on pulse oximetry and mixed venous oximetry [Abstract]. Anesthesiology 67:A171, 1987.

78. Barker SJ, Tremper KK. The effect of carbon monoxide inhalation on pulse oximeter signal detection. Anesthesiology 78:599–603, 1987.

79. Blair E. Clinical Hypothermia. New York: McGraw-Hill, 1964.

80. Danzl DF. Accidental hypothermia. In: Rosen P, Baker FJ, Barkin RM, Braen GR, Dailey RH, Levy RC, eds. Emergency Medicine: Concepts and Clinical Practice, 2nd ed. St Louis: CV Mosby, 1988:663–692.

81. Haskins SC. Hypothermia and its prevention during general anesthesia in cats. Am J Vet Res 42:856–861, 1981.

82. Gregory RT, Doolittle WM. Accidental hypothermia. Part II. Clinical implications of experimental studies. Alaska Med 15:48–52, 1973.

83. Miller JW, Danzl DF, Thomas DM. Urban accidental hypothermia: 135 cases. Ann Emerg Med 9:456–461, 1980.

84. Duguid H, Simpson RG, Stower JM. Accidental hypothermia. Lancet 9:1213–1219, 1961.

85. Thomas H. Fever. In: Rosen P, Baker FJ, Barkin RM, Braen GR, Dailey RH, Levy RC, eds. Emergency Medicine: Concepts and Clinical Practice, 2nd ed. St Louis: CV Mosby, 1988:309–320.

86. Callaham M. Heat illness. In: Rosen P, Baker FJ, Barkin RM, Braen GR, Dailey RH, Levy RC, eds. Emergency Medicine: Concepts and Clinical Practice, 2nd ed. St Louis: CV Mosby, 1988:693–717.

87. Gronert GA. Malignant hyperthermia. Anesthesiology 53:395–423, 1980.

88. Ayres SM, Keenan RL. The hyperthermic syndromes. In: Ayres SM, Grenvik A, Holbrook PR, Shoemaker WC, eds. Textbook of Critical Care. Philadelphia: WB Saunders, 1995:1520–1523.

89. Short CE, Paddleford RR. Malignant hyperpyrexia in the dog. Anesthesiology 39:462–463, 1973.

90. Bagshaw RJ, Cox RH, Knight DH, Detweiler DK. Malignant hyperthermia in a greyhound. J Am Vet Med Assoc 172:61–62, 1978.

91. de Jong RH, Heavner JE, Amory DW. Malignant hyperpyrexia in the cat. Anesthesiology 41:608–609, 1974.

92. Bellah JR. Suspected malignant hyperthermia after halothane anesthesia in a cat. Vet Surg 18:483–486, 1989.

93. McClure JJ. Malignant hyperthermia in the horse: Case report. Minn Vet 15:12–15, 1975.

94. Klein LV. Case report: A hot horse. Vet Anesth 2:41–44, 1975.

95. Keating WR. Direct effects of temperature on blood vessels: Their role in cold vasodilation. In: Hardy JD, Gagge AP, Stolwijk JAJ, eds. Physiological and Behavioral Temperature Regulation. Springfield, IL: Charles C Thomas, 1970:231–236.

96. McLellan SA, McClelland DBL, Walsh TS. Anaemia and red blood cell transfusion in the critically ill patient. Blood Rev 17:195–208, 2003.

97. Brown SA, Dusza K, Boehmer J. Comparison of measured and calculated values for colloid osmotic pressure in hospitalized animals. Am J Vet Res 55:910–915, 1994.

98. Couto CG. Spontaneous bleeding disorders. In: Bonagura JD, Kirk RW, eds. Kirk's Current Veterinary Therapy. Philadelphia: WB Saunders, 1995:457–461.

99. Griffin A, Callan MB, Shofer FS, Giger U. Evaluation of a canine D-dimer point-of-care test kit for use in samples obtained from dogs with disseminated intravascular coagulation, thromboembolic disease, and hemorrhage. Am J Vet Res 64:1562–1569, 2003.

100. Feige K, Kastner SBR, Dempfle CE, Balestra E. Changes in coagulation and markers of fibrinolysis in horses undergoing colic surgery. J Vet Med [A] 50:30–36, 2003.

101. Otto CM, Rieser TM, Brooks MB, Russel MW. Evidence of hypercoagulability in dogs with parvoviral enteritis. J Am Vet Med Assoc 217:1500–1504, 2000.

102. Davis CL, Chandler WL. Thromboelastography for the prediction of bleeding after transplant renal biopsy. J Am Soc Nephrol 6:1250–1255, 1995.

103. Hall HJ, Peters M, Eaton S, Pierro A. Hyperglycemia is associated with increased morbidity and mortality rates in neonates with necrotizing enterocolitis. J Pediatr Surg 39:898–901, 2004.

104. Finney SJ, Zekveld C, Elia A, Evans TW. Glucose control and mortality in critically ill patients. J Am Med Assoc 290:2041–2047, 2003.

105. Laird AM, Miller PR, Kilgo PD, Meredith JW, Chang MC. Relationship of early hyperglycemia to mortality in trauma patients. J Trauma 56:1058–1062, 2004.

106. Siegel JH, Fabian M, Smith JA, Kingston EP, Steele KA, Wells MR. Oxygen debt criteria quantify the effectiveness of early partial resuscitation after hypovolemic hemorrhagic shock. J Trauma 54:862–880, 2003.

107. Chiara O, Pelosi P, Segala M, et al. Mesenteric and renal oxygen transport during hemorrhage and reperfusion: Evaluation of optimal goals for resuscitation. J Trauma 51:356–362, 2001.

108. James JH, Luchette FA, McCarter FD, Fischer JE. Lactate is an unreliable indicator of tissue hypoxia in injury or sepsis. Lancet 354:505–508, 1999.

109. Rose BD, Post TW. Clinical Physiology of Acid-Base and Electrolyte Disorders. New York: McGraw-Hill, 2001.

110. Reeves RB, Park JS, Lapennas GN, Olszowka AJ. Oxygen affinity and Bohr coefficients of dog blood. J Appl Physiol 53:87–95, 1982.

111. Bartels H, Harms H. Sauerstoffdissoziationskurven des Blutes von Saugetieren. Pflugers Arch 268:334–365, 1959.

112. Smale K, Anderson LS, Butler PJ. An algorithm to describe the oxygen equilibrium curve for the Thoroughbred racehorse. Equine Vet J 26:500–502, 1994.

Section V
SELECTED ANESTHETIC AND ANALGESIC TECHNIQUES

Chapter 20

Local and Regional Anesthetic and Analgesic Techniques: Dogs

Roman T. Skarda and William J. Tranquilli

Introduction

The popularity of local anesthetic-induced neural blockade in dogs has increased over the past several years. A major driving force behind this increased usage is acceptance of the concept of blocking multimodal pathways to control animals' pain and suffering. Unlike most general anesthetics, which block the perception of pain by inducing anesthesia in an unconscious patient, local anesthesia and regional anesthesia completely block transmission of noxious impulses in a region of the body of a conscious patient. General anesthesia may be advantageous in dogs that are considered difficult to sedate and restrain for surgery and where complete immobilization and relaxation of the patient are required. Local and regional anesthesia also decreases the quantity of opioid and inhalation anesthetic required to obtain the desired plane of anesthesia intraoperatively.[1] Topical anesthesia, infiltration anesthesia, field blocks, selected nerve blocks of the head (anesthesia of the maxilla, upper teeth, eye and orbit, mandible, and lower teeth), anesthesia of the foot and leg (ring block, brachial plexus block, and intravenous regional anesthesia), multiple intercostal nerve blocks, lumbosacral epidural anesthesia, and continuous epidural anesthesia are all logical techniques for providing surgical analgesia and anesthesia in dogs that are considered at risk for inhalant or intravenous anesthesia (Table 20.1). Continuous interpleural analgesia and epidural opioid analgesia can be used to relieve postoperative pain following general anesthesia.

This chapter provides a general overview of the most commonly used local and regional anesthetic techniques for surgical and postoperative pain relief in dogs, emphasizing methodology, advantages, and disadvantages. The pharmacology of local anesthetic drugs, highlighting the mechanisms of action, relevant pharmacology and pharmacokinetics, toxicity, and potential drug interactions, are discussed in Chapter 14.

Topical Anesthesia

Many local anesthetics are effective when placed topically on mucous membranes and may be used in the mouth, tracheobronchial tree, esophagus, and genitourinary tract. Local anesthetics used topically include lidocaine (2% to 5%), proparacaine (0.5%), tetracaine (0.5% to 2.0%), butacaine (2%), and cocaine (4% to 10%). Preparations include injectables that are applied topically, cream, ointment, jelly, powder, and aerosol. Injectable preparations of lidocaine (0.5% to 5.0%), available in ampules and vials, with and without epinephrine (1:50,000 to 1:200,000), can be used for infiltration (0.5% to 1.0%) and nerve block (1% to 2%), and applied topically to mucous membranes (1% to 5%). Topical local anesthetic agents can relieve pain during cleaning or dressing of wounds, although their effect is highly variable.

Table 20.1. Classification and degree of required dexterity for producing local and regional anesthetic techniques in dogs.

Classification	Techniques	Required Manual Dexterity and Experience
Terminal anesthesia	Topical	+
	Intravenous regional anesthesia	++
Infiltration anesthesia	Subcutaneous, intramuscular injection	+
	Subpleural injection	++
	Ring block	+
Perineural anesthesia	Nerve blocks on the head	++
	Nerve blocks on the legs	+++
	Brachial plexus block	++
	Intercostal nerve block	+
Spinal anesthesia	Lumbosacral epidural anesthesia	++
	Continuous epidural anesthesia (catheter technique)	+++
	Lumbar subarachnoid anesthesia	+++
Postoperative analgesia	Epidural opioid analgesia	++
	Continuous epidural opioid analgesia (catheter technique)	+++
	Interpleural regional analgesia (catheter technique)	+++
Therapeutic analgesia	Anesthesia of the cervicothoracic ganglion	+++
	Anesthesia of the lumbar sympathetic ganglia	+++

+, little; ++, some; +++, considerable.

The lowest effective dose of topical anesthetic should always be used in order to prevent toxicity from excessive drug plasma concentrations.[2] Time between application of topical anesthetics and onset of anesthesia is generally longer, and pain relief less, than that achieved with infiltration anesthesia. A 2% to 4% solution of lidocaine used for topical anesthesia on mucous membranes produces effects in approximately 5 min and lasts for 30 min.

Local instillation of proparacaine (0.5%), tetracaine (0.5% to 1.0%), butacaine (2%), piperocaine (2%), oxybuprocaine (0.4%), or cocaine (1% to 4%) into the conjunctival sac anesthetizes the cornea and conjunctiva for short procedures (e.g., removal of hypertrophied gland of the third eyelid). Proparacaine (0.5%) has been advocated as an excellent topical anesthetic for examination of a painful eye, removal of foreign bodies, sutures, obtaining conjunctival scrapings, and subconjunctival injections.[3] Anesthesia occurs rapidly (1 to 6 min), lasts for 10 to 15 min after single instillation, and may last for up to 2 h after repeated instillation without untoward effects (e.g., irritation or epithelial damage).[4] A series of three to five instillations of 1 or 2 drops of proparacaine at approximately 1-min intervals may be necessary to produce satisfactory anesthesia of the cornea and conjunctiva. Topical anesthesia is very safe, is simple to apply, and can be repeated, although dogs may resent the application of cold solutions. Data on vascular uptake and maximum blood concentration are not available, large interpatient variability should be expected, and potential for bacterial contamination exists.[5]

Local anesthetic sprays (10% lidocaine or 14% to 20% benzocaine) anesthetize the mucosa up to a depth of 2 mm within 1 to 2 min after application. Anesthesia lasts for approximately 15 to 20 min. The movable nozzle (Jetco nozzle) of the spray can enable easy access to the site of application. Pressure on the nozzle with the forefinger delivers a specific quantity of the anesthetic each second (10 mg of lidocaine from a 10% lidocaine

spray can). The average expulsion rate from a benzocaine (Cetacaine) spray can is 200 mg/s.

Endotracheal tubes are frequently coated with local anesthetic jells but should not be lubricated with jelly containing 20% benzocaine hydrochloride. Topical sprays and ointments containing 14% to 20% benzocaine reproducibly cause dose-dependent methemoglobinemia. Preparations with over 8% benzocaine include Hurricane Spray (20%), Hurricane Topical Anesthetic Gel (20%) and Liquid (20%), Camphophenique Sting Relief Formula (20%), Dermoplast Anesthetic Pain Relief (20%), and Cetacaine Spray (14%).[6] Exposure of the tracheal mucosa to topical benzocaine oxidizes blood hemoglobin in dogs in proportion to the absorbed dose within 10 min. Methemoglobin cannot bind oxygen or carbon dioxide.[7] Dogs are usually asymptomatic when concentrations of methemoglobin are less than 20%, but show fatigue, weakness, dyspnea, and tachycardia at concentrations between 20% and 50%.[8] Laryngeal sprays containing benzocaine should be used with caution, and if signs of cyanosis and respiratory distress develop, methemoglobinemia should be considered. In general, benzocaine should be used sparingly and cautiously while continuously monitoring for cyanosis. Patients at risk of hypoxia after using benzocaine topical anesthesia should receive oxygen[6] and intravenous methylene blue (1.5 mg/kg) therapy.[8]

One of the oldest forms of topical anesthesia is superficial cooling. Ethyl chloride can be used to freeze a small local area of skin for punctures, skin biopsy, or incision of small abscesses. Ethyl chloride is sprayed on the skin for 3 to 7 s from an inverted bottle and a distance of 10 to 20 cm, with the jet stream aimed so that it meets the skin at an acute angle to lessen the shock of impact (Fig. 20.1). Surface anesthesia results from cooling (<4°C), which occurs during the evaporation process. Attempts to freeze large skin areas by using ethyl chloride are contraindicated be-

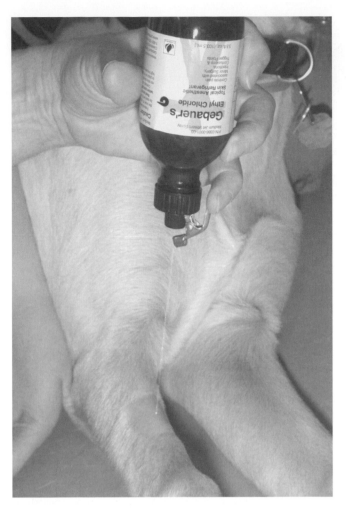

Fig. 20.1. Ethyl chloride is sprayed on the skin to produce surface anesthesia.

cause of the potential for frostbite. Ethyl chloride's brief action (<2 min), ability to produce a freezing sensation, and flammability when exposed to open flames and electric sparks (electrocauterization) limit its use. Inhalation of ethyl chloride should be avoided because it may produce narcotic and general anesthetic effects, or fatal coma with respiratory and cardiac arrest.

Pontocaine cream and a liposomal tetracaine preparation (0.5% tetracaine encapsulated into phospholipid vehicles) effectively penetrate human skin within 30 to 60 min of application, producing long-lasting (>4 h) analgesia.[9] The most clinically usable cream contains a 5% eutectic mixture of 2.5% lidocaine and 2.5% prilocaine (EMLA cream), which overcomes the human stratum corneum barrier within 1 h of topical application without adverse effects.[10] The usefulness of EMLA cream in dogs has been reported.[11]

Infiltration Anesthesia

Local infiltration of local anesthetics requires their extravascular placement by direct injection and may be the most reliable and safest of all the local anesthetic techniques (Table 20.1). Lido-

caine (0.5% to 2.0%) is the local anesthetic most often used for infiltration. Only sharp and sterile needles should be used. Local anesthesia can be produced by multiple intradermal or subcutaneous injections of 0.3 to 0.5 mL of local anesthetic solution by using a 2.5-cm, 22- to 25-gauge needle or by using a longer needle (3.75 to 5.0 cm) and slowly injecting local anesthetic while advancing the needle along the line of proposed incision (linear infiltration). Pain is minimal if the needle is advanced slowly into the first desensitized wheal and successive injections are made at the periphery of the advancing wheal. This technique assures that the dog senses only the initial needle insertion. Intradermal deposition of local anesthetic over a superficial abscess, cyst, or hematoma is a routine procedure. Infection along the filtration site will not occur if the needle has not entered the abscess. The amount of local anesthetic used for infiltration anesthesia depends on the size of the area to be anesthetized. Approximately 2 to 5 mg/kg of lidocaine or mepivacaine and 4 to 6 mg/kg of procaine without epinephrine may be used to diffuse into surrounding tissue from the site of injection and anesthetize the nerve fibers and endings. Large amounts of relatively dilute solutions are often infiltrated into operative sites. The lowest possible concentration of local anesthetic that will produce the desired effect should be administered. For example, an average dog (20 kg) will tolerate approximately 50 mL of 0.5% lidocaine without demonstrating signs of toxicity, whereas only 20 to 30 mL of 1% lidocaine or 10 to 15 mL of 2% lidocaine can be injected. The local anesthetic may be diluted in 0.9% sodium chloride solution (not with sterile water) to a 0.25% solution if a large volume of local anesthetic is needed for infiltration of a large operative area. The total dose of drug administered should be reduced by 30% to 40% in old dogs (>8 years) and sick or cachectic dogs in poor condition.[12]

Alternatively, approximately 5 to 8 mg/kg of local anesthetic with epinephrine (1:200,000) may be used for infiltration to produce local vasoconstriction, which reduces absorption rates (30%) and helps to maintain a high drug concentration at the nerve fiber, thus increasing the local anesthetic effect and duration (50%). Local anesthetics containing epinephrine should not be injected into tissues supplied by end arteries (e.g., ears and tail) or in thin and dark-skinned dogs (e.g., poodles) because of the risk of severe vasoconstriction, local ischemia, and necrosis. Epinephrine increases the potential risk of cardiac arrhythmias (e.g., sinus tachycardia, ventricular tachycardia, and ventricular fibrillation in a halothane-sensitized heart), although this has not been a problem when administered in conjunction with lidocaine in dogs. Hearts sensitized to ventricular arrhythmias with halothane do not develop serious ventricular arrhythmias when given lidocaine (1.3 to 7.9 mg/kg) containing epinephrine (0.3 to 1.9 mg/kg) in doses found in lidocaine-epinephrine mixtures used commonly for local anesthesia.[13] Subfascial and intra-arterial injections must be avoided.

Continuous-Infiltration Anesthesia

This can be accomplished by the use of a continuous catheter-insertion system and a disposable infusion pump (Fig. 20.2).[14] A sterile multipore catheter is placed within the surgical incision

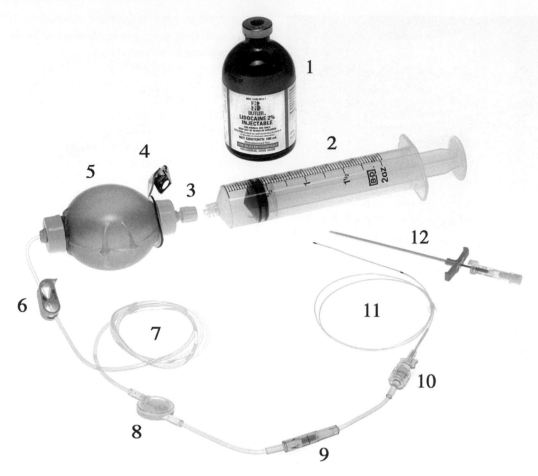

Fig. 20.2. Pain management system for continuous local anesthetic infiltration. The Pain Buster Soaker/ON-Q (I-Flow, Lake Forest, CA) provides continuous administration of local anesthetic into the surgery site for 1 to 5 days: (1) 100 mL of 2% lidocaine hydrochloride solution; (2) 60-mL syringe; (3) fill port with protection cap; (4) E-clip to secure the pump; (5) Pain Buster pump; (6) clamp; (7) pump tubing; (8) filter; (9) flow restrictor, 2-mL/h flow rate if placed in direct contact with the skin (31°C); (10) luer lock on the catheter connector; (11) radiopaque, fenestrated soaker catheter, with a 20-gauge, 59-cm long, 6.5–cm infusion segment; and (12) split-introducer sheath with the needle partially withdrawn from the needle guard.

(e.g., total ear-canal ablation with lateral bulla osteotomy [Fig. 20.3A], forelimb amputation [Fig. 20.3B], or median and lateral thoracotomies) at the end of the surgical procedure. The catheter is connected to an elastomeric reservoir infusion pump (Pain Buster Soaker system; Orthopedics, Vista, CA), which is filled with local anesthetic (i.e., lidocaine, mepivacaine, or ropivacaine) to its full capacity (65, 100, 270, or 335 mL) to deliver the local anesthetic at a constant rate (0.5, 2.0, 4.0, or 5.0 mL/h) for several days. The Pain Buster Soaker technique is generally well tolerated, producing good postoperative analgesia for up to 50 h, with no acute local anesthetic toxicity, hemodynamic instability, or breakthrough pain.[15] Side effects, such as nystagmus, restlessness, apprehension, and vomiting, are readily treated by removing the pump.

Field Block

This technique can be used for anesthetizing large areas. First, intradermal or subcutaneous linear infiltration is produced around the lesion as previously described. Local anesthetic is then deposited in the deeper tissues by passing the needle through the desensitized skin far enough to infiltrate the deep nerves supplying the area (Fig. 20.4).[16]

Intraperitoneal Infusion

The efficacy of intraperitoneal administration of either lidocaine (2%, 8.8 mg/kg with epinephrine 5 µg/mL), bupivacaine (0.75%, 2.2 mg/kg), or 0.9% sodium chloride solution, and additional subcutaneous injection of 2 mL of the assigned solution prior to incisional closure, has been evaluated for analgesia in 10 dogs upon completion of ovariohysterectomy.[17] Surgery was performed with the patient under general anesthesia (acepromazine-butorphanol-thiopental-isoflurane). No adverse side effects were observed. Pain scores, using the visual analogue scale (VAS), peaked for all groups at 0.5 h and returned to baseline by 18 h. Dogs in the bupivacaine group had significantly lower pain scores at 0.5 h than did the dogs in the 0.9% saline group. Butorphanol and/or acepromazine (0.22 mg/kg intramuscularly [IM] or intravenously [IV]) was given to provide supplemental analgesia to 7 of 10 dogs in the saline group, 4 of 10 dogs in the

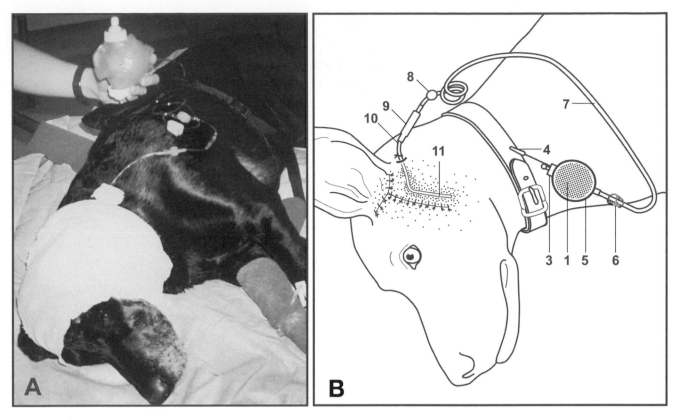

Fig. 20.3. Pain therapy by using the Pain Buster Soaker: black Labrador (39 kg) after total ear-canal ablation **(A)**. The Pain Buster pump is placed into a protective bag hanging beneath the neck. Lidocaine (2%) continuously infiltrates the wounds at a constant rate (2 mL/h) for several days. The numbers refer to the same system components as described in Fig. 20.2 **(B)**.

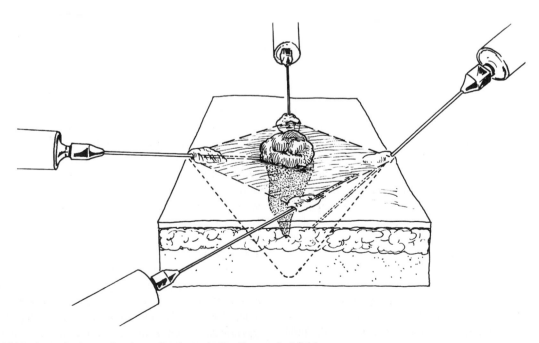

Fig. 20.4. Field block producing walls of anesthesia enclosing the surgical field.

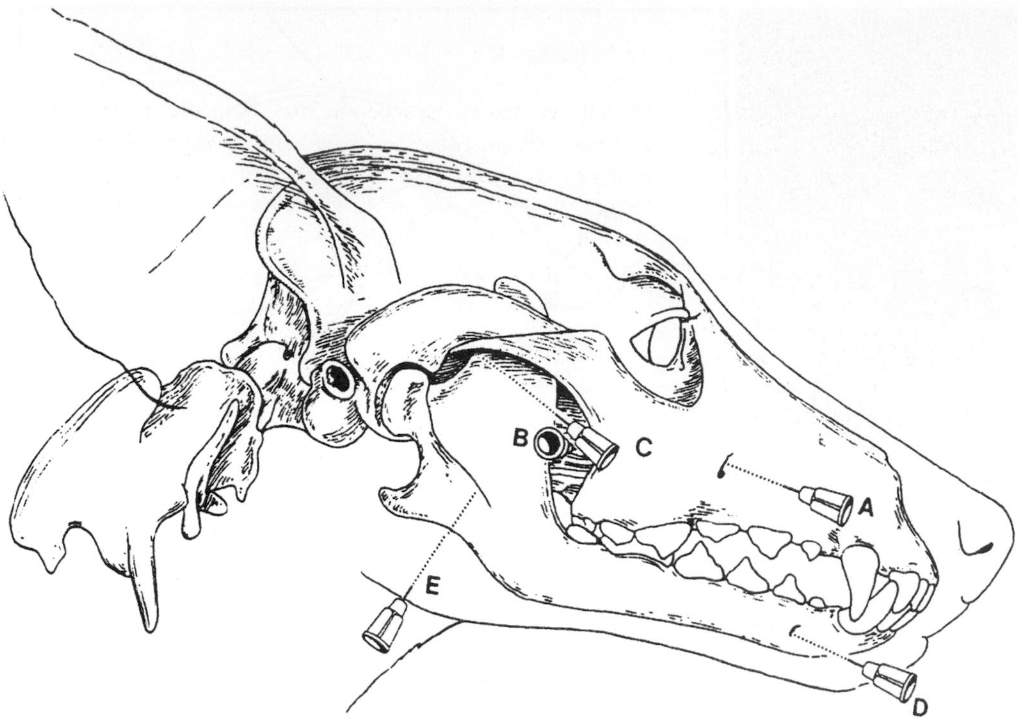

Fig. 20.5. Needle placement for producing nerve blocks on the head: infraorbital (A), maxillary (B), zygomatic, lacrimal, and ophthalmic (C), mandibular (E), and mental (D) nerves.

lidocaine group, and 2 of 10 dogs in the bupivacaine group. These findings can be interpreted as support for the use of intraperitoneal and subcutaneous bupivacaine for postoperative analgesia following ovariohysterectomy in dogs.[17,18]

Nerve Blocks

Injection of local anesthetic solution into the connective tissue surrounding a particular nerve produces loss of sensation (sensory nerve block) and/or paralysis (motor nerve block) in the region supplied by the nerves (regional anesthesia). Smaller volumes (1 to 2 mL) of local anesthetic are needed to produce nerve blocks when compared with a field block, thereby reducing the danger of toxicity.

Three supplemental methods of pain relief in 31 anesthetized dogs undergoing total ear-canal ablation with lateral bulla osteotomy have been compared.[19] The use of systemic opioids alone (e.g., oxymorphone, 0.05 mg/kg IV), intraoperative splash block, using bupivacaine (0.5% solution, 1.0 mg/kg per ear), and preoperative nerve block of the great auricular nerve (cervical nerve II) and the auriculotemporal nerve (cranial nerve V), using bupivacaine (0.5% solution, 0.5 mL per site), provided similar pain relief, although 33% of the dogs required additional analgesia or tranquilization after surgery. Rectal temperature, pulse rate, respiratory rate, and postoperative serum cortisol concentrations in dogs were not significantly different among groups ($P < 0.05$).

Regional Anesthesia of the Head

The administration of local anesthetic around the infraorbital, maxillary, ophthalmic, mental, and alveolar mandibular nerves provides valuable and practical advantages over general anesthesia when combined with effective sedation (Fig. 20.5). Each nerve may be desensitized by injecting 1 to 2 mL of a 2% lidocaine hydrochloride solution by using a 2.5- to 5-cm, 20- to 25-gauge needle.

The infraorbital nerve is desensitized at its point of emergence from the infraorbital canal. The needle is inserted either intraorally[20] or extraorally approximately 1 cm cranial to the bony lip of the infraorbital foramen.[21,22] The needle is advanced to the infraorbital foramen, which can be found between the dorsal border of the zygomatic process and the gum of the upper canine tooth (Fig. 20.5A). Successful injections desensitize the upper lip and nose, the roof of nasal cavity, and the surrounding skin up to the infraorbital foramen.

The maxillary nerve must be desensitized to completely desensitize the maxilla, upper teeth, nose, and upper lip. The needle is placed percutaneously along the ventral border of the zygomatic process approximately 0.5 cm caudal to the lateral canthus of the eye and is advanced into close proximity of the pterygopalatine fossa (Figs. 20.5B and 20.6). Local anesthetic is administered at the point where the maxillary nerve courses perpendicular to the palatine bone between the maxillary foramen and foramen rotundum.[20,21]

Eye and Orbit

Anesthesia of the eye and orbit is produced by desensitizing the ophthalmic division of the trigeminal nerve. General anesthesia for ophthalmic procedures has increased in popularity; however, retention of ocular reflexes during light and medium planes of general anesthesia in dogs can disturb the surgical field. Regional anesthesia, by anesthesia of ophthalmic nerves, produces immo-

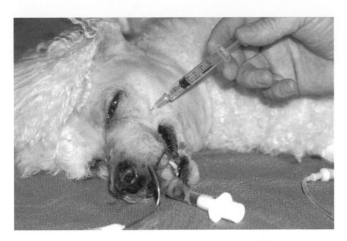

Fig. 20.6. Anesthesia of the maxillary nerve in a poodle (32 kg) after partial maxillectomy: site and direction of the inserted needle.

bility of the eye in addition to sensory anesthesia, and prevents the oculocardiac reflex, which can cause bradycardia, arrhythmias, and cardiac arrest as result of traction on the extrinsic muscles of the eye. A 2.5-cm, 22-gauge needle is inserted ventral to the zygomatic process at the level of the lateral canthus. The point of the needle should be approximately 0.5 cm cranial to the anterior border of the vertical portion of the ramus of the mandible. The needle is advanced medial to the ramus of the mandible in a mediodorsal and somewhat caudal direction until it reaches the lacrimal, zygomatic, and ophthalmic nerves at the orbital fissure (Fig. 20.5C). Deposition of 2 mL of local anesthetic at this site produces akinesia of the globe because of the proximity of the abducens, oculomotor, and trochlear nerves to

the ophthalmic nerve. Motor block is assessed by cessation of the following eye movements: laterally, caused by the lateral rectus muscle (abducens nerve); and upward, downward, medially, and laterally, caused by the superior, inferior, medial, and lateral rectus muscles, respectively (oculomotor nerve). The superior oblique muscle rotates the eye downward and laterally (oculomotor nerve), whereas the inferior oblique muscle rotates the globe upward and laterally (trochlear nerve).[23]

Retrobulbar or peribulbar anesthesia for local anesthesia of the eye runs the risk of direct subarachnoid injection, peribulbar hemorrhage, globe perforation, and intravascular injection.[5,23,24] When performing retrobulbar anesthesia, the risk of puncturing the globe is minimal if a 7.5-cm, 20-gauge needle is inserted at the lateral canthus through the anesthetized conjunctiva and is advanced past the globe toward the opposite mandibular joint until the base of the orbit is encountered.[20] When performing peribulbar anesthesia, the potential for puncturing ciliary and scleral blood vessels is minimal if a 5-cm curved needle (0.5-mm internal diameter) conformed to the roof of the orbit is inserted through the anesthetized conjunctival sac at the vertical meridian (Fig. 20.7).[25] Directing the needle away from the globe and toward the orbit also minimizes the risk of perforating the globe.

Injection of local anesthetic into the optic sheath can cause respiratory arrest attributable to the infiltration of local anesthetic into the subarachnoid space of the central nervous system (CNS).[24] The pressure generated by injection into the optic nerve sheath or intrascleral injection is three or four times that produced by injection into the retrobulbar adipose tissue (135 vs. 35 mm Hg).[24] Increased resistance encountered during retrobulbar block should serve as a warning, mandating redirection of the needle in order to prevent subarachnoid injection.

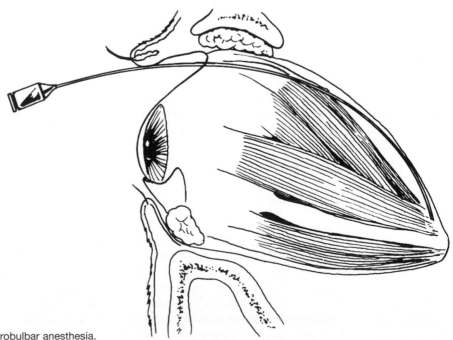

Fig. 20.7. Needle placement for producing retrobulbar anesthesia.

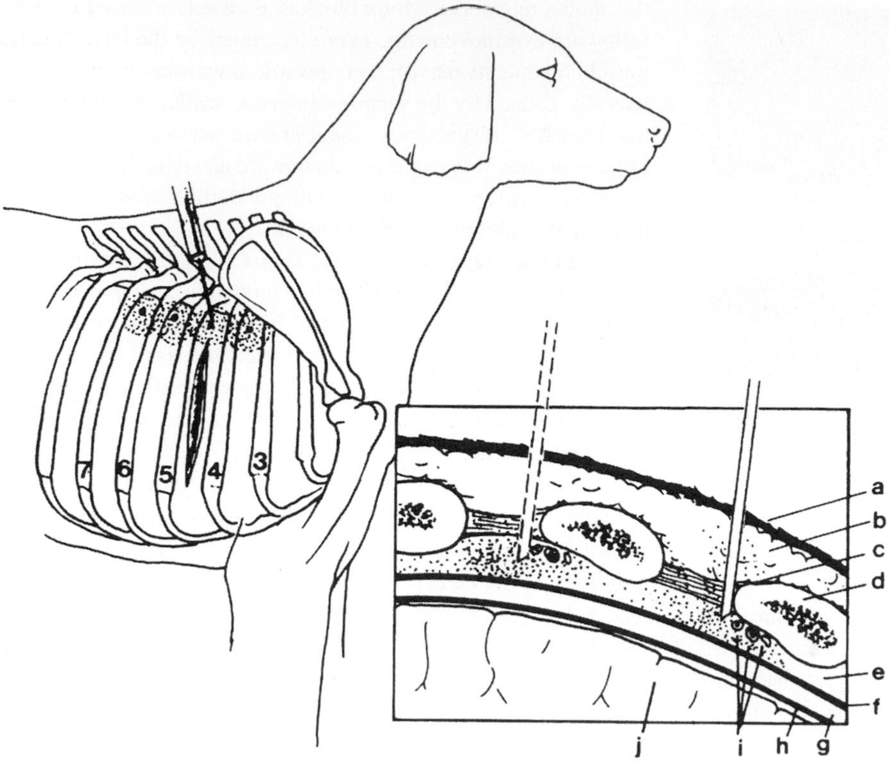

Fig. 20.8. Needle placement for inducing intercostal nerve blocks. **Inset:** (a) skin, (b) subcutaneous tissue, (c) intercostal muscles, (d) rib, (e) subcostal space, (f) pleura costalis and fascia, (g) interpleural space, (h) pleura pulmonalis, (i) intercostal artery, vein, and nerve, and (j) lung.

Lower Lip

This can be desensitized by percutaneously inserting a 2.5-cm, 22- to 25-gauge needle rostral to the mental foramen at the level of the second premolar tooth. Approximately 1 to 2 mL of local anesthetic is deposited in close proximity to the mental nerve (Fig. 20.5D).

Mandible and Lower Teeth

The mandible (including molars, premolars, canine, incisors, skin) and the mucosa of the chin and lower lip can be desensitized by injecting 1 to 2 mL of the local anesthetic in close proximity to the inferior alveolar branch of the mandibular nerve as it enters the mandibular canal at the mandibular foramen (Fig. 20.5E). A 2.5-cm, 22-gauge needle is inserted at the lower angle of the jaw approximately 0.5 cm rostral to the angular process and is advanced 1 to 2 cm dorsally along the medial surface of the ramus of the mandible to the palpable lip of the mandibular foramen.[20,22]

Intercostal Nerve Block

Intercostal nerve blocks may be used for relieving pain during and after thoracotomy, pleural drainage, and rib fractures, thereby minimizing the need for systemic analgesics that may depress respiration. They are not recommended for dogs with pulmonary diseases, which impair blood-gas exchange, or for dogs that cannot be observed for several hours after injection because of the potential for clinically delayed pneumothorax.

A minimum of two adjacent intercostal spaces both cranial and caudal to the incision or injury site are selectively blocked because of overlap of nerve supply.[26] The site for needle placement is the caudal border of the rib (R3-6) near the intervertebral foramen (Fig. 20.8). Approximately 0.25 to 1.0 mL of 0.25% or 0.5% bupivacaine hydrochloride per site, with or without epinephrine 1:200,000, is deposited. Small volumes and/or diluted local anesthetic solutions should be used as initial pain therapy so that the total dose does not exceed 3 mg/kg. Small dogs receive 0.25 mL/site, medium dogs 0.5 mL/site, and large dogs 1.0 mL/site. Postthoracotomy pain is generally controlled for 3 to 6 h after successful block.[26] Heart rate, respiratory rate, hematocrit, plasma protein, blood pH, arterial oxygen partial pressure (PaO_2), and arterial carbon dioxide partial pressure ($PaCO_2$) do not change significantly in halothane-anesthetized dogs after intercostal nerve block.[26,27] Prolonged analgesia may be achieved by repeated administrations of local anesthetics, although a patient may not tolerate multiple percutaneous injections. Intercostal nerve block produces relatively high blood concentrations of local anesthetic for a given dose;[28,29] therefore, the risk of toxic blood concentrations is greater.

Selective intercostal nerve block is easily performed because of the proximity of each nerve to its adjacent rib.[30] The intercostal nerves can be visualized beneath the parietal pleura during thoracotomy. This technique provides consistent analgesia and does not produce respiratory depression, with subsequent hypercarbia and hypoxemia, which is a more frequent problem in dogs administered intramuscular or intravenous opioids.[26,31] Because intercostal bupivacaine (0.5%, 0.5 to 1.0 mL) abolishes nociceptive input only from tissues supplied by the intercostal nerves,

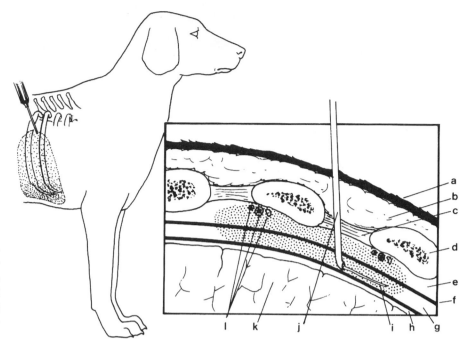

Fig. 20.9. Interpleural catheter placement. **Inset:** (a) skin, (b) subcutaneous tissue, (c) intercostal muscles, (d) rib, (e) subcostal space, (f) pleura costalis and fascia, (g) interpleural space, (h) pleura pulmonalis, (i) catheter, (j) Tuohy needle, (k) lung, and (l) intercostal artery, vein and nerve.

but not from the whole surgical site, additional analgesia with preoperatively administered epidural morphine (0.1 mg/kg) has been suggested to improve both intraoperative and immediate postoperative analgesia in dogs after thoracotomy.[32]

Interpleural Regional Analgesia

Interpleural injection of local anesthetics is a relatively new option for managing certain types of acute and chronic pain originating from thoracic and upper abdominal structures in humans.[33] Pain from rib fractures, metastasis to the chest wall, pleura, and mediastinum, mastectomy, chronic pancreatitis, cholecystectomy, renal surgery, abdominal cancer, and posthepatic neuralgia can be relieved by intermittent or continuous administration of local anesthetic into the pleural space through a catheter, without the systemic effects commonly observed after the use of parenterally administered (IM or IV) opioids.[34] Most clinical studies have been performed in patients recovering from gallbladder surgery. Less frequently, this technique has been used for pain relief in patients with multiple fractured ribs; other indications are uncommon.[35] Reports in the current literature provide evidence both supporting[36,37] and opposing[38–40] the effectiveness of postoperative pain management via interpleural analgesia after thoracotomy for pulmonary surgery in humans. The mechanisms of pain relief produced by interpleural analgesia are not fully understood, but at least three different sites of actions have been hypothesized: (a) retrograde diffusion of local anesthetic through the parietal pleura, causing intercostal nerve block;[41,42] (b) unilateral block of the thoracic sympathetic chain and splanchnic nerves;[43] and (c) diffusion of the anesthetic into the ipsilateral brachial plexus, resulting in a parietal block.[33]

The technique requires the insertion of a catheter into the pleural space of sedated or anesthetized dogs.[26,44–51] The catheter is placed into the pleural space either percutaneously or prior to closure of a thoracotomy (Fig. 20.9). Percutaneous placement of a catheter into the pleural space is difficult to perform on dogs with pleural fibrosis, because thickening of the pleura makes identification of the pleural space guesswork. The dog should be sedated, and the skin, subcutaneous tissues, periosteum, and parietal pleura over the caudal border of the rib should first be desensitized with 1 to 2 mL of 2% lidocaine solution, using a 2.5- to 5-cm, 20- to 22-gauge needle. A 5.0-cm × 1.4-mm outer diameter, 17-gauge Huber point (Tuohy) needle is then used for catheter placement. The stylet is removed and the needle filled with sterile saline until a meniscus is seen at the needle's hub. The needle is then advanced until a clicking sensation is perceived as the needle tip perforates the parietal pleura or until the meniscus disappears when the needle tip enters the pleural space (hanging-drop technique).

The hanging-drop technique for the identification of the subatmospheric pleural pressure is not always reliable because the meniscus may also disappear when the needle passes through the intercostal muscles. Alternatively, a freely moving 10-mL glass syringe is attached to the needle. The syringe and needle are then advanced as a unit. On entering the pleural space, the plunger of the syringe is drawn inward by the negative pressure of the interpleural space.[34] Some veterinarians place the catheter in the tissue plane superficial to the parietal pleura, close to or in the subcostal space (e in Fig. 20.9), in order to produce a more effective block attributable to a decreased loss of local anesthetic through thoracic drainage tubes.[35] A catheter (6- to 10-cm length of fenestrated medical grade silastic tubing, 2-mm inside diameter) can

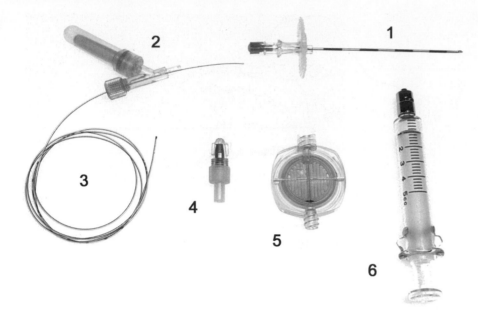

Fig. 20.10. Interpleural tray for continuous interpleural analgesia. The basic Pleurocert procedure set contains (1) Tuohy needle (1.7 × 80 mm, 16 gauge × 31/4 inches), (2) Y piece with control balloon, (3) radiopaque polyamide catheter (0.65 × 1.05 × 1000 mm), (4) screw connector, (5) luer lock antibacteria injection filter (0.2 μm), and (6) 5-mL glass syringe.

be introduced and advanced 3 to 5 cm beyond the needle tip with minimal resistance after the needle tip is placed subpleurally.

A technique has been developed to insert the catheter without disconnection to minimize the risk of pneumothorax.[52] The technique involves the use of a Tuohy needle to which a Y piece with a latex balloon and catheter is attached (Fig. 20.10). The needle is inserted until the balloon collapses under the negative pressure of the pleural cavity; the catheter is then advanced as required. The needle is then carefully withdrawn over the catheter, and the catheter is left in place.

Approximately 1 to 2 mg of bupivacaine/kg (0.5%, with or without 5 μg of epinephrine/mL) is injected over 1 to 2 min following negative aspiration of air or blood through the catheter. The catheter is then cleared with 2 mL of physiological saline solution. Bolus interpleural bupivacaine is effective in relieving postthoracotomy pain for 3 to 12 h.[26] The addition of epinephrine (5 μg/mL) to the local anesthetic solution may or may not increase the duration of analgesia and decrease the plasma concentration of the local anesthetic.

Complications, such as lung trauma, bleeding, and pneumothorax, are occasionally reported with the blind percutaneous insertion technique in humans.[53] The balloon technique is superior to other methods (i.e., loss-of-resistance technique, low-friction syringe-piston movement, and infusion technique). Sterile sets for single continuous interpleural analgesia are available that contain a Tuohy needle, catheter, control balloon, flat antibacterial injection filter, screw connector, screwdriver, and drape (Fig. 20.10).

A catheter can be placed in the open chest by inserting the Tuohy needle through the skin over the rib at a site that is at least two intercostal spaces caudal to the incision while care is taken to retract the lung. The catheter is then passed through the needle and placed 3 to 5 cm subpleurally under direct vision. Local anesthetic is injected in the usual manner. The ventral tip of the catheter is best anchored by using one encircling suture of surgical gut (3.0) in the intercostal space at the site of puncture.

Positioning of the catheter will affect the site of intercostal nerve blockade and is attributable to gravity-induced pooling of the local anesthetic within the interpleural space.[44,45,54] Dogs that recover from lateral thoracotomy should be placed with the incision side down. Dogs that have had a sternotomy should be placed in sternal recumbency for approximately 10 min to allow the local anesthetic to pool near the incision and adjacent intercostal nerves. The external portion of the catheter should be anchored with tape, sutured to the skin, and covered with a no-occlusive-type dressing that allows air circulation. Reportedly, analgesia produced by interpleural infusion in dogs is similar to analgesia produced by morphine (0.5 mg/kg subcutaneously) or selective intercostal nerve block with bupivacaine (0.5 mL of 0.5% bupivacaine per site), but lasts longer (3 to 12 h).[26] Dogs treated with 1.5 mg of interpleural bupivacaine/kg through an interpleural catheter do not demonstrate significant changes in heart rate, respiratory rate, hematocrit, plasma protein, blood pH, or $PaCO_2$.[26,49,50,51]

Studies have been performed to evaluate cardiovascular effects of low-dose interpleural bupivacaine (0.5%, 1.5 mg/kg), high-dose interpleural bupivacaine (0.5%, 3 mg/kg), and high-dose interpleural bupivacaine (0.5%, 3 mg/kg) with epinephrine 1:200,000 (5 μg/mL) in four dogs recovering from diazepam-ketamine-1.2% halothane and oxygen anesthesia.[47,49] The local anesthetic drugs were administered via an interpleural catheter (25 cm long) that was advanced through a 17-gauge needle at the left or right eighth intercostal space. Pneumothorax or any other pulmonary complication was not observed in any of the dogs evaluated radiographically. The low dosage rate (1.5 mg/kg) of 0.5% bupivacaine produced no significant ($P < 0.05$) alterations in heart rate, systolic, diastolic, and mean arterial blood pressure, cardiac output, and pulmonary arterial blood pressure, respiratory rate, and end-tidal carbon dioxide. Cardiac output, expressed as a percentage of change from baseline, was significantly higher in dogs receiving the low dosage (1.5 mg/kg) than dogs receiving the high dosage (3 mg/kg) of interpleural bupivacaine (126% ± 6% vs. 94% ± 6% change). Mean plasma concentrations of bupivacaine peaked 5 to 15 min after interpleural injection. Mean plasma concentrations of bupivacaine in individual dogs were variable and did not significantly ($P < 0.05$) differ among dogs treated with the low dose (1.5 mg/kg), high dose (3 mg/kg), and high dose (3 mg/kg) with epinephrine (1:200,000) of interpleural bupivacaine (0.5%).[49] Mean arterial blood pressure was decreased to 28 mm Hg in one dog 15 min after interpleural administration of 3 mg of bupivacaine/kg and was decreased to 37 mm Hg in one dog receiving 3 mg of bupivacaine/kg with epinephrine. This dog also demonstrated apnea for approximately 6 min and required positive-pressure ventilation. The maximum plasma concentration of bupivacaine in these hypotensive dogs was 3.4 and 3.6 µg/mL, respectively.[49] The high dosage rate (3 mg/kg) for interpleural administration is not recommended because it may cause hypotension in some individual animals. Careful patient monitoring is advised if dosages approach 3 mg/kg. The addition of epinephrine 5 µg/mL may not be of any advantage because it does not attenuate peak plasma concentrations.[49]

The effects of interpleural bupivacaine (0.5%, 1.5 mg/kg), intramuscular morphine (1.0 mg/kg), or interpleural morphine (0.1 mg/kg) have also been compared. Interpleural bupivacaine produced longer analgesia, less work of breathing, fewer blood-gas alterations, and earlier return to normal pulmonary function in the first 5 to 8 h after thoracotomy.[50] Interpleural administration of morphine (0.1 mg/kg) did not appear to provide any advantages in terms of analgesia or pulmonary function when compared with the intramuscular administration of morphine (1.0 mg/kg). These results differ from other experimental trials in dogs receiving either 0.5% bupivacaine (1.5 mg/kg) interpleurally, morphine (1.0 mg/kg) IM, or morphine (1.0 mg/kg) interpleurally.[51] Medium sternotomy significantly decreased pH, PaO_2, mean oxygen saturation of hemoglobin, and dynamic compliance; and significantly increased $PaCO_2$, alveolar-arterial difference in the partial pressure of oxygen, pulmonary resistance, and work of breathing. The effects of interpleural administration of bupivacaine and morphine were similar to effects of intramuscular administration of morphine and provided little or no additional benefit. It is not known what the effects of dilution by pleural fluid, such as blood and serum, and loss of local anesthetic through the thoracotomy tube are on overall efficacy. The dose of interpleural bupivacaine may have been inadequate in this study, considering that sternotomy may be more painful than intercostal thoracotomy.

The optimum total dose, concentration, or volume of interpleural bupivacaine in sick dogs have not been reported. Theoretically, one or two of the three branches of the phrenic nerve can be blocked, leaving the remaining branch(es) intact. Isolated contraction of the costal portion of the diaphragm without contraction of the crural portion may result in paradoxical respiration with negative intra-abdominal pressure.[46] The catheter is usually removed 24 h after thoracotomy when postoperative pain has normally decreased. Long-term use (over several weeks) of an interpleural catheter is possible if the catheter is subcutaneously tunneled.[55]

The administration of interpleural bupivacaine is greatly facil-

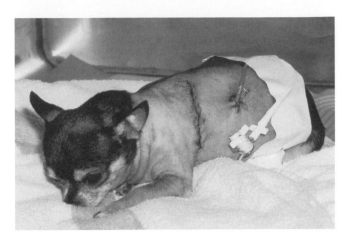

Fig. 20.11. Pain therapy in a Chihuahua (2 kg) recovering from left lateral thoracotomy and correction of a patent ductus arteriosus Botalli: 0.5% bupivacaine (1.5 mg/kg) was administered into a chest tube, which was placed interpleurally (total dose = 3 mg = 0.6 mL), and then the chest tube was cleared from the anesthetic with 0.6 mL of 0.9% sterile sodium chloride.

itated in dogs in which a chest tube has been placed for evacuation of air (Fig. 20.11). Interpleural regional analgesia has limitations but also several distinct advantages over the more traditional intercostal nerve block or the administration of parenteral opioids. The procedure is technically simple to perform. Only one needle stick is needed, in contrast to multiple sites of injection when performing an intercostal nerve block. Pain relief lasts longer and is less likely to produce CNS and respiratory depression than after the use of parenteral opioids. Interpleural administration of the local anesthetic (lidocaine or bupivacaine) approximately 30 min prior to removal of the chest tube helps to prevent pain associated with the tube removal.

Infection, tachyphylaxis to local anesthetic, high anesthetic blood concentration, systemic toxicity from local anesthesia, unilateral sympathetic block (evidenced as a Horner's syndrome) and increased subcutaneous skin temperature of the affected side, pleural effusion, phrenic nerve paralysis or paresis, and catheter-related complications (e.g., intrapulmonary placement of catheter) do not occur if the procedure is performed properly. Pain relief is minimal in people and dogs with a misplaced catheter, loss of local anesthetic in the chest tube, excessive bleeding into the pleural space, or altered diffusion within the parietal pleura after mechanical irritation by the surgical procedure.[56] A dilution of local anesthetic by pleural exudation appears to play a subordinate role in humans because a relationship between a loss of chest tube fluid and interpleural analgesic requirement or pain scores could not be demonstrated.[40] Care must be taken to avoid the serious potential complication of pneumothorax, particularly when this method is used bilaterally.[57]

Anesthesia of the Foot and Leg

Several techniques may be used to induce anesthesia of the foot and leg successfully: (a) infiltration of tissues around the limb by

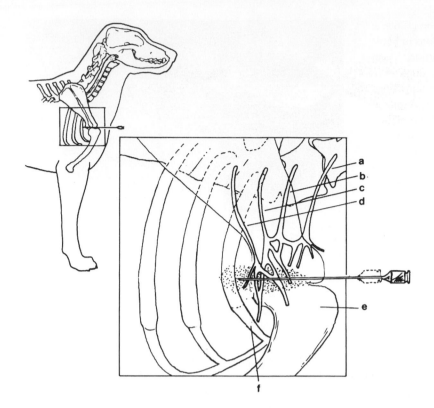

Fig. 20.12. Needle placement for brachial plexus block. **Inset:** ventral branches of (a) sixth, (b) seventh, (c) eighth cervical, and (d) first thoracic spinal nerves; (e) tuberosity of humerus; and (f) first rib.

using local anesthetic solution (ring block), (b) intra-articular injection of local anesthetic, (c) infiltration of the brachial plexus with local anesthetic solution (brachial plexus block), (d) injection of local anesthetic into an accessible superficial vein in an extremity that is isolated from the general circulation by placing a tourniquet proximal to the injection site (intravenous regional anesthesia), (e) perineural infiltration of sensory nerves in the limbs (nerve block), and (f) injection of local anesthetic solution into the lumbosacral epidural space to induce anesthesia of the hind legs,

Ring Block

Local infiltration and field block around the distal extremity may be performed with a 2- to 5-cm, 22- to 23-gauge standard needle. Intradermal wheals around a superficial lesion and subcutaneous infiltration around the limb are performed by using a short (<3 cm) and fine (23- to 25-gauge) needle.

Intra-articular Analgesia

A prospective study has compared the analgesic effect of the intra-articular administration of bupivacaine (0.5%, 0.5 mL/kg), preservative-free morphine (morphine sulfate [Duramorph] injection, USP; Elkins-Sinn, Cherry Hill, NJ) at a dose of 0.1 mg/kg diluted with 0.9% sodium chloride to a volume of 0.5 mL/kg or with 0.9% sodium chloride (0.5 mL/kg).[58] Dogs in the bupivacaine and morphine groups required less supplemental analgesia when morphine (0.5 mg/kg IM) at 6 and 24 h was used after cranial cruciate ligament repair than did the dogs in the 0.9% sodium chloride group. Intra-articular morphine provided some analgesia, as indicated by cumulative pain scores and measurement of pain threshold in both stifles by using a spring-

action load–measuring device (Pain Diagnostics and Thermography, Great Neck, NY), but not to the same level as intra-articular bupivacaine. Intra-articular morphine (0.1 mg/kg) did not produce the bradycardia, respiratory depression, or hypotension that might be observed after systemic administration of morphine. Ongoing inflammation is apparently needed for intra-articular opioids to produce noticeable antinociceptive effects.[59]

Brachial Plexus Block

Brachial plexus block is suitable for operations on the front limb within or distal to the elbow.[60–62] The technique should be done in well-sedated standing or laterally recumbent dogs. A 7.5-cm, 20- to 22-gauge needle is inserted medial to the shoulder joint and directed parallel to the vertebral column toward the costochondral junction (Fig. 20.12). In larger dogs, approximately 10 to 15 mL of 2% lidocaine hydrochloride solution with 1:200,000 epinephrine is injected slowly as the needle is withdrawn, if no blood is aspirated into the syringe, thereby placing local anesthetic in close proximity to the radial, median, ulnar, musculocutaneous, and axillary nerves. Gradual loss of sensation and motor function occurs within 10 to 15 min. Anesthesia lasts for approximately 2 h, and total recovery requires approximately 6 h.

A peripheral nerve stimulator can be used to accurately locate the radial, median, ulnar, musculocutaneous, and axillary nerves, thereby reducing the dose of local anesthetic for successful brachial plexus blockade in dogs.[62] One electrode (the alligator clip on the positively charged lead wire [red plug]) from the nerve locator is attached to the skin, while the other electrode (the alligator clip on the negatively charged lead wire [black plug]) is attached to the proximal portion of the insulated needle (0.72 × 10.8 mm, 22 gauge × 4.25 inches). A 20-mL syringe

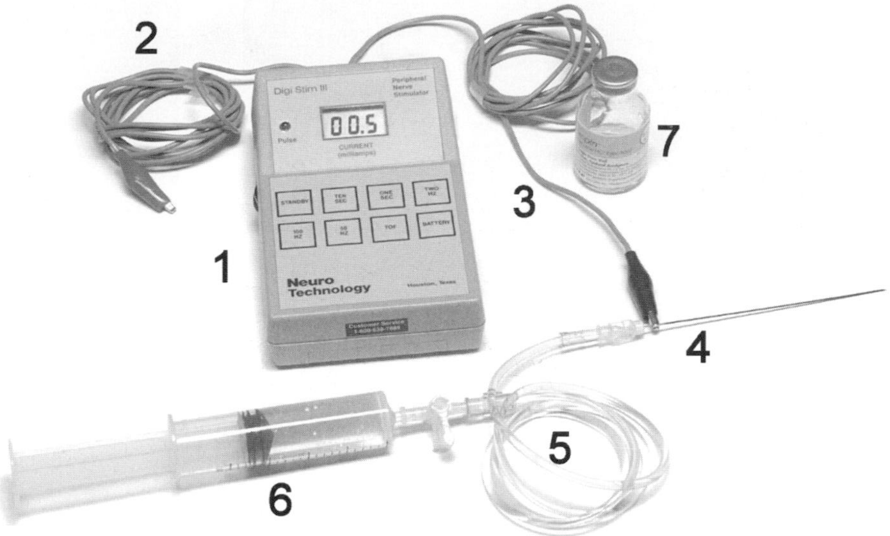

Fig. 20.13. (1) Peripheral nerve-stimulator used as an aid in accurately locating nerves when performing nerve-block procedures: The nerve locator is set at 2 Hz and low output (0.5 mA); the 0.5-mA current delivered to the patient is displayed; (2) the lead wire with red plug (+) and alligator clip for the patient's electrode; (3) the lead wire with black plug (−) and alligator clip for the needle; (4) Stimex insulated needle (22 gauge, 4.25 inches, 0.72 × 10.79 mm); (5) extension set; (6) 20-mL syringe with three-way stopcock, filled with (7) 0.2% ropivacaine hydrochloride.

containing the local anesthetic agent (2% lidocaine, 0.5% ropivacaine, or 0.5% bupivacaine, diluted with 0.9% sodium chloride solution to make a 0.375% concentration) is attached to a three-way stopcock, a fluid extension set, and the needle (Fig. 20.13). As the needle is inserted medial to the scapulohumeral joint toward the costochondral junction of the first rib, medial to the scapula but outside the thorax, the nerve stimulator is turned on to 2 Hz and 1.0 mA. As the paw begins to twitch, the needle is precisely placed to obtain maximal twitch with as little current (<0.5 mA) as possible. At this point, the syringe is aspirated to ensure that it is not in a blood vessel, and 0.1 to 0.2 mL of the anesthetic is injected until the twitch disappears. The technique is repeated three or more times, by fanning the needle dorsal and ventral from the initial placement. Direct deposition of the local anesthetic on the nerves at a maximum dose of 1.5 mg/kg of lidocaine, ropivacaine, or bupivacaine will produce good brachial plexus blockade. By using a nerve stimulator, a total dose of 4 mg of bupivacaine with 5 μg/mL of epinephrine was effective in providing anesthesia for middiaphyseal osteotomies of the humerus followed by intramedullary pin fixation in 11 of 12 dogs sedated with acepromazine and anesthetized with propofol.[62] Analgesia lasted for 11.1 ± 0.5 h.[62]

Brachial plexus block is relatively simple and safe to perform and produces selective anesthesia and relaxation of the limb distal to the elbow joint (Fig. 20.14). The relatively long waiting period (15 to 30 min) required to attain maximal anesthesia and some occasional failures to obtain complete anesthesia, particularly in fat dogs, are disadvantages of the technique.

Intravenous Regional Anesthesia

Intravenous regional anesthesia (IVRA) is a rapid and reliable method for producing short-term (<2 h) anesthesia of the extremities. The clinical value of IVRA in humans is well established. The IVRA technique is also known as *Bier block*.[63] Little information on clinical experiences with IVRA in dogs exists, even

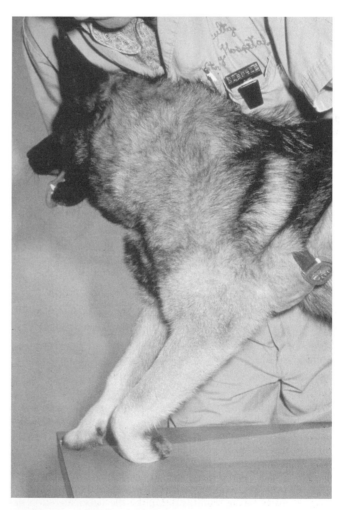

Fig. 20.14. Anesthesia of the brachial plexus of the left thoracic limb in a conscious dog.

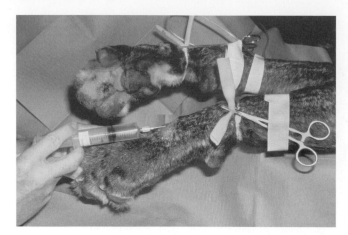

Fig. 20.15. Intravenous regional anesthesia in a sedated bullmastiff (80 kg) in right lateral recumbency for skin biopsies at the palmar paws of both front legs. A rubber tourniquet is placed distal to the carpus (right foot) and proximal to the carpus (left foot). The tourniquets are secured with hemostatic forceps, which are taped to the skin. Injection of 12 mL of 1% lidocaine hydrochloride solution (1.5 mg/kg per leg) into the cephalic vein is shown.

though it appears to be a simple, safe, and practical method for providing 60 to 90 min of regional anesthesia in an extremity distal to a tourniquet (Fig. 20.15).[64,65] The technique is best accomplished in dogs by placing an intravenous catheter in an appropriate and accessible vein (e.g., the cephalic or lateral saphenous vein) distal to the tourniquet. The limb is first desanguinated by wrapping it with an Esmarch bandage. A rubber tourniquet is placed around the limb proximal to the Esmarch bandage. The tourniquet must be tight enough to overcome arterial blood pressure.[66] Once the tourniquet is secured, the Esmarch bandage is unwrapped, and 2.5 to 5 mg/kg lidocaine is injected IV with light pressure. A period of 5 to 10 min is required to achieve maximum anesthesia before beginning the surgical procedure. Diluted concentrations (0.25% and 0.5%) of lidocaine produce adequate sensory blockade as long as the tourniquet is applied. By avoiding leakage and keeping the local anesthetic isolated in the limb, the incidence and severity of toxic symptoms are decreased and the percentage of successful blocks increased.[66] Complications resulting from blood-flow deprivation to the limb or from the dose of anesthetic used do not occur if the procedure is limited to 90 min.

Once the tourniquet is removed, sensation returns within 5 to 15 min and residual analgesia remains for up to 30 min. Minimal effects on heart rate, respiratory rate, or the electrocardiogram have been noted in dogs after removal of the tourniquet.[64] The site and mechanism of local anesthetic action in IVRA are unclear but may involve desensitization of major nerve trunks and/or sensory nerve endings.[67] Unlike the desensitization described in other nerve blocks, the onset of anesthesia and muscle paralysis begins distally and progresses proximally; thus, the local anesthetic should be injected as distally as possible in the limb to be anesthetized (Fig. 20.16). The blood-free surgery site

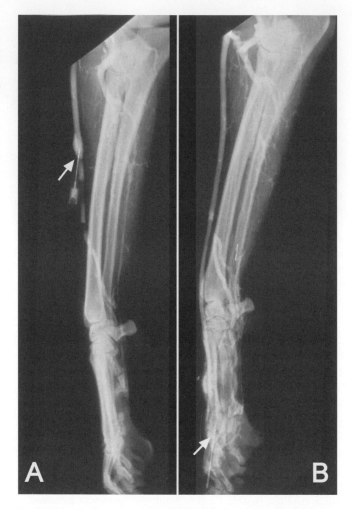

Fig. 20.16. Radiographs of the left forelimb of a German shepherd (35 kg). **A:** A mixture of 3 mL of 2% lidocaine hydrochloride solution and 3 mL of Omnipaque 300 was injected into the cephalic vein at a proximal site. Retrograde dissipation of the anesthetic was prohibited by venous valves; thus, anesthesia of the limb did not develop. **B:** The injection was repeated at a distal site 1 week later, thereby inducing anesthesia of the limb distal to the tourniquet. The *arrow* indicates the injection site.

is ideal for taking biopsy samples and removing a foreign body from the paws. Prolonged procedures (>90 min) may produce tourniquet-induced ischemia, which is associated with pain and increased blood pressure. If pain occurs, it is often difficult to control and requires induction of general anesthesia.[68] Reversible shock occurs if the tourniquet is removed after 4 h; and sepsis, endotoxemia, and death occur if the tourniquet is removed after 8 to 10 h. Bupivacaine should not be used for this technique because of the increased potential for cardiovascular collapse and death associated with its use IV.[69–72]

Nerve Blocks of the Limbs

Specific nerve blocks in the front limbs (radial, ulnar, median, and musculocutaneous nerves) and hind limbs (tibial, peroneal, and saphenous nerves) of dogs have been described.[73] These

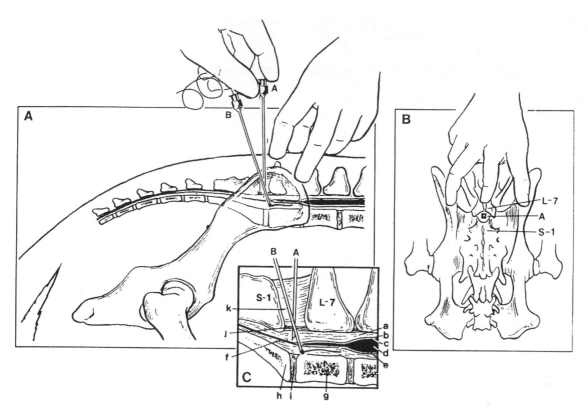

Fig. 20.17. **A:** Aseptic needle placement, using sterile surgical gloves, into the lumbosacral epidural space of a dog (A) and catheter placement for continuous epidural anesthesia using a local anesthetic and/or analgesia using an opioid (B). **B:** Dorsal view. Palpation of the dorsal spinous process of the L7 vertebra and dorsoiliac wings. **C:** Inset: (a) epidural space with fat and connective tissue, (b) dura mater, (c) arachnoid membrane, (d) spinal cord, (e) cerebrospinal fluid, (f) cauda equina, (g) seventh lumbar (L7) vertebra, (h) first sacral (S1) vertebra, (i) intervertebral disc, (j) interarcuate ligament (ligamentum flavum), and (k) interspinous ligament.

techniques are rarely used in clinical small animal practice because of difficulty in locating the proper site for injection of local anesthetic and the substitution of simpler methods (e.g., IVRA and epidural anesthesia).

Lumbosacral Epidural Anesthesia

This technique is noted for its simplicity, safety, and effectiveness, and is one of the most frequently used regional anesthetic techniques described for surgical procedures caudal to the umbilicus in dogs.[74–98] Epidural anesthesia is frequently recommended for cesarean section because, unlike other anesthetic techniques, it does not depress the puppies. The bitch remains awake and able to take care of her puppies immediately after surgery.

Dogs are generally sedated, tranquilized, or anesthetized to reduce fear and apprehension and then are placed either in sternal recumbency (for bilateral anesthesia) or in lateral recumbency (for ipsilateral anesthesia). The hind limbs can be extended cranially to maximally separate the lumbar vertebrae, making identification of the lumbosacral space easier.

The anesthetic procedure is not technically difficult when performed by an experienced clinician. The epidural space is located between the inner and outer layers of the dura mater (Fig. 20.17).

It contains nerves (cauda equina), fat, blood vessels, lymphatics, and occasionally the end of the spinal cord with its surrounding meninges (arachnoid and dura mater). The subarachnoid space contains cerebrospinal fluid (CSF). After a thorough surgical preparation, the local anesthetic solution is injected through a disposable 2.5- to 7.5-cm, 20- to 22-gauge spinal needle as a single dose or is injected through a catheter that is inserted at least 1.5 to 2.0 cm beyond the end of an 18- or 17-gauge Huber-point (Tuohy) or 18-gauge Crawford needle (continuous technique [Figs. 20.17 and 20.20]). A 2.5-cm, 22-gauge spinal needle is used for small dogs, a 3.8-cm, 20-gauge needle for medium-sized dogs, and a 7.5-cm 18-gauge needle for large dogs. Important landmarks for needle placement are easily identified in most dogs. The iliac prominences on either side of the spine are palpated by using the thumb and middle finger of one hand (Fig. 20.17). The spinous process of the seventh lumbar (L7) vertebra is located with the index finger. The lumbosacral (L7-S1) interspace should be palpated from both the cranial and caudal directions by moving the finger on the dorsal spinous processes of L6 to L7 and S2 to S1. This will help to avoid inadvertent placement of the needle into the L6 to L7 interspace. The needle must be placed correctly on the midline and caudal to the L7 spinous process, and is inserted until a distinct popping sensation is felt as the needle point penetrates the interarcuate ligament. Tail movement may indicate that the needle has engaged nerve tissue. The epidural space is best identified by the *loss-of-resistance test*, using either an air-filled or a saline-filled syringe. Deliberate injection of 3 to 4 mL of air into the epidural space of dogs weighing 20 to 27 kg results in bubble formation that can persist for 24 h. The bubbles, however, are not large or numerous enough to impede transfer of local anesthetic across the meninges and into the CSF, spinal roots, and cord, nor do they localize in any particular region (e.g., nerve roots); thus, subsequent injection of local anesthetic does not result in patchy anesthesia or inadequacies attributable to bubbles.[99] Subcutaneous crepitation may be felt at the site of skin penetration if air has been injected outside the epidural space.

After the needle has been placed, the stylet is removed from the needle hub and the stylet is carefully examined for CSF or blood smears. Also, the needle (or catheter) should be carefully inspected for flow of CSF or blood before the local anesthetic is administered. If inadvertent subarachnoid puncture occurs, as indicated by the presence of CSF, the procedure may either be abandoned or the intended epidural dose reduced by at least 50%. The presence of blood indicates penetration of the ventral venous plexus, after which the needle should be repositioned epidurally. Obtaining CSF at the L7 to S1 site is not uncommon, even though the subarachnoid space of dogs usually ends cranial to the lumbosacral interspace. The spinal cord and meninges in younger and smaller dogs may occasionally extend into the lumbosacral vertebral junction.[100] A subarachnoid injection may be made if CSF is encountered, with the precaution that 1 mL of local anesthetic per 10 kg of body weight is then injected over a 1-min period.[90,93] The reduced dose should avoid *total spinal anesthesia* with cardiovascular and respiratory depression or collapse. If blood is encountered, the needle is withdrawn and cleansed, and another attempt is made to place it into the epidural space. Intravascular injection of local anesthetic can cause systemic toxicity, which is characterized by convulsions, cardiopulmonary depression, and the absence of regional anesthesia[70,71,101] Inadvertent subarachnoid administration of small amounts (2 mL) of fresh autologous blood aspirated from the venous plexus during attempted lumbar epidural puncture in dogs may cause pelvic limb spasm. If this occurs, most dogs recover rapidly and demonstrate no signs of meningeal irritation, long-term neurological sequelae, or neuropathological changes.[102] To avoid excessive cranial advancement of neural blockade, it is also good practice to elevate the dog's head for approximately 5 min immediately after completion of the epidural administration of the anesthetic.

The shape and bevel orientation of the spinal needle affect the size of the dural defect. Large dural defects in humans may result in post–lumbar puncture headache attributable to a postulated increased CSF leak. The dural defect produced by a 22-gauge needle is smaller than that produced by a 22-gauge Quincke needle (27,400 vs. 39,400 μm^2). Likewise, a bevel orientation parallel rather perpendicular to the dural fibers causes smaller dural defects (39,400 vs. 73,300 μm^2), because the needle splits rather than cuts the longitudinal dural fibers.[103] It is also important to administer the calculated dose of local anesthetic at the body

temperature of the dog and slow enough (over 45 to 60 s) to avoid causing pain.

Local Anesthetic Drugs

A variety of local anesthetics of different concentrations and doses, and combinations of different local anesthetic drugs, have been used to produce epidural anesthesia in dogs and have induced a wide spectrum of sensory and motor blockades.[81,89,93,96,97,104–109] The selected local anesthetic and dosage (concentration and volume) depends on a dog's size, the desired extent of anesthesia, and the desired onset and duration of anesthetic effect. A test dose of 0.5 to 1.0 mL of 2% lidocaine hydrochloride solution produces almost immediate dilation of the external anal sphincter, followed by relaxation of the tail and ataxia of pelvic limbs, within 3 to 5 min. Approximately 1 mL of 2% lidocaine per 4.5 kg of body weight will completely anesthetize the pelvic limbs and posterior abdomen caudal to the first lumbar (L1) vertebra within 10 to 15 min after administration.[81] The flexor-pinch reflex of pelvic limbs will be absent in 5 to 10 min after injection.[77] Clinical experience indicates that the disappearance of the toe reflexes is associated with surgical anesthesia from midthorax to coccyx sufficient for abdominal surgery.[78] The latent period is prolonged to 20 to 30 min if 0.75% bupivacaine hydrochloride is administered and is attributable to the drug's low solubility and slow uptake by nervous tissue.[93] Good anesthesia for abdominal and orthopedic surgeries caudal to the diaphragm is generally achieved by administering 1 mL/5 kg (maximum, 20 mL) of 2% lidocaine or 0.5% bupivacaine, both with freshly added 1:200,000 epinephrine.

A reduced volume of 2% lidocaine (1 mL/6 kg) is generally satisfactory for epidural anesthesia in dogs for cesarean section. The reason for the (approximately 25%) decrease in dose requirement during pregnancy is unclear.[110] Several theories have been proposed: (a) distension of epidural veins, which decreases the size of the epidural space, and/or increase in the spread of local anesthetic;[111] (b) hormonal changes, which influence proteins that affect membrane sensitivity;[112] and (c) chronic exposure to progesterone, which alters the permeability of intercellular connective-tissue matrix, thereby facilitating diffusion of local anesthetics across the nerve sheath.[113] It is rarely necessary to inject more than 3 mg of lidocaine/kg of body weight for epidural anesthesia during cesarean section in dogs.

The anesthesia duration obtained from the deposition of epidural local anesthetic drugs primarily depends on the drug selected, the dermatomal level of anesthesia, and the presence or absence of epinephrine (Table 20.2). Postoperative analgesia (after general anesthesia) lasts longer when epidural anesthesia is performed at the end of surgery, and is attributable to a diminished intensity of the painful stimulus. Two percent solutions of procaine, lidocaine, and carbocaine have provided satisfactory anesthesia and muscle relaxation for 60 to 120 min. Epidural bupivacaine (0.75%) and etidocaine (1%) have induced surgical anesthesia for periods lasting from 4 to 6 h. Surgical anesthesia caudal to the last rib is produced and gradually converted into a phase of postoperative analgesia lasting for 24 h without affecting motor activity or cardiopulmonary function, if a combination of 0.7 to 1.0 mL/10-cm vertex-coccyx distance of 0.5% bupiva-

Table 20.2. Commonly used local anesthetic drugs and doses for peripheral and epidural block procedures in conscious dogs.

Local Anesthetic		Usual Doses (mg/kg)			Toxic Doses, IV (mg/kg)		Approximate Onset of Motor and Sensory Block (min)	Approximate Duration of Motor and Sensory Block (h)	Motor Block
Generic Name	Trade Name (Manufacturer)	Conc. (%)	With Epinephrine	Without Epinephrine	Convulsive	Lethal			
Ester linked									
Procaine	Novocaine (Withrop Laboratories)	1–2	8	6	36	100	10–15	0.5	±
Chloroprocaine	Nesacaine (Pennwalt)	1.0–1.5	8	6	—	—	7–15	0.5–1.0	±
Amide linked									
Lidocaine	Xylocaine (Astra Pharmaceutical Products)	0.5–2.0	7	5	11–20	16–28	10–15	1–2	+
Mepivacaine	Carbocaine (Breon Laboratories)	1–2	7	5	29	—	5–10	2.0–2.5	+
Bupivacaine	Marcaine (Breon Laboratories)	0.25–0.5	3	2	3.5–4.5	5–11	20–30	2.5–6.0	±
Ropivacaine	LEA 103 (Breon Laboratories)	0.5	5	3	4.9	—	5–15	2.5–4.0	+
Etidocaine	Duranest (Astra Pharmaceutical Products)	0.5–0.75	5	3	4.5	20	5–10	2–5	+++

Conc., concentration; IV, intravenous; ±, inconsistent motor nerve block; +, weak motor nerve block; +++, strong motor nerve block.

caine hydrochloride solution and 0.1 mg/kg of morphine hydrochloride is injected epidurally.[114]

The efficacy of bupivacaine and ropivacaine for producing lumbar epidural and subarachnoid anesthesia in dogs has been compared.[104] Various concentrations of ropivacaine (0.25%, 0.5%, 0.75%, and 1.0%) and bupivacaine (0.25%, 0.5%, and 0.75%) with a constant 3-mL epidural volume and 1-mL subarachnoid volume of ropivacaine and bupivacaine were assessed. Epidural blockade was also performed using solutions of ropivacaine and bupivacaine that contained epinephrine (1:200,000). There were no signs of adverse reactions, irreversible block, or other sequelae in any of the dogs studied. Onset of motor blockade (time from the completion of the injection until a dog's pelvic limbs cannot support weight) ranged from 1.7 to 4.1 min following subarachnoid injection. There were no differences in the onset of motor blockade between various anesthetic solutions. Duration of motor blockade (time from onset of motor blockade until the dog could support its own weight) ranged from 103 min (0.75% ropivacaine) to 163 min (0.75% bupivacaine). Solutions of 0.25% ropivacaine and 0.25% bupivacaine failed to induce complete loss of weight support following epidural injection. Onset of motor blockade varied between 5 and 9 min with the use of higher concentrations (>0.25%) and was inversely related to dose. Duration of motor blockade ranged from 141 min (0.5% ropivacaine) to 258 min (0.75% bupivacaine). The similar onset times for both drugs were related to their similar pKa (ropivacaine, 8.0; and bupivacaine, 8.1). The decreased motor-blocking potency of ropivacaine is consistent with its low lipid solubility. Epinephrine failed to prolong the duration of motor blockade for either drug. Little difference in vascular activity may exist between ropivacaine and bupivacaine when injected into the epidural space of dogs.[104]

A direct comparison between the effect of epidural bupivacaine and ropivacaine, using 0.5% and 0.75% solutions and 0.14- and 0.22-mL/kg volumes, on analgesia at the perineum (S3 dermatome), right and left hind-toe web (L5 to L7 dermatomes), flank (L2 to L5 dermatomes), and caudodorsal rib areas (T12 to L1 dermatomes), and associated cardiopulmonary effects (heart rate, systemic arterial blood pressure, pH, $PaCO_2$, PaO_2 bicarbonate, and base excess) in six dogs sedated with acepromazine (0.075 mg/kg IM) has been reported.[109] Sterile local anesthetic drugs were slowly administered (rate, 3 mL/min) into the epidural space at the lumbosacral junction via implantable vascular access ports.[115] The results of this study indicate that 0.22 mL/kg of 0.5% bupivacaine and ropivacaine produce greater anesthesia success at dermatomes L5 to L7 than does 0.5% at 0.14 mL/kg (>80% vs. <70% success), a similar extent of anesthesia, and mild cardiopulmonary changes. Varying the bupivacaine concentration did not affect the duration of perineal analgesia. Perineal analgesia with 0.5% and 0.75% ropivacaine has been reported to be slightly shorter than that achieved with 0.5% and 0.75% bupivacaine (115 to 140 vs. 137 to 145 min).[109]

Lidocaine and Bupivacaine Combination

The effects of epidural administration of lidocaine (2%, 5 mg/kg with epinephrine 1:200,000), bupivacaine (0.5%, 1.25 mg/kg with epinephrine 1:200,000), and lidocaine (2%, 2.5 mg/kg with epinephrine 1:200,0000) combined with bupivacaine (0.5%, 0.61 mg/kg with epinephrine 1:200,000) on the time of interdigital reflex loss, duration of analgesia and muscle relaxation, and cardiorespiratory effects in six dogs, weighing 5 to 10 kg, have been compared.[97] The combination of epidural bupivacaine with lidocaine achieves a shorter time to sphincter relaxation than does bupivacaine alone (23 ± 2 vs. 84 ± 23 s), longer analgesia than lidocaine alone (94 ± 8 vs. 54 ± 5 min), and longer muscle relaxation than either lidocaine (102 ± 8 vs. 59 ± 6 min) or bupivacaine (102 ± 8 vs. 57 ± 20 min). The combination of epidural lidocaine and bupivacaine produces minimal changes in arterial oxygen saturation, end-tidal carbon dioxide, respiratory and heart rates, and mean arterial blood pressure, and appears to be the best choice for maintaining anesthesia when surgical time is prolonged.[97]

Pharmacokinetics and Pharmacodynamic Properties

Local anesthetics injected epidurally may enter the CSF,[74,116] epidural venous blood, or lymph[80] and become partitioned in epidural fat. Epidurally administered drugs are dispersed by entering the lymphatic system by diffusion into the dural lymphatic vessels located at the level of the nerve roots, by leakage of local anesthetic drug out of the vertebral canal through the intervertebral foramina, and by vascular absorption and systemic redistribution.[117]

The pharmacokinetics of bupivacaine and ropivacaine after lumbar epidural administrations of either drug (0.75% solution, 3-mL volume with or without 1:200,000 epinephrine) in dogs have been determined.[70] Both drugs have a similar pharmacokinetic profile. Peak arterial concentrations of bupivacaine and ropivacaine occur within 5 to 10 min after injection and were less than 1 µg/mL. The addition of epinephrine did not consistently decrease the clearance (C_{max}) of either agent.

The disposition and pharmacological effects of bupivacaine[118] and, most recently, those of the S(−) isomer of bupivacaine[119] after intravenous and epidural administration in dogs have been reported. Bupivacaine (1.0 mg/kg IV) resulted in a mean ± standard deviation half-life of 34.5 ± 7.8 min, a mean plasma clearance of 20.2 ± 7.4 mL/kg/min, and a mean volume of distribution at a steady state of 0.7 ± 0.2 L/kg. After epidural administration of 0.5% bupivacaine (1.8 mg/kg), the peak plasma concentration was 1.4 ± 0.4 µg/mL approximately 5 min after administration. Onset and duration of anesthesia were 2.3 ± 2.2 min and 158 ± 49 min, respectively. The mean bupivacaine plasma concentration ranged between 0.2 and 1.4 µg/mL, and the half-life was 179 ± 34 min.[118] After intravenous administration of a 1-mg/kg dose of the S(−) isomer of bupivacaine (0.5%), the mean ± standard deviation half-life was 33.5 ± 17 min, the mean plasma clearance was 21 ± 11 mL/kg/min, and the mean volume of distribution at steady state was 0.8 ± 0.2 L/kg. Mean peak plasma concentration was 2.6 ± 0.7 µg/mL. Following epidural administration of the same dose peak plasma concentration decreased to 0.9 ± 0.5 µg/mL. Motor block began immediately after completion of epidural injection and lasted for 3 to 4 h.[119]

It has been shown that epidural anesthesia that extends as far cranially as the anterior thoracic dermatomes (T3 to T5) does not adversely change cardiovascular function, respiratory rate, arterial blood pH, and gas tensions (PaO_2 and $PaCO_2$) in conscious dogs or those sedated with methadone (0.8 mg/kg), acepromazine (0.3 mg/kg), or atropine (0.6 to 1.2 mg).[89] In awake healthy dogs, it is thought that compensation for markedly attenuated spinal sympathetic outflow during thoracic epidural anesthesia is accomplished by increasing endogenous vasopressin concentrations to support arterial blood pressure.[120,121] Severe hypotension (with mean arterial blood pressure < 60 mm Hg) can occur in aged and sick dogs with suppressed neurally mediated renin release or when endogenous vasopressin is prevented from acting on its vasopressin receptors.[79,121] Hypotension should be treated with intravenous crystalloid solutions (20 to 30 mL/kg) and/or a vasopressor (e.g., phenylephrine or ephedrine).[122] Hepatic and renal blood flow generally remains stable in dogs undergoing epidural anesthesia until the T1 to L3 spinal cord segments begin to be blocked. Arterial blood pressure can decrease to less than 30% to 40% of the preepidural anesthesia value with a high epidural block. Ephedrine (2.5 μg/kg/min) has been used successfully to rescue hypotensive dogs and return blood-flow values during high epidural anesthesia.[123]

High epidural anesthesia to the T1 myotomal level has been associated with increased intrathoracic volume at end expiration via an increase in intrathoracic tissue volume and the amount of gas in the lungs at end expiration (functional residual capacity).[124] It has been postulated that the increases in thoracic tissue volume are attributable to increases in intrathoracic blood volume. Thoracic epidural block before the production of experimental hemorrhagic shock has been advocated as potentially therapeutic.[95] Endocardial blood flow improves, and determinants of myocardial oxygen consumption decrease.[125]

Rectal temperature usually remains unchanged during epidural anesthesia in dogs. If hypothermia occurs after epidural injections, the cause might be redistribution of heat within the body.[126] In humans, fluctuation in skin temperature of the limbs (but not the trunk) and an absence of sweating (dogs have no sweat glands except in the paws)[127] may reflect changes in sympathetic activity after epidural nerve blockade.[94,128] Increased skin temperature in the pelvic limbs (1.2°C) and paws (2.0°C), coupled with decreased skin temperature in the thoracic limbs and thorax (−0.6°C), after bupivacaine lumbar epidural administration has been observed in conscious dogs.

Epidural anesthesia likely suppresses the markers of stress as represented by serum levels of andrenocorticotropic hormone, beta-endorphin, epinephrine, and norepinephrine.[120,129] In addition, epidural anesthesia may inhibit host-defense mechanisms against various microorganisms less than does general anesthesia.[130]

Adverse Effects

Adverse effects associated with epidural and subarachnoid anesthesia in dogs include (a) hypoventilation secondary to respiratory muscle paralysis, which is attributable to the spread of local anesthetic to the cervical spinal segments; (b) hypotension, Horner's syndrome (Fig. 20.18), and hypoglycemia caused by

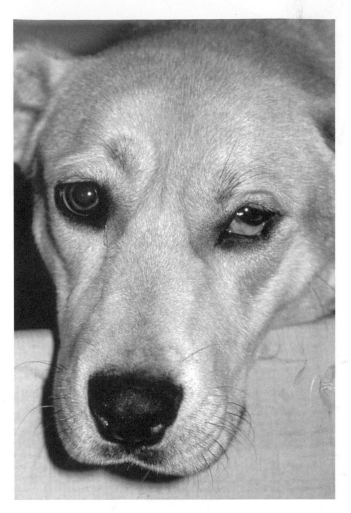

Fig. 20.18. Unilateral Horner's syndrome (i.e., ptosis, miosis, and enophthalmus) in a golden retriever (35 kg) with ipsilateral paresis of the left thoracic limb, after overdose (12 mL of 2% lidocaine) via lumbosacral epidural anesthesia.

sympathetic blockade; (c) Shiff-Sherrington–like reflexes; and (d) muscular twitches, coma, convulsion, and circulatory depression caused by toxic plasma concentrations of local anesthetic. Improper injection technique can cause delay in onset of anesthesia, unilateral hind-limb paresis, partial anesthesia of the tail or the perineal region, and sepsis.[131,132]

Although epidural anesthesia has been referred to as the ideal anesthetic procedure for bitches in dystocia,[77,133,134] respiratory depression can be a serious complication. Changes from a thoracic to a diaphragmatic (abdominal) pattern of breathing indicate at least partial motor block of the intercostal musculature, which may not be reflected by changes in arterial pH, PaO_2, or $PaCO_2$. The use of preblock oxygenation, proper doses of local anesthetic, and slight elevation of the head, neck, and thorax minimize this problem. The presence of paresis of the nictitating membrane of the eye (Fig. 20.18), which derives its sympathetic nerve supply from the first three thoracic spinal segments, is evidence that most, if not all, of the sympathetic outflow has been blocked by extensive epidural spread.

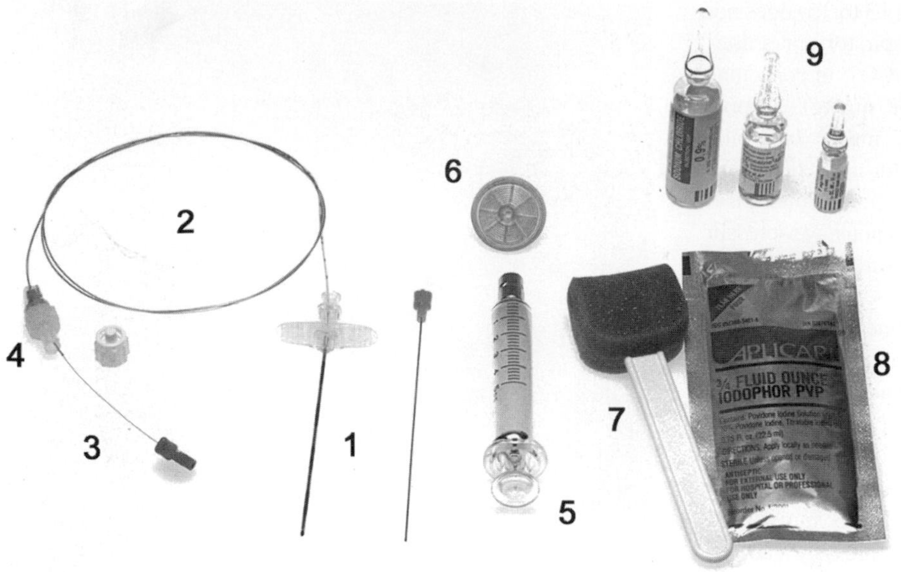

Fig. 20.19. Epidural trays for continuous epidural anesthesia. The basic sterile and single-use regional anesthesia delivery system contains (1) Tuohy needle (1.3 × 87 mm, 18 gauge × 31/2 inches), plastic hub, and detachable wing; (2) radiopaque (polytetrafluoroethylene) catheter with open end and stylet (0.9 × 1000 mm, 20 gauge × 36 inches); (3) catheter stylet; (4) catheter connector with luer plug; (5) 5-mL glass syringe; (6) epidural filter; (7) swabs; (8) iodine packet; and (9) 5 mL of lidocaine hydrochloride 1%, 1-mL epinephrine injection 1:200,000, and 10-mL sodium chloride injection 0.9%.

Anecdotal reports about delayed hair regrowth after epidural analgesia in dogs, though controversial, have been difficult to confirm. In one study, hair regrowth was complete after 4 months, and there was no difference in hair length among groups, indicating that neither epidural analgesia nor scrubbing or clipping seemed to affect hair regrowth in at least the limited number of dogs in this study.[135] In a more recent retrospective study, 8 of 72 dogs were reported to have delayed hair growth after epidural administration of morphine with or without bupivacaine.[136]

Complications with epidural anesthetic techniques can be prevented in most instances by following several basic rules, which include careful selection of drugs and dosage, aspiration before injection (to assure that the tip of the needle is not in a blood vessel or subarachnoid space), and injection of test doses.[96]

Absolute contraindications for epidural anesthetic techniques include infection at the lumbosacral puncture site, uncorrected hypovolemia, bleeding disorders, therapeutic or physiological anticoagulation, degenerative central or peripheral axonal diseases, and anatomical abnormalities that would make epidural anesthesia difficult. Bacteremia, neurological disorders, and minidose heparin therapy are relative contraindications. The benefits of epidural anesthesia often outweigh the risks.[137]

Continuous Epidural Anesthesia

The indications, advantages, contraindications, and complications associated with continuous epidural anesthesia in dogs are similar to those of the single-injection method. Additional advantages of continuous epidural anesthesia are the ability to tailor the anesthesia duration to the length of operation and to maintain a route for injecting epidural opioids during surgery and postoperatively.[86,114,138]

Despite numerous reports describing continuous epidural anesthesia in dogs, epidural catheters are not used routinely because of technical difficulties; the potential to damage the spinal cord, meninges, and nerves; the risk of infection; and catheter-related problems. Nevertheless, insertion of plastic catheters into the epidural space of dogs is relatively simple and safe, once practiced. Local anesthetics and/or opioids may be administered to produce continuous epidural anesthesia by placing a commercially available epidural catheter through an 18- or 17-gauge Huber-point (Tuohy) needle or 18-gauge Crawford needle into the epidural space (Fig. 20.19). Self-prepared sterile 20-gauge catheters (e.g., polyethylene tubing PE 160) may also be used.

A comprehensive selection of epidural products and accessories exists for use in people and can be adapted for dogs, thus making the technique in dogs easier and safer. Epidural trays contain an 8.7-cm, 18-gauge Tuohy needle and a 20-gauge catheter set with a radiopaque Teflon (polytetrafluoroethylene) catheter that resists kinking, with either an open rounded-tip or a closed-tip atraumatic catheter with lateral flow side ports, a thread-assist guidewire that eliminates the need for a stylet, a catheter connector that attaches quickly and securely without possibility of crushing the catheter, a luer-slip glass syringe, and a variety of syringes, needles, sterile preparation solutions, and sponges (Fig. 20.19). The theoretical advantages of the multiple side-port epidural catheter include even distribution of local anesthetic, less chance of clotting (because fibrin is less likely to collect on the side), and the ability to have a completely rounded and therefore atraumatic tip. Catheters should be placed, following strict aseptic technique, by using mask, gown, drapes, and prophylactic antibiotics. A skin preparation, using dry gauze dressings with or without antibiotic ointment (povidone iodine, Neosporin ointment [bacitracin, neomycin, and polymyxin B], or Bactroban ointment [mupirocin]), is very effective in preventing infection. A sterile 4 × 4-inch gauze or OpSite IV 3000 brand of dressing, which collects only minimal fluid underneath it, is tightly adhered to the skin and should be replaced daily or more often as needed to keep the wound dry. Plastic occlusive dressings are not ideal because they collect bacteria of normal skin

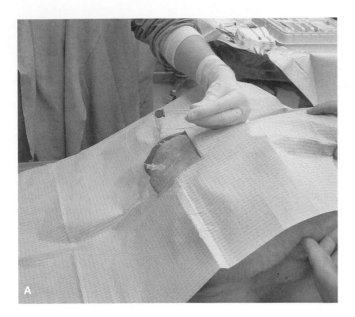

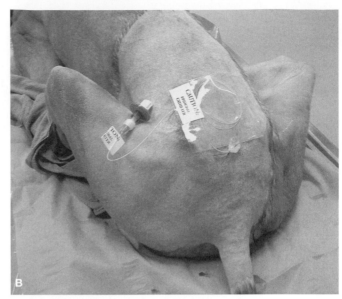

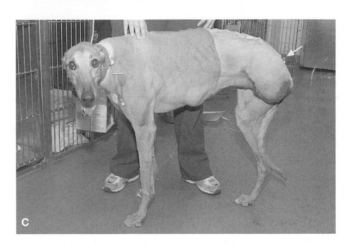

Fig. 20.20. A greyhound (30 kg) with a pathological fracture of the left distal tibia and middiaphysis fibula. **A:** A sterile fenestrated drape is placed over the surgically prepared lumbosacral area of the dog in sternal recumbency, with its hind legs extended cranially. A sterile wire-enforced epidural catheter is inserted into the Tuohy needle aseptically placed into the lumbar epidural space at the lumbosacral junction. **B:** The epidural catheter is advanced to the level of the first lumbar vertebra, is connected to the screw connector and antibacterial injection filter, and is then sutured to the skin. **C:** Administration of preservative-free morphine (0.1 mg/kg) (Astramorph PF, 0.5 mg/mL, total dose = 3 mg = 6 mL) into the epidural catheter rendered the dog pain free and with intact motor function for at least 18 h after limb amputation. The *arrow* points to the epidural catheter filter.

and wound secretions in constant exposure to the catheter site. The use of postoperatively administered systemic antibiotics is debated and is usually reserved for patients with a compromised immune system (e.g., diabetics). A thorough surgical preparation, using soap, antiseptic, or Hibiclens scrub (chlorhexidine cleanser), dramatically reduces the concentration of bacteria on the skin.

The Tuohy needle is placed into the epidural space between the L7 and S1 intervertebral space, similar to the single-injection epidural block technique. Catheterization is facilitated by first desensitizing the lumbosacral space with a small amount (2 mL) of 2% lidocaine. The Tuohy needle is inserted at a 15° to 45° angle from the vertical position with the bevel directed cranially (Figs. 20.17 and 20.20) and is advanced until the epidural space has been entered. The three techniques previously discussed—hanging drop, loss of resistance to air, and loss of resistance to saline—may be more readily performed in dogs that are positioned in sternal rather than lateral recumbency. Because the techniques may not always be ultimate proof that the needle has been placed epidurally, aspiration of the plunger before injection

should verify whether a vein has been entered. At this point, catheters with a stylet are preferred. A slight resistance is usually encountered when the catheter passes through the tip of the Tuohy needle. Special markings on the catheter denote the distance the catheter has been advanced. The catheter is advanced at least two to three markings beyond the hub of the needle, which ensures that at least 2 to 3 cm of catheter has entered the epidural space. Flushing the needle with saline, rotating the needle, and advancing the catheter while slowly withdrawing the needle help to thread the catheter into the epidural space. If these maneuvers fail, the needle and catheter should be withdrawn together. No attempt should be made to withdraw the catheter back through the needle, because this may sever the catheter. If this does occur, most authorities believe that no attempt should be made to retrieve a severed catheter.[105] Wire-reinforced catheters have been inserted epidurally to the anterior lumbar (L4)[139] or thoracic (T1)[116] vertebrae with minimal resistance and without coiling, turning on themselves, kinking, or knotting.

Tuohy needles have been epidurally placed at the second coccygeal (Co3 to Co2), third coccygeal (Co4 to Co3), or fourth coccygeal (Co5 to Co4) intervertebral space of dogs. A wire-reinforced catheter can then be threaded epidurally for up to 15 cm to reach the thoracic vertebrae.[117] Inserting a catheter for long distances increases the risk that the catheter tip may exit a paravertebral foramen. Fluoroscopy is recommended to facilitate catheter guidance.

A 20-cm-long intravenous catheter can be used to tunnel an epidural catheter subcutaneously if it is left in place for a prolonged period. Poor sterile technique when changing tubing and drugs is the most likely cause of catheters becoming infected. Such an infection is often heralded by radicular pain after bolus injections and decreasing analgesia, which generally precedes any sign of meningitis or systemic infection. The CSF (puncture site at C1-C2 to avoid going through an infected lumbar epidural space), epidural catheter (1-mL sterile 0.9% saline solution injected and withdrawn), and skin-insertion site should be cultured if an infection is suspected. After cultures have been obtained, the catheter is removed, and the patient is treated with systemic antibiotics.

Epidural Opioid Analgesia

Providing long-term analgesia while inducing minimal systemic effects is an important objective in medical care. Epidurally administered opiates (e.g., morphine) provide lengthy analgesia caudal to the umbilicus with very few systemic side effects.[30,32,107,136,138–154] A single epidural injection of 5 mg of morphine before major intra-abdominal surgery consistently relieves intraoperative and postoperative pain in people for at least 3 days.[155]

Preservative-free preparations of morphine (e.g., Duramorph PF [Elkins-Sinn, Cherry Hill, NJ] and Astramorph PF [Astra Pharmaceutical Products, Westborough, MA])[156,157] have not been associated with spinal cord histopathological changes. In contrast, parenterally administered morphine, which contains various preservatives—such as sodium bisulfite, metabisulfite, chlorbutanol, edetate disodium, formaldehyde, or phenol—has neurotoxic effects when placed directly on the spinal cord.[158] Any remaining opioid from single-dose vials that contain no bacteriostatic agents should be discarded.[145] Contraindications to epidural opioid analgesia are primarily associated with the epidural catheterization technique itself.

The presence of a large number of opiate receptors in the substantia gelatinosa of the dorsal horn of the spinal cord suggests that the administration of small doses of opioids into the epidural space should produce effective analgesia.[159] The administration of epidural opioids offers the advantage of producing more profound and prolonged analgesia with significantly smaller doses and less sedation than the analgesia produced by comparable parenterally administered (intramuscular or intravenous) opioids. Epidural opioids relieve somatic and visceral pain by selectively blocking nociceptive impulses without interfering with sensory and motor function or depressing the sympathetic nervous system (selective spinal analgesia).[159–165] Studies using subanalgesic doses of the μ-specific agonist (Tyr-D-Ala-Gly-NMe-Phe-Gly-ol [DAGO]) and the δ-specific agonist (D-Pen2-5-Enkephalin [DPDPE]) in cats have demonstrated a supra-additive interaction that significantly suppresses noxious stimuli.[166]

Morphine

The major advantages of selective nociceptive blockade by the use of epidural morphine are long-term pain relief without producing muscle paralysis or weakness, or significant hemodynamic effects. For example, a single dose of morphine (1 mg, diluted in 3 to 4 mL of physiological saline solution) administered via a catheter introduced into the epidural space between the lumbosacral vertebrae and advanced to the fourth and fifth lumbar vertebrae in dogs weighing 10 to 15 kg relieved pain caudal to the costal arch for up to 22 h without affecting heart rate, arterial blood pressure, pulmonary arterial pressure, cardiac output, systemic vascular resistance, PaO_2, mixed venous oxygen tension (PvO_2), $PaCO_2$, and arterial pH (pH_a).[139] Similarly, 0.1 mg of oxymorphone/kg in 3 mL 0.9% of sodium chloride solution administered epidurally in dogs via a catheter positioned between the lumbar L5 to L6 or L6 to L7 intervertebral space alleviated postthoracotomy pain for 10 h without affecting heart rate, respiratory rate, systolic and diastolic blood pressure, and PaO_2 and $PaCO_2$.[167]

The effects of epidural and intravenous morphine on analgesic effectiveness, vital signs, and cortisol and catecholamine concentrations in dogs (18 to 26 kg) after experimental thoracotomy have been compared.[168] Dogs were administered either 0.15 mg/kg of preservative-free morphine epidurally in 5 to 6 mL of 0.9% sodium chloride via a catheter 8 to 10 cm cranial to the entrance of the epidural space 30 to 40 min before the end of surgery or 0.15 mg/kg of morphine IV 5 to 10 min before the end of surgery. The efficacy of the opioid was increased if given before onset of pain. Dogs with epidural morphine administration demonstrated lower subjective pain scores and lower serum cortisol concentrations, plasma adrenaline and noradrenaline concentrations, noninvasive systolic arterial blood pressure, heart rates, and respiratory rates than did dogs with intravenous morphine for the first 10 h postoperatively.[168] A single epidural injection of morphine has been shown to be effective for up to 24 h in preventing physiological responses to postthoracotomy pain, one of the most severe causes of stress in the early postoperative period. In contrast, dogs given morphine IV often require supplemental morphine within 4 to 5 h.[143]

Epidural morphine (0.1 mg/kg diluted in 0.26 mL/kg of saline) decreases the minimum alveolar concentration of halothane and improves arterial blood pressure, cardiac index, stroke volume, left ventricular work, and pulmonary artery pressure in dogs.[169] The explanation for morphine's efficacy at such a low dose when given by the epidural route may be related to its low lipid solubility. Epidural administration of morphine (0.1 mg/kg) is typically one-tenth of the systemically administered dose, yet analgesia lasts significantly longer than that provided by other routes.

Postoperative evaluation of dogs undergoing major orthopedic surgery, using either a 100-μg/h transdermal fentanyl patch applied 24 h before surgery or epidural morphine (0.1 mg/kg) after induction of anesthesia, demonstrated a lower pain score with epidural morphine at 6 h after surgery than with transdermal fen-

Table 20.3. Physiochemical properties and doses of opioids for epidural analgesia in dogs.

Opioid	Molecular Weight of Base	pK^a (25°C)	Oil-water Partition Coefficient^a	Dose (mg/kg)	Approximate Time for Pain Relief (min)	Approximate Duration of Analgesia (h)
Morphine sulfate	285	7.9	1.42	0.05–0.15	30–60	10–24
Meperidine hydrochloride	247	8.5	38.8	0.5–1.5	10–30	5–20
Methadone hydrochloride	309	9.3	116	0.05–0.15	15–20	5–15
Oxymorphone hydrochloride	301	—	—	0.05–0.15	20–40	10–22
Fentanyl citrate	336	8.4	813	0.001–0.01	15–20	3–5

^{a}Octanol–pH 7.4 buffer partition coefficient.

tanyl. However, when all periods (6, 18, 30, and 42 h) after surgery were combined, analgesia with transdermal fentanyl was equivalent to that achieved with epidural morphine.[170]

Epidural administration of morphine sulfate (30 mg) in a multivesicular liposome (Depot Foam) formulation has also been evaluated.[171] Epidural morphine (5 mg and 30 mg), but not liposomes without morphine, produced potent analgesia, as measured by latency of thermally evoked skin twitch. The analgesic index (area under the time effect curve) was significantly greater in dogs treated with encapsulated morphine (30 mg) than in those treated with morphine sulfate (3 mg). The epidurally administered encapsulated morphine formulation produced significantly lower morphine concentrations in lumbar CSF and greater residency time than did epidural morphine. This study indicates that the action of epidural morphine can be extended by delivering higher doses of morphine (30 mg) in an encapsulated, persistent-release form.

Pharmacokinetic and Pharmacodynamic Properties

The physiochemical properties of opioids, particularly their lipid solubility, molecular weight, pK^a, and receptor-binding affinity, are important in determining their pharmacokinetic and pharmacodynamic properties and the onset and duration of analgesia (Table 20.3). Relatively hydrophilic morphine (oil-water partition coefficient, 1:42) remains in the CSF for longer periods, allowing rostral spread and analgesia distant from the site of injection (nonsegmental distribution of analgesia). For example, the lumbosacral epidural administration of 0.1 mg of morphine/kg has been reported to produce adequate postthoracotomy analgesia in dogs.[26,32,48,140,146]

Epidurally administered morphine is distributed by at least four different pathways: (a) transdural passage to the CSF and neural axis, (b) vascular uptake by epidural venous plexi and spinal radicular arteries, (c) lymphatic uptake, and (d) deposition into epidural fat.[117,141,172,173] The distribution in CSF, blood, and lymph of lumbar epidurally administered morphine (molecular weight, 285; and pKa, 7.9) into the lumbar area in dogs has been determined.[117] The fraction of morphine crossing the dura after epidural injection of 2 mg into a 30-kg dog has been calculated to be 0.3%.[117] Maximal morphine concentration in lumbar CSF ranged from 5 to 93 ng/mL and was reached 5 to 60 min after injection. Morphine clearance from the CSF was 106 min (mean

tß) independent of the dose.[117] In another study, the maximal concentration of a 0.1-mg/kg dose of morphine in cisternal CSF was 102.3 ± 28.0 ng/mL at 180 min after lumbar epidural administration.[141] The maximal concentration of morphine in serum of the same dogs was 95.7 ± 27.0 ng/mL at 31.0 ± 15.2 min.[141]

This large variability in CSF and plasma concentrations is a striking finding that emphasizes the need for adjusting the dose of epidural morphine for each patient. Practically, this can be accomplished by using an epidural catheter while observing the degree of analgesia and the severity of side effects. Pharmacodynamic studies evaluating the degree of analgesia and CSF and plasma drug concentrations of epidurally administered morphine support a spinal mechanism of action. These studies also indicate that rapid but short-lasting serum concentrations and delayed long-lasting CSF concentrations are often achieved with epidurally administered doses of morphine in dogs.

Oxymorphone

Oxymorphone, in comparison to morphine, is a relatively lipid-soluble opioid that binds more rapidly to opiate receptors in the spinal cord and has a smaller area of distribution in the CSF (segmental analgesia) (Table 20.3).

The analgesic and cardiorespiratory effects of epidurally administered bupivacaine (0.5%, 1.0 mg/kg), oxymorphone (0.1 mg/kg) in 0.75% bupivacaine (1 mg/kg), and intravenous oxymorphone (0.05 mg/kg) on halothane requirements have been evaluated.[150] There were no differences in end-tidal halothane requirements for dogs among the three groups. Respiratory depression was increased and heart rate was decreased with epidural oxymorphone-bupivacaine and intravenous oxymorphone treatments. Postoperative requirements of oxymorphone (0.05 mg/kg IV) were significantly less in dogs receiving the epidural oxymorphone-bupivacaine combination.[150]

The postoperative analgesic and cardiopulmonary effects of oxymorphone administered epidurally (0.05 mg/kg) and intramuscularly (0.15 mg/kg) or medetomidine administered epidurally (0.015 mg/kg) have also been evaluated in dogs undergoing pelvic or hind-limb orthopedic surgery.[174,175] The average duration of analgesia obtained with both epidural oxymorphone and medetomidine was 7 h, whereas intramuscular oxymorphone provided approximately 5 h of analgesia. All treatments decreased heart rate. There was no difference in arterial blood pressure with epidural and intramuscular oxymorphone, but pressure was increased with epidural medetomidine.

Butorphanol

Epidural butorphanol (0.25 mg/kg) administration in dogs reportedly reduces the inhalant anesthetic requirement (decreased isoflurane minimum alveolar concentration by 32%) without any cardiovascular and neurological side effects.[176] However, the rather brief analgesic action (80 min), as assessed by dogs not responding to toe-pinch stimulation of the hind limbs and forelimbs, limits the value of epidural butorphanol administration in clinical practice. Pharmacokinetic data from epidural butorphanol (0.25 mg/kg) administration in halothane-anesthetized dogs indicated that the maximum concentration of butorphanol and time to reach this concentration are 42.3 ng/mL at 13.9 min in blood and 18 ng/mL at 30 min in CSF. The authors concluded that the pharmacokinetic data suggest that analgesia is predominantly due to butorphanol's action on supraspinal structures following its vascular systemic absorption.[177]

Buprenorphine

The efficacy of epidural buprenorphine (4 μg/kg) versus epidural morphine (0.1 mg/kg) administered in a total volume of 0.2 mL/kg for postoperative pain relief in dogs undergoing cranial cruciate ligament rupture repair has been compared.[154] Epidural buprenorphine appeared to be as effective as epidural morphine for relief of postoperative hind-limb orthopedic pain in healthy dogs and may offer some advantages over morphine, such as lower abuse potential and reduced cost.[154]

Side Effects of Epidural Opioids

Potential side effects in patients include respiratory depression, dysphoria, urinary retention, delayed gastrointestinal motility, vomiting, rubbing of the face, and catheter-related problems such as catheter displacement, occlusion, and infection from chronic epidural catheterization.[145,158,178]

The analgesic efficacy, duration of action, and adverse side effects of epidurally administered morphine are dose related.[179] The most serious adverse effect is respiratory depression, which is biphasic. Respiratory depression has been attributed to the absorption of morphine into epidural veins and subsequent circulatory redistribution to the brain (early depression), and cephalad movement of morphine in CSF to the brain stem (late respiratory depression).[180] Lumbar epidural administration of excessive doses of morphine (20 mg of morphine sulfate in a 3-mL saline solution) in awake dogs (30 kg) increased $PaCO_2$ by 10 mm Hg at 1.5 to 2.0 h after administration, with no further ventilatory depression thereafter.[163] The maximal concentration of morphine in the CSF of these dogs was 64 ng/mL at 45 min after administration but gradually declined to 50% of maximum concentration at 6 h. The morphine concentration in arterial plasma was maximal at 30 min and declined to 20% of maximal by 6 h.

Administration of increasing concentrations (0.1 to 100.0 ng/mL) of morphine into the fourth ventricle or cisterna magna in awake dogs produced reduced tidal volume but not respiratory rate, suggesting that larger doses (20 mg) of epidural morphine can produce respiratory depression in dogs. This effect is most likely caused by the delivery of morphine to the brain-stem respiratory centers via the blood rather than via the CSF.[163] The time course of ventilatory depression following subarachnoid administration of morphine in dogs corresponded poorly with morphine concentration changes in the CSF.[164] Severe respiratory depression should not occur in dogs when therapeutic doses (0.1 mg/kg) of morphine are administered epidurally.

Preemptively administered epidural morphine with or without bupivacaine given to 242 dogs has produced mild respiratory and cardiovascular depression during anesthesia, whereas urinary retention, pruritus, and vomiting were seen in only seven, two, and six dogs, respectively. Six dogs vomited when a second dose of morphine was given epidurally the day after surgery.[136] Side effects are more common when intrathecal injection is performed as opposed to epidural injection, and side effects can usually be reversed by a low-dose intravenous infusion of naloxone, with minimal effect on the analgesia produced.[181]

Myoclonus[182–184] and neuroexitation[185,186] are very rarely observed complications in human patients after the epidural or intravenous administration of opioids. Similarly, involuntary muscle contractions in dogs, after either epidural or subarachnoid administration of preservative-free morphine, are extremely rare. Myoclonus and urinary retention have been reported in a 5-year-old German shepherd 90 min after subarachnoid injection of preservative-free morphine sulfate (0.15 mg/kg) diluted in 4 mL (0.1 mL/kg) of a sterile isotonic saline solution.[187] Muscle twitches started at the tail and then progressed to the hind limbs, trunk, and even partly the shoulders of the dog, which had just recovered from a 5-h oxymorphone-acepromazine-thiopental-isoflurane-oxygen anesthesia to complete a total hip-prosthesis surgery. The twitches became very strong with time and were not diminished by diazepam (0.2 to 1.0 mg/kg IV) or atracurium injected twice at 45-min intervals (0.2 and 0.1 mg/kg). The spasms were eventually controlled with pentobarbital administration (130 mg IV) and intermittent positive-pressure ventilation for 4 h.[188] The following day, the spasms were absent, but proprioceptive ataxia and hind-limb paresis, with urinary retention, persisted for another day. Bethanechol chloride (5 mg) was given by mouth every 8 h, and the bladder was emptied by catheterization once. The dog recovered over the next few days without further sequelae.[187]

In another report, a dog exhibiting hyperesthesia and extreme neuritis of the pelvic area and tail lasting 24 h slowly resolved over a 4-day period.[189] Overall, the incidence of severe complications was reported to be 0.75% in 365 dogs and 4 cats that received epidural morphine for a wide variety of procedures, including fracture repair or arthrodesis, limb and tail amputation, total hip replacement, thoracotomy, laparotomy, and laminectomy.[189]

Opioid-induced hyperalgesia, myoclonus, and seizures have been reproduced and studied extensively in rats.[182,183,190,191] Direct opioid receptor–mediated and nonopioid receptor–mediated excitatory and inhibitory mechanisms, metabolites (normorphine, morphine-3 glucuronide, and hydromorphone-3 glucuronide), and preservatives (sodium bisulfite) have all been implicated in these observed neurological side effects. Intrathecal naloxone has also been implicated in the potentiation of intrathecal morphine-induced hind-limb myoclonus and seizure activity in rats.[182]

Nonopioid Epidural Analgesia

Drugs from other classes—such as α-adrenoceptor agonists, N-methyl-D-aspartate (NMDA) receptor antagonists (e.g., ketamine), and serotonergic, cholinergic, and γ-aminobutyric acid (GABA) receptor agonists[192]—upon direct spinal administration in laboratory animals, have inhibited behaviors elicited by noxious stimuli.[193,194] With the exception of epidurally administered α$_2$-adrenoceptor agonists, such as xylazine,[147,148,195–200] medetomidine,[144,153,174,175,200,201] and NMDA receptor antagonist, such as ketamine,[202–207] there is little information on the clinical efficacy of nonopioid spinal analgesic drugs in dogs.

α$_2$-Adrenoceptor Agonists

Similar to morphine, the administration of α$_2$-agonists can produce a powerful effect on nociceptive processing by activating a dense population of α$_2$ receptors (i.e., α$_{2A}$, α$_{2B}$, α$_{2C}$, and α$_{2D}$) (heteroceptors) in the CNS and periphery.[208–210] In addition, some α$_2$-agonists can also activate imidazoline receptors (I$_1$ and I$_2$) and produce direct effects on sensory transmission (e.g., xylazine). Spinally administered α$_2$-agonists mediate analgesia by activating presynaptic α$_2$-adrenoceptors, which are located on primary afferent C fibers terminating in the superficial laminae of the dorsal horn of the spinal cord.[211] This activation induces G$_0$ proteins that decrease calcium influx, which results in a decreased release of neurotransmitters and/or neuropeptides (e.g., glutamate, substance P, neurotensin, calcitonin gene–related peptide, and vasoactive intestinal peptide), resulting in antinociception.[212,213] Activation of the α$_2$ heteroceptors, which are located postsynaptically on wide-dynamic-range projection neurons targeted by primary afferent fibers in the dorsal horn, results in hyperpolarization of neurons via G$_i$ protein–coupled potassium channels, producing postsynaptically mediated spinal analgesia.

Epidural Xylazine and Medetomidine

The effects of epidural xylazine on electroencephalogram (EEG) responses to surgical stimuli of varying intensity during experimental orthopedic procedures have been reported.[197,198] After epidural xylazine administration (L7-S1), anesthesia was maintained with isoflurane (end-tidal concentration, 1.5%) in oxygen. The EEG and hemodynamic variables (heart rate and mean arterial blood pressure) were evaluated at prestimulation, skin incision, removal of a bone graft from the dorsoiliac spine, opening and reaming of the medullary canal of the tibia for bone graft installation, and wound closure. Skin incision and removal of bone graft produced a significantly higher increase in α/δ ratio in the EEG in the saline group when compared with the xylazine group. In addition, the prestimulation 80% spectral edge frequency of the EEG in the xylazine group was significantly lower than in the saline group. The results of this study suggest that epidural xylazine (0.25 mg/kg) suppresses responses in the α/δ ratio to surgical stimulation and may exert its antinociceptive effect in dogs in part by a supraspinal action.[198]

The most obvious physiological effects of activating spinal α$_2$-adrenoceptors, other than their effect on altering nociceptive threshold, are bradycardia and hypotension.[200] Medetomidine (15 µg/kg) or xylazine (0.25 mg/kg) both produced similar cardiovascular and respiratory changes after lumbosacral epidural administration in dogs. Both drugs reduce heart rate, mean arterial blood pressure, and respiratory rate from baseline values. First-degree atrioventricular block was observed more often after xylazine administration (50% vs. 33%), whereas second-degree block was more frequently observed with the use of medetomidine (66% vs. 33%).[200]

Epidural medetomidine administration (0.015 mg/kg) reportedly produces analgesia lasting 7 to 8 h.[174,175] The duration of analgesia is comparable to that achieved with epidurally administered oxymorphone (0.05 mg/kg) for similar procedures. However, all medetomidine-treated dogs developed a decrease in heart rate and a transient increase in arterial blood pressure. Dogs typically develop second-degree atrioventricular block associated with sinus arrhythmia for a brief period during the first 20 min after medetomidine epidural injection.

Epidural Dexmedetomidine

Dexmedetomidine is the pharmacologically active D-isomer of medetomidine, a highly lipid-soluble α$_2$-receptor agonist[214] and, as such, is rapidly absorbed into the circulation and CNS. A dose-dependent effect of dexmedetomidine on antinociception and effects on respiratory function have been documented.[215] Different dose ranges of dexmedetomidine were used after each route of drug administration, with 4 to 6 days elapsing between the experiments. Dexmedetomidine by intrathecal (1, 3, or 10 µg), epidural (3, 15, and 50 µg), and intravenous (1, 3, and 10 µg/kg) routes produced a rapid dose-dependent increase in the thermal (60° ± 1°C for a maximum of 10 s) skin-twitch response latency at lumbar and thoracic areas and paw withdrawal to mechanical compression of the toes of the front and hind limbs. The dose required to reach 50% of maximal effect for skin-twitch response after intrathecal, epidural, and intravenous administration of dexmedetomidine was 1.8, 10, and 15 µg, respectively. The maximal effective dose produces approximately 90 min of hypoalgesia. The spinal effects do not appear to be associated with changes in behavioral alertness, motor function, or carbon dioxide response. Intravenous dexmedetomidine (1 to 10 µg) also elevates the nociceptive threshold significantly, as measured by thermal or mechanical nociceptive end points. In contrast to the spinal administration, however, intravenous dexmedetomidine produces dose-dependent sedation, significantly reduces heart and respiratory rates, and diminishes response to increased carbon dioxide. The α$_2$-adrenoceptor antagonist atipamezole (30 to 300 µg/kg IV), but not the opioid antagonist naloxone (30 µg/kg IV), antagonizes all of the observed effects of dexmedetomidine. These results suggest that spinally administered dexmedetomidine produces a powerful antinociceptive effect, mediated via α$_2$-adrenoceptors at the spinal level, whereas systemic redistribution of the drug produces sedation with significant cardiovascular and respiratory side effects.[215]

Ketamine

Ketamine has an analgesic action at many sites both centrally and peripherally. The mechanism of analgesic action of epidurally and intrathecally administered ketamine has not been clearly defined, and investigation into the contribution of supraspinal and/or spinal sites related to its analgesic and anesthetic action has not provided conclusive results. While reports regarding the efficacy of ketamine as a spinal analgesic are controversial, ketamine may block NMDA receptors and interact with subtypes of opioid, propionate, kainate, γ-aminobutyric acid A receptors,[216] and/or monoaminergic (serotonergic, noradrenergic, and dopaminergic) neural systems.[217] Ketamine also inhibits voltage-gated sodium-ion and potassium-ion channels, thereby suppressing myelinated nerve conduction.[218,219] Ketamine may reverse opioid tolerance by interacting with NMDA receptors, the nitric oxide pathway, and μ opioid receptors.[220] Evidence of the efficacy of ketamine for treatment of chronic pain in human patients has been reviewed and is considered moderate to weak.[221]

The analgesic action of epidurally injected ketamine has been assessed in anesthetized dogs by using cutaneous electrical stimulus (10 V) to the ischial and masseter muscle region.[204,205] The number of dogs responding to cutaneous electrical stimulation was significantly less following epidural ketamine-lidocaine administration than following epidural ketamine-saline administration. Similarly, the lumbosacral epidural injection of ketamine (20 mg/mL) at a dose of 2 mg/kg did not provide significant analgesia in dogs with chemically induced synovitis.[207]

The hemodynamic effects of ketamine when injected into the lumbosacral epidural space typically include increases in heart rate, mean arterial blood pressure, cardiac index, and stroke work index within 15 to 20 min.[205] It is not yet conclusive that epidural ketamine consistently decreases the requirement of inhalation anesthetics. Nevertheless, epidural and intrathecal doses of 1 to 3 mg of ketamine/kg of body weight have shown analgesic efficacy in canine studies.[202,203] Ketamine is rapidly distributed to the plasma and CSF (0.4 and 0.3 h, respectively) from the epidural space of dogs.[202]

Diazepam

Diazepam has been administered epidurally to dogs.[192] With a 2-mg/kg dose, the tail, perineum, anus, sacral, lumbar, abdomen, and hind limbs are desensitized and the hind limbs paralyzed for variable periods (50 to 100 min). Pulse rate is significantly increased, whereas skin temperature, rectal temperature, respiratory rate, mean arterial blood pressure, and central venous pressure are not affected. Neurological damage or toxicity, and inflammatory infiltration in histological preparations of the spinal cord, are not evident.[192] There has been little clinical use of benzodiazepines as analgesics when placed epidurally in dogs or other companion animals.

Ketorolac

Ketorolac (0.4 mg/kg) has been administered into the lumbar epidural space in dogs.[222,223] Gross necropsy revealed gastrointestinal ulceration of varying degrees in dogs administered epidural ketorolac. Histopathological analysis of the spinal cord and meninges revealed minimal focal leptomeningeal phlebitis in 25% of the dogs given this drug. Gastrointestinal ulceration induced by ketorolac is common and limits its use to a single injection. At present, both efficacy and safety need to be further evaluated before epidural administration of ketorolac or any other nonsteroidal anti-inflammatory drug can be recommended for clinical practice.[222,223]

Glucocorticoids

Glucocorticoids (e.g., prednisone, prednisolone, and methylprednisolone) are most commonly administered by systemic routes, either oral or injectable, to relieve pain and reduce inflammation. Perineural injection, either to spinal nerve roots or to peripheral nerves, to alleviate pain caused by nerve root disease or peripheral neuropathies is common in human patients.[224] The beneficial effects of epidurally administered betamethasone in a rat model of lumbar radiculopathy have been reported.[225] However, a series of lumbar epidural steroid injections for chronic back pain has produced life-threatening *Staphylococcus aureus* meningitis and cauda equina syndrome in one person[226] and transient blindness caused by retinal and vitreal hemorrhages from increased intracranial pressure in another person.[227] As of this writing, recommendations or dosages for the use of epidural glucocorticoids in dogs and other small companion animals have not been developed.

Epidural Drug Combinations

Epidural opioids (e.g., morphine or oxymorphone) with local anesthetics (e.g., lidocaine, bupivacaine, or ropivacaine) or α₂-adrenoceptor agonists (e.g., xylazine, medetomidine, or dexmedetomidine) have been administered to dogs before surgery to reduce general anesthetic requirements and provided intraoperative and postoperative pain control.

Local Anesthetics and Opioids

In rats, the combined intrathecal administration of morphine with lidocaine or bupivacaine reportedly produces antinociceptive effects that are more rapid in onset, last longer, and are greater in peak effect than when agents are administered alone at the same dose level.[228] Subsequently, several investigators have reported additive or synergistic effects of epidurally administered opioids and local anesthetics in people,[194,229–232] dogs,[30,107,151] and rats.[228] Although various local anesthetics and opioids have been administered epidurally in dogs, morphine, bupivacaine, and their combination effects have been the most critically evaluated.[93,107,118,140,169,233] For example, the epidural administration of morphine-bupivacaine provided longer-lasting analgesia and required a lower number of supplemental doses of analgesic agent than did morphine or saline alone. The times for rescue-oxymorphone administration in dogs treated with either epidural morphine alone, bupivacaine alone, the morphine-bupivacaine combination, or saline were 5.4, 9.1, 24, and 2.6 h, respectively.[107] Likewise, the coadministration of epidural lidocaine and fentanyl (100 μg in 0.3 mL of 0.9% sodium chloride with epinephrine 1:200,000) produces scrotal analgesia with faster onset

(1.3 ± 0.3 vs. 4.4 ± 0.4 min) and longer duration (143 ± 11 vs. 98 ± 8 min) than does lidocaine with epinephrine alone. The epidural coadministration of lidocaine and fentanyl consistently produces forelimb rigidity in dogs.[234]

α₂-Adrenoceptor Agonists and Opioids

Synergistic antinociceptive interactions have been observed between a variety of α₂-adrenoceptor and opioid receptor agonists.[235–237] The epidural administration of α₂-adrenoceptor agonists (xylazine or medetomidine) alone or in combination with morphine has gained some degree of use in veterinary practice during the last 5 years. A few studies documenting this synergy have been performed.

For example, dogs receiving low-dose epidural medetomidine (5 µg/kg) administration alone did not show evidence of analgesia, as evidenced by response to tail clamping. However, the addition of medetomidine to morphine prolonged the analgesia beyond that achieved with morphine alone (13.1 ± 3.1 vs. 6.3 ± 1.2 h), indicating a supra-additive effect with the administration of both drugs.[238] In another study, postoperative analgesia was assessed in dogs given either preservative-free morphine (0.1 mg/kg) or morphine (0.1 mg/kg) with medetomidine (5 µg/kg) via lumbosacral epidural injection.[153] Based on numerical rating scale, pain scores, posture, vocalization, and facial expression, epidurally administered morphine combined with medetomidine was associated with superior analgesic benefits when compared with morphine alone.

Ketamine and Opioids

In a more recent study, epidural ketamine (40 to 320 µg), morphine (0.6 to 160 µg), or fentanyl (0.16 to 10 µg), and a combination of 80 µg of ketamine with either morphine (2.5 to 80 µg) or fentanyl (0.04 to 10 µg) have all been assessed for analgesic properties.[238] Epidural ketamine produced only limited antinociception, whereas morphine and fentanyl exhibited a dose-related antinociception. Morphine's action was slow in onset and lasted long, whereas fentanyl had a fast onset and briefer action. In combination, ketamine improved maximal possible effect as well as duration of action of morphine-induced, but not fentanyl-induced, antinociception. Moreover, increasing doses of the highly lipophilic ketamine tended to decrease the maximal response of various doses of the highly lipophilic fentanyl. Competition, at least in part, for the same µ receptor or µ receptor subtypes, via P glycoprotein, could have been one mechanism by which higher doses of ketamine decreased the antinociceptive properties of fentanyl. These data indicate that ketamine and perhaps other drugs may actually have antagonistic effects with various opioids when coadministered in the epidural space to induce an analgesic action.[239]

Ganglion Blocks

Anesthesia of the cervicothoracic ganglion and lumbar sympathetic chain in dogs has been described to treat paralysis of the radial, facial, and trigeminal nerves and muscle and joint diseases:[240,241] 5 to 8 mL of 0.5% procaine hydrochloride solution has been administered in close proximity to the cervicothoracic ganglion and lumbar sympathetic chain without ill effects.

Conclusion

Local and regional anesthetic techniques in dogs have been used extensively to relieve the pain related to a variety of medical and surgical procedures. Appropriately selected topical, local, or regional (e.g., epidural) techniques can provide safe, effective, and reliable analgesia with minimal physiological alterations. Similarly, the interpleural administration of local anesthetic drugs or the epidural administration of opioids can provide unparalleled long-term relief of pain while preserving consciousness. Novel systems for the delivery of analgesics and other therapeutic modalities designed to be used with local anesthetics, opioids, and nonopioid analgesics may greatly facilitate the future management of perioperative pain in companion animals.[242]

References

1. Livingston A, Waterman AE, Chambers JP. Neurologic evaluation of effective post-operative pain therapy. In: Proceedings of the Chapter of Anaesthetics & Critical Care of the Australian College of Veterinary Scientists, 1994;226:189–202.
2. Ritchie JM, Cohen PJ. Local anesthetics: Cocaine, procaine and other synthetic local anesthetics. In: Goodman LS, Gilman AG, Gilman A, eds. The Pharmaceutical Basis of Therapeutics, 5th ed. New York: Macmillan, 1975:311–332.
3. Formstom C. Ophthaine (proparacaine hydrochloride): A local anesthetic for ophthalmic surgery. Vet Rec 1964;76:385.
4. Magrane WG. Investigational use of Ophthaine as a local anesthetic in ophthalmology. North Am Vet 1953;34:568–569.
5. Überreiter O. Zur Technik der Augenoperationen beim Hunde. Arch Wiss Prakt Tierheilkd 1937;74:235–332.
6. Severinghaus JW, Xu FD, Spellman MJ. Benzocaine and methemoglobin: Recommended actions. Anesthesiology 1991;74:385–386.
7. Harvey JW, Sameck JH, Burgard FJ. Benzocaine induced methemoglobinemia in dogs. J Am Vet Med Assoc 1979;175:1171–1175.
8. Paddleford RP, Krahwinkel DJ, Fuhr JE, et al. Experimentally induced methemoglobinemia in the dog following exposure to topical benzocaine HCl [Abstract]. In: Proceedings of the Second International Congress of Veterinary Anesthetists, Sacramento, CA, 1985:98–99.
9. Gesztes A, Mezei M. Topical anesthesia of the skin by liposome-encapsulated tetracaine. Anesth Analg 1988;67:1079–1081.
10. Ehrenstrom-Reiz GME, Reiz SLA. EMLA: A eutectic mixture of local anesthetics for topical anaesthesia. Acta Anaesthesiol Scand 1982;26:596–598.
11. Flecknell PA, Liles JH, Williamson HA. The use of lidocaine-prilocaine local anesthetic cream for pain-free venepuncture in laboratory animals. Lab Anim 1990;24:142–146.
12. Wilcke JR, Davis LE, Neff-Davis CA, et al. Pharmacokinetics of lidocaine and its active metabolites in dogs. J Vet Pharmacol Ther 1983;6:49–58.
13. Hamlin RL, Bishop MA, Hadlock DJ, et al. Effects of lidocaine, with or without epinephrine on ventricular rhythm. J Am Anim Hosp Assoc 1988;24:701–704.
14. Klein SM, Grant SA, Greengrass RA, et al. Interscalene brachial plexus block with a continuous catheter insertion system and a disposable infusion pump. Anesth Analg 2000;91:1473–1478.

15. Wolfe TM, Muir W. Local anesthetics: Pharmacology and novel applications. Compend Contin Educ Pract Vet 2003;25:916–927.

16. Ott RL. Local anesthesia in the dog. Fed Proc 1969;28:1450–1455.

17. Carpenter RE, Wilson DV, Evans AT. Evaluation of intraperitoneal and subcutaneous lidocaine and bupivacaine for analgesia following ovariohysterectomy in the dog [Abstract]. In: Proceedings of the Annual Scientific Meeting of the American College of Veterinary Anesthesiologists, Orlando, FL, 2002:15.

18. Carpenter RE, Wilson DV, Evans AT. Evaluation of intraperitoneal and incisional lidocaine or bupivacaine for analgesia following ovariohysterectomy in the dog. Vet Anaesth Analg 2004;31:46–52.

19. Buback JL, Boothe HW, Carroll GL, et al. Comparison of three methods for relief of pain after ear canal ablation in dogs. Vet Surg 1996;25:380–385.

20. Barth P. Die Leitungsanästhesie am Kopf des Hundes [PhD dissertation]. Zurich: Faculty of Veterinary Medicine, University of Zurich, 1948.

21. Frank ER. Dental anesthesia in the dog. J Am Vet Med Assoc 1928;73:232–233.

22. Gross ME, Pope ER, O'Brien D, et al. Regional anesthesia of the infraorbital and inferior alveolar nerves during noninvasive tooth pulp stimulation in halothane-anesthetized dogs. J Am Vet Med Assoc 1997;211:1403–1405.

23. Ahmad S, Ahmad A, Benzon HT. Clinical experience with the peribulbar block for ophthalmic surgery. Reg Anesth 1993;18:184–188.

24. Wang BC, Bogart BB, Hillman DE. Subarachnoid injection: A potential complication of retrobulbar block. Anesthesiology 1989;71:845–847.

25. Dietz O. Eine retro-bulbäre Anästhesie beim Hund zur Erzeugung einer Mydriasis. Berl Munch Tierarztl Wochenschr 1954;15:235–237.

26. Thompson SE, Johnson JM. Analgesia in dogs after intercostal thoracotomy: A comparison of morphine, selective intercostal nerve block, and interpleural regional analgesia with bupivacaine. Vet Surg 1991;20:73–77.

27. Gilroy BA. Effect of intercostal nerve blocks on post thoracotomy ventilation and oxygenation in the canine. J Vet Crit Care 1982;6:1–9.

28. Moore DC, Brindenbaugh LD, Thompson GE. Factors determining dosage of amide type local anesthetic drugs. Anesthesiology 1977;47:263–268.

29. Tucker GT. Pharmacokinetics of local anaesthetics. Br J Anaesth 1986;58:717–731.

30. Quandt JE, Rawlings CR. Reducing postoperative pain for dogs: Local anesthetic and analgesic techniques. Compend Contin Educ Pract Vet 1996;18:101–111.

31. Berg RJ, Orton EC. Pulmonary function in dogs after intercostal thoracotomy: Comparison of morphine, oxymorphone, and selective intercostal nerve block. Am J Vet Res 1986;47:471–474.

32. Pascoe PJ, Dyson DH. Analgesia after lateral thoracotomy in dogs: Epidural morphine vs. intercostal bupivacaine. Vet Surg 1993;22:141–147.

33. Kvalheim L, Reiestad F. Interpleural catheter in the management of postoperative pain [Abstract]. Anesthesiology 1984;61:A231.

34. Reiestadt F, Stromskag KE, Kjell E. Interpleural catheter in the management of postoperative pain: A preliminary report. Reg Anesth 1986;11:89–91.

35. Murphy DF. Interpleural analgesia. Br J Anaesth 1993;71:426–434.

36. Rosenberg PH, Scheinin BMA, Lepantalo MJA, et al. Continuous intrapleural infusion of bupivacaine for analgesia after thoracotomy. Anesthesiology 1987;67:811–813.

37. McIlvaine WB. Intrapleural anesthesia is useful for thoracic analgesia. Pro: Intrapleural anesthesia is useful for thoracic analgesia [Comment]. J Cardiothorac Vasc Anesth 1996;10:425–428.

38. Schneider RF, Villamena PC, Harvey J, et al. Lack of efficacy of intrapleural bupivacaine for postoperative analgesia following thoracotomy. Chest 1993;103:414–416.

39. Riegler FX. Intrapleural anesthesia is useful for thoracic analgesia. Con: Unreliable benefit after thoracotomy—Epidural is a better choice [Comment]. J Cardiothorac Vasc Anesth 1996;10:429–431.

40. Silomon M, Claus T, Huwer H, et al. Interpleural analgesia does not influence postthoracotomy pain. Anesth Analg 2000;91:44–50.

41. Stromskag KE, Reiestad F, Holmgvist EL, et al. Intrapleural administration of 0.25%, 0.375%, and 0.5% bupivacaine with epinephrine after cholecystectomy. Anesth Analg 1988;67:430–434.

42. Rocco A, Reiestad F, Gudmon J, et al. Intrapleural administration of local anesthetics for pain relief in patients with multiple rib fractures: Preliminary report. Reg Anesth 1987;12:10–14.

43. Morrow JS, Squier RC. Sympathetic blockade with interpleural analgesia [Abstract]. Anesthesiology 1989;71(3A):A662.

44. Riegler FX, Pelligrino DA, Vade Boncouer TR. An animal model of intrapleural analgesia [Abstract]. Anesthesiology 1988;69:A365.

45. Riegler FX, Vade Boncouer TR, Pelligrino DA. Interpleural anesthetics in the dog: Differential somatic neural blockade. Anesthesiology 1989;71:744–750.

46. Kowalski SE, Bradley BD, Greengrass RA, et al. Effects of interpleural bupivacaine (0.5%) on canine diaphragmatic function. Anesth Analg 1992;75:400–404.

47. Kushner LI, Trim CM. Evaluation of interpleural bupivacaine in dogs. In: Proceedings of the Veterinarian Midwest Conference, University of Illinois, Champaign-Urbana, 1993:12.

48. Conzemius MG, Brockman DJ, King LG, et al. Analgesia in dogs after intercostal thoracotomy: A clinical trial comparing intravenous buprenorphine and interpleural bupivacaine. Vet Surg 1994;23:291–298.

49. Kushner LI, Trim CM, Madhusudhan S, et al. Evaluation of the hemodynamic effects of interpleural bupivacaine in dogs. Vet Surg 1995;24:180–187.

50. Stobie D, Caywood DD, Rozanski EA, et al. Evaluation of pulmonary function and analgesia in dogs after intercostal thoracotomy and use of morphine administered intramuscularly or intrapleurally and bupivacaine administered intrapleurally. Am J Vet Res 1995;56:1098–1109.

51. Dhokarikar P, Caywood DD, Stobie D, et al. Effects of intramuscular or interpleural administration of morphine and interpleural administration of bupivacaine on pulmonary function in dogs that have undergone median sternotomy. Am J Vet Res 1996;57:375–380.

52. Sydow FW, Haindl H. Eine neue Technik der interpleuralen Blockade. Anesthetist 1990;39:280–282.

53. Symreng T, Gomez MN, Johnson B, et al. Intrapleural bupivacaine: Technical considerations and intraoperative use. J Cardiothorac Anesth 1989;3:139–143.

54. Vade Boncouer TR, Pelligrino DA, Riegler FX, et al. Interpleural bupivacaine in the dog: Distribution of effect and influence of injectate volume [Abstract]. Anesth Analg 1989;68(Suppl):S301.

55. Waldman SD. Subcutaneous tunneled intrapleural catheters in the long-term relief of upper quadrant pain of malignant origin: Description of a new technique and preliminary results [Abstract]. Reg Anesth 1989;4(Suppl 2):54.

56. Richardson J, Sabanathans, Shah RD, et al. Pleural bupivacaine placement for optimal postthoracotomy pulmonary function: A

prospective, randomized study. J Cardiothorac Vasc Anesth 1998;12:166–169.

57. Aguilar JL, Montero A, Vidal Lopez F, et al. Bilateral interpleural injection of local anesthetics. Reg Anesth 1989;14:93–94.
58. Sammarco JL, Conzemius MG, Perkowski SZ, et al. Postoperative analgesia for stifle surgery: A comparison of intra-articular bupivacaine, morphine, or saline. Vet Surg 1996;25:59–69.
59. Stein C, Millan MJ, Shippenberg TS, et al. Peripheral opioid receptors mediating antinociception in inflammation: Evidence for involvement of mu, delta and kappa receptors. J Pharmacol Exp Ther 1989;248:1269–1275.
60. Tufvesson G. Anestesi av plexus brachialis. Nord Veterinaermed 1951;3:183–193.
61. Nutt P. Brachial plexus analgesia in the dog. Vet Rec 1962;74:874–876.
62. Futema F, Fantoni DT, Costa Auler JO Jr, et al. A new brachial plexus block technique in dogs. Vet Anaesth Analg 2002;29:133–139.
63. Bier A. Über einen neuen Weg Lokalanästhesie an den Gliedmassen zu erzeugen. Arch Klin Chir 1908;86:1007–1016.
64. Küpper W. Die intravenöse Regionalanästhesie (BIER) beim Hund. Zentralbl Veterinarmed [A] 1977;24:287–297.
65. Webb AA, Cantwell SL, Duke T, et al. Intravenous regional anesthesia (Bier block) in a dog. Can Vet J 1999;40:419–421.
66. Grice SC, Eisenach JC, Prough DS. Intravenous regional anesthesia: Effect of tourniquet site and type on leakage under the tourniquet [Abstract]. Anesth Analg 1987;66(Suppl):S191.
67. Cotev S, Robin GC. Experimental studies on intravenous regional anaesthesia using radioactive lignocaine. Br J Anaesth 1966;38:936–939.
68. Chabel C, Russell LL, Lee R. Tourniquet-induced limb ischemia: A neurophysiologic animal model. Anesthesiology 1990;72:1038–1044.
69. Arthur GR, Feldman HS, Norway SB, et al. Acute IV toxicity of LEA-103, a new local anesthetic, compared to lidocaine and bupivacaine in the awake dog [Abstract]. Anesthesiology 1986;65:A182.
70. Arthur GR, Feldman HS, Covino BG. Comparative pharmacokinetics of bupivacaine and ropivacaine, a new amide local anesthetic. Anesth Analg 1988;67:1053–1058.
71. Pedigo NW, Walmsley PN, Kasten GW, et al. Relative cardiotoxicity of the long-acting local anesthetics bupivacaine and ropivacaine in dogs [Abstract]. Anesth Analg 1988;67(Suppl):S166.
72. Feldman HS, Arthur GR, Covino BG. Comparative systemic toxicity of convulsant and supraconvulsant doses of intravenous ropivacaine, bupivacaine and lidocaine in the conscious dog. Anesth Analg 1989;69:794–801.
73. Westhues M, Fritsch R. Local anesthesia. In: Animal Anesthesia. Edinburgh: Oliver and Boyd, 1964:114–119.
74. Rudin DO, Fremont-Smith K, Beecher HK. Permeability of dura mater to epidural procaine in dogs. J Appl Physiol 1951;3:388–398.
75. Bone JK, Beck JG. Epidural anesthesia in dogs. J Am Vet Med Assoc 1956;128:236–238.
76. Tufvesson G. Local anaesthesia in veterinary medicine. Sodertalje, Sweden: Astra International, 1963:36–43.
77. Evers WH. Epidural anesthesia in the dog: A review of 224 cases with emphasis on cesarean section. Vet Med Small Anim Clin 1968;63:1121–1124.
78. Klide AM, Soma LR. Epidural analgesia in the dog and cat. J Am Vet Med Assoc 1968;153:165–173.
79. Persson F. Epidural analgesia in dogs with special reference to intra-arterial blood pressure. Acta Vet Scand 1970;11:186–196.
80. Burfoot MF, Bromage PR. The effects of epinephrine on mepivacaine absorption from the spinal epidural space. Anesthesiology 1971;35:488–492.
81. Klide AM. Epidural anesthesia. In: Soma LR, ed. Textbook of Veterinary Anesthesia. Baltimore: Williams and Wilkins, 1971:450–467.
82. Lebeaux MI. Experimental epidural anaesthesia in the dog with lidocaine and bupivacaine. Br J Anaesth 1973;45:549–555.
83. Morikawa K, Bonica JJ, Tucker GT, et al. Effect of acute hypovolaemia on lignocaine absorption and cardiovascular response following epidural block in dogs. Br J Anaesth 1974;46:631–635.
84. Bradley RL, Withrow SJ, Heath RB, et al. Epidural anesthesia in the dog. Vet Surg 1980;9:153–156.
85. Pandey SK, Dass LL, Bhargava MK, et al. Evaluation of lidocaine HCl as a spinal anesthetic in dogs. Indian Vet J 1981;58:478–480.
86. Gerlach K, Bonath K, Ristic-Djuric Z, et al. Möglichkeiten der Langzeitanästhesie mit Bupivacaine und Langzeitanästhesie mit Morphine beim Hund mit Hilfe eines extraduralen Katheters. Fortschr Veterinarmed 1983;37:237.
87. Greitz T, Andreen M, Irestedt L. Haemodynamics and oxygen consumption in the dog during high epidural block with special reference to the splanchnic region. Acta Anaesthesiol Scand 1983;27:211–217.
88. Hally LE, Riedesel DH. Epidural anesthesia in the dog. Iowa State Vet 1983;45:45–48.
89. Nolte JG, Watney CG, Hall LW. Cardiovascular effects of epidural blocks in dogs. J Small Anim Pract 1983;24:17–21.
90. Dallman MJ, Mann FA. Epidural or spinal anesthesia for reduction of coxofemoral luxations in the dog. J Am Anim Hosp Assoc 1985;21:485–488.
91. Feldman HS, Hurley RJ, Covino BG. LEA-103 (Ropivacaine) a new local anesthetic: Experimental evaluation of spinal and epidural anesthesia in the dog, and sciatic nerve block in the rat [Abstract]. Anesthesiology 1986;65:A181.
92. Heath RB. The practicality of lumbosacral epidural analgesia. Semin Vet Med Surg (Small Anim) 1986;1:245–248.
93. Heath RB, Broadstone RV, Wright M, et al. Using bupivacaine hydrochloride for lumbosacral epidural analgesia. Compend Contin Educ Pract Vet 1989;11:50–55.
94. Peters J, Kousoulis L, Arndt JO. Effects of segmental thoracic extradural analgesia on sympathetic block in conscious dogs. Br J Anaesth 1989;63:470–476.
95. Shibata K, Yamamoto Y, Murakami S. Effects of epidural anesthesia on cardiovascular response survival in experimental hemorrhagic shock in dogs. Anesthesiology 1989;71:953–959.
96. Skarda RT. Local anesthesia in dogs and cats. In: Muir WW, Hubbell JAE, Skarda RT, eds. Handbook of Veterinary Anesthesia. Washington, DC: CV Mosby, 1989:100–119.
97. Cruz ML, Luna SPL, Clark RMO, et al. Epidural anaesthesia using lignocaine, bupivacaine or a mixture of lignocaine and bupivacaine in dogs. J Vet Anaesth 1997;24:30–32.
98. Jones RS. Epidural analgesia in the dog and cat [Review]. Vet J 2001;161:123–131.
99. Mikat-Stevens M, Stevens R, Schubert A, et al. Deliberate injection of air into the canine epidural space: A radiographic study [Abstract]. Anesth Analg 1989;68:194.
100. Fletcher TF. Spinal cord and meninges. In: Evans HE, Christensen GC, eds. Miller's Anatomy of the Dog, 2nd ed. Philadelphia: WB Saunders, 1979:947–962.
101. Liu P, Feldman HS, Covino BG. Comparative CNS and cardiovascular toxicity of various local anesthetic agents in awake dogs [Abstract]. Anesthesiology 1981;181:A156.

102. Ravindran RS, Tasch MD, Baldwin SJ, et al. Subarachnoid injection of autologous blood in dogs is unassociated with neurologic deficits. Anesth Analg 1981;60:603–604.

103. Sami HM, McNulty JA, Skaredoff MN, et al. The effect of spinal needle shape and bevel orientation on the size and shape of the dural defects: An SEM study in dogs. Anesthesiology 1989;71:A637.

104. Feldman HS, Covino BG. Comparative motor-blocking effects of bupivacaine and ropivacaine, a new amino amide local anesthetic, in the rat and dog. Anesth Analg 1988;67:1047–1052.

105. Hurley RJ, Arthur GR, Feldman HS, et al. The effects of epinephrine on the anesthetic and hemodynamic properties of ropivacaine and bupivacaine after epidural administration in the dog. Reg Anesth 1991;16:303–308.

106. Schmidt-Oechtering GU. Epidural anaesthesia in dogs and cats: Still an alternative to general anaesthesia [Abstract]. J Vet Anaesth 1993;20:40.

107. Hendrix PK, Raffe MR, Robinson EP, et al. Epidural administration of bupivacaine, morphine, or their combination for postoperative analgesia in dogs. J Am Vet Med Assoc 1996;209:598–607.

108. Duke T, Caulkett NA, Ball SD, et al. Comparative analgesic and cardiopulmonary effects of bupivacaine and ropivacaine in conscious dogs. In: Proceedings of the Annual Scientific Meeting of the American College of Veterinary Anesthesiologists, Dallas, TX, 1999:12.

109. Duke T, Caulkett NA, Ball SD, et al. Comparative analgesic and cardiopulmonary effects of bupivacaine and ropivacaine in the epidural space of the conscious dog. Vet Anaesth Analg 2000;27:13–21.

110. Butterworth JF IV, Walker FO, Lysak SZ. Pregnancy increases median nerve susceptibility to lidocaine. Anesthesiology 1990;72:962–965.

111. Bromage PR. Continuous lumbar epidural analgesia for obstetrics. Can Med Assoc J 1961;85:1136–1140.

112. Datta S, Lambert DH, Gregus J, et al. Differential sensitivities of mammalian nerve fibers during pregnancy. Anesth Analg 1983;62:1070–1072.

113. Gianetti A, Cerimele D. Effect of steroid hormones on the matrix of the dermis of the rat. In: Balazs EA, ed. Chemistry and Molecular Biology of the Intercellular Matrix, vol 3. London: Academic, 1970:1821–1827.

114. Bonath KH, Gerlach K, Ristic-Djuric Z, et al. Einfluss der extraduralen Langzeitanästhesie mit Bupivacaine und Langzeitanalgesie mit Morphin auf Kreislauf und Atmung des Hundes. Fortschr Veterinarmed 1983;37:237–239.

115. Remedios AM, Duke T. Chronic epidural implantation of vascular access ports in the cat lumbosacrum. Lab Sci 1993;43:262–264.

116. Usubiaga JE, Wikinski J, Wikinski R, et al. Transfer of local anesthetics to the subarachnoid space and mechanisms of epidural block. Anesthesiology 1964;25:752–759.

117. Durant PAC, Yaksh TL. Distribution in cerebrospinal fluid, blood, and lymph of epidurally injected morphine and insulin in dogs. Anesth Analg 1986;65:583–592.

118. Franquelo C, Toledo A, Manubens J, et al. Bupivacaine disposition and pharmacologic effects after intravenous and epidural administration in dogs. Am J Vet Res 1995;56:1087–1091.

119. Franquelo C, Toledo A, Manubens J, et al. Pharmacokinetics and pharmacologic effects of the S(−) isomer of bupivacaine after intravenous and epidural administration in dogs. Am J Vet Res 1999;60:832–835.

120. Stanek B, Schwartz M, Zimpfer M, et al. Plasma concentrations of noradrenaline and adrenaline and plasma renin activity during extradural blockade in dogs. Br J Anaesth 1980;52:305–311.

121. Peters J, Schlaghecke R, Thouet H, et al. Endogenous vasopressin supports blood pressure and prevents severe hypotension during epidural anesthesia in conscious dogs. Anesthesiology 190;73:694–702.

122. Butterworth JF IV, Piccione W Jr, Berrizbeitia LD, et al. Augmentation of venous return by adrenergic agonists during spinal anesthesia. Anesth Analg 1986;65:612–616.

123. Zhuang XL, Xu GH, Tong CY. Hemodynamic effects of ephedrine infusion on hypotension during epidural anesthesia in anesthetized dogs [Abstract]. Anesth Analg 1994;78(Suppl):S501.

124. Warner DO, Brichant JF, Ritman EL, et al. Epidural anesthesia and intrathoracic blood volume. Anesth Analg 1993;77:135–140.

125. Klassen GA, Bramwell RS, Bromage PR, et al. Effect of acute sympathectomy by epidural anesthesia on the canine coronary circulation. Anesthesiology 1980;52:8–15.

126. Sessler DI, Ponte J. Shivering during epidural anesthesia. Anesthesiology 1990;72:816–821.

127. Hammel HT, Wyndham CH, Hardy JD. Heat production and heat loss in the dog at 8–36°C environmental temperature. Am J Physiol (Lond) 1958;194:99–108.

128. Peters J, Breuksch E, Kousoulis L, et al. Regional skin temperatures after total sympathetic blockade in conscious dogs. Br J Anaesth 1988;61:617–624.

129. Kehlet H. Epidural analgesia and the endocrine-metabolic response to surgery(updates and perspectives. Acta Anaesthesiol Scand 1984;28:125–127.

130. Hole A, Unsgaard G, Breivik H. Monocyte functions are depressed during and after surgery under general anesthesia but not under epidural anesthesia. Acta Anaesthesiol Scand 1982;26:301–307.

131. Hall LW, Clarke KW. Veterinary Anesthesia, 8th ed. London: Bailliere Tindall, 1983:336–337.

132. Lumb WV, Jones EW. Veterinary Anesthesia, 2nd ed. Philadelphia: Lea and Febiger, 1984:407–408.

133. Goodger WJ, Levy W. Anesthetic management of cesarean section. Vet Clin North Am 1973;3:85–99.

134. Probst CW, Webb AI. Cesarean section in the dog and cat: Anesthetic and surgical techniques. In: Bojrab MJ, ed. Current Techniques in Small Animal Surgery. Philadelphia: Lea and Febiger, 1983:346–351.

135. Savas I, Saridomichelakis M, Galatos AD, et al. Does epidural analgesia affect hair re-growth in the lumbosacral region? A controlled study in 19 dogs (preliminary results). J Vet Anaesth 1998;25:58–59.

136. Troncy E, Junot S, Kerosack S, et al. Results of preemptive epidural administration of morphine with or without bupivacaine in dogs and cats undergoing surgery: 265 cases (1997–1999). J Am Vet Med Assoc 2002;221:666–672. Erratum in J Am Vet Med Assoc 2002;221:1149.

137. Yeager MP, Glass DD, Neff RK, et al. Epidural anesthesia and analgesia in high-risk surgical patients. Anesthesiology 1987;66:729–736.

138. Bonath KH, Saleh AS. Long term pain treatment in the dog by peridural morphine [Abstract]. In: Proceedings of the Second International Congress of Veterinary Anesthesiologists. Sacramento, CA: Veterinary Practice, 1985:161.

139. Knorr-Henn S. Epidurale Morphinwirkung auf Hämodynamik und Atemfunktionen des Hundes [PhD dissertation]. Giessen, Germany: Faculty of Veterinary Medicine, Justus-Liebig University, 1986.

140. Valverde A, Dyson DH, McDonell WN. Use of epidural morphine in the dog for pain relief. Vet Compend Orthop Traumatol 1989;2:55–58.

141. Valverde A, Dyson DH, Conlon P, et al. Cisternal CSF and serum concentrations of morphine following epidural administrations in the dog [Abstract]. In: Proceedings of the Veterinary Midwest Anesthesiologists' Conference, University of Illinois, Champaign-Urbana, 1990:12.

142. Valverde A, Conlon PD, Dyson DH, et al. Cisternal CSF and serum concentrations of morphine following epidural administration in the dog. J Vet Pharmacol Ther 1992;15:91–95.

143. Williams LL, Boudrieau RJ, Clark G, et al. Evaluation of epidural morphine in dogs for pain relief after hind limb orthopedic surgery [Abstract]. In: Proceedings of the Annual Scientific Meeting of the American College of Veterinary Anesthesiologists, New Orleans, LA, 1992:19.

144. Branson KR, Ko JCH, Tranquilli WJ, et al. Duration of analgesia induced by epidurally administered morphine and medetomidine in the dog. J Vet Pharmacol Ther 1993;16:369–372.

145. McMurphy RM. Postoperative epidural analgesia. Vet Clin North Am Small Anim Pract 1993;23:703–716.

146. Pascoe PJ, Dyson DH. Postoperative analgesia following lateral thoracotomy: Epidural morphine vs intercostal bupivacaine. In: Proceedings of the Annual Scientific Meeting of the American College of Veterinary Anesthesiologists, Las Vegas, NV, 1990:30.

147. Keegan RD, Greene SA. Cardiovascular effects of epidurally administered morphine and xylazine/morphine in isoflurane anesthetized dogs. In: Annual Scientific Meeting of the American College of Veterinary Anesthesiologists, Washington, DC, 1993:29.

148. Keegan RD, Greene SA, Weil AB. Cardiovascular effects of epidurally administered morphine and a xylazine-morphine combination in isoflurane-anesthetized dogs. Am J Vet Res 1995;56:496–500.

149. Quandt JE, Rawlings CR. Reducing postoperative pain for dogs: Local anesthetic and analgesic techniques. Compend Contin Educ Pract Vet 1996;18:101–111.

150. Torske KE, Dyson DH, Pettifer G. End tidal halothane concentration and postoperative analgesia requirements in dogs: A comparison between intravenous oxymorphone and epidural bupivacaine alone and in combination with oxymorphone. Can Vet J 1998;39:361–368.

151. Torske KE, Dyson DH, Conlon PD. Cardiovascular effects of epidurally administered oxymorphone and an oxymorphone-bupivacaine combination in halothane-anesthetized dogs. Am J Vet Res 1999;60:194–200.

152. Torske KE, Dyson DH. Epidural anesthesia and analgesia. Vet Clin North Am Small Anim Pract 2000;30:859–874.

153. Pacharinsak C, Greene SA, Keegan RD, et al. Postoperative analgesia in dogs receiving epidural morphine and medetomidine. Vet Anaesth Analg 2001;28:100–101.

154. Smith LJ, Kwang-An Yu J. A comparison of epidural buprenorphine with epidural morphine for postoperative analgesia following stifle surgery in dogs. Vet Anaesth Analg 2001;28:87–96.

155. Nègre I, Guéneron JP, Jamali SJ, et al. Preoperative analgesia with epidural morphine. Anesth Analg 1994;79:298–302.

156. Lanz E, Theiss D, Riess W, et al. Epidural morphine for postoperative analgesia: A double-blind study. Anesth Analg 1982;61:236–240.

157. Abouleish E, Barmada MA, Nemoto EM, et al. Acute and chronic effects of intrathecal morphine in monkeys. Br J Anaesth 1981;53:1027–1032.

158. Du Pen SL, Ramsey D, Chin S. Chronic epidural morphine and preservative-induced injury. Anesthesiology 1987;66:987–988.

159. Yaksh TL, Rudy TA. Analgesia mediated by a direct spinal action of narcotics. Science 1976;192:1357–1358.

160. Cousins MG, Mather LE. Intrathecal and epidural administration of opioids. Anesthesiology 1984;61:276–310.

161. Cousins MJ, Mather LE, Glynn CJ, et al. Selective spinal analgesia [Letter]. Lancet 1979;1:1141–1142.

162. Yaksh TL, Noueihed R. The physiology and pharmacology of spinal opioids. Annu Rev Pharmacol Toxicol 1985;25:433–462.

163. Pelligrino DA, Peterson RD, Henderson SK, et al. Comparative ventilatory effects of intravenous versus fourth cerebroventricular infusions of morphine sulfate in unanesthetized dog. Anesthesiology 1989;71:250–259.

164. Atchison SR, Durant PAC, Yaksh TL. Cardiorespiratory effects and kinetics of intrathecally injected D-ala2-D-leu5-enkephalin and morphine in unanesthetized dogs. Anesthesiology 1986;65:609–616.

165. Covino BG. Epidural morphine provides postoperative pain relief in peripheral vascular and orthopedic surgical patients: A dose-response study. Anesth Analg 1986;65:165–170.

166. Omote K, Nakagawa I, Kitahata LM, et al. The antinociceptive role of mu and delta opiate receptors and their interactions in the spinal dorsal horn of cats [Abstract]. Anesth Analg 1989;68(Suppl):S215.

167. Popilskis S, Kohn DI, Sanchez JA, et al. Comparison of epidural vs. intramuscular oxymorphone analgesia after thoracotomy in dogs. Vet Surg 1991;20:462–467.

168. Popilskis S, Kohn DF, Laurent L. Efficacy of epidural morphine versus intravenous morphine for post-thoracotomy pain in dogs. J Vet Anaesth 1993;20:21–25.

169. Valverde A, Dyson DH, Cockshutt JR, et al. Comparison of the hemodynamic effects of halothane alone and halothane combined with epidurally administered morphine for anesthesia in ventilated dogs. Am J Vet Res 1991;52:505–509.

170. Robinson TM, Kruse-Elliott KT, Markel MD, et al. A comparison of transdermal fentanyl versus epidural morphine for analgesia in dogs undergoing major orthopedic surgery. J Am Anim Hosp Assoc 1999;35:95–100.

171. Dragani JC, Rathbun ML, Yaksh TL, et al. Epidural encapsulated morphine in dogs: Analgesia and kinetics [Abstract]. In: Proceedings of the Annual Scientific Meeting of the American College of Veterinary Anesthesiologists, San Diego, CA, 1997:24.

172. Gourlay GK, Cherry DA, Plummer JL, et al. The influence of drug polarity on the absorption of opioid drugs into CSF and subsequent cephalad migration following lumbar epidural administration: Application to morphine and pethidine. Pain 1987;31:297–305.

173. Pelligrino DA, Peterson RD, Albrecht RF. Cisternal CSF morphine levels and ventilatory depression following epidural administration of morphine sulfate in the awake dog [Abstract]. Anesth Analg 1988;67(Suppl):S167.

174. Vesal N, Cribb PH. Analgesic and cardiopulmonary effects of epidural oxymorphone, epidural medetomidine and intramuscular oxymorphone in dogs: A clinical study [Abstract]. In: Proceedings of the Annual Scientific Meeting of the American College of Veterinary Anesthesiologists, Washington, DC, 1993:31.

175. Vesal N, Cribb PH, Frketic M. Postoperative analgesic and cardiopulmonary effects in dogs of oxymorphone administered epidurally and intramuscularly, and medetomidine administered epidurally: A comparative clinical study. Vet Surg 1996;25:361–369.

176. Troncy E, Cuvelliez SG, Blais D. Evaluation of analgesia and cardiorespiratory effects of epidurally administered butorphanol in isoflurane-anesthetized dogs. Am J Vet Res 1996;57:1478–1482.

177. Troncy E, Besner JG, Charbonneau R, et al. Pharmacokinetics of epidural butorphanol in isoflurane-anesthetized dogs. J Vet Pharmacol Ther 1996;19:268–273.

178. Du Pen SL, Peterson DG, Williams A, et al. Infection during chronic epidural catheterization, diagnosis, and treatment. Anesthesiology 1990;73:905–909.

179. Pybus DA, Torda TA. Dose-effect relationships of extradural morphine. Br J Anaesth 1982;54:1259–1262.

180. Kafer ER, Brown JT, Scott D, et al. Biphasic depression of ventilatory responses to CO_2 following epidural morphine. Anesthesiology 1983;58:418–427.

181. Rawal N, Schott U, Dahlstrom B, et al. Influence of naloxone infusion on analgesia and respiratory depression following epidural morphine. Anesthesiology 1986;66:194–201.

182. Shohami E, Evron S. Intrathecal morphine induces myoclonic seizures in the rat. Acta Pharmacol Toxicol 1985;56:50–54.

183. Shohami E, Evron S, Winstock M, et al. A new animal model for action myoclonus. Adv Neurol 1986;43:545–552.

184. Parkinson SK, Baily SL, Little WL, et al. Myoclonic seizure activity with high-dose spinal opioid administration. Anesthesiology 1990;72:743–745.

185. Frenk H, Watkins LR, Mayer DJ. Differential behavioral effects induced by intrathecal microinjection of opiates: Comparison of convulsive and cataleptic effects produced by morphine, methadone, and D-Ala2-methionine-enkephalinamide. Brain Res 1984;299:31–42.

186. Rozan JP, Kahn CH, Warfield CA. Epidural and intravenous-opioid-induced neuroexcitation. Anesthesiology 1995;83:860–863.

187. Kona-Boun J-J, Pibarot P, Quesnel A. Myoclonus and urinary retention following subarachnoid morphine injection in a dog [Review]. Vet Anaesth Analg 2003;30:257–264.

188. Kona-Boun J-J, Pibarot P, Quesnel A. Video clip about myoclonus in a German Shepherd associated with subarachnoid morphine. http://www.medvet.umontreal.ca/chuv/spasms.htm.

189. Wertz EM, Dunlop CI, Wagner AE, et al. Complications associated with epidural morphine in small animal anesthesia [Abstract]. In: Proceedings, Fifth International Congress of Veterinary Anesthesia, Guelph, Canada, 1994:163.

190. Yaksh TL, Harty GJ. Pharmacology of the allodynia in rats evoked by high dose intrathecal morphine. J Pharmacol Exp Ther 1987;244:501–507.

191. Yaksh TL, Harty GJ, Onofrio BM. High dose of spinal morphine produce [sic] a nonopiate receptor-mediated hyperesthesia: Clinical and theoretic implications. Anesthesiology 1886;64:590–597.

192. Kumar RVS, Ramakrisha O, Harapopal V, et al. The experimental use of diazepam for epidural anesthesia in dogs. Canine Pract 1994;19:20–23.

193. Yaksh TL, Stevens CW. Properties of the modulation of spinal nociceptive transmission by receptor selective agents. In: Dubner R, Gerhart GF, Bond MR, eds. Proceedings of the Fifth World Congress of Pain. Amsterdam: Elsevier, 1988:417–435.

194. Solomon RE, Gebhart GF. Synergistic antinociceptive interactions among drugs administered to the spinal cord. Anesth Analg 1994;78:1164–1172.

195. Greene SA, Keegan RD. Cardiovascular effects of epidurally administered xylazine in isoflurane-anesthetized dogs [Abstract]. In: Proceedings of the Annual Scientific Meeting of the American College of Veterinary Anesthesiologists, Washington, DC, 1993:27.

196. Greene SA, Keegan RD. Cardiovascular effects of epidurally administered xylazine in isoflurane-anesthetized dogs. Vet Surg 1995;24:283–289.

197. Otto KA, Piepenbrock S, Rischke B, et al. Effects of epidural xylazine on EEG responses to surgical stimulation in isoflurane-anesthetized dogs. In: Proceedings of the Annual Scientific Meeting of the American College of Veterinary Anesthesiologists, Atlanta, GA, 1995:10.

198. Otto KA, Piepenbrock S, Rischke B, et al. Effects of epidural xylazine on EEG responses to surgical stimulation during isoflurane anaesthesia in dogs. J Vet Anaesth 1997;24:33–38.

199. Rector E, Otto K, Kietzmann M, et al. Evaluation of the antinociceptive effect of xylazine after epidural administration in dogs under general anesthesia with isoflurane [in German]. Berl Munch Tierarztl Wochenschr 1997;10:15–23.

200. Sedighi MHR. A comparison of the haemodynamic effects of epidurally administered medetomidine and xylazine in dogs [Abstract]. Vet Anaesth Analg 2003;30:98.

201. Branson KR, Tranquilli WJ, Ko JCH, et al. Duration of analgesia induced by epidurally administered morphine and medetomidine in dogs [Abstract]. Vet Surg 1993;22:88.

202. Pedraz JL, Calvo MB, Gascon AR, et al. Pharmacokinetics and distribution of ketamine after extradural administration to dogs. Br J Anaesth 1991;67:310–316.

203. Baha F, Malbert CH. Effet de kétamine par voie intrathécale chez le chien. Rev Med Vet 1991;142:283–285.

204. Martin DD, Tranquilli WJ, Olson WA, et al. Analgesic action of epidural ketamine injection in isoflurane-anesthetized dogs [Abstract]. In: Proceedings of the Annual Scientific Meeting of the American College of Veterinary Anesthesiologists, Atlanta, GA, 1995:12.

205. Martin DD, Tranquilli WJ, Olson WA, et al. Hemodynamic effects of epidural ketamine in isoflurane-anesthetized dogs. Vet Surg 1997;26:505–509.

206. Iida H, Dohi S, Tanahashi T, et al. Spinal conduction block by intrathecal ketamine in dogs. Anesth Analg 1997;85:106–110.

207. Hamilton SM, Broadstone RV, Johnston SA. The evaluation of analgesia provided by epidural ketamine in dogs with chemically induced synovitis [Abstract]. In: Proceedings of the Annual Scientific Meeting of the American College of Veterinary Anesthesiologists, Orlando, FL, 2002:19.

208. Reddy SVR, Maderdrut JL, Yaksh TL. Spinal cord pharmacology of adrenergic agonist-mediated antinociception. J Pharmacol Exp Ther 1980;213:525–533.

209. Yaksh TL, Reddy SVR. Studies in the primate on the analgesic effects associated with intrathecal actions of opiate, α-adrenergic agonists, and baclofen. Anesthesiology 1981;54:451–467.

210. Millan MJ, Bervoets K, Rivet JM, et al. Multiple alpha-2 adrenergic receptor subtypes. II. Evidence for a role of rat alpha-2A adrenergic receptors in control of nociception, motor behavior and hippocampal synthesis of noradrenaline. J Pharmacol Exp Ther 1994;270:958–972.

211. Buerkle H, Yaksh TL. Pharmacological evidence for different alpha 2-adrenergic receptor sites mediating analgesia and sedation in the rat. Br J Anaesth 1998;81:208–215.

212. Takano M, Takano Y, Yaksh TL. Release of calcitonin gene-related peptide (CGRP), substance P (SP), and vasoactive intestinal polypeptide (VIP) from rat spinal cord: Modulation by α_2 agonists. Peptides 1993;14:371–378.

213. Eisenach J, Lysak S, Viscomi C. Epidural clonidine analgesia following surgery: Phase 1. Anesthesiology 1989;71:640–646.

214. Scheinin H, Virtanen R, Macdonald E, et al. Medetomidine: A novel alpha 2-adrenoceptor agonist: A review of its pharmacodynamic effects. Prog Neuropsychopharmacol Biol Psychiatry 1989;13:635–651.

215. Sabbe MB, Penning JP, Ozaki GT, et al. Spinal and systemic action of the α_2 receptor agonist dexmedetomidine in dogs: Antino-

ciception and carbon dioxide response. Anesthesiology 1994;80:1057–1072.

216. Kohrs R, Durieux ME. Ketamine: Teaching an old drug new tricks. Anesth Analg 1998;87:1186–1193.

217. Martin L, Smith D. Ketamine inhibits serotonin synthesis and metabolism in vitro. Neuropharmacology 1982;21:119–125.

218. Arhem P, Rydqvist B. The mechanism of action of ketamine on myelinated nerve membrane. Eur J Pharmacol 1986;126:245–251.

219. Benoit E, Carratu H, Dubois J, et al. Mechanism of action of ketamine in the current and voltage clamped myelinated nerve fiber of the frog. Br J Pharmacol 1986;87:291–297.

220. Takahashi H, Miyazaki M, Nanbu T, et al. The NMDA-receptor antagonist ketamine abolishes neuropathic pain after epidural administration in a clinical case. Pain 1998;75:391–394.

221. Hocking G, Cousins MJ. Ketamine in chronic pain management: Evidence-based review. Anesth Analg 2003;97:1730–1739.

222. Gallivan ST, Johnston SJ, Broadstone R, et al. The safety of epidurally administered ketorolac in dogs. [Abstract]. Vet Surg 1999;28:393.

223. Gallivan ST, Johnston SA, Broadstone RV, et al. The clinical, cerebrospinal fluid, and histopathologic effects of epidural ketorolac in dogs. Vet Surg 2000;29:436–441.

224. Abram SE. Neural blockade for neuropathic pain. Clin J Pain 2000;16(Suppl):S56–S61.

225. Hayashi N, Weinstein JN, Meller ST, et al. The effect of epidural injection of betamethasone or bupivacaine in a rat model of lumbar radiculopathy. Spine 1998;23:877–885.

226. Cooper AB, Sharpe MD. Bacterial meningitis and cauda equina syndrome after epidural steroid injections. Can J Anaesth 1996;43(5 Pt 1):471–474.

227. Victory RA, Hassett P, Morrison G. Transient blindness following epidural analgesia. Anaesthesia 1991;46:940–941.

228. Akerman B, Arwestrom E, Post C. Local anesthetics potentiate spinal morphine antinociception. Anesth Analg 1988;67:943–948.

229. Rucci FS, Cardamone M, Migliori P. Fentanyl and bupivacaine mixtures for extradural block. Br J Anaesth 1985;57:275–284.

230. Skerman JH, Thompson BA, Goldstein MT, et al. Combined continuous epidural fentanyl and bupivacaine in labour: A randomized study. Anesthesiology 1985;63:A450–454.

231. Gaffud MP, Bansal P, Lawton C, et al. Surgical analgesia for cesarean delivery with epidural bupivacaine and fentanyl. Anesthesiology 1986;65:331–334.

232. Maurette P, Bonada G, Djiane V, et al. A comparison between lidocaine alone and lidocaine with meperidine for continuous spinal anesthesia. Reg Anesth 1993;18:290–295.

233. Hussain SS, Kumar A. Physiological, haemocytological, biochemical and clinical effects of epidural morphine in dogs. Indian Vet J 1988;5:491–495.

234. Aminkov BY. Comparison between lidocaine alone and fentanyl with lidocaine for epidural anaesthesia in dogs. Rev Med Vet 1996;147:819–824.

235. Ossipov MH, Suarez LJ, Spaulding TC. Antinociceptive interactions between alpha$_2$-adrenergic and opiate agonists at the spinal level of rodents. Anesth Analg 1989;68:194–200.

236. Ossipov MH, Harris S, Lloyd P, et al. Antinociceptive interaction between opioids and medetomidine: Systemic additivity and spinal synergy. Anesthesiology 1990;73:1227–1235.

237. Omote K, Kitahata LM, Collins JG, et al. Interaction between opiate subtype and alpha-2 adrenergic agonists in suppression of noxiously-evoked activity of WDR neurons in the spinal dorsal horn. Anesthesiology 1991;74:737–743.

238. Branson KR, KØ JC, Tranquilli WJ, Benson J, Thurmon JC. Duration of analgesia induced by epidurally administered morphine and medetomidine in dogs. J Vet Pharmacol Ther 1993;16(3):369–372.

239. Hoffmann VL, Baker AK, Vercauteren MP, et al. Epidural ketamine potentiates epidural morphine but not fentanyl in acute nociception in rats. Eur J Pain 2003;7:121–130.

240. Dietz O. Die Anästhesie des Ganglion stellatum beim Hund. Zentralbl Veterinarmed 6:569–574, 1955.

241. Dietz O. Zur Grenzstrangblockade beim Tier. Arch Exp Veterinarmed 1957;11:310–330 and 349–385.

242. Wolfe TM, Bateman SW, Cole LK. Evaluation of a local anesthetic delivery system for the postoperative analgesic management of canine total ear canal ablation: A randomized, controlled, double-blinded study. Vet Anaesth Analg 2006;33:328–339.

Chapter 21

Local and Regional Anesthetic and Analgesic Techniques: Cats

Roman T. Skarda and William J. Tranquilli

Introduction

This chapter reviews the use of selective local and regional anesthetic and analgesic techniques in cats as an adjunct to light general anesthesia. The techniques are easily performed for diagnostic and surgical procedures to produce postoperative analgesia. A basic knowledge of the regional anatomy of the area to be desensitized and the pharmacology of drugs used to induce effective local anesthesia is required if the full potential of local anesthetic and analgesic techniques is to be realized.[1,2] Commonly used techniques in cats are topical anesthesia, local infiltration, nerve blocks (e.g., selective blockade of distal branches of nerves about the head, forelimb, and hind limb), brachial plexus block, intravenous regional anesthesia, epidural anesthesia, and epidural analgesia. Because of restraint problems, local and regional anesthetic techniques are typically administered to heavily sedated or anesthetized cats. A number of local anesthetic drugs that vary in potency, toxicity, and cost are available for these purposes. Most commonly, 0.5% to 2.0% lidocaine hydrochloride is used to anesthetize cats for 60 to 120 min, whereas 0.2% to 0.5% ropivacaine hydrochloride or 0.25% to 0.5% bupivacaine hydrochloride produce anesthesia for 240 to 360 min. The applied pharmacology of local anesthetic drugs in animals has been described in Chapter 14. Advantages of using regional anesthetic/analgesic techniques include (a) reduction of the required dose of general anesthetic drugs and thus minimal cardiopulmonary depression, (b) complete blockade of sensory and motor nerve fibers, and (c) prevention of the secondary (central) sensitization to pain. Preemptive analgesia theoretically (a) decreases the severity of pain during surgery, (b) reduces drug requirement for pain control, and (c) provides analgesia after surgery.[3-6]

Topical Anesthesia

Local anesthetics, either as lidocaine spray (10%, 100 mg/mL) or lidocaine hydrochloride solution, can be applied topically. One spray delivers 10 mg of lidocaine, which usually is sufficient to desensitize small areas of oral, nasal, and pharyngeal mucous membranes. Administration of 20 mg of lidocaine to the mucous membrane produces surface anesthesia up to 2 mm deep within 2 min, which lasts for about 15 min. Topical lidocaine (spray or instillation) is useful for minor diagnostic, therapeutic, and surgical procedures (e.g., endoscopy, placement of nasal catheters for tube feeding, foreign-body removal, biopsies, and repair of small mucosal wounds). Instillation of 1.0 mL of lidocaine (20 mg), ropivacaine (2 mg), or bupivacaine (2.5 mg) into the wound of skin incisions or lacerations provides good analgesia in cats (4 kg). These local anesthetics are ineffective when applied topically to intact skin. Sterile lidocaine jelly (2%, 20 mg/mL) provides good analgesia of the urethra during catheter placement, because lidocaine is absorbed across mucous membranes. The eutectic mixture of lidocaine and prilocaine (EMLA cream [lidocaine 2.5% and prilocaine 2.5%]) penetrates the stratum corneum of the skin. Cream is placed on the skin and covered with a clean dressing for at least 20 min to enable painless placement of arterial and venous catheters in nervous cats.[7] Proparacaine 0.5%, tetracaine 0.5%, or butacaine 2% can be applied topically to desensitize the cornea for 10 to 20 min. Repeated doses have been reported to prolong anesthesia up to 2 h without causing harmful effects.[8]

Infiltration Anesthesia

Local infiltration is primarily used for repair of superficial lacerations, cutaneous biopsy, and removal of dermal or subcutaneous tumors. Lidocaine hydrochloride (2 to 5 mg/kg), ropivacaine, or bupivacaine hydrochloride (3 mg/kg) is injected in the form of a subcutaneous bleb, line block, inverted V-block or triangular or rectangular pattern around a small tumor to be surgically removed, using a 25-gauge (G) × 0.6-inch needle or 22-G × 1-inch needle.[9] The dose of the local anesthetic should be carefully calculated to prevent toxicity. The syringe is aspirated before each injection and great care must be taken that the local

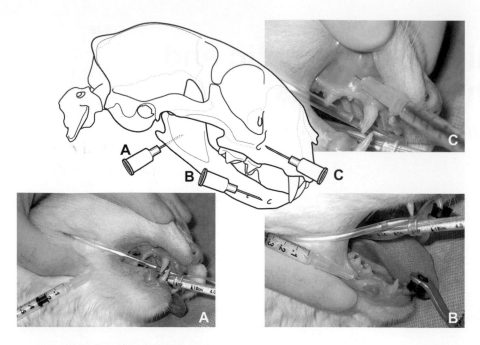

Fig. 21.1. Needle placement for nerve blocks of the head: **(A)** inferior alveolar (mandibular), **(B)** mental, and **(C)** infraorbital.

anesthetic is not inadvertently administered intravenously.[10–12] Sterile saline solution can be used to decrease the concentration and increase the volume of lidocaine (2 mL of a 1% solution instead of 1 mL of a 2% solution) to allow infiltration of a larger lesion. The total dose (20 mg) should be reduced by 30% to 50% in sick cats.

Regional Anesthesia of the Head

Commonly used nerve blocks to manage pain during and after surgical and dental procedures are the infraorbital, inferior alveolar and mental nerves (Fig. 21.1).[2,13,14] These nerves can be desensitized by injecting 0.1 to 0.3 mL of either 1.0% to 2.0% lidocaine, 0.2% to 0.5% ropivacaine, or 0.25% to 0.5% bupivacaine hydrochloride solutions, using a 30-G × 0.5-inch to 22-G × 1-inch needle.

Anesthesia of the Maxilla and Upper Teeth

The upper lip and muzzle, roof of the nasal cavity, soft and hard palates, and teeth in the upper dental arcade are supplied by sensory fibers of the infraorbital nerve. The nerve is blocked at the infraorbital foramen as it emerges from the infraorbital canal, ventral to the eye, approximately 1.0 cm dorsal to the third premolar at the junction of the maxilla and zygomatic arch. Improper identification of the infraorbital foramen and branching of a nerve proximal to the region of local anesthetic may cause failure to produce regional anesthesia.[13] The block is facilitated by angling the needle tip slightly medially. The needle is then advanced approximately 0.5 cm into the infraorbital canal, which is not a true canal in cats (Fig. 21.1C).

Anesthesia of the Mandible and Lower Teeth

The lower dental arcade, including the molars, canines, and incisors, and the skin and mucosa of the chin and lower lip are sup-

plied by sensory fibers of the mandibular nerve. The nerve can be easily blocked at the point of its entry into the mandibular canal at the mandibular foramen. The needle is inserted percutaneously at the ventromedial aspect of the ramus of the mandible, approximately 1.0 cm rostral to the angular process, and for a depth of 0.5 cm (Fig. 21.1A). In an alternative technique, the inferior alveolar nerve can be blocked intraorally, under the buccal fold.

The inferior alveolar nerve branches into the free rostral, middle, and caudal mental nerves, which supply sensory fibers to the lower lip and the medial half of the canine and three incisors. The mental nerve can be blocked at the mental foramina, caudal and ventral to the lower canine (Fig. 21.1B). The extremely small size of the mental foramina precludes the insertion of a needle or catheter into the termination of the mandibular canal.[13]

Anesthesia of the Limbs

Blockade of the distal branches of the radial, median, and ulnar nerves, blockade of cervical and thoracic nerves (brachial plexus block), and intravenous regional anesthesia are cost- and time-effective techniques for providing perioperative anesthesia and managing pain after surgical procedures of the forelimb in cats. In the hind limb, selective blockade of the common peroneal and tibial nerves is easily produced. Injection of the local anesthetic or opioid into the epidural space at the lumbosacral junction provides analgesia of the pelvic limbs and perineum.

Blockade of the Radial, Ulnar, and Median Nerves

Selective blockade of the distal branches of the radial, ulnar, and median nerves produces brief surgical anesthesia and postoperative analgesia after onychectomy or tenectomy. The nerve blocks are easily performed to supplement anesthesia or provide an alternative to wound irrigation with local anesthetic following ony-

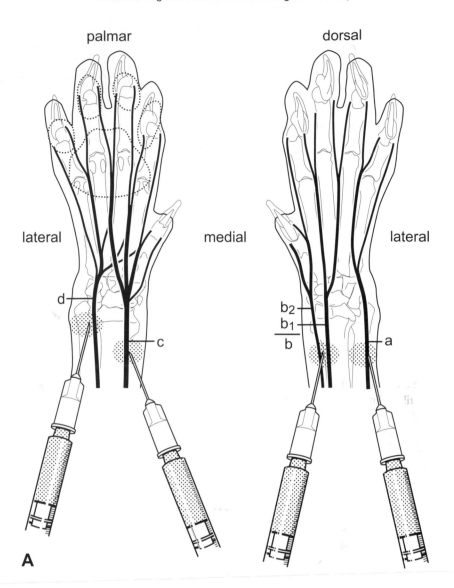

Fig. 21.2. A: Needle placement for nerve blocks on the foreleg: (a) dorsal branch of ulnar nerve, (b1) lateral branch and (b2) medial branch of superficial branch of radial nerve, (c) median nerve, and (d) palmar branch of the ulnar nerve.

A

chectomy.[15–21] The superficial branches of the radial nerve are blocked on the dorsomedial aspect proximal to the carpal joint. The palmar and dorsal cutaneous branches of the ulnar nerve are blocked just proximal and lateral to the accessory carpal bone. The median nerve is blocked proximal to the median carpal pad. A 22-G × 1-inch needle can be used, and approximately 0.3 mL of the anesthetic solution is administered subcutaneously at each site (Fig. 21.2A). In two alternative techniques, the local anesthetic (3 mg/kg body weight) is injected subcutaneously distal to the carpal joint to each of the dorsal and palmar proper digital nerves either as a four-point digital nerve block[22] or ring block.[23]

Blockade of the Common Peroneal and Tibial Nerves

Selective blockade of the distal branches of the common peroneal and tibial nerves produces perioperative and postoperative analgesia in the hind limb for onychectomy or tenectomy. The superficial branches of the common peroneal nerve are easily blocked by subcutaneous infiltration of the local anesthetic on

the dorsomedial aspect of the tarsus distal to the tarsal joint. The superficial branches of the tibial nerve are blocked by subcutaneous injection of the local anesthetic ventromedially and distally to the tarsal joint (Fig. 21.2B).

Brachial Plexus Block

Blockade of the ventral branches of the cervical (C6, C7, and C8) and thoracic (T1) spinal nerves can be used to anesthetize the forelimb and manage pain after surgical repair of the radius and ulna in cats.[14] The procedure is performed in well-sedated or anesthetized cats. A needle (22 G × 1 inch) is placed into the axillary space proximal to the shoulder, and approximately 0.5 mL of either 2% lidocaine (10 mg), 0.5% ropivacaine, or 0.5% bupivacaine (2.5 mg) is injected once the needle tip is cranial to the first rib and caudal to the cranial border of the scapula (Fig. 21.3). The same amount of the anesthetic is administered as the needle is withdrawn. The syringe is aspirated prior to each injection to avoid injection into the axillary artery and vein, which are close to the brachial plexus. The brachial plexus should not be

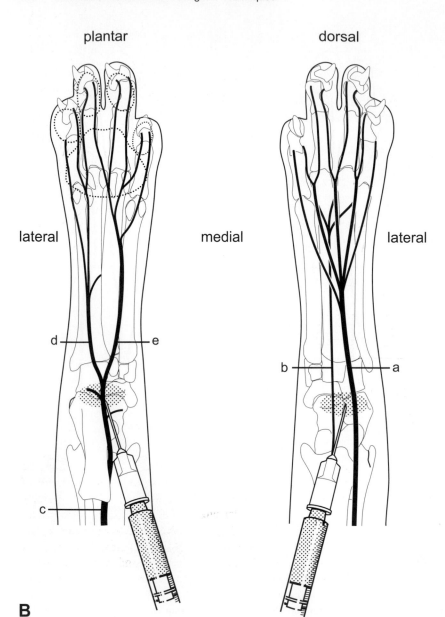

plantar   dorsal

lateral   medial   lateral

d   e

b   a

c

Fig. 21.3 (*continued*). **B:** Needle placement for nerve blocks on the hind leg: (a) superficial peroneal nerve, (b) deep peroneal nerve, (c) tibial nerve, (d) lateral plantar nerve, and (e) medial plantar nerve.

B

blocked bilaterally because of potential bilateral phrenic nerve blockade and subsequent compromised respiratory function.

Intravenous Regional Anesthesia

Intravenous regional anesthesia (IVRA) may be suitable for anesthetized cats undergoing surgery, including onychectomy, of the distal limbs. First, a 22-G × 1-inch intravenous catheter is inserted into the cephalic vein proximal to the carpus and with the catheter tip pointing distally.[24] Second, an inflatable blood pressure cuff (neonatal no. 2; Criticon, Tampa, FL) is placed proximal to the cephalic catheter and is inflated and maintained at 100 mm Hg greater than systolic pressure. Third, a second tourniquet, 6.25-mm rubber tubing, is tied above the elbow and left in place for 20 min. Lidocaine (1%, 3 mg/kg) is then injected into the distal cephalic venous catheter to anesthetize the entire limb distal to the tourniquet, as determined by lack of response to toe pinch.

After the tourniquet has been removed, analgesia still remains for approximately 20 min. No neurotoxicity or adverse hemodynamic or respiratory effects have been reported in cats breathing either a low (1.5%) or high (2.3%) concentration of isoflurane during IVRA. No adverse effects were noted during recovery from anesthesia 20 min after tourniquet removal.[24] The plasma lidocaine concentrations may vary. The reported highest mean lidocaine concentration was 2.8 ± 1.0 μg/mL after the injection of lidocaine (3 mg/kg) and was 3.1 ± 1.1 μg/mL after a second injection of lidocaine (3 mg/kg) 20 min later.[24] The model described simulated a 20-min onychectomy procedure per each front leg of the cat. Significant leakage under the tourniquet may occur, as determined by measurable venous plasma lidocaine concentrations (maximum, 4.42 μg/mL) prior to tourniquet release. Placement of the tourniquet and thus occlusion of blood supply distal to the tourniquet should be limited to 30 min to prevent complications (e.g., lameness or endotoxemia) (Fig. 21.4).

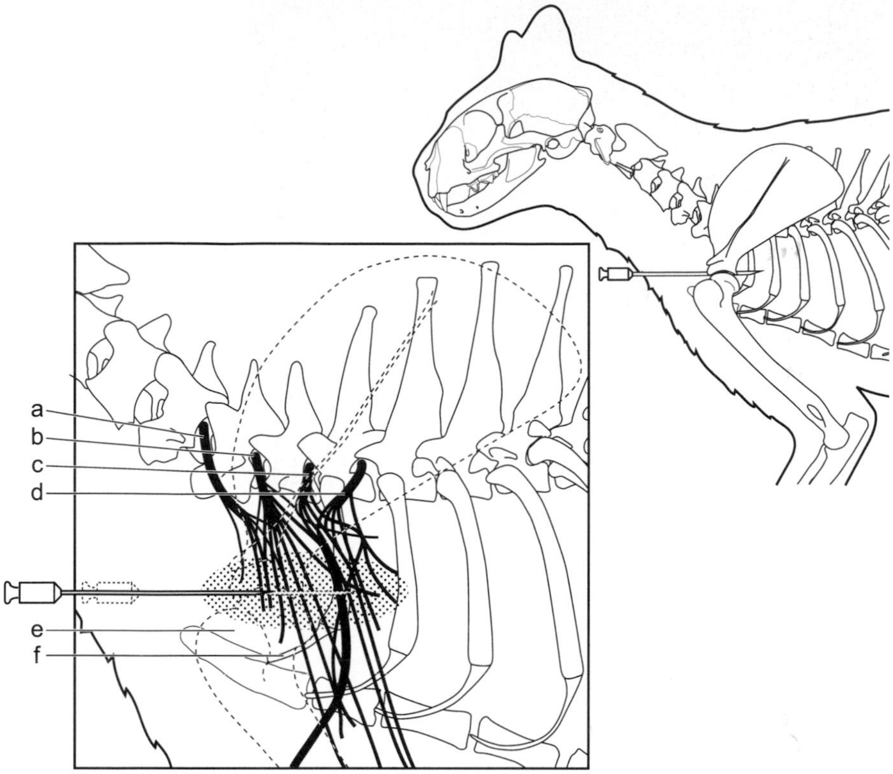

Fig. 21.3. Needle placement for brachial plexus block. **Inset:** ventral branches of (a) sixth, (b) seventh, and (c) eighth cervical, and (d) first thoracic spinal nerve; (e) tuberosity of humerus; and (f) first rib.

Intercostal Nerve Block

This technique is used to control pain following lateral thoracotomy, rib fractures, or pleural drainage. Two adjacent intercostal nerves, cranial and caudal to the incision site or wound (four sites in total), are blocked (Fig. 21.5). A needle (27 G × 1 inch) is inserted into the intercostal muscle close to the insertion of the epaxial muscles. The needle is directed dorsomedially and, using caution not to puncture the lung, its tip is walked off the caudal border of the rib. The syringe is aspirated before each injection of the anesthetic solution (3 mg/kg body weight), which is equally divided among the injection sites. Cats should be observed for development of pneumothorax during the first 30 min after the procedure. Cats with severe lung disease and those that rely on their intercostal muscles for maintaining ventilation and oxygen saturation must be monitored closely.[14]

Lumbosacral Epidural Anesthesia

Lumbosacral epidural anesthesia is safe and inexpensive and provides a reversible loss of sensation to a reasonably well-defined area of the body caudal to the diaphragm. This procedure is relatively easy to perform in heavily sedated or anesthetized cats.[25–27] Epidural injection of a local anesthetic may be used alone in cats that are at high risk of medical complications, that are aged, or that require immediate surgery of the rear quarter. The skin of the lumbosacral area is surgically prepared with an aseptic technique. A needle (22 G × 1 inch) is placed into the skin surface at the midline of the lumbosacral space. Except in obese cats, this space can be easily palpated halfway between the dorsoiliac wings and just caudal to the dorsal spinous process of the seventh lumbar vertebra. The needle is pushed ventrocaudally at a 45° angle to the dorsum to avoid pinching the seventh lumbar spinous process (Fig. 21.6). Resistance is encountered on reaching the ligamentum flavum. A distinct pop is usually felt when the needle is advanced through this ligament. Needle depth to reach the epidural space may vary from 6 to 25 mm (0.25 to 1.0 inch), depending on the cat's size. Further insertion of the needle will meet resistance, indicating the needle tip has encountered the bony floor of the vertebral canal, and thus necessitates the withdrawal of needle for 1 to 2 mm. The hub of the needle is observed for blood and cerebrospinal fluid (CSF). Because the dura sack terminates in the sacral area of cats, CSF may escape from the needle. If CSF is observed or aspirated, either the epidural injection is abandoned or only one-third to one-half of the original calculated dose of the drug is administered. Observation of blood within the needle indicates that the ventral venous sinus has been punctured; therefore, the needle should be removed. Intravascular injection of epidural drugs should be avoided to prevent toxicity. Lidocaine 2%, ropivacaine 0.2%, or bupivacaine 0.25% at the dose of 1.0 mL/4 kg produces analgesia up to the umbilicus area.[1,2,25] Analgesia usually lasts for at least 1 h with the use of lidocaine and 4 to 6 h with ropivacaine or bupivacaine injection. A regular local anesthetic dose (1.0 mL/4 kg) administered subarachnoidally (into the CSF) or a larger dose (>3 mL) administered epidurally produces a more cranial blockade that may be associated with decreased sympathetic activity and direct myocardial depression, and can cause

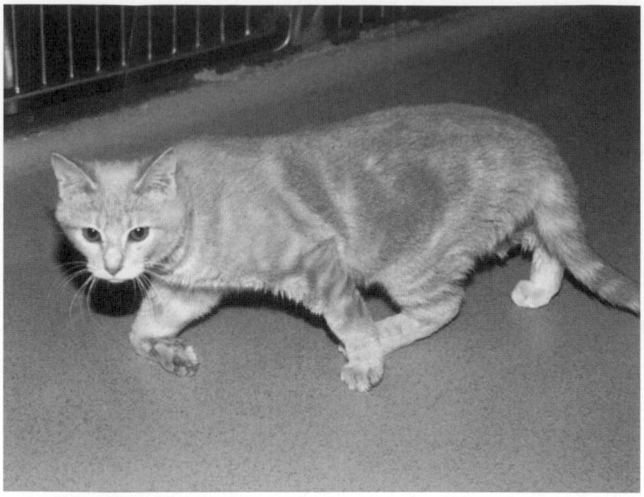

Fig. 21.4. Severe 18-h lameness of a cat, which had a rubber tourniquet in place above the right carpus during onychectomy for approximately 40 min.

hypotension, respiratory insufficiency, respiratory paralysis, and convulsions.

Epidural Opioid Analgesia

Preservative-free morphine (Astramorph/PF, 0.5 or 1.0 mg morphine/mL; or Duramorph, 0.5 or 1.0 mg morphine/mL) can be administered through a sterile needle or indwelling epidural catheter into the epidural space of cats to provide moderate to excellent intraoperative analgesia and postoperative pain control. An aseptic technique, as described for epidural injection of local anesthetic drugs, must be used. Placement of a vascular access device (access port model SLA-3.5H; Access Technologies, Division of Norfolk Medical Products, Skokie, IL) used as an indwelling epidural catheter in cats has been described (Fig. 21.6A).[28–30] In contrast to the administration of a local anesthetic drug by the epidural route, epidural morphine provides more prolonged analgesia (>6 h) with no effect on motor and sympathetic pathways.[31] The dose of morphine (0.1 mg/kg) must be calculated carefully and, to avoid inadvertent intravascular administration, the syringe should be aspirated before injection. A cat weighing 4 kg can be administered 0.4 mg morphine, which is 0.8 mL of Astramorph (0.5 mg/mL). If the needle tip has entered the intrathecal (subarachnoid) space, as recognized by free flow

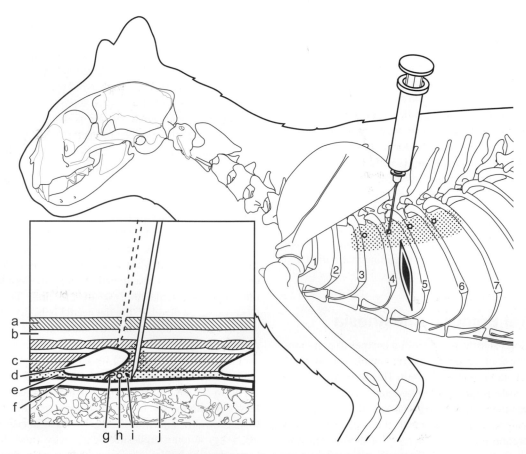

Fig. 21.5. Needle placement for inducing intercostal nerve blocks, showing the lateral aspect and the sagittal section **[inset]**: (a) skin, (b) subcutaneous tissue, (c) intercostal muscles, (d) rib, (e) subcostal space, (f) pleura costalis and fascia, (g) intercostal vein, (h) intercostal artery, (i) intercostal nerve, and (j) lung.

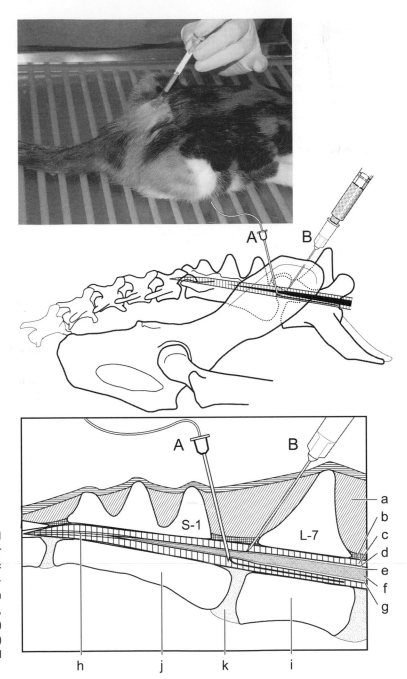

Fig. 21.6. Needle placement into the lumbosacral epidural space of the cat (B) and catheter placement for continuous epidural anesthesia by using a local anesthetic and/or analgesia by using an opioid (A). **Inset:** (a) interspinous ligament, (b) interarcuate ligament (ligamentum flavum), (c) epidural space with fat and connective tissue, (d) dura mater, (e) arachnoid membrane, (f) spinal cord, (g) cerebrospinal fluid, (h) cauda equina, (i) seventh lumbar (L7) vertebra, (j) first sacral (S1) vertebra, and (k) intervertebral disk.

of CSF from the needle hub or aspiration by the syringe,[32] the dose is reduced by 50% to 0.2 mg of morphine (0.4 mL of Astramorph). Administration of 0.05, 1.0, and 2.0 mg of epidural morphine per kilogram of body weight decreased the minimum alveolar isoflurane concentration requirements in cats by 21.4% ± 9.7%, 30.8% ± 9.6%, and 30.2% ± 6.8%, respectively.[33] Increasing the dose of morphine was not found to be significant, probably because of a saturation of opioid receptors with increasing doses of morphine. These cats demonstrated a significant decrease in systolic, mean and diastolic blood pressure, heart and respiratory rates, and arterial pH, whereas the arterial carbon dioxide tension increased with epidural morphine administration.[33] Mild hind-limb ataxia, but no excitement, licking, retch-

ing, or vomiting, was observed up to 60 min into recovery. Such side effects can be observed in nonanesthetized cats receiving epidural administration of morphine. Analgesia generally develops first, lasts longer, and is more profound in somatic areas of spinal cord segments, which are presumably exposed to the highest concentration of morphine.[34] The depressant effects of epidural morphine on the hemodynamic and respiratory centers are likely the result of interaction with opioid receptors in the central nervous system (general analgesia) after diffusion to the brain via the blood and CSF.

Analgesia and behavioral effects of epidural oxymorphone (0.025, 0.05, and 0.1 mg/kg mixed in 0.13 mL saline/kg) and saline placebo have been evaluated in four cats.[35] A spinal needle (22 G × 1.5 inches) was inserted into the epidural space at the lumbosacral junction, and the doses were given randomly to each cat anesthetized with isoflurane at 7-day intervals. Isoflurane was discontinued, and scores for pain, behavior, and sedation were recorded along with indirect blood pressure and respiratory rate at 30 and 60 min and hourly thereafter to 480 min. A noncrushing clamp was briefly placed 5 cm from the tail base to produce nociception at each time interval. No significant changes were observed in blood pressure, respiratory rate, behavior, or sedation of healthy cats. Analgesic effects were present for 52 ± 22 min in nontreated cats but increased to 332 ± 111 min with the highest oxymorphone dose (0.1 mg/kg).

Lumbosacral epidural injection of fentanyl (4 µg/kg) diluted to a total volume of 1 mL with physiological saline reportedly increases the pain threshold of the hind limb for up to 245 min after injection. No visible side effects or behavioral changes were observed, nor was analgesia detected in the forelimbs of these cats.[29] Epidural fentanyl injection was associated with a decrease in heart and respiratory rates and mean arterial blood pressure.[30] Epidural fentanyl also increased arterial PCO_2 and decreased arterial pH from 15 to 120 min after injection.[30] In these same studies, medetomidine (10 µg/kg) in 1 mL of saline significantly increased the pain threshold up to 245 min (hind limb) and 120 min (forelimb), respectively. Epidural medetomidine was associated with mild sedation and emesis in 12 of the 15 cats studied.[29] The hemodynamic profile during isoflurane (2.4%) anesthesia was a biphasic blood pressure response: first a significant increase (5 to 20 min after injection) and then a significant decrease (30 to 120 min after injection). Arterial PCO_2 and blood bicarbonate concentration were significantly increased, while arterial pH was significantly decreased for up to 2 h after epidural medetomidine administration.[30]

The N-methyl-D-aspartate (NMDA) receptor antagonistic action of ketamine may be useful in patients with chronic pathological pain states refractory to opioids, anticonvulsants, or antidepressants.[36] However, the safety of neuraxially administered ketamine remains unclear. No inflammatory reactions have been reported in animal studies when preservative-free ketamine has been used. Ketamine with benzethonium chloride preservative administered intrathecally has caused radicular demyelinization in rats.[37] Subpial vacuolar myelopathy[38] and focal lymphocytic vasculitis have been observed adjacent to the catheter tip in humans, but no neurological deficit or other histological changes were evident.[39]

Based on the observations to date, the epidural use of α_2-receptor agonists (xylazine and medetomidine), dissociative anesthetics (ketamine and tiletamine-zolazepam), and anti-inflammatory drugs (ketoprofen) cannot be advocated for routine epidural use in cats.[40]

Conclusion

Local and regional anesthetic techniques can safely be used in heavily sedated or anesthetized cats. The local and regional anesthetic and analgesic techniques described are compatible with systemically administered opioids (e.g., morphine, butorphanol,

and fentanyl patch), α_2-receptor agonists (e.g., xylazine and medetomidine), dissociative anesthetics (e.g., ketamine and tiletamine-zolazepam), anti-inflammatory drugs (e.g., ketoprofen), and/or inhalation anesthetic drugs (e.g., halothane, isoflurane, and sevoflurane). These techniques are both practical and effective when applying a multimodal pain-management strategy in cats.

References

1. Hall LW, Clarke KW. Anaesthesia of the cat. In: Veterinary Anaesthesia, 9th ed. London: Ballière-Tindall, 1991:337–338.
2. Skarda RT. Local anesthesia in dogs and cats. In: Muir WW III, Hubbell JAE, eds. Handbook of Veterinary Anesthesia, 2nd ed. St Louis: Mosby-Year Book, 1995:96–99.
3. Sackman JE. Pain: Its perception and alleviation in dogs and cats. Part I. The physiology of pain. Comp Contin Educ Pract Vet 1991;13:71–79.
4. Woolf CJ, Chong MS. Preemptive analgesia—treating postoperative pain by preventing the establishment of central sensitization. Anesth Analg 1993;77:362–379.
5. Pascoe P. Local and regional anesthesia and analgesia [Review]. Semin Vet Med Surg (Small Anim) 1997;12:94–105.
6. Muir WW, Woolf CJ. Mechanisms of pain and their therapeutic implication. J Am Vet Med Assoc 2001;219:1346–1356.
7. Flecknell PA, Liles JH, Williamson HA. The use of lignocaine-prilocaine local anaesthetic cream for pain-free venepuncture in laboratory animals. Lab Anim Sci 1990;24:142–146.
8. Duke T. Local and regional anesthetic and analgesic techniques in the dog and cat. Part I. Pharmacology of local anesthetics and topical anesthesia. Can Vet J 2000;41:883–884.
9. Duke T. Local and regional anesthetic and analgesic techniques in the dog and cat. Part II. Infiltration and nerve blocks. Can Vet J 2000;41:949–952.
10. Englesson S. The influence of acid-base changes on central nervous system toxicity of local anesthetic agents. I. An experimental study in the cats. Acta Anaesthesiol Scand 1974;18:79–87.
11. Chadwick HS. Toxicity and resuscitation in lidocaine or bupivacaine-infused cats. Anesthesiology 1985;63:385–390.
12. Nishikawa K, Fukuda T, Yukioka H, Fujimori M. Effects of intravenous administration of local anesthetics on the renal sympathetic nerve activity during nitrous oxide and nitrous oxide–halothane anaesthesia in the cat. Acta Anaesthesiol Scand 1990;34:231–236.
13. Gross ME, Pope ER, Jarboe JM, O'Brien DP, Dodam JR, Polkow-Haight J. Regional anesthesia of the infraorbital and inferior alveolar nerves during noninvasive tooth pulp stimulation in halothane-anesthetized cats. Am J Vet Res 2000;61:1245–1247.
14. Lemke KA, Dawson SD. Local and regional anesthesia. Vet Clin North Am Small Anim Pract 2000;30:851–855.
15. Benson GJ, Wheaton LG, Thurmon JC, Tranquilli WJ, Olson WA, Davis CA. Postoperative catecholamine response to onychectomy in isoflurane-anesthetized cats: Effects of analgesics. Vet Surg 1991;20:222–225.
16. Ko CH, Benson GJ, Tranquilli WJ. An alternative drug combination for use in declawing and castrating cats. Vet Med 1993;88:1061–1065.
17. Lin HC, Benson GJ, Thurmon JC, Tranquilli WJ, Olson WA, Bevill RF. Influence of anesthetic regimens on the perioperative catecholamine response associated with onychectomy in cats. Am J Vet Res 1993;54:1721–1724.

18. Carroll GL, Howe LB, Slater MR, et al. Evaluation of analgesia provided by postoperative administration of butorphanol to cats undergoing onychectomy. J Am Vet Med Assoc 1998;213:246–250.

19. Franks JN, Boothe HW, Taylor L, et al. Evaluation of transdermal fentanyl patches for analgesia in cats undergoing onychectomy. J Am Vet Med Assoc 2000;217:1013–1020.

20. Gellasch KL, Kruse-Elliot KT, Osmond CS, Shih AN, Bjorling DE. Comparison of transdermal administration of fentanyl versus intramuscular administration of butorphanol for analgesia after onychectomy in cats. J Am Vet Med Assoc 2002;220:1020–1024.

21. Winkler KP, Greenfield CL, Benson GJ. The effect of wound irrigation with bupivacaine on postoperative analgesia of the feline onychectomy patient. J Am Anim Hosp Assoc 1997;33:346–352.

22. Ringwood PB, Smith JA. Case of the month. J Am Vet Med Assoc 2000;217:1633–1635.

23. Matteson V. How to perform a ring block. Vet Technician 2000; June:341–356.

24. Kushner LI, Fan B, Shofer FS. Intravenous regional anesthesia in isoflurane anesthetized cats: Lidocaine plasma concentrations and cardiovascular effects. Vet Anaesth Analg 2002;29:140–149.

25. Klide AM, Soma LR. Epidural analgesia in the dog and cat. J Am Vet Med Assoc 1968;153:165–173.

26. Schmidt-Oechtering GU. Epidural anaesthesia in dogs and cats: Still an alternative to general anaesthesia. J Vet Anaesth 1993;20:40.

27. Hanson B. Epidural anesthesia and analgesia. In: Proceedings of the Predictable Pain Management Symposium. Orlando, FL: North American Veterinary Conference, 1996:49–55.

28. Remedios AM, Duke T. Chronic epidural implantation of vascular access catheters in the cat lumbosacrum. Lab Anim Sci 1993;43: 262–264.

29. Duke T, Cox AM, Remedios AM, Cribb PH. The analgesic effects of administering fentanyl or medetomidine in the lumbosacral epidural space of cats. Vet Surg 1994;23:143–148.

30. Duke T, Cox AK, Remedios AM, Cribb PH. The cardiopulmonary effects of placing fentanyl or medetomidine in the lumbosacral epidural space of isoflurane-anesthetized cats. Vet Surg 1994;23:149–155.

31. Pascoe PJ. Advantages and guidelines for using epidural drugs for analgesia. Vet Clin North Am Small Anim Pract 1992;22:421–423.

32. Yaksh TL, Noueihed R, Durant PAC. Studies of the pharmacology and pathology of intrathecally administered 4-anilopiperidine analogues and morphine in the rat and cat. Anesthesiology 1981;64:54–66.

33. Golder FJ, Pascoe PJ, Bailey CS, Ilkiw JE, Tripp LD. The effect of epidural morphine on the minimum alveolar concentration of isoflurane in cats. J Vet Anaesth 1998;25:52–56.

34. Tung AS, Yaksh TL. The antinociceptive effects of epidural opiates in the cat: Studies on the pharmacology and the effects of lipophilicity in spinal analgesia. Pain 1982;12:343–356.

35. Sawyer D, Striler E. Analgesia and behavioral responses to epidural oxymorphone in cats. In: Abstracts of the Proceedings of the Fifth International Congress of Veterinary Anesthesia, Guelph, Canada, 1994:209.

36. Hocking G, Cousins MJ. Ketamine in chronic pain management: An evidence-based review. Anesth Analg 2003;97:1730–1739.

37. Amiot P, Pallaci J, Vedrenne C, Pellerin M. Spinal toxicity of lysine acetylsalicylate and ketamine hydrochloride given by the intrathecal route in the rat [Abstract]. Ann Fr Anesth Reanim 1986;5:462.

38. Karpinsky N, Dunn J, Hansen L, Masliah E. Subpial vacuolar myelopathy after intrathecal ketamine: Report of a case. Pain 1997;73: 103–105.

39. Stotz M, Oehen HP, Gerber H. Histological findings after long term infusion of intrathecal ketamine for chronic pain: A case report. J Pain Symptom Manage 1999;18:223–228.

40. Torske KE, Dyson DH. Epidural analgesia and anesthesia. Vet Clin North Am Small Anim Pract 2000;30:871–874.

Chapter 22
Local and Regional Anesthetic and Analgesic Techniques: Horses

Roman T. Skarda and William J. Tranquilli

Introduction

Many diagnostic and surgical procedures are performed safely and humanely in horses by combining local anesthetic techniques with physical restraint and/or sedation. Sedation can be induced by drugs such as acepromazine, xylazine, or detomidine, either alone or in combination with morphine or butorphanol, among others, to facilitate handling of fractious horses.

The techniques in performing nerve and joint blocks vary considerably, depending on such factors as operative size; expected duration of surgery; size, temperament, and health of the patient; technical skill and personal preference of the veterinarian; and economics of time and material. Currently, the most common techniques used in horses are surface (topical) anesthesia, infiltration anesthesia, and a considerable number of peripheral nerve blocks (regional anesthesia). Peripheral nerve blocks, intra-articular and intrabursal injections, and local infiltrations (ring block) are commonly used to aid diagnosis of equine lameness and as a means of providing analgesia to a surgery site. Peripheral nerve blocks, which are performed at the end of an operation under general anesthesia, are helpful to control emergence excitement caused by pain in the recovery period. More complex infiltration techniques (e.g., cervicothoracic ganglion block or sympathetic ganglion block) are used by specialists to relieve vasoconstriction and pain. Similarly, central neural blockade techniques such as caudal epidural anesthesia, caudal subarachnoid anesthesia, segmental thoracolumbar epidural anesthesia, and thoracolumbar subarachnoid anesthesia are usually the province of specialists. Caudal epidural administration of morphine can provide bilateral analgesia over various sacral and thoracic (S5 to T9) dermatomes, with slow onset (6 to 8 h) and long duration of effect (17 to 19 h), and minimal sedation and cardiopulmonary effects in horses.

The technique of caudal epidural injection of local anesthetics, which traditionally is used to induce perineal analgesia in standing horses, has been markedly expanded in the recent years by the use of novel analgesics (opioids, α_2-adrenoceptor agonists, ketamine, and tramadol), and drug combinations. Motor nerve blockade induced by epidurally applied opiates or α_2-adrenoceptor agonists is minimal, whereas some relief of inflammatory, traumatic, perioperative, and chronic pain is possible. Ataxia, sedation, and cardiovascular side effects after epidural administration of opiates or α_2-adrenoceptor agonists can be reversed with antagonistic drugs (e.g., naloxone, yohimbine, or atipamezole). Additionally, the use of epidural catheters and accessories, which are commercially available in various epidural kits, greatly facilitates long-term analgesic drug administration in standing horses.

Improper injection technique contributes to inadequate anesthesia and complications. Each time a technique is performed, it will have its own rate of onset and duration, which is related to the specific local anesthetic used, neuroanatomy (thickness of the coverings of the nerve, arrangement of fibers within the mixed nerve, and blood supply to the area of injection), and personal interpretation of the animal's response.

The equipment for performing local anesthesia should include sharp and sterile needles, syringes in good working condition, sterile catheters and stylets, and sterile anesthetic solution. Chances of infection must be minimized by surgically preparing the injection sites, especially puncture sites into joints and epidural and subarachnoid spaces. Desired anesthetic effects without complications can be better obtained by using proper techniques, including aspiration before injection to avoid placing drug into the vascular system and avoidance of injections through or into inflamed tissues.

Choice of Local Anesthetic

The most commonly used local anesthetics in equine practice are 2% lidocaine (Xylocaine; Astra Pharmaceutical, Worcester, MA) or mepivacaine (Carbocaine-V; Winthrop Laboratories, New York, NY) hydrochloride (HCl) solution, both having an intermediate duration of action (1 to 2 h). In general, anesthesia begins most rapidly (within 3 to 5 min) during infiltration techniques and subarachnoid administration, followed in order of increasing onset time by minor nerve blockade (5 to 10 min), major nerve blocks, and epidural anesthesia (10 to 20 min).[1] The addition of epinephrine at concentration of 5 μg/mL (1:200,000) to the local anesthetic solution can improve the quality and duration of regional and epidural anesthesia. Ropivacaine is a novel local anesthetic recently evaluated in horses that provides local anesthesia for 3 to 6 h, similar to bupivacaine.

Regional Anesthesia

Anesthesia of the Head

The most frequently desensitized nerves of the head are the supraorbital, infraorbital, mandibular alveolar, and auriculopalpebral; other techniques, which desensitize the maxillary,[2,3] mandibular,[4,5] and ophthalmic nerves,[6,7] are not without danger and seldom used.

Eyelids

Anesthesia of the eyelids requires sensory denervation of four individual branches of the trigeminal (fifth) cranial nerve: the supraorbital (or frontal), lacrimal, zygomatic, and infraorbital. Voluntary closure of the eyelids (*palpebral akinesia*) is prevented by desensitizing the dorsal and ventral branches of the palpebral nerve (*auriculopalpebral nerve block*). A 1.5- to 2.5-cm, 22- to 25-gauge needle is used to inject local anesthetic without epinephrine to each of the listed nerves (Fig. 22.1).

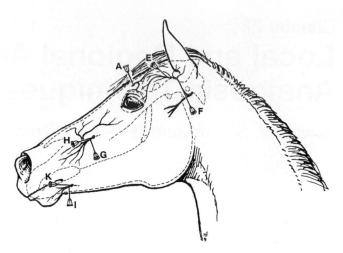

Fig. 22.1. Sites for needle placement to desensitize the supraorbital (A), auriculopalpebral (E and F), infraorbital (G and H), mental (I), and alveolar mandibular (K) nerves.

Upper Eyelid

The supraorbital (or frontal) nerve is the most commonly desensitized.[8,9] The nerve emerges through the supraorbital foramen, which can be easily palpated with the index finger about 5 to 7 cm dorsal to the medial canthus and in the center of an imaginary triangle formed by grasping the supraorbital process of the frontal bone with the thumb and middle finger and sliding medially (Fig. 22.2A). Approximately 2 mL of local anesthetic are injected subcutaneously over the foramen, 1 mL as the needle is inserted into the foramen and 2 mL as the needle is inserted to its full depth (2.5 cm) into the foramen (Fig. 22.2B). Successful administration of local anesthetic desensitizes the forehead, including the middle two-thirds of the upper eyelid and palpebral motor supply from the auriculopalpebral nerve (A in Fig. 22.3). Auriculopalpebral nerve block has no significant effect on intraocular pressure or peripheral corneal thickness in horses.[10]

The lateral canthus and lateral aspect of the upper eyelid are desensitized by administering local anesthetic to the lacrimal nerve.[9,11] The needle is inserted percutaneously at the lateral canthus and directed medially along the dorsal rim of the orbit (B in Fig. 22.4). A deep injection of 2 to 3 mL of the anesthetic at this site also desensitizes the lacrimal gland, local connective tissue, and temporal angle of the orbit (B in Fig. 22.3).

Medial canthal anesthesia is achieved by inserting the needle through the bony notch or irregularity on the dorsal rim of the orbit near the medial canthus and injecting 2 to 3 mL of local anesthetic around the infratrochlear nerve (C in Fig. 22.4). This procedure also desensitizes the nictitans, lacrimal organs, and connective tissues (C in Fig. 22.3).[9,11]

The lower two-thirds of the lower eyelid, skin, and connective tissue are desensitized by placing the needle subcutaneously on the lateral aspect of the bony orbit and supraorbital portion of the zygomatic arch (the site where the rim begins to rise), and infiltrating the zygomatic nerve with 3 to 5 mL of the anesthetic (D in Figs. 22.3 and 22.4).[9,11]

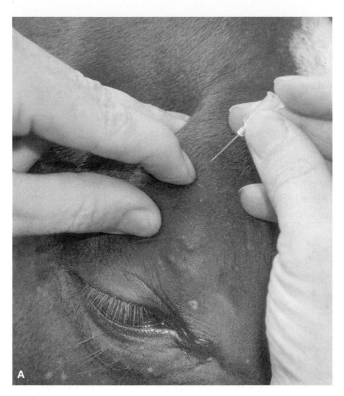

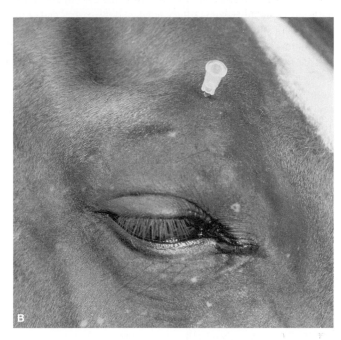

Fig. 22.2. **A:** Palpation of the supraorbital nerve. **B:** A 2.5-cm, 25-gauge needle is inserted into the supraorbital foramen.

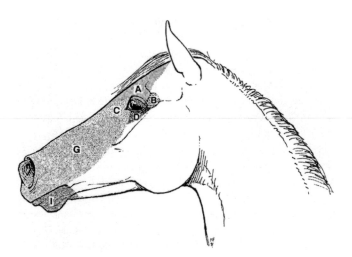

Fig. 22.3. Area of skin desensitization after blocking the supraorbital (A), lacrimal (B), infratrochlear (C), zygomatic (D), infraorbital (G), and mental (I) nerves.

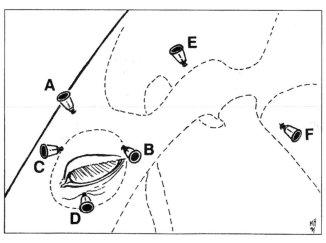

Fig. 22.4. Needle placement to supraorbital (A), lacrimal (B), infratrochlear (C), zygomatic (D), and (E and F) auriculopalpebral nerves.

Paralysis of the Orbicularis Oculi Muscles

Desensitization of the auriculopalpebral nerve is most frequently used for examination of the eye and temporary relief of eyelid spasms, since voluntary closure of the eyelids (akinesia) is prevented. The eyelids remain sensitive. In combination with topical anesthesia, this block is useful for removal of foreign bodies from the cornea and other ocular surgery. At least two injection sites have been suggested for paralyzing the palpebral musculature: either the most dorsal point of the zygomatic arch (E in Fig. 22.1)[4]

or the depression caudal to the mandible at the ventral edge of the temporal position of the zygomatic arch (F in Fig. 22.1).[11–13] In each location, the needle is placed subfascially, and 5 mL of the local anesthetic is administered in a fan-shaped manner.

Upper Lip and Nose

Anesthesia of the upper lip and nose requires a 2.5-cm, 20-gauge needle and deposition of 5 mL of local anesthetic to the infraorbital nerve as it emerges from the infraorbital canal (G in Fig.

22.1).[4,8] After displacing the flat levator labii superioris muscle dorsally, the bony lip of the infraorbital foramen can be palpated by the index finger about half the distance and 2.5 cm dorsal to a line connecting the nasomaxillary notch and the rostral end of the facial crest. Successful perineural infiltration of the local anesthetic at this site results in anesthesia of the entire anterior half of the face from the foramen rostrally (G in Fig. 22.3).

Upper Teeth and Maxilla
If a 5.0-cm, 20-gauge spinal needle is inserted into the infraorbital foramen and is advanced into the infraorbital canal for a depth of up to 3.5 cm (H in Fig. 22.1), the deposition of 5 mL of local anesthetic is adequate to desensitize the teeth as far as the first molar, the maxillary sinus, the roof of the nasal cavity, and the skin almost to the medial canthus of the eye.[14,15] Although local anesthesia can be produced for premolars and maxilla, extraction of these teeth and trephination of the maxillary sinus are more easily accomplished using general anesthesia.

Lower Lip
Anesthesia of the lower lip is induced by using a 2.5-cm, 22-gauge needle and successfully desensitizing the mental nerve rostrally to the mental foramen with 5 mL of local anesthetic. (I in Figs. 22.1 and 22.3).[4,13] The lateral border of the mental foramen is easily palpated at the horizontal ramus of the mandible in the middle of the interdental space, after the tendon of the depressor labii inferioris muscle is dorsally displaced.

Lower Incisors and Premolars
A 7.5-cm, 20-gauge spinal needle is inserted into the mental foramen and is advanced into the mandibular canal as far as possible in a ventromedial direction to inject 10 mL of local anesthetic to desensitize the mandibular alveolar nerve, thereby extending the area of anesthesia caudally as far as the third premolar (K in Fig. 22.1).[4,5,8,16] The technique is difficult, so extraction of teeth is better accomplished under general anesthesia.

Anesthesia of the Limbs
Regional anesthesia (peripheral nerve blocks),[1,17–32] intra-articular injection,[1,32–48] intrabursal injection[1,49–51] and local infiltration (ring block) are used to provide intraoperative and postoperative anesthesia to a surgery site and aid in accurate diagnosis, prognosis, and especially recommendation and treatment of equine lameness.

These techniques for the diagnosis of lameness are seldom used, however. Instead, review of the horse's medical history; observation of the horse at rest (standing normally with all feet on the ground); examination for exostosis or lumps; palpation of areas that are inflamed, enlarged, or seem sore; use of the hoof tester to determine painful areas or to determine whether the horse becomes more lame after a specific part of the leg has been manipulated; and observation of the horse in motion are relied upon in making the diagnosis. In some cases the diagnosis is not obvious, and nerve blocks and good-quality radiographs with adequate view are required to make a specific diagnosis. Rectal palpation of ovaries, uterus, aorta, iliac vessels, pelvis, kidney, and

viscera of a female and palpation of the inguinal canal of a stallion or gelding are additional examinations in cases of difficult diagnosis of hind-limb lameness. Restraint is best achieved physically with a twitch applied to the horse's upper lip and a man picking up the front leg on the same side as the operator.

To prevent infection, sterile syringes, needles, and local anesthetic should be used for each injection. Subcutaneous injections, as a minimum, require an alcohol preparation. Show-horse owners object to clipping and shaving of the site of needle penetration.[41] Intra-articular injections require a surgical scrub because of the risk of introducing contaminates; clipping the site is considered optional by many practitioners. Care must be taken not to place fingers on the end of the needle hub or especially on the tip of the syringe because of risk of contamination. To improve aseptic technique, it is wise to use surgical gloves when performing more complicated nerve and joint blocks.

Nerve blocks and intra-articular injections are performed first on the most distal branches of nerve trunks and joints, and proceed proximally with a systematic approach. Performing nerve blocks proximal to the carpus and tarsus is very uncommon. Proximal to the metacarpus, diagnostic anesthesia of the equine pectoral limb is nonspecific and best accomplished by joint anesthesia.[20] All corresponding digital nerves can be blocked on the hind limb as with the front limb (Figs. 22.5 and 22.6). A needle that is inserted in a distal to proximal direction and then attached to the syringe is less likely to break off if the horse makes a sudden leg movement. Adequate amounts of local anesthetic should be administered and enough time given for maximal effect. Post block examination is best accomplished by using deep digital pressure and pressure exerted by either a hoof tester, or a ballpoint pen for 1 to 2 s to test skin sensation distal to the block. Pressure from a blunt-tip instrument, such as a ballpoint pen, is preferable over a needle and avoids the production of numerous bleeding points.[26] The limb should be rubbed down and wrapped to prevent swelling and inflammation after the use of local anesthetic.

Local diagnostic blocks may fail or partially fail for several reasons, most common of which are incorrect anatomical deposition, inadequate anesthetic volume, dilution or hemodilution of anesthetic agent, presence of fibrous connective tissue inhibiting diffusion of anesthetic agent, multiple sites of pain, and the incorrectly perceived location of lameness.[48] Horses may become ataxic after nerve blockade in the limbs. Ataxia may lead to self-trauma because the horse may not know where the limbs are actually being placed.[31]

Digital Nerves
The palmar (or plantar) digital nerve is desensitized with the leg either bearing weight or elevated. It is palpated on the palmar (or plantar) aspect of the pastern medially and/or laterally midway between the coronary band and fetlock just palmar (or plantar) to the digital vein and artery (A in Figs. 22.5 and 22.6). A 2.5-cm, 25-gauge needle is inserted anteriorly to a depth equal to the length of the needle, and approximately 2 mL of local anesthetic is injected. Proper nerve blockade desensitizes the posterior one-third of the foot, including the navicular bursa, 5 to 10 min after the injection (Fig. 22.7A).

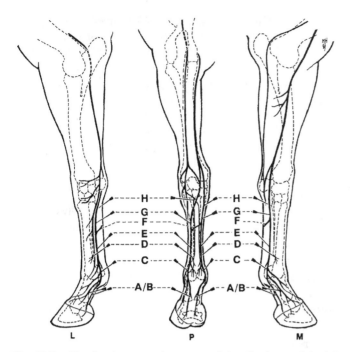

Fig. 22.5. Needle placement for nerves of the distal part of the left thoracic limb of the horse, lateral (L), palmar (P), and medial (M) views: lateral and medial palmar digital nerves (A), dorsal branches (B), lateral and medial palmar digital nerves (base sesamoid) (C), lateral and medial palmar nerves (D and G), lateral and medial palmar metacarpal nerves (E), communicating branch (F), and location of high suspensory block (H).

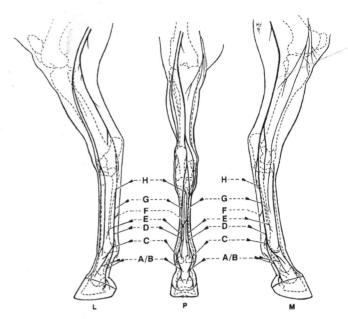

Fig. 22.6. Needle placement for nerves of the distal part of the left pelvic limb of the horse, lateral (L), plantar (P), and medial (M) views: lateral and medial plantar digital nerves (A), dorsal branches (B), lateral and medial plantar digital nerves (base sesamoid) (C), lateral and medial plantar nerves (D and G), lateral and medial plantar metatarsal nerves (E) communicating branch (F), and location of high suspensory block (H).

Anterior (or Dorsal) Digital Nerve Block

To block the dorsal or anterior digital nerve, which supplies sensory fibers to the anterior two-thirds of the hoof, the needle is directed anteriorly to the site of the posterior digital nerve and is inserted to a depth equal to the length of the needle while infiltrating subcutaneously 3 to 5 mL of local anesthetic (B in Figs. 22.5 and 22.6). All structures of the entire digit distal to the injection become anesthetized, including phalanges P1, P2, and P3; the proximal and distal interphalangeal joints; the entire corium; the dorsal branches of the suspensory ligament; and the distal extensor tendon.

Abaxial (Basilar) Sesamoidean Nerve Block

This can be done at the anterior and posterior digital nerves at the abaxial surface of the proximal sesamoids, to provide better analgesia of the pastern and proximal pastern joints (C in Figs. 22.5 and 22.6). Successful injections of 3 to 5 mL of local anesthetic subcutaneously at that site desensitize the entire foot distal to the injection, including the back of the pastern area and distal sesamoidean ligaments.

Low Palmar (or Plantar) Nerve Block

This is performed by injecting approximately 2 to 3 mL of local anesthetic at the following four points (four-point block) while the limb is bearing weight: the medial and lateral palmar or plantar nerves (D in Figs. 22.5 and 22.6) and the medial and lateral

palmar metacarpal or plantar metatarsal nerves (E in Figs. 22.5 and 22.6) distal to the communicating branch of the medial and lateral palmar or plantar nerves (F in Figs. 22.5 and 22.6). The injections are made between the flexor tendon and suspensory ligament (blocks medial and lateral palmar or plantar nerves) and between the suspensory ligament and the splint bone (blocks medial and lateral palmar metacarpal or plantar metatarsal nerves). This procedure desensitizes almost all structures distal to the fetlock and fetlock joint, except for a small area, dorsal to the fetlock joint, that is supplied by sensory fibers of the ulnar and musculocutaneous nerves (D in Fig. 22.7).

High Palmar (or Plantar) Nerve Block

Performing this block proximal to the communicating branch (F in Figs 22.5 and 22.6) of the medial and lateral palmar (or plantar) nerves assures that the palmar metacarpal (or plantar metatarsal) region, the fetlock, and all of the digits are desensitized (G in Figs. 22.5 and 22.6). A 3.75-cm, 22-gauge needle is placed subfascially into the groove between the suspensory ligament and deep flexor tendon on both the medial and the lateral sides approximately 5 cm distal to the carpometacarpal (carpometatarsal) joint, where 5 mL of the local anesthetic is injected.[52] The dorsal metacarpal (or metatarsal) region will still have sensation, but can be desensitized by injecting local anesthetic subcutaneously around the front of the cannon bone (ring block) (D + E in Fig. 22.7).

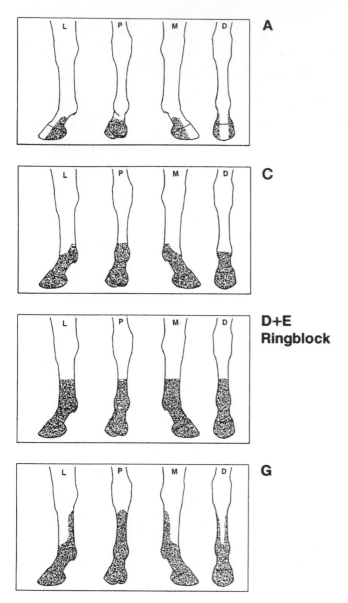

Fig. 22.7. Desensitized subcutaneous area after A, D, D + E, and G blockade.

High Suspensory Block

Deposition of 5 mL of local anesthetic solution to the medial and lateral palmar metacarpal (or plantar metatarsal) nerves (H in Figs. 22.5 and 22.6), which are subfascial between the superficial digital flexor tendon and the suspensory ligament, desensitizes the interosseous muscle (suspensory ligament) and inferior check ligament, the caudal aspect of the metacarpus (metatarsus), and the adjacent splint bones (G in Fig. 22.7).

Nerve Blocks Proximal to the Carpus

It is very uncommon to perform higher nerve blocks than the high suspensory block on the forelimb; however, to induce anesthesia of the carpus and distal forelimb, three nerves must be desensitized: the median, ulnar, and branches of the musculocutaneous nerve. The median nerve is desensitized on the medial

aspect of the forelimb, approximately 5 cm ventral to the elbow joint, by using a 3.75-cm, 20-gauge needle and injecting 10 mL of the anesthetic (A in Fig. 22.8). The ulnar nerve is desensitized by inserting a 2.5-cm, 22-gauge needle 10 cm proximal to the accessory carpal bone between the flexor carpi ulnaris and ulnaris lateralis muscles and injecting 5 mL of the anesthetic solution 1.5 cm deep beneath the fascia (B in Fig. 22.8). The medial cutaneous antebrachial nerve, a branch of the musculocutaneous nerve, is easily palpated just cranially to the cephalic vein at the anteromedial aspect of the forelimb halfway between the elbow and carpus. Approximately 10 mL of the anesthetic solution is deposited subcutaneously at that site by using a 2.5-cm, 22-gauge needle (C in Fig. 22.8).

Nerve Blocks Proximal to the Tarsus

It is very uncommon to do any higher blocks than the high suspensory block in the hind limb, but, to complete anesthesia of the hind limb from the tarsus distally, four nerves must be desensitized: tibial, saphenous, superficial peroneal (superficial fibular), and deep peroneal (deep fibular). The tibial nerve is desensitized by using a 2.5-cm, 22-gauge needle to inject 15 to 20 mL of local anesthetic subfascially between the combined tendons of the gastrocnemius muscle and superficial flexor tendon. Injection is best made on the medial aspect of the partially flexed limb, approximately 10 cm proximal to the point of the tarsus. Successful blockade desensitizes the posterior metatarsal region and most of the foot (A in Fig. 22.9). A ring block of the dorsal metatarsal region may be necessary to desensitize the anterolateral region. The saphenous nerve is desensitized by inserting a 2.5-cm, 22-gauge needle subcutaneously on the cranial or caudal aspect of the median saphenous vein, proximal to the tibiotarsal joint, and injecting 5 mL of the local anesthetic (B in Fig. 22.9). The medial aspect of the thigh and part of the metatarsal region will be anesthetized. The superficial and deep peroneal (fibular) nerves can be simultaneously desensitized by inserting a 3.75-cm, 22-gauge needle between the long and lateral digital extensor muscles approximately 10 cm proximal to the lateral malleolus of the tibia (C in Fig. 22.9). The superficial branch of the nerve is infiltrated subcutaneously with 10 mL of the local anesthetic. The needle is then advanced 2 to 3 cm to penetrate the deep fascia and to deposit 15 mL of the anesthetic around the deep branch. Anesthesia should include the anterolateral tarsal and metatarsal regions and the joint capsule of the tarsus.

Intra-articular Injections

Although arthrocentesis implies aspiration of synovial fluid, it allows for instillation of local anesthetic for the purpose of diagnostic anesthesia and use of therapeutic agents (e.g., saline flushes, antibiotics, hyaluronic acid, and anti-inflammatory drugs) as a therapy for certain diseases. The two most common local anesthetic agents used in intra-articular injections are mepivacaine and lidocaine HCl solution. Mepivacaine appears to cause less irritation than lidocaine for use in intra-articular injections.[53] Proper restraint, either physical or chemical, is indicated, and each horse should be considered potentially fractious.

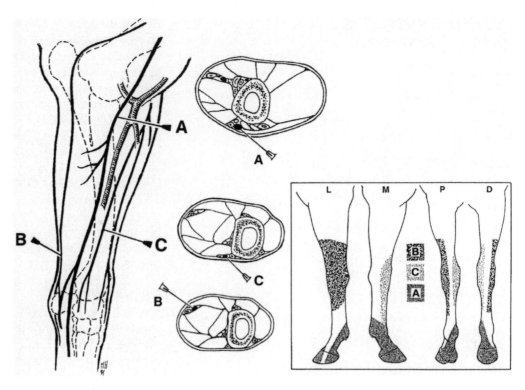

Fig. 22.8. Needle placement for median nerve (A), ulnar nerve (B), and musculocutaneous nerve (C); cross sections and desensitized subcutaneous areas of left forelimb. L, lateral; M, medial; P, palmar; and D, dorsal aspects.

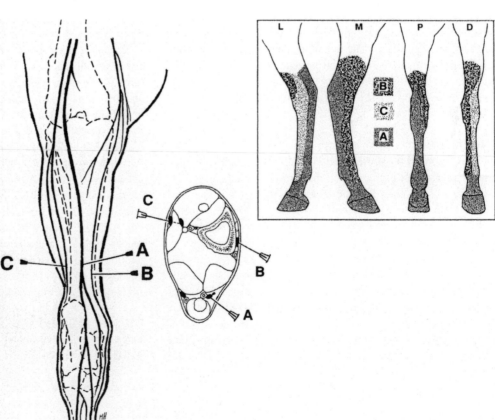

Fig. 22.9. Needle placement for tibial nerve (A), saphenous nerve (B), and peroneal nerve (C); cross sections and desensitized subcutaneous areas of left rear limb; L, lateral; M, medial; P, plantar; and D, dorsal aspects.

Podotrochlear (Navicular) Bursa Block

Numerous different techniques for injection of the navicular bursa have been described, but there is little conformity among these descriptions.[54] The procedure is best performed while the limb is bearing weight. The position of the navicular bone is highly predictable as a point 1.0 cm distal to the coronary band and halfway between the most dorsal and most palmar aspect of the coronary band. Irrespective of foot confirmation, anesthesia

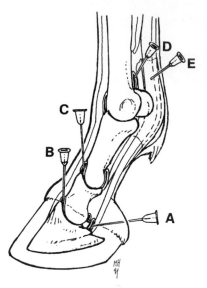

Fig. 22.10. Needle placement into the podotrochlear bursa (A), coffin joint (B), pastern joint (C), volar pouch of fetlock joint capsule (D), and digital flexor tendon sheath (E).

of the podotrochlear (navicular) bursa is induced by inserting a 5- to 7.5-cm, 18-gauge spinal needle through the digital pad between the bulbs of the heel until the needle strikes the bone along the midline at a point approximately at the level of the coronary band (A in Fig. 22.10). The needle is then slightly withdrawn until very little synovial fluid is aspirated, and 3 to 5 mL of local anesthetic is injected. Analgesia of the navicular bursa is more effective in desensitizing the dorsal margin of the sole than in desensitizing the angles of the sole.[55]

Coffin Block

Pain arising from the dorsal margin of the sole in horses can be attenuated by anesthesia of either the distal interphalangeal (coffin) joint (P2-P3) or palmar digital nerves.[56] The distal interphalangeal joint is desensitized with 5 to 10 mL of local anesthetic. A 3.75-cm, 18- to 20-gauge needle is inserted 1.5 cm proximal to the coronet approximately 2 cm lateral to the vertical center of the pastern and is directed obliquely ventral to the tendon toward the extensor process (B in Fig. 22.10). Anesthesia of the podotrochlear (navicular) bursa depends on diffusion of the local anesthetic through the suspensory ligament to the bursa, because the coffin joint and podotrochlear (navicular) bursa do not communicate. The combination of lidocaine HCl (20 mg/mL), epinephrine (0.012 mg/mL), and sodium penicillin (800,000 IU) must not be injected into the coffin joint of horses, because it can cause irreversible lameness through ossifying arthrodesis.[57]

Pastern Block

The proximal interphalangeal (pastern) joint (P1-P2) can be entered with ease by inserting a 3.75-cm, 20- to 22-gauge needle medially or laterally to the midline on the palpable epicondyles of P2, and injecting 5 to 8 mL of local anesthetic. The needle is directed vertically and inserted for approximately 2.5 cm (C in Fig. 22.10).

Fetlock Block

The metacarpophalangeal or metatarsophalangeal (fetlock) joint is one of the commonly and easily injected joints. A 3.75-cm, 20- to 22-gauge needle is inserted into the lateral pouch distal to the splint bone and dorsal to the annular ligament of the fetlock at a depth of approximately 0.5 to 1.5 cm (D in Fig. 22.10). When distended, this joint capsule may also be penetrated on the cranial surface of the joint. Approximately 8 mL of local anesthetic solution is injected.

Digital Flexor Tendon Sheath Block

This can be desensitized by inserting a 3.75-cm, 18- to 20-gauge needle to the distal end of the splint ("button") either medially or laterally cranial to the deep and superficial flexor tendons and caudal to the suspensory ligament, and injecting 10 mL of local anesthetic (E in Fig. 22.10).

Carpal Block

The radiocarpal (antebrachial carpal) and intercarpal (middle carpal) joints are the two most commonly injected carpal joints. The carpometacarpal joint communicates with the middle (intercarpal) joint and therefore does not require separate entry.[52] In one commonly used technique, the carpus is flexed and a 3.75-cm, 20-gauge needle is inserted on either side of the palpable extensor carpi radialis tendon to inject 5 to 10 mL of local anesthetic into each joint (A and B in Figs. 22.11 and 22.12). In an alternative method, which is used by many racetrack practitioners in standing horses, the needles are inserted perpendicularly through the skin on the posterolateral aspect of the radiocarpal and intercarpal joint spaces (C and D in Fig. 22.12). To locate the lateral site for penetration of the radiocarpal joint, the lateral digital extensor tendon and tendon of the ulnaris lateralis muscle are identified at the distal end of the ulna. These tendons narrow to form a depressed "V" anterior to the accessory carpal bone. The needle is then inserted approximately 1 to 2 cm distal to this V in the radiocarpal joint (C in Fig. 22.12). The intercarpal joint is approximately 2.0 to 2.5 cm distal to the first injection site (D in Fig. 22.12). The needles are inserted 1 to 2 cm until the joint spaces are encountered. Advantages of this technique include minimal risk of injuring the articular surfaces of the bones and injecting local anesthetic into a larger space of a more stable position of the leg from a safe lateral approach.[44,47]

Cubital (Elbow) Block

This is not a usual source of lameness, so it is rarely desensitized. A 5-cm, 18-gauge needle is inserted into the depression between the lateral epicondyle of the humerus and the lateral tuberosity of the radius at the anterior edge of the lateral collateral ligament (A in Fig. 22.13). Repeated flexion of the elbow joint greatly facilitates the identification of the palpable landmarks. The needle is directed obliquely in a caudomedial direction to reach the elbow joint at a depth of 3 to 4 cm; up to 20 mL of local anesthetic is required.

Olecranon Bursa Block

This is performed by inserting a 3.75-cm, 18-gauge needle caudal to the olecranon, directing the needle obliquely from proximal to distal and injecting about 10 to 15 mL of the local anesthetic (B in Fig. 22.13).

Bicipital Bursa Block

After the biceps brachii muscle is palpated, a 7.5-cm, 18-gauge spinal needle is inserted between the muscle and the proximal humerus from below and approximately 4 cm ventral and 2 cm posterior to the palpable anterior prominence of the lateral tuberosity of the humerus (C in Fig. 22.13). The needle is advanced up to 5 cm obliquely dorsomedial toward the opposite point of the shoulder to penetrate the bursa. At least 10 mL of local anesthetic is injected, and a 20-min period is allowed for maximal effect.

Shoulder Block

The scapula humeral (shoulder) joint can be difficult to enter because of its relative depth. Limb motion or muscle contraction must be prevented to avoid bending of a positioned needle. The tendon of the infraspinatus muscle can be palpated as a tense band extending from the scapula to the proximal humerus. A 7.5- to 12.5-cm, 18-gauge spinal needle is inserted just cranial to the tendon and between the palpable projections of the anterior and posterior parts of the lateral tuberosity of the humerus, and is directed to the opposite elbow (D in Fig. 22.13). Penetration from skin is up to 7.5 cm or until synovial fluid is aspirated. A volume of 30 mL or more of the anesthetic is injected. The shoulder joint may communicate with the bicipital bursa in some horses; therefore, injection of local anesthetic into the shoulder joint may diffuse the anesthetic to the bicipital bursa and improve a lameness associated with that structure.[45,46]

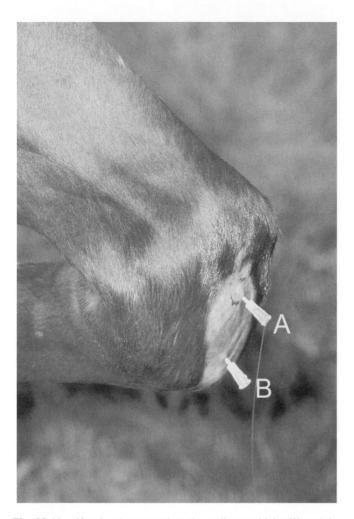

Fig. 22.11. Needle placement into the radiocarpal joint (A) and the intercarpal joint (B) of the right forelimb.

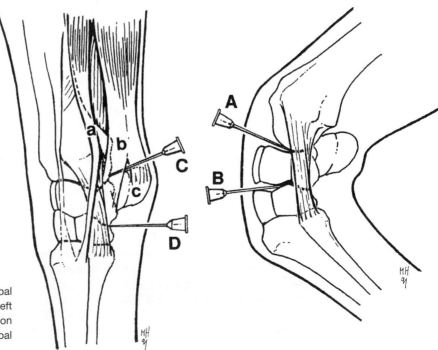

Fig. 22.12. Needle placement into the radiocarpal (A and C) and intercarpal (B and D) joints of the left forelimb (a, lateral digital extensor tendon; b, tendon of ulnaris lateralis muscle; and c, accessory carpal bone).

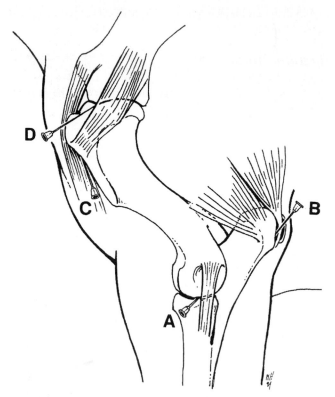

Fig. 22.13. Needle placement into the elbow joint (A), olecranon bursa (B), bicipital bursa (C), and shoulder joint (D) of the left forelimb.

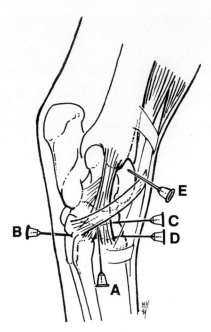

Fig. 22.14. Needle placement into the cunean bursa (A), tarsometatarsal space (B and D), distal intertarsal space (C), and tibiotarsal space (E) of the left hock joint; medial aspect.

Cunean Bursa Block

This block is more commonly performed in standardbreds and less commonly in horses that are ridden.[49,50] The cunean tendon is the tendon of the medial branch of the tibialis anterior muscle extending diagonally from anterior to posterior and inserting in the tarsal bone on the medial aspect of the tarsus (A in Fig. 22.14). A 2.5-cm, 22-gauge needle is inserted approximately 1.5 cm distal to the cunean tendon and then advanced between the cunean tendon and the tarsal bone to penetrate the bursa from distally. This approach is safe and, should the horse move, is less likely to break off the needle in the surrounding tissues. At least 10 mL of local anesthetic is frequently required and administered as the needle enters the skin, coming from under the tendon to fill the entire bursa after penetration (Fig. 22.15). One way to confirm the correct location of the block is to observe the increased intrabursal pressure causing local anesthetic to flow forcefully from the needle after removal of the syringe. A period of at least 20 min is required for maximum anesthetic effect.

Tarsal Block

Desensitizing the distal intertarsal and tarsometatarsal joints with local anesthetic improves lameness associated with early bone spavin. The tarsometatarsal joint is most easily entered by a 2.5-cm, 22-gauge needle on the posterior lateral aspect of the hock over the lateral head of the splint (metatarsal IV) (Fig. 22.16 and B in Fig. 22.14). The intertarsal joint is entered by a 2.5-cm, 22-gauge needle at a right angle to the skin ventral to the cunean ten-

don on the medial aspect of the tarsus (C in Fig. 22.14). Approximately 6 mL of local anesthetic solution is injected into the intertarsal joint space with pressure. Considerable resistance will be encountered, even with the needle placed in the joint. Sometimes the needle must be turned to be sure that the bevel is not against bone and allows for injection of the anesthetic solution. In an alternative method, a 2.5-cm, 22-gauge needle can be placed into the tarsometatarsal joint approximately 2.5 cm distal to the intertarsal joint while injecting the local anesthetic (D in Fig. 22.14). Communication between the distal intertarsal and tarsometatarsal joints is variable, but can be demonstrated by placing one needle in each of the two joints and observing the local anesthetic flowing from one needle after the anesthetic is injected into the other needle.[37,40] There is a higher pressure in the distal joint and, to get good dispersion of local anesthetic in both joints, both sites should be injected with local anesthetic solution.

Tibiotarsal Block

One of the most common joints in which arthrodesis is performed is the tibiotarsal (tarsocrural) joint. It is the easiest of all the equine joints to inject.[35] This joint is penetrated with a 3.75-cm, 18-gauge needle at the craniomedial aspect 2 to 3 cm ventral to the medial malleolus of the tibia on either the medial or lateral side of the saphenous vein (E in Fig. 22.14). The capsule is thin, superficial, and easily observed, and may also be distended caudomedially and craniolaterally in cases of tarsal osteoarthrosis (bone spavin).[37] The needle is inserted to a depth of less than 2 cm in a slightly dorsal direction toward the anterior medial aspect of the hock. Approximately 15 mL of local anesthetic is injected after synovial fluid is recovered on aspiration. Complete anesthe-

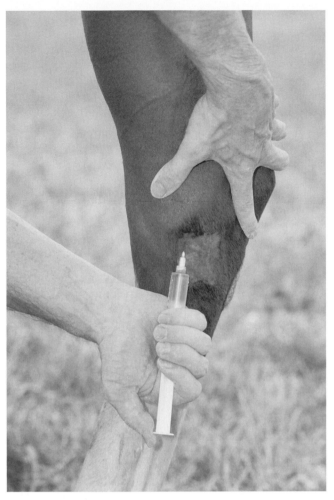

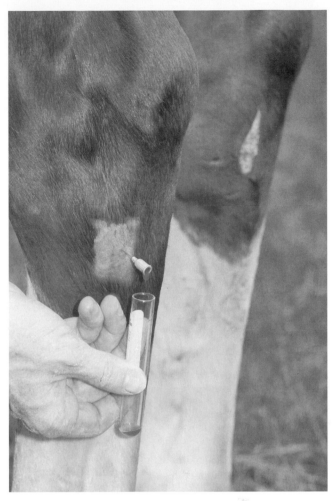

Fig. 22.15. Injection of local anesthetic (10 mL) into the cunean bursa of the right rear limb; medial aspect.

Fig. 22.16. Collection of fluid from the tarsometatarsal joint (left rear leg).

sia of the tibiotarsal joint has been achieved in healthy horses (250 to 680 kg) by intra-articular administration of 2 mL of 4% procaine HCl solution. The intra-articular concentration of procaine ranged from 3.7 to 5.4 mg of procaine/mL at 1 h after administration, which is above the anesthetic threshold concentration (0.2 mg/mL).[39]

Stifle Block

The stifle (genual) joint, which is the largest joint in the hind limb, consists of the femoropatellar and femorotibial joint spaces, which consist of medial and lateral pouches. The medial femoropatellar pouch is the common site where the stifle joint is injected for diagnostic blocks. It is most easily entered dorsal to the tibial crest between the middle and medial patellar ligaments (A in Fig. 22.17). The medial femoropatellar pouch enclosing the femoropatellar joint communicates with the medial femorotibial pouch of the femorotibial joint in most horses. The communicating opening, however, can be obstructed in an inflamed stifle joint, necessitating the injection of local anesthetic or medication into each individual compartment.[22] Entering the medial pouch of the femorotibial joint is technically difficult, but is accom-

plished between the medial patellar ligament and the medial collateral ligament approximately 4 cm dorsal to the proximal medial edge of the tibia (B in Fig. 22.17). The medial femorotibial pouch is chosen by some clinicians as the injection site because it is the area that is most likely to have injury and pain causing lameness. There is seldom an indication for injecting the lateral femorotibial pouch of the stifle joint because there is seldom injury in this area. The lateral femorotibial pouch can be entered and injected between the lateral patellar ligament and the lateral collateral ligament (C in Fig. 22.17). In some cases (approximately 25%), a communicating opening between the femoropatellar pouch and the lateral femorotibial pouch exists. A 5- to 7.5-cm, 18-gauge spinal needle is satisfactory for penetrating the joint capsule and injecting 30 to 40 mL of anesthetic into each pouch. To make the injection, it is best to feel around with the needle and insert it to a depth of 3 to 4 cm, until some resistance is encountered, during penetration of the joint capsule. Additional resistance is felt as local anesthetic solution is injected. A few drops of joint fluid can be recovered after some local anesthetic has been administered, but seldom is joint fluid aspirated before the injection of local anesthetic. It is important to use a

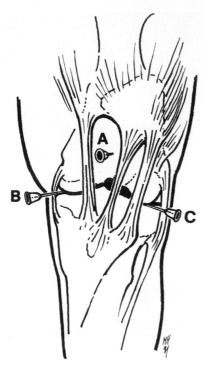

Fig. 22.17. Needle placement into the femoropatellar pouch (A), medial femorotibial pouch (B), and lateral femorotibial pouch (C) of the stifle joint.

larger rather than a smaller amount of local anesthetic and allow at least 20 min for maximal effect. Many horses will continue to improve for up to an hour after the injection. Any improvement in lameness is significant, because few horses are entirely sound after local anesthetic has been injected into the stifle joint. This is probably because most lameness involves the medial collateral ligaments and/or cruciate ligaments and structures adjacent to, but not inside, the joint capsule.

Coxofemoral Block

The coxofemoral (hip) joint is the most difficult of all joints to inject, so several approaches have been described.[22,35,36,43] The skin between the anterior and posterior eminences of the great trochanter of the femur is desensitized by injecting a small amount of local anesthetic. A wide-bored needle (3.75-cm, 14-gauge) is first inserted at that site, through which a thinner (15-cm, 18-gauge) and more flexible needle is inserted. The needle is then advanced anteromedially along the femoral neck until the joint capsule is penetrated (A in Fig. 22.18). The injection of 30 to 50 mL of local anesthetic is adequate, after synovial fluid is recovered on aspiration. Improvement in lameness should be assessed only after a minimum period of 30 min has passed to allow time for maximal anesthetic effect.

Trochanteric Bursa Block

The trochanteric bursa is located on the lateral aspect of the hip, between the anterior crest of the great trochanter of the femur and the middle gluteal muscle. The bursa is entered and injected by a 7.5-cm, 18-gauge needle, which is inserted 3 to 5 cm ventral to the anterior crest of the great trochanter and is directed dorsally and medially (B in Fig. 22.18). Synovial fluid is recovered by using continuous suction of a syringe that is attached to the needle, and then 10 to 15 mL of local anesthetic can be injected.

Anesthesia for Laparotomy

At least four techniques for obtaining anesthesia of the paralumbar and abdominal wall in standing horses have been described: (a) infiltration anesthesia, (b) paravertebral thoracolumbar anesthesia, (c) segmental dorsolumbar epidural anesthesia, and (d) segmental thoracolumbar subarachnoid anesthesia. Although infiltration of the incision line is the easiest and probably the most commonly used technique, any of these techniques may be used for abdominal surgery required for exploratory laparotomy, in-

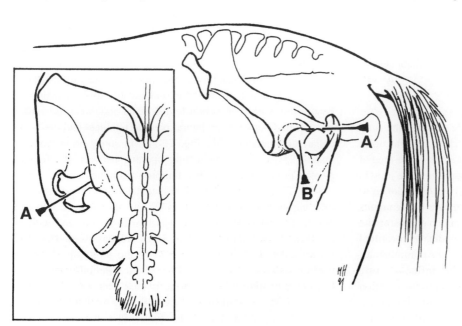

Fig. 22.18. Needle placement into the coxofemoral joint (A) and the trochanteric bursa (B).

testinal biopsy, ovariectomy, cesarean section, embryo transfer, castration of stallions with abdominal cryptorchidism, and liver or kidney biopsy.

Infiltration Anesthesia

Simple infiltration of the incision line (*line block*) is commonly used in equine practice. A 2.5-cm, 20-gauge or smaller needle is used for multiple subcutaneous injections of 1 mL of local anesthetic for each centimeter of incision. This can be repeated until the entire length of the desired incision is blocked. Pain is minimized by slow and continuous injections as the needle is inserted at the edge of the desensitized skin. This technique assures that the horse senses only the initial needle penetration. The needle can be advanced in multiple directions to produce a fan-shaped area of desensitization. Usually 10 to 15 mL of anesthetic is adequate for the skin and subcutaneous line block, whereas 50 to 150 mL of the anesthetic may be required to desensitize the deeper layers of muscle and peritoneum, depending on the area to be desensitized. A 7.5- to 10-cm, 18-gauge needle is used for deep deposition of the anesthetic. Toxicity is not to be expected with dosages of less than 250 mL of 2% lidocaine HCl solution, which is equivalent to 5 g, for infiltration of the paralumbar fossa in adult horses (500 kg),[2,58] whereas the intravenous bolus administration of much smaller doses (150 mL, 3 g/adult horse) may cause convulsions. At least 15 min should be allowed for maximal anesthetic effect. The primary advantages of local infiltration anesthesia are the ease of performing the technique and that precise knowledge of nerve location is not necessary. The disadvantages include disruption of normal tissue architecture, with excessive amount of fluid, hematoma, and trauma; incomplete anesthesia (particularly of the peritoneum); incomplete muscle relaxation of the deeper layers of the abdominal wall; toxicity after inadvertent injection into the peritoneal cavity; and increased cost and time required for long incisions (>1 m) as might be required for a cesarean section surgery.

Paravertebral Thoracolumbar Anesthesia

If a longer (>1 m) incision of the skin, musculature, and peritoneum of the midflank region is required, paravertebral thoracolumbar anesthesia (*paravertebral block*) can be used as an alternative to infiltration anesthesia.[7,59–61] This block is technically more difficult and less popular than other techniques, but can be accomplished in thin-muscled horses with palpable landmarks. The last thoracic (T18) and first and second lumbar (L1 and L2) spinal nerves are desensitized approximately 10 cm from the midline, after they have emerged from the intervertebral foramina and ramified into dorsal and ventral branches and their medial and lateral ramifications, respectively (Fig. 22.19). Approximately 10 mL of local anesthetic is injected to desensitize the lateral cutaneous branches of the dorsal spinal nerves T18, L1, and L2 subcutaneously at three sites: halfway between the last rib and the distal end of the first lumbar transverse process (for T18), between the first and second lumbar transverse processes (for L1), and between the second and third lumbar transverse processes (for L2). The injection sites for desensitizing the spinal nerves are easily identified by locating the third

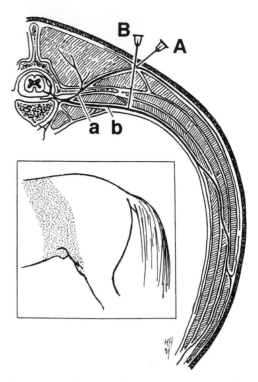

Fig. 22.19. Needle placement for paravertebral nerve blockades: A cranial view of a transection of the first lumbar vertebra at the location of the intervertebral foramen: (A) subcutaneous infiltration and (B) retroperitoneal infusion (a, dorsal branch, and b, ventral branch, of the L1 vertebral nerve). **Inset:** Desensitized subcutaneous area after blockade of T18, L1, and L2 vertebral nerves.

lumbar transverse process, which lies on a line between the most caudal extension of the last rib and perpendicular to the long axis of the spinal vertebrae.[61] The distance between the injection sites ranges from 3 to 6 cm (Fig. 22.20). After the skin is desensitized, a 7.5-cm, 18-gauge needle is inserted at each site to reach the ventral branches of T18, L1, and L2. The needle is first advanced until the peritoneum is punctured, which is indicated by either a loss of resistance to needle insertion or a slight sucking sound as air enters the needle. The point of the needle is then withdrawn to a retroperitoneal position, where a second deposit of 15 mL of local anesthetic is injected (B in Fig. 22.19). The advantages of paravertebral anesthesia when compared with infiltration anesthesia include the use of smaller doses of anesthetic, a wide and uniform area of anesthesia and muscle relaxation, and absence of local anesthetic from the operative wound margin, thus minimizing edema, hematoma, and possible interference with healing. The disadvantage is difficulty in performing the technique for the inexperienced practitioner. The fat and muscles in some horses almost put the transverse processes out of range of palpation, making the technique more time consuming or unpractical. There is some bowing of the back toward the desensitized side, making it more difficult to close the incision and navigate tissue landmarks. Inadvertent desensitization of the third lumbar spinal nerve, which carries motor fibers to the femoral and ischial nerves, causes loss of motor control of the ipsilateral pelvic limb.

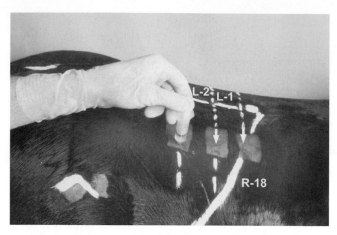

Fig. 22.20. Right thoracolumbar area of a standing adult horse with injection sites (arrows) for distal paravertebral block (R18, last rib; L1 and L2, spinous processes of first and second lumbar vertebrae). The dotted line transects the corresponding interspaces between spinous and transverse processes. Subcutaneous injection of L2 is shown. From Skarda.[3]

Segmental Dorsolumbar Epidural Anesthesia

This technique is not routinely used in horses because it is difficult to perform, requires a special catheter-stylet unit to catheterize the T18-L1 epidural space from the lumbosacral epidural space (Fig. 22.21),[62] and is associated with the risk of the catheter either kinking or curling within the epidural space. Catheter curling and injection of local anesthetic near spinal nerve roots contributing to femoral and ischial nerve outflow could result in motor nerve deficits in rear-limb function.

Segmental Thoracolumbar Subarachnoid Anesthesia

This is easier to master than segmental dorsolumbar epidural anesthesia. It produces the fastest and best-controlled surgical anesthesia of the flank in horses; however, special equipment and maintenance of aseptic technique are required.[63] A 17.5-cm, 17-gauge Huber-point Tuohy needle with stylet and with the bevel directed cranially is inserted into the subarachnoid space at the lumbosacral (L6-S1) intervertebral space (Fig. 22.22). This interspace is located 1 to 2 cm caudal of a line drawn between the cranial edge of each tuber sacral and the dorsal midline. Rectal palpation of the ventral lumbosacral eminence may be used to locate the L6-S1 intervertebral space.[63] The skin and lumbosacral fascia adjacent to the interspinous (L6-S1) ligaments are injected with 5 mL of 2% lidocaine HCl solution to help minimize pain during the puncture procedure. To prevent loss of motor control of the pelvic limbs, care must be taken not to inject the entire volume (5 mL) of local anesthetic into the subarachnoid space. The needle is advanced along the median plane perpendicularly to the spinal cord until entering the subarachnoid space. The stylet is removed, and 2 to 3 mL of cerebrospinal fluid (CSF) is aspirated. A Formocath polyethylene catheter (Becton-Dickinson, Rutherford, NJ), 100 cm long with a 0.095-cm outside diameter, reinforced with a stainless-steel spring guide (0.052-cm outside di-

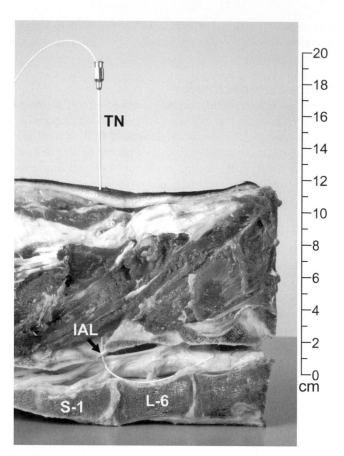

Fig. 22.21. Lateral view of sagittal section of the sixth lumbar (L6) and first sacral (S1) vertebrae. A 17.5-cm, 17-gauge Huber-point Tuohy needle (TN) is in place for catheterization of the lumbar epidural space. The arrow indicates the interarcuate ligament (IAL).

ameter), is passed through the needle and advanced approximately 60 cm to the midthoracic area. First the needle is withdrawn over the catheter, and then the spring guide is removed and the catheter is withdrawn a calculated distance to place its tip at T18-L1. Precise catheter positioning requires radiography for confirmation. A 23-gauge needle on a three-way stopcock is attached to the catheter, and 1.0 to 2.0 mL of CSF is removed. A small dose (1.5 to 2.0 mL) of a 2% mepivacaine HCl solution is injected through the catheter at a rate of approximately 0.5 mL/min. The previously collected CSF is used to remove the remaining local anesthetic from the catheter. Bilateral segmental anesthesia, extending from spinal cord segment T14 to segment L3, is maximal 5 to 10 min after injection and lasts 30 to 60 min. Surgical anesthesia is easily maintained by fractional bolus administration of 0.5 mL of the anesthetic at 30-min intervals or as needed (Fig. 22.23). The duration of anesthesia is determined by the decline of the subarachnoid mepivacaine concentration owing to absorption of drug into the systemic circulation and not due to hydrolysis of the drug within the CSF.[64]

Investigators have threaded a subarachnoid catheter to the thoracolumbar area in standing horses to use ketamine (12 to 15 mg/100 kg body weight [BW]) to produce segmental spinal block

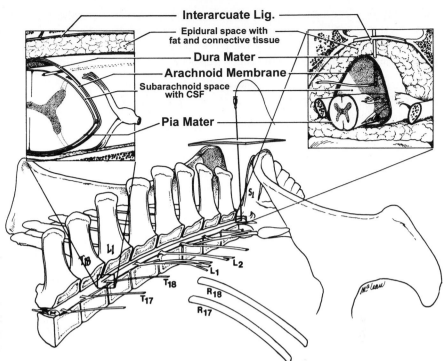

Fig. 22.22. Needle and catheter placement for thoracolumbar subarachnoid anesthesia. Cranial and left lateral aspects of the equine thoracolumbar and sacral vertebrae and their associated intraspinal structures with the tip of Huber point (Tuohy) needle, catheter, and steel spring guide in the subarachnoid space. CSF, cerebrospinal fluid. From Skarda and Muir.[63]

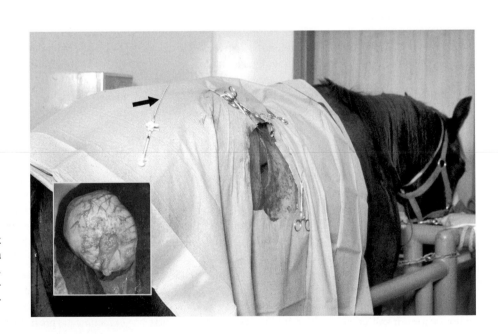

Fig. 22.23. Ovariectomy via left flank under segmental subarachnoid anesthesia (2 mL of 2% carbocaine hydrochloride). **Inset:** Granulosa cell tumor, 12.5-cm diameter. The arrow indicates the subarachnoid catheter.

between the T17 and L3 spinal nerves.[65] The analgesic effect of ketamine appeared after 5 to 10 min and lasted between 35 and 65 min. Horses did not react to surgical intervention on the abdominal wall and viscera, and significant changes in heart and respiratory rates, rectal temperature, and intestinal motility of horses were not observed after subarachnoid ketamine injection.[65]

There has been one report of lumbosacral subarachnoid catheterization in healthy horses that resulted in an acute inflammatory reaction after 12 h of catheterization, although there was no bacterial contamination.[66] The horses did not show any clinical signs of neurological dysfunction, such as ataxia, proprioception deficits, or changes in locomotor activity, and rectal temperature remained unchanged even though an inflammatory reaction in CSF occurred.

The advantages of thoracolumbar subarachnoid anesthesia as compared with dorsolumbar epidural anesthesia include simplicity of needle and catheter placements, minimal dosage, deposition of the anesthetic at nerve roots, rapid onset of anesthesia, and minimal physiological disturbance. The disadvantages include potential for traumatizing the conus medullaris, kinking and curling of the catheter in the subarachnoid space if the guidewire is recessed from the catheter tip, loss of motor control of the pelvic limbs and/or injecting the proper dose in a misplaced catheter, and meningitis after septic technique.

Caudal Anesthesia

Caudal epidural anesthesia, continuous caudal epidural anesthesia, and caudal subarachnoid anesthesia are possible techniques to produce regional anesthesia of the anus, perineum, rectum, vulva, vagina, urethra, and bladder in horses. Success in producing regional anesthesia of pelvic viscera and genitalia without losing locomotor function of the hind legs depends on cranial flow of local anesthetic to desensitize the caudal and the last three pairs of sacral nerves in the epidural space as they emerge either from the meninges (epidural technique) or the spinal cord (subarachnoid technique). In horses, the spinal cord and its meninges end in the midsacral region, and only the coccygeal nerves and the thin phylum terminale remain in the spinal canal.[67] The coccygeal nerves are not easily damaged at the site of needle penetration to produce caudal epidural blockade. Caudal subarachnoid blockade, however, requires the insertion of a spinal needle into the subarachnoid space at the lumbosacral intervertebral space and the passage of a catheter to the midsacral region; thus, the potential for trauma to the conus medullaris and nerve fibers by the needle or catheter exists. The neuroanatomy and effects of sensory, motor, and autonomic nerve blockade of various spinal cord segments are summarized in Table 22.1.[68,69]

Caudal Epidural Anesthesia

This is routinely used in horses because it is simple and inexpensive and requires no sophisticated equipment. The technique's use in horses was first described in 1925;[70] subsequently, many have reported its use for relieving pain and control of rectal tenesmus associated with irritation of the perineum, anus, rectum, and vagina during difficult labor; correction of uterine torsion, fetotomy, and various obstetric manipulations and surgical procedures such as amputation of the tail, rectovaginal fistula repairs, Caslick's closure (operation for pneumovagina), prolapsed rectum, urethrostomy; or anal, perineal, vulvar, and bladder procedures.[7,71–86]

The injection site is the epidural space between the first and second coccygeal vertebrae. The first coccygeal interspace (Co1-Co2) is identified as the first obvious midline depression caudal to the sacrum. It can generally be felt with the finger as the first movable coccygeal articulation when the tail is raised and lowered. The sacrococcygeal joint in many horses is fused and generally intersects with the midline and a line drawn over the back joining the two coxofemoral joints. The Co1-Co2 interspace may be more difficult to palpate in obese or well-developed horses, but generally lies at the most angular portion of the bend of the tail, approximately 5 cm cranial to the origin of the first tail hairs and the caudal fold of the tail. Correct needle placement requires the horse to be properly restrained and stand squarely with the croup symmetrical. In the standard technique, a 5- to 7.5-cm, 18-gauge spinal needle with fitted stylet is inserted through the disinfected skin in the center of the Co1-Co2 joint space while the needle is directed at almost right angles to the general contour of the croup or ventrocranially at an angle of approximately 10° to vertical. The needle is inserted in a median plane until it contacts the floor of the vertebral canal and is then withdrawn for approximately 0.5 cm to avoid injection into the intervertebral disk or ligamentous floor of the canal (E in Fig. 22.24). Painful reaction to the epidural needle is minimized if a 2.5-cm, 25-gauge needle is used to inject 2 to 3 mL of a 2% lidocaine HCl solution subcutaneously and adjacent to the interspinous and interarcuate ligaments. A popping sensation is often detected as the interarcuate ligament is penetrated. A hissing sound at the needle hub may often be heard upon penetration of the epidural space as air is drawn into the needle. Proper needle placement may be verified by applying 1 or 2 drops of local anesthetic to the needle and observing the drop(s) to be drawn into the epidural space by the negative pressure (*hanging-drop technique*) or confirmation can be made by resistance-free injection of 3 to 5 mL of air or local anesthetic solution (test dose), with no blood upon aspiration.

In the alternative technique, the spinal needle is inserted at the caudal part of the first intercoccygeal depression and directed cranioventrally at almost 30° to the horizontal plane until its point glides along the floor of the neural canal (F in Fig. 22.24). The spinal needle can be inserted to its full length (5 to 7.5 cm). Depth from skin surface to the neural canal varies between 3 to 7.5 cm, depending on the size and condition of the horse. The alternative technique is useful in horses that have fibrous connective tissue from previous epidural injections, which limits the diffusion of local anesthetic agents. However, unilateral analgesia is more likely to occur if the spinal needle has been inserted a considerable distance into the vertebral canal, allowing the needle tip to deviate from the midline, and if a small amount of local anesthetic has been given, to bathe the nerve roots primarily on one side of the spinal column.[7,87,88]

Epidural Local Anesthetics

Local anesthetics can provide profound relief from pain by inhibiting depolarization of the nerve membrane and conduction of nerve impulses. The amount of anesthetic injected is determined by considering the type of local anesthetic, the size and conformation of the horse, the depth of needle insertion into the vertebral canal (the actual distance of the needle bevel to the spinal cord), and the extent of regional anesthesia required (Fig. 22.25).

Lidocaine This has been shown to be most effective as an epidural analgesic. A mature mare (450 kg) may require a total of 6 to 8 mL of a 2% lidocaine HCl solution (0.26 to 0.35 mg/kg) to anesthetize the anus, perineum, rectum, vulva, vagina, urethra, and bladder. The order and magnitude of neural blockade are dose dependent but generally profound, and selective sensory blockade of nociceptive and motor fibers in dermatomes ranging from coccygeal to the second sacral vertebra is produced within 5 to 15 min and lasts 60 to 90 min. Additional local anesthetic should not be administered during this period, so as to prevent overdosing, which can result in marked ataxia and potentially recumbency, hypotension, and occasionally bradycardia from sympathetic blockade.[62,89–91]

Table 22.1. Neuroanatomy and action of caudal epidural analgesia.

Nerves	Ventral Branches	Spinal Cord Segment	Sensory	Motor	Parasympathetic	Sympathetic	
							Action
Caudal		Coccygeal	Most of the tail and skin between anus and tail root	Coccygeal muscle			
Caudal rectal (hemorrhoidal)		S5	Anal region, tail folds, and tail base	Coccygeus and levator ani externus muscle	Fibers in caudal rectal nerve		Straining in anorectal region due to excessive sympathetic stimulation
Middle rectal	Perineal nerve, caudal scrotal nerves, and labial nerves	S4, S5	Perineum, posterior croup, scrotum along its caudal aspects, and vulva without clitoris		Pelvic nerves, hypogastric plexus		Relaxation of bladder without sphincter, distal colon, rectum, and sexual organs
Pudendal	Dorsal nerve of penis, and deep perineal nerve	S4, S3, S2	Penis (corpus cavernosum and spongiosum); and clitoris and vulva	Perineal muscles fascia of ischiorectal fossa, and constrictor vulvae muscle		Retractor penis muscle	Prolapse of penis; and relaxation of vulva and vagina
Caudal gluteal	Caudal cutaneous femoral nerve	S2, S1	Lateral and posterior surfaces of hip and thigh	Extension of hip			
Cranial gluteal		S1, L6, L5	Lateral aspect of thigh	Flexor and abductors of hip		Splanchnic lumbar nerves (in part)	Relaxation of bladder and sphincter of bladder, distal colon, rectum, and sexual organs
Sciatic		S1, L6, L5	Middle to tibial region to foot	Flexor and abductors of hip; and flexor of stifle (in part) and extensors of hock and digit			Ataxia, and knuckling of hind fetlock

From Skarda,[68] p. 105.

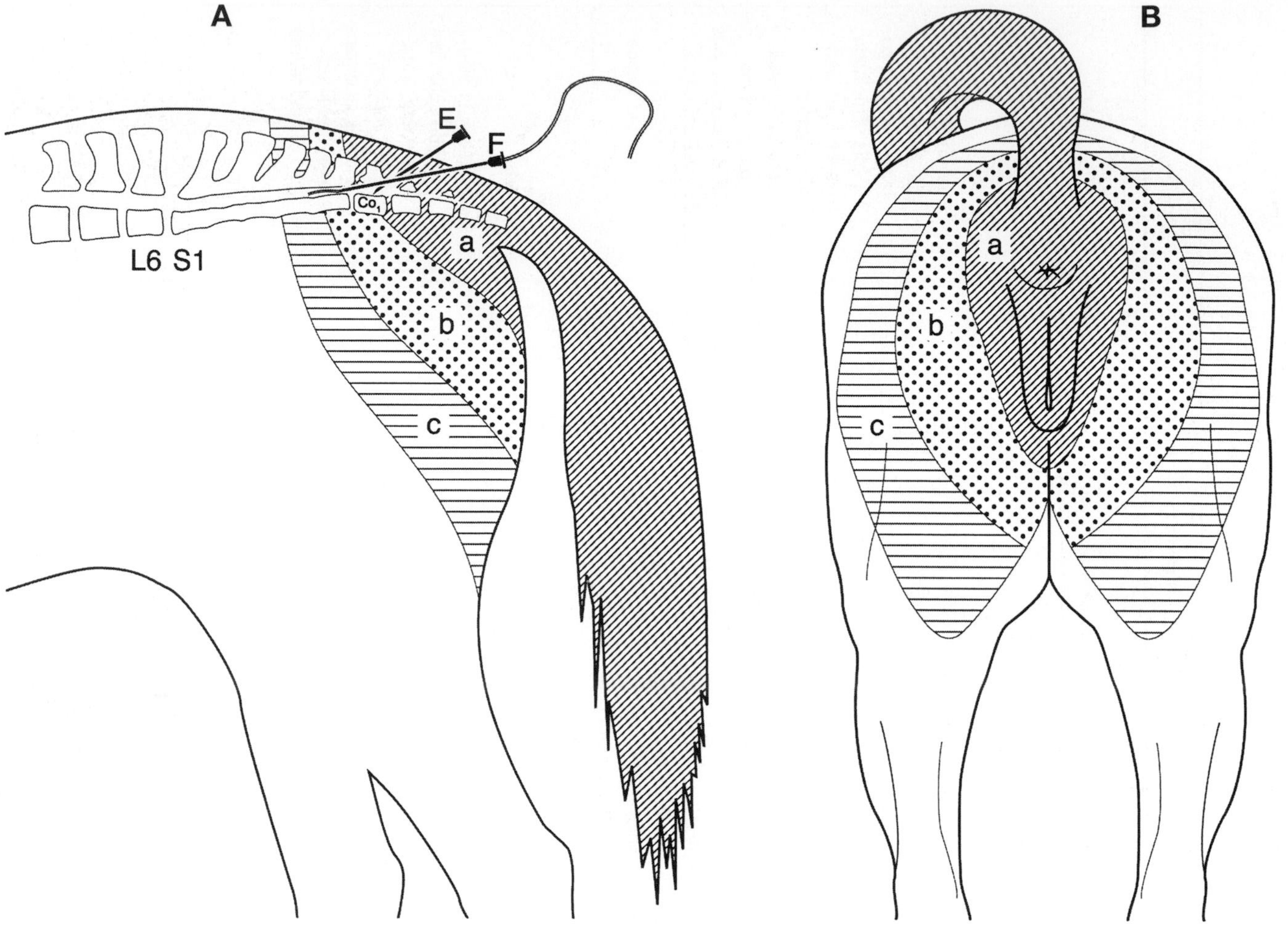

Fig. 22.24. Lateral **(A)** and caudal **(B)** drawings of the lumbosacral, sacral, and sacrococcygeal areas of a standing mare with marked loss of skin sensation from coccyx to S4 (a), coccyx to S3 (b), and coccyx to S2 (c), respectively, 60 min after epidural administration of ropivacaine (0.5% solution, 9 mL/500 kg body weight). Placement of spinal needle (E) and Tuohy needle (F) with the catheter for caudal epidural anesthesia. L6, sixth lumbar; S1, first sacral; and Co1, first coccygeal vertebrae. Modified from Skarda and Muir.[88]

Mepivacaine Mepivacaine HCl solution (2%) acts very similarly to lidocaine in producing caudal regional anesthesia in horses. Epidural injection of 60 to 100 mg of 2% mepivacaine HCl in aqueous solution (3 to 5 mL) at the caudal sacral (S5-C1 to S3) vertebrae (via catheter) can produce either unilateral or bilateral analgesia extending from spinal cord segment S1 to the coccyx in adult mares. Analgesia usually becomes evident in 20 min and lasts approximately 80 min.[62,92]

Ropivacaine This is the newest commercially available drug for use as a local and regional anesthetic. Its effect (0.5%, 8 mL/500 kg) has been evaluated when injected epidurally at the sacrococcygeal vertebral interspace in adult mares.[87,88] Lack of sensory perception to electrical stimulation (>40 mA) and absence of response to deep needle pricks extending from coccyx to S2 dermatomes indicated the presence of regional anesthesia. Epidurally administered ropivacaine induced variable analgesia extending bilaterally from the coccyx to S2 (three mares), coccyx to S3 (four mares), and coccyx to S4 (three mares), with minimal

sedation, ataxia, and cardiovascular and respiratory disturbances. Analgesia at the perineal area lasts 2 to 4 h.[88]

The efficacy of caudal (Co1-Co2) epidural administration of either 1% ropivacaine, 2% lidocaine, or a combination of 1% ropivacaine and 2% lidocaine for producing perineal anesthesia in mares has also been evaluated.[91] Local anesthetics were combined with adrenaline (1:200,000) and administered at a volume of 0.018 mL/kg. Perineal analgesia lasted 3 to 4.5 h. Three of the mares became recumbent: two that received lidocaine and one that received the combination of ropivacaine and lidocaine. It was concluded that the high incidence of ataxia and recumbency was probably attributable to the higher concentration (1% vs. 0.5%) of ropivacaine and admixture of adrenaline with these two local anesthetics.[91]

Bupivacaine The caudal epidural administration of hyperbaric bupivacaine (0.5%, 0.06 mg/kg BW) produces not only very rapid (<6 min) but prolonged (>5 h) bilateral perineal analgesia effects in adult horses.[93] Heart and respiratory rates, arterial

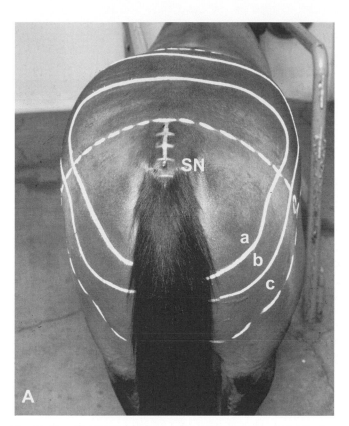

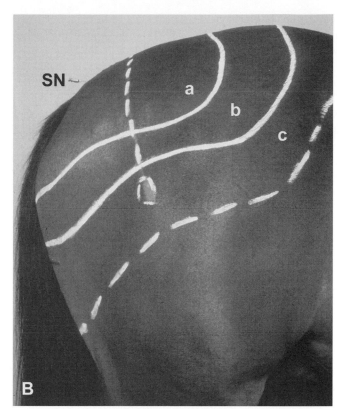

Fig. 22.25. Desensitized skin area in a standing horse 20 min after epidural injection of 6 mL (a), 8 mL (b), and 10 mL (c), respectively, of 2% carbocaine via a 15-cm, 18-gauge spinal needle inserted at the third coccygeal interspace to its full length horizontally (SN, spinal needle with stylet). Dorsocaudal **(A)** and lateral **(B)** aspects. From Skarda.[3]

blood pressure, and rectal temperature did not change after the epidural administration of bupivacaine.

Other Local Anesthetics   Other local anesthetics that have been used to achieve caudal epidural anesthesia in standing horses (weighing 500 kg) include 10 to 12 mL of 2% procaine HCl solution, 5 to 7 mL of 5% procaine HCl solution, and 3 to 5 mL of 5% hexylcaine HCl solution. The duration of anesthesia is dose related and ranges from 45 to 60 min for 2% procaine, 60 to 90 min for 5% procaine, and 90 to 120 min for 5% hexylcaine, respectively.[53] All of these local anesthetics provide relatively brief analgesia (45 to 120 min) and may necessitate readministration to enable completion of the procedure. If the needle is left in place and an injection cap is attached, additional amounts of local anesthetic can be administered to the desired effect.

Epidural α₂-Adrenoceptor Agonists

The caudal epidural administration of an α_2-adrenoceptor agonist, such as xylazine or detomidine, may be more appropriate for procedures requiring lengthy periods (>2 h) of analgesia. Following epidural administration, these agents bind to nonopioid receptors in the substantia gelatinosa layer of the spinal cord and produce spinal analgesia that can be attenuated by intravenous administration of α_2-antagonists such as atipamezole (0.1 mg/kg)[94–97] or yohimbine (0.05 mg/kg).[98,99] Because the equine

spinal cord terminates in the lumbosacral area, agents administered into the caudal epidural space must diffuse cranially to bind with receptors in the spinal cord. In addition, xylazine may have a direct local anesthetic effect on the cauda equina.[100]

Xylazine   This drug has been injected into the caudal epidural space of ponies[100–102] and horses[90,103–108] for a variety of diagnostic, obstetric, and surgical procedures performed in the anal and perineal regions. In the first report of epidural administration of xylazine in horses, a dose of 0.17 mg of xylazine per kilogram of BW, diluted to a volume of 10 mL by use of sterile 0.9% NaCl solution, was used.[103] This dosage was considered safe and effective for producing 2½ h of perineal analgesia in horses and infrequently induced ataxia of the pelvic limbs. Subsequent studies, assessing the analgesic effects of caudal epidural xylazine (0.25 mg/kg BW expanded to a 6-mL volume with 0.9% NaCl) injection have supported these initial observations.[106,107] Maximal dermatomal analgesic spread ranges from the first coccygeal to S3 spinal cord segments and usually lasts 2 to 3 h. Blockade of parasympathetic nerves may relax the genitalia and dilate the rectum.[107] Sedation and ataxia are minimal, and circulatory and respiratory variables—such as cardiac output, stroke volume, mean right atrial pressure, mean pulmonary artery pressure, systemic and pulmonary vascular resistance, oxygen consumption, core and rectal temperature, and arterial and mixed venous pH and gas tensions (partial pressure of oxygen [PO_2], and partial pressure of carbon dioxide [PCO_2])—do not change appreciably.[107]

Epidural xylazine (0.15 mg/kg) administration reportedly decreases the halothane requirement of horses by 35% in the thoracic limbs and by 40% in the pelvic limbs, supporting the involvement of α_2 receptors in spinal analgesia.[101,102] In a second study, a 1.5 minimum alveolar concentration of halothane alone and halothane with epidural xylazine (0.15 mg/kg BW diluted in 0.15 mL/kg of saline) administration did not induce a similar anesthetic response to hind-limb surgery.[108] Horses with epidural xylazine injection required less halothane (end-tidal halothane concentration, 0.9% vs. 1.4%) and inotropic support to maintain arterial blood pressure above 60 mm Hg and a higher cardiac index than did horses anesthetized with halothane alone.

Xylazine and Lidocaine   A mixture of lidocaine (0.22 mg/kg, 2% solution) and xylazine (0.17 mg/kg, 2% solution) can be safely used for long-lasting caudal epidural anesthesia in healthy adult horses.[90] This combination provides longer anesthesia of the perineum than does either drug given alone (5 h vs. 3 h), thereby minimizing the need for additional drugs. Pulse and respiratory rate are not altered appreciably, though some ataxia may be present. Usually sedation is not evident after the epidural administration of these doses of lidocaine–xylazine HCl. Although the combined use of lidocaine and xylazine at this dose range appears to have a wide margin of safety, there has been one report of a sudden collapse in the hindquarters of a thoroughbred mare (450 kg) undergoing urogenital surgery 90 min after completion of the epidural injection.[109] As would be expected, overdosing either of these agents can depress CNS, respiratory, and cardiovascular activity; can cause postural instability and/or recumbency; and can induce excitement in conscious horses.

Detomidine   Detomidine HCl (1%) at a dose of 60 µg of detomidine/kg BW, expanded to a 10-mL volume with sterile water, injected into the epidural space at the caudal sacral (S5 to S4) vertebrae (catheter technique) induces selective caudal analgesia and sedation (Fig. 22.26), mild ataxia, cardiopulmonary depression, and diuresis similar to the effects of intravenously or intramuscularly administered detomidine.[110–114] The analgesia induced with this technique can be variable, with bilateral spread from the coccyx as far cranially as T14 in some horses. Analgesia is often accompanied by mild ataxia and occasionally by buckling of the pelvic limbs. Horses appear deeply sedated and in a sleeplike state, evidenced by the lowering of their head and drooping of the upper eyelids. These signs are observed 5 min after drug administration and last 3 h. Doses of less than 30 µg of detomidine/kg BW appear ineffective in producing reliable analgesia, although the sedation produced can be greater than expected. Higher doses (>80 µg of detomidine HCl/kg) typically produce marked sedation, cardiopulmonary depression, increased frequency of second-degree atrioventricular heart block, renal diuresis, and recumbency, and cannot be recommended.[112] An initial dose of no more than 20 µg of detomidine HCl/kg BW should be used in horses that are debilitated.

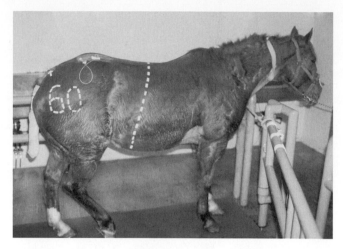

Fig. 22.26.   Desensitized skin area between T14 and coccyx and sedation in a standardbred mare (475 kg) 60 min after administration of 2.9 mL of 1% detomidine hydrochloride solution, diluted to a 10-mL volume with sterile water, into the epidural space of the first coccygeal intervertebral space. The epidural needle (white arrow) is left in position. A catheter is placed into the subarachnoid space at the lumbosacral intervertebral space for collection of cerebrospinal fluid (CSF). From Skarda and Muir.[110]

In general, results indicate that xylazine is perhaps a more desirable α_2-adrenoceptor agonist than is detomidine for inducing caudal epidural analgesia in horses. Xylazine exerts more potent antinociceptive action at the perineal dermatomes, with minimal cardiovascular depression, head ptosis, changes in pelvic limb position, and less renal diuresis.[114]

Should signs of rear-limb ataxia or motor blockade after caudal epidural administration of xylazine[109] or detomidine[115] develop, a tail-tie support is indicated until full hind-limb control is regained. Use of general anesthesia may be necessary to immobilize an excited horse completely. If general anesthesia is induced, anesthesia in horses given detomidine as a caudal epidural injection should be maintained with a lower concentration of inhalant. In one case report,[115] when a 364-kg, 15-month-old, sexually intact, cryptorchid male quarterhorse was positioned in standing stocks for castration, the horse unexpectedly collapsed to the floor, first to sternal and then into lateral recumbency, 15 min after epidural administration of 50 µg of detomidine HCl/kg at the first intercoccygeal space and infusion of 60 mL of 2% lidocaine in an inverted "L" pattern to desensitize the left flank.[115] Because the horse would not rise, general anesthesia was induced with intravenous diazepam (35 mg) and ketamine (750 mg). The horse was orotracheally intubated, and transported to the operating table. Anesthesia was maintained with halothane in oxygen (5 L/min) and surgery performed in the horse in dorsal recumbency. An expected smaller dose of halothane (<1.25%) was required to maintain a surgical plane of anesthesia in this horse, which recovered uneventfully 1 h and 55 min after discontinuation of halothane.[115]

α_2-Agonist–induced adverse side effects can be eliminated by the intravenous, epidural, or subarachnoid administration of α_2-adrenoceptor antagonists, such as atipamezole (Fig. 22.27), ida-

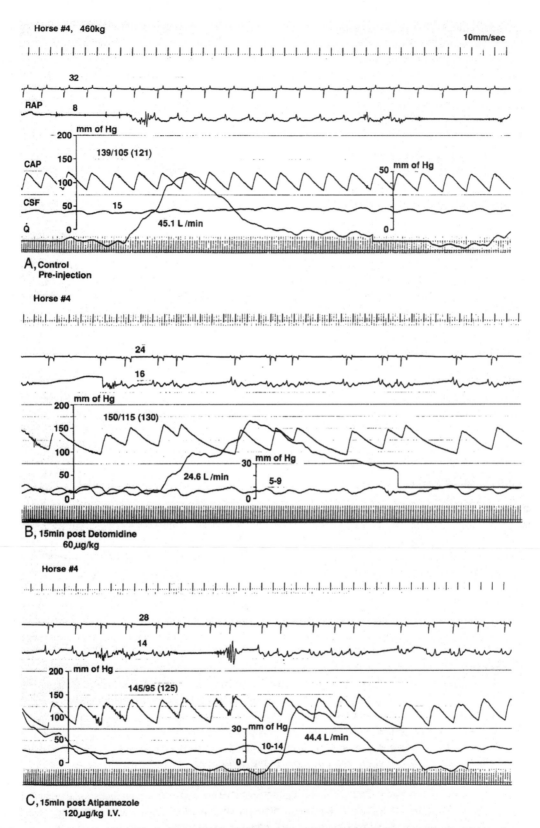

Fig. 22.27. Recording (10 mm/s) of lead II electrocardiogram (ECG), right atrial pressure (RAP), carotid arterial blood pressure (CAP), cerebrospinal fluid pressure (CSF), and cardiac output (Q) (thermodilution curve) before (control) **(A)**; 15 min after caudal epidural administration of 60 µg of detomidine hydrochloride solution per kilogram body weight, diluted to a 10-mL volume, using sterile water **(B)**; and 15 min after intravenous administration of 120 µg of atipamezole/kg **(C)**.

zoxan, yohimbine, or tolazoline.[94-98] The antagonistic effects of intravenous yohimbine (0.05 mg/kg BW) given after caudal (Co1-Co2) epidural administration of detomidine HCl solution (60 µg/kg BW) on antinociceptive, cardiorespiratory, and postural changes have been documented. Intravenously administered yohimbine rapidly reduced detomidine-induced perineal analgesia, reversed head ptosis, improved pelvic limb position, terminated sweating and diuresis, and antagonized detomidine-induced decreases in heart rate and cardiac output; but did not affect detomidine-induced decreases in respiratory rate.[98]

Medetomidine and Romifidine Medetomidine (15 µg/kg BW, diluted in 0.9% NaCl solution to 8 mL) injected into the epidural space at the first intercoccygeal vertebral space does not appear to produce surgical analgesia in the perineal region of adult horses.[116] Likewise, romifidine (80 µg/kg BW diluted in 0.9% NaCl solution to 8 mL) injection into the epidural space at the first intercoccygeal vertebral space has not resulted in a sufficient analgesic effect, even though signs of sedation (drooping of the lower lip and leaning the head against the stocks) are evident.[117] Based on the results of these studies, medetomidine and romifidine do not appear to be as efficacious as xylazine or detomidine when placed into the epidural space.

In summary, when choosing an α_2-adrenoceptor agonist for epidural analgesia, either 0.17 mg of xylazine/kg[103] or 60 µg of detomidine/kg[112] diluted in 10 mL of 0.9% NaCl solution has proven efficacious in achieving similar anesthesia of pelvic viscera and genitalia with minimal ataxia. With these doses, maximum analgesic effect should occur within 10 to 30 min and can last several hours. It is not advisable to redose during this time. If the needle is left in place and an injection cap is attached, additional amounts of local anesthetic or α_2-adrenoceptor agonist can be administered but should be regulated to keep the horse standing. In comparison, when relying solely on epidural local anesthetics, the duration of caudal analgesia is dose related and usually lasts 60 to 90 min with lidocaine (2%) or procaine (5%), and 90 to 120 min with either mepivacaine (2%) or hexylcaine (5%). Caudal epidurally administered local anesthetic solutions, when injected at recommended dosages, have minimal systemic side effects.

Epidural Ketamine
Ketamine is thought to produce analgesia primarily by its noncompetitive antagonism of *N*-methyl-D-aspartate (NMDA). High concentrations of ketamine may also produce local anesthetic-like effects by blocking sodium-ion channels.[118] The slow (1 min) injection of ketamine (0.5, 1.0, or 2.0 mg/kg BW) into the epidural space at the midsacral area (via a 17-gauge epidural catheter) has been reported to be effective in producing analgesia of the tail, perineum, and upper hind limb in horses.[119] Ketamine can be diluted in 0.9% NaCl solution and the volume adjusted to a final volume of approximately 10 mL for a 450-kg horse. Dosages of 0.5, 1.0, and 2.0 mg of ketamine/kg BW provide analgesia of the tail for 30, 50, and 80 min and in the perineum and upper hind limb for 30, 35, and 75 min, respectively. A sedative effect is also observed in a dose-response manner, with a

peak effect between 15 and 30 min after ketamine epidural deposition. Heart and respiratory rates, arterial blood pressure, arterial blood gases (PO_2 and PCO_2), and pH are generally unaffected when these doses of ketamine are used for epidural deposition.[119] Further studies are necessary to evaluate whether the analgesia produced by epidural ketamine is sufficient for surgery in horses.

The preemptive administration of ketamine (10%, 1.0 mg/kg BW, diluted with 0.9% NaCl solution to a total volume of 3.4 mL + [BW (kg) × 0.013]) into the epidural space at the midsacral vertebrae consistently reduced pain produced by a 10-cm skin incision in horses.[120] Cutaneous sensitivity was measured using von Frey filaments around the incision immediately after, 15 min after, and 2, 4, 6, and 8 h after suturing. When using this same method of assessing cutaneous sensitivity after skin incision, S+ ketamine (1.0 mg/kg BW, diluted with 0.9% NaCl solution to a total volume of 3.4 mL + [BW (kg) × 0.013]) reduced cutaneous sensitivity to mechanical stimuli for 75 min.[121] From these direct comparisons of the preemptive analgesic effects of epidurally administered S+ ketamine and racemic ketamine, it appears that both forms produce similar postincisional analgesic effects.[120,121]

Ketamine and Xylazine
A combination of ketamine (1.0 mg/kg) and xylazine (0.5 mg/kg) have been mixed in a syringe and injected into the epidural space at the first intercoccygeal (Co1-Co2) vertebral space in adult horses to produce good analgesia of the tail, perineal region, anus, and vulva. Analgesia is evident in 5 to 9 min and lasts on average 120 min.[122] The region of analgesia extends to the thigh and flank in some horses. As could be expected, the ketamine-xylazine combination usually induces mild sedation, as assessed by drooping of the head and the lower lip 20 min after injection. Heart and respiratory rates are often reduced after epidural drug administration.

Other Agents
Epinephrine
At a concentration of 5 µg/mL (1:200,000), epinephrine can be added to the local anesthetic solution to hasten the onset, prolong the duration, and improve the quality of epidural anesthesia. Carbonization of the base preparations of lidocaine increases pH and favors the anesthetic nonionic state and lipid solubility but does not demonstrate the theoretical advantage of increased diffusion and drug effect during caudal epidural anesthesia in horses.[89]

Alcohol
Alcohol (ethyl alcohol) has been injected into the caudal epidural space in horses to denervate coccygeal nerves and alter tail function, although its efficacy and safety for producing neurolysis in horses have not been reported. Axonal degeneration appears 20 min after injection and lasts several months to 1 year, depending on the completeness of neurolysis. Alcohol-induced alteration of tail motor function in horses can be diagnosed by electromyography and used as evidence to prosecute owners and exhibitors who may be inappropriately using this technique in show-ring

horses.[123] Inaccuracy of the technique and injection of excessive volumes of alcohol into the caudal epidural space produce painful paresthesias, neuritis, and paralysis of the bladder, rectum, and pelvic limb.

Continuous Caudal Epidural Anesthesia

Continuous caudal epidural anesthesia can be used in horses for extended surgery in the anal and perineal region, for obstetric procedures, and for relief of tenesmus.[124–128] A 10.2-cm, 18-gauge thin-walled Tuohy needle with stylet is aseptically inserted on the midline into the Co1-Co2 interspace. Pain from needle insertion is minimized with a subcutaneous wheal of 2 to 3 mL of 2% lidocaine HCl. Once through the skin, the needle, with the bevel pointed cranially, is directed at approximately 45° to vertical and advanced until an abrupt reduction in resistance to needle passage is noted, indicating piercing through the interarcuate ligament and entry into the vertebral canal. The injection of 5 mL of air or 2 to 3 mL of local anesthetic (test dose) should not encounter resistance. Apparently, the injection of 10 mL of sterile 0.9% NaCl solution into the epidural space does not greatly facilitate the advancement of an epidural catheter and is therefore not routinely recommended.[129] A commercially available 91.8-cm, 20-gauge Teflon epidural catheter with graduated markings and stylet or a medical-grade vinyl tubing (0.036-cm outside diameter) can be introduced into the needle and advanced cranially 2 to 4 cm beyond the tip of the needle (A in Fig. 22.28). The needle can then be removed from the catheter while the catheter is left in position. A catheter adapter (provided in the kit) or a three-way stopcock and 2.5-cm, 23-gauge needle is placed on the free end of the catheter for an injection port. A newer technique, which greatly facilitates epidural catheter insertion in horses, and has also been used by the author, involves the use of the Tuohy needle to which a Y piece with a latex balloon and catheter are attached (Fig. 22.29A). The needle is inserted until the balloon collapses under the negative pressure of the epidural space; the epidural catheter is then introduced into the needle from the other arm of the Y piece and advanced cranially as required (Fig. 22.29B). If the first of the four mark strips of the Teflon epidural catheter has reached the needle hub, the catheter has advanced 9 cm beyond the tip of the needle, thereby placing the epidural catheter tip at the midsacral S3 vertebral level in an adult horse (450 kg). The needle is then carefully removed while the catheter is left in position. A catheter adapter with luer lock (provided in the kit) is placed on the free end of the catheter, and an epidural filter (provided in the kit) is placed between the syringe and catheter adapter. All connections should be without leaks. The epidural catheter is sutured to the skin, and the skin-puncture site is covered with a sterile gauze, which is also sutured to the skin (Fig. 22.29C). Approximately 5 mL of anesthetic solution is then injected into the catheter over a 1-min period. Surgical anesthesia is easily maintained by fractional bolus administration of 3 mL of the anesthetic at 1-h intervals or as needed.

In an alternative, but more difficult, method, a 19.5-cm, 17-gauge Huber-point Tuohy needle with the bevel directed caudally is aseptically inserted into the epidural space at the lumbosacral (L6-S1) intervertebral space.[124] A Formocath polyethylene

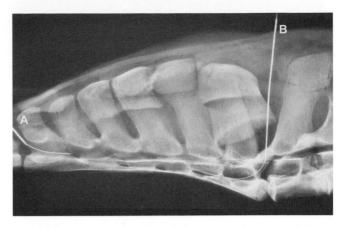

Fig. 22.28. Lateral radiograph of the sixth lumbar to second coccygeal area. **A:** A 10.2-cm, 18-gauge thin-walled Tuohy needle inserted at the Co1-Co2 interspace to insert a 20-gauge Teflon epidural catheter into the caudal (S5) sacral epidural space. **B:** A 19.5-cm, 17-gauge Huber-point Tuohy needle inserted at the lumbosacral (L6-S1) intervertebral space to insert a Formocath polyethylene catheter reinforced with a steel spring guide into the midsacral (S2-S3) epidural space.

catheter (0.095-cm outside diameter) reinforced with a stainless-steel spring guide is introduced into the needle and advanced 10 to 20 cm, to place the catheter tip at the caudal position of the sacral (S3 to S5) epidural space in an adult horse (450 kg) (B in Fig. 22.28).

A safe and convenient route for repeated administration of small fractional doses of the local anesthetic during surgery, while the tail is dorsally reflected for immobilization and surgical exposure, is the major advantage of the catheter technique when compared with the needle technique. In addition, the catheter tip is placed at the nerve roots of the pudendal and pelvic nerves, thus minimizing the dose of anesthetic required to produce caudal anesthesia. Fibrosis of the extradural space from repeated standard epidural blocks is avoided. The disadvantages of the catheter technique include greater cost of equipment, and complications from kinking and curling of the catheter and occlusion of the tip with fibrin. Optimal timing and amounts of repeated anesthetic doses, development of tachyphylaxis (acute tolerance to repeated injections), and augmented responses to long-term effects of repeated caudal epidural anesthesia in horses have not been reported.

Continuous Caudal Subarachnoid Anesthesia

This may be induced by repeated injections of local anesthetic solution (mepivacaine or ropivacaine) or α_2-adrenoceptor agonists (xylazine or detomidine) through a catheter introduced into the caudal subarachnoid space with a Tuohy needle (Fig. 22.30). The use of continuous caudal subarachnoid anesthesia in practice is limited owing to technical difficulty and potential trauma to the conus medullaris and nerve fibers by the needle or catheter, but it can be accomplished safely in horses while maintaining pelvic limb function with certain advantages when compared with epidural administration: Subarachnoid administration of local

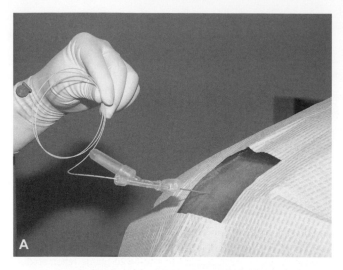

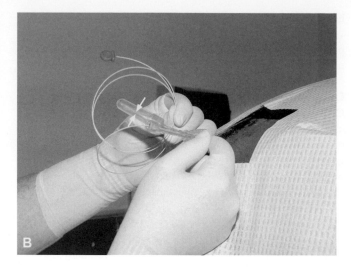

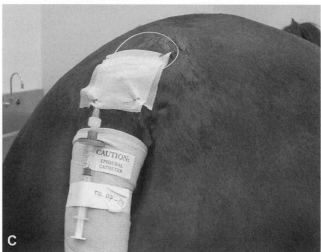

Fig. 22.29. **A:** A 10.2-cm, 18-gauge thin-wall Tuohy needle is inserted at the Co1-Co2 interspace. The needle is attached to a Y piece containing a latex balloon. The tip of a 91.8-cm, 20-gauge Teflon epidural catheter is inserted into the other free end of the Y piece. **B:** The Tuohy needle is inserted until the latex balloon collapses under the negative pressure of the epidural space (as indicated by the two arrows). The catheter is then advanced rostrally for a desired distance. **C:** The epidural catheter is sutured to the skin, and the skin-puncture site covered with a sterile gauze pad, which also is sutured to the skin.

anesthetics or α_2-adrenoceptor agonists requires approximately threefold less drug for a similar degree of caudal anesthesia, and the onset of anesthesia is twice as fast and the action lasts half as long as after epidural injection.[124]

The roots of the spinal nerves within the subarachnoid space are not covered by protective dural sheets and are more readily desensitized, making caudal subarachnoid analgesia the fastest and best-controlled surgical analgesia in horses. Incomplete or asymmetrical analgesia because of septa within the epidural space or inadequate dispersal of the anesthetic because of epidural fat is avoided.

In most adult horses, a 19.5-cm, 17-gauge Huber-point directional needle with the bevel directed caudally can be introduced through disinfected desensitized tissue at the lumbosacral (L6-S1) intervertebral space. Depth of needle penetration ranges from 11 to 14 cm in adult horses. When the needle point is judged to have passed through the tough interarcuate ligament (ligament flavum), by noticing an abrupt reduction in resistance to needle passage, the stylet is removed and approximately 1 mL of 2% carbocaine HCl solution or its equivalent is injected. The syringe

is filled with 2 mL of air and attached to the needle, which is then advanced continuously until a second sudden loss of resistance to air injection is noted, indicating that the dura has been penetrated. The subarachnoid space is then identified by free flow of CSF from the needle hub or aspiration of CSF. With full aseptic precaution, a 30-cm Formocath polyethylene catheter (0.062-cm outside diameter), reinforced with a stainless-steel spring guide, is passed and advanced approximately 25 cm to the midsacral region. The catheter tip cannot be advanced beyond this point, which is usually the end of the subarachnoid space (Fig. 22.30).

When using this technique, not more than 1.5 to 2.0 mL of 2% mepivacaine HCl is injected over a 3-min period (0.5 mL/min) to produce excellent bilateral caudal anesthesia from spinal cord segment S2 to coccyx within 5 to 10 min. Surgical anesthesia lasts approximately 0.5 to 1.5 h and is easily maintained by fractional bolus administration of 0.5 mL of the anesthetic at 30-min intervals or as needed.[124] A similar pattern of local anesthetic spread (faster absorption of drug from the epidural space and similar maximum venous plasma concentrations after epidural and subarachnoid injections) has been reported after midsacral epidural (S2-3 to

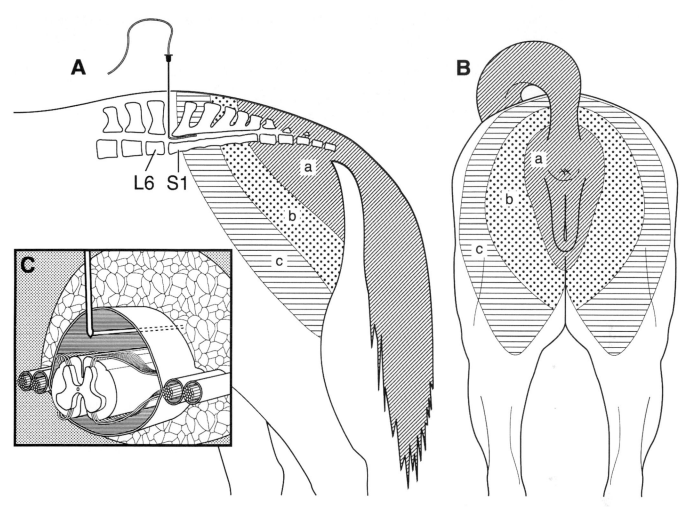

Fig. 22.30. Lateral **(A)** and caudal **(B)** drawings of the lumbosacral, sacral, and sacrococcygeal area of a standing mare with marked loss of skin sensation from coccyx to S4 (a), coccyx to S2 (b), and coccyx to S1, respectively, 30 min after midsacral subarachnoid administration of ropivacaine hydrochloride (0.2% solution, 5 mL/500 kg body weight). **C (inset):** A cranial–left lateral aspect of a transection of the first sacral vertebra at the location of the intervertebral foramen and its associated intraspinal structures with the tip of Huber-point (Tuohy) needle, catheter, and steel spring guide in the subarachnoid space. From Skarda and Muir.[110]

S5-Co1) and subarachnoid (S2-3) administration of mepivacaine HCl in aqueous solution (2%).[92] The venous plasma concentrations of mepivacaine determined during caudal epidural and subarachnoid analgesia did not produce measurable direct effects on heart rate, arterial blood pressure, arterial pH, and hematocrit.[92]

The analgesic, hemodynamic, respiratory, and behavioral alterations of horses after midsacral (S-2 to S-3) subarachnoid administration of ropivacaine (0.2%, 5 mL) HCl solution have been assessed.[130] Numerical scores of sedation, change in pelvic limb position, sweating in analgesic zones, urination, behavior, response to noise, and compliance with restraint were determined before and during a 5-h testing period (Fig. 22.30). Subarachnoidally administered ropivacaine induced variable analgesia extending bilaterally from coccyx to S1, with minimal sedation and change in pelvic limb position in standing mares. Perineal analgesia was attained in 7 min and lasted for over 3 h. Subarachnoid ropivacaine significantly reduced respiratory rates, but did not change heart rates, rectal temperature, arterial blood pressure,

packed cell volume, arterial gas tensions (PO_2 and PCO_2), pH, standard bicarbonate, and base excess from baseline values. These results demonstrate that ropivacaine (0.2% solution, 5 mL/500 kg BW) can be administered subarachnoidally at the midsacram (S2 to S3) to produce prolonged (>3 h) bilateral perineal analgesia with minimal changes in behavior and cardiopulmonary function in adult horses.

Similar to local anesthetic administration, detomidine HCl (1% solution), when administered at a dose of 30 µg/kg into the midsacral subarachnoid space, induces analgesia that extends from dermatome T15 to the coccyx within 10 to 15 min after injection (Fig. 22.31). Analgesia persists for over 2 h, with minimal ataxia, cardiopulmonary depression, and marked sedation in standing horses.[112] Yohimbine (50 µg/kg BW IV) or atipamezole (40 µg/kg BW IV) can be used to effectively reverse subarachnoidally administered detomidine-induced sedation with partial antagonism of detomidine-induced analgesia, ataxia, and cardiopulmonary depression (Fig. 22.32).[95–98]

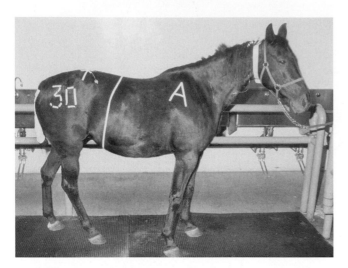

Fig. 22.31. Desensitized skin area between T16 and coccyx in a horse (460 kg) at 30 min after administration of 1.4 mL of 1% detomidine hydrochloride solution into the subarachnoid space of the midsacral (S2-S3) intervertebral space. The subarachnoid catheter (white arrow) is butterfly taped and sutured to the skin at the lumbosacral junction. Sedation was reversed 5 min after intravenous administration of 40 µg of atipamezole/kg.

There is likely to be further interest in the advantages obtained by the intrathecal use of combinations of local anesthetics with adrenoceptor agonists or opioids. An important component of analgesia produced by opiates and α_2-adrenoceptor agonists may be due to the inhibition of the release of neurotransmitters in the dorsal spinal cord from primary afferent terminals, thus preventing further propagation of nociceptive signals. Only preservative-free solutions should be administered into the subarachnoid space. Precise dosage (milligrams, milliliters, and specific gravity), catheter positioning, and aseptic technique are necessary to avoid serious complications such as meningitis, sciatic nerve dysfunction, rear-limb ataxia or motor blockade, recumbency, and cardiopulmonary depression or excitement in conscious horses.[131–133]

Epidural Opioid Analgesia

Numerous studies evaluating the epidural administration of opioids—including morphine, butorphanol, methadone, meperidine, tramadol, alfentanil, and U50488H—have been published in the veterinary literature in recent years.[134–144] Opioids can provide variable long-lasting analgesia when used alone or in combination with local anesthetics, α_2-adrenoceptor agonists, and/or ketamine. They have been used for both acute and chronic pain and have proven effective when administered preemptively, intraoperatively, or postoperatively.

Epidural Opioids

Morphine
Caudal epidural morphine administration has been considered a reasonable alternative for the relief of pain that does not respond to standard medication protocols.[134] In one of the earliest reports,

pain originating from an open luxation of the fetlock joint and comminuted fracture of the first phalanx in a 10-month-pregnant thoroughbred mare was relieved approximately 30 min after injection of 50 mg of morphine, diluted in 30 mL of 0.9% NaCl solution, into the epidural space at the sacrococcygeal interspace. It was judged that analgesia lasted 8 to 16 h, based on the mare's normal behavior (i.e., prolonged period of standing, no sweating, a normal appetite, and a normal heart rate). Analgesia was continued for 3 days by injecting additional morphine (0.2 mg/kg) into an epidural catheter (91.4 cm, 20 gauge) placed into the sacral epidural space by using an 8-cm, 16-gauge Tuohy needle.[134] In a second study, 50 to 100 µg of morphine/kg BW in 10 mL of 0.9% NaCl solution, injected into the epidural space at the first coccygeal interspace (Co1-Co2), produced analgesia lasting 17 to 19 h. Indirect arterial blood pressure, heart rate, respiratory rate, and rectal temperature did not change. Although the occurrence of pruritus (evident perineal wheals) in horses may be low, the author has observed this adverse side effect after the epidural use of morphine in horses (Fig. 22.33). Reportedly, epidural morphine (0.05 to 0.1 mg/kg BW) can produce segmental analgesia that preferentially affects the dorsal nerve branches of the lumbosacral plexus.[136] With higher doses (e.g., 100 µg/kg), epidural morphine may be accompanied by sedation and head drooping, while producing a more rapid onset, cranial spread, and longer duration. These effects are not typically observed with lower dose (e.g., 50 µg/kg) administration.[135]

Morphine (0.1 mg/kg BW) diluted in a volume of 20 mL of sterile water and administered into the epidural space at the first coccygeal (Co1-Co2) intervertebral space induces variable segmental analgesia extending from the coccyx to the thoracic dermatomes.[137–139] Analgesic action is greatest at the dermatomes closest to the epidural injection site. Analgesia (avoidance response, >40 V) in the perineal and sacral areas lasted for 5 h after the morphine injection. Head ptosis was observed within the first hour after administration of morphine, but no morphine-related changes in motor activity or behavior were observed.[140]

Butorphanol
This drug is often described as a κ opioid partial agonist and µ-antagonist and has been widely used as a systemic analgesic in many species, including horses. When butorphanol (0.08 mg/kg BW, in a total volume of 20 mL of sterile water) is injected into the first intercoccygeal epidural space in horses, no changes are observed in avoidance thresholds to noxious electrical stimulation of the dermatomes of the perineal, sacral, lumbar, and thoracic regions.[137–139] Changes are not evident in heart and respiratory rates, arterial blood pressure, rectal temperature, and motor activity. Further evidence of the minimal direct epidural analgesic effect of this opioid in horses includes its lack of effect, following caudal (Co1-Co2) epidural administration (0.05 mg/kg BW), on the minimum alveolar concentration (MAC) requirement of halothane.[143]

Methadone
This is a synthetic diphenylpropylamine opioid. A racemic mixture of levorotatory (L) and dextrorotatory (D) methadone is

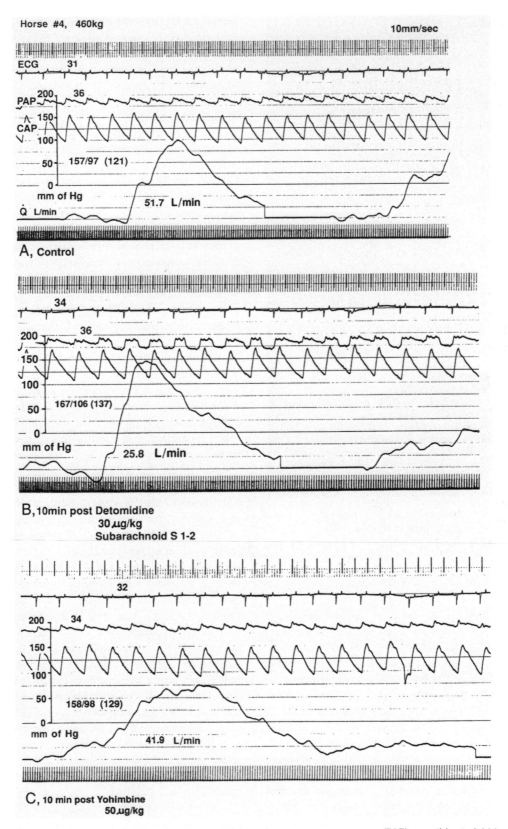

Fig. 22.32. Recording (10 mm/s) of lead II electrocardiogram (ECG), pulmonary artery pressure (PAP), carotid arterial blood pressure (CAP), and cardiac output (Q) (thermodilution curve) before (control) **(A)**, at 10 min after sacral (S1-S2) subarachnoid administration of 30 µg of detomidine hydrochloride solution/kg **(B)**, and at 10 min after intravenous administration of 50 µg of yohimbine/kg **(C)**.

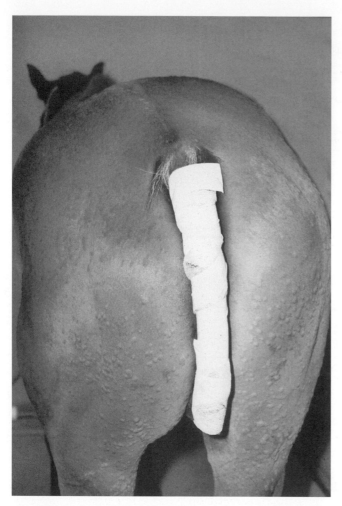

Fig. 22.33. Standardbred mare (470 kg) with multiple wheals over a body area extending from the coccyx to midthoracic region 20 min after caudal (Co1-Co2) epidural administration of morphine sulfate (0.15 mg/kg body weight) in 15 mL of 0.9% sodium chloride solution. Urticaria spontaneously cleared up 18 h later.

available in Europe for clinical use as an aqueous preservative-free solution (Heptadon, 10-mg ampullae; Ebewe Arzneimittel [BASF Pharma], Unterach, Austria). Olbrich and Mosing[144] have compared the effects of caudal epidural administration of methadone (0.1 mg/kg BW) and lidocaine (0.35 mg/kg BW), each diluted with sterile 0.9% NaCl solution to a total volume of 20 mL, on tolerance to thermal stimulation (62°C) of perineal, sacral, lumbar, and thoracic dermatomes. With both drugs, analgesia progressed from the coccyx to cranial in a time-related manner. Perineal analgesia was evident within 15 min of completing methadone or lidocaine injection. Analgesia of the flank region and 13th rib was observed 2 h after the methadone administration, and lasted for 2 and 3 h at the rib and flank, respectively. Perineal analgesia lasted 5 h after methadone injection, compared with 3 h following lidocaine. Analgesia was not produced at the lateral aspect of the crus and the coronary band of the pelvic limbs after methadone or lidocaine administration. Methadone-treated horses defecated and urinated normally, and

demonstrated no excitement, sedation, or ataxia. In contrast, epidural lidocaine caused moderate to severe hind-limb ataxia. Sweating occurred at the injection site and on the medial aspect of the hind limbs as early as 5 min after lidocaine injection in some horses.

Meperidine

This is a synthetic phenylpiperidine-derivative opioid and exerts the strongest local anesthetic effect among the clinically used opioids. Epidural injection of meperidine (Demerol 5%; Abbott Laboratories, North Chicago, IL) may be useful for inducing caudal epidural analgesia in standing conscious horses undergoing prolonged diagnostic, obstetric, or surgical procedures in the anal and perineal region. Meperidine (5%, 0.8 mg/kg BW) administered via epidural injection at vertebral levels extending from the sacrococcygeal intervertebral space to the fifth sacral vertebra induces bilateral analgesia extending from the coccygeal to first sacral dermatomes. The degree of sedation and ataxia induced is minimal (Fig. 22.34).[145,146] The mean onset of perineal analgesia in response to noxious electrical (<80 mA), thermal (<48°C), and skin-prick stimulation was 12 min after meperidine administration, with the analgesia lasting from 240 to over 300 min.[146] These results are supported by a second study, in which meperidine (5%, 0.6 mg/kg BW), administered epidurally between the first and second coccygeal vertebrae, induced bilateral perineal analgesia in less than 10 min. The analgesic effect lasted, on average, 4 h, with minimal cardiovascular effects, sedation, and motor blockade.[93]

Tramadol

This drug is a centrally acting synthetic analgesic drug with both an opioid and nonopioid mechanism of action. Tramadol (Silador or Sanofi; Tramadol Caraco Pharmaceutical Laboratories, Detroit, MI) is available as an injectable formulation for clinical use as an analgesic that does not cause the typical opioid side effects of respiratory depression, constipation, and sedation.[147] When administered epidurally in humans, tramadol is one-thirtieth as potent as morphine.[148] Tramadol (1.0 mg/kg BW) has been diluted in a total volume of 20 mL of sterile water and injected epidurally at the first intercoccygeal epidural space in adult horses. Analgesia (avoidance threshold, >40 V) is produced in the perineal and sacral areas within 30 min and provides analgesia for up to 4 h.[137–139] In comparison, complete perineal and sacral analgesia is present for 6 h after epidural injection of morphine (0.1 mg/kg BW) in an equal volume of sterile water (20 mL). Epidural morphine analgesia will typically last up to 5 h, indicating that at these doses epidural tramadol induces analgesia of faster onset but shorter duration than does epidural morphine.[139]

Alfentanil

Alfentanil (Alfenta; Janssen Pharmaceutical, Piscataway, NJ) is considered to be a highly lipid soluble and potent μ opioid analgesic. When injected into the caudal (Co1-Co2) epidural space of horses at a dosage of 0.02 mg/kg BW diluted to 20 mL of sterile water, alfentanil produced rapid (20 min), but minimal, perineal

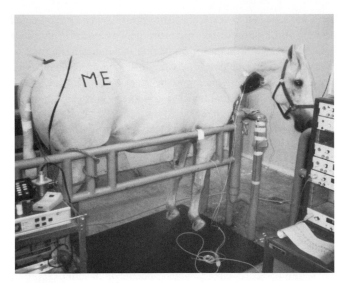

Fig. 22.34. Photograph of a healthy thoroughbred mare (615 kg) with marked area of loss of skin sensation between S1 and coccyx on the right side and sedation at 30 min after injection via needle of meperidine hydrochloride solution (5%; 0.8 mg/kg body weight) into the epidural space at the fifth sacral vertebra. The epidural needle with syringe attached is still in place. The ME indicates the epidural injection of meperidine.

and sacral analgesia without signs of CNS excitation.[137–139] The perineal and sacral analgesic effects induced by epidural alfentanil were considered minimal by the investigators.

Epidural Drug Combinations

Morphine and Detomidine

The combination of morphine (0.2 mg/kg) and detomidine (30 µg/kg) injected via a catheter inserted into the epidural space at the first intercoccygeal space and advanced to the lumbosacral region produces significant analgesia in experimentally induced hind-limb lameness (noticeable both at walk and at trot).[149,150] Results indicate that the epidural combination of morphine and detomidine can provide profound analgesia for equine hind-limb pain. The preoperative caudal epidural administration of morphine (0.2 mg/kg) and detomidine (30 µg/kg) has also been effective in decreasing lameness after painful bilateral stifle arthroscopy.[151] The systemic and local effects associated with long-term epidural catheterization and repeated morphine (0.2 mg/kg) and detomidine (0.03 mg/kg) administration (every 12 h) for 14 days revealed no difference in CSF values or spinal tissue inflammation or fibrosis in the control versus treatment horses.[152,153] Gross and histological examination of spinal tissue segments from the cervicothoracic, thoracolumbar, lumbosacral, and sacral spinal cord, and the catheter entry point itself, did not reveal evidence of adverse systemic effects of long-term epidural morphine-detomidine administration. However, a degree of lumbosacral and sacral spinal tissue inflammation and fibrosis was evident in catheterized horses, indicating that localized inflammation and fibrosis were likely catheter related and not drug related.[153]

Butorphanol and Lidocaine

Butorphanol (0.04 mg/kg) has been added to lidocaine (0.25 mg/kg) for injection into the caudal epidural space of adult mares.[142] When compared with the effects of epidural lidocaine (0.25 mg/kg BW) alone, the addition of butorphanol in nonsedated horses prolonged both cutaneous (fivefold longer) and visceral (eightfold longer) analgesia. A cranial extension of the cutaneous analgesia was also observed. However, horses demonstrated an unusual way of walking (high steps with pointed hoof) in their hind limbs (hyperkinesias), even though ataxia and weakness were not evident.[154]

Morphine and Romifidine

The analgesic, hemodynamic, and behavioral effects of caudal epidurally administered romifidine (30 or 60 µg/kg BW) combined with morphine (0.1 mg/kg BW) have also been evaluated in adult horses.[155] The analgesic effect induced was judged to be moderate. The duration of analgesia was dose dependent, with the 30-µg/kg dose providing 60 min of analgesia and the 60-µg/kg dose providing 90 min of analgesia when combined with 0.1 mg/kg of morphine. Intense sedation and moderate ataxia of the hind limbs were observed during the 4-h observation period. Heart and respiratory rates were decreased.[155]

Tiletamine and Zolazepam

Tiletamine is a phencyclidine derivative similar to ketamine, although more potent. Zolazepam is a benzodiazepine derivative licensed for use exclusively in combination with tiletamine in animals. The proprietary tiletamine-zolazepam combination (100 mg/mL [Telazol; Fort Dodge Laboratories, Fort Dodge, IA]) has been injected into the epidural space of horses at a dose of 0.5 and 1.0 mg/kg BW, diluted up to 5 mL in sterile water. Only a mild analgesic effect in response to threshold-to-pressure stimulation of the perineal area was observed.[156–158] Sedation was not observed and, although all horses remained standing, they were ataxic, demonstrating poor coordination of the hind limbs and fetlock flexion when they were walked out of the stocks. Muscle fasciculation and vigorous head-and-neck movements and dilated nares were observed in one mare 15 min after injecting the 1.0-mg dose of tiletamine-zolazepam/kg epidurally.

Tramadol and Fentanyl

A single caudal (Co1-Co2) epidural injection of a mixture of tramadol (1 mg/kg BW) and fentanyl (5 µg/kg BW) in 20 mL of sterile water reportedly induced analgesia in the perineal and sacral structures within 60 min of injection. Analgesia persisted for 12 to 18 h, with mild sedation and ataxia present in some horses.[159]

Although the pharmacological, pharmacokinetic, and clinical effects of epidurally coadministered local anesthetics, opioids, α_2-adrenoceptor agonists, and ketamine have not been fully characterized in horses, these drugs are increasingly being used by this route in an attempt to better manage equine pain. Further studies are necessary to determine the effectiveness of combining these drugs in the treatment of various soft tissue (e.g., perineal injury, lacerations, and septic arthritis) and orthopedic pain syn-

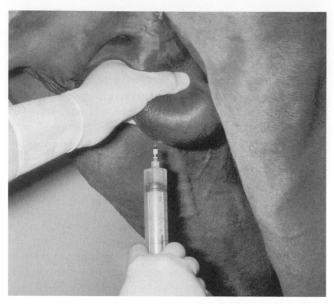

Fig. 22.35. Needle placement for right intratesticular injection in a standing horse.

dromes (e.g., fracture repair). When drug mixtures are used, the severity of pain should be assessed daily and the response to treatment recorded in the medical record.[128]

Anesthesia for Castration

One of the most commonly performed surgical procedures in general equine practice is castration. Regional anesthesia can be accomplished by injecting local anesthetic drug into the scrotum, testicle,[160,161] and spermatic cord.[162,163] Standing castrations are generally restricted to tractable yearlings and 2-year-olds. Proper restraint of the horse's head and sedation (e.g., tranquilizer-narcotic or sedative-narcotic combination) are required. The horse may be placed with its side against a wall and a twitch applied to its upper lip. The person holding the twitch should stand on the same side as the operator. The skin of the scrotum and prepuce is surgically prepared, and one of three techniques is used. In one technique, a 7.5-cm, 20-gauge needle is quickly inserted perpendicularly through the tensed skin of the scrotum, and 20 to 30 mL of local anesthetic is injected into the center of each testicle (Fig. 22.35). The local anesthetic should make the testicle firm and reach the inguinal canal within 90 s via lymph vessels for the blockade to begin.[160] Castration can usually be performed painlessly 10 min after the injection with no further use of the twitch. In a second method, percutaneous anesthesia of the spermatic cord is accomplished by inserting a 2.5-cm, 20-gauge needle into the cord as close to the external inguinal ring as possible, where 20 to 30 mL of local anesthetic is injected in a fan-shaped manner without perforating the skin, spermatic artery, and vein. The proposed incision line of the scrotal skin must also be infiltrated subcutaneously with 5 to 10 mL of the anesthetic because the scrotal skin is not desensitized by the deposition of anesthetic into the dartos or the substance of the testicle itself. The proce-

dures are repeated to desensitize the opposite spermatic cord and scrotum. Infiltration of the spermatic cord is less effective than intratesticular infiltration for producing local anesthesia for castration. In a third method, a 15-cm, 18-gauge needle is inserted into the testicle and directed into the spermatic cord while 30 mL of the anesthetic is being injected. The incision sites of the scrotal skin are also infiltrated. Since the testes are to be removed, damage to them is unimportant. More refractory horses are castrated under general anesthesia.[164]

Anesthesia of the Perineum

Regional anesthesia of the perineum enables perineal surgery, including urethrostomy, in standing horses. Perineal anesthesia is accomplished by desensitizing the superficial and deep (subfascial) branches of the perineal nerves. These branches arise on both sides of the anus and pass ventrally over the ischial arch to the scrotum. A 2.5-cm, 22-gauge needle is inserted approximately 2.5 cm dorsal to the ischial arch and 2.5 cm lateral to the anus in order to inject 5 mL of local anesthetic subcutaneously. A deeper subfascial injection of 5 to 7 mL of the anesthetic is then performed after the needle is directed dorsally 0.5 to 1.0 cm. The procedure is repeated at the opposite site.[165]

Anesthesia of the Penis or Vulva

The penis or vulva is anesthetized by desensitizing the ventral branches of the pudendal nerve. First the perineal nerves are desensitized as described above, and then a 5-cm, 20-gauge needle is inserted at the same site as for perineal nerve anesthesia and is advanced toward the midline to strike the ischiatic arch. Approximately 10 to 20 mL of local anesthetic is injected (Fig. 22.36).[166] The procedure is repeated at the opposite site.

Therapeutic Local Analgesia

Infiltration of sympathetic nerves by local anesthetic solution effectively interrupts reflex spasm of local vasculature and pain. The two common sites where the equine sympathetic nervous system is desensitized most effectively are the cervicothoracic (stellate) ganglion and the paralumbar sympathetic ganglia. Sensory and motor interruption does not result unless the thoracic or lumbar somatic nerves have been desensitized by faulty technique.

Cervicothoracic (Stellate) Ganglion Block

Infiltration of the cervicothoracic ganglion (CTG) in horses with local anesthetic solution is effective and therapeutically recommended for relief of vasoconstriction and pain in the head, neck, and front leg (Fig. 22.37). It can be successfully accomplished in horses with a variety of skin, muscle, nerve, and joint and tendon sheath diseases.[167,168] A single CTG blockade is effective in acute disorders, whereas two or three blockades are required for good results in chronic conditions of idiopathic shoulder lameness, radial nerve paralysis, and eczema of the head and neck.

The CTG is best reached from a cranial and paratracheal approach in a horse bearing equal weight with both thoracic limbs. The skin-puncture site is 12 to 17 cm dorsal to the intermediate

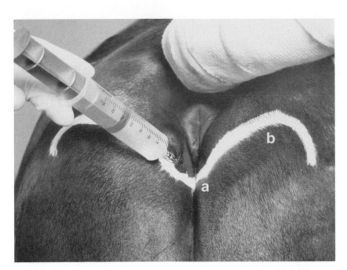

Fig. 22.36. Topographic anatomy for perineal and pudendal nerve block. The palpable ischiatic arch (a) and ischiatic tuberosity (b) are marked. Infiltration of the left pudendal nerve with local anesthetic is shown. From Skarda.[3]

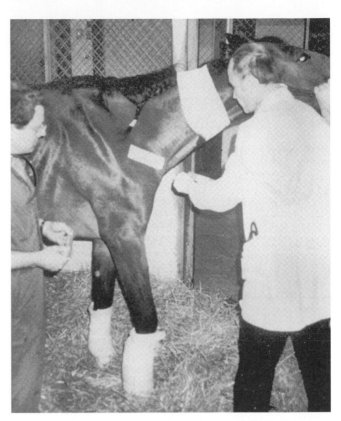

Fig. 22.37. Restraint of a thoroughbred mare (520 kg, 7 years old) during infiltration of the right-side cervicothoracic ganglion (CTG) with 1 g (100 mL of a 1% lidocaine hydrochloride solution) of lidocaine. Plasma lidocaine concentrations were 0.5 and 0.35 μg/mL at 30 and 60 min after injection. Pain relief from fetlock arthrodesis after comminuted P1 fracture and secondary osteomyelitis was evident by more weight bearing and food uptake for at least 3 days after CTG blockade.

tubercle of the humerus in the jugular furrow dorsal to the jugular vein and carotid artery. This area is aseptically prepared and infiltrated with 2 to 3 mL of local anesthetic solution. A 25-cm, 16-gauge needle is inserted through the desensitized skin and advanced horizontally or 5° dorsomedially until it impinges on the transverse process or body of the seventh cervical vertebra, and 2 to 3 mL of the anesthetic is injected (A in Fig. 22.38). The depth of needle penetration ranges from 10 to 15 cm, depending on the size of the musculus longus colli. The needle is first partially withdrawn and then reinserted more laterally and ventrally, thereby bypassing the seventh cervical vertebra and reaching the articulations of the first and second ribs (B in Fig. 22.38). The needle is then 15 to 20 cm from the surface of the skin.[169] After aspiration to be sure that the needle point has not entered a blood vessel, the pleural cavity, or subarachnoid space, approximately 50 mL of 1% lidocaine HCl in aqueous solution is injected with minimal resistance. This amount of anesthetic diffuses throughout the tissues surrounding the CTG. An additional 50 mL of lidocaine is injected during withdrawal of the needle for 5 to 10 cm to desensitize the sympathetic fibers between the CTG and the eighth cervical spinal nerve. Adequate sympathetic blockade is indicated by ipsilateral, increased subcutaneous temperature (up to 3°C) and profuse sweating of the head, neck, and thoracic limb; ipsilateral Horner's syndrome (e.g., ptosis, miosis, and enophthalmos) (Fig. 22.39A); and ipsilateral paresis. These signs are present 10 to 15 min after injection and last more than 75 min. The appearance of Horner's syndrome with no increase in subcutaneous temperature of the thoracic limb indicates that the CTG blockade has not been effective and sympathetic nerve supply to the thoracic limb has not been interrupted for therapeutic purposes.

Increased skin temperature is related to increased blood flow to muscle and cutaneous vascular beds and develops despite the cooling effect of profuse sweating. Factors responsible for sweating include blood supply and, hence, increased heat in the area, higher metabolism in sweat glands, and central stimulation caused by the horse's excitement. Horner's syndrome is caused by the interruption of the oculosympathetic pathway at the site of the CTG block and/or at the site of the ventral sympathetic roots between the eighth cervical and second thoracic spinal nerves.

Unilateral CTG blockade minimally changes heart rate, cardiac output, aortic blood pressure, and total peripheral resistance in conscious horses.[170] Maximal plasma concentrations of lidocaine after unilateral CTG blockade in adult horses have been reported, indicating that a toxic blood concentration was not present.[170] Ipsilateral laryngeal paralysis, decreased respiratory rates, and increased arterial carbon dioxide partial pressure ($PaCO_2$) are indicative of vagal inhibition. However, hypoventilation in resting horses is not severe enough to induce significant respiratory acidosis or hypoxemia. Potential serious complications are transitory brachial plexus and recurrent laryngeal nerve paralysis and pneumothorax. Bilateral CTG blockade is contraindicated in horses.

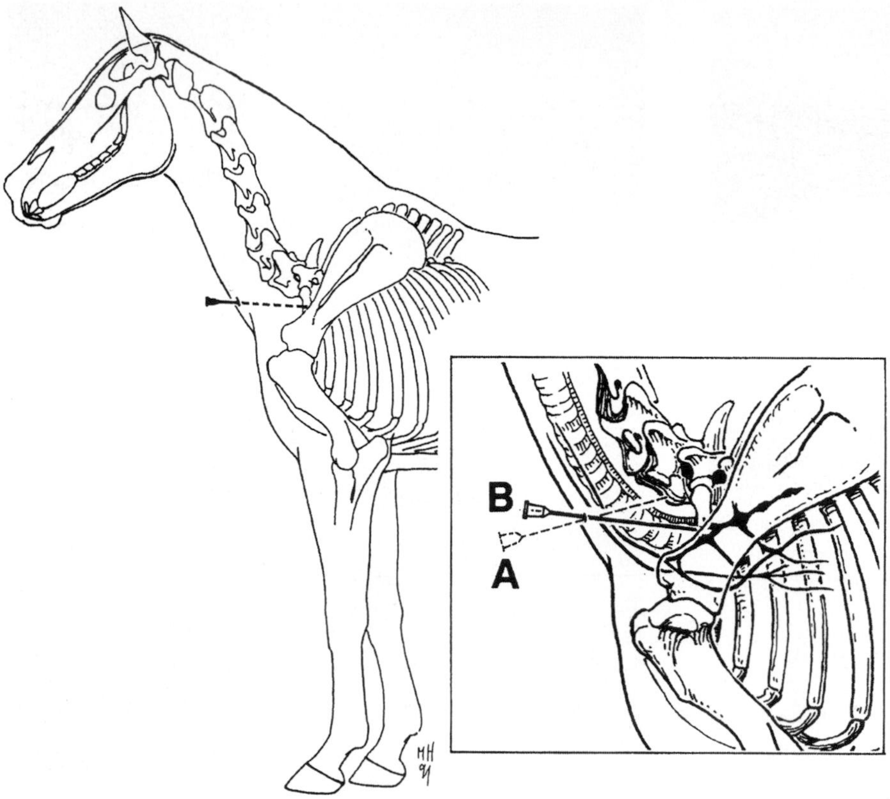

Fig. 22.38. Needle placement to seventh cervical vertebra (A) and cervicothoracic (stellate) ganglion (B) (left side).

Paravertebral Lumbar Sympathetic Ganglion Block

Infiltration of the lumbar sympathetic ganglia in horses with local anesthetic solution has been demonstrated as a therapeutic measure for myositis, periositis, coxitis, and paralysis of the fibular and penile nerves.[167,168] Although any of the interspaces between the 18th thoracic and fourth lumbar vertebrae may be used as possible sites to reach the lumbar sympathetic ganglia, the ideal puncture site is between the transverse processes of the second and third lumbar (L2 and L3) vertebrae, about 10 to 15 cm lateral to their spinous processes. This area is aseptically prepared and infiltrated with 2 to 3 mL of local anesthetic. A 25-cm, 18-gauge needle with a marker on the needle shaft is inserted through the desensitized skin and advanced until its tip contacts the transverse process of L2 or L3. The marker is used to note the depth of penetration (A in Fig. 22.40). The needle is partially withdrawn to the subcutaneous area and reinserted at approximately 45° from vertical for a calculated distance, which equals the distance between the marker (skin puncture) and the needle point plus an additional 5 to 8 cm (B in Fig. 22.40). The needle is correctly placed if there is no air from the peritoneal cavity or blood from a blood vessel upon needle aspiration and no resistance to the injection of local anesthetic results. Approximately 100 mL of 1% lidocaine HCl solution is slowly injected. This amount of anesthetic diffuses throughout the tissues surrounding the sympathetic trunk and two segments rostrally and caudally.

Adequate sympathetic blockade is recognized by profuse sweating and increased (up to 2.5°C) subcutaneous temperature of the ipsilateral pelvic limb within 10 min after injection. Nonsedated horses tolerate unilateral lumbar sympathetic ganglionic (ULSG) blockade well. Hemodynamic and respiratory alterations induced by unilateral ULSG blockade in horses are usually minor.[171] Potential complications include hematoma caused by puncture of blood vessels, intravascular injection, abdominocentesis, and needle breakage.

Novel Regional Analgesic Techniques

Intra-articular injection with morphine, abaxial nerve block with ketamine, and local application of 5% lidocaine patches are considered novel techniques to produce local and regional analgesia in horses.

Intra-articular Morphine

Intra-articular morphine might be a useful technique for pain relief after arthroscopic surgery. In a recent study, morphine sulfate (15 mg in 5 mL of 0.9% NaCl solution) containing 0.1% wt/vol sodium metabisulfite or 5 mL of 0.9% NaCl solution was injected into the left tibiotarsal joint of eight ponies, weighing 270 to 340 kg, to investigate whether intra-articular morphine inflames the joint and to determine the systemic absorption of morphine and its persistence intra-articularly after 24 h.[172] The peak

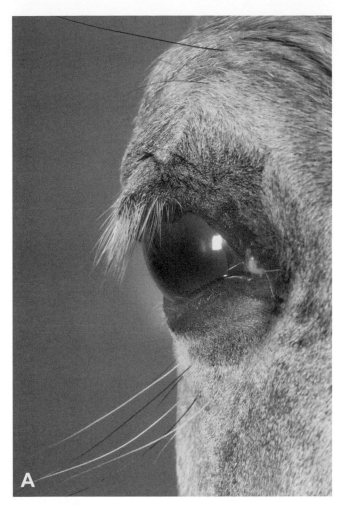
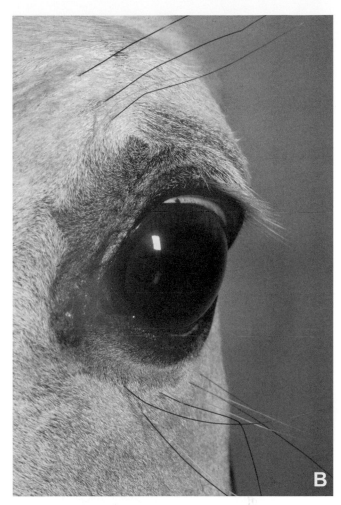

Fig. 22.39. Horner's syndrome as evidence of sympathetic blockade to the head 15 min after infiltration of the right cervicothoracic ganglion with 100 mL 1% lidocaine. **A:** Right eye with ptosis, miosis, and enophthalmos. **B:** Unaffected left eye.

mean plasma morphine concentration (7.1 µg/L) was determined 30 min after intra-articular morphine administration. Neither morphine nor its metabolites (morphine 3-glucuronide and morphine 6-glucuronide) were detected in plasma at 6 h while morphine was still detectable in the synovial fluid of each pony at 24 h after injection. There was no correlation between the concentration of morphine in plasma and in synovial fluid.[172]

Abaxial Nerve Block with Ketamine

The local analgesic effect of 5 mL of ketamine (1%, 2%, and 3% solution) injected as an abaxial sesamoid block has been assessed using a noxious thermal stimulus.[173] All horses injected with either 2% or 3% ketamine developed a rapid abaxial sesamoid block with a duration of action of 15 min. In horses injected with 1% ketamine, the failure rate was nearly 50%. Higher doses of ketamine may possess some local anesthetic properties by blocking sodium-ion and potassium-ion channels,

thereby stabilizing cellular membranes and obstructing nerve transmission.

Local Application of a 5% Lidocaine Patch

Lidocaine patch placement has been assessed for lameness localized to the carpus, fetlock, or distal limb. One or two patches of 5% lidocaine (Lidoderm; Endo Pharmaceuticals, Chadds Ford, PA) can be placed on the affected joints.[174] The area for patch placement should be clipped and then covered by the patch (10 × 14 cm). Patches contain 700 mg of lidocaine (50 mg/g adhesive) in an aqueous base with methylparaben and propylparaben as preservatives. Once the patch is applied, the joint should be bandaged. Transdermal lidocaine application appears to reduce pain in some horses. Mass spectrometry and enzyme-linked immunosorbent assays have not detected lidocaine in venous blood samples taken at 2, 4, 8, and 12 h after patch application, indicating that the systemic uptake of lidocaine is likely quite minimal.

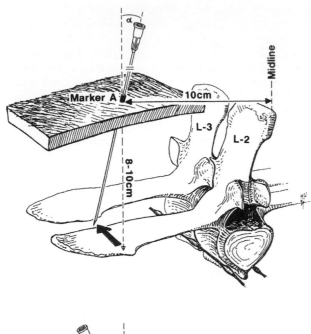

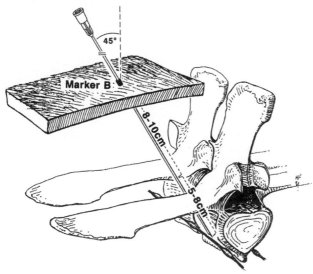

Fig. 22.40. Needle placement to lumbar sympathetic ganglia. Marker A: Needle tip at the L2 to L3 intertransverse space. Marker B: Right ganglionic chain.

References

1. Skarda RT. Local anesthetics and local anesthetic techniques in horses. In: Muir WW, Hubbell JAE, eds. Equine Anesthesia: Monitoring and Emergency Therapy. St Louis: CV Mosby, 1991:199–246.
2. Hall LW. Wright's Veterinary Anaesthesia and Analgesia, 7th ed. London: Ballière Tindall, 1971.
3. Skarda RT. Practical regional anesthesia. In: Mansmann RA, McAllister ES, Pratt PW, eds. Equine Medicine and Surgery, vol 1, 3rd ed. Santa Barbara, CA: American Veterinary, 1982:229–238.
4. Wittman F, Morgenroth H. Untersuchungen über die Leitungsanästhesie des Nervus infraorbitalis und des Nervus mandibularis bei Zahn- und Kieferoperationen. Festschrift fur Eugen Fröhner. Stuttgart, Germany: Von Ferdinand Enke, 1928:384–399.
5. Bressou C, Cliza S. Contribution à l'étude de l'anesthésie dentaire chez le cheval et chez le chien. Rec Med Vet 1931;107:129–134.
6. Lichtenstern G. Die Verwendung von Tropakokain in der tierärztlichen Chirurgie mit besonderer Berücksichtigung hinsichtlich seiner Verwendbarkeit in der Augapfelinfiltration beim Pferde. Berl Munch Tierarztl Wochenschr 1911;55:337–359.
7. Skarda RT. Practical regional anesthesia. In: Mansmann RA, McAllister ES, Pratt PW, eds. Equine Medicine, vol 1, 3rd ed. Santa Barbara, CA: American Veterinary, 1982:239–245.
8. Bolz W. Ein weiterer Beitrag zur Leitungsanästhesie am Kopf des Pferdes. Berl Munch Tierzartl Wochenschr 1930;46:529–530.
9. Manning JP, St Clair LE. Palpebral frontal and zygomatic nerve blocks for examination of the equine eye. Vet Med 1976;71:187–189.
10. Van der Woerdt A, Gilger BC, Wilkie DA, Strauch SM. Effect of auriculopalpebral nerve block and intravenous administration of xylazine on intraocular pressure and corneal thickness in horses. Am J Vet Res 1995;56:155–158.
11. Merideth RE, Wolf ED. Ophthalmic examination and therapeutic techniques in the horse. Compend Contin Educ 1981;3:S426–S433.
12. Rubin LF. Auriculopalpebral nerve block as an adjunct to the diagnosis and treatment of ocular inflammation in the horse. J Am Vet Med Assoc 1964;144:1387–1388.
13. Lindsay WA, Hedberg EB. Performing facial nerve blocks, nasolacrimal catheterization, and paranasal sinus centesis in horses. Vet Med 1991;86:72–83.
14. Eeckhout AVP. Un procédé pratique pour obtenir l'anesthésie complète des dents molaires supérieures chez le cheval. Ann Med Vet 1921;66:10–14.
15. Edwards JF. Regional anaesthesia of the head of the horse: An up-to-date survey. Vet Rec 1930;10:873–975.
16. Schönberg F. Anatomische Grundlagen für die Leitungsanästhesie der Zahnnerven beim Pferde. Berl Munch Tierarztl Wochenschr 1927;43:1–3.
17. Adams OR. Lameness in Horses, 3rd ed. Philadelphia: Lea and Febiger, 1974:91–112.
18. Pohlmeyer K, Redecker R. Die für die Klinik bedeutsamen Nerven an den Gliedmassen des Pferdes einschliesslich möglicher Varianten. Dtsch Tierarztl Wochenschr 1974;81:501–505, 537–541.
19. Zeller R. Die Lokalanästhesie bei der Lahmheitsuntersuchung. Berl Munch Tierarztl Wochenschr 1978;91:166–171.
20. Derksen FJ. Diagnostic local anesthesia of the equine front limb. Equine Pract 1980;2:41–47.
21. Gray BW, Engel HN, Rumph PF, LaFaver J, Brown BG, McKibbin JS. Clinical approach to determine the contribution of the palmar and palmar metacarpal nerves to the innervation of the equine fetlock joint. Am J Vet Res 1980;41:940–943.
22. Wheat JD, Jones K. Selected techniques of regional anesthesia. Vet Clin North Am Large Anim Pract 1981;3:223–246.
23. Worthman RP. Diagnostic anesthetic injections. In: Mansmann RA, McAllister ES, Pratt PW, eds. Equine Medicine and Surgery, 3rd ed. Santa Barbara, CA: American Veterinary, 1982:947–952.
24. Nyrop KA, Coffman JR, DeBowes RM, Booth LC. The role of diagnostic nerve blocks in the equine lameness examination. Compend Contin Educ 1983;5:S669–S676.
25. Colbern GT. The use of diagnostic nerve block procedures on horses. Compend Contin Educ 1984;6:611–619.
26. Ordidge RM, Gerring EL. Regional analgesia of the distal limb. Equine Vet J 1984;16:147–149.
27. Stashak TS. Diagnosis of lameness. In: Stashak TS, ed. Adams' Lameness in Horses. Philadelphia: Lea and Febiger, 1986:139–142, 659–661.

28. Gibson KT, Stashak TS. Effective techniques for localizing equine lameness. Vet Med 1989;84:992–996.

29. Gibson KT, Stashak TS. Using perineural anesthesia to localize equine lameness. Vet Med 1989;84:1082–1086.

30. Ford TS, Ross MW, Orsini PG. A comparison of methods for proximal palmar metacarpal analgesia in horses. Vet Surg 1989;18:146–150.

31. Gaynor JS, Hubbell JAE. Perineural and spinal anesthesia. Vet Clin North Am Equine Pract 1991;7:501–519.

32. Denoix MJM. Anesthésies semiologiques des régions proximales des membres. Swiss Vet 1991;8:12–22.

33. Van Pelt RW. Intra-articular injection of the equine carpus and fetlock. J Am Vet Med Assoc 1962;140:1181–1190.

34. Tufvesson G. Local Anaesthesia in Veterinary Medicine. Sodertalje, Sweden: Astra International, 1963.

35. Van Kruiningen HJ. Practical techniques for making injections into joints and bursae of the horse. J Am Vet Med Assoc 1963;143:1079–1083.

36. Brown MP, Valko K. A technique for intra-articular injection of the equine tarso-metatarsal joint. Vet Med Small Anim Clin 1980;75:265–270.

37. Gabel AA. Lameness caused by inflammation in the distal hock. Vet Clin North Am Large Anim Pract 1980;2:101–123.

38. Lindsay WA, Tayler SD, Walters JW. Selective intra-articular anesthesia as an aid in the diagnosis of bone spavin. J Am Vet Med Assoc 1981;178:297–300.

39. Wintzer HJ. Pharmacokinetics of procaine injected into the hock joint of the horse. Equine Vet J 1981;13:68–69.

40. Sack WO, Orsini PG. Distal intertarsal and tarsometatarsal joints in the horse: Communication and injection sites. J Am Vet Med Assoc 1981;179:355–359.

41. Byars TD, Brown C, Beisel D. Equine arthrocentesis. Equine Pract 1982;4:28–39.

42. Gibson KT, Stashak TS. Employing intra-articular anesthesia to detect joint lesions in lame horses. Vet Med 1989;84:1088–1092.

43. Moyer W. A Guide to Equine Joint Injection. Lawrenceville, NJ: Veterinary Learning Systems, 1986:1–32.

44. Belling TH. A better approach to intracarpal injections. Vet Med 1986;81:158–165.

45. Dyson S. Diagnostic technique in the investigation of shoulder lameness. Equine Vet J 1986;18:25–28.

46. Dyson S. Problems associated with the interpretation of results of regional and intra-articular anaesthesia in the horse. Vet Rec 1986;12:419–422.

47. Kiely RG, McMullan W. Lateral arthrocentesis of the equine carpus. Equine Pract 1987;9:22–24.

48. Schmotzer WB, Trimm KI. Local anesthetic techniques for diagnosis of lameness. Vet Clin North Am Equine Pract 1990;6:705–728.

49. Gabel AA. Diagnosis, relative incidence, and probable cause of cunean tendon bursitis-tarsitis of standardbred horses. J Am Vet Med Assoc 1979;175:1079–1085.

50. Gabel AA. Treatment and prognosis for cunean tendon bursitis-tarsitis of standardbred horses. J Am Vet Med Assoc 1979;175:1086–1088.

51. Lloyd KCK, Stover JM, Pascoe JR. A technique for catheterization of the equine antebrachiocarpal joint. Am J Vet Res 1988;49:658–662.

52. Ford TS, Ross MW, Orsini PG. Communication and boundaries of the middle carpal and carpometacarpal joints in horses. Am J Vet Res 1988;49:2161–2164.

53. Day TK, Skarda RT. The pharmacology of local anesthetics. Vet Clin North Am Equine Pract 1991;7:489–500.

54. Schramme MC, Boswell JC, Hamhougias K, Toulson K, Viitanen M. An in vitro study to compare 5 different techniques for injection of the navicular bursa in the horse. Equine Vet J 2000;32:263–267.

55. Schumacher J, Schumacher J, de Graves F, et al. A comparison of the effects of local analgesic solution in the navicular bursa of horses with lameness caused by solar or solar heel pain. Equine Vet J 2001;33:386–389.

56. Schumacher J, Steiger R, Schumacher J, et al. Effects of analgesia of the distal interphalangeal joint or palmar digital nerves on lameness caused by solar pain in horses. Vet Surg 2000;29:54–58.

57. Rijkenhuizen ABM. Complications following the diagnostic anesthesia of the coffin joint in horses. In: Proceedings, 15th European Society of Veterinary Surgery Congress. Bern: Klinik für Nutztiere und Pferde, 1984:7–13.

58. Heavner JE. Local anesthetics. Vet Clin North Am Large Anim Pract 1991;3:209–211.

59. Tillmann H. Zur Leitungsanästhesie bei Laparotomien am Pferd. Tierzartl Umschau 1949;4:302–303.

60. Goncalves AP. Anesthesia paravertebral lombar no cavalo (*Equus caballus*) [PhD dissertation]. Niteroi, Rio de Janeiro, Brazil: Faculdade de Veterinaria, Universidade Federal Fluminense, 1977.

61. Moon PF, Suter CM. Paravertebral thoracolumbar anaesthesia in 10 horses. Equine Vet J 1993;25:304–308.

62. Skarda RT, Muir WW. Segmental epidural and subarachnoid analgesia in horses: A comparative study. Am Vet Res 1983;44:1870–1876.

63. Skarda RT, Muir WW. Segmental thoracolumbar spinal (subarachnoid) analgesia in conscious horses. Am Vet Res 1982;43:2121–2128.5.

64. Skarda RT, Muir WW, Ibrahim AL. Spinal fluid concentrations of mepivacaine in horses and procaine in cows after thoracolumbar subarachnoid analgesia. Am J Vet Res 1985;46:1020–1024.5.

65. Bolte S, Inga C. Segmental subarachnoid analgesia with ketamine: An alternative for abdominal surgery in horses [Abstract]. In: Proceedings of the Fifth International Congress of Veterinary Anesthesia. Guelph, Canada: University of Guelph, 1994:141.5.

66. Natalini CC, Robinson EP. Effects of lumbosacral subarachnoid catheterization in horses. Vet Surg 1999;28:525–528.5.

67. Hopkins GS. The correlation of anatomy and epidural analgesia in domestic animals. Cornell Vet 1935;25:263–270.

68. Skarda RT. Local and regional analgesia. In: Short CE, ed. Principles and Practice of Veterinary Anesthesia. Baltimore: Williams and Wilkins, 1987:91–133.

69. Skarda RT. Local anesthetics and local anesthetic techniques in horses. In: Muir WW, Hubbell JAE, eds. Equine Anesthesia, Monitoring and Emergency Therapy. St Louis: CV Mosby, 1991:199–246.

70. Pape J, Pitzschk C. Versuche über extradurale Anästhesie beim Pferde. Arch Wiss Prakt Tierheilkd 1925;52:558–571.

71. McLeod WM, Frank ER. A preliminary report regarding epidural anesthesia in equines and bovines. J Am Vet Med Assoc 1927;72:327–335.

72. Cuillé J, Chelle P. L'anesthésie épidural chez les animaux domestiques. [Epidural anaesthesia in the domestic animal.] Rev Gen Med Vet 1931;40:393–445.

73. Srnetz A. Über Lokalanasthesie mit Percain beim Pferde. Prager Arch Tiermed Vergl Pathol 1931;11:207–211.

74. Brook GB. Spinal (epidural) anaesthesia in the domestic animals. Vet Rec 1935;15:549–608.

75. Krukowski SM. Epidural anesthesia in the cow and horse. Vet Med (Chicago) 1935;30:252–253.

76. Benesch F. Die Schmerzbetäubung in der Geburtshilfe und Gynäkologie der Haustiere. In: 13th World Veterinary Congress, vol 1. Zürich-Interlaken, Switzerland, 1938:377–385.

77. Brown TG. Discussion. In: Anaesthesia in Veterinary Practice. Vet Rec 1938;50:1617–1621.

78. Byrne MJ. Epidural anaesthesia. In: Anaesthesia in Veterinary Practice. Vet Rec 1938;50:1614–1618.

79. Barone R, Chayer R. Essais d'interprétation anatomique des anesthésies rachidiennes (épidurales et sous-durales) chez le cheval et le boeuf. Rev Med Vet 1950;101:27–43.

80. Heinze CD. Equine surgery: Variations in technique—Epidural anesthesia. Mod Vet Pract 1968;49:39–44.

81. Heath EH, Myers VS. Topographic anatomy for caudal epidural anesthesia in the horse. Vet Med Small Anim Clin 1972;67:1237–1239.

82. Slusher SH. Caudal epidural anesthesia in horses. Vet Med Small Anim Clin 1981;76:1773–1775.

83. Greene SA, Thurmon JC. Epidural analgesia and sedation for selected equine surgeries. Equine Pract 1985;7:14–19.

84. Laverty S, Pascoe JR, Ling GV, Lavoie JP, Ruby AL. Urolithiasis in 68 horses. Vet Surg 1992;21:56–62.

85. Hendrickson DA, Wilson DG. Laparoscopic cryptorchid castration in standing horses. Vet Surg 1997;26:335–339.

86. Grosenbaugh DA, Skarda RT, Muir WW. Caudal regional anaesthesia in horses. Equine Vet Educ 1999;11:98–105.

87. Skarda RT, Muir WW. Analgesic, hemodynamic and respiratory effects of caudal epidurally administered ropivacaine hydrochloride solution in mares [Abstract]. In: Proceedings of the Annual Meeting of the American College of Veterinary Anesthesiologists, Dallas, TX, 1999:14.

88. Skarda RT, Muir WW. Analgesic, hemodynamic and respiratory effects of caudal epidurally administered ropivacaine hydrochloride in mares. Vet Anaesth Analg 2001;28:61–74.

89. Schelling CG, Klein LV. Comparison of carbonated lidocaine and lidocaine hydrochloride for caudal epidural anesthesia in horses. Am J Vet Res 1985;46:1375–1377.

90. Grubb TL, Riebold TW, Huber MJ. Comparison of lidocaine, xylazine, and xylazine/lidocaine for caudal epidural analgesia in horses. J Am Vet Med Assoc 1992;201:1187–1190.

91. Luna SPL, Bueno SK, Cruz ML, Teixeiraneto FJ. Extradural anaesthesia using lidocaine, ropivacaine, hyperbaric lidocaine and a combination of lidocaine and ropivacaine in mares. Vet Anaes Analg 2000;27:57.

92. Skarda RT, Muir WW, Ibrahim AL. Plasma mepivacaine concentrations after caudal epidural and subarachnoid injection in the horse: Comparative study. Am J Vet Res 1984;45:1967–1971.

93. DeRossi R, Shapaio BF, Varela JV, Junqueira AL. Perineal analgesia and hemodynamic effects of epidural administration of meperidine or hypobaric bupivacaine in conscious horses. Can Vet J 2004;45:42–47.

94. Skarda RT, Muir WW, Carpenter JA. Antagonistic effects of atipamezole on epidurally administered detomidine-induced sedation, analgesia, and cardiopulmonary depression in horses [Abstract]. In: Proceedings of the Annual Scientific Meeting of the American College of Veterinary Anesthesiologists, Las Vegas, October 1990:9.

95. Skarda RT, Muir WW, Doerres-Phillips AJ. Antagonistic effects of atipamezole on subarachnoidally administered detomidine-induced sedation, analgesia, and cardiopulmonary depression in horses [Abstract]. In: Fourth International Congress of Veterinary Anaesthesiology, Utrecht, the Netherlands, 1991:15.

96. Skarda RT, Muir WW. Influence of atipamezole on effects of midsacral subarachnoidally administered detomidine in mares. Am J Vet Res 1998;59:468–478.

97. Skarda RT, Muir WW. Influence of intravenous yohimbine on caudal epidurally administered detomidine hydrochloride solution in mares [Abstract]. In: Proceedings of the Annual Meeting of the American College of Veterinary Anesthesiologists, Orlando, FL, 1998:25.

98. Skarda RT, Muir WW. Effects of intravenously administered yohimbine on antinociceptive, cardiorespiratory, and postural changes induced by epidural administration of detomidine hydrochloride solution to healthy mares. Am J Vet Res 1999;60:1262–1270.

99. Aziz MA, Martin GJ. Alpha agonist and local anesthetic properties of xylazine. Zentralbl Veterinarmed [A] 1978;25:181–188.

100. Fikes LW, Lin HC, Thurmon JC. A preliminary comparison of lidocaine and xylazine as epidural analgesics in ponies. Vet Surg 1989;18:85–86.

101. Doherty TJ, Rohrbach BW, Geiser DR. Epidural xylazine decreases halothane MAC in ponies [Abstract]. In: Veterinary Midwest Anesthesia Conference, Ohio State University, Columbus, 1996:24.

102. Doherty TJ, Geiser DR, Rohrbach BW. The effect of epidural xylazine on halothane minimum alveolar concentration in ponies. J Vet Pharmacol Ther 1997;18:246–248.

103. LeBlanc PH, Caron JP, Patterson JS, Brown M, Matta MA. Epidural injection of xylazine for perineal analgesia in horses. J Am Vet Med Assoc 1988;193:1405–1408.

104. LeBlanc PH, Caron JP. Clinical use of epidural xylazine in the horse. Equine Vet J 1990;22:180–181.

105. LeBlanc PH, Eberhart SW. Cardiopulmonary effects of epidurally administered xylazine in the horse. Equine Vet J 1990;22:389–391.

106. Skarda RT, Muir WW. Hemodynamic and respiratory effects of caudal epidurally administered xylazine hydrochloride solution in mares [Abstract]. In: Proceedings of the Annual Meeting of the American College of Veterinary Anesthesiologists, Atlanta, GA, 1995:19.

107. Skarda RT, Muir WW. Analgesic, hemodynamic and respiratory effects of caudal epidurally administered xylazine hydrochloride solution in mares. Am J Vet Res 1996;57:193–200.

108. Teixeira Neto FJ, McDonell W, Pearce S, Kerr C, Hurtig M, Durongphongtorn S. Evaluation of anesthesia maintained with halothane and epidural xylazine for hind limb surgery in horses. Vet Anaesth Analg 2001;28:107.

109. Chopin JB, Wright JD. Complication after the use of a combination of lignocaine and xylazine for epidural anaesthesia in a mare. Aust Vet J 1995;72:354–355.

110. Skarda RT, Muir WW. Physiologic responses after caudal epidural administration of detomidine in horses and xylazine in cattle. In: Short CE, Poznak AV, eds. Animal Pain. New York: Churchill Livingstone, 1992:292–315.

111. Skarda RT, Muir WW. Caudal analgesia induced by epidural or subarachnoid administration of detomidine hydrochloride solution in mares: A comparative study. In: Proceedings of the Annual Meeting of the American College of Veterinary Anesthesiologists, Washington, DC, 1993:20.

112. Skarda RT, Muir WW. Caudal analgesia induced by epidural or subarachnoid administration of detomidine hydrochloride solution in mares. Am J Vet Res 1994;55:670–680.

113. Skarda RT, Muir WW. Cardiovascular effects of caudal epidurally administered xylazine or detomidine HCl solution in mares: A comparative study [abstract]. In: Proceedings of the Fifth International Congress on Veterinary Anesthesiology, University of Guelph, Guelph, Canada, 1994:143.

114. Skarda RT, Muir WW. Comparison of antinociceptive, cardiovascular and respiratory effects, head ptosis, and position of pelvic limbs in mares after caudal epidural administration of xylazine and detomidine hydrochloride solution. Am J Vet Res 1996;9: 1338–1345.

115. Wittern C, Hendrickson DA, Trumble T, Wagoner A. Complications associated with administration of detomidine into the caudal epidural space in a horse. J Am Vet Med Assoc 1998;213:516–518.

116. Kariman A, Ghamsari SM, Mokhber-Dezfooli MR. Evaluation of analgesia induced by epidural administration of medetomidine in horses. J Faculty Vet Med, Tehran University 2001;56:49–51.

117. Kariman A. Cardiorespiratory and analgesic effects of epidurally administered romifidine in the horse [Abstract]. In: Proceedings of the Seventh World Congress on Veterinary Anaesthesiology, University of Bern, Bern, Switzerland, 2000:55.

118. Dowdy EG, Kaya K, Gocho Y. Some pharmacologic similarities of ketamine, lidocaine, and procaine. Anesth Analg 1973;52:839–842.

119. Gómez De Segura IA, De Rossi R, Santos M, San-Roman JL, Tendillo FJ. Epidural injection of ketamine for perineal analgesia in the horse. Vet Surg 1998;27:384–391.

120. Rédua MA, Valadão CAA, Duque JC, Balestrero LT. The preemptive effect of epidural ketamine on wound sensitivity in horses tested by using von Frey filaments. Vet Anaesth Analg 2002;29: 200–206.

121. Oleskovicz N, Vladão CAA, Farias A, Duque JCM. Pre-emptive epidural S+ ketamine in postincisional pain in horses [Abstract] In: Proceedings of the Eighth World Congress on Veterinary Anesthesiology, University of Tennessee, Knoxville, 2003:196.

122. Kariman A, Nowrouzian I, Bakhtiari J. Caudal epidural injection of a combination of ketamine and xylazine for perineal analgesia in horses [Abstract]. Vet Anaesth Analg 2000;27:115.

123. Colter SB. Electromyographic detection and evaluation of the tail alterations in show ring horses. In: Proceedings of the Sixth Annual Veterinary Medical Forum, American College Veterinary Internal Medicine, 1988:421–423.

124. Skarda RT, Muir WW. Continuous caudal epidural and subarachnoid anesthesia in mares: A comparative study. Am Vet Res 1983;44:2290–2298.

125. Greene EM, Cooper RC. Continuous caudal epidural anesthesia in the horse. J Am Vet Med Assoc 1984;184:971–974.

126. Greene EM, Cooper RC. Continuous caudal epidural anesthesia in the horse: An update. Proc Am Assoc Equine Pract 1985;31:409–414.

127. Ball MA, Cable CS, Kirker EJ. How to place an epidural catheter and indications for its use. Proc Am Assoc Equine Pract 1998;44:182–185.

128. Martin CA, Kerr CL, Pearce SG, Lansdowne JL, Boure LP. Outcome of epidural catheterization for delivery of analgesics in horses: 43 cases (1998–2001). J Am Vet Med Assoc 2003;222: 1394–1398.

129. Geernaert K, Hody JL, Adriaesen H, Van Steenberge A. Does epidural injection of physiological saline facilitate the advancement of catheters? Eur J Anaesthesiol 1993;10:349–351.

130. Skarda RT, Muir III WW. Analgesic, behavioral, and hemodynamic and respiratory effects of midsacral subarachnoidally administered ropivacaine hydrochloride in mares. Vet Anaesth Analg 2003;30: 37–50.

131. Cuillé J, Sendrail M. Analgésie cocainique par voie rachidienne. Rev Vet 1901;26:98–103.

132. Mettam AE. Surgical anaesthesia by the injection of cocaine into the lumbar subarachnoid space. Veterinarian (Lond) 1901;74: 115–121.

133. Saccani R. Cocainizzazione del midollo spinale negli animali domestici. Nuovo Ercolani 1901;11:272–274.

134. Valverde A, Little CB, Dyson DH. Use of epidural morphine to relieve pain in a horse. Can Vet J 1990;31:211–212.

135. Robinson EP, Moncada-Suarez JR, Felice L. Epidural morphine analgesia in horses [Abstract]. In: Proceedings of the Annual Meeting of the American College of Veterinary Anesthesiologists, Washington, DC, 1993:22.

136. Robinson EP. Preferential dermatomal analgesic effects of epidurally-administered morphine in horses. In: Bryden DI, ed. Animal Pain and Its Control. Sydney: University of Sydney, 1994:417–421.

137. Natalini CC, Robinson EP. Comparative evaluation of the analgesic effects of epidural morphine, alfentanil, butorphanol, tramadol, and U50488H in horses. In: Proceedings of the Annual Scientific Meeting of the American College of Veterinary Anesthesiologists, Dallas, TX, 1999:16.

138. Natalini CC, Robinson EP. Effects of epidural morphine, alfentanil, butorphanol, tramadol and U-50488H on heart rate, arterial blood pressure, respiratory rate, body temperature, and behavior in horses [Abstract]. In: Schatzmann U, ed. Proceedings of the Seventh World Congress on Veterinary Anaesthesiology. Bern: University of Bern, 2000:53.

139. Natalini CC, Robinson EP. Comparative evaluation of the analgesic effects of epidural morphine, alfentanil, butorphanol, tramadol and U50488H in horses. J Vet Anaesth Anal 2000;27:109.

140. Natalini CC, Robinson EP. Effects of epidural opioid analgesics on heart rate, arterial blood pressure, respiratory rate, body temperature, and behavior in horses. Vet Ther 2003;4:364–375.

141. Farny J, Blais D, Vaillancourt D, et al. Caudal epidural anesthesia with butorphanol in the mare [Abstract]. In: Proceedings, Fourth International Congress on Veterinary Anaesthesiology, Utrecht, The Netherlands, 1991:32.

142. Farny J, Blais D, Vaillancourt D, Bisaillon A, Garon O. Caudal epidural anesthesia with butorphanol and lidocaine in the mare [Abstract]. In: Proceedings of the Fifth International Congress of Veterinary Anesthesiologists, University of Guelph, Guelph, Canada, 1994:149.

143. Doherty TJ, Geiser DR, Rohrbach BW. Effects of high volume epidural morphine, ketamine and butorphanol on halothane minimum alveolar concentration in ponies. Equine Vet J 1997;29: 370–373.

144. Olbrich VH, Mosing M. A comparison of the analgesic effects of caudal epidural methadone and lidocaine in the horse. Vet Anaesth Analg 2003;30:156–164.

145. Skarda RT, Muir WW. Analgesic, hemodynamic, and respiratory effects of caudal epidural meperidine HCl solution in mares [Abstract]. In: Proceedings of the Annual Scientific Meeting of the American College of Veterinary Anesthesiologists, San Francisco, CA, 2000:31.

146. Skarda RT, Muir WW. Analgesic, hemodynamic, and respiratory effects induced by caudal epidural administration of meperidine hydrochloride in mares. Am J Vet Res 2001;62:1001–1007.

147. Raffa RB, Friederichs E, Reimann W, Shank RP, Codd EE, Vaught JL. Opioid and nonopioid components independently contribute to the mechanism of action of tramadol, an "atypical" opioid analgesic. J Pharmacol Exp Ther 1992;260:275–285.

148. Baraka A, Jabbur S, Ghabash M, Nader A, Khoury G, Sibai A. A comparison of epidural tramadol and epidural morphine for postoperative analgesia. Can J Anaesth 1993;40:308–313.

149. Sysel AM, Pleasant RS, Jacobson JD, Moll HD, Modransky PD, Warnick LD. Efficacy of an epidural combination of morphine and

detomidine in alleviating experimentally induced hindlimb lameness in horses. Vet Surg 1995;24:442.

150. Sysel AM, Pleasant RS, Jacobson JD, et al. Efficacy of an epidural combination of morphine and detomidine in alleviating experimentally induced hind limb lameness in horses. Vet Surg 1996;25:511–518.

151. Goodrich LR, Nixon AJ, Fubini SL, et al. Epidural morphine and detomidine decreases postoperative hindlimb lameness in horses after bilateral stifle arthroscopy. Vet Surg 2002;31:232–239.

152. Sysel AM, Pleasant RS, Sponenberg DP, et al. Systemic and local effects associated with long-term epidural catheterization and morphine/detomidine administration in the horse. Vet Surg 1995;24:442.

153. Sysel AM, Pleasant RS, Jacobson JD, et al. Systemic and local effects associated with long-term epidural catheterization and morphine-detomidine administration in horses. Vet Surg 1997;26:141–149.

154. Csik-Salmon J, Blais D, Vaillancourt D, Garon O, Bisaillon A. Utilisation du mélange lidocaine-butorphanol en anesthesie epidurale caudale chez la jument. Can J Vet Res 1996;60:288–295.

155. Natalini CC, Alves SDL, Polydoro AS, et al. Epidural administration of morphine combined with romifidine in horses [Abstract]. In: Proceedings of the Eighth World Congress of Veterinary Anesthesiologists, University of Tennessee, Knoxville, 2003:168.

156. Natalini CC, Robinson EP. Epidural administration of tiletamine/zolazepam in horses [Abstract]. In: Proceedings of the Annual Meeting of the American College of Veterinary Anesthesiologists, New Orleans, 2001:44.

157. Natalini CC, Alves SDL, Robinson EP. Epidural administration of tiletamine-zolazepam in horses. Vet Anaesth Analg 2002;29:109.

158. Natalini CC, Alves SDL, Guedes AGP, Polydoro AS, Brondani JT, Bopp S. Epidural administration of tiletamine/zolazepam in horses. Vet Anaesth Analg 2004;31:79–85.

159. Robinson EP, Natalini CC. Epidural anesthesia and analgesia in horses. Vet Clin Equine 2002;18:61–82.

160. Sarparanta L. Die Anwendung der Lokalbetäubung bei den Kastrationen. Finn Vet 1927;33:59–61.

161. Rieger H. Die testikuläre Injektion. Berl Munch Tierarztl Wochenschr 1954;67:107–109.

162. Matyschtschuk J. Beitrag zur Kastration am stehenden Pferd. Wien Tierarztl Wochenschr 1949;36:378–391.

163. Reed WD. Standing castration. In: Proceedings of the 14th Annual Meeting of the American Association of Equine Practitioners, Philadelphia, 1968:239–240.

164. Wriedt WD, Schebitz H, and Böhm D. Zur Kastration des Hengstes. Berl Munch Tierarztl Wochenschr 1979;92:41–42.

165. Magda JJ. Local anesthesia in operations on the male perineum in horses. Veterinariya 1948;25:34–36.

166. Magda JJ. Leitungsanästhesie des Pferdepenis. Sov Vet 1940;16:96–98.

167. Dietz O. Zur Grenzstrangblockade beim Tier. Arch Exp Veterinarmed 1958;11:310–330, 349–385.

168. Heidrich HD, Nöldner H. Üeber die Anwendung der Grenzstrang bzw: Stellatumblockade beim Pferd. Mh Vet Med 1963;18:58–61.

169. Skarda RT, Muir WW, Swanson CR, Hubbell JA. Cervicothoracic (stellate) ganglion block in conscious horses. Am J Vet Res 1986;47:21–26.

170. Skarda RT, Muir WW, Couri D. Plasma lidocaine concentrations in conscious horses after cervicothoracic (stellate) ganglion block with 1% lidocaine HCl solution. Am J Vet Res 1987;48:1092–1097.

171. Skarda RT, Muir WW, Hubbell JA. Paravertebral lumbar sympathetic ganglion block in the horse. In: Proceedings of the Second International Congress of Veterinary Anesthesiologists. Sacramento, CA: Veterinary Practice, 1985:160.

172. Raekallio M, Taylor PM, Johnson CB, Tulamo R-M, Ruprah M. The disposition and local effects of intra-articular morphine in normal ponies. J Assoc Vet Anaesth 1996;23:23–26.

173. Lopez-Sanroman FJ, Cruz JM, Santos M, Mazzini RA, Tabanera A, Tendillo FJ. Evaluation of the local analgesic effect of ketamine in the palmar digital nerve block at the base of the proximal sesamoid (abaxial sesamoid block) in horses. Am J Vet Res 2003;64:475–478.

174. Bidwell LA, Wilson DV, Caron JP. Systemic lidocaine absorption after placement of Lidoderm® patches on horses: Preliminary findings. In: Proceedings of the Veterinary Midwest Anesthesiology and Analgesia Conference, Indianapolis, IN, 2004:15.

Chapter 23

Local and Regional Anesthetic and Analgesic Techniques: Ruminants and Swine

Roman T. Skarda and William J. Tranquilli

Introduction

Local or regional analgesia is a preferred method in food animals because of accepted practice and economic necessity. Many surgical procedures are performed safely and humanely using a combination of physical restraint, mild sedation or tranquilization, and local or regional anesthesia. The techniques should provide reversible loss of pain to a limited body area with minimal effects on homeostasis. The standing position is optimal for a number of surgical procedures of ruminants, because it reduces the problems associated with bloat, salivation, recumbency-related regurgitation, and nerve or muscle damage.[1–4]

Local or infiltration analgesia is achieved by injecting a local anesthetic solution into the tissues at a surgical site, whereas regional analgesia is induced after perineural injection near major nerves. The most commonly used techniques in ruminants are surface (topical) anesthesia, infiltration anesthesia, nerve-block (conduction) anesthesia, epidural anesthesia, and intravenous regional anesthesia. Although local anesthetic drugs are routinely used, none has presently been approved by the Food and Drug Administration (FDA) for use in lactating dairy cows. Epidural morphine is safe and effective, and provides an alternative approach for treatment of pain after hind-limb orthopedic surgery.

Infiltration anesthesia, lumbosacral epidural anesthesia, and intratesticular injection are the most popular local anesthetic techniques in properly tranquilized pigs. The advantages of regional analgesia over general anesthesia include the need for minimal apparatus (e.g., syringe, needles, and drug) and little risk of toxic side effects. Several factors must be considered in the choice of a technique:[5]

1. The site, nature, and expected duration of surgery
2. The species, temperament, and health of the patient
3. Special requirements (such as minimum fetal depression during cesarean section)
4. The skill and experience of the veterinarian
5. The economics of time and materials

Local Anesthetics

A variety of local or regional anesthetic drugs can penetrate peripheral nerve barriers and provide reversible anesthesia with acceptable onset times and predictable duration.[5–9] The drugs vary as to the potency, toxicity, and cost, and none has been approved by the FDA for use in lactating dairy cows, although such agents are commonly used (Table 23.1). Lidocaine hydrochloride solu-

Table 23.1. Local analgesics

Agent (Generic Name)	Trade Name	Chemical Name	(Procaine = 1)	Potency (Procaine = 1)	Toxicity Dosage	Stability	Comments
Procaine	Novocaine (Winthrop Sterns, New York)	Para-aminobenzoic acid ester of diethylamino ethanol	1:1	1:1	1%–2% for infiltration and nerve block	Aqueous solutions are heat resistant; decomposed by bacteria	Hydrolyzed by liver and plasma esterase
Chloroprocaine	Nesacaine (Astra Pharmaceutical Products, Westboro, MA)	Para-amino-2 chlorobenzoic acid ester of B-diethyl amino ethanol	2.4:1	0.5:1	1%–2% for infiltration and nerve block	Multiple autoclaving accelerates hydrolysis and impairs potency	Immediate onset of action; 2-h duration with epinephrine
Lidocaine	Xylocaine (Astra Pharmaceutical Products, Westboro, MA)	Diethylaminoacet-2,6-xylidide	2:1	0.5%, 1:1; 1%, 1.4:1; 2%, 1.5:1	0.5%–2.0% for infiltration and nerve block; topically, 2%–4%	Aqueous solutions are thermostable; multiple autoclaving possible	Excellent penetrability; rate of onset twice as fast as procaine; 2-h duration with epinephrine
Mepivacaine	Carbocaine (Winthrop Laboratories, New York)	1-Methyl-2',6' pipecoloxylidide monohydrochloride	2.5:1	Less toxic than lidocaine	1%–2% for infiltration and nerve block	Resistant to acid and alkaline hydrolysis; multiple autoclaving possible	Absence of vasodilator effect makes addition of a vasoconstrictor unnecessary
Tetracaine	Pontocaine (Winthrop Laboratories, New York)	Parabutyl amino benzoyl dimethylamino-ethanol-HCl	12:1	10:1	0.1% for infiltration and nerve block; topically, 0.2%	Crystals and solutions should not be autoclaved	Slow onset of analgesia (5–10 min); 2-h duration; for eye installation
Hexylcaine	Cyclaine (Merck, Sharpe and Dohme, West Point, PA)	1-Cyclo-hexamino 2-propylbenzoate	1–2:1	2–4:1	0.5%–1.0% for infiltration; 2% for nerve block; 5% topically	Crystals and solutions are thermostable	Recommended for epidural and topical analgesia
Dibucaine	Nupercaine (CIBA Pharmaceutical Products, Summit, NJ)	α-Butyl-oxycinchoninic acid of diethylethylene-diamide	20:1	15:1	Topically, 0.1%	Thermostable but precipitation by alkalies	Slowly detoxified
Bupivacaine	Marcaine (Breon Laboratories, New York)	1-Butyl-2',6 pipe-coloxylidide-HCl	8:1	Greater margin of safety than lidocaine	0.25% for infiltration; 0.5% for nerve block; 0.75% for epidural block	Stable compound	Intermediate onset, lasting 4–6 h
Ropivacaine	Naropin (AstraZeneca LP, Wilmington, DE)	S-(-)-1-Propyl 2', 6'-pipecoloxylidide HCl monohydrate	8:1	Greater margin of safety than bupivacaine	0.2% for infiltration; 0.5% for nerve block; 0.75% and 1.0% for epidural block	Stable compound	Intermediate onset, lasting 4–6 h

tion has become the single agent of choice because of its intermediate anesthetic duration of 1½ to 3 h and the cost restrictions and limited space in a mobile-practice vehicle. The maximal dose of injected lidocaine should be limited to approximately 4 mg/kg of body weight (0.2 mL/kg of body weight without epinephrine) to avoid toxicity.

Patches of 5% lidocaine (Lidoderm; Endo Pharmaceuticals, Chadds Ford, PA) for transdermal delivery of lidocaine are available. Each patch (10 × 14 cm) contains 700 mg of lidocaine (50 mg per gram of adhesive) in aqueous base and methylparaben and propylparaben as preservatives. Although studies about the analgesic efficacy, pharmacology, and pharmacokinetics of trans-

dermal lidocaine in cattle have not been reported, two patches of 5% lidocaine applied around the fetlock joint have reduced local pain in cows (personal observation) (Fig. 23.1).

The addition of a vasoconstrictor, such as epinephrine at concentrations of 5 to 20 μg/mL (1:200,000 to 1:50,000), is occasionally incorporated or can be added to the commercial local anesthetic solution to increase intensity, prolong anesthetic activity, and reduce the potential for toxicity.[10] These concentrations may be obtained by adding 0.1 mL of 1:1000 (0.1 mg) epinephrine to 5 mL (1:50,000) and 20 mL (1:200,000) of local anesthetic solution. The use of local anesthetic drugs containing a vasoconstrictor often causes tissue necrosis along wound edges,

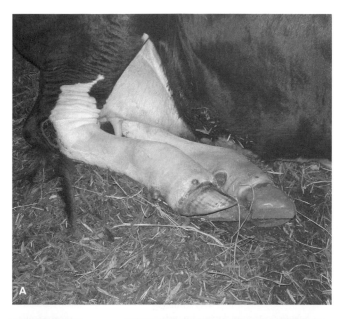

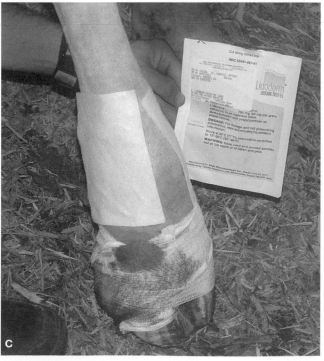

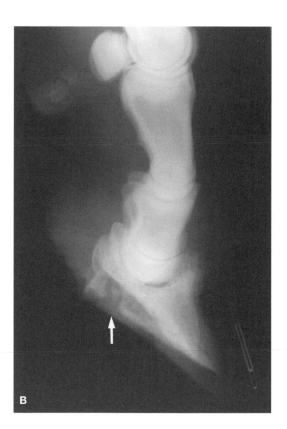

Fig. 23.1. Black-and-white Holstein cow, 4 years old, with sole abscess of the lateral claws and comminuted fracture of the lateral plantar process of digit IV of the right rear foot **(A)**. Radiograph of the distal phalanx (P3) confirms the fracture with articular involvement (*arrow*) and possible osteomyelitis and septic arthritis of the distal interphalangeal joint of digit IV, and pedal osteitis of the distal phalanx of digit IV **(B)**. A ring block, using 15 mL of 2% lidocaine, was performed at the midmetatarsal level, and the fractured plantar process of P3 was removed. An incision was made above the coronary band on the cranial aspect of the foot and connected to the opening of the abscess on the sole. Two gauze patches soaked in betadine solution were used to create a drain for the incision through the opening in the sole of the foot. Two 5% Lidoderm patches were placed over the metatarsals, one medially and one laterally **(C)**, and then the leg was wrapped with a bandage. Because the cow appeared more comfortable, was getting up easier without much encouragement, and was standing for longer periods after the transdermal lidocaine application, the Lidoderm patches were reapplied once a day for 3 additional days.

especially in thin-skinned animals, and it should be avoided for anesthesia of the teat and intravenous regional analgesia.

Adding hyaluronidase to lidocaine at a rate of 150 turbidity-reducing units per 25 mL will hasten the time of onset of infiltration anesthesia and shorten anesthesia, owing to increased permeability of the tissues.[10] The necessity for its use, other than in combination with procaine hydrochloride solution (1%), has been questioned with the introduction of newer local anesthetics with improved infiltration power. The enzyme enables smaller volumes of local anesthetic solution to be used. The combination of local anesthetics, epinephrine, and hyaluronidase produces prolonged anesthesia because of reduced uptake while maintaining the spreading action of hyaluronidase upon local anesthetics.[11] Accuracy in technique is still necessary because tissue fascial planes act as barriers. The greatest use of hyaluronidase is in ophthalmology (retrobulbar blocks) and local anesthetic nerve blocks for postoperative pain relief.

Regional Anesthesia of the Head

The most frequently desensitized nerves of the head are the auriculopalpebral, supraorbital, zygomaticotemporal (lacrimal), infraorbital, oculomotor, abducens, and trochlear. Many of these nerves are maxillary and ophthalmic branches of the trigeminal (fifth) cranial nerve.

Anesthesia of the Eye and Relaxation of the Globe

The neuroanatomy of ocular structures is complex. The globe, conjunctiva, nictitans, and most of the eyelids are supplied by sensory fibers of the ophthalmic division of the trigeminal nerve. The extraocular muscles are supplied by motor fibers of the trochlear nerve (superficial oblique muscle), the abducens nerve (lateralis rectus and retractor oculi muscles), and the oculomotor nerve. The oculomotor, trochlear, ophthalmic, and maxillary branches of the trigeminal and abducens nerves emerge from the foramen rotundum orbitale.

At present, topical and regional anesthetics are used to facilitate surgery of the eye and its associated structures. The eyelids (without anesthesia) are selectively paralyzed by desensitizing the auriculopalpebral branch of the facial nerve (akinesia). Anesthesia of the eye and orbit and immobilization of the globe are commonly achieved by retrobulbar injection of a local anesthetic or by using the Petersen technique (or its modification).[12]

For topical anesthesia, one or two drops of proparacaine hydrochloride (0.5%) solution are instilled in the eye. Pain associated with corneal disease is relieved in 30 s and for as long as 10 to 15 min.[13] In addition, blepharospasm caused by superficial irritation of the cornea is relieved, so examination of the eye or minor surgery is greatly facilitated. The FDA has approved the use of proparacaine in food animals to induce topical anesthesia for cauterization of corneal ulcers, removal of foreign bodies and suture from the cornea, and measurements of intraocular pressure (tonometry) when glaucoma is suspected. Other ophthalmic anesthetic solutions, such as Xylocaine [lidocaine] hydrochloride (4%) or tetracaine hydrochloride, are toxic to the corneal epithe-

lium, suppressing mitosis and reducing protective blink reflexes, and should not be used for treatment of the eye.[14]

Anesthesia and Akinesia of the Eyelids

The site for producing a linear subcutaneous infiltration (line block) is about 0.5 cm from the margin of the dorsal and ventral eyelids in adult cattle. Approximately 10 mL of a 2% lidocaine hydrochloride solution is administered at multiple sites, 0.5 cm apart, using a 2.5-cm, 22- or 25-gauge needle (Fig. 23.2A).

Paralysis of the eyelids (without analgesia) is commonly performed in cattle by selectively desensitizing the auriculopalpebral branch of the facial nerve (akinesia).[13] The nerve is sometimes palpable in a notch on the zygomatic arch, anterior to the base of the auricular muscles, where a 2.5-cm, 18- or 20-gauge needle is placed subcutaneously, and 5 to 10 mL of the anesthetic is deposited (Fig. 23.2B). The combination of topical anesthesia and auriculopalpebral akinesia is useful for removing foreign bodies from the cornea and conjunctival sac and for injecting medication into the bulbar subconjunctiva.

Anesthesia for Enucleation

In doing a retrobulbar block for enucleation or to facilitate surgery and radiation therapy in cattle with squamous cell carcinoma at the cornea, a 15-cm, 18-gauge needle with a fairly large bend (approximately 25-cm diameter) is used in adult cattle. Head restraint with a halter or nose grip is necessary. In small ruminants, a 3.75-cm, 22-gauge needle may be used.

The sites for lid penetration are at the superior, inferior, medial, or lateral orbital rim. The surgeon's index finger is used to deflect the globe and protect it from the needle point (Fig. 23.3A). When using the medial canthus approach, the medial wall of the bony orbit is felt. The needle is then inserted in the fornix of the conjunctiva cranial to the nictitans dorsomedial to the operator's finger until the orbital apex is encountered (Fig. 23.3B). Approximately 15 mL of a 2% lidocaine hydrochloride solution or equivalent is injected in small increments as the needle is advanced, thereby pushing initial structures from the needle point. The needle must not be fully inserted into the orbit to avoid penetration of the optic nerve sheath. Once the entire block is completed, the structures that will be desensitized include the optic nerve; the elevator palpebral muscles; the medial rectus, the dorsal rectus, the ventral rectus, and the inferior oblique muscles (all innervated by the oculomotor nerve); the superior oblique muscle (innervated by the fourth cranial nerve); the sensory part of the eye and adnexa (innervated by the fifth cranial nerve); the retractor oculi muscles; the lateral rectus muscle (innervated by the sixth cranial nerve); and the orbicularis oculi muscle (innervated by the seventh cranial nerve). A satisfactory retrobulbar nerve block should then accomplish anesthesia for whatever procedure would be desired for the eye and eyelids and will enable the proptosing of the eye for surgery on the cornea or enucleation.

Adverse effects that may result from retrobulbar injections include apnea,[15] orbital hemorrhages, direct pressure on the globe, penetration of the globe, damage to the optic nerve, initiation of the oculocardiac reflex, and injection into the optic nerve men-

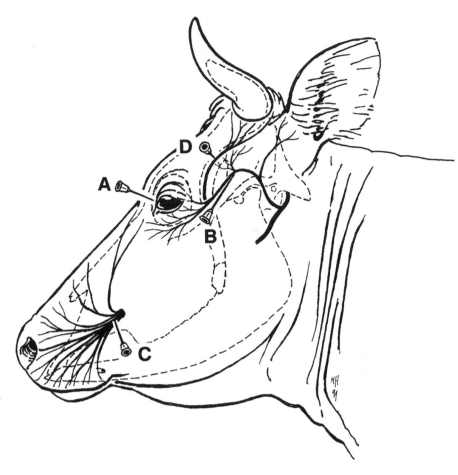

Fig. 23.2. Needle placement for infiltration of the eyelids (*A*) and nerve blocks on the head in cattle: auriculopalpebral (*B*), infraorbital (*C*), and cornual (*D*) branches of the zygomaticotemporal nerve.

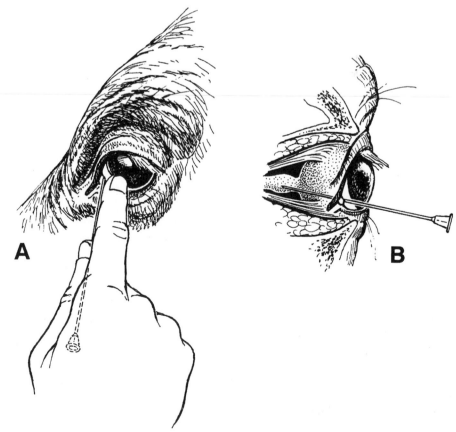

Fig. 23.3. Retrobulbar needle placement through the medial canthus **(A)** to the orbital apex **(B)** in cattle.

inges. Damage to the globe may be serious for procedures other than enucleation. If the optic nerve or optic foramen is penetrated and local anesthetic is injected beneath the meningeal covering, epidural or subarachnoid anesthesia of the brain may result, which can be fatal. Risk of subarachnoid (cerebrospinal fluid [CSF]) injection is minimized by aspiration check.

In performing the Peterson block,[16] the notch formed by the supraorbital process cranially, the zygomatic arch ventrally, and the coronoid process of the mandible caudally, is identified. A 2.5-cm, 22-gauge needle is inserted at this notch, and approximately 5 mL of a 2% lidocaine hydrochloride solution is injected subcutaneously. A 2.5-cm, 14-gauge needle (to serve as a cannula) is placed through the desensitized skin as far anterior and ventral as possible in the notch. A straight or slightly curved 10- to 12-cm, 18-gauge needle is inserted into the cannula in a horizontal and slightly posterior direction until it encounters the coronoid process of the mandible at approximately 2.5 cm through the skin. The cow's head is fully extended with frontal and nasal bones parallel to the ground. The needle with no syringe attached (to feel the bony landmarks) is gently manipulated anteriorly until its point passes medially in front of the coronoid process. The needle is then advanced to the pterygopalatine fossa rostral to the solid bony plate that is in close proximity to the orbitorotundum foramen at a depth of 7.5 to 10 cm (Fig. 23.4A). Penetration of the turbinates and nasopharynx must be avoided. Approximately 15 mL of the local anesthetic is injected under control of aspiration to ensure that the needle point has not entered the ventral maxillary artery. All of the important nerves (oculomotor, trochlear, and abducens) and the three branches of the trigeminal nerve (ophthalmic, maxillary, and mandibular) that emerge from the foramen orbitorotundum are desensitized 10 to 15 min after completion of the injection (Fig. 23.5).[17] A proper technique anesthetizes all the structures for sensory and motor function of the eye, except for the eyelid. The lid block is accomplished by desensitizing the auriculopalpebral branch of the facial nerve by withdrawing the needle to the subcutaneous tissue and reinserting it posteriorly for 5 to 7.5 cm lateral to the zygomatic arch, as an additional 5 to 10 mL of the anesthetic is injected (Fig. 23.4B). If the upper lid is involved in the surgical procedure, a line of infiltration with 10 mL of the local anesthetic should be made subcutaneously approximately 2.5 cm from the margin of the lid (Fig. 23.2A). The anesthetic is laid along its path while the needle is being advanced. Several different planes of anesthetic infiltration along the frontal crest are performed, so no matter where the nerve is coursing through that region, it should be desensitized by this fanning procedure.

As might be expected, some experience is required to strike a foramen that small at such great depth from the surface. To facilitate the Peterson procedure, a curved needle similar to that used for the retrobulbar block may be used. The concavity of the needle is kept caudal to facilitate the passage of the needle point rostral to the mandibular coronoid process. The needle is moved slightly back and forth, fanning across this area until some motor reaction and flinch of the animal's eye is determined.

When comparing the Peterson eye block and retrobulbar injection, it is apparent that the Peterson technique requires more skill to perform correctly, but is safer and more effective if done properly. There is less edema and inflammation than when eyelids and orbit are infiltrated. In addition, the risk of orbital hemorrhage, direct pressure on the globe, penetration of the globe, damage to the optic nerve, or injection into the optic nerve meninges is minimized with Peterson's technique.[18–21] Comparison of retrobulbar and Peterson nerve-block techniques via magnetic resonance imaging in bovine cadavers also indicates that the retrobulbar injection technique provides a greater distribution of a lipid contrast medium around the periorbital structures, the optic nerve, and in the ethmoid turbinates and nasopharynx, compared with the Peterson nerve-block technique, which primarily distributes the contrast medium in the perygopalatine fossa and only minimally in the surrounding structures.[22]

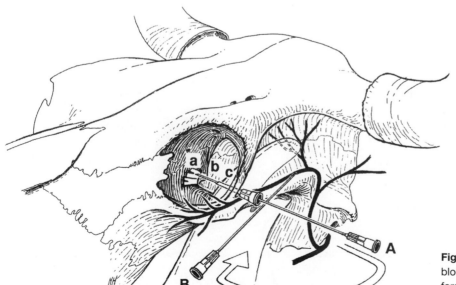

Fig. 23.4. Needle placement for Peterson eye block (A) and auriculopalpebral nerve block (B): a, foramen orbitorotundum; b, pterygoid crest; and c, coronoid process.

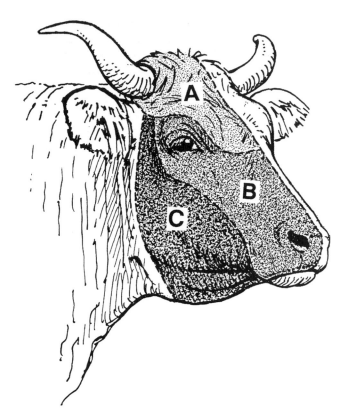

Fig. 23.5. Cutaneous areas of the bovine head supplied by sensory fibers from the ophthalmic (*A*), maxillary (*B*), and mandibular (*C*) nerves.

Both retrobulbar block and Peterson's technique prevent blinking for several hours. Antibiotic eye ointments of sterile saline solution should be applied to the cornea frequently during surgery and after orbital replacement of the globe to keep the cornea moist. Sunlight, dust, and wind in the eye must be avoided to prevent keratoconjunctivitis. Alternatively, the lids may be sutured together until motor activity of the lids returns. Local anesthetics in conventional concentrations should not produce nerve damage of clinical importance. Severe central nervous system (CNS) toxicity in both procedures, however, may arise from penetration of the turbinates and injection of local anesthetic solution into the optic nerve meninges and nasopharynx. The clinical signs of local anesthetic CNS toxicity include hyperexcitability, lateral recumbency, opisthotonus, tonic-clonic convulsions, respiratory arrest, and cardiac arrest.

Nasal Anesthesia

For repair of nasal lacerations in cattle and insertion of a nose ring in mature, ill-tempered bulls, nasal analgesia is required.[23,24] Bulls must be thoroughly restrained during the procedure and, if unruly, should be tranquilized before nasal analgesia is attempted. A 3.75-cm, 18-gauge needle is used for perineural injection of the infraorbital nerve at its point of emergence from the infraorbital canal. Difficult to palpate, the foramen is located rostral to the facial tuberosity on a line extending from the nasomax-

illary notch to the second upper molar (P2), which in adult animals is approximately 5 cm dorsal to P2. Approximately 20 to 30 mL of a 2% lidocaine hydrochloride solution is injected along a line rostral to the infraorbital foramen and superficial to the maxilla (Fig. 23.2C).

Anesthesia of the Horn

Anesthetic techniques for dehorning cattle and goats and for disbudding young kids have been described.[24–32] Considerable controversy exists over the ideal method for horn removal, quantification of dehorning-related pain, and consequently the necessity for regional analgesia for dehorning young calves. As early as the 1960s, behavioral, endocrine, and cardiac responses in young Friesian calves during and after dehorning with an electrical cauterizing dehorner either with or without sedation and analgesia (xylazine and butorphanol, intramuscularly [IM]), indicated that routine field use of local analgesia (corneal nerve block) improved the welfare of calves subjected to dehorning with a hot iron.[32]

Analgesia of the horn and base of the horn in cattle is achieved by desensitizing the cornual branch of the zygomaticotemporal (lacrimal) nerve, which is a portion of the ophthalmic division of the trigeminal nerve.[33,34] The zygomaticotemporal nerve leaves the lacrimal nerve within the orbit and passes through the temporal fossa dorsal to the zygomatic process of the squamous temporal bone and around the lateral edge of the frontal bone dorsal to the temporal muscle. At first it lies deep, but on the upper third of the lateral temporal ridge it lies relatively superficial, 7 to 10 mm deep. The zygomaticotemporal nerve supplies sensory fibers to the horn and surrounding skin, particularly on its caudal aspect, and the skin of the ear. The nerve can usually be palpated halfway between the lateral canthus and the horn (bud) between the thin frontalis muscle and temporal muscle. A 2.5-cm, 20-gauge needle is inserted ventromedially close to the frontal bone approximately 2 to 3 cm in front of the base of the horn, and 5 to 10 mL of a 2% lidocaine hydrochloride solution, depending on size, is injected (Fig. 23.2D). Needle penetration is from 1 cm in small cattle to 2.5 cm in large bulls. The cornual artery and vein are close to the site of block; thus, aspiration ensures that the needle point is not inadvertently intravascular. Cornual anesthesia should result unless anesthetic has been injected too deeply in the aponeurosis of the temporal muscle. With an adequately performed cornual nerve block, there is a blink response during infiltration and an ipsilateral lid droop because of the blockade of some branches of the auriculopalpebral nerve. In exceptional cases and in a fractured horn involving the frontal bone and sinuses,[34] a large posterior branch of the sinuum frontalis nerve maintains sensitivity of the cornual process. This nerve can be desensitized by using the Peterson eye-block technique.[16] Adult cattle and bulls with well-developed horns require extensive subcutaneous infiltration of the caudal aspect of the horn base to desensitize the cutaneous branches of the second cervical nerve.[16,25] Regional analgesia dissipates 3 to 4 h after use of a long-lasting local anesthetic (e.g., bupivacaine).[35] Thereafter, blood cortisol spikes may develop, and painful behavioral traits become evident.[36] In one study, combining corneal nerve block with wound cauterization substantially reduced the cortisol response for 1 day after dehorning, whereas dehorning alone caused marked cortisol response for nearly 7 h.[37] Intravenous administration of a nonsteroidal anti-inflammatory analgesic may also be useful in preventing acute postsurgical pain in dehorned calves. Systemic analgesia can be combined with regional analgesia to reduce the stress associated with dehorning.[38–40] In a study assessing the efficacy of the nonsteroidal anti-inflammatory drugs (NSAIDs), ketoprofen and adrenocorticotropic hormone, but not phenylbutazone, significantly reduced cortisol levels after local anesthetic administration and dehorning.[41] Pain was best mitigated after hot-iron dehorning in 4 to 8 week calves, with the combined effects of a local anesthetic (lidocaine) and an NSAID (ketoprofen) before dehorning, and an anti-inflammatory drug (ketoprofen) again 2 and 7 h after the procedure.[41] Similarly, the use of a corneal nerve block and intramuscular injection of ketoprofen at least 10 min prior to dehorning, combined with either the use of a butane burner or an electrical Rhinehart dehorning device, has proven efficacious in reducing pain-associated behavior.[42] Dairymen should be encouraged to dehorn calves at a young age to minimize the pain response. Based on elevated cortisol levels, scoop dehorning has been deemed unacceptable by some investigators.[43,44] Likewise, the dehorning of cattle while they are restrained with an electroimmobilizer may be painful on application and should not be relied on to produce appropriate analgesia for such an invasive procedure.[45]

The horns and bases of the horns in goats are supplied by the cornual branches of the zygomaticotemporal (lacrimal) and infratrochlear nerves. Goats are typically sedated with intramuscular xylazine (0.1 mg/kg) administration before regional analgesia is initiated. The cornual branch of the zygomaticotemporal (lacrimal) nerve is desensitized by inserting a 2.5-cm, 22-gauge needle halfway between the lateral canthus of the eye and lateral base of the horn as close as possible to the caudal ridge of the supraorbital process and 1.0 to 1.5 cm deep, with 2 to 3 mL of a 2% lidocaine hydrochloride solution in adult goats (Fig. 23.6A). A second injection is made halfway between the medial canthus of the eye and medial base of the horn to desensitize the cornual branch of the infratrochlear nerve. The needle is inserted dorsal and parallel to the dorsomedial margin of the orbit. The anesthetic is administered in a line, because this nerve is frequently branched (Fig. 23.6B).

Early disbudding of small horns (<1 cm in diameter at the base) in the first few days of life uses thermal cautery, whereas larger horns (>2 cm in diameter at the base) are removed by surgery. Hemorrhage should be controlled by ligating the cornual artery. Dehorning of goats that are 8 months of age or older opens the frontal sinus, which should be protected by a snug, but not too tight, sterile bandage for as long as 1 month. The bandage should not produce edema and postoperative pain over the dehorning site. An elliptical ring block around the base of the entire horn of mature goats should be laid for a cosmetic dehorning procedure. This technique produces excellent cosmetic appearance with minimal postoperative care.[46,47] Anesthesia of the nerve to the sinus mucosa and periosteum of the frontal sinus is impractical, because the nerve arises deep within the orbit and enters the

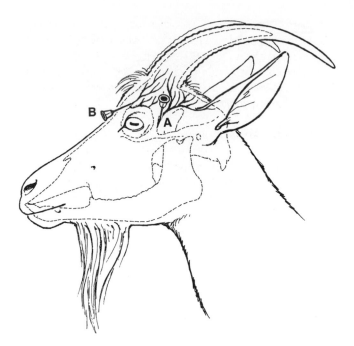

Fig. 23.6. Needle placement for desensitizing the cornual branches of the zygomaticotemporal (A) and infratrochlear nerve (B) in goats.

frontal bone without appearing superficial.[33] Sedation of the animal is required if the frontal sinus will be entered during horn removal.[28] General anesthesia should be used in mature goats with large horns. Owners should be advised that dehorning mature female goats late in gestation can induce abortion and that dehorning male goats used for breeding can temporarily alter their social status within a herd.[30]

Additional postoperative analgesia can be given by a single intravenous injection of flunixin meglumine (1 mg/kg of body weight). To alleviate pain during disbudding of young kids between 7 and 14 days of age, 0.5 mL of a 2% lidocaine hydrochloride solution is injected subcutaneously around the horn base (ring block). Toxic doses are more likely to administered accidentally after large areas of tissue have been infiltrated with 2% solutions of lidocaine, mepivacaine, procaine, and prilocaine or 0.5% bupivacaine. A total dose of 10 mg/kg (0.5 mL of a 2% solution/kg or 1 mL of a 1% solution/kg) of lidocaine should not be exceeded to prevent overdose. Inadvertent rapid intravenous infusions produce the most dramatic and rapid onset of symptoms. Apparent signs of toxicity include excitation, lateral recumbency, extensor rigidity, muscular twitching, dullness, generalized tonic-clonic convulsions, opisthotonus, and odontoprisis.[48,49] Coma, blindness, respiratory arrest, and cardiac arrest can occur with high plasma concentrations (>15 μg/mL) of lidocaine.

Anesthesia for Laparotomy

At least six techniques for inducing anesthesia of the paralumbar fossa and abdominal wall in standing ruminants have been described: (a) infiltration, (b) proximal paravertebral thoracolumbar, (c) distal paravertebral thoracolumbar, (d) segmental dorsolumbar epidural, (e) continuous lumbar segmental epidural, and (f) thoracolumbar subarachnoid anesthesia. Any of these techniques may be used for surgeries such as rumenotomy, cecotomy, correction of gastrointestinal displacement, intestinal obstruction and volvulus, cesarean section, ovariectomy, and liver or kidney biopsy, among others.[50,51]

Infiltration Anesthesia

Line Block

Simple infiltration of the incision line (line block) is the easiest and probably the most commonly used technique for producing analgesia of the flank in food animals. Multiple subcutaneous injections of 0.5 to 1.0 mL of a 2% lidocaine hydrochloride solution, 1 to 2 cm apart, are administered using a 2.5-cm, 20-gauge or smaller needle. Successive injections of 10 to 15 mL of the anesthetic are made slowly and continuously as the needle is inserted at the edge of the desensitized skin for the skin and subcutaneous line block. This is followed by inserting a 7.5- to 10-cm, 18-gauge needle through the desensitized skin and infiltrating the muscle layers and parietal peritoneum using 10 to 100 mL of the anesthetic, depending on the area to be desensitized (Fig. 23.7). Adult cattle (weighing 450 kg) safely tolerate 250 mL of a 2% lidocaine hydrochloride solution (5 g) for the line block, whereas in adult goats 10 mL of a 2% lidocaine hydrochloride solution (200 mg) should not be exceeded. It is common practice to dilute a 2% solution of the anesthetic with equal parts of sterile saline to make a 1% solution and decrease the total amount of drug by 50%.[49,50]

Inverted-7 or L Block

The inverted-7 or L block is a nonspecific regional analgesic technique in which up to 100 mL of a 2% lidocaine hydrochloride solution in adult cattle is injected into the tissues bordering the dorsocaudal aspect of the last rib and ventrolateral aspect of the lumbar transverse processes (Fig. 23.8). All nerves entering the surgical field are desensitized 10 to 15 min after administra-

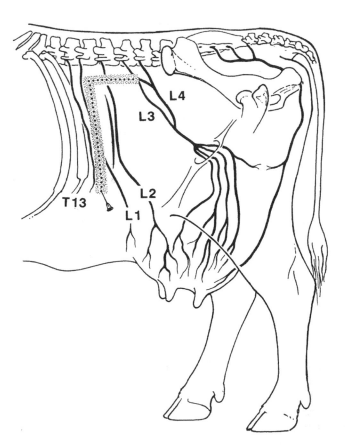

Fig. 23.8. Regional analgesia of the bovine flank by using the inverted-L infiltration pattern. T13 and L1 to L4 are ventral branches of 13th thoracic and first to fourth lumbar vertebral nerves.

tion of the anesthetic. Deposition of the anesthetic away from the incision site minimizes edema, hematoma, and possible interference with healing. The disadvantages of the inverted-7 or L block are similar to those of local infiltration anesthesia (line block) and include incomplete analgesia and muscle relaxation of the deep layers of the abdominal wall (particularly of the peritoneum), toxicity after injecting significant amounts of the anesthetic solution into the peritoneal cavity, and increased cost owing to larger doses of anesthetic and longer time required.

Proximal Paravertebral Thoracolumbar Anesthesia

The proximal paravertebral anesthesia is a good alternative to the inverted-7 or line block. The dorsal and ventral branches of the last thoracic (T13) and first and second lumbar (L1 and L2) spinal nerves are desensitized as they emerge from the intervertebral foramina (Fig. 23.9). The technique is also called the *Farquharson*,[52] *Hall*, or *Cambridge technique*.[53] In addition, the third and fourth (L3 and L4) lumbar spinal nerves can be desensitized if analgesia of the caudal most part of the paralumbar fossa for cesarean section or ipsilateral foreteat and mammary gland is desired.[54] However, weakness of the pelvic limb may be caused by desensitizing the L3 and L4 nerves, which carry motor fibers to the femoral and ischial nerves.

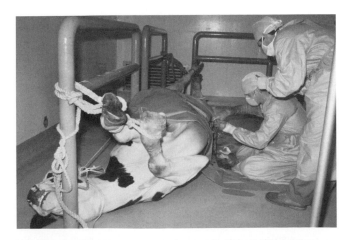

Fig. 23.7. Restraint of a 5-year-old Holstein cow, weighing 600 kg, in dorsolateral recumbency for right ventral abomasopexis. Approximately 25 mL of a 2% lidocaine hydrochloride solution desensitized a 15-cm abdominal incision line. From Skarda,[5] p. 630.

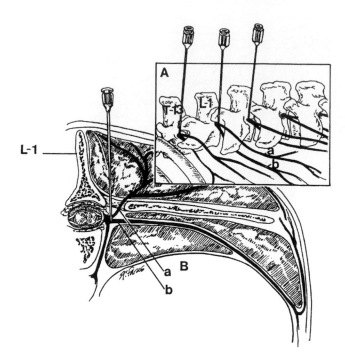

Fig. 23.9. Needle placement for proximal paravertebral nerve block in cattle. **A:** Left lateral aspect of thoracolumbar vertebrae T13 to L4 with needle tip placed at spinal nerves T13, L1, and L2. **B:** Cranial view of a transection of the first lumbar vertebra at the location of the intervertebral foramen: *a*, dorsal branch; and *b*, ventral branch of L1 vertebral nerve. From Skarda,[5] p. 631.

In cattle, the skin overlying the spinal column on the side to be desensitized is clipped, surgically scrubbed, and disinfected. The skin at the most obvious parts of the transverse processes of L1, L2, and L3 at a point 2.5 to 5.0 cm from the dorsal midline is identified and desensitized by injecting 2 to 3 mL of a 2% lidocaine hydrochloride solution, using a short and comparatively fine needle (2.5-cm, 20-gauge). If the T13 and L1 transverse processes cannot be palpated, the distance between the more prominent transverse processes of L2 and L3 is measured to mark the anterior sites at which the needle is to be introduced to desensitize nerves L1 and T13, respectively. The cranial aspect of the transverse processes will usually be on a same cross-sectional plane with the intervertebral foramina, so palpation of the most cranial border of the transverse process of L2 is of value in locating the L1-L2 intervertebral foramen, from which the first lumbar (L1) spinal nerve emerges.

A 1.25-cm, 14-gauge needle (to serve as a cannula) is first inserted into the desensitized skin to minimize skin resistance during insertion of a stout 4.25- to 15-cm, 18-gauge spinal needle. The needle is passed ventrally until its point encounters the transverse process of L2 or the intertransverse (L1-L2) ligament. Small amounts (2 to 3 mL) of the anesthetic are injected as the needle is advanced to counteract spasm of the longissimus dorsi muscle and prevent bending of the long needle. When contact is made with bone, the needle is walked off the cranial edge of the transverse process of L2 and advanced approximately 1 cm to pass through the intertransverse fascia. The penetration of the in-

tertransverse fascia can usually be felt. Approximately 10 to 15 mL of a 2% lidocaine hydrochloride solution is injected with little resistance to desensitize the ventral branch of L1. The needle is withdrawn 1 to 2.5 cm to above the fascia and dorsal surface of the transverse process. An additional 5 mL of the anesthetic is injected with slight resistance to desensitize the dorsal branch of L1. To desensitize T13 and L2, the needle is inserted cranial to the transverse processes of L1 and L3, its tip walked off the cranial edges of the transverse processes to a depth comparable to the previous injection site, and the nerves desensitized similarly to L1.

In sheep and goats, T13, L1, and L2 are desensitized similarly to the cattle method, but 2.5 to 3.0 cm off the midline and with less anesthetic (2 to 3 mL/site). Full anesthesia develops in approximately 10 min and lasts 1½ h. Signs of successful nerve blockade include anesthesia of the skin, increased skin temperature because of hyperemia after paralysis of cutaneous vasomotor nerves, and scoliosis toward the desensitized side caused by paralysis of paravertebral muscles.

When compared with infiltration analgesia, proximal thoracolumbar paravertebral block offers a wide and uniform area of analgesia and muscle relaxation. Analgesia is developed from the 13th rib caudal to the tuber coxae and ventrally to the fold of the flank. The incision site is not disrupted. Disruption occurs with an infiltration block when excessive amount of anesthetic is injected into the tissues and multiple skin punctures by the needle produce hemorrhage and trauma. With an infiltration block, a considerable amount of time is required to desensitize an area of approximately 45 cm, as would be required in a cesarean section. If an incision this long is necessary, a paravertebral nerve block could be done much more quickly and in a more professional and impressive manner. The technique relies on finding landmarks, but it is not at all difficult in thin, bony cows with easily palpable transverse processes. The four major disadvantages of the thoracolumbar paravertebral nerve block are (a) its technical difficulty, particularly in fat cattle and some beef cattle in which the lumbar transverse processes are not easily palpated; (b) arching of the spine due to paralysis of back muscles, which bow out toward the area of incision after unilateral blockade, making the closure of the incision more difficult; (3) the risk of penetrating vital structures such as the aorta and thoracic longitudinal vein on the left side and the caudal vena cava on the right side; and (4) loss of motor control of the pelvic limb caused by caudal migration of local anesthetic to the femoral nerves.

Distal Paravertebral Thoracolumbar Anesthesia

A lateral approach to the dorsal and ventral rami of spinal nerves T13, L1, and L2 in cattle has been used. The technique is also called the *Magda, Cakala,* or *Cornell technique.*[55] The skin is clipped and disinfected at the distal ends of the first lumbar (L1), second lumbar (L2), and fourth lumbar (L4) transverse processes, and 10 to 20 mL of a 2% lidocaine hydrochloride solution is injected in a fan-shaped infiltration pattern ventral to each transverse process, using a 7.5-cm, 18-gauge needle (Fig. 23.10). The needle is withdrawn a short distance and reinserted slightly

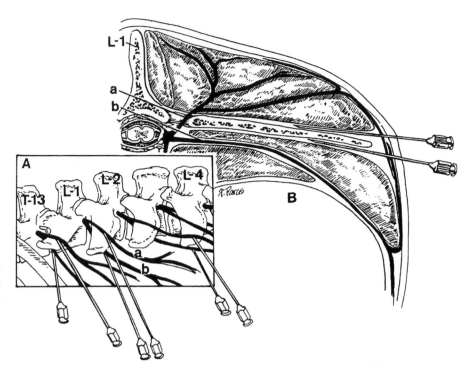

Fig. 23.10. **A:** Left lateral aspect of needle placement for distal paravertebral nerve block in cattle to block dorsal (*a*) and ventral (*b*) rami of spinal nerves T13, L1, and L2. **B:** Cranial view of the transaction of the first lumbar vertebra at the location of the intervertebral foramen. From Skarda,[5] p. 633.

dorsal and caudal to the transverse process to inject additional 5 mL of the anesthetic and desensitize the cutaneous branch of the dorsolateral branches. The procedure is repeated for the second and fourth lumbar transverse processes.

Distal paravertebral anesthesia as compared with proximal paravertebral anesthesia offers the advantages of using more routinely sized needles, lack of scoliosis, lack of risk of penetrating a major blood vessel (e.g., the aorta or the posterior vena cava), minimal weakness in the pelvic limb, and minimal ataxia. On the other hand, disadvantages of the technique are the larger doses of the anesthetic needed and variations in efficiency, particularly if the nerves follow a variable anatomical pathway.

Segmental Dorsolumbar Epidural Anesthesia

Although not an easy technique to perform, injection of local anesthetic into the epidural space either between the first and second lumbar (L1 and L2) vertebrae or, less commonly, between the last thoracic (T13) and first lumbar (L1) vertebrae in cattle has been employed to desensitize a number of nerve roots as they emerge from the dura covering the spinal cord and produce a belt of anesthesia around the animal's trunk while maintaining control of the limbs (Fig. 23.11). This type of spinal block may be referred to as *segmental dorsolumbar epidural anesthesia* or *Arthur block.*[56] The technique was first described in 1948;[56] subsequently, many have reported its use.[57–61] Cattle must be thoroughly restrained during the procedure.

In the standard technique, the skin area caudal to the T13 or L1 spinous process and contralateral to the flank region to be desensitized is aseptically prepared, and 2 to 4 mL of a 2% lidocaine hydrochloride solution is injected subcutaneously and adjacent to the interspinous (T13-L1 or L1-L2) ligaments to minimize pain during the puncture procedure. The first lumbar (L1-L2) interver-

tebral space in cattle is located 1.5 to 2.0 cm caudal to an imaginary line drawn across the back from the cranial edge of the transverse process of the second lumbar (L2) vertebrae. The dorsal lumbar processes and the depression between them can occasionally be palpated. A 1.25-cm, 14-gauge needle to facilitate penetration of an 11.25-cm, 18-gauge spinal needle with stylet is inserted at that site. The needle is advanced through the interosseous canal, which is formed by the arches of spinous processes T13 and L1, cranially and caudally, and the intervertebral articular processes laterally, until an abrupt reduction in needle passage is noted, indicating piercing through the interarcuate ligament and entry into the vertebral canal (Fig. 23.12). The spinal needle is inserted for a distance of 8 to 12 cm while being directed ventrally and medially at an angle of 10° to 15° with the vertical, at which point the needle has reached the epidural space. The spinal needle can be inserted through the muscle with relative ease, but encounters a slight increase in resistance during the insertion process at the interspinous and interarcuate ligaments.

Withdrawal and redirection of the needle are necessary if the needle point impinges against the bony arches of T13 and L1 or L1 and L2, respectively. The needle is properly placed into the epidural space if no blood or CSF flows from the needle hub or is obtained upon aspiration. Because of the negative pressure in the epidural space, a sucking sound is heard as air enters the needle immediately after penetration of the interarcuate ligament. This negative epidural pressure may vary between heifers (−10 mm Hg) and lactating (−17 to −20 mm Hg) or pregnant (−15 mm Hg) cows, but the epidural pressure will be negative in all cattle.[62] Most often, the epidural space is identified by the loss-of-resistance method.[39] This means that first a marked resistance to injection of saline or air is encountered when the point of the needle enters the interarcuate ligament, and resistance completely

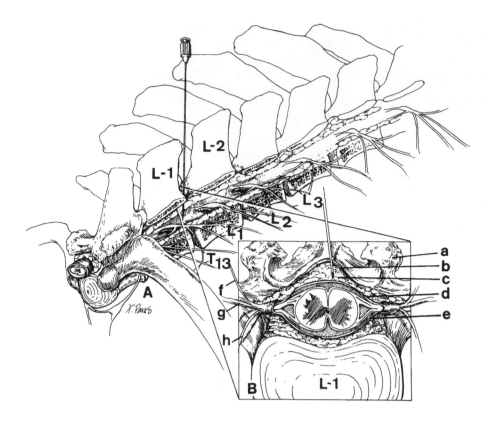

Fig. 23.11. Needle placement for segmental dorsolumbar epidural analgesia in cattle. **A:** Cranial and left lateral aspect of the thoracolumbar vertebrae and their associated spinal nerves T13 to L3 with needle tip placed at the L1 to L2 intervertebral space. **B:** Cranial view of a transection of the first lumbar vertebra at the location of the intervertebral foramen, showing the relation of the structures inside the spinal canal: *a*, articular process; *b*, interarcuate ligament; *c*, epidural space with fat and connective tissue; *d*, dura mater; *e*, arachnoid membrane; *f*, dorsal branch; *g*, ventral branch of first lumbar [L1] spinal nerve; and *h*, ramus communicans. From Skarda,[5] p. 634.

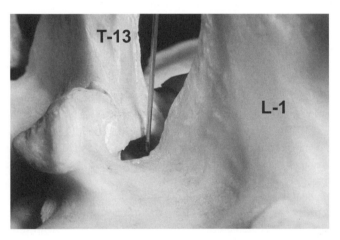

Fig. 23.12. The 11.25-cm, 18-gauge spinal needle is directed ventrally and medially of approximately 10° from vertical to enter the neural canal via intervertebral space, which is surrounded by the bases of the spinous processes cranially and caudally and by the intervertebral articular processes laterally (T13, thirteenth thoracic; and L1, first lumbar vertebra).

disappears after the point of the needle has passed through the ligament. An alternative method is to place a few drops of saline or local anesthetic solution in the hub of the needle and observe the drops being aspirated into the needle by the subatmospheric pressure of the epidural space (hanging-drop method).[63,64] If bleeding occurs, the stylet is placed into the needle, and the needle is withdrawn after 2 to 3 min. If the dura is inadvertently punctured and CSF is obtained, segmental thoracolumbar subarachnoid anesthe-

sia may be performed or the procedure terminated. After piercing through the interarcuate ligament, approximately 8 mL of either a 2% lidocaine hydrochloride solution or a 5% procaine hydrochloride solution can be injected in an average 500-kg cow. This amount of anesthetic is sufficient to desensitize the T13, L1, and L2 dermatomes within 7 to 20 min with a duration of 45 min to 2 h.[59] The needle must not be manipulated further, but should be removed immediately after injection in order to avoid damage to the spinal cord and meninges (Fig. 23.13).

Factors that influence epidural spread and duration of anesthesia include age, extradural fat, pregnancy, venous circulation, and variables that are under the direct control of the anesthetist, such as positioning of the patient, choosing the site for epidural puncture, orientation of the needle bevel, and determining the volume. Although there is considerable disagreement among authors about the ultimate mode of action of epidural anesthetics, spread of the anesthetic solution within the epidural space is the first event after injection. The epidural space at the thoracolumbar (T13-L1) or first lumbar (L1-L2) intervertebral space in cattle cannot be reached by the spinal needle if the interarcuate ligament is ossified because of old age (>8 years).[65]

The typical effects of segmental blockade in young ruminants reflect a predominantly paravertebral site of action, whereas the widespread anesthesia produced by injection of small volumes in elderly cattle indicates a more intense action within the subarachnoid space itself. The dura becomes more permeable to local anesthetics with age because of a progressive increase in the size and number of arachnoid villi, thereby providing a larger area through which local anesthetic can diffuse into the subarachnoid space. The epidural local anesthetic dose needs to be reduced

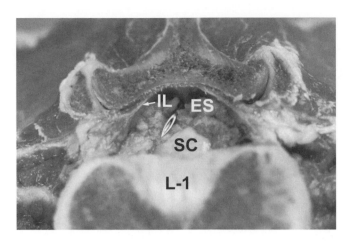

Fig. 23.13. Cranial view of a transection of the first lumbar (L1) vertebra at the location of the intervertebral foramen of an adult cow, with needle tip placed for unilateral (right side) segmental dorsolumbar epidural anesthesia. ES, epidural space with fat and connective tissue; SC, spinal cord; and L1, first lumbar vertebra.

slightly in old patients. Similarly, migration of epidural anesthetics is enhanced by distension (engorgement) of epidural veins in full-term pregnancy and increased quantities of fat in obesity. Selective anesthesia on one side of the spinal column is achieved by placing the needle tip within the epidural space across the midline and injecting small volumes of the anesthetic to the nerve roots on the contralateral side (Fig. 23.13). Bilateral anesthesia is achieved by administering either a larger volume of the anesthetic or a regular dose through a needle with its tip placed within the epidural space in the median plane dorsal to the spinal cord, and desensitizing the nerve roots on both sides. The bevel of the spinal needle is directed cranially to limit the caudal flow of the anesthetic, thereby minimizing the risk of loss of motor control of the pelvic limbs.

The area of segmental anesthesia is a function of total mass (volume × concentration) of drug injected. Increasing the volume or concentration will increase the area desensitized. In general, a single injection of a 2% or 3% lidocaine hydrochloride solution (10 mL), 4% or 5% procaine hydrochloride solution (10 mL), or a 2% tubocaine hydrochloride (10 to 15 mL) into the epidural space at the T13-L1 intervertebral space induced satisfactory anesthesia and relaxation of the abdominal wall and flank for operations such as rumenotomy and cesarean section, with the animal standing. Anesthesia develops approximately 10 min after injection and lasts approximately 2 h. Onset and duration of anesthesia vary widely between local anesthetic drugs and are influenced by several factors. (Table 23.1).

Segmental spread of anesthesia is improved by increasing the volume of the solution injected, whereas a more rapid onset of analgesia and motor blockade, greater frequency of adequate analgesia, greater depth of motor blockade, and longer periods of analgesia are better achieved by increasing the concentration of the anesthetic. The extent of cranial and caudal migration of dye (0.12% new methylene blue in 0.9% saline), rather than diffusion through meninges to CSF, after injection into the first interlum-

bar epidural space has been evaluated in cattle.[66] As can be expected, the number of stained vertebrae and amount of epidural fat and dura mater were greater in cows administered 10 mL compared with 5 mL of solution. However, the number of stained vertebrae in the 5-mL group was comparable to the number of dermatomes with bilateral analgesia after administration of the larger volume (10 mL) of local anesthetic (procaine), suggesting a wider distribution in the epidural space than provision of actual dermatomal analgesia.

Extradural fat content and venous circulation have also been shown to influence the spread and the pharmacokinetics of 5 mL of xylazine in 0.9% sodium chloride (NaCl) solution when injected into the dorsolumbar (L1-L2) epidural space.[67,68] A wider area of segmental analgesia with faster onset and longer analgesia was obtained with xylazine when injection was made deeper under the epidural fat. In comparison, the more superficial administration of xylazine between the periosteum and epidural fat produced uneven distribution of analgesia in the right and left flanks with a slower onset and shorter period of analgesia and sedation.[68]

Various flank surgeries, including cecotomy, cesarean section, laparoscopy, omentopexy, rumenotomy, duodenotomy, and fistulization, have been performed during dorsolumbar (L1-L2) epidural anesthesia achieved with either lidocaine, xylazine, or a combination of both drugs.[60,61] The injection depth used was about 9 mm deeper than the epidural entrance depth (8 cm). The number of analgesic dermatomes increased after injection of epidural xylazine (0.05 mg/kg) when compared with the epidural injection of lidocaine (0.2 mg/kg) alone.[60] The combination of 0.025 mg/kg of xylazine and 0.1 mg/kg of lidocaine was very effective in producing regional analgesia of the flank when performing standing laparotomy in conscious cattle.[60,61]

The antagonistic efficacy of atipamezole (0.025 mg/kg in 0.9% NaCl) given by either the intravenous or epidural route, 30 min after the onset of segmental thoracolumbar analgesia induced by the epidural injection of xylazine at the first lumbar intervertebral space, has been documented.[69] The wide range of segmental analgesia and slower-developing ataxia was considered evidence of xylazine diffusion into the CSF. Atipamezole given by either route (intravenous or epidural) reversed analgesia at the flank, as well as sedation. However, the flank area became desensitized again after intravenous atipamezole administration and remained so for nearly 2 h. Ataxia was more rapidly reversed by epidural atipamezole administration than by intravenous injection.[69] Although the mechanism by which epidurally administered xylazine produces analgesia remains controversial, the results of this study support an analgesic action being mediated by α_2-adrenergic receptors, not by a local anesthetic effect. Analgesia at the flank was completely reversed by atipamezole (0.025 mg/kg intravenously [IV] or epidurally), a specific and potent α_2-adrenergic receptor antagonist. Furthermore, α_2-adrenergic receptors and α_2-adrenergic receptor mRNAs have been identified on the dorsal and ventral root fibers and spinal cord of calves.[70]

As for knowing exactly where the local anesthetic block occurs following epidural administration, the critical CSF concentration of local anesthetic required to eliminate response to deep needle-prick stimulation at the thoracolumbar T13 to L1 dermatomes has been assessed.[71,72] The subarachnoid threshold concentration of procaine was reached after repeated epidural injections, but not after a single administration, indicating that segmental lumbar epidural anesthesia in cattle may be primarily due to analgesia of dura-covered roots outside the epidural space (paravertebral site), and to be minimally, if at all, dependent on desensitization of nerves within the subarachnoid space.

Finally, segmental spread of anesthesia is improved by a fast injection, but the advantage of a larger segmental area of analgesia is offset by a shorter duration, increased occurrence of incomplete analgesia, and high frequency of the patient's discomfort upon injection, which is probably attributable to transient elevation of CSF pressure. The rate of injection should be slow—a volume of 10 mL given over approximately 10 s.

Selective unilateral segmental (T13-L3) epidural anesthesia in cattle has been associated with decreases in arterial blood pressure and total peripheral resistance, with no changes in stroke volume, left ventricular stroke work, and left ventricular minute work. Increases in heart rate and cardiac output are typical.[73] Increases in cardiac output are believed to be caused by an increase in heart rate secondary to the decreased vascular resistance. Respiratory rate; arterial and mixed-venous pH, oxygen, and carbon dioxide tensions; oxyhemoglobin saturation; oxygen content; oxygen transport; and oxygen uptake remain unaltered, indicating that the sympathetic blockade caused by thoracolumbar epidural injection is well tolerated in nonsedated healthy cattle.[73]

The advantages of segmental dorsolumbar epidural anesthesia as compared with proximal and distal paravertebral anesthesia include the use of a single injection of a small quantity of anesthetic and uniform analgesia and relaxation of the skin, musculature, and parietal peritoneum. The disadvantages include difficulty in performing the technique, potential for trauma to the spinal cord or venous sinuses, and loss of motor control of the pelvic limbs; also, there is the potential for a more profound physiological disturbance owing to overdose or subarachnoid injection.

Continuous Lumbar Segmental Epidural Anesthesia

Continuous lumbar epidural anesthesia in cattle can be achieved by aseptically placing a catheter into the epidural space (Fig. 23.14). A 10.2-cm, 18-gauge thin-walled Tuohy needle with stylet is inserted into the epidural space at the thoracolumbar (T13-L1) interspace as previously described. This space is identified with reference to the last rib (T13) and the cranial edge of the transverse process of the first lumbar (L1) vertebra.[74] A small quantity of local anesthetic solution (2 to 3 mL) is injected along the track of the needle. The distance from the skin to the thoracolumbar (T13-L1) epidural space may vary between 8 and 12 cm, depending on size. Injection of 5 mL of air should not encounter resistance. If no CSF or blood flows from the needle, 1 mL of a 2% lidocaine hydrochloride solution is injected into the thoracolumbar epidural space during a 10-s period to avoid pain caused by impingement of the catheter and stylet at the spinal cord. After the bevel in the epidural space is directed caudally, a

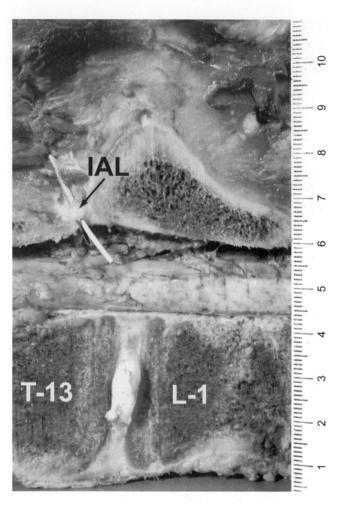

Fig. 23.14. Paramedian sagittal section of the thoracolumbar area of an adult cow with needle placement for catheterization of the lumbar epidural space (T13, thirteenth thoracic; and L1, first lumbar vertebra). IAL, interarcuate ligament.

commercially available 91.8-cm, 20-gauge Teflon epidural catheter with graduated markings and stylet is introduced into the needle and advanced caudally 3 to 5 cm beyond the tip of the needle. The needle is removed from the catheter while the catheter is left in position and sutured to the skin at the site of emergence from the skin.

Injection of approximately 6 mL of a 2% lidocaine hydrochloride solution or a 5% procaine hydrochloride solution at the anterior portion of the lumbar (L1 to L2) area should produce unilateral or bilateral anesthesia extending from spinal cord segments T12 to L4 of adult cows. Analgesia is achieved 10 to 20 min after completion of the injection and lasts 1 h to 1 h 40 min.[74] A more caudal spread of epidural block can be expected with an injection of local anesthetic more caudal than L2. An overdose of local anesthetic (>6 mL) to the L2 area or a regular dose of anesthetic at a more caudal level than L2 should be avoided to prevent anesthesia of the femoral and sciatic nerves and thus loss of pelvic limb function.[74] The reason for unilateral analgesia could be attributable to placement of the epidural catheter at the nerve roots on one side, minimal circumferential

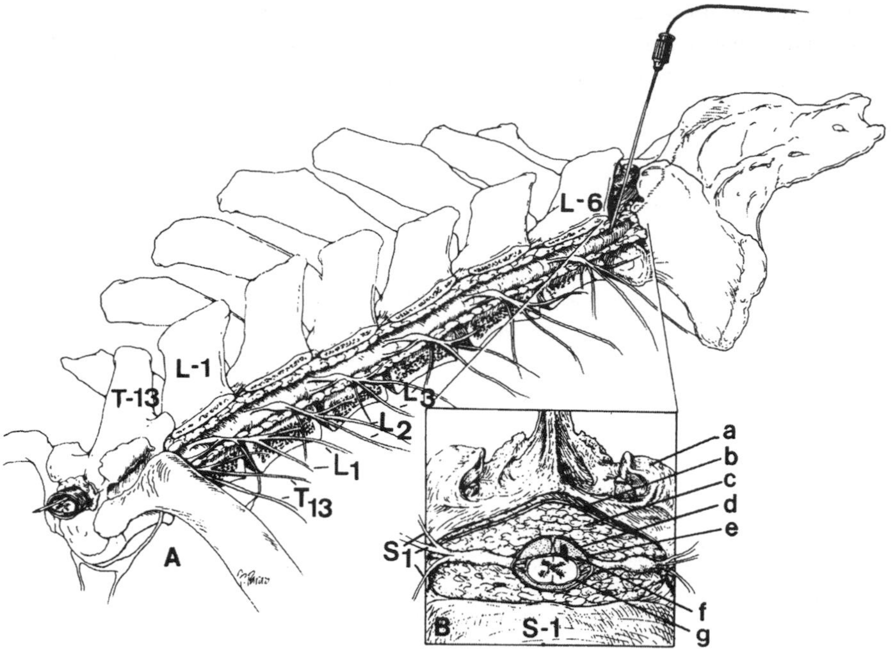

Fig. 23.15. Needle and catheter placement for thoracolumbar subarachnoid analgesia in cattle. **A:** Cranial and left lateral aspect of the bovine thoracolumbar and sacral vertebrae and their associated spinal nerves T13 to L3, with needle tip placed at the lumbosacral intervertebral space. **B:** Cranial view of a transection of the first sacral vertebra at the location of the intervertebral foramen, showing the relation of the structures inside the spinal canal: *a*, articular process; *b*, interarcuate ligament; *c*, epidural space with fat and connective tissue; *d*, dura mater; *e*, arachnoid membrane; *f*, subarachnoid space with cerebral spinal fluid and needle tip; and *g*, pia mater. From Skarda,[5] p. 635.

dissipation (overflow) of local anesthetic around the dura mater spinalis, and lateral escape of the local anesthetic from the epidural space through patent intervertebral foramina.

In comparison to segmental epidural anesthesia, produced by injection of local anesthetic through a spinal needle, continuous segmental epidural anesthesia offers the advantages of providing a route for repeated small fractional maintenance doses of local anesthetic drug, making the extent of anesthesia more readily controlled and producing a lower frequency of accidental subarachnoid administration of local anesthetic. The reported disadvantages of the catheter technique include higher frequency of postanesthetic myositis, caused by the larger bore and blunter needle, higher frequency of unilateral blockade, unpredictability of whether ipsilateral or contralateral anesthesia develops, and lack of analgesia after passage of the catheter tip into the paravertebral space.

Thoracolumbar Subarachnoid Anesthesia

In cattle, this is performed by aseptically introducing a catheter into the subarachnoid space at the lumbosacral (L6-S1) intervertebral space and advancing it to the thoracolumbar (T13-L1) intervertebral space (Fig. 23.15).[74–77] Although the dorsal subarachnoid space in cattle can be penetrated at the thoracolumbar (T13-L1) and first lumbar (L1-L2) intervertebral spaces, dura puncture at these sites is not recommended because of potential trauma to the spinal cord. Cattle must be well restrained in a stock to facilitate the catheterization procedure. The skin at the lumbosacral (L6-S1) intervertebral space and lumbosacral fascia adjacent to the interspinous (L6-S1) ligaments are injected with approximately 5 mL of a 2% lidocaine hydrochloride solution, using a 15-cm, 18-gauge spinal needle. The space is located 1 to 2 cm caudal of a line drawn between the cranial edge of each tuber sacrale and the dorsal midline.

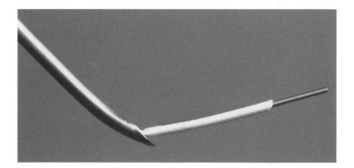

Fig. 23.16. The tip of a 17-gauge Huber-point Tuohy needle with Formocath polyethylene catheter (0.095-cm outside diameter), reinforced with a stainless-steel spring guide (0.05-cm outside diameter).

A larger-bore (17.5-cm, 17-gauge) Huber-point Tuohy needle with stylet is inserted at the desensitized L6-S1 site and is advanced along the median plane perpendicular to the spinal cord until the needle enters the subarachnoid space. The bevel of the needle is directed cranially, the stylet is removed, and 2 to 3 mL of CSF is aspirated. Occasionally, it is necessary to make several minor adjustments before the needle is satisfactorily positioned into the subarachnoid space. Redirection of the needle is required if CSF cannot be obtained, and should be accomplished after almost complete withdrawal of the needle to prevent bending it. Upon CSF aspiration, a Formocath polyethylene catheter 80 to 100 cm long with a 0.095-cm outside diameter, reinforced with a stainless-steel spring guide (0.05-cm outside diameter), is passed through the needle (Fig. 23.16) and advanced approximately 60 cm to the midthoracic area. Minimal resistance to catheter advancement and no movement of the patient indicate proper technique, without kinking and curling of the catheter and no trauma to the spinal nerve roots within the subarachnoid space. The needle is withdrawn over the catheter; then the spring guide is removed and a catheter adapter or a 23-gauge needle with a three-way stopcock is attached to the catheter. The catheter is then gently withdrawn a calculated distance to place its tip at T13-L1.

The catheter must never be withdrawn after advancing it through the spinal needle because withdrawal may shear off the catheter within the subarachnoid space.[75,78] The following measurements are made to place the catheter tip at the T13-L1 intervertebral space: (a) the total length of the catheter (T), (b) the distance BC between the skin surface (B) and the subarachnoid puncture site (C), and (c) the distance CD between the lumbosacral (C) and thoracolumbar (D) intervertebral space: ($T = AB + BC + CD$). The length of the free end of the external catheter and the skin surface (AB) equals the total length of the catheter minus the distance from entering the skin to the tip of the subarachnoidally placed catheter: $AB = T - (BC + CD)$. The average distance between the palpable lumbosacral (L6-S1) and thoracolumbar (T13-L1) intervertebral spaces was approximately 45 cm in adult cows.[75] Proper subarachnoid positioning of the catheter can be radiographically confirmed if the guidewire is left in position (Fig. 23.17).

A small dose (1.5 to 2.0 mL) of a 2% lidocaine hydrochloride solution or a 5% procaine hydrochloride solution is injected at a rate of approximately 0.5 mL/min. Surgical anesthesia extending from spinal cord segment T9 to L3 on one or both sides is maximal 5 to 10 min after injection and lasts for 20 min to 1 h 20 min.[75] The absorption of drug into the systemic circulation determines the decline of subarachnoid anesthetic concentration and thus the duration of subarachnoid analgesia. The spinal fluid concentration necessary for analgesia is approximately 200-μg procaine/mL in calves and adult cows,[65,71] and is easily maintained by fractional bolus administration of 0.5 mL of the anesthetic at 30-min intervals or as needed. In vitro measurements of the rate of hydrolysis of procaine in spinal fluid taken from adult cows did not detect changes in the spinal fluid concentration of procaine after a 2-h incubation (37°C).[72]

When compared with dorsolumbar epidural analgesia, the advantages of thoracolumbar subarachnoid analgesia include simplicity of needle and catheter placements, anesthetic deposition at nerve roots (and thus a minimal dose requirement), minimal physiological disturbance, and small doses for maintenance of analgesia. A disadvantage of the catheter technique is the unpredictability of whether ipsilateral or contralateral analgesia develops. The cause for the one-sided block has not been investigated, but could be attributable to minimal circumferential dissipation (overflow) of local anesthetic around the pia mater spinalis after placement of the catheter at the ventral surface of the spinal cord, where it could be trapped between the trabecula and dorsal longitudinal ligament. Kinking and curling of the catheter are readily determined by lack of CSF aspiration and avoidance responses of cattle. Accidental vascular puncture and faulty catheter positioning make the technique ineffective for producing abdominal analgesia of the flank region. Thoracolumbar subarachnoid anesthesia is not readily applicable for field use because it requires special equipment, precise dosage administration and catheter placement, and maintenance of sterility.

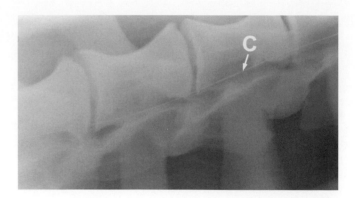

Fig. 23.17. Radiograph of the caudal lumbar vertebrae of an adult Holstein cow (630 kg) with a catheter (C) in the subarachnoid space; a lateral oblique view.

Anesthesia for Obstetric Procedures and Relief of Rectal Tenesmus

At least four techniques are advocated in ruminants for pain relief and muscle relaxation during obstetric manipulations and surgical procedures involving the tail, perineum, anus, rectum, vulva, vagina, prepuce, and skin and scrotum. These techniques include the caudal epidural, continuous caudal epidural, sacral paravertebral, and pudendal nerve blocks. Any of these techniques may be used for a number of surgical procedures, such as suturing tears in the perineum and vulva, reconstruction of the perineum (Gotze's operation), retraction of the uterine cervix, reduction of prolapsed uterus, ovariectomy, and embryotomy. These techniques may also be used as adjunctive treatments for controlling rectal tenesmus associated with irritation of the perineum, anus, rectum, and vagina. Properly performed blocks do not desensitize femoral and ischial nerves, thereby preserving pelvic limb function. These techniques are not applicable to pigs.

Caudal Epidural Anesthesia

Because this technique is simple and inexpensive, and requires no sophisticated equipment, it is routinely used in cows, sheep, and goats. Needle placement is either at the sacrococcygeal (S5-Co1) or more commonly at the first coccygeal (Co1-Co2) interspace, beyond the termination of the spinal cord and meninges (Fig. 23.18).[79,80] Only the coccygeal nerves, the thin phylum terminale, the vasculature, and epidural fat and connective tissue remain in the spinal canal at the site of needle penetration, and these structures are not easily damaged when using aseptic technique.[80] The location of the Co1-Co2 interspace is easily identified by elevating and lowering the tail and palpating the depression and movement between the respective vertebrae. The Co1-Co2 interspace is larger and more easily penetrated than the S5-Co1 site. The S5-Co1 interspace may be ossified in older cows and is not so easily detectable in fat cows.[81]

The skin over the Co1-Co2 joint space is disinfected and desensitized with small amount (2 to 3 mL) of local anesthetic to ensure minimal movement during insertion of a 3.75- to 5-cm, 18-gauge needle. The epidural needle is inserted in a median

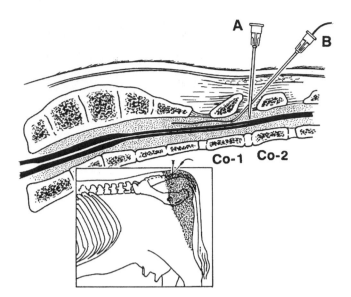

Fig. 23.18. Needle placement for caudal epidural analgesia and catheterization of the sacral epidural space in cattle. Co1, first coccygeal; and Co2, second coccygeal vertebra. The desensitized subcutaneous area after caudal blockade is *stippled*: epidural needle placement (*A*) and epidural catheter placement (*B*).

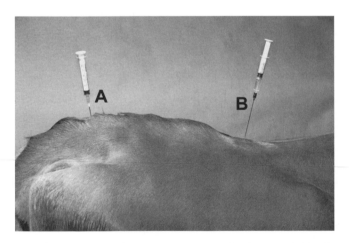

Fig. 23.19. *A:* A 3.75-cm, 18-gauge needle is placed into the epidural space at the first coccygeal (Co1-Co2) intervertebral space of a Jersey cow (460 kg). *B:* A 15-cm, 20-gauge spinal needle is placed into the epidural space at the lumbosacral (L6-S1) intervertebral space.

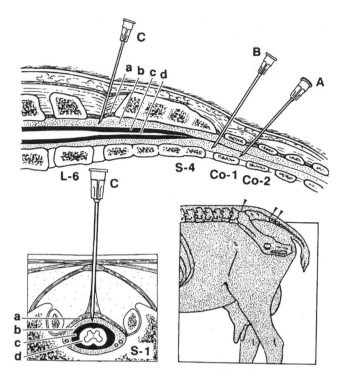

Fig. 23.20. Needle placement for caudal epidural analgesia (*A* and *B*) and lumbosacral epidural analgesia (*C*) in goats: L6, sixth lumbar; S4, fourth sacral; Co1, first coccygeal; and Co2, second coccygeal vertebra. A cranial view of a transection of the first sacral vertebra at the location of the intervertebral foramen is shown in the **bottom left inset**: *a*, interarcuate ligament; *b*, epidural space; *c*, subarachnoid space; and *d*, spinal cord. The desensitized subcutaneous area after anterior epidural anesthesia is *stippled* and often extends to the umbilicus of the goat and is shown in the **bottom right inset**.

plane until it contacts the floor of the vertebral canal while it is directed either at right angle to the general contour of the croup or ventrocranially at an angle of approximately 10° to vertically (Fig. 23.19A). The needle is then withdrawn approximately 0.5 cm from the ligamentous floor or intervertebral disk to place its tip in the epidural space of the neural canal. Aspiration of a few drops of the anesthetic from the hub into the needle and minimal resistance to injection of the anesthetic indicate that the bevel is placed epidurally.

Production of caudal anesthesia depends on the total dose (volume × concentration) of the anesthetic administered. When 1 mL of a 2% lidocaine hydrochloride solution per 100 kg of body weight is injected at a rate of 1 mL/s, the area of anesthesia extends cranially to the middle of the sacrum and ventrally over the perineum to the inner aspect of the thigh. Proper techniques should desensitize the pelvic viscera and genitalia, and paralyze the tail and abolish abdominal contractions.[82] However, locomotor function of the hind legs and uterine motility remain unaffected. Maximal anesthesia may require 10 to 20 min and can be expected to last 30 min to 2½ h.

Caudal epidural anesthesia in sheep and goats can be extremely useful for tail docking in lambs and for intravaginal obstetric procedures.[83,84] A 2.5- to 3.75-cm, 18-gauge needle is inserted epidurally at Co1-Co2 or S5-Co1 (Fig. 23.20), and no more than 1 mL of a 2% lidocaine hydrochloride solution per 50 kg of body weight is injected. Careful aseptic precautions similar to the technique in cattle must be used. Although a 2% lidocaine hydrochloride solution is now almost universally used, the addition of 0.125 mL of 1:80,000 epinephrine per milliliter of anesthetic can suppress the tone and motility of the tail for longer than 1 h.[85]

Adjusting the pH of a 2% lidocaine hydrochloride solution from 6.3 to 6.9 by the addition of 1 mL of 8.4% sodium bicarbonate solution (1 mEq) to 10 mL of lidocaine has little or no effect on the time of onset and duration of caudal epidural anesthesia in cattle.[86]

Caudal Epidural Analgesia with α₂-Adrenergic Agonists

α_2-Adrenoceptor agonists, such as xylazine, detomidine, medetomidine, and clonidine, have been injected into the caudal epidural space of cattle in an attempt to produce prolonged analgesia (2 to 3 h) of perineal/or flank areas, which is satisfactory for most surgical or obstetric procedures in cattle and llamas.[87–109]

With the exception of bupivacaine, local anesthetic drugs, such as procaine, lidocaine, and mepivacaine, when administered into the epidural space at the first coccygeal (Co1-Co2) or sacrococcygeal (S3-Co1) intervertebral space, provide perineal analgesia accompanied by muscle paralysis (30 min to 2¹/₂ h) and may have to be readministered to enable completion of prolonged surgical procedures. In contrast to the effects of local anesthetics, the α_2-adrenoceptor agonists produce analgesia with minimal proprioception deficits or motor nerve blockade.

Caudal Epidural Xylazine

Perineal analgesia lasts significantly longer (up to 3 h) in cattle after injection of 0.05 mg of xylazine/kg of body weight, diluted to a 5-mL volume with sterile water into the epidural space at the Co1-Co2 intervertebral space, than when lidocaine is injected.[88–90,97,102,106] However, side effects, such as sedation, mild ataxia, bradycardia, hypotension, respiratory acidosis, hypoxemia, and ruminal amotility, are routinely observed in conscious standing cattle when xylazine is given epidurally.[93,95,98,102] These side effects can be partially reversed by intravenous administration of tolazoline (0.3 mg/kg), an α_2-adrenoceptor antagonist, while not diminishing the desirable local (S3 to the coccyx) analgesic effects.[94] Nonetheless, care must be taken to limit the volume of xylazine and its rostral spread to the femoral and sciatic nerves. Xylazine appears to exhibit some direct local anesthetic sensory and motor nerve–blocking actions in addition to its spinal cord α_2-adrenoceptor–mediated analgesic effects.

Xylazine hydrochloride (0.05 mg/kg in 5 mL) diffuses from the caudal epidural space into the CSF of adult cattle and can produce a degree of subarachnoid nerve-root anesthesia.[90,91] Xylazine is not detectable in bovine plasma, however, making it doubtful that its presence within the subarachnoid space after epidural administration is secondary to absorption of xylazine from the bloodstream.[91] Because uterine motility can increase after epidural xylazine administration, this technique is not recommended for providing analgesia during obstetric procedures in pregnant ruminants or fetotomy procedures.[89]

As might be expected, the degree of analgesia, sedation, and ataxia is dose dependent with sacrococcygeal epidural xylazine administration. With increased doses of xylazine (50, 70, 100 µg/kg), perineal analgesia and marked systemic effects (e.g., sedation, decreased heart and respiratory rates, and decreased rumen motility and bloat) have been prolonged. Further increases of the xylazine dose (120 µg/kg) extend analgesia to the udder without affecting the flank, along with marked sedation, sternal decubitus, ptyalism, and ptosis.[96,100]

Irreversible paralysis in three cows and a near fatal apnea in one calf after epidural administration of xylazine have been reported.[106] Although necropsy of the recumbent cows demonstrated marked demyelinization of the lumbar spinal cord, it is not clear whether the preservative in the xylazine, or the drug itself, produced the demyelinization. Further studies are needed to determine whether analgesia induced by epidurally or subarachnoidally administered xylazine may, in part, be due to demyelinization of the spinal cord.

Caudal Epidural Xylazine and Lidocaine

By reducing the dose of xylazine to 0.03 mg/kg of body weight and adding a 2% lidocaine hydrochloride solution to a total volume of 5 mL, a more useful epidural anesthetic action may be achieved when performing procedures such as rumenotomy, cesarean section, correction of vaginal or uterine prolapse, repairs of perineal lacerations and rectovestibular fistulae, and removal of vaginal tumors.[97] The xylazine-lidocaine combination extends analgesia as far cranially as the T13 and L1 spinal segments, thereby covering the tail, perineum, udder, and flank areas. Surgical analgesia is attained in 3 to 4 min after drug administration and lasts for about 1 h 40 min, with a moderate degree of ataxia.[97] Although the combination of xylazine and lidocaine typically produces sedation and mild ataxia, the analgesia lasts longer than that achieved with either xylazine or lidocaine alone.[103]

Caudal epidural anesthesia has also been used in llamas on occasion. Either 2% lidocaine (0.22 mg/kg), 10% xylazine (0.17 mg/kg) diluted with 2 mL of sterile water, or the combination of 2% lidocaine (0.22 mg/kg) and 10% xylazine (0.17 mg/kg) have been injected into the epidural space at the sacrococcygeal (S5-Co1) junction.[104,105] Duration of analgesia is extended with the combination of xylazine and lidocaine to nearly 3¹/₂ h compared with just over 1 h with lidocaine alone. Mild sedation is often apparent 20 min after epidural xylazine administration, and at this dose lasts approximately 30 min.[105]

Caudal Epidural Detomidine

Both the epidural administration and the intramuscular administration of detomidine (40 µg/kg) in cattle appear to induce comparable degrees of analgesia of the perineum and flank, moderate sedation and ataxia, hypertension, cardiopulmonary depression, and ruminal hypermotility.[107] Consequently, the epidural administration of detomidine does not appear to be more or less advantageous or disadvantageous than intramuscular administration.

Caudal Epidural Medetomidine

The analgesic, cardiovascular, and respiratory effects of epidural medetomidine (15 µg/kg diluted in 5 mL of 0.9% NaCl) injection at the first or second coccygeal intervertebral space in adult cattle has been evaluated.[108] Medetomidine induced perineal analgesia within 5 to 10 min, which lasted nearly 7 h, but was accompanied by mild to moderate sedation. The degree of medetomidine-induced analgesia was more pronounced and the duration longer than that achieved with a standard epidural dose of lidocaine. Two of six cows became recumbent, but were easily coaxed to stand. Salivation was evident, as was the increased frequency of urination after medetomidine. Heart and respiratory rates were decreased, but arterial blood pressure remained unchanged.[108]

Caudal Epidural Clonidine Epidural clonidine administration can produce profound antinociception in people, cattle, sheep, goats, pigs, and horses without the sensory or motor blockade of local anesthetics.[109–119] Although epidurally and intrathecally administered clonidine has been successfully employed as an analgesic in human patients for treatment of acute postoperative pain and in patients tolerant to intrathecally administered opiates, its use has been somewhat limited because of its short-acting analgesic effect and accompanying sedation, hypotension, bradycardia, and respiratory depression.[120,121]

Caudal Epidural Ketamine

Ketamine alone has been administered into the epidural space at the first intercoccygeal (Co1-Co2) space of cattle. It induces dose-dependent depression (0.5, 1.0, and 2.0 mg/kg) of pain stimulus in the tail, vulva, anus, and perineum, but not in the hind-limb area, and produces minimal sedation, ataxia, cardiopulmonary effects, and changes in rumen function.[122,123] The 0.5-mg/kg dose produced lack of response to stimulation of the tail only, whereas 1 mg/kg produced variable analgesia, lasting 55 min in the tail and 15 min in the anus and perineum, but having no effect in the vulva. The 2-mg/kg dose of ketamine produced analgesia in all regions tested, lasting 1 h 15 min in the anus and perineum, 1 h 20 min in the vulva, and up to 1 h 40 min in the tail, but this dose was accompanied by moderate sedation and ataxia in two cows. At these doses, ketamine did not induce any analgesia in the hind limbs.[122]

In a similar study, cattle were injected with 5, 10, and 20 mL of 5% ketamine at the first intercoccygeal (Co1-Co2) space.[123] Dose-dependent analgesia without sedation was observed at the tail and perineum 5 min after all three doses. Analgesia lasted from 20 min (low dose) to 1 h (high dose). Moderate ataxia was observed with the 20-mL dose of ketamine. One cow became recumbent after a 20-mL ketamine dose administration. Respiratory rate, mean arterial blood pressure, rumen motility, and rectal temperature were not affected.[123]

Continuous Caudal Epidural Anesthesia

This is indicated in cattle and sheep with prolapse of the vagina and/or rectum, which can provoke severe continuous straining. The technique in cattle is simply performed by inserting a fine catheter into the epidural space at S5-Co1 or Co1-Co2 through a 7.5-cm, 16- or 17-gauge needle, which is either a thin-walled Huber-point directional needle or a Hustead needle.[124,125] The skin and the needle track are desensitized. After a stab incision on the midline is made to minimize resistance to the passage of the somewhat blunt needle, the spinal needle with stylet in place and bevel directed cranially is advanced for 5 to 8 cm while being directed at approximately 45° to vertical until resistance to needle passage is abruptly reduced. The stylet from the needle is removed, and a test dose of 2 to 3 mL of anesthetic is injected with

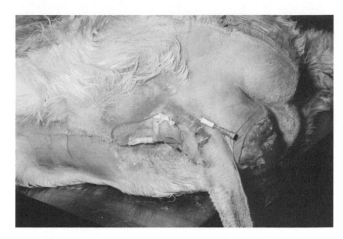

Fig. 23.21. An epidural catheter with adapter in a calf with rectal prolapse.

almost no resistance, assuring proper placement of the needle in the epidural space.

A 30-cm medical-grade vinyl epidural catheter (0.036-cm outside diameter) with gradual markings is introduced into the canal through the needle and advanced cranially 3 to 4 cm beyond the tip of the needle (Fig. 23.18B). The needle is then withdrawn, leaving the catheter in position. Approximately 3 to 5 mL of a 2% lidocaine hydrochloride solution is injected into the catheter at 4- to 6-h intervals or whenever the animal shows signs of straining. The catheter adapter or 23-gauge needle and three-way stopcock are placed on the free end of the catheter. The catheter can be used for many hours of infusion if it is sutured to the skin puncture site with adhesive tape. The sterility of the free end of the catheter is maintained by using protective sterile gauze (Fig. 23.21).

Alcohol epidural injection can be used for long-term demyelinization of nerve roots in sheep and goats. First, only 0.5 to 1.0 mL of a 2% lidocaine hydrochloride solution per 50 kg of body weight is injected epidurally at Co1-Co2 or S5-Co1, and the extent of caudal analgesia is noted to ensure that the level of rostral spread does not extend to the sciatic or femoral nerve roots. After full sensation has returned, a mixture of equal volumes of 70% to 95% ethyl or isopropyl alcohol and a 2% lidocaine hydrochloride solution is injected at the same site, using a similar volume and injection rate as the previous injection.

Analgesia of the pelvic and perineal area and paralysis of the tail should result and last from a few days to several months, depending on the time required for remyelinization of the nerves.[126] The alcohol technique is not practical in cattle because the prolonged flaccidity of the tail may lead to buildup of manure and urine in the perineal area, with subsequent dermal excoriation and maggot infestation during fly season. The problems of alcohol epidural anesthesia in sheep and goats with docked tails are similar to, but less serious than, those in cattle. The chronic flaccid tail may possibly become inflamed, necrotic, and purulent, leading to a fly strike in the rectal area. Prolonged rear-limb paralysis from the demyelinization of sciatic and femoral nerve roots can result from overdosing on alcohol epidural anesthetic.

Sacral Paravertebral Anesthesia

Sacral paravertebral injection is advocated to relieve rectal tenesmus associated with rectal prolapse without sciatic nerve dysfunction.[127,128] This technique is associated with minimal risk of the animal's lying down and maintenance of motor function of the tail. Success of the technique depends on blockade of the pelvic splanchnic nerve (medial hemorrhoidal nerve) and caudal rectal nerve (caudal hemorrhoidal nerve), which supply sensory fibers to the anus, vulva, and vagina. The third, fourth, and fifth sacral spinal nerves (S3, S4, and S5) are major components of the pelvic splanchnic and caudal rectal nerves and are desensitized at the emergence from the sacrum on both sides of the spine in cattle and sheep. In males, S3 supplies motor fibers to the retractor penis muscle and, in order to prevent preputial prolapse, must not be desensitized. With the animal in standing restraint and good control of anterior, posterior, and lateral movement, the skin of the dorsal sacral area is cleansed and disinfected. Hair removal is optional. The general anatomical site of sacral foramina S3, S4, and S5 is identified approximately 1.0 to 1.5 cm from the dorsal midline of the vertebral crest or usually just lateral to the border of the crest.

Nerve S5 is at the sacrococcygeal (S5-Co1) junction. Nerves S4 and S3 exit from the S4 and S3 foramina, 3 and 6 cm cranial to the S5 foramen in yearling-to-adult cattle. A 5- to 7.5-cm, 16- or 18-gauge needle, preferably with stylet, is inserted ventrally to a depth just beyond where it enters the foramen (Fig. 23.22). A stab incision through the desensitized skin facilitates the insertion of the needle. A 2% lidocaine hydrochloride solution (5 to 10 mL) is injected into a 1-cm-diameter area within each dorsal foramen to desensitize both the dorsal and ventral rami of that nerve. Anesthesia of the anus, vulva, and vagina can be expected within 10 min after completion of injection and typically lasts for approximately 2 h. No unfavorable sequelae associated with urination and defecation should occur, because urinary bladder sphincter tone and motor function of the tail are maintained, although the motor function of the anal sphincter is slightly reduced. Sensation to the clitoris is unaffected.

Long-term anesthesia (up to 5 weeks) of the sacral area, as determined by observing no avoidance responses to deep needle prick to skin and muscle, may be produced by the administration of 1 to 2 mL of 70% to 95% ethyl or isopropyl alcohol to S3, S4, and S5, without the unfavorable sequelae associated with alcohol epidural anesthesia.[127,128] Caudal epidural analgesia with a 2% lidocaine hydrochloride solution greatly facilitates the subsequent alcohol paravertebral technique.

Bilateral sacral (S3, S4, and S5) paravertebral analgesia can be produced in sheep and goats similarly to that in cattle by using a 7.5-cm, 18-gauge needle, except that the volume of lidocaine, alcohol, and alcohol-anesthetic mixture is reduced to 1 to 2 mL per injection site.

The advantage of sacral paravertebral anesthesia when compared with epidural anesthesia is relief of straining without sciatic nerve dysfunction, thereby maintaining pelvic limb function and viability of the tail. The disadvantages are technical difficulty and paraphimosis in bulls if S3 is chronically desensitized with alcohol.

Desensitization of the Internal Pudendal (Pudic) Nerves

This technique is used either in standing males for penile analgesia and relaxation distal to the sigmoid flexure and examination of prolapsed penis[129,130] or in standing females for relief of straining caused by uterine prolapse or chronic vaginal prolapse.[131,132] The internal pudendal nerve block is useful in the surgical management of a number of surgical procedures, including repair of uterovaginal prolapse; cervicovaginopexy; anorectal prolapse (rectopexy); ablation of anorectal, perianal, and intra-anal tumors, polyps, and abscesses; and catheterization for dislodging urethral calculi.[131] The technique involves desensitizing the internal pudendal nerve fibers of the ventral branches (S3 and S4) and the anastomotic branch of the middle hemorrhoidal nerve (S3 and S4), using an ischiorectal fossa approach. With cattle restrained in a standing position, the lesser sciatic foramen is identified by rectal palpation as a soft circumscribed depres-

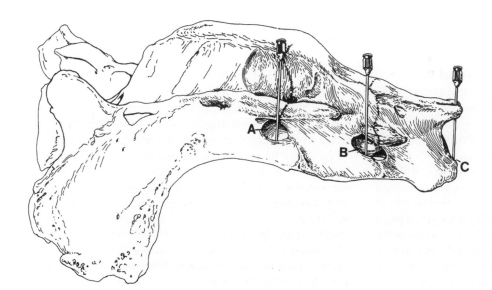

Fig. 23.22. Needle placement for sacral paravertebral analgesia in cattle. Third (*A*), fourth (*B*), and fifth (*C*) sacral foramen. From Skarda,[5] p. 640.

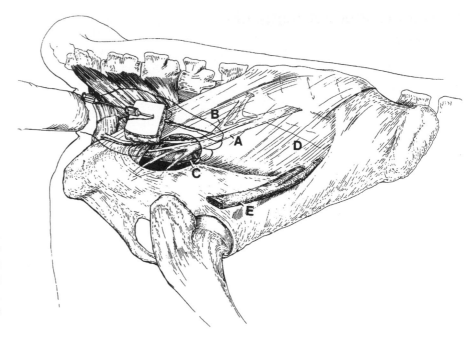

Fig. 23.23. Needle placement to the internal pudendal nerve in cattle. The position of the hand palpating the internal pudendal nerve (*A*) on the right side is shown. Caudal rectal nerve (*B*), internal pudendal artery (*C*), sacrosciatic ligament (*D*), and sciatic nerve (*E*). From Skarda,[5] p. 641.

sion in the sacrosciatic ligament. The foramen is less than a hand's breadth (5 cm) cranial to the anus. The pulsation of the internal pudendal artery can be felt a finger's width ventral to the internal pudendal nerve in the fossa.

The skin over the ischiorectal fossa on both sides is disinfected and desensitized with 2 to 3 mL of a 2% lidocaine hydrochloride solution. A 1.25-cm, 14-gauge needle to serve as a cannula for an 8.25-cm, 18-gauge spinal needle is inserted through the desensitized skin. The longer needle is then inserted via cannula for a distance of approximately 5 to 7 cm slightly downward until it contacts the internal pudendal nerve at the deepest point of the ischiorectal fossa (Fig. 23.23). The position of the needle point is verified by rectal digital palpation. Up to 25 mL of the local anesthetic solution (2% or 3% lidocaine hydrochloride) is injected around the nerve. The needle is then partially withdrawn and directed 2 to 3 cm more caudodorsally, where an additional 10 mL of the anesthetic is deposited at the cranial border of the foramen to desensitize the muscular branches and caudal rectal nerve (middle hemorrhoidal nerve).[129,133] The position of the hands is reversed, and the procedure is repeated on the opposite side of the pelvis. Pudendal nerve block is effective after 30 min and should last for 2 to 4 h. The addition of hyaluronidase (150 IU) and epinephrine (1:10,000) to the local anesthetic reduces the anesthetic required (20 mL) and increases the duration of anesthesia.[134] Success with the pudendal nerve block depends on locating pelvic landmarks.

A relatively simple technique for approaching the internal pudendal nerve in sheep from the lateral side has been described.[135] A finger is placed into the rectum to locate the slitlike sciatic foramen. A 3.75-cm, 18-gauge needle is then inserted through the corresponding skin site, and its point is advanced to the foramen. A 2% lidocaine hydrochloride solution (3 to 5 mL) is de-

posited at the foramen. The needle is withdrawn, and the injection site is massaged. The procedure is repeated on the opposite side while keeping the finger in the rectum.

When compared with caudal epidural anesthesia, the advantages of internal pudendal nerve desensitization are that sciatic nerve function and tail tone are maintained and that the volume of local anesthetic needed to desensitize the nerve supply to the penis by the epidural technique invariably causes posterior paralysis. Ballooning of the vagina may also aid in retention after it is repositioned in cows with prolapse.[131] The disadvantages of internal pudendal nerve block are lack of cervical analgesia and the necessity of identifying the injection sites by rectal palpation. The bull's penis should be protected from injury by replacing it into the prepuce and taping or purse stringing the external preputial orifice.

Desensitization of the Dorsal Nerve of the Penis

The dorsal nerve of the penis as it passes over the ischial arch may be desensitized for penile anesthesia and relaxation as an alternative technique to the internal pudendal nerve block.[136] The skin adjacent to the penile body approximately 10 cm ventral to the anus and 2.5 cm from the midline is infiltrated with 2 to 3 mL of a 2% lidocaine hydrochloride solution, using a fine needle (22 to 25 gauge). A 4-cm, 20-gauge needle is then inserted through the desensitized skin and advanced for 5 to 7 cm to contact the pelvic floor. Aspiration assures that the needle tip is not placed into the dorsal artery of the penis. While the needle is withdrawn for approximately 1 cm, the region is infiltrated with 20 to 30 mL of a 2% lidocaine hydrochloride solution. The procedure is repeated on the opposite side of the penis. Analgesia and paralysis of the penis are expected within 20 min and should last for 1 to 2 h.

Anterior Epidural Anesthesia

Introduction

Anterior epidural anesthesia is advocated for all procedures caudal to the diaphragm. The anesthetic solution, dosed at 1 mL/4.5 kg of body weight, is injected into the epidural space either at the lumbosacral (L6-S1) junction (lumbosacral epidural anesthesia) or at the sacrococcygeal (S5-Co1) or first intercoccygeal (Co1-Co2) space, using a larger volume of the anesthetic ranging from 40 mL to 150 mL in adult cattle and 5 mL to 25 mL in calves (high caudal epidural anesthesia). The site for needle placement at the lumbosacral site in lighter, immature cattle, sheep, and goats is usually palpable as a depression on the midline caudal to a line joining the anterior border of the ilium on each side (Fig. 23.20C), so injection is made at this site. The lumbosacral space in swine is the only practical injection site for inducing epidural anesthesia, making lumbosacral epidural block the most commonly used form of regional analgesia in swine. The sacrococcygeal or first intercoccygeal space is the injection site of choice in adult cattle and bulls for producing anterior block because the technique is relatively simple and trauma to the spinal cord and meninges are avoided. These structures end cranial to the site of injection, and the risk of injecting the local anesthetic into the subarachnoid space is almost nonexistent.

Proper techniques by either the lumbosacral or coccygeal approach should provide analgesia of the perineal region, the entire inguinal region, the flanks, and the abdominal wall up to the umbilicus. Cranial spread of the anesthetic affects the pelvic limb function by desensitizing the sixth lumbar (L6) and first and second sacral (S1 and S2) spinal nerves (sciatic supply), the fifth and sixth lumbar (L5 and L6) spinal nerves (obturator and femoral supply), and more cranial nerves. Depending on the degree involved, the dysfunction of hind limbs ranges from mild ataxia to complete posterior paralysis. Injury (e.g., hip dislocation) during onset (ataxia) or recovery must be avoided and can be prevented if the animals are restrained in sternal recumbency with their hind legs roped together proximal to the tarsus until recovery is complete, as determined by normal tail function. A major difficulty in producing anterior epidural anesthesia is the uncertainty of the precise extent of paralysis produced. Many factors have been shown to affect the cranial spread of the anesthetic within the epidural space. The major determinants are the size and age of the animal, the presence and size of abdominal mass (pregnancy), and other variables that can be controlled by the anesthetist, namely, positioning the patient, choosing the site of epidural puncture, orientation of the needle bevel, determining the volume and concentration of the anesthetic solution, and speed of injection.[65]

Increasing the dose (volume × concentration) increases the area desensitized. In general, the cranial extent of sensory blockade associated with epidural administration of lidocaine or mepivacaine in calves, goats, and juvenile pigs is not as far cranial as the dye-solution migration observed immediately after euthanasia.[137,138]

As stated previously, with the use of local anesthetic drugs, increasing the volume will improve segmental spread, whereas increasing the concentration will provide a more rapid onset of analgesia and motor nerve inhibition, greater frequency of adequate anesthesia, greater intensity of motor blockade, and a longer duration of effects.[65] A greater area of epidural anesthesia may be achieved by a relatively fast injection. However, the advantage of a large segmental area of anesthesia is offset by the higher frequency of patient discomfort upon injection because of transient elevation of CSF pressure and a relatively fast vascular and lymphatic absorption of the anesthetic, thereby reducing the duration and increasing the occurrence of incomplete block. Gravity has a more definite role in the spread of subarachnoid anesthesia than it does in epidural anesthesia; however, with both techniques, a more rapid onset to maximal segmental analgesia, a longer effect, and a more intensive motor nerve inhibition are achieved on the dependent side. Gravity also allows for unilateral anesthesia in sheep and goats owing to preferential escape of the anesthetic solution toward the paravertebral region. The cephalic spread of anesthesia after epidural or subarachnoid injection of specifically prepared hyperbaric solutions is limited in animals kept in a sitting position. Pregnant animals generally require a reduced dose per kilogram of body weight of the local anesthetic for satisfactory epidural and subarachnoid anesthesia. This may be attributable to decreased volume of the epidural space caused by distension of epidural veins (engorgement), increased sensitivity of neural tissue owing to hormonal changes, and a faulty overestimation of the lean body mass.

Migration of the anesthetic is enhanced by transmission of intra-abdominal pressure (pregnancy) and respiratory-induced intrathoracic pressure. Elderly cattle (over 8 years) with progressively occluded intervertebral foramina may require a smaller volume of the anesthetic than younger cattle with open intervertebral foramina.[65]

Lumbosacral Epidural Anesthesia in Swine

The technique of epidural block is relatively easy to master in well-sedated pigs and is most commonly employed to facilitate cesarean section; repair of rectal, uterine, or vaginal prolapse; repair of umbilical, inguinal, or scrotal hernias; surgery of scirrhous cord; and surgery of the prepuce, penis, or rear limbs.[139–155] Epidural anesthesia, however, is contraindicated in pigs with known cardiovascular disease, bleeding disorders, and shock or toxemic syndromes, because of sympathetic blockade and consequent depression of blood pressure.[145,149] The use of sedatives that produce ataxia, partial recumbency, and hypotension should be avoided. Use of a weighing crate, chute, or hog snare is generally necessary to restrain a pig properly. Chemical restraint is required in some instances. A small pig is restrained on its breast or side, whereas a large sow or boar is preferably injected while it is still standing.

The site for the needle placement is on the midline immediately caudal to the spinous process of the last lumbar (L6) vertebra (Fig. 23.24). The injection site is felt as a palpable depression a distance caudal to the transverse line between the cranial prominences of the wing of the ilium (iliac crest) on either side, 0.5 to 1.5 cm in pigs weighing 10 to 50 kg and 1.5 to 2.5 cm in pigs weighing 50 kg or more. In large pigs in which the iliac

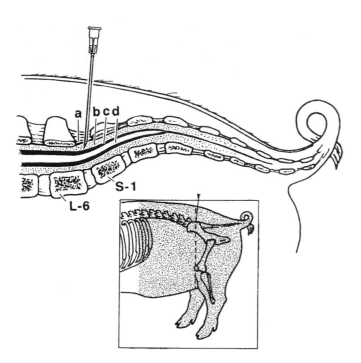

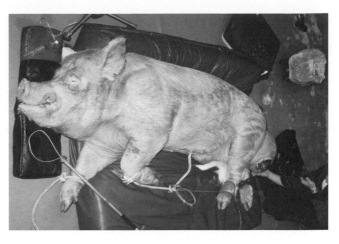

Fig. 23.25. Restraint of a 3-year-old Yorkshire hog, weighing 325 kg, in lateral recumbency. Anesthesia and relaxation distal to the midthoracic region developed after injection of 20 mL of a 2% lidocaine hydrochloride solution into the epidural space at the lumbosacral intervertebral space. From Skarda,[5] p. 645.

Fig. 23.24. Needle placement for anterior lumbosacral epidural anesthesia in pigs: L6, sixth lumbar vertebra; S1, first sacral vertebra; *a*, interarcuate ligament; *b*, epidural space; *c*, subarachnoid space; and *d*, spinal cord. The desensitized subcutaneous area after epidural anesthesia is *stippled*.

wings are not palpable, a vertical line through the patella may be used as a guide to locate the lumbosacral space 2 to 3 cm caudal to the vertical line.[142,145,146,150] The tissues over the space are thoroughly cleansed, disinfected, and infiltrated with 3 to 5 mL of a 2% lidocaine hydrochloride solution.

A 14-gauge needle can be used to support and guide the spinal needle. The appropriate spinal needles used vary between 6 to 8 cm, 20 gauge for pigs weighing 10 to 20 kg and 10 to 16 cm, 18 gauge for pigs weighing over 100 kg. The needle, preferentially with stylet and the bevel directed cranially, is inserted at the lumbosacral space by using an angle of approximately 20° caudal to the vertical. Penetration depends on the size and condition of the pig, and may be up to 2 to 4 cm in pigs weighing between 10 and 20 kg and 4 to 10 cm in pigs weighing between 20 and 100 kg. For heavy boars and sows, a 10- to 15-cm spinal needle should be selected. The needle passes through a definite area of resistance as it encounters the interarcuate ligament. Penetration of the ligament by the needle tip is often felt as a slight pop and is associated with sudden movements by the animal indicating entrance into the vertebral canal. The lumbosacral aperture in pigs is relatively large (1.5 × 2.5 cm) and allows for some margin of error. The subarachnoid space containing CSF is comparatively small at the lumbosacral-intervertebral space and is not easily penetrated at that site. The spinal cord ends anterior to the sixth lumbar (L6) vertebrae and is unlikely to be traumatized by the needle.

The dose of anesthetic is calculated by either weight or length of the pig. Anesthesia caudal to the umbilicus can be expected after injecting 1 mL of a 2% lidocaine hydrochloride solution per 4.5 kg of body weight at a rate of approximately 1 mL/2 to 3 s.[53] Anesthesia should occur within 10 min, and recovery should be complete at the end of the second hour. Similar results have been achieved by using a smaller dose, such as 1 mL per 7.5 kg for pigs weighing up to 50 kg and an additional 1 mL for every 10-kg increase in weight.[139,140] Good results have been obtained for laparotomy of pregnant sows by using a 2% lidocaine hydrochloride solution with epinephrine (5 to 12.5 µg/mL) and calculating the dosage as 1 mL for the first 40 cm of back length as measured from the base of the tail to the occipital protuberance, and an additional 1.5 mL of 2% lidocaine for each additional 10 cm.[141,148] Regardless of the weight or length, the dose should be adjusted to the pig's condition and the surgical procedure (Fig. 23.25). A maximum dose of 20 mL of 2% lidocaine is suggested as the upper limit: 4 mL/100 kg, 6 mL/200 kg, and 8 mL/300 kg of body weight for standing castrations; and 10 mL/100 kg, 15 mL/200 kg, and 20 mL/300 kg of body weight for cesarean sections.[139]

The sedative, analgesic, and immobilizing effects of xylazine and detomidine, when injected into the lumbosacral (L6-S1) epidural space of pigs, were evaluated and compared during a 2-h test period.[151] Epidural xylazine (2 mg/kg in 5 mL 0.9% NaCl solution) induces immobilization and bilateral analgesia extending from the anus to the umbilicus within 5 min after completion of injection and persists for at least 2 h. Epidural detomidine (500 µg/kg in 5 mL 0.9% NaCl solution) induces sedation and lateral recumbency, but minimal analgesia caudal to the umbilicus, within 10 min after completion of injection. Atipamezole (200 µg/kg IV) immediately reverses xylazine-induced and detomidine-induced sedation, whereas xylazine-induced analgesia and hindlimb immobilization are not antagonized by atipamezole.

In large sows undergoing elective cesarean sections, 1 mg/kg of 10% xylazine in 10 mL of 2% lidocaine injected at the lumbosacral space induces excellent analgesia extending from the anus to the umbilicus and produces rear-limb paralysis, as evidenced by a "sitting dog" posture, 5 to 8 min after completion of injection.[152] The intravenous administration of 0.003 mL/kg of a Telazol (tiletamine-zolazepam) mixture (50 mg/mL of tiletamine and zolazepam each) with ketamine (50 mg/mL) and xylazine (50 mg/mL) immobilizes the forequarters. This mixture safely immobilizes sows. Palpebral and corneal reflexes are maintained with only minimal changes in heart rate, respiratory rate, and mean arterial blood pressure. The rear limbs may be affected for as long as 7 to 8 h after epidural injection with the xylazine-lidocaine mixture. Sows are usually able to walk normally 12 h after surgery. Piglets appeared healthy, without signs of sedation or tranquilization.[152]

Epidural anesthesia can be used with general anesthesia to reduce the injectable or inhalation anesthetic requirements. The cardiopulmonary and analgesic effects of epidurally administered lidocaine (5 mg/kg of body weight), alfentanil (5 µg/kg), and xylazine (0.2 mg/kg) in pigs anesthetized with 1% to 1.2% end-tidal isoflurane anesthesia have been compared.[153–155] Lidocaine provides 45 min to 1 h of analgesia and is associated with decreases in heart rate, respiratory rate, systolic arterial blood pressure, tidal volume, minute volume, core temperature, pH_a, arterial oxygen partial pressure, and total carbon dioxide, and increases in pulmonary capillary wedge pressure, arterial carbon dioxide partial pressure, and bicarbonate-ion concentration. Epidural alfentanil has no analgesic effect. Epidural xylazine provided 1 1/2 h of analgesia and decreased core temperature and tidal volume, offering the most desirable actions in isoflurane-anesthetized pigs.[155]

Studies on the effects of epidurally and intrathecally administered drugs on blood flow of the spinal cord have been suggested as a part of their toxicological assessment.[156] To investigate the effect of epidural administration of incremental doses of clonidine (3, 10, and 30 µg/kg, each dose given in a volume of 5 mL) via a lumbar epidural catheter, on regional and central blood flow and hemodynamics, 11 anesthetized pigs, weighing 20 to 23 kg, were studied.[118] Lumbar epidural clonidine (3 µg/kg, a dose of clinical interest) did not affect regional blood flow to the spinal cord, brain, and cerebellum. Higher doses (10 and 30 µg/kg) of epidural clonidine produced local vasoconstriction, with a reduction in flow of 25% to 35% in the lumbar and thoracic spinal cord, 61% in the adrenal gland, and 78% in skeletal muscles.

Further interest in pain management is likely to encourage the development of new epidural techniques, emphasizing reduced frequency of injections and localized absorption of drug molecules at the injection site. For example, the effect of 4 mL of poloxamer gel (25%) containing 2% lidocaine hydrochloride or 2% ibuprofen sodium on the duration of analgesia after lumbar (L4 to L6) epidural administration via a catheter has been evaluated.[157] The gel solutions are highly viscous at room temperature, but liquid at refrigeration temperature, enabling injection of a cold-fluid solution that forms a gel in situ at a physiological temperature. In this study, antinociceptive response as assessed by observing the motor function and the nociceptive reflex–withdrawal response to painful pressure stimulation on the feet lasted 1 h longer and was more effective over time in comparison with routine epidural lidocaine injection. With the lidocaine gel, motor blockade in hind limbs lasted 1 1/2 h longer than with normal lidocaine solution. Epidurally administered ibuprofen in gel or solution prolonged analgesia, almost by 100%, when compared with ibuprofen administered IV. Analgesia was, however, not prolonged after ibuprofen epidural gel injection when compared with the epidural solution. The gel formulation apparently prolonged the systemic absorption of lidocaine and ibuprofen and increased the epidural availability of lidocaine, but not ibuprofen, for epidural analgesia. Only minor inflammatory changes in tissues of the epidural space were observed after epidural poloxamer gel injection in pigs.[157]

Epidural anesthesia is a good choice in swine, with low morbidity and mortality, minimal CNS depression, and rapid recovery being its advantages. A rapid recovery is important for sows on a farm if they are to nurse pigs or are to be sold for slaughter before other complications develop. A rapid recovery also enables pathogen-free sows to leave the clinic as soon as the piglets do.[158] Epidural anesthesia can also be used with general anesthesia to reduce inhalant or injectable anesthetic requirements.[144]

Lumbosacral epidural anesthesia that extends anterior to the last rib is generally safe in pigs, although complications may arise from overdose. These include cardiovascular and respiratory collapse, transient loss of consciousness, tremors, convulsions, vomiting, and meningitis associated with septic technique.

Anterior Epidural and Subarachnoid Anesthesia in Small Ruminants

Anterior analgesia produced by epidural and subarachnoid spinal nerve blocks provides excellent surgical conditions for cesarean section; intra-abdominal, pelvic, or hind-limb surgery; and udder surgery in small ruminants. The technique may be accomplished by injecting local anesthetic into either the epidural or the subarachnoid space at the lumbosacral intervertebral space.[159–164]

With full aseptic precautions, in adult sheep and goats, a 6- to 7-cm, 20-gauge spinal needle with a fitted stylet is inserted on the midline halfway between the last lumbar (L6) and first sacral (S1) vertebrae at approximately 90° to the skin (Fig. 23.20C). The site for needle placement is usually palpable as a depression on the midline just caudal to a line joining the anterior border of the ilium on each side. Penetration of the interarcuate ligament is often associated with a sudden movement of the animal owing to pain or the lack of resistance either to further needle passage or to the injection of 5 mL of air, indicating that the vertebral space has been entered.

First, an attempt is made to aspirate CSF into a syringe. If CSF is not withdrawn, it can be assumed that the dura has not been punctured, and epidural injection is made with 1 mL of a 2% lidocaine hydrochloride solution per 4.5 kg of body weight. Posterior paralysis and anterior analgesia extending a fourth of the distance from the pubis to the umbilicus can be expected within 2 to 10 min and last as long as 2 h. The dose of lidocaine recommended for epidural anesthesia in the sheep may vary from a low of 8 to 15 mL of 1.5% lidocaine hydrochloride solution with 1:100,000 epinephrine, depending on the size of the sheep,[53] to 1 mL of 2% solution per 5 kg.[164]

Anterior Epidural Anesthesia in Small Ruminants

Sedation with xylazine (0.1 mg/kg IM) followed 5 min later by lumbosacral analgesia induced by administration of 2% lidocaine (0.18 to 0.24 mg/kg) and xylazine (0.05 mg/kg) into the lumbosacral epidural space for umbilical surgery in dairy calves has been investigated.[161]

Supplemental local infiltration of lidocaine cranial to the umbilicus was required in five of six calves in dorsal recumbence to provide adequate analgesia. Calves maintained adequate cardiac output, stroke volume, and oxygen delivery, but were hypotensive throughout the surgery and after placement into sternal recumbency. Reversal of xylazine-induced sedation with tolazoline (1 mg/kg IV) caused transient (30 s) sinus bradycardia and sinus arrest for up to 6 s and second-degree atrioventricular block (Mobitz type 1), accompanied by severe systemic arterial hypotension (20 to 30 mm Hg). The anesthetic protocol may be useful when respiratory compromise or costs are concerns, and the surgical procedure can be completed in less than 1 h. Caution should be exercised when tolazoline (an α_1-antagonist and α_2-antagonist) is administered IV to reverse xylazine-induced sedation in neonatal calves, because profound hypotension may occur.

Xylazine and detomidine are α_2-adrenoceptor agonists commonly used in small ruminants. When the analgesic effects of epidurally and IM administered xylazine (0.3 mg/kg) or detomidine (20 µg/kg) in healthy sheep (1 to 3 years old) were compared, the epidural administration of either drug produced a greater degree of analgesia in the tail, perineum, hind limbs, and flank region than did similar doses of xylazine or detomidine administered IM.[165] Analgesia was observed within 2 min of each drug administration, with no difference in onset time of analgesia. Epidural xylazine produced complete analgesia of the tail, perineum, hind limbs, flank, thoracic wall, and forelimbs, whereas epidural detomidine produced only mild to moderate analgesia of these regions. Analgesia lasted longer after epidural xylazine (1½ h) than after intramuscular xylazine (30 min), intramuscular detomidine (30 min), or epidural detomidine (30 min). Sedation was evident, and all sheep became recumbent after the epidural injection of xylazine. Ataxia developed after the intramuscular administration of either drug, but was more pronounced after epidural administration. Changes in pulse and respiratory rates, rectal temperature, ruminal motility, and hematologic and biochemical parameters were transient. In a similar study, the cardiovascular and respiratory effects of epidural versus intravenous xylazine (0.2 mg/kg) in sheep were compared.[166] No changes were observed in heart rate, arterial blood pressure, cardiac output, pH_a, arterial carbon dioxide partial pressure, and arterial and mixed-venous oxygen content after epidural xylazine administration, whereas the intravenous route of xylazine produced significant decreases in mean and diastolic arterial blood pressure, arterial oxygen partial pressure, and oxygen saturation.

Analgesic effects have been assessed after the lumbosacral (L6-S1) epidural administration of xylazine (2%, 0.4 mg/kg, diluted with 0.9% NaCl) in rams. Analgesia was evident in the hind limb and perineum in 2 to 3 min and provided analgesia up to the midthoracic (T5 to T6) vertebrae 10 min after drug administration.[167] Analgesia and motor nerve blockade lasted from 2 h to 2 h 20 min and from 3 h to 4 h 40 min, respectively. Side effects included bradycardia, tachypnea, decreased minute volume, and metabolic alkalosis.[167]

In a similar study, the analgesic effects of xylazine (0.07 mg/kg, diluted in 2.5 mL of sterile water) injected into the epidural space at the sacrococcygeal or lumbosacral sites in 22 ewes (body weight range, 60 to 85 kg) suffering from dystocia (vaginal prolapse and emphysematous fetuses) were evaluated.[168] Analgesia of the flank was appropriate for caesarean section 40 to 50 min after xylazine administration at either the sacrococcygeal or the lumbosacral epidural sites. Sedation was not observed in any of the ewes. Neither vaginal nor rectal prolapse recurred. The alleviation of tenesmus was attributed in part to the prolonged analgesic action achieved by epidural xylazine injection.

A combination of 2% xylazine (0.07 mg/kg) mixed with 2% lidocaine (0.5 mg/kg) administered into the sacrococcygeal epidural space has also produced effective caudal analgesia in sheep with preparturient vaginal or cervicovaginal prolapse.[169] This epidural mixture has been used for replacement and retention of rectal, cervical, and uterine prolapse in postpartum ewes.[170] There was no evidence that epidural xylazine-lidocaine caused premature labor.[171] The combined epidural injection of xylazine and lidocaine has been considered by some investigators as an improvement over lidocaine epidural injection alone, primarily because of the lack of abdominal straining for at least 1 day after prolapse replacement.

The epidural coadministration of an α_2-adrenoceptor agonist and opioid appears to shorten the onset time while prolonging the duration of antinociception. For example, in one study, 10 min after completion of injection, xylazine (0.2 mg/kg) administered epidurally alone produced a lack of response to electrical stimulation that lasted for 1½ h, whereas a xylazine-fentanyl combination produced antinociceptive effects in 5 min that lasted 5 h. The cardiopulmonary effects, which were measured after epidural xylazine-fentanyl injection, included decreases in cardiac output, cardiac work, arterial and mixed-venous pH, and bicarbonate values.[172]

Following the acute and chronic lumbar epidural administration of preservative-free and antioxidant-free solutions of morphine (Astramorph/PF [0.5 or 1.0 mg of morphine/mL] and Infumorph 500 [25 mg of preservative-free morphine sulfate sterile solution/mL]) and hydromorphone (Dilaudid-HP [10 mg of hydromorphone hydrochloride/mL]), there was no change in CSF chemistry or hematology, or damage to spinal nerves, arachnoid, pia, or spinal cord tissues. In one portion of the study, three ewes receiving either morphine or hydromorphone developed hind-limb weakness with progressive deterioration of motor and reflex function, hypersensitivity to touch in the flanks, dermatomal flank irritation (scratching and licking, progressing to abrasions), discomfort with injection, catheter-related side effects, and severe neurological damage. Some spinal cord compression was common in all ewes, whereas partial spinal cord necrosis was observed in 50% of ewes after the 30-day epidural use of concentrated morphine and hydromorphone.[173]

Anterior Subarachnoid Anesthesia in Small Ruminants

If spinal fluid is aspirated into the syringe or drips from the hub after needle placement, it is obvious that the dorsal epidural space, the dura, and arachnoid meninges have all been punctured and the subarachnoid space has been entered. Under these circumstances, half the epidural dose (0.5 mL/4.5 kg) can be injected at a rate of approximately 1 mL every 2 to 3 s. Posterior paralysis occurs in 1 to 3 min. With the reduced dose, anesthesia may extend to the last rib, similar to epidural administration of 2% lidocaine but lasting 1 to 1¹/₂ h (Fig. 23.26).

Gravity, not diffusion of drug in the CSF, determines the spread of anesthesia. For bilateral anesthesia, the animal is placed on its back immediately after administration of the anesthetic and removal of the needle; for unilateral anesthesia, the animal is maintained in lateral decubitus with its affected side dependent. Although epidural anesthesia and subarachnoid anesthesia in small ruminants are useful techniques and easily performed, careful observation of patients after injection and proper positioning must be maintained in order to avoid complications.[174]

A few studies have evaluated the actions of α_2-agonists placed into the subarachnoid space of small ruminants. The analgesic effects of intrathecally (subarachnoid) applied xylazine and clonidine placed into the cervical region of the spinal cord of sheep have been studied.[175,176] Xylazine and clonidine both produced dose-dependent analgesia of the forelimbs, with slow onset and maximum effect observed after 45 min to 1 h. Clonidine appeared to be twice as potent as xylazine, with doses of 3, 6, and 12 µg of clonidine being similar to 5, 10, and 25 µg of xylazine.

The antinociceptive and physiological effects of xylazine (50 µg/kg) and detomidine (10 µg/kg) administered subarachnoidally at the lumbosacral space in sheep indicate that xylazine produces a higher threshold rise, faster onset, and longer threshold enhancement than does detomidine.[177] Atipamezole at doses of 5 µg/kg and 2.5 µg/kg, when administered IV at maximum threshold effects produced by xylazine and detomidine, did not affect the resulting antinociception as assessed by electrical stimulation.[177]

It should be appreciated that serious side effects may result from injecting the full epidural dose into the subarachnoid space, thereby rapidly advancing the anesthetic through lumbar, thoracic, cervical, and cranial subarachnoid spaces. Likewise, it is not safe to withdraw the needle from the subarachnoid space to the epidural space and proceed with an epidural injection. A dura hole may be patent for many hours and, if spinal anesthesia is considered, a deliberate technique of subarachnoid injection using 1.5 to 2.0 mL of Heavy Nupercaine (1:200 dibucaine in 6% glucose) in adult sheep has been recommended.[53]

CSF morphine concentration at the brain stem can increase when lumbar epidural morphine is administered adjacent to a dural puncture. Following dural puncture at the lumbar vertebrae with either a 25-gauge Whitacre needle or an 18-gauge Tuohy needle, the concentrations of morphine in CSF sampled at the cisterna magna 6 h after epidural morphine administration were 154 ± 32 and 405 ± 53 ng/mL, respectively.[178] These values are 7 and 20 times larger than without dural puncture. These findings highlight the potential for delayed respiratory depression when epidural morphine is injected after a dural puncture.

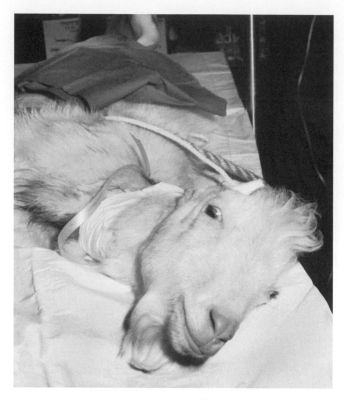

Fig. 23.26. Restraint of an 8-year-old female Nubian goat, weighing 80 kg, in lateral recumbency during lumbosacral subarachnoid anesthesia (the right hind foot was amputated).

As a general rule, the subarachnoid administration of lipophilic opioids produces CSF distribution different from CSF distributions of hydrophilic opioids. For example, when morphine (2 mg), hydromorphone (1 mg), methadone (2 mg), naloxone (1 mg), and [^{14}C]sucrose (5 µCi), in 100-µL dosing solution, were coadministered into the lumbar subarachnoid space or right lateral ventricle of sheep, their distribution into the lumbar subarachnoid space or right lateral ventricle varied greatly.[179] Morphine, hydromorphone, and [^{14}C]sucrose were detected in lumbar CSF at 1¹/₂ h to 1 h 45 min after lateral ventricle injection, whereas hydromorphone and [^{14}C]sucrose were detected in lateral ventricle CSF 50 min after lumbar subarachnoid injection. In contrast, methadone was not detected in ventricle CSF after lumbar subarachnoid injection, nor was it detected in lumbar CSF after ventricle administration. Methadone, being a highly lipophilic opioid, exerts its effect predominantly on tissues near the site of injection.

A number of studies have evaluated the effects of subarachnoid administration of α_2-agonists, ketamine, and local anesthetics or combinations thereof in small ruminants.[180–183] The assessment of the analgesic, ataxic, sedative, cardiopulmonary, and systemic effects of ketamine (3 mg/kg), xylazine (0.1 mg/kg), or lidocaine (2.5 mg/kg) after subarachnoid injection (L6-S1) in goats is one such study.[180] Subarachnoidally administered xylazine produced various degrees of analgesia of the tail, perineum, hind limbs, flanks, and caudodorsal rib areas, which were characterized by a slower onset and longer duration than the effects of ketamine or lidocaine. However, subarachnoid xylazine also caused clinical relevant bradycardia, hypotension, and respiratory depression, whereas ketamine and lidocaine did not significantly affect the cardiovascular and respiratory systems of goats.

The effects of the α_2-agonist romifidine alone or in combination with ketamine have also been evaluated following subarachnoid injection.[181] After the intrathecal administration of the romifidine and ketamine, analgesia of the tail, perineum, and hind limbs reportedly occurred in 35 s and lasted for at least 2 h. These results indicate a possible synergistic analgesic interaction between intrathecally administered α_2-agonists and ketamine. Goats also demonstrated moderate to complete weakness of the hindquarters after injection of this combination, whereas heart and respiratory rates and arterial blood pressure were decreased and central venous pressure was increased.[181] Although postoperative analgesia in food animals is often ignored, the increased interest in the use of local anesthetics, α_2-adrenoceptor agonists, ketamine, and opioids by the epidural and subarachnoid routes as a means of prolonging perioperative analgesia is encouraging.[176,181–185]

Complications from Anterior Epidural and Subarachnoid Anesthesia

Complications may arise from faulty anterior epidural and subarachnoid anesthesia and lack of patient management. These complications can include loss of consciousness, convulsions, respiratory paralysis, hypotension, and hypothermia after overdose,[186,187] and possibly headache after dural puncture (unknown in nonverbal species). Respiratory paralysis is caused by desensitization of motor nerves supplying the intercostal muscle and/or by desensitizing the phrenic nerves supplying the diaphragm. Animals with severe hypotension show signs of distress, collapse, tachycardia or bradycardia, weak pulse, and shallow, rapid respiration. Therapy is comprised of rapid fluid infusion; raising the animal's hindquarters above the level of the heart to prevent pooling of blood in the hindquarters and to improve venous return, cardiac output, and arterial blood pressure; and supporting respiration by intubation, positive-pressure ventilation, and oxygen administration. In addition, the use of α_1-adrenergic agonists (e.g., methoxamine, metaraminol, ephedrine, and phenylephrine) has been recommended to constrict the epidurally or subarachnoidally induced dilation of vascular beds in splanchnic and pelvic viscera and muscles of the pelvic limbs. The routine use of metaraminol (5 mg IM) during epidural anesthesia in sheep has been advocated, and, if hypotension is severe, 5- to 10-mg of methoxamine can be given IV.[53] The use of ephedrine in pregnant ewes is advantageous because it preserves uterine blood flow.[188] Hypothermia is caused by a patient's inability to shiver. Heat lamps and warm blankets are useful in warming patients.

Teat and Udder Anesthesia of Cows

Introduction

The udder is supplied from fibers of the genitofemoral nerves, which have their origin from the third and fourth lumbar spinal

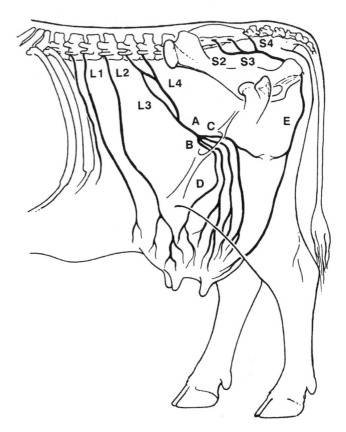

Fig. 23.27. Schematic illustration of the nerve supply to a cow's udder: *A*, inguinal nerve; *B*, internal anterior nerve; *C*, posterior inguinal nerve; *D*, external inguinal nerve; and *E*, perineal inguinal nerve. L1 to L4 are ventral branches of the first to fourth lumbar vertebral nerves. S2, S3, and S4 are ventral branches of the second, third, and fourth sacral vertebral nerves.

cord segments.[189] Cranially, the skin and some glandular tissue of the forequarters are supplied by the ilioinguinal (L2) and iliohypogastric (L1) nerves. Caudally, the udder is supplied by the mammary branch of the pudendal nerve and distal branch of the perineal nerve, which originate from the second, third, and fourth sacral spinal cord segments (Fig. 23.27). Milk secretion is under hormonal control, as there are no secretory nerves to the udder.

Teat analgesia is required for repair of teat lacerations and injuries that most commonly affect the orifice. For this reason, local anesthesia (ring block, inverted-V block, teat cistern infusion, and intravenous regional anesthesia of the teat) is adequate for most surgical procedures, using either physical restraint or chemical tranquilization.[19,190] Xylazine on its own as a sedative and analgesic is very effective for minor procedures, but its use in advanced gestation may be contraindicated. Standing restraint is advantageous because it prevents udder trauma; however, asepsis and safety to the operator must not be compromised. General anesthesia is rarely necessary for udder surgery except perhaps for udder amputation.

Paravertebral block of the first, second, and third lumbar (L1,

L2, and L3) spinal nerves or segmental lumbar epidural block of these nerves may be used for surgical procedures of the foreudder and foreteats. Both techniques have been described as difficult and often result in cows lying down. Using the perineal nerve block in standing ruminants, surgical procedures may be performed on the caudal-most teats and escutcheon areas of the udder. However, most surgical procedures of the caudal teats and body of the udder require high caudal epidural anesthesia or lumbosacral epidural anesthesia. Both techniques have been described, and there is no advantage to using one technique over the other in performing udder surgery. If high caudal epidural anesthesia is the method used for major udder surgery, up to 150 mL of a 2% lidocaine hydrochloride solution may be required to extend the analgesia to L1 in adult cows. Analgesia can be expected within 10 to 15 min and lasts 1 to 1½ h.

Ring Block of the Teat

After thoroughly cleansing the entire teat and teat base, physical restraint is used (e.g., holding the nose or using a flank strap, rope around the legs, or dorsal tail elevation). An elastic band may be applied firmly around the base of the teat to prevent diffusion of local anesthetic up into the udder. The tourniquet is not applied for removal of supernumerary teats. A 1.5-cm, 25-gauge needle is inserted subcutaneously transverse to the direction of the teat to deposit 4 to 6 mL of a 2% lidocaine hydrochloride solution in the form of a peripheral ring block (Fig. 23.28A). The solution is then massaged into the tissues. The technique provides adequate analgesia of the teat distal to the tourniquet within 10 min and lasts for approximately 2 h. Minor procedures, such as laceration repair, perforating fistula, nonperforating laceration, wart removal, teat removal in gangrenous mastitis, teat-obstruction opening, and fistula and supernumerary teat removal, are facilitated when using ring block. The technique is simple and inexpensive, and cows remain standing. Potential complications are prevented by using aseptic technique and safety during infiltration.

Inverted-V Block of the Teat

As an alternative to the ring block, a 1.5-cm, 25-gauge needle and 4 to 6 mL of local anesthetic solution are used to infiltrate the skin and muscularis of the surgical site by using an inverted-V pattern (Fig. 23.28B). Adequate analgesia for repairs of lacerations or fistulas or for removing warts in standing cows is achieved by this technique. Again, physical restraint and tranquilization are required for aseptic technique and safety during infiltration.

Teat-Cistern Infusion

Infusion of the teat cistern with local anesthetic is recommended for procedures that require anesthesia of the mucous membrane lining of the cistern. Although the muscularis, subcutaneous layers, and skin are not desensitized by this technique, procedures such as removal of teat polyps, opening of contracted sphincters, and opening of the spider teats may be facilitated. Combined with adequate physical restraint and chemical tranquilization, the cistern is milked out and the orifice thoroughly cleansed with al-

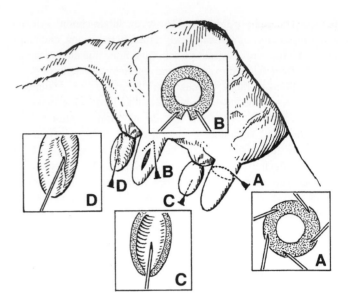

Fig. 23.28. Needle placement for bovine ring block (*A*), inverted-V block (*B*), teat-cistern infusion (*C*), and intravenous regional teat block (*D*).

cohol. A narrow gauze bandage or suture is placed as high up on the teat as possible to act as a tourniquet, preventing milk from entering the teat and diluting the anesthetic agent. To fill the teat, a teat cannula is introduced and approximately 10 mL of a 2% lidocaine hydrochloride solution is infused (Fig. 23.28C). Anesthesia develops in 5 to 10 min; thereafter, the remaining lidocaine is milked out and the tourniquet is removed.

Intravenous Regional Anesthesia of the Teat

This technique provides anesthesia of the entire teat distal to a preplaced tourniquet. The technique is best accomplished in recumbent cows. A tourniquet is placed around the base of the teat as described for teat cistern infusion. Any superficial teat vein distal to the tourniquet may be used for injection of 5 to 7 mL of a 2% lidocaine hydrochloride solution or its equivalent by using a 2.5-cm, 22- to 25-gauge needle (Fig. 23.28D). Digital pressure and gentle massage are applied to the site of injection to prevent hematoma formation. Analgesia of the teat distal to the tourniquet occurs within 3 to 5 min and persists for the time the tourniquet is applied. Sensation returns to the teat 5 to 10 min after tourniquet removal. Restraint and aseptic technique are critical.

Perineal Nerve Block

Desensitization of the perineal nerve facilitates repair of laceration and removal of supernumerary teats or warts in the caudal-most udder or escutcheon area.[189] The nerve is readily desensitized by injecting 5 to 7 mL of a 2% lidocaine hydrochloride solution into the subcutaneous and subfascial tissues at the ischial arch approximately 2 cm lateral to the midline on both sides.[191] The technique does not inhibit wound healing, but it is more difficult technically than local infiltration.

Anesthesia of the Foot

Introduction

Anesthesia of the foot may be induced by (a) infiltrating the tissues around the limb with local anesthetic solution (ring block), (b) injecting local anesthetic solution into an accessible superficial vein in an extremity isolated from circulation by placing a tourniquet on the animal's leg (intravenous regional anesthesia), (c) desensitizing specific nerves (regional analgesia, anesthesia of the brachial plexus, and epidural anesthesia), and (d) using general anesthesia in especially fractious animals or procedures requiring complete immobilization for asepsis and safety during operation.

Ring Block

Many practitioners consider the ring block or infiltration of local anesthetic from skin to bone, encircling the digit at the junction of the proximal and middle of the metatarsus or metacarpus, to be the most reliable way of anesthetizing the digit.[192] A 2.5-cm, 25-gauge needle may be used to inject approximately 15 mL of a 2% lidocaine hydrochloride solution at several sites: deep and superficial to the flexor tendons and in a partial circle around medially and laterally to the extensor tendons. The area between the anterior and posterior injection sites may be divided into thirds; the anesthetic may be injected at one-third to two-thirds of the distance between them. The technique does not require precise anatomical knowledge of the limb. The ring block increases the risk of inducing pyogenic bacteria from multiple injection sites, however, and is often only partially successful.

Intravenous Regional Anesthesia

Intravenous regional anesthesia (IVRA) is a simple and safe method for producing analgesia of the digit in cattle, small ruminants, and pigs, and can be substituted for the cumbersome local infiltration or nerve-block procedures. It is ideal for digital surgery, in which the amount of bleeding at the surgical site must be reduced. In cattle, the technique involves placing either an elastic bandage, a tourniquet of stout rubber tubing, or an inflatable cuff (inflation pressure, >200 mm Hg or 26.7 kPa) proximal[193,194] or distal to the tarsus,[194–196] proximal to the elbow,[197–199] and proximal[193,200] or distal to the carpus to obstruct the arterial inflow.[196,201] In the pelvic limb, a rolled bandage is placed in the depression on either side of the limb between the Achilles tendon and the tibia to increase the pressure on the underlying vessels.[193–195]

IVRA is best performed on the leg of an animal that has been cast and restrained in lateral recumbency with the particular limb uppermost, but alternatively it can be induced in a raised leg of a sedated animal standing.[202] In the thoracic limb, the skin over the prominent common dorsal metacarpal vein, plantar metacarpal vein, or radial vein distal to the tourniquet is clipped, shaved, and disinfected (Fig. 23.29A). The cranial branch of the lateral saphenous vein or lateral plantar digital vein is a suitable site for injection in the pelvic limb (Fig. 23.29B). A 2.5-cm to 3.75-cm, 20- or 22-gauge needle with syringe attached is inserted either in proximal or in distal direction as close to the surgical site as possible. In adult cattle, 30 mL of a 2% lidocaine hydrochloride solution (without epinephrine) is injected as rapidly as possible.[193–195,201,203] Smaller volumes (3 to 10 mL) of lidocaine are adequate for IVRA in small ruminants and pigs.[196]

The needle is removed from the vein, and digital pressure and gentle massage are applied to the site of injection to prevent development of subcutaneous hematoma. Anesthesia of the limb distal to the tourniquet develops after 5 min, is optimal in 10 min, and persists for the period the tourniquet is left in place. Analgesia occurs latest in the interdigital region. Ischemic necrosis, severe lameness, and edema are not expected to occur if the tourniquet is applied for less than 2 h.[193,194] Few surgical procedures require this length of time. Usually, an operation is completed in 10 to 30 min, when the tourniquet may be safely released. Sensation and motor function return to the leg within 10 min after tourniquet release, and no signs of cardiovascular or CNS toxicity are likely.[193,200,204,205] After tourniquet removal, partial analgesia may persist for an additional 30 min or longer. Evidence of lidocaine toxicity has rarely been reported in cattle if the tourniquet has remained in place for 20 min or more. Maximal venous plasma concentration of lidocaine after tourniquet release was 1.5 µg/mL,[195] which is less than that considered to be toxic.

A measurable concentration of lidocaine in jugular venous blood in buffalo calves (102 ± 9.4 kg) was demonstrated after infusion of a 2% lidocaine hydrochloride solution (4 mg/kg body weight) into the dorsal digital vein, despite tourniquet occlusion.[206] The lidocaine concentration progressively rose after injection to 2.9 and 3.67 µg/mL at 30 min and 1 h, and was further increased to 6.9 ± 0.9 µg/mL at 5 min after tourniquet release. Salivation, tremors, and rapid pulse have occurred in cattle after early tourniquet removal (<20 min). Symptoms of lidocaine toxicity—including CNS symptoms and signs such as convulsions and seizures, profuse salivation, and hypotension in cattle—may occur if a large bolus of lidocaine hydrochloride (6 to 8 mg/kg) is injected into the systemic circulation. Toxicity in early tourniquet removal is avoided if the tourniquet is loosened for 10 to 15 s and retightened for 2 to 3 min, and this procedure is repeated several times.[207] In cases of local sepsis in the distal limb in cattle, combined use of IVRA and antibiotics has been described.[208] It is advised, however, to limit the dose of sodium penicillin to 100,000 IU dissolved in 15 to 20 mL of a 2% lidocaine hydrochloride solution to prevent thrombosis of the veins distal to the tourniquet. Swelling of the forelimb and long-lasting lameness (25 days) in 18% of a group of water buffalo calves (85 to 100 kg of body weight) has been reported after IVRA, when 400,000 IU of benzyl penicillin was diluted in 12 to 15 mL of an 8% to 12% procaine hydrochloride solution and injected into the radial vein distal to a tourniquet.[197] Microthrombosis of digital veins might have been produced in these animals by salt formation of procaine penicillin and benzyl penicillin.[209] In any case, animals should be carefully observed for changes in respiratory and pulse rates during the first 10 min after tourniquet release.

Advantages of IVRA when compared with ring block or regional nerve blocks are that it requires no precise anatomical knowledge of the limb and only a single injection is made, thereby reducing tissue trauma, contamination of fascial planes

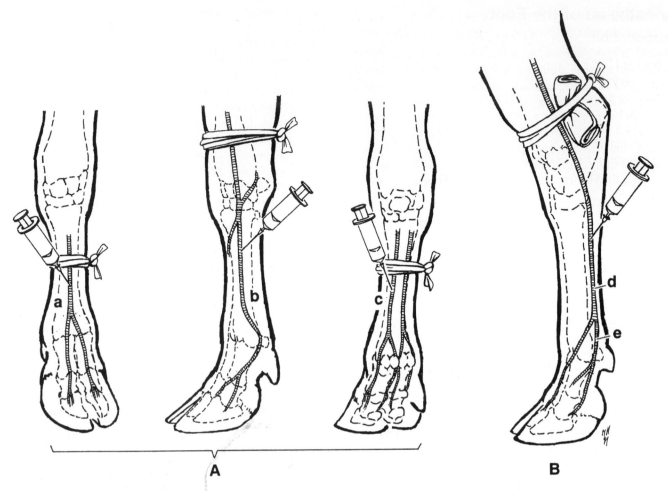

Fig. 23.29. Tourniquet and needle placement for intravenous regional analgesia of the bovine forelimb **(A)** and rear limb **(B)**: *a*, dorsal metacarpal vein (dorsal view); *b*, radial vein (medial view); *c*, plantar metacarpal vein (palmar view); *d*, cranial branch of lateral saphenous vein; and *e*, lateral plantar digital vein.

or tendon sheaths, and time required for producing digital analgesia. In addition, the amount of bleeding at the surgical site is reduced during application of the tourniquet. One disadvantage of IVRA is an approximately 7% inexplicable failure rate, with particular lack of analgesia in the interdigital area, even when the technique is performed correctly without hematoma formation at the puncture site.

Regional Anesthesia of the Thoracic Limb

Brachial Plexus Block

Anesthesia of the brachial plexus in cattle can be achieved by desensitizing the ventral roots of the sixth, seventh, and eighth cervical (C6, C7, and C8) and first and second thoracic (T1 and T2) spinal nerves as they pass over the lateral aspect of the middle third of the first rib, thereby inducing loss of sensation distally and including the elbow joint.[136] The skin-puncture site is 12 to 14 cm cranial to the acromion of the scapula and lymph node. This area is surgically scrubbed and infiltrated with 2 to 3 mL of local anesthetic solution. The animal's head is held away from the side to be injected. A 16-cm, 18-gauge needle, preferably with stylet, is inserted through the desensitized area and pushed horizontally or 5° ventrocaudally until it impinges at the lateral surface of the first rib, where approximately 10 mL of a 1% or 2% lidocaine hydrochloride solution containing 1:200,000 epinephrine (to delay absorption and diminish the risk of toxicity) or equivalent is injected. The needle is first withdrawn 5 to 10 cm, and then its tip is redirected 1.5 cm more distal to the first injection site, where an additional 10 mL of the anesthetic is deposited. Two to three more injections are made similarly until a band of anesthetic 6 to 8 cm long has been injected along the rib and ventral to the initial site. The needle is correctly placed if there is no air, blood, or CSF upon needle aspiration. Onset of analgesia and loss of motor power are gradual, with maximal effects achieved 15 to 20 min after injection and lasting 1 1/2 to 2 h.

Digital Nerve Block

The nerves in the digits of cattle are not easily located distal to the carpus and tarsus because of tense skin and subcutaneous fibrous tissue. However, individual nerves can be desensitized.

To produce analgesia distal to the carpus, the median nerve, the ulnar nerve, the medial antebrachial nerve (a cutaneous branch of the musculocutaneous nerve), and the dorsal antebrachial nerve (a cutaneous branch of the radial nerve) must be desensitized.[8,136,210] Local infiltration of the skin and subcutis can be used effectively where massive extensive muscle mass proximal to the carpus prohibits perineural injection.

The median nerve may be desensitized by injecting 10 to 20 mL of a 2% lidocaine hydrochloride solution beneath the fascia approximately 5 cm distal to the elbow anterior to the flexor carpi radialis muscle on the posterior radius. The nerve lies deep, but it can be palpated and perineurally infiltrated at that site by using a 5-cm, 18- to 20-gauge needle (Fig. 23.30C).

The ulnar nerve can occasionally be palpated approximately 10 cm (a hand's breadth) above the accessory carpal bone at the posterolateral (volar-lateral) surface of the radius. Approximately 5 mL of a 2% lidocaine hydrochloride solution is injected underneath the superficial fascia in a groove between the flexor carpi ulnaris and ulnaris lateralis muscle by using a 5-cm, 20-gauge needle (Fig. 23.30B). The resulting median and ulnar nerve blocks desensitize the medial-posterior aspect of the metacarpus and posterior aspect of the digits.[136] The medial and dorsal antebrachial nerves supply sensory fibers to the medial and dorsal aspects of the carpus and, in conjunction with the median and ulnar nerves, the limb distal to the carpus. The cutaneous medial and dorsal antebrachial nerves may be desensitized anteriorly approximately 10 cm above the carpus by injection of 20 mL of a 2% lidocaine hydrochloride solution in a band 4 to 6 cm wide adjacent to the dorsal radius just anterior to the cephalic vein (Fig. 23.30A).

Alternatively, anesthesia can be produced from the midmetacarpus distally by desensitizing four nerves at the midmetacarpal area (four-point block): the dorsal metacarpal nerve (a superficial branch of the radial nerve), the medial palmar nerve (a continuation of the median nerve), and the dorsal and palmar branches of the ulnar nerve.[211] A 1.25-cm, 22-gauge needle may be used to inject 5 mL of a 2% lidocaine hydrochloride solution at each site. The needle point is directed proximally to prevent its breaking in the event the animal should kick and pull the leg away. The dorsal metacarpal nerve is desensitized by subfascial injection of the anesthetic medial to the medial digital extensor tendon (Fig. 23.31A). The medial palmar nerve is desensitized at the medial aspect of the superficial flexor tendon in the groove between the superficial flexor tendon and the suspensory ligament (Fig. 23.31B). The dorsal branch and the lateral palmar branch of the ulnar nerve are desensitized by perineural infiltration on the lateral aspect of the limb just anterior and posterior to the suspensory ligament (Fig. 23.31C and D).

Anesthesia of the Interdigital Region

For interdigital anesthesia of the front and hind feet, the branches of the medial dorsal and palmar (plantar) axial digital nerves must be desensitized. Using a 5-cm, 16- or 18-gauge needle, 5 to 10 mL of a 2% lidocaine hydrochloride solution is injected at a depth of 3.5 to 5.0 cm to infiltrate the soft region proximal to the junction of the claws on both the dorsal and the volar aspects of the first phalanx (pastern) (Fig. 23.30D). This method should ad-

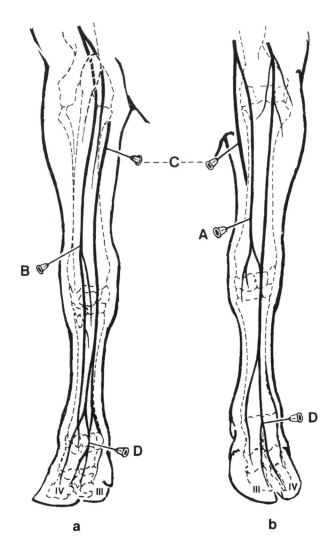

Fig. 23.30. Needle placement for desensitizing the musculocutaneous (A), ulnar (B), median (C), and axial digital III and IV (D) nerves of the left forelimb in cattle: a, caudolateral; and b, dorsomedial aspects.

equately desensitize all the dorsal and palmar (plantar) axial digital nerves for removal of interdigital fibromas (corns). Alternatively, a 10-cm, 18-gauge needle can be inserted at a 90° angle to the skin on the dorsum of the pastern, and the middle of the interdigital space can be infiltrated from a single injection site by using 15 to 20 mL of the anesthetic solution.

Regional Anesthesia of the Pelvic Limb

Nerve blocks of the pelvic limb in cattle have seldom been emphasized because IVRA and epidural anesthesia may be conveniently used for anesthesia of the hind legs. Regional anesthesia of the tarsus and distally can be produced by desensitizing the common peroneal nerve and tibial nerve.[212] Both nerves are continuations of the sciatic nerve. A 3- to 5-cm, 18- to 20-gauge needle with approximately 20 mL of a 2% lidocaine hydrochloride solution are used at each site, inducing anesthesia within 10 to 20

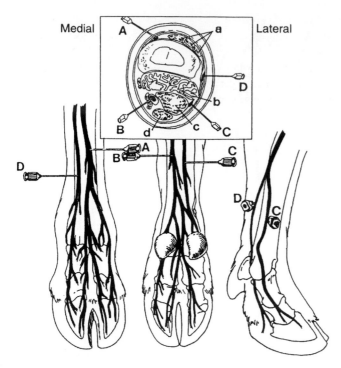

Fig. 23.31. Needle placement for midmetacarpal nerve blocks on the right forefoot in cattle. Dorsal metacarpal nerve (*A*), medial palmar nerve (*B*), lateral palmar branch of the ulnar nerve (*C*), and dorsal branch of the ulnar nerve (*D*): dorsal aspect **(left)**, palmar aspect **(center)**, lateral aspect **(right)**, and cross-sectional aspect **(inset)**. **Inset:** *a*, extensor tendons; *b*, interosseous ligament; *c*, deep digital flexor tendon; and *d*, superficial digital extensor tendon. From Skarda,[5] p. 655.

min. The common peroneal nerve is desensitized just caudal to the posterior edge of the lateral condyle of the tibia deep to the aponeurotic sheath of the biceps femoris muscle (Fig. 23.32A). The tibia nerve is desensitized at a point approximately 10 cm above the tuber calcis between the gastrocnemius tendon and the deep digital flexor tendon on the medial aspect of the limb (Fig. 23.32B). Alternatively, anesthesia distal to the tarsus is produced by desensitizing four nerves (four-point block): the lateral and medial plantar metatarsal nerves (both are continuations of the tibial nerve) and the superficial and deep branches of the peroneal nerve.[136,210,211,213] The superficial peroneal nerve lies superficial to the extensor tendons, and the deep peroneal nerve lies deep on the metatarsus; the lateral and medial plantar metatarsal nerves lie superficial in a fibrous sheath containing artery and vein lateral and medial to the flexor tendons, respectively. A 2.5-cm, 22-gauge needle with approximately 5 mL of a 2% lidocaine hydrochloride solution is used at each site, just above the middle of the junction between the proximal and middle third of the metatarsus.

The superficial peroneal nerve is desensitized subcutaneously on the dorsal surface of the metatarsal bone in the proximal third of the metatarsus (Fig. 23.33A). The deep peroneal nerve is desensitized in the midmetatarsal region beneath the extensor tendons (Fig. 23.33B). Traditionally, the deep peroneal nerve is ap-

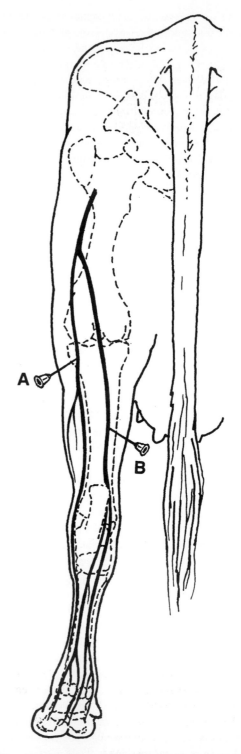

Fig. 23.32. Needle placement for desensitizing the common peroneal nerve (*A*) and tibial nerve (*B*) in cattle: caudal aspect.

proached by placing a 22-gauge needle under the extensor tendons from the lateral side. Alternatively, a 2.5-cm, 25-gauge needle can be placed through the extensor tendon by using slow injection with considerable pressure. Penetration of the dorsal metatarsal artery must be avoided.

The medial and lateral plantar metatarsal nerves are desensi-

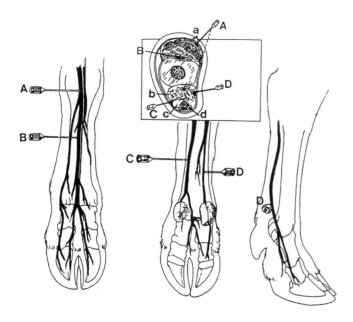

Fig. 23.33. Needle placement for midmetatarsal nerve blocks on the right hind foot in cattle: superficial peroneal nerve (*A*), deep peroneal nerve (*B*), medial plantar metatarsal nerve (*C*), and lateral plantar metatarsal nerve (*D*): dorsal aspect **(left)**, plantar aspect **(center)**, lateral aspect **(right)**, and cross-sectional aspect **(inset)**. **Inset:** *a*, extensor tendons; *b*, interosseous ligament; *c*, deep digital flexor tendon; and *d*, superficial digital flexor tendon). From Skarda,[5] p. 657.

tized approximately 5 cm above the fetlock in the groove between the suspensory ligament and flexor tendons on the medial and lateral aspects of the limb (Fig. 23.33C and D). Adequate analgesia for claw amputation can be expected after the four-point block. However, if sensation to the bulb of the heels after injection still remains, it is advisable to repeat the perineural infiltration not only of the lateral and medial plantar metatarsal nerves, but also of the deep peroneal nerve, which supplies sensory fibers to the interdigital area and bulb of the heels.

The advantages of specific nerve blocks in the foot as compared with general anesthesia are fewer complications associated with regional anesthesia and immediate ambulation of the animal after surgery. The most obvious disadvantage of regional anesthesia is that it requires a good knowledge of the anatomy of the region. Multiple injections are required for each region. Analgesia is often incomplete, probably owing to anastomotic, collateral, or recurrent nerve branches.[213] The use of general anesthesia may be advantageous in fractious animals that require complete immobilization. In addition, the use of general anesthesia avoids the necessity of injection of the local anesthetic into inflamed tissue, which is often painful and ineffective and can cause the spread of infection or absorption of toxins.

Intra-articular Anesthesia

Arthrocentesis may be considered for diagnostic work in conjunction with examination of joint fluid, but intra-articular analgesia is seldom used, although it is an inexpensive means of providing site-specific analgesia.[214]

In a recent study, 2% lidocaine (40 mg, 2 mL) was chosen for preincisional intra-articular administration, whereas postclosure intra-articular 0.5% bupivacaine (10 mg, 2 mL) was used because of its longer-lasting action in adult sheep undergoing stifle arthrotomy during general anesthesia.[215,216] Intra-articular lidocaine plus bupivacaine provided analgesia for 3 to 7 h postoperatively.

Anesthesia for Castration

Castration of bulls, sheep, goats, and pigs is one of the most commonly performed surgical procedures in general practice. Optimal methods for pain control during castration are controversial. The operation may be performed by using chemical restraint and regional anesthesia with animals in either the standing or cast position, or by using general anesthesia induced by intravenous or intratesticular injection of a barbiturate or dissociative. The choice of method to be used largely depends on the species and the opportunity to observe the animal after castration. Regional anesthesia can be induced by intratesticular injection of local anesthetic solution in all food animals.

The scrotum should be cleansed with a detergent antiseptic solution, and the proposed line of incision subcutaneously infiltrated with 3 to 5 mL of a 2% lidocaine hydrochloride solution. The anesthetic is injected as the skin is tensed over the testicle and is pulled on the needle.

In bulls and boars, a 3.75- to 7.5-cm, 16- to 18-gauge needle is first inserted through the skin below the tail of the epididymis and then pushed quickly into the center of the testicle by using an angle of approximately 30° from perpendicular without puncturing the side or bottom (Fig. 23.34). The anesthetic (10 to 15 mL per 200 kg of body weight) is injected into the substance of each testicle. The anesthetic is said to enter lymph vessels quickly and to desensitize the sensory fibers in the spermatic cord.[217]

In bull calves, rams, and bucks, a smaller needle (2.5 to 3.75 cm, 20 gauge) is used to enable easy flow between 2 and 10 mL, depending on the size of the animal, of a 2% lidocaine hydrochloride solution to the center of the testicle and to minimize backflow through the needle tract. The bulk of the anesthetic quickly passes from the testes up the spermatic cord via the lymph vessels into the blood, so the administration of an excessive dose must be avoided or intoxication will occur. Intratesticular injection of 3 to 15 mL of a 2% lidocaine hydrochloride solution can be satisfactory for castration in male pigs up to approximately 5 months of age. Additionally, 2 to 5 mL of the anesthetic is injected subcutaneously beneath the scrotum as the needle is withdrawn. General anesthesia, however, is more suitable for older pigs.

Because the distribution and effectiveness of lidocaine into the testicle of piglets have been questioned, the distribution of 0.4 mL of radioactive [^{14}C]lidocaine with 5 mg of adrenaline/mL injected into each testis and subcutaneously in the scrotum of six male piglets has been evaluated.[218] Autoradiograms show radioactivity in the testes, distally where the subcutaneous injection was made, and in the entire length of the spermatic cord 10 min after completion of the injection.

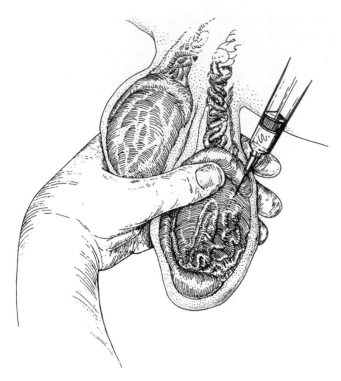

Fig. 23.34. Needle placement for right testicular injection in a bull calf. From Skarda,[5] p. 659.

In another study, to reduce pain associated with ring castration, local anesthetic (2% lidocaine) was injected into three sites around the scrotal neck (1 mL into the anterior-medial surface and 0.5 mL into each lateral surface) of lambs about 6 weeks of age 5 to 10 s before rubber-ring castration.[219] Injecting lidocaine (1 mL) into each testis through the caudal pole after ring application did not reduce cortisol levels associated with ring castration and docking, however.[220] In two other studies in calves, the intravenous administration of the anti-inflammatory ketoprofen (3 mg/kg of body weight) was considered more effective than the injection of 8 to 9 mL of 2% lidocaine into each testis during castration to alleviate the associated stress response.[221,222] Systemic analgesia with ketoprofen was considered more effective in reducing inflammatory responses associated with castration than either local or epidural anesthesia.

Intratesticular Injection

A sclerosing agent (Chem-Cast) may be painlessly injected into the testes of bull calves weighing less than 70 kg in order to destroy the testicular tissue within 60 to 90 days without edema, hemorrhage, or unacceptable necrosis.[223] The recommended dose is 1 mL per testicle in calves weighing up to 45 kg and 1.5 mL per testicle in calves weighing 46 to 68 kg. As compared with surgical castration and mechanically crushing the cord (Burdizzo method), chemical castration is simple and fast; it lacks the high risk of infection associated with surgical castration, and it contributes to improved weight gain. There is no withdrawal time for nontesticular tissues obtained from calves treated with Chem-Cast.[223]

Conclusion

Presently, sufficient clinical work has been done to establish the usefulness, safety, and limitations of local and regional anesthesia techniques in ruminants and swine. Generally speaking, the rational use of a 2% lidocaine hydrochloride solution provides economic and good intraoperative analgesia with rapid recovery and minimal side effects. The systemic administration of an NSAID (e.g., ketoprofen IV) may also be considered for relieving both intraoperative and postoperative pain and stress commonly observed after surgical procedures, such as dehorning and castration.

References

1. Ames NK, Riebold TW. Anesthesia in cattle. In: Proceedings of the 11th Annual Convention of the American Association of Bovine Practitioners, 1978:75–77.
2. Thurmon JC, Benson GF. Anesthesia in ruminants and swine. In: Howard J, ed. Current Veterinary Therapy: Food Animal Practice. Philadelphia: WB Saunders, 1981:58–89.
3. Trim CM. Sedation and general anesthesia in ruminants. Bovine Pract 16:137–144, 1981.
4. Cox VS, McGrath CJ, Jorgensen SE. The role of pressure damage in pathogenesis of the downer cow syndrome. Am J Vet Res 43:26–31, 1982.
5. Skarda RT. Techniques of local analgesia in ruminants and swine. Vet Clin North Am Food Anim Pract 2:621–663, 1986.
6. Booth NH. Local anesthetics. In: Jones LH, Booth NH, McDonald LE, eds. Veterinary Pharmacology and Therapeutics, 4th ed. Ames: Iowa State University Press, 1977:417–436.
7. Heavner JE. Local anesthetics. Vet Clin North Am 3:209–221, 1981.
8. Lumb WV, Jones EW. Veterinary Anesthesia, 2nd ed. Philadelphia: Lea and Febiger, 1984.
9. Link RP, Smith JC. Comparison of some local anesthetics in cattle. J Am Vet Med Assoc 129:306–309, 1956.
10. Moore DC. An evaluation of hyaluronidase in local and nerve block analgesia: A review of 519 cases. Anesthesiology 11:470–484, 1950.
11. Watson D. Hyaluronidase. Br Anaesth 71:422–425, 1993.
12. Hare WCD. A regional method for the complete anaesthetization and immobilization of the bovine eye and its associated structures. Can J Comp Med 21:228–234, 1957.
13. Rubin LF, Gelatt KN. Analgesia of the eye. In: Soma LR, ed. Veterinary Anesthesia. Baltimore: Williams and Wilkins, 1971:489–499.
14. Cust RE. Anaesthesia and akinesia. In: Blogg JR, ed. The Eye in Veterinary Practice. North Melbourne, Australia: VS Supplies, 1975:169–178.
15. Ramakrishna O. Apnoea following retrobulbar block in cattle. Indian Vet J 72:97–98, 1995.
16. Peterson DR. Nerve block of the eye and associated structures. J Am Vet Med Assoc 118:145–148, 1951.
17. Maksimovic B. Akinesie des M. orbicularis palpebrum bei Rindern. Vet Arch 20:75–78, 1950.
18. Schreiber J. Die anatomischen Grundlagen der Leitungsanästhesie beim Rind. I. Die Leitungsanästhesie der Kopfnerven. Wien Tierarztl Wochenschr 42:129–153, 1955.
19. Gibbons WJ. Local anesthesia in bovine practice. Mod Vet Pract 40:36–39, 1959.

20. Gabel AA. Practical technics for bovine anesthesia. Mod Vet Pract 45:39–44, 1964.

21. Elmore RG. Food-animal regional anesthesia: Bovine blocks—Ocular. Vet Med Small Anim Clin 75:1760–1762, 1980.

22. Pearce SG, Kerr CL, Boure LP, Thompson K, Dobson H. Comparison of the retrobulbar and Peterson nerve block techniques via magnetic resonance imaging in bovine cadavers. Am Vet Med Assoc 223:852–855, 2003.

23. Monke DR. Local nasal anesthesia in the bull. Vet Med Small Anim Clin 76:389–393, 1981.

24. Steiner A, von Rotz A. Die wichtigsten Lokalanästhesien beim Rind: Eine Übersicht. Schweiz Arch Tierheilk 145:262–271, 2003.

25. Browne TG. The technique of nerve-blocking for dehorning cattle. Vet Rec 50:1336–1337, 1938.

26. Wheat JD. New landmark for cornual nerve block. Vet Med 45:29–30, 1950.

27. Elmore RG. Food-Animal Regional Anesthesia. Edwardsville, KS: Veterinary Medicine, 1981.

28. Vitums A. Nerve and arterial blood supply to the horns of the goat with reference to the sites of anesthesia for dehorning. J Am Vet Med Assoc 125:284–286, 1954.

29. Spoulding CE. Procedures for dehorning the dairy goat. Vet Med Small Anim Clin 72:228–230, 1977.

30. Bowen JS. Dehorning the mature goat. J Am Vet Med Assoc 171:1249–1250, 1977.

31. Baker JS. Dehorning goats. Bovine Pract 2:33–39, 1981.

32. Grondahl-Nielsen C, Simonsen HB, Lund JD, Hesselholt M. Behavioural, endocrine and cardiac responses in young calves undergoing dehorning without and with the use of sedation and analgesia. Vet J 158:14–20, 1999.

33. Lauwers H, DeVos NR. The nerve supply of the horn of the ox with regards to the course of the ophthalmic nerve. Vlaams Diergeneeskd Tijdschr 35:451–464, 1966.

34. Butler WF. Innervation of the horn region in domestic ruminants. Vet Rec 80:490–492, 1967.

35. McMeekan CM, Mellor DJ, Stafford KJ, Bruce RA, Ward RN, Gregory NG. Effects of local anesthesia of 4 to 8 hours' duration on the acute cortisol response to scoop dehorning in calves. Aust Vet J 76:281–285, 1998.

36. Sylvester SP, Mellor DJ, Stafford KJ, Bruce RA, Ward RN. Acute cortisol responses of calves to scoop dehorning using local anaesthesia and/or cautery of the wound. Aust Vet J 76:118–122, 1998.

37. Sutherland MA, Mellor DJ, Stafford KJ, Gregory NG, Bruce RA, Ward RN. Effect of local anesthetic combined with wound cauterisation on the cortisol response to dehorning in calves. Aust Vet J 80:165–167, 2002.

38. McMeekan CM, Stafford KJ, Mellor DJ, Bruce RA, Ward RN, Gregory NG. Effects of regional analgesia and/or a non-steroidal anti-inflammatory analgesic on the acute cortisol response to dehorning in calves. Res Vet Sci 64:147–150, 1998.

39. Faulkner PM, Weary DM. Reducing pain after dehorning in dairy calves. J Dairy Sci 83:2037–2041, 2000

40. Boandl KE, Wohlt JE, Carsia RV. Effects of handling, administration of a local anesthetic, and electrical dehorning on plasma cortisol in Holstein calves. J Dairy Sci 72:2193–2197, 1989.

41. Sutherland MA, Mellor DJ, Stafford KJ, Gregory NG, Bruce RA, Ward RN. Cortisol responses to dehorning of calves given a 5-h local anaesthetic regimen plus phenylbutazone, ketoprofen, or adenocorticotropic hormone prior to dehorning. Res Vet Sci 73:115–123, 2002.

42. Lissemore K, Milligan B, DeHaan A, Millman S, Duffield T. Strategies to minimize response following dehorning in dairy calves [Abstract]. In: Proceedings of the 23rd World Buiatrics Congress, Quebec, Canada, July 11–16, 2004:168.

43. Stillwell G, Saraiva Lima M, Capitão E, Nunes T. Evaluation of the effect of local anaesthesia and local anaesthesia associated with analgesia on the levels of cortisol after hot-iron, chemical, or scoop dehorning [Abstract]. In: Proceedings of the 23rd World Buiatrics Congress, Quebec, Canada, July 11–16, 2004:173.

44. Kattesh HG, Doherty TJ, Welborn MG, Saxton AM, Morrow JL, Dailey JW. Behavioral and physiological responses of calves to dehorning using a long-lasting local anesthetic [Poster]. In: Proceedings of the Eighth World Congress of Veterinary Anesthesia, Knoxville, TN, 2003:215.

45. Carter PD, Johnston NE, Corner LA, Jarrett RG. Observations on the effect of electro-immobilisation on the dehorning of cattle. Aust Vet J 60:17–19, 1983.

46. Wallace CE. Cosmetic dehorning. In: Amstutz HE, ed. Bovine Medicine and Surgery, 2nd ed, vol 2. Santa Barbara, CA: American Veterinary, 1980:1240–1244.

47. Hague BA, Hooper RN. Cosmetic dehorning in goats. Vet Surg 26:332–334, 1997.

48. Scarratt WK, Troutt HF. Iatrogenic lidocaine toxicosis in ewes. J Am Vet Med Assoc 188:184–185, 1986.

49. Morishima HO, Pedersen H, Finster M, et al. Toxicity of lidocaine in adult, newborn, and fetal sheep. Anesthesiology 55:57–61, 1981.

50. Gibbons WJ, Catcott EJ, Smithcors JF, eds. Bovine Medicine and Surgery. Wheaton, IL: American Veterinary, 1970.

51. Oehme FW, Prier JE, eds. Textbook of Large Animal Surgery. Baltimore: Williams and Wilkins, 1974.

52. Farquharson J. Paravertebral lumbar anesthesia in the bovine species. J Am Vet Med Assoc 97:54–57, 1940.

53. Hall LW, Clarke KW. Veterinary Anaesthesia, 9th ed. Eastbourne, UK: Balliere Tindall, 1991.

54. Arnold JP, Kitchell RL. Experimental studies of the innervation of the abdominal wall of cattle. Am J Vet Res 18:229–240, 1957.

55. Cakala S. A technique for the paravertebral lumbar block in cattle. Cornell Vet 51:64–67, 1961.

56. Arthur GH. Some notes on a preliminary trial of segmental epidural anesthesia of cattle. Vet Rec 68:254–256, 1956.

57. Buchholz JH. Beitrag zur extraduralen Anästhesie bei den Haustieren unter besonderer Berücksichtigung der Frage, ob die Injektionsstelle für die extradurale Anästhesie kranialwärts verschoben werden kann [Master's thesis]. Giessen, Germany: University of Giessen, 1948.

58. Heeschen W. Erfahrungen mit der lumbalen Extraduralanästhesie (Segmentalanästhesie) bei Laparatomien am stehenden Rind. Dtsch Tierarztl Wochenschr 6:146–152, 1968.

59. Skarda RT, Muir WW. Segmental lumbar epidural analgesia in cattle. Am J Vet Res 40:52–57, 1979.

60. Taguchi K, Yamagishi N, Yamada H. Xylazine-induced thoracolumbar epidural analgesia in cows: Effects of diluent volume of xylazine and a combination of xylazine and lidocaine. In: Proceedings of the 20th World Buiatrics Congress, Sidney, Australia, vol 2, 1998:841–844.

61. Lee I, Yamagishi N, Oboshi K, Ayukawa Y, Sasaki N, Yamada H. Clinical use of modified dorsolumbar epidural anesthesia in cattle [Abstract]. In: Proceedings of the 23rd World Buiatrics Congress, Quebec, Canada, July 11–16, 2004:167.

62. Lee I, Yamagishi N, Oboshi K, Yamada H, Ohtani M. Multivariate regression analysis of epidural pressure in cattle. Am J Vet Res 63:954–957, 2002.

63. Dogliotti AM. A new method of block anesthesia. Segmental peridural spinal anesthesia. Am J Surg 20:107–118, 1933.

64. Gutierrez A. Anesthesia metamerica peridural. Rev Chir (Buenos Aires) 11:665–685, 1932.

65. Skarda RT. Lumbar epidural and subarachnoid analgesia in cattle, horses, and humans: A comparative study [Postdoctoral thesis]. Zurich: University of Zurich, 1984.

66. Lee I, Soehartono RH, Yamagishi N, Taguchi K, Yamada H. Distribution of new methylene blue injected into the dorsolumbar epidural space. Vet Anaesth Analg 28:140–145, 2001.

67. Lee I, Yamagishi N, Oboshi K, Yamada H. Effect of epidural fat on xylazine-induced dorsolumbar epidural analgesia in cattle. Vet J 65:330–332, 2003.

68. Lee I, Yamagishi N, Oboshi K, Yamada H. Eliminating the effect of epidural fat during dorsolumbar epidural analgesia in cattle. Vet Anaesth Analg 31:86–89, 2004.

69. Lee I, Yamagishi N, Oboshi K, Yamada H. Antagonistic effects of intravenous or epidural atipamezole on xylazine-induced dorsolumbar epidural analgesia in cattle. Vet J 166:194–197, 2003.

70. Lee I, Hikasa Y, Yamagishi N, Oboshi K, Yamada H. The binding and acting sites of epidural alpha 2-adrenergic agonists. Personal communication, 2003.

71. Skarda RT, Yeary RA, Muir WW, Burt JK. Appearance of procaine in spinal fluid during segmental epidural analgesia in cows. Am J Vet Res 42:639–646, 1981.

72. Skarda RT, Muir WW, Ibrahim AL. Spinal fluid concentration of mepivacaine in horses and procaine in cows after thoracolumbar subarachnoid analgesia. Am J Vet Res 46:1020–1024, 1985.

73. Skarda RT, Muir WW. Hemodynamic effects of unilateral segmental lumbar epidural analgesia in cattle. Am J Vet Res 40:645–650, 1979.

74. Skarda RT, Muir WW, Hubbell AEJ. Comparative study of continuous lumbar segmental epidural and subarachnoid analgesia in Holstein cows. Am J Vet Res 50:39–44, 1989.

75. Skarda RT, Muir WW. Segmental thoracolumbar subarachnoid analgesia in cows. Am J Vet Res 42:632–638, 1981.

76. Skarda RT, Muir WW. Effects of segmental subarachnoid analgesia on arterial blood pressure, gas tensions and pH in adult conscious cows. Am J Vet Res 42:1747–1750, 1981.

77. Skarda RT, Muir WW. Hemodynamic and respiratory effects of segmental subarachnoid analgesia in adult Holstein cows. Am J Vet Res 43:1343–1348, 1982.

78. Brown S. Fractional segmental spinal anesthesia in poor risk surgical patients: Report of 600 cases. Anesthesiology 13:416–428, 1952.

79. McLeod WM, Frank ER. A preliminary report regarding epidural analgesia in equines and bovines. J Am Vet Med Assoc 72:327–335, 1928.

80. Hopkins GS. The correlation of anatomy and epidural analgesia in domestic animals. Cornell Vet 25:263–270, 1935.

81. Elmore RG. Food-animal regional anesthesia: Bovine blocks— Epidural. Vet Med Small Anim Clin 75:1017–1029, 1980.

82. Numans SR, Havinga E. Die Wirkungsweise der Lokalanästhetika bei der Epiduralinjektion. Rec Trav Chim 62:497–502, 1943.

83. Linzell JL. Some observations on general and regional anaesthesia in goats. In: Graham-Jones O, ed. Small Animal Anaesthesia. London: Pergamon, 1964.

84. Bradley WA. Epidural analgesia for taildocking in lambs. Vet Rec 79:787–788, 1966.

85. Rulcker C. Lignocaine hydrochloride with and without adrenaline for epidural analgesia in cattle. Vet Rec 77:1180–1182, 1965.

86. Riebold TW, Hawkins JK, Crisman RO. Effect of buffered lidocaine on epidural anesthesia in cattle. In: Short CE, Poznak AV, eds. Animal Pain. New York: Churchill-Livingstone, 1992:303–306.

87. Caron JP, LeBlanc PH. Epidural analgesia in cattle using xylazine [Abstract]. In: Proceedings of the American College of Veterinary Anesthesiologists, San Francisco, 1988. http://www.pubmedcentral.nih.gov/articlerender.fcgi?artid=1255581.

88. Caron JP, LeBlanc PH. Caudal epidural analgesia in cattle using xylazine. Can J Vet Res 53:486–489, 1989.

89. Ko JCH, Althouse GC, Hopkins SM, Jackson LL, Evans LE, Smith RP. Effects of epidural administration of xylazine or lidocaine on bovine uterine motility and perineal analgesia. Theriogenology 32:779–786, 1989.

90. Skarda RT, Sams RA, St Jean G. Plasma and spinal fluid concentrations of xylazine in cattle after caudal epidural injection [Abstract]. In: Proceedings of the Annual Meeting of the American College of Veterinary Anesthesiologists, New Orleans, Louisiana, 1989:27.

91. Skarda RT, Sams RA, St Jean G. Plasma and spinal fluid concentrations of xylazine in cattle after caudal epidural injection [Abstract]. Vet Surg 19:319–320, 1990.

92. St Jean G, Skarda RT, Muir WW, Hoffsis GF. Caudal epidural analgesia induced by xylazine administration in cows. Am J Vet Res 51:1232–1236, 1990.

93. Zaugg JL, Nussbaum M. Epidural injection of xylazine: A new option for surgical analgesia of the bovine abdomen and udder. Vet Med 85:1043–1046, 1990.

94. Skarda RT, St Jean G, Muir WW. Influence of tolazoline on caudal epidural administration of xylazine in cattle. Am J Vet Res 51:556–560, 1990.

95. Skarda RT, Muir WW. The physiologic responses after caudal epidural administration of xylazine in cattle and detomidine in horses. In: Short CE, Poznak AV, eds. Animal Pain. New York: Churchill-Livingstone, 1992:24–34.

96. Gomez de Segura IA, Tendillo FJ, Marsico F. Alpha-2 as a regional anaesthetic in the cow [Abstract]. In: Proceedings of the Fourth International Congress of Veterinary Anaesthesia, Utrecht, The Netherlands, 1991:111.

97. Nowrouzian I, Ghamsari SM. Field trials of xylazine/lidocaine HCl via epidural in cows [Abstract]. Proceedings of the Fourth International Congress of Veterinary Anaesthesia, Utrecht, The Netherlands, 1991:365.

98. Caulkett NA, Cribb PN, Duke T. Xylazine epidural analgesia for cesarean section in cattle. Can Vet J 34:674–676, 1993.

99. Caulkett NA, Cribb PN, MacDonald DG, Fretz PB, Janzen ED. Xylazine hydrochloride epidural analgesia: A method of providing sedation and analgesia to facilitate castration of mature bulls. Compend Contin Educ Food Anim 15:1155–1159, 1993.

100. Gomez de Segura IA, Tendillo FJ. Alpha-2 agonists for regional anaesthesia in the cow. J Vet Anaesth 20:32–33, 1993.

101. Rehage J, Kehler W, Scholz H. Experiences with the use of xylazine for sacral epidural anesthesia in cattle [in German]. Dtsch Tierarztl Wochenschr 101:14–16, 1994.

102. Chevalier HM, Provost PJ, Karas AZ. Effect of caudal epidural xylazine on intraoperative distress and post-operative pain in Holstein heifers. Vet Anaesth Analg 31:1–10, 2004.

103. Grubb TL, Riebold TW, Crisman RO, Lamb LD. Comparison of lidocaine, xylazine, and lidocaine-xylazine for caudal epidural analgesia in cattle. Vet Anaesth Analg 29:64–68, 2002.

104. Grubb TL, Riebold TW, Huber MJ. Evaluation of lidocaine, xylazine, and a lidocaine/xylazine combination for epidural anesthesia in the llama [Abstract]. In: Proceedings of the Annual Meeting of the American College of Veterinary Anesthesiologists, 1992:16.

105. Grubb TL, Riebold TW, Huber MJ. Evaluation of lidocaine, xylazine, and a lidocaine/xylazine combination for epidural anesthesia in the llama [Abstract]. Vet Surg 22:88, 1993.

106. George LW. Pain control in food animals. In: Steffey EP, ed. Recent Advances in Anesthetic Management of Large Domestic Animals. Ithaca, NY: International Veterinary Information Service, 2003:A0615.1103. http://www.ivis.org.

107. Prado ME, Streeter RN, Mandsager RE, Shawley RV, Claypool PL. Pharmacologic effects of epidural versus intramuscular administration of detomidine in cattle. Am J Vet Res 60:1242–1247, 1999.

108. Lin HC, Trachte EA, DeGraves FJ, Rodgerson DH, Steiss JE, Carson RL. Evaluation of analgesia induced by epidural administration of medetomidine to cows. Am J Vet Res 59:162–167, 1998.

109. Kalia PK, Madan R, Batra RK, Latha V, Vardhan V, Gode GR. Clinical study on epidural clonidine for postoperative analgesia. Indian J Med Res 83:550–552, 1986.

110. Glynn C, Dawson D, Sanders R. A double-blind comparison between epidural morphine and epidural clonidine in patients with chronic non-cancer pain. Pain 34:123–128, 1988.

111. De Rossi R, Bucker GV, Varela JV. Perineal analgesic actions of epidural clonidine in cattle. Vet Anaesth Analg 30:64–71, 2003.

112. Eisenach JC, DeKock R, Klimscha W. Alpha$_2$-adrenergic agonists for regional anesthesia: A clinical review of clonidine (1984–1995). Anesthesiology 83:655–674, 1996.

113. Eisenach JC, Dewan DM, Rose JC, Angelo JM. Epidural clonidine produces antinociception, but not hypotension, in sheep. Anesthesiology 66:496–501, 1987.

114. Eisenach JC, Grice SC. Epidural clonidine does not decrease blood pressure or spinal blood flow in awake sheep. Anesthesiology 68:335–340, 1988.

115. Eisenach JC, Castro MI, Dewan DM, Rose JC. Epidural clonidine analgesia in obstetrics: Sheep studies. Anesthesiology 70:51–56, 1989.

116. Castro MI, Eisenach JC. Pharmacokinetics and dynamics of intravenous, intrathecal, and epidural clonidine in sheep. Anesthesiology 71:418–425, 1989.

117. Smith BD, Baudendistel LJ, Gibbons JJ, Schweiss JF. A comparison of two epidural α$_2$-agonists, guanfacine and clonidine, in regard to duration of antinociception, and ventilatory and hemodynamic effects in goats. Anesth Analg 74:712–718, 1992.

118. Gordh T Jr, Feuk U, Norlén K. Effect of epidural clonidine on spinal cord blood flow and regional and central hemodynamics in pigs. Anesth Analg 65:1312–1318, 1986.

119. Valadão CAA, Dória RGS, Fariass A, Duque JCM, Almeida RM, Castro-Neto A. Comparative study of epidural xylazine and clonidine in horses [Abstract]. In: Proceedings of the Eighth World Congress of Veterinary Anesthesia, Knoxville, TN, 2003:197.

120. Coombs DW, Saunders RL, Lachance D, Savage S, Ragnarsson TS, Jensen LE. Intrathecal morphine tolerance: Use of intrathecal clonidine, DADLE, and intraventricular morphine. Anesthesiology 62:358–363, 1985.

121. Penon C, Ecoffey C, Cohen SE. Ventilatory response to carbon dioxide after epidural clonidine injection. Anesth Analg 72:761–764, 1991.

122. Marsico F, Nascimento PRL, de Paula AC, et al. Epidural injection of ketamine for caudal epidural analgesia in the cow. J Vet Anaesth 26:27–31, 1999.

123. Lee I, Yoshiuchi T, Yamagishi N, et al. Analgesic effect of caudal epidural ketamine in cattle. J Vet Sci 4:261–264, 2003.

124. Bierschwal CJ. A technic for continuous epidural anesthesia in the bovine. Vet Med 55:44–46, 1960.

125. Elmore RG. Food-animal regional anesthesia: Bovine blocks—Continuous epidural analgesia. Vet Med Small Anim Clin 75:1174–1176, 1980.

126. Kuzucu EY, Derrick WS, Wilber SA. Control of intractable pain with subarachnoid alcohol block. J Am Med Assoc 195:541–544, 1966.

127. Noordsy JL. Sacral paravertebral alcohol nerve block as an aid in controlling chronic rectal tenesmus in cattle. Vet Med Small Anim Clin 77:797–801, 1982.

128. Adjanju JB. Alcohol block of the distal ventral sacral nerves of the bovine species as a method of controlling rectal tenesmus [Master's Thesis]. Manhattan, KS: Kansas State University, 1975.

129. Noordsy JL. Bovine surgery 1976. In: Proceedings of the Ninth International Congress on Cattle Disease, Paris, 1976:21–30.

130. Larson LL. The internal pudendal (pudic) nerve block for anesthesia of the penis and relaxation of the retractor penis muscle. J Am Vet Med Assoc 123:18–27, 1953.

131. Deshmukh SE, Deshpande KS. Internal pudendal nerve block in cows. Indian Vet J 57:73–75, 1980.

132. Misra SS. Studies on clinical use of pudic-nerve block in bovine. In: Proceedings of the Fourth International Congress of Veterinary Anaesthesia, Utrecht, The Netherlands, 1991:108.

133. Habel RE. A source of error in the bovine pudendal nerve block. J Am Vet Med Assoc 128:16–17, 1956.

134. Bhokre AP, Deshpande KS. Experimental study on effect of hyaluronidase in pudic nerve block in bovines. Indian Vet J 56:872–874, 1979.

135. McFarlane IS. The lateral approach to the pudendal nerve block in the bovine and ovine. J S Afr Vet Assoc 34:73–76, 1963.

136. Westhues M, Fritsch R. Animal Anesthesia, vol 1. London: Oliver and Boyd, 1964:171–181.

137. Johnson RA, Lopez MJ, Hendrickson DA, Kruse-Elliott KT. Cephalad distribution of three differing volumes of new methylene blue injected into the epidural space in adult goats. Vet Surg 25:448–451, 1996.

138. Lopez MJ, Johnson R, Hendrickson DA, Kruse-Elliott KT. Craniad migration of differing doses of new methylene blue injected into the epidural space after death of calves and juvenile pigs. Am J Vet Res 58:786–790, 1997.

139. Eibl K. Die Lumbalanästhesie in der täglichen Praxis bei Jungbullen und Schweinen. Munch Tierarztl Wochenschr 86:145–148, 1935.

140. Getty R. Epidural anesthesia in the hog: Its technique and applications. In: American Veterinarians Medical Association Scientific Proceedings of the 100th Annual Meeting, New York, 1966:88–98.

141. Strande A. Epidural anaesthesia in young pigs: Dosage in relation to the length of the vertebral column. Acta Vet Scand 9:41–49, 1968.

142. Booth NH. Anesthesia in the pig. Fed Proc 28:1547–1552, 1969.

143. Anderson IL. Anaesthesia in the pig. Aust Vet J 49:474–477, 1973.

144. Runnels LJ. Practical anesthesia and analgesia for porcine surgery. In: Proceedings of the American Association of Swine Practitioners, March 1976:80–87.

145. Benson GJ, Thurmon JC. Anesthesia of swine under field conditions. J Am Vet Med Assoc 174:594–596, 1979.

146. Trim CM. Epidural analgesia in swine. Vet Anesth 8:23–25, 1980.

147. Elmore RG. Food-animal regional anesthesia: Porcine blocks—Lumbosacral (epidural). Vet Med Small Anim Clin 76:387–388, 1981.

148. Framstad T, Austad R, Knaevelsrud T. Epidural anesthesia of sows: Techniques and dosage for obstetric procedures. Nord Veterinaertidsskrift 102:363–369, 1990.

149. Framstad T, Knaevelsrud T. Effect on pulse rate and blood pressure of premedication and epidural anaesthesia in the sow. J Vet Anaesth 19:32–36, 1992.

150. Skarda RT. Techniques of local analgesia in ruminants and swine. Vet Clin North Am Food Anim Pract 12:579–626, 1996.

151. Ko JCH, Thurmon JC, Benson JG, Tranquilli WJ. Evaluation of analgesia induced by epidural injection of detomidine and xylazine in swine. J Vet Anaesth 19:56–60, 1993.

152. Ko JCH, Thurmon JC, Benson JG, Tranquilli WJ. A new drug combination for use in porcine cesarean sections. Vet Med Food Anim Pract 88:466–472, 1993.

153. Pera AM, Mascias A, Criado A, Barreiro A, Dinev D, Tendillo FJ. Cardiopulmonary and analgesic effects of epidural lidocaine, alfentanil and xylazine in pigs anesthetized with isoflurane [Abstract]. In: Proceedings of the Annual Meeting of the American College of Veterinary Anesthesiologists, New Orleans, 1992:10.

154. Pera AM, Mascias A, Criado A, Barreiro A, Dinev D, Tendillo FJ. Cardiopulmonary and analgesic effects of epidural lidocaine, alfentanil and xylazine in pigs anesthetized with isoflurane [Abstract]. Vet Surg 22:86, 1993.

155. Tendillo FJ, Pera AM, Mascias A, et al. Cardiopulmonary and analgesic effects of epidural lidocaine, alfentanil, and xylazine in pigs anesthetized with isoflurane. Vet Surg 24:73–77, 1995.

156. Yaksh TL. Effects of spinally administered agents on spinal cord blood flow: A need for further studies. Anesthesiology 59:173–175, 1983.

157. Paavola A, Tarkkila P, Xu M, Wahlstrom T, Yliruusi J, Rosenberg P. Controlled release gel of ibuprofen and lidocaine in epidural use: Analgesia and systemic absorption in pigs. Pharm Res 15:482–487, 1998.

158. Miniats OP, Jol D. Gnotobiotics pigs: Derivation and rearing. Can J Comp Med 42:428–437, 1978.

159. Grono LR. Spinal anaesthesia in the sheep. Aust Vet J 42:58–59, 1966.

160. Hopcroft SC. Technique of epidural anaesthesia in experimental sheep. Aust Vet J 43:213–214, 1967.

161. Lewis CA, Constable PD, Huhn JC, Morin DE. Sedation with xylazine and lumbosacral epidural administration of lidocaine and xylazine for umbilical surgery in calves. J Am Vet Med Assoc 214:89–95, 1999.

162. Vesal N, Oloumi MM. A preliminary comparison of epidural lidocaine and xylazine during total intravenous anaesthesia in Iranian fat-tailed sheep. Zentralbl Veterinarmed [A] 45:353–360, 1998.

163. Hendrickson DA, Kruse-Elliott KT, Broadstone RV. A comparison of epidural saline, morphine, and bupivacaine for pain relief after abdominal surgery in goats. Vet Surg 25:83–87, 1996.

164. Gray PR. Anesthesia in goats and sheep. I. Local analgesia. Compend Contin Educ Pract Vet 8:S33–S39, 1986.

165. Abdel-Wahed RE. Epidural versus systemic administration of alpha₂ agonists in sheep [Abstract]. In: Proceedings of the Eighth World Congress of Veterinary Anesthesia, Knoxville, TN, 2003:216.

166. Aminkov B, Pascalev M. Cardiovascular and respiratory effects of epidural vs intravenous xylazine in sheep. Rev Med Vet 149:69–74, 1998.

167. Aminkov B, Hubenov HD. The effect of xylazine epidural anaesthesia on blood gas and acid-base parameters in rams. Br Vet J 151:579–585, 1995.

168. Scott PR, Gessert ME. Evaluation of extradural xylazine injection for caesarean operation in ovine dystocia cases. Vet J 154:63–67, 1997.

169. Gessert ME, Scott PR. Combined xylazine and lidocaine caudal epidural injection in the treatment of ewes with preparturient vaginal or cervico-vaginal prolapse. Agri-Practice 16:15–17, 1995.

170. Scott PR, Sargison ND, Penny CD, Pirie RS. The use of combined xylazine and lignocaine epidural injection in ewes with vaginal or uterine prolapses. Theriogenology 43:1175–1178, 1995.

171. Scott PR, Gessert ME. Management of post-partum cervical uterine or rectal prolapses in ewes using caudal epidural xylazine and lignocaine injection. Vet J 153:115–116, 1997.

172. Aminkov BY, Dinev D, Pascalev M. The anti-nociceptive and cardiopulmonary effects of extradural fentanyl-xylazine in sheep. Vet Anaesth Analg 29:126–132, 2002.

173. Coombs DW, Colburn RW, DeLeo JA, Hoopes PJ, Twitchell BB. Comparative spinal neuropathology of hydromorphone and morphine after 9- and 30-day epidural administration in sheep. Anesth Analg 78:674–681, 1994.

174. Clutton RE, Boyd C, Ward JL, Sponenberg DP. Fatal body positioning during epidural anesthesia in a ewe. Can Vet J 30:748–750, 1989.

175. Waterman A, Livingston A, Bouchenafa O. Analgesic effects of intrathecally-applied alpha 2-adrenoceptor agonists in conscious, unrestrained sheep. Neuropharmacology 27:213–216, 1979.

176. Waterman AE, Livingston A, Bouchenafa O, et al. Analgesic actions of alpha 2 adrenergic agonist drugs administered intrathecally in conscious sheep [Abstract]. In: Proceedings of the Third International Congress of Veterinary Anaesthesia, Brisbane, Australia, 1988:41.

177. Haerdi-Landerer M Ch, Schlegel U, Neiger-Aeschbacher G. Antinociceptive effect of intrathecally applied alpha₂ agonists (xylazine and detomidine) in sheep and the response to atipamezole [Abstract]. Vet Anaesth Analg 30:88, 2003.

178. Swenson JD, Wisniewski M, McJames S, Ashburn MA, Pace NL. The effect of prior dural puncture on cisternal cerebrospinal fluid morphine concentrations in sheep after administration of lumbar epidural morphine. Anesth Analg 83:523–525, 1996.

179. Payne P, Gradert TL, Inturrisi CE. Cerebrospinal fluid distribution of opioids after intraventricular and lumbar subarachnoid administration in sheep. Life Sci 59:1307–1321, 1996.

180. DeRossi R, Junqueira AL, Beretta MP. Analgesic and systemic effects of ketamine, xylazine, and lidocaine after subarachnoid administration in goats. Am J Vet Res 64:51–56, 2003.

181. Aithal HP, Amarpal, Kinjavdekar P, Pawde AM, Pratap K. Analgesic and cardiopulmonary effects of intrathecally administered romifidine or romifidine and ketamine in goats (Capra hircus). J S Afr Vet Assoc 72:84–91, 2001.

182. Kinjavdekar P. Spinal analgesia with α₂-agonists and their combination with ketamine and lidocaine in goats [PhD dissertation]. Izatnagar, India: IVRI Deemed University, 1998.

183. Kinjavdekar P, Singh GR, Amarpal, Pawde AM, Aithal HP. Effect of subarachnoid xylazine and medetomidine on hemodynamics and ECG in goats. J Vet Med [A] 46:271–275, 1999.

184. Pablo LS. Epidural morphine in goats after hindlimb orthopedic surgery. Vet Surg 22:307–310, 1993.

185. Waterman AE, Kyles AE, Livingston A. Spinal activity of analgesics in sheep [Abstract]. In: Proceedings of the Fourth Inter-

national Congress of Veterinary Anaesthesia, Utrecht, The Netherlands, 1991:37.

186. Lebeaux M. Sheep: A model for testing spinal and epidural agents. Lab Anim Sci 25:629–633, 1975.

187. Nelson DR, Ott RS, Benson GJ. Spinal analgesia and sedation of goats with lidocaine and xylazine. Vet Rec 105:278–280, 1979.

188. Ralson DH, Shnider SM, de Lorimer AA. Effects of equipotent ephedrine, metaraminol, mephentermine, and methoxamine on uterine blood flow on the pregnant ewe. Anesthesiology 40:354–370, 1974.

189. St Clair LE. The nerve supply to the bovine mammary gland. Am J Vet Res 3:10–16, 1942.

190. Noordsy JL. Food Animal Surgery. Bonner Springs, KS: Veterinary Medical, 1978.

191. Getty R. Sisson and Grossman's the Anatomy of the Domestic Animals, 5th ed. Philadelphia: WB Saunders, 1975.

192. Greenough PR. Development of an approach to lameness examination in cattle. Vet Clin North Am Food Anim Pract 1:3–11, 1985.

193. Prentice DE, Wyn-Jones G, Jones RS, Jagger DW. Intravenous regional anaesthesia of the bovine foot. Vet Rec 94:293–295, 1974.

194. Estill CT. Intravenous local analgesia of the bovine lower leg. Vet Med Small Anim Clin 72:1499–1502, 1977.

195. Elmore RG. Food-animal regional anesthesia: Bovine blocks—Intravenous limb block. Vet Med Small Anim Clin 75:1835–1836, 1980.

196. Knight AP. Intravenous regional anesthesia of the bovine foot. Bovine Pract 1:14–15, 1980.

197. Manohar M, Kumar R, Tyagi RPS. Studies on the intravenous retrograde regional anaesthesia of the forelimb in buffalo calves. Br Vet J 127:401–407, 1971.

198. Kumar R, Manohar M, Tyagi RPS. The fate of intravascularly infused regional anesthesia: A radiographic investigation. J Am Vet Radiol Soc 14:87–92, 1973.

199. Tyagi RPS, Kumar R, Manohar M. Studies on intravenous retrograde regional anaesthesia for the forelimbs of ruminants. Aust Vet J 49:321–324, 1973.

200. Jones RS, Prentice DE. Some observations on intravenous anaesthesia of the bovine foot [Abstract]. Proc Assoc Vet Anaesth Gr Br Ir 5:13–17, 1974.

201. Fehlings K. Intravenöse regionale Anästhesie an der V. digitalis dorsalis communis III: Eine brauchbare Möglichkeit zur Schmerzausschaltung bei Eingriffen an der Vorderzehe des Rindes. Dtsch Tierarztl Wochenschr 87:4–7, 1980.

202. Surborg H. Aspects of treatment of severe claw disease in a large animal practice. Bovine Pract 19:227–229, 1984.

203. Weaver AD. Intravenous local anesthesia of the lower limb in cattle. J Am Vet Med Assoc 160:55–57, 1972.

204. Antalovsky A. Technik der intravenösen Schmerzausschaltung im distalen Gliedmassenbereich beim Rind. Vet Med (Praha) 7:413–420, 1965.

205. Bogan JA, Weaver AD. Lidocaine concentrations associated with intravenous regional anesthesia of the distal limb of cattle. Am J Vet Res 39:1672–1673, 1978.

206. Gogoi SN, Nigam JM, Peshin PK, Sharifi D, Patil DB. Studies on intravenous regional analgesia of the hind limb in the bovine. Zentralbl Veterinarmed [A] 38:544–552, 1991.

207. Skarda RT. Local and regional anesthesia. In: Short CE, ed. Principles and Practice of Veterinary Anesthesia. Baltimore: Williams and Wilkins, 1987:91–133.

208. Steiner A, Ossent P, Mathis GA. Die intravenöse Stauungsanästhesie/Antibiose beim Rind: Indikationen, Technik, Komplikationen. Schweiz Arch Tierheilkd 132:227–237, 1990.

209. Kraus SJ, Green RL. Pseudoanaphylactic reactions with procaine penicillin. Cutis 17:765–767, 1976.

210. Taylor JA. The applied anatomy of the bovine foot. Vet Rec 72:1212–1215, 1960.

211. Raker CW. Regional analgesia of the bovine foot. J Am Vet Med Assoc 128:238–239, 1956.

212. Collin CW. A technic to produce analgesia of the hind digits of cattle. Vet Rec 75:833–834, 1963.

213. Jalaluddin AM, Rao SV. Diagnosis of lameness in the ox by means of nerve blocks. Indian Vet J 49:1246–1256, 1972.

214. Tufvesson G. Local Anesthesia in Veterinary Medicine. Stockholm: Astra International, 1963.

215. Shafford HL, Mallinckrodt CH, Turner AS, Hellyer PW. Intraarticular lidocaine and bupivacaine in sheep undergoing stifle arthrotomy. Vet Anaesth Analg 28:103–104, 2001.

216. Shafford HL, Hellyer PW, Turner AS. Intra-articular lidocaine plus bupivacaine in sheep undergoing stifle arthrotomy. Vet Anaesth Analg 31:20–26, 2004.

217. Rieger H. Die Testiculäre Injektion. Berl Munch Tierarztl Wochenschr 67:107–109, 1954.

218. Ranheim B, Haga AH, Andersen S, Ingebrigsten K. Distribution of radioactive lidocaine injected into the testes in piglets: Preliminary results [Abstract]. In: Proceedings of the Eighth World Congress of Veterinary Anesthesia, Knoxville, TN, 2003:200.

219. Sutherland MA, Mellor DJ, Stafford KJ, et al. Acute cortisol responses of lambs to ring castration and docking after the injection of lignocaine into the scrotal neck or testes at the time of ring application. Aust Vet J 77:738–741, 1999.

220. Graham MJ, Kent JE, Molony V. Effects of four analgesic treatments on the behavioural and cortisol responses of 3-week old lambs to tail docking. Vet J 153:87–97, 1997.

221. Earley B, Crowe MA. Effects of ketoprofen alone or in combination with local anesthesia during castration of bull calves on plasma cortisol, immunological, and inflammatory responses. J Anim Sci 80:1044–1052, 2002.

222. Ting ST, Earley B, Hughes JM, Crowe MA. Effect of ketoprofen, lidocaine local anesthesia, and combined xylazine and lidocaine caudal epidural anesthesia during castration of beef cattle on stress responses, immunity, growth, and behavior. J Anim Sci 81:1281–1293, 2003.

223. Miller RE. An efficient and safe method of castration for the bovine by the intratesticular injection of Chem-Cast. Bovine Proc 15:156–159, 1983.

Chapter 24

Acupuncture

Roman T. Skarda and Maria Glowaski

Introduction

A veterinarian's training often leads to skepticism of Eastern traditional medical practices because of the apparent conflicts with Western scientific methodology and the feeling that Eastern medical practice is somewhat faith based. It is important that novices to *traditional Chinese medicine* (TCM) understand that much of the theory and vocabulary, although similar to Western terminology, have little direct correlation. Much of the practice of TCM developed before the advent of Western medical science and publication of medical textbooks, so a simplified method had to be devised for the practice of TCM based on diagnostic and treatment strategies observable on the external surfaces of the body. Consequently, it is best to think of the description of acupuncture points and TCM diagnostics as metaphors or teaching aids rather than anatomical or pathophysiological correlates to Western medicine.

Treatment strategies have evolved over millennia of trial and error in many species and represent a consensus among TCM practitioners as to what is effective. Current Western medical teaching is that TCM is complementary to Western medicine rather than a replacement for it. Acupuncture is traditionally viewed as one treatment modality among several used by TCM practitioners.

Most Western acupuncture charts show transpositional acupuncture points and meridians on animals, meaning the points are adapted from anatomical correlates on the human body. This creates some interesting adaptations, since animal anatomy (especially horses) varies considerably from humans. Some acupuncturists prefer to use the points described for animals in the early Chinese veterinary texts. These may or may not be aligned with modern points. They are difficult for many Westerners to learn because the names are in Chinese and often describe the anatomy in terms of natural objects (rivers, branches, etc.). Some acupuncturists only use points located on the distal limbs. These are often referred to as *Ting* points and are the ends of the meridians and are usually extremely painful when needled (like sticking needles under fingernails), so they would be expected to produce a pronounced response.

Any patient being treated with acupuncture should be evaluated using the standards of care established for Western-based veterinary medicine. This includes a thorough physical examination, chest auscultation, blood work if necessary, and any other diagnostics that are required. Failure to maintain this standard of care could lead to malpractice. Acupuncture is often used in conjunction with Western treatments such as surgery or pharmacological therapy. It is recommended that written refusal of a Western-based standard of care be obtained from clients who seek to use acupuncture exclusively. Such clients have caused much concern and ethical debate among veterinarians.

History

Acupuncture is an integral part of an ancient Chinese system of medicine that has been used for more than 2500 years to treat diseases and relieve pain. According to tradition, acupuncture is based on a philosophy of balance and unity between the universe, living beings, and energy flow that penetrates everywhere and everything. Any imbalance, disruption, or energy-flow blockage within the body can cause disease or pain. The main concept and philosophy of acupuncture is to return the body to a harmonized, balanced state.

The numerous techniques and approaches to acupuncture reflect a variety of medical traditions and schools from China, Korea, Japan, Vietnam, and other Eastern countries. Some of these approaches focus on points located on traditional acupuncture meridians that crisscross the body surface. Other methods focus on points located on the ear (auricular acupuncture) or hands or feet (Korean hand acupuncture [*Su-Jok*]). In general, it is believed that the ears, hands, and feet are micromodels of the entire body, with areas that represent the body parts, organs, meridians, and acupuncture points. These micromodels have the same principles of energy flow as the whole body. An explanation that has been offered for this phenomenon is a principle of the fractalization (similarity) of living and nonliving things in which small parts have the same shape as the whole.[1] No matter what method of acupuncture is used, it must be applied to specific points to achieve analgesia or other beneficial regional or systemic effects.

Modern research on the basic mechanisms of acupuncture started in the People's Republic of China in 1949, where Mao Zedong encouraged the practice of acupuncture. Ten years later, acupuncture was introduced in the former Soviet Union, where further research was initiated. The practices and research results remained essentially unknown to most Western scientists and physicians. This typically reflected a failure to publish articles in English, along with a lack of interest in the Western research community.[2]

Interest in acupuncture surged in the United States in the early 1970s, in part, because James Reston, a *New York Times* reporter covering President Richard Nixon's trip to China, developed acute appendicitis. After his postoperative pain was treated with acupuncture, he described his experience on the front page of the newspaper, igniting an interest in acupuncture in the Western medical community.[3] Subsequently, American and European physicians visiting China witnessed surgeries in which the only anesthetic used was acupuncture. A number of articles in newspapers and magazines about the use of acupuncture instead of general anesthesia followed. Basic research on acupuncture's mechanisms in Western societies started in 1976 after the endorphin hypothesis of acupuncture's mechanism of action was introduced. Further advancement of acupuncture research was prompted by introduction of functional magnetic resonance imaging (fMRI) and positron-emission tomographic scanning, which revealed the relation between acupuncture stimulation and activation of certain brain structures.[4–8] Interest in the United States led the National Institutes of Health to create the National Center for Complementary and Alternative Medicine (NCCAM), which has funded basic and clinical acupuncture studies.

In 1997, the World Health Organization issued a list of human medical conditions that may benefit from treatment with acupuncture. Applications include prevention and treatment of postoperative and chemotherapy-associated nausea and vomiting, treatment of pain, therapy for alcohol and other drug addiction, treatment of asthma and bronchitis, and rehabilitation from neurological damage such as that caused by stroke.[9] Scientific information on the effectiveness of acupuncture for veterinary disorders is limited. The effectiveness of treatment is based on a consensus among veterinarians commonly performing acupuncture in specific species.

Skepticism about the effectiveness of acupuncture therapy in humans and animals remains among some Western medical practitioners. Some factors contributing to this skepticism are (a) the scientific basis of acupuncture remains unclear, (b) the philosophical basis of acupuncture is difficult for a modern industrial society to accept, (c) the operational language is unusual, and (d) the traditional system of acupuncture points does not correspond to Western concepts of anatomy or neurology. Moreover, traditional Chinese acupuncture remains a mix of philosophy and science and teaches that many factors can profoundly influence the outcome of the treatment. In addition to the signs related to the disease, a practitioner might consider a patient's gender and psychological profile, the season, the time of the day, and even the environment in which the treatment is administered.[10–18] Because of these differences, it is believed that the efficacy of interventions may differ substantially among patients with similar symptoms, and thus it is difficult to standardize procedures. Scientific exploration of these factors remains limited. Another problem associated with acupuncture studies is defining an adequate placebo as a control intervention for them. Some trials compare acupuncture with drugs, and others use *sham acupuncture* (acupuncture at random spots on the body surface that are thought to be inactive). There is substantial controversy, however, about the use of sham acupuncture as a control treatment because the procedure itself can provide neurohormonal and clinical effects, though usually of lower effectiveness compared with treatment at defined acupuncture points.[19]

Basic Concepts

The theory of TCM, of which acupuncture is one part, is complex and beyond the scope of this review. Unlike Western biomedical science, TCM does not make a distinction between physical, mental, and emotional components of life. Moreover, it considers a being as an integral part of the universe. It is believed that everything within the universe, including animals, obeys the same laws. Therefore, health and disease result from balance or imbalance.

Organs and Meridians

Most modern acupuncture schools teach meridian theory. However, early practitioners (and some modern practitioners) do not recognize meridians or do not agree on their path. Meridians are most useful in remembering locations of points, although they are used in developing treatment protocols. Meridians were identified based on observations in a small percentage of people who are extremely sensitive to acupuncture. A meridian can describe the course of a tingling or burning sensation along a path that roughly corresponds to the meridian. Most of the meridians are not obviously associated anatomically with nerve pathways, although many of the relationships observed seem to be explained by the way peripheral nerves enter the spinal cord and neural pathways converge in the brain. For example, many people that have heart attacks describe a pain across the chest and down the arm. The heart meridian courses down the chest and arm. The pain (origin in the heart muscle) is felt in the arm because some of the afferent fibers enter the spinal cord near the location of afferents from the thoracic limb. Other observations indicate that distant areas of the body have complementary effects because many areas in the somatosensory cortex of the brain colocalize. Associations between internal organs and meridians (and superficial points) are very common and make sense if the concept of referred pain is understood.

The theory of traditional Chinese acupuncture recognizes 12 main meridians with corresponding organs in the human body. In addition, eight so-called *curious meridians* can be distinguished. Most acupuncture "organs" have names similar to organs of Western medicine but only an approximate correlation with physiological functions and anatomical structures. Organs, as seen in ancient Chinese traditions, are functional systems rather than anatomical structures, with broader and sometimes peculiar physiological functions and anatomical representations. For example, two traditional acupuncture organs, namely, "triple warmer" and "pericardium" ("heart governor"), do not have a distinct anatomical representation at all. All meridians and organs are connected and related to one another directly or indirectly according to various rules and principles:

- Each organ has a corresponding meridian with acupuncture points located along it.
- Meridians travel inside the body and on the body's surface and are connected to one another and organs by a complex network of accessory collateral connections.
- The function of the meridians is to regulate and modify the corresponding organ or group of related organs. It is believed that meridians can control pain along the areas they traverse.

Points

In Chinese acupuncture, points are called *xue*, which means "cave" or "hole."[20,21] In Chinese acupuncture tradition and language, the names of points are important and informative. Western acupuncture practitioners rarely use Chinese names because of unfamiliarity with the Chinese language. Instead, the points are identified by number and capital letter abbreviation of the meridian to which they belong: 365 classic points are located along the meridians and at least the same number of extrameridian points. The exact location of the points is important, because, according to classic theory, even small deviations from the intended location can nullify the response. The distance of acupoints to anatomical landmarks is usually described as *cun*.

Investigation into the anatomy and physiology of acupuncture points has resulted in a hypothesis that most recognized acupuncture points coincide with tissues that are capable of eliciting a strong neurohumoral response when irritated. These include nerves, neurovascular complexes, Golgi tendon apparatuses, and other sensitive tissues. Stimulation of these tissues might cause acute and intense irritation that triggers endogenous analgesic, immune, and behavior-adapting systems to be activated, resulting in the clinical effectiveness of acupuncture.

Point Location

Several factors have been associated with precise location of acupuncture points:

- Points are located in a small hollow or depression on the skin surface.
- Acupuncture points are usually tender compared with the surrounding area, and a response (probably associated with

discomfort) can often be elicited with deep palpation. Human patients describe a feeling of slight pain or numbness radiating circumferentially for at least a centimeter when the point is pressed.

- A subjective roughness or stickiness can be appreciated when an acupuncture point is brushed slightly with the finger.[21]
- A specific feeling called the *De-Qi* sensation is usually felt by human patients, and the acupuncturist feels a change in the resistance to needle movement, when a needle stimulates an acupuncture point.

In humans, the De-Qi sensation may be described as soreness, numbness, warmth, heaviness, or distension around the area where a needle is inserted. Sometimes this sensation radiates along the pathway of the meridian to which the stimulated point belongs. An experienced practitioner also feels tightness and some heaviness in the fingers when the needle hits the point.[22] This change in needle resistance coupled with the animal's reaction to needle placement is what most veterinary acupuncturists rely on to assess the attainment of De-Qi sensation. Most human and veterinary acupuncturists consider De-Qi sensation to be crucial in achieving the effect of acupuncture.[22–24]

The descriptions of the diameter and depth of acupuncture points vary among various species. Traditionally, the size depends on the individual point, the patient's condition, the time of day, and possibly the season. The depth depends on the amount of hair on the patient, skin thickness (e.g., the thin skin of cats versus the rather thick skin of stallions), location of the point, and duration of the disease.[21,22] In veterinary acupuncture, most clinically used points in most species are believed to be 3 to 15 mm below the skin surface.

Point Stimulation

Traditional Chinese acupuncture teaches that each point has specific functions and indications for use. For example, stimulation of certain acupuncture points distant from the source of pain can provide analgesia, whereas stimulation of inappropriately selected points in close proximity to the source of pain might be ineffective or even aggravate the symptoms. Stimulation of site-specific acupoints usually induces spatially restricted analgesia. Although this aspect of acupuncture has yet to be studied in detail, Benedetti et al.[25] demonstrated that, in people, placebo or treatment expectation provides an analgesic response with a highly spatial presentation, which is completely abolished by systemic naloxone administration. These data indicate that this type of analgesic response is mediated by endogenous opioid release but that the effect is regional rather than systemic. Acupuncture might manifest a similar mechanism of action. Li et al.[26] demonstrated that acupuncture stimulation of the ipsilateral Huantiao (GB 30) point, which is traditionally thought to be effective in treating pain in the lower limbs, including sciatica pain, significantly inhibits nociceptive responses of spinal dorsal horn neurons evoked by stimulation of the sural nerve in rats. In contrast, stimulation of the contralateral Huantiao (GB 30) and some other points produce much less, if any, inhibition.

Cho et al.,[5] using functional MRI, demonstrated a correlation between activation of specific areas of the brain and corresponding acupoint stimulation predicted by ancient acupuncture literature. In this study, acupuncture points belonging to the bladder meridian and located on the foot were stimulated. These points are traditionally related to the eyes and visual function. The investigators also demonstrated activation or deactivation of signal intensity in the visual cortex. A subsequent study confirmed this finding and demonstrated activation of visual and auditory cortex caused by electroacupuncture stimulation of eye-related points and ear-related points, respectively.[8] However, electroacupuncture at sham points also elicited activation in the auditory cortical zone, suggesting that acupuncture-induced activation of medial occipital cortex and superior temporal gyrus may not be an acupoint-specific phenomenon.

Point specificity was also questioned in another functional MRI study by Cho et al.,[27] where meridian and sham acupuncture were both involved in the transmission and perception of pain. Meridian acupuncture demonstrated more profound pain control than did sham-point stimulation, but the effect may not have been entirely point specific. Point specificity, as stated in traditional acupuncture literature and demonstrated by clinical practice and some experimental studies, is not fully supported by other studies and therefore remains a controversial issue. For any species being treated with acupuncture therapy, only careful systematic research using site-, organ-, and function-specific acupuncture points with carefully selected sham control points can resolve this issue.

Mechanisms of Analgesic Action

Starting in the 1960s, Western-trained Chinese physicians began to study acupuncture analgesia, particularly acupuncture-induced physiological changes in the central nervous system (Fig. 24.1). This, and subsequent research in Western countries, resulted in the discovery of several plausible mechanisms of acupuncture analgesia, receptors, and several endogenous opioids involved in the process; hence, a comprehensive hypothesis of acupuncture analgesia was formed. Experimental studies on animals and clinical studies on humans have since identified numerous clinical and physiological responses to acupuncture stimulation.

Comprehensive Mechanism Theory

Based on a review of hundreds of modern scientific studies on acupuncture analgesia, Pomeranz and Stux[2] proposed a comprehensive mechanism of action for acupuncture analgesia. The basis for the theory is that three mechanisms contribute to acupuncture analgesia:

1. Acupuncture needles stimulate type I and type II afferent nerves or A-δ fibers in muscles, all of which send impulses to the anterolateral tract of the spinal cord. At the spinal cord, pain is blocked presynaptically by the release of enkephalin and dynorphin, preventing pain messages from ascending in the spinothalamic tract.

2. Acupuncture stimulates midbrain structures by activating cells in the periaqueductal gray matter and the raphe nucleus.

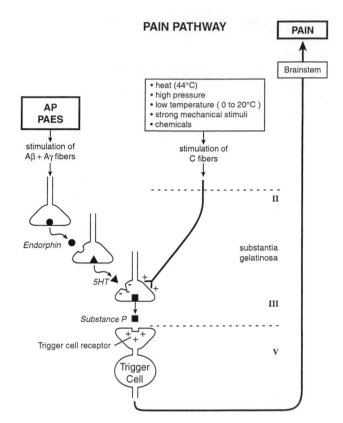

PAIN PATHWAY

Fig. 24.1. Pain pathway and mechanism of inhibition by acupuncture (AP) and percutaneous acupuncture electrical stimulation (PAES). The release and binding of endorphin and serotonin (5-hydroxytryptamine [5HT]) inhibits substance P release in the substantia gelatinosa that normally mediates pain transmission within the spinal cord.

They in turn send descending signals through the dorsolateral tract, causing the release of the monoamines norepinephrine and serotonin in the spinal cord. These neurotransmitters inhibit pain presynaptically and postsynaptically by reducing transmission of signals through the spinothalamic tract (diffuse noxious inhibitory control).

3. Stimulation in the pituitary-hypothalamic complex provokes systemic release of ß-endorphin into the bloodstream from the pituitary gland. Its release is accompanied by the release of adrenocorticotropic hormone.

The National Institutes of Health and National Commission for Complementary and Alternative Medicine have also suggested three possible mechanisms of action for acupuncture:

1. Conduction of electromagnetic signals that may start the flow of endogenous analgesic compounds and immune system cells to specific areas of the body that are injured.
2. Activation of the opioid systems in central nervous system and peripheral tissues.
3. Changes in brain chemistry, sensation, and involuntary bodily functions.

These mechanisms are supported by the observations that conditions that have the best responses to acupuncture include pain,

Fiber spectra profile of a sensory nerve

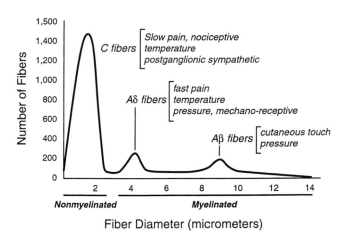

Fig. 24.2. Different-diameter nerve fibers have differing characteristics enabling waveform stimulation neuroselectivity. Large-diameter myelinated (A-ß) fibers can respond to high, 100-Hz stimulus, whereas small nonmyelinated (C) fibers respond to low-frequency stimulation (2 to 10 Hz).

immune-related dysfunctions, and visceral dysfunctions. Conditions that are not reversible, functional conditions (end-stage disease) often respond poorly to acupuncture, although occasionally symptomatic improvement may be observed.

Nociceptors

A-δ fibers are activated by pinprick, pressure, thermal manipulation, and high-threshold ergo receptors in muscles. A-δ fibers provide rapid, precisely located identification of noxious stimu-

lation without affective response. Some of these fibers terminate on the rostral reticular formation and thalamus. From there, they pass forward to the arcuate nucleus of the hypothalamus and on to the prefrontal cortex.[24] Myelinated A-δ fibers are considered the most likely candidates for conveying acupuncture stimuli, but other fibers, including nonmyelinated C fibers and A-ß fibers, may contribute (Fig. 24.2). C fibers, which are ontogenetically older, produce pain described as slow, deep, throbbing, and dull. This sort of pain is often accompanied by a strong affective component. Therefore, noxious stimulation by the C-fiber system leads to a perception of pain that is poorly localized but has considerable behavioral and emotional impact. These fibers primarily make synaptic contacts in substantia gelatinosa in lamina II. Different kinds of fibers are involved in different components of the De-Qi sensation.[28] Because different modalities of acupuncture stimulation produce different types of De-Qi sensation, they may trigger diverse brain networks, based on their activation of various types of afferent input.[6]

The Brain

Acupuncture influences on regional brain activity were elaborated by Wu et al.,[7] who reported that acupuncture at two major points, Zusanli (ST 36 [Fig. 24.3]) and Hegu (LI 4 [Fig. 24.3]), activates the hypothalamus and nucleus accumbens on functional MRI and deactivates the rostral part of the anterior cingulate cortex, amygdala, and hippocampal complex. In contrast, control stimulation by superficial needling that did not elicit the De-Qi sensation did not alter regional brain activity. Therefore, acupuncture at major points with strong analgesic properties seems to activate structures of the descending antinociceptive pathway and to deactivate multiple limbic areas subserving pain association.

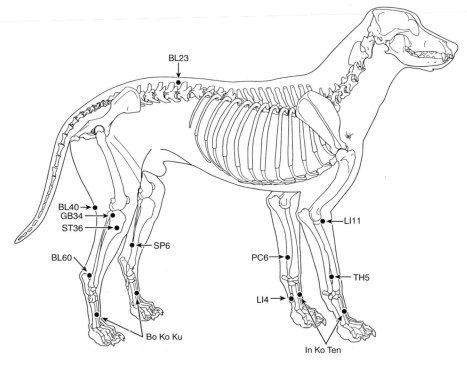

Fig. 24.3. The anatomical location of various acupuncture points, including the Zusanli (ST-36) and Hegu (LI-4) points, that can produce analgesia in dogs.

Other Potential Mechanisms

Acupuncture not only provokes release of endogenous opioids from central nervous system stores, but may also activate other analgesic mechanisms. For example, acupuncture may relieve pain by modulating the hypothalamic-limbic system.[4,8] Biella et al.[4] used positron-emission tomographic scans in healthy volunteers who were not experiencing any pain to evaluate regional cerebral blood flow in response to classic manual acupuncture stimulation of the Zusanli (ST 36) and Qize (LU 5) acupuncture points. The researchers demonstrated activation of the left anterior cingulum, the insulae bilaterally, the cerebellum bilaterally, the left superior frontal gyrus, and the right medial and inferior frontal gyri. Several imaging studies indicate that the same structures are activated by acute and chronic pain.[29–32] *Placebo acupuncture* (needles inserted superficially into nonacupuncture points 1 cm lateral to each acupoint and then immediately extracted) also produced a degree of cerebral activation, but at areas differing from those activated by traditional acupuncture points. Cho et al.[27] had similar results. All the structures that were activated by acupuncture are also involved in nociceptive processing and play a role in the concept of the *neuromatrix* as proposed by Melzack.[33] Biella et al.[4] proposed that, according to this concept, acupuncture can be thought of as a conflicting message in the pain neuromatrix, unbalancing it and thus modifying the perception of pain.

An interesting theory has been proposed suggesting an important integrative role of connective tissue in the mechanism of action of acupuncture.[34] Langevin and Yandow[35] found 80% correspondence between acupuncture points and the location of intramuscular connective tissue planes in postmortem tissue sections. According to this theory, needle manipulations lead to the development of coupling between needle and tissue, with subsequent transduction of the mechanical signal to a cellular response that may underlie some of the therapeutic effects of acupuncture both locally and distally.

Acupuncture analgesia leads to development of tolerance when applied continuously or repeatedly over short time intervals. It would be reasonable to speculate that when acupuncture stimulation releases endogenous opioids to exert an analgesic effect, it also provokes the release of antianalgesic substances. Cholecystokinin is a powerful antagonist of the analgesic effect of acupuncture, and cholecystokinin antisense RNA increases the analgesic effect induced by acupuncture.[36–40]

Many studies have focused on the analgesic effects of acupuncture and the role of endogenous opioids in acupuncture analgesia. However, acupuncture stimulation produces a much broader spectrum of systemic responses, including altering the secretion of neurotransmitters and neurohormones and changing the central and peripheral regulation of blood flow. There are also data suggesting that acupuncture alters immune function and accelerates nerve regeneration.[24,41,42] The mechanisms of these physiological responses remain unclear.

Types of Acupuncture

Invasive methods include skin penetration with an acupuncture needle with subsequent manual stimulation of needles, electroacupuncture, or chronic intradermal needle insertion. These methods are considered *dry needle* techniques. Drugs can be injected into acupoints, a technique considered *wet needle* acupuncture or *aquapuncture*. Noninvasive methods include acupressure, transcutaneous electrical stimulation, moxibustion, and application of various stimulating patches and pellets.

Because the traditional theory of acupuncture is based on the concept that diseases are caused by an imbalance of Qi, the goal of needle insertion is, in the context of TCM, to disperse excessive Qi or to replenish it. These two goals can be achieved by several means: applying needles of different sizes or lengths, using needles made of different material, changing the direction of needle insertion, selecting different points for stimulation, and so forth. For strong stimulation, a bigger needle, more intense needle manipulation, or directing the needle tip against the hypothetical energy flow along the meridian is believed to disperse the excessive energy, whereas for mild stimulation, a smaller needle, gentle and more superficial needle insertion, or directing the needle toward the energy flow is used to replenish it. Manual stimulation techniques can be altered to provide the desired effect by using strong vertical up-and-down movements, rotational movements, or mild vibrating movements, for example. Some practitioners believe that selecting the proper acupuncture maneuvers and appropriate points is key to producing a satisfactory therapeutic effect. Consistent with this theory, Chen et al.[43] demonstrated that different manual needling maneuvers provide different responses on tail-flick latency and vocalization threshold in rats.

Electrical Stimulation

Electrical stimulation of acupuncture points (*electroacupuncture*) was developed as an alternative to manual stimulation of acupuncture points. Electrical stimulation has several advantages in that it (a) is less painful than manual stimulation, (b) requires less practitioner time directly spent with the patient, (c) provides better analgesia, and (d) facilitates standardization.[44] Transcutaneous and percutaneous electrostimulation are now the most common types of acupuncture analgesia performed in people (Fig. 24.4).[45]

In humans, the De-Qi sensation depends on the type of acupuncture stimulation. Manual stimulation produces mainly soreness, fullness, and distension, whereas electroacupuncture generally produces tingling and numbness. Kong et al.[6] report that manual acupuncture manipulations decrease fMRI signals, in contrast to electroacupuncture stimulation, which generally increases MRI signal intensity. Both types of stimulation, however, produce analgesia. Therefore, various stimulation modalities seem to trigger different brain networks, depending on how acupoints are stimulated. How various stimulation modalities influence brain networks in companion animal species such as dogs and cats has not been evaluated.

Electroacupuncture with high-frequency stimulation (100 to 200 Hz) provides rapid-onset analgesia that is not cumulative and cannot be blocked by naloxone. This type of analgesia is probably mediated by norepinephrine, serotonin, and dynorphins.[46] In contrast, low-frequency stimulation (2 to 4 Hz) and medium-

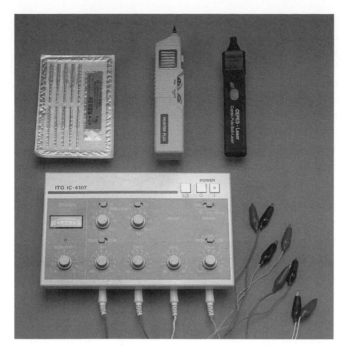

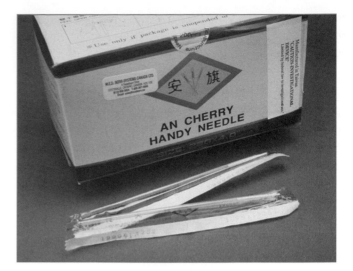

Fig. 24.5. Most good-quality needles are manufactured in China, Japan, or South Korea. They should be sterilized at 120°C for 30 min at 15 pounds of pressure before each use, especially for percutaneous acupuncture electrical stimulation therapy.

Fig. 24.4. A package of ten sterile acupuncture needles (top left) for single use. Pointer-plus handheld unit for electrically locating and stimulating transcutaneous points (transcutaneous electrical nerve stimulation) (top middle). Acu-Vet unit for stimulating acupuncture points transcutaneously (top right). Electroacupuncture Unit IC 4107 for locating and stimulating acupuncture points percutaneously (percutaneous acupuncture electrical stimulation). There is little standardization of acupuncture equipment because it is manufactured in several different countries.

frequency stimulation (15 to 30 Hz) produce an analgesic effect that is reversed by naloxone (and therefore presumably mediated by enkephalin and endorphins), have a tendency to accumulate, and last at least 1 h after treatment ceases.[44,46] Reportedly, antinociception induced by low-frequency stimulation is mediated by both μ opioid and δ opioid receptors; high-frequency electroacupuncture stimulation induces antinociception mediated by κ opioid receptors; and medium-frequency stimulation (e.g., 30 Hz) induces antinociception mediated by all three opioid receptor types.[47]

Needles

Most modern acupuncture needles are made of stainless steel, although needles made of gold or silver are also available (Fig. 24.5). Most acupuncture needles are between 1.3 and 12.7 cm long and range from 26 to 36 gauge in diameter. The tips of the needles are rounded and thus separate fibers rather than cutting tissues. For this reason, even capillary bleeding from an acupuncture site is rare unless a needle accidentally penetrates a vessel. In the treatment of human patients, special needles have been developed for intradermal use, auricular acupuncture, and hand and foot acupuncture.

Veterinary Acupuncture

Probably the most commonly treated species is the dog, although historically, equine acupuncture was more widely used because horses were important for the daily survival of people (similar to the history for Western veterinary medicine). Dogs tend to be cooperative, and most relax during the treatment. If an animal becomes severely distressed, it is unlikely that the treatment will have the desired effect. The most commonly treated problems are related to the musculoskeletal system. It is important for beginners to recognize that pain and disuse in many musculoskeletal diseases—especially chronic degenerative diseases, including low-grade intervertebral disk disease—often wax and wane. This coupled with the placebo effect would suggest that some of patients treated (whether with acupuncture or nonsteroidal anti-inflammatory drugs [NSAIDs]) should improve, at least for a while. One should be careful to not interpret a positive response as possession of superior TCM skills. However, some scientific evidence supports the use of acupuncture alone or in conjunction with other Western treatments such as NSAIDs.[48,49] Other common uses for acupuncture in canine patients include treatment of signs associated with chronic diseases such as cancer, nervous system degeneration, and organ failure, such as chronic renal disease. Unless functional tissue is present, reversal of the course of disease is unlikely. Acupuncture cannot miraculously regenerate tissue. Owners should be educated on what the treatment capabilities are of any form of therapy before administering it.[50]

Based on experiences with horses and needles, it would not be expected that they are good patients for acupuncture. However, horses tend to relax with treatment and often do not respond much to needle placement. The veterinary acupuncturist should use common sense, and care is required anytime one is working around a large animal capable of lethal force. For example, although acupuncture points are described all over the equine body, few practitioners routinely use points between or behind the rear legs.

Equine acupuncture is commonly used as a treatment for medical colic, lameness, performance issues, and behavioral problems. One should realize that using acupuncture as the sole treatment for a surgical colic likely constitutes malpractice unless the owners do not consent to surgery. Western therapies should always be used when they are considered the established standard of care. Acupuncture is being increasingly used for the symptomatic treatment of postoperative ileus in horses with little documentation of its efficacy.

Acupuncture has been used in almost all species. Although species-specific diagrams may not be available, an understanding of anatomy will often help veterinary acupuncturists locate the transpositional points. Theory remains the same except that one should realize that there are relative differences in the normal characteristics of different species. Before agreeing to treat any species, acupuncturists must weigh the perceived benefits and the potential distress induced in transport and treatment. Some zoos consult with acupuncturists because the animals are frequently handled and can be safely restrained by keepers in a relatively stress-free manner. On the other hand, animals that never leave their familiar surroundings may be severely stressed by the whole exercise.

Owners should be informed about the complications and contraindications to treatment.[50] Complications are rare, but include infection, tissue or organ trauma, and needle breakage. Acupuncture needles are extremely flexible and strong, so breakage is rare. It is more common for hypodermic needles to break. An animal's behavior can change after treatments, so owners should be educated on what to expect. Some practitioners have suggested that acupuncture treatment can be problematic in cancer patients. Increased blood flow and needle trauma might spread cancer. However, many people find acupuncture useful for symptomatic treatment of paraneoplastic conditions. Acupuncture-associated stress and physiological responses can cause extremely ill animals to decompensate. It is suggested that very ill animals be treated very conservatively at first until they can tolerate more aggressive treatment. Implants for chronic acupoint stimulation (e.g., gold beads) should not be used when animals are subject to prepurchase examinations (mostly horses). The beads will show up on radiographs and are usually diagnostic for preexisting lameness. Pregnancy can be a contraindication to acupuncture, because it is believed that stimulating points distal to the elbow and knee may induce labor.

Application in a Perioperative Setting

Perioperative acupuncture and related techniques have been advocated for preoperative sedation, to reduce intraoperative opioid use, and to decrease postoperative pain. There is compelling evidence that acupuncture reduces postoperative nausea and vomiting in human patients, and it has been used to decrease vomiting associated with opioid administration to dogs. It may also stabilize cardiac function and ameliorate some consequences of anesthesia and surgery.

Mann[51] proposed the theory that diseased organs have a reduced response threshold to stimuli, whereas a considerable stimulus is needed to alter the function of a healthy organ. Therefore, just the small stimulus of an acupuncture needle may treat severe disease, whereas a comparable stimulus normally produces little or no effect in healthy volunteers.[51] To some extent, then, perioperative acupuncture contradicts a traditional principle of acupuncture philosophy in that its goal is to achieve an abnormal insensitivity to pain and reduced awareness and concern. Perioperative acupuncture can be divided into three components: preoperative preparation, intraoperative acupuncture-assisted anesthesia, and postoperative care.

Preoperative Preparation

The goals of preoperative preparation with acupuncture are to optimize the conditions for patients, reduce preoperative anxiety, and trigger release of endogenous opioids to enhance analgesia. One way that acupuncture might help preoperative preparation is by producing relaxation and sedation. For example, Ekblom et al.[52] demonstrated that although acupuncture did not produce intraoperative and postoperative analgesia for dental surgery in humans, it caused significant relaxation and drowsiness. Ulett et al.[44,53] reported that electroacupuncture to classic acupoints is associated with a deep calming effect. In people, postoperative pain intensity and consumption of postoperative analgesics both correlate with the amount of anxiety that patients experience.[54,55]

Intraoperative Assisted Anesthesia

Reduction in volatile anesthetic or opioid requirement is a clinically important outcome because it can reduce anesthetic toxicity and duration of recovery. Evidence suggests that inadequately treated pain, even during general anesthesia, activates nociceptive pathways.[56] Subsequent release of local mediators then primes the nociceptive system and aggravates postoperative pain.[57] To the extent that intraoperative acupuncture inhibits activation of nociceptive pathways and provides analgesia, it may similarly reduce postoperative pain and the requirement for postoperative opioids.

It is important to emphasize that acupuncture does *not* provide true anesthesia or unconsciousness, because it preserves all normal sensory, motor, and proprioception sensations. It does not provide adequate muscle relaxation or suppress autonomic reflexes caused by intra-abdominal visceral pain.[58] Instead, acupuncture produces analgesia and sedation as long as patients are cooperative.[59–63] For these reasons, acupuncture cannot be recommended for use as a sole anesthetic technique in veterinary patients.

Acupuncture is relatively safe and, in combination with conventional anesthetic techniques, can reduce the required dose of opioids. It has been suggested that acupuncture facilitates more comfortable postoperative conditions than does anesthesia alone.[60,64] Questionable results, however, were obtained by Sim et al.[58] in a blinded, randomized, placebo-controlled study on the effect of electroacupuncture on intraoperative alfentanil and morphine consumption during gynecologic surgery. Patients received true acupuncture or placebo acupuncture (continued throughout surgery), or they received no preoperative treatment and acupuncture postoperatively (continued for 45 min). Intraoperative alfentanil consumption was similar in the acupuncture and control groups but was significantly greater ($P = 0.024$) in the group that received acupuncture postoperatively. This finding may indicate a treatment-expectation placebo effect accompanied by endogenous opioid release in both control and preoperative acupuncture groups, rather than an acupuncture effect, although endogenous opioid concentrations were not measured. Acupuncture-induced postoperative analgesia in the preoperative acupuncture group was obvious during the first 6 to 12 h postoperatively. However, cumulative 24-h, patient-controlled analgesia consumption of morphine was not significantly less in the acupuncture-treated groups than in the placebo groups. The inability of acupuncture to reduce the 24-h morphine consumption can possibly be explained by the analgesic effect of a single electroacupuncture session lasting only 2 to 3 h.[65]

Acupuncture might decrease volatile anesthetic requirements. In an experimental setting, electroacupuncture produces a small, but statistically significant, reduction in halothane requirement in anesthetized dogs.[66] Similar results have been recently observed by Culp et al.[67] when using electroacupuncture during isoflurane anesthesia but not when using manual needle stimulation. Electroacupuncture therapy decreased isoflurane requirement (minimum alveolar concentration) by 10%. An advantage of evaluating acupuncture during general anesthesia is that it enables full blinding without resorting to sham stimulation. In three volunteer studies, anesthetic requirement with and without acupuncture was determined by the Dixon up-and-down method and defined by the average desflurane concentration required to prevent purposeful movement of the extremities in response to noxious electrical stimulation.[68–70] The first study was a crossover, double-blinded, placebo-controlled study in which Greif et al.[68] showed that transcutaneous electrical stimulation of the lateralization-control point near the ear tragus reduces anesthetic requirement for acute noxious stimulation by 11% ± 7%. Acupuncture stimulation was initiated after induction of general anesthesia. In the second study, Taguchi et al.[70] found that acupuncture initiated after induction of general anesthesia reduced desflurane requirement by 8.5% ± 7%. Auricular acupuncture was performed after induction of general anesthesia with needles placed at the Shen Men, thalamus, tranquilizer, and master cerebral points on the right ear. In the third volunteer trial, Morioka et al.[69] tested the hypothesis that electroacupuncture at the Zusanli (ST 36), Yanglingquan (GB 34), and Kunlun (BL 60) acupuncture points on the leg decreased anesthetic requirement during electrical noxious stimulation on the thighs. Desflurane requirement on the acupuncture (4.6% ± 0.6%) and control (4.6% ± 0.8%) days did not differ. Acupuncture significantly reduced anesthetic requirement in two of these three volunteer trials, but neither reduction was clinically important. This conclusion is consistent with that of a recent clinical study in which patients given acupuncture-assisted anesthesia required even more volatile anesthetic than did patients in the control group.[71] Available data therefore indicate that acupuncture has little, if any, effect on anesthetic requirement. As might be expected, manual stimulation of classic acupuncture points during surgery did not influence pain scores or change intraoperative or postoperative analgesic requirements.[72]

Postoperative Pain Control

Acupuncture and related techniques can potentially serve as important adjuvants for pain control and for relieving opioid-related adverse effects during the postoperative period. However, controversial results, dissimilar study designs, and diverse modes of acupuncture-point stimulation make it difficult to evaluate the clinical importance of perioperative acupuncture analgesia across a wide array of species. The results of few randomized, controlled clinical trials on acupuncture-related postoperative pain relief have been published in English. Interpretation of these available studies is complicated by the fact that acupuncture success depends on numerous factors, including adequate patient selection and the acupuncturist's knowledge and skill level.

Christensen et al.[73] demonstrated that postoperative analgesic requirement or pain was not reduced in human patients receiving electroacupuncture before and during hysterectomy. However, in this study, patients were also given relatively high doses of meperidine for induction and intraoperative pain control. Opioid-induced analgesia may have masked the putative benefit of electroacupuncture.

In another study, acupuncture increased intraoperative discomfort, postoperative pain, and consumption of analgesic after dental surgery.[52] In this study, local anesthesia was supplemented by preoperatively or postoperatively administered acupuncture with manual stimulation. Both acupuncture groups had increased consumption of pain medication and greater pain rating postoperatively than did the control group.[52] In addition, patients from the preoperative acupuncture group needed more local anesthetic than did patients from the other groups and expressed more distress during the surgical procedure. However, patients in both acupuncture groups demonstrated significant mental relaxation. There are several potential explanations for these conflicting results: (a) The relaxing effect of acupuncture might blunt the activation of a natural endogenous pain-inhibiting system. (b) The vasodilatation induced by acupuncture might have caused faster washout of the local anesthetic. (c) The investigators might have used suboptimal acupoint selection and stimulation technique.

In contrast, in a randomized, double-blinded, placebo-controlled trial, Lao et al.[74] demonstrated the efficacy of acupuncture for reducing pain and postoperative analgesic consumption after a similar oral surgery. The stimulated acupoints and technique selected for this study were similar to those selected for the previous study. An experienced acupuncturist performed the procedure, in contrast to the previous study, where the level of expertise of the person performing acupuncture was not disclosed (it is not uncommon that acupuncture for research purposes is performed by inexperienced personnel). Acupuncture or a noninsertion placebo treatment was administered twice: immediately after the surgical procedure and after the patient reported moderate pain. The results showed that pain-free postoperative time was significantly longer in the acupuncture group (173 min) than in the placebo group (94 min) ($P = 0.01$), and the average

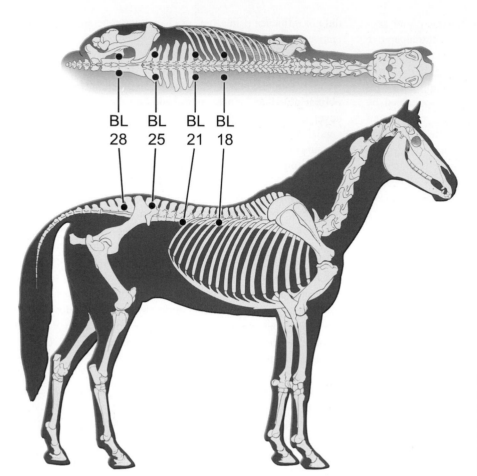

BL
28

BL
25

BL
21

BL
18

Fig. 24.6. Equine Shu points located bilaterally 3 to 6 cm lateral to the midline can be used to induce visceral analgesia in horses with colic and visceral organ disease or dysfunction. Horses are typically treated at these points with percutaneous acupuncture electrical stimulation for colic pain.

pain medication consumption was significantly less in the acupuncture group.

As previously mentioned, in human patients, point selection and mode of stimulation perform important roles in the outcome of acupuncture for postoperative pain relief. It seems that different components of postoperative pain respond to different combinations of acupuncture points. *Shu* points of the internal organs are located bilaterally 3 cm lateral to the posterior midline. Shu points are associated with the viscera and traditionally have been used for treatment of internal organ diseases.[20] Stimulation of these points may alleviate pain associated with visceral organ dysfunction (Fig. 24.6).[20] For example, consumption of supplemental morphine is reduced by 50% and the incidence of postoperative nausea is reduced by 20% to 30% in acupuncture patients undergoing upper or lower abdominal surgery.[60] In this controlled, double-blinded study, intradermal needles were inserted paravertebrally in Shu points. All needles were inserted while patients were in the preinduction area. In addition to less morphine consumption and postoperative nausea, patients with intradermal acupuncture had better pain relief than did controls ($P < 0.05$). Plasma cortisol and epinephrine concentrations were 30% to 50% less in the acupuncture group during recovery and on the first postoperative day ($P < 0.01$).

Transcutaneous electrical nerve stimulation (TENS) near the incision site significantly reduces postoperative pain.[75] However, this treatment seems to be most effective for the superficial cutaneous component of postoperative pain, leaving the deep visceral pain component largely intact. It seems likely that high-frequency TENS near the incision site mainly stimulates specific afferent nerve fibers instead of triggering endogenous opioid-release mechanisms.[76,77] Combining TENS and stimulation of viscera-associated Shu points in the treatment plan is therefore promising for reducing postoperative superficial and deep visceral pain, respectively.

Both high-frequency and low-frequency electroacupuncture at the Zusanli (ST 36) point performed 20 min immediately before induction of anesthesia reduces morphine consumption after abdominal surgery in human patients.[61] This point is traditionally considered effective for the treatment of abdominal disorders. The high-frequency acupuncture group had a 61% reduction in 24-h patient-controlled analgesia morphine consumption. Pain scores postoperatively did not significantly differ between groups, but cumulative morphine consumption for the first 24 h, number of patient-controlled analgesia demands, and intervals for the first request for analgesic were significantly less in both the high-frequency and low-frequency electroacupuncture groups. The aforementioned parameters were also reduced in the sham-acupuncture group compared with the control group, although they were greater than in the acupuncture groups. This is not surprising because sham acupuncture seems to have an analgesic effect in 40% to 50% of patients compared with 60% to 70% for real acupuncture and 30% to 35% for placebo (control).[78] The extrapolation or translation of human clinical trial findings to veterinary patients is controversial, although similar responses and mechanisms of action are plausible.

Acupuncture for the treatment of postoperative nausea and vomiting is one of its most common and investigated uses in human patients. This application has not been adequately assessed for use in animals during the perioperative period to date. Acupuncture may reduce nausea and vomiting through endogenous ß-endorphin release into the cerebral spinal fluid or through a change in serotonin transmission via activation of seritonergic and noradrenergic fibers.[79,80] The exact mechanisms have yet to be established.

Miscellaneous Perioperative Uses

Cardiopulmonary Resuscitation

In a study using 35 dogs anesthetized with halothane, acupuncture reversed cardiovascular depression induced by morphine and halothane. Acupuncture at point Jen Chung (GV 26) significantly increased cardiac output, stroke volume, heart rate, mean arterial pressure, and pulse pressure while simultaneously significantly decreasing total peripheral resistance and central venous pressure. The authors concluded that stimulation of the GV 26 acupoint could be helpful in resuscitating patients whose cardiovascular system is depressed by opioids and volatile anesthetics.[81]

GV 26 (also called Renzhong) is in the midline of the nasal philtrum, one-third of the way from the nose to the edge of the upper lip. The point is in the center of the horizontal line joining the lower edge of the nostrils. GV 26 has many clinical uses, the best known being its use in emergencies (coma, shock, apnea, anesthetic emergencies, drowning, etc.).

In human patients, the Neiguan (P 6) point has long been considered a primary point for treatment of various cardiovascular diseases.[21] It has been shown to be effective as an adjunct therapeutic modality in conservative treatment of severe angina pectoris.[82] Electroacupuncture at Neiguan (P 6) was effective in maintaining the hemodynamics and cardiac contractility in anesthetized open-chest dogs.[83] End-diastolic volume was maintained and even slightly increased in comparison with the control group, in which end-diastolic volume gradually decreased over 11/2 h; stroke volume and cardiac output also slightly increased compared with the control group. The end-systolic pressure and end-systolic elastance increased markedly in the Neiguan (P 6) acupuncture group. No analogous data support acupuncture-induced cardiovascular benefits in human patients, an obvious prerequisite to clinical application of the technique.

Impaired Intestinal Function

A major side effect of general anesthesia and opioid administration for postoperative pain control is the impairment of intestinal function.[84] To the extent that intraoperative and postoperative acupuncture for pain relief decreases perioperative opioid consumption, it may be beneficial for indirectly speeding postoperative recovery of intestinal function.[60] Acupuncture treatment has also been shown to promote postoperative recovery of impaired intestinal function after abdominal surgery in people.[85] Acupuncture for the treatment of ileus in horses is becoming more common, and practitioner consensus indicates that it may be effective in some horses.

General Principles of Acupuncture Analgesia

Patient Selection

Acupuncture in people is more effective in young adults than in the elderly. Small children are usually poor candidates for acupuncture-assisted anesthesia and analgesia with needles simply because they are rarely willing to cooperate with the acupuncturist. The same can probably be said for veterinary patients. However, choosing patients wisely and having their owner's consent and help will improve the chances for successful therapy. Obviously, acupuncture is not suitable for moribund preoperative patients because acupuncture is less effective in decompensated patients.[11]

Point Selection

According to traditional Chinese theory, certain rules and principles are generally applied when selecting points for acupuncture treatment. First, appropriate meridians should be selected, and then appropriate points on these meridians should be stimulated. For example, for postoperative pain control, a meridian that passes through the surgical area or close to the surgical area is usually selected. Also, according to the *organ phenomena* concept of TCM, the lung commands the skin. Consequently, stimulation of acupuncture points on the lung meridian can provide analgesia for surgical skin incisions. Similarly, the liver meridian commands the eyes, making the liver meridian ideal for ophthalmologic surgery. Whether these relationships hold true for acupuncture therapy in companion animal species is speculative.

Needling of points that easily produce a strong De-Qi sensation is thought to provide better analgesia. Conversely, analgesia is often poor at needling points that produce weak De-Qi response or in which the sensation is difficult to obtain. When selecting acupuncture points, one must consider convenience as well as the patient's comfort. Points located below the knee or elbow are usually selected during surgery. Points located on the ear are often selected for acupuncture during the perioperative period. After the locus point is identified, auxiliary points may be added.[28]

Summary

Acupuncture is increasingly being incorporated into veterinary medicine and more specifically pain management.[86] Acupuncture and related analgesic techniques are being widely used in conventional human medical settings, as well. Accordingly, the number of owners willing to use or specifically request acupuncture techniques for their pets is likely to increase. However, despite more than 30 years of research, the exact mechanisms of action and efficacy of specific acupuncture techniques have yet to be completely established. Consequently, considerable controversy remains about the role of acupuncture in both human and veterinary clinical medicine. Nevertheless, it should be remembered that the *how* is not as important to the patient as is the *outcome*. Although an exact explanation for the mechanisms may not yet exist, it seems reasonable to continue to explore acupuncture's potential as an adjuvant to proven analgesic and anesthetic techniques in both people and animals.

References

1. Bouevitch V. Microacupuncture systems as fractals of the human body. Med Acupunct 2003;14:14–16.
2. Pomeranz B, Stux G, eds. Scientific Bases of Acupuncture. Berlin: Springer-Verlag, 1987.
3. Reston J. Now, let me tell you about my appendectomy in Peking. New York Times, July 26, 1971:A1, A6.
4. Biella G, Sotgiu ML, Pellegata G, Paulesu E, Castiglioni I, Fazio F. Acupuncture produces central activations in pain regions. Neuroimage 2001;14:60–66.
5. Cho ZH, Oleson TD, Alimi D, Niemtzow RC. Acupuncture: The search for biologic evidence with functional magnetic resonance imaging and positron emission tomography techniques. J Altern Complement Med 2002;8:399–401.
6. Kong J, Ma L, Gollub RL, et al. A pilot study of functional magnetic resonance imaging of the brain during manual and electroacupuncture stimulation of acupuncture point (LI-4 Hegu) in normal subjects reveals differential brain activation between methods. J Altern Complement Med 2002;8:411–419.
7. Wu MT, Hsieh JC, Xiong J, et al. Central nervous pathway for acupuncture stimulation: Localization of processing with functional MR imaging of the brain: Preliminary experience. Radiology 1999; 212:133–141.
8. Wu MT, Sheen JM, Chuang KH, et al. Neuronal specificity of acupuncture response: A fMRI study with electroacupuncture. Neuroimage 2002;16:1028–1037.
9. National Institutes of Health (NIH). Acupuncture. NIH Consensus Statement, 1997;15(5):3. http://consensus.nih.gov/cons/107/107_statement.pdf.
10. Bossut DF, Page EH, Stromberg MW. Production of cutaneous analgesia by electroacupuncture in horses: Variations dependent on sex of subject and locus of stimulation. Am J Vet Res 1984;45:620–625.
11. Masayoshi H. Ryodoraku Treatment: An Objective Approach to Acupuncture. Osaka: Naniwasha, 1990.
12. Quan LB. Optimum Time for Acupuncture: A Collection of Traditional Chinese Chronotherapeutics. Jinan: Shandong Science and Technology, 1988.
13. Bossut DF, Mayer DJ. Electroacupuncture analgesia in naive rats: Effects of brainstem and spinal cord lesions, and role of pituitary-adrenal axis. Brain Res 1991;549:52–58.
14. Bossut DF, Mayer DJ. Electroacupuncture analgesia in rats: Naltrexone antagonism is dependent on previous exposure. Brain Res 1991;549:47–51.
15. Bossut DF, Huang ZS, Sun SL, Mayer DJ. Electroacupuncture in rats: Evidence for naloxone and naltrexone potentiation of analgesia. Brain Res 1991;549:36–46.
16. Astin JA, Marie A, Pelletier KR, Hansen E, Haskell WL. A review of the incorporation of complementary and alternative medicine by mainstream physicians. Arch Intern Med 1998;158:2303–2310.
17. Eisenberg DM, Davis RB, Ettner SL, et al. Trends in alternative medicine use in the United States, 1990–1997: Results of a follow-up national survey. J Am Med Assoc 1998;280:1569–1575.
18. Wang SM, Peloquin C, Kain ZN. Attitudes of patients undergoing surgery toward alternative medical treatment. J Altern Complement Med 2002;8:351–356.
19. Vincent C, Lewith G. Placebo controls for acupuncture studies. J R Soc Med 1995;88:199–202.
20. Ellis A, Wiseman N, Boss K. Grasping the Wind. Brookline, MA: Paradigm, 1989.
21. De Morant GS. Chinese Acupuncture (L'Acuponcture Chinoise). Brookline, MA: Paradigm, 1994.
22. Lin JG. Studies of needling depth in acupuncture treatment. Chin Med J (Engl) 1997;110:154–156.
23. Vincent CA, Richardson PH, Black JJ, Pither CE. The significance of needle placement site in acupuncture. J Psychosom Res 1989;33:489–496.
24. Ernst E, White A. Acupuncture: A Scientific Appraisal. Oxford: Butterworth-Heinemann, 1999.
25. Benedetti F, Arduino C, Amanzio M. Somatotopic activation of opioid systems by target-directed expectations of analgesia. J Neurosci 1999;19:3639–3648.
26. Li CY, Zhu LX, Ji CF. Relative specificity of points in acupuncture analgesia. J Tradit Chin Med 1987;7:29–34.
27. Cho Z-H, Son YD, Han J-Y, et al. fMRI neurophysiological evidence of acupuncture mechanisms. Med Acupunct 2003;14: 16–22.
28. Wang KM, Yao SM, Xian YL, Hou ZL. A study on the receptive field of acupoints and the relationship between characteristics of needling sensation and groups of afferent fibres. Sci Sin [B] 1985;28:963–971.
29. Casey KL. Forebrain mechanisms of nociception and pain: Analysis through imaging. Proc Natl Acad Sci USA 1999;96:7668–7674.
30. Derbyshire SW, Jones AK, Gyulai F, Clark S, Townsend D, Firestone LL. Pain processing during three levels of noxious stimulation produces differential patterns of central activity. Pain 1997;73:431–445.
31. Andersson JL, Lilja A, Hartvig P, et al. Somatotopic organization along the central sulcus, for pain localization in humans, as revealed by positron emission tomography. Exp Brain Res 1997;117: 192–199.
32. Peyron R, Laurent B, Garcia-Larrea L. Functional imaging of brain responses to pain: A review and meta-analysis (2000). Neurophysiol Clin 2000;30:263–288.
33. Melzack R. From the gate to the neuromatrix. Pain 1999;82(Suppl 6):S121–S126.
34. Langevin HM, Churchill DL, Cipolla MJ. Mechanical signaling through connective tissue: A mechanism for the therapeutic effect of acupuncture. FASEB J 2001;15:2275–2282.
35. Langevin HM, Yandow JA. Relationship of acupuncture points and meridians to connective tissue planes. Anat Rec 2002;269:257–265.
36. Han J. Central neurotransmitters and acupuncture analgesia. In: Pomeranz B, Stux G, eds. Scientific Bases of Acupuncture. Berlin: Springer-Verlag, 1987:7–33.
37. Han JS, Li SJ, Tang J. Tolerance to electroacupuncture and its cross tolerance to morphine. Neuropharmacology 1981;20:593–596.
38. Han JS. Cholecystokinin octapeptide (CCK-8): A negative feedback control mechanism for opioid analgesia. Prog Brain Res 1995;105: 263–271.
39. Han JS, Ding XZ, Fan SG. Cholecystokinin octapeptide (CCK-8): Antagonism to electroacupuncture analgesia and a possible role in electroacupuncture tolerance. Pain 1986;27:101–115.
40. Tang NM, Dong HW, Wang XM, Tsui ZC, Han JS. Cholecystokinin antisense RNA increases the analgesic effect induced by elec-

troacupuncture or low dose morphine: Conversion of low responder rats into high responders. Pain 1997;71:71–80.

41. Pomeranz B. Acupuncture research related to pain, drug addiction and nerve regeneration. In: Pomeranz B, Stux G, eds. Scientific Bases of Acupuncture. Berlin: Springer-Verlag, 1987:35–52.

42. Chen YS, Yao CH, Chen TH, et al. Effect of acupuncture stimulation on peripheral nerve regeneration using silicone rubber chambers. Am J Chin Med 2001;29:377–385.

43. Chen ZQ, Xu W, Yan YS, Chen KY. Different effects of reinforcing and reducing manipulations in acupuncture assessed by tail-flick latency, vocalization threshold and skin temperature in the rat. J Tradit Chin Med 1987;7:41–45.

44. Ulett GA, Han S, Han JS. Electroacupuncture: Mechanisms and clinical application. Biol Psychiatry 1998;44:129–138.

45. Han JS, Terenius L. Neurochemical basis of acupuncture analgesia. Annu Rev Pharmacol Toxicol 1982;22:193–220.

46. Cheng RSS. Neurophysiology of acupuncture analgesia. In: Pomeranz B, Stux G, eds. Scientific Bases of Acupuncture. Berlin: Springer-Verlag, 1987:53–78.

47. Chen XH, Geller EB, Adler MW. Electrical stimulation at traditional acupuncture sites in periphery produces brain opioid-receptor-mediated antinociception in rats. J Pharmacol Exp Ther 1996;277:654–660.

48. Vas J, Mendez C, Perea-Milla E, et al. Acupuncture as a complementary therapy to the pharmacological treatment of osteoarthritis of the knee: Randomised controlled trial. BMJ 2004;329:1216.

49. Berman BM, Lao L, Langenberg P, Lee WL, Gilpin AM, Hochberg MC. Effectiveness of acupuncture as adjunctive therapy in osteoarthritis of the knee: A randomized, controlled trial. Ann Intern Med 2004;141:901–910.

50. Flemming DD, Scott JF. The informed consent doctrine: What veterinarians should tell their clients. J Am Vet Med Assoc 2004;224:1436–1439.

51. Mann F. Acupuncture: The Ancient Chinese Art of Healing and How It Works Scientifically. New York: Vintage, 1972.

52. Ekblom A, Hansson P, Thomsson M, Thomas M. Increased postoperative pain and consumption of analgesics following acupuncture. Pain 1991;44:241–247.

53. Ulett GA. Conditioned healing with electroacupuncture. Altern Ther Health Med 1996;2:56–60.

54. Lim AT, Edis G, Kranz H, Mendelson G, Selwood T, Scott DF. Postoperative pain control: Contribution of psychological factors and transcutaneous electrical stimulation. Pain 1983;17:179–188.

55. Scott LE, Clum GA, Peoples JB. Preoperative predictors of postoperative pain. Pain 1983;15:283–293.

56. Melzack R, Coderre TJ, Katz J, Vaccarino AL. Central neuroplasticity and pathological pain. Ann NY Acad Sci 2001;933:157–174.

57. Grubb BD. Peripheral and central mechanisms of pain. Br J Anaesth 1998;81:8–11.

58. Sim CK, Xu PC, Pua HL, Zhang G, Lee TL. Effects of electroacupuncture on intraoperative and postoperative analgesic requirement. Acupunct Med 2002;20:56–65.

59. Wang SM, Kain ZN. Auricular acupuncture: A potential treatment for anxiety. Anesth Analg 2001;92:548–553.

60. Kotani N, Hashimoto H, Sato Y, et al. Preoperative intradermal acupuncture reduces postoperative pain, nausea and vomiting, analgesic requirement, and sympathoadrenal responses. Anesthesiology 2001;95:349–356.

61. Lin JG, Lo MW, Wen YR, Hsieh CL, Tsai SK, Sun WZ. The effect of high and low frequency electroacupuncture in pain after lower abdominal surgery. Pain 2002;99:509–514.

62. Stener-Victorin E, Waldenstrom U, Nilsson L, Wikland M, Janson PO. A prospective randomized study of electro-acupuncture versus alfentanil as anaesthesia during oocyte aspiration in in-vitro fertilization. Hum Reprod 1999;14:2480–2484.

63. Wang B, Tang J, White PF, et al. Effect of the intensity of transcutaneous acupoint electrical stimulation on the postoperative analgesic requirement. Anesth Analg 1997;85:406–413.

64. Kho HG, van Egmond J, Zhuang CF, Lin GF, Zhang GL. Acupuncture anaesthesia: Observations on its use for removal of thyroid adenomata and influence on recovery and morbidity in a Chinese hospital. Anaesthesia 1990;45:480–485.

65. Christensen PA, Noreng M, Andersen PE, Nielsen JW. Electroacupuncture and postoperative pain. Br J Anaesth 1989;62:258–262.

66. Tseng CK, Tay AA, Pace NL, Westenskow DR, Wong KC. Electroacupuncture modification of halothane anaesthesia in the dog. Can Anaesth Soc J 1981;28:125–128.

67. Culp LB, Skarda RT, Muir WW III. Comparisons of the effects of acupuncture, electroacupuncture, and transcutaneous cranial electrical stimulation on the minimum alveolar concentration of isoflurane in dogs. Am J Vet Res 2005;66:1364–1373.

68. Greif R, Laciny S, Mokhtarani M, et al. Transcutaneous electrical stimulation of an auricular acupuncture point decreases anesthetic requirement. Anesthesiology 2002;96:306–312.

69. Morioka N, Akca O, Doufas AG, Chernyak G, Sessler DI. Electroacupuncture at the Zusanli, Yanglingquan, and Kunlun points does not reduce anesthetic requirement. Anesth Analg 2002;95:98–102.

70. Taguchi A, Sharma N, Ali SZ, Dave B, Sessler DI, Kurz A. The effect of auricular acupuncture on anaesthesia with desflurane. Anaesthesia 2002;57:1159–1163.

71. Kvorning N, Christiansson C, Beskow A, Bratt O, Akeson J. Acupuncture fails to reduce but increases anaesthetic gas required to prevent movement in response to surgical incision. Acta Anaesthesiol Scand 2003;47:818–822.

72. Gupta S, Francis JD, Tillu AB, Sattirajah AI, Sizer J. The effect of pre-emptive acupuncture treatment on analgesic requirements after day-case knee arthroscopy. Anaesthesia 1999;54:1204–1207.

73. Christensen PA, Rotne M, Vedelsdal R, Jensen RH, Jacobsen K, Husted C. Electroacupuncture in anaesthesia for hysterectomy. Br J Anaesth 1993;71:835–838.

74. Lao L, Bergman S, Hamilton GR, Langenberg P, Berman B. Evaluation of acupuncture for pain control after oral surgery: A placebo-controlled trial. Arch Otolaryngol Head Neck Surg 1999;125:567–572.

75. Smith CM, Guralnick MS, Gelfand MM, Jeans ME. The effects of transcutaneous electrical nerve stimulation on post-cesarean pain. Pain 1986;27:181–193.

76. Melzack R. Prolonged relief of pain by brief, intense transcutaneous somatic stimulation. Pain 1975;1:357–373.

77. Melzack R, Wall PD. Acupuncture and transcutaneous electrical nerve stimulation. Postgrad Med J 1984;60:893–896.

78. Lewith GT, Machin D. On the evaluation of the clinical effects of acupuncture. Pain 1983;16:111–127.

79. Clement-Jones V, McLoughlin L, Tomlin S, Besser GM, Rees LH, Wen HL. Increased beta-endorphin but not met-enkephalin levels in human cerebrospinal fluid after acupuncture for recurrent pain. Lancet 1980;2:946–949.

80. Stein DJ, Birnbach DJ, Danzer BI, Kuroda MM, Grunebaum A, Thys DM. Acupressure versus intravenous metoclopramide to prevent nausea and vomiting during spinal anesthesia for cesarean section. Anesth Analg 1997;84:342–345.

81. Lee DC, Clifford DH, Lee MO, Nelson L. Reversal by acupuncture of cardiovascular depression induced with morphine during halothane anaesthesia in dogs. Can Anaesth Soc J 1981;28:129–135.

82. Richter A, Herlitz J, Hjalmarson A. Effect of acupuncture in patients with angina pectoris. Eur Heart J 1991;12:175–178.

83. Syuu Y, Matsubara H, Kiyooka T, et al. Cardiovascular beneficial effects of electroacupuncture at Neiguan (PC-6) acupoint in anesthetized open-chest dog. Jpn J Physiol 2001;51:231–238.

84. Kurz A, Sessler DI. Opioid-induced bowel dysfunction: Pathophysiology and potential new therapies. Drugs 2003;63:649–671.

85. Wan Q. Auricular-plaster therapy plus acupuncture at zusanli for postoperative recovery of intestinal function. J Tradit Chin Med 2000;20:134–135.

86. Skarda R. Complementary and alternative pain therapy. In: Muir WW III, Gaynor JS, eds. Handbook of Veterinary Pain Management. St Louis: CV Mosby, 2002:281–322.

Chapter 25
Rehabilitation and Palliative Analgesia

Dianne Dunning and Duncan X. Lascelles

Introduction

Companion animal rehabilitation is a rapidly growing area aimed at improving supportive care in veterinary patients. In the veterinary setting, rehabilitation is essentially akin to the human-oriented profession of physical therapy. Similar to physical therapy, rehabilitation uses physical and mechanical methods such as light, heat, cold, water, electricity, massage, and exercise to improve function and reduce pain and morbidity in a variety of conditions, including orthopedic and neurological disease. Other terms commonly used to describe rehabilitation are physical rehabilitation, physical therapy, and physiotherapy. Because pain and discomfort may be elicited by some techniques on occasion, therapists should be prepared to administer an appropriate analgesic, if necessary. Advanced training and certification in rehabilitation are available for certified veterinary technicians, physical therapists, and veterinarians. Practice acts vary from state to state, with most requiring that animal rehabilitation be supervised and in some cases implemented by a veterinarian.

Until recently, rehabilitation has not played an important role in the management of a pain in veterinary medicine.[1] Standard postoperative care has focused on basic nursing and support care, confinement, and pharmaceutical intervention. With the incorporation of rehabilitation into overall supportive care and pain management, many patients are recovering sooner and more completely from medical, surgical, and traumatic events. To date, however, the benefits of nondrug therapies in the management of pain, including those of rehabilitation, have been relatively undocumented in the veterinary literature.[2,3] Similarly, the analgesic effects and overall benefits of therapies such as acupuncture and electroacupuncture, acupressure, and transcutaneous electrical nerve stimulation are relatively undefined. Despite this lack of experimental scientific evidence for their efficacy, clinical experience in veterinary patients suggests that the use of such therapeutic modalities in conjunction with drug therapy can be beneficial. The desired clinical outcome is better control of discomfort and reduction in the overall pharmacological requirement of patients.

Therapeutic Modalities

Seven therapeutic modalities are used to decrease pain, reduce inflammation, and stimulate normal healing responses in veterinary patients: (1) local hypothermia and hyperthermia, (2) passive range-of-motion activity, (3) massage, (4) therapeutic exercise, (5) hydrotherapy, (6) ultrasound, and (7) electrical stimulation. In this chapter, the indications and contraindications, along with the methods of action and application are discussed for each therapeutic modality commonly used in companion animal rehabilitation.

Local Hypothermia

Local hypothermia therapy, or cryotherapy, entails the application of therapeutic cold to a musculoskeletal tissue. Common forms of therapeutic cold include commercial available reusable ice and gel packs, continuously circulating cold-water blankets, homemade ice packs and towels, ice massage, and cold-water hydrotherapy. The application of local hypothermia is indicated in the acute (<72 h) postinjury period to ameliorate inflammation, irritation, pain, swelling, and edema. The primary purported method of action of cryotherapy is via vasoconstriction, which reduces arterial and capillary blood flow, thereby minimizing fluid leakage and edema. Because cryotherapy also decreases enzyme activity and metabolism in tissues, it is effective against local inflammation in periarticular and articular tissues.[4] Analgesia is provided by alteration of sensory nerve conduction and skeletal muscle relaxation.[5,6]

The cooling effects of local hypothermia on deeper tissues are less profound and unpredictable, depending on the application method, the initial temperature of the treated area, and the duration of treatment.[7] Regardless, application of local hypothermia should be limited to multiple short sessions (5 to 15 min up to four times daily) to prevent reflex vasodilation and edema.[6–9] Overzealous cryotherapy causing a 10.0°C (18.0°F) or more decrease in tissue temperature may cause protein degradation, local hyperemia, epithelial and nerve damage, and muscle atrophy and contracture. The use of local hypothermia should be avoided in hypothermic animals. If body core temperature is further dropped, peripheral vasoconstriction and increased blood pressure may ensue. Furthermore, cryotherapy is contraindicated in people and presumably animals that have diabetes mellitus, ischemic injuries, vasculitis, or indolent wounds.

Local Hyperthermia

This technique uses heat to promote capillary dilation and increase capillary hydrostatic pressure, permeability, and filtration. The cellular and vascular changes produced by heat also stimulate inflammation and invigorate wound healing. Tissues treated with local hyperthermia increase in temperature, which causes a local histamine release while simultaneously enhancing cellular metabolism.[10] Heat therapy provides pain relief by increasing blood flow and capillary permeability, decreasing edema, increasing local metabolic rate, increasing extensibility of collagen in articular and ligamentous tissues, and decreasing muscle tension and spasm, as well as providing general relaxation.[4,11–13]

Common forms of therapeutic heat used in veterinary medicine include the application of hot packs, warm towels, warm-water blankets, therapeutic ultrasound, circulating warm-water baths, and hydrotherapy units. The therapeutic protocol for heat is similar to that for cryotherapy, with application durations varying from 15 to 20 min, two to four times a day. Other types of less frequently used heat therapy include incandescent, infrared, ultraviolet, and microwave radiation, all of which require special equipment and training.

As the primary method of action of heat therapy is inflammatory, local hyperthermia should be used only once acute inflammation has subsided, typically 24 to 72 h after injury or surgery. Heat therapy is indicated to remove the inflammatory mediators and edema present in the peri-injury site tissues. It is important to note that local hyperthermia has a narrow therapeutic temperature window (40° to 45°C [104° to 113°F]) and warrants careful monitoring.[10,14,15] Care should be taken not to prematurely apply heat too soon after a traumatic injury, because that can induce vascular leakage, exacerbate the inflammatory response, augment edema and seroma formation, and potentiate hemorrhage and pain.[10,14,15] Local hyperthermia has few indications in the immediate postoperative period and should be combined with other forms of physical therapy (massage or exercise) in the later stages of convalescence (>72 h after surgery). Therapeutic heat is also contraindicated in neurological or vascularly impaired patients.[10,14,15] Direct nerve injury from local hyperthermia and burns is possible, especially with prolonged application or the use of electric heating pads.

Passive Range of Motion

Passive range of motion (PROM) exercise refers to the controlled movement of the limbs and joints in flexion, extension, adduction, and abduction by the therapist with no effort being exerted by the animal.[16] The goals of PROM are to stretch and manipulate the periarticular structures of the appendicular skeleton to maintain normal joint ROM while preventing soft tissue and muscle contracture.[16] Experimental evidence evaluating the effects of prolonged immobilization and restricted weight bearing on canine cartilage reveals chondrocyte atrophy and deterioration of the supportive matrix, which in many cases is irreversible.[1] In addition to direct benefits to cartilage, PROM improves blood flow and sensory awareness of the affected joints and limbs. However, PROM is not a replacement for normal weight bearing and the superior affects of voluntary active movement. In comparison to PROM, active exercise produces superior cartilage, better prevents muscle atrophy, and improves muscle strength and endurance.[1,17]

PROM should be instituted immediately after surgery and continued until the patient begins to ambulate within normal limits. If the animal has decreased ROM, as documented by goniometry, the PROM exercises can be prolonged to improve the function of the limb. Typically, PROM is performed with the animal in relaxed lateral recumbency. The joint or joints are flexed or extended to their nonpainful end point and held for 10 to 30 s and returned to a normal or functional standing position. These cycles are repeated for 10 to 15 complete cycles of flexion and extension. Caution should be taken not to overstretch the periarticular tissues, because overzealous PROM may tear the joint capsule and surrounding tissues and result in pain and unintentional fibrous scar formation. Contraindications to the use of PROM include unstable fractures, luxations, hypermotile joints, or skin graphs.

Therapeutic Massage

This involves the manual or mechanical manipulation of soft tissues and muscle by rubbing, kneading, or tapping. Benefits of massage include increased local circulation, reduced muscle spasm, attenuation of edema, and breakdown of irregular scar tissue formation. The method of action of this therapeutic technique is based on both reflexive and mechanical effects. The reflexive effects are due to stimulation of peripheral receptors, which produces the central effects of relaxation while simultaneously producing muscular relaxation and arteriolar dilation. The mechanical effects are due to increased lymphatic and venous drainage removing edema and metabolic waste, increased arterial circulation enhancing tissue oxygenation and wound healing, and manipulation of restrictive connective tissue enhancing ROM and mobility.

The most common techniques of massage used in veterinary medicine are effleurage, pétrissage, cross fiber, and tapotement. *Effleurage* (Latin, *effluere*, "to flow out") is a form of superficial or light stroking massage and is generally used in the beginning of all massage sessions to relax and acclimatize the animal. *Pétrissage* is characterized by deep kneading and squeezing of muscle and surrounding soft tissues. *Cross fiber* is also a deep massage that is concentrated along lines of restrictive scar tissue and designed to promote normal ROM.[9,18] This type of massage has limited use in veterinary medicine because it requires sedation of the animal during therapy and most often temporarily exacerbates lameness because of an inflammatory response to the tissue manipulation. *Tapotement* involves the percussive manipulation of soft tissues with cupped hand or massage equipment and is most commonly used to relax spastic muscle contraction or enhance postural drainage for respiratory conditions. Contraindications to massage therapy include unstable or infected fractures or tissue and the direct manipulation of a malig-

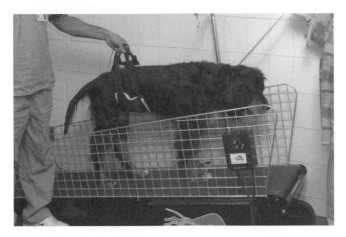

Fig. 25.1. A dog undergoing therapeutic exercise by walking on elevated treadmill.

nancy. In most instances, massage is an indispensable therapy when animals are in intensive care and have restricted mobility.[10]

Therapeutic Exercise

The potential for catastrophic failure associated with uncontrolled activity has previously limited the role of therapeutic exercise in the recovery of veterinary patients, particularly in postoperative orthopedic animals. Controlled active therapeutic exercise, however, may be safely performed in most cases, even orthopedic, when closely assisted and attended to by the therapist or the attentive owner. The benefits of therapeutic exercise are abundant. Exercise helps build strength, muscle mass, agility, coordination, and cardiovascular health. In addition, therapeutic exercise may be used as a preventive measure to improve general health, reduce obesity, and increase performance in all veterinary patients.[1,18] Prior to initiating therapy, all animals must be fully evaluated and assessed, because it is imperative to match the intensity of the activities to the animal's level of function and ability. Included in the repertoire of controlled active exercise are assisted standing; facilitated walking; prolonged, momentary, and repeated sits and downs; stair walking; walking on inclines and hills; and weight shifting (Fig. 25.1).[1,18] When performed appropriately and in consultation with the primary-care clinician or surgeon, these activities can be performed early in the postoperative recovery period and modified and intensified to promote cardiovascular and musculoskeletal fitness.

Aquatic Based Rehabilitation

Aquatic based therapeutic techniques for veterinary patients include local therapeutic massage with warm or cold water, underwater treadmill exercise, and swimming. Massage in water is particularly beneficial for postoperative animals, because it is an efficacious method for removing lymphedema from extremities. Water-based massage is also relaxing and effective for cleansing surgical incisions. Cold-water hydrotherapy may be employed as soon as a surgical incision has established a fibrin seal, which is generally within 24 h of surgery. This form of hydrotherapy is a

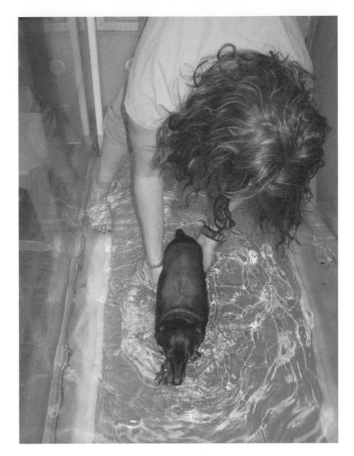

Fig. 25.2. A dog undergoing aquatic based therapeutic rehabilitation to reduce concussion during exercise.

relatively low tech–high yield form of rehabilitation in that it requires little equipment, other than a washtub and a hose.

Increasing the water depth and the temperature to 30°–32°C (86°–90°F) provides a nongravitation environment that is ideal for performing nonconcussive active-assisted exercise such as underwater treadmill and swimming activity (Fig. 25.2).[19] The natural properties of water provide both buoyancy and resistance, which can be manipulated to improve limb mobility, joint ROM, gait, and cadence.[6] Caution should be used with any water exercise in order to minimize the risk of aspiration or drowning. It is wise to acclimatize animals to water before initiating any therapy regimen.[1,18]

Therapeutic Ultrasound

The method of action of therapeutic ultrasound is based on the delivery of energy to tissue in the form of acoustic vibrations. Sound waves can produce both physiological heat and cellular inflammation.[18] The net physiological effects of ultrasound may be divided into two categories: thermal and nonthermal.[18] The *thermal* effects of ultrasound increase connective tissue extensibility and vascularity and provide a form of temporary nerve blockage, thus promoting muscular relaxation and pain relief. The *nonthermal* effects of ultrasound include the acceleration and compressing of the inflammatory phase of healing; an in-

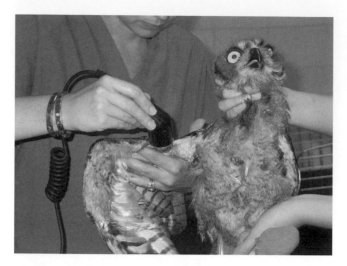

Fig. 25.3. Therapeutic ultrasound therapy in a bird to reduce scar tissue and enhance tendon healing.

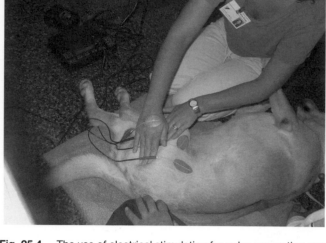

Fig. 25.4. The use of electrical stimulation for pulse generation over weakened muscle groups to enhance contraction in a dog.

crease in local circulation; a decrease in edema; an increase in endorphins, enkephalins, and serotonin; and the stimulation of collagen synthesis and bone growth.[20] Therapeutic ultrasound is primarily indicated in the treatment of chronic scar tissue and indolent decubital ulcers. It may also be effective for palliation of muscle spasms and for enhanced tendon healing (Fig. 25.3).[18,20] Contraindications for the use of therapeutic ultrasound include tissue infection or inflammation. Prior to its application, therapeutic ultrasound should be thoroughly investigated because there is a wide variety of continuous-wave or pulsed-wave delivery modes, wave intensities, and therapy regimens to choose from.[18,20] Complications are associated with operator inexperience and error that can produce excessive heat, free radicals, and subsequent tissue destruction.[18,20]

Electrical Stimulation

This entails the delivery of electrical current to a selected treatment area.[21] Common uses for electrical stimulation include muscle reeducation, pain palliation, and edema reduction.[21] There are a variety of waveforms and devices available, varying in cost and versatility. The nomenclature is quite confusing and does little to improve one's understanding of the fundamentals of electrical stimulation. Essentially, however, there are two forms: neuromuscular electrical stimulation (NMES) and transelectrical nerve stimulation (TENS).

NMES is indicated in animals that are neurological, debilitated, recumbent, or immobile or need prolonged joint immobility. It prevents disuse atrophy and improves limb performance by recruiting contracting fibers and increasing maximum contractible force of affected muscles.[18] The electrical stimulation device consists of a simple pulse generator and electrodes, which are placed over selected weakened or paralyzed muscle groups to create an artificial contraction (Fig. 25.4).[18] Pulse amplitude, rate, and cycle length may be varied to suit the comfort of the patient.[18] Muscular pain and edema may also be reduced because of improved blood flow.[18] Combining neuromuscular stimulation

with PROM exercises improves joint ROM and prevents muscle contracture and is particularly indicated in fractures of the distal femur of young dogs.[18] This technique has proven effective in promoting muscle reeducation after prolonged disuse.

TENS has been used widely to identify neural stimulators that modify pain. Electrical stimulation to alter pain sensation involves the application of an electrical current to a sensory nerve. There are various suggestions as to the mechanism(s) responsible for altered pain sensation: the gate control theory, which involves the increased activity of the sensory afferents causing presynaptic inhibition of pain transmission; an endogenous opiate release; the counterirritant theory; and the placebo effect.[22] In most patients, altered pain sensation via TENS is probably due, in part, to all of the aforementioned mechanisms. TENS should be considered an adjunctive pain management modality, to be combined with other pain-management techniques rather than as a sole therapy to control pain.

Summary

Implementing rehabilitation as part of a multimodal analgesic regimen will augment pain management and facilitate veterinary patients' recovery and return to function. The nature of any rehabilitation program is influenced by factors such as facilities, equipment, and trained personnel.[8] It should be appreciated that one does not always need advanced training and equipment to perform physical therapy in animals. Most patients will experience improved recoveries with simple fundamental techniques such as massage, cold packing, PROM, and controlled exercise regimens.

References

1. Manning A, Rush J, Ellis D. Physical therapy for the critically ill veterinary patient. Part II. The musculoskeletal system. Comp Contin Educ Pract Vet 1997;19:803–807.

2. Deng G, Cassileth B, Yeung K. Complementary therapies for cancer-related symptoms. J Support Oncol 2004;2:419–426.

3. Nadler SF. Nonpharmacologic management of pain. J Am Osteopath Assoc 2004;104:S6–S12.

4. Anderson GI. Fracture disease and related contractures. Vet Clin North Am 1991;21:845–857.

5. Hodges C, Palmer R. Postoperative physical therapy. In: Harari J, ed. Surgical Complications and Wound Healing. Philadelphia: WB Saunders, 1993:389–405.

6. Payne J. General management considerations for the trauma patient. Vet Clin North Am Small Anim Pract 1995;25:1015–1029.

7. Meeusen R, Lievens P. The use of cryotherapy in sports injuries. Sports Med 1986;3:398–414.

8. Downer A, Spear V. Physical therapy in the management of long bone fractures in small animals. Vet Clin North Am 1975;5:157–164.

9. Taylor R, Lester M. Physical therapy in canine sporting breeds. In: Bloomberg M, ed. Canine Sports Medicine and Surgery. Philadelphia: WB Saunders, 1998:265–275.

10. Langer G. Physical therapy in small animal patients: Basic principles and application. Comp Contin Educ Pract Vet 1984;6:933–936.

11. Taylor R. Postsurgical physical therapy: The missing link. Comp Contin Educ Pract Vet 1992;14:1583–1593.

12. Millis DL, Levine D. The role of exercise and physical modalities in the treatment of osteoarthritis. Vet Clin North Am 1997;27:913–930.

13. Gentry S, Mann F. Postoperative care of canine and feline orthopedic patients. J Am An Hosp Assoc 1993;29:146–150.

14. Taylor RA. Postsurgical physical therapy: The missing link. Comp Contin Educ Pract Vet 1992;14:1583–1594.

15. Payne JT. General management considerations for the trauma patient. Vet Clin North Am Small Anim Pract 1995;25:1015–1029.

16. Coby L. Range of motion. In: Tiser, ed. Therapeutic Exercise: Foundations and Techniques. Philadelphia: FA Davis, 1989:20–23.

17. Manning AM, Rush J, Ellis DR. Physical therapy for critically ill veterinary patients. Part II. The musculoskeletal system. Comp Contin Educ Pract Vet 1997;19:803–807.

18. Taylor R. Postsurgical physical therapy: The missing link. Comp Contin Educ Pract Vet 1992;12:1583–1594.

19. Cider A, Schaufelberger M, Sunnerhagen K, Andersson B. Hydrotherapy: A new approach to improve function in the older patient with chronic heart failure. Eur J Heart Fail 2003;5:527–535.

20. Walsh W, Huckle J, Bliss J, et al. Can low-intensity pulsed ultrasound be used to augment tendon-bone healing? In: Proceedings of 49th Annual Meeting of the Orthopedic Research Society [Abstract], New Orleans, 2003.

21. Johnson J, Levine D. Electrical stimulation. In: Millis D, Levine D, Taylor R, eds. Canine Rehabilitation and Physical Therapy. Philadelphia: WB Saunders, 2004:289–302.

22. Devor M. Pain mechanisms. Neuroscientist 1996;2:233–244.

Section VI
ANESTHESIA, ANALGESIA, AND IMMOBILIZATION OF SELECTED SPECIES AND CLASSES OF ANIMALS

Chapter 26
Dogs and Cats

Richard M. Bednarski

Introduction

The selection of a particular anesthetic regimen is predicated upon the patient's physical status and temperament, the type of procedure for which anesthesia is being considered, anticipation of perioperative pain, the familiarity with anesthetic drugs, the type of facility and available equipment, the personnel available for assistance, and the cost of anesthetic drugs. There is no single best method for anesthetizing dogs or cats, and familiarity with just one anesthetic technique at best limits a veterinarian's ability to perform the myriad of surgical and diagnostic procedures commonly performed in a modern veterinary practice. A debilitated dog or cat undergoing extensive repair of a fractured limb will require a different anesthetic regimen than one undergoing routine neutering, one requiring short-term restraint for radiography, or a geriatric patient requiring extensive dental manipulations.

General anesthesia is characterized by muscle relaxation, unconsciousness, amnesia, and analgesia. Rarely does a single drug provide all of these elements at safe doses. Inhalation anesthetics come closest to satisfying all of these conditions, but even they are more useful when coadministered with anesthetic adjunctive drugs such as opioids, local anesthetics, or neuromuscular junction–blocking agents. As a general rule, when formulating an anesthetic plan, it is best to consider using relatively low doses of several different drugs rather than a large dose of a single drug. For example, apnea resulting from a large bolus of propofol can be eliminated, or its duration shortened, by prior administration of acepromazine, opioids, or α_2-adrenergic agonists, which allow administration of a lower propofol dose.[1] The opioid drugs, although important components of modern anesthetic regimens, by themselves do not produce general anesthesia.[2] Muscle rigidity, salivation, and long recoveries associated with large dosages of ketamine can be lessened when it is combined in reduced doses with opioids, α_2-adrenergic agonists, and central muscle relaxants such as benzodiazepines.[3]

Any chemical restraint or general anesthetic plan must include a provision to control pain if it is present or anticipated. A good analgesic regimen should include drugs sufficient to ensure analgesia during and after the procedure. The one thing that should not vary among anesthetic procedures is the degree of vigilance associated with monitoring an anesthetized dog or cat. Early warning of impending anesthetic difficulty is the single most important factor responsible for decreasing anesthetic-related morbidity and mortality.

Preanesthetic Considerations

Recording a thorough history (Table 26.1) and conducting the physical examination are the most important components of a preanesthetic evaluation. Even young, seemingly healthy, animals presented for routine procedures such as neutering require both. These animals may have never been previously examined by a veterinarian, and congenital disorders, severe parasitism, or heartworm disease may be discovered.

Signalment

Anesthesiologists are often queried about "sensitivity to anesthesia" in a variety of dog and cat breeds. Although several breed-associated anesthesia concerns have been documented, all breeds have been successfully anesthetized by using standard anesthetic regimens, and most reports of "sensitivities" are anecdotal. One well-documented breed-associated anesthetic concern is the altered pharmacokinetics of barbiturates and other anesthetic drugs in sight hounds.[4] Another is brachycephalic breeds and their associated airway anatomical malformations. Since toy breeds have

Table 26.1. Signalment and history, including questions of organ system function

A. Signalment
   1. Age
   2. Breed
   3. Gender
B. Body weight
C. Duration of ongoing complaint
D. Concurrent medications
   1. Angiotensin-converting enzyme inhibitors
   2. H$_2$ blockers
   3. Antibiotics: aminoglycosides
   4. Cardiac glycosides
   5. Phenobarbital
   6. Nonsteroidal anti-inflammatory drugs
   7. Calcium channel blockers
   8. Beta blockers
   9. Tricyclic antidepressants
E. Signs of organ system disease
   1. Diarrhea
   2. Vomiting
   3. Polyuria-polydipsia
   4. Seizures and personality change
   5. Exercise intolerance
   6. Coughing and stridor
   7. Weight loss and loss of body condition
F. Previous anesthesia and allergies
G. Duration since last meal

Table 26.2. Preanesthesia physical examination

A. Body weight and body condition
   1. Obesity
   2. Cachexia
   3. Dehydration
B. Cardiopulmonary
   1. Heart rate and rhythm
   2. Auscultation
      Heart sounds and murmurs
      Breath sounds
   3. Capillary refill time
   4. Mucous membrane color
      Pallor
      Cyanosis
   5. Pulse character
C. Central nervous system and special senses
   1. Temperament
   2. Seizure, coma, and stupor
   3. Vision and hearing
D. Gastrointestinal
   1. Parasites
   2. Abdominal palpation
E. Hepatic
   1. Icterus
   2. Abnormal bleeding
F. Renal
   1. Palpate kidneys and bladder
G. Integument
   1. Tumors
   2. Flea infestation
H. Musculoskeletal
   1. Lameness
   2. Fractures
I. Pain Assessment

a greater surface area–body mass ratio and have a relatively greater metabolic rate, they require careful attention to maintenance of body heat and blood glucose concentrations. Additionally, they require a relatively greater dose of drugs on a per-kilogram basis. Generally, there are no gender-related differences in the response to anesthesia. However, a history of the estrous cycle will often identify recent estrus and thus alert the clinician to the concerns associated with an enlarged and vascularized uterus. This would potentially cause concern regarding blood loss during an ovariohysterectomy. Additionally, the owner of an intact female animal should be queried about the possibility of their animal being pregnant because the stress of surgery and anesthesia may adversely affect the fetus(es).

Age is an important anesthetic consideration. Generally, the very young (less than 11 weeks) and the aged (more than 80% of the expected life span) do not biotransform anesthetic drugs as rapidly as do young, healthy patients.[5] Healthy geriatric patients may only require 25% to 50% of the dose of sedatives, hypnotics, tranquilizers, and opioids given to comparable young healthy animals.

History

In addition to questions concerning organ system function (Table 26.1), the owner should be queried regarding any previous anesthetic episodes, past and present illnesses, and past and current medication history, including history of heartworm prophylaxis.[6] The time elapsed since the last feeding should be noted.

Physical Examination

The preanesthetic physical examination should be thorough, with all body systems considered (Table 26.2). Any abnormality discovered by physical examination or suggested by the medical history should be followed with appropriate laboratory or other suitable diagnostic testing. The assessment of an animal's temperament is critical. Vicious or aggressive dogs will require a different approach to anesthesia than quiet, relaxed individuals.

Laboratory Evaluation

The minimum preanesthetic laboratory data required for young healthy dogs are hematocrit and plasma protein. These tests are easy, quick, and inexpensive. Hematocrit is an indicator of hemoglobin concentration, which directly relates the ability of the blood to transport oxygen to the tissues. As a general rule, a hematocrit of less than 20% indicates the need for perioperative administration of blood or, if available, a hemoglobin-based oxygen-carrying solution. Hemoglobin concentration (g/dL) can be approximated by dividing the hematocrit by 3.

For elective procedures in middle-aged to older animals, or animals treated chronically with medications that could alter liver or renal function (e.g., nonsteroidal anti-inflammatory drugs, phenobarbital, or antineoplastic chemotherapeutics), a complete blood count, urinalysis, and biochemistry profile should be performed. Other tests should be performed (e.g., thoracic radiographs and/or echocardiography) if the history or physical examination suggests specific organ system disease. A minimum laboratory database prior to emergency anesthesia should include packed cell volume, total protein, and electrolytes (sodium, potassium, and chloride).

Physical Status

Many factors (e.g., age, breed, concurrent disease, surgical procedure, surgeon skill, and available equipment) contribute to the overall anesthetic risk for a given patient. One risk factor is the physical status of the patient. A convenient system of status classification for veterinary patients has been adapted from the American Society of Anesthesiologists.[7] In general, physical status I and II patients appear to be at less risk for anesthetic complications. Physical statuses III through V are usually at greater anesthetic risk. However, this is not to imply that category I and II patients are at no risk from unanticipated anesthetic mishaps (Table 26.3).

Patient Preparation

Fasting

Healthy dogs and cats should be fasted for at least 6 h prior to being anesthetized, if possible. Water can be allowed until just prior to anesthesia. Dogs and cats less than 8 weeks old and those weighing less than 2 kg should not be fasted longer than 1 or 2 h, because they are at a greater risk of perianesthetic hypoglycemia. They should receive dextrose-containing intravenous fluids during any prolonged anesthesia (longer than 15 min) and/or serial blood glucose measurements should be performed until fully recovered.

Patient Stabilization

When possible, life-threatening physiological disturbances should be corrected prior to anesthesia (Table 26.4). However, this may not always be possible, and anesthesia should never be delayed if immediate surgical or medical intervention is the only way to save the patient's life.

Venous Access

Advantages to inserting an intravenous catheter into a peripheral vein include the following: Tissue-toxic drugs such as thiopental can be administered without fear of perivascular administration, intravenous fluid administration is facilitated, and the circulation is immediately accessible for administration of emergency drugs. The most common site for catheter insertion in dogs and cats is the cephalic vein. The lateral and medial saphenous veins are also easily accessible and may be preferred if surgery is performed on the head or thoracic limbs. The jugular vein can also be used, especially if longer-term indwelling catheters are being placed. Typically, an over-the-needle style of catheter is most suitable for perianesthetic use. A 20-gauge, 2-inch catheter is

Table 26.3. Physical status classification of veterinary patients

ASA Status Level	Patient Description
I	Normal healthy patient
II	Non-incapacitating systemic disease (e.g., obesity, mild dehydration, and simple fractures)
III	Severe systemic disease not incapacitating (e.g., compensated renal insufficiency, stable congestive heart failure, controlled diabetes mellitus, or cesarean section)
IV	Severe systemic disease that is a constant threat to life (e.g., gastric dilation and volvulus)
V	Moribund, not expected to live 24 h irrespective of intervention (e.g., severe uncompensated systemic disturbance)

ASA, American Society of Anesthesiologists.
Procedures performed under emergency conditions are denoted by placing an *E* behind the physical status number.

Table 26.4. A list of conditions that should be corrected prior to anesthesia

A. Severe dehydration
B. Anemia or hypoproteinemia
   Packed cell volume < 20 with acute blood loss
   Albumin < 2.0 g/dL
C. Acid-base and electrolyte disturbances
   pH < 7.2
   Potassium < 2.5–3.0 or > 6.0
D. Pneumothorax
E. Cyanosis
F. Oliguria or anuria
G. Congestive heart failure
H. Severe, life-threatening cardiac arrhythmias

suitable for most dogs and cats weighing more than 2 kg, and a 22-gauge, 1.25-inch catheter is suitable for those that are smaller. An 18-gauge catheter can be used in medium to large dogs if more rapid fluid administration is anticipated or needed.

Intravenous Fluids

The purpose of perianesthetic administration of intravenous fluids is to maintain vascular volume and adequate cardiac preload, which can be decreased as a result of increased vascular capacitance associated with anesthetic drugs, blood loss, and insensible fluid loss. In healthy patients without metabolic disease, a balanced electrolyte solution such as lactated Ringer's solution is most suitable for routine use since most fluid loss during anesthesia is isotonic. A patient's disease process may warrant the use of other fluids, such as normal saline, those containing dextrose, or a colloid solution, such as whole blood, packed red cells or other hemoglobin-based oxygen carrier, plasma, or a plasma expander.[8] The routine crystalloid administration rate for dogs and cats is 10 mL · kg^{-1} · h^{-1}. This rate can be decreased to 5 mL · kg^{-1} · h^{-1} for the second and subsequent hours of anesthesia if the surgical procedure is associated with minimal blood loss. Preexisting cardiac disease (e.g., mitral valve insufficiency) may warrant reduced fluid administration rates so as to not cause potentially fatal pulmonary edema.

Several styles of fluid administration sets are available. An administration set with a 10-drop/mL calibration is most convenient for patients weighing more than 5 kg. For smaller patients, a calibrated 60-drop/mL drip chamber enables a more precise estimation of proper fluid rate. If very small volumes of fluid are given, or precise volume measurement is desired, a syringe pump may be used. It is convenient to calculate the number of drops per minute necessary to deliver the calculated hourly fluid amount. The following example uses a 10-drop/mL drip set in a 25-kg dog at a rate of 10 mL · kg^{-1} · h^{-1}:

25 kg · 10 mL/kg/h = 250 mL/h
250 mL/h · 10 drops/mL = 2500 drops/h
2500 drops/h ÷ 60 min = 42 drops/min

A danger of perioperative fluid administration to very small animals is inadvertently administering too much fluid by improperly adjusting the drip rate. This can be particularly problematic in cats because they have a relatively small plasma volume relative to their size. A mechanical infusion pump or measured volume administration set will assist with delivery of the correct fluid amount.

The Anesthetic Plan

Several things should be considered when formulating an anesthetic plan (Table 26.5). In general, the anesthetic or chemical restraint technique rely primarily on local anesthesia, injectable anesthesia, or inhalation anesthesia. These techniques frequently overlap. For example, inhalation anesthesia is usually initiated with injectable anesthetics. Local anesthetic nerve blocks are typically accompanied by general anesthesia.

The remainder of the discussion regarding the choice of anesthetic drugs assumes the reader has reviewed and has a familiarity with the pharmacology of the various anesthetic drugs.[9,10] Although the drug combinations described are suitable for a variety of patients, the reader should refer to the appropriate sections of this text or consult a veterinary anesthesiologist if questions remain about how to anesthetize and monitor specific patients.

Short-Term Anesthesia (Less than 15 Minutes)

Several drugs are available for short-term anesthesia or chemical restraint (Tables 26.6 to 26.9). Immobilization for a short duration not requiring strong analgesia (radiography, suture removal, otoscopic examination, etc.) can be performed most simply with intravenous injectable drugs such as thiopental, propofol, or the ketamine/diazepam combination. These drugs induce rapid and predictable short-term loss of consciousness. Thiopental is relatively inexpensive and is suitable for short-term restraint of most

Table 26.5. Considerations for selecting an anesthetic plan

A. Procedure to be performed
   Duration
      <15 min
      15 min to 1 h
      >1 h
   Type of procedure
      Minor medical or surgical
      Major invasive surgery
   Anticipated perioperative pain
B. Available assistance and equipment
   Assistance
      Ventilatory assist or control
      Restraint
   Equipment
      Anesthetic machine
   Type of inhalation anesthetic
   Appropriate monitoring devices
C. Patient's temperament
   Quiet, relaxed, or calm
   Nervous and/or excitable
   Vicious
   Moribund or comatose
D. Physical status
   ASA categories I through V
E. Breed
   Sight hound
   Brachycephalic
   Toy

ASA, American Society of Anesthesiologists (see Table 26.3).

healthy dogs and cats. A disadvantage to its use as a sole anesthetic is that relatively large doses are required, full recovery can take up to 1 h, and recovery can be associated with ataxia and disorientation. These undesirable characteristics are reduced when its administration is preceded by a tranquilizer such as acepromazine or a sedative such as medetomidine. Another disadvantage is that it must be administered intravenously, a problem with fractious or uncooperative animals. Perivascular thiopental administration is associated with local tissue inflammation, pain, and potential tissue necrosis. Perivascular administration should be attended to by infiltrating the area with a crystalloid fluid (e.g., 0.9% sodium chloride) volume equal to three to five times the volume of perivascularly administered thiopental. Additionally, a local anesthetic such as lidocaine and an anti-inflammatory (e.g., methylprednisolone) may be infiltrated near the site of perivascular injection. Another important side effect of thiopental is the significant respiratory depression that can accompany its use. Alternatives to thiopental include propofol, etomidate, and the combinations of diazepam and ketamine or tiletamine and zolazepam (Telazol). The duration of action following a 1-bolus dose of these drugs is generally less than 15 min. Because of its rapid plasma clearance, multiple boluses of propofol, or a propofol infusion, can be used to prolong the duration of restraint without significantly prolonging the duration of recovery.[11]

Table 26.6. Sedatives and tranquilizers

Drug	Dosage (mg/kg)[a]	Comments
Acepromazine	0.025–0.2 IV, IM, SC (3–4 mg maximum)	Mild to moderate sedation of 1- to 2-h duration
Xylazine	0.3–2.2 IV, IM	Moderate to deep sedation, analgesia; 20 min to 1 h
Medetomidine	Dogs, 0.005–0.05 IV, IM Cats, 0.05–0.12 IV, IM	Similar effects to xylazine but 1- to 3-h duration
Diazepam	0.2–0.4 IV, IM	Most useful when combined with other sedatives, opioids, or ketamine Avoid IM in cats and small dogs
Midazolam	0.1–0.3 IV, IM, SC	Similar to diazepam but also useful IM or SC

IM, intramuscular; IV, intravenous; and SC, subcutaneous.
[a]Generally the low end of the dosage range is used IV and in sick or debilitated patients.

Table 26.7. Opioids and opioid combinations

Drug(s)	Dosage (mg/kg)[a]	Comments
Oxymorphone	0.05–0.1 IV, IM, SC	Excitement when used alone in young healthy dogs Duration of analgesia is 1–4 h
Morphine	0.2–0.6 IM, SC	Same as for oxymorphone
Hydromorphone	0.1–0.2 IV, IM, SC	Same as for oxymorphone
Butorphanol	0.2–0.4 IV, IM, SC	Opioid agonist/antagonist Minimal sedation when used alone Duration of analgesia is <1 h in dogs and up to 2–3 h in cats
Buprenorphine	0.005–0.01 IV, IM, SC, PO	Partial opioid agonist with approximately 6-8-h duration
Acepromazine-opioid	0.05–0.1 IV, IM Use dosage ranges for opioids listed above	Can be combined in same syringe Sedation lasts 15 min to 1 h
Midazolam-opioid	0.2–0.3 IV, IM Use dosage ranges for opioids listed above	Can be combined in same syringe Sedation lasts 15–40 min Generally produces poor results in young, healthy animals Not recommended for immobilization of vicious or difficult to handle animals Better quality restraint in older or debilitated animals
Xylazine-opioid	0.4–0.6 IV, IM Use dosage ranges for opioids listed above	Both drugs are reversible; sedation lasts 30–40 min Observe for bradycardia Useful for immobilization of difficult to handle or vicious animals
Medetomidine-opioid	Dogs, 0.001–0.002 IM Use dosage ranges for opioids listed above Cats, 0.004–0.006 IM Use lower end of dosage ranges for opioids listed above	Both drugs are reversible; sedation lasts 30 min to 1 h Observe for bradycardia Useful for immobilization of difficult to handle or vicious animals

IM, intramuscular; IV, intravenous; PO, oral; and SC, subcutaneous.
[a]Use low end of opioid dosage in cats.

Table 26.8. Cyclohexylamines and cyclohexylamine combinations

Drug(s)	Dosage (mg/kg)	Comments
Ketamine	2.0–10.0	Not useful alone in dogs
	IV, IM	Useful restraint in cats lasts 5–30 min
Ketamine-diazepam	5.5/0.20	Diazepam and midazolam are equally effective in this combination
and ketamine-midazolam	IV	Useful restraint lasts 5–10 min
		Poor muscle relaxation
Ketamine-xylazine	10.0/0.7–1.0	Useful restraint lasts 20–40 min
	IM	
Ketamine-acepromazine	10.0/0.2	Useful restraint lasts 20–30 min
	IM	
Tiletamine-zolazepam	2.0–8.0	Limited shelf-life after reconstitution
(Telazol)	IV, IM	Useful restraint for 20 min to 1 h
Telazol-ketamine-xylazine[a]	Cats	Long recoveries
	0.022 mL/kg	
Medetomidine-ketamine-	Cats	Good immobilization
opioid	0.03–0.06/5.0	Medetomidine and opioid can be reversed
	Use opioid dose	Can be used without opioid for restraint alone
	listed in previous table	
	Dogs	
	0.015–0.03/3.0	
	Use opioid dose listed	
	in previous table	

IM, intramuscular; and IV, intravenous.
[a]Reconstitute Telazol powder with 4 mL ketamine (100 mg/mL) and 1 mL xylazine (100 mg/mL).

Table 26.9. Injectable anesthetic drugs[a]

Drug	Dosage (mg/kg)	Comments
Thiopental	8.0–20.0	Use lower dosage after premedication
	IV	
Methohexital	3.0–8.0	Muscle rigidity
	IV	Best if preceded by a tranquilizer or sedative
		Duration 3–5 min
Etomidate	0.5–2.0	Duration 5–10 min
	IV	Myoclonus, gagging/retching
Propofol	4.0–6.0	Duration 5–10 min after single-bolus dose
	IV	Apnea for several minutes with rapid injection
	CRI,[b] 0.2–0.8	
	mg/kg/min	
Alphaxalone	1.0–15.0	Use lower dosages after premedication and for anesthetic induction and larger dosages for longer
	IV, IM	term immobilization

IM, intramuscular; and IV, intravenous.
[a]Injectable combinations using ketamine are listed in Table 26.8.
[b]Constant-rate infusion.

Dissociative-anesthetic combinations (ketamine-diazepam or tiletamine-zolazepam) produce less muscle relaxation than thiopental or propofol. They also are associated with increased salivation and dysphoria upon recovery. However, dissociative-anesthetic combinations generally produce less respiratory and cardiovascular depression than other available short-acting injectable anesthetics. Muscle relaxation and recovery quality are improved and salivation lessened when dissociatives are given with or preceded by a tranquilizer or sedative.[12]

Sedative/opioid combinations are suitable for short-term restraint for minimally invasive procedures or those procedures not requiring general anesthesia. An advantage is that one or both of

Table 26.10. Antagonists of various classes of anesthetic drugs

Drug	Dosage (mg/kg)
Alpha$_2$	
Yohimbine	0.1
	IV, IM
Atipamezole	0.04–0.5
	IM[a]
Benzodiazepine	
Flumazenil	0.01–0.2
	IV[b]
Opioid	
Naloxone	0.002–0.02
	IV, IM[c]

IM, intramuscular; and IV, intravenous.

[a]Dosage in milligrams is equal to five times the previously administered dosage of medetomidine.

[b]Begin with lowest dosage and repeat, if necessary, to effect.

[c]Use lowest dosage for "partial" reversal and highest dosage for complete reversal (refer to text for explanation).

these components can be reversed, enabling a rapid return to preanesthetic mentation and function (Table 26.10). Propofol or thiopental can be added to the regimen when complete immobilization or general anesthesia is necessary.

Alphaxalone is a neurosteroid anesthetic drug that produces hypnosis and muscle relaxation by enhancing GABA$_A$ receptor ion conduction. Immobilization is characterized by excellent muscle relaxation and hypnosis in dogs and cats. It is solubilized in cyclodextran and thus does not induce histamine release as did the Cremaphor vehicle used in Saffan (alphaxalone and alphadolone). It can be administered intravenously or intramuscularly, and its duration of action is dose dependent. It is compatible for use following commonly used preanesthetic sedatives and tranquilizers.[13]

The relatively cumbersome nature of inhalation anesthesia makes it inconvenient for use in very short procedures. However, the rapid induction and recovery associated with isoflurane and sevoflurane make them suitable for short-term anesthesia, particularly in neonates or those animals with severe organ system compromise. Mask induction with inhalant anesthetics should be preceded by preanesthetic administration whenever possible to reduce the stress and anxiety (and catecholamine release) associated with the initial breathing of high concentrations of inhalant anesthetics.

Intermediate-Term Anesthesia (15 Minutes to 1 Hour)

For procedures of intermediate duration that do not require good analgesia, thiopental, ketamine/diazepam, and propofol can be used and redosed to effect. Typically, one-third to one-half of the induction dose is administered slowly to prolong the anesthetic effect. Thiopental and ketamine/diazepam should not be redosed many times. Their initial duration of action following bolus administration primarily depends on redistribution away from the

brain to other tissues, such as muscle. However, when these tissues are saturated with drug, redistribution greatly slows, and metabolism becomes the rate-limiting factor for awakening. Propofol, because of its relatively rapid clearance and large volume of distribution, can be administered repeatedly to dogs by using small boluses or by constant-rate infusion (Table 26.9).

Invasive surgical procedures such as feline onychectomy or canine and feline gonadectomy typically require 15 min to 1 h of anesthesia, accompanied by good perioperative analgesia. Several options are available (Table 26.8). A combination of Telazol, ketamine, and xylazine is suitable for cats, although its use has been associated with prolonged recoveries.[14] An alternative is the combination of medetomidine, ketamine, and an opioid. Inclusion of an α_2-adrenergic agonist in the combinations suggests that partial antagonism of the anesthetic and analgesic effects with atipamezole is possible, if required. Inhalation anesthesia is also appropriate for procedures of intermediate duration and may be the most convenient. Inhalant anesthetic delivery of this duration usually requires intubation and careful monitoring, but has the benefit of enabling a rapid adjustment of the depth of anesthesia should anesthetic conditions change unexpectedly (e.g., loss of blood or respiratory arrest).

Long-Term Anesthesia (Longer Than 1 Hour)

Long procedures are best managed with inhalation anesthesia. Awakening from sevoflurane and isoflurane anesthesia is predictably rapid. Even sick and debilitated patients recover from prolonged periods of inhalation anesthesia relatively quickly, and liver or renal impairment does not directly affect drug clearance. Injectable anesthesia using intramuscularly or intravenously administered drugs has been described.[15–18] Those techniques that involve infusion of propofol and opioid combinations along with reversible tranquilizers or sedatives are most suitable for prolonged anesthesia because of propofol's predictably rapid clearance. Those techniques involving nonreversible drugs are less suited for prolonged immobilization because of the attendant prolonged recovery. Most anesthetic techniques are associated with some degree of respiratory depression and a loss of the protective swallowing reflex, so tracheal intubation and a means to assist ventilation are essential to reducing anesthetic risk.

Premedication

Inhalation anesthesia can be initiated without premedication; however, administration of a sedative, tranquilizer, opioid, or combination of these drugs is recommended prior to induction (Tables 26.6 and 26.7). Preanesthetic drugs aid in restraint, reduce apprehension, decrease the quantity of potentially more dangerous drugs used to produce general anesthesia, facilitate induction, enhance perioperative analgesia, and reduce arrhythmogenic autonomic reflex activity. Premedications are usually administered intramuscularly or subcutaneously 15 to 20 min before induction. The choice of premedication depends on signalment, temperament, physical status, concurrent disease, the procedure to be performed, and personal preference (Table 26.11). For procedures associated with postoperative pain, premedication should include an

Table 26.11. Suggestions for premedication in dogs and cats[a]

Dogs	Premedication
Young normal healthy	Acepromazine
	Xylazine
	Medetomidine
	Any of the above with an opioid agonist if moderate to severe perioperative pain is anticipated; any of the above with butorphanol or buprenorphine if less intense pain is anticipated or for moderate restraint
Aggressive/vicious	Acepromazine–opioid agonist
	Medetomidine–opioid agonist
	Xylazine–opioid agonist
Geriatric	Acepromazine (low end of dosage range)
	Midazolam-opioid
Painful procedures	Acepromazine–opioid agonist
	Midazolam–opioid agonist
Cats	Acepromazine-opioid (low dosage)
	Ketamine (low dosage)
	Ketamine (low dosage–acepromazine)
	Xylazine or medetomidine (young and healthy)
	Telazol (low dosage)

[a]These drugs or drug combinations should be administered between 15 and 30 min prior to anesthetic induction.

analgesic such as an opioid or α_2-adrenergic agonist and possibly a nonsteroidal anti-inflammatory drug. Fewer analgesics are typically needed postoperatively when analgesics are administered preemptively.[19] Repeated patient assessment following surgery is needed to assess the adequacy of analgesia, and additional analgesics should be administered when needed.

Induction

Induction is most easily accomplished in most animals with propofol, etomidate, dissociative anesthetic–benzodiazepine combinations, or thiopental (Table 26.9). Advantages to an intravenous method of induction include rapid loss of consciousness and ability to quickly intubate endotracheally. Alternatives to these rapid intravenous induction protocols include higher-dose intramuscular dissociative anesthetic–benzodiazepine administration, chamber or mask inhalant induction, or high-dose intravenous opioid induction. These techniques can be useful in special circumstances, but for routine use in healthy dogs and cats their disadvantages generally outweigh their advantages.

Chamber/Mask

One disadvantage to chamber and mask induction is the associated waste-gas pollution. Another is the struggling and associated stress during the induction phase.[20] Mask induction is most easily accomplished in moribund animals and small tractable dogs. Prior tranquilization or sedation enhances the quality and speed of induction.[21] Isoflurane and sevoflurane are the most suitable inhalants because they produce a relatively rapid induction.[22] Relatively high oxygen flow rates (4 L/min for chamber and 3 L/min for mask) and vaporizer settings (3% to 5% isoflurane and 5% to 7% sevoflurane in healthy animals) are used. The use of nitrous oxide is not necessary during chamber or mask induc-

tion.[23] With chamber induction, once the animal loses its righting reflex and is unresponsive to the chamber being tilted from side to side, the animal is removed from the chamber and induction is continued using an appropriately sized mask and the vaporizer setting used during the chamber phase. Mask induction (not preceded by a chamber) is begun by exposing the animal to the mask and oxygen. The inhalation concentration is slowly increased to 3% to 5% for isoflurane and 5% to 7% for sevoflurane. This is accomplished with a non-rebreathing or rebreathing circuit by gradually increasing the vaporizer setting over 2 to 4 min. Use of a non-rebreathing anesthetic system (e.g., the Bain coaxial system [see Chapter 17]) will facilitate a more rapid induction because the time-consuming exchange of the room air in the reservoir bag, breathing circuit, and carbon dioxide absorber of a circle system with anesthetic-laden gas from the vaporizer is not necessary.

Intravenous High-Dose Opioid Induction

A disadvantage to opioid induction is the attendant relatively slow loss of consciousness. Advantages include good cardiovascular stability (although severe bradycardia may be seen when anticholinergics are not coadministered) and the attenuation of the stress response associated with anesthesia and surgery. Opioid induction works best in debilitated dogs and is not recommended in cats or young healthy dogs that are not well sedated. Incremental doses of an opioid agonist (Table 26.7) are alternated with small incremental doses of diazepam or midazolam (Table 26.6) until the dog can be intubated.

Anesthetic Maintenance

The maintenance phase of anesthesia begins when unconsciousness is induced and ends with discontinuation of anesthetic deliv-

Table 26.12. Vaporizer settings[a]

Drug	Induction Phase (%)	Maintenance Phase (%)
Halothane	3	1–2
Isoflurane	3	1.5–2.5
Sevoflurane	4–5	2–4

[a]Listed vaporizer settings assume a fresh-gas flow of 1 to 2 L/min during the induction phase (first several minutes following induction with injectable drug), and a fresh-gas flow of 10 mL/kg/min during the maintenance phase. Low-flow system vaporizer settings are typically 1 to 2% higher. Refer to text for discussion of mask or chamber induction.

ery. After the loss of consciousness, a properly sized cuffed endotracheal tube or alternative airway is usually inserted to enable assisted ventilation, if necessary, and protect against aspiration of oropharyngeal contents. Adequate cardiovascular function is rapidly verified and the anesthetic vaporizer turned on. The initial and subsequent anesthetic vaporizer settings (percentage concentration of inhalant) vary with the condition of the patient, the type of breathing circuit used, and the fresh-gas flow rate (Table 26.12). The relatively high fresh-gas flow rate and vaporizer setting that are initially used after induction are decreased to maintenance settings when the patient nears the desired anesthetic plane (usually when palpebral reflex disappears and the heart rate begins to decrease). The vaporizer setting is adjusted according to signs of anesthetic depth. The most useful signs of anesthetic depth in dogs and cats include a combination of muscle tone (assessed by opening the mouth its full extent), heart and respiratory rates, and systemic blood pressure. All but systemic blood pressure are easily and inexpensively monitored and should be performed routinely. Other monitors that may be used include a pulse oximeter and a capnometer. Pulse oximetry noninvasively provides an estimate of hemoglobin's oxygen saturation (normal $\geq 95\%$). This information along with packed cell volume or hemoglobin concentration indicates the oxygen content of arterial blood. A capnometer noninvasively assesses ventilation by monitoring respiratory rate and end-tidal expired (related to arterial) carbon dioxide partial pressure. End-tidal CO_2 monitors can also identify problems with the gas delivery system such as malfunctioning one-way valves and exhausted CO_2 absorbent, especially when graphic display of the CO_2-time profile is provided (i.e., capnogram).

The Anesthetic Record

This is part of the permanent patient record and should include notation of patient status; the anesthetic drugs used, including time of administration; dose and effect; duration of the surgery; and notation of significant perioperative events. Ideally, heart rate, respiratory rate, blood pressure, and any other variables monitored should be recorded at regular intervals (5 to 10 min). Recording these data at regular intervals creates a visual aid that assists in determining the change in patient status during the anesthetic period. For example, a steadily increasing heart rate accompanied by a steadily decreasing blood pressure during a 15-min interval could signal hypotension caused by fluid loss or excessive anesthetic depth. This is easily observed on the anesthetic record but may not be noticed without the visual prompt of the data recorded over time.

Perioperative Analgesia

Concurrent administration of various analgesic drugs during inhalation anesthesia is useful to enhance intraoperative and postoperative analgesia. These drugs can be continued into the postanesthetic period to maintain analgesia. Infusions of low doses of ketamine, lidocaine, opioids, and their combinations have been described as adjuncts to inhalation anesthesia (Table 26.13).[24–26] When using these drugs, the concentration of inhalant anesthetic can often be significantly reduced. Increased respiratory depression is a concern, and the adequacy of ventilation should be closely monitored.

Recovery

Recovery begins when the procedure for which a patient has been anesthetized is finished, and the anesthetic drugs have been discontinued. Patient status should be monitored regularly during recovery until the patient is conscious, extubated, and heart rate, respiratory rate, and body temperature have returned to normal. Young healthy animals undergoing routine procedures usually do not need supplemental oxygen during recovery. However, contin-

Table 26.13. Drugs and drug combinations administered by constant-rate infusion to enhance intraoperative analgesia

Drug(s)	Infusion Rate	Comments
Ketamine	2–10 µg/kg/h	Useful as an adjunct to other perioperative analgesics
Fentanyl	1–5 µg/kg/h	Useful alone or with other perioperative analgesics; first administer loading dose of 2 µg/kg
Lidocaine	40 µg/kg/min	Useful as an adjunct to other perioperative analgesics; loading dose of 2 mg/kg
Morphine-lidocaine-ketamine	0.24/0.3/0.06 mg/kg/h[a]	Useful alone or with other perioperative analgesics

[a]To 1 L of crystalloid, add 24 mg morphine, 300 mg lidocaine, and 60 mg ketamine. Administer at 10 mL/kg/h intraoperatively. Concentration can be adjusted (increased) to fit postoperative maintenance fluid rates.

uous use of pulse oximetry is helpful to identify unexpected postanesthetic hypoxemia. Hypoxemia caused by respiratory depression, atelectasis-related ventilation/perfusion mismatch, and/or rapidly decreased fraction of inspired oxygen (e.g., near 100% oxygen to 21% room air) is easily addressed if detected early. If nitrous oxide was used during anesthetic maintenance, the breathing circuit should be repeatedly flushed with oxygen and the patient allowed to breathe an oxygen-enriched gas mixture for 5 to 10 min after discontinuation of nitrous oxide. This helps prevent the diffusion hypoxia that can develop if the inspired oxygen concentration suddenly decreases while nitrous oxide is rapidly moving from the blood into the alveolar gas. Sick or debilitated dogs and cats benefit from supplemental oxygen during recovery, particularly if hypothermic, because shivering can significantly increase oxygen consumption. The tracheal tube cuff should be deflated and untied when a patient is disconnected from the anesthetic machine. This permits extubation in the event that the patient rapidly awakens and begins chewing, but care should be exercised when moving the animal to the recovery area so premature accidental extubation does not occur. If an esophageal stethoscope or temperature probe was used, it should be removed at this time. Dogs and cats should be extubated as soon as the swallowing reflex occurs, unless there is a specific contraindication to removing the tracheal tube at this time (e.g., brachycephalic airway syndrome). Dogs and cats should never be left to recover unobserved. Recover patients in a well-ventilated area to minimize exhaled anesthetic gas pollution of the workspace.

Occasionally, a dog or cat will awaken suddenly from anesthesia, become disoriented, and will vocalize, paddle, and appear incoherent. This sudden arousal can be caused by emergence delirium or pain, and it is important to distinguish between them. Emergence delirium occurs most frequently in non-premedicated animals and in particular those awakening rapidly from anesthesia. With emergence delirium, the dog or cat will typically soon become quiet and more comfortable, usually within 10 min. A quiet, reassuring voice and restraint are all that are usually necessary to guide the animal through this period of excitement. If pain is believed to be the cause of the rough recovery, rapid-acting opioid analgesics (e.g., fentanyl) should be administered intravenously. Postoperative pain control is managed best with preanesthetic analgesic administration of relatively long-lasting analgesics, local anesthetics, and attention to signs of pain.

Dogs or cats receiving perioperative fluids can develop a fully distended or overdistended urinary bladder that can cause signs of discomfort. If a full bladder is palpated, it can be gently expressed before recovery. Occasionally, a low dose of acepromazine (0.03 to 0.05 mg/kg intravenously) is necessary to quiet an excited animal.

Perioperative Hypothermia

Because of the loss of normal thermoregulatory core-to-periphery temperature gradients and impaired central thermoregulatory responses, some decrease in core body temperature is unavoidable during anesthesia and surgery. The patient's temperature should be monitored, especially if supplemental heat sources are used (e.g., forced warm-air systems), because accidental hyperthermia is possible. It is more effective to prevent hypothermia rather than trying to warm a hypothermic patient during recovery, because skin vasoconstriction in response to hypothermia inhibits warming of blood near the body surface. Anesthetic-induced vasodilation facilitates warming and heat gain. Insulating and warming devices should be used during anesthesia and recovery.[27] Devices that are available for warming patients include circulating warm-water heating blankets, infrared heat lamps, incubators, and circulating warm-air blankets. Electric heating pads should never be used, because they have been associated with severe burns.[28] These burns usually are manifest from several days to 1 week after contact with the heating pad. The burn pattern often traces the pattern of the heating wire within the blanket. Care must be used with heat lamps or surgical gloves filled with warm water, because they also have produced thermal burns by being placed too close to unprotected skin. An advantage of using warm water and forced-air heating blankets is that temperature is uniform over their entire surface, and their maximum temperature is well below 105°F, the maximum safe patient heating-source interface.[29] Warming will be hastened if the patient's limbs are cocooned within the warming device. Incubators are convenient for warming small dogs and cats, and, if needed, supplemental oxygen can also be introduced through the incubator during the warming period. A circulating warm-air blanket that cocoons the patient is the most effective device for maintaining body temperature and perioperative warming.[29,30]

Delayed Anesthetic Recovery

Occasionally, a dog or cat that received several drugs during the anesthetic episode will remain mildly hypothermic and unresponsive. In these instances, consideration should be given to antagonism of reversible drugs (α_2-adrenergic agonists or opioids) that were given as part of the anesthetic regimen. Relatively small intravenous boluses of naloxone (2 to 3 µg/kg) can be used to reverse the central nervous system and thermoregulatory depression associated with the opioids while leaving opioid analgesia mostly intact.

Severe hypoglycemia is an easily corrected problem that can result in delayed anesthetic recovery. Blood glucose concentration should be measured if hypoglycemia is suspected, and intravenous dextrose-containing fluids given until blood glucose concentrations normalize. Arterial hypotension associated with blood loss or poor cardiac function cause altered mentation and slow recovery. Periodic measurement of arterial blood pressure during recovery, especially in debilitated patients, is warranted. Hypercarbia ($PaCO_2$ approaching 100 mm Hg) associated with respiratory-depressant anesthetic and adjunctive drugs may cause severe mental impairment and possibly respiratory arrest. Use of capnometry or arterial blood-gas analysis during the anesthetic and recovery period helps facilitate early detection and correction of respiratory depression. Occasionally, animals with undiagnosed, compensated central nervous system disease (e.g., hydrocephalus) may decompensate under anesthesia, resulting in impaired brain function. Prevention of hypercarbia, hypoxemia, and hypotension and rapid implementation of resuscitative measures (e.g., mannitol and controlled ventilation) may limit brain injury and speed recovery. Many problems that lead to delayed recovery from anesthesia can be prevented or otherwise managed with appropriate patient monitoring during and after anesthetic drug delivery.

References

1. Kojima K, Nishimura R, Mutoh T, Hong SH, Mochizuki M, Sasaki N. Effects of medetomidine-midazolam, acepromazine-butorphanol, and midazolam-butorphanol on induction dose of thiopental and propofol and on cardiopulmonary changes in dogs. Am J Vet R 2002;63:1671–1679.

2. Hall R, Szlam F, Hug C. The enflurane sparing effect of alfentanyl in dogs. Anesth Analg 1987;66:1287–1291.

3. Haskins S, Farver T, Patz J. Cardiovascular changes in dogs given diazepam and diazepam-ketamine. Am J Vet Res 1986;47:795–798.

4. Robinson EP, Sams RA, Muir WW. Barbiturate anesthesia in greyhound and mixed-breed dogs: Comparative cardiopulmonary effects, anesthetic effects, and recovery rates. Am J Vet Res 1986; 47:2105–2112.

5. Short C. Drug disposition in neonatal animals. J Am Vet Med Assoc 1984;184:1161–1162.

6. Seahorn J, Robertson S. Concurrent medications and their impact on anesthetic management. Vet Forum 2002;119:50–67.

7. Dripps RD, Lamont A, Eckenhoff JE. The role of anesthesia in surgical mortality. J Am Med Assoc 1961;178:261–266.

8. Kudnig S, Mama K. Perioperative fluid therapy. J Am Vet Med Assoc 2002;221:1112–1121.

9. Ilkiw J. Injectable anesthesia in dogs. Part I. Solutions, doses and administration. In: Gleed RD, Ludders JW, eds. Recent Advances in Veterinary Anesthesia and Analgesia: Companion Animals. Ithaca, NY: International Veterinary Information Service, 2002. http://www.ivis.org.

10. Ilkiw J. Injectable anesthesia in dogs. Part 2. Comparative Pharmacology. In: Gleed RD, Ludders JW, eds. Recent Advances in Veterinary Anesthesia and Analgesia: Companion Animals. Ithaca, NY: International Veterinary Information Service, 2002. http://www.ivis.org.

11. Nolan AM, Reid J. Pharmacokinetics of propofol administered by infusion in dogs undergoing surgery. Br J Anaesth 1993;70:546–551.

12. Smith JA, Gaynor JS, Bednarski RM, Muir WW. Adverse effects of administration of propofol with various preanesthetic regimens in dogs. J Am Vet Med Assoc 1993;202:1111–1115.

13. Muir W, Lerche P, Wiese A, et al. The cardiorespiratory safety and anesthetic effects of alfaxan CD RTU when administered alone or in combination with preanesthetic medications in dogs [Abstract]. In: Veterinary Midwest Anesthesia and Analgesia Conference, April 17–18, 2004. Indianapolis, IN, 2004.

14. Williams LS, Levy JK, Robertson SA, Cistola AM, Centonze LA. Use of the anesthetic combination of tiletamine, zolazepam, ketamine, and xylazine for neutering feral cats. J Am Vet Med Assoc 2002;220:1491–1495.

15. Hughes JM, Nolan AM. Total intravenous anesthesia in greyhounds: Pharmacokinetics of propofol and fentanyl: A preliminary study. Vet Surg 1999;28:513–524.

16. Ilkiw JE, Pascoe PJ. Effect of variable-dose propofol alone and in combination with two fixed doses of ketamine for total intravenous anesthesia in cats. Am J Vet Res 2003;64:907–912.

17. Ilkiw JE, Pascoe PJ. Cardiovascular effects of propofol alone and in combination with ketamine for total intravenous anesthesia in cats. Am J Vet Res 2003;64:913–915.

18. Mendes G, Selmi A. Use of a combination of propofol and fentanyl, alfentanil, or sufentanil for total intravenous anesthesia in cats. J Am Vet Med Assoc 2003;223:1608–1613.

19. Woolf CF, Chong M. Preemptive analgesia: Treating postoperative pain by preventing the establishment of central sensitization. Anesth Analg 1993;77:362–379.

20. Mutoh T, Nishimura R, Kim H. Rapid inhalation induction of anesthesia by halothane, enflurane, isoflurane, and sevoflurane and their cardiopulmonary effects in dogs. J Vet Med Sci 1995;57:1007–1013.

21. Mutoh T, Nishimura R, Sasaki N. Effects of medetomidine-midazolam, midazolam-butorphanol, or acepromazine-butorphanol as premedicants for mask induction of anesthesia with sevoflurane in dogs. Am J Vet Res 2002;63:1022–1028.

22. Lerche P, Muir WW, Grubb T. Mask induction of anaesthesia with isoflurane or sevoflurane in premedicated cats. J Small Anim Pract 2002;43:12–15.

23. Mutoh T, Nishimura R, Sasaki N. Effects of nitrous oxide on mask induction of anesthesia with sevoflurane or isoflurane in dogs. Am J Vet Res 2001;62:1727–1733.

24. Wagner A, Walton J, Hellyer P, Gaynor JS, Mama KR. Use of low doses of ketamine administered by constant rate infusion as an adjunct for postoperative analgesia in dogs. J Am Vet Med Assoc 2002;221:72–75.

25. Muir W, Wiese A, March P. Effects of morphine, lidocaine, ketamine, and morphine-lidocaine-ketamine drug combination on minimum alveolar concentration in dogs anesthetized with isoflurane. Am J Vet Res 2003;64:1155–1160.

26. Nunes de Moraes A, Dyson D, O'Grady M, McDonell WN, Holmberg DL. Plasma concentrations and cardiovascular influence of lidocaine infusions during isoflurane anesthesia in healthy dogs and dogs with subaortic stenosis. Vet Surg 1998;27:486–497.

27. Imrie MM, Hall GM. Body temperature and anaesthesia. Br J Anaesth 1990;64:346–354.

28. Swaim SF, Lee AH, Hughes KS. Heating pads and thermal burns in small animals. J Am Anim Hosp Assoc 1989;25:156–162.

29. Hynson J, Sessler DI. Comparison of intraoperative warming devices [Abstract]. Anesth Analg 1991;72:S118.

30. Machon R, Raffe M, Robinson E. Warming with a forced air warming blanket minimizes anesthetic-induced hypothermia in cats. Vet Surg 1999;28:301–310.

Chapter 27

Horses

John A. E. Hubbell

Introduction

Anesthesia in adult horses is complicated by a relatively unique set of problems associated with their temperament, large body mass, and thoracoabdominal anatomy. Thus, although an understanding of the pharmacology of the drugs used is essential for safe anesthetic practice, the knowledge base must not stop there. Prolonged recumbency is an unnatural position for horses. This, coupled with horses' seeming desire to escape unfamiliar situations by running, makes induction and recovery from anesthesia difficult. Particularly challenging are those situations when an injured or painful horse must be anesthetized.[1,2] In addition, the potential for inadequate muscle blood flow and deleterious changes in cardiopulmonary function associated with lateral and dorsal recumbency must be understood. A number of studies have been published examining perioperative morbidity and mortality in horses.[3–6] The reported mortality rates associated with elective equine anesthesia range from 0.1% to 1.0%, with higher incidences reported for emergency and out-of-hours procedures.[3] The largest study performed to date indicates that there are statistically significant differences in the incidence of mortality dependent on the person performing the anesthesia and the person performing the surgery.[3] Other factors cited include age (high risk in the very young and low risk for young adults, with increasing risk with age), duration of surgery (higher risk for longer surgery), type of surgery (fractures at higher risk), timing of surgery (outside of "normal hours" at greater risk), the drugs used for sedation prior to anesthesia (greatest risk when no drugs are used; reduced risk for acepromazine and greater risk for

romifidine administration), and the use of inhalant anesthetics (increased risk with inhalant anesthetic induction, and increased risk of inhalant anesthesia when compared with total intravenous anesthesia).[3] The studies reported to date have not examined the effect of monitoring techniques (arterial blood pressure and arterial blood gases) or the other anesthetic adjuncts that could be used (e.g., controlled ventilation or use of vasopressors). These techniques and adjuncts may play a major role in the safety of any anesthetic; thus, any discussion that does not take them into account is incomplete. This chapter focuses on practical aspects of handling horses and the use of specific drugs, alone and in combination.

Physical Restraint

Prior to the development of appropriate sedatives, tranquilizers, and other anesthetics, physical restraint was a primary method by which practitioners accomplished the treatment and the completion of some surgical and diagnostic techniques. With the advent of useful anesthetics, the reliance on physical restraint has diminished, but the techniques remain an integral part of safe equine practice. Physical restraint may be as innocuous as taking hold of a horse's halter or picking up a patient's leg to limit movement. In most situations, some level of physical restraint is combined with appropriate drugs to induce a tractable patient. The method of physical restraint should be based on (a) the age, size, and temperament of the horse; (b) its physical status; (c) the number and training of available personnel; and (d) the duration and nature of the procedure.

Methods of Drug Delivery

Anesthetics are administered to horses by topical, oral, subcutaneous, intramuscular, epidural, intravenous, and inhalant routes. The effective application of anesthetics topically is probably limited to the eye and mucous membranes. Oral formulations for tranquilization can be drenched or mixed with feed but are somewhat unpredictable because the potential for limited consumption and absorption makes it difficult to predict the timing and magnitude of the effects produced. Intramuscular injection is more effective than subcutaneous injection. Sedatives and tranquilizers are often administered intramuscularly because of ease of administration, longer action, and a decrease in the intensity of deleterious side effects when compared with intravenous administration. Disadvantages of intramuscular administration of drugs include delayed onset of action, decreased intensity of effect, and (because a larger quantity of drug is required) increased cost. Epidural or spinal injection of drugs can be used for analgesia. Drugs used by the epidural route include the local anesthetics, α_2-adrenergic agonists, and opioid receptor agonists. The intravenous route is preferred by most veterinary practitioners. Sedatives, tranquilizers, and injectable anesthetics (barbiturates and ketamine) can be administered intravenously. Intravenous injection induces rapid onset of action, higher peak intensity of effect, briefer action, and a greater ability to titrate the desired effect by repeated administration. Inhalation anesthesia (e.g., halothane, isoflurane, or sevoflurane) requires the constant administration of drug that is delivered in oxygen.

Equipment

The equipment required for the delivery of anesthetic to equine patients varies from a syringe and needle to expensive inhalation anesthetic systems equipped with ventilators. Most equine anesthesia is performed as short-term anesthesia in the field. In this setting, the ability to supplement the inspired oxygen concentration of patients is usually limited. In the absence of the ability to supplement inspired oxygen, time of recumbency should be limited to 1 h. Oxygen supplementation benefits all anesthetized patients. Methods of supplementing oxygen in the field include the use of insufflation and the use of a demand valve. Insufflation is performed by inserting a tube into the horse's nose. Oxygen can be supplied in a small tank equipped with a pressure-reducing valve and flowmeter. Flow should be set at a minimum of 15 L/min in order to be effective.[7] A size-E oxygen cylinder contains approximately 650 L of oxygen when full, so it can supply 40 to 45 min of oxygen at 15 L/min flow. If apnea occurs, the flow rate can be increased and a breath can be delivered by occluding the nostrils until the thoracic wall rises appropriately, and then releasing the nostrils to allow exhalation. Alternatively, a demand valve (Fig. 27.1) can be used. A demand valve delivers oxygen by one of two mechanisms. When the horse inhales, the demand valve is triggered and delivers oxygen at high flow rates. The increased airway pressure generated by exhalation shuts the demand valve off. In the absence of ventilation, the demand valve can be triggered by the operator by pushing a button. The button is released upon appropriate chest expansion, the flow stops, and the patient exhales. A demand valve can be used with a tube that is inserted in the nostril and advanced in the airway (if the nostrils are occluded) but is best used in combination with an appropriately placed endotracheal tube.

Oxygenation should be maximized if extended anesthesia is contemplated. The best way to provide optimal oxygenation is to use an anesthetic machine in combination with an endotracheal tube that allows the airway to be sealed. Anesthetic machines for adult horses provide for the delivery of high oxygen concentrations (greater than 95%) whether or not inhalation anesthetics are being used. Oxygen flow rates to maintain high inspired-oxygen concentrations depend on a horse's metabolic rate but are in the range of 2 to 5 L/min in adult horses.

Endotracheal tubes are helpful both in the field and in more so-

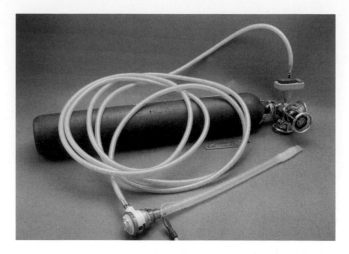

Fig. 27.1. A demand valve coupled with an oxygen source such as a size-E tank can be used for resuscitation in case of respiratory or cardiovascular collapse. The demand valve is connected to a 12- to 14-mm (internal diameter) endotracheal tube placed via the nostril into the pharynx. One hand is used to activate the demand valve while the other is used to occlude the airway by squeezing the area just caudal to the nostrils. End inflation by releasing the trigger mechanism at the point when a normal thoracic excursion has been completed. Repeat this maneuver four to six times a minute until spontaneous respiration resumes.

phisticated settings where inhalation anesthetics are employed. To be effective, endotracheal tubes should seal the airway. This is usually done by inflating a cuff. Endotracheal tubes are usually placed orally. The use of a bite block, easily made with 2-inch polyvinyl chloride pipe, will extend the life of the tube. Endotracheal tubes can also be placed via the ventral meatus of the nasal cavity. This route is particularly useful for intraoral surgery. Smaller endotracheal tubes should be used. Prior to anesthesia, the halter should be checked to ensure that it is appropriately applied and sufficiently strong to withstand the forces generated during induction and recovery.

Safe anesthesia in horses depends on maintaining relatively light levels of anesthesia, which is sometimes difficult to assess. Should the horse move, maintaining control is important until additional anesthetic can be administered. The use of a chest rope (Fig. 27.2) and casting harness or hobble system enables control of movement. A hobble system is easily devised by using a 35- to 40-foot length of 1-inch cotton rope. Soft, larger-diameter rope is preferred because the chance of a rope burn is minimized.

Some anesthetic techniques require only drugs, needles, syringes, and the ability to make a venipuncture. The placement of an intravenous catheter increases the safety of anesthesia by assuring venous access, ensuring (with proper placement) that medications are given intravenously, and reducing the number of venipunctures to one. Anesthetic agents, particularly the thiobarbiturates and to a lesser extent guaifenesin, are irritating and can cause tissue destruction when administered extravascularly. The relative guarantee of venous access is important when administering anesthetic agents, because of the dilemmas faced when an

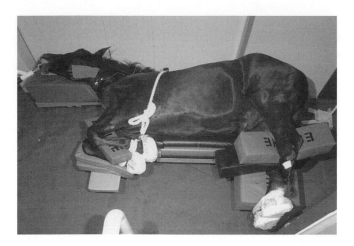

Fig. 27.2. A horse placed in right lateral recumbency for surgery. All ventral surfaces are padded with foam rubber. The front and rear legs are separated with pads in an attempt to reduce venous compression. A chest rope is used to position the front legs. The position reduces the "lever arm" effect of the front legs and reduces pressure on the weight supporting the shoulder. The chest rope should not be overtightened because respiration could be impeded.

anesthetic agent is administered to no apparent effect. The lack of effect could be caused by perivascular injection of the drug, administration of an inadequate dose, or an idiosyncratic reaction of the patient. The presence of a properly placed catheter ensures that the drug was administered intravascularly and enables administration of additional drug if required. Useful catheter sizes for horses are 10 to 14 gauge for adult horses and 14 to 20 gauge for foals. The jugular vein is the usual site for catheterization. In the absence of patent jugular veins, the median, cephalic, lateral thoracic, or saphenous veins can be used. In those settings where inhalation anesthesia of horses for longer than 1 h is routine and frequent, additional equipment is required. The maintenance of adequate arterial blood pressure in horses has been shown to correlate with a reduced number of postanesthetic complications.[8] Arterial blood pressure can be measured inexpensively using an aneroid manometer following aseptic placement of a catheter (18 to 22 gauge) in a peripheral artery. Aneroid manometers enable the estimation of mean arterial blood pressure.[9] At more expense, some monitors with blood pressure transducers enable measurement of systolic, mean, and diastolic blood pressures and may automatically display these values digitally. The maintenance of a mean arterial blood pressure greater than 60 to 70 mm Hg is associated with a reduction in postoperative complications, so the use of such devices and the correction of hypotension when it occurs are necessary, particularly in horses anesthetized for 45 min or longer.[6,10] Appropriate padding helps to prevent pressure injury to muscle tissues. Commercially available foam-rubber pads, air mattresses, and water mattresses can be used for this purpose.

Preparation of Patients

A physical examination should be performed prior to the administration of any anesthetic drug. If a horse is only to be tranquil-

ized, a brief physical examination should emphasize the cardiovascular and respiratory systems. If recumbency is to be induced, a more complete physical examination should be performed. A thorough evaluation of the respiratory system is warranted. Physical signs of respiratory disease include cough, discharge at the nostrils or eyes, submandibular lymph node enlargement, fever, and increases in respiratory rate. Auscultation should be performed over both sides of the thorax. Occlusion of the nostrils or the use of a plastic rebreathing bag to stimulate deep breathing enables a better evaluation of breath sounds. Palpation of the trachea and larynx may elicit a cough. Incipient respiratory disease can be further evaluated by performing a white blood cell count, and counts in excess of 12,000 to 14,000 cells/mL are cause for further evaluation. Serum fibrinogen levels can also be used as an index of systemic inflammation. Horses with respiratory infections should be allowed 3 weeks to recover prior to elective procedures. Many horses present with subclinical respiratory disease. General anesthesia has been associated with depression of immune function. A horse with subclinical respiratory disease could develop overt disease following anesthesia.

Respiratory stridor is another cause for concern. Most anesthetics cause relaxation of the muscles of the upper airway, particularly the nostrils.[11] Relaxation of these muscles may allow the nostrils to sag inward on inhalation, partially occluding the airway. A tracheostomy should be performed prior to the induction of anesthesia if there is severe upper-airway obstruction or if the nasal cavity will be occluded as part of the surgery. For example, surgical techniques for removal of the nasal septum and ethmoid hematomas require the placement of an absorbent pack in the nasal cavity in order to effect hemostasis. A tracheostomy is required because horses are obligate nasal breathers.

The cardiovascular system is evaluated clinically by auscultating for heart sounds, palpating peripheral pulses, evaluating the color of mucous membranes, and assessing capillary refill time and skin turgor. Physical signs of cardiovascular abnormalities may include exercise intolerance, distension of the jugular veins with and without jugular pulses, and pallor. Cardiac auscultation must be performed in a quiet environment. Heart rate should be determined, and the presence or absence of pauses noted. Pauses should disappear if the horse is exercised briefly. Occasional pauses can be evaluated further with an electrocardiogram. Common physiological rhythm variations in horses include first-degree heart block, second-degree heart block, sinus arrest or sinoatrial block, and variably configured P waves. The most common arrhythmia of clinical significance in horses is atrial flutter or fibrillation. A presumptive diagnosis of atrial flutter can be made by auscultating heart sounds of various intensities that occur at irregular rates. The palpation of pulses of varying strengths occurring at irregular intervals provides more evidence. A diagnosis of atrial fibrillation can be confirmed with an electrocardiogram. Atrial and ventricular premature contractions are occasionally observed in horses prior to surgery. Atrial premature contractions seem to have little significance. Premature ventricular contractions, particularly if they occur at a rate faster than three per minute, should be evaluated further. Cardiac murmurs can be ausculted in a relatively high percentage of adult horses.[12]

Most soft systolic murmurs (grade III out of VI or less) are interpreted as innocent flow murmurs in the absence of other signs of cardiac disease. Potential sources of significant murmurs in horses include ventricular septal defects, mitral valve insufficiency, and aortic insufficiency.

Neuromuscular function, in particular the presence or absence of ataxia, should be evaluated to anticipate possible problems with recovery from anesthesia. Other pertinent factors would include a history of "tying up" (rhabdomyolysis) or hyperkalemic periodic paralysis.

Following a complete physical examination of the animal and documentation of its medical history, ancillary tests and procedures should be performed as indicated by the physical status and history. The determination of packed cell volume and plasma total protein is easy and inexpensive, and it provides baseline information about the oxygen-carrying capacity and hydration status of the patient.

Some surgical procedures, such as ovariectomy, are facilitated if food is withheld for 24 to 48 h prior to anesthesia. A prolonged fast does not seem to be necessary for other procedures. Gastric emptying occurs rapidly in horses; thus, a 4- to 6-h period of withholding food should be adequate. Access to water should be maintained. It has been suggested that horses anesthetized at higher altitudes benefit from a longer period without food because of their propensity for gas distension. The shoes should be removed or at least covered to decrease the chance that the horse will lacerate itself on recovery. Before induction, the horse's mouth should be rinsed to remove foreign material.

Standing Chemical Restraint

A wide variety of agents have been used to produce chemical restraint in standing horses (Table 27.1). Current practice has evolved to the point where three groups of agents are commonly used: phenothiazines, α_2-adrenergic agonists, and opioid receptor agonists. Butyrophenone tranquilizers were reported to be effective in horses, but more recent reports suggest significant undesirable adverse effects that prevent their recommendation.[13,14] Diazepam is used as a muscle relaxant in horses, but the level of

sedation produced is not profound enough to be useful for restraint.[15] Chloral hydrate is a sedative-hypnotic that was widely used for sedation and anesthesia prior to the availability of inhalation anesthetics. The best use of chloral hydrate was for augmentation of the effects of other sedatives and tranquilizers in particularly obstreperous horses. Chloral hydrate is given intravenously and produces severe tissue necrosis if given perivascularly. Chloral hydrate is not currently available in pharmaceutical preparations suitable for horses.

Phenothiazine Tranquilizers

These produce calming and a relaxed state from which horses can be aroused. Phenothiazine tranquilizers can be administered orally, intramuscularly, and intravenously to horses. The two drugs that are in common use are promazine and acepromazine. Phenothiazines produce tranquilization by blocking the action of neurotransmitters both centrally and peripherally. As in other species, hypotension caused by α_1-adrenergic blockade can be produced. Hypotension is of particular concern in nervous or excitable horses or in horses that have sustained blood loss or are dehydrated. The respiratory effects of phenothiazines are minimal and are generally limited to decreases in respiratory rate. Persistent penile paralysis can occur after phenothiazine administration to horses. The mechanism of the effect is unknown. Penile paralysis is uncommon but remains a consideration. Treatment should include support of the penis to prevent or reduce swelling. Benztropine mesylate may be effective in resolving penile paralysis:[16] 8 mg of benztropine was administered to two adult horses, and paralysis resolved within 10 min.[16] Benztropine is used in the treatment of Parkinson's disease and is believed to have central anticholinergic effects.

Acepromazine is available as a 1% solution (10 mg/mL) for parenteral injection. The onset of effect of acepromazine occurs within 15 to 30 min of administration. The duration of tranquilization following administration depends on the dose but may persist for 6 to 10 h. Acepromazine produces calming, with minimal muscle relaxation or ataxia. Acepromazine does not produce analgesia but may potentiate other drugs such as the opioids that are analgesics. Acepromazine will not transform an aggressive

Table 27.1. Drugs used for standing chemical restraint, for analgesia, and as preanesthetics

Drug	Dose and Route	Onset of Effect	Comments
Acepromazine	0.02–0.05 mg/kg IM, IV	30–40 min IV, IM	Use cautiously in stressed or hypotensive horses
Xylazine	0.5–1.0 mg/kg IV	3–5 min IV	Ataxia produced, head-down posture
	1.0 –2.2 mg/kg IM	10–20 min IM	Start with a low dose and repeat as needed
Detomidine	0.01–0.02 mg/kg IV	3–5 min IV	Ataxia produced, head-down posture
	0.02–0.04 mg/kg IM	10–20 min IM	Start with a low dose and repeat as needed
			Can be given orally
Butorphanol	0.01–0.03 mg/kg IV	3–5 min	Usually used in combination with a sedative or tranquilizer
Morphine	0.3–0.5 mg/kg IV	3–5 min	Sedate with xylazine or detomidine prior to administering morphine
			Potential for excitement.
			Reversible with naloxone

IM, intramuscularly; IV, intravenously; and PO, per os (orally).

horse into a docile one but will reduce the animal's awareness and response to external stimuli. Increasing the dose does not ensure a more pronounced effect, because approximately 30% to 40% of horses administered acepromazine do not attain the desired effect. Acepromazine is used as an aid to training, to produce standing restraint, and prior to transportation because it is long acting, inexpensive, and does not produce severe ataxia. The most reliable indication that a horse has been sedated with acepromazine is extrusion of the penis from the sheath.[17] Other signs include some drooping of the eyelids and slight protrusion of the third eyelid. Contraindications to the use of acepromazine would include the previously mentioned blood-loss or shocklike state, because of the α_1-adrenergic antagonist effects of acepromazine. The resulting hypotension is particularly prone to occur after intravenous administration of acepromazine and can cause syncope and recumbency. Treatment includes the intravenous administration of large volumes of polyionic fluids. Known bleeding disorders are another contraindication to acepromazine, because phenothiazines can inhibit platelet function.

α_2-Adrenoceptor Agonists

These drugs produce sedation, analgesia, and muscle relaxation when administered intravenously or intramuscularly to horses. The three α_2-adrenoceptor agonists currently available for equine use in the United States are xylazine, detomidine, and romifidine, with medetomidine used in other countries.[18] The effects of the drugs are similar, but detomidine is approximately 80 to 100 times more potent than xylazine and its action lasts twice as long. Romifidine has a duration of action similar to detomidine, and its sedative effects are less profound than those of either xylazine or detomidine. α_2-Adrenergic agonists are used for the temporary relief of colic pain, as adjuncts to general anesthesia, and alone and in combination with other drugs for standing chemical restraint. Xylazine and detomidine have also been administered epidurally to produce regional analgesia.[19,20] α_2-Adrenergic agonists reach peak effect in 3 to 5 min after intravenous administration and within 10 to 15 min of intramuscular administration. Oral administration is usually saved for occasions when a horse is not amenable to injections because of inconsistent effects. Oral (sublingual) administration of detomidine has been shown to produce profound sedation 45 min after administration.[21]

Sedation with α_2-adrenergic agonists is characterized by profound depression, with the horse assuming a head-down posture. The horse may attempt to head press. The eyelids and lips droop, and the horse may sway because of the muscle relaxation and ataxia produced. The muscles of the nostrils relax, which may lead to snoring or potentially obstruction in predisposed horses. Normal horses rarely become recumbent following α_2-adrenergic agonist administration, but they may be difficult to move because of ataxia and muscle relaxation. α_2-Adrenergic agonists may have more pronounced effects in foals, so the dose should be reduced. As in other species, the administration of α_2-adrenergic agonists is characterized by decreases in cardiac output, primarily caused by increases in vascular resistance and decreases in heart rate. α_2-Adrenergic agonists may induce or exacerbate first-degree and second-degree atrioventricular blockade.

Respiration is depressed, but the effect is usually not apparent unless other drugs are coadministered or anesthesia is induced. The frequency and volume of urination are increased after administration of α_2-adrenergic agonists. In adult horses, serum glucose levels increase and serum insulin levels decrease.[22] The effects of α_2-adrenergic agonists can be antagonized by the administration of yohimbine, atipamezole, or tolazoline.[23]

α_2-Adrenergic agonists are frequently used in horses with abdominal pain to facilitate evaluation and for pain relief. By repeated evaluation and general consensus, α_2-adrenergic agonists are the most effective available drugs for the treatment of colic pain.[24,25] The use of α_2-adrenergic agonists is controversial, however, because in addition to relieving colic pain, they cause decreases in intestinal propulsive activity. Thus, although the pain is controlled, the resolution of the cause of the abdominal pain may be slowed. The duration of the reduction in propulsive activity approximates the duration of sedation. A rational approach is to administer small doses of α_2-adrenergic agonists intravenously and frequently reevaluate the patient, and then readminister the drug as necessary. Xylazine may be more useful in this setting than detomidine because xylazine has a briefer action, prompting more frequent reevaluation.

Opioid Receptor Agonists

Opioids have been used to produce analgesia and augment chemical restraint in horses. Because of their ability to cause nervousness and excitability, opioids are most frequently used in combination with sedatives or tranquilizers to produce standing chemical restraint. Butorphanol, a synthetic opioid agonist-antagonist, is approved for treatment of abdominal pain in horses. Butorphanol is less apt to cause excitement than are opioid agonists but can cause nervousness and ataxia at higher doses. Both the analgesia and nervousness produced by opioid agonists and agonists-antagonists can be reversed by naloxone, an opioid antagonist. Caution should be used, however, because the duration of effect of some opioid agonists, such as morphine, may be longer than that of the antagonist. This could lead to renarcotization (resumed excitement) 4 to 6 h after narcotic administration. Such excitement responds to the administration of additional antagonist or a tranquilizer. The clinical use of opioids is discussed in the Standing Chemical Restraint section. A myriad of potential combinations can be used to produce standing chemical restraint, but most combine a sedative-tranquilizer with an opioid.

Acepromazine and Xylazine Combination

This combination has been used to improve tranquilization with some reduction in deleterious side effects.[26] Reduced doses of both drugs are used, typically 0.02 to 0.03 mg/kg of acepromazine and 0.2 to 0.5 mg/kg of xylazine. The drugs can be combined in the same syringe and are usually given intravenously. The reduced dose of xylazine produces less ataxia and less of a head-down posture than would be seen with xylazine alone (given in a higher dose). Thus, the horse stands more squarely on all four feet. The combination produces faster onset and longer action than either agent given alone. The suppliers of xylazine caution against its coadministration with tranquilizers.

Sedative/Tranquilizer-Opioid Combinations

The combination of xylazine and butorphanol has been investigated.[27] When combined, the dose of xylazine is usually reduced because butorphanol provides some analgesia with few deleterious cardiovascular side effects. Because of the reduced dose of xylazine, the horse is usually less ataxic. Occasionally, horses twitch and jerk their heads after being given this combination. Head pressing may occur. The drugs can be given in combination in the same syringe. The analgesia produced is not sufficient to perform a skin incision, so local anesthetic blockade may be needed. Butorphanol has also been used in combination with detomidine.[28]

The combination of α_2-adrenergic agonists and morphine has been used to produce standing chemical restraint for surgery.[29,30] Morphine should not be given until a horse is fully sedate, because of the potential for excitement. Within 5 min of morphine administration, the horse assumes a head-down, sawhorse position. The placement of a nose twitch and elevation of the head may be helpful in stabilizing patients on all four feet. Although analgesia is produced, horses remain sensitive to touch, so the technique is usually combined with local blockade. Both drugs are potentially reversible using an α_2-adrenergic antagonist (e.g., yohimbine or tolazoline) and an opioid receptor antagonist (e.g., naloxone). As mentioned, occasionally, renarcotization (excitement or nervousness) occurs following administration of the combination, owing to the long half-life of morphine in horses. The excitement can be abated by administration of a narcotic antagonist or simply by tranquilizing the patient.

Analgesia

The recognition and management of pain has long been a part of equine practice. The goals of pain management cover a wide range from simply reducing the inflammation and discomfort of mild arthritis to the ordeal of exerting control over a violent, thrashing mare with a distended abdomen. Traditional approaches to providing analgesia include the administration of nonsteroidal anti-inflammatory drugs (NSAIDs), local anesthetics, and many of the drugs used for standing chemical restraint (α_2-adrenergic agonists and opioids). Other drugs, not classically considered analgesics, such as steroids, orgotein, methocarbamol, and polysulfated glycosaminoglycans, are used because they are anti-inflammatory and, as such, may increase the comfort of individuals. In addition, acupuncture has been reported to relieve back pain in exercising horses and to reduce the anesthetic requirement for other drugs.[31,32]

Pain is infrequently mentioned as a presenting complaint by horse owners. Most gait abnormalities occur when an animal alters its locomotion in order to reduce pain. The pain is localized by progressively and selectively desensitizing regions and structures until the gait abnormality is altered or resolved. Once localized, the source of the pain is investigated with imaging modalities and is modified or, if possible, removed. Alternatives to removal include the administration of systemic analgesics or sensory denervation. Colic represents another presenting pain sign. Frequently, the response to analgesic administration aids in the

determination of the severity of the disease. Mild episodes of colic are initially treated with NSAIDs. If the analgesia produced by NSAIDs is insufficient, short-acting α_2-adrenergic agonists are used to provide analgesia and facilitate further diagnostic procedures. The response to α_2-adrenergic agonist administration and the information gleaned from diagnostic procedures are used to determine the severity of the disease and whether an abdominal exploratory surgery is required. The use of α_2-adrenergic agonists and opioids in colic treatment is limited by their effects on gastrointestinal motility. The reductions in motility and increases in sphincter tone may slow the resolution of hypomotile states and contribute to postoperative ileus. Other drugs (lidocaine and ketamine) and therapeutic modalities (acupuncture) are being investigated to determine their utility in producing analgesia for colic pain with fewer overall side effects.

A number of NSAIDs have been approved for use in horses (Table 27.2).[33] Phenylbutazone administered orally and intravenously is widely used for the treatment of inflammation and pain associated with acute and chronic musculoskeletal injuries and conditions. Phenylbutazone administration enables some unsound horses to live apparently comfortable lives and may permit performance in horses that cannot otherwise compete. For this reason, phenylbutazone administration in many racing jurisdictions is limited to a maximum allowable plasma concentration. Phenylbutazone and other NSAIDs are also used to provide perioperative analgesia for orthopedic and other surgery. Ketoprofen, flunixin meglumine, naproxen, meclofenamic acid, and diclofenac are additional NSAIDs approved for use in horses in the United States. These other drugs are primarily used as alternatives to phenylbutazone for selected indications. Flunixin meglumine is also used for relief of the pain associated with colic. Diclofenac is approved for topical administration as a liposome-based topical cream. It is approved for control of pain and inflammation associated with osteoarthritis of the tarsal, carpal, and distal joints. Renal failure, gastrointestinal ulceration, diarrhea, hypoproteinemia, and anemia are reported side effects of NSAID administration.[34,35] The incidence of side effects is dose dependent and is greatest in foals, in hypovolemic animals, and when the drugs are administered for extended periods. Anecdotal evidence suggests that some NSAIDs are more effective when given in combination, but the relevant scientific literature is limited.[36] A number of NSAIDs with increased selectivity for the inhibition of inducible prostaglandin synthesis have been developed for other species. The development and use of similar compounds for horses is minimal and will probably be limited by cost.

The use of local and regional analgesic techniques in horses is increasing. Local anesthetic agents are frequently used in equine dentistry, in the diagnosis of lameness, and to desensitize areas for standing surgery. Local anesthetics are also increasingly being used in combination with general anesthesia to reduce central sensitization, reducing the requirements for postoperative analgesia. The epidural or spinal administration of local anesthetics desensitizes the perineum for surgery or obstetric manipulations. The epidural administration of α_2-adrenergic agonists and opioids, alone and in combination with local anesthetics, pro-

Table 27.2. Nonsteroidal anti-inflammatory drugs used for analgesia

Drug	Dose and Route	Dosing Interval	Comments
Phenylbutazone	2.2–4.4 mg/kg IV, PO	8–12 h	Very irritating given perivascularly
Flunixin meglumine	1.1 mg/kg IV, PO, IM	12–24 h	Infrequently used IM because of local reactions
Ketoprofen	2.2 mg/kg IV	12–24 h	Once daily for 5 days
Meclofenamic acid	2.20 mg/kg PO	24 h	Approved but not marketed for horses
Naproxen	10 mg/kg PO	24 h	Approved but not marketed for horses
Carprofen	0.7 mg/kg IM	24 h	Less than 25% of the dog dose

IM, intramuscularly; IV, intravenously; and PO, per os (orally).

vides analgesia for the perineum and hindquarters of increased duration with less muscle relaxation and ataxia.[37] Detomidine has been used to produce analgesia as far rostrad as the 14th thoracic dermatome without producing recumbency, indicating selectivity for inhibiting pain over motor fibers.[20] The placement of a catheter in the epidural space allows for repeat administration, extending repeated administration for as long as 14 days.[38]

Intravenous Anesthesia

A number of injectable drug combinations have been used to produce anesthesia in horses (Table 27.3).[39] The most commonly used agents include the thiobarbiturates, ketamine, and guaifenesin or diazepam in combination. It is paramount that horses be calmed prior to the induction of anesthesia. The administration of appropriate doses of preanesthetic agents, primarily phenothiazines and α_2-adrenergic agonists, not only produces calm, sedate patients, but allows for a reduced dose of anesthetic. The maxim to "never anesthetize an excited horse" should serve as a warning. Intravenous anesthesia is commonly used because of the ambulatory nature of equine practice.

Although all anesthetized horses benefit from oxygen supplementation, intravenous anesthesia can usually be safely produced in healthy horses for periods up to 1 h without oxygen supplementation.

Cyclohexamine anesthetics (ketamine and tiletamine) produce a state that has been called *dissociative anesthesia* and is characterized by comparatively good cardiopulmonary support and short duration. Heart rate, arterial blood pressure, and cardiac output are well maintained. Although respiration is depressed, with a characteristic apneustic breathing pattern, apnea is infrequent. The main complication of cyclohexamine anesthesia is poor to inadequate skeletal muscle relaxation. Cyclohexamine anesthetics should *not* be given to horses unless a profound degree of skeletal muscle relaxation is present. Skeletal muscle is usually relaxed by the administration of an α_2-agonist and diazepam or guaifenesin. A commonly used technique for the production of intravenous anesthesia is the combination of xylazine (1.0 mg/kg intravenously [IV]) with ketamine (2.2 mg/kg IV).[40] Xylazine should be given 3 to 5 min prior to ketamine to ensure the horse is sedate and muscle relaxation is evident. Horses become recumbent within 90 to 120 s of ketamine administration,

Table 27.3. Drugs used for induction and maintenance of anesthesia in sedate horses

Drug	Dose	Comments
Ketamine	1.5–2.0 mg/kg IV	Horses must be maximally relaxed prior to administration
		Relaxation can be produced with xylazine, diazepam, or guaifenesin
Thiopental	4–6 mg/kg IV with guaifenesin	Potential for apnea with administration of large boluses
	7–12 mg/kg without guaifenesin	Use with guaifenesin to allow a reduction in dose
Guaifenesin	50 mg/kg IV, to effect	Primarily a muscle relaxant
		Do not use alone
		Use in sedate horses in combination with ketamine or thiopental
Diazepam	0.06–0.1 mg/kg IV	Primarily a muscle relaxant
		Used primarily with ketamine
Tiletamine-zolazepam	0.7–1.0 mg/kg IV	Horse should be fully sedate before administration
		Produces 30 min of anesthesia with good muscle relaxation
		Hypoventilation may occur
"Triple-drip" (mixture of guaifenesin 5%, ketamine 0.1%, and xylazine 0.05%)	2 mL/kg/h	Not used for induction in adult horses
		Used to extend xylazine-ketamine or xylazine-diazepam-ketamine anesthesia
		Monitor ventilation and the degree of muscle relaxation

IM, intramuscularly; IV, intravenously; and PO, per os (orally).

are anesthetized for approximately 15 to 20 min, and stand within 30 to 45 min after induction. Horses that are not completely sedated prior to ketamine administration may not lie down or may stay recumbent only briefly.[41] Recoveries from xylazine-ketamine anesthesia are generally smooth, with horses requiring a single attempt to stand. The addition of diazepam (0.05 to 0.1 mg/kg IV) to xylazine-ketamine anesthesia shortens the time to induction and makes it more predictable, improves muscle relaxation, and extends anesthesia time approximately 5 min.[42,43] Guaifenesin can also be used to augment muscle relaxation. Xylazine-ketamine anesthesia can be extended by readministering half of the original dose of each agent, by administering boluses of thiobarbiturates (thiopental, 1.0 mg/kg IV), or by the administration of guaifenesin.[44] The combination of xylazine (1.0 mg/kg IV) with a commercially available cyclohexamine combination of tiletamine and zolazepam (Telazol, 1.0 to 1.5 mg/kg IV) produces somewhat longer-term anesthesia (25 to 35 min) with improved muscle relaxation and greater respiratory depression.[45] Zolazepam is a benzodiazepine tranquilizer (similar to diazepam) that relaxes skeletal muscle. The recoveries from xylazine-tiletamine-zolazepam anesthesia are not as smooth as those following xylazine-ketamine anesthesia. The use of a combination of detomidine, ketamine, and tiletamine-zolazepam in xylazine-sedated horses has been described.[46] Tiletamine-zolazepam powder (500 mg) is reconstituted with 4 mL of 100 mg/mL of ketamine and 1 mL of 10 mg/mL of detomidine. This combination is administered at a dose of 1 mL/150 kg body weight and produces a smooth induction and approximately 40 min of recumbency with minimal analgesic effect. These combinations can be used for induction of anesthesia prior to the administration of inhalant anesthetic agents. Neither ketamine, diazepam, nor tiletamine-zolazepam are approved for use in horses.

Thiobarbiturates can be used to produce short-term or long-term intravenous anesthesia in horses. Horses should be sedated prior to thiobarbiturate administration because this allows for a reduction of dose. The dose can be further reduced if guaifenesin is administered prior to or in combination with a barbiturate. Induction of anesthesia with thiobarbiturates in non-premedicated horses is often stormy. Induction and recovery can be smoothed by prior administration of a sedative or tranquilizer. The larger the dose of thiobarbiturate, the more likely that apnea will occur. Anesthesia from a single barbiturate bolus lasts approximately 15 to 20 min, with recovery occurring within 45 to 60 min. More than one attempt to stand may be required, and there may be a period of ataxia. Recovery is usually acceptable if the total intravenous dose of thiobarbiturate is less than 7 mg/kg. The use of thiobarbiturates as the *sole* anesthetic agent has been largely supplanted by other techniques, although thiopental is still frequently used in combination with other agents (guaifenesin) or to induce anesthesia that is maintained with inhalant agents.

Guaifenesin is a centrally acting skeletal muscle relaxant that produces mild sedation and variable analgesia. Guaifenesin is intravenously administered in 5%, 10%, and 15% concentrations given to effect (50 to 100 mg/kg). Frequently, a pressurized de-

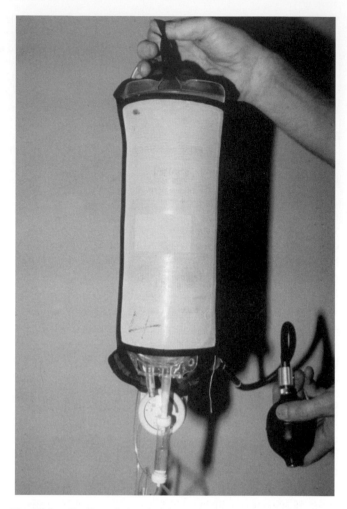

Fig. 27.3. Guaifenesin is administered in large volumes. The use of a pressure bag shortens the time of delivery, facilitating induction of anesthesia.

livery system is used because large volumes must be administered rapidly (Fig. 27.3). Higher concentrations of guaifenesin are difficult to store and may be associated with hemolysis.[47] Guaifenesin should *not* be given alone, because it does not provide sufficient analgesia for surgery. Guaifenesin is usually administered in combination with agents that produce analgesia (xylazine and ketamine) or a hypnotic state (thiobarbiturates). Guaifenesin is incorporated in many anesthetic techniques because it allows a dose reduction in sedatives and anesthetics that produce greater cardiopulmonary depression. Guaifenesin produces profound skeletal muscle relaxation with comparatively minimal depression of arterial blood pressure and cardiac output. Diaphragmatic function is minimally depressed, but arterial pH and blood gases are affected when recumbency is produced. Horses should be sedated prior to the start of guaifenesin infusion. Guaifenesin can be mixed with thiobarbiturates (0.2% to 0.3% thiopental, 2 to 3 g, in 1 L of guaifenesin), enabling a reduction in the dose of thiobarbiturate required. The combination is administered rapidly, to effect. Once recumbency has been produced, the rate of administration is slowed or stopped, depending on the depth of anesthesia required. The induction dose produces anesthesia that lasts 15 to 25 min. If longer periods are required, additional guaifenesin-thiopental can be administered. Alternatively, guaifenesin can be administered to effect (buckling of the knees and lowering of the head), followed by a bolus of thiobarbiturate (thiopental, 3 to 4 mg/kg) or ketamine (1.5 to 2.2 mg/kg). This latter technique enables a more accurate prediction of when recumbency will occur.

The combination of an α_2-adrenergic agonist, guaifenesin, and ketamine has been used to produce anesthesia in horses or as a method of extending the anesthesia produced by other techniques (Table 27.3).[48] One combination is formulated by combining 500 mg of xylazine, 2000 mg of ketamine, and 50 g of guaifenesin in 1 L of sterile water. Anesthesia is usually induced by administering xylazine and then ketamine, as previously described, but may be induced by rapidly administering the combination to effect (approximately 1 to 2 mL/kg) followed by an infusion of 2.2 mL/kg/h for maintenance. This combination provides useful anesthesia with good muscle relaxation. Respiratory depression and bradycardia are primary concerns and should be monitored carefully. Additionally, the appearance of the eyeball helps in determining whether a horse is appropriately anesthetized. Patients should have a brisk palpebral reflex, occasional nystagmus should be present, and the eye should appear wet, which is evidence of tear production. Recovery from anesthesia is generally good.

Inhalation Anesthesia

Inhalation anesthetics, which are frequently used for maintenance of general anesthesia in horses, are occasionally used for induction of anesthesia in foals following nasotracheal intubation, while adult horses are more safely induced with an intravenous technique. Halothane, isoflurane, and sevoflurane are commonly used clinically. Nitrous oxide is not recommended because of the difficulties in maintaining adequate oxygenation in recumbent horses. Nitrous oxide diffuses into closed gas spaces (intestinal gas) and enlarges them, predisposing horses to bloat and ileus. Inhalation anesthetics are usually delivered in oxygen via a sealed airway, thus optimizing the inspired concentration of oxygen. The administration of inhalation anesthetic agents to horses requires specifically designed large animal anesthetic machines and precision, out-of-the-circle vaporizers. Inhalation anesthesia is usually used for horses that are anesthetized for longer than 45 min and for those that have cardiovascular or respiratory compromise. Inhalant administration requires vigilant monitoring of anesthetic depth and cardiopulmonary function. The anesthetic effects produced by various inhalant anesthetics are very similar.[49] Inhalant anesthetics are cardiopulmonary depressants.[50] Cardiac output may be somewhat better maintained with isoflurane and sevoflurane, but arterial blood pressure may be lowered. Respiratory depression is comparable, but horses breathing isoflurane or sevoflurane may breathe more slowly. Horses awaken most rapidly after sevoflurane administration followed by isoflurane and then halothane, relative to the solubility coefficients of the drugs.[51,52] This may alter the management of the latter part of the anesthetic period in that the administration of sevoflurane or isoflurane may have to be continued longer than for halothane in order to assure that a horse does not attempt to rise too quickly following the termination of the procedure.

Monitoring and Perianesthetic Supportive Care

Monitoring is the key to safe anesthetic practice. The American College of Veterinary Anesthesiologists has developed a set of guidelines for anesthetic monitoring that call for routine assessment and recording of indices of circulation, oxygenation, and ventilation at regular intervals (assessment every 5 min and recording at least every 10 min).[53] Horses are specifically mentioned, with the suggestions that a continuous electrocardiogram and a noninvasive blood flow or blood pressure monitor and/or direct monitor of arterial blood pressure be employed in horses anesthetized for longer than 45 min and/or horses anesthetized with inhalant anesthetics. Documentation of all drugs administered and the dose, time, and route of their administration along with a regular recording of the monitored variables complete the anesthetic record. In addition to these indices, anesthetic depth should be regularly assessed, and appropriate adjustments made as necessary. Documentation, through the development of an anesthetic record, of the physical status of the patient and the drugs administered, and periodic evaluations of the drug's cardiopulmonary effects, are necessary, not only for safe anesthesia but also to help minimize the veterinarian's liability should complications arise that result in examination of the methods used. Horses that have lost blood or are in shock should be aggressively treated with intravenous fluids prior to induction of anesthesia.

Physical methods of monitoring (no equipment required) usually suffice for short-term anesthesia. The skills required for physical monitoring of anesthesia parallel those skills required to perform a physical exam. The eye is of particular interest. During surgical levels of anesthesia with inhalants, horses have a dull palpebral reflex (the eyes close slowly when the eyelashes are stimulated) and a strong corneal reflex (the eyes close rapidly when pressure is applied to the cornea). Nystagmus can be present, but it is usually slow and the eye should be moist. Spontaneous blinking or rapid nystagmus are signs of light planes of anesthesia. Eye signs are not helpful during anesthesia with the cyclohexamine anesthetics (ketamine and tiletamine), because these agents cause rapid nystagmus, blinking, and tearing, irrespective of the anesthetic plane. For longer anesthetic periods, particularly those where hypotension or respiratory depression is expected, arterial blood pressure should be measured. The maintenance of mean arterial blood pressure higher than 60 mm of Hg has been identified as a critical factor in preventing postanesthetic myopathies in horses.[6,54] The preferred method of measurement of arterial blood pressure is the use of an indwelling arterial catheter and a measuring device that indicates pressure in millimeters of mercury (mm Hg). Blood pressure alterations are a reasonably good index of anesthetic depth in addition to their use in the assessment of cardiovascular status. Blood pressure falls as anesthesia deepens and increases as anesthesia lightens. Mean arterial blood pressure should range between 60 and 90 mm Hg during anesthesia. A mean arterial blood pressure lower than 60 mm Hg is associated with the loss of autoregulation of blood flow to some vascular beds and should be avoided.[6] Hypotension is treated by decreasing the delivery of anesthetics (if possible), administering intravenous fluids (crystalloids and colloids), and administering vasoactive drugs. If the anesthetic plane is appropriate, the rate of fluid administration should be increased. The maintenance rate of fluid administration during anesthesia ranges from 5 to 10 mL/kg/h. Fluids can be rapidly administered with a pump if hypotension occurs. Fluid rates should be decreased if the packed cell volume falls below 20% or the total protein concentration falls below 3.5 g/dL. Hypovolemia in the presence of low packed cell volume and total protein must be corrected by using blood or blood products.

Hypotension that does not respond to fluid therapy is treated with inotropic or vasoactive agents such as dobutamine or ephedrine. Dobutamine is a synthetic catecholamine that increases cardiac output and arterial blood pressure by increasing the strength of myocardial contractions.[55] Dobutamine is administered slowly (infused) to effect and then titrated to maintain a desired arterial blood pressure. Signs of overdose include tachycardia, hypertension, and supraventricular and ventricular premature arrhythmias. The infusion should be reduced or discontinued if signs of toxicity occur. Dobutamine has a brief effect, so its effects decrease rapidly when it is discontinued. Ephedrine produces similar effects increasing arterial blood pressure and cardiac output.[56] Ephedrine is given as an intravenous bolus and produces effects that persist for 20 to 30 min or longer. The administration of calcium solutions may produce increases in arterial blood pressure particularly if ionized calcium levels are marginal or decreased.[57]

Anesthetized horses hypoventilate to varying degrees. The compromises produced by hypoventilation are generally well tolerated during briefer anesthetic periods (less than 45 min) in healthy horses. The compromises become more critical as anesthesia lengthens or if disease is present. Horses anesthetized for longer than 45 to 60 min benefit from oxygen supplementation and may benefit from assisted ventilation. Other maneuvers, including the application of positive end-expiratory pressure, the use of bronchodilators, and selective ventilation, have been investigated but have not been widely adopted.[58–60] In the absence of arterial blood-gas analysis, oxygen should be supplemented during prolonged anesthesia. Arterial blood-gas analysis can help identify horses that are hypoventilating or shunting pulmonary blood flow and thus direct therapeutic interventions.

Acute bouts of hyperkalemic periodic paralysis have been reported during anesthesia.[61,62] In addition, laryngeal and pharyngeal dysfunction has been reported that could compromise airway function.[63] Chronic treatment of hyperkalemic periodic paralysis with acetazolamide seems to be effective in reducing the incidence of hyperkalemia, but patients predisposed to the disease are at increased risk. Signs of hyperkalemia in anesthetized horses include protrusion of the third eyelid, muscle fasciculations, bradycardia, and electrocardiographic changes, including flattening of P waves, tenting of T waves, and widening of the QRS complex. Hypotension may be present. Anticholinergics are frequently ineffective in the treatment of bradycardia. Initial treatment should include the administration of calcium-containing solutions such as calcium gluconate to counteract the cellular effects of hyperkalemia. Large quantities of potassium-deficient fluids should be administered intravenously to reduce potassium levels by dilution. Two other methods of reducing serum potassium levels include the administration of sodium bicarbonate and the use of glucose-containing solutions with dextrose.

Recovery

This is a critical phase of equine anesthesia but in many ways the least controllable.[64] As a horse awakens from anesthesia, it may try to rise prematurely and subsequently fall, creating excitement. This excitement may lead to further attempts to stand with poor results. Ideally, horses regain consciousness within 10 to 20 min of anesthetic discontinuation, roll to sternal recumbency for a brief period, and then rise. Most horses return to standing within 1 h of anesthetic drug discontinuation. Attempts to speed the recovery process usually cause horses to have a prolonged period of unsteadiness once they stand. Recovery should only be prompted if a horse had cardiopulmonary embarrassment while anesthetized. In this instance, rolling the horse into sternal recumbency during recovery improves oxygenation. Insufflation or the use of a demand valve can also support oxygenation.[7] Horses that try to rise too quickly can be sedated with small doses of intravenous xylazine (0.2 mg/kg). Laryngospasm is infrequent in horses. Some anesthetists prefer to leave the endotracheal tube in place until a horse is standing. Others remove the endotracheal tube when a horse begins to swallow (in lateral recumbency). It is important that horses swallow when the endotracheal tube is removed so that the soft palate is replaced in its normal position under the epiglottis. Occasionally, particularly after dorsal recumbency, congestion of the nasal passage causes snoring. Congestion can be alleviated by the intranasal administration of phenylephrine prior to recovery or the passage of a 30- to 40-cm-long, 10- to 14-mm (internal diameter) endotracheal tube (Fig. 27.4) into the nasopharynx via the ventral meatus.[65] The tube is tied to the halter to prevent aspiration and is removed after the horse stands.

Presumably, smoother recoveries are facilitated by placing horses in a quiet, darkened environment. Good footing is important. As a horse tries to stand, it needs to be able to plant its feet and not have them slip. The horse can be aided to its feet by attaching head and tail ropes. In stalls specifically designed for recovery, strong metal rings can be attached to opposite walls. The head and tail ropes can be passed through the rings (Fig. 27.5), removing the supporting personnel from the immediate area of the horse.

Horses that fail to rise within 90 min of the end of anesthesia should be evaluated further. Potential causes include weakness, rhabdomyolysis, or neurogenic paralysis. Weakness may be the result of residual tranquilization or electrolyte abnormalities

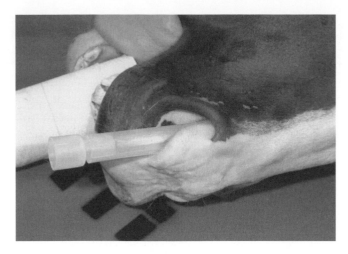

Fig. 27.4. A 12- to 14-mm (internal diameter) endotracheal tube can be inserted into the pharynx via the ventral meatus to reduce respiratory stridor during recovery. The tube can be placed at any point during anesthesia, tied to the halter during recovery, and then removed when the horse is standing. A piece of polyvinylchloride pipe used as an aide for orotracheal intubation is shown.

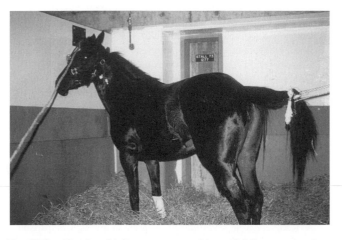

Fig. 27.5. Head and tail ropes are used to assist the recovery from anesthesia. The ropes are run through strong rings that are attached to opposite walls of the recovery stall. This allows some support and control of the horse's movements once it stands without placing assisting personnel in a position where they might be injured. The horse needs to move its head to balance itself as its stands, so the head rope should not be pulled until the animal is standing.

(hypocalcemia or hyperkalemia). Rhabdomyolysis and neurogenic paralysis are difficult to differentiate. Horses often attempt to stand but cannot or stand on three legs if a single limb is affected. Orthopedic injury should be ruled out. The treatment of rhabdomyolysis and neurogenic paralysis is similar and essentially supportive. Intravenous fluids are indicated to promote perfusion and assure urine formation to minimize the chances for myoglobinuric renal failure. Acepromazine in small doses can be administered to calm horses and to promote peripheral perfusion.

Small doses of diazepam (0.02 to 0.04 mg/kg IV) can reduce muscle cramping. The muscle relaxant dantrolene and nonsteroidal anti-inflammatory agents have also been advocated. Unaffected weight-bearing limbs should be wrapped with support bandages. Horses that have a single limb affected usually can stand and have a good prognosis for recovery. Prolonged recumbency worsens the prognosis. Early aggressive treatment is required for a successful outcome.

References

1. Hubbell JAE, Hinchcliff KW, Schmall LM, Muir WW, Robertson JT, Sams RA. Anesthetic, cardiorespiratory, and metabolic effects of four intravenous anesthetic regimens induced in horses immediately after maximal exercise. Am J Vet Res 2000;61:1545–1552.
2. Rankin DC, Greene SA, Keegan RD, Weil AB, Schneider RK, Bayly WM. Anesthesia of horses with a combination of detomidine, zolazepam, tiletamine, and isoflurane immediately after strenuous treadmill exercise. Am J Vet Res 1999;60:743–748.
3. Johnston GM, Eastment JK, Wood JLN, Taylor PM. The confidential enquiry into perioperative equine fatalities (CEPEF): Mortality results of phases 1 and 2. Vet Anaesth Analg 2002;29:159–170.
4. Young SS, Taylor PM. Factors influencing the outcome of equine anaesthesia: A review of 1314 cases. Equine Vet J 1993;25:147–151.
5. Mee AM, Cripps PJ, Jones RS. A retrospective study of mortality associated with general anaesthesia in horses: Elective procedures. Vet Rec 1998;142:275–276.
6. Mee AM, Cripps PJ, Jones RS. A retrospective study of mortality associated with general anaesthesia in horses: Emergency procedures. Vet Rec 1998;142:307–309.
7. Mason DE, Muir WW, Wade W. Arterial blood gas tensions in horses during recovery from anesthesia. J Am Med Vet Assoc 1987; 190:989–994.
8. Grandy JL, Steffey EP, Hodgson DS, Woliner MJ. Arterial hypotension and the development of postanesthetic myopathy in halothane anesthetized horses. Am J Vet Res 1987;48:192–197.
9. Riebold TW, Evans TE. Blood pressure measurements in the anesthetized horse: Comparison of four methods. Vet Surg 1985;14: 332–337.
10. Klein L. A review of 50 cases of postoperative myopathy in the horse: Intrinsic and management factors affecting risk. Proc Am Assoc Equine Pract 1978;24:89–95.
11. Lavoie JP, Pascoe JR, Kurpershoek CJ. Effects of xylazine on ventilation in horses. Am J Vet Res 1992;53:916–920.
12. Kriz NG, Hodgson DR, Rose RJ. Prevalence and clinical importance of heart murmurs in racehorses. J Am Vet Med Assoc 2000;216: 1441–1445.
13. Lees P, Serrano L. Effects of azaperone on cardiovascular and respiratory functions in the horse. Br J Pharmacol 1976;56:263–269.
14. Dodman NH, Waterman E. Paradoxical excitement following the intravenous administration of azaperone in the horse. Equine Vet J 1979;11:33–35.
15. Muir WW, Sams RA, Huffman RH, Noonan JS. Pharmacodynamic and pharmacokinetic properties of diazepam in horses. Am J Vet Res 1982;43:1756–1762.
16. Wilson DV, Nickels FA, Williams MA. Pharmacologic treatment of priapism in two horses. J Am Vet Med Assoc 1991;199:1183–1184.
17. Ballard S, Shults T, Kownacki AA, Blake JW, Tobin T. The pharmacokinetics, pharmacological responses, and behavioral effects of acepromazine in the horse. J Vet Pharmacol Ther 1982;5:21–31.

18. Wagner AE, Muir WW, Hinchcliff KW. Cardiovascular effects of xylazine and detomidine in horses. Am J Vet Res 1991;52:651–657.

19. LeBlanc P, Caron JP, Patterson JS, Brown M, Matta MA. Epidural injection of xylazine for perineal analgesia in horses. J Am Vet Med Assoc 1988;193:1405–1408.

20. Skarda RT, Muir WW. Caudal analgesia induced by epidural or subarachnoid administration of detomidine hydrochloride solution in mares. Am J Vet Res 1994;55:670–680.

21. Ramsay EC, Geiser D, Carter W, Tobin T. Serum concentrations and effects of detomidine delivered orally to horses in three different mediums. Vet Anaesth Analg 2002;29:219–222.

22. Tranquilli WJ, Thurmon JC, Benson GJ, et al. Hyperglycemia and hypoinsulinemia during xylazine-ketamine anesthesia in Thoroughbred horses. Am J Vet Res 1984;45:11–14.

23. Gross ME, Tranquilli WJ. Use of alpha 2-adrenergic receptor antagonists. J Am Vet Med Assoc 1989;195:378–381.

24. Kalpravidh M, Lumb WV, Wright M, Heath RB. Effects of butorphanol, flunixin, levorphanol, morphine, and xylazine in ponies. Am J Vet Res 1984;45:217–223.

25. Muir WW, Robertson JT. Visceral analgesia: Effects of xylazine, butorphanol, meperidine, and pentazocine in horses. Am J Vet Res 1985;38:2081–2084.

26. Muir WW, Skarda RT, Sheehan WC. Hemodynamic and respiratory effects of a xylazine-acetylpromazine drug combination in horses. Am J Vet Res 1979;30:1518–1522.

27. Robertson JT, Muir WW. A new analgesic drug combination in the horse. Am J Vet Res 1983;44:1667–1669.

28. Clarke KW, Paton BS. Combine use of detomidine with opiates in the horse. Equine Vet J 1988;20:331–334.

29. Muir WW, Skarda RT, Sheehan WC. Hemodynamic and respiratory effects of xylazine-morphine sulfate in horses. Am J Vet Res 1979; 40:1417–1420.

30. Dyson DH, Pascoe PJ, Viel L, Staempfli H, Baird JD, Stevenson E. Comparison of detomidine hydrochloride, xylazine and xylazine plus morphine in horses: A double blind study. Equine Vet Sci 1987; 7:211–215.

31. Martin BB, Klide AM. Use of acupuncture for the treatment of chronic back pain in horses: Stimulation of acupuncture points with saline solution injections. J Am Vet Med Assoc 1987;190:1177–1183.

32. Skarda RT, Tejwani GA, Muir WW. Cutaneous analgesia, hemodynamic and respiratory effects, and beta-endorphin concentration in spinal fluid and plasma of horses after acupuncture and electroacupuncture. Am J Vet Res 2002;63:1435–1442.

33. Lees P, Higgins AJ. Clinical pharmacology and therapeutic uses of non-steroidal anti-inflammatory drugs in the horse. Equine Vet J 1985;17:83–96.

34. Gunson DE, Soma LR. Renal papillary necrosis in horses after phenylbutazone and water deprivation. Vet Pathol 1983;20:603–610.

35. Traub-Dargatz JL, Bertone JJ, Gould DH, Wrigely RH, Weiser MG, Forney SD. Chronic flunixin meglumine therapy in foals. Am J Vet Res 1988;49:7–12.

36. Semrad SD, Sams RA, Harris ON, Ashcraft SM. Effects of concurrent administration of phenylbutazone and flunixin meglumine on pharmacokinetic variables and in vitro generation of thromboxane B2 in mares. Am J Vet Res 1993;54:1901–1905.

37. Sysel AM, Pleasant RS, Jacobson JD, et al. Efficacy of an epidural combination of morphine and detomidine in alleviating experimentally induced hindlimb lameness in horses. Vet Surg 1995;25:511–518.

38. Sysel AM, Pleasant RS, Jacobson JD, et al. Systemic and local effects associated with long-term epidural catheterization and morphine-detomidine administration in horses. Vet Surg 1997;26:141–149.

39. Matthews NS, Hartsfield SM, Cornick JL, Williams JD, Beasley A. A comparison of injectable anesthetic combinations in horses. Vet Surg 1991;20:268–273.

40. Muir WW, Skarda RT, Milne DW. Evaluation of xylazine and ketamine hydrochloride for anesthesia in horses. Am J Vet Res 1977;38:195–201.

41. Trim CM, Adams JG, Hovda LR. Failure of ketamine to induce anesthesia in two horses. J Am Vet Med Assoc 1987;190:201–202.

42. Butera ST, Moore JN, Garner HE, Amend JF, Clarke LL, Hatfield DG. Diazepam/xylazine/ketamine combination for short term anesthesia in the horse. Vet Med Small Anim Clin 1978;73:490, 495–499.

43. Brock N, Hildebrand SV. A comparison of xylazine-diazepam-ketamine and xylazine-guaifenesin-ketamine in equine anesthesia. Vet Surg 1990;19:468–474.

44. McCarty JE, Trim CM, Ferguson, D. Prolongation of anesthesia with xylazine, ketamine, and guaifenesin in horses: 64 cases (1986–1989). J Am Vet Med Assoc 1990;197:1646–1650.

45. Hubbell JAE, Bednarski RM, Muir WW. Xylazine and tiletamine-zolazepam anesthesia in horses. Am J Vet Res 1989;50:737–742.

46. Muir WW, Lerche P, Robertson JT, et al. Comparison of four drug combinations for total intravenous anesthesia of horses undergoing surgical removal of an abdominal testis. J Am Vet Med Assoc 2000;217:869–873.

47. Grandy JL, McDonell WN. Evaluation of concentrated solutions of guaifenesin for equine anesthesia. J Am Vet Med Assoc 1980;176: 619–622.

48. Greene SA, Thurmon JC, Tranquilli WJ, Benson GJ. Cardiopulmonary effects of continuous intravenous infusion of guaifenesin, ketamine, and xylazine in horses. Am J Vet Res 1986;47:2364–2367.

49. Steffey EP, Howland, D. Comparison of circulatory and respiratory effects of isoflurane and halothane anesthesia in horses. Am J Vet Res 1980;41:821–825.

50. Grosenbaugh DA, Muir WW. Cardiorespiratory effects of sevoflurane, isoflurane, and halothane anesthesia in horses. Am J Vet Res 1998;59:101–106.

51. Whitehair KJ, Steffey EP, Willits NH, Woliner MJ. Recovery of horses from inhalation anesthesia. Am J Vet Res 1993;54: 1693–1702.

52. Matthews NS, Hartsfield SM, Mercer D, Beleau MH, MacKenthun A. Recovery from sevoflurane anesthesia in horses: Comparison to isoflurane and effect of postmedication with xylazine. Vet Surg 1998;27:480–485.

53. American College of Veterinary Anesthesiologists. Suggestions for monitoring anesthetized veterinary patients. J Am Vet Med Assoc 1995;206:936–937.

54. Hennig GE, Court MH. Equine postanesthetic myopathy: An update. Compend Contin Educ Pract Vet 1991;13:1709–1716.

55. Swanson CR, Muir WW, Bednarski RM, Skarda RT, Hubbell JAE. Hemodynamic responses in halothane-anesthetized horses given infusions of dopamine or dobutamine. Am J Vet Res 1985;46: 365–370.

56. Grandy JL, Hodgson DS, Dunlop CI, Chapman PL, Heath RB. Cardiopulmonary effects of ephedrine in halothane-anesthetized horses. J Vet Pharmacol Ther 1989;12:389–396.

57. Grubb TL, Benson GJ, Foreman JH, et al. Hemodynamic effects of ionized calcium in horses anesthetized with halothane or isoflurane. Am J Vet Res 1999;60:1430–1435.

58. Wilson DV, Soma LR. Cardiopulmonary effects of positive end-expiratory pressure in anesthetized mechanically ventilated ponies. Am J Vet Res 1990;51:734–739.

59. Robertson SA, Bailey JE. Aerosolized salbutamol (albuterol) improves PaO$_2$ in hypoxaemic anaesthetized horses: A prospective clinical trial in 81 horses. Vet Anaesth Analg 2002;29:212–218.

60. Nyman G, Frostell C, Hedenstierna G, Funkquist B, Kvart C, Blomqvist H. Selective mechanical ventilation of dependent lung regions in the anaesthetized horse in dorsal recumbency. Br J Anaesth 1987;59:1027–1034.

61. Robertson SA, Green SL, Carter SW, Bolon BN, Brown MP, Shields RP. Postanesthetic recumbency associated with hyperkalemic periodic paralysis in a quarter horse. J Am Vet Med Assoc 1992;201:1209–1212.

62. Bailey JE, Pablo L, Hubbell JAE. Hyperkalemic periodic paralysis during halothane anesthesia in a horse. J Am Vet Med Assoc 1996;208:1–7.

63. Carr EA, Spier SJ, Kortz GD, Hoffman EP. Laryngeal and pharyngeal dysfunction in horses homozygous for hyperkalemic periodic paralysis. J Am Vet Med Assoc 1996;209:798–803.

64. Hubbell JAE. Recovery from anaesthesia in horses. Equine Vet Educ 1999;11:160–167.

65. Lukasik VM, Gleed RD, Scarlett JM, et al. Intranasal phenylephrine reduces post-anesthetic upper airway obstruction in horses. Equine Vet J 1997;29:236–238.

Chapter 28
Ruminants

Thomas W. Riebold

Introduction

As in other species, sedation and anesthesia are often required for surgical or diagnostic procedures in ruminants. The decision to induce general anesthesia may be influenced by a ruminant's temperament and its specific anatomical and physiological characteristics. Ruminants usually accept physical restraint well and that, in conjunction with local or regional anesthesia, is often sufficient to enable completion of many procedures. Other diagnostic and surgical procedures that are more complex require general anesthesia.

In addition to discussing techniques for cattle, goats, and sheep, anesthetic techniques for South American camelids, primarily llamas and alpacas, are discussed. South American camelids do not accept restraint as well as domestic ruminants and often require sedation before local or regional anesthesia. Although they have some unique species characteristics regarding anesthesia, many of the principles and techniques used in food-animal and equine anesthesia also apply to South American camelids. Except for differences in size, anesthetic management of alpacas and llamas is similar.

Preanesthetic Preparation

Considerations for preanesthetic preparation include fasting, assessment of hematologic and blood chemistry values, venous catheterization, and estimation of body weight. Domestic ruminants have a multicompartmental stomach with a large rumen that does not empty completely. South American camelids have a stomach divided into three compartments.[1] Each species, therefore, is susceptible to complications associated with recumbency and anesthesia: tympany, regurgitation, and aspiration pneumonia. To reduce the risk associated with these potential complications, calves, sheep, goats, and camelids should be fasted 12 to 18 h and deprived of water for 8 to 12 h prior to anesthesia. Adult cattle should be fasted 18 to 24 h and deprived of water for 12 to 18 h. In nonelective cases, this is often not possible, and precautions should be taken to avoid aspiration of gastric fluid and ingesta. Fasting neonates is not advisable because hypoglycemia may result. Fasting and water deprivation will decrease the likelihood of tympany and regurgitation by decreasing the volume of fermentable ingesta. Fasting can also cause bradycardia in cattle.[2] Additionally, pulmonary functional residual capacity may be better preserved in fasted anesthetized ruminants.[3] Although gas does not appear to accumulate in the first compartment of anesthetized camelids, these precautions are recommended to decrease the incidence of regurgitation. Even with these precautions, some ruminants will become tympanitic, whereas others will regurgitate.

Hematologic and blood chemistry values may be determined before anesthesia. Results should be compared with reference values.[4-7] Venipuncture and catheterization of the jugular vein are often performed prior to anesthesia. Adult cattle require 12- to 14-gauge catheters, whereas 16-gauge catheters are appropriate for adult camelids, calves, and large goats and sheep, and 18-gauge catheters are appropriate for juvenile camelids, sheep, and goats. Physical restraint during venipuncture or catheterization varies and can consist of a handler holding the animal's halter or use of head gates and chutes for adult cattle and llamas. If a camelid is fractious, grasping its ear may be helpful. Turning the animal's head to either side may hinder venipuncture and catheter placement in goats and camelids. Infiltration of local anesthetic to desensitize skin structures at the site of catheterization is recommended.

Camelids do not have a jugular groove. The jugular vein lies deep to the sternomandibularis and brachiocephalicus muscles, ventral to cervical vertebral transverse processes, and superficial to the carotid artery and vagosympathetic trunk within the carotid sheath for most of its length.[8-10] Beginning at a point about 15 cm caudal to the ramus of the mandible, the rostral course of the jugular vein is separated from the carotid artery by the omohyoideus muscle. The bifurcation of the jugular vein is located at the intersection of a line drawn caudally along the ventral aspect of the body of the mandible and another line connecting the base of the ear and the lateral aspect of the cervical transverse processes. Venipuncture or catheterization can be performed at the bifurcation or at any point caudal to it. Because of the close proximity of the carotid artery to the jugular vein, one must confirm that the vein has been catheterized and not the artery. After occlusion of the vessel, one will be unable to see the jugular vein distend; however, the vein can be palpated particularly rostrally and more easily in females and altered males because their skin is thinner. On occasion, one will be able to see the jugular vein distend on crias and juvenile camelids. Camelids can have four to five jugular venous valves that prevent flow of venous blood into the head when the head is lowered during grazing.[8] Contact with jugular venous valves may prevent catheterization; a site caudal to the point where the valve was contacted should be used.

For accurate drug administration, the animal must be weighed. It is easy to overestimate the body weight of camelids because they are fairly tall, and their long hair coat obscures their body condition. Adult male llamas usually weigh 140 to 175 kg, occasionally reaching or exceeding 200 kg. Adult female llamas usually weigh 100 to 150 kg but may occasionally exceed 200 kg. Adult male alpacas usually weigh 60 to 100 kg, and adult female alpacas usually weigh 50 to 80 kg. The body weight of crias and small juveniles may be determined on a bathroom scale.

Anticholinergics are usually not administered to domestic ruminants prior to induction of anesthesia. They do not consistently decrease salivary secretions unless used in higher doses given frequently. Anticholinergics, while decreasing the volume of secretions, make them more viscous and difficult to clear from the trachea. The usual doses of atropine used to prevent bradycardia in domestic ruminants (0.06 to 0.1 mg/kg intravenously [IV]) do not prevent salivation during anesthesia. Camelids are prone to increased vagal discharge during intubation or painful stimuli during surgery. Atropine administration (0.02 mg/kg IV or 0.04 mg/kg intramuscularly [IM]) is recommended to prevent bradyarrhythmia and will also decrease salivary secretions.[11] Glycopyrrolate (0.005 to 0.01 mg/kg IM or 0.002 to 0.005 mg/kg IV) may be substituted for atropine.[12,13]

Sedation/Restraint

Drugs traditionally used to tranquilize and/or sedate ruminants include acepromazine, the α_2-agonists such as xylazine, detomidine, medetomidine, and romifidine; pentobarbital, chloral hydrate, diazepam, and midazolam.

Acepromazine is the most commonly used phenothiazine derivative tranquilizer in veterinary anesthesia. It is not commonly used in ruminants but can be used in a manner similar to its use in horses. In general, though, lower doses of acepromazine are required for cattle than for horses. The usual doses of acepromazine used in sheep and goats are 0.03 to 0.05 mg/kg IV and 0.05 to 0.1 mg/kg IV,[14] which may increase the risk of regurgitation during anesthesia.[14] Acepromazine should not be injected into the coccygeal vein. The close proximity of the coccygeal ar-

tery makes the risk of inadvertent intra-arterial injection possible, with subsequent loss of the tail. Acepromazine can also cause prolapse of the penis and is contraindicated in debilitated and hypovolemic patients.

Xylazine, detomidine, romifidine, and medetomidine induce sedation by stimulating the central α_2-adrenoceptors. Xylazine is often used to sedate or, in higher doses, restrain (recumbency and heavy sedation) ruminants. There appears to be some variation in response between species and within a species. Xylazine is a more potent sedative in ruminants than in horses.[15] Goats appear to be more sensitive to xylazine than are sheep,[13,14,16] with cattle appearing to be of intermediate sensitivity when compared with sheep and goats. South American camelids appear to be intermediate between cattle and horses in sensitivity to xylazine, and alpacas appear to be less sensitive to xylazine than are llamas. Hereford cattle are more sensitive to xylazine than are Holstein cattle,[17] and anecdotal evidence indicates that Brahmans are perhaps the most sensitive of cattle breeds.[18] Extreme environmental conditions can cause cattle to have a pronounced and prolonged response to xylazine.[19] Variation in response to the analgesic effects of xylazine between breeds of sheep has been reported.[20,21] Detomidine has been used to a lesser extent in ruminants but provides sedation and/or analgesia in domestic ruminants not unlike that obtained in horses. Medetomidine and romifidine have been used to a lesser extent in ruminants.

Although complete data are not available on the cardiovascular and respiratory effects of xylazine in camelids, bradycardia[22] typically occurs as it does in other species.[17,23–25] Poorly trained or berserk male camelids tend to be less responsive, and debilitated individuals are more depressed by sedative doses of xylazine. Xylazine causes hyperglycemia and hypoinsulinemia in cattle and sheep.[26–31] Hypoxemia and hypercarbia are common side effects in domestic ruminants,[14,17,22,32] and sheep are at risk of developing pulmonary edema.[33] Xylazine has an oxytocin-like effect on the uterus of pregnant cattle[34] and sheep.[35] Detomidine may not have this same effect on the gravid uterus[36] and would appear to be the α_2-agonist of choice for sedating pregnant cattle or sheep.

The degree of sedation or restraint produced by α_2 agents depends on the dose and overall animal temperament. Low doses of xylazine (0.015 to 0.025 mg/kg IV or IM) typically provide sedation without recumbency in domestic ruminants.[12,13] Higher doses (0.1 to 0.2 mg/kg IV) provide sedation without recumbency in camelids.[37] Detomidine can be given at 2.5 to 10.0 μg/kg IV in cattle[13,36,38,39] and at 10 to 20 μg/kg in sheep[14] to provide standing sedation for approximately 30 to 60 min. Medetomidine has been given at a dose of 5 μg/kg IV to cattle[39] or at 10 μg/kg IM to llamas[40] for brief periods of standing sedation with minimal analgesia.

Higher doses of xylazine will induce recumbency, heavy sedation, or possibly light planes of general anesthesia in domestic ruminants and camelids. Xylazine (goats, 0.05 mg/kg IV or 0.1 mg/kg IM;[13,14,41] sheep, 0.1 to 0.2 mg/kg IV or 0.2 to 0.3 mg/kg IM;[13,14,41] and cattle, 0.1 mg/kg IV or 0.2 mg/kg IM[18]) will induce recumbency for approximately 1 h. Xylazine (0.3 to 0.4 mg/kg IV) usually induces 20 to 30 min of recumbency in llamas.[8–11,37] Alpacas may require an increased dose, approximately 10% to 20%, to achieve the same result.[42] A high dose of detomidine, 30 µg/kg IV, will produce recumbency in sheep. This dose is equivalent to xylazine at 0.15 mg/kg IV, medetomidine at 10 µg/kg IV, or romifidine at 50 µg/kg IV.[43] In llamas, detomidine in doses as high as 40 µg/kg IV provides mild sedation but not restraint.[37] Medetomidine given at 10 µg/kg IV induces recumbency in cattle.[39] When given at 20 to 30 µg/kg IM to llamas, medetomidine provides profound sedation and recumbency lasting up to 120 min.[40] Higher doses of all α_2 agents can be expected to induce longer periods of recumbency in all species.

Sedation following administration of α_2-adrenoceptor agonists can be reversed by α_2-adrenoceptor antagonists. When yohimbine is given at 0.12 mg/kg IV, its efficacy varies in cattle[44,45] whereas it is somewhat ineffective in sheep.[46] Higher doses of yohimbine (1.0 mg/kg IV) will generally reverse xylazine sedation in sheep.[47] Tolazoline is usually given at 0.5 to 2.0 mg/kg IV,[45] but at 2.0 mg/kg IV it can cause hyperesthesia in cattle[48,49] and at doses of 4 mg/kg can cause seizurelike activity in llamas.[50] Tolazoline can induce unwanted cardiovascular effects such as transient bradycardia, sinus arrest, and hypotension.[51] Idazoxan can be given at doses of 0.05 mg/kg IV to sheep[46] and calves to reverse xylazine sedation.[51] Atipamezole at doses varying from 20 to 60 µg/kg IV has been used to reverse medetomidine sedation in calves.[13,52,53]

Yohimbine (0.12 mg/kg IV) has been used in llamas in combination with 4-aminopyridine (0.3 mg/kg IV) to produce complete recovery from xylazine sedation.[22] Its use singly in camelids is also effective, and it can be administered at 0.12 mg/kg IV.[37] If sufficient arousal does not occur, additional yohimbine can be given. Tolazoline is also effective for reversing xylazine sedation in camelids. When given at the recommended equine dose to camelids, tolazoline causes severe complications: transitory apnea, cardiac arrest, seizurelike activity, depression, and vague signs of abdominal pain, followed by death within 24 h. One method of administering tolazoline to healthy camelids is to give 50% of the calculated dose (1.0 to 2.0 mg/kg IV) initially and the remainder if reversal is inadequate.[37] In most instances, the initial dose (1.0 mg/kg IV) of tolazoline is adequate for sufficient arousal. Following tolazoline administration at the full calculated dose of 2.0 mg/kg IV, opisthotonus can occur in some animals. After excitement subsides, recovery is usually uneventful.

Doxapram, an analeptic, has also been used to enhance the arousal response from yohimbine or tolazoline: 1.0 mg/kg IV has been somewhat effective in cattle[54] but ineffective in llamas at 2.0 mg/kg IV.[22]

Pentobarbital (2 mg/kg IV) has been used in cattle for standing sedation and tranquilization.[55] Caution must be exercised to avoid inducing excitement. Pentobarbital provides moderate sedation for 30 min and mild sedation for an additional 60 min. Chloral hydrate or chloral hydrate–magnesium sulfate solutions can be used to sedate ruminants.[18] These drugs must be injected slowly IV to avoid tissue necrosis. Diazepam (0.25 to 0.5 mg/kg IV) injected slowly will provide 30 min of sedation without analgesia in sheep and goats.[14,41] Midazolam (0.4 to 0.6 mg IM[56,57] or 0.3 mg/kg IV[58]) will provide sedation and recumbency in

sheep and goats for 10 to 20 min. Midazolam given at 1.0 mg/kg IM[56] or 0.6 mg/kg IV[58] can induce recumbency and heavy sedation in goats. Increasing the midazolam dose to 1.2 mg/kg IV lengthens recumbency for up to 30 min.[57]

Butorphanol is an opioid agonist-antagonist that provides sedation and analgesia in camelids and domestic ruminants. It is often given at 0.1 to 0.2 mg/kg IM in camelids[59] and at 0.05 to 0.5 mg/kg IM in sheep and goats.[14,60,61] Ataxia and dysphoria have been reported following butorphanol administration (0.1 to 0.2 mg/kg IV) in sheep.[61]

Combinations of xylazine and butorphanol have been used in camelids and domestic ruminants to provide neuroleptanalgesia. Doses are 0.01 to 0.02 mg/kg IV of each drug administered separately to domestic ruminants and 0.2 mg/kg IV of each drug for camelids (M. J. Huber, personal communication, 1993). Action lasts approximately 1 h. Combinations of butorphanol, xylazine, and ketamine have also been used together in restraining camelids.[62] This combination is prepared by adding 100 mg (1 mL) of xylazine and 10 mg (1 mL) of butorphanol to 10 mL of ketamine. It is administered at 1 mL/40 pounds IM to alpacas and at 1 mL/50 pounds IM to llamas.[62] At this dose, recumbency occurs within 5 min and lasts approximately 25 min. Other combinations of butorphanol, xylazine, and ketamine have also been reported.[63] Given IV at 0.22 to 0.33 mg/kg xylazine, 0.22 to 0.33 mg/kg ketamine, and 0.077 to 0.11 mg/kg butorphanol, this combination is more predictable.[63] Animals will become recumbent, and analgesia lasts for 15 to 20 min. Administering a partial dose of ketamine will lengthen the analgesia. When this combination is given IM, the dose range is increased to 0.22 to 0.55 mg/kg for xylazine, 0.22 to 0.55 mg/kg for ketamine, and 0.055 to 0.11 mg/kg for butorphanol.[63] Onset occurs within 10 min, and the recumbency is extended to approximately 45 min.

Induction

Ruminants are not always sedated prior to induction of anesthesia. Atraumatic physical restraint can be used in lieu of sedatives in some circumstances. Because ruminants seldom experience emergence delirium, sedation during the recovery period is not required. In some instances, though, sedation is required to make handling of these animals, primarily adult bulls, safer during the induction period. Sedation will tend to lengthen the recovery period from general anesthesia[38] and increase the likelihood of regurgitation.[14]

General anesthesia can be induced by either injectable or inhalation techniques. Available drugs include thiobarbiturates, ketamine, guaifenesin, tiletamine-zolazepam, propofol, pentobarbital, halothane, isoflurane, and sevoflurane. Anesthesia can be induced in small ruminants, weighing less than 50 to 100 kg, either by mask with halothane, isoflurane, or sevoflurane or with injectable techniques. Anesthesia can be induced in larger animals with either intravenous or intramuscular techniques. Anesthesia can also be induced with halothane, isoflurane, or sevoflurane by mask in small or debilitated camelids or in camelids restrained with xylazine-ketamine, tiletamine-zolazepam, etc. Mask induction in healthy untranquilized adult camelids is usually not attempted because application of the mask may provoke spitting. Addition of nitrous oxide (50% of total flow) to the inspired inhalant-gas mixture will speed induction. During induction, lower concentrations of halothane (3%), isoflurane (3%), or sevoflurane (4%) are administered when patients weigh less than 25 kg. Higher concentrations are used with larger patients.

Barbiturates

The thiobarbiturates thiopental and thiamylal have been used extensively in veterinary anesthesia, alone and in combination with guaifenesin. Used separately, they quickly induce anesthesia. Muscle relaxation is relatively poor but still sufficient to accomplish intubation. The acid-base status and physical status of patients affect the actions of these drugs. Acidemia increases the nonionized fraction (the active portion) of the drug, increasing its activity and thus decreasing the dose required.[64] In addition, the heart, brain, and other vital organs receive a larger portion of cardiac output when patients are in shock.[65] Because patients in shock are often acidemic, altered kinetics and hemodynamics can cause a relative overdose.

Recovery from induction doses of thiobarbiturates is based on redistribution of the drug from the brain to other tissues in the body. Metabolism of the agent continues for some time following recovery until final elimination occurs. Maintenance of anesthesia with thiobarbiturates is not recommended because saturation of tissues causes recovery to be dependent on metabolism and recovery will be prolonged. Concurrent use of large doses of nonsteroidal anti-inflammatory drugs (NSAIDs) may be contraindicated because recovery can be delayed as thiobarbiturate is displaced from protein.[66]

Thiopental can be given at a dose of 6 to 10 mg/kg IV and will provide approximately 10 to 15 min of anesthesia. Camelids often require additional thiopental for tracheal intubation. Thiamylal is administered in similar fashion although in slightly lower doses, usually 25% to 30% less.

Pentobarbital has been used to anesthetize domestic ruminants but is no longer commonly used. If the situation arises in which it is used, the dose is 20 to 25 mg/kg IV, half given rapidly and the remainder to effect. When given at an anesthetic dose, pentobarbital causes profound respiratory depression and is not an effective analgesic. Sheep appear to metabolize pentobarbital more quickly than other species.[14] Recovery in domestic ruminants is usually prolonged, and other anesthetic techniques are more appropriate.

Ketamine

This agent stimulates the limbic system, causing dysphoria, hallucinations, and excitement, in addition to tonic-clonic muscle activity when used alone in horses. Those same traits characterize its use in ruminants, although perhaps not to the same extent as in horses. It also provides mild cardiovascular stimulation. Although ketamine does not eliminate the swallowing reflex, tracheal intubation can be accomplished in most ruminants.

Ketamine will induce immobilization and incomplete analgesia when given alone, but it is usually combined with a sedative or tranquilizer. Most commonly, xylazine or diazepam is recom-

mended, although the availability of detomidine offers another alternative. Xylazine (0.1 to 0.2 mg/kg IM) can be given, followed by ketamine (10 to 15 mg/kg IM), to smaller domestic ruminants.[14,41,67] In goats, it is preferable to use the lower dose of xylazine followed by ketamine.[14,41] Anesthesia usually lasts about 45 min and can be prolonged by injection of 3 to 5 mg/kg IM of ketamine. The longer duration of action of xylazine obviates the need for its readministration in most cases. Alternatively, intravenous xylazine (0.03 to 0.05 mg/kg) followed by ketamine (3 to 5 mg/kg), or intramuscular xylazine (goats, 0.1 mg/kg; and sheep, 0.2 mg/kg) followed by intravenous ketamine (3 to 5 mg/kg), can provide anesthesia lasting up to 15 to 20 min.[14] Adult cattle can be anesthetized for short periods with xylazine (0.1 to 0.2 mg/kg IV) followed by ketamine (2.0 mg/kg IV).[68] The lower dose of xylazine is used when cattle weigh more than 600 kg.[68] Anesthesia lasts approximately 30 min but can be prolonged for 15 min with additional ketamine (0.75 to 1.25 mg/kg IV).[68] When evaluated in sheep, xylazine (0.1 mg/kg IV) and ketamine (7.5 mg/kg IV) provided anesthesia lasting 25 min while decreasing cardiac output, mean arterial pressure, and peripheral vascular resistance.[69] Medetomidine has been combined with ketamine to induce anesthesia in calves. Because medetomidine (20 µg/kg IV) is much more potent that xylazine, lower doses of ketamine (0.5 mg/kg IV) can be used.[53] However, a local anesthetic block at the surgical site may be required when ketamine is used at this dose.[53] When using α_2-agonist–ketamine combinations, anesthesia can be reversed with α_2-adrenoceptor antagonists without much excitement during recovery.

Diazepam (0.1 mg/kg IV) followed immediately by ketamine (4.5 mg/kg IV) can be used in most domestic ruminants. Muscle relaxation is usually adequate for tracheal intubation, although the swallowing reflex may not be completely obtunded. Anesthesia usually lasts 10 to 15 min following diazepam-ketamine administration, with recumbency of up to 30 min. Higher doses of diazepam (0.25 to 0.5 mg/kg IV) with ketamine (4.0 to 7.5 mg/kg IV) have also been used in sheep and provide the same duration of anesthesia.[14,41,69] Investigations into the cardiopulmonary effects of diazepam (0.375 mg/kg IV) and ketamine (7.5 mg/kg IV) in sheep have shown a decrease in cardiac output and an increase in peripheral vascular resistance without arterial pressure being affected.[69] Midazolam has been substituted for diazepam in goats and is given at 0.4 mg/kg IM followed by ketamine at 4.0 mg/kg IV after recumbency occurs (approximately 15 min). Anesthesia lasts approximately 15 min.[56]

Xylazine (0.25 to 0.35 mg/kg IM) and ketamine (6.0 to 10.0 mg/kg IM, 15 min later) usually provide 30 to 60 min of recumbency in camelids.[8,11] The simultaneous administration of xylazine (0.44 mg/kg IM) and ketamine (4.0 mg/kg IM) usually provides restraint for 15 to 20 min.[10,70] Higher doses of xylazine (0.8 mg/kg IM) and ketamine (8.0 mg/kg IM) given simultaneously usually induce anesthesia within 5 min, and the duration of anesthesia provided is approximately 30 min.[70] Anesthesia depth varies with the amount given and the camelid's temperament but is usually sufficient for minor procedures such as suturing lacerations, draining abscesses, or applying casts. When any of these combinations provides insufficient anesthetic depth, supplemental local anesthesia may be required in order to complete the surgery. Tracheal intubation may not be possible. However, these combinations heavily sedate (if not anesthetize) and immobilize the patient, facilitating venipuncture and administration of additional anesthetic agent or application of a face mask to increase the anesthesia depth when necessary. Xylazine (0.25 mg/kg IV) and ketamine (3.0 to 5.0 mg/kg IV) may be administered 5 min apart to obtain a more uniform response and sufficient anesthesia depth for tracheal intubation.[8] Diazepam (0.1 mg/kg IV) and ketamine (4.5 mg/kg IV) as used for domestic ruminants produces recumbency that lasts approximately 20 min but does not reliably provide enough muscle relaxation for tracheal intubation in camelids.

Guaifenesin

This agent is a centrally acting skeletal muscle relaxant that exerts its effect at the internuncial neurons in the spinal cord and at polysynaptic nerve endings.[71] It can be used alone to induce recumbency in domestic ruminants and camelids, but this usage is not recommended because it imparts little, if any, analgesia.[72] Addition of ketamine or thiobarbiturate to guaifenesin solution improves induction quality and decreases the volume required for anesthetic induction. Muscle relaxation is improved when compared with induction with ketamine alone or the thiobarbiturates given alone. Typically, 5% guaifenesin solutions are used. Hemolysis can occur with 10% guaifenesin solutions.[73] Commonly, these solutions are given rapidly to effect, either by gravity and large-gauge catheter or by pressurizing the bottle. The calculated volume dose when using 5% guaifenesin solution is 2.0 mL/kg. The amount of ketamine added to guaifenesin varies but is commonly 1.0 g/50 g of guaifenesin. The amount of thiobarbiturate added to guaifenesin varies but is commonly 2.0 g/50 g of guaifenesin. For convenience, guaifenesin-based mixtures may be injected with large syringes rather than administered by infusion to camelids and small ruminants.

Following induction, guaifenesin-based solutions (with thiopental or ketamine) can be infused to effect to maintain anesthesia. If desired, xylazine can also be added to ketamine-guaifenesin solutions for induction and maintenance of anesthesia in cattle[68,74] and sheep.[75] Final concentrations are guaifenesin, 50 mg/mL; ketamine, 1 to 2 mg/mL; and xylazine, 0.1 mg/mL. This solution is infused at 0.5 to 1.0 mL/kg IV for induction. Anesthesia is maintained by infusion of the mixture at 1.5 mL/kg/h for calves,[74] 2 mL/kg/h for adult cattle,[68] and 2 mL/kg/h for sheep,[75] although the final administration rate will vary with case requirements. If the procedure requires more than 2 mL/kg of the guaifenesin-ketamine-xylazine mixture in order to complete the surgery, the amount of xylazine added should be decreased by at least 50% because its action may last longer than that of the other two agents in the mixture. Alternatively, a solution with a final concentration of guaifenesin (50 mg/mL), ketamine (1 mg/mL), and xylazine (0.05 mg/mL) can be formulated and infused at 2.0 mL/kg/h IV for maintenance to avoid the potential cumulative effects of xylazine overdose. Because ruminants may regurgitate during xylazine-ketamine-guaifenesin anesthesia, intubation is highly recommended.

Tiletamine-Zolazepam

A proprietary combination of equal parts of tiletamine (a dissociative anesthetic agent similar to, but more potent than, ketamine) and zolazepam (a potent benzodiazepine sedative similar to diazepam) is available for use as an anesthetic agent in cats and dogs. When used alone, tiletamine induces poor muscle relaxation and causes excitement during recovery. The addition of zolazepam to tiletamine modifies these effects. As with ketamine, the swallowing reflex remains but is obtunded. Like ketamine-benzodiazepine combinations, this combination provides slight cardiovascular stimulation, causing the heart rate to increase.[76] Elimination of tiletamine and zolazepam is not uniform, with variation occurring for each drug's clearance among species. Differential clearance of the two drugs can affect recovery quality.[76]

In many respects, tiletamine-zolazepam can be considered to be similar to ketamine premixed with diazepam. When used alone in horses, it provides unsatisfactory anesthesia.[77] Muscle relaxation is poor, and recovery is characterized by excitement. However, when combined with a sedative such as xylazine, it can be used successfully in horses. Because of differences in temperament between horses and domestic ruminants and camelids, tiletamine-zolazepam can be used successfully in most ruminants with or without xylazine. However, addition of xylazine to tiletamine-zolazepam will lengthen and enhance the overall anesthetic effect.

Tiletamine-zolazepam given at 4.0 mg/kg IV causes minimal cardiovascular alteration in calves and provides anesthesia of 45- to 60-min duration.[78] Xylazine (0.1 mg/kg IM) followed immediately by tiletamine-zolazepam (4.0 mg/kg IM) produces onset of anesthesia within 3 min, and anesthesia duration of approximately 1 h.[79] Calves are fully recovered approximately 130 min after injection. Increasing xylazine to 0.2 mg/kg IM increases duration of anesthesia and recumbency and the incidence of apnea.[79] Xylazine can also be administered at a lower dose of 0.05 mg/kg IV followed by tiletamine-zolazepam at 1.0 mg/kg IV to induce anesthesia of shorter duration.[68]

Tiletamine-zolazepam given at 12.0 mg/kg IV in sheep has provided approximately 2.5 h of surgical anesthesia, with a total recumbency time of 3.2 h.[80] More recent investigations in sheep have shown that tiletamine-zolazepam, dosed at 12 to 24 mg/kg IV, causes cardiopulmonary depression, with anesthesia of approximately 40 min.[81] Rather than using these relatively large doses, it is more appropriate to decrease the initial dose of tiletamine-zolazepam to 2.0 to 4.0 mg/kg IV and administer additional tiletamine-zolazepam as required to prolong anesthesia. Butorphanol (0.5 mg/kg IV) combined with tiletamine-zolazepam (12 mg/kg IV) given either simultaneously or 10 min apart induces 25 to 50 min of anesthesia in sheep, with mild cardiopulmonary depression.[82] Tiletamine-zolazepam (4.0 mg/kg IM) can immobilize llamas for up to 2 h.[83] The length of recumbency is unaffected by administration of flumazenil, indicating that the duration of action is more likely influenced by tiletamine than by zolazepam.[83] Cardiovascular function is preserved although hypercarbia and hypoxemia can occur in some animals. Airway reflexes are maintained. Local anesthesia may still be required for some surgical procedures.[83] In camelids, tiletamine-zolazepam (2.0 mg/kg IV) alone provides 15 to 20 min of anesthesia and 25 to 35 min of recumbency.[37] Anesthesia depth is adequate to intubate nasally, but muscle relaxation is poor and oral intubation is difficult.

Propofol

This nonbarbiturate, nonsteroidal hypnotic agent can be used to provide brief periods of anesthesia (5 to 10 min). The recommended dose is 4.0 to 6.0 mg/kg IV for the induction of domestic ruminants.[14,84–86] Induction is smooth, as is recovery. If injected too rapidly, apnea may occur. Slow administration will prevent this complication. A 2-mg/kg IV dose has been used to induce anesthesia in camelids.[87] However, tracheal intubation is often difficult at this dose, and additional propofol is usually needed. A light plane of anesthesia can be maintained with a constant infusion of propofol at 0.4 mg/kg/min IV.[87] The approximate time from discontinuation of propofol infusion to sternal recumbency is 10 to 15 min.[87] The use of infusion pumps enables a more precise propofol administration.

Maintenance

Tracheal intubation is recommended in all ruminants and camelids because it provides a secure airway and prevents aspiration of salivary and ruminal contents if active or passive regurgitation occurs. In lightly anesthetized ruminants, active regurgitation can occur during intubation[11,68] whereas passive regurgitation can occur at any time during anesthesia due to relaxation of the cardia. Because rumen contents contain more solid material than do the gastric contents of monogastric animals, there is greater potential for ingesta to obstruct the larynx while the more fluid portion drains from the mouth. Consequently, patients that are not intubated are at higher risk of aspiration of rumen contents. Intubated animals that have regurgitated during anesthesia are also at risk following extubation. Treatment involves removal of ingesta from the buccal cavity or buccal lavage prior to extubation. If active regurgitation has occurred, anesthesia depth should be rapidly increased and the airway quickly protected to prevent aspiration.

Several techniques can be used for intubation. Adult cattle can be intubated blindly or with digital palpation. Following insertion of a mouth speculum or the use of gauze loops, the animal's head and neck are hyperextended to make the orotracheal axis approach 180°. An endotracheal tube of appropriate size is inserted and manipulated into the larynx (Table 28.1). If that technique is unsuccessful, the anesthetist's hand should be inserted into the mouth with the tube. After the epiglottis is located and depressed, a finger can be placed between the arytenoid cartilages and the tube inserted into the trachea. If desired, an equine nasogastric tube can be inserted into the larynx and serve as a guide for the endotracheal tube. Depending on the size of the animal and the individual's arm, the airway might be obstructed when this technique is performed, so it is important that intubation is prompt. If the technique requires more than 1 min, the hand and arm should be withdrawn from

Table 28.1. Sizes of endotracheal tubes needed for ruminants and camelids of various body weights

Body Weight (kg)	Endotracheal Tube Size (mm i.d.)	
	Oral	Nasal
<30	4–7	4–6
30–60	8–10	6–8
60–100	10–12	8–10
100–200	12	10–12
200–300	14–16	
300–400	16–22	
400–600	22–26	
>600	26	

i.d., internal diameter.

the oral cavity to allow the animal to ventilate before the attempt at intubation is continued.

When blind orotracheal intubation is unsuccessful in calves or other small ruminants, a laryngoscope with a 250- to 350-mm blade is required. Visibility of the larynx is improved by hyperextending the animal's head and neck to make the orotracheal axis approach 180°. Using suction or gauze on a sponge forceps to swab the pharynx will improve visibility if secretions are an impediment. Attempting intubation when the anesthetic plane is insufficient may provoke active regurgitation. With adequate depth of anesthesia, this reflex is eliminated. The epiglottis is depressed so that the larynx is visible. The endotracheal tube should be placed in the oral pharynx and inserted into the larynx during inspiration. If desired, a stylet (e.g., a 1-m 0.5-cm stylet[88] or a large male dog urinary catheter) can be inserted through the endotracheal tube. The stylet should be about 1.5 times the length of the endotracheal tube. The stylet is placed through the larynx, and the endotracheal tube is then passed beyond the end of the stylet into the trachea.

Blind oral intubation is more difficult in sheep and goats, and intubation is best performed with laryngoscopy. To perform blind oral intubation, the animal's head and neck are extended after placement of the endotracheal tube in the oral pharynx. The larynx can be palpated and the tube directed into the larynx.[41] Members of both of these species have active laryngeal reflexes that may be obtunded by topical application of 2% lidocaine. This can be performed with an adjustable pattern plant sprayer[89] or with a syringe. The use of cetacaine® is not recommended because overdosage can easily occur and because benzocaine-based local anesthetics can cause methemoglobinemia.[90] After desensitization of the larynx, intubation can be performed with the same technique used in calves. Oral intubation performed in camelids is similar to that used in domestic ruminants. Blind oral intubation is usually unsuccessful, and laryngoscopy with a 250- to 350-mm laryngoscope is recommended. Desensitization of the larynx is usually not required.

Blind nasotracheal intubation has been described in awake or mildly sedated calves, although it requires an endotracheal tube one size smaller than that used orally.[91] The technique in calves is very similar to that described for foals and is useful for induction of inhalation anesthesia or to facilitate oral surgery. Particular attention is needed to ensure that the tube is directed into the ventral meatus. Following placement of the tube in the nasopharynx, the calf's head and neck are extended to facilitate passage into the larynx. The tube is secured in place and connected to the anesthetic-delivery system connected to the anesthetic machine.

Nasotracheal intubation is also possible in sheep[38] and camelids,[92] although it requires an endotracheal tube one size smaller than that used orally. Camelids are prone to epistaxis, so the use of a lubricant that contains phenylephrine is recommended. Blind nasal intubation is technically easier than blind oral intubation, but nasal intubation under laryngoscopic control is technically more difficult than orotracheal intubation. Even though nasotracheal intubation can be more difficult, it offers the option of the animal recovering with the endotracheal tube in place as a method of preventing airway obstruction during recovery. The endotracheal tube is advanced with slow gentle pressure through the external nares into the ventral meatus. An obstruction encountered at approximately 10 cm in adults is usually the middle meatus. An obstruction encountered more caudally, approximately 25 cm in adults, is likely the nasopharyngeal diverticulum.[92] In either case, the tube should be withdrawn and redirected. If the endotracheal tube cannot be redirected past the nasopharyngeal diverticulum, placement of a prebent stylet into the tube to direct its tip ventrally is usually effective.

After the endotracheal tube has been advanced into the nasopharynx, the camelid's head and neck should be extended and the tube manipulated into the larynx. If the tube will not enter the larynx, placing the prebent stylet in the endotracheal tube to direct the tube tip ventrally into the larynx instead of the esophagus is helpful. Although visibility of the larynx is somewhat limited, oral laryngoscopy will aid intubation and confirm correct placement of the tube.

Endotracheal intubation can be confirmed with several techniques. Initially, they include visualization of the endotracheal tube passing into the larynx. When transparent endotracheal tubes are used, water-vapor condensation will appear and then disappear during each breath. One can feel gas being expelled from the tube during exhalation, and, when the endotracheal tube is connected to the anesthesia machine, synchrony between movement of the rebreathing bag and the thorax will be noted. Finally, if a capnograph is available, carbon dioxide will be detected in exhaled gas.

Anesthesia in ruminants can be maintained with halothane, isoflurane, or sevoflurane. Although methoxyflurane can be used in small domestic ruminants and camelids, induction and recovery are prolonged. Liver failure has been reported in hyperimmunized goats subjected to halothane anesthesia,[93] but a study performed in young healthy goats showed that halothane or isoflurane is unlikely to cause hepatic injury.[94] The NSAID flunixin meglumine should not be used immediately before or after methoxyflurane anesthesia because renal failure may result.[95] It would appear that the use of this combination of drugs should be avoided in all species, including ruminants.

Conventional small animal anesthesia machines can be used to anesthetize ruminants weighing less than 60 kg. Conventional human anesthesia machines or small animal machines with expanded soda lime canisters are adequate for animals weighing up to 200 kg. Conventional large animal anesthesia machines can be used to anesthetize cattle weighing over 200 kg. Anesthesia is usually induced with 3% to 5% halothane, 3% to 5% isoflurane, or 4% to 6% sevoflurane and with oxygen flow rates of 20 mL/kg/min. Anesthesia is induced in animals of lesser body weight by using agent concentrations at the lower end of the range. Anesthesia is usually maintained with 1.5% to 2.0% halothane, 1.5% to 2.5% isoflurane, or 2.5% to 3.5% sevoflurane with oxygen flow rates reduced to 12 mL/kg/min. These vaporizer settings correspond to end-expired anesthetic concentrations of 1.25 to 1.5 minimum alveolar concentration (MAC) and should be adequate for ruminants that were not sedated prior to induction. Ruminants that have been sedated prior to induction can usually be maintained on end-expired anesthetic concentrations of 1.0 to 1.25 MAC, although final concentrations may vary depending on the sedative used. Because domestic ruminants have a respiratory pattern characterized by rapid respiratory rate and small tidal volume (with more dead-space ventilation), higher vaporizer settings (e.g., 2% to 3% halothane) may be required to better maintain anesthesia in spontaneously breathing patients.

Supportive Therapy

This is an important part of anesthetic practice. As veterinarians become more familiar with use of the anesthetic drugs, longer and more involved surgical procedures are attempted. As duration and difficulty increase, the likelihood of complications can also increase. Attention to supportive therapy in anesthetized ruminants and camelids can decrease the incidence of complications and improve outcome. Supportive therapy includes patient positioning, fluid administration, mechanical ventilation, cardiovascular support, and good monitoring techniques.

Patient Positioning

Improper positioning and padding of anesthetized horses have been implicated as causes of postanesthetic myopathy and/or neuropathy.[96] A similar situation may occur in adult cattle. Postanesthetic myopathy does not appear to readily occur in calves, goats, sheep, and South American camelids. Anesthetized ruminants should be positioned on a smooth, flat, padded surface. Larger adult cattle require either water beds, dunnage bags, or 10-cm high-density foam pads, whereas 5-cm-thick pads are sufficient for sheep, goats, and South American camelids. Patients positioned in dorsal recumbency should be balanced squarely on their back with both gluteal areas bearing equal weight. The forelegs and hind legs should be flexed and relaxed. External support should be placed under the maxilla to prevent hyperextension of the neck.

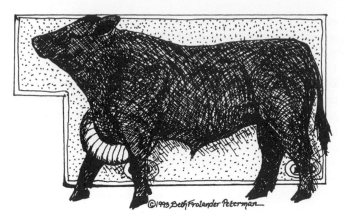

Fig. 28.1. Cattle positioned in lateral recumbency should be placed on padding with an inner tube placed over the dependent foreleg and that leg drawn cranially. Support should be placed under the nondependent foreleg and hind leg so they are parallel to the table.

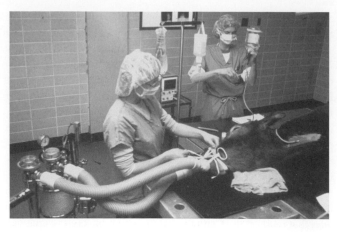

Fig. 28.2. Position of the head and neck to enable fluid to drain from the oral cavity.

Adult cattle in lateral recumbency should have an automobile inner tube (valve stem pointed down) placed under the shoulder of the dependent foreleg to help minimize pressure on the radial nerve as it traverses the musculospiral groove of the humerus. The point of the elbow should be positioned at 5 o'clock in the inner tube for cattle in right lateral recumbency or at 7 o'clock for cattle in left lateral recumbency. In addition, the dependent foreleg is drawn anteriorly so that the weight of the thorax rests on the triceps rather than on the humerus. Nonelastic tape covering the portion of the inner tube not under the shoulder will prevent overexpansion of that section of inner tube and will help to ensure shoulder support (Fig. 28.1). The other three legs are positioned perpendicular to the body, with the uppermost legs elevated and parallel to the table surface. Support of these legs will improve venous drainage and prevent injury to the brachial plexus. The head and neck are maintained in a slightly extended position, with the head resting on a pad or Turkish towel (Fig. 28.2). If possible, the patient's head should be positioned so that salivary secretions and gastric contents, if regurgitation occurs, will drain from the mouth and not wick between the animal's head and the pad and contact the eye. The dependent eye should be closed prior to placing the head on the padding, and bland ocular ointment should be instilled in the other eye. Camelids have prominent eyes, so special attention should be given to the dependent eye to avoid injury. Use of circulating warm-water heating blankets or convective warm-air blowers should be considered to prevent hypothermia in juvenile cattle, sheep, camelids, and goats. Adults are not as likely to become hypothermic, so the use of warm-water heating blankets is not required.

Fluid Administration

Fluid administration during anesthesia is important to correct preexisting dehydration, if present, provide volume to offset anesthesia-related vasodilatation, and provide maintenance needs. A balanced electrolyte solution is preferred. Lactated Ringer's solution, Normosol-R,® or the equivalent are most commonly used and are administered rapidly (10 to 25 mL/kg/h) in hypotensive patients. After hypotension is corrected, fluid administration may be slowed to 4 to 6 mL/kg/h. Although ruminants salivate copiously while anesthetized, replacement of bicarbonate is usually not required. Other fluids (e.g., saline) may be given when indicated. To increase fluid delivery rate when needed, two administration sets can be connected to one catheter with a Y connector, multiple catheters can be placed, a peristaltic pump can be used, or the fluid source may be pressurized. For convenience, fluids packaged in 3-L or 5-L bags can be used for large-volume administration. When administering large volumes of fluid, serial determinations of hematocrit and plasma total solids should be performed to prevent hemodilution and pulmonary edema. Hematocrit should remain above 25% and plasma total solids above 4 g/dL. Plasma or whole blood transfusion should be considered for hypoproteinemic or anemic individuals. Administration of sodium bicarbonate is indicated for correction of severe metabolic acidemia as determined by analysis of blood gas or total carbon dioxide.

Respiratory Supportive Therapy

Although anesthetized South American camelids ventilate well, domestic ruminants tend to hypoventilate while anesthetized. Mechanical ventilation should be considered when the procedure will exceed 1.5 h and is indicated to prevent hypoventilation in individuals that will not maintain sufficient alveolar ventilation. To minimize the effects of mechanical ventilation on the cardiovascular system, inspiratory time should be no more than 2 to 3 s, inspiratory pressure should be 20 to 30 cm of water, tidal volume should be 13 to 22 mL/kg, and respiratory rate should be 6 to 10 breaths/min. Hypocarbia alone can cause bradycardia in ruminants. In the absence of blood-gas analysis, overall minute volume should be decreased if unexplained bradycardia occurs.

During intravenous anesthesia, ruminants also benefit from supplemental oxygen. If the animal is intubated, the endotracheal tube can be connected to a demand valve. This piece of equipment is connected to an oxygen source that enables the patient to breathe spontaneously.[97] Compression of a button on the demand valve enables the anesthetist to "sigh" the patient. Because demand valves are designed for humans, there is an increase in the work of breathing associated with their use in large animals.[98] Intubated ruminants can also be insufflated with oxygen (5 L/min for small ruminants and 15 L/min for adult cattle). A flowmeter is connected to an oxygen source, and the tubing from the flowmeter is then inserted into the endotracheal tube.[99]

Cardiovascular Supportive Therapy

Hypotension has been implicated as a cause of either postanesthetic myopathy or neuropathy.[96,100,101] To help avoid these postanesthetic complications in ruminants, normotension should be maintained during anesthesia. Hypotension may be corrected simply by adjusting anesthetic depth. Although vasopressors can be used to correct hypotension, expansion of vascular volume either with rapid fluid administration or with the use of inotropes is a better alternative. Inotropes are preferred because they can increase stroke volume and cardiac output. Calcium borogluconate (23% solution) may also increase myocardial contractility and can be given as a slow infusion (0.5 to 1.0 mL/kg/h IV) to effect. Calcium administration may cause bradycardia, however, necessitating the use of a chronotrope if hypotension persists. Ephedrine, a mixed α and β sympathomimetic drug, can be used at 0.02 to 0.06 mg/kg IV to increase blood pressure simply by increasing cardiac contractility.[102] Lack of response at low doses can indicate excessive depth of anesthesia. Dobutamine, a synthetic β-agonist, can also be used to improve cardiac output. At low doses, it increases myocardial contractility and, at higher doses, heart rate as well.[103] Dobutamine is preferred over dopamine because hemodynamics improve, with smaller increases in heart rate.[104] It is infused at 1.0 to 2.0 μg/kg/min IV to effect.[103] Use of an infusion pump is recommended for convenience and consistency. After correction of hypotension, infusion rate can often be decreased for maintenance.

Monitoring

As with any species, good anesthetic techniques require monitoring to ensure that drug administration meets the animal's requirements and to prevent excessive insult to the cardiovascular, respiratory, nervous, and musculoskeletal systems, thereby decreasing the risk of complications. Monitoring includes techniques that require the tactile, visual, and hearing skills of the anesthetist, as well as the more sophisticated techniques that require instrumentation. Attention is directed to three systems: the cardiovascular, respiratory, and central nervous systems. Ideally, one monitors variables that respond rapidly to changes in anesthetic depth, which gives the anesthetist time to alter anesthetic administration before the anesthetic plane becomes either excessive or insufficient. While monitoring is done constantly, most variables are recorded at 5-min intervals. In many instances, monitoring equipment is used to aid evaluation of physiological responses to anesthesia and, therefore, anesthetic depth. Use of these instruments can make evaluation more precise and the selection of ancillary drugs more rational.

Variables that can be used to monitor the cardiovascular system are heart rate, pulse pressure (pulse strength), color of mucous membranes, and capillary refill time. In healthy anesthetized adult cattle, the heart rate is usually 60 to 90 beats/min. Animals that have received an anticholinergic will have an increased heart rate. The normal heart rate for calves, sheep, and goats varies with age. Juveniles will have a heart rate of 90 to 130 beats/min, which decreases as they mature. The normal heart rate for adult anesthetized camelids after the administration of an anticholinergic is 80 to 100 beats/min. For anesthetized juvenile camelids after the administration of an anticholinergic, it is 100 to 125 beats/min. The heart rate may exceed the normal range at the beginning of anesthesia, because of excitement associated with induction or hypotension, but, most often, it returns to the normal range within 10 to 20 min. In compromised patients, the heart rate begins to approach the normal range during anesthesia as oxygen, fluid, and analgesic support begin to stabilize the patient. The heart rate usually decreases as anesthesia depth increases, although that response can be masked by prior administration of anticholinergics.

Pulse pressure can be ascertained at several locations and should be full and bounding. The common digital, caudal auricular, radial, and saphenous arteries are commonly palpated. The facial artery can be palpated in young calves, but it becomes more difficult to do so as an animal ages. Because most anesthetic agents depress the cardiovascular system and overdosage causes the heart to function less effectively as a pump, diminished pulse pressure is indicative of increased anesthetic depth. Pulse pressure should be strong and palpated at different locations for comparison. Noting the amount of turgor present in the vessel during diastole can give an indication of diastolic pressure. If the vessel is easily collapsed by digital pressure during diastole, then diastolic pressure and, therefore, systolic and mean pressure can be assumed to be low even though pulse pressure may feel adequate.

Mucous membranes should be pink, although the mucous membranes of some ruminants and camelids are pigmented, making assessment difficult. Cyanosis must also be noted, although animals breathing oxygen and an inhalation agent may be apneic for several minutes before cyanosis occurs. Because at least 5 g/dL of reduced hemoglobin is required before cyanosis can be detected, severely anemic animals may not show this sign. Flushed mucous membranes are associated with vasodilatation, which can be caused by hypercarbia, halothane, α-adrenergic antagonists, or histamine release, or may be associated with postural hypostatic congestion.[105] Brick-red mucous membranes are associated with endotoxic shock. Following digital compression to blanch an area of the gum, capillary refill should occur in 1 to 2 s. Both of these variables give an indication of tissue perfusion. Excessive depth of anesthesia will cause the mucous membranes to become pale and capillary refill time to increase. By combining data from these variables, one can qualitatively assess adequacy of blood pressure. For example, if an animal has a normal heart rate, strong pulse pressure, pink mucous membranes, and short capillary refill time, and its peripheral arteries are not easily collapsed by digital pressure during diastole, then one can assume that blood pressure is in the normal range. Conversely, if pulse pressure is weak, mucous membranes are pale, capillary refill time is prolonged, and the peripheral arteries are easily occluded by digital pressure, then the animal's blood pressure is below normal and either anesthesia depth is excessive and/or cardiovascular support is needed.

The respiratory system is evaluated by monitoring respiratory rate and tidal volume. Spontaneous breathing rates are usually 20 to 30 breaths/min or higher in adult cattle; calves, sheep, and goats usually have respiratory rates of 20 to 40 breaths/min. Awake cattle have a decreased tidal volume when compared with horses.[106] That relationship persists in anesthetized cattle and other domestic ruminants in that they have a decreased tidal volume when compared with other species. Tidal volume is estimated by observing the amount the rebreathing bag empties during inspiration. Increasing the anesthetic depth can usually be expected to cause tidal volume and eventually respiratory rate to decrease. Normal values for respiratory rate in anesthetized camelids are 15 to 30 breaths/min for adults and 20 to 35 breaths/min for juveniles. Camelids tend to ventilate reasonably well when breathing spontaneously as judged by analysis of blood gas and respiratory gas during sevoflurane, isoflurane, or halothane anesthesia.

The central nervous system can be monitored by observation of ocular reflexes. The palpebral reflex disappears with minimal anesthesia depth in cattle, sheep, and goats and is usually of no value during anesthesia. The globe will rotate as anesthetic depth changes in cattle[3,39,107] (Fig. 28.3). The eyeball is normally centered between the palpebrae in awake cattle in lateral recumbency. As anesthesia is induced, the eyeball rotates ventrally, with the cornea being partially obscured by the lower eyelid. As anesthesia deepens, the pupil becomes completely hidden by the lower eyelid; this sign indicates stage III, plane 2 to 3 anesthesia. A further increase in anesthetic depth is accompanied by dorsal rotation of the eyeball. Dorsal movement is complete when the cornea is centered between the palpebrae; this sign indicates deep surgical anesthesia with profound muscle relaxation. During recovery, the eyeball rotates in reverse order to that during induction.[3,39,107] The globe does not rotate in response to changes in anesthesia depth in goats, sheep, or South American camelids. Usually, the palpebral reflex of the dorsal eyelid of camelids remains during surgical anesthesia. However, if the camelid can move its ventral eyelid without tactile stimulation, anesthetic depth is decreasing and eventually limb movement will occur.[37] Nystagmus usually does not occur during anesthesia of domestic ruminants or camelids. When it does occur, it cannot be correlated with changes in anesthesia depth. The corneal reflex should always be present.

Some ruminants will display involuntary swallowing motions under anesthesia without exhibiting other signs of insufficient anesthesia depth. This reflex may indicate that anesthesia depth is somewhat light but still appropriate. Response to pain from the surgical procedure can also be used to estimate anesthesia depth. In some instances, camelids may respond by showing a more active palpebral reflex. Purposeful movement in all species indicates insufficient depth of anesthesia. An increase in arterial pressure associated with the surgical manipulation does not necessarily indicate inadequate anesthesia if purposeful movement does not occur.

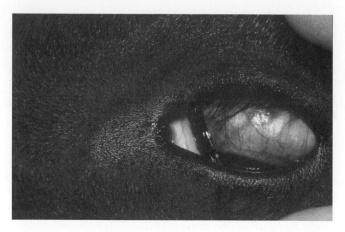

Fig. 28.3. Ocular rotation in a downward direction is indicative of surgical anesthesia.

Electrocardiography (ECG) is used with either standard limb leads (I, II, and III) or a dipole lead for detection of cardiac rate and rhythm disturbances. The lead that has the largest amplitude should be selected. A recorder is optional and useful because it enables one to record an ECG at the beginning of the case for future reference. Most ECG units emit an audible tone whenever a QRS complex is detected. Anesthetists should learn to always listen to the audible rhythm in the background during the case, especially during distractions. Because an ECG gives no information regarding blood pressure or pulse strength, emphasis should be placed on monitoring pulse and arterial pressure instead of relying solely on the ECG.

Mean arterial pressure provides an accurate variable for assessing anesthesia depth. In most instances, changes in anesthesia depth become evident quickly through increases or decreases in blood pressure. Additionally, it is a more definitive variable than monitoring pulse pressure alone. Monitoring pulse pressure determines the difference between systolic and diastolic pressure. An animal with systolic and diastolic pressures of 120/90 mm Hg will have pulse pressure similar to that of another animal with pressures of 90/60 mm Hg. However, a large difference exists in mean pressure or perfusion pressure. The former animal will have a mean pressure of about 100 mm Hg, whereas the latter will have a mean pressure of about 70 mm Hg. Since animals with low mean pressure during anesthesia are more at risk of developing complications, identification of this situation is important.[100,101] Normal arterial pressure values in anesthetized cattle are systolic pressure, 120 to 150 mm Hg; diastolic pressure, 80 to 110 mm Hg; and mean pressure 90 to 120 mm Hg; and are typically greater than in standing cattle.[108] Normal values for systolic and diastolic pressure in sheep, goats, and camelids are 90–120/60–80 mm Hg. Normal values for mean pressure in sheep, goats, and camelids are 75 to 100 mm Hg. However, if camelids are aroused by painful stimuli, mean arterial pressure may approach 150 mm Hg. Arterial pressure can be monitored either indirectly or directly. Indirect methods of determining arterial pressure require the use of various infrasonic and ultrasonic devices to detect blood flow in peripheral arteries. Doppler and

Dinamap® devices can be used with cuffs wrapped around the tail of cattle and the limbs of sheep and goats,[18] or around the tail or the limbs of South American camelids.[10] The cuff diameter should be 40% of limb or tail circumference.[109] Direct methods require catheterization of an artery and use of a pressure transducer and amplifier or an aneroid manometer to determine pressure values. A transducer system determines systolic, diastolic, and mean arterial pressures. An aneroid manometer can be substituted for the pressure transducer and amplifier, but only the mean pressure can be obtained.[110] Mean pressure changes rapidly in response to changes in anesthetic depth, and even the use of this rather simple system enables anesthetists to make appropriate responses.

Percutaneous arterial catheterization is easily performed in most ruminants and is relatively free of complications.[110,111] The caudal auricular, saphenous, and common digital arteries are most commonly catheterized vessels when over-the-needle Teflon (polytetrafluoroethylene) catheters are used. Passage of this type of catheter through the unbroken skin will often damage the catheter, making arterial placement difficult. Thus, incising the skin or piercing it with a slightly larger needle at the catheterization site is recommended.[111] A skin incision is usually unnecessary when the caudal auricular artery is catheterized, because the skin is relatively thin in that location and the artery is often inadvertently pierced because the skin is relatively immobile in that area. For adults, 3- to 5-cm 18- to 20-gauge catheters are used, with 2.5- to 3-cm 20- to 22-gauge catheters used in juveniles. An extension set with stopcock is used to connect the arterial catheter to a syringe containing heparinized (2.0 units/mL) saline and a piece of noncompliant tubing attached to the pressure transducer or aneroid manometer. After the arterial catheter is removed, digital pressure is maintained at the site to prevent hematoma formation. If desired, a pressure bandage can be used.

Central venous pressure can be determined to assess venous return, myocardial function, and the need for fluid replacement. This is a good variable to use—along with serial determinations of hematocrit, plasma total solids, and urine production—in evaluating fluid replacement but often provides little information regarding changes in anesthesia depth. Normal values are 5 to 10 cm of water pressure.

Normal values for arterial blood-gas analysis are similar to those for other species.[5,6] Respiratory gas can be analyzed to determine end-tidal carbon dioxide and inhalant anesthetic concentration. Because domestic ruminants have a respiratory pattern characterized by small tidal volume, end-expired gas might not be sufficiently representative of alveolar gas and accurate results might not be obtained. End-tidal gas analysis is more accurate when assessing carbon dioxide during controlled ventilation. Anesthetic analyzers that use optical low-spectrum infrared measurement cannot distinguish between methane and halothane in expired gas of herbivores and will report falsely increased concentrations of halothane, and to a lesser degree isoflurane, in the anesthetic circuit.[112] The presence of methane does not affect analyzers that use high-spectrum infrared measurement or piezoelectric measurement.[112] Analyzers that use low-spectrum infrared measurement can be used in herbivores by intermittently (every 15 to 30 min) placing a small container of activated charcoal in the sample path to adsorb halothane.[113] Methane will pass through the charcoal without adsorption and be measured. After removing the charcoal container from the sample path, one can subtract the concentration of background methane from the displayed value to determine halothane or isoflurane concentration.

Recovery

Ruminants and South American camelids recover well from general anesthesia and seldom experience emergence delirium, make premature attempts to stand, or sustain injuries. When an α_2-agonist is used as part of the anesthetic regimen, an α_2-antagonist can be used to hasten recovery.[13,22,39,44,45,49,53,89,114]

Domestic ruminants should not be extubated until the laryngeal reflex has returned. Orally intubated camelids should not be extubated until the animal is swallowing, coughing, and actively trying to expel the endotracheal tube. Precautions should be taken to prevent camelids from damaging or aspirating the endotracheal tube. If a patient has regurgitated, the buccal cavity and pharynx should be lavaged to prevent aspiration of the material. In these instances, the endotracheal tube should be withdrawn with the cuff inflated in an attempt to remove any material that may have located to the trachea. Since camelids are obligate nasal breathers,[92] gas exchange must be confirmed after extubation; the airway commonly becomes obstructed during the transition from oral endotracheal intubation to nasal breathing and, in severe cases, can necessitate tracheotomy. The endotracheal tube of nasally intubated camelids can be removed after they stand. Although ruminants recover well from general anesthesia with minimal assistance, an attendant should be available.

Intraoperative Complications

Fortunately, major complications do not occur often during or following well-planned anesthesia in ruminants. However, one must be vigilant so that the unexpected occurrence of a complication can be recognized and effectively treated. As is the case in anesthesia of all species, potential complications are better prevented, and therefore emphasis should be placed on formation and implementation of a rational anesthetic regimen. Airway obstruction, apnea, and hypothermia are diagnosed and treated in a manner similar to the ways in which other domestic species are diagnosed and treated.

Although anesthetized camelids do not appear to become tympanitic, fermentation of ingesta and the animal's inability to eructate ruminal content often cause tympany during anesthesia. As tympany develops, more pressure is placed on the diaphragm, decreasing functional residual capacity and impeding ventilation.[115] In addition, tympany increases the risk of regurgitation. Therapy involves passage of a stomach tube to decompress the rumen. On occasion, one will be unable to pass the stomach tube into the rumen. In these difficult cases, placing the animal in sternal recumbency will aid the procedure. When that is not possible, the rumen can be decompressed with a 12-gauge needle inserted through the abdominal wall. Fortunately, ruminal tympany is usually of the nonfrothy type, and decompression is easily accomplished. External pressure placed on the rumen will help expel gas from the orogastric tube. Ruminal tympany can also occur during the use of nitrous oxide, which tends to accumulate in gas-filled viscus.[116] Discontinuation of nitrous oxide administration along with decompression of the rumen is recommended.

Connective tissue is not as fibrous in ruminants' lungs, and therefore excessive airway pressure can cause pneumothorax and emphysema more easily than in horses.[117] Signs include dyspnea and increased resistance to inspiration because of tension pneumothorax. It is treated by placement of a chest tube and aspiration of the gas. It is much easier to prevent than treat. Do not use excessive airway pressure (>30 cm of water) when "sighing" animals or when using controlled ventilation.

Cardiac arrhythmias usually do not occur in anesthetized ruminants. Atrial fibrillation can occur in cattle as a sequela to metabolic derangement secondary to gastrointestinal obstruction. Atrial fibrillation usually resolves when the primary problem is corrected. Because cattle are amenable to physical restraint and local anesthesia, corrective surgery is often performed without general anesthesia. Diagnosis can be confirmed with ECG. The oculocardiac reflex is a well-recognized reflex in most animals and can be treated similarly in ruminants.[116,118] Cardiac arrest is treated with similar techniques commonly used in horses.[119–121]

Postoperative Complications

Because ruminants and camelids tend to recover well from general anesthesia, long-bone fractures, cervical fractures, or other catastrophic injuries seldom occur. Should they occur, therapy is based on severity of the fracture and the economic value of the animal. Postoperative myopathy-neuropathy can occur in larger cattle but is not a problem in calves, sheep, goats, or camelids. The problem is recognized when muscle weakness or motor nerve dysfunction are observed, with some animals being unable to stand. Therapy is symptomatic, with intravenous fluids administered to maintain hydration, acid-base status, and electrolytes; along with analgesics, NSAIDs, and vitamin E–selenium compounds as indicated. Slinging the animal may be helpful but can increase muscle damage. Myopathy may take several days to resolve and can be life-threatening. Again, it is better to prevent muscle or nerve damage by positioning anesthetized animals properly and avoiding excessive depth of anesthesia.

A less common cause of delayed recovery is muscle weakness caused by neuromuscular blockade. Because ruminants have very low levels of pseudocholinesterase, metabolism of succinylcholine is slow, causing prolonged effects of this drug.[122] Neuromuscular blockade may also be caused by interaction of anesthetics and aminoglycoside antibiotics[123] or by incomplete reversal of nondepolarizing muscle relaxants.[124] Muscle relaxants are rarely administered to ruminants.

Thrombophlebitis can occur after perivascular injection of irritating compounds, although usually not with the frequency or severity that occurs in horses, and is treated similarly.[125] Corneal ulcers can also occur following anesthesia.[126]

Aspiration pneumonia occurs after regurgitation of rumen or gastric contents and subsequent inhalation of the material. Active regurgitation might cause the material to be inhaled deeply into the pulmonary tree, initiating bronchospasm and physical obstruction of the airways. Signs include dyspnea and, depending on severity, cyanosis. If the patient survives the initial insult, pneumonia is certain. Broad-spectrum antibiotics, anti-inflammatory therapy, etc., are indicated.[127] Silent or passive regurgitation can occur with the same results, except that there usually is not as much particulate material in the regurgitant. Similar treatment is instituted. Because of the potential severity of this complication, prevention must be emphasized. Tracheal intubation is recommended, and, if not possible, the occiput should be elevated to encourage fluids to drain from the mouth rather than into the trachea[38] (Fig. 28.2).

Analgesia

Providing postoperative analgesia is an important component of veterinary anesthesia. There are very few approved drugs for provision of analgesia in domestic ruminants and none approved for use in South American camelids. Drugs that have been used in other species include the NSAIDs, carprofen, flunixin, phenylbutazone, and ketoprofen; the opioids and opiates, butorphanol, buprenorphine, fentanyl, and morphine; and lidocaine and ketamine. Although α_2-agonists can provide analgesia, their behavioral effects usually limit their use in ruminants. When applicable, local anesthetic agents can be used to desensitize structures and tissue.[128] Epidural administration of local anesthetic agents and opioids and opiates may be appropriate for some procedures.

Flunixin, which is approved for use in cattle, is dosed at 1.1 to 2.2 mg/kg IV per day. Carprofen can be given at 0.7 mg/kg IV daily.[129] When given at 4.0 mg/kg, therapeutic levels are maintained for at least 72 h.[129] Ketoprofen can be dosed at 3.3 mg/kg IV daily.[129] Phenylbutazone is recommended at a dose of 2.2 mg/kg orally every 48 h.[129] Withdrawal times following the use of NSAIDs in ruminants are not well defined either for meat or for milk, and caution must be exercised to prevent residues from entering the food supply.[129] More latitude is available when administering NSAIDs to ruminants used in biomedical research.

Use of all the NSAIDs carries the risk of ulcer formation in the third gastric compartment of South American camelids. When extended use of these agents is anticipated, it is recommended—in an effort to determine the minimal dose needed to provide analgesic effect—that dosage amount and frequency be decreased after the desired effect is obtained. Flunixin is commonly used for analgesia in South American camelids. The dose range is 0.5 to 1.1 mg/kg IV given once daily.[130] Flunixin has been given at 1.1 mg/kg twice daily. Phenylbutazone is less commonly used in camelids. When used, it is administered in a manner similar to that in domestic ruminants (i.e., 2.2 mg/kg orally every 48 h).[131] Ketoprofen has also been used in llamas at a dose of 1 to 2 mg/kg IV once daily.[132]

Opioids have been used to provide analgesia to domestic ruminants and South American camelids. Most commonly, either butorphanol (0.05 to 0.2 mg/kg IM four times a day) or morphine (0.5 to 0.1 mg/kg IM four times a day) has been recommended.[13] The effect for both drugs lasts 3 to 6 h. The use of other opioids, such as buprenorphine, fentanyl (both injectable and transdermal), hydromorphone, and oxymorphone, may be considered in dosages similar to those used in canine or equine patients.[133-136] The dose may be adjusted if the behavioral effects become problematic (i.e., too much sedation, dysphoria, or locomotor activity).

Epidural opioids have been used extensively to provide analgesia in companion animals[133,134,137,138] and in horses.[139] Morphine, which is the most commonly used agent, is typically administered at a dose of 0.1 mg/kg to ease postoperative abdominal and orthopedic pain and to prevent tenesmus in horses[139] and camelids.[37] Analgesia begins in 30 to 60 min, with the action lasting 12 to 24 h. Injection is typically through the sacrocaudal space but can also be made at the lumbosacral space. A ruminant or camelid that becomes recumbent should be placed in sternal recumbency. As in other species, the lumbosacral space is caudal to a line connecting the anterior border of the wings of the ileum. In camelids, one can usually easily palpate the spinous process of the last lumbar vertebra and direct the needle caudal to it to enter the space. The spinous process of the first sacral vertebra is much smaller than that of the last lumbar vertebra and is difficult to palpate. Usually, an 18-gauge 7-cm spinal needle is adequate. If the injection is made at the lumbosacral space, one must aspirate prior to injection to ensure that the intrathecal space has not been entered. Dose requirements are 50% to 70% less when an agent is given intrathecally compared with epidural injection. If cerebrospinal fluid is obtained, the analgesic dose must be decreased or the needle must be withdrawn for epidural placement of the drug.

Infusions of ketamine and lidocaine have been used to provide analgesia in large and small animal patients. Ketamine is effective in small animal patients when administered at a loading dose of 0.5 mg/kg IV followed by an infusion at 10 µg/kg/min.[140] Ketamine has also been given alone at 6.6 to 13.3 µg/kg/min IV in horses[141] and at 40 µg/kg/min in camelids without untoward behavioral effects.[142] If desired, a loading dose of 0.5 mg/kg can also be used in ruminants. Systemic lidocaine administration has been effective in reducing overall anesthetic requirements in animals under inhalation anesthesia.[143-145] The reported lidocaine loading dose ranges from 2.5 to 5.0 mg/kg IV to be followed by an infusion of 50 to 100 µg/kg/min.[143,145]

Provision of general anesthesia and analgesia to domestic ruminants and South American camelids for complex diagnostic and surgical procedures can be very rewarding. Although each species may exhibit unique characteristics, meeting the challenges of anesthetizing a wide variety of ruminants and camelids contributes greatly to the overall veterinary care of these species.

References

1. Vallenas A, Cummings JF, Munnell JF. A gross study of the compartmentalized stomach of two new-world camelids, the llama and guanaco. J Morphol 143:399–424, 1971.
2. McGuirk SM, Bednarski RM, Clayton MK. Bradycardia in cattle deprived of food. J Am Vet Med Assoc 196:894–896, 1990.
3. Tranquilli WJ. Techniques of inhalation anesthesia in ruminants and swine. Vet Clin North Am Food Anim Pract 2:593–619, 1986.
4. Lassen ED, Pearson EG, Long PO, Schmotzer WB, Kaneps AJ, Riebold TW. Serum biochemical values in llamas: Reference values. Am J Vet Res 47:2278–2280, 1986.
5. Latimer KS, Mahaffey EA, Prasse KW, eds. Duncan and Prasse's Veterinary Laboratory Medicine: Clinical Pathology, 4th ed. Ames: Iowa State University Press, 2003:331–342.
6. Kaneko, J, Harvey JW, Bruss ML. Clinical Biochemistry of Domestic Animals, 5th ed. San Diego: Academic, 1997:890–894.
7. Kramer JW. Normal hematology of cattle, sheep, and goats. In: Feldman BF, Zinkl JG, Jain NC, eds. Schalm's Veterinary Hematology, 5th ed. Philadelphia: Lippincott Williams & Wilkins, 2000: 1075–1088.
8. Fowler ME. Medicine and Surgery of the South American Camelid. Ames: Iowa State University Press, 1989.
9. Amsel SI, Kainer RA, Johnson LW. Choosing the best site to perform venipuncture in a llama. Vet Med 82:535–536, 1987.
10. Heath RB. Llama anesthetic programs. Vet Clin North Am Food Anim Pract 5:71–80, 1989.
11. Riebold TW, Kaneps AJ, Schmotzer WB. Anesthesia in the llama. Vet Surg 18:400–404, 1989.
12. Short CE. Preanesthetic medications in ruminants and swine. Vet Clin North Am Food Anim Pract 2:553–566, 1986.
13. Carroll GL, Hartsfield SM. General anesthetic techniques in ruminants. Vet Clin North Am Food Anim Pract 12:627–661, 1996.
14. Taylor PM. Anaesthesia in sheep and goats. In Pract 13:31–36, 1991.
15. Greene SA, Thurmon JC. Xylazine: A review of its pharmacology and use in veterinary medicine. J Vet Pharmacol Ther 11:295–313, 1988.
16. Gray PR, McDonell WN. Anesthesia in goats and sheep. Part I. Local analgesia. Compend Contin Educ Pract Vet 8(Suppl): S33–S39, 1986.
17. Raptopoulos D, Weaver BMQ. Observations following intravenous xylazine administration in steers. Vet Rec 114:567–569, 1984.
18. Trim CM. Special anesthesia considerations in the ruminant. In: Short CE, ed. Principles and Practice of Veterinary Anesthesia. Baltimore: Williams and Wilkins, 1987:285–300.
19. Fayed AH, Abdalla EB, Anderson RR, Spencer K, Johnson HD. Effect of xylazine in heifers under thermoneutral or heat stress conditions. Am J Vet Res 50:151–153, 1989.
20. Ley S, Waterman A, Livingston A. Variation in the analgesic effects of xylazine in different breeds of sheep. Vet Rec 126:508, 1990.
21. O'Hair KC, McNeil JS, Phillips YY. Effects of xylazine in adult sheep. Lab Anim Sci 36:563, 1986.
22. Riebold TW, Kaneps AJ, Schmotzer WB. Reversal of xylazine-induced sedation in llamas using doxapram or 4-aminopyridine and yohimbine. J Am Vet Med Assoc 189:1059–1061, 1986.
23. Aouad JI, Wright EM, Shaner TW. Anesthesia evaluation on ketamine and xylazine in calves. Bov Pract 2:22–31, 1981.
24. Campbell KB, Klavano PA, Richardson P, Alexander JE. Hemodynamic effects of xylazine in the calf. Am J Vet Res 40:1777–1780, 1979.
25. Freire ACT, Gontijo RM, Pessoa JM, Souza R. Effect of xylazine on the electrocardiogram of the sheep. Br Vet J 137:590–595, 1981.
26. Symonds HW. The effect of xylazine upon hepatic glucose production and blood flow rate in the lactating dairy cow. Vet Rec 99:234–236, 1976.
27. Symonds HW, Mallison CB. The effect of xylazine and xylazine followed by insulin on blood glucose and insulin in the dairy cow. Vet Rec 102:27–29, 1978.

28. Eichner RD, Prior RL, Kvasnicka WG. Xylazine-induced hyperglycemia in beef cattle. Am J Vet Res 40:127–129, 1979.

29. Brockman RP. Effect of xylazine on plasma glucose, glucagon and insulin concentration in sheep. Res Vet Sci 30:383–384, 1981.

30. Muggaberg J, Brockman RP. Effect of adrenergic drugs on glucose and plasma glucagon and insulin response to xylazine in sheep. Res Vet Sci 33:118–120, 1982.

31. Thurmon JC, Nelson DR, Hartsfield SM, Rumore CA. Effects of xylazine hydrochloride on urine in cattle. Aust Vet J 54:178–180, 1978.

32. Hopkins TJ. The clinical pharmacology of xylazine in cattle. Aust Vet J 48:109–112, 1972.

33. Uggla A, Lindqvist rA. Acute pulmonary oedema as an adverse reaction to the use of xylazine in sheep. Vet Rec 113:42, 1983

34. LeBlanc MM, Hubbell JAE, Smith HC. The effect of xylazine hydrochloride on intrauterine pressure in the cow and the mare. In: Proceedings of the Annual Meeting of the Society of Theriogenology, 1984:211–220.

35. Jansen CAM, Lowe KC, Nathanielsz PW. The effects of xylazine on uterine activity, fetal and maternal oxygenation, cardiovascular function, and fetal breathing. Am J Obstet Gynecol 148:386–390, 1984.

36. Jedruch J, Gajewski Z. The effect of detomidine hydrochloride (Domosedan) on the electrical activity of the uterus in cows. Acta Vet Scand Suppl 82:189–192, 1986.

37. Riebold TW. Anesthesia in South American Camelids. In: Proceedings of American College of Veterinary Anesthesiologists/International Veterinary Academy of Pain Management/Academy of Veterinary Technician Anesthetists Meeting, Phoenix, AZ, 2004:155–169.

38. Hall LW, Clarke KW. In: Veterinary Anaesthesia, 9th ed. Philadelphia: Bailliére Tindall, 1991:236–259.

39. Greene SA. Protocols for anesthesia of cattle. Vet Clin North Am Food Anim Pract 19:679–693, 2003.

40. Waldridge BM, Lin HC, DeGraves FJ, Pugh DG. Sedative effects of medetomidine and its reversal by atipamezole in llamas. J Am Vet Med Assoc 211:1562–1565, 1997.

41. Gray PR. Anesthesia in goats and sheep. Part II. General anesthesia. Compend Contin Educ Pract Vet 8(Suppl):S127–S135, 1986.

42. Cebra CK, Tornquist SJ. Meta-analysis of glucose tolerance in llamas and alpacas [Abstract]. In: Proceedings of the Fourth European Symposium on South American Camelids, Goettingen, Germany, 2004:27.

43. Celly, CS, McDonell WN, Black WD, Young S. The comparative hypoxaemic effect of four alpha 2 adrenoceptor agonists (xylazine, romifidine, detomidine and medetomidine) in sheep. J Vet Pharmacol Ther 20:464–471, 1997.

44. Kitzman JV, Booth NH, Hatch RC, Wallner B. Antagonism of xylazine sedation by 4-aminopyridine and yohimbine in cattle. Am J Vet Res 43:2165–2169, 1982.

45. Thurmon JC, Lin HC, Tranquilli WJ, et al. A comparison of yohimbine and tolazoline as antagonist xylazine sedation in calves [Abstract]. Vet Surg 18:170–171, 1989.

46. Hsu WH, Hanson CE, Hembrough FB, Schaffer DD. Effects of idazoxan, tolazoline, and yohimbine on xylazine-induced respiratory changes and central nervous system depression in ewes. Am J Vet Res 50:1570–1573.

47. Ko JCH, McGrath CJ, Jacobson JD. Effects of atipamezole and yohimbine on medetomidine-induced central nervous system depression and cardiorespiratory changes in lambs [Abstract]. Vet Surg 23:79, 1994.

48. Ruckenbusch Y, Toutain PL. Specific antagonism of xylazine effects on reticulo-rumen motor function in cattle. Vet Med Rev 5:3–12, 1984.

49. Young DB, Shawley RV, Barron SJ. Tolazoline reversal of xylazine-ketamine anesthesia in calves [Abstract]. Vet Surg 18:171, 1988.

50. Read MR, T Duke, AR Toews. Suspected tolazoline toxicosis in a llama. J Am Vet Med Assoc 216:227–229, 2000.

51. Lewis CA, Constable PD, Hun JC, Morin DE. Sedation with xylazine and lumbosacral epidural administration of lidocaine and xylazine for umbilical surgery in calves. J Am Vet Med Assoc 214:89–95, 1999.

52. Doherty TJ, Ballinger JA, McDonell WN, Pascoe PJ, Valliant AE. Antagonism of xylazine-induced sedation by idazoxan in calves. Can J Vet Res 51:244–248, 1987.

53. Raekallio M, Kivalo M, Jalanka, Vaisio O. Medetomidine/ketamine sedation in calves and its reversal with atipamezole. J Vet Anaesth 18:45–47, 1991.

54. Zahner JM, Hatch RC, Wilson RC, Booth NH, Kitzman JV, Brown J. Antagonism of xylazine sedation in steers by doxapram and 4-aminopyridine. Am J Vet Res 45:2546–2551, 1984.

55. Valverde A, Doherty TJ, Dyson D, Valliant AE. Evaluation of pentobarbital as a drug for standing sedation in cattle. Vet Surg 18:235–238, 1989.

56. Stegmann GF. Observations on the use of midazolam for sedation, and induction of anaesthesia with midazolam in combination with ketamine in the goat. J S Afr Vet Assoc 69:89–92, 1998.

57. Stegmann GF, Bester L. Sedative-hypnotic effects of midazolam in goats after intravenous and intramuscular administration. J Vet Anaesth Analg 28:49–55, 2001.

58. Kyles AE, Waterman AE, Livingston A. Antinociceptive activity of midazolam in sheep. J Vet Pharmacol Ther 18:54–60, 1995.

59. Barrington GM, Meyer TF, Parish SM. Standing castration of the llama using butorphanol tartrate and local anesthesia. Equine Pract 15:35–39, 1993.

60. O'Hair KC, Dodd KT, Phillips YY, Beattie RJ. Cardiopulmonary effects of nalbuphine hydrochloride and butorphanol tartrate in sheep. Lab Anim Sci 38:58–61, 1988.

61. Waterman AE, Livingston A, Amin A. Analgesic activity and respiratory effects of butorphanol in sheep. Res Vet Sci 51:19–23, 1991.

62. Abrahamsen EJ. General anesthesia in field or practice. In: Proceedings of Current Veterinary Care and Management of Llamas and Alpacas. Columbus: Ohio State University, 2004:181–183.

63. Abrahamsen EJ. Sedation and chemical restraint of camelids. In: Proceedings of Current Veterinary Care and Management of Llamas and Alpacas. Columbus: Ohio State University, 2004: 25–26.

64. Rouse S. Pharmacodynamics of thiobarbiturates. Vet Anesth 5:22–26, 1978.

65. Pascoe PJ. Emergency care medicine. In: Short CE, ed. Principles and Practice of Veterinary Anesthesia. Baltimore: Williams and Wilkins, 1987:558–598.

66. Chaplin MD, Roszkowski AP, Richards RK. Displacement of thiopental from plasma proteins by nonsteroidal anti-inflammatory agents. Proc Soc Exp Biol Med 143:667–671, 1973.

67. Blaze CA, Holland RE, Grant AL. Gas exchange during xylazine-ketamine anesthesia in neonatal calves. Vet Surg 17:155–159, 1988.

68. Thurmon JC, Benson GJ. Anesthesia in ruminants and swine. In: Howard JC, ed. Current Veterinary Therapy 3: Food Animal Practice. Philadelphia: WB Saunders, 1993:58–76.

69. Coulson NM. The cardiorespiratory effects of diazepem/ketamine and xylazine/ketamine anesthetic combinations in sheep. Lab Anim Sci 39:591–597, 1989.

70. DuBois WR, Prado TM, Ko JCH, Mandsager RE, Morgan GL. A comparison of two intramuscular doses of xylazine-ketamine combination and tolazoline reversal in llamas. J Vet Anaesth Analg 31:90–96, 2004.

71. Grandy JL, McDonell WN. Evaluation of concentrated solutions of guaifenesin for equine anesthesia. J Am Vet Med Assoc 176:619–622, 1980.

72. Thurmon JC. Injectable anesthetic agents and techniques in ruminants and swine. Vet Clin North Am Food Anim Pract 2:567–592, 1986.

73. Wall R, Muir WW. Hemolytic potential of guaifenesin in cattle. Cornell Vet 80:209–216, 1990.

74. Thurmon JC, Benson GJ, Tranquilli WJ, Olson WA. Cardiovascular effects of intravenous infusion of guaifenesin, ketamine, and xylazine in Holstein calves [Abstract]. Vet Surg 15:463, 1986.

75. Lin HC, Tyler JW, Welles EG, Spano JS, Thurmon JC, Wolfe DF. Effects of anesthesia induced and maintained by continuous intravenous administration of guaifenesin, ketamine, and xylazine in spontaneously breathing sheep. Am J Vet Res 54:1913–1916, 1993.

76. Tracy CH, Short CE, Clark BC. Comparing the effects of intravenous and intramuscular administration of Telazol. Vet Med 83:104–111, 1988.

77. Hubbell JAE, Muir WW. Xylazine and tiletamine-zolazepam anesthesia in horses. Am J Vet Res 50:737–742, 1989.

78. Lin HC, Thurmon JC, Benson GJ, Tranquilli WJ, Olson WA. The hemodynamic response of calves to tiletamine-zolazepam anesthesia. Vet Surg 18:328–334, 1989.

79. Thurmon JC, Lin HC, Benson GJ, et al. Combining Telazol and xylazine for anesthesia in calves. Vet Med 84:824–830, 1989.

80. Conner GH, Coppock RW, Beck CC. Laboratory use of CI-744, a cataleptoid anesthetic, in sheep. Vet Med Small Anim Clin 69:479–482, 1974.

81. Lagutchik MS, Januszkiewicz AJ, Dodd KT, Martin DG. Cardiopulmonary effects of a tiletamine-zolazepam combination in sheep. Am J Vet Res 52:1441–1447, 1991.

82. Howard BW, Lagutchik MS, Januszkiewicz AJ, Martin DG. The cardiovascular response of sheep to tiletamine-zolazepam and butorphanol tartrate anesthesia. Vet Surg 19:461–467, 1990.

83. Klein LV, Tomasic M, Olsen K. Evaluation of Telazol in llamas [Abstract]. Vet Surg 19:316–317, 1990.

84. Waterman AE. Use of propofol in sheep. Vet Rec 122:260, 1988.

85. Nolan AM, Reid J, Welsh E. The use of propofol as an induction agent in goats [Abstract]. J Vet Anaesth 18:53–54, 1991.

86. Handel IG, Weaver BMQ, Staddon GE, Cruz Madorran JI. Observation on the pharmacokinetics of propofol in sheep. In: Proceedings of the Fourth International Congress of Veterinary Anesthesia, Utrecht, The Netherlands, 1991:143–154.

87. Duke T, Egger CM, Ferguson JG, Frketic MM. Cardiopulmonary effects of propofol infusion in llamas. Am J Vet Res 58:153–156, 1997.

88. Hubbell JAE, Hull BL, Muir WW. Perianesthetic considerations in cattle. Compend Contin Educ Pract Vet 8:92–102, 1986.

89. Kinyon GE. A new device for topical anesthesia. Anesthesiology 56:154–155, 1982.

90. Lagutchik MS, Mundie TG, Martin DG. Methemoglobinemia induced by a benzocaine-based topically administered anesthetic in eight sheep. J Am Vet Med Assoc 201:1407–1410, 1992.

91. Quandt JE, Robinson EP. Nasotracheal intubation in calves. J Am Vet Med Assoc 209:967–968, 1996.

92. Riebold TW, Engel HN, Grubb TL, et al. Anatomical considerations during intubation of the llama: The presence of a nasopharyngeal diverticulum. J Am Vet Med Assoc 204:779–783, 1994.

93. O'Brien TD, Raffe MR, Cox VS, Stevens DL, O'Leary TP. Hepatic necrosis following halothane anesthesia in goats. J Am Vet Med Assoc 189:1591–1595, 1986.

94. McEwan M-M, Gleed RD, Ludders JW, Stokol T, Del Piero F, Erb HN. Hepatic effects of halothane and isoflurane anesthesia in goats. J Am Vet Med Assoc 217:1697–1700, 2000.

95. Mathews K, Doherty T, Dyson D, Wilcock B, Valliant A. Nephrotoxicity in dogs associated with methoxyflurane anesthesia and flunixin meglumine analgesia [Abstract]. Can Vet J 31:766–771, 1990.

96. White NA. Postanesthetic recumbency myopathy in horses. Compend Contin Educ Pract Vet 4(Suppl):S44–S52, 1982.

97. Riebold TW, Evans AT, Robinson NE. Evaluation of the demand valve for resuscitation of horses. J Am Vet Med Assoc 176:1736–1742, 1980.

98. Watney GCG, Watkins SB, Hall LW. Effects of a demand valve on pulmonary ventilation in spontaneously breathing, anaesthetized horses. Vet Rec 117:358–362, 1985.

99. Gabel AA, Heath RB, Ross JN, et al. Hypoxia: Its prevention in inhalation anesthesia in horses. In: Proceedings of the American Association of Equine Practitioners, 1966:179–196.

100. Cribb PH. The effects of prolonged hypotensive isoflurane anesthesia in horses: Post-anesthetic myopathy [Abstract]. Vet Surg 17:164, 1988.

101. Grandy JL, Steffey EP, Hodgson DS, Woliner MJ. Arterial hypotension and the development of postanesthetic myopathy in halothane-anesthetized horses. Am J Vet Res 48:192–197, 1987.

102. Grandy JL, Hodgson DS, Dunlop CI, Chapman PL, Heath RB. Cardiopulmonary effects of ephedrine in halothane-anesthetized horses. J Vet Pharmacol Ther 12:389–396, 1989.

103. Daunt DA. Supportive therapy in the anesthetized horse. Vet Clin North Am Equine Pract 6:557–574, 1990.

104. Tranquilli WJ, Greene SA. Cardiovascular medications and the autonomic nervous system. In: Short CE, ed. Principles and Practice of Veterinary Anesthesia. Baltimore: Williams and Wilkins, 1987:426–454.

105. Manley SV. Monitoring the anesthetized horse. Vet Clin North Am Large Anim Pract 3:111–134, 1981.

106. Gallivan GJ, McDonell WN, Forrest JB. Comparative ventilation and gas exchange in the horse and cow. Res Vet Sci 46:331–336, 1989.

107. Thurmon JC, Romack FE, Garner HE. Excursion of the bovine eyeball during gaseous anesthesia. Vet Med Small Anim Clin 63:967–970, 1968.

108. Matthews NS, Gleed RD, Short CE. Cardiopulmonary effects of general anesthesia in adult cattle. Mod Vet Pract 67:618–620, 1986.

109. Grandy JL, Hodgson DS. Anesthetic considerations for emergency equine abdominal surgery. Vet Clin North Am Equine Pract 4:63–78, 1988.

110. Riebold TW, Evans AT. Comparison of simultaneous blood pressure determinations by four methods in the anesthetized horse. Vet Surg 14:332–337, 1985.

111. Riebold TW, Brunson DB, Lott RA, Evans AT. Percutaneous arterial catheterization in the horse. Vet Med Small Anim Clin 75:1736–1742, 1980.

112. Moens YP, Gootjes P, Lagerweij E. The influence of methane on the infrared measurement of halothane in the horse. J Vet Anaesth 18:4–7, 1991.

113. Gootjes P, Moens YP. A simple method to correct infrared measurement of anaesthetic vapour concentration in the presence of methane. J Vet Anaesth 24:24–25, 1997.

114. Kruse-Elliott KT, Riebold TW, Swanson CR. Reversal of xylazine-ketamine anesthesia in goats [Abstract]. Vet Surg 16:321, 1987.

115. Masewe VA, Gillespie JR, Berry JD. Influence of ruminal insufflation on pulmonary function and diaphragmatic electromyography in cattle. Am J Vet Res 40:26–31, 1979.

116. Lumb WV, Jones EW. In: Veterinary Anesthesia, 2nd ed. Philadelphia: Lea and Febiger, 1984:75–99 and 213–239.

117. Heath RB. General anesthesia in ruminants. In: Jennings PB, ed. The Practice of Large Animal Surgery. Philadelphia: WB Saunders, 1984:202–204.

118. Short CE, Rebhun WC. Complications caused by the oculocardiac reflex during anesthesia in the foal. J Am Vet Med Assoc 176:630–631, 1980.

119. Muir WW, Bednarski RM. Equine cardiopulmonary resuscitation. Part I. Compend Contin Educ Pract Vet 5(Suppl):S228–S234, 1983.

120. Muir WW, Bednarski RM. Equine cardiopulmonary resuscitation. Part II. Compend Contin Educ Pract Vet 5(Suppl):S287–S295, 1983.

121. Hubbell JAE, Muir WW, Gaynor JS. Cardiovascular effects of thoracic compression in horses subjected to euthanasia. Equine Vet J 25:282–284, 1993.

122. Tavernor WD. Muscle relaxants. In: Soma LR, ed. Veterinary Anesthesia. Baltimore: Williams and Wilkins, 1971:111–120.

123. Adams HR, Teske RH, Mercer HD. Anesthetic-antibiotic relationships. J Am Vet Med Assoc 169:409–412, 1976.

124. Hildebrand S. Neuromuscular blocking agents in equine anesthesia. Vet Clin North Am Equine Pract 6:587–606, 1990.

125. Courley KTT. Fluid therapy for horses with gastrointestinal disease. In: Smith BP, ed. Large Animal Internal Medicine, 3rd ed. St Louis: CV Mosby, 2002:682–694.

126. Whitley RD, Vygantas DR. Ocular trauma. In: Smith BP, ed. Large Animal Internal Medicine, 3rd ed. St Louis: CV Mosby, 2002:1159–1164.

127. Ames TR, Baker JC, Wikse SE. The bronchopneumonias (respiratory disease complex of cattle, sheep, and goats). In: Smith BP, ed. Large Animal Internal Medicine, 3rd ed. St Louis: CV Mosby, 2002:551–570.

128. Skarda RT. Local and regional anesthesia in ruminants and swine. Vet Clin North Am Food Anim Pract 12:579–626, 1996.

129. George LW. Pain control in food animals. In: Steffey EP, ed. Recent Advances in Anesthetic Management of Large Domestic Animals. Ithaca, NY: International Veterinary Information Service, 2003:A0615.1103. http://www.ivis.org/advances/Steffey_Anesthesia/george/chapter_frm.asp? LA=1.

130. Navarre CB, Ravis WR, Nagilla R, et al. Pharmacokinetics of flunixin meglumine in llamas following a single intravenous dose. J Vet Pharmacol Ther 24:361–364, 2001.

131. Navarre CB, Ravis WR, Nagilla R, Simpkins A, Duran SH, Pugh DG. Pharmacokinetics of phenylbutazone in llamas following single intravenous and oral doses. J Vet Pharmacol Ther 24:227–231, 2001.

132. Navarre CB, Ravis WR, Campbell J, Nagilla R, Duran SH, Pugh DG. Stereoselective pharmacokinetics of ketoprofen in llamas following intravenous administration. J Vet Pharmacol Ther 24:223–226, 2001.

133. Wagner AE. Opioids. In: Muir WW, Gaynor JS, eds. Handbook of Veterinary Pain Management. St Louis: CV Mosby, 2002:164–183.

134. Pascoe PJ. Opioid analgesics. Vet Clin North Am Small Anim Pract 30:757–772, 2000.

135. Bennett RC, Steffey EP. Use of opioids for pain and anesthetic management in horses. Vet Clin North Am Equine Pract 18:47–60, 2002.

136. Zimmel DN. How to manage pain and dehydration in horses with colic. In: Proceedings of the 49th Annual Meeting of the American Association of Equine Practitioners, New Orleans, LA, 127–131.

137. Torske KE, Dyson DH. Epidural analgesia and anesthesia. Vet Clin North Am Small Anim Pract 30:859–874, 2000.

138. Gaynor JS, Mama KR. Local and regional anesthetic techniques for alleviation of perioperative pain. In: Muir WW, Gaynor JS, eds. Handbook of Veterinary Pain Management. St Louis: CV Mosby, 2002:261–280.

139. Robinson EP, Natalini CC. Epidural anesthesia and analgesia in horses. Vet Clin North Am Equine Pract 18:61–82, 2002.

140. Wagner AE, Walton JA, Hellyer PW, Gaynor JS, Mama KR. Use of low doses of ketamine administered by constant rate infusion as an adjunct for postoperative analgesia in dogs. J Am Vet Med Assoc 221:72–75, 2002.

141. Matthews NS, Fielding CL, Swinebroad EL. How to use a ketamine constant rate infusion in horses for analgesia. Proc Am Assoc Equine Pract 50:227–228, 2004.

142. Schlipf JW Jr, Eaton K, Fulkerson P, Riebold TW, Cebra C. Constant rate infusion of ketamine reduces minimum alveolar concentration of isoflurane in alpacas [Abstract]. In: Proceedings of American College of Veterinary Anesthesiologists/International Veterinary Academy of Pain Management/Academy of Veterinary Technician Anesthetists Meeting, Phoenix, AZ, 2004:58.

143. Doherty TJ, Frazier D. Effect of intravenous lidocaine on halothane minimum alveolar concentration in ponies. Equine Vet J 30:300–303, 1998.

144. Valverde A, Doherty TJ, Hernandez J, Davies W. Effect of lidocaine on the minimum alveolar concentration of isoflurane in dogs. J Vet Anaesth Analg 31:264–271, 2004.

145. Redua MA, Doherty T, Castro-Queiroz P, Rohrbach BW. Effect of intravenous lidocaine and ketamine on isoflurane minimum alveolar concentration in goats [Abstract]. In: Proceedings of American College of Veterinary Anesthesiologists/International Veterinary Academy of Pain Management/Academy of Veterinary Technician Anesthetists Meeting, Phoenix, AZ, 2004:56.

Chapter 29
Swine

John C. Thurmon and Geoffrey W. Smith

Introduction

Swine (*Sus scrofa domestica*) present a special challenge to immobilization and anesthesia. A thorough understanding of their physiological response to mechanical restraint, anesthesia, and surgery is essential for their safe handling.

Pigs come in all sizes. They range from piglets (0.5 to 3 kg) and miniatures (10 to 30 kg) to individuals that can weigh in excess of 400 kg. Most research is conducted in pigs weighing less than 50 kg, as is most field and hospital surgery. Exceptions include cesarean sections in mature sows and surgery in large boars.

The pig's anatomical structure is not conducive to manual restraint, especially when it has grown large. The pig's body is shaped such that, in the wild, it can scurry through underbrush and escape through small openings in an effort to elude its enemies. No part of its body is easily grasped for restraint.

Pigs have only a few superficial veins (primarily on the dorsolateral surface of their ears) into which an injection can be made. As a result, drugs injected by the intramuscular route have become popular for immobilization and for induction of anesthesia. Intramuscular injections must be made with needles in excess of 3 cm in length. Shorter needles may result in injection into fatty tissue, delaying drug absorption into the bloodstream and delivery to the central nervous system (CNS). Injection into fatty tissue is one of the most common reasons for alteration of the expected response to an intended intramuscular injection of an anesthetic.

Most discussions are directly related to the importance of swine as an agricultural entity because individual market pigs have limited economic value. Valuable breeding stock is an exception. The overall value of individuals and the species as a whole increases when we consider their selective breeding potential and contribution to medical research. Pigs are physiologically more closely related to humans than are most other species. Because of this similarity, swine play an important role in human medical research. The cardiopulmonary system and other organ systems, including the skin and gastrointestinal tract, are similar to those in humans. Thus, pigs have become widely used as laboratory research animals. This has increased in recent years with the advent of genetic research directed toward various human diseases.

Several publications have reviewed anesthetic and analgesic techniques in swine for research purposes.[1-4] Domestic or commercial species (i.e., food-producing swine) have undergone genetic alterations that impact their reaction to stress and other responses to surgery and anesthesia. Veterinarians should be familiar with these variations so as to minimize the occurrence of preventable emergencies (e.g., malignant hyperthermia).

Sexual maturity occurs at approximately 6 months of age. Body weight among breeds is highly variable. Studies comparing three miniature breeds of pigs at 4 months of age clearly revealed a significant difference in heart weight to body weight ratio. When measured under the same conditions, cardiovascular parameters were significantly different among these pigs.[5] This suggests that biological measurements should not be extrapolated among breeds or from one age to another. This variability implies the need for more information regarding the norm for various ages, sizes, breeds, and genders.

Preparation for Anesthesia

Elective surgery involving the abdominal organs is made easier when mature pigs are starved for 12 to 24 h. It is less stressful for an isolated pig that can see and have nose contact with its fellow penmates while food is being withheld. Gastrointestinal gas will rapidly accumulate in improperly starved pigs. A full abdomen can produce enormous pressure on the diaphragm, decreasing pulmonary functional residual capacity and decreasing alveolar ventilation, as well as complicating intra-abdominal organ manipulation. This is particularly true when surgery is 2 to 3 h long. Bloat will often develop in nonfasted pigs receiving an anticholinergic. The consequences of these alterations are complicated by deep general anesthesia and any position associated with a head-down tilt. Pigs are often restrained by hoisting them by their rear legs. The head-down position can interfere with breathing already depressed by the anesthetic. When surgery is completed, the pig should be placed in an independent stall until it has completely recovered from anesthesia. Otherwise, penmates may cannibalize the recovering pig.

Sows presented for cesarean surgery are often hypotensive. If labor has been prolonged, it is not uncommon for them to be suffering from shock. It is wise to administer large amounts of balanced electrolyte fluids and antibiotics prior to surgery. Sows under these circumstances are not good candidates for extradural or subarachnoid analgesia. Either may lead to hypotension, and heavy fluid loading combined with ephedrine or phenylephrine is recommended. Fluid loading is often a difficult chore, because large peripheral veins are scarce in most breeds. An exception is mature Landrace sows (Fig. 29.1).

Restraint

Baby pigs and small potbellied pigs are easily restrained by placing one hand over their back and the other under their sternum. Rough handling, particularly during hot weather, should be avoided because it can easily cause overheating and acute death. Mature swine may be restrained with a soft cotton rope looped around the maxilla just behind the upper canine teeth. A steel-cable hog snare is also used for this purpose but is painful, and pigs soon learn to avoid its placement. Head catches similar to those designed for cattle and small ruminants can be used, but because of the shape of the pig's head and neck, a considerable amount of pressure must be exerted on the squeeze to secure the head. This excessive pressure can result in airway occlusion. A pig in the head squeeze must be observed closely to ensure that its airway remains functional.

A mobile device commonly used for restraint is a webbed-top stanchion. This apparatus is preferred over most commercial devices because it can be used to restrain pigs of all sizes. If the device is of sufficient size, several pigs can be placed on it at one time for anesthetic induction or other minor procedures. Extradural injection is easily performed when a pig is restrained in the webbing. Furthermore, the stanchion can serve as an operating table for minor elective procedures. Nylon webbing is easily sterilized by using a cold antiseptic solution or by steaming. The cart is mobile and can be used to weigh the patient and transport it into the surgery room for induction of anesthesia. Other devices are available but are expensive and designed to accommodate only one pig at a time. The size of the pig that can be restrained is also limited.

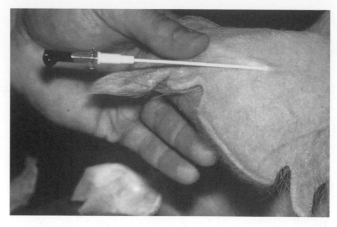

Fig. 29.1. Cannulation of the central ear vein of a Landrace sow with a 16-gauge catheter. A rubber band has been placed tightly around the base of the ear to engorge the veins so they are more easily identified.

Injection Sites

Pigs have a proclivity to store body fat. Thus, any injection intended for intramuscular deposition must be made with a needle that will reach muscular tissue. It is not desirable to inject into the ham muscles of pigs destined for human food. Although subcutaneous injections can be made, the pig's tight skin prevents injection of large volumes other than in the flank region and lateral side of the neck immediately posterior to the ear. The blood supply to fatty tissue is poor, and drug uptake and distribution from this tissue are very slow. Clinically, this often conveys a misconception about drug efficacy. The convenience of intramuscular injection is attractive, but if the drug is injected into fat, drug onset will be delayed and recovery will be prolonged. The possibility of injection into fatty tissue detracts from intramuscular injection technique in swine. This problem is frequently encountered in potbellied pigs when injections are made either in the neck or rump areas (Figs. 29.2 and 29.3).

For induction of anesthesia, intravenous injection is preferred, but the accessibility of veins is sparse in some breeds. In Landrace swine, the auricular veins are usually large and easily cannulated. Most injections are made in the central or ventrolateral auricular veins. The major artery is located on the dorsolateral aspect of the ear. Injection of an anesthetic (e.g., barbiturates) into the artery can cause tissue slough of the distal end of the ear. Using a tourniquet, it is possible to raise the cephalic vein located on the dorsomedial aspect of the forelimb between the elbow and carpus. However, this is often difficult in a struggling pig. A single needle puncture is almost essential; otherwise, a hematoma will often form, resulting in venous constriction.

In the rear limb, the femoral vein is prominent. Patient restraint for injection is a problem that often cannot be overcome unless a sedative is given. The medial and lateral saphenous veins are seldom used because of their small size and the difficulty of patient restraint when attempting vena puncture. The jugular vein can be entered if appropriate restraint is applied, but only if the vein is well cannulated should an anesthetic be injected. Of con-

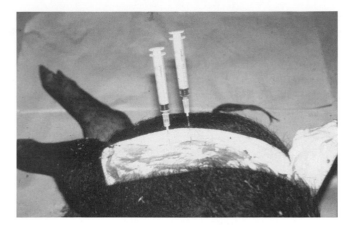

Fig. 29.3. Injection into the rump of an adult potbellied pig requires at least a 1.5-inch needle for intramuscular drug deposition.

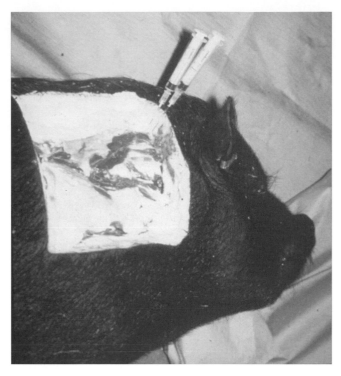

Fig. 29.2. Injection into neck region of an adult potbellied pig requires at least a 1.5-inch needle to reach muscle tissue.

cern is the close proximity of the carotid artery. An alternative to the jugular vein is the anterior vena cava. Entrance is made in the jugular furrow just lateral to the manubrium sterni, with the needle directed at the opposing shoulder. The right side is usually selected for vena cava puncture, even though the left side can be used. Injections should be given slowly. The anterior vena cava puncture is primarily used for blood-sample collection and is not recommended for anesthetic drug administration.

Tracheal Intubation

The technique of inserting a tube into each individual nostril, connected by a Y piece (Carlen's adaptor) and attached to the anesthetic rebreathing system, should be discouraged. This method does nothing to protect the airway from aspiration of vomitus. Further, any attempt to ventilate an apneic pig with nasal intubation can result in gastric distension (meteorism) and displacement of the diaphragm anteriorly. Functional lung capacity is decreased, increasing the likelihood of hypoxemia. The importance of tracheal intubation cannot be overemphasized. It provides a means of alveolar ventilation and protects the airway and lungs from aspiration of foreign material.[6]

Two primary body positions, dorsal or sternal recumbency, are used for tracheal intubation. The technique that best serves the anesthetist should be chosen. Once proficiency has been gained, body position is of little or no importance. Placing pigs in sternal recumbency appears to be best for those anesthetists that have had little or no experience. Gauze strips or small cotton ropes are placed behind the upper and lower canine teeth to open the pig's mouth. A mouth wedge designed specifically for swine may be

used with or without gauze strips. The pig's head should be extended, but excessive extension will make the arytenoid cartilages (i.e., laryngeal opening) more difficult to identify and in some cases can actually occlude the airway. For pigs weighing more than 50 kg, a laryngoscope with a 205-mm blade with an extension (4 to 8 cm long) is desirable. Although some anesthetists use the blade tip to depress the epiglottis, it is more desirable to set the blade so that when the handle is raised the tip of the blade displaces the base of the epiglottis ventrally, providing maximal exposure of the laryngeal opening. A local anesthetic (e.g., 1 to 3 mL of a 2% to 4% solution of lidocaine sprayed directly into the laryngeal opening) will relieve laryngeal spasms and coughing when intubating a lightly anesthetized pig. Succinylcholine (1 to 2 mg/kg intravenously [IV]) may be given, but this drug may trigger malignant hyperthermia in susceptible swine. Furthermore, because the rimaglottidis is so small and because the mouth cannot be opened widely, a plastic guide stylet (three times the length of the endotracheal tube) placed a short distance into the trachea can be safely used to guide the endotracheal tube through the larynx. Only cuffed tubes should be used in mature swine. When using a guide tube, it must be held stationary as the endotracheal tube is being inserted over it. A stiff stylet that is advanced deeply into the respiratory passages can injure the bronchial and peribronchial tissues. Tension pneumothorax could be a sequela.

A quick review of the anatomy of the pig's larynx (Fig. 29.4A and B) illustrates the tortuous course a tube must take to pass through the larynx and reach the trachea. When passing the tube without the aid of a stylet in a pig placed in a sternal position, the natural tube curvature is placed so that the tip is ventral. As the tube is advanced, it will meet resistance when the tip contacts the posterior floor of the larynx. At this point, rotate the tube 180° and apply minimal pressure. A correctly sized tube will be felt to start its descent into the trachea, at which time it should again be rotated back to its original position (i.e., with the curvature dorsal and the tip ventral). Some individuals with extremely fat jowls (e.g., large potbellied pigs) can often best be intubated while in lateral or dorsal recumbency (Fig. 29.4C). These posi-

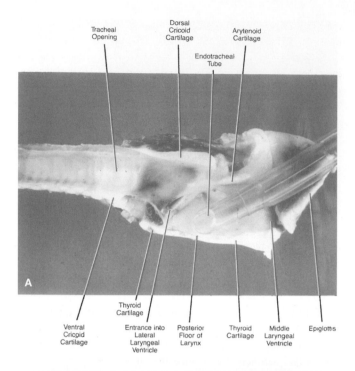

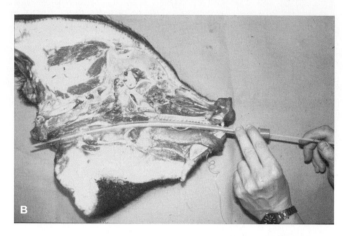

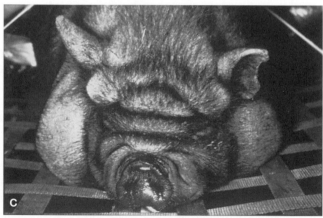

Fig. 29.4. **A:** A sagittal view of a pig's larynx and trachea. Note the acute angle between posterior portion of the larynx and the tracheal opening. Passage of the endotracheal tube is often difficult because of the entrapment of its tip in the floor of the larynx. Prior placement of a guide stylet through the tracheal opening will prevent entrapment of the endotracheal tube in the middle laryngeal ventricle just anterior to the thyroid cartilage and the posterior floor of the larynx anterior to the cricoid cartilage when the tube is passed into the trachea. **B:** A sagittal view of a potbellied pig's head with the endotracheal tube being positioned with the aid of a guide stylet. Note the small oral passageway and the tortuous route the tube must take through the larynx to finally enter the trachea. **C:** Potbellied pigs are often difficult to intubate, especially when extremely brachycephalic.

tions allow for a more direct route through the larynx and into the trachea. The size of the endotracheal tube is important. Practically, one should have three sizes at hand: the one thought to be correct, one size larger, and one size smaller. Tube sizes will range from 3 to 4 mm for piglets up to 16 to 18 mm in large boars or sows (Table 29.1).

Traumatic intubation that injures the delicate laryngeal mucosa can have a serious consequence. Formation of a hematoma or generalized laryngeal edema may go unnoticed, only to become evident when the tube is removed during recovery. Under all circumstances, the tube should not be removed until the pig is indicating laryngotracheal tube awareness as it awakens (e.g., coughing) or otherwise rejects the tube. A light spray of 2% to 4% lidocaine into the laryngeal opening just prior to or at the time of tube removal will often prevent laryngospasm after tube withdrawal.

The use of a laryngeal mask airway for induction of anesthesia with inhalation anesthetics eliminates the requirement for IV

Table 29.1. Endotracheal tube sizes for swine.

Swine size	Tube size (mm)
Piglets	3–5
10–15 kg	5–7
20–50 kg	8–10
100–200 kg	10–14
Larger pigs	16–18

injected drugs for induction, thus eliminating a major step in the anesthetic process of swine.[7] This technique was initially designed for people and has not been evaluated for use with artificial ventilation, which requires sealing of the upper airway. Endotracheal intubation is not technically difficult for experienced individuals.

Anesthetic Induction, Monitoring, and Recovery

Induction and Monitoring

The thiobarbiturates are the standard to which other injectable anesthetics are compared. Two other major classes of anesthetics that are commonly used in swine are the dissociatives (e.g., ketamine) and the inhalants. Induction drug popularity ebbs and flows but in large part is governed by proper preanesthetic medication. As in other species, so long as pigs are not overdosed, the chosen induction drug or drugs are of minimal importance.

The thiobarbiturates are considered monoanesthetics but are poor analgesics. The anesthetic dose is very close to the apneic dose. Repeated injection will saturate tissues and prolong recovery. There is no specific antagonist for barbiturates. Some drug combinations will provide better laryngeal relaxation than do barbiturates. A combination that provides good laryngeal relaxation consists of guaifenesin, ketamine, and xylazine (triple drip).

When anesthesia is being induced with an inhalant (e.g., halothane or isoflurane) in oxygen, there is a minimal amount of time to complete the intubation procedure once the nose cone is removed. Until regular breathing and signs of surgical anesthesia occur, the nose cone should be kept in place. Thus, the general procedure is to remove the nose cone, open the pig's mouth and quickly spray the laryngeal opening with lidocaine, replace the nose cone, and continue with inhalant administration. For intubation, the laryngeal opening is exposed and identified with a laryngoscope, and the tube put in place by one of two methods described earlier. After proper positioning of the tube, the cuff is inflated so that when a pressure of 18 to 20 cm H_2O is applied to the rebreathing circuit, a slight escapement of air can be heard from the pig's mouth.

Apnea is simply dealt with by rhythmically squeezing the rebreathing bag four to eight times per minute or by the use of an Ambu resuscitator bag when the patient is not connected to an anesthetic-rebreathing system. With the latter, either oxygen or ambient air can be used. Excessive ventilation will decrease blood carbon dioxide (CO_2) concentration and may prolong apnea. Experience gained in intubating pigs will increase an anesthetist's confidence and proficiency. Furthermore, an assistant who understands the anatomy of the pig's airway and appreciates the importance of keeping the pig's head and neck properly positioned is essential for a clean, safe, tracheal intubation.

The bispectral index (BIS) is a variable derived from an electroencephalogram that has been reported to be a measure of the hypnotic component of the anesthetic state. It has been used in people and animals to provide a measure of anesthetic depth. In swine, BIS values have a poor correlation with anesthetic depth and do not predict changes in arterial blood pressure or heart rate.[8,9] Nor have bispectral index values been useful for predicting recovery from either sevoflurane or propofol anesthesia.[9] It appears that BIS values should not be solely relied on to monitor anesthesia depth in swine.

Care During Recovery

Apnea resulting from laryngeal hematoma, edema, and/or spasms can occur and quickly cause death once the endotracheal tube is removed. Spraying the larynx with a modest amount of phenylephrine (Neosynephrine) prior to tube removal may be helpful in decreasing vascular congestion and edema formation in some cases. Thus, monitoring respiration and other signs during recovery is of the utmost importance. Less vigilant monitoring is required once a pig has gained its righting reflex and can maintain sternal position. Difficulty in breathing and restlessness accompanied by hypoxemia are usually the first signs of a traumatic recovery that must be dealt with at once, because time is crucial. Laryngeal edema can be treated by reintubation, but attempting to intubate a struggling pig is usually futile. If the intravenous catheter is still in place, the pig can be reanesthetized and an endotracheal tube quickly positioned to support ventilation. In extreme emergencies, it may be more efficient and less time consuming to quickly perform a tracheostomy after local anesthetic infiltration of tissues around the trachea.

It is important to keep piglets warm during recovery. If the chest or abdomen has been opened for any length of time in small pigs, it is essential to prevent further loss of body temperature and provide a source of external heat by covering the pig with a blanket or by using a warm-air–circulating device. Wrapping the extremities in bubble sheeting, the type used to pack fragile items for shipment, is helpful. Also, a sheet of this material between the patient and a cold surgical tabletop will help maintain body temperature. Warm fluids should be administered whenever possible.

Postoperative pain should be treated with appropriate analgesics. α_2-Adrenoceptor agonists, opioids, and local anesthetics can be administered alone or in combination to induce analgesia. These drugs have also been injected alone and in combination in the epidural space to provide postoperative analgesia. Opioid agonist-antagonists that can be injected parenterally in pigs to relieve postoperative pain include pentazocine (0.4 to 0.5 mg/kg intramuscularly [IM]), butorphanol (0.1 to 0.5 mg/kg IM or IV), nalbuphine (0.15 to 0.2 mg/kg IM), and buprenorphine (0.1 to 0.2 mg/kg IM or IV). Transdermal fentanyl patches that deliver 50 or 100 µg/h can also be used to control postoperative pain for 3 to 4 days.

Injectable Drugs

Parasympatholytic Drugs

The anticholinergic drugs atropine sulfate and glycopyrrolate are commonly used in swine. Because bradycardia is seldom a problem in anesthetized swine, the main use of these drugs is to inhibit excessive salivation. Neither drug is routinely required. Generally, the pig has a heart rate faster than 80 beats/min. Under clinical situations, a heart rate faster than 120 beats/min is not uncommon. Anticholinergics increase heart rate and thus myocardial work and oxygen consumption. Tachycardia can lead to a variety of other arrhythmias and, if not properly dealt with, can end in cardiac arrest. Preexisting bradycardia (i.e., heart rates below 50 beats/min) should be treated with either atropine (0.02 to 0.04 mg/kg IM) or glycopyrrolate (0.005 to 0.01 mg/kg IM) prior to anesthesia induction. Unlike cats and cattle, swine will respond to anticholinergics with a drier mouth. The airway will be drier and intubation easier. The major contraindication to this class of drugs is an existing tachycardia, as may be seen in patients with fever, extreme excitement, or hyperthyroidism.

Because swine occasionally vomit during the recovery period, glycopyrrolate would seem to be the anticholinergic of choice. This drug tends to decrease gastric fluid secretion and acid content and, unlike atropine, promotes gastric emptying. Further, glycopyrrolate is a large quaternary ammonia compound and does not readily cross the blood-brain barrier. In people, glycopyrrolate is considered to be about twice as potent an antisialagogue as atropine and has a longer action.[10]

Ataractics (Tranquilizers)

Phenothiazine derivatives are not as effective in swine as in many other species. Although tranquilized swine are easier to approach, they will still resist mechanical restraint vigorously. It seems that the most effective tranquilizer in swine is azaperone (a butyrophenone derivative). Most tranquilizers offer little or no analgesia. Thus, their use in anesthetizing swine is limited unless they are combined with other drugs that induce analgesia and depress CNS activity. For example, Innovar-Vet (droperidol and fentanyl) will provide reasonable calming if administered in pigs experiencing pain. However, if aroused, pigs often sneeze and appear to become more excited after drug injection. When Innovar-Vet is combined with xylazine, sedation is more pronounced, and pigs often lie quietly for some time. However, pigs will often respond vigorously to painful manipulation. Veterinary practitioners have reportedly given extremely large doses of phenothiazine tranquilizers along with local analgesics to induce intense quiescence in older sows undergoing cesarean section. The use of these high doses can induce intense vascular alpha-receptor blockade, resulting in hypotensive shock, and should be discouraged. Many of these sows fail to recover, even though their piglets reportedly recover satisfactorily. The use of high doses of a tranquilizer as a substitute for an anesthetic is improper in any species.

Butyrophenone tranquilizers include droperidol, fluanisone, and azaperone. Although azaperone is often used as a preanesthetic, its predominant use (2.5 mg/kg IM) is to prevent fighting and anxiety among newly mixed pigs. Large doses will induce deep tranquilization and hypotension. The recommended intramuscular dose of azaperone for preanesthetic tranquilization ranges from 2 mg/kg in older, large swine to 8 mg/kg in young swine for purposes of immobilization. The use of droperidol as a sedative in pigs has also been described. A dose of 0.3 mg/kg IM induced sedation within 5 min, with a duration of about 2 h.[11]

The benzodiazepines (i.e., minor tranquilizers) are useful in swine but expensive. Although there are many benzodiazepine derivatives, diazepam and midazolam are most frequently used in North America. Reportedly, flurazepam (2 mg/kg IV),[12] lorazepam (0.1 mg/kg IV),[13] brotizolam (1 to 10 mg/kg orally),[14] and zolazepam (a component of Telazol) produce good effects in swine. Benzodiazepines induce hypnosis, sedation, and muscle relaxation, but little or no analgesia. Thus, they are generally combined with an anesthetic or strong analgesic to enhance anesthetic action. Diazepam (1 to 10 mg/kg IM or 0.5 to 2.0 mg/kg IV) is usually combined with ketamine and xylazine or with an inhalant for its additive muscle-relaxing and sedative effects. Diazepam, as is true of most benzodiazepine derivatives, will decrease anesthetic requirement even though it is not a strong analgesic. When given in large doses, benzodiazepines prolong recovery. This is particularly true in older sows and boars given large intramuscular doses. Midazolam, unlike diazepam, is water soluble and may be given by either the intravenous route or intramuscular route without causing severe pain. The dose ranges from 0.1 to 0.5 mg/kg, with 0.5 mg/kg IM providing adequate sedation for conducting minor procedures in swine.[11] Midazolam is approximately twice as potent as diazepam.

Sedation can be achieved with intranasally injected midazolam (0.2 or 0.4 mg/kg).[15] Midazolam induces significant calming and sedation within 3 to 4 min. The optimal intranasal dose of midazolam to induce rapid and reliable sedation in laboratory piglets is approximately 0.2 mg/kg.

Flumazenil is a specific benzodiazepine antagonist. The minimal effective dose for reversal of diazepam or midazolam has not been established in swine. Clinical experience suggests that a dose of 1 part flumazenil to 13 parts of a benzodiazepine agonist will adequately antagonize lingering sedation and muscle relaxation (e.g., if 1.3 mg/kg of diazepam is given, 0.1 mg/kg of flumazenil is required). When using this ratio, flumazenil demonstrates good efficacy in antagonizing the residual muscle-relaxing actions of zolazepam in mature swine.

α_2-Adrenoceptor Agonists

The α_2-adrenoceptor agonists available for veterinary use include xylazine, detomidine, romifidine, and medetomidine. However, only xylazine has been used to any great extent in swine. Although xylazine is an extremely potent sedative in other animal species, it is not in swine. After injection of xylazine or detomidine, some sedation is apparent. Pigs will usually lie down in 10 to 15 min but, when approached, will rapidly rise and flee. Thus, in swine, xylazine is usually combined with other drugs. For example, xylazine and ketamine have become a popular anesthetic drug combination for use in swine. The dose of xylazine ranges from 1 to 2 mg/kg administered either IM or IV. The intravenous dose of detomidine or medetomidine is 40 µg/kg, whereas the intramuscular dose of either agent is reportedly 80 µg/kg. Sedation from α_2-adrenoceptor agonists can be effectively antagonized with either yohimbine (0.15 to 0.2 mg/kg IV) or tolazoline (2 to 4 mg/kg IV). Atipamezole, which is also a very effective α-adrenoceptor antagonist, has been used at doses ranging from 200 to 300 µg/kg IM to reverse α_2-agonist effects in pigs.[16]

In isoflurane (1.3% end-tidal sample)-anesthetized swine (15 to 35 kg), studies designed to test the analgesic effects of xylazine, medetomidine, and detomidine revealed that xylazine (2 mg/kg) and medetomidine (40 µg/kg), but neither detomidine (40 µg/kg) nor the α_2-antagonist atipamezole (200 µg/kg), provided short-term analgesia.[17] All α_2-agonists increased blood pressure. Of interest, atipamezole administration increased blood pressure, apparently as a result of an increase in heart rate, that persisted throughout the postanesthetic observation period. These results suggest that α_2-agonists provide only short-term analgesia and that their use as preemptive analgesics may not be an appropriate choice.

α_2-Agonist Epidural Analgesia

Xylazine has both α_1 and α_2 activity, whereas detomidine acts predominately at α_2-adrenoceptors. Both alpha-subtype receptors are located in the dorsal horn of the spinal cord.[18,19] Also, analgesia can be induced by both α_1- and α_2-adrenergic agonists when injected intrathecally.[20] This finding supports the speculation that xylazine-induced analgesia is mediated in part by α-adrenoceptor stimulation. The ratio of α_1- to α_2-adrenoceptors in the spinal cord of domestic swine has not been determined. Xylazine induces more profound analgesia than does detomidine in this species.[19] In pigs receiving either intrathecal xylazine or detomidine, the response is different after a pure α_2-antagonist (e.g., atipamezole) is administered. In detomidine-treated pigs, sedation, analgesia, and immobilization are quickly abolished after intravenous injection of atipamezole. In xylazine-treated pigs, however, sedation is abolished, but loss of motor and sensory responses posterior to the site of xylazine injection remains.[19] Seemingly, this indicates the presence of a xylazine-induced spinal local analgesic effect. This has also been reported in horses and cattle.[21-23] Although epidural injection of either xylazine or detomidine induces some sedation, analgesia, and immobilization, the intensity of analgesia appears to be greater with xylazine. Xylazine's superior analgesic action could be mediated by either its α_1-adrenoceptor activity located in the dorsal horn of the spinal cord and/or a local analgesic effect independent of α-adrenoceptor stimulation.[19]

With this knowledge, sows weighing from 150 to 225 kg scheduled for a cesarean section can be given an epidural injection of 10 mL of 2% lidocaine containing xylazine at a dose of 0.5 to 1.0 mg/kg. The onset of sedation, analgesia, and rear-limb immobilization are rapid. Complete immobilization of the rear quarters lasts for approximately 3 to 4 h. Sows will lie quietly for over 1 h, at which time some front-limb movement may occur. Even though there is some xylazine-induced sedation, the forelimbs should be tethered. Piglets are lively when delivered and experience no difficulty in breathing. Lingering sedation can be effectively antagonized with either yohimbine (0.15 to 0.2 mg/kg IV), tolazoline (2 to 4 mg/kg IV), or atipamezole (200 to 300 µg/kg IM). Veterinarians skilled in the technique of epidural injection will find this a useful anesthetic regimen for use in swine when analgesia posterior to the umbilicus and mild sedation are both required.

Barbiturates

Because barbiturates are given primarily by intravenous injection in the ear vein, dilute solutions are preferred (i.e., 5% concentration or less). Perivascular injection will often cause sloughing of the skin surrounding the vessel. The thiobarbiturates (i.e., thiopental and thiamylal) and oxybarbiturates can be used in swine either by a repeated bolus technique or by continuous infusion.[24,25] If properly ventilated, pigs will survive extraordinarily large doses over time, but recovery may be extremely long. Because of their rapid onset and shorter duration of action in

swine, thiobarbiturates (e.g., thiopental) are preferred over oxybarbiturates (e.g., pentobarbital). The effect of a barbiturate may be enhanced with xylazine (1 to 2 mg/kg), ketamine (2 to 4 mg/kg), a benzodiazepine (e.g., diazepam, 2 to 4 mg/kg), or another tranquilizer (e.g., azaperone, 2 to 4 mg/kg). When a barbiturate is used alone for more than a brief period of surgical anesthesia, the patient's trachea should be intubated, and a means of instituting positive pressure ventilation must be at hand. An Ambu bag will serve this purpose well because it may be used to ventilate with ambient air or oxygen. Properly ventilated pigs can tolerate three times the surgical dose of a barbiturate. Death of swine from barbiturates is usually a direct result of respiratory arrest.

Pentobarbital is vaguely classed as a short-acting barbiturate, but when dosed repeatedly or administered as a constant infusion, recovery will be prolonged. The anesthetic dose of pentobarbital ranges from 20 to 40 mg/kg IV. When given as a continuous infusion, the recommended dose is 5 to 15 mg $\cdot$ k^{-1} $\cdot$ h^{-1}.[24,25] Xylazine will decrease the anesthetizing dose of pentobarbital measurably, as will diazepam or ketamine.[24]

Pentobarbital is an extremely effective anticonvulsant. Diazepam can be given for this purpose but has a shorter period of action and is much more expensive. In addition, dysphoria, often seen in swine recovering from ketamine administration, can be controlled with pentobarbital (6 to 10 mg/kg IV or IM). When possible, the smaller dose is given slowly IV. When intravenous injection is not possible, the larger dose (10 mg/kg) diluted to 3% or less with saline or water may be given IM. When administered IM as a dilute solution, pentobarbital should be injected deeply into a large muscle mass. In commercial swine, the most appropriate site for intramuscular injection is the neck muscle just caudal to the ear.

Commercially available thiobarbiturates are sold as desiccated powders and solubilized with either distilled water or saline. Concentrations of 2.5% to 5% are preferred. Until the removal of thiamylal from the market, it was the most widely used barbiturate in veterinary patients, including swine. Thiobarbiturates are characterized as being ultra-short-acting. This is somewhat of a misnomer inasmuch as duration of action correlates directly with total dose. More correctly stated, these barbiturates have a more rapid onset of action than oxybarbiturates.

The thiobarbiturates are more soluble in blood and tissue than are the oxybarbiturates (e.g., pentobarbital). Thus, the induction dose is less and recovery time is shorter after a single bolus injection of thiobarbiturate. As with the oxybarbiturates, thiobarbiturates are sometimes used as monoanesthetics. Analgesia is minimal until deep planes of anesthesia occur. As previously stated, the dose for deep surgical anesthesia is very close to the apneic dose. The induction dose of either thiopental or thiamylal ranges from 10 to 20 mg/kg IV. The higher dose is given in unpremedicated young swine and the lower dose in sedate or tranquilized swine. To a large extent, the dose depends on the degree of analgesia and immobilization required. For example, procedures that are pain free, such as radiography, require a minimal dose. The dose also depends on the physical condition of the patient and availability of respiratory support equipment. When thiamylal or thiopental is used as a continuous infusion to maintain anesthesia, the recommended dose is 3 to 6 mg · kg^{-1} · h^{-1} IV.[24,25]

Because the swallowing reflex remains intact after induction with a dissociative (e.g., ketamine or tiletamine), a small dose of thiopental (4 to 6 mg/kg IV) can be used to abolish laryngeal reflexes that interfere with endotracheal intubation. Specific antagonists for barbiturates are unavailable at this time. However, after ensuring a patent airway, an analeptic such as doxapram (0.50 to 1.0 mg/kg IV) can be used to stimulate breathing. This effect can be short-lived in patients that have received large doses of a barbiturate. Under such circumstances, mechanical ventilation should be initiated and continued until the pig reinitiates spontaneous breathing.

Injectable anesthetic drug combinations, because of ease of administration and economic concerns, have become extremely important in swine destined for short-term anesthesia. An important study used 46 mature swine to compare the effects of several anesthetic combinations. One group was given azaperone (1.0 mg/kg IM) and ketamine (2.5 mg/kg IM), a second group received etomidate (200 µg/kg IV) followed by midazolam (100 µg/kg IM), and a third group was given ketamine (2 mg/kg IM) and midazolam (100 µg/kg IM). The remainder of the pigs (n = 15) were given pentobarbital (15 to 20 mg/kg IV). Clinical comparison of the foregoing drug combinations with pentobarbital alone clearly revealed that pentobarbital caused more respiratory depression and a higher complication rate than all the other drug combinations.[26] Pentobarbital caused severe respiratory depression. Apnea occurred in two pigs and was fatal in one. Positive-pressure ventilation with oxygen was required in three other pigs to sustain pulmonary function. It seems that, although pentobarbital is a useful injectable anesthetic, surgical anesthesia with this drug requires close patient observation and ventilatory support. As a matter of fact, when pentobarbital is used alone, veterinarians should be prepared to deal with apnea; otherwise, anesthetic catastrophes are inevitable. In summary, the thiobarbiturates are useful in swine, but they cannot be recommended as monoanesthetics for prolonged surgery without controlled ventilation and/or when rapid patient recovery is required.

Methohexital is an ultra-short-acting methylated oxybarbiturate that is approximately three times as potent as thiopental. It is usually prepared in a 2.5% solution. In veterinary practice, it has been used primarily in sight hounds because of its brief action. It has proven an effective induction anesthetic in many species when administered IV. It may also be given to maintain anesthesia by continuous infusion. However, it induces muscle fasciculations during induction, and recovery is often described as rough in swine not receiving preanesthetic medication (e.g., xylazine or azaperone). Methohexital is used most often to induce anesthesia, followed by maintenance with an inhalant. As with the thiobarbiturates, the dose varies considerably and depends on the type and amount of preanesthetic given. In healthy, unpremedicated, commercial swine, the dose ranges from 6 to 10 mg/kg IV. In potbellied pigs, one-half to two-thirds the dose recommended for commercial swine appears to be appropriate.

Recovery from a single anesthetizing dose of methohexital is usually complete in 20 to 30 min. As with all barbiturates, respiratory depression and apnea are the most serious problems encountered when high doses are injected rapidly IV or when repeat doses are given. The necessity for repeat administration has been largely resolved under field conditions by providing complete analgesia with local infiltration of the surgical site or epidural injection of a local anesthetic. Lidocaine (2%) is a reasonable choice for local infiltration and often enables completion of minor surgery as the pig recovers from barbiturate-induced unconsciousness.

Dissociatives

Drugs disconnecting higher brain centers (thalamocortical) from lower centers (limbic systems) are referred to as *dissociative* anesthetics. The first dissociative used in veterinary anesthesia was phencyclidine hydrochloride. Although its use in swine and bears gained some popularity, illicit use as a street drug resulted in its removal from the medical market. Subsequently, tamer and perhaps less addictive derivatives were synthesized: ketamine and tiletamine. These drugs have become popular for anesthesia induction and brief surgical procedures when combined with α$_2$-agonists, opioids, and/or benzodiazepines.

Ketamine, an extremely popular and widely used anesthetic in people and animals, and its predecessor, phencyclidine, are often referred to as "pig tranquilizers" by uneducated individuals. Attempts to use these agents as monoanesthetics in swine have not induced effective surgical anesthesia. On the other hand, when combined with opioids, benzodiazepines, and or α$_2$-agonists, the level of anesthesia and analgesia increases. Such drug combinations can be used to provide both long-term and short-term anesthesia in swine. Typically, prolonged anesthesia and analgesia requires coadministration of sedative and analgesic drugs. Without added sedation and analgesia, recoveries can be extremely rough and prolonged.[27]

Tiletamine is available only in a proprietary compound (Telazol). This drug combination consists of a 1:1 mixture of tiletamine and zolazepam. The latter is a benzodiazepine similar to diazepam but more potent. Anesthesia induced with dissociatives is characterized by incomplete muscle relaxation, often referred to as a *cataleptoid state*. Zolazepam tends to relieve this problem by providing muscle relaxation but does not seem to add measurably to analgesia.

Dissociative-induced analgesia appears to result in part from its action on N-methyl-D-aspartate (NMDA) and opioid receptors. However, attempts to antagonize ketamine's action with naloxone have not been effective.[28] During ketamine anesthesia, the patient's eyes remain open and the swallowing reflex usually remains intact. However, this does not prevent the patient from aspirating vomitus should vomiting occur during anesthesia. Vomition can be a real threat when pigs are not properly fasted. In people, ketamine-induced analgesia has been described as intense.[29] From clinical and laboratory observations, ketamine does not appear to induce analgesia in swine of the same magnitude as that described in people.[30]

Because ketamine induces excessive salivation in swine, it seems logical to administer an anticholinergic (atropine, 0.04 mg/kg IM). However, the use of atropine should be avoided in patients with tachycardia or fever. When given IM at a dose of 10 to 12 mg/kg, ketamine will immobilize swine in approximately 5 min. Although xylazine does not provide good muscle relaxation or sedation when given alone, it will greatly enhance the anesthetic effects of ketamine. The xylazine dose range is 2 to 3 mg/kg IM or 1 to 2 mg/kg IV. When combined with ketamine, xylazine improves analgesia and muscle relaxation.[4] When necessary, anesthesia can be prolonged in healthy patients by using 2 to 4 mg/kg of ketamine and 0.5 to 1.0 mg/kg of xylazine mixed in the same syringe and injected slowly IV. When an auricular vein can be cannulated prior to induction, ketamine should be administered IV. A smaller dose is required (4 to 6 mg/kg). Recovery is quicker and excitement during recovery is less likely to occur with the lower intravenous dose. Excitement during recovery is most often seen in old, mature sows and boars but is less likely when xylazine is a part of the anesthetic regimen.

Because physical restraint is frequently difficult in mature swine, the intramuscular route is often used to immobilize large patients. A drug combination that reportedly works well when administered IM is ketamine (4 mg/kg), oxymorphone (0.15 mg/kg), and xylazine (4 mg/kg). If an intravenous injection can be made, the dose of each drug is decreased by one-half.[4,31] This drug combination, although expensive, offers relatively good analgesia and muscle relaxation. Recovery is generally smooth and can be hastened with naloxone and yohimbine administration. It should be remembered that oxymorphone and xylazine reversal antagonizes postoperative analgesia and sedation. An excitatory response may ensue.

Ketamine (6 to 8 mg/kg) and xylazine (1 to 2 mg/kg) drawn into the same syringe may be safely used to anesthetize large boars for castration. One-half of the drug combination is injected deep into the center of each testicle. Rapid castration removes the remaining drug contained in the testicle, promoting a rapid recovery. Large doses of pentobarbital have also been administered intratesticularly for the same purpose, but recoveries are considerably longer.

The 5-mL vials of Telazol contain 250 mg of tiletamine and 250 mg of zolazepam. Zolazepam is similar to diazepam but is water soluble and more potent than diazepam. As previously mentioned, zolazepam has a central muscle-relaxant action that partially relieves the cataleptoid state induced by a dissociative. Excessive or repeat dosing of Telazol can cause prolonged recovery, particularly in older swine and other large species. Telazol is approved only for intramuscular use in dogs and cats but has been widely used in other species, including swine.

Telazol alone does not provide enough CNS depression and analgesia for most surgical procedures but can be an effective anesthetic in swine when combined with the proper adjunct. Presently, xylazine is the most popular drug for this purpose. α_2-Agonists have been shown to decrease the requirement for inhalant anesthesia by as much as 90%. Telazol (6.6 mg/kg IM) combined with xylazine (2.2 mg/kg IM) immobilizes 20- to 30-kg pigs in 1 to 2 min, and the anesthetic time extends up to approximately 1 h. Tracheal intubation is easily performed.[32] These drugs can be mixed in the same syringe for easier administration. Prolonged recoveries have been experienced in old sows and

boars when given the dose reported for 20- to 30-kg pigs. Extended recoveries are more likely when this drug regimen is administered IM or after redosing to extend anesthesia. Prolonged recovery appears to be due in large part to zolazepam's lingering effects. Consequently, smaller intravenous doses are recommended for older swine (Telazol, 2.2 to 4.4 mg/kg; and xylazine, 1.1 mg/kg). When using the intravenous route, anesthesia may be safely extended by giving one-half the original dose as required.

Telazol and xylazine have been used extensively to immobilize collared peccaries (*Tayassu tajacu*) and feral swine (*Sus scrofa*) for several years. This drug combination, when precisely combined, is one of most effective immobilizing compounds for swine when injected IM. Of interest is a study that shows that a 1:1 mixture of Telazol and xylazine (100 mg Telazol + 100 mg xylazine/mL) effectively and safely immobilizes wild collared peccaries as well as feral domestic swine (*Sus scrofa*). The mixture dose of 4 to 5 mg/kg IM was effective in both species. Immobilization time was rapid (4 to 5 min), and recovery times ranged from 54 to 78 min.[33]

Another report has suggested that a combination of Telazol and xylazine effectively and safely immobilized the babirusa species (*Babyrousa babyrussa*).[34] Anesthesia in females required a higher induction dose than did that in males. Xylazine was administered first in females at a dose of 1.88 ± 0.37 mg/kg IM, whereas males received 1.22 ± 0.16 mg/kg IM. After xylazine premedication, anesthesia was induced with Telazol at a dose of 2.2 mg/kg in females and 1.7 mg/kg IM in males. This anesthetic combination is reported to have rapidly induced immobilization, analgesia, and good muscle relaxation. However, supplemental ketamine was given to prolong anesthesia, when required. The sedative and muscle-relaxing actions of xylazine and zolazepam were safely and rapidly antagonized by yohimbine (0.15 mg/kg IM) and flumazenil (1 mg/20 mg of zolazepam IM), respectively. Interestingly, atipamezole (200 to 300 µg/kg IM) appears to be a more effective α_2-antagonist in swine than does yohimbine.

Injectable Drug Combinations

Telazol-Ketamine-Xylazine (TKX)

Zolazepam appears to be responsible for the posterior weakness observed in recovering mature swine when Telazol is given IM in anesthetic doses. To minimize this problem, the dissociative content in the Telazol mixture can be increased by adding ketamine. Xylazine is also added to increase the sedative and analgesic effects of the mixture. In an unused vial of Telazol, 2.5 mL of ketamine (100 mg/mL) and 2.5 mL of xylazine (100 mg/mL) are added to dissolve the powder. This mixture provides 100 mg of dissociative/mL (tiletamine plus ketamine) and 50 mg/mL each of xylazine and zolazepam. In this mixture, zolazepam constitutes only 25% of the total drug dose rather than the 50% found in the proprietary mixture.

For commercial swine, the recommended dose of this drug combination is 1 mL/35 to 75 kg IM, depending on the anesthetic depth required. For sedation and light anesthesia, potbellied pigs appear to require a smaller dose, approximately one-half that given to commercial swine. Anesthesia may be extended by injecting one-half the intramuscular dose slowly IV to avoid apnea or by administering either halothane or isoflurane in oxygen from a nose cone. The inhalation anesthetic requirement is greatly decreased with this drug mixture.

In growing swine weighing 20 to 45 kg under field conditions, three injectable general anesthetic drug combinations were compared, including azaperone (2 mg/kg IM) + metomidate (10 mg/kg intraperitoneally); tiletamine + zolazepam (6 mg/kg IM) + xylazine (2 mg/kg IM); and tiletamine + zolazepam + ketamine + xylazine (TKX, 1 mL/45 kg IM) (as described previously). Clinical observations, plus pinprick and ease of drug mixture, were used to evaluate anesthetic effectiveness.[35] Although this study did not find any significant differences between the three anesthetic protocols, past experience and reports have clearly shown that TKX is superior to all combinations evaluated. Preparation of drug mixtures should not be considered a major disadvantage when such mixtures better provide for smooth induction, good analgesia, muscle relaxation, and rapid recovery.

In another study, four anesthetic drug combinations were evaluated in swine. These combinations included TKX (Telazol, 4.4 mg/kg IM; ketamine, 2.2 mg/kg IM; and xylazine, 2.2 mg/kg IM); TX (Telazol, 4.4 mg/kg IM; and xylazine, 2.2 mg/kg IM); T2X (Telazol, 4.4 mg/kg IM; and xylazine, 4.4 mg/kg IM); and KX (ketamine, 8 mg/kg IM; and xylazine, 4 mg/kg IM). These drug combinations were evaluated for restraint and induction of surgical anesthesia in 40 swine, 10 in each group. All drug combinations were drawn up singularly, mixed in a single syringe, and administered as a single intramuscular injection. All combinations were reportedly safe and satisfactory for anesthesia induction in swine of this age (6 to 8 months). However, the TKX and T2X combinations were preferred.[36]

Because of the popularity of potbellied pigs as companion animals, practitioners are occasionally asked to perform selected surgical and diagnostic procedures on these swine (e.g., hoof trim, hernia repair, ovariohysterectomy, castration, cesarean section, and ultrasound for pregnancy diagnosis). The potbellied pig's body appears to be sturdily built but is heavily covered with fatty tissue, and drug injection can be problematic. Table 29.2 lists a variety of drugs and combinations used in this breed of swine. For predictable response, care must be taken to ensure the anesthetic drugs are deposited into muscle and not fat when intramuscular injection is attempted.

Guaifenesin-Ketamine-Xylazine (Triple Drip)

This drug combination is prepared by adding 2 mg of ketamine and 1 mg of xylazine to each milliliter of 5% guaifenesin prepared in 5% dextrose in water. The drug combination must be administered IV. This can be a major problem because of the absence of accessible auricular veins in some individuals. The induction dose ranges from 0.67 to 1.0 mL of the mixture per kilogram. The average anesthetic maintenance dose is 2.2 mL · $kg^{-1} · h^{-1}$. Using a standard intravenous delivery set (15 drops = 1 mL), the maintenance dose is calculated as follows: (kilograms of body weight) $\times$ (2.2 mL · $kg^{-1} · h^{-1}$) $\times$ 15 drops/mL divided by 60 = drops/min and when divided again by 60 =

drops/s. In a 150-kg sow, induction would require approximately 100 to 150 mL, depending on the rate of injection. Maintenance would be calculated as follows: 150 $\times$ 2.2 $\times$ 15 = 4950 drops/h divided by 60 = 83 drops/min, divided by 60 again = approximately 1.4 drops/s. This dosage rate is sufficient for the average sow. Sows that have been in prolonged labor usually require a smaller dose. On the other hand, young, vigorous sows, in labor for only a short time, may require an increased dose. Animal response will serve as a guide to dose requirement. As with any injectable mixture, it should be given to effect as measured by monitoring of vital signs.

Induction and recovery from this anesthetic mixture are rapid (recovery occurring in 30 to 45 min). Recovery time can be decreased by intravenous injection of a specific xylazine antagonist (e.g., yohimbine, 0.06 to 0.1 mg/kg; or tolazoline, 2 to 4 mg/kg). When the α_2-antagonist is given, postoperative analgesia is diminished. Rapid arousal to the antagonist suggests that xylazine is most likely responsible for residual anesthetic effect during recovery following continuous infusion of triple drip.

Triple drip used for cesarean section provides excellent relaxation and analgesia. Piglets are only minimally depressed. Clearly, neonatal depression is directly related to the total dose of triple drip prior to fetal delivery. Surgical speed is of the essence. Xylazine likely is responsible for neonatal respiratory depression. This speculation is based on clinical observations that piglets will quickly commence breathing after a small dose of an α_2-antagonist is administered. A minimal dose of doxapram (i.e., 0.25 to 0.5 mg/kg) can also be used to stimulate breathing once the airway is cleared.[4]

Medetomidine-Butorphanol-Ketamine

The intramuscular administration of MBK (atropine, 25 µg/kg, and medetomidine, 80 µg/kg; combined with butorphanol, 200 µg/kg, and ketamine, 10 mg/kg) has also provided appropriate anesthesia and analgesia for short-term surgical procedures in pigs.[37] Anesthesia induction is rapid and is sufficient to support surgical procedures for at least 30 to 45 min. Recovery is generally smooth but can be effectively and quickly reversed with atipamezole (240 µg/kg IM), if necessary. This combination was reportedly less cardiorespiratory depressive and more profoundly analgesic than a combination consisting of xylazine (2 mg/kg), butorphanol (200 µg/kg), and ketamine (10 mg/kg) given IM. The loss of response to painful stimuli was greater with MBK than with XBK. The authors suggest that MBK may be a superior drug combination for brief surgical analgesia/anesthesia. This combination has also been used in potbellied pigs when rapid recovery is desired.

Inhalation Anesthetics

The inhalants are safe anesthetics for swine other than for those individuals susceptible to malignant hyperthermia. Because of the equipment required for administration, inhalants can only be used practically within hospitals. Halothane and isoflurane have been the primary inhalants used in swine. Enflurane, an isomer of isoflurane, is of limited use without appropriate premedica-

Table 29.2. Doses of preanesthetic and anesthetic induction drugs used in potbellied pigs.[65]

Drug	Dose (mg/kg)	Route	Comments
Preanesthetic drugs			
Acepromazine	0.10–0.45	IM	Slow onset of action, 20–30 min to peak effect; no analgesia; maximum dose, 15 mg
Xylazine	1.0–2.0	IM	Minimal sedation; may cause vomiting before surgery or during recovery; administer with atropine to block increased vagal tone; will offset hyperalgesic effect produced by thiobarbiturates
Diazepam	0.5–1.0	IV	Effective central muscle relaxant; high doses produce ataxia and recumbency
	4.0–8.0	IM	
Fentanyl citrate and droperidol	1.0 mL/10 kg	IM	Administer with atropine 20–30 min before induction; excitement and goose-stepping may occur
Azaperone	0.23–2.5	IM	Light sedation produced
Induction drugs			
Ketamine	20	IM	Poor analgesia and muscle relaxation
Tiletamine-zolazepam (Telazol)	4.4	IM	Inadequate for intubation; rough recovery, characterized by vocalization, excessive salivation, and paddling motions
Thiobarbiturates			
Thiopental or	10–20	IV	Concentration should be 5% or less; administered one-half as rapid bolus to unpremedicated pigs; supplemental doses prolong recovery
Thiamylal	6–18	IV	
Injectable drug combinations			
Acepromazine plus	0.5	IM	Onset of recumbency within 5 min; unreliable; recovery in 65 to 80 min
Ketamine	15.0 (given 20 min after acepromazine injection)		
Diazepam plus	1.0–2.0	IM	Analgesia not as profound as with xylazine-ketamine; smooth recovery; mix together in one syringe
Ketamine	10–18		
Xylazine plus	2.2	IM	Mix together in one syringe to administer; good induction combination; intubation easily performed; acceptable short-term anesthesia with smooth recovery
Tiletamine-zolazepam (Telazol)	4.4		
Atropine plus	0.044	IM	Similar to the xylazine-tiletamine-zolazepam combination; smooth recovery in 2 h
Xylazine plus	4.4		
Tiletamine-Zolazepam (Telazol)	6.0		
Xylazine[a] Ketamine Tiletamine-Zolazepam (Telazol)	1 mL/75 kg	IV	Anesthesia can be maintained with 0.5 mL/75 kg IV; must be given slowly (over 60 s) to minimize respiratory depression
Xylazine[a] Ketamine Tiletamine-Zolazepam (Telazol)	1 mL/25 kg	IM	Good induction combination; intubation possible; recovery smoother than tiletamine-zolazepam alone; 80-min duration
Atropine plus	0.025	IM	Mix together in one syringe; rapid induction of anesthesia and good analgesia; suitable for minor surgery; duration approximately 30–45 min; recovery smooth and rapid but can be reversed with atipamezole (0.24 mg/kg IM)
Medetomidine plus	0.08		
Butorphanol plus	0.2		
Ketamine	10.0		
Xylazine	2.20	IV	Mix together in one syringe; suitable for short-term anesthesia and minor surgery; rapid and shallow breathing; duration approximately 20–30 min; smooth, rapid recovery; all doses may be doubled for administration IM
Ketamine	2.0		
Oxymorphone	0.075		
GKX for swine (triple drip)[b]	0.5–1.0 mL/kg (to induce); 2.0 mL/kg/h to maintain anesthesia	IV	Decrease induction dose 50% if tranquilizer or sedative is administered; administer atropine IM before induction; rapid recovery after discontinuing GKX infusion; recovery may be hastened by administration of yohimbine (0.125 mg/kg IV)
Inhalation agents			
Isoflurane	To effect	Inhalation	Recommended for young or sick pigs; recovery rapid
Sevoflurane	To effect	Inhalation	Recommended for young or sick pigs; recovery rapid

IM, intramuscularly; IV, intravenously.

[a]Make the combination by reconstituting tiletamine-zolazepam (Telazol) with 2.5 mL of ketamine (100 mg/mL) and 2.5 mL of xylazine (100 mg/mL). Each milliliter of the resultant combination will contain 50 mg of tiletamine, 50 mg of zolazepam, 50 mg of ketamine, and 50 mg of xylazine.

[b]The solution contains 50 mg/mL of glycerol guaiacolate, 2 mg/mL of ketamine, and 1 mg/mL of xylazine. The combination should be mixed in the desired quantity immediately before use, because of the potential diminished potency of the mixture during storage. The concentration of drugs in this mixture varies among species.

From Wertz and Wagnert.[65]

tion. High inspired concentrations of enflurane can cause a seizurelike response.

Desflurane is an isomer of isoflurane and is nonflammable. It is more volatile than either halothane or isoflurane. Because of this physical characteristic, it requires a special vaporizer for its administration. These vaporizers are extremely expensive and limit desflurane's use primarily to people and possibly swine research. Because its solubility in blood is much lower than that of the other halogenated drugs, induction of anesthesia and recovery are very rapid and depth can be readily regulated. In swine, desflurane's minimal alveolar concentration (MAC) is somewhere between 8% and 10%.

Isolated perfused-lung studies have shown that halogenated anesthetics decrease pulmonary vasoconstrictor response to alveolar hypoxia. The results of studies in intact animals have been less convincing. More importantly, sevoflurane at a clinical dose (1 MAC) had no clinically significant effect on hypoxic-pulmonary vasoconstriction in anesthetized piglets.[38] This suggests that, at clinical doses, sevoflurane and likely other inhalants are extremely safe to use in healthy swine.

In some circumstances, nitrous oxide (N_2O) can be used to enhance the effects of other inhalants (e.g., halothane and isoflurane). Normobaric extrapolation studies reveal that an inspired concentration of nearly 200% would be required for complete anesthesia in swine.[39] The requirement for high concentrations of N_2O to decrease the inhaled concentration of the major anesthetic can aggravate hypoxic conditions. Rapid movement of N_2O from the blood to the alveoli at the termination of anesthesia, when the pig is permitted to breathe ambient air, can also cause diffusion hypoxia. Thus, to avoid this potential complication, pigs should be permitted to breathe a high concentration of oxygen for 5 to 10 min after discontinuing N_2O administration.

Isoflurane has a broad safety margin. It is more insoluble in blood and tissue than is halothane. This physical property is highly desirable because it produces a more rapid induction and recovery. The anesthetic depth is easily regulated. Both inhalants quickly cross the placental barrier and depress the fetus. Isoflurane is more desirable when performing cesarean section. After delivery and once breathing is initiated, piglets rapidly eliminate isoflurane from body tissues. CNS depression disappears rapidly. Although halothane is less expensive, the recovery time of neonates is longer. Because of their high vapor pressures, newer inhalants should be administered only from equipment designed specifically for their use. Their high vapor pressures and relatively small safety margins prohibit use by the open-drop method.

The physical characteristics of halothane and isoflurane are similar enough that they may be administered from the same precision vaporizer designed specifically for either drug. For example, isoflurane can be administered from a properly cleaned and calibrated halothane vaporizer. Regardless of which anesthetic is chosen, for adult swine it should be administered in oxygen from a circle or a to-and-fro rebreathing system. Anesthetic machines and delivery systems designed for people or small animals are adequate for most adult swine weighing up to 150 kg, provided the soda lime is fresh and actively absorbing CO_2.

In sedated sows, anesthesia may be safely induced with an inhalant and properly fitted nose cone. Generally, the machine is set to deliver 4 to 8 L of oxygen and 3% to 5% isoflurane. When anesthesia has been induced, the trachea should be intubated. Oxygen flow and anesthetic concentration are gradually decreased. For maintenance, oxygen flow ranges from 1 to 3 L/min. Halothane maintenance concentration ranges from 1.5% to 2.5% (mean, 2%), whereas 2% to 3% isoflurane (mean, 2.5%) is usually required to maintain surgical anesthesia.

N_2O can be used to speed induction of anesthesia. When N_2O is part of the anesthetic induction regimen, pigs are permitted to breathe oxygen and either halothane or isoflurane via nose cone. When signs of sedation appear (i.e., usually 3 to 4 min), N_2O is quickly entrained with oxygen so that it contributes 60% to 70% of the fresh gas inflow (e.g., 2 L of oxygen and 4 L of N_2O) into the breathing system. Because of its high concentration gradient, it moves rapidly from the alveoli to the bloodstream. This technique increases the alveolar concentrations of oxygen (i.e., initially, hyperoxic effect) and the primary anesthetic (e.g., halothane or isoflurane). This increase in concentration gradient of the inhalant increases the rapidity of movement from the alveoli to blood and thus increases the induction speed. This phenomenon is referred to as the *second gas effect*. When induction is complete, N_2O delivery is either decreased to less than 70% of total fresh gas flow or discontinued altogether.

Carbon Dioxide in Oxygen

CO_2 in oxygen can be used to induce anesthesia effectively in piglets. However, induction and surgical time should be restricted to 10 min or less. Most veterinarians are concerned about the humane treatment of all animals. For example, the processing of piglets (i.e., castration, tail docking, and ear notching) involves painful procedures. Because processed pigs are generally destined for human consumption, the use of most injectable anesthetics is not approved to relieve pain associated with processing procedures. Thus, when general anesthesia is used for this purpose, it must be safe, simple, economic, effective, and leave no tissue residues. Further, the anesthetic must have a rapid onset and allow rapid recovery. An anesthetic technique using CO_2 (a natural body by-product of metabolism) and oxygen has been developed to meet these requirements: 50% oxygen and 50% CO_2 (2 L/min oxygen and 2 L/min CO_2) administered by nose cone with a simple mechanical device is illustrated in Fig. 29.5. When assessing this device in 34 piglets, the mean time to inducing unconsciousness was approximately 31 s, whereas processing required 33 s. After CO_2 was discontinued, recovery was complete in 28 s. The time for induction processing and recovery was an average of 92 s.[40] The cost per piglet was less than 4 cents. This same technique has proven effective and safe in other neonatal species (e.g., lambs and kids).

In a later report, inhalation of CO_2 (90%) for 60 s in piglets induced anesthesia rapidly. Muscular response lasts for 13 to 30 s during the induction process. CNS suppression lasts for approximately 1 min after removal from CO_2 inhalation. A study designed to compare halothane 5% in oxygen and 80% CO_2 in 20%

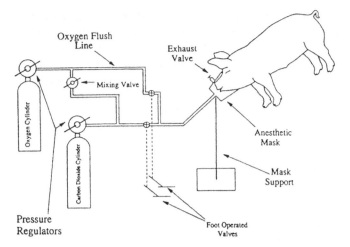

Fig. 29.5. Schematic drawing illustrating a device used to administer a 50:50 carbon dioxide–oxygen mixture to anesthetize piglets. The device uses a combination regulator-flowmeter to deliver gas flows to an anesthetic mask. Line pressures of 50 psi and flow rates of 1 L/min each of oxygen and carbon dioxide are adequate for rapid anesthetization of piglets, relieving pain associated with piglet processing (e.g., castration, tail docking, and ear notching). From Thurmon and Benson.[4]

oxygen revealed that anesthesia with the CO_2-oxygen combination induced surgical anesthesia rapidly and safely. Castration was performed without any reaction.[41] However, the 50:50 combination of CO_2-oxygen each flowing at a rate of 2 L/min delivered via a tightly fitted mask appears to be a more rational and safer use of CO_2 for short-term anesthesia of piglets.

Xenon gas is known to have anesthetic properties in people. To determine its efficacy and safety in swine, nine Pietrain, malignant hyperthermia–sensitive swine, anesthetized with pentobarbital, were mechanically ventilated with 70% xenon for 2 h.[42] Heart rate, mean arterial pressure, cardiac output, body temperature, arterial and mixed venous blood gases, plasma catecholamines, and lactate were measured at 10-min intervals during xenon-oxygen ventilation after a 30-min xenon-washout period. This study next used halothane (1% inspired) and succinylcholine (3 mg/kg IV). During the xenon phase of the study, no changes characteristic of malignant hyperthermia were observed. In contrast, 20 min after administration of halothane and succinylcholine, all swine developed a fulminating and fatal malignant hyperthermic episode. Clearly, xenon anesthesia does not trigger malignant hyperthermia in susceptible swine. In contrast, desflurane, inhaled in repeatedly increasing concentrations, caused fulminating malignant hyperthermia in large white pigs genetically selected for development of this condition.[43]

Less Commonly Used Injectable Drugs

Opioids

These have been used in swine as adjuncts with other drugs to induce and maintain surgical anesthesia. They have also been used as constant infusions for maintenance. The first commercially available opioid drug combination was fentanyl and droperidol in a concentration of 0.4 and 20 mg/mL, respectively (Innovar-Vet). Pigs may become excited after Innovar-Vet injection. Salivation is often excessive unless atropine has been given. A major problem with this combination is the difference in drug half-life between the two drugs. That of fentanyl is quite short, whereas that of droperidol is rather long. Thus, the use of a specific opioid antagonist (e.g., naloxone) is ineffective in shortening a prolonged recovery because deep droperidol tranquilization often remains after the action of fentanyl has waned. In such situations, pigs may respond violently if a high degree of postoperative pain persists. Innovar-Vet (1 mL/13 to 14 kg IM) combined with ketamine (11 mg/kg IM) will induce satisfactory anesthesia for 20 to 30 min in young swine.[1,2,44]

High-dose opioid infusion is commonly used for anesthesia in cardiovascular research because opioids have minimal effect on cardiovascular function.[45,46] Fentanyl is most often used for this purpose. In people, fentanyl can be administered IV in a wide range of doses (50 to 150 µg/kg). Even with high doses, the hemodynamic stability is excellent.[29] Opioid anesthesia in swine has been maintained with fentanyl at a constant infusion of 45 to 90 µg · kg^{-1} · h^{-1}. The dose requirement in swine appears to be larger than for humans and most other species.[47] Fentanyl has been safely administered at a dose as high as 200 µg/kg/h in pigs.

Mild tranquilization will generally prevent muscle rigidity after an intravenous opioid bolus and before infusion is commenced. In people, chest muscle rigidity following fentanyl administration is referred to as *woody chest syndrome*. Clinical experience suggests this may also occur in swine. Severe muscle rigidity can be completely eliminated by the use of a muscle relaxant.

The two opioids most commonly used in swine are buprenorphine and fentanyl. Buprenorphine can be dosed at 0.01 mg/kg IV or IM to provide analgesia for 6 h, whereas a dose of 0.02 mg/kg IV or IM provides analgesia for up to 12 h. Significant analgesia is generally not observed with doses less than 0.01 mg/kg.[48] Although buprenorphine is effective for controlling pain following surgery, its efficacy in ameliorating pain associated with chronic inflammation, organ failure, or systemic disease is questionable. Transdermal fentanyl patches may also be used for postoperative analgesia in swine. Serum concentrations of fentanyl reach a maximum of 0.5 to 1.5 ng/mL by 36 to 48 h after applying a patch designed to deliver 50 or 100 µg of fentanyl per hour.[49,50] The 50-µg/h patch (but not the 25-µg/h patch) provided postoperative analgesia comparable to buprenorphine given at 0.01 mg/kg IM for 3 to 4 days.[50] Buprenorphine is generally recommended when short-term analgesia is needed. Since buprenorphine must be redosed every 8 to 12 h, fentanyl patches are preferred when longer pain control is necessary (e.g., after a thoracotomy).

Generally speaking, an opioid antagonist should be given only when an opioid severely depresses ventilation. In most instances, an agonist-antagonist (e.g., butorphanol or nalbuphine) can be given to restore ventilation while retaining some degree of analgesia.[51] The half-life of nalbuphine in people ranges from 3 to 6 h. However, fentanyl respiratory depression reversed by nalbuphine antagonism has been reported to recur in 2 to 3 h.[29] A similar situation could be expected in swine following butorphanol administration after long-term fentanyl infusion. Naloxone (0.5 to 2 mg/kg IV or IM) effectively antagonizes the residual effects of fentanyl.

Propofol

This is an isopropylphenol derivative administered only intravenously. This nonbarbiturate is supplied in an aqueous solution of 10% soybean oil, 2.5% glycerol, and 1.2% purified egg phosphatide in a concentration of 10 mg/mL.[52] The drug is approximately twice as potent as thiopental and perhaps half as potent as methohexital. In people, consciousness returns more rapidly after a single injection or a constant infusion than with either thiamylal or thiopental. The residual CNS effect is less than that of the barbiturates. The clearance from plasma at a rate greater than the hepatic blood flow suggests that tissue sequestration plays an important role in its short duration of action.[29] Propofol is often described as a hypnotic offering only minimal analgesia. As a result, it is generally used for anesthesia induction or combined with a strong analgesic (e.g., an opioid or α_2-adrenoceptor agonist). Propofol has been used in combination with azaperone and thiopental in pigs, but none of these drugs provide good analgesia. When propofol is used alone as an induction agent in dogs, the dose ranges from 6 to 8 mg/kg IV. Rapid injection may cause apnea. In swine, deep sedation can be maintained with a constant infusion of 4 to 10 mg $\cdot$ kg^{-1} $\cdot$ h^{-1}. Propofol infused at a rate of 12 mg $\cdot$ kg^{-1} $\cdot$ h^{-1} did not trigger malignant hyperthermia in susceptible swine.[53]

Cardiovascular studies have been performed in piglets after the administration of propofol at 7.5, 15, and 30 mg $\cdot$ kg^{-1} $\cdot$ h^{-1}.[54] Mean arterial pressure decreases approximately 25% with no dose difference. Heart rate and left ventricular pressure were unchanged from control. Propofol appears to be a relatively safe hypnotic for use in newborn piglets. Because propofol has such a minimal influence on heart function, a combination of low doses of propofol and fentanyl may be a useful anesthetic in neonatal pigs.

Medetomidine (20 to 40 μg/kg) and propofol (2 to 4 mg/kg) induces a light plane of anesthesia in 30- to 60-kg pigs. Xylazine (1 to 2 mg/kg) appears to be a reasonable substitute for medetomidine. Neither medetomidine nor xylazine are as effective in swine as they are in most other species. When combined with propofol, though, α_2-agonists provide a degree of analgesia commensurate with a light plane of anesthesia. Because propofol does not have a preservative, the possibility of bacterial contamination is a real threat if the entire vial is not used soon after opening. A scrupulously sterile technique must be used after the heat-sealed vial has been opened. If the drug is to be stored for later use, complete sterility is essential.

Alphaxalone and Alphadalone (Saffan)

Saffan is a neurosteroid anesthetic that has been used in swine for some time in Europe and Canada. Anesthetic response to this drug combination is brief, lasting only 10 to 15 min when a dose of 5 to 6 mg/kg is injected IV. The dose can be decreased by ad-

ministering xylazine (1 to 2 mg/kg IM) or azaperone (4 mg/kg IM). The latter will prolong recovery time. Saffan anesthesia may be prolonged by repeated intravenous injection of doses ranging from 2 to 4 mg/kg. This drug combination has been used without incident in swine susceptible to malignant hyperthermia. Alfaxan-CD (hydroxypropyl–beta-cyclodextrin [HPCD]) has recently been introduced in Australia as an anesthetic for use in dogs and cats. This new neurosteroid preparation does not cause histamine release because the carrier solution has been changed from Cremaphor EL (a polyethoxylated castor oil) to a cyclodextrin.[55]

Etomidate

This is a carboxylated imidazole compound unrelated to other injectable anesthetics. It is a relatively poor analgesic and muscle relaxant, and is often classified as a sedative hypnotic when given in low doses (e.g., 2 to 4 mg/kg). Etomidate maintains cardiovascular stability but suppresses adrenocortical activity in people.[56] It does not trigger malignant hyperthermia in susceptible swine.[57] Etomidate in clinically recommended doses causes hemolysis in dogs.

When pigs have been sedated with either xylazine (1 to 2 mg/kg IM or IV) or azaperone (2 to 4 mg/kg IM), analgesia and recovery time are prolonged after etomidate administration. Azaperone premedication prolongs recovery more, but the degree of analgesia is less than with the coadministration of xylazine and etomidate. Etomidate induction (0.6 mg/kg IV) followed by ketamine infusion at a rate of 10 mg $\cdot$ kg^{-1} $\cdot$ h^{-1} has been used to maintain anesthesia in experimental swine.[24]

Metomidate

Metomidate (4 mg/kg IV), which is a hypnotic similar to etomidate, provides rather stable cardiovascular function. In Europe, it has often been used in combination with azaperone (2 to 4 mg/kg IM) to anesthetize swine. Azaperone is given as a preanesthetic, and metomidate is used to maintain anesthesia by repeat injection at 15- to 30-min intervals.[58] The metomidate dose can be doubled to prolong anesthesia. Under such circumstances, it must be administered slowly to prevent apnea. Anesthesia with minimal analgesia has been maintained by continuous infusion of azaperone (2 mg $\cdot$ kg^{-1} $\cdot$ h^{-1}) and metomidate (8 mg $\cdot$ kg^{-1} $\cdot$ h^{-1}). Metomidate (15 mg/kg) has also been given by intraperitoneal injection.[1] However, because this route of administration is often accompanied by peritonitis and intra-abdominal adhesions, peritoneal injections are discouraged and should no longer be recommended. Because metomidate provides poor analgesia, a local analgesic (e.g., lidocaine), an α_2-agonist, or an opioid is often administered concomitantly with metomidate and azaperone.

α-Chloralose

This drug has been used exclusively in the research laboratory. It is a poor analgesic, and hypnosis is usually accompanied by spontaneous leg movement. Blood pressure is unchanged or increased. Heart rate is usually increased, and respiratory depression does not occur until large doses are administered.

α-Chloralose is relatively insoluble, and onset of effect is slow, requiring approximately 15 to 20 min. α-Chloralose (55 to 86 mg/kg) can be combined with morphine (0.3 to 0.9 mg/kg) to improve overall anesthesia. However, continuous limb paddling still often occurs in pigs given this drug combination. Ketamine (5 to 10 mg/kg IV or IM) and butorphanol (0.5 mg/kg IV or IM) can also be combined with α-chloralose in an effort to enhance the overall anesthetic and analgesic actions of this drug.[1]

Malignant Hyperthermia

It was not until the early 1970s that E. W. Jones reported the occurrence of an unusual metabolic condition in swine.[59] Prior to that report, healthy swine leaving the farm for market by truck and arriving dead were diagnosed as having *soft watery pork* (i.e., *pale soft exudative pork*) syndrome. As people and swine with the disease were observed more closely, the condition later became known as *malignant hyperthermia*. The condition is characterized by striated muscle deterioration. Since that time, pigs with this genetic peculiarity have been identified in most swine breeds. Malignant hyperthermia has also been diagnosed in other species, including dogs, horses, cats, birds, deer, and other wild animals. In wild species, the syndrome is frequently referred to as *capture myopathy*. However, of all the mammalian species, malignant hyperthermia is most commonly encountered in swine.

Malignant hyperthermia is most prevalent in individuals of breeds having a high ratio of muscle to total body mass and rapid growth.[60,61] Breeding for these market characteristics appears to have played a major role in increasing swine's predisposition to developing malignant hyperthermia. The breeds most frequently carrying this genetic alteration are Pietrain, Landrace, spotted swine, large white, and Hampshire (not necessarily in this order). Although malignant hyperthermia may occur in other breeds, the incidence is encountered less frequently in the Duroc breed.[62] In highly susceptible individuals, malignant hyperthermia may be triggered by the stress of restraint for blood sampling, castration, and other processing procedures in market swine. Malignant hyperthermia has been observed in young boars pursuing gilts that were unreceptive to breeding, particularly under hot summer conditions. Individuals arising from parentage with a strong inherent predisposition to malignant hyperthermia were very common at one time, particularly in the Landrace breed.

Malignant hyperthermia in swine is caused by an inherited autosomal recessive disorder that causes a single amino-acid mutation in the porcine ryanodine receptor 1 gene (*RYR1*). This ryanodine receptor is a calcium-release channel, and susceptible swine are not capable of controlling calcium efflux from inside the sarcoplasmic reticulum.[63] With the advent of rapid genetic testing to detect the presence of this gene in swine, the incidence of malignant hyperthermia has declined dramatically, although it is still present in the domestic swine population.

The incidence of malignant hyperthermia in potbellied pigs is unknown. It can be expected to be small or nonexistent because this breed has a high ratio of fat to body mass. Potbellied pig deaths attributed to this condition may actually be caused by the stress of restraint. Halothane anesthesia in thousands of potbellied pigs over the last 2 decades has not uncovered a single death that could be attributed to malignant hyperthermia. Presently, anesthetic-related deaths attributed to MH in this species of swine appear to be speculative.

The occurrence of malignant hyperthermia is associated with a sudden increase in muscle oxygen requirement and, thus, lactate production. Body temperature increases, as does respiration rate. Metabolic acidosis is accompanied by muscular contraction, sympathetic activation, and increased muscle cellular permeability. Initially, serum magnesium, calcium, phosphorus, and potassium ion concentrations are increased. These changes are followed by a decrease in serum potassium and calcium ion concentrations. Myoglobinuria often appears shortly thereafter if the affected animal does not succumb.

Clinically, the syndrome in swine is characterized by rapid onset of tachycardia, hyperthermia, muscle rigidity (i.e., activation of limb extensor muscles), tachypnea progressing to dyspnea, and finally apnea. A rapidly increasing end-tidal CO_2 concentration is the most revealing clinical sign of impending malignant hyperthermia. In the later stages of the syndrome, tachycardia is accompanied by dysrhythmias that lead to bradycardia and finally cardiac arrest. Current findings indicate that metabolic status during malignant hyperthermia is characterized by an increased oxygen demand ischemia of the heart and skeletal muscle. Insufficient coronary blood flow and increased metabolism as a result of tachycardia and increased concentrations of catecholamines are dominant factors contributing to the dramatic alteration in cardiac performance during porcine malignant hyperthermia.[64] When tachycardia is accompanied by malignant arrhythmias, treatment success is unlikely. Most patients will die regardless of treatment.

In susceptible swine, clinical signs appear shortly after exposure to halothane. An exception to this occurs when swine have been given a phenothiazine tranquilizer (e.g., acetylpromazine) and anesthesia is induced with a thiobarbiturate (e.g., thiopental). Under such circumstances, the onset is delayed when anesthesia is continued with a halogenated hydrocarbon (e.g., halothane) or a halogenated ether (e.g., isoflurane). However, malignant hyperthermia may occur in susceptible swine when the effects of the tranquilizer and/or the barbiturate have waned. Thus, it is important to understand that time of onset of the syndrome is influenced by drugs used in various anesthetic regimens and is not always an acute response to halothane or succinylcholine administration. Succinylcholine injected into susceptible swine can easily trigger the syndrome, whereas nondepolarizing muscle relaxants (e.g., pancuronium) are less likely to do so.

Prevention and Treatment

The drug used most commonly to prevent and treat malignant hyperthermia in swine is dantrolene (Dantrium, 2 to 5 mg/kg IV). This muscle relaxant is also an antipyretic. It suppresses calcium ion release but does not appear to inhibit uptake of calcium by muscle tissue cells. Even though it acts directly within muscle cells, its depressant effect on respiratory muscle function is minimal. The use of dantrolene has proven to be a valuable prophylactic treatment for malignant hyperthermia in susceptible swine and people.

Dantrolene is dosed orally (5 mg/kg) 8 to 10 h prior to surgery. There is evidence that the drug should be repeated (3 to 5 mg/kg IV) preoperatively and postoperatively should surgery be prolonged. When a known triggering drug has been used to maintain anesthesia (e.g., halothane or isoflurane), the patient should be monitored closely for 1 day postoperatively.

Symptomatic treatment includes rapid termination of the inhalant, changing of the anesthetic machine rubber goods (i.e., hoses and rebreathing bag), or switching to a clean machine for administering 100% oxygen, procaine (1 to 2 mg/kg IV), intravenous corticosteroids, sodium bicarbonate (2 to 4 mEq/kg IV) if severe metabolic acidosis is present, and body cooling. Whole body cooling may be achieved with an ice water–alcohol mixture and cold fluids IV, orally, or by infusion per rectum.

Anesthetic drugs least likely to trigger malignant hyperthermia in susceptible swine include thiopental, propofol, etomidate, metomidate, and epidural anesthesia. In highly susceptible swine, restraint for intravenous or epidural drug injection can precipitate the syndrome. In susceptible swine, preanesthetic medications (e.g., acetylpromazine) known to inhibit the malignant hyperthermia syndrome should be administered IM prior to anesthesia induction.

References

1. Thurmon JC, Tranquilli WJ. Anesthesia for cardiovascular research. In: Stanton HC, Mersmann HJ, eds. Swine in Cardiovascular Research, vol 1. Boca Raton, FL: CRC, 1986:39–59.

2. Riebold TW, Thurmon JC. Anesthesia in swine. In: Tumbleson ME, ed. Swine in Biomedical Research, vol 1. New York: Plenum, 1986:243–254.

3. Swindle MM. Anesthesia and analgesia. In: Swindle MM, ed. Surgery, Anesthesia, and Experimental Techniques in Swine. Ames: Iowa State University Press, 1998:33–64.

4. Thurmon JC, Benson GJ. Anesthesia in ruminants and swine. In: Howard J, ed. Current Veterinary Therapy 3: Food Animal Practice. Philadelphia: WB Saunders, 1993:58–76.

5. Smith AC, Spinale FG, Swindle MM. Cardiac function and morphology of Hanford miniature swine and Yucatan miniature and micro swine. Lab Anim Sci 40:47–50, 1990.

6. Thurmon JC, Benson GJ. Special anesthesia considerations of swine. In: Short CE, ed. Principles and Practice of Veterinary Anesthesia. Baltimore: Williams and Wilkins, 1987:308–322.

7. Wemyss-Holden SA, Porter SA, Baxter P, Rudkin GE, Maddern GJ. et al. The laryngeal mask airway in experimental pig anesthesia. Lab Anim 33:30–34, 1999.

8. Haga HA, Tevik A, Moerch H. Bispectral index as an indicator of anaesthetic depth during isoflurane anaesthesia in the pig. J Vet Anaesth 26:3–7, 1999.

9. Martin-Cancho M, Carrasco-Jimenez MS, Lima JR, Ezquerra LJ, Crisostomo V, Uson-Gargallo J. Assessment of the relationship of bispectral index values, hemodynamic changes, and recovery times associated with sevoflurane or propofol anesthesia in pigs. Am J Vet Res 65:409–416, 2004.

10. Cohn MS, Lichtiger M. Premedications. In: Lichtiger M, Moya F, eds. Introduction to the Practice of Anesthesia, 2nd ed. Hagerstown, MD: Harper and Row, 1978:13.

11. Bustamante R, Valverde A. Determination of a sedative dose and influence of droperidol and midazolam on cardiovascular function in pigs. Can J Vet Res 61:246–250, 1997.

12. Ochs HR, Greenblatt DJ, Eichelkraut W, Bakker C, Gobel R, Hahn N. Hepatic vs. gastrointestinal presystemic extraction of oral midazolam and flurazepam. J Pharmacol Exp Ther 243:852–856, 1987.

13. Pender KS, Pollack CV, Woodall BN, Parks BR. Intraosseous administration of lorazepam: Same-dose comparison with intravenous administration in the weanling pig. J Miss State Med Assoc 1991: 365–368.

14. Danneberg P, Bauer R, Boke-Kuhn K, Hoefke W, Kuhn FJ, Lehr E, Walland A. General pharmacology of brotizolam in animals. Arzneimittelforschung 36(3A):540–551, 1986.

15. Lacoste L, Bouquet S, Igrand P, Caritez JC, Carretier M, Debaene B. Intranasal midazolam in piglets: Pharmacodynamics (0.2 vs 0.4 mg/kg) and pharmacokinetics (0.4 mg/kg) with bioavailability determination. Lab Anim 34:29–35, 2000.

16. Nishimura R, Hwiyool K, Matasunaga S, et al. Antagonism of medetomidine sedation by atipamezole in pigs. J Vet Med Sci 54: 1237–1240, 1992.

17. Tendillol FJ, Mascias A, Santos M, Segura IA, San Roman F, Castillo-Olivares JL. Cardiopulmonary and analgesia effects of xylazine, detomidine, medetomidine, and the antagonist atipamezole in isoflurane-anesthetized swine. Lab Anim Sci 46:215–219, 1996.

18. Giron LT, McCann SA, Crist-Orlando SG. Pharmacological characterization and regional distribution of alpha-noradrenergic binding sites of rat spinal cord. Eur J Pharmacol 115:285–290, 1985.

19. Ko JCH, Thurmon JC, Benson GJ, Tranquilli WJ, Olson WA. Evaluation of analgesia induced by epidural injection of detomidine or xylazine in swine. J Vet Anaesth 19:56–60, 1992.

20. Yaksh TL. Pharmacology of spinal adrenergic system which modulate spinal nociceptive processing. Pharmacol Biochem Behav 22:845–856, 1985.

21. LeBlanc PH, Caron JP, Patterson JS, Brown M, Matta MA. Epidural injection of xylazine for perineal analgesia in horses. J Am Vet Med Assoc 193:1405–1408, 1988.

22. Fikes LW, Lin HC, Thurmon JC. A preliminary comparison of lidocaine and xylazine as epidural analgesics in ponies. Vet Surg Anesth 18:5–86, 1989.

23. Ko JCH, Althouse GC, Hopkins SM, Jackson LL, Evans LE, Smith RP. Effects of epidural administration of xylazine or lidocaine on bovine uterine motility and perineal analgesia. Theriogenology 32:786–797, 1989.

24. Worek FS, Blumel G, Zaravik, J, Zimmerman GJ, Pfeiffer UJ. Comparison of ketamine and pentobarbital anesthesia with the conscious state in a porcine model of Pseudomonas aeruginosa septicemia. Acta Anesth Scand 32:509–515, 1988.

25. Swindell MM, Smith AC, Hepburn BJS. Swine as models in experimental surgery. J Invest Surg 1:65–79, 1988.

26. Clutton RE, Blissitt KJ, Bradley AA, Camburn MA. Comparison of three injectable anesthetics techniques in pigs. Vet Rec 141: 140–146, 1997.

27. Boschert K, Flecknell PA, Fosse FT, et al. Ketamine and its use in the pig: Recommendations of the consensus meeting on ketamine anesthesia in pigs, Bergin, 1994. Lab Anim 30:209–219, 1996.

28. Reich DL, Silvay, G. Ketamine: An update on the first twenty-five years of clinical experience. Can J Anaesth 36:186–197, 1989.

29. Stoelting RK. Pharmacology and Physiology in Anesthetic Practice, 2nd ed. Philadelphia: JB Lippincott 1991:134–147.

30. Thurmon JC, Nelson DR, Christie GJ. Ketamine anesthesia in swine. J Am Vet Med Assoc 160:1325–1330, 1972.

31. Breese CE, Dodman NH. Xylazine-ketamine-oxymorphone: An injectable anesthetic combination in swine. J Am Vet Med Assoc 184:182–183, 1984.

32. Thurmon JC, Benson GJ, Tranquilli WJ, Olson WA, Tracy CH. The anesthetic effects of Telazol and xylazine in pigs: Evaluating clinical trials. Vet Med 83:841–845, 1988.

33. Gabor TM, Hellgren EC, Silvy NJ. Immobilization of collared peccaries (*Tayassu tajacu*) and feral hogs (*Sus scrofa*) with Telazol and xylazine. J Wildl Dis 33:161–164, 1997.

34. James SB, Cook RA, Raphael BL, et al. Immobilization of babirusa (*Babyrousa babyrussa*) with xylazine and tiletamine/zolazepam and reversal with yohimbine and flumazenil. J Zoo Wildl Med 30:521–525, 1999.

35. Henrikson H, Jensen-Waern M, Nyman G. Anesthetics for general anesthesia in growing pigs. Acta Vet Scand 36:401–411, 1995.

36. Ko JC, Williams BL, Rogers ER, Pablo LS, McCaine WC, McGrath CJ. Increased xylazine dose-enhanced anesthetic properties of Telazol-xylazine combination in swine. Lab Anim Sci 45:290–294, 1995.

37. Sakaguchi M, Nishimura R, Sasaki N, Ishiguro T, Tamura H, Takeuchi A. Anesthesia induced in pigs by use of a combination of medetomidine, butorphanol, and ketamine and its reversal by administration of atipamezole. Am J Vet Res 57:529–534, 1996.

38. Kerbaul F, Bellezza M, Guidon C, et al. Effects of sevoflurane on hypoxic pulmonary vasoconstriction in anesthetized piglets. Br J Anesth 85:440–445, 2000.

39. Tranquilli WA, Thurmon JC, Benson GJ. Anesthetic potency of nitrous oxide in young swine (*Sus scrofa*). Am J Vet Res 46:58–60, 1985.

40. Thurmon JC, Lin HC, Curtis SE. Carbon dioxide and oxygen anesthesia for castration of baby pigs [Abstract]. In: 71st Conference of Research Workers in Animal Disease, Chicago, Illinois, November 5–6, 1990:34.

41. Kohler I, Moens Y, Busato A, Blum J, Schatzmann U. Inhalation anaesthesia for castration of piglets: CO_2 compared to halothane. Zentralbl Veterinarmed A 45:625–633, 1998.

42. Froeba G, Marx T, Pazhur J, et al. Xenon does not trigger malignant hyperthermia in susceptible swine. Anesthesiology 91:1047–1052, 1999.

43. Bonome Gonzalez C, Alvarez-Refojo F. Malignant hyperthermia in a pig anesthetized with desflurane. Rev Esp Anestesiol Reanim 48:81–84, 2001.

44. Benson GJ, Thurmon JC. Anesthesia of swine under field conditions. J Am Vet Assoc 174:594–596, 1979.

45. Merin RG, Verdouw PD, Jong JW. Myocardial functional and metabolic responses to ischemia in swine during halothane and fentanyl anesthesia. Anesthesiology 56:84–92, 1982.

46. Schuman RE, Swindle MM, Knick BJ, Case CL, Gelette PC. High dose narcotic anesthesia using sufentanil in swine for cardiac catheterization and electrophysiologic studies. J Invest Surg 7:243–248, 1994.

47. Kleinsasser A, Linder KH, Hoermann C, Schaefer A, Keller C, Loeckinger A. Isoflurane and sevoflurane anesthesia in pigs with a preexistent gas exchange defect. Anesthesiology 95:1422–1426, 2001.

48. Rodriguez NA, Cooper DM, Risdahl JM. Antinociceptive activity of and clinical experience with buprenorphine in swine. Contemp Top Lab Anim Sci 40:17–20, 2001.

49. Wilkinson AC, Thomas ML, Morse BC. Evaluation of a transdermal fentanyl system in Yucatan miniature pigs. Contemp Top Lab Anim Sci 40:12–16, 2001.

50. Harvey-Clark CJ, Gilespie K, Riggs KW. Transdermal fentanyl compared with parenteral buprenorphine in post-surgical pain in swine: A case study. Lab Anim 34:386–398, 2000.

51. Baily PL, Clark NJ, Pace NL, et al. Antagonism with postoperative opioid-induced respiratory depression: Nalbuphine versus naloxone. Anesth Analg 66:1109–1114, 1987.

52. Sebel PS, Lowdon JD. Propofol: A new intravenous anesthetic. Anesthesiology 67:260–277, 1989.

53. Raff M, Harrison GG. The screening of propofol in MH swine. Can J Anaesth 36:186–197, 1989.

54. Graham MR, Thiessen DB, Mutch WA. Left ventricular systolic and diastolic function is unaltered during propofol infusion in newborn swine. Anesth Analg 86:717–723, 1998.

55. Carpenter RE, Grimm KA, Tranquilli WJ, et al. Preliminary report on the use of alfaxalone for anesthetic induction in goats [Abstract]. In: Veterinary Midwest Anesthesia and Analgesia Conference Proceedings, Indianapolis, Indiana, April 23–24, 2005:10.

56. Fragen RJ, Shanks CJ, Molteni A, Abram MJ. Effects of etomidate on hormonal responses to surgical stress. Anesthesiology 61:652–656, 1984.

57. Suresh MS, Nelson TE. Malignant hyperthermia: Is etomidate safe? Anesth Analg 64:420–424, 1985.

58. Svendsen P, Carter AM. Blood gas tensions, acid-base status and cardiovascular function in miniature swine anesthetized with halothane and methoxyflurane or intravenous metomidate hydrochloride. Pharmacol Toxicol 64:88–93, 1989.

59. Jones EW, Nelson TE, Anderson IL, Kerr DD, Burnap TK. Malignant hyperthermia of swine. Anesthesiology 36:42–51, 1972.

60. Gronert GA, Milde GH, Theye RA. Dantrolene in porcine malignant hyperthermia. Anesthesiology 44:488–495, 1976.

61. Gronert GA. Malignant hyperthermia. Anesthesiology 53:395–423, 1980.

62. Wagner AJ. The porcine stress syndrome. Vet Med Rev 1:68–77, 1972.

63. MacLennan DH, Phillips MS. Malignant hyperthermia. Science 256:789–794, 1992.

64. Roewer N, Dziadzka A, Greim C, Kraas E, Schulte am Esch J. Cardiovascular and metabolic responses to anesthetic-induced malignant hyperthermia in swine. Anesthesiology 83:141–159, 1995.

65. Wertz EM, Wagnert AE. Anesthesia in potbellied pigs. Compend Contin Educ 17:369–382, 1995.

Chapter 30
Laboratory Animals

Paul A. Flecknell, Claire A. Richardson, and Aleksandar Popovic

Introduction

Anesthesia of laboratory animals provides some unique challenges to veterinary anesthetists. In addition to working with less familiar species, the constraints of particular research projects may limit the anesthetic and analgesic options available. Some of the anesthetic regimens proposed by investigators may be unfamiliar to anesthetists who have worked only in a clinical environment; for example, the use of chloralose or urethane. Finally, the duration of anesthesia required may range from a matter of seconds (e.g., for blood sampling) to several days for some neurophysiological studies. Although these factors may seem daunting, the involvement of veterinary anesthetists in this field is essential if we are to help promote both high standards of anesthesia and high standards of animal welfare. Many laboratory-animal facilities employ veterinarians specialized in laboratory-animal medicine, and it is always advisable to contact them prior to offering advice or becoming directly involved in providing assistance to a research group.

Selecting an Anesthetic Regimen

In addition to the usual factors to be considered when selecting an anesthetic regimen, a further issue when working with laboratory species is the potential interactions between the anesthetic and the particular research protocol. It is important to discuss the proposed anesthetic regimen with the research group concerned and try to indicate any specific pharmacological properties of the anesthetic that are likely to be relevant. This may require a detailed literature search. A variety of strategies may be needed to identify relevant information—note that some product development work will have been conducted in laboratory species, but that the agent may be referred to by its original manufacturer's drug identifier (e.g., propofol as ICI 35 168). If it is determined that interactions could occur, it is important to place them in the overall context of the research protocol. In addition, do not overlook the importance of high standards of perioperative care and minimizing the general effects of anesthesia. These include respiratory depression, producing hypoxia, hypercapnia, and acidosis; cardiovascular depression with reduction in cardiac output and alterations in organ blood flow; and depression of thermoregulation, causing hypothermia and consequent changes in metabolism and cardiovascular function.

If an animal is undergoing surgical procedures, then the effects of surgical stress are almost unavoidable and will have profound and long-lasting effects on the animal's metabolism and endocrine system.[1]

General Considerations

The majority of laboratory animals will be young, healthy adults, although in some circumstances animals with intercurrent disease will be encountered. Laboratory-facility veterinarians should be able to provide information on the health status of the animals and the incidence of clinical and subclinical disease. Most facilities require that animals undergo a period of acclimatization, usually for 1 to 2 weeks, prior to their use in research procedures. This provides an excellent opportunity for habituation to handling and restraint. It also provides time for the anes-

Table 30.1. Physiological data for rodents and rabbits.

	Mouse	Rat	Rabbit	Guinea Pig	Hamster	Gerbil
Adult body weight (g)	25–40	300–500	2000–6000	700–1200	85–150	85–150
Body temperature (°C)	37.5	38	38	38	37.4	39
Respiratory rate (breaths/min)	80–200	70–115	40–60	50–140	80–135	90
Heart rate (beats/min)	350–600	250–350	135–325	150–250	250–500	260–300

thetist and the animal-care staff to assess the behavior and temperament of animals, perform a general clinical examination, and obtain background data such as growth rate and food and water consumption. This information is of considerable value when assessing postoperative recovery. Some basic biological data are provided in Tables 30.1 and 30.2.

Rodents and Rabbits

Small rodents and rabbits do not vomit, so there is generally no need to withhold food or water prior to anesthesia. Withholding food from small rodents for prolonged periods can be detrimental because it can predispose them to hypoglycemia. Rabbits and guinea pigs are more likely to develop postoperative gastrointestinal disturbances if food is withheld. In anesthetized guinea pigs, small quantities of food are often found in the mouth, but this is not prevented by withholding food.

Nonhuman Primates

Both Old World and New World primates may vomit during induction or recovery from anesthesia, so withdrawal of food for 8 h and water for 2 to 3 h preoperatively is advisable. Note that these animals may eat bedding or other material in their cages, so withdrawing food does not guarantee an empty stomach.

Preanesthetic Medication

Rodents and Rabbits

Since anesthesia in rodents is often induced by using an anesthetic chamber, or by using an injection of drugs by the intraperitoneal or subcutaneous routes, preanesthetic medication is not often given. In rabbits, induction with a volatile agent delivered via a face mask may be considered, but a sedative agent (e.g., diazepam or acepromazine) should be administered because animals often find this procedure stressful.[2,3] Even when volatile agents are not used, since rabbits are easily stressed when handled and restrained, use of sedatives or tranquilizers can have significant benefits. Administration of the drug before removal from the animal's home cage or pen is advisable. Suitable agents are listed in Table 30.3. Preanesthetic sedation may also be considered advisable if isoflurane is to be administered to guinea pigs, because this agent appears to be an irritant in this species.

When only immobilization is required, rather than anesthesia, high doses of some of the agents listed in Table 30.3 may be effective, but often low doses of anesthetic combinations (e.g., ketamine-medetomidine) are more useful.

Preanesthetic medication with an analgesic may be advisable in all of these species, as part of a perioperative pain-management

Table 30.2. Physiological data for nonhuman primates.

	Marmoset	Rhesus Macaque
Average adult body weight	500 g	8–12 kg
Body temperature (°C)	38.5–40.0	39
Respiratory rate (breaths/min)	50–70	35
Heart rate (beats/min)	225	150

regimen (see the section on Effective Pain Control), and dose rates of suitable analgesics are listed in Table 30.4.

As in other species, atropine or glycopyrrolate can be administered to reduce bronchial and salivary secretions, although this is rarely needed in rodents that are free of respiratory infection. However, these agents may be useful in protecting the heart from vagal inhibition caused by some surgical procedures (e.g., handling of the viscera, or carotid cannulation that may involve direct vagal manipulation). It is advisable to use glycopyrrolate in rabbits because atropine is often relatively ineffective in this species.[4]

Nonhuman Primates

The use of preanesthetic medication in Old World primates (macaques and baboons) has been considered essential because of concerns for the safety of the staff involved. However, the change in emphasis in husbandry techniques so that primates are well socialized and may accept intravenous injection increases the anesthetic options that can be selected. If animal-care staff advises that chemical restraint is needed, then ketamine can be administered to immobilize an animal so that it can then be handled safely. Drug administration may be facilitated by use of a cage design that allows the animal to be confined for injection, or the animal can be trained to stand and accept the injection. As an alternative to the dissociative anesthetics, sedatives and tranquilizers can also be used in nonhuman primates, but these are not always effective in preventing aggression. Medetomidine should be used with great care in nonhuman primates because its sedative effects are less predictable and some animals may suddenly become alert and bite their handlers. When combined with ketamine, animals are immobilized and a medium plane of anesthesia is produced.[5] As in other species, atipamezole can be administered to reverse the effects of medetomidine. Although the effects of ketamine still remain, recovery is generally rapid.

The use of ketamine in New World monkeys such as mar-

Table 30.3. Preanesthetic agents for use in rodents and rabbits.

Drug	Species	Dose Rate	Effect
Acepromazine	Rat, guinea pig	2.5 mg/kg IP or SC	Sedation, but still active
	Mouse, hamster, gerbil	3–5 mg/kg IP or SC	
	Rabbit	1 mg/kg SC or IM	Sedated, often immobilized
Acepromazine + butorphanol	Rabbit	0.5 mg/kg + 1.0 mg/kg IM or SC	Sedation, often immobilized, some analgesia
Atropine	Mouse, hamster, gerbil, rat, guinea pig	40 µg/kg SC or IM	Reduced bronchial and salivary secretions, inhibits vagal responses, ineffective in many rabbits
Diazepam	Mouse, hamster, gerbil, guinea pig	5 mg/kg IP	Sedation
	Rat	2.5 mg/kg IP	
	Rabbit	1–2 mg/kg IM	
Glycopyrrolate	Rabbit	0.01 mg/kg IV or 0.1 mg/kg SC or IM	Reduced bronchial and salivary secretions, inhibits vagal responses
Innovar-Vet (fentanyl-droperidol)	Rabbit	0.22 mL/kg IM	Sedation and analgesia; often sufficiently immobilized for minor surgical procedures
	Mouse	0.5 mL/kg IM	
	Hamster	1.5 mL/kg IM	
	Guinea pig	0.4 mL/kg IM	
Hypnorm (fentanyl-fluanisone)	Mouse, hamster, gerbil, rat, guinea pig	0.5 mL/kg SC or IP	Sedation and analgesia; often sufficiently immobilized for minor surgical procedures
	Rabbit	0.3–0.5 mL/kg SC or IM	
Medetomidine	Mouse, hamster, rat	30–100 µg/kg SC or IP	Sedation and some analgesia, immobilized at higher dose rates
	Rabbit	100–500 µg/kg SC or IP	
Midazolam	Mouse, hamster, gerbil, guinea pig	5 mg/kg IP	Sedation
	Rat	2.5 mg/kg IP	
	Rabbit	1–2 mg/kg IM	
Xylazine	Mouse, hamster, rat	5 mg/kg SC or IM	Sedation and some analgesia, immobilized at higher dose rates
	Rabbit	2.5 mg/kg SC or IM	

IM, intramuscularly; IP, intraperitoneally; IV, intravenously; SC, subcutaneously.

Table 30.4. Suggested analgesic dose rates for rodents and rabbits[a].

Analgesic	Mouse	Rat	Rabbit	Guinea Pig	Hamster	Gerbil
Buprenorphine	0.1 mg/kg SC per 6–12 h	0.01–0.05 mg/kg SC per 6–12 h	0.01–0.05 mg/kg SC	0.05 mg/kg SC	0.1 mg/kg SC	0.1 mg/kg SC
Butorphanol	2 mg/kg SC per 4 h	2 mg/kg SC per 4 h	0.1–0.5 mg/kg SC	2 mg/kg SC	?	?
Carprofen	10 mg/kg SC	5 mg/kg SC	4 mg/kg SC once daily or 1.5 mg/kg PO daily	2.5 mg/kg	?	?
Flunixin	2.5 mg/kg SC twice daily	2.5 mg/kg SC twice daily	1.1 mg/kg SC twice daily	?	?	?
Meloxicam	5 mg/kg SC per 4 h	1–2 mg/kg SC or 4 mg/kg PO	0.2 mg/kg SC daily	?	?	?
Morphine	2–5 mg/kg SC	2–5 mg/kg SC per 4 h	2–5 mg/kg SC or IM per 4 h	2–5 mg/kg SC or IM per 4 h	?	?
Oxymorphone	?	0.2–0.3 mg/kg SC	0.1–0.2 mg/kg IM or IV	?	?	?
Pethidine	10–20 mg/kg SC or IM per 2–3 h	10–20 mg/kg SC or IM per 2–3 h	10 mg/kg SC or IM per 2–3 h	10–20 mg/kg SC or IM	?	?

IM, intramuscularly; IV, intravenously; PO, per os (orally); SC, subcutaneously.
[a]Dose rates are based largely on uncontrolled clinical trials and a limited range of procedures and so are likely to be subject to revision. A "?" indicates that information is insufficient to make a firm recommendation of an appropriate dose.

Table 30.5. Preanesthetic agents for use in nonhuman primates.

Drug	Species	Dose Rate
Alphaxalone-alphadolone	Marmoset	12–18 mg/kg IM
Ketamine	Rhesus macaque	5–25 mg/kg IM

IM, intramuscularly.

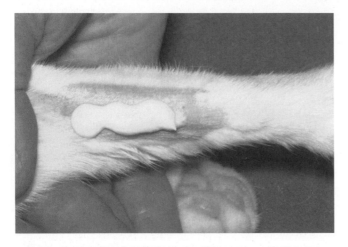

Fig. 30.1. Application of local anesthetic cream (EMLA Cream; AstraZeneca, London) to the skin overlying the cephalic vein of a cat. Local anesthetic cream should be applied 45 min to 1 h prior to venipuncture.

mosets has been associated with muscle damage. This is probably related to the low pH of ketamine (3 to 4) and its injection into the relatively small muscle mass of these animals. Similar effects have been seen in small rodents. Although an even larger volume of injectate is required, alphaxalone-alphadolone is well tolerated and appears to be nonirritant. It produces deep sedation, and additional drug can be given intravenously to deepen anesthesia.[6,7] Dose rates of suitable agents are listed in Table 30.5.

Special Considerations with Other Species in a Research Environment

Cats

Cats should be well socialized and thus easy to restrain for intravenous administration of anesthetic agents. They may resent insertion of over-the-needle catheters and may struggle in response to venipuncture. This can be avoided by using local anesthetic cream as shown in Fig. 30.1.[8] This mixture of lignocaine and prilocaine produces full-skin-thickness anesthesia, but requires 45 min to 1 h of contact time and needs to be covered with a dressing. An alternative approach is to administer a sedative.

Dogs

Early socialization of laboratory-bred dogs is important, because they will then be easy to handle and restrain for injection of anesthetics. Like cats, they may resent insertion of over-the-needle catheters and may struggle in response to venipuncture. Use of

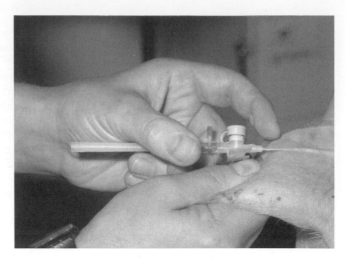

Fig. 30.2. Placement of an over-the-needle catheter into the ear vein of a pig. A local anesthetic cream may be applied to the ear 4 min to 1 h prior to venipuncture.

EMLA Cream (lidocaine 2.5% and prilocaine 2.5%) can prevent discomfort during venipuncture or catheter placement. Alternatively, a range of different sedatives can be administered as preanesthetic medication.

Pigs

Laboratory-bred pigs (usually minipigs) should have been socialized to be accustomed to human contact. They can be readily trained to accept some degree of restraint, enabling intramuscular injection of a sedative combination to immobilize them. If trained to accept restraint in a sling, then the ear can be anesthetized with EMLA Cream and a catheter placed for intravenous induction of anesthesia (Fig. 30.2). Many pigs, particularly those reared under farm conditions, may be apprehensive and difficult to approach. Such animals should be immobilized or heavily sedated. Drug administration is easier if a long needle (3 to 4 cm) is attached using extension tubing to a syringe so that, after the catheter is placed, the drug can be injected without the need for physical restraint of the animal.

Sheep

Few sheep are bred specifically for research purposes; after a few weeks of acclimatization, however, they may become more tractable and approachable than those housed on farms.

Handling, Restraint, and Routes of Drug Administration

Small animals should be handled with care. Habituation to handling during acclimatization will facilitate future restraint and reduce the stress to the animal and operator during the administration of anesthetics. It is important to make animals aware about our intentions before attempting to handle them, especially if they are asleep, in order to minimize stress and also avoid bite injuries.

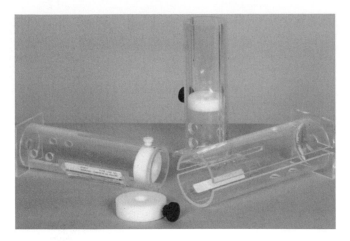

Fig. 30.3. Rodent restraint tubes. Mice and rats may be placed in these tubes to facilitate venipuncture.

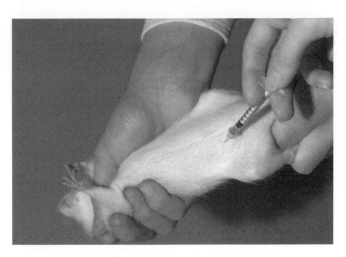

Fig. 30.4. Intraperitoneal injection of a rat. The rat is restrained in dorsal recumbency by an assistant. An injection is made into its lower left abdominal quadrant.

Anesthetics or analgesics may cause discomfort, irritation, and/or ulceration of the skin, mucous membranes, vascular endothelium, or muscles if they are irritant (e.g., low or high pH), cold (straight from the refrigerator) and/or administered by an inappropriate route (e.g., pentobarbital by intramuscular route).

Intravenous injection or placement of intravenous catheters for anesthetic administration in conscious rodents may be challenging even for experienced operators. The use of physical methods (e.g., restraint tubes) or volatile anesthetics for induction may provide the desired restraint to facilitate this task (Fig. 30.3).

Rodents

The intraperitoneal route of administration is the easiest approach for small rodents, because larger amounts of fluids may be administered. However, errors during administration by this route are quite common (e.g., intravisceral, subcutaneous, or administration into the adipose tissue).[9] Such errors may cause organ damage or delayed onset of action of the anesthetic agent. Injections are usually made into the left lower abdominal quadrant. Rodents are restrained in dorsal recumbency, as shown in Fig. 30.4.

Most of the commercially available analgesic and anesthetic agents are available in high concentrations, so that only very small volumes would be required for injection in small rodents. Precise dosing is easier if insulin syringes (50 IU, 0.5 mL) are used. Alternatively, a commercial preparation can be diluted to provide a more accurately administered volume. For intravenous administration, butterfly needles or over-the-needle catheters with or without extension sets may be used for initial induction and anesthetic maintenance by infusion, as shown in Fig. 30.5.

Hamsters

Animals can be held in both hands, immobilizing the head to avoid being bitten (Fig. 30.6). Alternatively, grasp the loose skin around the neck and back region firmly (Fig. 30.7). The saphenous vein may be used for intravenous administration. For other routes, see Table 30.6.

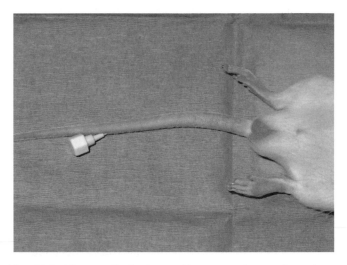

Fig. 30.5. An anesthetized rat with an over-the-needle catheter placed in its lateral tail vein.

Gerbils

Gerbils are generally easy to handle and can be scooped into the palm of a hand. Alternatively, they can be picked up gently at the base of the tail, but grasping the distal end of the tail might detach skin. Gerbils dislike being picked up and turned onto their backs. The lateral tail or saphenous veins may be used for intravenous administration. For other routes of administration, see Table 30.6.

Guinea Pigs

Guinea pigs are easily lifted by grasping them gently around the thorax and shoulders with one hand while supporting the hindquarters with the other hand (Fig. 30.8). Aural, saphenous, or penile veins (only under anesthesia) may be used for intravenous administration. For other routes, see Table 30.6.

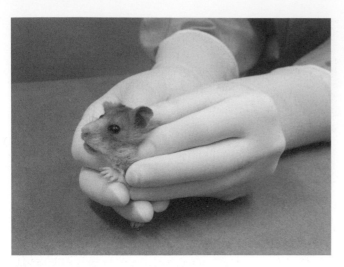

Fig. 30.6. Hamster restraint. The hamster is held in both hands with its head immobilized.

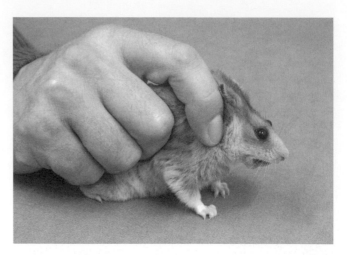

Fig. 30.7. Hamster restraint. The hamster is grasped firmly by the loose skin around its neck and back.

Mice

Mice are not as easily habituated to restraint as other rodents, and there are great variations between different strains. Some are relatively docile and easy to catch, whereas others may be extremely active. Mice are usually grasped by the base of the tail and lifted from the cage (Fig. 30.9). When placed on a nonslip surface such as a cage lid or laboratory coat, they can be grasped by the loose skin overlying the animal's back, with the tail restrained between the operator's fingers (Fig. 30.10). This form of restraint is particularly suitable for intraperitoneal, intramuscular, and subcutaneous administration of drugs. For administration details, see Table 30.6.

Rats

The easiest and most humane way to lift a rat is with one hand supporting the hind quarters and the other hand supporting the head, with the thumb under the foreleg and mandible (Fig. 30.11). Rats can be grasped using the loose skin overlying the neck and back, if necessary. For administration details, see Table 30.6.

Rabbits

Gently approach the rabbit in the cage or floor pan and grasp the skin of the neck and back firmly, supporting the abdomen and hind legs with the other hand (Fig. 30.12). When carrying rabbits, the head is kept between the arm and the chest of the handler (Fig. 30.13). Wrapping the rabbit in a towel or a purpose-designed restraint device may facilitate handling and is particularly helpful when performing intravenous injections (Fig. 30.14). For administration details, see Table 30.6.

New World Primates (Marmosets and Tamarins)

If well socialized, these animals can be easily restrained for mask induction of anesthesia or for intramuscular or subcutaneous administration of drugs. Intravenous administration, using the lateral tail vein, requires firm restraint and is often easier after administration of a sedative or tranquilizer. If animals resent restraint, they may bite, so protective gloves may be required to protect the operator (Fig. 30.15).

Table 30.6. Routes of injection for rodents and rabbits.

Injection Site	Species	Location	Needle Size (Gauge)	Precautions
Intramuscular	Rodents	Quadriceps or posterior thigh muscles	25–27	Muscle mass is very small, avoid sciatic nerve
	Rabbits	Quadriceps, dorsal lumbar, or posterior thigh muscles	24–27	Avoid sciatic nerve
Intravenous	Mice and rats	Lateral tail or saphenous vein	24–28	
	Rabbits	Marginal ear vein, cephalic or saphenous vein	23–25	Use a local anesthetic cream (EMLA Cream) prior to injection
Subcutaneous	Rodents	Interscapular or inguinal region	21–25	Highly viscous liquids may cause discomfort and are difficult to inject
	Rabbits	Interscapular or flanks	21–25	

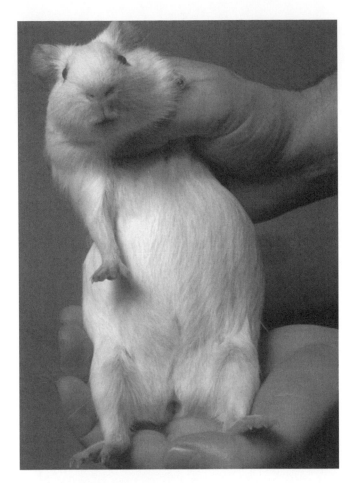

Fig. 30.8. Guinea pig restraint. The guinea pig is grasped gently around its thorax and shoulders with one hand while the other hand supports its hindquarters.

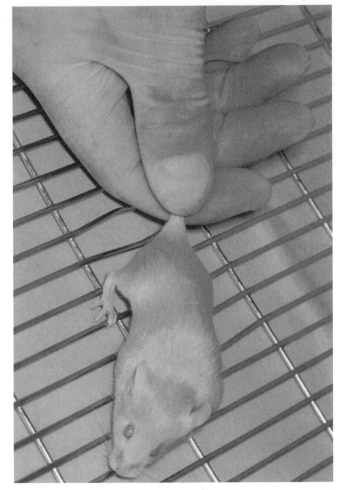

Fig. 30.9. Mouse restraint. The mouse is grasped by the base of its tail.

Old World Primates (Rhesus Macaques and Baboons)

If well socialized, these animals may be restrained by their familiar handler to enable intramuscular injections (into the quadriceps) or intravenous administration (into the saphenous or cephalic veins). Animals that are apprehensive or resent handling should be sedated using ketamine. Face-mask induction of anesthesia or intravenous administration of anesthetics can then be performed more easily.

Inhalational Anesthetic Agents

Diethyl Ether

This anesthetic, which was widely used in laboratory rodents, was delivered in a simple apparatus, with liquid anesthetic placed on a swab in an anesthetic chamber. These delivery systems provided no consistency in terms of induction concentration, and the agent itself has been shown to be irritant and stressful.[10] It has now largely been replaced with other agents that are delivered using more controlled methods. In addition to animal-welfare considerations, ether is explosive when mixed with oxygen or air.

Halothane

This can be used to provide safe and effective anesthesia in most laboratory species. Its effects on the cardiovascular and other body systems are broadly similar to those seen in companion and farm animals. In guinea pigs, it has been reported to cause hepatic injury,[11] although it is well tolerated in this species, in contrast to isoflurane and sevoflurane. Halothane is often preferred to isoflurane for neurophysiological studies (e.g., the electroencephalograph) because halothane's effects on some central nervous system activity at comparable planes of anesthesia are less pronounced.[12]

Isoflurane

This is now one of the most widely used inhalational agents for laboratory animals. Its popularity has been enhanced by its relative lack of metabolism. It is therefore thought to be less likely to interfere with drug pharmacokinetic and pharmacodynamic studies in anesthetized animals and less likely to have longer-term effects as a result of induction of liver microsomal enzyme systems. It is important to emphasize to research workers that other factors, such as changes in regional blood flow as a result of

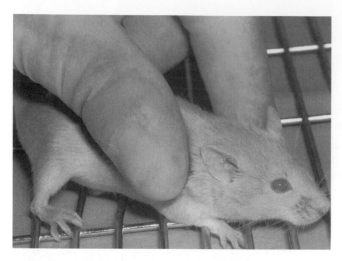

Fig. 30.10. Mouse restraint. The mouse is placed on a cage lid and then grasped by the loose skin overlying its back.

isoflurane administration, also can influence their studies. However, the rapid induction and recovery from anesthesia and ease of change of anesthetic depth make it suitable for both very short term and long term anesthetic protocols in a range of different species. As in companion animals, isoflurane can be combined with other agents (e.g., alfentanil) to provide a balanced anesthetic regimen with reduced nonspecific effects on body systems.

Desflurane

This has not been extensively used in laboratory species, although details of minimum alveolar concentration (MAC) and other characteristics of this agent are available.[13] It has similar effects in laboratory species as in companion animals and can be used to provide stable anesthesia with rapid induction and recovery. It appears to be better tolerated for anesthetic induction in rabbits than are other volatile agents.[3]

Sevoflurane

Use of sevoflurane is limited at present, but its popularity is likely to increase as it becomes more widely available in veterinary clinical practice. In addition, the speed and quality of induction and recovery and the ability to rapidly adjust anesthetic depth make it an attractive agent for a range of different studies. In guinea pigs, it appears to have much more variable effects than in other rodents. High concentrations may be required to maintain a surgical plane of anesthesia, and high mortality has been reported.

Nitrous Oxide

As in other animal species, nitrous oxide cannot produce anesthesia when used alone because its MAC value exceeds 100%. It can be used as part of a balanced anesthetic regimen to reduce the concentration of other anesthetic agents required. However, since MAC in small rodents exceeds 200%, the effects are relatively small. Since nitrous oxide is not absorbed by activated charcoal gas–scavenging units, it may be more convenient to avoid its use

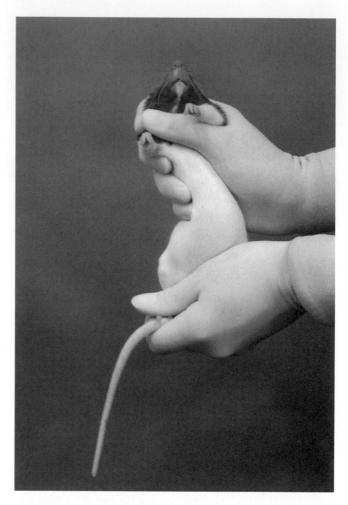

Fig. 30.11. Rat restraint. The rat is grasped with one hand supporting its hindquarters and one hand supporting its head, with the thumb under its foreleg and mandible.

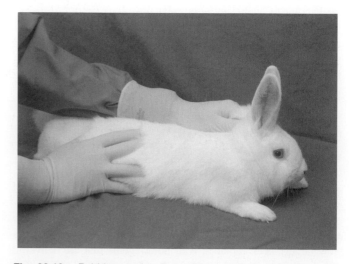

Fig. 30.12. Rabbit restraint. The rabbit is initially grasped by the skin of its neck and back.

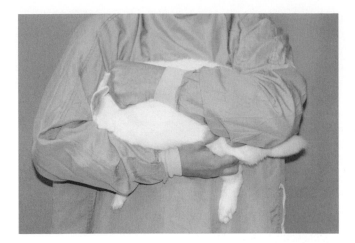

Fig. 30.13. Rabbit restraint. The rabbit is carried with its head between the handler's arm and chest.

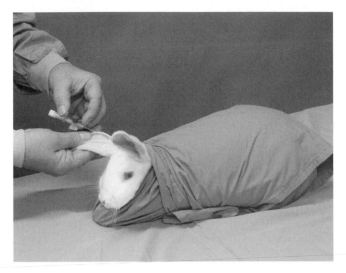

Fig. 30.14. Rabbit restraint. The rabbit is wrapped in a surgical drape to facilitate venipuncture.

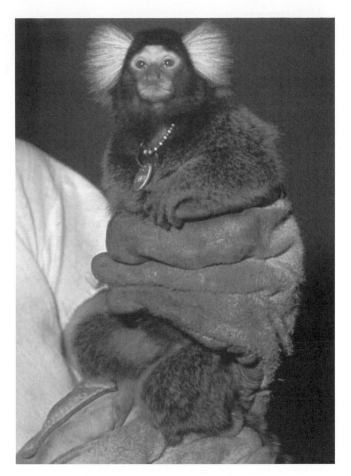

Fig. 30.15. Marmoset restraint. The handler is wearing protective gloves.

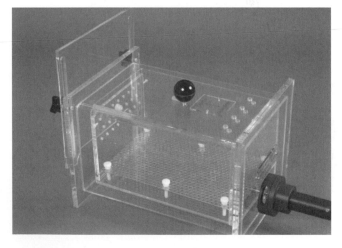

Fig. 30.16. Rodent anesthetic chamber (available from Harvard Instruments, South Natick, MA). This particular design enables effective scavenging of waste anesthetic gases.

altogether. In specific circumstances, for example, during prolonged anesthesia for neurophysiological studies, where the effects of anesthetic agents can be critical, its small contribution to depth of anesthesia and analgesia can be significant.

Delivery Systems

A major advantage of using volatile anesthetics in small mammals is the ease of administration using an anesthetic-induction chamber (Fig. 30.16). Ideally, chambers of different sizes should be available (e.g., for animals weighing less than 100 g and for animals weighing up to 1 kg). To reduce the period of involuntary excitement during induction, the chamber should be filled rapidly, with the maximum safe induction concentration of the agent. Since all anesthetic vapors are heavier than air, the anesthetic gas should be introduced at the bottom of the chamber and

excess gas ducted from the top. After loss of consciousness, the animal can then be removed from the chamber, and maintained by using a face mask, at a reduced concentration of agent. Providing effective gas scavenging when a face mask is being used can be difficult, but several systems are available commercially that assist with this, for example, the double-mask system.

Anesthesia can also be induced by face mask, and this can be a rapid and convenient technique when using sevoflurane in rats and mice. As mentioned earlier, volatile anesthetics generally provoke a breath-holding response in rabbits that is often associated with violent struggling unless preanesthetic agents are given. After sedation, the animal should be observed carefully during administration of the anesthetic and the mask removed briefly if breath holding occurs.

Nonhuman primates and other larger animals will generally be heavily sedated or completely immobilized with preanesthetic medication if a volatile agent is to be administered for anesthesia induction.

Some laboratory-animal units are equipped to provide only air as the carrier gas, and this is inadvisable. All of the currently available agents produce some degree of respiratory depression, but hypoxia can be prevented by delivery in oxygen. During recovery from anesthesia, oxygen should continue to be provided until the animal has begun to regain consciousness. If this is not done, then severe hypoxia can occur in some individuals.

Injectable Agents

Rodents and Rabbits

One noteworthy difference relating to the use of injectable anesthetics in small rodents in comparison to companion and farm animals is the difficulty of intravenous access. This results in anesthetic combinations often being administered as single injections by the intraperitoneal, subcutaneous, or intramuscular route, rather than intravenously, to effect. Although this is a simple and rapid means of producing anesthesia, it has inevitable consequences in relation to the safety of certain anesthetic agents, especially those in which the anesthetic dose is close to the lethal dose. Since there is considerable variation between different strains of rodents in their response to anesthetic agents,[14] anesthetic combinations that either have a broad safety margin or are wholly or partially reversible are preferred.

The small body size and high metabolic rate of rodents can result in relatively high dose rates of some anesthetic agents being required to achieve unconsciousness. When coupled with the relative lack of efficacy of agents such as ketamine, this can lead to very high dose rates being administered (e.g., 100 mg/kg ketamine). Since the drug formulations for veterinary use are normally optimized to give convenient volumes for a dog or a cat, the volume per kilogram of drug to be injected into a mouse can be relatively very high, and, if given intramuscularly, can damage tissue and cause pain on initial injection. Anesthetic combinations that are most widely used in rodents and rabbits are discussed below, and suggested dose rates are listed in Table 30.7.

Ketamine cannot be used as the sole anesthetic agent in rodents and rabbits, but when combined with sedatives such as acepromazine, or sedative analgesics such as medetomidine, varying planes of anesthesia can be produced. In small rodents, combinations with tranquilizers often produce only light anesthesia, which is insufficient for surgical procedures, whereas combinations with α_2-agonists such as medetomidine and xylazine produce surgical planes of anesthesia. In contrast, in rabbits, combinations of ketamine with acepromazine and diazepam often produce surgical planes of anesthesia. The likely effects of these various combinations are also listed in Table 30.7.

The use of medetomidine or xylazine with ketamine has the advantage that the sedative-analgesic component of the combination can be reversed with α_2-antagonists such as atipamezole. Since this anesthetic combination produces cardiovascular and respiratory depression, in addition to other systemic effects such as hyperglycemia and diuresis, it is strongly advised to administer the antagonist as a routine. Reversing the α_2-agonist will, of course, reduce the level of postoperative analgesia provided, so that additional agents (e.g., carprofen or buprenorphine) should be administered, if this has not already been done.

In guinea pigs, the effects of ketamine and xylazine and/or medetomidine are more variable, and surgical anesthesia may not be produced.[15] In all species, if the plane of anesthesia is insufficient, then administering additional doses of the combination may have unpredictable effects. It is preferable to administer a low concentration of an inhalant anesthetic (e.g., isoflurane) to deepen anesthesia. This same approach can be used to prolong the period of surgical anesthesia. As an alternative, the surgical field can be infiltrated with local anesthetic. As in other species, it is inadvisable to administer atropine routinely when using high doses of α_2-agonists. Severe hypertensive effects causing mortality have been reported in rats.

Tiletamine in combination with zolazepam (Telazol) has been recommended as an anesthetic for use in rodents and rabbits. As with ketamine–benzodiazepine combinations, the depth of anesthesia produced is not always sufficient to enable surgical procedures to be undertaken. Combining the mixture with xylazine increases anesthetic depth, but the effects are still variable.

Etorphine-methotrimeprazine (Immobilon), fentanyl-fluanisone (Hypnorm), and fentanyl-droperidol (Innovar-Vet) have all had their use in rodents and rabbits described.[16,17] All of these agents produce immobility and profound analgesia when used alone, but also cause significant respiratory depression. Fentanyl-fluanisone, when combined with midazolam or diazepam, produces surgical anesthesia in all species. Attempts to develop similar mixtures with the other commercially available neuroleptanalgesic combinations have been less successful.[18,19]

Fentanyl-fluanisone-midazolam has the advantage that it can be mixed and administered as a single injection, but the active components must be diluted with sterile water before being combined. The mixture is stable for several weeks, but on occasion can crystallize. If this is noted, the mix should be discarded. The fentanyl component can be reversed by using naloxone, but this also reverses all analgesic effects of the combination. It is preferable to reverse the fentanyl with a mixed agonist-antagonist such as butorphanol, nalbuphine, or the partial agonist buprenorphine.[20] This reverses any respiratory depression, although full recovery may be prolonged because of the sedative effects of the midazolam and fluanisone. Flumazenil will reverse the midazolam, but its relatively short half-life means that resedation can occur.

Table 30.7. Anesthetic and related drugs for use in rodents and rabbits[a].

Drug	Dose Rate	Effect	Anesthesia Duration (min)	Sleep Time (min)
Anesthetic and related drugs for use in mice				
Fentanyl-fluanisone and diazepam	0.3 mL/kg IM + 5 mg/kg IP	Surgical anesthesia	30–40	120–240
Fentanyl-fluanisone and midazolam[b]	10 mL/kg IP	Surgical anesthesia	30–40	120–240
Ketamine and medetomidine	75 mg/kg + 1 mg/kg IP	Surgical anesthesia	20–30	60–120
Ketamine and xylazine	80 mg/kg + 10 mg/kg IP	Surgical anesthesia	20–30	60–120
Tiletamine-zolazepam	80–100 mg/kg IM	Immobilization		60–120
Tribromoethanol	240 mg/kg IP	Surgical anesthesia	15–45	60–120
Anesthetic and related drugs for use in rats				
α-Chloralose	55–65 mg/kg IP	Light anesthesia	480–600	Nonrecovery only
Chloral hydrate	400 mg/kg IP	Light/surgical anesthesia	60–120	120–180
Fentanyl-fluanisone and diazepam	0.3 mL/kg IM + 2.5 mg/kg IP	Surgical anesthesia	20–40	120–240
Fentanyl-fluanisone and midazolam[b]	2.7 mL/kg IP	Surgical anesthesia	20–40	120–240
Ketamine and medetomidine	75 mg/kg + 0.5 mg/kg IP	Surgical anesthesia	20–30	120–240
Ketamine and xylazine	75 mg/kg + 10 mg/kg IP	Surgical anesthesia	20–30	120–240
Tiletamine-zolazepam	40–50 mg/kg IP	Light anesthesia	15–25	60–120
Urethane	1000 mg/kg IP	Surgical anesthesia	360–480	Nonrecovery only
Anesthetic and related drugs for use in rabbits				
Alphaxalone-alphadolone	6–9 mg/kg IV	Light anesthesia	5–10	10–20
Fentanyl-fluanisone and diazepam	0.3 mL/kg IM + 2 mg/kg IP or IV	Surgical anesthesia	20–40	60–120
Fentanyl-fluanisone and midazolam[b]	0.3 mL/kg IM + 2 mg/kg IM or IV	Surgical anesthesia	20–40	60–120
Ketamine and acepromazine	50 mg/kg IM + 1 mg/kg IM	Surgical anesthesia	20–30	60–120
Ketamine and medetomidine	15 mg/kg SC + 0.25 mg/kg SC	Surgical anesthesia	20–30	90–180
Ketamine and xylazine	35 mg/kg IM + 5 mg/kg IM	Surgical anesthesia	20–30	60–120
Propofol	10 mg/kg IV	Light anesthesia	5–10	10–15
Thiopentone	30 mg/kg IV	Surgical anesthesia	5–10	10–15
Anesthetic and related drugs for use in guinea pigs				
Alphaxalone-alphadolone	40 mg/kg IP	Immobilization		90–120
Fentanyl-fluanisone and diazepam	1 mL/kg IM + 2.5 mg/kg IP	Surgical anesthesia	45–60	120–180
Fentanyl-fluanisone and midazolam[b]	8 mL/kg IP	Surgical anesthesia	45–60	120–180
Ketamine and medetomidine	40 mg/kg + 0.5 mg/kg IP	Moderate anesthesia	30–40	90–120
Ketamine and xylazine	40 mg/kg + 5 mg/kg IP	Surgical anesthesia	30	90–120
Anesthetic and related drugs for use in hamsters				
Fentanyl-fluanisone and midazolam[b]	4 mL/kg	Surgical anesthesia	20–40	60–90
Ketamine and medetomidine	100 mg/kg + 0.25 mg/kg IP	Surgical anesthesia	30–60	60–120
Ketamine and xylazine	100–200 mg/kg +10 mg/kg IP	Surgical anesthesia	30–60	90–150
Anesthetic and related drugs for use in gerbils				
Fentanyl-fluanisone and midazolam[b]	8 mL/kg	Surgical anesthesia	20	60–90
Ketamine and medetomidine	75 mg/kg + 0.5 mg/kg IP	Medium anesthesia	20–30	90–120
Ketamine and xylazine	50 mg/kg + 2 mg/kg IP	Immobilization		20–60

IM, intramuscularly; IP, intraperitoneally; IV, intravenously; SC, subcutaneously.

[a]Note that considerable between-strain variation occurs, so dose rates should be taken only as a general guide.

[b]Dose (mL/kg) of a mixture of 1 part Hypnorm (fentanyl-fluanisone) plus 2 parts water for injection, and 1 part midazolam (5-mg/mL initial concentration).

In rabbits, the combination is best administered separately—fentanyl-fluanisone initially to produce sedation, analgesia, and peripheral vasodilation. This makes placement of an intravenous catheter, for example, in the marginal ear vein, simple and enables slow intravenous administration of the midazolam to produce the desired effects.

In rats, rabbits, and guinea pigs, mixtures of potent opioids (e.g., fentanyl or sufentanil) can be combined with medetomidine or other α_2-agonists to produce surgical anesthesia. In some instances, the addition of a benzodiazepine improves the degree of muscle relaxation.[20] These combinations have the advantage that they can be completely reversed by using specific antagonists.

Thiobutabarbital (Inactin) has been extensively used to provide medium-term to long-term anesthesia in rats. It is considered to have minimal effects on the cardiovascular system; in many respects, however, it resembles other barbiturates, producing reduction in cardiac output and organ blood flows.[21]

Urethane is a hypnotic agent that produces long-lasting and stable anesthesia with minimal cardiovascular and respiratory system depression. Urethane provides good narcosis and muscle relaxation, but the analgesic component may not be adequate. It is commonly used in terminal experiments for central and peripheral neural function studies where reflex responses should be preserved. When administered intraperitoneally, the most common route used, it has profound endocrine and metabolic effects, producing superficial damage and necrosis of intra-abdominal organs and massive leakage of plasma into the peritoneal cavity.[22] The onset of the aforementioned effects is rapid. Similar effects have not been observed when urethane was administered by subcutaneously, intravenously, or intra-arterially. Urethane is a carcinogenic and potentially mutagenic anesthetic agent therefore it should only be used if other suitable alternatives are not available and only for terminal (non recovery) studies.

Chloralose is used to provide long-lasting anesthesia, particularly in studies in which maintenance of cardiovascular responses is required. α-Chloralose is a hypnotic, and the anesthesia depth produced may be insufficient to enable surgical procedures to be undertaken. Induction and recovery from chloralose are very prolonged, so the agent is normally used only for terminal procedures. To avoid problems associated with a prolonged onset of action, anesthesia is often induced using another agent (e.g., isoflurane). Following intravenous cannulation and any other surgical procedures, chloralose is then administered.

Although now rarely used in farm-animal anesthesia, chloral hydrate, because of its minimal effects on the cardiovascular system, is still used to anesthetize laboratory animals. It is also used in neuropharmacology studies, because it is thought to have a reduced likelihood of interacting with other compounds. It produces medium-duration anesthesia. The anesthesia depth varies between different strains of rodent and can be sufficient for surgical procedures to be undertaken.[23,24] In some strains of rat, chloral hydrate can cause postanesthetic ileus, which can be fatal.[25] Using a dilute solution of chloral hydrate (36 mg/mL) can reduce the incidence of ileus.

Tribromoethanol (Avertin) is a hypnotic that produces surgical anesthesia in rats and mice that lasts approximately 15 to 20 min.

It has become extremely popular for anesthesia of mice for embryo transfer and for the production of transgenic animals, and has been reported to be safe and effective.[26] However, if improperly prepared or poorly stored, tribromoethanol can cause gastrointestinal disturbances. More recently, it has been reported that tribromoethanol can cause low-grade peritoneal irritation, even when correctly prepared and stored.[27,28] In view of these potential adverse effects, tribromoethanol is better replaced with other anesthetic combinations.

Nonhuman Primates

A very extensive range of anesthetic agents can be used in these species (Table 30.8). In most Old World primates, ketamine is administered initially to provide restraint. It is then possible to place an intravenous catheter and use an intravenous induction agent such as propofol, thiopental, or alphaxalone-alphadolone. Alternatively, anesthesia can be induced by using an inhalant anesthetic delivered via face mask. All of the currently used inhalant agents can be used safely and effectively in primate species.

As with other species, balanced anesthetic regimens—for example, ketamine as a preanesthetic medication, induction with propofol, followed by maintenance with sevoflurane, perhaps together with an opioid infusion—can provide stable anesthesia for many hours. However, body systems should be monitored carefully, and it is often advisable to intubate and assist ventilation if opioid infusions are used.

As mentioned earlier, ketamine has been reported to cause muscle necrosis in New World primates, so alphaxalone-alphadolone can be used as an alternative. Anesthesia can be deepened by further doses administered intravenously.[7] Alternatively inhalational agents can be used or propofol by continuous infusion.

Monitoring and Intraoperative Care

It is particularly important to provide high standards of perioperative care with laboratory animals, since not only can problems such as hypothermia prolong recovery, they cause widespread physiological effects that may interfere with particular research objectives. As in veterinary clinical practice, one staff member may need to act as both anesthetist and surgeon, so detailed clinical monitoring may be lacking. Use of electronic monitoring devices can therefore be of considerable value. The type of monitoring used should be selected based on the species, duration of anesthesia, type of surgery, and assessment of the degree of risk of complications or emergencies. Use of such devices is straightforward in Old World nonhuman primates, rabbits, and other large species, but is complicated by the small body size of other laboratory species. Small size is associated with a rapid heart rate (>300 beats/min) that may exceed the upper limits of some monitors, and the low signal strength may not be detectable. In addition, small body size limits such procedures as invasive blood-pressure monitoring and makes most noninvasive devices ineffective. Some equipment is now available that can function despite these problems, and routine electronic monitoring is becoming increasingly commonplace.

Table 30.8. Anesthetics and related drugs for use in nonhuman primates[a].

Anesthetic and Related Agents	Dose Rate	Effect
Alphaxalone-alphadolone	10–12 mg/kg IV	Surgical anesthesia
	12–18 mg/kg IM	Immobilization, anesthesia
Ketamine/diazepam	15 mg/kg IM + 1 mg/kg IM	Surgical anesthesia
Ketamine/xylazine	10 mg/kg IM + 0.5 mg/kg IM	Surgical anesthesia
Propofol	7.5–12.5 mg/kg IV	Surgical anesthesia

IM, intramuscularly; IV, intravenously.
[a]Note that considerable between-animals and between-species variation occurs so dose rates should only be taken as a general guide.

Assessment of Respiratory Function

Clinical observation of respiratory rate and pattern is relatively straightforward, but can be complicated by placement of surgical drapes, especially in small rodents. In these smaller species, the anesthetic circuit will not normally contain a reservoir bag, so observation of bag movements cannot be used to monitor respiration. Unfortunately, many electronic monitors do not respond to the relatively small respiratory movements and low tidal volumes, especially when used with animals weighing less than 200 g. In these small mammals, direct observation of respiratory rate and pattern may be the only option available.

In common with other species, the pattern, rate, and depth of anesthesia vary both with anesthetic depth and with the anesthetic regimen used. With inhalant anesthetics and the majority of injectable regimens, respiratory rate falls. Typical respiratory rates during anesthesia are 50 to 100 breaths/min for small rodents and 30 to 60 breaths/min for rabbits. Since many of these animals show a very marked stress-related tachypnea prior to induction, assessment of the degree of respiratory depression should either be based on estimates of normal resting rate (Table 30.1) or established by observing the animals preoperatively when undisturbed. A reduction to less than 50% of the estimated normal respiratory rate should cause concern. Gradual changes in rate, rather than a sudden reduction, are more usual, so keeping an anesthetic record is advisable.

The adequacy of oxygenation and heart rate can be assessed by using a pulse oximeter, but the high heart rates in rodents may exceed the upper limits of the monitor. A monitor with an upper limit of at least 350 beats/min is needed, and successful operation may also depend on the type of probe used. It is advisable to try several instruments, probes, and probe positions to find the most reliable combination. In the authors' experience, a signal can usually be obtained from across the hind foot in rodents or across the base of the tail. In rabbits, the toe, tail, tongue, and ear are also useful. In particular, the use of an angled probe placed in the mouth has proven particularly reliable.

End-tidal carbon dioxide is difficult to measure in small mammals. The gas volume sampled by side-stream capnographs may be very large in relation to the animal's tidal volume, and mainstream capnographs introduce too much equipment dead space into the anesthetic-breathing circuit. In rabbits and Old World primates, equipment designed for pediatric use in people usually functions well (Fig. 30.17).

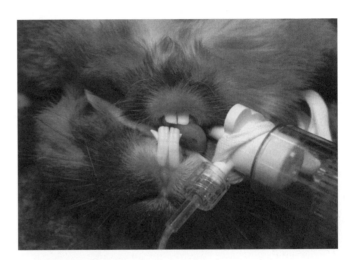

Fig. 30.17. An anesthetized rabbit. There is a low dead-space connector (Portex; Smiths Medical, Hythe, Kent, England) on the end of the endotracheal tube, with a side-port connector for capnograph connection.

Maintenance of a patent airway may be assisted by placement of an endotracheal tube, but the small size of many laboratory species makes this technically difficult. Intubation of nonhuman primates is relatively straightforward when using a small Macintosh blade or other curved design. Alternatively, a Soper or Wisconsin blade can be used to visualize the larynx (Fig. 30.18). The animal can be positioned either in sternal recumbency or on its back, depending on the preferences of the anesthetist. A cuffed 4-mm tube can be placed in a 7- to 8-kg Rhesus monkey. An introducer can be used to help pass the tube through the vocal cords, and laryngospasm can be prevented by spraying the cords with lidocaine. Stimulation of the larynx in a lightly anesthetized animal can provoke violent coughing and occasionally vomiting, so it is important to ensure that the animal is sufficiently deeply anesthetized before intubation is attempted.

Rabbits can also be intubated relatively easily by using either an otoscope to visualize the larynx or a blind technique. Prior to intubation, the animal should breathe 100% oxygen for 1 to 2 min. Uncuffed endotracheal tubes should be used to maximize the airway diameter; a 3- to 3.5-mm-diameter tube is usually suitable for a 3- to 4-kg rabbit. Tubes with a diameter of less than

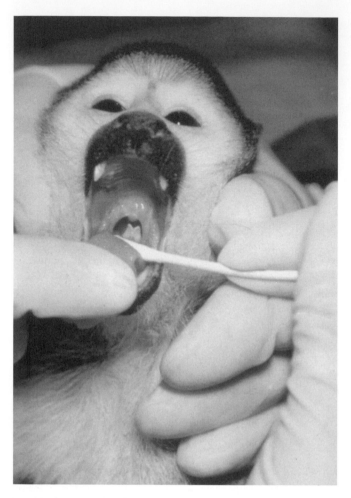

Fig. 30.18. An immobilized squirrel monkey with a view of its larynx prior to intubation.

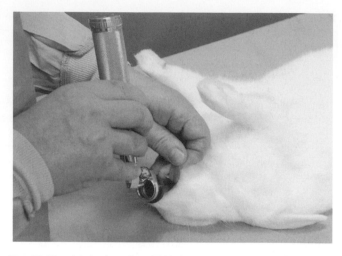

Fig. 30.19. Intubation of a rabbit's larynx by using an otoscope. The rabbit is in dorsal recumbency, and oxygen is administered for at least 2 min through a face mask prior to intubation.

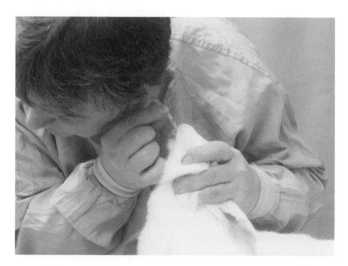

Fig. 30.20. Intubation of a rabbit by using the "blind technique." The rabbit is in ventral recumbency, and oxygen is administered for at least 2 min prior to intubation. To intubate, the endotracheal tube is placed in the rabbit's mouth to the level of its larynx. On inspiration, the endotracheal tube is gently advanced into the larynx in the direction of the loudest breath sounds.

2.5 mm are required for very small rabbits (<800 g), and these should be purchased from specialist suppliers.

When an otoscope is used, the rabbit is positioned on its back, its mouth opened, and its tongue pulled forward into the gap between the incisors and premolars, taking care not to injure the tongue on the edges of the incisors (Fig. 30.19). The otoscope speculum should be inserted into the gap between teeth on the opposite side of the mouth to the tongue and advanced until the end of the soft palate or the larynx is visible. In some animals, the epiglottis will be positioned behind the soft palate, hiding the larynx from view. To expose the larynx, the introducer is used to reposition the epiglottis and soft palate. The larynx should then be sprayed with local anesthetic. The introducer is then advanced through the otoscope speculum, through the larynx, and into the trachea. The otoscope is removed and the endotracheal tube threaded onto the introducer and into the trachea. The introducer is then withdrawn.

To place a tube using the blind technique, the rabbit is positioned on its chest, with its head and neck extended upward (Fig. 30.20). The endotracheal tube is introduced into the gap between the incisors and premolars and advanced into the pharynx. When the larynx is reached, some increase in resistance is felt. The tube

can then be advanced into the larynx and trachea—this is usually accompanied by a slight cough. In some cases, the tube passes into the esophagus and will need to be withdrawn and repositioned. Passage of the tube is often assisted by gently rotating it through 45° as it is advanced into the larynx. The tube position can be monitored by listening at the end of the tube—if breath sounds can be heard, the tube is in the pharynx or the trachea. As an alternative to intubation, a laryngeal mask can be used.[29] This technique is easier to master than endotracheal intubation, but assisted ventilation may not be effective. If only oxygen supplementation is required, a nasal catheter can be passed and positioned in the back of the pharynx.

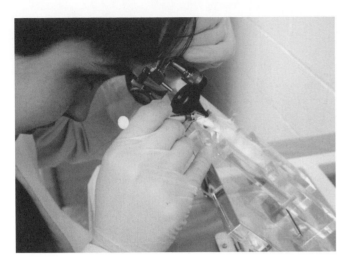

Fig. 30.21. A rodent workstand (available from Hallowell EMC, Pittsfield, MA) designed to facilitate endotracheal intubation in mice and rats.

Intubation of small rodents is made easier if a specialized apparatus is used. A technique using a modified otoscope speculum to visualize the larynx and an over-the-needle catheter as the endotracheal tube is relatively easy to master. Although a variety of other methods have been described, the modified otoscope (Fig. 30.21) enables rapid, atraumatic intubation and is supplied together with an instructional video.

After intubation, animals can be maintained on an appropriate anesthetic circuit; for example, a purpose-made low-dead-space T piece for small rodents, or a pediatric T piece or unmodified Bain's circuit for rabbits or nonhuman primates.

Assessment of Cardiovascular Function

Clinical monitoring of the cardiovascular system is difficult in small rodents because of their size. Peripheral pulse is difficult or impossible to palpate, and even when the thorax is palpated, since heart rate is frequently greater than 250 beats/min, accurate heart rate cannot be assessed. In rabbits and guinea pigs, the chest can be auscultated, but this is difficult in smaller rodents. An esophageal stethoscope can be used in rabbits. When using electronic monitoring equipment, the upper rate limits (often 250 or 300 beats/min) are often exceeded, and some instruments will not detect the low-amplitude electrocardiographic signal.

Other clinical assessments, such as use of capillary refill time, are practicable and useful in rabbits and primates. In all species, assessment of the color of the mucous membranes enables some assessment of peripheral perfusion. Arterial blood pressure can be measured by using noninvasive systems in nonhuman primates and larger rabbits or by using pediatric-sized cuffs or specially designed veterinary equipment. Blood pressure can be measured in this way in rats, using a tail cuff, but special apparatus is required. Invasive blood-pressure monitoring is possible in all species, but surgical exposure of the vessel is needed in rodents, which tends to limit use of this technique to nonrecovery procedures. In rabbits, an over-the-needle catheter can be placed

in the central ear artery, and, in primates, the femoral artery can be catheterized by using a Seldinger technique.

Blood volume in all of these species is approximately 70 mL/kg of body weight, so small rodents will have very low total blood volumes (e.g., 2 mL for a 30-g mouse). It is therefore critically important to minimize blood loss by careful surgical technique and to monitor blood loss by accurate weighing of swabs and assessing other losses at the surgical site.

Thermoregulation

Small mammals have an increased surface area to body weight ratio that results in rapid cooling during anesthesia. Maintaining body temperature and careful monitoring to ensure this is being achieved effectively are therefore critically important. Hypothermia can cause much delayed recovery from anesthesia and, if severe, can cause cardiac arrest. Rectal temperature should be monitored with an electronic thermometer. The probe size of less expensive instruments is usually appropriate for animals weighing 250 g or more, but specialist instruments are needed for very small rodents (e.g., mice and hamsters). To reduce loss, the area of fur shaved during preparation of the surgical site should be minimized, and use of skin disinfectants should be limited to the minimum necessary to maintain asepsis. Animals should be placed on a heating pad maintained at 37° to 39°C. It is important that measures to maintain body temperature are continued into the postoperative period.

Emergencies

All of the measures for coping with anesthetic emergencies applicable to companion animals can be used in laboratory species, but as with many other techniques, small body size can limit or complicate some of these procedures. To assist ventilation if an animal has not been intubated, its head and neck should be extended, its tongue pulled forward, and its chest squeezed between the anesthetist's thumb and forefinger. If the tongue is difficult to grasp, it can be rolled forward using a cotton-wool bud (Q-tip). When an animal has been intubated, respiration can be assisted relatively easily. Attempting to assist ventilation by using a face mask is usually unsuccessful, but in small rodents a soft piece of rubber tubing can be placed over the nose and mouth, and the lungs inflated by gently blowing down the tube. Doxapram (5 to 10 mg/kg intravenously, intramuscularly, or subcutaneously) can also be administered to stimulate ventilation. Oxygen should always be administered with doxapram administration if this is not already being provided.

As mentioned earlier, since total blood volume is low in small rodents, every effort should be made to minimize blood loss. If fluid therapy is required, this can be delivered via an over-the-needle catheter in the tail vein of rats, the medial tarsal vein in guinea pigs, or the marginal ear vein, cephalic vein, or jugular vein in rabbits. The cephalic or saphenous veins can be used in nonhuman primates, and the lateral tail vein can be used in marmosets. If whole blood is required, then a suitable donor may be available in the research facility. All of the commonly available fluid products can be administered safely to small mammals and other laboratory species. In smaller rodents in which intravenous access is not practicable, intraperitoneal or subcutaneous administration of warmed electrolyte solutions can slowly replace fluid deficits, but will be of minimal benefit if rapid hemorrhage is occurring. In these smaller species, placement of an intraosseous catheter can provide an alternative route for fluid replacement. If cardiac arrest occurs, external cardiac massage and emergency drugs such as epinephrine can be used when attempting resuscitation.

Postoperative Care

If possible, a separate recovery area should be provided, because this makes it easier to provide an optimal environment during this period. It also encourages individual attention and special nursing, if those are required.

Most of the commonly used anesthetics will continue to cause some degree of respiratory depression in the immediate postoperative period. In addition to continuing to monitor respiratory function, care must be taken that respiratory obstruction does not occur. Small rodents and rabbits may attempt to hide and push into the corner of a recovery cage, and this can result in airway obstruction. Also, when allowed to recover in a group, rodents may huddle together, which can decrease oxygen availability for the animals at the bottom of the group. Although recovery is often more rapid after use of inhalational agents, significant hypoxia (oxygen saturation of less than 70%) can occur, and this should be prevented by maintaining the animal in an oxygen-enriched environment, either by using a face mask or by delivering oxygen into the incubator until respiratory function is judged to be normal.

It is also important that measures to maintain normal body temperature are continued in the recovery period. This can often be achieved by allowing small animals to recover in a pen or cage in a recovery room (maintained at a high ambient temperature, with supplemental heating of the cage as necessary) or inside an incubator. A temperature of 25° to 30°C is needed for adult animals and 35° to 37°C for neonates. If an incubator is unavailable, heating pads and lamps should be provided. Care must be taken not to overheat the patient, and a thermometer should be placed next to the animal to monitor the temperature in its immediate environment.

During recovery from anesthesia, animals should be provided with bedding, such as synthetic sheepskin (Fig. 30.22). If this is not available, then toweling or a blanket should be used. Sawdust or wood shavings are unsuitable because this type of bedding will often stick to an animal's eyes, nose, and mouth. Tissue paper is often provided as bedding for small rodents, but it is relatively ineffective because animals usually push it aside during recovery from anesthesia and end up lying in the bottom of a plastic cage soiled with urine and feces.

Drinking water should be available, but care must be taken that this not be spilled, because, if the animal's skin becomes wet, it will lose heat rapidly. Small rodents are usually accustomed to using water bottles, so this is rarely a problem, but it can present difficulties with rabbits, guinea pigs, ferrets, and larger species.

It may also be judged necessary to provide fluid therapy post-

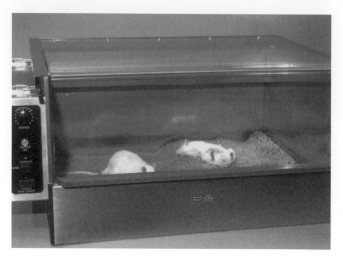

Fig. 30.22. Rats recovering from anesthesia in an incubator. Rats are provided with dry synthetic bedding.

operatively. This can be given by intravenous infusion in larger animals, but it is most convenient in small rodents to give warmed (37°C) subcutaneous or intraperitoneal dextrose-saline at the end of surgery (Table 30.9).

Food should be provided for most laboratory species immediately after they regain consciousness. Animals should be encouraged to eat as soon as possible, and this can often be achieved by providing highly palatable foods. A mash made by soaking pelleted diet in warm water is often rapidly consumed by small rodents, providing both additional fluid as well as food intake.

When monitoring the recovery of nonhuman primates, an additional concern is ensuring the safety of staff because of the potentially serious consequences of being bitten by a primate. The use of propofol sedation during recovery, so that animals can be allowed to regain consciousness in a controlled manner, can be helpful. After completion of surgery, the anesthetic (e.g., isoflurane) is discontinued and recovery of reflexes monitored. After return of the pedal withdrawal response and increase in jaw tone, propofol can be administered intravenously to deepen anesthesia slightly. Having produced a stable plane of light anesthesia, the animal either can be extubated when jaw tone returns or moved from the operating area to its recovery cage. Deep sedation or light anesthesia can be continued with incremental doses of propofol. The intravenous catheter can then be removed and the animal allowed to recover completely. Recovery from propofol is normally smooth, rapid, and associated with a less prolonged period of ataxia than is, for example, isoflurane. An alternative is either to maintain the primate on sevoflurane or to switch to this agent at the end of surgery. In our experience, recovery from this agent is smooth and rapid.

Pain Assessment

If analgesics are to be administered appropriately, then it is essential that attempts are made to assess the severity of postoperative pain. Only when this is done can one determine whether an

Table 30.9. Volumes of fluid for administration to rodents and rabbits[a].

Route	Mouse	Rat	Rabbit	Guinea Pig	Hamster	Gerbil
Intraperitoneal (mL)	2	5	50	20	3	2–3
Subcutaneous (mL)	1–2	5	30–50	10–20	3	1–2

[a]Volumes are suggested rates for adult animals. All fluids should be warmed to body temperature prior to administration.

appropriate dose of analgesic has been administered. Pain assessment is also essential to judge whether an appropriate type of analgesic has been selected, when to repeat dosing, and when to discontinue therapy.

Unfortunately, assessing pain in laboratory species is difficult. At present, the only practical option may be to judge the likely pain intensity based on the type of surgery and skill of the surgeon and use this to formulate an analgesic protocol. As with anesthesia selection, the aims of the particular research project should be considered when selecting the analgesic. Attempts should still be made to assess pain, and, since this is a rapidly developing field, it is important to continue to monitor the scientific literature for new information. Analgesic efficacy clearly varies considerably between different strains of rodents,[30] and this reinforces the need for pain-scoring systems.

At the time of writing, pain-scoring schemes have been developed for rats, following abdominal surgery.[31] In this species, back arching, contraction of the abdominal muscles, staggering and falling (not related to anesthetic recovery), and twitching of the skin overlying the back and abdomen all appear to be pain related. If more than one or two back arches, abdominal contractions, or staggers are seen in a 5-min period, then additional analgesia may be required. Illustrative material is available from www.digires.co.uk. In mice, similar behaviors have been noted (S. Wright-Williams, personal communication), as has a reduction in normal activities such as climbing (A. Karas, personal communication), but these behaviors have not yet been developed into a formal pain-scoring system. Some rabbits also show abdominal contractions after laparotomy, but changes in postoperative behavior in this species appear to be much more variable and to be markedly inhibited in some animals by the presence of an observer. Virtually no information is available regarding pain-related behavior in guinea pigs, hamsters or gerbils, or nonhuman primates.

In rats and probably other small rodents, analgesic efficacy can be assessed retrospectively by evaluating food and water intake and body weight. Body weight, food intake, and water intake decreases after many types of surgery in several different strains of rat, and administration of analgesics reduces this effect.[32,33] However, changes are not always consistent, particularly in juvenile animals.[34]

Pain Alleviation

Since all of the analgesic agents available for use in animals and people have been developed and tested for safety and efficacy in laboratory animals, likely effective doses can be suggested for

Table 30.10. Suggested analgesic dose rates for nonhuman primates (marmosets and rhesus macaques)[a].

Analgesic	Dose Rate
Buprenorphine	0.005–0.01 mg/kg IM or IV, per 6–12 h
Carprofen	2–4 mg/kg SC per 24 h
Meloxicam	0.1 mg/kg PO per 24 h

IM, intramuscularly; IP, intraperitoneally; IV, intravenously; SC, subcutaneously.

[a]Dose rates are based largely on uncontrolled clinical trials and a limited range of procedures and so are likely to be subject to revision.

most agents. However, the assessments of efficacy made during drug development are often based on tests that rely on acute painful stimuli (e.g., brief noxious heat or pressure). These differ from clinical pain. The dose rates suggested in Tables 30.4 and 30.10 are based on clinical experience, published data that incorporated a means of assessing postoperative pain, or data from analgesimetric assays, such as the late-phase formalin test, that are believed to be more relevant to clinical pain.[35]

Nonsteroidal Anti-inflammatory Drugs

All of the nonsteroidal anti-inflammatory drugs (NSAIDs) available for use in animals or people can be administered to laboratory species. The general considerations related to their use in other species apply equally to laboratory species; however, since most laboratory animals undergoing surgery are young, healthy adults, concerns related to preexisting disease are often minimal. Of the agents available, the oral preparation of meloxicam is of particular value because it is highly palatable to many small rodents and to nonhuman primates, particularly if added to a favorite foodstuff. The duration of action of NSAIDs in rodents and rabbits is uncertain, but carprofen and meloxicam appear to have duration of at least 8 and possibly 24 h.

Opioids

These are effective at alleviating postoperative pain, but some species-specific side effects have been reported. In nonhuman primates, butorphanol has been reported to cause a relatively greater degree of respiratory depression than occurs in other species.[5] Buprenorphine causes very little depression of respiration at clinically relevant dose rates, so is recommended as the partial agonist of choice in nonhuman primates. Opioids may also cause sedation or excitement, with their effects varying considerably in different animal species. The effects on behavior also depend on the drug dose that has been administered. Morphine sedates rats, but produces excitement in mice and, at high doses, a characteristic elevated and rigid tail (the Straub tail response). Although an effective analgesic, buprenorphine use in some strains of rat in some research institutes has been reported to cause pica, manifested as compulsive eating of bedding material. This is most severe when inappropriately high drug doses are administered,[36] but can also be seen at lower dose rates. Although the problem can be prevented by housing the animals on grid floors,[37] it may represent abdominal discomfort or nausea, so, if seen, an alternative analgesic should be used for that particular strain of animal. This side effect does not occur consistently, and, in view of the prolonged duration of action and safety of buprenorphine, this analgesic is often considered the opioid analgesic of choice in rats and other laboratory species.[35] A suggested analgesic dose of buprenorphine for use in nonhuman primates is listed in Table 30.10.

Effective Pain Control

Whatever the choice of analgesic regimen, it is important to administer sufficient drug to relieve pain effectively. If pain is not controlled effectively as rapidly as possible, such control can become progressively more difficult to achieve. This is one reason why preoperative administration of analgesics before elective surgery is advocated. In addition to providing more effective pain relief, it also may reduce the dose of anesthetic required. Experience with small rodents and rabbits has shown that the use of buprenorphine in this way enables the concentration of isoflurane or halothane needed for surgical anesthesia to be reduced by 25% to 50%. Care should be taken when using injectable anesthetics administered intraperitoneally or intramuscularly. As discussed earlier, in these circumstances the dose of anesthetic cannot be adjusted to meet individual requirements, and it is clear that opioids can potentiate the effects of anesthesia.[38] In view of the difficulty of adjusting the dose of injectable anesthetic, it is probably better to administer opioid analgesics postoperatively. When using neuroleptanalgesics, the opioid component will provide analgesia that can conveniently be partially reversed with the administration of buprenorphine or butorphanol. The latter opioid provides better reversal, but has a short duration of action, so either an additional dose should be given, or it should be combined with a NSAID.

As in other species, in many circumstances combinations of different agents can be particularly effective: for example, local nerve block at the time of repair of a thoracotomy, coupled with the administration of systemic opioids and NSAIDs, followed by repeated administration of opioids and NSAIDs, as required.[39] As the degree of pain subsides, the opioids can be reduced and pain controlled solely with NSAIDs. Suggested NSAID dosages for use in nonhuman primates are listed in Table 30.10.

Anesthesia of Neonatal Rodents

Neonatal rodents can be safely and effectively anesthetized with inhalant anesthetics, such as isoflurane.[40] The majority of in-

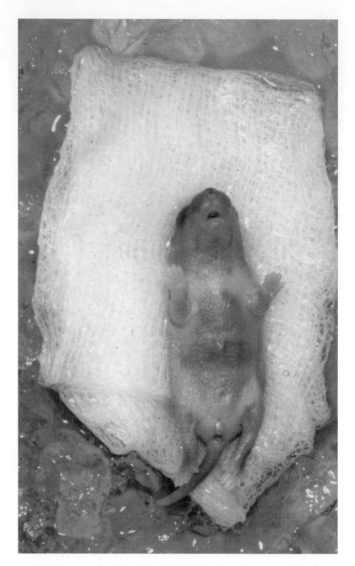

Fig. 30.23. A rat pup placed on a gauze swab with crushed ice.

jectable anesthetics may be associated with a high mortality, but fentanyl-fluanisone can be used in neonatal and juvenile rats.[41] Hypothermia is still used as an anesthetic technique in some research laboratories. Reducing body temperature to around 4° to 5°C by placing newborn rodents in a refrigerator or on crushed ice immobilizes them and slows their cardiac and respiratory function to virtually undetectable levels (Fig. 30.23). At these temperatures, nerve conduction is slowed or completely blocked, so that it is assumed that surgery can be performed without the animals experiencing pain or distress.[42] The technique remains controversial, but mortality is low when this approach is used. In the authors' opinion, this approach should be used only when alternative methods have been shown to be unsuitable.

Fetal Surgery

The majority of descriptions of fetal surgery rely on anesthesia of the mother to produce sufficient anesthesia in the fetus, although it may also be useful to infiltrate the surgical site in the fetus with local anesthetic to prevent movement in response to surgery. The fetus probably cannot perceive pain,[43] but nociceptor activation may produce changes in the central nervous system that can alter pain perception after birth or otherwise alter development.[44] It is therefore recommended that local anesthesia be used in the fetus, and that anesthetic regimens that cross the placenta be used in the mother.

References

1. Kehlet H (1989) Surgical stress: The role of pain and analgesia. Br J Anaesth 63:189–195.
2. Flecknell PA, Liles JH (1996) Halothane anaesthesia in the rabbit: A comparison of the effects of medetomidine, acepromazine and midazolam on breath-holding during induction. J Vet Anaesth 23:11–14.
3. Hedenqvist P, Roughan JV, Antunes L, Orr HE, Flecknell PA (2001) Induction of anaesthesia with desflurane and isoflurane in the rabbit. Lab Anim 35:172–179.
4. Olson ME, Vizzutti D, Morck DW, Cox AK (1993) The parasympatholytic effects of atropine sulphate and glycopyrrolate in rats and rabbits. Can J Vet Res 57:254–258.
5. Horn WA (2001) Primate anaesthesia. Vet Clin North Am Exot Anim Pract 4:239–266.
6. Green CJ, Halsey MJ, Precious S, Simpkin S (1978) Alphaxalone-alphadolone anesthesia in laboratory animals. Lab Anim 12:85–89.
7. Whelan G, James MF, Samson NA, Wood NI (1999) Anaesthesia of the common marmoset (Callithrix jacchus) using continuous intravenous infusion of alphaxalone/alphadalone [sic]. Lab Anim 33:24–29.
8. Flecknell PA, Liles JH, Williamson HA (1990) The use of lignocaine-prilocaine local anaesthetic cream for pain-free venepuncture in laboratory animals. Lab Anim 24:142–146.
9. Morton DB, Jennings M, Buckwell A, et al. (2000) Refining procedures for the administration of substances. Lab Anim 35:1–41.
10. De Haan M, van Herck H, Tolboom JB, Beynen AC, Remie R (2002) Endocrine stress response in jugular-vein cannulated rats upon multiple exposure to either diethyl-ether, halothane/O_2/N_2O or sham anaesthesia. Lab Anim 36:105–114.
11. Shenton JM, Chen J, Uetrecht JP (2004) Animal models of idiosyncratic drug reactions. Chem Biol Interact 150:53–70; Author reply, 167–168.
12. Antunes LM, Roughan JV, Flecknell PA (2003) Comparison of electroencephalogram activity and auditory evoked response during isoflurane and halothane anaesthesia in the rat. Vet Anaesth Analg 30:15–23.
13. Eger EI (1992) Desflurane animal and human pharmacology: Aspects of kinetics, safety, and MAC. Anesth Analg 75(4 Suppl): S3–S7; Discussion, S8–S9.
14. Lovell DP (1986) Variation in barbiturate sleeping time in mice. 1. Strain and sex differences. Lab Anim 20:85–90.
15. Nevalainen T, Pyhala L, Voipio HM, Virtanen R (1989) Evaluation of anaesthetic potency of medetomidine-ketamine combination in rats, guinea pigs and rabbits. Acta Vet Scand 85:139–143.
16. Flecknell PA (1996) Laboratory Animal Anaesthesia, 2nd ed. San Diego: Elsevier.
17. Flecknell PA, Mitchell M (1984). Midazolam and fentanyl-fluanisone: Assessment of anaesthetic effects in laboratory rodents and rabbits. Lab Anim 18:143–146.
18. Whelan G, Flecknell PA (1994) The use of etorphine/methotrimeprazine and midazolam as an anaesthetic technique in laboratory rats and mice. Lab Anim 28:70–77.
19. Whelan G, Flecknell PA (1995) Anaesthesia of laboratory rabbits using etorphine/methotrimeprazine and midazolam. Lab Anim 29:83–89.
20. Hu C, Flecknell PA, Liles JH (1991) Fentanyl and medetomidine anaesthesia in the rat and its reversal using atipamazole [sic] and either nalbuphine or butorphanol. Lab Anim 26:15–22.
21. Holstein-Rathlou N-H, Christensen P, Leyssac PP (1982) Effects of halothane–nitrous oxide inhalation anesthesia and Inactin on overall renal and tubular function in Sprague-Dawley and Wistar rats. Acta Physiol Scand 114:193–201.
22. Maggi CA, Meli A (1986) Suitability of urethane anesthesia for physiopharmacological investigations in various systems. Part 1: General considerations. Experientia 42:109–113. Part 2: Cardiovascular system. Experientia 42:290–297. Part 3: Other systems and conclusions. Experientia 42:531–537.
23. Sisson D, Siegel J (1989) Chloral hydrate anaesthesia: EEG power spectrum analysis and effects on VEPs in the rat. Neurotoxicol Teratol 11:51–56.
24. Field KJ, White WJ, Lang CM (1993) Anaesthetic effects of chloral hydrate, pentobarbitone and urethane in adult male rats. Lab Anim 27:258–269.
25. Fleischmann RW, McCracken D, Forbes W (1977) Adynamic ileus in the rat induced by chloral hydrate. Lab Anim Sci 27:238–243.
26. Papaioannou VE, Fox JG (1993) Efficacy of tribromoethanol anesthesia in mice. Lab Anim Sci 43:189–192.
27. Zeller W, Meier G, Burki K, Panoussis B (1998) Adverse effects of tribromoethanol as used in the production of transgenic mice. Lab Anim 32:407–413.
28. Reid WC, Carmichael KP, Srinivas S, Bryant JL (1999) Pathologic changes associated with use of tribromoethanol (Avertin) in the Sprague Dawley rat. Lab Anim Sci 49:665–667.
29. Smith JC, Robertson LD, Auhll A, March TJ, Derring C, Bolon B (2004) Endotracheal tubes versus laryngeal mask airways in rabbit inhalation anesthesia: Ease of use and waste gas emissions. Contemp Top Lab Anim Sci 43:22–25.
30. Mogil JS, Wilson SG, Bona K, et al. (1999) Heritability of nociception. I. Responses of 11 inbred mouse strains on 12 measures of nociception. Pain 80:67–82.
31. Roughan JV, Flecknell PA (2001) Behavioural effects of laparotomy and analgesic effects of ketoprofen and carprofen in rats. Pain 90:65–74.
32. Liles JH, Flecknell PA (1994) A comparison of the effects of buprenorphine, carprofen and flunixin following laparotomy in rats. J Vet Pharmacol Ther 17:284–290.
33. Flecknell PA, Roughan J, Stewart R (1999). A comparison of the effects of oral or subcutaneous carprofen or ketoprofen following laparotomy in the rat. Vet Rec 144:65–67.
34. Roughan JV, Flecknell PA (2003) Evaluation of a short-duration behaviour-based post-operative pain scoring system in rats. Eur J Pain 7:397–406.
35. Roughan JV, Flecknell PA (2002) Buprenorphine: A reappraisal of its antinociceptive effects and therapeutic use alleviating post-operative pain in animals. Lab Anim 36:322–343.
36. Clarke JA, Myers PH, Goelz MF, Thigpern JE, Forsythe DB (1997) Pica behavior associated with buprenorphine administration in the rat. Lab Anim Sci 47:300–303.
37. Jacobson C (2000) Adverse effects on growth rates in rats caused by buprenorphine administration. Lab Anim 34:202–206.

38. Roughan JV, Burzaco Ojeda O, Flecknell PA (1999) The influence of pre-anaesthetic administration of buprenorphine on the anaesthetic effects of ketamine/medetomidine and pentobarbitone in rats and the consequences of repeated anaesthesia. Lab Anim 33:234–242.

39. Kehlet H, Wilmore DW (2002) Multimodal strategies to improve surgical outcome. Am J Surg 183:630–641.

40. Danneman P, Mandrell T (1997) Evaluation of five agents/methods for anesthesia of neonatal rats. Lab Anim Sci 47:386–395.

41. Clowry GJ, Flecknell PA (2000) The successful use of fentanyl/fluanisone ("Hypnorm") as an anaesthetic for intracranial surgery in neonatal rats. Lab Anim 34:260–264.

42. Budnick B, McKeown ML, Wiederholt WC (1981) Hypothermia-induced changes in rat short latency somatosensory evoked potentials. Electroencephalogr Clin Neurophysiol 51:19–31.

43. Mellor DJ, Gregory NJ (2003) Responsiveness, behavioural arousal and awareness in fetal and newborn lambs: Experimental, practical and therapeutic implications. NZ Vet J 51:2–13.

44. Vanhatalo S, van Nieuwenhuizen O (2000) Fetal pain? Brain Dev 22:145–150.

Chapter 31
Exotic and Zoo Animal Species

Rachael E. Carpenter and David B. Brunson

Introduction

This chapter reviews anesthesia and immobilization of a wide array of selected species commonly found in zoos and wildlife parks, as well as a number of exotic species that have a special role in either animal agriculture or as companion animals. In some instances, species have been included in this chapter because of the unique challenges they present when endeavoring to capture or anesthetize them either in the wild or captured environment.

Flying Mammals: Bats

Bats should be handled with thick leather gloves to prevent one from being bitten.[1] Bats harbor a number of viruses that can cause human illnesses and even death. Therefore, sedation and anesthesia are recommended if extensive handling is necessary. Fruit bats (*Eidolon helvum*) have been sedated with a phenothiazine tranquilizer (intramuscular [IM] chlorpromazine, 2.5 mg/100 g). After the tranquilizer has taken effect, the bat can be mounted on a restraining board with wings extended and an inhalant anesthetic administered by mask. Other methods of chemical restraint include IM xylazine (2 to 3 mg/kg) administration, which will provide 30 to 40 min of sedation. Ketamine can be given IM at a dose of 10 to 20 mg/kg along with this dose of xy-lazine to provide more complete immobilization with muscle relaxation and a quiet recovery. Medetomidine (50 μg/kg IM) has also been combined with ketamine (5 mg/kg IM) for short-term immobilization. Telazol (tiletamine-zolazepam) may be a good alternative for injectable immobilization at an IM dose of 8 to 10 mg/kg.[2] Intraperitoneal (IP) pentobarbital injection at a dose of 0.05 mg/g of body weight has been used in a number of genera of bats (*Rhinolophus*, *Hipposideros*, *Tadarida*, *Molussus*, *Eptesicus*, *Chilonycteris*, and *Artibeus*) to implant electrodes surgically on the round window of the cochlea or in the brain. Smaller doses (0.03 to 0.045 mg/g) have been used for *Myotis lucifugus* and *Pleocotus townsendii*.[3,4]

Isoflurane or sevoflurane delivered by mask or into an induction chamber can be safely used to anesthetize bats. Following mask induction, megachiropterous can be intubated (2- to 3-mm internal diameter [ID]) to maintain anesthesia. When intubating bats, care must be taken to avoid lacerations from teeth and direct contact with saliva. Intravenous (IV) access is feasible via the brachial vessels overlying the distal humerus.[2]

Terrestrial Mammals

Armadillos

There are ten living genera of armadillos. *Dasypus novemcinctus*, the most common, weighs 4 to 5 kg as an adult. Armadillos should be caught close to the base of the tail to avoid the hind claws. Because armadillos can incur a large oxygen debt, they may lie completely still without breathing for long periods. Armadillos also have the ability to recover spontaneously from repeated episodes of ventricular fibrillation.[5] Anesthetics may be administered into the subcarpal tissues or the spinal muscles by inserting a needle between two bands slightly to one side of the midline. The site should be thoroughly cleansed to avoid danger of abscess formation.

Neuroleptanalgesic combinations (e.g., fentanyl-droperidol, 0.20 to 0.25 mL/kg IM) appear to produce sufficient depression and analgesia for surgery.[6] Longer procedures have been performed with slow IV infusion of thiopental.[7] Infused over a period of 1 h, 5 mL of 0.5% solution is adequate and safe for most adults. The usual dosage is 5 to 6 mg · kg^{-1} · h^{-1}. Alternatively, pentobarbital (25 mg/kg IV) has been administered via the superficial femoral vein.[8] Half the dose is given rapidly, followed by the remainder to effect. Apnea and breath holding are not reported to be a problem with this technique. Injections can be made into the two prominent superficial femoral veins. The femoral vein is the only accessible superficial vein that can be easily catheterized. Midline cesarean section has been performed with local infiltration of lidocaine.

Telazol (8.5 mg/kg IM), xylazine (1 mg/kg) with ketamine (7.5 mg/kg), and medetomidine (75 µg/kg) with ketamine (7.5 mg/kg) have been evaluated for their anesthetic actions following IM administration. All three combinations induced anesthesia within 5 min.[9] Armadillos were immobilized for approximately 45 min, with recovery requiring 2 to 3 h. When atipamezole was used to antagonize medetomidine, recovery was shortened to 15 min or less.[9]

Inhalation anesthesia with isoflurane or sevoflurane is easily achieved with a closed induction chamber. Premedication with IM atropine sulfate (total dose, 0.1 mg) can be used to diminish secretions. A soft polyethylene endotracheal tube 4- to 8-mm ID is easily placed through the laryngeal opening with the use of a laryngoscope. Following intubation, anesthesia may be maintained with isoflurane concentrations in the range of 1.5% to 2.5% delivered via a rebreathing system using a precision vaporizer.

Wild Rodents

Chinchillas are easily removed from their cages by grasping them by the base of the tail and lifting them off their feet. Anesthesia can be induced with either 1.5% to 2.5% halothane or isoflurane or 2.5% to 4.0% sevoflurane. Old reports indicate that the IM administration of 15 mg of meperidine approximately 30 min prior to surgery, followed by 1% subcutaneous (SC) lidocaine solution injected along the proposed line of incision, provides adequate analgesia and sedation for cesarean section in chinchillas.[10] Recovery is rapid, and the young suckle within minutes after delivery. Midazolam or diazepam (5 mg/kg) plus ketamine (15 to 20 mg/kg) administered IM also produces relaxation and analgesia for up to 2 h. Thiopental sodium in dilute solution can also be administered IV to effect for minor surgical procedures. Epidural anesthesia has been used for cesarean section because the lumbosacral fossa is easily located and is comparatively large.[11] Epidural anesthesia techniques are similar to those used for dogs and cats and can be achieved with local anesthetics such as lidocaine. In a 2004 study, an IM combination of midazolam (1.0 mg/kg), medetomidine (0.05 mg/kg), and fentanyl (0.02 mg/kg) was compared with the IM injection of either xylazine (2.0 mg/kg) with ketamine (40.0 mg/kg) or medetomidine (0.06 mg/kg) with ketamine (5.0 mg/kg) to assess combination anesthetic actions in chinchillas. The xylazine-ketamine and medetomidine-ketamine combinations provided longer surgical tolerance, but overall the midazolam-medetomidine-fentanyl combination was preferred because it induced less cardiopulmonary depression and achieved good anesthesia with the potential for complete reversal.[12]

Squirrels are best anesthetized with isoflurane or sevoflurane administered into an induction chamber. Ketamine (10 to 20 mg/kg) is the most commonly used injectable anesthetic in gray and fox squirrels. It provides adequate immobilization for physical examination and diagnostic procedures. A combination of medetomidine and ketamine has also been used to immobilize squirrels (Table 31.1).

In prairie dogs, ketamine (100 to 150 mg/kg) plus xylazine (20 mg/kg) administered IV produces 1.5 to 2.0 h of satisfactory surgical anesthesia.[13] Xylazine can be administered 10 min prior to ketamine or may be given in the same syringe at the same time. For longer periods of anesthesia, inhalant anesthetics can also be administered via a mask or following endotracheal intubation. Because prairie dogs are obligate nasal breathers, they need to only have their nose in the mask for induction and maintenance of inhalant anesthesia. Visualization of the larynx is difficult without the use of a modified otoscope or laryngoscope. If all that is required is a short period of sedation, a lower dose of ketamine (40 mg/kg) can be combined with acepromazine (0.4 mg/kg) and administered IM.[14] Butorphanol (2 mg/kg subcutaneously) or buprenorphine (0.02 mg/kg SC) may be used to produce analgesic effects in prairie dogs. Marmots are similar to prairie dogs and have been successfully anesthetized with combinations of xylazine-ketamine, medetomidine-ketamine, and xylazine-Telazol.[15]

Agoutis are large, excitable, agile rodents that can injure themselves or handlers if not carefully restrained. Ketamine alone (25 to 35 mg/kg) has been used to immobilize agoutis.[16] Ketamine can be coadministered with analgesics or sedative-analgesics for painful procedures. As might be expected, xylazine, phenothiazine tranquilizers, and fentanyl-droperidol alone are not as effective. Inhalant anesthetics (isoflurane or sevoflurane) delivered via a face mask or by endotracheal tube produce good surgical anesthesia following ketamine immobilization.

The coypu (nutria) is difficult to restrain for IV injection. They have no readily accessible superficial veins. Endotracheal intubation can be performed in anesthetized animals with a slightly flexible tube containing a curved stylet. Intubation can be performed without visualization of the laryngeal opening. Animals weighing 3 to 5 kg require a 5-mm-ID endotracheal tube. Upon insertion, apnea may occur. Following intubation, anesthesia can be maintained with any inhaled anesthetic. In early investigations, chloralose (80 mg/kg) and pentobarbital (40 mg/kg) were administered IP for sedation but did not provide adequate surgical anesthesia at these dosages. Ketamine (10 to 20 mg/kg) plus 2 mg of xylazine have been assessed together in 4- to 5-kg nutria for tail amputation surgery. Prolonged anesthesia was produced by 20 mg/kg of ketamine, whereas 10 mg/kg was insufficient for surgery.[17] Administration of medetomidine (0.1 mg/kg IM) plus ketamine (5 mg/kg IM) induces rapid anesthesia in nutria (Table 31.1). Immobilization lasts for approximately 40 to 60 min. Atipamezole (0.5 to 0.7 mg/kg IM) will awaken animals within 5 to 10 min of administration. The atipamezole dose should be four- to fivefold the dose of medetomidine. Atropine (0.1 mg/kg) is effective as a preanesthetic to decrease salivary secretions.

Voles have been anesthetized for nearly 3 h with pentobarbital at an IP dose of 0.06 mg/g of body weight. Surgical anesthesia can be induced for 15 to 20 min in meadow voles with a 0.06- to 0.09-mg/g dose of pentobarbital injected IM. In recent years, the use of IM or IP pentobarbital for anesthesia has been supplanted with injectable combinations and the use of inhalant anesthetics in most rodent species. Additional information on the dosing of ketamine-medetomidine combinations in wild rodents (e.g., squirrels) is listed in Table 31.1.

Table 31.1. Species and medetomidine and ketamine intramuscular dosages used for immobilization of nondomestic mammals

Species	Medetomidine (µg/kg)	Ketamine (mg/kg)	Plane[a]	Documentation[b]
Insectivora				
Hedgehog (*Erinaceus euro paeus*)	100	5	2	+
Primate				
Baboon (*Papio hamadryas*)	100	5	1–2	+
Chimpanzee (*Pan troglodytes*)	50	5	3	++
Common marmoset (*Callithrix jacchus*)	100	5	1–2	
Cotton-headed tamarin (*Saguinus oidipus*)	100	5	2–3	++
Emperor tamarin (*Saguinus imperator*)	100	5	2–3	++
Lar gibbon (*Hylobates lar*)	70	3	2	+
Lowland gorilla (*Gorilla gorilla*)	50	5	3	+
Red-bellied tamarin (*Saguinus labiatus*)	100	5	2	
Rodentia				
Brown squirrel (*Sciurus vulgaris*)	100	5	1	+
Norwegian lemming (*Lemmus lemmus*)	200–300	—	2–3	+
Nutria (*Myocastor coypus*)	100	5	2–3	+++
Camivora				
Amur leopard (*Panthera pardus orientalis*)	60–80	2.5–3.0	3	++
Blue fox (*Alopex lagopus*)	50	2.5	3	+++
Brown bear (*Ursus a. arctos*)	50	2	3	+
Ferret (*Mustela putorius*)	100	5	2	+
Golden cat (*Felis temmincki*)	80–100	3–4	3	++
Jaguar (*Panthera onca*)	60–80	2.5	3	+
Lion (*Panthera leo*)	60–80	2–3	3	+
Lynx (*Lynx lynx*)	80–100	2.5–3.5	3	++
Maned wolf (*Chrysocyon brachyurus*)	80	2.5	3	+
Mink (*Mustela vision*)	100	5	1–2	+
Pine marten (*Martes martes*)	100	5	2	+
Polar bear (*Thalarctos maritimus*)	30	2.5	3	++
Red panda (*Ailurus fulgens*)	80–100	2.5–4.0	2–3	+
Snow leopard (*Panthera uncía*)	60–80	2.5–3.0	3	+++
Ermine (*Mustela erminea*)	100	5	2–3	++
Sun bear (*Helarctos malayanus*)	60–80	2–3	2–3	+
Tiger (*Panthera tigris*)	60–80	2.5	3	+
Wolf (*Canis lupus*)	60–100	3–5	3	++
Wolverine (*Gulo gulo*)	100	5	3	++
Perissodactyla				
Przewalski's wild horse (*Equus przewalski*)	60–80	1.5–2.0	2–3	+
Artiodactyla				
Alpine ibex (*Capra i. ibex*)	80–140	1.5	2–3	+++
Axis deer (*Axis axis*)	50	1–2	2	++
Bactrian camel (*Camelus bactrianus*)	40	—	I	+
Barbary sheep (*Ammotragus lervia*)	100–140	1.5	2–3	++
Blackbuck (*Antilope cervicapra*)	200–300	1.5–2.0	2–3	+
Chamois (*Rupicapra r. rupicapra*)	70–100	1.5–2.0	2–3	+++
Fallow deer (*Dama dama*)	100–150	2.0–2.5	2–3	++
Forest reindeer (*Ranifer tarandus fennicus*)	60–80	0.6–0.8	2–3	+++
Guanaco (*Lama guanicoe*)	60–100	1.5–2.0	2–3	+
Himalayan tahr (*Hemitragus jeinlahicus*)	80–100	1.5	2–3	++
Llama (*Lana glama*)	50	1	2	+
Markhor (*Capra falconeri rnegaceros*)	60–100	1.5–2.0	2–3	+++
Moose (*Alces alces*)	60	1.5	2	+
Mouflon (*Ovis musimon*)	125	2.5	2	+
Pére David's deer (*Elaphurus davidianus*)	30	1	3	+
Red deer (*Cervus elaphus*)	50	1.5	3	++

(continued)

Table 31.1. Species and medetomidine and ketamine intramuscular dosages used for immobilization of nondomestic mammals (*continued*)

Species	Medetomidine (µg/kg)	Ketamine (mg/kg)	Plane[a]	Documentation[b]
Reindeer (*Rangifer tarandus tarandus*)	30	1	3	++
Rocky mountain goat (*Oreamnos americanus*)	60–80	1.5	2–3	+++
Roe deer (*Capreolus capreolus*)	50	1–2	2	++
Wapiti (*Cervus canadensis*)	60–80	1.5–2.0	2–3	+
White-tailed deer (*Odocoileus virginianus*)	60–80	1.5–2.0	2–3	++
Wisent (*Bison bonasus*)	50–80	1.5–2.5	2–3	+
Yak (*Bos mutus grunninens*)	70–100	2–3	2–3	+
Marsupiala				
Red-neck wallaby (*Macropus rufogriseus*)	100	5	2–3	+

[a](1) Insufficient, animal sedated but able to struggle considerably or get up; (2) moderate, deep sedation but occasional muscle tension or mild struggling when handled; and (3) complete immobilization, good muscle relaxation and no arousal after handling or nociceptive stimuli.

[b]Subjective evaluation of how reliable the given recommendations are, ranging from + (least reliable) to +++ (most reliable).

Modified from Jalanka and Koeken.[135]

Mustelids

A metal or Plexiglas tube is convenient for restraining mink. The dimensions of the tubes will vary according to the size of the mink being restrained.[18] One end of the tube is covered with hardware cloth, with the other remaining open. The mink is inserted headfirst into the tube. Vaccinations or other injections can be administered SC or IM on the inner surface of the hind leg while the animal is restrained. Anesthesia has been induced with carbon dioxode–oxygen mixtures (1:1), but isoflurane or sevoflurane administration is obviously preferable for chamber inductions. Maintenance of anesthesia with halothane or isoflurane by use of rebreathing or non-rebreathing delivery systems is preferred. In field situations, mink and polecats have been successfully immobilized and anesthetized with a combination of ketamine (10 mg/kg IM) and medetomidine (0.20 mg/kg IM) for radio-transmitter implantation. Induction was achieved in less than 4 min, and immobilization lasted from 28 to 54 min.[19] Older reports indicate that reserpine (0.036 to 0.05 mg) can be administered orally in feed to render mink less nervous and excitable.[20] Apparently, there is a wide margin of safety with few cumulative toxic effects.

For ferrets, anesthesia is commonly induced with sevoflurane or isoflurane in an induction chamber. Atropine (0.04 mg/kg) can be administered either SC or IM prior to induction. To maintain anesthesia, inhalants are then delivered via a mask or through an endotracheal tube. Injectable mixtures for producing short periods of anesthesia in ferrets include ketamine (26 mg/kg IM) plus acepromazine (0.22 mg/kg IM), ketamine alone (20 to 30 mg/kg IM) to produce light surgical anesthesia for 40 to 60 min, Althesin (12 to 15 mg of total steroid/kg IM), which is a 3:1 mixture of alphaxalone with alphadolone acetate, to produce 15 to 30 min of light anesthesia, and Telazol at a dose of 5 to 10 mg/kg IM. A mixture of Telazol (250 mg tiletamine and 250 mg zolazepam) solubilized in 4 mL of ketamine (400 mg) and 1 mL of 10% xylazine (100 mg/mL) designed for use in exotic cats can be used in ferrets and feral cats at a dose of 0.03 to 0.04 mL/kg IM.

This mixture has been used for castrations, declawing, and intra-abdominal surgery.[21,22] Medetomidine (0.1 mg/kg IM) can also be combined with ketamine (5 mg/kg IM) to induce a short period of anesthesia in ferrets (Table 31.1).

In general, rapid-acting volatile anesthetics such as isoflurane or sevoflurane are preferred for anesthetizing skunks. For small skunks, a transparent plastic disposable bag is an ideal container for induction with sevoflurane or isoflurane. Anesthesia is induced while the skunk is in the bag, and the surgery is performed through a small opening cut in the bag. Once immobilized, the skunk is removed and the bag is discarded. This procedure should be performed in a well-ventilated room to minimize human exposure to anesthetic gases and skunk musk. The best age for removal of the scent glands in skunks appears to be 5 to 6 weeks of age, when the skunk's weight is about 2 pounds.[23] If inhalant anesthesia is not feasible, pentobarbital can be administered IP to induce anesthesia by using a 2-mL syringe and 25-gauge needle; the usual dose ranges for adult skunks are 15 to 30 mg/kg.

An anesthetic technique for wild skunks caught in traps using a 9-foot pole syringe has been described.[24] The operator stands at a distance while making an IM injection and thus facilitates handling without exposure to musk or possibly being bitten. With this technique, pentobarbital solution has been administered IM at the rate of 20 mg/kg of body weight. Skunks are less likely to expel musk if the operator is slow and deliberate. Skunks that expel musk usually direct it at the pole syringe when the drug is injected. The immobilizing combination of ketamine (16 mg/kg IM) plus xylazine (8 mg/kg IM) has also been effective in skunks. Anesthesia is usually induced in less than 3 min with immobilization lasting approximately 30 min.[25]

Stoat (*Mustela erminea*) and weasel (*Mustela nivalis*) are extremely fierce and difficult to handle. They will bite through thick leather gloves and, if held tightly, may be asphyxiated.[26] A satisfactory and nontraumatic method of inducing anesthesia is to place these animals in a Plexiglas induction chamber (10 × 4

× 4 inches) attached to the end of the cage by means of a removable slide. A 2½-inch-diameter hole connects the box to the cage. The animal is easily coaxed into this box. Isoflurane or sevoflurane is then introduced into the box via the fresh gas line from the vaporizer. Safe induction concentrations range from 2.5% to 4.0%. Once the animal is unable to right itself, it can be removed from the chamber and inhalant anesthesia maintained at lower concentrations by using a face mask or via delivery through an endotracheal tube. The intubation technique is similar to that used for ferrets. Light surgical anesthesia can be maintained with 1.5% to 2.0% concentrations of isoflurane or 2% to 3% sevoflurane. Alternately, medetomidine (0.1 mg/kg IM) plus ketamine (5 mg/kg IM) has been used to immobilize stoats with variable success (Table 31.1).

Badgers (*Taxidea taxus*), which have a ferocious disposition, have been successfully immobilized with phencyclidine, acepromazine, chlorpromazine, or succinylcholine administration. Ketamine appears to be the most satisfactory drug for immobilizing the European badger (*Meles meles*).[27] The average effective dose is 20 mg/kg IM, and repeated smaller doses are sometimes administered. Complete recovery occurs in 90 to 180 min, depending on the total dose administered. A number of studies have evaluated anesthetic combinations in badgers in comparison with ketamine alone (20 mg/kg). The addition of midazolam with lower doses of ketamine (10 to 15 mg/kg) did not improve anesthesia, nor did the combination of medetomidine (80 µg/kg) with only 5 mg/kg of ketamine.[28] The combination of butorphanol, medetomidine and ketamine appeared to improve overall muscle relaxation and anesthesia, however.[29] Following immobilization with either IM administered ketamine (15 to 25 mg/kg) plus xylazine (0.5 to 1.0 mg/kg) or Telazol (8 to 12 mg/kg) plus xylazine (0.5 to 1.0 mg/kg), anesthesia can be maintained with isoflurane or sevoflurane delivered through a mask or endotracheal tube.

Wild Procyonids

Members of this family include the ring-tailed cat, raccoon, coatimundi, mountain coati, lesser panda, and giant panda. Anesthetic techniques used in these species are primarily based on experience gained in the immobilization and anesthesia of raccoons. These anesthetic techniques would appear applicable for most procyonids. Intravenous anesthesia is not practical because of difficulty in restraining these species. Ketamine or Telazol have been used extensively and are made more efficacious when supplemented with an α₂-agonist (e.g., xylazine or medetomidine). A phenothiazine (acepromazine) or benzodiazepine (diazepam) tranquilizer can also be combined with ketamine. When ketamine has been used alone at a dose of 20 to 30 mg/kg IM, induction takes 3 to 7 min, and recovery can be expected to occur in 45 to 90 min. A combination of a lower dose of ketamine (10 mg/kg IM) with xylazine (2 mg/kg IM) or other α₂-agonist is more often used to immobilize wild procyonids today. Induction occurs in 3 to 5 min after IM injection. Anesthesia appears adequate, lasts for 15 to 20 min, and can be prolonged by administering one-quarter to one-half of the original combination dose IM or by the administration of isoflurane or sevoflurane via a face mask or an endotracheal tube. Medeto-

midine (0.1 mg/kg IM) can also be combined with ketamine (4 mg/kg IM) to immobilize wild red pandas.

Telazol has been used in a variety of procyonids for chemical restraint and short, minor surgical procedures. A dose of 10 mg/kg IM induces anesthesia lasting for 20 to 60 min. With this dose, reflexes (including the palpebral, corneal, pinnal, pharyngeal, and laryngeal) should persist.[30]

Wild and Feral Canids

In the mid–20th century, these species were usually immobilized by using dart guns with drugs such as nicotine, phencyclidine, etorphine, or succinylcholine. These drugs are rarely used today, having been replaced with various dose combinations of ketamine (e.g., 10 mg/kg IM) plus xylazine (e.g., 2 mg/kg IM) or plus medetomidine (0.1 mg/kg IM) (Table 31.1). With these dosages of ketamine and α₂-agonists, induction time averages 5 to 10 min. Anesthesia usually lasts 15 to 20 min, and recovery is complete in approximately 30 min. Medetomidine alone (0.025 to 0.1 mg/kg IM) can be used to produce dose-dependent sedation and immobilization of many wild canids. Nevertheless, for safety reasons, ketamine is commonly administered with medetomidine to ensure immobilization. The dose of ketamine used should never be less than 2.5 mg/kg IM for immobilizing any wild carnivore. Once captured, wild canids can be anesthetized with inhalants in the same manner as domesticated dogs. Anesthesia is commonly induced with the animal in a squeeze cage. An injectable tranquilizer, narcotic, and/or ketamine or Telazol is administered, followed by administration of an inhalant such as isoflurane or sevoflurane. Coyotes and other wild carnivores caught in steel traps often injure themselves struggling. A cloth-covered diazepam tablet was described in the 1960s for attachment to the trap. The tablet would hopefully be ingested by the coyote after capture, with the intent of calming the animal and preventing additional self-inflicted harm.[31]

Wild Felids

Throughout the latter half of the 20th century, many species of nondomesticated cats have been immobilized with high doses of ketamine alone (Table 31.2).[32] However, salivation, muscle rigidity, and convulsions can occur with ketamine immobilization alone. Combinations of ketamine (10 to 20 mg/kg IM) and xylazine (2 mg/kg IM) can be used to induce short periods of anesthesia (i.e., 5 to 20 min) in most wild felids. Additional doses can be given when necessary to prolong anesthesia. Xylazine alone has been used to immobilize wild cats at a dose ranging from 1 to 3 mg/kg of body weight, but it should be understood that large felids immobilized with xylazine alone can be easily aroused by auditory, visual, and physical stimuli. Medetomidine in combination with ketamine has also been used to immobilize a variety of wild felids (Table 31.1). For many decades now etorphine (M-99) has also been used successfully to immobilize African lions and other wild cats.[33] For a 100-kg lion, the suggested total dose of M-99 is approximately 0.5 mg. In adult lions, tremors associated with M-99 injection can be controlled with acepromazine administration (total dose, 25 to 30 mg). Appropriate doses of Telazol (1.5 to 5.0 mg/kg IM) will usually induce anesthesia in large fe-

Table 31.2. Use of intramuscular ketamine in nondomesticated cats

Species	Sex	Age in Years (M = Months)	Weight (kg)	Dose of Ketamine (mg/kg)	Onset Time (min)
Ocelot (*Felis pardalis*)	F	12	8	5	NM
	F	12	8	6	NM
	F	14	8	14	10
Serval (*Felis serval*)	M	8 M	11	9	10
	F	4	9	15	NM
Leopard cat (*Felis bengalensis*)	M	10 M	3	14	NM
	M	10 M	3	8	U
	F	10 M	2	11.5	U
	F	10 M	1	15	10
	M	10 M	2	25	8
Clouded leopard (*Neofelis nebulosa*)	M	15	18	8.5	U
Chinese leopard (*Pan therapardus Japonensis*)	F	3.5	38	15	7 (C)
Black leopard (*Panthera pardus*)	F	13	54	15	19
Margay (*Felis wiedii*)	F	7	3	15	NM
Jaguar (*Panthera onca*)	F	14	60	13	10
	M	5	83	18	U
Cheetah (*Acinonyx jubatus*)	M	7	34	8	U
	M	7	33	11	NM
	M	7	34	12	U
	M	7	34	11.5	8 (C)
	M	10	42	9.5	6
	M	12	30.5	10	6
Puma (*Felis concolor*)	F	12	24	11	7
	F	12	24	11	14
	M	8 M	27	15	U
	M	8 M	27	18	U
	F	6	23	22	3
	M	14	50	18	8
	M	2	30	15	7
	M	2	58	20	13
	M	2.3	45	18	U
	M	2.5	56	25	8
Lion (*Panthera leo*)	F	12	150	10	U
	M	2	140	18	6
	M	3	163	14	U (C)
	F	2	95	20	5 (C)
Tiger (*Panthera tigris*)	M	15	130	7	7
	F	7	110	14	9

C, convulsions observed; NM, not measured; U, unsafe to handle.

lids within 2 to 5 min, providing 15 to 30 min of immobilization and analgesia. The coadministration of atropine with dissociative anesthetics generally prevents excessive salivation. Some tigers may be more sensitive to Telazol than others. Reported adverse reactions to Telazol in tigers and other large cats include prolonged muscle rigidity and an inability to stand for several days after recovery.

Historically (mid–20th century), succinylcholine chloride had been used for immobilization of a large variety of wild species, including large cats such as African and North American mountain lions (*Felis concolor*).[34] With the availability of newer drugs

and combinations for immobilization of wild and feral animals, succinylcholine alone is no longer considered an acceptable immobilizing drug.

Relatively high doses of meperidine and promazine have been used as preanesthetics in some large cats, such as ocelots, leopards, and lions. In lions, 11 mg/kg of meperidine or 4.4 to 9.0 mg/kg of promazine has been used to achieve sedation.[35,36] SC and IM injections are facilitated by use of a squeeze cage. Once sedation is evident, a tourniquet can be applied to the tail to help locate the caudal vein for IV injection of the injectable anesthetic.

When compared with smaller domestic cats, big cats appear to

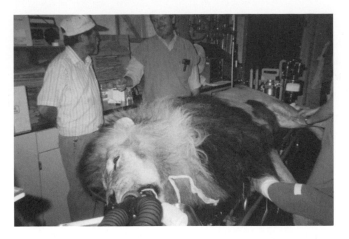

Fig. 31.1. Adult male lion anesthetized with isoflurane. Indirect blood pressure was measured at 5-min intervals by using an oscillometric device and cuff placement around the metatarsal artery. Fluid administration is important during long procedures and will assure a ready venous access for drug administration.

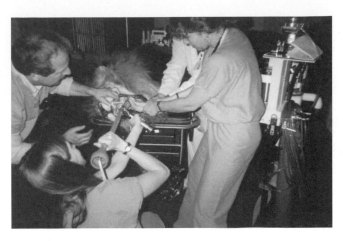

Fig. 31.2. Large animal cuffed endotracheal tube is passed into the trachea for delivery of inhalation anesthetic to an adult tiger. Flow rates of 5 to 6 L/min are recommended. The tube should be secured in place to prevent movement and laryngeal trauma.

require less anesthetic per kilogram to produce surgical anesthesia. For example, when combined with medetomidine (0.03 mg/kg IM), the required dose of ketamine is reportedly only 2.5 mg/kg IM for immobilization of tigers and lions (Table 31.1). Certain reflexes may persist, and the recovery period is usually longer for larger cats. The rate and character of ventilation are important criteria for assessing depth of anesthesia. Fewer than 10 breaths per minute is cause for concern. To avoid the need to use larger doses of general anesthetic in large undomesticated cats, it is suggested that local anesthetics be employed, whenever possible, to desensitize tissues and structures prior to surgical manipulation. Additional information on various injectable drug combinations in large cats, including propofol IV administration, has been published.[37–39]

Whenever possible, inhalational anesthesia with isoflurane or sevoflurane is preferred for longer periods of general anesthesia of large felids. A more precise control of anesthesia depth is provided, and the animal will have a more rapid emergence upon completion of the procedure (Fig. 31.1). If the procedure is expected to be of considerable duration, endotracheal intubation is preferable to mask delivery of the inhalant. Tracheal intubation in large cats can be achieved with or without a laryngoscope (Fig. 31.2). Large lions and tigers require a medium Cole tapered tube or an 18- to 24-mm-ID cuffed tube commonly used in small adult horses. Before the endotracheal tube is positioned in the trachea, the larynx should be sprayed with lidocaine to decrease the likelihood of laryngeal spasms.

Wild and Feral Swine

Wild and feral hogs have been captured by placing α-chloralose on corn or in mixtures of flour, peanut butter, sardines, and syrup. The feeding site should be baited for several days prior to using the drugged bait. When one teaspoonful of methocel per cup is added to dampened shelled corn, it causes the relatively insolu-

ble α-chloralose to adhere to the corn. The maximum safe dosage for feral hogs is about 2.2 g/10 kg of body weight, and the minimum effective dose is about 2.2 g/40 kg. One cup of bait with 2 g of α-chloralose appears to be effective.[40] Bait should be removed after the trapping operation, because the bait is potentially dangerous to other wildlife. Once captured and restrained, wild swine and javelinas can be anesthetized with a dissociative such as ketamine or a barbiturate such as thiopental (10 mg/kg IV). Adult peccaries and feral hogs have been successfully immobilized with a 1:1 mg mixture of Telazol (100 mg) and xylazine (100 mg). This mixture has provided adequate anesthesia and analgesia to perform short surgical procedures.[41] Once adequate restraint or immobilization has been achieved, anesthetic techniques used in domestic breeds of pigs are effective in wild and feral swine.

Wild Ruminants

Bovidae Species

Prior to the availability of modern immobilizing drugs, Beale and Smith[42] reported on the use of 6 to 10 mg/45 kg of succinylcholine chloride to immobilize pronghorn antelope. Xylazine (1 to 3 mg/kg) or carfentanil was also commonly employed for sedation and capture of antelope and other wild ruminants in the latter half of the 20th century.[43] Carfentanil has often been combined with a tranquilizer, as was reported for its use in roan antelope immobilized with 11 to 13 μg/kg when combined with 0.75 mg/kg of azaperone.[44] Intramuscular immobilizing doses of fentanyl, etorphine, and xylazine employed in African antelopes and other wild Bovidae species are listed in Table 31.3. Xylazine alone and in combination with ketamine has also been used extensively for the immobilization of many captive and free-ranging Bovidae ruminants. For example, in the 1980s, captive dorcas gazelles were immobilized by using xylazine (0.25 mg/kg IM) and ketamine (12 mg/kg IM) prior to electroejaculation and

Table 31.3. Immobilizing intramuscular doses of drugs in several African Bovidae species

Species	Age	Sex	Body Weight (kg)	Immobilized Approx. Total Times	Immobilized No. of Animals	Fentanyl	Immobilon LA (Large Animal) Etorphine	+ Acepromazine	Xylazine	Nalorphine	Diprenorphine
Bongo	Adult	M	300	5	2	70	4.4–4.9	18–20	75	200	6.0
Boocercus euryceros	Adult	F	220	12	5	40	2.45–2.94	10–20	50	120	3.6
	Immature	M	50	2	1	10	—	—	10	30	—
			80	2	2	15	—	—	10	45	—
Zebra duiker	Adult	M/F	15	18	4	3.0	—	—	2.5–6.0	10	—
Cephalophus zebra	2 weeks	M	1.0	1	1	1.0	—	—	—	2.5	—
Red flanked duiker	Adult	M/F	9	9	4	2.0	—	—	2.0	6.0	—
Cephalophus rufilatus	Immature	M	5	3	1	1.0	—	—	1.0	2.5	—
Jentink's duiker	Adult	M	80	5	1	15	—	—	10	50	—
Cephalophus jentinkii											
Maxwell's duiker	Adult	M/F	5.0	11	4	1.0–1.5	—	—	1.0–1.5	3–4	—
Cephalophus maxwellii											
Yellow-back duiker	Adult	M/F	65	11	4	15–20	—	—	10–20	50	—
Cephalophus sylvicultor											
Black duiker	Adult	M	15	3	1	3	—	—	3	10	—
Cephalophus niger											
Eland	Adult	F	300	4	1	—	2.94	12	50	—	3.6
Taurotragus oryx	Immature	M/F	150–200	14	6	—	1.96	8	40–50	—	2.4
	Immature	M	120	4	2	15–20	1.46	6	20–40	50	2.0
	Immature	F	60	1	1	12	—	—	12	30	—
Beisa oryx	Immature	M/F	150	16	5	30	1.96–2.45	8–10	20–30	80	2.4–3.0
Oryx beisa											
Harnessed antelope	Adult	M/F	20	3	3	4.0	—	—	4	10	—
Tragelaphus scriptus											
Coke's hartebeeste	Adult	M/F	180	5	3	—	1.47	6	20–30	—	2.0
Alcelaphus buselaphus cokei											
Impala	Adult	M/F	30–50	8	5	10	—	—	10	25	—
Aepyceros melampus											
Wildebeest	Adult	M/F	180–200	17	5	—	1.47–1.96	6–8	20–30	—	2.0–2.5
Connochaetes tourinus	Immature	F	70	3	1	—	0.49	2	10	—	0.6
Defassa waterbuck	Adult	M	320	5	2	50	1.96–2.94	8–12	40–50	125	2.4–3.6
Kobus defassa											
Thomson's gazelle	Adult	M/F	18	5	3	5.0	—	—	5.0	12.5	—
Gazella thomsonii											
Buffalo	Near adult	F	375	3	1	—	2.45	10	25	—	3.0
Syncerus caffer											

From Haigh.[136]

sperm collection.[45] More recently, a number of wild Bovidae species have been successfully immobilized and/or anesthetized with combinations incorporating medetomidine and ketamine with an opioid in an effort to further enhance the analgesic and anesthetic actions of this combination.[46,47] When necessary, atipamezole can be administered at a ratio fivefold the medetomidine dose to help prevent resedation in the field and possible predation.[48]

To capture bighorn sheep, etorphine has been used at a dose of approximately 22 μg/kg IM.[49] The IM injection of acepromazine (total dose, 15 mg in adults) after capture prolongs the effect of etorphine and facilitates handling. Injection of cyprenorphine effects rapid recovery from the effects of etorphine. It is recommended that cyprenorphine or diprenorphine be administered in a dose 2¹/₂ times the amount of etorphine and that half be administered IV and half IM to smooth recovery and decrease the likelihood of renarcotization. Xylazine has been used alone to immobilize bighorn sheep, with total effective dosages ranging from 350 mg for adult males to 250 mg for adult females. Long recoveries resulted in some deaths before the procedure was shortened and the anesthesia made safer by reversal with the administration of idazoxan, an α_2-antagonist.[50] To tranquilize bighorn sheep in a captive environment, diazepam can be mixed at a dose of approximately 13 mg per each kilogram of feed fed to the sheep.

The domestic buffalo (*Bubalus bubalis*) is raised mainly in Asia as a producer of meat and milk. It is only distantly related to the American bison (*Bison bison*). Most anesthetic techniques for the buffalo have been inferred from work with cattle. Several studies have shown considerable variation between species, however. The effects of xylazine on water buffalo calves at doses of 0.22 and 0.44 mg/kg IV and 0.44 mg/kg IM were assessed in the late 1970s.[51] Recovery times were dose related and varied from 65 to 130 min for the IV doses, whereas the IM dose produced an average of 150 min of recumbency. Administration of 0.04 mg/kg of atropine IM reduces salivary secretions and bradycardia observed with xylazine administration. Ketamine (2.0 mg/kg IV) has been combined with chlorpromazine (2.0 mg/kg IM) to anesthetize water buffalo calves. Pretreatment with chlorpromazine increases the duration of analgesia and recovery time beyond that achieved with ketamine alone. Short-term surgical procedures (5 to 10 min) with this drug combination have been performed in calves.[52]

The use of guaifenesin (165 mg/kg IV) alone in water buffalo calves to produce complete immobilization causes significant hypotension. Cardiovascular and respiratory effects produced by high doses of guaifenesin are generally undesirable.[53] An anesthetic mixture used as early as the 1960s consisted of chloral hydrate (30 g), magnesium sulfate (15 g), and thiopental (2.5 g) in 1000 mL of distilled water.[54] Thirty minutes after the SC administration of atropine, the mixture was administered IV at approximately 2.0 mL/kg. Anesthesia was deemed adequate for 15 to 25 min following the initial injection and could be prolonged by additional injections. Newer methods of providing short periods of injectable anesthesia rely on the combination of ketamine with α_2-agonists and other tranquilizers, such as diazepam and triflupromazine, to enhance muscle relaxation and improve overall

safety.[55] In one study, a 0.1-mg/kg IV dose of detomidine was combined with 0.1 mg/kg dose of diazepam IV and 3 mg/kg of ketamine IV for 15 min of excellent anesthesia.[56] Inhalant anesthesia has also proven satisfactory in water buffalo and is preferred for longer-lasting anesthesia when the appropriate facilities and delivery equipment are available at the zoo facility or wildlife park.

Bison (*Bison bison*) are generally dangerous and difficult to handle, and heavy equipment is required in order to restrain mature animals. Capture equipment is necessary to catch free-roaming animals. Early reports (1960s) indicate captured bison being administered chloral hydrate (250 mg/kg) to achieve deep surgical anesthesia. More recently, reports of bison immobilization have emphasized the IM use of α_2-agonist agents (e.g., xylazine or medetomidine) with either potent opioids (e.g., carfentanil) or Telazol, a dissociative and benzodiazepine proprietary mixture.[57,58] The use of combinations incorporating xylazine or medetomidine with Telazol has caused some concerns regarding rumenal tympany. The anesthetic and physiological effects of these combinations have been effectively antagonized with the administration of α_2-antagonists: tolazoline (for xylazine) and atipamezole (for medetomidine).[58] Once bison have been restrained and/or immobilized by physical or chemical methods, IV and inhalant techniques commonly used in large domestic cattle can be effective in providing short periods of general anesthesia.

Cervidae Species

Over three decades ago, reports on the effects of IM injections of 0.3 mg/kg up to 9 mg/kg of xylazine in red, fallow, and spotted deer were published.[59–61] With clinically effective doses of xylazine, sedation begins within 3 to 10 min and usually lasts 1 to 2 h. A degree of analgesia is produced, but supplementation with a local or regional anesthetic was required for surgery. During the onset of sedation, there is some salivation, but regurgitation of ruminal contents or ruminal tympany has been rare. Alterations in respiratory rhythm, ranging from transient apnea to a Cheyne-Stokes respiration, are typically observed with the higher doses of xylazine and have been frequently encountered in red deer, moose, sitatunga (marshbuck), and Barbary sheep. Xylazine had also been used alone to immobilize captive white-tailed deer in the 1970s.[62] Induction times were shorter in fawns and freshly trapped deer. Immobilization was prolonged with doses above 3 mg/kg, and it was recommended that higher doses than this should not be used. In general, xylazine alone produces good sedation and analgesia in wild Cervidae species, but, with lower doses, immobilization and muscle relaxation are sometimes insufficient for handling.

When given alone, the dose of ketamine for most deer species ranges from 10 to 20 mg/kg IM. More recently, two of the more common drug mixtures for immobilizing wild deer are ketamine-xylazine and Telazol-xylazine. Medetomidine has also been combined with ketamine at varying doses to immobilize several species of deer and other Cervidae species (Table 31.1). Atipamezole can be used to antagonize medetomidine-ketamine–induced immobilization of captive and wild deer at approximately fivefold the administered dose of medetomidine (Table 31.4).

Table 31.4. Total atipamezole intramuscular doses and atipamezole-medetomidine ratios (wt/wt) in selected ruminant species to reverse medetomidine-ketamine–induced immobilization

Species	n	Atipamezole (μg/kg)		Atipamezole-Medetomidine Ratio (wt/wt)	
		Median	Min.–Max.	Median	Min.–Max.
Alpine ibex	70	543	152–833	5.0	1.7–7.1
Barbary sheep	10	298	142–417	3.7	2.9–5.0
Chamois	41	328	197–653	5.0	3.0–7.1
Forest reindeer	41	309	185–522	5.0	3.0–7.0
Himalayan tahr	29	345	143–658	5.0	4.0–5.6
Markhor	62	409	194–698	5.0	4.0–5.6
Rocky Mountain goat	22	315	114–714	5.0	2.5–5.8
White-tailed deer	25	294	160–435	5.0	2.7–6.0

From Jalanka and Koeken.[135]

Potent opioids can also be used to immobilize many species of captive wild deer and other wild ruminants. In the 1970s, for fallow and other species of deer, IM administered mixtures of etorphine (2 mg/100 kg) with xylazine (30 mg/100 kg) or fentanyl (0.3 to 0.66 mg/kg) with xylazine (0.5 to 1.3 mg/kg) were proven to be quite reliable and effective.[63,64]

For tranquilization of deer prior to transportation, chlorpromazine can be administered IM at a dose of 4.4 mg/kg. Good results have also been obtained in elk with this dose. Full effect occurs in about 1 h and lasts for 16 to 24 h. When used as preanesthetics prior to injectable or inhalant anesthetics, phenothiazine tranquilizers should be injected IM at least 1 h in advance. In the 1990s, longer-lasting neuroleptics began to be administered IM in wild ruminants to provide days or even weeks of taming effects.[65] Zuclopenthixol acetate (1 mg/kg) and decanoate (10 mg/kg) provide 3 to 4 days and 10 to 20 days of calming effect, respectively. The action of perphenazine enanthate (1 mg/kg) typically lasts 7 to 10 days, whereas pipothiazine palmitate (5 mg/kg) reportedly provides 2 to 4 weeks of calming action.

The reaction of deer to IV barbiturate anesthesia varies greatly. Deer must be watched closely during the recovery period. Salivation and bloating are common problems. If pentobarbital is to be used, it should be preceded by atropine administration, and the animal should be deprived of feed and water for 1 day prior to induction. In a series of approximately 50 deer anesthetized with pentobarbital, one death and several cases of postoperative pneumonia, caused by regurgitation of rumen contents, occurred.[66] To eliminate such complications, endotracheal intubation is recommended during general anesthesia of deer, as in other ruminants. In general, high-dose barbiturate anesthesia alone cannot be recommended for most wild ruminant species.

As with Bovidae species, the oral ingestion of diazepam alone has been used to produce sedation and muscle relaxation for capture of wild Cervidae.[67] The dose ranges from 125 to 250 g/10 kg of feed. The effects vary depending on the amount ingested but may persist for several days. Maximum effect occurs 4 to 8 h after ingestion. Sedated individuals should be separated from nontranquilized animals if possible, because the latter may injure less alert deer. As tranquilization deepens, animals eat less, making this sedation technique somewhat self-limiting.

Succinylcholine chloride or gallamine has been used to immobilize North American elk (*Cervus canadensis*), but these muscle relaxants may cause bloating and severe respiratory depression and can no longer be recommended. Newer methods include the use of potent opioids, such as carfentanil, or the use of α_2-agonist plus ketamine combinations to immobilize or anesthetize elk.[68] Intranasal xylazine administration as a novel method of calming and reducing stress in captured elk appears promising, as well.[69]

A number of drugs have been used to immobilize and anesthetize caribou, including fentanyl (0.3 to 0.6 mg/kg IM), xylazine (0.25 to 0.5 mg/kg IM), and azaperone (0.5 to 1.2 mg/kg IM).[70] Etorphine (0.02 to 0.1 mg/kg IM) has also proven effective in caribou when combined with acepromazine (0.02 to 0.1 mg/kg IM). Xylazine alone produces long-lasting immobility in moose. Sedate animals require constant supervision. A mixture of xylazine (0.15 to 0.5 mg/kg) and fentanyl (0.15 to 0.5 mg/kg) delivered by dart syringe has proven effective in the helicopter-assisted capture of moose.[64] Hyaluronidase (150 to 300 NF units) added to the IM anesthetic mixture decreases the induction times by 36% to 45%.

Camelids

Large Camelidae can be reliably sedated with xylazine. IM doses ranging from 0.4 to 0.9 mg/kg have been used in Arabian and Bactrian camels. In most instances, once sedation is evident, there is no resistance to positioning and manipulation of feet. Sedation usually begins within 10 min and can vary in duration from 45 min to 5 h. Larger doses produce sedation for as long as 1 day. Regurgitation of rumen contents and ruminal tympany are not common, and recovery is unaccompanied by struggling and excitement.[71] Sedation in Bactrian camels that is achieved with xylazine doses of 0.25 to 0.50 mg/kg IM has been antagonized with doxapram administration (0.05 to 0.13 mg/kg IV).[72] In earlier reports (1960s) of camel anesthesia, premedication with IM chlorpromazine (1 mg/kg) reportedly decreased the dose of chloral hydrate or pentobarbital sodium necessary to induce anesthesia while prolonging its duration.[72] Satisfactory IV anesthesia has been achieved in adult camels with a combination of chlorpromazine (0.5 mg/kg IM), pentobarbital (total dose, 2.0 g IV), and 2.5 g/50 kg of body weight of chloral hydrate administered IV. Anesthesia can be prolonged with supplemental IV doses of pentobarbital when using this combination. In recent years, camels are more typically immobilized with xylazine (e.g., 0.15 mg/kg IM) plus ketamine (e.g., 2.5 mg/kg IM) combinations.[73]

For laparotomy and rumenotomy procedures, regional analgesia can be used in camels by infiltration of 2% lidocaine in a reverse-seven pattern along the caudal edge of the last rib and the distal tips of the lumbar transverse processes. Epidural anesthesia can also be attempted in camels with the animals fastened in the sitting position. Injection is made with a 5-cm needle at the sacrococcygeal or first coccygeal space, with the needle slanted forward about 45° from vertical. Administration of 12 to 16 mL of 2% lidocaine produces analgesia of the anus, udder, vagina, scrotum, and hind limbs. Administration of 50 mL of 2% lidocaine in adult camels anesthetizes the hindquarters and abdominal somatic tissues up to the level of the umbilicus.

A mixture of guaifenesin (110 mg/kg) and thiopental (4.4 mg/kg) has been administered IV to induce anesthesia in camels. For short-term (1 h or less) maintenance of general anesthesia, 5% guaifenesin in 5% dextrose plus thiopental (2 mg/mL) is administered to effect. As with other large domesticated ruminants, once intubated, inhalant anesthetics such as halothane, isoflurane, or sevoflurane can be used to maintain longer periods of anesthesia.[74]

Giraffes

Some investigators feel that xylazine alone is unsuitable for restraint of giraffes.[75] When combined with etorphine, however, results are more satisfactory. The sedative-anesthetic effects of this drug combination can be antagonized with the coadministration of diprenorphine (2 to 4 mg total dose IV) and an α_2-antagonist such as yohimbine (0.1 to 0.15 mg/kg IV) or tolazoline (1.0 mg/kg IV). Administration of etorphine alone has been used for surgical analgesia and restraint of adult reticulated giraffes (*Giraffa camelopardalis reticulata*)[76] but is usually administered IM (total dose of 2.5 mg) along with xylazine (0.3 mg/kg IM) or acepromazine (total dose, 30 mg IM). This combination produces recumbency and, when supplemented with an additional 1 mg of etorphine, produces surgical analgesia. Carfentanil has been combined with xylazine and ketamine has been combined with medetomidine to immobilize free-ranging giraffes safely.[77,78]

Perissodactyls

Wild and Feral Equids

Etorphine (0.017 mg/kg IM) alone or in combination with acepromazine (0.04 mg/kg IM) has been used to restrain captive wild asses for electroejaculation procedures.[45,79] Carfentanil, administered in similar doses of 0.015 to 0.033 mg/kg IM, has been used to immobilize zebras (*Equus burchelli*) and Mongolian wild (Przewalski's) horses.[80–82] Immobilization usually occurs within 10 min after carfentanil injection. Xylazine (0.6 mg/kg IM) is often used as a synergist to decrease both the dose requirement of carfentanil (0.02 mg/kg IM) or etorphine and narcotic-induced muscle rigidity.[83] Following carfentanil injection, mild tachycardia, hypertonia, and hyperthermia have been observed in some wild horses. Severe physiological disturbances have been observed in domestic horses after the coadministration of xylazine (1 mg/kg IM) and carfentanil (0.015 mg/kg IM).[80] These changes were characterized by a hypermetabolic state including tachycardia, vigorous muscle activity, tachypnea, and increased rectal temperature. One horse was euthanized because of the onset of severe pulmonary edema that was unresponsive to treatment.[80] The authors speculated that these untoward responses may have been the result of insufficient dosage. Medetomidine (0.06 to 0.08 mg/kg IM) combined with ketamine (1.5 to 2.0 mg/kg IM) has also been used to immobilize wild horses effectively (Table 31.1). This combination produces good muscle relaxation, and recovery is rapid and complete after IV or SC administration of atipamezole. Generally speaking, once sedated, wild Equidae may be given injectable and inhalant general anesthetics in the same manner and dosages as domesticated horses.

Rhinoceros

In the 1960s, white rhinoceros (*Dicerus simus simus*) were typically immobilized with a mixture of morphine and chlorpromazine administered IM.[84] The doses used were approximately 1.5 g of morphine, 175 mg of scopolamine, and 725 mg of chlorpromazine. Complete immobilization required 30 to 45 min in a 1600-kg animal. A variation of this mixture was made by substituting diethylthiambutene for morphine. For a 1400-kg animal, the dose of diethylthiambutene was approximately 3.0 g. These mixtures were also used successfully to immobilize black rhinoceros. Other combinations used to immobilize black rhinoceros included (a) etorphine and acepromazine, (b) etorphine, acepromazine, and azaperone, or (c) etorphine and azaperone (Table 31.5).[85] In the late 1970s, carfentanil alone was used to immobilize rhinos. The total IM dose ranges from 1.0 to 1.5 mg in juveniles to 2.5 to 3.0 mg in adults. These doses achieve deep sedation. The effects of carfentanil can be readily antagonized with diprenorphine.[86] Recommended carfentanil dosages and adjunctive drugs for immobilizing rhinoceros and a variety of other wild African species are listed in Table 31.6. Recent reports of anesthesia in rhinoceros species have emphasized the sensitivity of these animals to potent opioids and the safety concerns accompanying their use.[87] To reduce the etorphine dose requirement, a combination of etorphine with detomidine and ketamine has been successfully used to immobilize an adult one-horned rhinoceros repeatedly for semen collection.[88] In captive white rhinos conditioned to repeated handling, the administration of a combination of butorphanol (total dose, 70 mg) and azaperone (total dose, 100 mg) alone can produce heavy sedation to light anesthesia (animals became recumbent) for laparoscopy.[89]

Table 31.5. Drug immobilization data on 11 black rhinoceros in East Africa

| | | Intramuscular Doses (mg) of Drugs (with µg/kg in Parentheses) | | | | | | Elapsed Time (min) from Injection to: | | | |
| | | Analgesic | | Neuroleptic | | Antidote | | | | | |
Sex	Weight (kg)[a]	Etorphine	Fentanyl	Acepromazine	Azaperone	Nalorphine	Route	Ataxia	Down	Antidote	Up
Female	818 E	2.0 (2.44)		25.0 (30.5)		200.0 (244.5)	IM	7	15	118	126
Male	1185 A	2.0 (1.69)		20.0 (16.8)	250.0 (210.9)	200.0 (168.7)	IM	5	25	258	270
Male	1085 A		20.0[b] (18.43)	10.0 (9.2)	300.0 (276.5)			7			
		2.0[c] (1.84)		20.0 (18.4)		300.0 (276.5)	IM		7	63	81
Male	1196 A	2.0 (1.76)		25.0 (21.7)		300.0 (250.8)	IM	5	25	170	177
Male	955 E	2.0 (2.09)		25.0 (26.1)	200.0 (209.5)			8	18	Drowned in lake	
Male	1033 A	2.0 (1.93)		25.0 (24.2)	200.0 (193.6)	300.0 (290.4)	IM	7	42	74	77
Male	700 E	2.0 (2.86)		25.0 (35.7)	200.0 (285.7)	250.0 (357.1)	IM	5	12	66	79
Female	400 E	1.0 (2.50)		20.0 (25.0)	200.0 (250.0)	200.0 (250.0)	IM	7	12	46	55
Male	600 E	2.0 (3.33)			350.0 (583.3)	200.0 (333.3)	IM	7	13	60	65
Male	750 E	2.5 (3.33)			400.0 (533.3)	250.0 (333.3)	IM	4	9	51	63
Female	820 E	2.25 (2.74)			400.0 (487.8)	180.0 (219.5)	IM	5	10	65	77

[a]A, actual weight; E, estimated weight; IM, intramuscular.
[b]First syringe, little effect other than slight ataxia after 28 min.
[c]Second syringe.
From Denney.[85]

Table 31.6. Recommended intramuscular dosage of carfentanil (Wildnil) and additives for the immobilization of 19 free-ranging wild animal species

| | Analgesic (Narcotic) | | | Additive | | | | Analgesic Antagonist | | | |
| | Adult Body Weight (kg) | Carfentanil | | Xylazine | | Azaperone | | Naloxone | | Cyprenophine | |
		Dosage Rate (µg/kg)	Total Dose[a] (mg)	Dosage Rate (µg/kg)	Total Dose[a] (mg)	Dosage Rate (µg/kg)	Total Dose[a] (mg)	Multiplication Factor	Total Dose[b] (mg)	Multiplication Factor	Total Dose[b] (mg)
African elephant	5000	1	5	—	—	—	—	6–10	40	10–12	50
Square-lipped rhinoceros	2000	1	2	—	—	100	200	6–10	16	10–12	20
Black rhinoceros	1000	1.5	1.5	—	—	150	150	8–10	10	10–12	12
Giraffe	1000	3(1.5)[d]	3(l.5)[d]	40	40	100	100	3–4	12	4–5	15
African buffalo	700	5	3.5	50	35	150	105	2–3	10	3–4	12.5
Eland	800	8	6.4	200	160	300	240	2–3	15	3–4	20
Roan antelope	250	10	2.5	100	25	300	75	2–3	7	3–4	10
Blue wildebeest	220	8	1.75	80	17.5	240	52.5	2–3	5	3–4	6
Black wildebeest	150	8	1.2	80	12	240	36	2–3	3.5	3–4	5
Red hartebeest	140	10	1.4	100	14	300	42	2–3	4	3–4	5
Tsessebe	140	10	1.4	100	14	300	42	2–3	4	3–4	5
Blesbok	90	10	0.9	100	9	300	27	2–3	2.5	3–4	3.5
Common waterbuck	240	10	2.4	100	24	300	72	2–3	7	3–4	8
Greater kudu	260	10	2.6	100	26	300	78	2–3	7	3–4	8
Gemsbok	180	10	1.8	100	18	300	54	2–3	5	3–4	7
Impala	50	7	0.35	100	5	300	15	3–4	1.4	4–5	1.7
Springbok	35	10	0.35	100	3.5	300	10.5	3–4	1.4	4–5	1.7
Steenbok	12	10	0.12	100	1.2	300	3.6	3–4	0.4	4–5	0.5
Warthog	80	12.5	1	100	8	300	24	3–4	4	4–5	5
Burchell's zebra[c]											

[a]Analgesic or additive total dose = analgesic rate × body weight.

[b]Analgesic antagonist total dose = analgesic total dose × multiplication factor.

[c]Carfentanil was not recommended for zebras. Etorphine is recommended as the principal immobilizing agent.

[d]Numbers in parentheses denote noncasting dosage levels for giraffes.

The dosages listed are for free-ranging wild animals. Wild animals adapted to captive conditions usually require lower dosages.

When a short induction period is required, the carfentanil dosage rate can be drastically increased.

Carfentanil can be used without an additive. In cases of excitable species and warthogs, a mixture (cocktail) with a sedative is recommended. Xylazine is preferred.

Although diprenorphine is not listed as an antagonist, it can be used with equal success in dosages slightly less than those cited for cyprenorphine. Nalorphine hydrobromide can also be used as an antagonist.

From DeVos.[86]

Elephants

Several sedatives and anesthetics have been used to immobilize and anesthetize elephants. As early as the 1950s, meperidine hydrochloride was reportedly administered IV at the dose of 2.2 mg/kg to help in the manipulation of an elephant's painful fracture.[90] In the 1960s, there was a report of Indian elephants being anesthetized with pentobarbital IV administered through the middle auricular vein.[91] Beginning in the 1970s, elephants were more commonly immobilized with etorphine administration. The IM dose of etorphine for the African elephant varies from a total dose of 4 to 8 mg, or approximately 1.5 mg/1000 kg of body weight. Hyaluronidase can be combined with etorphine to enhance drug uptake from the IM injection site.[92] A commercial mixture of etorphine-acepromazine (Immobilon LA: 2.45

mg/mL of etorphine and 10 mg/mL of acepromazine) has been used to sedate and control adult Asian elephants. A 2004 report has further confirmed the usefulness and safety of this combination in adult Asian elephants by providing 30 to 60 min of recumbency and neuroleptanesthesia for placement of radio collars on free-ranging animals.[93] The average IM dose of Immobilon LA administered was 3.3 mL, with a range of 6 to 11 mg of etorphine and 25 to 45 mg of acepromazine in ten adult wild elephants.[93] The dose recommendation was based on an unusual measurement: 1 mL/4 ft of shoulder height. Immobilon LA appears to induce more predictable narcotization than does etorphine alone.[94] Nevertheless, etorphine administration (total IM doses ranging from 4 to 6 mg) in African elephants (*Loxodanta africana*) ranging in weight from 2700 to 6000 kg usually produces either sternal or lateral recumbency.[95] The latter is preferred because sternal recumbency reduces ventilation by placing great pressure on the diaphragm. A simple method of providing intermittent positive-pressure ventilation following etorphine immobilization of elephants in the field has been described.[96] This technique of constructing a portable ventilator with the use of two high-flow demand valves and a Y piece of a large animal anesthesia circuit dramatically increased arterial oxygen partial pressure (PaO_2) from 40 to 366 mm Hg in one elephant.[96] It should be appreciated that large elephants may become immobilized in the standing position when the lower dose (total dose, 4 mg) of etorphine is used. If this occurs, elephants may be administered acepromazine to improve sedation and immobilization. Again, although etorphine alone can immobilize adult African elephants satisfactorily, the addition of acepromazine (total dose, 25 to 50 mg) will usually enhance and prolong the tranquil state.

Adult Asian and African elephants can be sedated for air or other modes of transport in the field with the administration of either xylazine (total dose, 100 to 175 mg) or azaperone (total dose, 120 mg).[97] Elephants usually remain standing in cages and are somnolent. Injections of xylazine can be repeated at the same dose rate at approximately 3-h intervals to maintain standing sedation during air transport.[98] Medetomidine has also been assessed as a sedative in Indian elephants at a dose of 3 to 5 µg/kg IM. Sedation was evident on average in 6 min and lasted 1 h 6 min with the 3-µg/kg dose and 2 h 14 min with the 5-µg/kg dose. The head drooped, and the tail and trunk became flaccid. Bradycardia was common, and hypothermia developed in some animals.[99]

A report on repeated inhalation anesthesia of an African elephant was published by Dunlop et al. in 1994.[100] Food was withheld for 1 day and water for 12 h prior to induction. Chemical restraint and sternal recumbency were induced with 0.0017 mg/kg of etorphine administered IM. Atropine (0.04 mg/kg IM) was administered prior to an additional 0.0006 mg/kg etorphine administered IV. Following the second dose of etorphine, the elephant was placed in lateral recumbency. A stomach tube was placed into the larynx by digital palpation, as is done in adult cattle. A 40-mm-ID cuffed endotracheal tube was passed into the trachea by using the stomach tube as a guide, the cuff was inflated, and the endotracheal tube was connected to two large animal breathing circuits joined in parallel at the Y piece. Initially, each machine was set to deliver 5% isoflurane in 15 L/min of oxygen. After 45 min, the two vaporizers were reset to deliver 2% to 3% isoflurane in 5 L of oxygen/min. Anesthesia was maintained for 2 h 35 min, at which time end-tidal isoflurane concentration ranged from 1.05 to 1.15 vol%. At the completion of surgery, isoflurane administration was discontinued. Diprenorphine was administered IV 25 to 40 min later, and the elephant stood unaided within 3 to 4 min.[100]

In another report by Gross et al.,[101] an Asian elephant was anesthetized for cesarean section for removal of a dead fetus. Excitement was observed in this elephant shortly after the IV injection of atropine. Azaperone (0.035 mg/kg IM) premedication had been followed 1 h 30 min later by a 0.05 mg/kg IV dose of atropine. Within 1 min of atropine injection, the elephant began swaying, kicking, and moving in an agitated manner around the stall. Normally responsive to commands, the elephant refused to obey verbal direction. When this behavior had not abated after 30 min, an additional dose of azaperone (0.018 mg/kg IM) was administered. Within 15 min, the elephant became calm and responsive to commands, and anesthesia was then induced with etorphine (0.002 mg/kg IV). Following intubation, anesthesia was maintained with two large animal anesthetic machines arranged in parallel delivering 100% oxygen and was supplemented with additional doses of etorphine when necessary. The authors speculated that the excitement observed following atropine administration was caused primarily by atropine rather than by a drug interaction with azaperone. Atropine has often been used in elephants, and suggested dosages vary from 0.11 mg/kg IM to 0.01 mg/kg IV. As with domestic animals, differences in sensitivity to the effects of atropine on the central nervous system may exist in elephants, especially when preexisting pathology or abnormal physiological conditions are present.[101] Information on the use of carfentanil for immobilization of free-ranging elephants and other species is listed in Table 31.6. Information on the use of etorphine in captive elephants and other species is listed in Table 31.7.

Hippopotamus

Relatively little information is available on restraint and anesthesia of hippopotamus. These large artiodactyls live in and around rivers and shallow lakes and have raised eyes and nostrils that enable them to float partially submerged while viewing and breathing. Their nostrils have valves, and a hippopotamus can remain completely submerged for up to 4 min. Large males may weigh up to 2800 kg. Etorphine can be administered IM at a total dose of 2 to 6 mg alone to produce sedation and anesthesia. Adult captive hippopotamus have been administered etorphine (1 to 5 mg/kg) in combination with xylazine (70 to 80 µg/kg IM) or acepromazine (20 µg/kg IM) to produce chemical restraint. Immobilization can be reversed with the administration of either diprenorphine (3 µg/kg IM) or naltrexone (150 to 180 µg/kg IM). Reversal reportedly occurs more rapidly with naltrexone administration (4 vs. 21 min).[102] Animals will often seek the safety of their water pools once injected and should be kept away from water when immobilization procedures are attempted in a zoo or wildlife-park facility. Phencyclidine (0.6 to 1.1 mg/kg IM) has also been combined with xylazine or acepromazine to immobilize free-ranging animals in large African parks. Many animals have been injected while in the water or near it. It is reported that animals that remain in water will float to the surface once sedated. These animals can be safely roped and hauled to the shore. Animals have remained immobilized for approximately 40 min after injection with these drug mixtures.[30]

Primates

Primates present many unique problems regarding their capture and restraint. When kept in a zoo or other management facility, it is beneficial to perform routine procedures on primates with as little stress to the animal as possible. Consequently, many primates are being conditioned to cooperate with handlers voluntarily for routine blood draws, tranquilization, and administra-

Table 31.7. Intramuscular (IM) etorphine (M991) restraint of large, feral animals kept in captivity

Family Groups	Suggested IM Drugs and Dosage	Comments on Other Drugs	Other Comments
Kangaroos and wallabies	Etorphine 0.1 mg per 20 lb body wt	Phenothiazine-derivative tranquilizers are not effective for restraint.	
	Etorphine 1 mg per 200 lb	Succinylcholine is effective but hazardous.	No longer recommended.
Elephants	Etorphine 1 mg per 2000 lb body wt given intramuscularly		If this dosage is ineffective, further attempts for restraint should not be made for 1 day; then the dosage can be increased by half the original dosage.
Zebras and other wild equines	Etorphine 1 mg per 200 lb body wt. Can be mixed with acepromazine 2 mg per 100 lb body wt	Phenothiazine tranquilizers are ineffective as sole restraint agents.	Care must be exercised not to cause severe exertion and excitement in these animals. A tie-up syndrome has been seen in sedentary individuals that were exerted.
Camels and llamas	Etorphine 2 mg per 500 lb body wt		Emprosthotonic reflexes have occurred.
Tapir	Etorphine 1 mg per 100 lb body wt		
Elk and large deer	Etorphine 1 mg per 100 lb body wt		This drug is not very effective in small deer.
Giraffes	Etorphine 3 mg per 400 lb body wt		Etorphine has variable effect on giraffes. A relatively high dose is suggested because of the effectiveness of the antagonist, cyprenorphine.
American bison	Etorphine 1 mg per 200 lb body wt		Great care must be taken with herds because of their tendency to charge a single downed animal and human handlers.

From Sedgwick and Acosta.[137]

tion of IV medications and anesthetics.[103] Outside of the laboratory situation, traditional capture and restraint techniques typically have to be employed as a prelude to anesthetizing nonhuman primates.

Oral benzodiazepines can be used to facilitate handling but may produce unpredictable levels of sedation in many individuals.[104] Oral sedation of chimpanzees can be successfully accomplished with Telazol (15 mg/kg) mixed with orange juice or other liquids.[105] An alternative sedative technique relies on the use of potent oral and/or transmucosal opioids for sedation. Chimpanzees have also been successfully sedated with droperidol (1.25 to 2.5 mg orally) followed by the transmucosal administration of carfentanil (2.0 µg/kg). Within 40 min of carfentanil exposure, chimps will usually become sedate enough to allow IM hand injection of an anesthetic regimen like naltrexone-tiletamine-zolazepam.[106] A lollipop formulation of fentanyl (intended dose, 10 to 15 µg/kg) has also been used to sedate captive orangutans (*Pongo pygmaeus*) and gorillas (*Gorilla gorilla*) successfully but was found to be unreliable in chimpanzees (*Pan troglodytes*).[107]

Medetomidine-ketamine combinations can be used to restrain a wide variety of primate species. This combination induces a rapid induction, stable immobilization, excellent relaxation, and calm recoveries.[108–111] α_2-Agonist–dissociative combinations have the advantage of being easily antagonized with atipamezole. Telazol can also be used alone or in combination with an α_2-agonist to immobilize primates.

Captive primates are increasingly being trained to present their arms for IV injections so that anesthetic induction agents such as propofol are can be used for induction and maintenance.[104] Inhalant anesthetics are often used for maintenance of longer periods of anesthesia. Most primate species are easily intubated by using a laryngoscope and proper positioning. It is important to note that primates have a very short trachea relative to many other mammals and care should be taken not to intubate a mainstem bronchus.

Ursids

Several anesthetic techniques have been used for capturing, immobilizing, and anesthetizing bears. In the 1960s, investigators reported on the use of α-chloralose mixed with honey to capture black bears (*Ursus americanus*) in the field. The effective dose for wild bears is 2 g per 3 to 8 kg of feed. Recovery usually occurs between 8 and 10 h from the time of ingestion.[112] More recently, a number of favorable reports have been published on the use of carfentanil mixed in small volumes of honey (5 to 20 mL) administered incrementally to captured bears.[113–115] This appears to be a promising technique for immobilizing a number of bear species. The dose range for ingested carfentanil ranges from 7 to 17 µg/kg. The mean dose requirement is 8 to 10 µg/kg. Muscle rigidity and oxygen desaturation were evident in some bears, and, in one study, diazepam was administered to alleviate muscle rigidity.[113] Anesthesia in bears was effectively reversed with naltrexone administration at a ratio of 100 mg/mg of carfentanil ingested. A rapid return to mobility resulted within 10 min of naltrexone administration.

Ketamine and xylazine combined in a ratio of approximately 2:1 on a per-milligram basis produces good anesthesia in captive and wild black bears (*Ursus americanus*). The optimum dose range is 4.5 to 9.0 mg/kg of ketamine and 2.0 to 4.5 mg/kg of xylazine when injected IM. Smaller bears appear to be induced more quickly. Supplemental injections have been used to maintain tractability for as long as 31 h.[116] Free-ranging polar bears (*Ursus maritimus*) can be immobilized with a concentrated solution of ketamine (200 mg/mL) plus xylazine (200 mg/mL). Cubs apparently require approximately 3 mg of each drug per kilogram of body weight, whereas adults require 7 mg/kg.[117] Relatively low doses of medetomidine (0.03 to 0.06 mg/kg IM) and ketamine (2.5 to 4.0 mg/kg IM) have also been used to immobilize brown and polar bears (Table 31.1). More recently, free-ranging bears have been immobilized with a combination of either xylazine or medetomidine with Telazol. These studies indicate that either xylazine (2 mg/kg IM) plus Telazol (3 mg/kg IM) or medetomidine (50 µg/kg IM) plus Telazol (2 mg/kg IM) provide rapid, smooth, reliable immobilization with adequate analgesia that is reversible with atipamezole.[118–121]

As early as the 1960s, bears were being successfully anesthetized with thiopental, thiamylal, or pentobarbital sodium administered IV in the cephalic or saphenous vein. A squeeze cage facilitates the procedure. If this is not available, the caged animal is offered a favorite food; when it reaches for the food, the paw is grasped by an assistant wearing gloves. A rope is tied around the limb to act as a tourniquet and to distend the vein. With this technique, 715 mg of pentobarbital provided surgical anesthesia for a 35-kg Malayan sun bear for 2 h.[122] Reportedly, an average IV dose of 13.5 mg/kg of pentobarbital enables safe handling and minor surgery of American and Himalayan black bears.[123] Following induction with an IV thiobarbiturate, anesthesia is maintained with either isoflurane or sevoflurane administered via a muzzle mask or endotracheal tube–delivery method. Inhalants are the preferred drugs for maintaining anesthesia for long procedures because they provide good reliable muscle relaxation and more rapid emergence.[115] As with most large carnivorous animals, endotracheal intubation can be easily accomplished.

Marsupials

Care should be used when catching and restraining kangaroos, because the claws on their hind limbs are well developed and sharp. Occasionally, a kangaroo will bite or claw with its forepaws. For field capture of macropods in the 1970s and 1980s, ketamine (3.0 mg/kg) was often combined with etorphine (0.005 mg/kg) and administered IM for immobilization.[124] Immobilization usually occurred within 3 to 4 min after injection. Ketamine has also been combined with xylazine (8 mg/kg IM of each) to induce satisfactory anesthesia.[125] Alternatively, Althesin has been administered at the rate of 15 mg of total steroid per kilogram IM for anesthesia and good muscle relaxation.

Generally, phenothiazine tranquilizers have a slow onset of action in marsupials, and effects may last for 2 to 3 days. For this reason, benzodiazepine tranquilizers such as midazolam (0.2 mg/kg IM) have been considered a better and safer class of drugs for tranquilization of marsupials.[124] Because macropods are prone to trauma-related injuries and capture myopathy, a smooth and rapid induction is paramount. The two ideal combinations that are currently used are medetomidine-ketamine and tiletamine-zolazepam to achieve a rapid, smooth induction. Medetomidine-ketamine holds the advantage of rapid reversal with atipamezole, as well. Doses of medetomidine range from 40 to 70 µg/kg IM mixed with 4 to 7 mg/kg of ketamine IM for most kangaroo species.[2] As is typical, the recommended dose of atipamezole is fivefold the medetomidine dose administered. The Telazol dose varies from 2 to 8 mg/kg for a wide range of macropod species. Once anesthetized with either combination, ketamine (1 to 2 mg/kg) can be administered IV to prolong anesthesia. Propofol can also be administered IV to effect (6 to 8 mg/kg) to achieve additional anesthesia. Larger kangaroos can be somewhat difficult to intubate.[2]

Red and gray kangaroos have been anesthetized by IV administration of thiopental in the recurrent tarsal vein. Small kangaroos (tammar wallabies and quokkas) are often anesthetized with thiopental (28 mg/kg IV), intubated, and maintained with an inhalant in oxygen.[126] The rat kangaroo (*Potorous tridactylus* Kerr), or potoroo, is a small species that can be picked up by the tail. It will bite, kick, and scratch if not handled carefully. A large plastic tube can be devised (6-inch diameter by 13 inches long) with a slot in the end gate to enable access to the tail for venipuncture. The vein, located at the lateral aspect of the base of the tail, can be distended with a tourniquet. It has been appreciated for several decades that rat kangaroos may have a lower tolerance to thiopental and pentobarbital anesthesia than many other kangaroo species.[127] Several drugs and older anesthetic protocols successfully used for inducing anesthesia in marsupials are listed in Table 31.8.

Possums and gliders belong to several marsupial families. Of these marsupials, the most common species in captivity is the sugar glider. These small marsupials are best anesthetized with isoflurane in a chamber or mask. Alternatively, both ketamine (20 mg/kg IM) alone or Telazol (5 to 6 mg/kg IM) alone can be

Table 31.8. Sedation and anesthesia of marsupials

Agent	Dose and Route	Species and Comments
Azaperone, 40 mg/mL	2–4 mg/kg by IM injection	Tranquilization in large macropods
Diazepam, 5 mg/mL	2–4 mg/kg IM or IV	All marsupials; tranquilization or anticonvulsant
Diazepam	Oral (in feed) 2 mg/kg	Tranquilization in all marsupials
Acepromazine	0.1 mg/kg IM	Indications of some delayed effect (lasts some days); needs quiet and dark for some hours to have maximum effect
Ketamine HCl	20 mg/kg IM	Monotremes for light surgical anesthesia
	25 mg/kg IM	Anesthesia (light) in dasyurids, macropods, wombat, koala
	30–50 mg/kg IM	Phalangers for light anesthesia; variable; give 30 mg/kg first and then, if insufficient, give additional 20 mg/kg
Thiopental	20 mg/kg as 2.5% or 5% solution (exactly as small animals) by IV injection	All marsupials (tail veins usually easy to use)
Alphaxolone, 9 mg/mL Alphadolone, 3 mg/mL	0.25–0.5 mL/kg IV to effect	Macropods and phalangers; short duration, can top up; recover fast
Halothane	Inhalation to effect	Bell jar for tiny dasyurids; anesthetic machine and mask or tube in larger species
Etorphine and combinations	0.5 mL of "large animal Immobilon" per large kangaroo by IM projectile	Only for capture; restricted availability; can cause excitement and self-injury
Ketamine-xylazine	5 mg/kg ketamine; 2 mg/kg xylazine in same projectile	Capture of macropods

IM, intramuscular; IV, intravenous.
Adapted from Reddacliff.[138]

used. Ketamine (20 to 25 mg/kg IM) and fentanyl-droperidol (0.75 to 1.0 mL/kg IM) have both been used to immobilize opossums satisfactorily for handling.[128] Over the years, both inhalants and pentobarbital sodium have been commonly used to anesthetize this marsupial. Pentobarbital at a dose of 36 mg/kg, produces satisfactory anesthesia when administered IV. IP injection, which is less reliable and provides a narrower margin of safety, is no longer recommended. α-Chloralose has also been safely used in opossums to produce long periods of anesthesia. Induction is achieved with thiopental administered IV, followed by α-chloralose administered at a dose of approximately 12 mg IV every 2 h.

Inhalants can be administered via a closed system or via a mask once an opossum is adequately sedate.[129] For prolonged procedures, thiopental can be given for induction of anesthesia and intubation, followed by administration of isoflurane or sevoflurane. For smaller possum species, as for sugar gliders, chamber induction with a fast-acting inhalant anesthetic (isoflurane or sevoflurane) is the preferred technique, but depression of the central nervous system may be difficult to assess when possums are stressed (enter into a physiological sleep) and become nonresponsive to external stimuli. For larger possum species, as well as koalas, Telazol can be given in a dose range of 4 to 10 mg/kg IM or 1 to 3 mg/kg IV.[130] In free-ranging mountain possums, Telazol was dosed IM as high as 20 to 30 mg/kg for rapid immobilization.[131] In another report, surgical anesthesia was achieved in possums with 5 mg/kg IM of xylazine combined with ketamine at 20 to 30 mg/kg IM.[132] Koalas have also been immobilized safely and rapidly with alphaxalone-alphadolone (Althesin) at doses of 3 to 6 mg/kg IM or 1 to 2 mg/kg IV.[2,133]

Insectivora

Hedgehogs

Hedgehogs and other insectivores, such as tenrecs, shrews, and moles, are easily anesthetized with isoflurane or sevoflurane in oxygen in an induction chamber or box. Anesthesia can be maintained with the inhalant delivered via a face mask or endotracheal tube at a concentration ranging from 0.5% to 1.5% for isoflurane and 2.5% to 3.5% for sevoflurane. Hedgehogs can be intubated relatively easily. The most commonly used injectable anesthetic is ketamine (5 to 20 mg/kg IM), alone or in combination with diazepam (0.5 to 2.0 mg/kg IM), xylazine (0.5 to 1.0 mg/kg IM), or medetomidine (100 μg/kg IM) (Table 31.1). Telazol can also be effective at a dose of 1 to 5 mg/kg IM. Hypothermia is a real threat because of the hedgehog's small body size. Fluids can be given IV or SC in the loose tissue beneath the spines. SC fat may account for up to 50% of the hedgehog's body weight and can cause delayed absorption of fluids and anesthetics when injected in this tissue. IM injections require a needle length sufficient to extend through fatty subcutaneous tissues. Either buprenorphine (0.01 mg/kg) or butorphanol (0.2 to 0.4 mg/kg IM or SC) can be administered to provide analgesic therapy following surgery.[134]

References

1. Church JCT, Noronha RFX. The use of the fruit bat in surgical research. East Afr Med J 42:348, 1965.
2. Pye GW. Marsupials, insectivore and chiropteran anesthesia. Vet Clin North Am Exot Anim Pract 4:211, 2001.
3. Grinnell AD. The neurophysiology of audition in bats: Intensity and frequency parameters. J Physiol 167:38, 1963.
4. Suga N. Single unit activity in cochlear nucleus and inferior colliculus of echolocating bats. J Physiol 172:449, 1964.
5. Hoff HE, Coles SK, Szabuniewicz M, McCrady JD. The respiratory heart rate relationship in the armadillo. Cardiovasc Res Cent Bull 21:37, 1982.
6. Szabuniewicz M, McCrady JD. Some aspects of the anatomy and physiology of the armadillo. Lab Anim Care 19:843, 1969.
7. Anderson JM, Benirschke K. The armadillo in experimental biology. Lab Anim Care 16:202, 1966.
8. Wampler SN. Husbandry and health problems of armadillos, *Dasypus novemcinctus*. Lab Anim Care 19:391, 1969.
9. Fournier-Chambrillon C, Vogel I, Fournier P, de Thoisy B, Vie JC. Immobilization of free-ranging nine-banded and great long-nosed armadillos with three anesthetic combinations. J Wildl Dis 36:131, 2000.
10. Hayes FA. Modifications for cesarian section in chinchillas. Vet Med 50:367, 1955.
11. Riddell WK. Caudal anesthesia in canine surgery. J Small Anim Med 1:159, 1952.
12. Henke J, Baumgartner C, Roltgen I, Eberspacher E, Erhardt W. Anaesthesia with midazolam/medetomidine/fentanyl in chinchillas (*Chinchilla lanigera*) compared to anaesthesia with xylazine/ketamine and medetomidine/ketamine. J Vet Med [A] Physiol Pathol Clin Med 51:259, 2004.
13. Roslyn J, Thompson JE Jr, DenBesten L. Anesthesia for prairie dogs. Lab Anim Sci 29:542, 1979.
14. Johnson D. Prairie dog medicine and surgery. In: Atlantic Coast Veterinary Conference Proceedings, 2004:1.
15. Beiglbock C, Zenker W. Evaluation of three combinations of anesthetics for use in free-ranging alpine marmots (*Marmota marmota*). J Wildl Dis 39:665, 2003.
16. Bacher JD, Potkay S, Baas JE. An evaluation of sedatives and anesthetics in the agouti (*Dasyprocta* spp.). Lab Anim Sci 26:195, 1976.
17. Van Foreest A. Use of ketamine/xylazine combination for tail amputation in nutria. J Zoo Anim Med 11:19, 1980.
18. Hummon OJ. A device for the restraint of mink during certain experimental procedures. J Am Vet Med Assoc 106:104, 1945.
19. Fournier-Chambrillon C, Chusseau JP, Dupuch J, Maizeret C, Fournier P. Immobilization of free-ranging European mink (*Mustela lutreola*) and polecat (*Mustela putorius*) with medetomidine-ketamine and reversal by atipamezole. J Wildl Dis 39:393, 2003.
20. Lafortune JG, Rheault JPE. Essai d'évaluation clinique de la reserpine (Serpasil) chez le vison. Can J Comp Med Vet Sci 24:243, 1960.
21. Ko JCH, Thurmon JC, Benson GJ. An alternative drug combination for use in declawing and castrating cats. Vet Med 88:1061, 1993.
22. Cantwell S. Ferret, rabbit and rodent anesthesia. Vet Clin North Am Exot Anim Pract 4:169, 2001.
23. Barry JA. Removal of scent glands in skunks. MSU Vet 19:77, 1958.
24. Verts BJ. A device for anesthetizing skunks. J Wildl Manage 24:344, 1960.
25. Lopez-Gonzalez CA, Gonzalez-Romero A, Laundre JW, et al. Field immobilization of pygmy spotted skunks from Mexico. J Wildl Dis 34:186, 1998.
26. Healey P. A simple method for anaesthetizing and handling small carnivores. J Inst Anim Tech 18:37, 1967.
27. Mackintosh CG, MacArthur JA, Little TWA, Stuart P. The immobilization of the badger. Br Vet J 132:609, 1976.
28. Thornton PD, Newman C, Johnson PJ, et al. Preliminary comparison of four anaesthetic techniques in badgers (*Meles meles*). Vet Anaesth Analg 32:40, 2005.
29. de Leeuw AN, Forrester GJ, Spyvee PD, Brash MG, Delahay RJ. Experimental comparison of ketamine with a combination of ketamine, butorphanol and medetomidine for general anaesthesia of the Eurasian badger (*Meles meles* L.). Vet J 167:186, 2004.
30. Wallach JD, Boever WJ. Diseases of Exotic Animals: Medical and Surgical Management. Philadelphia: WB Saunders, 1983:469.
31. Balser DS. Tranquilizer tabs for capturing wild carnivores. J Wildl Manage 29:438, 1965.
32. Hime JM. Use of ketamine hydrochloride in non-domesticated cats. Vet Rec 95:193, 1974.
33. Wallach JD, Frueh R, Lentz M. The use of M.99 as an immobilizing and analgesic agent in captive wild animals. J Am Vet Med Assoc 151:870, 1967.
34. Hornocker MG, Craighead JJ, Pfeiffer EW. Immobilizing mountain lions with succinylcholine chloride and pentobarbital sodium. J Wildl Manage 29:880, 1965.
35. Clifford DH. Observations on effect of preanesthetic medication with meperidine and promazine on barbiturate anesthesia in an ocelot and a leopard. J Am Vet Med Assoc 133:459, 1958.
36. Clifford DH, Stowe CM Jr, Good AL. Pentobarbital anesthesia in lions with special reference to preanesthetic medication. J Am Vet Med Assoc 139:111, 1961.
37. Tomizawa N, Tsujimoto T, Itoh K, Ogino T, Nakamura K, Hara S. Chemical restraint of African lions (*Panthera leo*) with medetomidine-ketamine. J Vet Med Sci 59:307, 1997.
38. Epstein A, White R, Horowitz IH, Kass PH, Ofri R. Effects of propofol as an anaesthetic agent in adult lions (*Panthera leo*): A comparison with two established protocols. Res Vet Sci 72:137, 2002.
39. Miller M, Weber M, Neiffer D, Mangold B, Fontenot D, Stetter M. Anesthetic induction of captive tigers (*Panthera tigris*) using a medetomidine-ketamine combination. J Zoo Wildl Med 34:307, 2003.
40. Austin DH, Peoples JH. Capturing hogs with alpha chloralose. In: Proceedings of the 21st Annual Conference of the Southeast Association Game and Fish Commission, New Orleans, 1967.
41. Gabor TM, Heligren EC, Silvy NJ. Immobilization of collared peccaries (*Tayassu tajacu*) and feral hogs (*Sus scrofa*) with Telazol and xylazine. J Wildl Dis 33:161, 1997.
42. Beale DM, Smith AD. Immobilization of pronghorn antelopes with succinylcholine chloride. J Wildl Manage 31:840, 1967.
43. Gaukler VA, Kraus M. Zur Immobilisierung von Wildwiederkauern mit Xylazin (Bay Va 1470). Zool Garten 38:1, 1970.
44. Hofmyer JM. Immobilization of black rhinos, eland and roan antelope with R33799. Report, Etosha Ecological Institute, Okaukuejo via Outjo, Namibia, October, 1978.
45. Howard JG, Pursel VG, Wildt DE, Bush M. Comparison of various extenders for freeze-preservation of semen from selective captive wild ungulates. J Am Vet Med Assoc 179:1157, 1981.
46. Citino SB, Bush M, Grobler D, Lance W. Anaesthesia of roan antelope (*Hippotragus equinus*) with a combination of A3080, medetomidine and ketamine. J S Afr Vet Assoc 72:29, 2001.

47. Chittick E, Horne W, Wolfe B, Sladky K, Loomis M. Cardiopulmonary assessment of medetomidine, ketamine, and butorphanol anesthesia in captive Thompson's gazelles (*Gazella thomsoni*). J Zoo Wildl Med 32:168, 2001.

48. Bush M, Raath JP, Phillips LG, Lance W. Immobilisation of impala (*Aepyceros melampus*) with a ketamine hydrochloride/medetomidine hydrochloride combination, and reversal with atipamezole hydrochloride. J S Afr Vet Assoc 75:14, 2004.

49. Logsdon HS. Use of drugs as a capture technique for desert bighorn sheep [PhD dissertation]. Fort Collins: Colorado State University, 1969.

50. Jorgenson JT, Samson J, Festa-Bianchet M. Field immobilization of bighorn sheep with xylazine hydrochloride and antagonism with idazoxan. J Wildl Dis 26:522, 1990.

51. Peshin PK, Kumar A. Physiologic and sedative effects of xylazine in buffaloes. Indian Vet J 56:864, 1979.

52. Pathak SC, Nigam JM, Peshin PK, Singh AP. Anesthetic and hemodynamic effects of ketamine hydrochloride in buffalo calves (*Bubalis bubalis*). Am J Vet Res 43:875, 1982.

53. Singh J, Sobti VK, Kohli RN, Kumar VR, Khanna AK. Evaluation of glyceryl guaiacolate as a muscle relaxant in buffalo calves. Zentralbl Veterinarmed [A] 28:60, 1981.

54. Johari MP, Sharma SP. General anaesthesia in buffaloes by intravenous use of chloral-thiopentone sodium mixture. Indian J Vet Sci 32:235, 1962.

55. Sharma AK, Kumar N, Dimri U, et al. Romifidine-ketamine anaesthesia in atropine and triflupromazine pre-medicated buffalo calves. J Vet Med [A] Physiol Pathol Clin Med 51:420, 2004.

56. Pawde AM, Amarpal, Kinjavdejar P, Aithal HP, Pratap K, Bisht GS. Detomidine-diazepam-ketamine anaesthesia in buffalo (*Bubalus bubalis*) calves. J Vet Med [A] Physiol Pathol Clin Med 47:175, 2000.

57. Kock MD, Berger J. Chemical immobilization of free-ranging North American bison (*Bison bison*) in Badlands National Park, South Dakota. J Wildl Dis 23:625, 1987.

58. Caulkett NA, Cattet MR, Cantwell S, Cool N, Olsen W. Anesthesia of wood bison with medetomidine-zolazepam/tiletamine and xylazine-zolazepam/tiletamine combinations. Can Vet J 41:49, 2000.

59. Kloppel G. Zur Immobilisation von Zoo- und Wiltieren. Kleintierpraxis 14:203, 1969.

60. Hime JM, Jones DM. The use of xylazine in captive wild animals. In: Sonderdruck aus Verhandlungsbericht des XI Internationalen Symposiums uber die Erkrankugen der Zootiere, Budapest. London: Zoological Society of London, 1970.

61. Honich M. Untersuchungen uber wirtung van BAY Va 1470 biem wild [Abstract]. In: Twelfth International Symposium on Diseases of Zoo Animals, Budapest. Budakeszi, Hungary: Laboratory for Game Diseases, Ministry of Agriculture, 1970.

62. Roughton RD. Xylazine as an immobilizing agent for captive white-tailed deer. J Am Vet Med Assoc 167:574, 1975.

63. Harrington R. Immobilon-rompun in deer. Vet Rec 94:362, 1974.

64. Haigh JC, Stewart RR, Frokjer R, Hauge T. Capture of moose with fentanyl and xylazine. J Zoo Anim Med 8:22, 1977.

65. Read M. Long acting neuroleptic drugs [online]. In: Heard D, ed. Zoological Restraint and Anesthesia, 2002. Available from http://www.ivis.org.

66. Wolff WA, Davis RW, Lumb WV. Chloral hydrate-halothanenitrous oxide anesthesia in deer. J Am Vet Med Assoc 147:1099, 1965.

67. Thomas WD. Chemical immobilization of wild animals. J Am Vet Med Assoc 138:263, 1961.

68. Miller MW, Wild MA, Lance WR. Efficacy and safety of naltrexone hydrochloride for antagonizing carfentanil citrate immobilization in captive Rocky Mountain elk (*Cervus elaphus nelsoni*). J Wildl Dis 32:234, 1996.

69. Cattet MR, Caulkett NA, Wilson C, Vandenbrink T, Brook RK. Intranasal administration of xylazine to reduce stress in elk captured by net gun. J Wildl Dis 40:562, 2004.

70. Haigh JC. Capture of woodland caribou in Canada. In: Proceedings of the American Association of Zoo Veterinarians, Knoxville, TN, 1978:110.

71. Custer R, Kramer L, Kennedy S, Bush M. Hematologic effects of xylazine when used for restraint of Bactrian camels. J Am Vet Med Assoc 171:899, 1977.

72. Said AH. Some aspects of anaesthesia in the camel. Vet Rec 76:550, 1964.

73. White RJ, Bali S, Bark H. Xylazine and ketamine anaesthesia in the dromedary camel under field conditions. Vet Rec 120:110, 1987.

74. Singh R, Peshin PK, Patil DB, et al. Evaluation of halothane as an anaesthetic in camels (*Camelus dromedaries*). Zentralbl Veterinarmed [A] 41:359, 1994.

75. Bush M, Ensley PK, Mehren K, Rapley W. Immobilization of giraffes with xylazine and etorphine hydrochloride. J Am Vet Med Assoc 169:884, 1976.

76. Williamson WM, Wallach JD. M99-induced recumbency and analgesia in a giraffe. J Am Vet Med Assoc 153:816, 1968.

77. Bush M, de Vos V. Observations on field immobilization of free-ranging giraffe (*Giraffa camelopardalis*) using carfentanyl and xylazine. J Zoo Wild Anim Med 18:135, 1987.

78. Bush M, Grobler DG, Raath JP, Phillips LG Jr, Stamper MA, Lance WR. Use of medetomidine and ketamine for immobilization of free-ranging giraffes. J Am Vet Med Assoc 218:245, 2001.

79. Seidel VB, Straub G, Carlo WR, Effert W. Anasthesie, Hamatologie und Biochemie beim Kiang (*Equus hemionus kiang*, Moorcroft, 1981). In: Sonderdruck aus Verhandlungsbericht des XXIV Internationalen Symposiums uber die Erkrankungen der Zootiere, Veszprem, Hungary, 1982.

80. Shaw ML, Carpenter JW, Leith DE. Complications with the use of carfentanil citrate and xylazine hydrochloride to immobilize domestic horses. J Am Vet Med Assoc 206:833, 1995

81. Allen JL. Renarcotization following carfentanil immobilization of nondomestic ungulates. J Zoo Wildl Med 20:423, 1989.

82. Allen JL. Immobilization of Mongolian wild horses (*Equus przewalski przewalski*) with carfentanil and antagonism with naltrexone. J Zoo Wildl Med 23:422, 1992.

83. Plotka ED, Seal US, Eagle TC, Asa CS, Tester JR, Siniff DB. Rapid reversible immobilization of feral stallions using etorphine hydrochloride, xylazine hydrochloride and atropine sulfate. J Wildl Dis 23:471, 1987.

84. Harthoorn AM, Player IC. The narcosis of the white rhinoceros: A series of eighteen case histories. Tijdschr Diergeneeskd 89:225, 1964.

85. Denney RN. Black rhinoceros immobilization utilizing a new tranquillizing agent. East Afr Wildl J 7:159, 1969.

86. De Vos V. Immobilization of free-ranging wild animals using a new drug. Vet Rec 103:64, 1978.

87. Portas TJ. A review of drugs and techniques used for sedation and anaesthesia in captive rhinoceros species. Aust Vet J 82:542, 2004.

88. Atkinson MW, Hull B, Gandolf AR, Blumer ES. Repeated chemical immobilization of a captive greater one-horned rhinoceros (*Rhinoceros unicornis*), using combinations of etorphine, detomidine and ketamine. J Zoo Wildl Med 33:157, 2002.

89. Radcliffe RW, Ferrell ST, Childs SE. Butorphanol and azaperone as a safe alternative for repeated chemical restraint in captive white rhinoceros (*Ceratotherium simum*). J Zoo Wildl Med 31:196, 2000.

90. Counsilman JW. Demerol hydrochloride as an anesthetic for an elephant. North Am Vet 35:835, 1954.

91. Anderson IL. Tutu poisoning in two circus elephants. NZ Vet J 16:146, 1968.

92. Osofsky SA. A practical anesthesia monitoring protocol for free-ranging adult African elephants (*Loxodonta africana*). J Wildl Dis 33:72, 1997.

93. Dangolla A, Silva I, Kuruwita VY. Neuroleptanalgesia in wild Asian elephants (*Elphas maximus maximus*). Vet Anaesth Analg 31:276, 2004.

94. Bongso TA, Perera BMAO. Observations on the use of etorphine alone and in combination with acepromazine maleate for immobilization of aggressive Asian elephants (*Elephas maximus*). Vet Rec 102:339, 1978.

95. Wallach JD, Anderson JL. Oripavine M99 combinations and solvents for immobilization of the African elephant. J Am Vet Med Assoc 153:793, 1968.

96. Horne WA, Tchamba MN, Loomis MR. A simple method of providing intermittent positive-pressure ventilation to etorphine-immobilized elephants (*Loxodonta africana*) in the field. J Zoo Wildl Med 32:519, 2001.

97. Stegmann GF. Etorphine-halothane anesthesia in two five-year-old African elephants (*Loxodonta africana*). J S Afr Vet Assoc 70:164, 1999.

98. Bongso TA. Use of xylazine for the transport of elephants by air. Vet Rec 107:492, 1980.

99. Sarma B, Pathak SC, Sarma KK. Medetomidine: A novel immobilizing agent for the elephant (*Elephas maximus*). Res Vet Sci 73:315, 2002.

100. Dunlop CI, Hodgson DS, Cambre RC, Kenny DE, Martin HD. Cardiopulmonary effects of three prolonged periods of isoflurane anesthesia in an adult elephant. J Am Vet Med Assoc 205:1439, 1994.

101. Gross ME, Clifford CA, Hardy DA. Excitement in an elephant after intravenous administration of atropine. J Am Vet Med Assoc 205:1437, 1994.

102. Ramsay EC, Loomis MR, Mehren KG, Boardman WS, Jensen J, Geiser D. Chemical restraint of the Nile hippopotamus (*Hippopotamus amphibious*) in captivity. J Zoo Wildl Med 29:45, 1998.

103. Laule GE, Bloomsmith MA, Schapiro SJ. The use of positive reinforcement training techniques to enhance the care, management, and welfare of primates in the laboratory. J Appl Anim Welf Sci 6:163, 2003.

104. Horne WA. Primate anesthesia. Vet Clin North Am Exot Anim Pract 4:239, 2001.

105. Knottenbelt MK, Knottenbelt DC. Use of an oral sedative for immobilization of a chimpanzee (*Pan troglodytes*). Vet Rec 126:404, 1990.

106. Kearns KS, Swenson B, Ramsay EC. Oral induction of anesthesia with droperidol and transmucosal carfentanil citrate in chimpanzees (*Pan troglodytes*). J Zoo Wildl Med 31:185, 2000.

107. Hunter RP, Isaza R, Carpenter JW, Koch DE. Clinical effects and plasma concentrations of fentanyl after transmucosal administration in three species of great ape. J Zoo Wildl Med 35:162, 2004.

108. Selmi AL, Mendes GM, Figueiredo JP, Barbudo-Selmi GR, Lins BT. Comparison of medetomidine-ketamine and dexmedetomidine-ketamine anesthesia in golden-headed lion tamarins. Can Vet J 45:481, 2004.

109. Williams CV, Glenn KM, Levine JF, Horne WA. Comparison of the efficacy and cardiorespiratory effects of medetomidine-based anesthetic protocols in ring-tailed lemurs (*Lemur catta*). J Zoo Wildl Med 34:163, 2003.

110. Kalema-Zikusoka G, Horne WA, Levine J, Loomis MR. Comparison of the cardiorespiratory effects of medetomidine-butorphanol-ketamine and medetomidine-butorphanol-midazolam in patas monkeys (*Erythrocebus patas*). J Zoo Wildl Med 34:47, 2003.

111. Vie JC, DeThoisy B, Fournier-Chambrillon C, Genty C, Keravec J. Anesthesia of wild red howler monkeys (*Alouatta seniculus*) with medetomidine/ketamine and reversal by atipamezole. Am J Primatol 45:399, 1998.

112. Stafford SK, Williams LE Jr. Data on capturing black bears with alpha-chloralose. In: Proceedings of the 22nd Annual Conference of the Southeastern Association of Game and Fish Commissioners, Baltimore, MD, 1968.

113. Ramsay EC, Sleeman JM, Clyde VL. Immobilization of black bears (*Ursus americanus*) with orally administered carfentanil citrate. J Wildl Dis 31:391, 1995.

114. Mortenson J, Bechert U. Carfentanil citrate used as an oral anesthetic agent for brown bears (*Ursus arctos*). J Zoo Wildl Med 32:217, 2001.

115. Mama KR, Steffey EP, Withrow SJ. Use of orally administered carfentanil prior to isoflurane-induced anesthesia in a Kodiak brown bear. J Am Vet Med Assoc 217:546, 2000.

116. Addison EM, Kolenosky GB. Use of ketamine hydrochloride and xylazine hydrochloride to immobilize black bears (*Ursus americanus*). J Wildl Dis 15:253, 1979.

117. Lee J, Schweinsburg R, Kernan F, Haigh J. Immobilization of polar bears (*Ursus maritimus*, Phipps) with ketamine hydrochloride and xylazine hydrochloride. J Wildl Dis 17:331, 1981.

118. Cattet MR, Caulkett NA, Lunn NJ. Anesthesia of polar bears using xylazine-zolazepam-tiletamine or zolazepam-tiletamine. J Wildl Dis 39:655, 2003.

119. Cattet MR, Caulkett NA, Polischuk SC, Ramsay MA. Reversible immobilization of free-ranging polar bears with medetomidine-zolazepam-tiletamine and atipamezole. J Wildl Dis 33:611, 1997.

120. Onuma M. Immobilization of sun bears (*Helarctos malayanus*) with medetomidine-zolazepam-tiletamine. J Zoo Wildl Med 34:202, 2003.

121. Caulkett NA, Cattet MR. Physiological effects of medetomidine-zolazepam-tiletamine immobilization in black bears. J Wildl Dis 33:618, 1997.

122. Fowler ME. Extracting canine teeth of a bear. J Am Vet Med Assoc 137:60, 1960.

123. Clarke NP, Huheey MJ, Martin WM. Pentobarbital anesthesia in bears. J Am Vet Med Assoc 143:47, 1963.

124. Keep JM. Marsupial anaesthesia. Proc Postgrad Committee Vet Sci Univ Sydney 36:123, 1978.

125. Wilson GR. Intramuscular anaesthesia in the red kangaroo. Aust Vet Pract 6:51, 1976.

126. Richardson KC, Cullen LK. Anesthesia of small kangaroos. J Am Vet Med Assoc 179:1162, 1981.

127. Cisar CF. The rat kangaroo (*Potorous tridactylus*): Handling and husbandry practices in a research facility. Lab Anim Care 19:55, 1969.

128. Feldman DB, Self JL. Sedation and anesthesia of the Virginia opossum. Lab Anim Sci 21:717, 1971.

129. Luschei ES, Mehaffey JJ. Small animal anesthesia with halothane. J Appl Physiol 22:595, 1967.

130. Vogelnest L. Chemical restraint of Australian native fauna. Proc Postgrad Committee Vet Sci Aust Wildl Univ Sydney 327:149, 1999.

131. Viggers KL, Lindenmayer DB. The use of tiletamine hydrochloride and zolazepam hydrochloride for sedation of the mountain brush-tail possum, *Trichosurus caninus* Ogilby (Phalangeridae: Marsupialia). Aust Vet J 72:215, 1995.

132. Keller LS, Drozdowicz CK, Rice L, Bowman TA, Lang CM. An evaluation of three anaesthetic regimes in the gray short-tailed opossum (*Monodelphis domestica*). Lab Anim 22:269, 1988.

133. Tribe AT, Middleton D. Anesthesia of native mammals and birds. Proc Postgrad Committee Vet Sci Aust Wildl Univ Sydney 104:789, 1999.

134. Smith AJ. General husbandry and medical care of hedgehogs. In: Bonagura J, ed. Kirk's Current Veterinary Therapy XIII. Philadelphia: WB Saunders, 2000:1128.

135. Jalanka HJ, Koeken BO. The use of medetomidine, medetomidine-ketamine combinations and atipamezole in nondomestic mammals: A review. J Zoo Wildl Med 21:259, 1990.

136. Haigh JC. The immobilization of Bongo (*Boocercus eurycus*) and other African antelopes in captivity. Vet Rec 98:237, 1976.

137. Sedgwick CJ, Acosta AL. Capture drugs. Mod Vet Pract 50:32, 1969.

138. Reddacliff G. Therapeutic index: Marsupials. Proc Postgrad Committee Vet Sci Univ Sydney 39:1037, 1978.

Chapter 32

Chemical Immobilization of Free-Ranging Terrestrial Mammals

Nigel A. Caulkett and Jon M. Arnemo

Introduction

Chemical immobilization of free-ranging wildlife can be challenging. The nature of the procedure dictates that veterinarians must ignore many of the principals that underlie good anesthetic practice in other settings. It is generally not possible to access the patients for a preanesthetic physical examination or laboratory work. Physical status of the patients cannot be accurately assessed, and generally animals are assumed to be healthy. Even if physical status and anesthetic risk could be determined, generally only a few effective protocols are available. Induction of anesthesia in wildlife can be extremely stressful, and stress-related conditions or injuries can result. Free-ranging wildlife are subject to environmental hazards and are often at risk for hypothermia or hyperthermia. Appropriate supportive care, such as controlled ventilation, intravenous fluid therapy, or inotropic support, is often not possible in field situations. Veterinarians may be required to work on species for which there is very little information about their physiology or pharmacological response to drugs. Extrapolation between similar species may be required, but can result in unexpected complications. Issues of human safety also must be considered. Given the challenges that are encountered during wildlife capture, it is not surprising that morbidity and mortality of animals can be high and injury to people engaged in the capturing procedure common.

Wildlife anesthesia should be a cooperative effort between biologists and veterinarians. A team approach is invaluable and draws on the strengths of different backgrounds and training. Veterinarians can play an important role in protocol development, monitoring, supportive care, and stress reduction. Additionally, because procedures performed on wildlife are becoming more invasive, provision of appropriate analgesia is an important emerging role of veterinary care.

This chapter focuses on the major principals of wildlife capture and handling. It includes some drug recommendations for commonly encountered wildlife, but it is beyond the scope of a single chapter to provide complete dose recommendations for terrestrial mammals. The *Handbook of Wildlife Chemical Immobilization* is a very complete synopsis of currently recommended dosages in most terrestrial mammals.[1] The handbook is a valuable reference for anyone involved in wildlife capture. The authors have retained parts of the original chapter from the third edition of *Lumb and Jones' Veterinary Anesthesia*, written by Leon Nielsen, in this revised edition, and we acknowledge his contribution.

Field Anesthesia
General Considerations

Wildlife capture is often required for research purposes. Capture events should be carefully planned because, with careful forethought, complications can be anticipated and treatments better prepared. Capture sites may be preplanned and chosen based on their suitability. The capture can be planned at an appropriate time of the year when environmental hazards are minimized. For example, ungulates may be captured in late winter or spring to decrease the risk of hyperthermia and enable tracking in snow or visualization of animals in deciduous forest. Often individual animals are not targeted, and the capture team can choose any animal in a relatively safe capture environment. It is generally possible to adhere to strict pursuit times. If it is not absolutely necessary to capture the target animal, pursuit can be terminated to decrease the risk of stress-related disease, such as exertional myopathy. Current literature and experts in the field can be consulted prior to the capture event to ensure the most suitable technique is used. It may be possible to close areas to the public where wildlife are captured. Finally, appropriate equipment for monitoring and supportive care should be obtained and taken into the field.

Wildlife capture, in management situations, takes place in a much less controlled environment, which may be more hazardous. It is becoming increasingly common to have to deal with wildlife in urban environments that contain many hazards. Public safety and crowd control can be issues. Management-related capture may be required at any time of the day or night and any time of the year. Generally, a chase cannot be terminated, and injury or myopathy may result. In most situations, attempts at capture must continue until the animal is under control or destroyed. These situations arise quickly and usually must be resolved quickly. Often the personnel involved in capture are wildlife managers such as wardens or conservation officers. A limited choice of drugs may be available. In these situations, it is important to use drug combinations with a rapid onset and a high margin of safety. Wildlife managers often need to deal with a variety of species, and ideally a drug combination should be used that is effective in a wide range of species.

Terrain

Choosing an ideal location for wildlife capture may not always be possible. Ideally, the capture site should be open enough to enable good visualization of the animal during the induction period. Particular attention should be paid to bodies of water, because some species may enter the water after drug administration and be at risk of drowning. Obvious risks are associated with mountainous terrain (Fig. 32.1). Forest can be a particular hazard because animals may be very difficult to track beneath a forest canopy. Telemetry darts may be useful in these situations. Some species, such as black bears and mountain lions, may climb trees to escape capture. Equipment should be available to cushion their fall or to facilitate removing the animal from the tree. In an urban environment, particular attention must be paid to traffic. It is often advisable to enlist the help of law enforcement officers for crowd and traffic control.

Weather

Weather conditions may dictate whether wildlife capture is possible. Helicopter work is generally not possible in high winds or foggy conditions. Snow and rain can lead to hypothermia, partic-

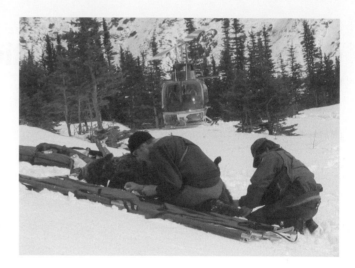

Fig. 32.1. Mountainous terrain carries the risk of sudden weather changes, avalanches, loss of the animal under the forest canopy, and falls from cliffs or steep slopes.

ularly if wind is also present to enhance convective heat loss. Smaller mammals may be particularly prone to hypothermia. Several of the drug regimens used for wildlife capture can impede thermoregulation and lead to hypothermia or hyperthermia.[2,3] Hyperthermia is a serious complication that can be difficult to treat in field situations. When possible, captures should be planned for the cooler hours of the day. In remote locations, sudden changes in weather may also be a hazard to personnel. It is important to keep track of current and changing conditions during planned events. Capture for management purposes may occur at any time. Provision should be made to prevent heat loss and actively cool animals, if required.

Equipment

Logistics and space limitations generally dictate what type of equipment can be carried in a field situation. It is often difficult to carry all but the most necessary pieces. Fortunately, there are compact ambulatory monitors suitable for field use. Hypoxemia is a common complication of wildlife anesthesia, particularly with ruminants.[4–10] Oxygen is fundamental supportive care during anesthesia. Aluminum E and D cylinders, combined with a sturdy regulator and flowmeter, are ideal for field use (Fig. 32.2). Often, nasal insufflation of oxygen is adequate to treat hypoxemia. In some situations, equipment for ventilatory support is also recommended. It is difficult to carry a wide range of emergency drugs or an adequate volume of crystalloid fluids to treat shock. A basic emergency kit containing epinephrine, atropine, lidocaine, and reversal agents should always be carried. Equipment for airway support should also be included in an emergency kit. Ruminants are predisposed to ruminal tympany. It is wise to carry a suitably sized tube or hose to facilitate rumen desufflation. Equipment should also be carried to treat lacerations and other incidental injuries. Equipment should be carefully chosen to withstand use in a field situation and to be as lightweight and compact as possible.

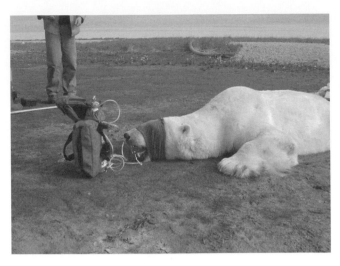

Fig. 32.2. Portable oxygen cylinders and sturdy regulators will greatly facilitate oxygen delivery in field situations.

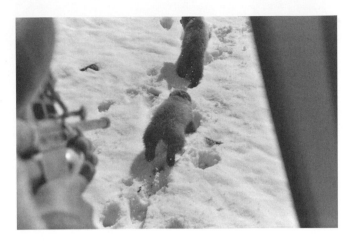

Fig. 32.3. A skilled pilot is required for effective aerial capture. Everyone working around helicopters should receive appropriate training.

Capture Technique

An animal may be captured initially by physical or chemical means. The choice of capture technique depends on the species, the terrain, the facilities, and the experience of the capture crew. Many species of ungulates can be effectively captured and handled by experienced teams with physical techniques such as net guns.[11–13] Physical restraint can be very stressful for wild animals, and methods need to be developed to reduce stress. Sedatives or anesthetics can be used to decrease the stress of handling once animals have been netted.[13] Net gunning can cause high rates of mortality if it is performed by inexperienced personnel. The risk to capture personnel can also be high. Jessup et al.[14] reported that, over a 12-year period in New Zealand, there were 127 helicopter crashes and 25 human fatalities during net-gun capture of red deer. These figures stress the need for experienced pilots and capture personnel. The terrain may dictate the choice of capture technique (Fig. 32.3). Grizzly bears can be effectively darted from a helicopter in open Alpine areas. This technique is less effective in forested parts of their range. In forested areas, it is often safer to capture the animal first with a snare or culvert trap, followed by remote delivery of anesthetics. The use of physical restraint will confine an animal's movements during the induction of anesthesia. Physical restraint can induce greater stress than chemical restraint.[15] Generally, physical restraint should be of brief duration to avoid stress-related complications.

Target and Nontarget Species

Prior to embarking on a capture session, it is important to become as familiar as possible with the target species. This can include a search of current literature and texts. Ideally, experts in the field should be consulted to determine the most suitable technique and supportive care for the target species. In research-related captures, it may not be a particular individual that requires capture (i.e., a certain gender or age class may be the target). This gives researchers some leeway to choose animals in an ideal capture situation. Nontarget animals may include capture of the right species, but the wrong gender or age class. If traps are used, nontarget species may be caught. Researchers need to anticipate which nontarget species may be trapped and be familiar with the best current techniques for anesthesia of these species. Wildlife managers need to be familiar with techniques for all the species that they may encounter in their work. In management situations, a technique that facilitates anesthesia in a variety of species is often preferable.

Other Hazards

A number of hazards can be encountered during anesthesia of free-ranging wildlife. It is important to perform a risk assessment prior to embarking on a project. Potential risks should be identified and steps taken to reduce risk. The target species can pose a risk. There are the obvious risks of serious injury from large carnivores. Ungulates can also act aggressively, and injury may also occur from flailing limbs or heads in lightly anesthetized animals. Smaller carnivores can inflict serious injuries if they are not handled properly. It is important to know how a species will act in a stressful situation. It is also important to leave an exit for the animal and an exit for the capture personnel. Many species carry zoonotic disease, so capture personnel should be aware of potential zoonotic disease and handle the animal in an appropriate manner.

A firearm backup is important with more dangerous species (Fig. 32.4). The primary person performing the backup should be trained and experienced in the use of firearms, and an appropriate firearm should be used. If firearms are commonly used, all members of the capture team should receive firearm safety training. Similar training is advisable for people using dart rifles or dart pistols. Since helicopters can be hazardous, appropriate training and protective equipment, such as helmets, will help to minimize the risk of injury.

The environment itself can be hazardous. Capture may occur

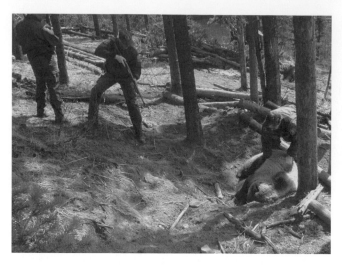

Fig. 32.4. A firearm backup is vital when potentially dangerous animals are approached. In this picture, one fish-and-wildlife officer is focused on the target bear. The other officer is scanning the vicinity for other bears.

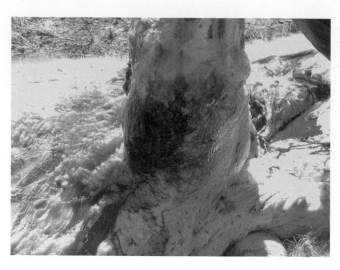

Fig. 32.5. Postmortem image of a hematoma caused by a high-velocity injection of Telazol into the forelimb of a polar bear. The drug was delivered via an explosive discharge mechanism.

in remote locations. In these situations, capture personnel must be prepared to look after themselves if they cannot return to a base area. A method of communication with rescue services may need to be established. In some environments, weather can change rapidly and will often dictate whether capture can take place. There are hazards specific to the terrain and region; for instance, capture personnel should receive avalanche training before working in mountainous regions with an avalanche risk. It is important to anticipate risks in any environment.

Pharmaceuticals used for wildlife anesthesia can present a serious human health hazard because of their high potency and concentrated formulations. Potent narcotics, such as carfentanil, etorphine, and thiafentanil, can induce serious toxicity in people.[16] These drugs must be handled with extreme caution. Protective clothing, such as disposable gloves or face shields, should be used to prevent skin or mucous membrane contact. A pharmacological antagonist should be available to treat human exposure. Potent narcotics receive a great deal of attention, but any concentrated sedative or anesthetic must be treated with respect. Medetomidine can be formulated at a concentration of 10 mg/mL (Zalopine; Orion Pharma Animal Health, Turku, Finland) for use in wildlife. Dexmedetomidine, which is used at a dose of 1 to 2 µg/kg in people,[17] is approximately twice as potent as medetomidine, because levomedetomidine has no clinical effects.[18] This dose would be equivalent to 2 to 4 µg of medetomidine per 1 kg of body weight or a total of 150 to 300 µg in a 75-kg person. The high end of this dose range is equivalent to 0.03 mL of Zalopine. Obviously, there is the risk of toxicity from exposure to a very low volume of Zalopine. Telazol (tiletamine-zolazepam) is another immobilizing mixture that can be delivered in a concentrated form and therefore must also be handled with caution. Everyone working on a capture team should be trained in first aid, and equipment should be available to provide respiratory and airway support in the hands of trained personnel.

Prior to any capture, it is advisable to meet with local medical personnel and discuss an evacuation and treatment plan in the face of drug exposure. A meeting of this nature will familiarize physicians and emergency medical services personnel with the drugs that are being used and the potential treatments. In the event of an emergency, this can save valuable time and someone's life.

Remote Drug-Delivery Equipment

Wildlife capture often requires remote drug delivery, often over relatively long distances. Generally, it is difficult to deliver drugs accurately at distances greater than 40 m. There have been major advances in the equipment available for remote drug delivery. It is important to realize that these systems have the potential to produce serious injury or death if they are used inappropriately. The major sources of injury arise from dart-impact trauma, high-velocity injection of dart contents, and inaccurate dart placement (Fig. 32.5). Dart-impact trauma results from dispersion of energy on dart impact. Impact kinetic energy is represented by the following equation: $KE = 1/2M \times V^2$, where M = mass of the dart and V = velocity.[1] High velocity is the major factor that will cause trauma. A good general rule is to use the lowest velocity that will provide an accurate trajectory at a given distance. Practice with a darting system at a variety of distances is vital to minimize velocity. The other major factor is the mass of the dart. Darts with a lower mass will have less impact energy at a given velocity. This should be a consideration in the choice of a darting system, particularly when dealing with smaller animals that are more prone to trauma.

Inaccurate dart placement can cause injury. This most frequently occurs if darts penetrate the abdomen, thorax, or vital structures of the head and neck. The major factors that can lead to inaccurate dart placement include a lack of practice with the

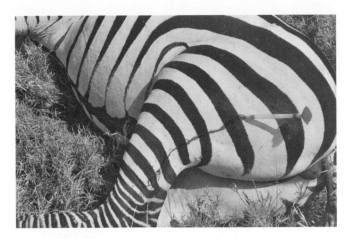

Fig. 32.6. In most species, darts should be placed in the large muscle mass of the hind limb. This facilitates drug absorption and decreases the risk of trauma to vital structures.

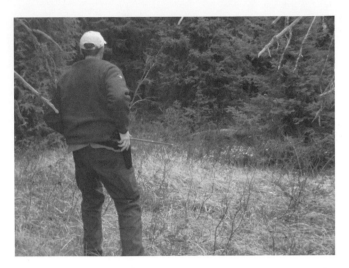

Fig. 32.7. The pole syringe is useful for drug delivery in caged or trapped animals. It can be used cautiously, as in this image, to facilitate additional drug administration in lightly anesthetized, but recumbent, animals.

darting system, an attempt to place a dart over an excessive range, and inherent inaccuracy of the darting system.

The final source of injury is related to high-velocity injection of dart contents. Systems that expel drug via an explosive charge can disrupt tissue and produce trauma. These systems should only be used on large, well-muscled animals (Fig. 32.6). Injection volume should be minimized to decrease the degree of tissue trauma. When possible, the use of darts that deliver their contents via compressed air should be considered to minimize trauma. The choice of system depends on the range required, the dart size, and individual characteristics of the target animal. The next section is a general discussion of remote delivery equipment. A more complete review can be found elsewhere.[19] A further review and manufacturer information can be found in the *Handbook of Wildlife Chemical Immobilization.*[1]

Pole Syringe

This is a simple device that can be used to extend reach for injection. In its simplest form, the pole is an extension of the syringe plunger, with the barrel of the syringe covering the end of the pole. It is typically used on confined animals (e.g., animals confined in traps or cages) or can be used to top up anesthesia in recumbent, but lightly anesthetized, animals. It is generally used on approach to the animal before initial contact is made (Fig. 32.7).

Pole syringes vary in length, but generally do not exceed 3 or 4 m. These can be simple homemade devices that consist of a disposable syringe attached to the tip of a wooden or plastic pole, or they may be commercial products. Commercial pole syringes come in a variety of designs. It is generally advantageous to select a pole syringe that can be disassembled into segments for transport and storage. Another factor to consider is ease of cleaning. Some devices use a disposable syringe that facilitates the use of proper aseptic technique. It is preferable to select a device that has a variety of syringe heads to facilitate accurate delivery of a variety of volumes.

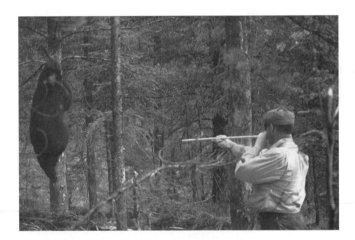

Fig. 32.8. Blowguns are useful for distances of up to 10 m. They are quiet and produce minimal trauma to animals. They are most useful in caged, snared, or treed animals.

Blowgun

This is the most basic of all remote drug-delivery systems. By blowing into a 1- to 2-m pipe, a trained operator can accurately propel a lightweight (3 to 5 mL) drug dart up to 10 or 15 m. The blowgun is useful as a short-range, limited-volume, drug-delivery system. It is commonly used in zoo work, wildlife rescue, and urban animal-control work (Fig. 32.8). The blowgun is nearly silent, uncomplicated to use and maintain, and well suited for immobilization of smaller animals. Because of their light weight, limited mass, and low velocity, blowgun darts cause minimal impact damage and tissue trauma. The discharge mechanism in most blowgun darts is compressed air or butane gas (Fig. 32.9). Practice with the blowgun is required before range and accuracy can be attained. Leaky darts can be hazardous to the op-

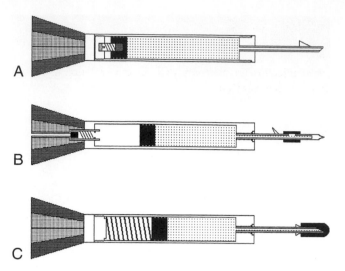

Fig. 32.9. A: Dart with explosive discharge mechanism. **B:** Dart with air-activated drug-discharge mechanism. **C:** Dart with coil spring–activated drug-discharge mechanism.

erator, and pressurized darts should be carefully inspected before loading. Several excellent systems are commercially available, but they can also be manufactured inexpensively from disposable syringes and plastic or conduit pipes.

Power Projection Systems

A variety of systems are commercially available to propel darts up to 50 m. Rifles are available that propel the dart via a .22-caliber powder charge, carbon dioxide (CO_2) gas, or compressed air. Pistols generally use CO_2 or compressed air.

Powder-Charged Projectors

These systems use the gas expansion from a fired .22-caliber charge to propel the drug dart. There are two basic types of this projector. The first uses different .22-caliber charges to compensate for various distances. The Palmer rifle (Palmer Chemical and Equipment, Douglasville, GA) is a good example of this technology. It is very important that the correct charge be used for the dart size and distance, and that the manufacturer's recommendations are followed. The use of long-range charges at short distances can produce serious trauma. Dart velocity may also be regulated by pushing the dart farther down the barrel of the projector. The farther the dart is moved toward the muzzle, the lower will be its velocity. A rod with markings for different settings and distances is useful for consistency in positioning the dart in the barrel. This method can be useful when darting at short distances.

The second type of powder projector vents the gas from a single blank .22-caliber charge through a ported velocity control. By adjusting the velocity control, the range of the dart can be regulated in accordance with dart size and distance. This system affords greater versatility and faster operation in cases where the distance to the animal may change frequently or suddenly. It requires practice at a variety of settings to become an effective

marksperson, and the velocity control must be kept clean to maintain consistency and accuracy. Paxarms (Timaru, New Zealand) and Pneu-Dart (Williamsport, PA) manufacture systems that use this technology.

Compressed Gas–Powered Projectors

These systems typically use compressed air or CO_2 to propel darts 5 to 50 m. They are manufactured in the form of pistols, rifles, and pistol grips that can be attached to a blowgun, and are available from a variety of companies worldwide. CO_2-powered projectors use gas from a CO_2 cartridge to propel the drug dart. Only fresh CO_2 cartridges should be used. Projectors should be stored according to the manufacturer's recommendations because some units must be stored cocked to preserve the O-rings.

Compressed air–powered projectors use compressed air from a tank or pump to propel the dart. A control valve and/or gauge on the projector, pump, or tank provide a means of regulating the air pressure for dart size and distance. Air-propulsion systems are often used in connection with blowgun components and to propel lightweight drug darts short to medium distances.

Darts

Darts must deliver their contents into a muscle group on impact. There are three major systems in common use to facilitate drug injection. Choice of these systems will depend on the situation and the size of the animal. Darts that use an explosive discharge mechanism can produce considerable muscle trauma and should be reserved for large, well-muscled animals.

Explosive Discharge Mechanisms

These darts have an aluminum or plastic body into which a small explosive cap is placed between the plunger and the tail. Upon impact, a firing pin inside the cap is forced forward, against the resistance of a spring, detonating the charge. The expanding gas pushes the plunger forward, and the drug is expelled through the needle. The speed of injection, 0.001 s, may cause tissue damage.[19] The explosive caps are very sensitive to moisture and must be kept dry. When placed in the dart, the cap must have its open end against the tail. If it is turned around, detonation and expulsion of the drug will occur at the moment the projector is fired (Fig. 32.9).

If reusable darts are used, the fit of the dart should be tested by inserting the dart in the muzzle. If it slides in and out with ease, the dart is not deformed and can be loaded. If the dart jams in the muzzle, the dart barrel is deformed and should not be reloaded. With repeated use, the dart barrel may expand where the aluminum is weakened by the threads cut into it. This is caused by the high pressure created in the dart when gases from the explosive charge push the plunger forward at great speed. All of the darts with explosive discharge mechanisms inject through the tip of the needle. The needle should be barbed so that it stays in the animal during injection. If there is no barb or if the barb is removed, the force of the frontal expulsion of the drug is often sufficiently powerful to drive the dart out of the animal with only partial injection.

Air-Activated Mechanisms

These darts consist of an aluminum or plastic body into which air is introduced through a one-way valve in the tail piece and compressed behind the plunger. At impact, a silicone seal is displaced, exposing a port in the side of the needle. The plunger is pushed forward by air pressure, and the drug is expelled through the port (Fig. 32.9). Depending on the type and usage, plastic darts can be used repeatedly, but will eventually begin to leak or lose air pressure. In extreme cold, the drug may freeze inside the dart; therefore, darts should be kept warm in a secure container placed in an inside pocket or in a heated vehicle or helicopter until used.

Spring-Activated Discharge Mechanisms

These darts consist of an aluminum or plastic body that contains a coil spring behind the plunger. After the drug is loaded into the front of the dart, a rubber seal is placed over the needle tip. The tail piece with the coil spring is then screwed into the dart, compressing the spring behind the plunger. Upon impact, the needle tip penetrates the rubber seal, and the coil spring pushes the plunger forward, expelling the drug (Fig. 32.9).

Pharmacology

Ideal Drug Combination

Wildlife immobilization has progressed a great deal in recent years. A variety of drugs are available to facilitate capture and handling, and new techniques continue to develop. If an ideal drug combination could be developed, it would need to possess most of the properties listed here:

Rapid Onset of Activity

A rapid effect is one of the most important attributes required in a capture drug. The induction period is a hazardous time. Handlers and bystanders may be at risk of injury if induction is prolonged. Rapid onset will limit the risks of trauma, hyperthermia, and possibly capture myopathy. Ideally, the animal should be immobilized within 1 to 5 min after injection. Practically, most current combinations can take longer than 5 min to induce anesthesia.

High Margin of Safety

Drugs used for wildlife capture must have a high margin of safety. It is difficult to transport supportive equipment into the field; therefore, capture drugs should produce minimal cardiopulmonary depression. Wild animals are not weighed prior to capture, and it is not uncommon to overestimate weight. Capture drugs must have a high therapeutic index to decrease the risk of mortality from overdose.

Handler Safety

Precautions must always be taken to avoid exposure to potent drugs. Ideally, drugs should be relatively safe to handle, with minimum risks of intoxication if the handler contacts the drug. The ability to antagonize the effects of the drug is also desirable in field situations.

Small Volume of Delivery

Capture drugs should be potent and concentrated enough to facilitate delivery at low volumes (ideally, <3 mL). This decreases the risk of injection trauma from high-velocity injection and facilitates accurate dart flight.

Narcosis

The animal should loose consciousness and be unaware of its surroundings.

Ability to Antagonize Immobilization

Free-ranging wildlife often live in an environment full of potential hazards, so they must be cared for until they are fully awake. A pharmacological antagonist should be available because the ability to antagonize immobilization will speed recovery and is also of value in emergency situations. Because it can be difficult to provide supportive care, complications such as hyperthermia can become life threatening, and antagonism of immobilization may be the only viable option in managing unexpected complications.

Versatility

Wildlife managers often deal with a variety of species. Thus, an ideal drug combination could be used, with predictable effects, in a wide range of species. This limits the variety of drugs required to be kept on hand and leads to familiarity with the effects of the combination most commonly used.

Drug Stability

Wildlife capture may need to be performed in a wide range of ambient temperatures. Ideally, drugs should remain stable, in solution, over a wide range of ambient temperatures.

Analgesia

In recent years, it has become more common to perform potentially painful procedures during wildlife handling. These procedures can include ear tagging, tooth removal, biopsies, and even surgery for abdominal or subcutaneous implant placement. These situations dictate that appropriate intraoperative and postoperative analgesia must be provided.

Paralytic Agents

These have been used in wildlife capture for thousands of years. Remote delivery of curare was used by South American hunters to procure game. Early work by wildlife researchers used nondepolarizing muscle relaxants, such as tubocurarine and gallamine. Succinylcholine, a depolarizing muscle relaxant, has also been used for wildlife capture. Nicotine alkaloids stimulate autonomic ganglia to produce paralysis.

All neuromuscular junction–blocking agents produce immobilization via paralysis of skeletal muscle. The dosage must be adequate to provide a locomotor block, while sparing diaphragmatic function. Obviously, this technique has a very narrow margin of safety. Animals immobilized with paralytic agents are conscious and under considerable stress. The use of paralytics, as the sole agent for wildlife capture, is considered inhumane and is no longer acceptable. Fortunately, a variety of safer and more humane techniques are available to facilitate wildlife capture and handling.

Opioids

A variety of opioids have been used for wildlife capture. Opioids can be used in a wide range of species, but are particularly effective in ungulates. The opioids produce analgesia and sedation, but lack muscle-relaxant properties. They have been used alone or, more often, with the addition of a neuroleptic agent, the inclusion of which potentiates the opioid, produces a smoother induction by counteracting the excitatory state associated with opioid induction, and decreases muscle rigidity. Opioids are predictable in action, act relatively fast, and can be reversed with the administration of a suitable antagonist. If not reversed, the duration of immobilization is lengthy, often several hours, during which the animal is at risk from opioid-induced respiratory depression and environmental hazards. Underdosing of opioids can result in a prolonged induction time, characterized by central nervous system (CNS) excitation, which can cause hyperthermia, exhaustion, lost animals, and/or death of the animal. The side effects of opioid-induced immobilization include

1. Excitation after administration, resulting in aimless running, pacing, or walking, which may lead to hyperthermia or capture myopathy[20]
2. Regurgitation of ruminal content or vomiting, with the risk of regurgitation increased when carfentanil is combined with xylazine[21]
3. Severe respiratory depression and hypoxemia[4,8]
4. Muscle rigidity[20]
5. Renarcotization[20,22,23]

Many of these drugs are extremely potent and must be handled carefully to avoid accidental human exposure.[16,24,25]

Carfentanil

This has been used for wildlife captures since the early 1980s. The commercial preparation, produced by ZooPharm (Fort Collins, CO), is available at a concentration of 3 mg/mL. Carfentanil is approximately 8000 times as potent as morphine, making the commercial preparation very effective at low volumes of administration. Carfentanil is particularly useful in ungulates, but has also been used in large carnivores.[1,26–28] Advantages of carfentanil include a rapid onset of activity, reliability, potency, and reliable reversal if an appropriate antagonist is used. The use of carfentanil alone can cause muscle rigidity; therefore, it is often combined with a sedative agent with muscle-relaxant properties, such as xylazine.[20] There are disadvantages of using this combination in moose, because the addition of xylazine to carfentanil may produce an increased incidence of aspiration pneumonia.[21]

Carfentanil has a relatively long action. Carfentanil-induced immobilization should be antagonized with an appropriate antagonist. If the duration of the antagonist is shorter than that of carfentanil, renarcotization can result. Naltrexone should be used for reversal of carfentanil, because renarcotization has been reported following antagonism with naloxone, diprenorphine, and nalmefene.[22,23] Other adverse effects of carfentanil-based combi-

nations include respiratory depression, hypoxemia, hypertension, CNS excitation, and hyperthermia.[4,8,29]

Etorphine

Etorphine hydrochloride has been used successfully in many species, but has been particularly effective in ungulates, rhinoceroses, and elephants. Etorphine, which is approximately $2\frac{1}{2}$ times less potent than carfentanil, can be used alone or in combination with a suitable neuroleptic synergist. Induction course, induction time, and immobilization duration are dose dependent. Underdosing can cause excitation, with associated problems. At optimum doses, the first effects may be observed 3 to 8 min after intramuscular injection. The full effect may be reached in 20 to 30 min. Recovery is slow (up to 7 or 8 h) if no antagonist is given. When an antagonist is administered, animals will recover in 1 to 3 min after intravenous injection and in 5 to 10 min following intramuscular injection. The most serious side effect is respiratory depression. For that reason, an animal should not be kept immobilized longer than necessary, and drug effect should be reversed as soon as possible. Other side effects are often dose or species dependent and may include excitement, muscle tremors, convulsions, regurgitation, bloat, bradycardia, tachycardia, hypertension, hyperthermia, and renarcotization.

Thiafentanil (A-3080)

This is a potent narcotic that has some potential advantages over carfentanil. Thiafentanil is approximately 6000 times as potent as morphine (vs. 8000 for carfentanil)[30] and has a higher therapeutic index than carfentanil in some species (48 vs. 16 in domestic ferrets).[30] The major advantages of thiafentanil are a more rapid onset and a briefer action than carfentanil, which should result in a lower incidence of renarcotization.[30] Thiafentanil is not yet commercially available, but its use has been described in a variety of species.[5,30–33] It has been used alone or in combination with α_2-adrenergic agonists.[31–33] Side effects are similar to those of other narcotics and include respiratory depression and hypoxemia.[31] Reports have detailed the use of thiafentanil combined with medetomidine and ketamine.[5,32] This is a promising combination that appears to be efficacious and have fewer side effects than does high-dose narcotic anesthesia.[5,32]

Opioid Antagonists

A major advantage of opioid-based anesthesia is the ability to antagonize the opioid and rapidly reverse immobilization. To be effective, the antagonist should outlast the agonist drug and ideally be highly selective for the desired receptor type(s). Three drugs are commonly used for this purpose: naltrexone, naloxone, and diprenorphine. Naltrexone is probably the most versatile drug, with the lowest risk of renarcotization.

Naltrexone

This is commercially available in a 50-mg/mL concentration. It is a pure opioid antagonist that will produce rapid antagonism of μ opioid receptor agonists. The major advantage of naltrexone is that it will produce reliable antagonism of longer-acting opioids, such as carfentanil. A study comparing carfentanil reversal with nalmefene, diprenorphine, and naltrexone demonstrated renarcotization with diprenorphine and nalmefene.[22] Naltrexone has been recommended at a dose of 100:1 (naltrexone-carfentanil). The drug is active following intramuscular and intravenous administration. A more rapid antagonism will occur if the drug is administered intravenously.

Naloxone

Naloxone hydrochloride is a pure narcotic antagonist (i.e., it has no known agonistic properties). It may be used to reverse the effects of all the aforementioned opioids, and reversal occurs within 1 to 3 min of intravenous injection. Naloxone has a short half-life; therefore, animals may revert to a state of immobilization within a few hours and require repeated treatment with naloxone. Renarcotization has been noted in field studies that used naloxone as an antagonist for carfentanil.[23] A low dose of naloxone (2 µg/µg carfentanil intravenously) has been shown to improve oxygenation while maintaining immobilization in elk.[4]

Diprenorphine

Diprenorphine hydrochloride (M50-50; Lemmon, Sellersville, PA) is the antagonist used to reverse the effects of etorphine. While relative to etorphine as an antagonist, it does have agonistic properties of its own. Reversal is rapid following intravenous injection, with animals becoming ambulatory in 1 to 3 min. If the antagonist is injected intramuscularly, reversal takes longer (up to 15 to 20 min). Side effects are rare, although overdosing may cause continued immobilization because of its partial agonist activity. Following accidental human exposure to etorphine, diprenorphine hydrochloride should not be used as an antagonist because of its agonist effects. Naloxone or naltrexone are the preferred human antagonists.

Cyclohexamines

These produce a state of dissociative anesthesia. Phencyclidine hydrochloride was the first drug in this class used for wildlife capture. The cyclohexamines, used alone, produce muscle rigidity or twitching. Other side effects are hyperthermia, excessive salivation, catecholamine release, and convulsions. The cyclohexamines act fast, have a relatively wide margin of safety, and depress respiration and circulation only moderately at optimum doses. Laryngeal reflexes are somewhat preserved with these agents.

Cyclohexamines may be used alone in some species, but the effects of the addition of a benzodiazepine or α_2-adrenergic agonist will be additive or synergistic with the cyclohexamine, produce a smoother induction and recovery, and alleviate the muscle rigidity common to dissociative anesthesia.[2] The cyclohexamines have been used in a wide variety of species, but are particularly known for their effectiveness in carnivores, bears, primates, and birds. There are no known antagonists for this class of drugs. The drugs in this category include ketamine and the tiletamine-zolazepam combination (Telazol; Fort Dodge Laboratories, Fort Dodge, IA).

Ketamine

Ketamine hydrochloride is a dissociative anesthetic commercially available in 10-, 50-, and 100-mg/mL aqueous solutions.

Since these concentrations may be too low for efficient delivery to larger species, it may be lyophilized and reconstituted at 200 mg/mL. Ketamine should never be used as the sole immobilizing agent. A tranquilizer-sedative should be used in almost all cases to reduce or prevent its hypertonic effects. Ketamine has been used successfully in many species, and doses vary widely from one species to another. Induction time and immobilization duration are dose and species dependent. At optimum doses, the first effects are observed in 2 to 5 min following intramuscular injection, with the full effects reached in 5 to 10 min. Immobilization usually lasts from 45 min to 2 h. Side effects of ketamine immobilization may include convulsions, catatonia, apnea, excessive salivation, and hyperthermia as a consequence of catatonia. Many of these side effects can be negated by adding a benzodiazepine or α_2-adrenergic agonist. Medetomidine-ketamine has some advantages over xylazine-ketamine because a lower dose of ketamine is usually required.[34] This will result in smaller injection volumes and the ability to antagonize the medetomidine with fewer adverse side effects from the remaining ketamine. Ketamine-based combinations are unreliable in bears. Sudden recoveries have been encountered with xylazine-ketamine and medetomidine-ketamine in brown and polar bears.[34,35]

Tiletamine-Zolazepam

A commercial preparation of tiletamine, a dissociative anesthetic, and zolazepam, a benzodiazepine drug, is available as a freeze-dried powder (Telazol). It is effective in a variety of species and, at optimum doses, first effects may be noticeable within 1 or 2 min of intramuscular injection, with full effects reached within 15 to 30 min. The induction is usually smooth, with good muscle relaxation and somatic analgesia. The duration varies with species, but may persist for several hours. Because tiletamine and zolazepam are metabolized at different rates, the quality of emergence and duration of recovery may be affected. Recovery occurs in 3 to 8 h in most cases, but may be prolonged in some species.

Tiletamine-zolazepam combinations may cause hypertension and increase heart rate and cardiac output. Other effects are salivation, occasional muscle rigidity, and hyperthermia (particularly if the mixture is combined with an α_2-adrenergic agonist).[35–38] Telazol has been used alone in a variety of species.[39] It is very effective in carnivores, and recovery tends to be smooth, but can be prolonged. The use of Telazol alone in ungulates can result in rough recoveries. Reconstitution of Telazol with an α_2-adrenergic agonist will decrease the volume injected, enhance analgesia, and decrease recovery times following antagonism of the α_2-adrenergic agonist.[35–38] These combinations will produce a better quality of immobilization and recovery, particularly in ungulates.[7,40,41] Generally, the addition of an α_2-adrenergic agonist will greatly decrease Telazol requirements. In polar bears, the Telazol requirement was reduced by up to 75%.[35,36]

α_2-Adrenergic Agonists

These are CNS depressants with sedative, muscle relaxant, and analgesic properties. Used alone, α_2-adrenergic agonists produce unreliable immobilization. They are best used in combination with opioids or dissociative anesthetics. When used in high dosages, α_2-adrenergic agonists may critically depress respiration and circulation. Commonly encountered side effects include hypoxemia in ungulates and hypertension with or without bradycardia.[6–9,34,36,37,42] These agents can also contribute to ruminal tympany and regurgitation in ungulates.[7,21] In very excited animals, they do not produce a satisfactory level of immobilization. They also disrupt thermoregulatory mechanisms, leading to hyperthermia or hypothermia.[2,36,37] Recovery, without reversal, from high doses is usually prolonged and difficult. In field situations, it is generally recommended that the effects of α_2-adrenergic agonists be antagonized at the completion of the procedure.

Xylazine

This is commonly available in 20- and 100-mg/mL aqueous solutions. It is also available as a powder and as 300-mg/mL solution specifically for wildlife capture. The 20-mg/mL solution is too dilute to be useful for remote injection.

When administered alone, xylazine does not produce reliably immobilized free-ranging wildlife. Its effectiveness appears to be decreased in excited or stressed animals. It may appear to induce a recumbent sleeplike or anesthetic-like state; however, stimulation may cause rapid arousal with defense responses intact. In calm animals, the initial effect may be seen within 4 to 5 min of intramuscular injection, with full effect reached within 15 to 20 min. Adverse effects can include hypoxemia, bradycardia, hypotension, ruminal tympany, and decreased thermoregulatory ability.

Xylazine has been used effectively as a synergist with opioids and cyclohexamines. The inclusion of xylazine has decreased dose requirements of the primary immobilizing drugs, produced a faster and smoother induction, and countered some of the undesirable side effects of these drugs. The response to high doses of xylazine may conceal a recovery from the primary immobilizing drug and place workers at risk if the animal is suddenly aroused by noises, touch, or other stimulation.

The effects of xylazine may be reversed with the administration of an α_2-adrenergic antagonist. In general, 1 mg of atipamezole is required to antagonize 10 mg of xylazine. If xylazine is used in combination with a cyclohexamine, its effects should not be reversed before the animal has metabolized a significant fraction of the latter drug, in order to avoid the side effects of the cyclohexamine.

Xylazine is typically used intramuscularly for wildlife immobilization. Intranasal administration of xylazine can be beneficial to decrease stress and struggling following net-gun capture.[13] This route has a rapid onset of activity and is simple to administer in physically restrained animals.[13]

Detomidine

Detomidine hydrochloride is available in a 10-mg/mL solution. The effects of detomidine have been well studied in horses, but information on its use for immobilization of captive and free-ranging wild animals is somewhat limited. It has been combined with etorphine in rhinoceros and has proven to be effective in ze-

bras when combined with carfentanil and ketamine.[43,44] The action of detomidine is much like that of xylazine. Its effects may be reversed by an appropriate α_2-adrenergic antagonist. In general, 1 to 3 mg of atipamezole should be used to antagonize 1 mg of detomidine.

Medetomidine

Medetomidine hydrochloride is a potent α_2-adrenergic agonist that has proven to be a very useful drug for wildlife capture. The 1-mg/mL formulation is suitable for use in small mammals, but is too dilute for use in larger species. Medetomidine is also available in 10 mg/mL (Zalopine; Orion Pharma Animal Health) and 20 mg/mL (ZooPharm) concentrations. The latter concentrations are adequate for capture of most large land mammals. Medetomidine will produce sedation, analgesia, and muscle relaxation. The drug should not be used alone because, as with xylazine, immobilization is unreliable. Medetomidine can be combined with a low dose of ketamine or Telazol. A relatively low dose of the dissociative drug is required with medetomidine, and antagonism of medetomidine with atipamezole (at three to five times the medetomidine dose) will hasten recovery.[34] Side effects of medetomidine include hypertension, bradycardia, and hypoxemia.[7,8,34,36,42,44] Hypoxemia may be particularly pronounced in ruminants.[7] Medetomidine can also impair thermoregulatory ability, resulting in hyperthermia.[35,36]

Romifidine

A fourth α_2-adrenergic agonist, romifidine, at 10 mg/mL (Sedivet; Boehringer Ingelheim Vetmedica, St. Joseph, MO) has been developed for use in domestic animals. Its action is similar to the other α_2-adrenergic agonists. There is minimal data on the use of romifidine in free-ranging mammals.

α_2-Adrenergic Antagonists

The utility of α_2-agonist–induced sedation is greatly increased by the availability of antagonists. Several competitive antagonists are used in wildlife work. Atipamezole is the most selective of the three antagonists currently used and can be used in all species. There are species dependent differences in response to yohimbine and tolazoline.[2] Yohimbine, for example, is not particularly effective in wild bovids, and either tolazoline or atipamezole is preferred in these species. Antagonists should generally be administered intramuscularly unless the situation is emergent. CNS excitement, tachycardia, and hypertension may be seen with intravenous administration.[34,45] Animals may arouse rapidly from immobilization following intravenous administration of atipamezole.[7,35,42] With potentially dangerous species, this may not allow adequate time to retreat to a safe distance.

Atipamezole

This is the most specific and potent α_2-adrenergic antagonist currently available. It is typically used to antagonize medetomidine at three to five times the medetomidine dose administered.[34] It is equally effective in the antagonism of xylazine (1 mg of atipamezole per 10 mg of xylazine) and detomidine (1 to 3 mg of atipamezole per 1 mg of detomidine).

Yohimbine

Yohimbine hydrochloride is an effective α_2-adrenergic antagonist for reversal of xylazine in a variety of species. Some species may respond reliably, whereas others may show no or only partial recovery. Yohimbine may cause tachycardia, hypertension, and CNS excitement. At clinical doses, it does not produce effective antagonism of medetomidine.

Tolazoline

This has proven to be an effective α_2-adrenergic antagonist in some wild and domestic species. High dosages of tolazoline may produce systemic hypotension, and tachycardia has been observed in sheep.[2] Tolazoline is effective in bison and other bovids where yohimbine lacks efficacy.

Drug Combinations

It is uncommon to use single agents for wildlife capture. Typically, agents are combined either for their synergistic effects or to counter adverse side effects. The combination of an opioid with an α_2-adrenergic agonist has already been discussed. Xylazine-ketamine has been used for many years and has the advantage of versatility (i.e., it is effective in many ungulate and carnivore species). The major disadvantages of xylazine-ketamine are the large volume required and the residual effects of ketamine if xylazine is antagonized soon after administration. Medetomidine-ketamine shares the versatility of xylazine-ketamine, with the advantages of decreased volume and lower ketamine requirement. Antagonism of medetomidine will likely cause fewer side effects from residual ketamine, because the overall amount of dissociative anesthetic administered is lower.[34]

Medetomidine-ketamine is useful in a wide range of species.[34] It should be used cautiously, or its use avoided, in bears, because sudden recoveries have been reported in brown bears and polar bears.[34,35] Xylazine-Telazol and medetomidine-Telazol can be delivered in small volumes and are useful in a wide range of wildlife species. Antagonism of the α_2-adrenergic agonist will hasten recovery. Time to sternal recumbency and standing is generally more rapid after antagonism of medetomidine compared with xylazine.[6,35–38] This is probably the result of a lower Telazol dose required in the medetomidine-Telazol combination, when compared with xylazine-Telazol.[6,37]

Neuroleptic Drugs

Neuroleptic agents such as acepromazine and droperidol have been used as adjunctive agents in wildlife capture for many years. Typically, they have been used in combination with potent opioids such as etorphine. A more recent application of these agents is the use of long-acting tranquilizers to facilitate translocation of wild animals. Long-acting neuroleptics have been developed to treat human psychosis. Depending on the formulation, these drugs may have effects for days to weeks. These drugs will produce an overall reduction in stress of handling, which should decrease the incidence of trauma and myopathy and facilitate adaptation to a novel environment. Typically, these agents are phenothiazines, butyrophenones, or benzodiazepines.[46] A short-

acting agent, such as haloperidol, may be combined with a long-acting agent, such as perphenazine enanthate, to produce rapid onset of action and prolonged activity.[46]

Perphenazine Enanthate

Perphenazine is a phenothiazine derivative that is formulated in a sesame oil vehicle. The onset of perphenazine is 12 to 16 h, and its effects can last up to 10 days. The use of this drug has been reported in a variety of species, including red deer and Przewalski's horses.[47,48] Flight distance is decreased in red deer, and animals maintain better body condition than controls.[47] In Przewalski's horses, the drug has been used to effectively decrease dominance aggression during the establishment of a bachelor herd.[48]

Zuclopenthixol Acetate

This is a thioxanthine derivative that has been used in a variety of species and will have effects lasting 3 to 4 days.[47,49–51] Treated animals have a decreased flight distance and are easier to manipulate. Animals spend more time eating and drinking compared with controls and have been observed to spend less time pacing. A dose of 1 mg/kg has been used in most studies. Occasionally, extrapyramidal signs have been noted at this dose.[51] These signs usually resolve without treatment.[51]

The Capture Event

Precapture Planning

Before undertaking any wildlife capture, an appropriate plan of action must be devised for the capture procedure. The species should be researched to determine the most effective and current technique for capture. A decision needs to be made as to the use of physical or chemical restraint. Logistical considerations are important. In remote areas, communication and evacuation plans must be established. Equipment must be carefully selected for use in the field. Drug needs must be anticipated, and it is generally wise to budget for at least 50% more drug than is actually needed for the target animals. This will help to offset any drug wasted from lost darts or poor dart placement.

In the immediate recapture period, the target animal is located and weight is estimated. The terrain, weather, and situation must be evaluated to determine whether capture will be attempted. Most commonly, the drug dart is loaded after the target animal has been located and observed; however, there may be times when it is more practical to load the darts beforehand. Drug doses may be calculated for specific sizes or age groups, and the darts are preloaded and marked accordingly. However, metal darts should not be kept loaded for longer than a 12-h period because of the possibility that corrosive action of the drugs may impair the injection mechanism and damage the dart. Preloaded darts with air-activated discharge mechanisms should not be pressurized because they have a tendency to leak, or lose pressure, if armed for an extended period. Choose darts that are lightweight and have barbed needles of an appropriate length for the target animal.

Generally, the animal will need to be approached to within a distance of 30 to 40 m for accurate drug delivery. There are many methods to facilitate approaching to within this distance. Animals may be stalked, approached in a vehicle or helicopter, or trapped or snared prior to approach. Trapping has the advantage of limiting movement during the capture event, but it may prove to be more stressful than helicopter capture.[14] Pursuit of animals should generally be limited to no more than 2 to 5 min. The incidence of capture myopathy, hyperthermia, and trauma will increase with prolonged chase times. In management situations, pursuit may often be required until the animal is captured. It is beyond the scope of this chapter to consider species-specific considerations. It is advisable to include experienced personnel on the capture team and to consult with experienced wildlife managers, biologists, and veterinarians to determine anticipated complications, animal behavior when stressed, and the current approaches to dealing with the target species.

Induction

Many factors may influence induction time. These include the drug dose received, the animal's physical condition, its age and gender, and its sensitivity to the immobilizing drug. Dart placement is probably the most important determinant of induction time. To facilitate quick absorption of the drug, the muscle masses of the neck, shoulder, or hindquarter must be injected (Fig. 32.6). Animals that are excited or stressed can have induction times that are considerably longer than in calm animals.

Some animals will put on considerable fat deposits prior to denning and fasting and must be dealt with in a different manner during these times. Brown bears, for example, can generally be darted in the hindquarter when they emerge from spring dens. In the fall, these animals have considerable fat deposits overlying the rump and must be darted in the shoulder or neck. As soon as the dart is placed, the time should be recorded, and the animal must be carefully observed to ensure that it is not lost during the induction period.

Induction is a dangerous time during which animals may be lost or injured. If a helicopter was used in pursuit, it will need to back off to a safe distance where an animal can be observed, but not stressed. The helicopter may need to steer an animal away from potential hazards such as cliffs or water. Time to sternal recumbency and head down should be recorded.

Initial approach to an animal can be dangerous. The animal should be observed from a safe distance to determine that there is no purposeful movement. When α_2-adrenergic agonist–based protocols are used (e.g., medetomidine-ketamine or xylazine-tiletamine-zolazepam), the animal's head or limbs should not move prior to approach. If tiletamine-zolazepam alone or narcotics are used, there may be some involuntary movement in adequately immobilized animals. Once it has been determined that the animal is safe to approach, it should be cautiously approached accompanied by a firearm backup, if necessary. It is important to leave safe exits for the capture team and the animal. To gauge the animal's response, auditory stimulation such as clapping or shouting should be employed as the animal is approached. If there is no response to auditory stimulation, the response to tactile stimulation should be gauged. It is advisable to

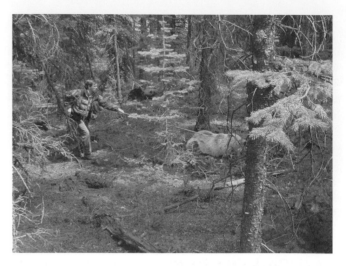

Fig. 32.10. Initial contact should be made from a safe distance. In this picture, a pole syringe is being used to initiate contact with a grizzly bear.

use a stick or pole syringe to extend reach when stimulating the animal (Fig. 32.10). When it is safe, the palpebral reflex and airway can be checked. A set of vital signs, including rectal temperature, respiratory rate, and heart rate, should be monitored. The animal's eyes can be lubricated with an ophthalmic solution or gel, and a blindfold can be placed to decrease visual stimulation. At this point, hobbles may be considered to limit movement in the event of sudden recovery in ungulates.

Monitoring and Supportive Care

Following capture, the animal should be positioned to avoid pressure points and ensure optimum ventilation. Carnivores may be positioned in lateral or sternal recumbency, but ruminants should be positioned in sternal recumbency whenever possible. The head and neck should be extended to maintain a patent airway. A stretcher system may be employed to facilitate movement of the animal and to keep it elevated above the ground. Vital signs should be monitored every 5 to 10 min. Ideally, continuous monitoring as with a pulse oximeter should be used. Painful procedures such as tooth extraction or biopsies should be performed soon after induction when the animal is in the deepest plane of anesthesia. If animals are manipulated to determine body mass, it is best to do this during a deep plane of anesthesia because the stimulus can result in arousal.[52]

Hypoxemia is not uncommon during wildlife anesthesia.[4–10,29,31,36,42] Hypoxemia, in the face of hyperthermia, is a particularly serious situation, because hyperthermia increases tissue oxygen demand. This can increase the risk of exertional myopathy or cause acute mortality. Hypoxemia can often be prevented or treated in the field with the administration of supplemental oxygen. The animal should be monitored for hypoxemia, ideally with a pulse oximeter. A multisite sensor applied to the tongue generally provides a good signal. Normal hemoglobin saturation should be 95% to 98%, and below 85% is considered hypoxemic. If a pulse oximeter is not available, the mucous membranes

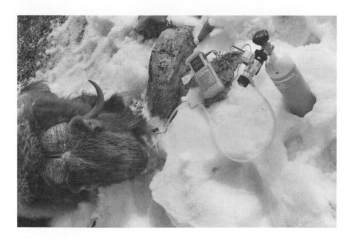

Fig. 32.11. A nasal catheter is being used to deliver supplemental inspired oxygen to an anesthetized musk ox. The oxygen flow is adjusted to try to achieve a desired percentage of hemoglobin saturation of 95% or more.

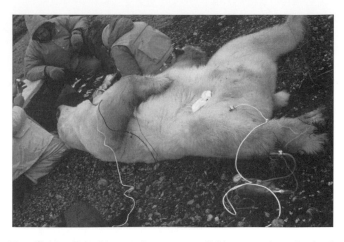

Fig. 32.12. Portable monitors are available to perform in-depth physiological monitoring during wildlife capture. In this image, a monitor is used to measure direct arterial pressure and electrocardiographic status in a polar bear.

should be monitored for cyanosis. Severely hypoxemic animals are often tachycardic. Tachycardia, followed by severe bradycardia (heart rate, <30 beats/min) is often a warning sign that hypoxemia is very severe and the heart may soon fail.

The use of supplemental inspired oxygen should be considered in hypoxemic animals. Portable equipment is available to facilitate oxygen delivery. An ambulance-type regulator (Easy Reg; Precision Medical, Northampton, PA) and an aluminum D cylinder is lightweight, portable and sturdy. It can provide a 10-L/min flow for up to 30 min. An E cylinder will provide this flow for 1 h or more. A nasal catheter can be used in most animals. The catheter should be threaded as far as the medial canthus of the eye. The flow rate should be adjusted to maintain a saturation of greater than 95% (Fig. 32.11).

Heart rate and pulse quality should be monitored every 5 min. The auricular artery is easily palpated in many ungulate species. If the auricular artery cannot be palpated, a femoral pulse can be used. Equipment is available to measure direct or indirect blood pressure and electrocardiographic status in the field (Fig. 32.12).

In ruminants, maintenance in sternal recumbeny will help to prevent ruminal tympany. If ruminal tympany is a problem, the animal may be rocked gently to stimulate eructation. A rumen tube can be used, but may predispose the animals to regurgitation and aspiration. Generally, if ruminal tympany is severe, it is advisable to finish the procedure quickly and antagonize the anesthetic agents. If α_2-adrenergic agonists have been used, the administration of tolazoline, yohimbine, or atipamezole will stimulate ruminal activity and facilitate the correction of tympany.

Rectal temperature should be monitored every 5 to 10 min. Ungulates are particularly prone to hyperthermia, especially after a long chase. Rectal temperatures higher than 40°C are cause for concern, and attempts should be made to cool the animal. Cold water sprayed on the animal or snow packed into the inguinal and axillary regions may help. Rectal temperature higher than 41°C is an emergency and should be treated aggressively. It is difficult to cool large animals actively, and often the best option with severe hyperthermia is to antagonize the immobilizing agents and allow the animal to recover. Hyperthermic animals should receive supplemental inspired oxygen to offset any hypoxemia and reduce the likelihood of anaerobic tissue metabolism.

Anesthesia depth should be closely monitored. Some drug combinations have proven to be unreliable in bears. Xylazine-ketamine and medetomidine-ketamine are unreliable, and sudden recoveries may be encountered.[34,35] The use of these combinations is best avoided in most situations. Factors that increase the risk of sudden arousal include loud noise, and distress vocalization of offspring is particularly dangerous. Other factors include movement of a bear (i.e., changing the body position or location of the anesthetized animal) or painful stimuli such as tooth extraction. Techniques for monitoring anesthesia depth will depend on the agent used. Tiletamine-zolazepam will produce reliable anesthesia with predictable signs of recovery. As anesthesia lightens, spontaneous blinking will occur. Carnivores often develop chewing and paw movements. They will start to lift their head and may attempt to raise themselves with their forelimbs. Animals with significant head movement generally require a top-up dose of tiletamine-zolazepam or ketamine unless they are to be left to recover. Top-up or small additional doses of tiletamine-zolazepam can significantly prolong recovery and should be used only if longer than 30 min of additional downtime is required. Ketamine is a better choice if 5 to 20 min of additional time is needed.

With xylazine-ketamine or medetomidine-ketamine, head lifting or limb movement signals that the animal is extremely lightly anesthetized and should not be approached or manipulated. Increased intensity of the palpebral reflex or nystagmus are generally good indicators that the animal is lightly anesthetized. When procedures on the animal have been completed, the area should be cleared of equipment, and personnel should retreat to a safe area and observe the recovery.

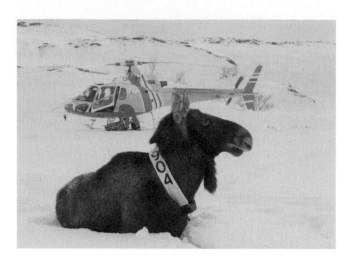

Fig. 32.13. Since modern antagonists can work very rapidly, it is always important to have an avenue of escape with potentially dangerous animals.

Recovery

Considerations for recovery vary, depending on the choice of drug and the situation. In most situations, a reversible technique is desirable. If a reversible technique is not used, the animal should be observed until it can ambulate. Prior to reversal, equipment should be removed from the capture site, and personnel should retreat to a safe distance. The animal should be placed in a comfortable position and its airway cleared. A final set of vital signs are obtained and monitoring equipment removed. Typically, one person remains with the animal and a backup person, if required. Antagonists are administered intramuscularly unless there is an immediate need for rapid recovery. The animal's recovery should be observed from a safe distance (Fig. 32.13).

Human Safety

Many hazards to human safety are inherent in wildlife immobilization. Potent narcotics have received considerable attention because of the risk of intoxication from very small volumes. However, any agent used for wildlife capture should be treated with caution and respect. The most important piece of safety equipment is the latex glove. Gloves should be worn whenever drugs are handled; indeed, it is good practice to wear gloves throughout the capture procedure.

Wildlife anesthesia should never be performed by a single person. At least two people should be present whenever potent drugs are handled, and everyone working on the capture team should be trained in cardiopulmonary resuscitation and first aid. Loading and charging of darts is a time of high risk for exposure to drugs, during which the use of face shields may be considered to prevent contamination of mucous membranes. Darts should be charged under a protective cover to decrease the risk of accidental drug exposure. Antagonists, such as naloxone, should be immediately available if they are indicated for treating human exposure.

Dart-delivery equipment should be handled with care and only by trained individuals. Darts have the potential to induce significant tissue injury and death. Firearm safety rules apply to darting equipment, and individuals handling this equipment should be appropriately trained.

Helicopters present a significant hazard. Wildlife capture requires a very skilled pilot to decrease risk of injury to the target animal and the capture personnel.[53] Anyone working around a helicopter must receive training in helicopter safety.

The target animal can present a risk to personnel. This risk is obvious with large carnivores, but ungulates can also present a significant risk that can be greatly increased if they are cornered or protecting young. Many deer species undergo a period of rut during the breeding season, during which stags are often more aggressive. The best way to avoid injury is to work with people who are familiar with animal behavior and to leave an escape route for the animal and personnel. As previously mentioned, a firearm backup should be available when working with dangerous animals.

During capture, the focus tends to be on the captured animal. It is always important to be aware of the surroundings because other animals may approach the capture team. This is particularly important with social carnivores, such as lions. It is also important with bears, particularly if members of a family group are captured. In these situations, an armed lookout should be posted to protect the capture team.

Complications Related to Wildlife Capture

Physical Trauma

During immobilization and capture, physical injuries such as contusions, lacerations, abrasions, punctures, and fractures may be inflicted on an animal accidentally or by mishandling. Minor injuries can be treated successfully in the field, but fractures and other serious conditions are difficult to treat effectively and often require that the animal be euthanized.

Minor lacerations may be cleaned, treated with a topical antibiotic ointment, and protected with an insect repellant. An appropriate antibiotic may be given intramuscularly to help prevent infection. Closure may be considered for large lacerations, which should be cleaned and debrided as much as possible. These lacerations are often contaminated, and, if they are closed, appropriate drainage and administration of long-acting antibiotics must be considered.

Physical trauma may be prevented by taking notice of any hazard in the environment that may cause injury to the animal during capture and by careful handling. Traps, snares, nets, or other forms of manual capture or restraint that are used should be appropriate for the species and set by trained individuals.

Hyperthermia

This is commonly encountered during wildlife capture. The most immediate sign is a critical rise in body temperature to above 41°C. Other symptoms include rapid shallow breathing, panting, and weak, rapid, or irregular heart rate. Ultimately, animals can convulse and die. Causative factors of hyperthermia in-

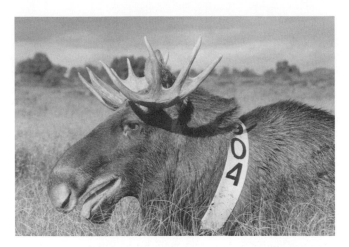

Fig. 32.14. Ungulates are particularly prone to hypoxemia during immobilization. Treatment of hyperthermia is difficult in the field; therefore, antagonism of immobilization is often the best option.

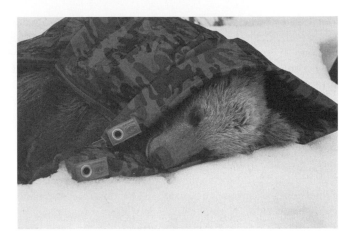

Fig. 32.15. Young animals, such as this brown bear cub, should be insulated from the ground and covered to reduce heat loss.

clude high ambient temperatures, excessive muscular exertion from prolonged pursuit, and interference with normal thermoregulatory mechanisms by α_2-adrenergic agonists. Treatment in the field may include moving the animal into shade or spraying it with cold water. Packing ice or snow around the animal and/or cold-water enemas may also be indicated. The use of supplemental inspired oxygen should be considered to optimize arterial oxygen content. Treatment is often not effective, and generally the best option in field situations is to complete procedures rapidly and administer antagonists (Fig. 32.14).

The risk of hyperthermia may be reduced by avoiding immobilization or capture on very warm days or by limiting activities to the coolest part of the day. It is best to avoid prolonged pursuit, keep stress to a minimum, and use the least severe method of physical restraint. Protecting animals from high ambient temperatures and direct exposure to the sun can also reduce hyperthermia.

Hypothermia

This is a concern when animals are immobilized when ambient temperatures are low. It occurs most commonly in young animals, animals with small body masses, and animals in poor body condition. Hypothermia is characterized by decrease in body temperature to below 35°C. If untreated, hypothermia may result in prolonged recovery, acidosis, and arrhythmias. Causative factors of hypothermia include low ambient temperature, evaporative cooling, wetness, precipitation, and drugs, such as α_2-adrenergic agonists, that impair thermoregulation. Supportive procedures consist of an immediate attempt to increase body temperature by drying a wet animal, covering the animal, and providing external heat sources such as hot-water bottles (Fig. 32.15).

Bloat

Bloat during wildlife capture is commonly caused by ruminal atony associated with the administration of α_2-adrenergic agonists and other drugs that alter gastrointestinal motility. The re-

sult is the inability to relieve gases from the rumen or stomach through normal eructation. The impact of bloat can be reduced by placing the immobilized animal in sternal recumbency with the neck extended and the head forward, permitting saliva and any regurgitated material to drain. Smaller animals can be moved from side to side over the brisket, and their front quarters can be elevated. If positioning does not relieve the bloat, inserting a lubricated and properly sized tube via the esophagus into the rumen will relieve pressure. The last resort to relieve abdominal pressure is emergency trocharization of the rumen. Generally, bloat will resolve following the administration of an α_2-adrenergic antagonist or recovery from drug effects. In the face of severe bloat, procedures should be completed rapidly or discontinued, and drug effects rapidly reversed.

Exertional Myopathy

Most free-ranging animals exert themselves infrequently only to escape danger. They are not conditioned for running at full effort over long distances. Chasing wild animals with a helicopter or motor vehicle imposes a tremendous amount of stress. The effects of sympathetic exhaustion from sustained stress, combined with intense muscular exertion, are the causative factors of various life-threatening syndromes known as *exertional myopathy*.[54–56]

Intense sustained muscular exertion associated with capture pursuit or resisting physical restraint leads to the production and buildup of lactate in muscle cells and metabolic acidosis. Severe lactate accumulation may cause metabolic dysfunction or death of skeletal muscle cells, resulting in the release of intracellular potassium ions (K^+), calcium ions (Ca^{2+}), and myoglobin. High concentrations of myoglobin in the plasma and ultrafiltrate within the renal tubules can cause acute renal failure. Hyperkalemia and acidosis cause arrhythmias and circulatory failure.

Exertional myopathy is difficult to treat, so prevention is of utmost importance. Capture myopathy may be prevented by reducing and minimizing capture stress, fear, and exertion. Chase time should be limited to 2 min and capture efforts not resumed for at least 1 day once capture has failed. Visual and auditory stimulation, handling, and restraint of the captured animal are kept to a minimum. One should provide a stress-free postcapture environment. Captured wild animals should not be handled or stressed for at least 6 weeks following capture. Four common clinical syndromes of exertional myopathy have been identified: acute death syndrome, delayed peracute death syndrome, ataxic-myoglobinuric syndrome, and muscle-rupture syndrome.

Acute Death Syndrome

With the *acute death syndrome* form of exertional myopathy, the animal appears depressed and weak and remains recumbent after reversal. Breathing is rapid and shallow, heart rate is rapid and weak, and hypotension persists, progressing to shock signs and/or death within 3 to 4 h. Causative factors include exhaustion, lactic acidemia, hypoglycemia, and hyperthermia. Supportive procedures consist of fluid therapy to increase blood volume and pressure, restore electrolyte balance, correct acidosis, and increase renal perfusion and diuresis.

Delayed Peracute Death Syndrome

In this syndrome, the animal appears to be in reasonably good condition after the initial capture episode. However, when stressed again (usually 1 day after the initial capture episode), it dies of ventricular fibrillation and cardiac arrest. The pathogenesis of this syndrome is believed to be muscle destruction and potassium release, sensitizing the heart to catecholamines and arrhythmias.

Ataxic-Myoglobinuric Syndrome

This condition is characterized by ataxia, brownish urine, and possibly death within hours or days after capture. Increased levels of serum glutamic-oxaloacetic transaminase (SGOT), creatine phosphokinase (CPK), lactate dehydrogenase (LDH), and blood urea nitrogen (BUN) are associated with lesions in skeletal muscles and kidneys. Death may occur acutely or within 4 to 5 days from kidney failure following myoglobin-mediated tubular destruction. Some animals may survive this syndrome, provided appropriate supportive therapy is instituted.

Muscle-Rupture Syndrome

The first signs of this syndrome can be observed within 1 to 2 days after capture. The animal seems unable to support weight on its hind legs. Hocks are hyperflexed, and CPK, LDH, and SGOT levels are increased, but the BUN level is normal (Fig. 32.16). The animal will usually die within 3 or 4 weeks. On necropsy, there are extensive, light-colored areas in the large muscles used for escape (fight-or-flight response).

Respiratory Depression and Hypoxemia

Hypoxemia is common during wildlife anesthesia and immobilization.[4–10,29,31,36,42] Major causative factors include respiratory depression from immobilizing agents (particularly potent narcotics), ventilation-perfusion mismatching, airway obstruction, and other factors. Immediately after initial contact with a down animal, steps must be taken to ensure a patent airway (Fig.

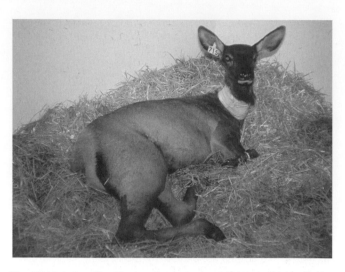

Fig. 32.16. An elk with muscle rupture syndrome and hyperflexion of the hocks.

32.17). Severe hypoxia can cause hypotension, arrhythmias, and death. Hypoxemia in the face of hyperthermia can rapidly result in tissue hypoxia.

The best treatment for hypoventilation is endotracheal intubation and controlled ventilation with supplemental inspired oxygen. This can be difficult in field situations, particularly with very large animals. Partial reversal of narcotics has been used successfully to treat respiratory depression.[4]

Ventilation-perfusion mismatching will generally respond to supplemental inspired oxygen.[6,9] Hypoxemia caused by hypoventilation will also respond to supplemental inspired oxygen, although arterial CO_2 partial pressure will remain elevated and respiratory academia untreated.[29] In the field, the simplest way to treat hypoxemia is to administer supplemental inspired oxygen via a nasal cannula.[6] The animal should be monitored with a pulse oximeter and oxygen flow adjusted to maintain a saturation of peripheral oxygen (SpO_2) greater than 90%. Other causes of hypoxemia include aspiration and pneumothorax (secondary to dart penetration of the thoracic cavity). Pneumothorax might be treatable with thoracocentesis, so equipment should be carried to perform thoracocentesis in the field.

Capture-Associated Mortality

Chemical immobilization of free-ranging mammals is a form of veterinary anesthesia conducted under the most extreme circumstances. The anesthetic risk in wild animals undoubtedly is highly influenced by the capture protocol that is applied. Typically, most deaths are observed in the early phase of a large capture project before the methods have been refined, drug doses have been adjusted, and the immobilization team has gained experience. Moreover, an increased risk of mortality may be seen when captures are carried out for specific purposes like health evaluation of animals under environmental or pathogenic stress. Mortalities caused by capture and anesthesia of free-ranging mammals can be grouped into three different categories. The first is direct effects

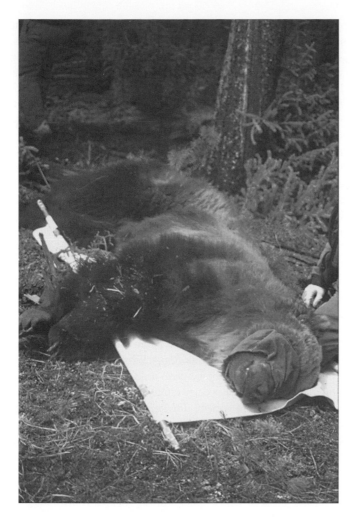

Fig. 32.17. Airway management and supportive care in a grizzly bear. The head and neck have been extended to achieve a clear airway. The bear has been placed on a flat surface and insulated from the ground. After eye lubrication, a blindfold is placed to decrease visual stimuli.

of the immobilizing drug itself (e.g., respiratory depression, shock, hyperthermia, and asphyxia caused by tympany or vomiting). The second group, indirect effects (e.g., drowning, pneumothorax due to misplacement of darts, and trauma from dart impact), might be a direct consequence of the drug used (e.g., etorphine often induces hyperthermia, which may cause the animal to seek water actively for cooling, with drowning as a possible sequela). Finally, the third category is secondary effects caused by the capture process (e.g., trauma from traps, long-term effects from chasing or stress, separation of family groups, and various problems with radio collars or implantable transmitters). Secondary effects have nothing to do with the anesthetic risk per se and should be treated as a separate entity.

In his review of stress and capture myopathy in artiodactylids, Spraker[55] stated that a mortality rate greater than 2% during trapping is unacceptable. This should be the rule of thumb when a large number (>100) of free-ranging animals are being anesthetized or captured (e.g., a mortality rate greater than 2% during

chemical immobilization requires that the anesthetic protocol be reevaluated). By using immobilizing drugs and doses with proven safety, proper remote drug-delivery systems, and established capture methods and techniques, an experienced capture team should be able to minimize the risk of mortality.

Considerations for Commonly Anesthetized Free-Ranging Wildlife

This section deals with general recommendations and considerations for representative species. The species have been chosen because they are commonly encountered or extensively studied. Readers are referred to the *Handbook of Wildlife Chemical Immobilization* for complete dosing information and a reference list by species.[1] Dosages required for immobilization of free-ranging animals are generally higher than those required in captive individuals.[57] This factor must be kept in mind when dosages are planned for wildlife capture, or a relative underdose may occur. Injection site and method of drug delivery can also affect dose requirements. A comparison of hand injection versus dart delivery demonstrated that 50% more drug was required when animals were darted.[58] Method of capture, season, and potentially the gender of an animal can also alter drug dose requirements.

American and Northern European Species
White-Tailed Deer (Odocoileus virginianus) *and Mule Deer* (Odocoileus hemionus)
These species are commonly encountered in management situations. Mature white-tailed deer can weigh 60 to 150 kg, and mature mule deer usually weigh 75 to 135 kg.[1] They are not particularly difficult to anesthetize if they are kept reasonably calm during immobilization. Excited or stressed deer tend to be less affected by the sedative actions of α_2-adrenergic agonists and often require higher dosages. Common complications include trauma, hyperthermia, and capture myopathy. Ruminal tympany is not commonly encountered during anesthesia of these species. Hypoxemia is not uncommon with narcotic-based or α_2-adrenergic agonist–based protocols, and supplemental inspired oxygen should be considered.[8]

A variety of techniques have been used to induce immobilization. White-tailed deer can be anesthetized with 2.2 mg/kg of xylazine combined with 4.4 mg/kg of Telazol.[40,59] This combination is equally effective on mule deer, and immobilization can be partially antagonized with 0.1 to 0.2 mg/kg of yohimbine. A dosage of 0.1 mg/kg of medetomidine combined with 2.5 mg/kg of ketamine will produce a good quality of immobilization in mule deer and white-tailed deer.[8] Atipamezole administered at three to five times the medetomidine dose will effectively antagonize immobilization.

North American Elk (*Red Deer*, Cervus elaphus)
Elk or red deer may be captured via physical or chemical means. If physical capture (net gunning) is used, sedation can be quickly induced with intranasal xylazine.[13] Mature elk weigh approximately 230 to 318 kg, and red deer weigh 60 to 180 kg.[1] Chemical immobilization can be induced with narcotics or

α_2-adrenergic agonists combined with dissociatives. Complications are similar to those expected with other deer species. Elk should be monitored for ruminal tympany and hyperthermia. Hypoxemia is common in anesthetized elk, especially during immobilization with xylazine-carfentanil or xylazine-Telazol.[4,6] Hypoxemia can be effectively treated by partial antagonism of drugs or by administration of supplemental oxygen.

Elk can be immobilized with 10 µg/kg of carfentanil combined with 0.1 mg/kg of xylazine.[1,4] Immobilization can be antagonized with naltrexone. Alternatively, a mixture of 0.4 mg/kg of xylazine and 3 mg/kg of Telazol is also effective.[41,60] Immobilization with this combination can be partially antagonized with 0.125 mg/kg of yohimbine.

Red deer are smaller than elk, but the considerations for immobilization are similar. The drugs of choice for red deer capture are 0.11 mg/kg of medetomidine with 2.2 mg/kg of ketamine.[61] In this combination, medetomidine should be antagonized with 0.5 mg/kg of atipamezole. An alternative drug combination is 2.5 mg/kg of xylazine with 2.5 mg/kg of Telazol.[1] However, because of the long elimination time of Telazol, recoveries can be prolonged.

Moose (Alces alces)

Moose are the largest member of the deer family, with adult males averaging 500 kg.[1] They are found in the northern latitudes of Europe, Russia, and North America. Moose in the far northern latitudes of these regions may reach a much larger body mass (up to 800 kg). Their large size necessitates the use of potent drug combinations to maintain a low drug volume. The use of carfentanil-xylazine has been recommended as in other deer species.[62] The addition of xylazine to carfentanil decreases the incidence of muscle rigidity, but also increases the risk of regurgitation and aspiration pneumonia.[21] For this reason, if carfentanil is used in moose, it should be administered as the sole agent at a dose of 10 µg/kg. In addition to the risk of regurgitation, moose are at risk for hyperthermia and capture myopathy.

In Europe, moose have been effectively immobilized with 60 µg/kg of medetomidine combined with 1.5 mg/kg of ketamine.[34,63] Immobilization can be antagonized with 0.3 mg/kg of atipamezole. Currently, the drug of choice for free-ranging moose is etorphine alone at a dose of 7.5 mg per adult and half this dose in calves.[64] Xylazine (1.5 mg/kg)-Telazol (3 mg/kg) has been used in management situations. Immobilization with this combination can be partially antagonized with yohimbine or tolazoline.

Fallow Deer (Dama dama)

A variety of techniques have been used to anesthetize fallow deer, often with unreliable effects. Adult fallow deer weigh approximately 40 to 100 kg.[1] Currently, the recommended drug combination for fallow deer is 0.1 mg/kg of medetomidine with 1.0 mg/kg of Telazol.[65]

American Bison (Bison bison) and European Bison (Bison bonasus)

Bison range in size from 350 to 1000 kg, with the largest subspecies being the wood bison (Bison bison athebascae) found in northern Canada.[1] The large size of these animals dictates that potent, concentrated drugs be used to facilitate delivery of the smallest drug volume possible. Bison are prone to bloat and regurgitation. Fasting can decrease the risk of these complications, but obviously this is not possible in free-ranging animals. Hypoxemia is another major complication,[7] but can generally be managed with supplemental oxygen. A dosage of 5 µg/kg of carfentanil combined with 0.07 mg/kg of xylazine can be used to immobilize North American and European bison.[23,66] Naltrexone should be used to antagonize carfentanil in bison, because renarcotization has been encountered with naloxone.[23,66] Alternatively, 0.06 mg/kg of medetomidine combined with 1.2 mg/kg of Telazol, or 3 mg/kg of Telazol combined with 1.5 mg/kg of xylazine can be used to anesthetize bison.[7] Xylazine-Telazol is best reserved for small, calm animals because the volume can become too large. Ketamine (2.5 mg/kg) combined with 0.08 mg/kg of medetomidine has been used effectively in European bison.[34]

Caribou (Reindeer, Rangifer tarandus)

Caribou can be very difficult to immobilize and often have higher drug dose requirements compared with related species.[67] Their speed and agility make them a difficult target for remote drug delivery. Rangifer species range in size from 80 to 300 kg, with woodland caribou being the largest subspecies.[1] The drug combination of choice for reindeer and caribou is 0.1 mg/kg of medetomidine with 2.5 mg/kg of ketamine.[34] These doses are not effective in free-ranging woodland caribou. In these animals, 0.2 to 0.25 mg of medetomidine with ketamine is recommended.[68]

Pronghorn Antelope (Antilocapra americana)

Pronghorn antelope can be extremely difficult to immobilize. They often have very high drug dose requirements, and immobilization is often unreliable with α_2-adrenergic agonist or dissociative-based protocols. Hyperthermia is a common complication.

Pronghorn antelope usually weigh 40 to 50 kg.[1] The current combination of choice is 0.05 mg/kg of carfentanil combined with 1.0 mg/kg of xylazine.[69] Although not yet available, thiafentanil alone and thiafentanil-xylazine have proven to be superior to other drug combinations for pronghorn antelope capture.[33]

Baird's Tapir (Tapir bairdii)

This is one of three New World tapir species. Adult animals, which weigh 200 to 300 kg,[1] have been effectively anesthetized with a total dose of 2 mg of etorphine in combination with 8 mg of acepromazine.[70] This combination often results in hypoxemia and, since the animals are often captured at night, an increased human safety risk is associated with the use of potent narcotics.[70] An alternative technique is to use 0.2 mg/kg of butorphanol combined with 0.4 mg/kg of xylazine. This technique is effective in calm animals and will induce approximately 30 min of recumbency.[71] Immobilization can be prolonged with 1 mg/kg of ketamine given intravenously. The mixture can be antagonized with 0.2 mg/kg of naltrexone plus 0.125 mg/kg of yohimbine.

Brown Bear (Ursus arctos)

Brown bears range across parts of North America, Europe, and Asia. Adult bears generally weigh between 100 and 325 kg.[1] Most brown bears are captured in spring or early summer. Body weights are 80 to 100 kg for adult females and 140 to 240 kg for adult males. In the autumn, body weights increase by up to 40% as animals prepare for hibernation.

A variety of techniques can be used to immobilize brown bears. Telazol is routinely used for management of brown bears in North America. Reversible combinations are desirable in certain situations, particularly in free-ranging sows with cubs. Telazol (or Zoletil), 7 to 9 mg/kg, will produce reliable immobilization, but can also result in prolonged recoveries.[72] Injection volume requirements are high, necessitating the use of large darts that can produce excessive tissue trauma. Xylazine (2 mg/kg) combined with Telazol (3 mg/kg) is effective. This combination is partially reversible with yohimbine or atipamezole, but some residual sedation will probably remain. Animals immobilized with this mixture will benefit from supplemental inspired oxygen, since hypoxemia is common.[38] Medetomidine (M) combined with Telazol (TZ) will produce reliable immobilization. This combination has been used effectively on European brown bears. These are the standard doses used for fieldwork (spring and early summer) on Scandinavian brown bears: yearlings (15 to 45 kg), 1.25 mg M + 62.5 mg TZ; small bears (2 to 3 years, 45 to 70 kg), 2.5 mg M + 125 mg TZ; adult females and small males (70 to 120 kg), 5 mg M + 250 mg TZ; adult males (120 to 200 kg), 10 mg M + 500 mg TZ; and large males (>200 kg), 15 mg M + 750 mg TZ. The M-TZ ratio is kept constant so that doses can be split or combined. For reversal, atipamezole at 5.0 mg per 1.0 mg of medetomidine is given intramuscularly.[73]

Polar Bear (Ursus maratimus)

Polar bears can have substantial body-fat deposits throughout the year. The shoulder and neck are the best sites for drug delivery. Male polar bears can be large and heavy. Body weights greater than 500 kg are not uncommon. To keep drug volume and dart size to a minimum, concentrated drug combinations are required. Once anesthesia is induced, the bears should be positioned carefully to avoid compartment syndrome caused by excessive pressure on the limbs. Polar bears enter a hypometabolic state during the summer. At that time of the year, the bears are fasting and body temperature is decreased (34° to 35°C), so immobilizing drug requirements may also be decreased. In areas where large numbers of polar bears congregate, reversible anesthetic protocols should be considered. This decreases the risk of predation from other bears. Reversible protocols should also be considered for mother bears with cubs. One drug choice is 8 to 10 mg/kg of Telazol,[74] which produces reliable immobilization, but can also lead to prolonged recoveries. Volume requirements are high, which can produce excessive tissue trauma and necessitate the use of large darts. Xylazine (2 mg/kg)-Telazol (3 mg/kg) will also induce effective immobilization.[37] This mixture, which can be delivered at approximately half the volume of Telazol alone, is potentially reversible with yohimbine or atipamezole. However, reversal of this mixture is not reliable, probably be-

cause of residual Telazol sedation. Animals immobilized with this mixture will benefit from supplemental inspired oxygen. Medetomidine (75 µg/kg)-Telazol (2.2 mg/kg) is very effective in polar bears. This combination produces reliable immobilization with a rapid onset,[35,36] can be delivered in a small volume, and is readily reversible with atipamezole (administered at four times the medetomidine dose).

Black Bear (Ursus americanus)

Black bear females weigh 92 to 140 kg, and males weigh approximately 115 to 270 kg.[1] Generally, these bears have a more placid nature than brown bears, and Telazol dose requirements are lower. The bear may be snared or captured in a culvert trap prior to drug administration. Physical capture of the bear will facilitate drug administration and limit mobility on anesthesia induction. One drug choice is 4 to 6 mg/kg of Telazol, which produces reliable immobilization and can be delivered at a relatively low volume in most bears.[75] Xylazine-Telazol is also effective in black bears at the same dose described for brown and polar bears (2 mg/kg of xylazine with 3 mg/kg of Telazol).[76] This dose could possibly be lowered, but further work is needed to determine the optimal dose for this species. Medetomidine (52 µg/kg)-Telazol (1.7 mg/kg) is also effective.[42] This combination produces a rapid onset of immobilization and can be delivered in a small volume. It is readily reversible with atipamezole administered at four times the medetomidine dose.

Lynx (Felis lynx and Lynx canadensis)

European and North American lynx can be treated in a similar manner. Female European lynx weigh 16 to 18 kg, and males weigh 21 to 23 kg. North American lynx weigh 5.1 to 17.2 kg.[1] Lynx are often captured by physical means prior to immobilization. Medetomidine (0.2 mg/kg)-ketamine (5 mg/kg) is considered the drug combination of choice in European lynx.[34,77] This dose can be reduced by 50% in captive lynx.[77] Telazol is an alternative mixture that can be administered to lynx at 5 mg/kg.[78]

Mountain Lion (Felis concolor)

Mountain lions are commonly anesthetized for translocation by wildlife managers. It is common to tree mountain lions prior to dart placement. Hounds can be effectively trained to pursue and tree them. The current drug combination of choice for mountain lion capture is 2 mg/kg of ketamine combined with 75 µg/kg of medetomidine.[79] This mixture is readily reversible with atipamezole. Telazol has been used alone at a dose of 8 mg/kg; however, recoveries can be prolonged.[39] Xylazine-Telazol has been effectively used by wildlife managers. Initial results suggest that a dose of 2 mg/kg of xylazine combined with 3 mg/kg of Telazol will anesthetize mountain lions effectively.

Jaguar (Panthera onca)

The jaguar is the largest New World felid, weighing 64 to 114 kg. Jaguars may be baited or captured by physical means prior to immobilization. Telazol has been described for immobilization of jaguars at a recommended dose of 4 to 8 mg/kg.[39,80] This dose can be supplemented with 1 to 2 mg/kg of ketamine, as needed.

The use of medetomidine (70 µg/kg)-ketamine (2.5 mg/kg) has also been described in captive animals.[34]

Wolverine (Gulo gulo)

Wolverines are found in the northern latitudes of Europe, Russia, and North America. Males are typically 50% heavier than females, and normal body weight ranges are 9 to 11 kg in adult females and 14 to 16 kg in adult males. Wolverines can be immobilized from a helicopter or in the den. Standard doses for capture are 3 mg of medetomidine combined with 75 mg of ketamine for adult females and 4 mg of medetomidine and 100 mg of ketamine for adult males. Inductions are rapid, and there are no major clinical side effects. Effective reversals are achieved with 5 mg of atipamezole per 1 mg of medetomidine. Alternatively, 175 mg of Telazol can be used to immobilize adult wolverines.[81]

Gray Wolf (Canis lupus)

Gray wolves are widely distributed throughout the northern hemisphere. Males typically weigh 25% more than females. Average body weights in Scandinavian gray wolves are 40 kg for adult females and 50 kg for adult males. Occasionally, adult males will be much heavier (especially in North America). Gray wolves are immobilized from a helicopter or after being captured in a snare or a leg-hold trap. The drug of choice is Telazol. A standard dose of 500 mg can be used for all animals weighing more than 25 kg. Anesthesia inductions are rapid, but recoveries are prolonged and may take 4 to 6 h. Medetomidine-ketamine should be used with care for immobilization of wolves from a helicopter because some animals tend to develop severe hyperthermia (41° to 42°C) with this combination.[82]

Wild Boar (Sus scroffa)

Eurasian wild pigs or wild boars are indigenous to Europe, Asia, and North Africa, and have been introduced into North America, Australia, and New Zealand. Wild boars are captured in traps and immobilized from a short distance with a tranquilizing pistol or blowgun. For brief procedures, 0.1 mg/kg of medetomidine with 0.2 mg/kg of butorphanol and 5 mg/kg of ketamine have been recommended.[83] Effective reversal is achieved by using 5 mg of atipamezole per 1 mg of medetomidine. Combinations of medetomidine-butorphanol-Telazol can also be used to anesthetize wild boars, but recoveries are more prolonged.[84]

African and Asian Species

Tiger (Panthera tigris)

Eight different subspecies of tiger have been recognized, although some may only represent morphological variations. Small populations of tigers are found in India, Southeast Asia, and southeast Russia. Tigers usually weigh 100 to 160 kg (adult females) or 180 to 260 kg (adult males).[85] Commonly, 70 µg/kg of medetomidine combined with 3 mg/kg of ketamine is used.[1] Effective reversal is achieved with 5 mg of atipamezole per 1 mg of medetomidine. An alternative drug combination is 0.8 mg/kg of xylazine combined with 11 mg/kg of ketamine.[86,87] Xylazine can be antagonized with 0.125 mg/kg of yohimbine, but because of the high dose of ketamine, reversals are not as effective as with medetomidine-ketamine. Telazol has caused several adverse reactions in tigers and should be used with caution and only when other drugs are unavailable.[1,88]

Lion (Panthera leo)

Five subspecies of lion are recognized. Lions are found on the African continent from South Sahara to South Africa. A remnant population exists in India. Body weights range from 120 to 180 kg in adult females to 150 to 240 kg in adult males.[85] There are two excellent drug combinations for immobilization and anesthesia of lions. For brief procedures, 70 µg/kg of medetomidine combined with 2.5 mg/kg of ketamine can be used.[1] Inductions are rapid, and analgesia and muscle relaxation are good. Due to the low dose of ketamine, animals may demonstrate sudden unexpected recoveries and should be closely monitored.[89] Immobilization can be prolonged by administration of additional ketamine at 1.5 mg/kg.[1] Telazol alone at a dose of 4 to 5 mg/kg can be used, but recoveries usually take several hours.[1,90] Low-dose Telazol (0.8 mg/kg) in combination with medetomidine (50 µg/kg) has also been successfully used for capture of lions.[91] Inductions are smooth, immobilization complete, muscle relaxation good, analgesia adequate for minor procedures, and the anesthetic actions last approximately 1½ h. Atipamezole can be used to reverse the effects of medetomidine, and it is recommended that 5 mg of atipamezole per 1 mg of medetomidine be administered to ensure that sedation does not recur.[1]

Leopard (Panthera pardus)

Seven subspecies are currently recognized. Leopards are found in Africa south of the Sahara and in South Asia. Scattered populations are in North Africa, Arabia, and the Far East. Leopards weigh 30 to 70 kg. Males are typically 50% heavier than females.[85] Medetomidine (70 µg/kg)-ketamine (3 mg/kg) is usually sufficient and the combination most commonly used.[1] However, higher doses (0.1 and 5 mg/kg, respectively) of these two drugs may be needed to achieve complete anesthesia in cage-trapped leopards. Atipamezole, at 5 mg per 1 mg of medetomidine, can be used for reversal of immobilization.[1] Telazol alone at 5 to 8 mg/kg, or xylazine at 1 mg/kg in combination with ketamine at 8 to 11 mg/kg, can also be used to immobilize leopards.[1]

Cheetah (Acinonyx jubatus)

Two subspecies of cheetah are recognized: the African cheetah and the Asian cheetah (nearly extinct). Cheetahs weigh 39 to 65 kg. Males are typically 15% heavier than females.[85] Recommended drugs for immobilization are medetomidine at 70 µg/kg combined with ketamine at 3 mg/kg.[1] If necessary, additional ketamine (2 mg/kg) can be given. For reversal, 5 mg of atipamezole per 1 mg of medetomidine can be administered. Another combination for reversible anesthesia is 50 µg/kg of medetomidine and 1.5 mg/kg of Telazol. These doses have been used on free-ranging African leopards and were modified from a study on zoo animals.[92] Atipamezole at 5 mg per 1 mg of medetomidine is effective for anesthesia reversal in captive leopards, but sedation, lasting up to 4 h, can persist in some captive animals. This raises concerns about the use of this combination in free-ranging animals that must be released shortly after the anesthetic event.[92] Alternative combinations include 3 mg/kg of Telazol alone or 0.5 mg/kg of xylazine with 6 to 8 mg/kg of ketamine.

Plains Zebra (Equus burchelli)

Zebras are indigenous only to Africa. The plains or common zebra is distributed widely in eastern and southern Africa, with more than half a million animals in the Serengeti–Masai Mara ecosystem of Tanzania and Kenya. Three subspecies are recognized. Plains zebras weigh 200 to 340 kg.[85] Two other zebra species, mountain zebras (Equus zebra) and Grevy's zebras (Equus grevyi), are endangered and are restricted to small populations on the continent. Most recommended drug combinations for immobilization of zebras involve the use of etorphine.[1,93,94] In free-ranging plains zebra etorphine (4 to 7 mg for males and 3 to 4 mg for females) combined with either azaperone (40 to 60 mg), xylazine (40 to 60 mg), acepromazine (30 mg), or detomidine (5 to 10 mg) will induce recumbency. Immobilization is often not complete, and blindfolding is recommended. Complete muscle relaxation is difficult to obtain, and paddling, shivering, and sweating are often seen. Respiratory depression is a common side effect in zebras during chemical immobilization. Hyperthermia is another major complication, particularly if induction is prolonged. Hemoglobin saturation and rectal temperature should be closely monitored. Supplemental oxygen, equipment for intubation and ventilation, and water for cooling should be available, as well as emergency drugs (e.g., respiratory stimulants and benzodiazepines in case of convulsions). Upon induction, zebras can be positioned either in sternal or lateral recumbency. Recently, a comparison of three combinations was carried out:[95]

1. 6 mg of etorphine with 80 mg of azaperone for males, and 4 mg of etorphine with 80 mg of azaperone for females
2. 5 mg of etorphine with 5 mg of medetomidine for males and females
3. 3 mg of etorphine with 150 mg of ketamine and 10 mg of detomidine for males and females

All combinations induced complete immobilization with lateral recumbency; however, hypoxemia ($SpO_2 < 85\%$) occurred in most animals. Rapid reversal was achieved with standard doses of antagonist drugs (e.g., diprenorphine and atipamezole).[1] Preliminary results indicate that etorphine-ketamine-detomidine is superior to the other two combinations. Zebra skin is thin, and lightweight darts with low impact energy should be used to avoid penetration wounds. Dart wounds often bleed profusely, and prophylactic antibiotic treatment is recommended.

African Buffalo (Syncerus caffer)

The African buffalo is indigenous to Africa south of the Sahara. Two subspecies are recognized, Cape buffalo and forest buffalo, with intermediate forms. Large males weigh up to 800 kg and females up to 750 kg.[85] Recommended drugs are 8 to 10 mg of etorphine combined with 150 to 200 mg of azaperone for adult bulls and 6 to 8 mg of etorphine combined with 150 mg of azaperone for adult cows.[94] Diprenorphine at 2.4 mg per 1 mg of etorphine is used for reversal.[94] Etorphine (at the same doses for

males and females) can also be combined with xylazine (70 to 80 mg for bulls and 40 to 60 mg for cows). A standard dose of yohimbine is used for reversal of xylazine effects.[1]

African Elephant (Loxodonta africana)

African elephants are found south of the Sahara. Two subspecies are recognized: savannah elephant and forest elephant (some authorities classify them as different species). Savannah elephants may reach 4000 to 6500 kg, and forest elephants are significantly smaller.[85] Females are usually two-thirds of male weight within a given geographical area. Etorphine at 8 to 12 mg is the drug of choice for adult African elephants.[94] Azaperone at 70 to 100 mg can be added in the dart, but may prolong recovery, and animals may struggle to rise following reversal. The recommended dose is 14 to 20 mg of etorphine for bulls and 10 to 15 mg for cows. Hyaluronidase at 1000 to 3000 IU has been added in the dart to hasten induction. Preferred darting sites are the rump or shoulders; areas near the ears and trunk should be avoided. Elephants are large and difficult to handle. To avoid respiratory compromise, they should not be allowed to remain in sternal recumbency following induction.[1,94] Breathing through the trunk must be unimpaired, and dart wounds should be flushed with an antimicrobial solution to prevent abscessation. Diprenorphine at 3 to 4 mg per 1 mg of etorphine given intravenously is commonly used to reverse etorphine immobilization.

Giraffe (Giraffa camelopardalis)

Giraffes are found in Africa south of the Sahara. Nine subspecies are recognized. Males and females may reach a height of 4.9 to 5.2 and 4.3 to 4.6 m, respectively, and weigh up to 1800 and 1180 kg, respectively.[85] The current capture philosophy for giraffes is to administer a high dose of immobilizing drug to facilitate induction in the shortest possible time and then quickly antagonize the drugs after physical restraint has been achieved.[1,94] Immobilization of giraffes should not be attempted without prior consultation with an experienced handler. Blood pressure must be maintained in a normal range to supply blood to the brain. The head should be held at all times, from initial recumbency to the point where it is starting to recover.[1,94] Etorphine-azaperone is the recommended drug combination for giraffe anesthesia.[94] Doses are 10 to 12 mg of etorphine and 40 to 60 mg of azaperone for adult bulls and 8 to 10 mg of etorphine and 40 mg of azaperone for adult cows. Hyaluronidase (2000 IU) has been added in the dart to hasten induction. Reversal is achieved by administration of diprenorphine at 2.4 mg per 1 mg of etorphine. Preliminary trials indicate that thiafentanil (15 to 18 mg for bulls and 10 to 14 mg for cows) may be superior to etorphine in giraffes, with induction times as quick as 3 min. A medetomidine-ketamine regimen with doses based on shoulder height, followed by atipamezole, has been used for reversible immobilization of free-ranging giraffes.[96] However, the results of trials in the Kruger National Park have been inconclusive regarding the efficacy of this combination, which is currently under continued evaluation.[94]

White Rhinoceros (Ceratoterium simium)

The white rhinoceros is endangered and is found in scattered populations in South and Northeast Africa. Males weigh 2200 kg and females 1600 kg.[94] The recommended drug combination is etorphine combined with detomidine, xylazine, or azaperone. Dose recommendations vary between researchers and areas. Etorphine at 3 to 4 mg and detomidine at 10 to 20 mg for adults seem to be superior to other combinations.[1,94] Hyaluronidase at 2000 IU should be added to the drug mixture to shorten induction. White rhinoceroses are prone to significant respiratory depression following etorphine administration, so close monitoring is necessary. The standard protocol in Africa is to administer 10 to 15 mg of nalorphine intravenously immediately to all immobilized animals. Respiration can also be improved by intravenous administration of 300 to 400 mg of doxapram. Reversal is achieved by 75 to 150 mg of naltrexone, with one-third of the dose given intramuscularly and two-thirds intravenously.[1,94] Detomidine and xylazine can be reversed by standard doses of yohimbine or atipamezole.

Black Rhinoceros (Diceros bicornis)

The black rhinoceros is also critically endangered and is found in tiny, isolated populations in Africa from the Cape to Kenya. Males weigh 850 to 1000 kg, and females average 880 kg.[94] The recommended drug combination for immobilization is etorphine (2 to 4 mg) combined with either azaperone (50 to 150 mg), detomidine (10 to 15 mg), or xylazine (60 to 100 mg).[94] Black rhinoceros are less sensitive to the effects of etorphine than are white rhinoceroses, and the highest safe dose should be used to produce shorter induction times, especially in rough terrain.[94] Hyaluronidase, at 2000 IU, should be added in the dart to hasten induction. Although hypoxia does not appear to be a problem in the majority of black rhinoceros, they should be monitored for signs of respiratory depression.[1,94] Sternal recumbency is preferred, but the animals can be kept in lateral recumbency, if necessary. Body position should be changed every 30 min to avoid ischemia of dependent tissues. Naltrexone at 75 to 150 mg or diprenorphine at 2.4 mg per 1 mg of etorphine can be used for reversal. Reversal may rapidly arouse potentially aggressive animals. When used, detomidine and xylazine can be reversed by standard doses of either yohimbine or atipamezole.

African Wild Dog (Lycaon pictus)

The African wild or hunting dog is an endangered species found in fragmented populations in Southern and East Africa. Males and females are of similar size and weigh 20 to 32 kg.[85] Recommended drugs are medetomidine at 100 μg/kg and ketamine at 5 mg/kg, followed by atipamezole at 5 mg per 1 mg of medetomidine for reversal.[94] Fentanyl-xylazine has also been recommended in African wild dogs.[90] Severe hypoxia may develop, so the dogs should be closely monitored. For reversal, naltrexone is superior to naloxone. Xylazine effects can be antagonized with either atipamezole or yohimbine.[94]

Spotted Hyena (Crocuta crocuta)

There are four species in the hyena family: spotted hyena, striped hyena, brown hyena, and aardwolf. The best known of the hyenas is the spotted hyena, which is distributed in Sub-Saharan Africa except the Congo rain forest and the far south. Males

weigh 45 to 60 kg and females 55 to 82 kg. Telazol at 5 mg/kg has been recommended for immobilization.[1,92] However, recent experiences show that 8 to 12 mg/kg of ketamine combined with 0.5 to 1.0 mg/kg of xylazine or 100 μg/kg of medetomidine combined with 5 mg/kg of ketamine is superior to Telazol alone. These combinations produce a smoother anesthesia with less salivation and excitement (Dr. Markus Hofmeyr, personal communication). Atipamezole can be used to antagonize medetomidine effects, whereas yohimbine or atipamezole are equally effective for xylazine reversal.

References

1. Kreeger TJ, Arnemo JM, Raath JP. Handbook of Wildlife Chemical Immobilization. Fort Collins, CO: Wildlife Pharmaceuticals, 2002.
2. Klein LV, Klide AM. Central α_2 adrenergic and benzodiazepine agonists and their antagonists. J Zoo Wildl Med 20:138–153, 1989.
3. Cattet MRL, Caulkett NA, Stenhouse GB. Anesthesia of grizzly bears using xylazine-zolazepam-tiletamine or zolazepam-tiletamine. Ursus 14:88–93, 2003.
4. Moresco AM, Larsen RS, Sleeman JM, Wild MA, Gaynor JS. Use of naloxone to reverse carfentanil citrate–induced hypoxemia and cardiopulmonary depression in Rocky Mountain wapiti (Cervus elaphus nelsoni). Zoo Wildl Med 32:81–89, 2001.
5. Citino SB, Bush M, Grobler D, Lance W. Anaesthesia of roan antelope (Hippotragus equinus) with a combination of A3080, medetomidine and ketamine. J S Afr Vet Assoc 72:29–32, 2001.
6. Read MR, Caulkett NA, Symington A, Shury TK. Treatment of hypoxemia during xylazine-tiletamine-zolazepam immobilization of wapiti. Can Vet J 42:661–664, 2001.
7. Caulkett NA, Cattet MRL, Cantwell S, Cool N, Olse W. Anesthesia of wood bison with medetomidine-Telazol and xylazine-Telazol combinations. Can Vet J 41:49–53, 2000.
8. Caulkett NA, Cribb PH, Haigh JC. Comparative cardiopulmonary effects of carfentanil-xylazine and medetomidine-ketamine in mule deer and mule deer/white-tailed deer hybrids. Can J Vet Res 64:64–68, 2000.
9. Read MR. A review of alpha2 adrenoceptor agonists and the development of hypoxemia in domestic and wild ruminants. J. Zoo Wildl Med 34:134–138, 2003.
10. Heard DJ, Olsen JH, Stover JS. Cardiopulmonary changes associated with chemical immobilization and recumbency in white rhinoceros (Ceratotherium simum). J Zoo Wildl Med 23:197–200, 1992.
11. Kock MD, Jessup A, Clark RK, Franti CE. Effects of capture on biological parameters in free-ranging bighorn sheep (Ovis canadensis): Evaluation of drop-net, drive-net, chemical immobilization and the net gun. J Wildl Dis 23:641–651, 1987.
12. Kock MD, Jessup A, Clark RK, Franti CE, Weaver RA. Capture methods in five subspecies of free-ranging bighorn sheep: An evaluation of drop-net, drive-net, chemical immobilization, and the net gun. J Wildl Dis 23:634–640, 1987.
13. Cattet MRL, Caulkett NA, Wilson C, Vandenbrink T, Brook RK. Intranasal administration of xylazine to reduce stress in elk captured by net gun. J Wildl Dis 40:562–565, 2004.
14. Jessup DA, Clark RK, Weaver RA, Kock MD. The safety and cost-effectiveness of net-gun capture of desert bighorn sheep (Ovis canadensis nelsoni). J Zoo Anim Med 19:208–213, 1988.
15. Cattet MRL, Christison K, Caulkett NA, Stenhouse GB. Physiologic responses of grizzly bears to different methods of capture. J Wildl Dis 39:649–654, 2003.

16. Wax PM, Becker CE, Curry CS. Unexpected gas casualties in Moscow: A medical toxicology perspective. Ann Emerg Med 41:700–705.

17. Belleville JP, Ward DS, Bloor BC, Maze M. Effects of intravenous dexmedetomidine in humans. I. Sedation, ventilation, and metabolic rate. Anesthesiology 77:1125–1133, 1992.

18. Kallio A, Ponkilainen R, Scheinin H. Effects of dexmedetomidine, a selective alpha 2-adrenoceptor agonist on hemodynamic control mechanisms. Clin Pharmacol Ther 46:33–42, 1989.

19. Bush M. Remote drug delivery systems. J Zoo Wildl Med 23:159–180, 1992.

20. Haigh JC. Opioids in zoological medicine. J Zoo Wildl Med 21:391–413, 1990.

21. Kreeger TJ. 2000. Xylazine-induced aspiration pneumonia in Shira's moose. Wildl Soc Bull 28:751–753.

22. Allen JL. Renarcotization following carfentanil immobilization of nondomestic ungulates. J Zoo Wildl Med 20:423–426, 1989.

23. Kock MD, Berger J. Chemical immobilization of free-ranging North American bison in Badlands National Park, South Dakota. J Wildl Dis 23:625–633, 1987.

24. Anonymous. Veterinary surgeon's Immobilon death "accidental." Vet Rec 98:144, 1976.

25. Parker J, Haigh JC. Human exposure to immobilizing agents. In: Nielsen L, Haigh JC, Fowler ME, eds. Chemical Immobilization of North American Wildlife. Milwaukee: Wisconsin Humane Society, 1983:119–136.

26. Haigh JC, Lee LJ, Schweinsburg RE. Immobilization of polar bears with carfentanil. J Wildl Dis 19:140–144, 1983.

27. Mama KR, Steffey EP, Withrow SJ. Use of orally administered carfentanil prior to isoflurane-induced anesthesia in a Kodiak brown bear. J Am Vet Med Assoc 217:546–549, 2000.

28. Ramsay EC, Sleeman JM, Clyde VL. Immobilization of black bears (Ursus americanus) with orally administered carfentanil citrate. J Wildl Dis 31:391–393, 1995.

29. Schumacher J, Citino, SB, Dawson R. Effects of a carfentanil-xylazine combination on cardiopulmonary function and plasma catecholamine concentrations in female bongo antelopes. Am J Vet Res 58:157–161, 1997.

30. Stanley TH, McJames SW, Kimball J, Port JD, Pace NL. Immobilization of elk with A-3080. J Wildl Manage 52:577–581, 1988.

31. Jansen DL, Rath JP, de Vos V, Anderson JM. Immobilization and physiological effects of the narcotic A-3080 in impala (Aepyceros melampus). J Zoo Wildl Med 24:11–18, 1993.

32. Grobler D, Bush M, Jessup D, Lance W. Anaesthesia of gemsbok (Oryx gazelle) with a combination of A3080, medetomidine and ketamine. J S Afr Vet Assoc 72:81–83, 2001.

33. Kreeger TJ, Cook WE, Piche CA, Smith T. Anesthesia of pronghorns using thiafentanil or thiafentanil plus xylazine. J Wildl Manage 65:25–28, 2001.

34. Jalanka HH, Roeken BO. The use of medetomidine, medetomidine-ketamine combinations, and atipamezole in nondomestic mammals: A review. J Zoo Wildl Med 21:259–282, 1990.

35. Cattet MRL, Caulkett NA, Polischuk SC, Ramsay MA. Anesthesia of polar bears with zolazepam-tiletamine, medetomidine-ketamine, and medetomidine-zolazepam-tiletamine. J Zoo Wildl Med 30:354–360, 1999.

36. Caulkett NA, Cattet MRL, Caulkett JM, Polischuk SC. Comparative physiological effects of Telazol, medetomidine-ketamine, and medetomidine-Telazol in polar bears (Ursus maritimus). J Zoo Wildl Med 30:504–509, 1999.

37. Cattet MRL, Caulkett NA, Lunn NJ. Anesthesia of polar bears using xylazine-zolazepam-tiletamine or zolazepam-tiletamine. J Wildl Dis 39:655–664, 2003.

38. Cattet MRL, Caulkett NA, Stenhouse GB. Anesthesia of grizzly bears using xylazine-zolazepam-tiletamine or zolazepam-tiletamine. Ursus 14:88–93, 2003.

39. Schobert E. Telazol use in wild and exotic animals. Vet Med 82:1080–1088, 1987.

40. Murray SSL, Monfort SL, Ware L, McShea WJ, Bush M. Anesthesia in female white-tailed deer using Telazol and xylazine. J Wildl Dis 36:670–675, 2000.

41. Millspaugh JJ, Brundige GC, Jenks JA, Tyner CL, Hustead DR. Immobilization of rocky mountain elk with Telazol and xylazine hydrochloride, and antagonism by yohimbine hydrochloride. J Wildl Dis 31:259–262, 1995.

42. Caulkett NA, Cattet MRL. Physiological effects of medetomidine-zolazepam-tiletamine immobilization in black bears (Ursus americanus). J Wildl Dis 33:618–622, 1997.

43. Kock MD, Morkel P, Atkinson M, Foggin C. Chemical immobilization of free-ranging white rhinoceros (Ceratotherium simum simum) in Hwange and Matobo National Parks, Zimbabwe, using combinations of etorphine (M99), fentanyl, xylazine and detomidine. J Zoo Wildl Med 26:207–219, 1995.

44. Klein L, Citino SB. Comparison of detomidine/carfentanil/ketamine and medetomidine/ketamine anesthesia in Grevy's zebra. In: Proceedings, Joint Conference of the American Association of Zoo Veterinarians, Wildlife Disease Association, and American Association of Wildlife Veterinarians, East Lansing, Michigan, 1995:290–293.

45. Caulkett NA, Duke T, Cribb PH. Cardiopulmonary effects of medetomidine-ketamine in domestic sheep (Ovis ovis) maintained in sternal recumbency. J Zoo Wildl Med 27:217–226, 1996.

46. Ebedes H. The use of long-acting tranquilizers in captive wild animals. In: McKenzie A, ed. The Capture and Care Manual: Capture, Care, Accommodation and Transportation of Wild African Animals. Pretoria: Wildlife Decision Services and the South African Veterinary Foundation, 1993:71–99.

47. Diverio S, Goddard PJ, Gordon IJ, Elston DA. The effect of management practices on stress in farmed red deer (Cervus elaphus) and its modulation by long-acting neuroleptics: Behavioural responses. Appl Anim Behav Sci 36:363–376, 1993.

48. Atkinson MW, Blumer ES. The use of a long-acting neuroleptic in the Mongolian wild horse (Equus przewalskii przewalskii) to facilitate the establishment of a bachelor herd. In: Proceedings of the Annual Meeting of the American Association of Zoo Veterinarians, Houston, Texas, 1997:199–200.

49. Shury TK. Use of azaperone with zuclopenthixol acetate for tranquilization of free ranging wood bison and immobilization with carfentanil and xylazine. In: Proceedings of the Annual Meeting of the American Association of Zoo Veterinarians, Omaha, Nebraska, 1998:408–409.

50. Clippinger TL, Citino SB, Wade S. Behavioral and physiologic response to an intermediate-acting tranquilizer, zuclopenthixol, in captive Nile lechwe (Kobus megaceros). In: Proceedings of the Annual Meeting of the American Association of Zoo Veterinarians, Omaha, Nebraska, 1998:38–40.

51. Read M, Caulkett N, McCallister M. Evaluation of zuclopenthixol acetate to decrease handling stress in wapiti. J Wildl Dis 36:450–459, 2000.

52. Cattet MRL, Caulkett NA, Streib KA, Torske KE, Ramsay MA. Cardiopulmonary response of anesthetized polar bears to suspension by net and sling. J Wildl Dis 35:548–556, 1999.

53. Jessup DA. The use of the helicopter in the capture of free roaming wildlife. In: Nielsen L, Haigh JC, Fowler ME, eds. Chemical Immobilization of North American Wildlife. Milwaukee: Wisconsin Humane Society, 1982:289–303.

54. Harthoorn AM. Physical aspects of both mechanical and chemical capture. In: Nielsen L, Haigh JC, Fowler ME, eds. Chemical Immobilization of North American Wildlife. Milwaukee: Wisconsin Humane Society, 1982:63–71.

55. Spraker TR. Stress and capture myopathy in artiodactylids. In: Fowler ME, ed. Zoo and Wild Animal Medicine: Current Therapy 3. Philadelphia: WB Saunders, 1993:481–488.

56. Williams ES, Thorne T, Exertional myopathy. In: Fairbrother A, Locke LL, Hoff GL, eds. Noninfectious Diseases of Wildlife, 2nd ed. London: Manson, 1996:181–193.

57. Heard DJ. Chemical immobilization of felids, ursids, and small ungulates. Vet Clin North Am Exot Anim Pract 4:267–298, 2001.

58. Ryeng KA, Arnemo JM, Larsen S. Determination of optimal immobilizing doses of a medetomidine hydrochloride and ketamine hydrochloride combination in captive reindeer. Am J Vet Res 62:119–126, 2001.

59. Beringer J, Hansen LP, Wilding W, Fischer J, Sheriff SL. Factors affecting capture myopathy in white-tailed deer. J Wildl Manage 60:373–380, 1996.

60. Caulkett N, Haigh JC. Anesthesia of North American deer. In: Heard D, ed. Zoological Restraint and Anesthesia. Ithaca, NY: International Veterinary Information Service, 2004. Document B0171.0404. http://www.ivis.org.

61. Arnemo JM, Moe R, Søli NE. Chemical capture of free-ranging red deer (Cervus elaphus) with medetomidine-ketamine. Rangifer 14:123–127, 1994.

62. Seal US, Schnitt SM, Peterson RO. Carfentanil and xylazine for immobilization of moose (Alces alces) on Isle Royale. J Wildl Dis 21:48–51, 1985.

63. Arnemo JM, Kreger TJ, Soveri T. Chemical immobilization of free-ranging moose. Alces 39:243–253, 2003.

64. Arnemo JM, Ericsson G, Øen EO, et al. Immobilization of free-ranging moose (Alces alces) with etorphine or etorphine-acepromazine-xylazine in Scandinavia (1984–2003): A review of 2754 captures. In: Joint Conference of the American Association of Zoo Veterinarians, American Association of Wildlife Veterinarians, and Wildlife Disease Association, 2004:519–520.

65. Fernandez-Moran J, Palomeque J, Peinado, VI. Medetomidine/tiletamine/zolazepam and xylazine/tiletamine/zolazepam combinations for immobilization of fallow deer (Cevus dama). J Zoo Wildl Med 31:62–64, 2000.

66. Haigh JC, Gates CC. Capture of wood bison (Bison bison athebascae) using carfentanil-based mixtures. J Wildl Dis 31:37–42, 1995.

67. Arnemo JM, Aanes R, Oystein OS, Caulkett NA, Rettie WJ, Haigh JC. Reversible immobilization of free-ranging Svalbard reindeer, Norwegian reindeer and woodland caribou: A comparison of medetomidine-ketamine and atipamezole in three subspecies of Rangifer tarandus. In: Proceedings of the Wildlife Disease Association Conference, June, Grand Teton National Park, Wyoming, 2000.

68. Caulkett NA, Rettie JW, Haigh JC. Immobilization of free ranging woodland caribou (Rangifer tarandus caribou) with medetomidine-ketamine and reversal with atipamezole. In: Proceedings of the Annual Meeting of the Association of Wildlife Veterinarians, November, Puerto Vallarta, Mexico, 1996:389–393.

69. Kreeger TJ, Lanka R, Smith T, Smeltzer T. Anesthesia of pronghorns in an urban environment using carfentanil and xylazine. In: 18th Biennial Pronghorn Antelope Workshop, 1999:69–73.

70. Paras-Garcia A, Foerster CR, Hernandez SM, Leandro D. Immobilization of free-ranging Baird's tapirs (Tapirus bairdii). In: Proceedings of the Annual Meeting of the American Association of Zoo Veterinarians, 1996:12–17.

71. Foerster SH, Bailey JE, Aguilar R, Loria DL, Foerster CR. Butorphanol/xylazine/ketamine anesthetic protocol for the immobilization of free-ranging Baird's tapirs in Costa Rica. J Wildl Dis 36:335–341, 2000.

72. Taylor WP Jr, Reynolds HV III, Ballard WB. Immobilization of grizzly bears with tiletamine hydrochloride and zolazepam hydrochloride. J Wildl Manage 53:978–981, 1989.

73. Arnemo JO, Brunberg S, Ahlqvist P, et al. Reversible immobilization and anesthesia of free-ranging brown bears (Ursus arctos) with medetomidine-tiletamine-zolazepam and atipamezole: A review of 575 captures. In: Proceedings of the Annual Meeting of the American Association of Zoo Veterinarians, 2001:234–236.

74. Stirling IC, Spencer C, Andriashek D. Immobilization of polar bears (Ursus maritimus) with Telazol in the Canadian arctic. J Wildl Dis 25:159–168, 1989.

75. Gibeau ML, Paquet PC. Evaluation of Telazol for immobilization of black bears. Wildl Soc Bull 19:400–402, 1991.

76. Caulkett N, Cattet MRL. Anesthesia of bears. In: Heard D, ed. Zoological Restraint and Anesthesia. Ithaca, NY: International Veterinary Information Service, 2002. Document B0143.0302. http://www.ivis.org.

77. Arnemo JM, Linnell JDC, Wedul SJ, Ranheim B, Odden J, Andersen R. Use of intraperitoneal radio-transmitters in lynx (Lynx lynx) kittens: Anesthesia, surgery and behavior. Wildl Biol 5:245–250, 1999.

78. Poole KG, Mowat G, Slough BG. Chemical immobilization of lynx. Wildl Soc Bull 21:136–140, 1993.

79. Schumacher J, et al. Comparative cardiopulmonary effects of ketamine-medetomidine and ketamine-xylazine in cougars (Felis concolor). In: Proceedings of the American Association of Zoo Veterinarians, Columbus, Ohio, 1999:45–46.

80. Deem SL. Capture and immobilization of free-living jaguars (Panthera onca). In: Heard D, ed. Zoological Restraint and Anesthesia. Ithaca, NY: International Veterinary Information Service, 2002. Document B0183.0102. http://www.ivis.org.

81. Golden HN, Schultz BS, Kunkel KE. Immobilization of wolverines with Telazol from a helicopter. Wildl Soc Bull 30:492–497, 2002.

82. Arnemo JM, Ahlqvist P, Liberg O, Sand H, Segerström P, Wabakken P. A new drug combination for reversible immobilization of free-ranging gray wolves. In: Proceedings of the World Wolf Congress, Banff, Canada, September 25–28, 2003:64.

83. Arnemo JM. Chemical immobilization and anaesthesia of wild boars. Orion Pharma Animal Health, Turku, Finland. DDA News 1:4, 2004.

84. Enqvist KE, Arnemo JM, Lemel J, Truvé J. Medetomidine/tiletamine-zolazepam and medetomidine/butorphanol/tiletamine-zolazepam: A comparison of two anesthetic regimens for surgical implantation of intraperitoneal radiotransmitters in free-ranging juvenile European wild boars (Sus scrofa scrofa) [Extended abstract]. In: Proceedings of the American Association of Zoo Veterinarians and International Association of Aquatic Animals Medical Joint Conference, New Orleans, Louisiana, September 17–21, 2000:261–263.

85. MacDonald D. The New Encyclopedia of Mammals. Oxford: Oxford University Press, 2001.

86. Goodrich JM, Kerlet LL, Schleyer BO, et al. Capture and chemical anesthesia of Amur (Siberian) tigers. Wildl Soc Bull 29:533–542, 2001.

87. Smith JLD, Sunquist ME, Tamang KM, Rai PB. A technique for capturing and immobilizing tigers. J Wildl Manage 47:255–259, 1983.

88. Sarma KK. Tiletamine-zolazepam as general anaesthetic in Royal Bengal tigers. Indian Vet J 79:677–679, 2002.

89. Quandt SKF. The pharmacology of medetomidine in combination with ketamine hydrochloride in African lions (*Panthera leo*) [Thesis]. Pretoria: University of Pretoria, 1992.

90. McKenzie AA, ed. The Capture and Care Manual. Pretoria: Wildlife Decision Support Services and the South African Veterinary Foundation, 1993.

91. Fahlman Å, Loveridge A, Wenham C, Foggin C, Arnemo JM, Nyman G. Reversible anaesthesia of free-ranging lions (*Panthera leo*) in Zimbabwe. J S Afr Vet Assoc 76:187–192, 2005.

92. Deem SL, Ko JC, Citino SB. Anesthetic and cardiorespiratory effects of tiletamine-zolazepam-medetomidine in cheetahs. J Am Vet Med Assoc 213:1022–1026, 1998.

93. Walzer C. Equidae. In: Fowler ME, Miller RE, eds. Zoo and Wild Animal Medicine, 5th ed. St Louis: WB Saunders, 2003:578–586.

94. Kock MD, Meltzer D, Burroughs R, eds. Chemical Capture and Physical Restraint of Wild Animals: A Training and Field Manual for African Species. Zimbabwe Veterinary Association Wildlife Group and International Wildlife Veterinary Services, 2006:124-125.

95. Arnemo JM, Wiik H. Chemical immobilization of zebras. Orion Pharma Animal Health, Turku, Finland. DDA News 2:3–4, 2004.

96. Bush M, Grobler DG, Raath JP, Phillips LG, Stamper MA, Lance WR. Use of medetomidine and ketamine for immobilization of free-ranging giraffes. J Am Vet Med Assoc 218:245–249, 2001.

Chapter 33

Aquatic Mammals

David B. Brunson

General Considerations

Marine mammals, which are air-breathing animals that have evolved for a primarily aquatic environment, include seals, sea lions, walruses, whales, cetaceans, polar bears, sea otters, and manatees. These animals have highly adapted physiology that presents unique anesthetic challenges.

Drug delivery is difficult for several reasons. Animals that live in a cold aquatic environment have heavy fur coats, thick blubber, or fat layers for insulation. Remote drug delivery requires special considerations for the site, depth, and method of drug injection. Intravenous (IV) access is usually very limited even on immobilized or anesthetized animals.

The pulmonary systems are highly developed to facilitate rapid oxygen and carbon dioxide exchange, as well as breath holding. Marine mammals frequently have short upper airways with extensive cartilaginous support down to the small bronchioles. They also take large breaths (tidal volumes), which aids in rapid gas exchange.

Seals breathe episodically in sleep. Higher centers in the brain modulate the central rhythm generator both positively and negatively for breathing. During episodic breathing, these modulating influences alternate in a fashion that produces periods of apnea alternating with periods of relatively high-frequency ventilation.[1] If seals are awoken during high-frequency ventilation, their breathing immediately slows.

Marine mammals have a highly developed dive reflex. This is a complicated physiological adaptation that is characterized by breath holding (apnea), decreased heart rate, and shunting of blood to critical aerobic organs. During a dive, peripheral tissues either reduce metabolic functions or function by hypoxic or anaerobic pathways. The implication for anesthesia is that absorption may be unpredictable or slower if central nervous system (CNS) depressants are administered intramuscularly during breath holding or during activation of the dive reflex. Once breathing is initiated, blood flows to the periphery. Darting or drug administration should be timed to occur during active ventilation and avoided during apnea.

Much is still unknown regarding specific marine mammal species and their physiological adaptations. Most immobilization and anesthetic information is obtained through observations during field capture or during medical management of captive animals. Thus, much of what we know is anecdotal and observational rather than from blinded, well-controlled studies of the drugs and animal physiology. As a result, when an anesthetic technique works well, it is adopted and used repeatedly. On the other hand, when even a single immobilization or anesthetic management is associated with either ineffective or adverse effects, the drugs are frequently abandoned. This chapter attempts to provide guidance to readers on what has been used successfully and cautions where information is still limited. For each species and situation, chemical capture, restraint, and anesthetic procedures should be carefully researched, planned, and executed. Networking with individuals experienced with the species and working conditions will increase the chances of a successful outcome. Generally, marine mammals should not be darted with an anesthetic while remaining in their aquatic environment, because they can dive out of sight and drown.

Cetaceans

Porpoises and whales breathe through a modified nasal orifice, called the *blowhole*, located on the dorsum of the head just anterior to the cranial vault. It appears on the surface as a single, transversely crescentic opening with a forward-facing concavity. It is closed by a muscular nasal plug and opens through the action of forehead muscles. Normally under water it remains closed. In porpoises, ventral to the blowhole are vestibular and tubular air sacs connected to the paired nares, which begin a few centimeters down the respiratory passage. A septum divides the nares for 10 to 12 cm, after which the respiratory passage becomes single again just above the glottis. The larynx forms an arytenoepiglottal tube giving a direct opening from the internal nares to the lungs, thus enabling the animal to breathe only through the blowhole (Fig. 33.1). Approximately 10 cm from the base of the larynx, the trachea branches into a separate right bronchus which, at about 15 cm, bifurcates into two main bronchi. It is important, when a porpoise is intubated, that the endotracheal tube not extend into the bronchus. To ensure proper

1. Blowhole
2. Cranium
3. Cerebral hemisphere
4. Cerebellum
5. Bony nares
6. Nasal cavity
7. Glottis
8. Nasopharyngeal sphincter
9. Esophagus
10. Arytenoid cartilage
11. Cricoid cartilage
12. Trachea
13. Eparterial bronchus
14. Tracheal cartilages
15. Thyroid cartilage
16. Epiglottic cartilage
17. Hyoid bone
18. Tongue
19. Oral cavity
20. Palate
21. Oropharyngeal sphincter

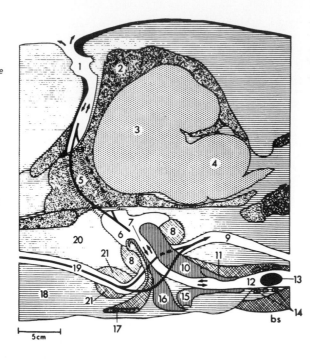

Fig. 33.1. Sagittal view of the head and neck of the bottlenose dolphin. From Nagel et al.[36]

placement, the tube should be measured and marked prior to placement.

Porpoises can take one full respiration in 0.3 s. With a tidal volume of 5 to 10 L, the flow rates through the air passages range from 30 to 70 L/s during expiration and inspiration. Porpoises breathe two or three times each minute. Each breath is deep (approximately 80% tidal air). After inspiration, the animal holds an apneustic plateau for 20 to 30 s, followed by rapid exhalation and inspiration.

Preanesthetic treatment with anticholinergics is recommended. Bradycardia, which is frequently observed during anesthesia, may be produced by strong parasympathetic stimulation or the effects of sedatives or analgesics. An IV or intramuscular (IM) dosage of 0.02 mg/kg is recommended.

Sedation and analgesia have been studied in porpoises to identify drugs that produce minimal respiratory depression. Sedation with diazepam has produced variable results. As in many mammalian species, benzodiazepines appear to have mild sedative effects, with minimal respiratory or cardiovascular depression. The primary use of these drugs should be for their antianxiety and the synergistic effects with other CNS depressants, such as opioids. Diazepam or midazolam at 0.05 to 0.1 mg/kg IV has been used safely in cetaceans.[2]

The relatively short-acting opioid meperidine hydrogen chloride (HCl) provides moderate restraint in cetaceans, without obvious deleterious effects. Three dosages of meperidine HCl have been studied in several species of cetaceans and pinnipeds (Table 33.1). The IM dosages evaluated were 0.11, 0.23, or 0.45 mg/kg administered by hand syringe.[3] Restraint was achieved rapidly, with maximum effect occurring 20 min after IM injection and lasting for 2 to 3 h. Analgesia appeared to last as long as 4 h and was sometimes accompanied by restoration of appetite in animals suffering physical discomfort. The higher doses increased

sedation and analgesia without noticeably depressing respiration. Based on the results of this study, the recommended initial dose of meperidine is 0.2 mg/kg IM when sedating cetaceans. If deemed necessary, higher dosages can be used safely, however.

Porpoises can be intubated while awake but intubation is more easily accomplished after sedation or induction of unconsciousness. Porpoises have relatively large airways. A 24- to 30-mm equine endotracheal tube with an inflatable cuff can be used. The mouth is held open with towels by assistants. The hand is inserted into the pharynx and grasps and pulls the larynx anteroventrally from the normal intranarial position. The endotracheal tube is then guided into the trachea by inserting two fingers into the glottis and passing the tube along the palm of the hand. A method of introducing the endotracheal tube through the blowhole has been described for use in smaller cetaceans, like *Delphinus delphis* and *Stenella styx*.[4] For induction without thiopental, 3.5% isoflurane or halothane is administered for 5 to 15 min via a mask or endotracheal tube, after which 1.0% to 1.25% is used to maintain surgical anesthesia. If thiopental is used to induce anesthesia before intubation, 1.5% to 2.0% isoflurane or halothane is sufficient for maintenance. Sevoflurane should be an excellent inhalant anesthetic for cetaceans. Because of its lower blood-gas solubility, it equilibrates faster than isoflurane, thus hastening induction and recovery. The lower potency of sevoflurane requires higher vaporizer settings for induction and maintenance. Expected settings would be 4.5% to 5.0% for mask induction and 2.25% to 2.75% for maintenance.

Induction can be achieved by the IV administration of thiopental at 10 mg/kg or propofol at 4 to 6 mg/kg via one of the tailfluke veins. These dosage recommendations are for unsedated animals. Lower dosages should be used if an animal is already sedated or debilitated. Injection of thiopental alone (10 mg/kg IV) produces 10 to 15 min of light anesthesia followed by 45 min

Table 33.1. Meperidine dosage used in dolphins and whales.

Species	Total number of restraints	Meperidine		
		0.11 mg/kg	0.23 mg/kg	0.45 mg/kg
Bottlenose dolphin	74	2	62	10
Pilot whale	4		2	2
Killer whale	4		2	2
White-sided dolphin	3		3	
False killer whale	10		9	1
Common dolphin	1		1	

of respiratory depression, during which the animal may require artificial ventilation. A dose of 15 to 25 mg/kg IV produces surgical anesthesia for 10 to 25 min, with respiratory depression lasting 1 to 2½ h. Sensitivity to barbiturates has been further demonstrated following high doses of intraperitoneal pentobarbital (10 to 30 mg/kg), which has reportedly caused respiratory failure and death.[5] Consequently, this technique is no longer recommended. Likewise, because plasma cholinesterase levels may be extremely low or absent in bottlenose dolphins (*Tursiops truncatus*), the use of succinylcholine to induce muscular paralysis is not recommended.

The heart rate during general anesthesia is typically 100 to 120 beats per minute (beats/min). During delivery of 100% oxygen, arterial pH averages 7.35, partial pressure of oxygen (PaO_2) is maintained at 100 to 200 mm Hg, and partial pressure of carbon dioxide ($PaCO_2$) is 35 to 50 mm Hg. In conscious cetaceans breathing ambient air, arterial PaO_2 reportedly ranges from 65 to 98 mm Hg, and $PaCO_2$ ranges from 40 to 60 mm Hg.

Cessation of tail-fluke movements indicates surgical anesthesia and occurs after loss of strong corneal and eyelid reflexes. The swimming reflex is considered the best criterion for assessing the depth of anesthesia. Reflexes typically observed when assessing depth of anesthesia in porpoises include (1) the palpebral reflex, (2) corneal reflex, (3) swallowing in response to tactile stimulation of the pharynx, (4) retraction of the tongue, (5) reflex movements of the body when the anus is distended, (6) tail movements, (7) movements of the pectoral flippers in response to surface stimulation, (8) movement of the blowhole after stimulation of the nares or vestibular sacs, and (9) vaginal or penile movements when the area is manipulated.

During the recovery period, the endotracheal tube is kept in position until the blowhole reflex returns. This usually requires 15 to 45 min after cessation of inhalant administration. Timing the removal of the endotracheal tube is critical. Extubation should occur only after the animal is capable of breathing on its own, as manifested by movements of the blowhole and thorax, and by struggling, coughing, and/or bucking. When the endotracheal tube is removed, the larynx must be placed in its normal intranarial position. If the animal does not exhale through the blowhole within 3 min or if the heart rate falls below 60 beats/min, the endotracheal tube must be reinserted and the animal ventilated for a few more minutes. In water, porpoises are near neutral in buoyancy. Out of

water, it is more difficult for them to breathe and maintain circulation. For this reason, animals should be returned to water as soon as possible following recovery from anesthesia.

Local anesthesia can be used to provide analgesia for minor painful procedures. Using structural landmarks, a method has been devised for anesthetizing the lower jaw of the bottlenose dolphin.[6] With this procedure, its teeth can be extracted and age determined by counting dentine layers in sections of etched teeth. The toxic doses of various local anesthetics have not been determined in cetaceans, so one should use the smallest dose necessary to desensitize tissues or structures prior to surgery or invasive diagnostic procedure.

Toothed and Balen Whales

Chemical immobilization and anesthesia have been attempted in large cetaceans. Killer whales have been sedated with meperidine and midazolam for minor procedures coupled with local anesthesia. Sedation has been attempted in removing an embedded rope in a free-ranging North Atlantic right whale. The adult male was estimated to be 50 feet long and weigh 40,000 kg. Each attempt at sedation was separated by at least 2 weeks. The dosage was increased on each attempt, with the final attempt producing mild sedation. Based on killer whale experiences and initial ineffective attempts with lower dosages, the most effective dose of midazolam was determined to be 0.025 mg/kg IM. The meperidine dose was set at 0.17 mg/kg IM. Four doses were administered to the whale over 2 h 43 min for a total dose of 40 g of meperidine and 4 g of midazolam. Although the whale never stopped swimming, its respiratory frequency decreased and diving behavior ceased.[7]

Pinnipedia

Pinniped species are made up of the otarids (eared seals), phocids (true seals), and odobenids (walruses). The physical characteristics vary widely among these groups. Size is especially variable, and body weight should be estimated carefully based on species, age, and gender. As a group, these animals have highly efficient respiratory systems. The alveolar exchange in seals has been measured at approximately 46% as compared with terrestrial mammals, where the alveolar exchange is usually in the range of 12% to 16%. In species that can be physically restrained or sedated with benzodiazepine tranquilizers (diazepam or midazolam, 0.1 mg/kg IM), induction with gas anesthetics is recommended. Mask inductions with isoflurane or sevoflurane can be very fast, occurring in as little as three to four breaths because of high alveolar exchange and the low solubility of these anesthetic gases.

During anesthesia of pinnipeds, their temperature should be continuously monitored via esophageal or rectal probe. Hyperthermia or hypothermia can occur during physical restraint, sedation, anesthesia, and handling outside of the normal aquatic environment. It is important to be prepared to support body temperature by either warming or cooling the animal, as necessary. Assessment of ventilation requires the use of both carbon dioxide monitoring and pulse oximetry. A Doppler flow detector can also be an important tool in assessing peripheral perfusion.

Odobenidae (Walruses)

Walruses are very challenging to anesthetize. Adult males weight up to 3000 pounds (1360 kg). High mortality rates have been reported with the use of opioids and dissociative anesthetics but are most likely the result of severe respiratory and circulatory compromise when the animals are out of the water and under anesthesia. Respiratory arrest has been commonly reported during immobilization with potent opioids. Even with ventilatory support, these large animals may develop circulatory failure during anesthesia.

Captive walruses have been immobilized with a combination of midazolam (0.1 mg/kg) and meperidine (2.2 mg/kg). To prevent vagal induced bradycardia, the use of atropine (0.04 mg/kg) is also recommended. The recommended injection sites for IM injections are the hip and epaxial muscles. A long needle (3 to 4 inches) must be used to ensure effective IM drug absorption.

IV access is difficult, but vascular access can be obtained via the epidural venous sinus. Needle placement is identical to placement of epidural needles or catheters via the lumbosacral space. With the walrus in sternal recumbency, the wings of the ileums can be palpated. The needle should be perpendicular to the skin. For large walruses, a 6-inch-long spinal needle is required. Easy aspiration of blood with a syringe indicates proper depth and placement. Epidural IV access can be used for administration of fluid, emergency drugs, and anesthetics. Small boluses of propofol (40 to 60 mg) can be used to relax muscles and facilitate endotracheal intubation. During inhalant anesthesia, emergency drugs can be administered via the endotracheal tube when IV access is not available.

During the onset of immobilization and anesthesia, heart rate is usually between 80 and 100 beats/min. As anesthesia deepens, heart rate slows to around 60 beats/min. Apnea is common during anesthesia and immobilization. Ventilatory support is essential when working with walruses.

Intubation is easiest with the walrus in sternal recumbency with head extended. Despite their large size, walruses have small oral cavities. Digital palpation of the larynx and direct placement of the endotracheal tube is possible once the animal is relaxed and the mouth pulled open by an assistant.

Isoflurane can be used to maintain general anesthesia in walruses. Oxygen flow rates and vaporizer settings are similar to those recommended for equine anesthesia. The oxygen flow rate should be at least 4 L/min to ensure adequate delivery of anesthetic and oxygen.

When used alone, meperidine has been administered by IM injection at dosages ranging from 0.23 to 0.45 mg/kg. In this dose range, sedation/restraint is usually moderate, without apparent detrimental effects.[3]

Otariidae (Sea Lions and Fur Seals)

Attempts to sedate seals and sea lions have met with variable success. As is the case for most wildlife, sedatives alone should not be relied on for immobilization. Additionally, species response may vary with the use of phenothiazine and benzodiazepine tranquilizers.[8] Nevertheless, the use of tranquilizers is beneficial in the overall management of Otariidae because tranquilizers decrease the overall anesthetic dose requirement and adverse side effects when combined with dissociatives or opioids.

Ringed seals and sea lions have been immobilized with ketamine alone (4.5 to 11.0 mg/kg IM).[9] However, because of the concern for excessive salivation, animals with respiratory problems should not be given high doses of ketamine alone. Atropine (total dose, 0.3 to 0.6 mg) can be given concurrently to prevent excessive salivation. Phocid seals have been successfully anesthetized with a combination of ketamine (1.5 mg/kg) and diazepam (0.05 mg/kg) IM or IV.[10] This protocol is preferred over ketamine (2 mg/kg) alone because the ketamine dose can be decreased and induction and recovery are generally smoother. Apparently, Weddell seals (Leptonychotes weddelli) can be safely immobilized with relatively low doses of ketamine (2 mg/kg IM) prior to induction with a gas anesthetic.[11]

Southern elephant seals (Mirounga leonina) are generally so lethargic that they can be injected at close range with a pole syringe.[12] A 16- to 18-gauge needle up to 4 inches long is needed to penetrate the skin and underlying blubber. Although succinylcholine (2.5 mg/kg) has been used to immobilize seals rapidly,[12] it should not be used without concurrent analgesic or anesthetic drug administration and ventilatory support.

For IV injections, sea lions are best restrained in a squeeze cage to enable access to a protruding flipper. A vein on the ventral aspect of the flipper, approximately 3 cm anterior to its posterior edge, can be used for IV administration. Thiopental or thiamylal can be given at the rate of 2.2 to 4.4 mg/kg to produce anesthesia.[13] Barbiturates should be given rapidly to minimize struggling and to produce relaxation. Alternatively, isoflurane or halothane can be administered by means of a face mask to induce anesthesia. Sea lions can hold their breath for as long as 5 min. When they do breathe, their air intake is enormous and rapid. For this reason, the respiratory pattern during anesthetic induction is not an accurate gauge of CNS depression. Once the animal is induced, the trachea is easily intubated for further inhalant administration. Concentrations of 0.75% to 1.5% are usually sufficient to maintain anesthesia.

Northern sea lions have been successfully anesthetized with Telazol (tiletamine-zolazepam). The recommended dose range is

1.8 to 2.5 mg/kg IM. The effective dose may vary from one animal to another. Tiletamine-zolazepam doses of more than 2.5 mg/kg IM can be fatal in sea lions. Hypothermia is commonly observed in animals that receive higher doses (2.5 mg/kg IM or larger).[14]

Several anesthetic regimens have been described for inducing anesthesia in California sea lions (*Zalophus californianus*).[15] The first combination consists of atropine (0.02 mg/kg) given IM 10 min prior to medetomidine (0.14 mg/kg IM) and ketamine (2.5 mg/kg IM) administration. Sea lions of all ages and weights (13.5 to 145.0 kg) have been anesthetized with this mixture. Following IM injection, induction time ranges from 9 to 17 min, whereas anesthesia time ranges from 17 to 57 min.[15] It should be noted that the standard 1.0-mg/mL concentration of medetomidine is too dilute and expensive for this technique and may limit its use. Reversal with atipamezole at a dosage of 0.2 mg/kg IM can hasten and reduce recovery time.[15]

In a similar study using 1.0 mg/kg IM of Telazol, the medetomidine dosage was reduced by half to 0.07 mg/kg IM. Induction time was reduced to approximately 5 min, while anesthesia/immobilization with this mixture averaged nearly 30 min. The disadvantages of this anesthetic regimen include prolonged ataxia, weakness, and some disorientation during recovery. Typically, this combination will provide a rapid induction with a reliable plane of anesthesia. Recovery can be hastened with atipamezole at a dosage of 0.2 mg/kg IM.[16]

Young California sea lion pups that are hand caught can be induced by mask technique alone using either isoflurane or sevoflurane. Induction and recovery times average under 10 min when using isoflurane alone to maintain anesthesia.[17] Relaxation is evident within a few minutes of administration of isoflurane by mask.

Premedication with IM meperidine (0.23 to 0.45 mg/kg) apparently provides little restraint of sea lions, while causing profound respiratory depression. Consequently, low dosages are advised when using meperidine for analgesia or as part of the immobilization technique in this species of seals.[3]

Steller sea lions have been darted using Telazol delivered via a carbon dioxide–powered blowpipe. The average dose administered was 2.3 mg/kg IM. Approximately one-third of the animals required additional CNS depression with isoflurane to achieve anesthesia. Following induction, all animals were intubated and maintained on isoflurane in oxygen. If apneustic breathing was observed after Telazol injection, doxapram was used to stimulate breathing and aid in induction of inhalant anesthesia.[18] Young Steller sea lion pups and yearlings caught by trained scuba divers have become severely hypothermic (<90°F [<32°C]) when anesthetized immediately after snaring, emphasizing the importance of monitoring temperature closely when working with this species.[18]

Both ketamine (2.1 mg/kg IM) and Telazol (1.1 mg/kg IM) have been used to immobilize fur seals. Individual animal response to these drugs appears to be highly variable, however. The dose requirement for satisfactory levels of anesthesia and immobilization appears to be less than for most other species of seals. Few side effects have been observed when using low doses of these drugs, aside from mild tremors caused by ketamine, and respiratory depression or prolonged apnea caused by tiletamine-zolazepam. When working with fur seals, relatively low doses of ketamine or Telazol can be quite effective, especially for animals in good body condition.[19]

Phocids (True Seals)

Phocidae or true seals include northern hemisphere seals such as the harbor, gray, bearded, and hooded seals. The southern hemisphere seals include monk, crabeater, Weddell, leopard, Ross, and elephant seals. Many of these species have been studied in free-ranging environments and are commonly included in zoological parks and aquariums.

Southern elephant seals have been extensively studied, and multiple anesthetic techniques have been used successfully. Telazol has been administered to over 1000 southern elephant seals without acute fatality. Older and better-conditioned animals appear to have faster recoveries, and no gender differences have been noted. Apnea has been observed in some animals, but typically lasts less than 5 min.[20] A 1-mg/kg IM dose of Telazol is considered both safe and effective in this species.[21] Telazol administration at a dose under 0.5 mg/kg IV will produce anesthesia in 30 s or less. Anesthesia achieved with IV Telazol, even at this low dose, will range from 15 to 20 min.[22]

Ketamine alone can be administered to elephant seals at doses ranging from 2 to 8 mg/kg IM. At a dose of 8 to 9 mg/kg IM, immobilization should occur in 15 min. The dosage required depends greatly on which sedative is used in conjunction with ketamine. An IM dose of 0.4 to 0.5 mg/kg of xylazine has been combined with 5 to 6 mg/kg of ketamine for short periods of immobilization.[23] Alternatively, diazepam can be dosed at 0.3 mg/kg IM with 8 mg/kg IM of ketamine. Lower doses of xylazine (0.4 mg/kg) or diazepam (0.1 mg/kg) can also be given IV to supplement muscle relaxation during ketamine anesthesia. Medetomidine (0.013 mg/kg IM) has also been combined with ketamine (2 mg/kg IM) to enhance muscle relaxation during immobilization.[24]

In a study on the use of antagonists and stimulants to reverse sedation in elephant seals, yohimbine (0.06 mg/kg IM) reversed xylazine sedation better than did doxapram, whereas 4-aminopyridine actually prolonged recovery.[25] Doxapram (0.5, 1, 2, and 4 mg/kg IV) caused a dose-dependent increase in the depth and rate of ventilation, which began within 1 min, peaked after 2 min, and lasted for up to 5 min. The 2-mg/kg dose appeared to be both safe and effective. Higher dosages (4 mg/kg) caused arousal and shaking in some seals. Administration of doxapram via the endotracheal tube was an unreliable route of drug delivery.[25]

Butorphanol has been evaluated as an analgesic in young elephant seals at a dosage of 0.055 mg/kg IM.[26] The dosage was conservative and produced minimal observable effects. A complete evaluation of this opioid's analgesic efficacy in seals requires additional use and observation. Similarly, published reports of anesthetics in many phocids is sparse, making dosage recommendations based on efficacy and safety difficult. For example, when 30 Weddell seals were administered Telazol at IM doses ranging from 100 to 300 mg, only 16 were fully immobilized, while 7 were moderately sedate and 7 were only lightly sedated. However, nearly 25% of the animals in the study died. The cause of mortality is unknown and likely not due solely to either the drugs or dosages used.[27]

Several IM drugs or drug mixtures have been described for use in gray seals. These include ketamine (6 mg/kg) and diazepam (0.3 mg/kg), which produced adequate immobilization;[28] tiletamine-zolazepam (1 mg/kg); and carfentanil (0.01 mg/kg) with ketamine (5 mg/kg) and xylazine (1 mg/kg).[29] Each of these drug combinations was reportedly effective in immobilizing gray seals.

Sirenia (Manatees)

Many minor procedures can be performed with proper physical restraint. Local anesthetic infiltration should be used for procedures that are painful. Captive manatees are removed from the water by draining the pool or elevating the bottom of the holding tank. While out of the water, manatees should be sprayed with water to avoid skin drying and should be kept out of the sun to prevent skin burning. They should be held in sternal recumbency because the tail is potentially dangerous if placed in dorsal or lateral recumbency. The tail can be restrained by people and foam pads.

Sedation with midazolam generally works well. A dosage of 0.045 mg/kg IM is recommended. For light general anesthesia and restraint, the combination of midazolam (0.066 mg/kg IM) and meperidine (up to 1.0 mg/kg IM) is effective. Flumazenil and naloxone are effective antagonists for this combination.[30]

Nasal-tracheal intubation is easily accomplished with the aid of a fiberoptic endoscope, which is placed in one nasal passage while the endotracheal tube is passed via the opposite nasal passage. Manual or mechanical ventilation is recommended to maintain the carbon dioxide level within normal limits during general anesthesia. Isoflurane or sevoflurane are appropriate anesthetics for maintenance with expected vaporizer settings of 1.5% to 2.5%.

Carnivora

Polar Bears

Since polar bears can have substantial fat deposits throughout the year, the shoulder and neck are the best sites for IM drug delivery. Male polar bears can be large and heavy. Body weights of greater than 500 kg are not uncommon. Because of their large size and drug requirements, potent drug combinations are required to keep drug volume and dart size to a minimum. Immobilized polar bears should be positioned to avoid excessive pressure on limb muscles because such pressure has caused muscle swelling and lameness. During the summer, polar bears enter a hypometabolic state that is characterized by fasting and decreased body temperature (93° to 95°F [34° to 35°C]). Immobilizing drug requirements may also be decreased during the summer. In areas where large numbers of polar bears congregate, reversible anesthetic protocols should be considered because they will decrease the risk of predation by other bears. Reversible protocols should also be considered for mother bears with cubs.

Polar bears immobilized with Telazol typically keep their heads out of the water better than bears immobilized with opioids. This is probably due to muscle extension with the use of dissociative anesthetic versus the relaxed curled body position associated with the use carfentanil or etorphine.

Mature polar bears can be darted with 22-caliber blank powered projectors and explosive-discharge darts. A needle up to 10 cm long is necessary to ensure the IM injection of drugs. Polar bears are notorious for pretending to be immobilized and have been known to awaken suddenly when approached. Always use caution when approaching this species.

Immobilization drug choices include dissociatives and opioids. Because Telazol is available in a lyophilized form, it can be reconstituted with an α_2-agonist, keeping the total volume lower than with ketamine. Dosages of 8 to 10 mg/kg of Telazol will produce reliable immobilization, but can also result in prolonged recoveries.[31] Used alone, the volume requirements are high, making the use of a large dart necessary. The greater mass of a large volume and the dart itself are more likely to produce excessive tissue trauma and animal injury when the projectile penetrates tissue. For this reason, an IM combination of xylazine (2 mg/kg) and Telazol (3 mg/kg) is preferred as it has approximately half the volume requirement of Telazol alone. Additionally, partial reversal can be accomplished by administration of either yohimbine or atipamezole. When rapid reversal of this mixture is not achieved, it is probably due to residual zolazepam sedation.

A similar anesthetic regimen consists of the IM injection of 75 µg/kg of medetomidine mixed with 2.2 mg/kg of Telazol.[32] This combination has a rapid onset of action and can be delivered IM in a small volume to free-ranging polar bears. To reduce volume, medetomidine (1 mg/mL) can be lyophilized and reconstituted to a concentration of 6 mg/mL. The IM dosage range reported for this mixture was 1.2 to 7.7 mg/kg. In all bears, the total volume injected was always less than 10 mL. The average dose of medetomidine injected was 0.07 mg/kg, whereas the average dose of Telazol injected was 2.3 mg/kg. This regimen resulted in an average anesthesia time of approximately 3 h. When medetomidine was reversed with atipamezole (0.24 mg/kg IM), recovery time was reduced to an average of 6 min.[32] Medetomidine coadministration substantially reduced the volume requirement of Telazol while providing analgesia. If Telazol is used alone, dosage requirement increases from under 2.5 to 5 mg/kg IM. With the medetomidine-tiletamine-zolazepam mixture, bears become ataxic in 1 to 3 min, typically sit in 4 to 5 min, and become recumbent shortly thereafter. Maximal effects are usually seen in 20 min. The duration is dose dependent, with recumbency lasting approximately 2 h.[32] Following immobilization, the suspension of polar bears in a cargo net can cause acute hypertension (up to a 50% increase in mean arterial pressure), hypoxemia, and evidence of stress. Cargo nets can restrict both ventilation and circulation. Bears should be transported on a rigid platform rather than lifted in a net.[33]

Opioids can provide for some sedation and analgesia, as well as immobilization. Fentanyl, carfentanil, and etorphine have all been used to immobilize polar bears. The published mean IM dosage for fentanyl in polar bears is 0.44 mg/kg. Unless concentrated forms of fentanyl become available, the volume needed is usually too large for the practical use of this drug in adult bears. Fentanyl reportedly provides better muscle relaxation than etorphine. Naloxone can be dosed at 25 mg per 10 mg of fentanyl or 25 mg per 0.5 mg of etorphine for rapid reversal (within 10 min).[34]

Sea Otters

Numerous combinations have been assessed in sea otters, including Telazol, butorphanol-diazepam, oxymorphone-acepromazine-diazepam, azaperone-fentanyl-diazepam, and fentanyl-diazepam. Of these, the most effective combinations appear to be fentanyl (0.1 mg/kg) with either acepromazine or diazepam (0.22 mg/kg) IM.[35]

Manual restraint and nets are often effective for capture and examination. Hand injection can be used in these situations. If manual restraint is feasible, mask induction with either isoflurane or sevoflurane works well. Altered thermoregulation may cause body temperature to increase during capture. Otters should be transported in well-ventilated cages that are iced to help keep animals cool during transport.

Experience in sedating sea otters after the 1989 Valdez oil spill resulted in the recommendation of combined fentanyl (0.05 to 0.1 mg/kg IM) and diazepam (0.1 mg/kg IM) as the preferred technique in this species. It should be noted that many other immobilizing mixtures were used only a few times, and the mortality rate for all anesthetized sea otters was extremely high because of oil exposure.[35]

Other drug combinations used successfully to sedate, immobilize, or anesthetize sea otters include Telazol alone (2 mg/kg IM); ketamine (2.5 mg/kg IM) and medetomidine (0.25 mg/kg IM); ketamine (10 mg/kg IM) and midazolam (0.25 mg/kg IM); ketamine (1.5 mg/kg IM) and xylazine (1.5 mg/kg IM); and etorphine (0.03 to 0.05 mg/kg IM) with diazepam (0.06 mg/kg IM).

References

1. Milsom WK, Harris MB, Reid SG. Do descending influences alternate to produce episodic breathing? Respir Physiol 110:307–317, 1997.
2. Meshcherskii RM, Meniailov NV, Shepeleva IS, et al. Narcotization of dolphins without blocking their own respiration [in Russian]. Zh Evol Biokhim Fiziol 14:410–411, 1978.
3. Joseph BE, Cornell LH. The use of meperidine hydrochloride for chemical restraint in certain cetaceans and pinnipeds. J Wildl Dis 24:691–694, 1988.
4. Rieu M, Gautheron B. Preliminary observations concerning a method for introduction of a tube for anaesthesia in small delphinids. Life Sci 7:1141–1146, 1968.
5. Lily JC. Man and Dolphin. New York: Doubleday, 1961.
6. Ridgway SH, Green RF, Sweeney JC. Mandibular anesthesia and tooth extraction in the bottlenosed dolphin. J Wildl Dis 11:415–418, 1975.
7. Brunson DB, Rowles TK, Gulland FM, et al. Technique for drug delivery and sedation of a free-ranging North Atlantic Right Whale (*Balenea glacialis*). In: Proceedings of the American Association of Zoo Veterinarians [AAZV], 2002:320–322.
8. Hubbard RC, Poulter TC. Seals and sea lions as models for studies in comparative biology. Lab Anim Care 18(Suppl):288–297, 1968.
9. Beraci JR. An appraisal of ketamine as an immobilizing agent in wild and captive pinnipeds. J Am Vet Med Assoc 163:574–577, 1973.
10. Beraci JR, Skirnisson K, St Aubin DJ. A safe method for repeatedly immobilizing seals. J Am Vet Med Assoc 179:1192–1193, 1981.
11. Hochachka PW, Liggins GC, Quist J, et al. Pulmonary metabolism during diving: Conditioning blood for the brain. Science 198: 831–834, 1977.
12. Ling JK, Nicholls DG, Thomas CDB. Immobilization of southern elephant seals with succinylcholine chloride. J Wildl Manage 37: 468–479, 1967.
13. Tidgway SH, Simpson JG. Anesthesia and restraint for the California seal lion, *Zalophus californianus*. J Am Vet Med Assoc 155:1059–1063, 1969.
14. Loughlin TR, Spraker T. Use of Telazol to immobilize female northern sea lions (*Eumetopias jubatus*) in Alaska. J Wildl Dis 25:353–358, 1989.
15. Haulena M, Gulland FM, Calkins DG, Spraker TR. Immobilization of California sea lions using medetomidine plus ketamine with and without isoflurane and reversal with atipamezole. J Wildl Dis 36:124–130, 2000.
16. Haulena M, Gulland FM. Use of medetomidine-zolazepam-tiletamine with and without atipamezole reversal to immobilize captive California sea lions. J Wildl Dis 37:566–573, 2001.
17. Heath RB, DeLong R, Jameson V, Bradley D, Spraker T. Isoflurane anesthesia in free ranging sea lion pups. J Wildl Dis 33:206–210, 1997.
18. Dabin W, Beauplet G, Guinet C. Response of wild subantarctic fur seal (*Arctocephalus tropicalis*) females to ketamine and tiletamine-zolazepam anesthesia. J Wildl Dis 38:846–850, 2002.
19. Field IC, Bradshaw CJ, McMahon CR, Harrington J, Burton HR. Effects of age, size and condition of elephant seals (*Mirounga leonine*) on their intravenous anaesthesia with tiletamine and zolazepam. Vet Rec 151:235–240, 2002.
20. Baker JR, Fedak MA, Anderson SS, Arnbom T, Baker R. The use of a tiletamine-zolazepam mixture to immobilize wild grey seals and southern elephant seals. Vet Rec 126:75–77, 1990.
21. McMahon CR, Burton H, McLean S, Slip D, Bester M. Field immobilisation of southern elephant seals with intravenous tiletamine and zolazepam. Vet Rec 146:251–254, 2000.
22. Woods R, McLean S, Burton HR. Pharmacokinetics of intravenously administered ketamine in southern elephant seals (*Mirounga leonina*). Comp Biochem Physiol [C] 123:279–284, 1999.
23. Gales NJ, Burton HR. Prolonged and multiple immobilizations of the southern elephant seal using ketamine hydrochloride or ketamine hydrochloride-diazepam combinations. J Wildl Dis 23:614–618, 1987.
24. Woods R, McLean S, Nicol S, Burton H. Chemical restraint of southern elephant seals (*Mirounga leonine*): Use of medetomidine, ketamine and atipamezole and comparison with other cyclohexamine-based combinations. Br Vet J 152:213–224, 1996.
25. Woods R, McLean S, Nicol S, Burton H. Antagonism of some cyclohexamine based drug combinations used for chemical restraint of southern elephant seals (*Mirounga leonina*). Aust Vet J 72:165–171, 1995.
26. Nutter F, Haulena M, Bai SA. Preliminary pharmacokinetics of single dose intramuscular butorphanol in elephant seals (*Mirounga angustirostris*). In: Abstracts of the Proceedings of the American Association of Zoo Veterinarians/American Association of Wildlife Veterinarians [AAZV/AAWV] Joint Conference, 1998:372–373.

27. Phelan JR, Green K. Chemical restraint of Weddell seals (*Leptonychotes weddellii*) with a combination of tiletamine and zolazepam. J Wildl Dis 28:230–235, 1992.

28. Baker JR, Anderson SS, Fedak MA. The use of a ketamine-diazepam mixture to immobilize wild grey seals (*Halichoerus grypus*) and southern elephant seals (*Mirounga leonine*). Vet Rec 123:287–289, 1988.

29. Baker JR, Gatesman TJ. Use of carfentanil and a ketamine-xylazine mixture to immobilize wild grey seals (*Halichoerus grypus*). Vet Rec 116:208–210, 1985.

30. Walsh M, Bossart G. Manatee medicine. In: Fowler ME, Miller E, eds. Zoo and Wild Animal Medicine: Current Therapy, 4th ed. Philadelphia: WB Saunders, 1999:507–516.

31. Haigh JC, Stirling I, Broughton E. Immobilization of polar bears (*Urus maritimus* Phipps) with a mixture of tiletamine hydrochloride and zolazepam hydrochloride. J Wildl Dis 21:43–47, 1985.

32. Caulkett NA, Cattet MRL, Caulkett JM, Polischuk SC. Comparative physiologic effects of Telazol, medetomidine-ketamine, and medetomidine-Telazol in polar bears (*Ursus maritimus*). J Zoo Wildl Med 30:504–509, 1999.

33. Cattet MRL, Caulkett NA, Streib KA, Torske KE, Ramsay MA. Cardiopulmonary response of anesthetized polar bears to suspension by net and sling. J Wildl Dis 35:548–556, 1999.

34. Patenaude RP. Evaluation of fentanyl citrate, etorphine hydrochloride, and naloxone hydrochloride in captive polar bears. J Am Vet Med Assoc 175:1006–1007, 1979.

35. Sawyer DC, Williams TD. Chemical restraint and anesthesia of sea otters affected by the oil spill in Prince William Sound, Alaska. J Am Vet Med Assoc 208:1831–1834, 1996.

36. Nagel EL, Morgane PJ, McFarland WL. Anesthesia for the bottlenose dolphin *Tursiops truncatus*. Science 146:1591–1593, 1964.

Chapter 34
Birds

John W. Ludders and Nora S. Matthews

Introduction

The principles and practices of avian anesthesia depend on an understanding of avian anatomy, physiology, and pharmacology. This chapter focuses on the avian pulmonary and cardiovascular systems because they are of the utmost importance in the anesthetic management of birds; where appropriate, however, other organ systems are discussed. Although drugs are discussed in general terms, and more specifically for ratites, this chapter is not a compendium of drugs and doses useful for anesthetic management of all species of birds. For such a compendium the reader is referred to the list of suggested readings at the end of this chapter.

Form and Function
Pulmonary System

The avian pulmonary system is very different from that of the mammalian system. A brief description of avian pulmonary anatomy and physiology will help to explain earlier misconceptions and current realities regarding the effects of anesthetics on birds, especially inhalant anesthetics. The avian respiratory system consists of two separate and distinct functional components: a component for ventilation (conducting airways, air sacs, thoracic skeleton, and muscles of respiration), and a component for gas exchange (parabronchial lung).

Ventilation Component
Larynx and Trachea

The avian larynx protrudes into the pharynx as a somewhat heart-shaped mound and consists of four laryngeal cartilages: the cricoid, procricoid, and the right and left arytenoid cartilages.[1] Unlike mammals, the thyroid and epiglottic cartilages are absent in birds.[1] In birds, the larynx functions as a barrier to foreign material entering the airway, opens the glottis during inspiration, assists in swallowing, and may modulate sound production.[1]

In all avian species the tracheal cartilages form complete rings, but there are significant species-related variations in tracheal anatomy.[1] For example, the emu and ruddy duck have an inflatable saclike diverticulum (tracheal sac) that opens from the trachea.[1] In the emu the sac arises from the ventral surface of the trachea approximately three-quarters of the way down the neck, where there is a slitlike opening created by the incomplete tracheal rings ventrally (Fig. 34.1).[1] The caudal end of the sac may extend almost to the level of the sternum. This sac is present in both sexes and is responsible for the characteristic booming call of the emu.

In the ruddy duck the sac opens in a depression on the dorsal wall of the trachea immediately caudal to the larynx, thus lying between the trachea and esophagus.[1] In this bird the sac is found

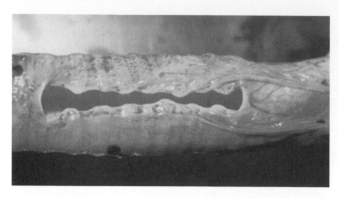

Fig. 34.1. Tracheal slit of an emu (*Dromaius novaeholllandiae*). From J. A. Smith, DVM, DACVA; with permission.

only in the male and may act as a sounding board for the bill-drumming display of the male.[1]

The male of many anseriform species (waterfowl such as ducks and mergansers) has a unique anatomical feature of the trachea—the tracheal bulbous expansion—which is a bulblike structure in the trachea, and its exact function has not been determined.

A double trachea, found in some penguins and petrels, consists of a median septum dividing part of the trachea into right and left channels.[1] In both groups of birds the septum extends cranially from the bronchial bifurcation, but the length of the septum is quite variable. For example, in the jackass penguin the septum extends to within a few centimeters of the larynx, whereas in the rockhopper penguin the septum is only 5 mm long.[1]

Some species of birds have complex tracheal loops or coils that, depending on the species, may be located in the caudal neck, within the keel, or within the thorax and the keel (Fig. 34.2). Studies in cranes have demonstrated that tracheal coiling enables these birds to produce extremely loud calls by using very low driving pressures.[2]

The fact that birds generally have relatively long necks, not to mention tracheal loops and coils, has important implications for the functional morphology of the trachea, especially tracheal dead space. Studies indicate that the typical bird trachea is 2.7 times longer than that of comparably sized mammals, but because the bird trachea is 1.29 times wider, the tracheal resistance in birds and mammals is comparable.[1] Tracheal dead-space volume is increased in birds to about 4.5 times that of comparably sized mammals, but the relatively low respiratory frequency of birds, approximately one-third that of mammals, ensures that the effect of the larger tracheal dead-space volume is decreased.[1] As a result the minute tracheal ventilation rate is only about 1.5 to 1.9 times that of mammals.[1]

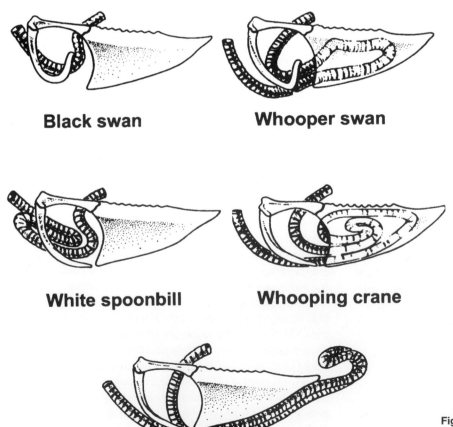

Black swan

Whooper swan

White spoonbill

Whooping crane

Helmeted curassow

Fig. 34.2. Different forms of tracheal loops: black swan (*Cygnus atratus*), whooper swan (*Cygnus cygnus*), white spoonbill (*Platalea leucorodia*), whooping crane (*Grus americana*), and helmeted curassow (*Crax Pauxi*). Adapted from McLelland.[1]

Syrinx

The syrinx, the sound-producing organ in birds, is located at the junction of the trachea and mainstem bronchi. Its shape, size, and location are extremely variable among avian species. For a thorough review of this anatomical structure the reader is referred to the work by A. S. King.[3] The location and structure of the syrinx explain why gas flowing through the trachea, especially during positive-pressure ventilation, can produce sound in an intubated bird.

Bronchi

The bronchial system of birds consists of three orders of branching: a primary bronchus (extrapulmonary and intrapulmonary), secondary bronchi, and tertiary bronchi (parabronchi), the latter of which, along with the periparabronchial mantle of tissue, forms the gas-exchange tissues of the lung.[4]

The primary bronchus enters the lung ventrally and obliquely at the junction of the cranial and middle thirds of the lung, and then passes dorsolaterally to the lung surface, where it turns caudally in a dorsally curved course until at the caudal lung margin it opens into the abdominal air sac.[5] Under the low columnar, pseudostratified epithelium of the primary bronchi is a well-developed internal circular smooth muscle layer and longitudinally oriented smooth muscles that respond to a variety of stimuli and can change the internal diameter of the primary bronchus.[6] Acetylcholine, pilocarpine, and histamine induce strong contraction of the bronchial smooth muscle, whereas atropine blocks their effects but has no effect when given alone.[7]

Secondary Bronchi

Any bronchus arising from a primary bronchus is a secondary bronchus, and in most birds the secondary bronchi are arranged into four groups: medioventral, mediodorsal, lateroventral, and laterodorsal secondary bronchi.[4] The medioventral secondary bronchi arise from the primary intrapulmonary bronchus close to where it enters the lung, and these secondary bronchi occupy the ventral surface of the lung.[8] The mediodorsal, lateroventral, and laterodorsal secondary bronchi arise from the caudal curved portion of the primary intrapulmonary bronchus. Between the medioventral group of secondary bronchi and the three remaining groups of secondary bronchi, depending on the species, is a section of primary bronchus devoid of secondary bronchi.[4] For a short distance the secondary bronchi have the same histological structure as the primary bronchus, but subsequently develop simple squamous epithelium.[9,10] There are single small circular bands of smooth muscle over which there is ciliated epithelium.[6] Many of the medioventral and lateroventral secondary bronchi open into the cervical, clavicular, cranial thoracic, or abdominal air sacs.

Air Sacs

Birds have nine air sacs: two cervical, an unpaired clavicular, two cranial and two caudal thoracic, and two abdominal air sacs. The air sacs are thin-walled structures composed of simple squamous epithelium covering a thin layer of connective tissue, although close to the secondary bronchial openings into the air sacs are groups of ciliated cuboidal and columnar cells.[4] The air sacs are vessel poor and as such do not significantly contribute to gas exchange in birds.[11] To a varying extent, depending on the species, diverticula from the air sacs aerate the cervical vertebrae, some of the thoracic vertebrae, vertebral ribs, sternum, humerus, pelvis, and head and body of the femur.[4]

The air sacs functionally serve as bellows to the lungs by providing tidal air flow to the relatively rigid avian lung.[12] Based on their bronchial connections, air sacs are grouped into a cranial group consisting of the cervical, clavicular, and cranial thoracic air sacs, and a caudal group consisting of the caudal thoracic and abdominal air sacs.[13] The volume is distributed approximately equally between the cranial and caudal groups of air sacs.[14] During ventilation, all air sacs are effectively ventilated, with the possible exception of the cervical air sacs, and the ratio of ventilation to volume is similar for each air sac.[14]

Muscles of Respiration and the Thoracic Skeleton

In birds, unlike in mammals, both inspiration and expiration are active processes requiring muscular activity (Table 34.1). With contraction of the inspiratory muscles the internal volume of the thoracoabdominal cavity increases (Fig. 34.3), and since the air sacs are the only significant volume-compliant structures within the body cavity, volume changes occur mainly in the air sacs.[14] Pressure within the air sacs becomes negative relative to ambient atmospheric pressure, and air flows from the atmosphere into the pulmonary system, specifically into the air sacs and across the gas-exchange surfaces of the lungs.

Gas-Exchange Component

Tertiary Bronchi

The basic unit for gas exchange is the tertiary bronchus or parabronchus and its mantle of surrounding tissue. The parabronchi, which connect the two main sets of secondary bronchi, are long, narrow tubes that display only a mild degree of anastomosing (Fig. 34.4).[8] A network of smooth muscle surrounds the entrances to the parabronchi, and this smooth muscle, upon electric stimulation of the vagus nerve, can contract and cause narrowing of the openings to the parabronchi.[15] The inner surfaces of the tubular parabronchi are pierced by numerous openings into chambers called atria that are separated from each other by interatrial septa (Fig. 34.5). The atrial openings also are surrounded by bundles of smooth muscle.[4] Since the avian lung is richly innervated with vagal and sympathetic nerves, efferent and afferent pathways might exist for controlling pulmonary smooth muscle, and with it the flow of air through the parabronchial lung, in response to a variety of stimuli.[13] Arising from the floor or abluminal surface of the atria are funnel-shaped ducts, the infundibula, that lead to air capillaries. The air capillaries measure 3 to 10 μm in diameter and form an anastomosing three-dimensional network intimately interlaced with a similarly structured network of blood capillaries.[4,5] It is within this mantle of interlaced air and blood capillaries, this periparabronchial tissue, that gas exchange occurs.

The small radius of curvature of air capillaries is associated with very high surface tensions that work against their anatomical and gas-exchange integrity, but their functional integrity is

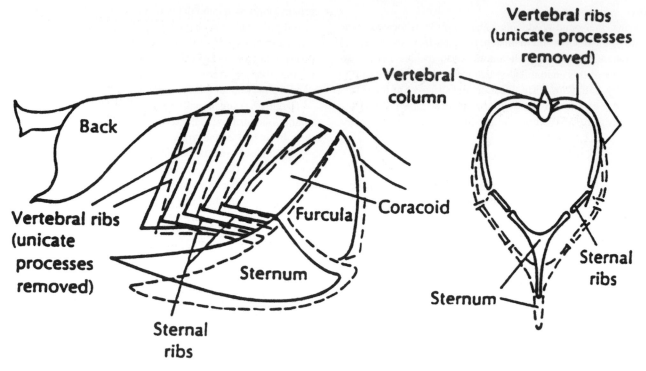

Fig. 34.3. Changes in the position of the thoracic skeleton during breathing in a bird. The *solid lines* represent thoracic position at the end of expiration, whereas the *dotted lines* show the thoracic position at the end of inspiration. From Fedde,[184] with permission.

Table 34.1. Muscles of respiration in birds.

Inspiratory Muscles	Expiratory Muscles
Principal	**Principal**
M. scalenus	Mm. intercostales interni (in 3rd & 6th spaces)
Mm. intercostales interni (in 2nd space)	Mm. intercostales externi (in 5th & 6th spaces)
Mm. intercostales externi (except in 5th & 6th spaces)	M. costosternalis par minor
M. costosternalis pars major	M. obliquus externus abdominis
M. levatores costarum	M. obliquus internus abdominis
Accessory	M. rectus abdominis
M. serratus profundus	M. transversus abdominis
	Mm. costoseptales
	Accessory
	M. serratus superficialis pars cranialis et caudalis
	M. rhomboideus superficialis
	M. rhomboideus profundus
	M. latissimus dorsi
	Mm. iliocostalis et longissimus dorsi

Adapted from Fedde.[188]

maintained by surfactant and by anatomical details that contribute to the rigidity of the avian lung. Surfactant is a lipoproteinaceous material produced by squamous respiratory cells, and it forms a trilaminar substance unique to birds.[16] Not only does surfactant cover surfaces of the atria, infundibula, and air capillaries, but it is also found in outgrowths of squamous respiratory cells that form at the abluminal surface of the cells and extend through clefts between blood capillaries to reach other air capil-

laries. In addition to this network, squamous respiratory cells appear to project processes—retinacula—that bridge to the opposite side of air capillaries.[16] All of this results in an intricate intercapillary anastomosing network that firmly anchors the air capillary system to the blood capillaries and forms the structural basis for the rigid avian lung that has a constant volume during all phases of ventilation.[4,16,17]

There are two types of parabronchial tissue in the avian lung:

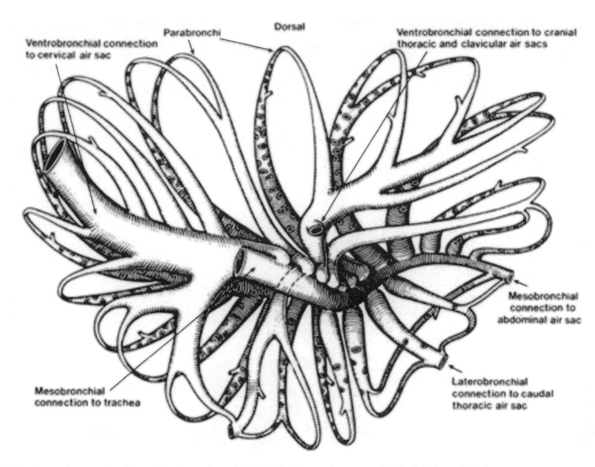

Ventrobronchial connection
to cervical air sac

Parabronchi

Dorsal

Ventrobronchial connection to cranial
thoracic and clavicular air sacs

Mesobronchial
connection to
abdominal air sac

Mesobronchial
connection to trachea

Laterobronchial
connection to caudal
thoracic air sac

Fig. 34.4. Two views of secondary bronchi and parabronchi in the right lung of a goose. **A:** Medial view of the lung.

paleopulmonic and neopulmonic. The paleopulmonic parabronchial tissue consists of essentially parallel, minimally anastomosing parabronchi and is found in all birds (Fig. 34.6A). By comparison, neopulmonic parabronchial tissue is a meshwork of anastomosing parabronchi located in the caudolateral portion of the lung; its degree of development is species dependent (Fig. 34.6B and C).[4] Penguins and emus have only paleopulmonic parabronchi. Pigeons, ducks, and cranes have both paleopulmonic and neopulmonic parabronchi, with the neopulmonic accounting for 10% to 12% of the total lung volume.[13] In fowl-like birds and song birds the neopulmonic parabronchi are more developed and may account for 20% to 25% of the total lung volume.[13] Although the paleopulmonic and neopulmonic parabronchi are histologically indistinguishable from each other, the direction of gas flow within the two types differs.

During inspiration and expiration the direction of gas flow in the paleopulmonic parabronchi is unidirectional, whereas in the neopulmonic parabronchi it is bidirectional (Fig. 34.7).[13,14] The unidirectional flow of gas through the intrapulmonary primary bronchus, the secondary bronchi, and the paleopulmonic parabronchi is governed by processes of aerodynamic valving and not by mechanical valving mechanisms.[18–25] Aerodynamic valving occurs as a consequence of the orientation of secondary bronchial and air sac orifices to the direction of gas flow, elastic pressure

differences between the cranial and caudal group of air sacs, and gas convective inertial forces.[18,20,21,23,25,26] The potential advantage of unidirectional gas flow to birds is discussed later.

A cross-current model of gas exchange describes the relationship between gas and blood flows within the avian lung. In birds there is no equivalent of alveolar gas because parabronchial gas continuously changes in composition as it flows along the length of the parabronchus.[27] The degree to which capillary blood is oxygenated and carbon dioxide is eliminated depends on where along the length of the parabronchus the blood contacts the blood-gas interface. As a result the gas composition of arterial blood is formed by the mixing of streams of end-capillary blood of widely varying gas composition.[28] In addition, blood perfusing the inspiratory end of the parabronchus can equilibrate with gas entering the parabronchus that has a high partial pressure of oxygen. The overall result is that the partial pressure of carbon dioxide in end-parabronchial gas ($PECO_2$) can exceed the arterial carbon dioxide partial pressure ($PaCO_2$). In like manner, the partial pressure of oxygen in end-parabronchial gas (PEO_2) can be lower than the arterial oxygen partial pressure (PaO_2).[29–31] This potential overlap of the ranges of blood and gas partial pressures for both carbon dioxide and oxygen, which cannot occur in the mammalian alveolar lung, demonstrates the high gas-exchange efficiency of the avian lung.[29,30]

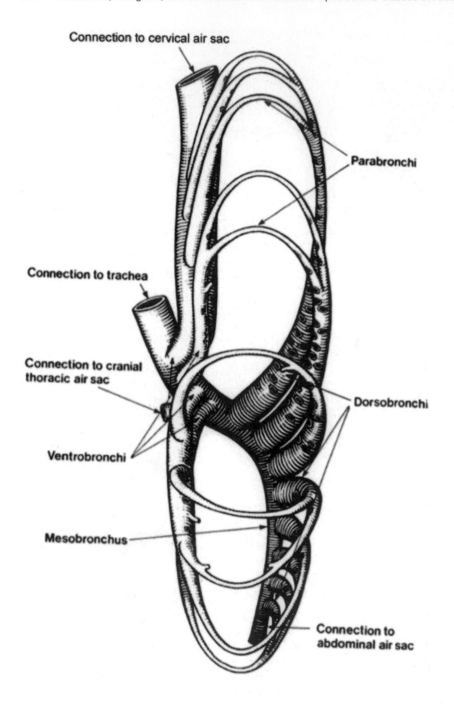

Connection to cervical air sac

Parabronchi

Connection to trachea

Connection to cranial thoracic air sac

Dorsobronchi

Ventrobronchi

Mesobronchus

Connection to abdominal air sac

Fig. 34.4. *(continued)* **B:** Dorsal view of the lung. From Brackenbury,[185] with permission.

A number of factors limit gas-exchange efficiency in the avian lung, including mismatching of ventilation and perfusion, diffusion barriers, heterogeneity within the lung, and postpulmonary shunts.[29,31] It is generally assumed that diffusion is the primary gas transport mechanism in air capillaries,[32] but small amounts of iron oxide particles (mean diameter, 0.18 μm) have been found in air capillaries, indicating that there is some convective transport of aerosol to the atria and the initial portions of the infundibula.[33] The gas-exchange efficiency of the avian lung usually is not apparent under resting conditions (Table 34.2), but becomes readily apparent under conditions of exercise or stress, such as during flight at altitude or hypoxia.[31,34–37]

Despite its relative efficiency, the avian lung does have some

limitations. By using casting methods and gas-washout techniques, the specific volume (respiratory gas volume per unit body mass) of the avian respiratory system is estimated at between 100 and 200 mL/kg (by comparison, the specific volume for dogs is 45 mL/kg).[14] However, in birds the gas volume in the parabronchi and air capillaries is only 10% of the total specific volume, whereas that in the mammalian lung is 96% of the total specific volume. Because the ratio of residual gas volume to tidal volume is so much smaller in birds than in mammals, it has been suggested that cyclic changes in parabronchial gas flow, such as reversal of gas flow, could produce significant and intolerable cyclic changes in parabronchial gas exchange somewhat analogous to breath holding.[12] The unidirectional flow of gas within

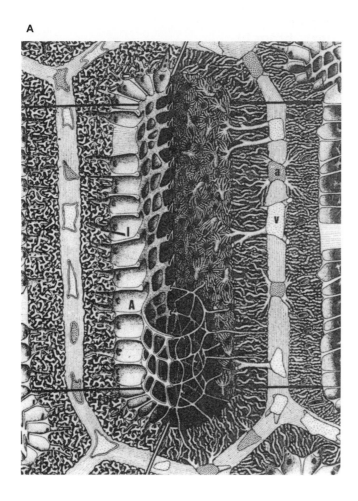

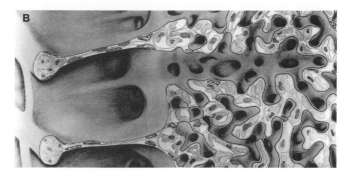

Fig. 34.5. Three-dimensional drawings of a parabronchus and an atrium. **A:** Sagittal section of a parabronchus. On the left side are atria with infundibula departing from them and the three-dimensional air capillary meshwork arising from the infundibula. On the right side within the interparabronchial septa are the arterioles (dense stippling) from which the capillaries originate and run radially to the lumen. The infundibula lie between the capillaries, which are surrounded by a well-developed three-dimensional air capillary network. **B:** Atrium and infundibulum. At the left, two of the circular smooth muscle bundles surrounding the lumen of the parabronchus are shown in cross section. The atria are separated by this septa running horizontally and vertically. Originating from each atrium, a few infundibula pass perpendicularly into the parabronchial mantle. At the right, an infundibulum is shown in longitudinal section with air capillaries arising from it at all levels. The air capillaries cross-link and interlace, making up a three-dimensional meshwork around the blood capillaries. The very thin epithelium of the air capillaries and its surfactant film are shown as a single dark line. From Duncker,[6] with permission from Elsevier Science and Professor Duncker; digital images kindly provided by Professor Duncker. A, atrium; a, arteriole; I, infundibulum; and v, venule.

the avian lung solves this problem. In addition, it appears that the volume of parabronchial gas available for gas exchange may be larger than anatomical studies would indicate and may be due to factors such as cardiogenic mixing or pulsations of blood flow within the pulmonary capillaries.[12]

Control of Ventilation

Birds have many of the same physiological components for respiratory control as mammals, such as a central respiratory pattern generator, central chemoreceptors that are sensitive to partial pressure of carbon dioxide (PCO_2), and many similar peripheral chemoreceptors.[38] Birds have a unique group of peripheral receptors located in the lung, called intrapulmonary chemoreceptors (IPCs), that are vagal respiratory afferents inhibited by high lung PCO_2 and excited by low lung PCO_2, and that provide phasic feedback for the control of breathing, specifically the rate and depth of breathing.[38–41] They are not mechanoreceptors and are insensitive to hypoxia.[42,43] This is not to imply, however, that IPCs are the sole receptors stimulated by inhaled gas containing even low partial pressures of carbon dioxide, as arterial and central chemoreceptors also are stimulated.[44]

There may be species differences in carbon dioxide responsiveness depending on the ecological niche that a given species occupies. The carbon dioxide responsiveness of IPCs in chickens, ducks, emus, and pigeons is greater than the responsiveness

of IPCs of burrowing owls, a species of bird that lives underground, where the concentration of carbon dioxide is higher than that of aboveground-dwelling birds.[45,46]

Cardiovascular System

The avian heart is a four-chambered muscular pump that separates venous blood from arterial blood. Birds have larger hearts, larger stroke volumes, lower heart rates, and higher cardiac output than do mammals of comparable body mass.[47] Birds also have higher blood pressures than do mammals.[47,48] The atria and ventricles are innervated by sympathetic and parasympathetic nerves.[48] Norepinephrine and epinephrine are the principal sympathetic neurotransmitters, whereas acetylcholine is the principal parasympathetic neurotransmitter. Excitement and handling can increase the concentration of norepinephrine and epinephrine, especially the latter, in the heart and blood.[48] This has significant implications for the anesthetic management of birds because inhalant anesthetics, especially halothane, sensitize the myocardium to catecholamine-induced cardiac arrhythmias. Hypoxia, hypercapnia, and anesthetics, the last depending on the type and dose, all can depress cardiovascular function.

The conduction system of the avian heart consists of the sinoatrial node, the atrioventricular node (and its branches), and Purkinje fibers.[49] Two groups of animals can be identified by the depth and degree to which Purkinje fibers ramify within the ven-

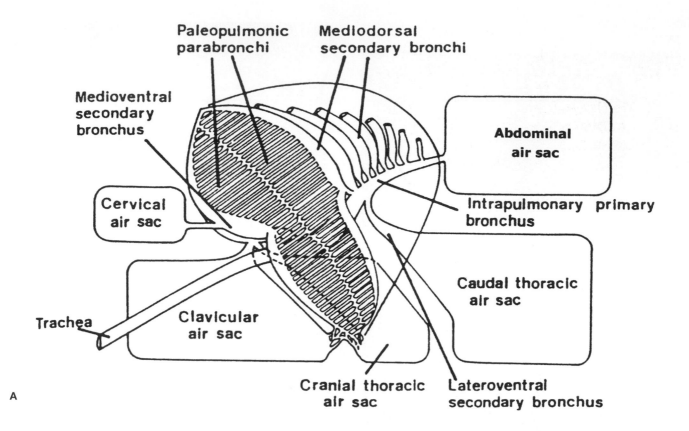

A

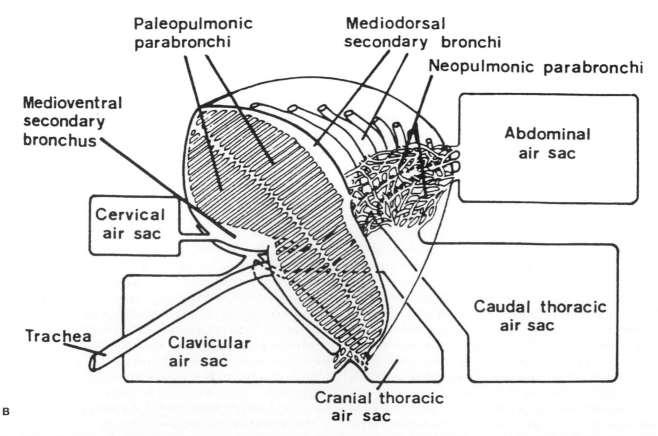

B

Fig. 34.6. Drawings of paleopulmonic and neopulmonic lungs. **A:** The paleopulmonic lung found in penguins and emus. **B:** The paleopulmonic and neopulmonic lungs found in storks, ducks, and geese.

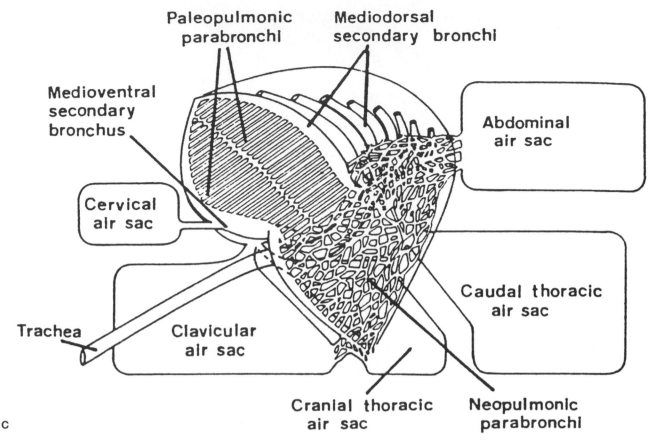

Fig. 34.6. (*continued*) **C:** The paleopulmonic lung and more highly developed neopulmonic lung found in chickens, sparrows, and other song birds. From Fedde,[13] with permission.

tricular myocardium, and the pattern of ramification is classified as type 1 or 2.[50] The pattern of Purkinje fiber distribution within the ventricular myocardium is responsible for the QRS morphology of the electrocardiogram (ECG). In birds, Purkinje fibers completely penetrate the ventricular myocardium from endocardium to epicardium, and the pattern of ventricular activation is described as type 2b, a pattern that may facilitate synchronous beating at high heart rates.[51] ECG characteristics have been described for a number of avian species, and the salient features of the avian ECG are summarized in Table 34.3.[49,51–55]

Renal Portal System

The avian kidney receives venous blood from the legs through the renal portal circulation, as well as arterial blood through the arterial circulation.[56,57] The flow of afferent venous blood, unlike in other nonmammalian vertebrates, is not obligatory, since blood can either perfuse the renal parenchyma or bypass it and enter the central circulation (Fig. 34.8). A unique valvelike structure, the shape of which ranges from a thin membrane to a thickened funnel with one or many openings depending on the species, is located within the external iliac vein at the point where the efferent renal vein joins the external iliac vein.[57] The valve contains smooth muscle innervated by cholinergic and adrenergic nerves. Epinephrine causes the valve to relax, whereas acetyl-

choline causes it to contract. When the valve contracts (closes), venous blood from the legs perfuses the kidney, but when the valve is relaxed (open), the venous blood is directed to the central circulation. The control of renal valve activity is complex, and its function is not fully understood.

Form and Function: Implications for Anesthetic Management

Air Sacs

The air sacs of birds are vessel poor and do not significantly participate in gas exchange. For this reason they do not play a major role in the uptake of inhalant anesthetics, nor, as has been suggested, do they accumulate or concentrate anesthetic gases.[58] Indeed, a study of anesthetized spontaneously breathing pigeons found that the concentration of isoflurane in the abdominal air sacs was always lower than the concentration measured at the end of the endotracheal tube.[59]

Fluidic Valving and Mechanical Positive-Pressure Ventilation

During positive-pressure ventilation, it is possible that the direction of gas flow within the avian lung may be reversed, but such a reversal does not affect gas exchange, since the efficiency of the

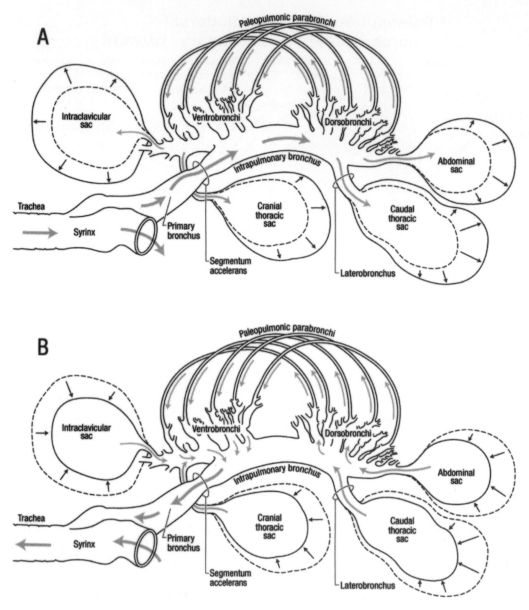

Fig. 34.7. Schematic representation of the right paleopulmonic lung and air sacs of a bird and the pathway of gas flow through the pulmonary system during inspiration and expiration (the neopulmonic lung has been removed for purposes of clarity). **A:** Inspiration. **B:** Expiration. Adapted from Fedde[13] and Brown et al.,[186] with permission.

cross-current model does not depend on the direction of flow.[14] Studies in which blood gases were collected from mechanically, bidirectionally ventilated birds did not show an adverse effect of mechanical ventilation on gas exchange.[60,61]

Effects of Anesthesia and Body Position on Ventilation

As mentioned earlier, the avian lung is very efficient at gas exchange, but this efficiency is compromised by anesthesia. A number of causative factors are probably responsible. In mammalian species, it has been amply demonstrated that injectable and inhalant anesthetics, through their effects on the central nervous system and peripheral chemoreceptors, significantly depress ven-

tilatory responses to hypoxia and hypercapnia.[62–64] Since birds have many of the same mechanisms for controlling ventilation as mammals, it seems reasonable to assume that anesthetics will similarly depress avian ventilatory control mechanisms. A number of studies have shown that inhalants depress the responsiveness of a number of peripheral control mechanisms that directly or indirectly affect ventilation.[65–67]

Barbiturates depress ventilation in birds, but birds retain the ability to respond to inspired carbon dioxide.[68,69] Furthermore, electromyograms from cocks lightly anesthetized with pentobarbital demonstrated that inspiratory and expiratory muscles of ventilation were equally depressed by the anesthetic.[70] Muscle relaxation is a feature of general anesthesia, and the degree

Table 34.2. Gas-exchange variables in awake resting birds.

Variable	Pigeon	Domestic Fowl	Pekin Duck	Muscovy Duck (*Cairina moschata*)	Common Starling (*Sturnus vulgaris*)	Black Duck (*Anas rubripes*)
Weight (kg)	0.38	1.6	2.38	2.16	0.08	1.03
M_{O2} (mmol · min^{-1})	0.35	1.09	1.67	—	0.13	0.84
f_{resp} (min^{-1})	27	23	8 to 15	10	92	27
V_T (mL)	7.5	33	16 to 98	69	0.67	30
V_E (l · min^{-1})	0.204	0.760	0.807 to 0.910	0.700	0.061	0.79
Q (l · min^{-1})	0.127	0.430	0.423 to 0.973	0.844	—	—
PaO_2 (Torr)	95	87	93 to 100	96	—	—
$PaCO_2$ (Torr)	34	29	34 to 36	36	—	—

M_{O2}, oxygen consumption; f_{resp}, respiratory frequency; V_T, tidal volume; V_E, minute ventilation; Q, cardiac output; PaO_2, arterial oxygen partial pressure; $PaCO_2$, arterial carbon dioxide partial pressure. Adapted from Powell and Scheid.[30]

of relaxation depends on the anesthetic. Because inspiratory and expiratory muscle activity is essential for ventilation in birds, any depression of muscle activity will affect ventilatory efficiency.

The position of a bird during anesthesia can significantly affect ventilation. As early as 1896, it was recognized that ventilation was reduced in birds placed on their backs.[71] A number of factors contribute to this phenomenon, not the least of which is the weight of the abdominal viscera compressing the abdominal air sacs and thus reducing their effective volume.

In summary, a number of factors regulating ventilation are affected by anesthetics. By understanding how anesthetics affect these control mechanisms, appropriate adjustments can be made in anesthetic management, thus minimizing or eliminating anesthetic-induced deleterious effects on pulmonary function in anesthetized birds.

Lung Gas Volume, Anesthesia, and the Dive Response

During anesthesia the lack of a significant functional residual volume within the lung limits the period of time that a bird can remain apneic. During induction of anesthesia in birds, especially waterfowl, apnea and bradycardia can occur and last for 3 to 5 min. Anesthetic gases are not required to elicit this response, as it can occur when a mask is placed snugly over a bird's beak and face. This response has been referred to as a *dive response*, but it is actually a stress response that appears to be mediated by stimulation of trigeminal receptors in the beak and nares, at least in diving ducks.[72–74] During the stress response, blood flow is preferentially distributed to the kidneys, heart, and brain.[75] This stress response makes safe induction of anesthesia in these birds a challenge. This response may be ameliorated by the use of premedicants such as diazepam or midazolam.

Unidirectional Ventilation: Implications for Anesthesia and Artificial Respiration

Because of the flow-through nature of the avian respiratory system, birds can be ventilated by flowing a continuous stream of

gas through the trachea and lungs, and out through a ruptured or cannulated air sac.[76,77] This same technique can be used to induce and maintain anesthesia in birds.[76,78–80] This technique also offers an effective means by which to ventilate and resuscitate an apneic bird or a bird with an obstructed airway.[81,82] In one study in which arterial blood gases were compared before and after cannulation of the clavicular air sac in ducks, the arterial blood gases (PaO_2 and $PaCO_2$) remained unchanged by air sac cannulation.[83] Despite the lack of change in blood gases, tidal volume increased significantly, and a doubling of minute ventilation was coupled with a slight but insignificant increase in respiratory frequency. However, a report involving sulfur-crested cockatoos (*Cacatua galerita*) suggests that the clavicular air sac may not be an appropriate route for air sac cannulation and delivery of anesthetic gas in all avian species.[78] In this latter study, anesthesia could not be maintained when isoflurane was insufflated through the clavicular air sac

Intramuscular Injections and the Renal Portal System

For walking birds, intramuscular injections are most commonly administered in the pectoral muscles and in the leg muscles for flying birds. Because birds have a renal portal system, there has been some concern that injections in the leg muscles might result in rapid elimination of drug through the kidneys and diminished anesthetic response.[84] The renal portal system may play an important role in those situations in which drug efficacy depends on a constant blood level, as is the case for antimicrobial drugs. In a study of pigeons that were injected with flumequine in the pectoral and leg muscles, significant differences in bioavailability were found between the two injection sites, but whether this was caused by the renal portal system or by differences in blood flow was undetermined.[85] Although the renal portal system may be an important variable in antimicrobial therapy, its effect on anesthetic drugs injected into the leg muscles is probably unimportant. Injectable anesthetics are given to effect, and if a first dose does not produce the desired result, an additional smaller dose can be given to achieve the desired effect.

Table 34.3. Avian electrocardiogram configurations and characteristics.

	Parakeet						Parrot						Pigeon						Owl					
	Iᵃ	II	III	aVR	aVL	aVF	I	II	III	aVR	aVL	aVF	I	II	III	aVR	aVL	aVF	I	II	III	aVR	aVL	aVF
P wave	+	+	+	−	±	+	+	+	+	−(80%) ±(20%)	+(20%) ±(80%)	+	+(88%) ±(12%)	+	+(43%) ±(57%)	−	±	+	+	+	+	−	−	+
VD		QS or rS	RS or QS or rS	qR or R or QR	QR or R or qR	rS or QS or RS	R (50%) QS (30%) RS (20%)	QS or rS	QS or rS	R or qR	R or qR	QS or rS	rS or qs	rS or QS	rS or QS or qR	R or qR	R or qR or QS	rS or QS						
T wave	UI	+	+	−	−	+	Var.	+	+	−	−	+	±	+	+	−	−	+	AB	+ or AB	+ or AB	− or AB	− or AB	+ or AB
MEA	−118° (−90° to −162°)						−86° (−83° to −108°)						−92° (−83° to −99°)						−102° (−81° to −127°)					

VD, ventricular depolarization; +, positive wave; −, negative wave; ±, biphasic wave; UI, unidentifiable; Var. = variable; AB, absent; MEA, mean electrical axis.
ᵃElectrocardiogram leads.

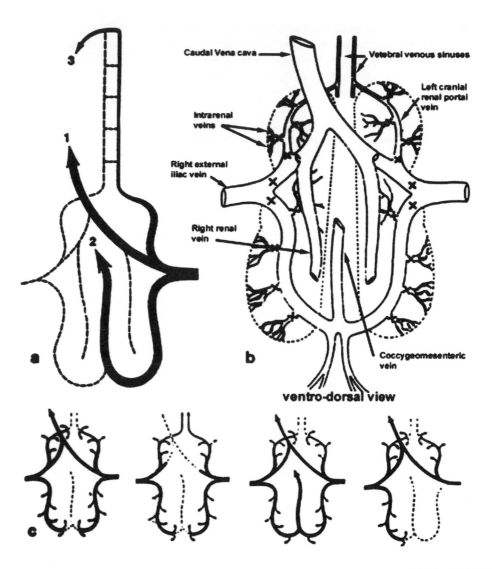

Fig. 34.8. Ventral views of renal portal shunts, portal sphincters, and variations in portal blood flow. **a:** The three renal portal shunts as marked on the left kidney: *1*, through the portal valve to the caudal vena cava; *2*, through the caudal renal portal vein to the caudal mesenteric vein; and *3*, through the cranial renal portal vein to the internal vertebral venous sinuses. Shunts 1 and 2 can function individually, or all three collectively, to bypass of the kidney completely. **b:** Numerous combinations of vasoconstriction (marked by *crosses*) result in highly varied patterns of blood flow. **c:** Selected examples of routes of blood flow through the avian kidney. From Johnson,[187] with permission.

In the figure labels: Caudal Vena cava, Vetebral venous sinuses, Left cranial renal portal vein, Intrarenal veins, Right external iliac vein, Right renal vein, Coccygeomesenteric vein, ventro-dorsal view.

General Considerations for Anesthesia

Physical Examination

Every bird should be given a thorough physical examination prior to anesthesia. A number of excellent texts describe in detail the techniques for physical examination and what to look for in specific avian species.[86–88] In general, quiet observation of a bird in its cage provides a great deal of information. A bird's awareness of, and attention to, its surrounding environment, body form and posture, feather condition, and respiratory rate all provide clues to its physical condition. Birds should be removed from their cage and examined, with particular attention given to the nares and mouth. A stethoscope with a pediatric head should be used to auscultate the heart and lungs. At the same time the sharpness of the keel should be determined because this is a good indicator of muscle mass and body fat.

Acclimation

When possible a bird should be allowed to acclimate to the clinic or hospital environment prior to anesthesia. A bird brought into a new environment will be stressed. Time allows the bird to calm down after the initial physical examination and also gives the veterinarian time to evaluate the results of blood work. It is not unusual that once a bird has acclimated to the new environment, other signs of disease may become apparent that were masked at first presentation.

Fasting

Fasting of birds prior to anesthesia and surgery has been controversial. Arguments against fasting stem from a concern that fasted birds will become hypoglycemic because of their high metabolic rate and poor hepatic glycogen storage.[89,90] However, because of the hazards associated with regurgitation in minimally fasted birds, some practitioners recommend that avian species, regardless of size, be fasted overnight.[91] A reasonable approach is to hold an avian patient off food long enough for the upper gastrointestinal tract to empty, usually overnight in large birds and 4 to 6 h in smaller birds.[92] Experience with waterfowl, cranes, and ratites also suggests that in these birds an overnight fast is not deleterious and reduces the incidence of regurgitation-associated problems. In an emergency a bird with a full crop should be held upright during induction with a finger positioned just below the mandible so as to block the esophagus.[92] Once the bird is anesthetized, the crop can be emptied by placing a finger covered with gauze over the choanal slits to prevent food from entering the nasal cavity and then milking the food contents out of the crop and esophagus.[92] At the end of anesthesia the oral cavity should be checked for and cleaned of food material to prevent aspiration.

Physical Restraint

Proper physical restraint is an important part in the handling and anesthetic management of any bird. Improper capture or restraint can cause physical trauma, including wing or leg fractures. Because birds cannot dissipate heat through the skin, they can become stressed and easily overheated with prolonged restraint. Psittacine owners often judge the expertise of a veterinarian by his or her ability to restrain their bird without bruising it around the face. In general, a bird must be restrained so that the wings and legs are controlled and not allowed to flap or kick about. For long-necked birds such as herons and cranes, the neck must also be controlled so as to avoid head, eye, and neck trauma.

Proper restraint is also necessary to protect personnel working around birds. Each avian species has its own unique and effective mechanisms for defense. Birds of prey will use their talons and inflict severe physical trauma on a handler or assistant, and the risk of infection from such wounds is quite real. Although most birds of prey do not bite, some, such as great horned owls, will use their talons and beak to great effect. Psittacines have very strong beaks that can cause severe soft tissue injury. Cranes and herons will use their long, pointed beaks in a spearing manner, and they seem to focus on handlers' eyes. Understanding the physical characteristics and defensive means of birds is crucial to provide restraint that is safe both for the bird and for the people working with the bird.

Injectable Anesthetics

Injectable anesthetics are used frequently to anesthetize birds. Among the many advantages associated with their use are their low cost, ease of use, and the rapidity with which anesthesia can be induced. In addition, expensive equipment is not required for delivery or maintenance of anesthesia, and pollution of the work environment is not an issue. However, inherent disadvantages associated with the use of injectables include great species and individual variation among birds in terms of dose and response, difficulty in delivering a safe volume to small birds, ease in overdosing by any route, difficulty in maintaining surgical anesthesia without severe cardiopulmonary depression, and the potential for prolonged and violent recoveries.[90]

Pharmacological Considerations

Pharmacological principles that apply to mammals also apply to birds. Pharmacokinetics describe the absorption, distribution, biotransformation, and excretion of a drug. Pharmacokinetics are also used to estimate dose and assess the suitability of a route of administration. The fate of a drug in the body, including protein binding, volume of distribution, biotransformation, and excretion, differs from species to species because the relationship between biotransformation and excretion is determined by metabolic factors and genetics.[93] A frequent assumption is that all birds are similar and pharmacologically belong to one group. This assumption can lead either to limited efficacy or to intoxication even among closely related species.[93] Veterinarians do have alternative methods available to determine safe, yet effective, doses for drugs used in birds. Allometric scaling and the concepts of physiological time are recognized and accepted alternatives for determining drug doses in lieu of pharmacokinetic data.[93–96] More important, the general principles underlying allometric scaling serve as a rational basis for understanding how drug doses are affected by body mass or metabolic rate. A simple, but specific, example puts these principles and concepts into a clinically relevant perspective. Dosing guidelines for the use of ketamine in birds reflect the allometric concept that drug doses are inversely related to body mass. For example, a recommended dose for ketamine in a small psittacine weighing under 100 g is 0.07 to 0.10 mg/g intramuscularly (IM), whereas a bird weighing over 500 g would receive 0.03 to 0.06 mg/g IM.[97]

There is very little information about the pharmacodynamics of drugs commonly used in birds. It is known that there can be significant differences in response among avian species given the same drug.[85,98] For example, the commercially available form of ketamine consists of a racemic mixture of the *levo*isomers and *dextro*isomers of ketamine. In great horned and snowy owls this racemic mixture characteristically induces chemical restraint and anesthesia of poor quality.[98] When great horned owls receive only the *d* form of ketamine, anesthesia induction is smoother and there are fewer cardiac arrhythmias, whereas the *l* form of ketamine is associated with inadequate muscle relaxation, with cardiac arrhythmias, and with excited behavior during recovery.[98] Whether these differences are due to differing pathways for drug metabolism among birds, production of pharmacologically active metabolites, or differences in types of receptors or receptor sensitivity is not known.

Injection Sites

Commonly used subcutaneous injection sites include the area over the back between the wings, the wingweb, and the skinfold in the inguinal region. The pectoral and thigh muscles can be used for intramuscular injections. The ulnaris vein, dorsal metatarsal vein, and jugular vein can be used for intravenous injections, as well as for catheterization. In general the right jugular vein is larger and easier to visualize than the left jugular vein and is an easy vessel to draw blood from or to catheterize.

Drugs

Ketamine, diazepam, and xylazine have been used to induce anesthesia of relatively short duration. Ketamine produces a state of catalepsy and can be given by any parenteral route. Doses range from 10 to 200 mg/kg, depending on species and route of administration. Drugs such as diazepam or xylazine have been combined with ketamine in order to prolong or improve the quality of anesthesia, to provide muscle relaxation, or to provide additional analgesia. When used alone, ketamine is suitable for chemical restraint for minor surgical and diagnostic procedures, but is not a suitable general anesthetic for major surgical manipulations.[99,100] Higher doses of ketamine only serve to prolong its action while decreasing its margin of safety.[99]

Diazepam is an anxiolytic and anticonvulsant with excellent muscle-relaxant properties. As with all anxiolytics, it lacks analgesic properties and should not be viewed as providing additional analgesia when combined with primary anesthetics such as ketamine. Diazepam can be used to tranquilize a bird prior to mask induction with an inhalant anesthetic, thus reducing the stress and struggling associated with anesthetic induction. An important feature of diazepam is that its action is brief and recovery is not prolonged.

Midazolam is a more potent, longer-acting benzodiazepine that has been used in birds. In Canada geese, midazolam (2 mg/kg IM) induced adequate sedation for purposes of radiography, and the effective sedation lasted up to 20 min after injection.[101] Mean arterial blood pressure remained stable, and arterial blood gases, which were measured in a select number of birds, were unchanged from baseline values.[101] In a study of quail (*Colinus virginianus*), midazolam at a dose of 6 mg/kg injected IM produced heavy sedation in nine of ten birds and mild sedation in one. Time to peak onset of sedation was 10 min after administration and, as judged by heart and respiratory rates, cardiopulmonary function was unaltered.[102] Midazolam appears to be a safe drug that can be used to facilitate induction of anesthesia or to provide a variable period of sedation for minor non-painful procedures such as radiography. In raptors and pigeons the effects of midazolam last for several hours after the termination of anesthesia. Although complications associated with prolonged recovery have not been reported, it can be considered an undesirable feature of any drug.

Xylazine, an α_2-adrenergic agonist with sedative and analgesic properties, has been used for minor surgical and diagnostic procedures. It has profound cardiopulmonary effects, including second-degree heart block, bradyarrhythmias, and increased sensitivity to catecholamine-induced cardiac arrhythmias. To enhance its sedative and analgesic properties, xylazine is frequently combined with other anesthetic drugs, such as ketamine. When used alone in high doses, xylazine is associated with respiratory depression, excitement, and convulsions in some species.[103] Hypoxemia and hypercapnia were observed in Pekin ducks given xylazine and a combination of xylazine and ketamine.[104]

To hasten recovery or to treat an overdose following the use of an α_2-adrenergic agonist such as xylazine, an α_2-adrenergic antagonist such as tolazoline, yohimbine, or atipamezole can be used. Turkey vultures anesthetized with a combination of xylazine and ketamine regained consciousness approximately 4 min after tolazoline (15 mg/kg) was given intravenously (IV).[105] Red-tailed hawks anesthetized with a combination of xylazine and ketamine recovered from anesthesia significantly faster after receiving yohimbine than did birds not receiving the antagonist.[106] In addition, a yohimbine dose of 0.1 mg/kg was effective and found not to cause profound cardiopulmonary changes.[106] In pigeons the effects of anesthesia with a combination of medetomi-

dine, butorphanol, and ketamine were incompletely reversed with atipamezole injected IM 1 h after the ketamine was injected; arousal occurred within 10 min of injection.[107]

Propofol has been used in a variety of birds, including chickens, pigeons, barred owls and rheas, red-tailed hawks and great horned owls, canvasback and mallard ducks, barn owls, Hispaniolan parrots, common buzzard and tawny owls, spectacled and king eiders, and wild turkeys.[108–118] Its effects are characterized by a rapid onset of action, but the speed of recovery can be variable and is species dependent. As is characteristic of the drug, it can produce hypoventilation or apnea and hypoxemia. In chickens and pigeons, propofol produced respiratory depression and apnea, and the lethal dose appears to be close to the induction dose in these species.[108,109] In red-tailed hawks and great horned owls, propofol not only decreased effective ventilation, but recovery was reported to be prolonged, with some birds exhibiting moderate to severe excitatory central nervous system signs.[111] In Hispaniolan parrots anesthetized with propofol, recovery times were prolonged when compared with isoflurane anesthesia.[116] In wild turkeys induced (5 mg/kg) and maintained (0.05 mg/kg/min) with propofol, apnea was observed for 10 to 30 s after induction, and the respiratory rate was significantly decreased at 4 min after its administration and throughout the period of infusion; two male turkeys developed severe transient hypoxemia, one at 5 and the other at 15 min after induction.[118] The average time to standing after discontinuation of propofol infusion was 11 min.[118]

Surgical anesthesia can be maintained for relatively long periods (1 to 12 h) by using intermediate to long-acting barbiturates or combinations of drugs with intermediate durations of effect. Pentobarbital can be used to produce anesthesia of several hours' duration with a dose of 25 to 30 mg/kg IV.[119] Since it requires 10 to 15 min for full onset of action, the drug should be administered initially as a bolus consisting of half the total dose and the remainder titrated over several minutes until the desired plane of anesthesia is achieved.

Phenobarbital is a long-acting barbiturate and produces anesthesia lasting for as long as 1 day when administered at 130 mg/kg.[119] Its onset of action is very slow, requiring as much as 30 min before surgical anesthesia is achieved. As is true for pentobarbital, additional doses of phenobarbital can be administered as needed to deepen the plane of anesthesia, but there is a narrow margin between anesthesia and severe cardiac depression and death.

Equithesin is a combination of pentobarbital, chloral hydrate, and magnesium sulfate. It does not produce a surgical plane of anesthesia when used alone, but does produce surgical anesthesia lasting for as long as 90 min when combined with diazepam.[58]

Local Anesthetics

These have been used in birds with unfortunate consequences, including seizures and cardiac arrest.[119] The problem is related to the small size of some avian species and inappropriate doses.[90] For example, 0.1 mL of 2% lidocaine administered IM or subcutaneously (SC) to a 30-g parakeet is equivalent to 67 mg/kg, which is a gross and toxic overdose for any animal. Lidocaine can be used in birds for local anesthesia, but the dose must not exceed 4 mg/kg, which is a dose that is difficult to achieve in very small birds unless the drug is diluted. Although local anesthetics provide sufficient local analgesia, they do nothing for stress induced by physical restraint and handling of an awake bird.

Opioids

In birds the lack of an anthropocentric type of response to pain does not necessarily mean that they do not perceive pain or that pain does not cause them distress. It may be that the behavior or physiological variables associated with pain in birds have not been adequately characterized, and there are a number of reasons for this. The problem of recognizing pain in birds has been confused by research looking at the effects of opioids in birds. In contrast to studies of the analgesic effects of opioids in mammals, the objective of opioid studies in birds has been to evaluate the effect on learned behavior, not analgesia per se.[109,120–123] The results of the few studies that have evaluated the analgesic effects of opioids in birds are conflicting. In one study, morphine produced hyperalgesia, whereas, in another, it produced analgesia.[124,125] The results of one study in chickens indicated that motor deficits associated with the administration of morphine may mask the analgesic effects of the drug.[126] More recent studies of μ opioid receptor agonists suggest that their analgesic effects can be variable. For example, fentanyl (0.01 and 0.02 mg/kg IM) was rapidly absorbed when given to white cockatoos (*Cacatua alba*) weighing 572 ± 125 g, and its elimination half-life was 1.2 to 1.4 h.[127] In the same study, fentanyl was given at 0.02 mg/kg IM or 0.2 mg/kg SC and, in terms of response to pain, there was no difference in response times between saline injection and fentanyl at 0.02 mg/kg, even though for 2 h plasma levels were at concentrations considered to be analgesic in humans.[127] The dose at 0.2 mg/kg provided significant analgesia in some birds, but this dose required a large volume (approximately 2.3 mL per 572-g bird) and caused excitement in some birds.[127]

In African gray parrots, buprenorphine (0.1 mg/kg IM), a partial μ opioid receptor agonist, had no analgesic effects when compared with saline.[128] These studies suggest that, for analgesia in birds, μ opioids have little clinical efficacy. κ-Receptor agonist opioids, such as butorphanol, appear to be effective analgesics in birds possibly because κ opioid receptors account for 76% of the radiolabeling of pigeon forebrain tissues.[129] Butorphanol has been shown to produce analgesia in cockatoos and African gray parrots.[128,130,131]

Inhalant Anesthetics

Inhalant anesthetics, especially isoflurane and sevoflurane, are considered the anesthetics of choice for use in birds, and they offer several advantages for patient management not provided by injectable drugs. Advantages include rapid induction and recovery (especially when inhalant anesthetics with low blood-gas solubility are used, such as isoflurane and sevoflurane); easier control of anesthetic depth; the concurrent use of oxygen with inhalants, which provides respiratory support; and fast recovery that does not depend on metabolic pathways. A disadvantage is that the delivery of the potent inhalants requires special equip-

ment, such as a source of oxygen, a vaporizer, a breathing circuit, and a mechanism for scavenging waste anesthetic gases, although these are widely available in veterinary practices.

Breathing Circuits and Fresh Gas Flows

Non-rebreathing circuits, such as the Bain circuit or Norman elbow, are ideal for use in birds because they offer minimal resistance to spontaneous patient ventilation. An additional advantage to the plastic Bain circuit when used in very small birds is that it is light. When a non-rebreathing circuit is used, oxygen flows should be two to three times minute ventilation, or 150 to 200 mL $\cdot$ kg^{-1} $\cdot$ min^{-1}.

Induction Techniques

The variety of techniques for inducing gas anesthesia in birds are limited only by an anesthetist's imagination. Birds can be induced with commercially available small animal masks or with homemade masks fabricated from plastic bottles, syringe cases, syringes, or breathing-hose connectors. Mask induction techniques can be used in a wide variety of birds of various sizes, from the very small up to, and including, the emu. Mask induction is unsatisfactory in adult ostriches, even if they are debilitated.

Other techniques include the use of plastic bags or chambers. Birds can be induced by inserting their heads into plastic bags (preferably clear plastic) into which oxygen and anesthetic vapor are introduced via a non-rebreathing circuit. Plastic bags have been used to enclose a bird cage completely in order to induce anesthesia in a bird that is difficult to manage.[132]

An anesthetic chamber can be used to induce anesthesia. A disadvantage to this technique is that the anesthetist is not in physical contact with the bird and cannot get a feel for how the bird is responding to the anesthetic. In addition, birds can injure themselves as they pass through stage II (involuntary excitement) anesthesia.

Whatever inhalant induction technique is used, anesthetists must take precautions to control and eliminate anesthetic-gas pollution in the work environment. If a mask is used, it should fit snugly over the bird's beak and face or over its entire head. If a plastic bag or chamber is used, it should be free of leaks. Once induction is completed, the bag or chamber must be removed from the area without "dumping" the contents into the workplace environment.

Intubation

Any bird larger than 100 g (e.g., a cockatiel) can be intubated.[133] However, unique anatomical features that can interfere with intubation, such as the median tracheal septum found in some penguins or the large bills of toucans and flamingos, must be kept in mind while planning an intubation strategy. The glottis is easy to visualize in most birds and, depending on the size of the bird, the larynx and trachea are easily intubated. Some birds are difficult to intubate either because of their unique oropharyngeal anatomy or because of their size. Psittacine species, especially the smaller birds such as parakeets, can be difficult to intubate because of the awkward location of the glottis at the base of the humped, fleshy tongue.[134]

Intubation in small birds is not without risk. Tubes with very small internal diameters can impose significant resistance to ventilation, a feature that becomes an even greater hazard when an endotracheal tube develops a partial or complete obstruction caused by a mucus plug. During anesthesia, especially when an anticholinergic is not used, mucus production can be copious, and because of the drying effects of the inspired cold and dry gases, the mucus becomes thick and tenacious. Obstruction of an endotracheal tube can be detected by observing the bird's pattern of ventilation. As the airway becomes occluded, the duration of the expiratory phase is prolonged. An artificial sigh usually confirms the presence of an obstruction because the air sacs fill in a seemingly normal manner, but they empty slowly or not at all. This problem can be corrected quickly by extubating the bird and cleaning the tube or replacing it altogether. Airway noises may be heard as the tube becomes more obstructed with mucus. An anticholinergic, such as atropine (0.04 mg/kg) or glycopyrrolate (0.01 mg/kg), reduces mucus production and minimizes the formation of mucus plugs.

During intubation, care must be exercised not to traumatize the trachea. The tube should not fit tightly, and if the endotracheal tube has a cuff, it either should not be inflated or must be inflated with extreme care. Since the trachea is composed of complete rings of cartilage an overly inflated cuff can traumatize and even rupture the tracheal mucosa and rings. Damage to the trachea may not become evident until 5 to 7 days after intubation, when the processes of healing and fibrotic narrowing of the trachea cause signs of dyspnea. When an endotracheal tube cuff is overinflated, the tracheal rings may rupture longitudinally rather than circumferentially.

Minimum Anesthetic Concentration

The minimum alveolar concentration that produces anesthesia in mammals exposed to noxious stimuli is referred to as *MAC*. It is a measure that provides a description of concentration and effect, it can be used to quantify factors that influence anesthetic requirements, and it is a term equally applicable to all inhalation anesthetics.[135] As defined, MAC is not appropriate for discussions concerning inhalation anesthesia in birds because it presupposes the presence of an alveolar lung. In birds, MAC has been defined as the *minimal anesthetic concentration* required to prevent gross purposeful movement in a bird subjected to a painful stimulus.[61]

Although the avian pulmonary system anatomically and physiologically differs from the mammalian pulmonary system, MAC values (Table 34.4) for halothane, isoflurane, and sevoflurane in birds are similar to MAC values reported for mammals.[61,136–140,141,142] This lends support to the observation that different species or classes of animals do not show large variations in effective concentrations for inhalant anesthetics.[143]

Halothane, Isoflurane, and Sevoflurane

A number of inhalant anesthetics, including chloroform, cyclopropane, ether, methoxyflurane, and halothane, have been used to induce general anesthesia in birds.[144–147] Although these drugs are historically interesting, this review focuses on halothane,

Table 34.4. Minimal anesthetic concentration (MAC) for halothane, isoflurane, and sevoflurane in birds[a].

Bird	Halothane	Isoflurane	Sevoflurane
Cockatoo	—	1.44%[130]	—
Chicken	0.85%[138]	1.25%[140]	2.21%[139]
Duck	1.05%[136]	1.32%[137]	—
Sandhill crane	—	1.35%[61]	—

Superscripts are reference numbers.

isoflurane, and sevoflurane, the most commonly used inhalant anesthetics at this time. Of these three inhalants, isoflurane is preferred for anesthesia in birds. Its introduction has revolutionized avian medicine and surgery because it is well tolerated by birds of all sizes.[97]

Halothane, isoflurane, and sevoflurane, at all end-tidal anesthetic concentrations and in a dose-dependent manner, depress ventilation.[61,136–140,148] More specifically, as the concentration of anesthetic increases, the partial pressure of carbon dioxide increases significantly. *Anesthetic index* (AI), a measure of the tendency for an inhalant anesthetic to cause respiratory depression and apnea, is derived by dividing the end-tidal concentration of an anesthetic at apnea by the MAC for the anesthetic.[149] The lower the AI is for an anesthetic, the greater is its depressant effect on ventilation. In ducks anesthetized with halothane the AI was found to be 1.51 or lower, whereas the AI for ducks anesthetized with isoflurane was 1.65.[136,137] These AI values are considerably lower than those reported for dogs, cats, or horses, and suggest that halothane and isoflurane depress ventilation more in birds than in mammals.[150–152]

The effect of halothane on blood pressure can be variable. In chickens and ducks, increasing concentrations of halothane can cause a decrease in mean arterial blood pressure, or no change.[136,138,153] In contrast, isoflurane appears to consistently cause a dose-dependent decrease in mean arterial blood pressure, possibly because of isoflurane-associated peripheral vasodilation.[61,137,153,154] Sevoflurane has been reported to decrease blood pressure in chickens, but only during controlled ventilation did the blood pressure decrease in a dose-dependent fashion, whereas this did not occur during spontaneous ventilation, probably because of the attendant hypercapnia.[139,140]

In mammals, positive-pressure ventilation depresses mean arterial blood pressure by creating positive intrathoracic pressures that compress the great vessels, thus impeding the venous return of blood to the heart. In sandhill cranes anesthetized with isoflurane, mean arterial blood pressure was actually higher during positive-pressure ventilation than it was during spontaneous ventilation.[61] Such is not the case in chickens anesthetized with sevoflurane.[140]

Cardiac arrhythmias frequently occur in animals, including birds, anesthetized with halothane. Cardiac stability is one of the perceived advantages of isoflurane and sevoflurane and is one of the reasons why they have so readily gained wide acceptance in clinical avian practice. However, in a study in which an electric fibrillation model was used to investigate the myocardial irritant effects of isoflurane and halothane, isoflurane was found to lower the threshold for electric fibrillation more than halothane.[154] The reasons for the discrepancy between clinical experience and the result of this study are not clear, but hypoventilation, which is common during general inhalant anesthesia, may be a contributing factor. Not only does hypoventilation make it difficult to control the plane of anesthesia, it can have a variety of adverse effects on cardiopulmonary function through direct or indirect mechanisms. For example, in ducks held at a constant end-tidal halothane concentration of 1.5% and in which $PaCO_2$ was varied from 40 to 80 mm Hg, unifocal and multifocal cardiac arrhythmias occurred in six of the 12 ducks.[155] The mean $PaCO_2$ at which arrhythmias developed was 67 ± 12 mm Hg and in five of six ducks with arrhythmias, the arrhythmias disappeared after carbon dioxide inhalation was terminated.[155] For these reasons, ventilation in birds should be assisted or controlled during general inhalant anesthesia.

Nitrous oxide can be used as an adjunct to general anesthesia in birds, but is not suitable for use as the sole anesthetic.[144] One study suggests that nitrous oxide (50%) may decrease the concentration of isoflurane necessary to maintain a suitable plane of anesthesia by only 11%.[156] As with other anesthetic gases and vapors, nitrous oxide is not uniquely sequestered or concentrated in the air sacs. The considerations for using nitrous oxide are the same as for its use in mammals, such as adequate pulmonary function and delivery of sufficient oxygen to meet a patient's metabolic demands. The minimum fraction of inspired oxygen that should be provided is generally accepted to be 30%. The use of nitrous oxide may pose problems in some avian species. For example, diving birds such as pelicans have subcutaneous pockets of air that do not communicate with the respiratory system, and the use of nitrous oxide in these birds can cause subcutaneous emphysema.[157]

Adjuncts to General Anesthesia

Muscle paralytics may prove to be very useful in the anesthetic management of birds, especially during long surgical procedures requiring adequate muscle relaxation and immobility. All too often a bird only appears to be adequately anesthetized, lying still on the surgical table, with complete muscular relaxation, slow respiration, closed eyelids, and relaxed feathers. The bird may accept a surgical scrub and draping, and a skin incision may be completed, when suddenly the patient displays unequivocal signs of being unsuitably anesthetized for surgery by throwing itself about on the table with flopping wings and neck.[134]

Atracurium is a nondepolarizing muscle relaxant with short duration of effect and minimal cardiovascular effects. The neuromuscular and cardiovascular effects of atracurium given to 24 anesthetized chickens have been reported.[158] The effective dose associated with 95% twitch depression in 50% of the birds ($ED_{95/50}$) was calculated to be 0.25 mg/kg, and the $ED_{95/95}$ was calculated to be 0.46 mg/kg. The duration of action for the 0.25-mg/kg dose was 34.5 ± 5.8 min, whereas it was 47.8 ± 10.3 min at the highest dose of 0.45 mg/kg. Edrophonium (0.5 mg/kg IV) reversed the effects of atracurium. There were small but statistically significant changes in cardiovascular variables in that heart rate decreased and blood pressure increased after atracurium was administered, but these changes were considered unimportant clinically.[158]

Because birds have skeletal muscles that control pupillary diameter, neuromuscular paralytics have been used to produce mydriasis. In a study of three paralytics (d-tubocurarine, pancuronium, and vecuronium) and two autonomic drugs (atropine and phenylephrine) used with or without a surface-acting penetrating agent (either saponin or benzalkonium chloride) and administered to adult cockatoos (*Cacatua sulphurea*), African gray parrots (*Psittacus erithacus*), and blue-fronted Amazon parrots (*Amazona aestiva*), vecuronium produced the most consistent and greatest pupillary dilatation in all three species with the fewest systemic side effects.[159] More recently, in juvenile double-crested cormorants (*Phalacrocorax auritus*), vecuronium alone and in combination with atropine and phenylephrine were evaluated as mydriatics.[160] The cormorants were treated with each of four drug regimens: 1% atropine; vecuronium (total, 0.16 mg/eye); atropine with vecuronium; and atropine plus 2.5% phenylephrine, followed by vecuronium. The regimen of atropine, phenylephrine, and vecuronium provided the most consistent dilation, with larger average pupil size and longer average duration; no side effects from vecuronium were observed in these birds.[160]

Monitoring

Birds must be monitored during anesthesia. Physiological variables to monitor include respiratory rate and tidal volume, oxygenation, heart rate and rhythm, body temperature, and muscle relaxation. Both respiratory rate and tidal volume should be monitored during anesthesia in order to assess the adequacy of ventilation and the depth of anesthesia. Respiratory frequency by itself can be misleading as to the adequacy of ventilation and anesthetic depth. High respiratory frequencies in an anesthetized bird do not necessarily indicate that the bird is lightly anesthetized and hyperventilating. More often, high respiratory rates are associated with small tidal volumes and a greater proportion of dead space ventilation rather than effective ventilation.[61]

Ventilation can be monitored by watching the frequency and degree of motion of the sternum or movements of the breathing circuit reservoir bag. Capnography can also be used to monitor ventilation in birds, but accurate sampling of airway gas may require adjustments in sampling flow rate or technique.[161] When monitoring ventilation in birds, respiratory pauses longer than 10 to 15 s should be treated by lightening the plane of anesthesia and ventilating the bird by either periodically squeezing the reservoir bag or using a positive-pressure mechanical ventilator. Birds can be mechanically ventilated, and although the direction of gas flow through the avian pulmonary system may be reversed, gas exchange is not affected adversely.[61,162] During positive-pressure ventilation, airway pressure should not exceed 15 to 20 cm H_2O pressure to prevent volotrauma to the air sacs. Ventilation also can be assessed by noting the color and capillary refill time of mucous membranes. The color of the cere, beak, or bill, as well as coloration on the head, can give an indication of the adequacy of cardiopulmonary function.

Pulse oximeters can be used to monitor oxygenation, but the typical pulse oximeter is designed to measure oxygenated and deoxygenated mammalian hemoglobin, not avian hemoglobin. Although pulse oximeters may track trends in oxygenation, they tend to underestimate oxygenation levels at high oxygen saturation levels and overestimate oxygenation levels at lower saturation levels because of the differences between avian and mammalian hemoglobin.[163]

The heart is an electromechanical pump, and the blood vessels are the conduits for its output. The adequacy of pump function can be assessed by monitoring mucous membrane color and refill time as noted earlier, as well as monitoring the ECG and blood pressure, and by palpating peripheral pulses. An ECG is used to monitor the electric activity of the heart. Standard bipolar and augmented limb leads can be used to monitor and record the avian ECG. To assure adequate skin contact for an interference-free signal, ECG clips can be attached to hypodermic needles inserted through the skin at the base of each wing and through the skin at the level of each stifle. An alternative technique is to attach the ECG clips to stainless-steel wires that have been inserted through the prepatagium of each wing and the skin at the lateral side of each stifle. The wire size selected depends on the size of the bird. In birds larger than 500 g, 20- or 22-gauge wire can be used. Appropriately sized hypodermic needles are used to insert the wires through the skin.

Pump function can be assessed by monitoring the pulsations of blood through a peripheral artery or by monitoring blood pressure. Arterial blood pressure in birds larger than 4 kg can be monitored directly, but this technique is not feasible in smaller birds. The Doppler flow probe is an effective device for monitoring blood flow in small birds, and blood flow or blood pressure in either moderately sized or large birds. With the Doppler probe secured in position over a peripheral artery, pulse rate and rhythm can be determined. The probe can be placed over a digital artery, and a sphygmomanometer attached to a cuff placed around the leg can be used to measure arterial blood pressure indirectly.

Body temperature should be monitored for a number of reasons. The stress associated with anesthesia and surgery is minimized when birds are maintained at or near their normal body temperature. During anesthesia, it is not unusual to see major fluctuations in body temperature, but hypothermia is the most common problem, and one that decreases the amount of anesthetic needed to maintain anesthesia, causes cardiac instability, and prolongs recovery. In well-insulated birds (feathers, drapes, and heating pads), hyperthermia can occur and also cause cardiac instability and an increased oxygen demand. Body temperature can be reliably monitored with an electronic thermometer and a long, flexible thermistor probe inserted into the esophagus to the level of the heart. Temperature monitored from the cloaca can vary significantly over time, owing to movements of the cloaca that affect the position of the thermometer or a thermistor probe. Body temperature can be adjusted by inserting or removing pads or blankets between the bird and cold surfaces, using circulating warm-water blankets (not electric heating pads), maintaining a light plane of surgical anesthesia, raising or lowering the environmental temperature, or wetting the bird's legs with alcohol.

According to a report involving Hispaniolan Amazon parrots the most effective method for maintaining body temperature was a forced-air warming device.[164] Even though such a device may not prevent an initial drop in core body temperature, it appears to maintain body temperature within a clinically acceptable range.[164]

Recovery

Precautions should be taken to protect birds while they recover from anesthesia. Birds must be kept from flopping uncontrollably, because this can lead to serious neck, wing, or leg injuries. Struggling and flopping behavior can be prevented by lightly wrapping a bird with a towel, but wrapping poses its own hazards. If a bird is wrapped too tightly, sternal movements will be impeded and breathing will be difficult, if not impossible. Wrapping can lead to excessive retention of body heat and cause hyperthermia. If a bird has not been fasted prior to anesthesia, regurgitation can occur during recovery. Keeping a bird intubated during the recovery phase helps to maintain an open airway.

Ratites

Ratites have been raised for commercial purposes for almost 100 years, and there is an extensive base of knowledge concerning the commercial management of these birds. Little information is available about anesthesia because in their native countries where the value of individual birds is low, they are not usually presented for extensive veterinary care. In general, young ratites (ostriches weighing under 30 kg and emus weighing under 18 kg) may be treated with the same considerations as given to other birds because the same problems of hypoglycemia, hypothermia, hypotension, and hypoventilation tend to occur. Hypoglycemia and hypothermia do not appear to be common in adult birds, but restraint and handling are more difficult.

Restraint

Restraint of adult ratites is challenging, so it is important to work with personnel, such as the owner, who are experienced in handling adult birds. Adult ostriches may average 114 kg and stand 6 feet tall. They can move very quickly, peck accurately at objects, and have large-toed feet with which they can strike forward. Most farm-raised birds have been handled, and information about the bird's individual temperament can be obtained from the owner or handler. As with other birds, they can be hooded to facilitate handling. Hoods can be made from surgical stockinette, and the head can be manually restrained (Fig. 34.9). Distracting the bird by allowing it to peck at a shiny object, which is held firmly to prevent ingestion, may be sufficient for completing minor procedures. The ostrich can be herded into a corner or chute by using a solid object such as a sheet of plywood or a large pad, or by holding one wing at the base of the humerus and pushing the bird in front of the handler. It is important always to work from behind or beside the bird to remain out of forward striking range of the feet. If the bird is recumbent, as can occur after sedation, it is best to transport the bird in sternal recumbency with it sitting on its hocks. This position enables control of

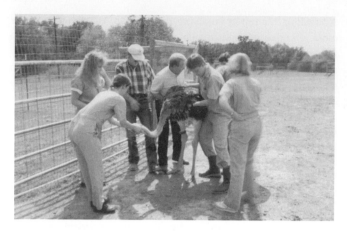

Fig. 34.9. Manual restraint, including hooding, of an ostrich.

the feet. In smaller birds, the handler may be able to restrain the bird safely by stepping over its back, grasping the hocks from behind, and folding the legs up to the body.

Injections and Catheter Placement

Intramuscular injections are best given into the large muscle mass of the thigh. Although ratites are reported to have a renal portal system, drugs are effective when given in this location.[165] Intravenous injections can be given into the jugular vein. As is generally true for all birds, the right jugular is more prominent than the left jugular. Routinely placing a catheter (14 gauge, 10 cm) in the jugular vein is recommended in order to prevent hematoma formation from repeated needle sticks. In ostriches, the branchial vein may also be used for injections and catheterization (18 gauge, 3.0 to 4.5 cm).[166] In emus, because of their vestigial wings, the brachial vein is very difficult to use, but the metatarsal vein can be used. The thick, cornified skin on the lower limbs of the ostrich makes it difficult to use the metatarsal vein.

Preoperative Assessment

Performing a good physical examination and preoperative assessment in an adult ostrich can be challenging and is often impossible. It is an unfortunate fact that a bird's state of health cannot be judged reliably by its behavior. Ill adult ostriches may appear to be quite normal and active. Some blood work is needed, preferably a complete blood count and chemistry profile. Acid-base imbalances and dehydration should be corrected before any bird is anesthetized. Normal hematologic and chemistry values have been reported.[167–170] It is important to get an accurate weight. Visual estimation of body weight is difficult because the feathers may conceal a very thin bird. Other preparations for anesthesia will depend on a bird's temperament and the facilities and personnel available. Adult ostriches and emus are routinely fasted overnight, but water is not withheld.

Preanesthetics

Although a wide variety of tranquilizers and sedatives have been used as preanesthetics in ratites (Tables 34.5 and 34.6), a caveat is necessary before discussing the effects of preanesthetics in

ratites.[170–176] Almost all of the information relating drug and effect has been generated from clinical cases. Much of the variability in response to anesthetics is owing to variations in drug requirements imposed by disease conditions, as well as a lack of controlled studies. In point of fact, only one study reports dose effects for anesthetics in ratites.[176] In addition the practical problems of restraint impose restrictions on the acquisition of clinical data. For these reasons the following should be taken as guidelines derived from clinical experience and studies.

For healthy, large ratites, premedication with xylazine (1 to 2 mg/kg IM) appears to facilitate handling, placement of catheters, and induction of anesthesia. This dose of xylazine would produce excessive cardiovascular depression in a sick bird, which emphasizes the importance of an accurate preoperative assessment. Diazepam (0.4 to 1.0 mg/kg IM) is especially effective in sick or debilitated ratites, or may be combined with xylazine in healthy ratites. Midazolam (0.4 mg/kg IM) also appears to be an effective preanesthetic.

Induction of Anesthesia

Ketamine appears to induce the most reliable and smoothest inductions in ratites, especially when combined with diazepam or following xylazine or midazolam premedication (Tables 34.5 and 34.6).[177] Intravenous injection rapidly induces anesthesia and enables anesthetists to titrate the drug dose to achieve a desired effect. However, this may not be possible in fractious birds or where there is little assistance for restraint. Doses for intramuscular injection may be metabolically scaled by using an intermediate value between passerine and nonpasserine birds.[178] Induction with tiletamine-zolazepam, either IM or IV, produces satisfactory results, but recoveries are rough and prolonged.[179] Carfentanil has been used for induction, but induction and recovery are reported to be rough.[173] In smaller ratites and debilitated birds, mask induction with isoflurane is effective and fairly smooth. In contrast, mask induction in adult ostriches, even if they are debilitated, is not recommended because induction can take as long as 30 to 45 min.

Intubation

Intubation of ratites is similar to that for many other avian species. The larynx is readily accessible, the beak opens widely, and there is no epiglottis. Although the tracheal rings are complete, portions of the trachea are collapsible, so some caution must be used when advancing the endotracheal tube. In an ostrich with a collapsed trachea, intubation was successfully performed following induction with diazepam (0.3 mg/kg IV) and ketamine (7 mg/kg IV).[180] Depending on their size, ostriches can be intubated with endotracheal tubes with internal diameters of 10 to 18 mm, whereas emus generally require endotracheal tubes measuring 9 to 14 mm. Careful inflation of the cuff is usually necessary to enable good ventilation of adult ratites. The tracheal cleft in emus (Fig. 34.1), which is more highly developed in females but present in both sexes, does not complicate intubation. The cleft does make effective positive-pressure ventilation difficult, but this problem can be overcome by placing a tight wrap (e.g., Vetrap) around the distal third of the neck.

Table 34.5. Induction drugs, procedure, body weight, ASA class, heart and respiratory rates, blood pressure (systolic/diastolic, mean) and complications in nine ostriches anesthetized at the College of Veterinary Medicine, Texas A&M University, 1992.

Induction[a]	Procedure	Wt (kg)	ASA Class	HR (beats/min)				BP (mm HG) Systolic/Diastolic Mean				RR (beats/min)				Complications
				15[b]	30	45	60	15	30	45	60	15	30	45	60	
Diaz, 0.35 mg/kg IM and IV Ket, 6.3 mg/kg IV	Enterotomy	79	4E	45	45	45	40	100/75 85	85/76 78	90/65 75	80/55 65	10	10	10	10	Cardiac arrest Hypovolemia Anemia
Diaz, 0.5 mg/kg IM Ket, 6.6 mg/kg IV	Skin graft	91	2	45	45	45	60	NA[c]	165/125 145	150/100 130	165/120 145	10	10	10	10	None reported
Iso, mask	Proventriculotomy	30	3	68	60	68	60	70/20 30	60/20 30	90/27 45	115/30 45	8	8	8	8	Anemia Blood transfusion
Xyl, 3.6 mg/kg IM Ket, 16.5 mg/kg IM	Tendon repair	112	2	60	60	58	80	NA	230/215 225	225/205 215	250/230 240	15	6	8	8	None reported
Diaz, 0.2 mg/kg IV Ket, 16.4 mg/kg IV	Proventriculotomy	95	4E	35	35	38	35	NA	NA	205/175 185	210/190 200	8	8	8	8	Bradycardia
Xyl, 3.2 mg/kg IM Ket, 16.4 mg/kg IM	Phacofragmentation	87	1	40	45	75	65	NA	NA	130/70 88	130/60 82	6	6	6	6	None reported
Xyl, 1.9 mg/kg IM Diaz, 0.1 mg/kg IV Ket, 7.1 mg/kg IV	Proventriculotomy	106	3	60	95	90	85	NA	NA	NA	110/95 105	10	10	10	10	Bradycardia in recovery
Xyl, 3.5 mg/kg IM Ket, 17.7 mg/kg IM Diaz, 0.1 mg/kg IV Ket, 2.6 mg/kg IV	Proventriculotomy	85	2	70	70	68	68	65/45 50	105/85 95	115/95 105	NA	16	16	16	16	None reported
Mid, 0.57 mg/kg IM Ket, 6.8 mg/kg IV	Cast application	88	2	65	48	48	50	NA	90/50 65	120/72 95	145/195 120	10	10	10	10	None reported

HR, heart rate; BP, blood pressure; RR, respiratory rate.
[a]Diaz, diazepam; Ket, ketamine; Iso, isoflurane; Xyl, xylazine; Mid, midazolam; IM, intramuscularly; IV, intravenously.
[b]Minutes of anesthesia.
[c]NA, data not available.

Table 34.6. Induction drugs, procedures, body weight, ASA class, heart and respiratory rates, blood pressure (systolic/diastolic, mean) and complications in ten emus anesthetized at the College of Veterinary Medicine, Texas A&M University, 1992.

Induction[a]	Procedure	Wt (kg)	ASA Class	HR (beats/min)				BP (mm HG) Systolic/Diastolic Mean				RR (beats/min)				Complications
				15[b]	30	45	60	15	30	45	60	15	30	45	60	
Diaz, 0.37 mg/kg IM Ket, 7.3 mg/kg IV	Egg bound	41	2	155	150	145	125	NA[c]	50/40 45	75/45 62	110/60 95	12	12	12	12	Hypotension
Diaz, 0.56 mg/kg IM Ket, 14.8 mg/kg IV	Proventriculotomy	27	3E	58	60	72	58	135/60 88	125/95 108	115/90 105	100/80 90	15	15	15	15	None reported
Mid, 0.4 mg/kg IM Ket, 1 mg/kg IV	Egg bound	40	2	135	125	90	122	NA	NA	88/40 52	100/55 75	14	14	14	14	None reported
Azaperone, 2.7 mg/kg IM Ket, 3.8 mg/kg IV	Skin graft	26	2	50	30	30	40	NA	NA	NA	NA	8	8	8	8	Bradycardia
Diaz, 1.0 mg/kg IM Ket, 10 mg/kg IV	Wound debridement	31	2	85	65	70	65	NA	NA	NA	NA	10	10	10	10	None reported
Diaz, 1.0 mg/kg IV Ket, 19 mg/kg IV	Tracheal endoscopy	21	4	105	110	140	142	175/105	182/125	200/130	170/130	15	17	17	15	None reported
Diaz, 0.7 mg/kg IM Ket, 6.7 mg/kg IV	Endoscopy	45	2	92	92	80	70	NA	NA	NA	NA	6	6	10	8	Regurgitation at recovery
Xyl, 4.5 mg/kg IM Ket, 21 mg/kg IM	Papilloma removal	35	2	20	30	40	40	NA	128/100 115	150/125 135	140/130 135	10	10	10	10	Bradycardia
Diaz, 0.5 mg/kg IV Ket, 7.0 mg/kg IV	Endoscopy		2	100	130	90	125	120/155 175	195/140 160	170/115 135	155/100 120	25	25	32	32	None reported
Xyl, 4.7 mg/kg IM Ket, 25 mg/kg IM	Osteotomy	17	2	40	35	35	32	128/70 95	100/50 65	100/40 48	80/40 50	12	12	12	12	None reported

HR, heart rate; BP, blood pressure; RR, respiratory rate.
[a]Diaz, diazepam; Ket, ketamine; Mid, midazolam; Xyl, xylazine; IM, intramuscularly; IV, intravenously.
[b]Minutes of anesthesia.
[c]NA, data not available.

Maintenance and Monitoring

Maintenance of anesthesia with isoflurane in oxygen and delivered from a precision vaporizer is recommended. The breathing circuit should be appropriate for the size of the ratite. Emus and ostriches under 130 kg can be maintained on a small animal breathing circuit. Larger ostriches can be maintained on a large animal breathing circuit. Ventilation of the larger ratites is recommended for two reasons. First, ventilation, as judged by respiratory rate and analysis of arterial blood for carbon dioxide, appears to be markedly depressed by anesthetic induction drugs. Second, ventilation appears to facilitate the uptake of inhalant anesthetics. Despite high vaporizer settings (3% to 5%), it may take 30 to 60 min to stabilize the plane of anesthesia. The reasons for this are not completely clear. A large respiratory volume (approximately 15 L in a 70- to 100-kg bird) certainly contributes, but ostriches may have a functional shunting system, which affects uptake of anesthetic gas.[181] Unlike flighted birds, in which increased ventilation tends to be linked to the increased muscular activity of flight, ostriches pant to cool themselves. Apparently this mechanism enables ostriches to cool themselves without effectively hyperventilating.[181]

Because of their larger size, ratites are generally easier to monitor than other avian species. An ECG should be used, with the leads positioned by attaching one electrode to the neck, one to a wing fold, and the third electrode near the keel or on the opposite wing. Standardizing the placement of leads can be difficult because of the large size, tight skin, and surgical incision sites.

Blood pressure can be measured directly or indirectly. Indirect measurement with an oscillometric technique or a Doppler flow probe can be accomplished in emus and ostriches. The cuff is placed on the leg above the tarsus over the tibial artery. In ostriches, direct arterial blood pressure can be monitored with a catheter placed in the brachialis or ulnaris artery of the wing or in the metatarsal artery of a pelvic limb (Fig. 34.10). In emus, since the wing is vestigial, the brachial artery is very small and difficult to catheterize, so the pedal artery must be used. The transducer is zeroed at the level of the keel. Normal blood pressure values for awake or anesthetized ratites have not been reported. Ostriches have been observed to have high blood pressures (Tables 34.5 and 34.6) that increase over time during anesthesia and are not the result of hypoxia, hypercarbia, or a light plane of anesthesia. In fact, if the pressures are not higher than those expected in anesthetized normal small animals, hypovolemia or anesthetic depression of cardiovascular function should be suspected. In emus, blood pressures appear to be somewhat lower than in ostriches. Tourniquet-induced hypertension has been reported in an ostrich undergoing surgery for removal of a sequestrum on the tarsometatarsal bone. Immediately after tourniquet release, blood pressure decreased from approximately 240 to 175 mm Hg.[182]

Oxygen saturation of hemoglobin can be monitored with a pulse-oximeter probe placed on the upper or lower beak. Oxygen-hemoglobin dissociation differs among species. The oxygen-hemoglobin dissociation curve for birds is qualitatively similar to that for mammals, but there are quantitative differences.[12] For this reason, the accuracy of pulse oximetry in birds

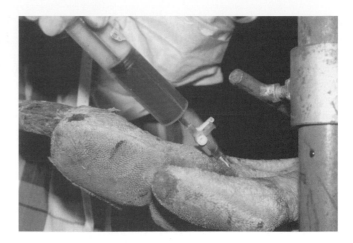

Fig. 34.10. Catheter in the digital artery of an ostrich for measuring arterial blood pressure and collecting arterial blood samples for analysis of pH, arterial carbon dioxide partial pressure ($PaCO_2$), and arterial oxygen partial pressure (PaO_2).

Table 34.7. Arterial blood-gas values from nine ostriches anesthetized with isoflurane and mechanically ventilated[a].

pH	CO_2	O_2	HCO_3	BE	TV	Beats/min
7.53	24.1	471	20	0.6	13 mL/kg	11
(0.06)	(3.9)	(97)	(2.4)	(2.4)	(1)	(3)

[a]Values were corrected for body temperature by using a Ciba Corning blood-gas analysis machine. Arterial blood samples were taken approximately 30 min after the induction of anesthesia. Values shown are mean, with standard deviation in parentheses. BE, base excess; TV, tidal volume.

Table 34.8. Arterial blood-gas values from ten emus anesthetized with isoflurane and breathing spontaneously[a].

pH	CO_2	O_2	HCO_3	BE
7.20	56.7	355	20.1	−7.0
(0.08)	(2.9)	(24)	(0)	(4)

[a]Values were corrected for body temperature by using a Ciba Corning blood-gas analysis machine. Arterial blood samples were taken approximately 30 min after the induction of anesthesia. Values shown are mean, with standard deviation in parentheses. BE, base excess.

is unknown. Clinical experience indicates that saturation of peripheral oxygen (SpO_2) and PaO_2 are generally high.

Rate and depth of ventilation can be monitored as a measure of anesthetic depth, in the same manner as for other avian species. During controlled ventilation, tidal volumes of 10 to 13 mL/kg, respiratory rates of 8 to 16 breaths/min, and inspiratory pressures of 10 to 15 cm of water have been used for controlled positive-pressure ventilation. These settings effectively ventilate or slightly hyperventilate ostriches, as judged by analysis of PaO_2 and carbon $PaCO_2$ (Tables 34.7 and 34.8). Similar settings are used for emus, but because of the greater difficulty in collecting arterial blood-gas samples, correlation with mechanical ventilation has not been reported.

Muscle relaxants appear to be effective in ratites. Both atracurium (0.3 mg/kg IV) and vecuronium (0.08 mg/kg IV) have been used during general anesthesia. Duration of effect appears to be similar to that in mammalian species. A peripheral nerve stimulator, with its electrodes placed on the proximal and distal ends of the wing, can be used to assess the block.

Recovery

Recoveries from inhalant anesthesia are generally prolonged, even when every attempt has been made to maintain a light anesthetic plane or decrease the anesthetic plane in the later stages of surgery. Weaning from the ventilator is also slow, and ventilation is often maintained with an Ambu-bag (bag valve mask), or similar device, after disconnection and while moving to the recovery area. Ratites usually undergo recovery in a darkened, padded area, or a well-bedded stall. In the ideal setting a ratite recovery box would be small and narrow, yet tall enough to allow the bird to stand, and would be padded to protect its head. Manual restraint as a means of controlling recovery of adult ratites is dangerous and is not recommended.

Complications

Many of the complications, such as bradycardia associated with visceral manipulation, do not require treatment or are manageable. It is not clear whether the high incidence of complications is typical of ratites or is due to health-related factors, since many of the birds are debilitated. Cardiac problems are particularly common and include bradycardia (heart rate under 30 beats/min), atrial and ventricular premature beats, cardiac fibrillation, and cardiac arrest.[183] Bradycardia usually responds to glycopyrrolate (0.01 mg/kg) or reversal with yohimbine when xylazine has been used. This high incidence of complications points out the need for good preoperative assessment, stabilization of the patient prior to anesthesia, and adequate intra-anesthetic monitoring.

Summary

Anesthetic management of birds is an art and a science. There is a pressing need for pharmacokinetic and dose-response studies of drugs commonly used in avian anesthesia. Without this scientific information, anesthesia will continue to be limited by anecdotal information and clinical judgment.

References

1. McLelland J. Larynx and trachea. In: King AS, McLelland J, eds. Form and Function in Birds, vol 4. London: Academic, 1989:69–103.
2. Gaunt AS, Gaunt SLL, Prange HD, et al. The effects of tracheal coiling on the vocalizations of cranes (Aves; Gruidae). J Comp Physiol 1987;161:43–58.
3. King AS. Functional anatomy of the syrinx. In: King AS, McLelland J, eds. Form and Function in Birds, vol 4. London: Academic, 1989:105–192.
4. McLelland J. Anatomy of the lungs and air sacs. In: King AS, McLelland J, eds. Form and Function in Birds, vol 4. London: Academic, 1989:221–279.
5. Duncker H-R. Structure of avian lungs. Respir Physiol 1972;14:44–63.
6. Duncker H-R. Structure of the avian respiratory tract. Respir Physiol 1974;22:1–19.
7. King AS, Cowie AF. The functional anatomy of the bronchial muscle of the bird. J Anat 1969;105:323–336.
8. Scheid P, Piiper J. Gas exchange and transport. In: Seller TJ, ed. Bird Respiration, vol 1. Boca Raton, FL: CRC, 1987:97–129.
9. Hodges RD. The Histology of the Fowl. London: Academic, 1974.
10. King AS, McLelland J. Birds: Their Structure and Function, 2nd ed. London: Bailliere Tindall, 1984:110–144.
11. Magnussen H, Willmer H, Scheid P. Gas exchange in air sacs: Contribution to respiratory gas exchange in ducks. Respir Physiol 1976;26:129–146.
12. Scheid P. Mechanisms of gas exchange in bird lungs. Rev Physiol Biochem Pharmacol 1979;86:137–186.
13. Fedde MR. Structure and gas-flow pattern in the avian respiratory system. Poult Sci 1980;59:2642–2653.
14. Scheid P, Piiper J. Respiratory Mechanics and air flow in birds. In: King AS, McLelland J, eds. Form and Function in Birds, vol 4. London: Academic, 1989:369–391.
15. Barnas GM, Mather FB, Fedde MR. Response of avian intrapulmonary smooth muscle to changes in carbon dioxide concentration. Poult Sci 1978;57:1400–1407.
16. Klika E, Scheuermann DW, De Groodt-Lasseel MH, et al. Anchoring and support system of pulmonary gas-exchange tissue in four bird species. Acta Anat (Basel) 1997;159:30–41.
17. Klika E, Scheuermann DW, De Groodt-Lasseel MH, et al. An SEM and TEM study of the transition of the bronchus to the parabronchus in quail (Coturnix coturnix). Ann Anat 1998;180:289–297.
18. Banzett RB, Butler JP, Nations CS, et al. Inspiratory aerodynamic valving in goose lungs depends on gas density and velocity. Respir Physiol 1987;70:287–300.
19. Banzett RB, Nations CS, Wang N, et al. Pressure profiles show features essential to aerodynamic valving in geese. Respir Physiol 1991;84:295–309.
20. Brown R, Kovacs C, Butler J, et al. The avian lung: Is there an aerodynamic expiratory valve? J Exp Biol 1995;198:2349–2357.
21. Butler JP, Banzett RB, Fredberg JJ. Inspiratory valving in avian bronchi: Aerodynamic considerations. Respir Physiol 1988;72:241–255.
22. Jones JH, Effmann EL, Schmidt-Nielsen K. Control of air flow in bird lungs: Radiographic studies. Respir Physiol 1981;45:121–131.
23. Kuethe DO. Fluid mechanical valving of air flow in bird lungs. J Exp Biol 1988;136:1–12.
24. Scheid P, Piiper J. Aerodynamic valving in the avian lung. Acta Anaesthesiol Scand Suppl 1989;90:28–31.
25. Wang N, Banzett RB, Butler JP, et al. Bird lung models show that convective inertia effects inspiratory aerodynamic valving. Respir Physiol 1988;73:111–124.
26. Banzett RB, Lehr JL. Gas exchange during high-frequency ventilation of the chicken. J Appl Physiol 1982;53:1418–1422.
27. Scheid P, Piiper J. Analysis of gas exchange in the avian lung: Theory and experiments in the domestic fowl. Respir Physiol 1970;9:246–262.
28. Piiper J, Scheid P. Comparative physiology of respiration: Functional analysis of gas exchange organs in vertebrates. Int Rev Physiol 1977;14:219–253.

29. Piiper J, Scheid P. Gas exchange in avian lungs: Models and experimental evidence. In: Bolis L, Schmidt-Nielsen K, Maddrell SHP, eds. Comparative Physiology. Amsterdam: North-Holland, 1973: 161–185.

30. Powell FL, Scheid P. Physiology of gas exchange in the avian respiratory system. In: King AS, McLelland J, eds. Form and Function in Birds, vol 4. London: Academic, 1989:393–437.

31. Powell FL, Hopkins SR. Comparative physiology of lung complexity: Implications for gas exchange. News Physiol Sci 2004;19:55–60.

32. Powell FL. Diffusion in avian lungs. Fed Proc 1982;41:2131–2133.

33. Stearns RC, Barnas GM, Walski M, et al. Deposition and phagocytosis of inhaled particles in the gas exchange region of the duck, Anas platyrhynchos. Respir Physiol 1987;67:23–36.

34. Faraci FM, Kilgore DL, Fedde MR. Oxygen delivery to the heart and brain during hypoxia: Pekin duck vs bar-headed goose. Am J Physiol 1984;247:R69–R75.

35. Faraci FM, Kilgore DL, Fedde MR. Blood flow distribution during hypocapnic hypoxia in Pekin ducks and bar-headed geese. Respir Physiol 1985;61:21–30.

36. Black CP, Tenney SM. Oxygen transport during progressive hypoxia in high-altitude and sea-level waterfowl. Respir Physiol 1980;39:217–239.

37. Shams H, Scheid P. Efficiency of parabronchial gas exchange in deep hypoxia: Measurements on the resting duck. Respir Physiol 1989;77:135–146.

38. Gleeson M, Molony V. Control of breathing. In: King AS, McLelland J, eds. Form and Function in Birds, vol 4. London: Academic, 1989:439–484.

39. Hempleman SC, Rodriguez TA, Bhagat YA, et al. Benzolamide, acetazolamide, and signal transduction in avian intrapulmonary chemoreceptors. Am J Physiol Regul Integr Comp Physiol 2000;279:R1988–1995.

40. Shoemaker JM, Hempleman SC. Avian intrapulmonary chemoreceptor discharge rate is increased by anion exchange blocker 'DIDS'. Respir Physiol 2001;128:195–204.

41. Hempleman SC, Adamson TP, Begay RS, et al. CO_2 transduction in avian intrapulmonary chemoreceptors is critically dependent on transmembrane Na^+/H^+ exchange. Am J Physiol Regul Integr Comp Physiol 2003;284:R1551–R1559.

42. Hempleman SC, Burger RE. Receptive fields of intrapulmonary chemoreceptors in the Pekin duck. Respir Physiol 1984;57:317–330.

43. Barnas GM, Mather FB, Fedde MR. Are avian intrapulmonary CO_2 receptors chemically modulated mechanoreceptors or chemoreceptors? Respir Physiol 1978;35:237–243.

44. Fedde MR, Nelson PI, Kuhlmann WD. Ventilatory sensitivity to changes in inspired and arterial carbon dioxide partial pressures in the chicken. Poult Sci 2002;81:869–876.

45. Hempleman SC, Burger RE. Comparison of intrapulmonary chemoreceptor response to PCO_2 in the duck and chicken. Respir Physiol 1985;61:179–184.

46. Kilgore DL Jr, Faraci FM, Fedde MR. Ventilatory and intrapulmonary chemoreceptor sensitivity to CO_2 in the burrowing owl. Respir Physiol 1985;62:325–339.

47. Grubb BR. Allometric relations of cardiovascular function in birds. Am J Physiol 1983;245:H567–H572.

48. Sturkie PD. Heart and circulation: Anatomy, hemodynamics, blood pressure, blood flow. In: Sturkie PD, ed. Avian Physiology, 4th ed. New York: Springer-Verlag, 1986:130–166.

49. Sturkie PD. Heart: Contraction, conduction, and electrocardiography. In: Sturkie PD, ed. Avian Physiology, 4th ed. New York: Springer-Verlag, 1986:167–190.

50. O'Callaghan MW. Regulation of heart beat. In: Phillipson AT, Hall LW, Pritchard WR, eds. Scientific Foundations of Veterinary Medicine. London: William Heinemann Medical Books, 1980; 303–312.

51. Keene BW, Flammer K. ECG of the month. J Am Vet Med Assoc 1991;198:408–409.

52. Kisch B. The electrocardiogram of birds (chicken, duck, pigeon). Exp Med Surg 1951;9:103–124.

53. Lumeij JT, Stokhof AA. Electrocardiogram of the racing pigeon (Columba livia domestica). Res Vet Sci 1985;38:275–278.

54. Zenoble RD. Electrocardiography in the parakeet and parrot. Compend Contin Educ 1981;3:711–716.

55. Zenoble RD, Graham DL. Electrocardiography of the parakeet, parrot and owl. In: Proceedings of the Annual Meeting of the American Association of Zoo Veterinarians, 1979:42–45.

56. Palmore WP, Ackerman N. Blood flow in the renal portal circulation of the turkey: Effect of epinephrine. Am J Vet Res 1985;46:1589–1592.

57. Burrows ME, Braun EJ, Duckles SP. Avian renal portal valve: A reexamination of its innervation. Am J Physiol 1983;245:H628–634.

58. Christensen J, Fosse RT, Halvorsen OJ, et al. Comparison of various anesthetic regimens in the domestic fowl. Am J Vet Res 1987; 48:1649–1657.

59. Hellebrekers LJ, Sap R, van Wandelen RM. Spontaneous ventilation versus intermittent positive pressure ventilation in birds. In: Fourth International Congress of Veterinary Anaesthesia, August 25–30, Utrecht, The Netherlands, 1991:81.

60. Piiper J, Drees F, Scheid P. Gas exchange in the domestic fowl during spontaneous breathing and artificial ventilation. Respir Physiol 1970;9:234–245.

61. Ludders JW, Rode J, Mitchell GS. Isoflurane anesthesia in sandhill cranes (Grus canadensis): Minimal anesthetic concentration and cardiopulmonary dose-response during spontaneous and controlled breathing. Anesth Analg 1989;68:511–516.

62. Pavlin EG, Hornbein TF. Anesthesia and the control of ventilation. In: Cherniak NS, Widdicombe JG, eds. Handbook of Physiology. Sect 3: The Respiratory System. Vol 2: Control of Breathing. Bethesda, MD: American Physiological Society, 1986:793–813.

63. Hirshman CA, McCullough RE, Cohen PJ, et al. Hypoxic ventilatory drive in dogs during thiopental, ketamine, or pentobarbital anesthesia. Anesthesiology 1975;43:628–634.

64. Hirshman CA, McCullough RE, Cohen PJ, et al. Depression of hypoxic ventilatory response by halothane, enflurane and isoflurane in dogs. Br J Anaesth 1977;49:957–963.

65. Bagshaw RJ, Cox RH. Baroreceptor control of heart rate in chickens (Gallus domesticus). Am J Vet Res 1986;47:293–295.

66. Molony V. Classification of vagal afferents firing in phase with breathing in Gallus domesticus. Respir Physiol 1974;22:57–76.

67. Pizarro J, Ludders JW, Douse MA, et al. Halothane effects on ventilatory responses to changes in intrapulmonary CO_2 in geese. Respir Physiol 1990;82:337–347.

68. Osborne JL, Mitchell GS. Ventilatory responses during arterial homeostasis of PCO_2 at low levels of inspired carbon dioxide. In: Piiper J, ed. Respiratory Function in Birds, Adult and Embryonic. Berlin: Springer-Verlag, 1978:168–174.

69. Osborne JL, Mitchell GS. Regulation of arterial PCO_2 during inhalation of CO_2 in chickens. Respir Physiol 1977;31:357–364.

70. Fedde MR, Burger RE, Kitchell RL. Electromyographic studies of the effects of bodily position and anesthesia on the activity of the respiratory muscles of the domestic cock. Poult Sci 1964;43: 839–846.

71. King AS, Payne DC. Normal breathing and the effects of posture in *Gallus domesticus*. J Physiol (Lond) 1964;174:340–347.

72. Woakes AJ. Metabolism in diving birds: Studies in the laboratory and the field. Can J Zool 1988;66:138–141.

73. Butler PJ. The exercise response and the "classical" diving response during natural submersion in birds and mammals. Can J Zool 1988;66:29–39.

74. Jones DR, Furilla RA, Heieis MRA, et al. Forced and voluntary diving in ducks: Cardiovascular adjustments and their control. Can J Zool 1988;66:75–83.

75. Jones DR, Bryan RM Jr, West NH, et al. Regional distribution of blood flow during diving in the duck (*Anas platyrhynchos*). Can J Zool 1979;57:995–1002.

76. Burger RE, Lorenz FW. Artificial respiration in birds by unidirectional air flow. Poult Sci 1960;39:236–237.

77. Burger RE, Meyer M, Graf W, et al. Gas exchange in the parabronchial lung of birds: Experiments in unidirectionally ventilated ducks. Respir Physiol 1979;36:19–37.

78. Jaensch SM, Cullen L, Raidal SR. Air sac functional anatomy of the sulphur-crested cockatoo (*Cacatua galerita*) during isoflurane anesthesia. J Avian Med Surg 2002;16:2–9.

79. Whittow GC, Ossorio N. A new technic for anesthetizing birds. Lab Anim Care 1970;20:651–656.

80. Wijnberg ID, Lagerweij E, Zwart P. Inhalation anaesthesia in birds through the abdominal air sac, using a unidirectional, continuous flow. In: Fourth International Congress of Veterinary Anaesthesia, August 25–30, 1991, Utrecht, The Netherlands, 1991:80.

81. Harrison GJ. Selected surgical procedures. In: Harrison GJ, Harrison LR, eds. Clinical Avian Medicine and Surgery. Philadelphia: WB Saunders, 1986:577–595.

82. Rosskopf WJ. Surgery of the avian respiratory system. In: Proceedings of the American College of Veterinary Surgeons, 1988: 373–382.

83. Rode JA, Bartholow S, Ludders JW. Ventilation through an air sac cannula during tracheal obstruction in ducks. J Assoc Avian Vet 1990;4:98–102.

84. Clark CH, Thomas JE, Milton JL, et al. Plasma concentrations of chloramphenicol in birds. Am J Vet Res 1982;43:1249–1253.

85. Dorrestein GM, van Miert AS. Pharmacotherapeutic aspects of medication of birds. J Vet Pharmacol Ther 1988;11:33–44.

86. Fowler ME, Miller RE. Zoo and Wild Animal Medicine, 5th ed. Philadelphia: WB Saunders, 2003.

87. Cooper JE. Birds of Prey: Health and Disease, 3rd ed. Oxford: Blackwell Science, 2002.

88. Ritchie BW, Harrison GJ, Harrison LR. Avian Medicine: Principles and Application. Lake Worth, FL: Wingers, 1994.

89. Altman RB. Avian anesthesia. Compend Contin Educ 1980;2: 38–42.

90. Franchetti DR, Klide AM. Restraint and anesthesia. In: Fowler ME, ed. Zoo and Wild Animal Medicine. Philadelphia: WB Saunders, 1978:359–364.

91. Harrison GJ. Pre-anesthetic fasting recommended. J Assoc Avian Vet 1991;5:126.

92. Sinn LC. Anesthesiology. In: Zantop DW, ed. Avian Medicine: Principles and Application, abridged ed. Lake Worth, FL: Wingers, 1997:589–599.

93. Dorrestein GM. The pharmacokinetics of avian therapeutics. Vet Clin North Am Small Anim Pract 1991;21:1241–1264.

94. Boxenbaum H. Interspecies scaling, allometry, physiological time, and the ground plan of pharmacokinetics. J Pharmacokinet Biopharm 1982;10:201–227.

95. Schmidt-Nielsen K. Scaling: Why Is Animal Size So Important? Cambridge: Cambridge University Press, 1991.

96. Sedgwick CJ, Pokras MA. Extrapolating rational drug doses and treatment periods by allometric scaling. In: Proceedings of the 55th Annual Meeting of the American Animal Hospital Association, 1988:156–157.

97. McDonald S. Common anesthetic dosages for use in psittacine birds. J Assoc Avian Vet 1989;3:186–187.

98. Redig PT, Larson AA, Duke GE. Response of great horned owls given the optical isomers of ketamine. Am J Vet Res 1984;45:125–127.

99. McGrath CJ, Lee JC, Campbell VL. Dose-response anesthetic effects of ketamine in the chicken. Am J Vet Res 1984;45:531–534.

100. Salerno A, van Tienhoven A. The effect of ketamine on heart rate, respiration rate and EEG of white leghorn hens. Comp Biochem Physiol [C] 1976;55:69–75.

101. Valverde A, Honeyman VL, Dyson DH, et al. Determination of a sedative dose and influence of midazolam on cardiopulmonary function in Canada geese. Am J Vet Res 1990;51:1071–1074.

102. Day TK, Roge CK. Evaluation of sedation in quail induced by use of midazolam and reversed by use of flumazenil. J Am Vet Med Assoc 1996;209:969–971.

103. Samour JH, Jones DM, Knight JA, et al. Comparative studies of the use of some injectable anaesthetic agents in birds. Vet Rec 1984; 115:6–11.

104. Ludders JW, Rode J, Mitchell GS, et al. Effects of ketamine, xylazine, and a combination of ketamine and xylazine in Pekin ducks. Am J Vet Res 1989;50:245–249.

105. Allen JL, Oosterhuis JE. Effect of tolazoline on xylazine-ketamine–induced anesthesia in turkey vultures. J Am Vet Med Assoc 1986;189:1011–1012.

106. Degernes LA, Kreeger TJ, Mandsager R, et al. Ketamine-xylazine anesthesia in red-tailed hawks with antagonism by yohimbine. J Wildl Dis 1988;24:322–326.

107. Atalan G, Uzun M, Demirkan I, et al. Effect of medetomidine-butorphanol-ketamine anaesthesia and atipamezole on heart and respiratory rate and cloacal temperature of domestic pigeons. J Vet Med [A] 2002;49:281–285.

108. Lukasik VM, Gentz EJ, Erb HN, et al. Cardiopulmonary effects of propofol anesthesia in chickens (*Gallus gallus*). J Assoc Avian Vet 1997;11:93–97.

109. Fitzgerald G, Cooper JE. Preliminary studies on the use of propofol in the domestic pigeon (*Columba livia*). Res Vet Sci 1990;49: 334–338.

110. Clippinger TL, Platt SR, Bennett RA, et al. Electrodiagnostic evaluation of peripheral nerve function in rheas and barred owls. Am J Vet Res 2000;61:469–472.

111. Hawkins MG, Wright BD, Pascoe PJ, et al. Pharmacokinetics and anesthetic and cardiopulmonary effects of propofol in red-tailed hawks (*Buteo jamaicensis*) and great horned owls (*Bubo virginianus*). Am J Vet Res 2003;64:677–683.

112. Machin KL, Caulkett NA. Evaluation of isoflurane and propofol anesthesia for intraabdominal transmitter placement in nesting female canvasback ducks. J Wildl Dis 2000;36:324–334.

113. Machin KL, Caulkett NA. Cardiopulmonary effects of propofol and a medetomidine-midazolam-ketamine combination in mallard ducks. Am J Vet Res 1998;59:598–602.

114. Mama KR, Phillips LG Jr, Pascoe PJ. Use of propofol for induction and maintenance of anesthesia in a barn owl (*Tyto alba*) undergoing tracheal resection. J Zoo Wildl Med 1996;27:397–401.

115. Mikaelian J. Intravenously administered propofol for anesthesia of the common buzzard (*Buteo buteo*), the tawny owl (*Strix aluco*),

and the barn owl (*Tyto alba*). In: Proceedings of the First Conference of the European Committee of the Association of Avian Veterinarians, Vienna, 1991:97–101.

116. Langlois I, Harvey RC, Jones MP, et al. Cardiopulmonary and anesthetic effects of isoflurane and propofol in Hispaniolan Parrots (*Amazona ventralis*). J Avian Med Surg 2003;17:4–10.

117. Mulcahy DM, Tuomi P, Larsen SR. Differential mortality for male spectacled eiders (*Somateria fischeri*) and king eiders (*Somateria spectabilis*) subsequent to anesthesia with propofol, bupivacaine, and ketoprofen. J Avian Med Surg 2003;17:117–123.

118. Schumacher J, Citino SB, Hernandez K, et al. Cardiopulmonary and anesthetic effects of propofol in wild turkeys. Am J Vet Res 1997;58:1014–1017.

119. Fedde MR. Drugs used for avian anesthesia: A review. Poult Sci 1978;57:1376–1399.

120. Leander JD, McMillan DE. Meperidine effects on schedule-controlled responding. J Pharmacol Exp Ther 1977;201:434–443.

121. Leander JD. Opioid agonist and antagonist behavioural effects of buprenorphine. Br J Pharmacol 1983;78:607–615.

122. France CP, Woods JH. Morphine, saline and naltrexone discrimination in morphine-treated pigeons. J Pharmacol Exp Ther 1987; 242:195–202.

123. Herling S, Valentino RJ, Solomon RE, et al. Narcotic discrimination in pigeons: Antagonism by naltrexone. Eur J Pharmacol 1984;105:137–142.

124. Hughes RA. Codeine analgesic and morphine hyperalgesic effects on thermal nociception in domestic fowl. Pharmacol Biochem Behav 1990;35:567–570.

125. Bardo MT, Hughes RA. Shock-elicited flight response in chickens as an index of morphine analgesia [Brief communication]. Pharmacol Biochem Behav 1978;9:147–149.

126. Rager DR, Gallup GG Jr. Apparent analgesic effects of morphine in chickens may be confounded by motor deficits. Physiol Behav 1986;37:269–272.

127. Hoppes S, Flammer K, Hoersch L, et al. Disposition and analgesic effects of fentanyl in white cockatoos (*Cacatua alba*). J Avian Med Surg 2003;17:124–130.

128. Paul-Murphy JR, Brunson DB, Miletic V. Analgesic effects of butorphanol and buprenorphine in conscious African grey parrots (*Psittacus erithacus erithacus* and *Psittacus erithacus timneh*). Am J Vet Res 1999;60:1218–1221.

129. Mansour A, Khachaturian H, Lewis ME, et al. Anatomy of CNS opioid receptors. Trends Neurosci 1988;11:308–314.

130. Curro TG, Brunson DB, Paul-Murphy J. Determination of the ED50 of isoflurane and evaluation of the isoflurane-sparing effect of butorphanol in cockatoos (*Cacatua* spp.). Vet Surg 1994;23:429–433.

131. Paul-Murphy J, Ludders JW. Avian analgesia. Vet Clin North Am Exot Anim Pract 2001;4:35–45.

132. Bednarski RM, Ludders JW, LeBlanc PH, et al. Isoflurane–nitrous oxide–oxygen anesthesia in an Andean condor. J Am Vet Med Assoc 1985;187:1209–1210.

133. Klide AM. Avian anesthesia. Vet Clin North Am 1973;3:175–186.

134. Sedgwick CJ. Anesthesia of caged birds. In: Kirk R, ed. Current Veterinary Therapy VII. Philadelphia: WB Saunders, 1980: 653–656.

135. Eger EI II. Anesthetic Uptake and Action. Baltimore: Williams and Wilkins, 1974.

136. Ludders JW. Minimal anesthetic concentration and cardiopulmonary dose-response of halothane in ducks. Vet Surg 1992;21: 319–324.

137. Ludders JW, Mitchell GS, Rode J. Minimal anesthetic concentration and cardiopulmonary dose response of isoflurane in ducks. Vet Surg 1990;19:304–307.

138. Ludders JW, Mitchell GS, Schaefer SL. Minimum anesthetic dose and cardiopulmonary dose response for halothane in chickens. Am J Vet Res 1988;49:929–932.

139. Naganobu K, Fujisawa Y, Ohde H, et al. Determination of the minimum anesthetic concentration and cardiovascular dose response for sevoflurane in chickens during controlled ventilation. Vet Surg 2000;29:102–105.

140. Naganobu K, Ise K, Miyamoto T, et al. Sevoflurane anaesthesia in chickens during spontaneous and controlled ventilation. Vet Rec 2003;152:45–48.

141. Eger EII. Isoflurane: A Compendium and Reference, 2nd ed. Madison, WI: Anaquest, 1985.

142. Steffey EP. Inhalation anesthetics. In: Thurmon JC, Tranquilli WJ, Benson GJ, eds. Lumb & Jones' Veterinary Anesthesia, 3rd ed. Baltimore: Williams and Wilkins, 1996:297–329.

143. Quasha AL, Eger EI II, Tinker JH. Determinations and applications of MAC. Anesthesiology 1980;53:315–334.

144. Arnall L. Anaesthesia and surgery in cage and aviary birds (I). Vet Rec 1961;73:139–142.

145. Dolphin RE, Olsen DE. Anesthesia in the companion bird. Vet Med Small Anim Clin 1977;72:1761–1765.

146. Gandal CP. Avian anesthesia. Fed Proc 1969;28:1533–1534.

147. Myers RE, Stettner LJ. Safe and reliable general anesthesia in birds. Physiol Behav 1969;4:277.

148. Korbel R. Comparative investigations on inhalation anesthesia with isoflurane (Forene) and sevoflurane (SEVOrane) in racing pigeons (*Columba livia* Gmel., 1789, var. *domestica*) and presentation of a reference anesthesia protocol for birds [in German]. Tierarztl Prax Ausg K Klientiere Heimtiere 1998;26:211–223.

149. Regan MJ, Eger EI II. Effect of hypothermia in dogs on anesthetizing and apneic doses of inhalation agents: Determination of the anesthetic index (Apnea/MAC). Anesthesiology 1967;28: 689–700.

150. Steffey EP, Howland D Jr. Isoflurane potency in the dog and cat. Am J Vet Res 1977;38:1833–1836.

151. Steffey EP, Howland D Jr. Potency of enflurane in dogs: Comparison with halothane and isoflurane. Am J Vet Res 1978;39: 573–577.

152. Steffey EP, Howland D Jr, Giri S, et al. Enflurane, halothane, and isoflurane potency in horses. Am J Vet Res 1977;38:1037–1039.

153. Goelz MF, Hahn AW, Kelley ST. Effects of halothane and isoflurane on mean arterial blood pressure, heart rate, and respiratory rate in adult Pekin ducks. Am J Vet Res 1990;51:458–460.

154. Greenlees KJ, Clutton RE, Larsen CT, et al. Effect of halothane, isoflurane, and pentobarbital anesthesia on myocardial irritability in chickens. Am J Vet Res 1990;51:757–758.

155. Naganobu K, Hagio M, Sonoda T, et al. Arrhythmogenic effect of hypercapnia in ducks anesthetized with halothane. Am J Vet Res 2001;62:127–129.

156. Korbel R, Burike S, Erhardt W, et al. Effect of nitrous oxide application in racing pigeons (*Columba livia* Gmel., 1789, var. *dom.*): A study using the airsac perfusion technique. Isr J Vet Med 1996; 51:133–139.

157. Reynolds WT. Unusual anaesthetic complication in a pelican. Vet Rec 1983;113:204.

158. Nicholson A, Ilkiw JE. Neuromuscular and cardiovascular effects of atracurium in isoflurane-anesthetized chickens. Am J Vet Res 1992;53:2337–2342.

159. Ramer JC, Paul-Murphy J, Brunson D, et al. Effects of mydriatic agents in cockatoos, African gray parrots, and Blue-fronted Amazon parrots. J Am Vet Med Assoc 1996;208:227–230.

160. Loerzel SM, Smith PJ, Howe A, et al. Vecuronium bromide, phenylephrine and atropine combinations as mydriatics in juvenile double-crested cormorants (*Phalacrocorax auritus*). Vet Ophthalmol 2002;5:149–154.

161. Edling TM, Degernes LA, Flammer K, et al. Capnographic monitoring of anesthetized African grey parrots receiving intermittent positive pressure ventilation. J Am Vet Med Assoc 2001;219:1714–1718.

162. Pettifer GR, Cornick-Seahorn J, Smith JA, et al. The comparative cardiopulmonary effects of spontaneous and controlled ventilation by using the Hallowell EMC Anesthesia WorkStation in Hispaniolan Amazon parrots (*Amazona ventralis*). J Avian Med Surg 2002;16:268–276.

163. Schmitt PM, Gobel T, Trautvetter E. Evaluation of pulse oximetry as a monitoring method in avian anesthesia. J Avian Med Surg 1998;12:91–99.

164. Rembert MS, Smith JA, Hosgood G, et al. Comparison of traditional thermal support devices with the forced-air warmer system in anesthetized Hispaniolan Amazon parrots (*Amazona ventralis*). J Avian Med Surg 2001;15:187–193.

165. Fowler ME. Comparative clinical anatomy of ratites. J Zoo Wildl Med 1991;22:204–227.

166. Bezuidenhout AJ, Coetzer DJ. The major blood vessels of the wing of the ostrich (*Struthio camelus*). Onderstepoort J Vet Res 1986;53:201–203.

167. Levi A, Perelman B, Waner T, et al. Haematological parameters of the ostrich (*Struthio camelus*). Avian Pathol 1989;18:321–327.

168. Levy A, Perelman B, Waner T, et al. Reference blood chemical values in ostriches (*Struthio camelus*). Am J Vet Res 1989;50:1548–1550.

169. Palomeque J, Pinto D, Viscor G. Hematologic and blood chemistry values of the Masai ostrich (*Struthio camelus*). J Wildl Dis 1991;27:34–40.

170. Stoskopf MJ, Beall FB, Ensley PK, et al. Immobilization of large ratites: Blue necked ostrich and double wattled cassowary with hematologic and serum chemistry data. J Zoo Anim Med 1982;13:160–166.

171. Jacobson ER, Ellison GW, McMurphy R, et al. Ventriculostomy for removal of multiple foreign bodies in an ostrich. J Am Vet Med Assoc 1986;189:1117–1119.

172. Fowler JD, Bauck L, Cribb PH, et al. Surgical correction of tibiotarsal rotation in an emu. Companion Anim Pract 1987;1:26–30.

173. Cornick JL, Jensen J. Anesthetic management of ostriches. J Am Vet Med Assoc 1992;200:1661–1666.

174. Ensley DK, Launer DP, Blasingame JP. General anesthesia and surgical removal of a tumor-like growth from the foot of a double-wattled cassowary. J Zoo Anim Med 1984;15:35–37.

175. Honnas CM, Jensen J, Cornick JL, et al. Proventriculotomy to relieve foreign body impaction in ostriches. J Am Vet Med Assoc 1991;199:461–465.

176. van Heerden J, Keffen RH. A preliminary investigation into the immobilising potential of a tiletamine/zolazepam mixture, metomidate, a metomidate and azaperone combination and medetomidine in ostriches (*Struthio camelus*). J S Afr Vet Assoc 1991;62:114–117.

177. Grubb B. Use of ketamine to restrain and anesthetize emus. Vet Med Small Anim Clin 1983;78:247–248.

178. Sedgwick CJ, Pokras MA, Kaufman G. Metabolic scaling: Using estimated energy costs to extrapolate drug doses between different species and different individuals of diverse body sizes. In: Proceedings of the Annual Meeting of the American Association of Zoo Veterinarians, 1990:249–254.

179. Schobert E. Telazol use in wild and exotic animals. Vet Med 1987;82:1080–1088.

180. Jones JH. Pulmonary blood flow distribution in panting ostriches. J Appl Physiol 1982;53:1411–1417.

181. Schmidt-Nielsen K. Temperature regulation and respiration in the ostrich. Condor 1969;71:341–352.

182. Cornick SJL, Martin GS, Tulley TN, et al. Tourniquet induced hypertension in an ostrich. J Am Vet Med Assoc 1995;207:344–346.

183. Matthews NS, Burba DJ, Cornick JL. Premature ventricular contractions and apparent hypertension during anesthesia in an ostrich. J Am Vet Med Assoc 1991;198:1959–1961.

184. Fedde MR. Respiration. In: Sturkie PD, ed. Avian Physiology, 4th ed. New York: Springer-Verlag, 1986:191–220.

185. Brackenbury JH. Ventilation of the lung-air sac system. In: Seller TJ, ed. Bird Respiration, vol 1. Boca Raton, FL: CRC, 1987:39–69.

186. Brown RE, Brain JD, Wang N. The avian respiratory system: A unique model for studies of respiratory toxicosis and for monitoring air quality. Environ Health Perspect 1997;105:188–200.

187. Johnson OW. Urinary organs. In: King AS, McLelland J, eds. Form and Function in Birds, vol 1. London: Academic, 1979:183–235.

188. Fedde MR. Respiratory muscles. In: Seller TJ, ed. Bird Respiration, vol 1. Boca Raton, FL: CRC, 1987:3–37.

Chapter 35
Reptiles, Amphibians, and Fish

Darryl J. Heard and Mark D. Stetter

Introduction

Successful herptile (reptile and amphibian) anesthesia requires an understanding of anatomy and physiology in health and disease.[1,2,3] Most herptiles are physiologically resilient, capable of surviving severe hypoxemia and hypothermia that would rapidly kill other vertebrates.[1,3] Survival into the immediate postoperative period is an inadequate measure of the safety of an anesthetic regimen. Physiological disruptions incurred by poor drug selection and anesthetic technique may not be immediately obvious.

As in all animals, physical restraint alone is inhumane for performing painful procedures even if the animal does not physically respond. During strenuous exercise, the muscles of reptiles and amphibians rapidly produce large amounts of lactic acid due to anaerobic metabolism.[4] Lactic acidemia occurs in apparently immobile, bound reptiles due to isometric muscle contractions and has been incriminated in mortality of translocated crocodiles.[4] The use of hypothermia for immobilization is controversial. It is questionable whether it induces altered mentation sufficient for painful diagnostic and surgical procedures; furthermore, hypothermia impairs drug metabolism, digestion, and immune function.[5]

Biology, Anatomy, and Physiology

Herptile biology (herpetology) is comprehensively described by Pough et al. and Zug et al.[1,3] The approximately 4600 living amphibian species are divided into the Gymnophiona (caecilians, 165 species), Anura (frogs and toads, 4100 plus), and Urodela (salamanders and newts, 415).[1] There are approximately 7150 reptile species.[1] Most are squamates (lizards, snakes, and amphisbaenians, 6850 species), followed by chelonians (turtles and tortoises, 260), crocodilians (crocodiles, alligators, caiman, and gharial, 22), and tuatara (2 species).[1]

Herptiles maintain their body either at a specific set-point temperature or within the range between an upper and a lower set point (preferred optimum temperature).[1] As ectotherms, they are reliant on external or environmental heat sources for thermoregulation. Amphibians generally prefer lower environmental temperatures. Water loss increases in amphibians as temperature increases. Set-point temperatures change seasonally and differ between the sexes. Body temperatures are higher during food digestion, pregnancy, and bacterial infections.[1]

Although frogs, toads, and salamanders have one ventricle, it is functionally divided, and blood tends to remain unmixed.[2] Pulmonary arterial branches supply the skin to support its respiratory function. In submerged amphibians, pulmonary gas exchange is absent, and systemic blood flow to the skin is increased for gas exchange. Squamate and chelonian hearts are also anatomically three-chambered, but are functionally five-chambered.[1] The heart has two inflow routes (the right and left atria) and three outflows (the pulmonary artery and the left and right aortic arches). Both heart chambers are completely divided in crocodilians and, although the left aortic arch originates from the right ventricle, a foramen connects both arches.[2] This foramen enables both aortic arches to carry unmixed oxygenated blood from the lungs. During the dive response, pulmonary blood flow decreases, and most of the right ventricular output is ejected into the left aortic arch and bypasses the lungs.[2]

Amphibian hearts are found in the cranial third of the coelomic cavity. Lizard cardiac location ranges from between the forelimbs (e.g., iguanas, chameleons, skink, and water dragons) to almost the middle of the body (e.g., monitor lizards and tegu).[6] Snake hearts are usually located 20% to 25% of body length from the head. This position is influenced by the animal's predominant lifestyle, the distance being ranked arboreal < terrestrial < aquatic.[7] To determine cardiac location, the snake is placed in dorsal recumbency, and the ventral scale movement over the heart is visualized. Allowing light to reflect off the ventral scales facilitates this. The shell surrounds the chelonian heart. Crocodile hearts are found on the midline in the cranial third of the coelomic cavity.

Heart rate is influenced by temperature, body size, metabolism, respiratory state, and the presence or absence of painful stimuli.[8] It varies inversely with temperature except at the extremes of temperatures studied. In lizards, an increase in body temperature of 10°C, over the range 20° to 40°C, increases heart rate by a factor of approximately 2.0 to 2.5.[8] Heart rates are often higher during heating than cooling, inversely related to body size, and decreased during apnea.[8]

The lungs are only one of several respiratory structures in amphibians.[1,3] In most adults and larvae, the highly vascularized, moist skin is the major respiratory surface. The buccopharyngeal cavity is also often heavily vascularized and is a minor gaseous exchange surface. Amphibians use buccal pumping to force air into the lungs. Gills are the major respiratory structures in larvae and a few adult salamanders.

The left lung is vestigial in snakes except boas and pythons, and two regions are present: the vascular lung and an air sac.[1] The vascular lung in the anterior part of the body is folded into chambers, providing a large surface area for gas exchange. The air sac posterior to the vascular lung regulates airflow and may extend through most of the coelomic cavity. Although reptile lung volume is greater than that of a comparably sized mammal, gaseous exchange surface area is less.[1]

Reptiles do not have a true diaphragm, but do use a negative-pressure pumping system to ventilate.[1,9] Both inspiration and expiration are active.[9] Inhalation occurs by thoracic cavity expansion that lowers lung pressure, causing passive airflow into the lungs. The ventilatory cycle airflow is biphasic, commencing with exhalation followed by inhalation.[9] There are two main respiratory patterns: (a) single breaths interspersed by periods of breath holding and (b) episodes of consecutive lung ventilations followed by long apneic periods lasting from a few minutes to more than an hour. In general, aquatic animals exhibit an episodic breathing pattern, whereas terrestrial herptiles breathe in single breaths. Also, aquatic herptiles usually have longer apneic periods.[9] There is normally a pause after the relaxation phase of

ventilation, sometimes for several minutes before initiation of exhalation. Ventilatory responses to both hypoxemia and hypercapnia are temperature dependent.[9] The hypoxic threshold increases as body temperature rises.

In chelonians, the dorsal surface of the lung is attached to the carapace, and the ventral surface is joined to a connective-tissue sheet attached to the viscera.[1] Exhalation occurs when the viscera is forced upward against the lungs. Extension and retraction of the legs increase the coelomic cavity volume. This enables the viscera to fall ventrally, pulling the lungs down, increasing lung volume and drawing air inward. Extension and retraction of the legs can also be used to ventilate an apneic chelonian. The crocodilian liver, posterior to the lungs, acts as a plunger for compression and expansion.[1] Abdominal muscles pull the liver forward during expiration to compress the lungs. Conversely, during inhalation, the diaphragmaticus muscles attached to the pelvis pull the liver caudally. Connective tissues attach the liver to the lungs.

Physical Restraint

Amphibians

All amphibians secrete a variably potent toxin from dorsal skin glands. Most require direct contact with mucous membranes for absorption. To prevent intoxication, as well as injury to patient skin, amphibians should be handled with talc-free latex gloves that have been washed in clean water. The gloves decrease abrasion and prevent contact with the oils and other substances present on human skin. Some amphibians will bite. When not being handled, amphibians are confined to clean plastic containers that contain water from the animal's enclosure (Fig. 35.1). Plastic bags are useful to facilitate examination and procedures such as radiography of agile animals, which may also be restrained with small, moist, foam pads. Large anurans may be grasped with one hand placed immediately anterior to the back legs, while the other hand grips around the front legs (Fig. 35.2). Salamanders are grasped immediately behind the forelegs and then in front of the hind legs. Their tails are fragile and may break away. Caecilians, sirens, and amphiumas are difficult to restrain without using some form of chemical restraint. A snake tube may be used for examination and induction.

Nonvenomous Snakes

Aggressive snakes should be approached from behind using a piece of newspaper, a leather glove, or a towel to prevent the animal from biting. Many snakes detect infrared heat and, therefore, a warm hand. Handling of food items such as birds and small mammals prior to handling snakes should be avoided. The snake's head is grasped at its base while supporting the rest of the body. Tame snakes may be gently lifted from below, but it will be necessary to restrain the head for manipulation for anesthesia. Large snakes require multiple handlers and are preferably restrained in large cloth bags.

Venomous Snakes

Venomous snakes are restrained by experienced handlers, and at least two people are always present. Induction is performed in a

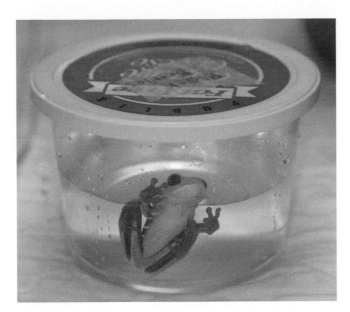

Fig. 35.1. A red-eyed tree frog confined in a clear plastic container containing a solution of tricaine methane sulfonate (MS-222) for induction of anesthesia. The container prevents escape while still allowing the animal to be monitored.

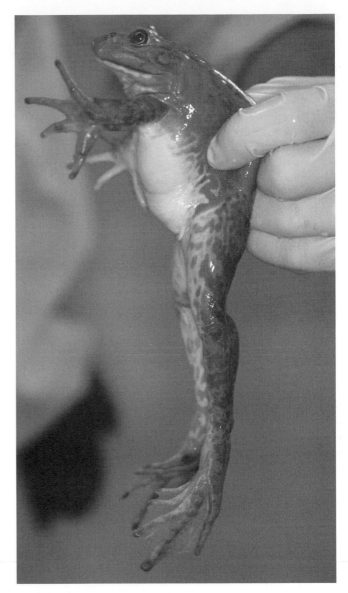

Fig. 35.2. A physical restraint technique for a large anuran such as this American bullfrog.

room that allows easy personnel movement and no hiding places in the event of an escape. Snake tongs and hooks are used to transfer animals from transport containers to either a Plexiglas tube, squeeze cage, or induction chamber. Fast, agile snakes are either transferred from container to induction chamber through a snake tube or anesthetized in their transport containers. Head restraint will not necessarily prevent handler envenomation.

Snake tubes made of clear, shatterproof plastic are used for restraint during either physical examination or anesthetic induction. The snake is placed on the floor with no obstructions. The tube is held with tongs and placed in front of the snake, which is either gently coerced with a snake hook or allowed to move freely into the tube. Once it advances sufficiently far into the tube, the handler grasps its body and the tube and prevents any retrograde movement. The tube diameter is carefully selected to allow the snake easy movement, but prevent it from turning around. The tube may be connected to the anesthetic breathing system for induction with an inhalant anesthetic. Squeeze cages are constructed of clear plastic and usually possess a foam pad into which the snake is compressed. Multiple holes are drilled through the squeeze wall to enable intramuscular (IM) injection. Induction chambers are made of clear plastic, have a solid lid that can be locked, and an inlet and outlet for the inhalant anesthetic and carrier gas.

Turtles and Tortoises

Although most chelonians are gentle and easy to handle, they may bite either in response to pain or when they feel threatened. Large tortoises will damage fingers and hands that interfere with the rapid leg retraction during a startle response. Aquatic chelonians will bite and scratch and are restrained at either the lateral

or caudal shell margins. Soft-shelled and common snapping turtles will reach their heads back almost two-thirds the length of their carapace. All sea turtles have the potential to deliver a major bite to the handler and, when removed from the water, will vigorously flap their flippers.

Lizards

All lizards will bite. Large lizards will also scratch and whip with their tails. Small lizards are restrained in a plastic bag or with a towel. Inappropriate tail restraint may elicit tail autotomy (shedding). Gecko skin is fragile and easily torn during restraint. The Gila monster and beaded lizard are venomous. Iguanas are immobilized for short periods by gently pressing down on their eyes and will "revive" spontaneously in response to loud noises and position changes.

Crocodiles, Alligators, Caiman, and Gharial

All crocodilians bite, whip their tail, and roll to escape physical restraint. They can sweep their head 180° from side to side and are preferably approached from behind. Small crocodilians are grasped around the neck and at the base of the tail. A towel may be used temporarily to blind the animal and hold it to the handler's body. In small animals, the neck grip includes a foreleg to reduce rolling. Medium to large crocodilians are very dangerous. In captivity, these animals can be induced with food or training to enter a physical restraint device. If an animal is semiconfined, a zip tie may be placed over the upper and lower jaws and the mouth tied closed. The jaw opening force is much less than the closing force, so it is relatively easy to keep the mouth closed. Once this is accomplished, a rope is placed around the neck to include a forelimb, and the animal is hauled onto land. A physical restraint board will facilitate handling and transportation (Fig. 35.3). The mouth is taped closed using electricians tape because it is less injurious to the skin and appears more resilient in a wet environment than are other tapes. Care is taken to prevent occlusion of the nares at the tip of the maxilla. In many crocodilians, teeth protruding outside the jaw can still lacerate an unwary handler if the animal swings its head. Prolonged restraint with the mouth closed will result in dehydration, even if the animal is allowed to immerse. Very large crocodilians are preferably chemically immobilized with a remote delivery device before handling. This is not only for personnel safety, but also to reduce lactic acidemia, as discussed previously. Particular care must be taken in narrow-snouted crocodilians (e.g., gharial) to not fracture the jaws.

Preanesthetic Preparation

Values for respiration rate, heart rate, and temperature are determined for reference. Accurate admission weight and subsequent daily weighing are essential patient care. The shell is included in the body weight of chelonians when calculating drug dosages. Minimal diagnostic testing includes blood collection for packed cell volume, total protein, and glucose. Blood glucose levels are generally lower (30 to 100 mg/dL) than those observed in mammals. Anesthesia is preferably performed in the morning to allow monitoring and ventilation during regular work hours if recovery is prolonged. A herptile anesthetic patient is maintained within its preferred optimum temperature during the perianesthetic period (25° to 30°C for amphibians and temperate and aquatic reptiles, and ≥30°C for tropical species). Although regurgitation and aspiration are unlikely to cause problems, perioperative fasting is recommended because of impaired digestion.

Premedication

Prolonged parenteral drug clearance generally precludes the use of sedatives and tranquilizers that cannot be reversed with an antagonist. Parasympatholytics are not indicated to reduce secretions. α_2-Adrenergic agonists alone produce minimal to no sedation and questionable restraint. Benzodiazepines, particularly midazolam, appear to be effective and useful adjuncts to anesthesia

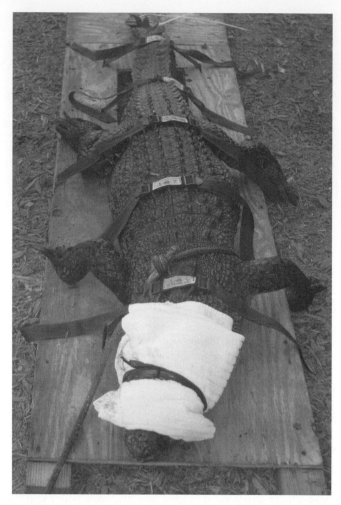

Fig. 35.3. A New Guinea crocodile physically restrained using a home-made restraint board. Note the use of a towel to cover the eyes and ears to reduce external stimuli.

in some, but not all, water turtles, lizards, and crocodilians.[10–13] The effects of benzodiazepines can be reversed with flumazenil.

Opioids and nonsteroidal anti-inflammatory drugs are administered preoperatively when pain is present or likely to occur. Generally, the same drugs and dosages can be used as those used in mammals, but dosing is less frequent because of relatively prolonged drug clearance. Unlike birds, reptiles appear refractory to the analgesic effects of butorphanol, but responsive to morphine, meperidine, and buprenorphine.[14–17] Further research to evaluate analgesic pharmacology and perianesthetic regimens in reptiles and amphibians is needed.[18]

Local Anesthesia

This approach can be an alternative to general anesthesia in reptiles restrained for procedures involving superficial and accessible sites (e.g., the limbs of lizards and chelonians). Small-volume syringes and small-gauge needles are used for accurate drug dosing. The toxic dosages of most local anesthetics do not appear to have been investigated in most nonmammalian species.

Parenteral Anesthesia: Administration Routes

Historically, IM injections into the muscles of the anterior body have been used to reduce drug passage through the kidneys via the renal portal system. However, studies in turtles and green iguanas demonstrate that only a small proportion of hind-limb venous return passes through the kidney.[19,20] Consequently, it is unlikely the IM injection site has much influence on drug anesthetic activity.[20] Furthermore, posterior IM injection offers the advantages of increased personnel safety, a larger muscle mass for injection, and more injection-site options.[20] An exception is the circulation of the green iguana. Blood from the ventral caudal (coccygeal) vein of the green iguana does appear to enter the renal portal system. Consequently, drugs with a very high first-pass tubular excretory rate should not be administered by this route in this species. In snakes, IM injections are administered into the paravertebral musculature, whereas the pectoral and triceps muscles are used in chelonians and lizards, respectively. Distal limb injection is avoided because irritant solutions will cause tissue necrosis and sloughing. The forearms of chelonians appear particularly susceptible. Crocodilians have calcified cutaneous structures (osteoderms) concentrated on the dorsum and flanks that will block IM injection.[21]

Intravenous (IV) and intraosseous injection sites are described in Tables 35.1 and 35.2, respectively. Intravenous access in amphibians is primarily limited to the ventral abdominal vein. Vascular access is difficult in snakes, and jugular vein catheterization requires surgical dissection.[21] In medium to large snakes, the palatine vein can be catheterized, but the palatine teeth preclude its use in the induction period (Fig. 35.4). Intracardiac injection is unnecessary, potentially traumatic, and delivers high drug concentrations directly to the endocardium and coronary flow. Ventral coccygeal vein injection using a 27-gauge needle is possible, but even in large snakes is difficult.

The jugular vein of tortoises and freshwater turtles is bilaterally located at the level of the auricular scale on the dorsolateral surface of the neck. The vein is catheterized using an over-the-needle catheter (18 to 24 gauge) either percutaneously or after surgical dissection. However, most awake chelonians resist extension of the neck and head required to access this vessel. Tame Galapagos tortoises may allow jugular vein injection though a 19- or 23-gauge butterfly catheter if they are first distracted with food, neck scratching, or a water spray. The subcarapacial vessels are composed of branches from the jugular vein. They are located in the midline underneath the carapace. The dorsal cervical sinuses of sea turtles can be used for catheterization with a through-the-needle catheter.[22] The venous plexus on the inside of the forearm of tortoises is unsuitable for catheterization and anesthetic infusion. However, the dorsal coccygeal vein is readily accessible in small to large chelonians. To facilitate access, large tortoises and turtles are gently turned on their backs to cause them to tail curl. Care is taken to prevent being kicked by the hind legs, and the site is cleaned and disinfected to prevent bacterial contamination from feces. A 16- to 18-gauge over-the-needle catheter can be placed in this vessel in large tortoises and turtles (Fig. 35.5).

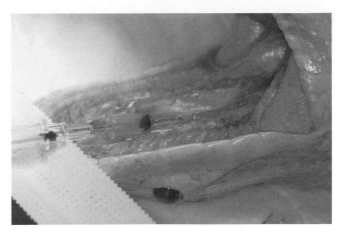

Fig. 35.4. Placement of an 18-gauge over-the-needle catheter in the palatine vein of an anesthetized Burmese python. The handler must take great care to avoid being injured by the palatine teeth that lie parallel to the vessel. After removal of the catheter, pressure and gauze must be applied for several minutes to provide hemostasis.

Intraosseous catheterization of the distal humerus has been described in sea turtles.[22] Intraosseous catheterization of the femur, tibia, or humerus is performed in lizards following lidocaine infiltration of the cannulation site (Fig. 35.6). Correct placement is assessed by palpation, ease of injection, absence of subcutaneous edema at the injection site, and radiography. In lizards, either the ventral coccygeal (Fig. 35.7) or abdominal veins can be used for injection. The ventral coccygeal vein has been recommended for aggressive lizards and is approached from either the ventral or ventrolateral tail surface (Fig. 35.8). The cephalic vein is located on the dorsal surface of the forearm and may be catheterized after local anesthetic infiltration and surgical dissection. The ventral coccygeal vein can be catheterized percutaneously in larger lizards and crocodilians. The technique involves turning the tail to the side at an acute angle to enable placement of an over-the-needle catheter. The catheter can then be inserted at an acute angle in the ventral midline or from the ventrolateral aspect of the tail (Fig. 35.9).

Parenteral Drugs

Dissociative Anesthetics

The major disadvantages of ketamine include poor muscle relaxation, inadequate analgesia, prolonged recovery, the high dosage requirement for surgical anesthesia, and large injection volume.[23–27] Repetitive administration may result in drug accumulation and prolonged recovery. Advantages to ketamine include a relatively brief effect and some analgesia, and it can be administered intramuscularly. In herptiles, ketamine produces hypertension and tachycardia, bradypnea, and hypoventilation.[23,25,28] Ketamine dosage is reduced, and immobilization quality is improved by combining ketamine with either an α-adrenergic agonist or a benzodiazepine.[10,21,29–32] The α-adrenergic agonists are typically reversed with the antagonist atipamezole to shorten re-

Table 35.1. Vascular access in amphibians and reptiles

Amphibians	Ventral abdominal vein–Located in the midline immediately under the skin and may occasionally be identified by using transillumination. Use a 25- to 27-gauge needle and be careful to avoid penetrating the underlying viscera.
	Ventral coccygeal vein–Located in the ventral midline of the tail. Use a 22- to 27-gauge needle. Insert the needle less than one-third of the distance from cloaca to tail. Apply gentle aspiration until either bone or blood is encountered. If unsuccessful, reposition the needle either cranially or caudally
	Heart–Indicated for emergencies. Not recommended for routine injection.
Crocodilians	Ventral coccygeal vein–Insert the needle in the ventral midline of the tail. Insert a 22- to 25-gauge, 1.5- to 3.0-inch needle (Fig. 35.9) less than one-third of the distance from cloaca to tail. Apply gentle aspiration until either bone or blood is encountered. If unsuccessful, reposition the needle either cranially or caudally. This vessel may also be approached laterally by directing the needle at the vertebral body and "walking" it to the vessel on the ventral aspect of the bone.
	Dorsal coccygeal vein–Located dorsal to the vertebrae in the midline. Insert a 22- to 25-gauge 1.5- to 3.0-inch needle less than one-third of the distance from cloaca to tail. Apply gentle aspiration until either bone or blood is encountered. If unsuccessful, reposition the needle either cranially or caudally.
	Supravertebral sinus–This vessel lies immediately dorsal to the spinal canal and is not recommended for anesthetic administration because of the potential for drug to be accidentally administered into the spinal fluid.
Squamata Snakes	Palatine vein (medium to large snakes)–Located medial to the palatine teeth in the roof of the mouth (Fig. 35.4). Take care to prevent injury to fingers.
	Jugular vein–The right is larger than the left. Make an incision four to seven scutes cranial to the heart at the junction of the ventral scutes and the right lateral body scales. Identify the vein by using blunt dissection just medial to the tips of the ribs.[49]
	Coccygeal vein–Located on the ventral midline of the tail. Insert a 22- to 27-gauge needle less than one-third of the distance from cloaca to tail to avoid the hemipenes in males and the anal sacs. Apply gentle aspiration until either bone or blood is encountered. If unsuccessful, reposition the needle either cranially or caudally.
	Heart–Indicated for emergencies. Not recommended for routine injection.
Lizards	Cephalic vein–Located on the dorsal (anterior) surface of the distal foreleg. Make a skin incision from the elbow distal and medial over the dorsal forearm to enable visualization of the vein.[49]
	Ventral abdominal vein–Located in the ventral midline, it may be entered percutaneously or following a small skin incision in the midline to visualize the vessel.
	Coccygeal vein–Located in ventral midline of tail (Figs. 35.8). Insert the needle sufficiently caudal to the cloaca to avoid the hemipenes in males and the anal sacs. The vessel is entered either directly from the ventral midline or laterally. The needle is inserted ventral to the transverse processes and advanced until the vertebral body is contacted. While gentle suction is applied with the syringe, the needle is "walked" ventrally around the vertebral body until the vessel is identified. It may also be approached laterally as described in crocodilians.
Chelonia (tortoises and turtles)	Jugular vein–Located on lateral surface of neck at the level of the auricular scale. In some animals, it may be percutaneously catheterized. In hypovolemic or hypotensive animals, a longitudinal skin incision is required for visualization. Positive-pressure ventilation may assist distension of the vessel for catheterization.
	Dorsal coccygeal vein–Located in midline, dorsal to the vertebrae (Fig. 35.5). To facilitate injection, turn the animal gently on its back to cause it to curl its tail onto its plastron. Clean the injection site of feces and other debris. Take care to avoid being kicked by large tortoises. Insert the needle in the midline and advance it until bone is contacted. Gentle suction will enable identification of the vessel.
	Dorsal cervical sinus (sea turtles)–Located on the dorsolateral surface of the neck just under the palpable dorsal neck muscles.

covery time. In gopher tortoises, medetomidine-ketamine combinations produce marked hypertension, tachycardia, and prolonged apnea.[30] The latter results in hypoxemia and hypercapnia if the animal is not ventilated. Intravenous atipamezole administration is not recommended because of potential transient asystole, bradyarrhythmias, and profound hypotension.[30]

Tiletamine and zolazepam (Telazol) is not indicated for use in most herptiles because of its long duration of effect (≥24 h). However, it does offer the advantage of potency and the ability to produce a high drug concentration, thereby reducing injection

dosage. This is useful when immobilizing large aggressive reptiles (e.g., pythons, monitor lizards, and crocodilians).

Propofol

This is the anesthetic induction agent of choice when preinduction vascular access has been attained. Its main advantage is that it is rapidly metabolized and thus has a relatively brief effect. In iguanas, propofol (10 mg/kg intraosseously) produces short-term immobilization, but is associated with prolonged apnea.[33] Subsequent clinical experience indicates this dosage is excessive.

Table 35.2. Techniques and sites for intraosseous catheterization in amphibians and reptiles.[a]

Order	Site
Anura (frogs and toads)	Distal femur–Flex stifle, curve in the distal femur, usually enables the catheter to be introduced proximal to the joint.
Squamata (lizards)	Distal femur–Flex stifle, curve in the distal femur, usually enables the catheter to be introduced proximal to the joint (Fig. 35.6).
	Proximal tibia–Differentiate it from the lateral fibula. Pass the catheter through the tibial crest and pass the needle to the medial surface of the leg as it is passed into the bone.
	Proximal humerus–Place the catheter either into the greater tubercle or slightly medial to it.
Chelonia	
Tortoises and Turtles	Carapace-plastron bridge–Pass the needle at an acute angle through the bony bridge between the plastron and the carapace. The catheter usually enters the coelomic cavity rather than the intramedullary space.
Sea turtles	Distal humerus–Place the animal in sternal recumbency. From the front, grasp left or right foreflipper, insert the needle in the distal one-quarter of the medial aspect of the humerus at an angle of about 30° to 45° from parallel. Insert the needle as far distal as possible without entering the joint capsule. Turtle bone is very dense, so it is difficult to introduce a catheter.

[a]In all but the smallest patients, spinal needles are recommended to prevent blockage of the needle bore with a bone plug. Measuring half the length of the bone approximates needle length. All intraosseous catheter sites are cleaned and aseptically prepared for introduction of the needle. The bone selected for catheterization is firmly grasped in one hand, and the needle inserted with a twisting of the wrist. Successful placement is indicated by a sudden change in resistance and rapid advancement of the needle, a "grating" feeling as the needle passes through medullary bone, and ease of infusion of a test injection of heparinized saline. Intraosseous catheters can remain in place for 3 days before removal.

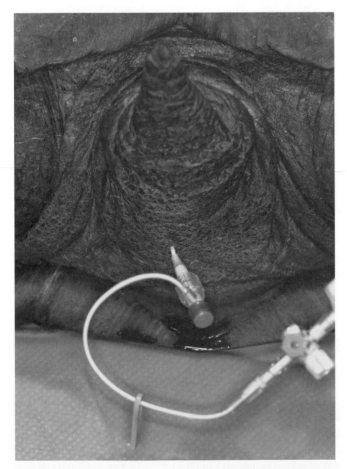

Fig. 35.5. A subadult Galapagos tortoise with a 16-gauge over-the-needle catheter placed in the dorsal coccygeal vein for administration of propofol.

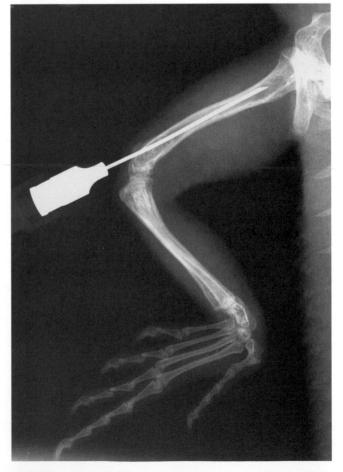

Fig. 35.6. This radiograph of the femur of a bearded dragon demonstrates the placement of an intraosseous catheter for fluid administration.

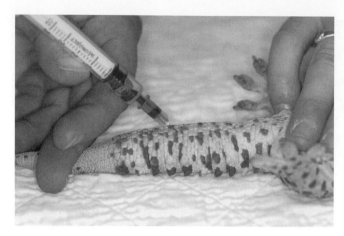

Fig. 35.7. The ventral midline approach for accessing the ventral coccygeal vein in a physically restrained Tokay gecko.

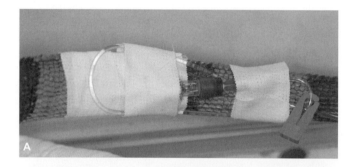

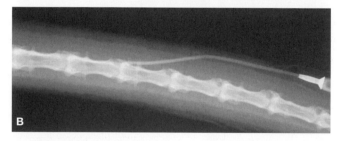

Fig. 35.8A and B. An intravenous catheter placed in the coccygeal vein of a green iguana. This vessel can also be catheterized in other large lizard species and crocodilians.

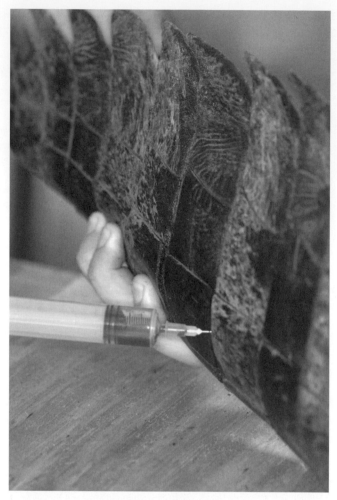

Fig. 35.9. A lateral approach technique for accessing the ventral coccygeal vein in the tail of a New Guinea crocodile.

To reduce the adverse cardiopulmonary effects, it is recommended that propofol be administered in small boluses to effect. In herptiles, time between boluses may need to be 2 to 5 min or more to allow sufficient time for maximum effect.

The muscle relaxants succinylcholine, gallamine, and rocuronium have been used to restrain and immobilize chelonians and crocodilians.[34,35] The major advantages of succinylcholine are small injection volume, relatively short recovery, and low cost. A major disadvantage is that it produces muscle contractions that cause pain, distress, hyperkalemia, and myoglobinuria. Further, paralysis of the respiratory muscles produces apnea and hypoxemia. Since succinylcholine depends on hepatic and/or circulating pseudocholinesterases for metabolism and excretion, liver dysfunction makes duration of recovery unpredictable. Phallus prolapse, with associated trauma, is a frequent complication in male reptiles administered muscle relaxants. The nondepolarizing muscle relaxants offer the advantage of reversal with neostigmine. However, because there are alternative induction and immobilization regimens, neuromuscular blocking drugs are not recommended for immobilization of herptile species.

Inhalant Anesthesia

This is used for maintenance because of ease of control of anesthetic depth, reasonably rapid recovery, and predictability of effects across different species. Induction and recovery are generally slower in herptiles than mammals and often unpredictable. Low cardiac output that delays anesthetic removal from the alveoli would be expected to promote a rapid induction.[8] However, this effect is counterbalanced by an inefficient respiratory system and low alveolar ventilation.[36] Furthermore, cardiac shunts (particularly in aquatic and semiaquatic species) may bypass either part or all lung tissue.[8,36] To hasten inhalation anesthetic induction, it is recommended herptiles be at their preferred optimum body temperature, that they be ventilated after being intubated to improve alveolar ventilation, that high vaporizer settings be used initially until anesthetic depth is achieved, and that inhalant anesthetics with low tissue solubility be used. To promote rapid recovery, provide ventilation with room air, ensure the animal is at an appropriate temperature, begin lowering vaporizer settings 10 to 20 min before completion of the procedure, and use inhalant anesthetics with low tissue solubility.[37]

Herptiles at their preferred optimum temperature appear to have similar anesthetic requirements as mammals.[38,39] Hypothermic reptiles require a lower maintenance anesthetic setting than at their preferred optimum temperature. Since metabolic rates of reptiles are much lower than those of mammals, oxygen requirement and carbon dioxide production are also much less.[36] Nitrous oxide enhances the induction rate and reduces the requirement for other inhaled anesthetics.[38] As expected, sevoflurane administration to desert tortoises and black-throated monitors produces more rapid induction and recovery than does isoflurane.[38,40] Both isoflurane and sevoflurane produce dose-dependent cardiopulmonary depression.[17,40,41]

Manufactured masks or syringe cases are used for inhalant anesthetic induction in lizards and occasionally tortoises. Clear plastic endotracheal tubes ($\geq$2-mm internal diameter) are used for intubation in small reptiles ($\geq$0.5 to 2.0 kg). For very small patients, tubes are constructed from either over-the-needle (18 to 20 gauge) or urinary catheters. However, mucous plugs may act as one-way valves allowing air into the lungs, but not back out, causing respiratory tract hyperinflation. Adequate time must also be allowed between breaths for effective exhalation through very small diameter tubes.

The herptile glottis is located at the base of the tongue and is closed except during exhalation and inspiration. The glottal opening of the green sea turtle is difficult to visualize because of caudally directed pharyngeal spines. The chameleon trachea is very short and flexible. Intubation is facilitated by direct application of local anesthetic to the glottis. Gentle ventral traction on the lower jaw will cause the mouth to open. Alternatively, aggressive herptiles will often open their mouth in response to gentle tapping on their rostrum. Once open, the mouth is prevented from closing with a mouth gag. In small to medium-sized herptiles, a rubber cooking spatula is used to prevent oral cavity and teeth damage. Time is allowed for the glottis to open before insertion of the endotracheal tube. Alternatively, the bevel of the lubricated endotracheal tube is used to gently open the closed glottis. After intubation, a mouth gag constructed of wrapped gauze squares is placed in the mouth. In small herptiles, attaching the animal's head, endotracheal tube, and breathing system to a tongue depressor reduces the possibility of the endotracheal tube accidentally being either twisted or removed.

In crocodilians, at the base of the tongue is a gular flap that must be ventrally displaced to visualize the glottis. After anesthetic induction, the animal's head is hyperextended, and the lower jaw gently pulled downward to enable placement of a mouth gag. A piece of pinewood makes a good mouth gag because the teeth can sink into it without causing damage.

Perioperative Monitoring and Supportive Care

Anesthetic Depth

Increasing depth toward a surgical plane of anesthesia is assumed when muscle tone (e.g., jaw muscle or cloacal sphincter) decreases, palpebral and corneal reflexes are obtunded, and there is no response to a noxious stimulus. In general, the corneal and cloacal reflexes are not lost at surgical anesthetic levels. Palpebral and corneal reflexes are not elicited in snakes and some lizard species because a spectacle protects the cornea. A fixed dilated pupil (unresponsive to light) and no corneal reflex (when previously present) are cross-species indicators of either excessive anesthetic depth or brain-stem hypoperfusion. Respiration rate and depth are not usually useful in assessing anesthetic depth because most herptiles become either apneic or bradypneic at a surgical anesthetic plane. During inhalant anesthetic induction, snakes relax from the head to tail and recover in the opposite direction. Hence, the absence of a response to either a tail or cloacal pinch suggests that an adequate surgical anesthetic plane has been achieved. Similarly, the toe and cloacal pinch response is used to monitor anesthetic depth in amphibians, lizards, and chelonians. The palpebral or corneal response can also be used in chelonians and most lizards. Heart rate and arterial blood pressure will increase in response to a painful stimulus, and sudden increases in these physiological variables often indicate decreased anesthetic depth.

Thermoregulation

During the perianesthetic period, herptiles have an impaired thermoregulatory ability. External heat sources include warm-water or forced-air blankets and radiant heat lamps. Although hypothermia prevention is important, hyperthermia is more likely to cause trauma and death. It is recommended that body temperatures not exceed 35°C. Burns may occur if a herptile is allowed to remain either on a hot surface or under a closely placed heat lamp. Thermal injury is more likely to occur in dehydrated animals with poor peripheral perfusion. Amphibians are prone to dehydration at higher temperatures (>30°C), so their skin must not be allowed to dry out.

Cardiovascular Monitoring and Supportive Care

In herptiles, heart sounds are not usually externally auscultated. The electrocardiograms resemble those of mammals, with clearly defined P, QRS, and T components.[36] In reptiles, an SV wave may precede the P wave.[36] Standard lead positions are used. However, traditional positioning will not provide adequate wave deflections in herptiles with low signal voltages. Electrodes are placed in the cervical region in lizards with hearts located at the pectoral girdle.[6] In snakes, the electrodes are placed two heart lengths cranial and caudal to the heart.[6] In tortoises and turtles, the cranial leads are placed on the skin between the neck and the forelimbs.[6] To improve signal detection, a stainless-steel suture is passed through the skin and attached to the electrodes.

Doppler flow-detection contact sites include the ventral aspect of the tail base, the carotid and femoral arteries, and directly over the heart. The chelonian carotid artery is located ventral to the jugular vein on the lateral surface of the neck. It is covered by a layer of muscle and usually not visible. In chelonians, a pencil probe placed at the thoracic inlet will detect flow in either the heart or the major arteries. In an emergency, placement of a probe over the eye may detect ocular arterial flow in large chelonians. A probe placed either down the esophagus or into the cloaca and directed dorsally may also detect arterial flows.

Some reptiles have underdeveloped circulatory reflexes because they usually remain horizontal (e.g., aquatic and terrestrial snakes). To prevent orthostatic hypotension in these animals, positional changes are made slowly, normal body position (usually horizontal and sternal) is maintained, and hypovolemia and hypotension are aggressively treated.

Vascular access is described above and in Tables 35.1 and 35.2. Subcutaneous administration of fluids is not appropriate for correction of deficits or hemorrhage in the perianesthetic period. Balanced electrolyte solutions are used for routine fluid administration. An argument has been made against the use of lactated Ringer's solution in reptiles because of the prolonged half-life of lactate.[42] It is suggested that a 1:1 combination of 5% dextrose and a nonlactated multiple-electrolyte solution such as Normosol-R (CEVA Laboratories, Overland Park, KS) or Plasma Lyte (Baxter Health Care, Deerfield, IL) be used.[42] Isotonic dextrose solution (5%) or combinations are indicated when hypoglycemia is present or expected. When necessary for transfusion, blood is collected into heparinized syringes and administered soon after collection. Small-volume infusers are essential for accurate fluid infusion in small anesthetized patients.

Respiratory Monitoring and Supportive Care

Auscultation of the respiratory tract is made difficult by the presence of scales in squamates and the shell in chelonians. To improve sound transmission, use a good-quality stethoscope and place a moistened paper towel between the stethoscope diaphragm and the skin. An esophageal stethoscope will also detect respiratory sounds.

There are two schools of thought when analyzing ectotherm blood-gas samples.[9] One believes the values should be corrected back to a common body temperature, usually 37°C. Arterial pH decreases consistently and systematically with increasing temperature in virtually all ectothermic vertebrates. Another group recommends analyzing and interpreting the sample at the animal's body temperature. Arterial blood samples are difficult to obtain in most herptiles. The preferable sampling site is the carotid artery because it reflects blood flowing to the brain.[43] Because of the presence of shunting and the multiple functional chambers, cardiac samples do not accurately reflect carotid arterial blood values.

Transmission pulse oximetry is made difficult by the lack of suitable placement sites. Reflectance pulse-oximeter sensors can be placed in either the esophagus or the cloaca of anesthetized animals. Diethelm et al.[44] evaluated pulse oximetry in green iguanas. Oxyhemoglobin and deoxyhemoglobin absorbencies at 660 and 940 nm were determined to be similar to those of human hemoglobin in vitro. A reflectance probe was placed in the esophagus and the measured saturation of peripheral oxygen (SpO_2) was compared with arterial oxygen saturation (SaO_2) values calculated from arterial oxygen partial pressure (PaO_2) in blood samples obtained from the abdominal aorta. There were no significant differences between SpO_2 and SaO_2 values, and it was concluded that pulse oximetry is an excellent tool for monitoring pulse rate and oxygen saturation in iguanas. The study abstract does not mention how the SaO_2 values were calculated and does not address methemoglobin concentrations.[44] Another recent study in green iguanas showed no relationship between calculated hemoglobin saturations and those obtained from a pulse oximeter.[17]

Most reptiles appear to develop either apnea or marked bradypnea and hypoventilation when anesthetized. Hence, it is usually necessary to provide ventilation during anesthesia. The respiration rate required is very low (<4 breaths/min) and the tidal volume of reptiles is usually larger than that of mammals of a comparable size. Further research is necessary to determine optimum ventilation, whether spontaneous or assisted, in anesthetized reptiles. The presence of cardiac shunts in reptiles renders capnography inaccurate because end-tidal carbon dioxide partial pressure ($ETCO_2$) values do not reflect arterial carbon dioxide partial pressure ($PaCO_2$) levels.[9]

Resuscitation

This follows the same sequential guidelines used in mammalian patients. The low metabolic rates and low oxygen requirement of most herptiles allows a prolonged "window" of time in which resuscitation can be successful. The author (D.H.) has revived an iguana after 30 min of apparent asystole.

Anesthetic Recovery

Inhalant anesthetic administration is discontinued 15 to 20 min before the end of a surgical procedure. If indicated, additional analgesics are administered at this time. When a procedure is completed, the reptile is transported to the recovery site. Care is taken to prevent orthostatic hypotension by maintaining the animal horizontal and avoiding rapid changes in body position. The endotracheal tube is maintained in position until spontaneous respirations or attempts to remove the endotracheal tube are noted. The endotracheal tube is connected to a bag valve mask and ventilated with room air to facilitate return to spontaneous ventilation.[37] Amphibian patients are transferred with no anesthetic to clean tank water. The animal is provided with a heat source, and cloacal temperature is monitored. Hyperthermia and burns are prevented as discussed above. Prolonged recovery may be due to delayed hepatic biotransformation or renal excretion of parenteral anesthetic drugs, pulmonary shunting preventing removal of inhalant anesthetics, hypothermia, hypoglycemia, and severe metabolic disturbances (i.e., acidemia, hyperkalemia, hyponatremia, or hypocalcemia).

Selected Anesthetic Protocols

It is recommended that all amphibians and reptiles undergoing surgery and/or potentially painful procedures receive an analgesic(s) in the perioperative period.[15,16] Anesthetic protocols are outlined in Table 35.3.

Table 35.3. Recommended anesthetic regimens for amphibians and reptiles.[a]

Amphibians	Tricaine methane sulfonate (MS-222).[45] Buffer a 0.02% to 0.2% (0.2 to 2 g/L) solution with sodium bicarbonate 1 to 3 g/L to a pH of 7.0 to 7.4. Immerse the animal until it is anesthetized (20 to 30 min) and then wash its surfaces with clean water. If supplemental anesthetic is required, immerse the animal in half-strength solution or drape it with towels soaked in solution. Alternatively, intubate it and maintain it with inhalant anesthetic in oxygen. Recovery should be in clean water from the animal's habitat.
	Topical isoflurane (3 mL of isoflurane + 3.5 mL of water-soluble gel + 1.5 mL of water, mixed thoroughly in a serum tube).[46] Apply dorsally (0.025 mL/kg for aquatic and 0.035 mL for terrestrial animals). Induce anesthesia in a clear plastic container and remove the animal from the container once the animal's righting response is lost. Wipe off all gel with a moist towel. The animal can be intubated and maintained with inhalant anesthetic in oxygen. Recovery should be in clean water from animal's habitat.
	Clove oil anesthetic bath.[47] Make it immediately before use: 0.30 mL of clove oil (eugenol: minimum, 85%; and specific gravity, 1.038 to 1.060) per liter of dechlorinated water and agitate for 4 min. Immerse the amphibian in a shallow tray for 15 min and then wash off the liquid. Gastric prolapse is common.
Crocodilians	Propofol (3 to 5 mg/kg IV). Intubate and ventilate (2 to 4 breaths/min) with either isoflurane (2% to 3%) or sevoflurane (4% to 5%) in oxygen (± nitrous oxide).
	Tiletamine-zolazepam (4 to 6 mg/kg IM). Wait 30 to 45 min and then intubate and ventilate (2 to 4 breaths/min) with either isoflurane (2% to 3%) or sevoflurane (4% to 5%) in oxygen (± nitrous oxide).
	Medetomidine-ketamine (100 to 200 µg/kg + 5 to 10 mg/kg IM, higher dosages in juveniles). Intubate and ventilate (2 to 4 breaths/min) with either isoflurane or sevoflurane in oxygen (± nitrous oxide).[21] Reverse medetomidine with atipamezole (500 µg/kg IM).
Lizards	Propofol (3 to 5 mg/kg IV, IO). Intubate and ventilate (2 to 4 breaths/min) with either isoflurane or sevoflurane (4% to 5%) in oxygen (± nitrous oxide).
	Mask induction with isoflurane (5%) or sevoflurane (7%). Intubate and ventilate (2 to 4 breaths/min) with either isoflurane (2% to 3%) or sevoflurane (4% to 5%) in oxygen (± nitrous oxide).
	Lidocaine (1%) desensitization of the glottis. Wait 2 to 3 min and then intubate and ventilate (2 to 4 breaths/min) with either isoflurane (2% to 5%) or sevoflurane (4% to 7%) in oxygen (± nitrous oxide),
	Tiletamine-zolazepam (4 to 6 mg/kg IM, IV, IO). Intubate and ventilate (2 to 4 breaths/min) with either isoflurane (1% to 3%) or sevoflurane (3% to 5%) in oxygen (± nitrous oxide).
	Medetomidine-ketamine (150 µg/kg: 10 to 15 mg/kg IM, IV, IO). Intubate and ventilate (2 to 4 breaths/min) with either isoflurane (1% to 3%) or sevoflurane (3% to 5%) in oxygen (± nitrous oxide).
Nonvenomous Snakes	Lidocaine (1%) desensitization of glottis. Wait 2 to 3 min and then intubate and ventilate (2 to 4 breaths/min) with either isoflurane (5%) or sevoflurane (7%) in oxygen (± nitrous oxide); maintain with either isoflurane (2% to 3%) or sevoflurane (3% to 5%) in oxygen (± nitrous oxide).
	Large snakes (pythons and boas): tiletamine-zolazepam (3 to 5 mg/kg IM) or medetomidine-midazolam (30 µg/kg–0.3 mg/kg). Wait 45 min and then intubate and ventilate (2 to 4 breaths/min) with either isoflurane (3%) or sevoflurane (5%) in oxygen (± nitrous oxide); maintain with either isoflurane (2% to 3%) or sevoflurane (3% to 5%) in oxygen (± nitrous oxide).
	Propofol (3-5 mg/kg IV), ventral coccygeal vein. Intubate and ventilate (2 to 4 breaths/min) with either isoflurane (3%) or sevoflurane (5%) in oxygen (± nitrous oxide); maintain with either isoflurane (2% to 3%) or sevoflurane (3% to 5%) in oxygen (± nitrous oxide).
Venomous Snakes	Induction-chamber isoflurane (5%) or sevoflurane (7%). Wait until the animal loses its righting reflex and then intubate and ventilate (2 to 4 breaths/min); maintain with either isoflurane (2% to 3%) or sevoflurane (4% to 5%) in oxygen (± nitrous oxide).
	Tiletamine-zolazepam (3 to 5 mg/kg IM, with the snake in squeeze cage). Intubate and ventilate (2 to 4 breaths/min); cover the fangs with a syringe case; maintain with either isoflurane (2% to 3%) or sevoflurane (4% to 5%) in oxygen (± nitrous oxide).
	Place the snake in Plexiglas tube, and use tongs and forceps to open its mouth; lidocaine (1%) desensitization of glottis. Wait 2 to 3 min and then intubate and ventilate (2 to 4 breaths/min) with either isoflurane (5%) or sevoflurane (7%) in oxygen (± nitrous oxide); cover the fangs with a syringe case; maintain with either isoflurane (2% to 3%) or sevoflurane (3% to 5%) in oxygen (± nitrous oxide).
Tortoises and Turtles	Propofol (3 to 5 mg/kg) IV, dorsal coccygeal or jugular vein. Intubate and ventilate (2 to 4 breaths/min); maintain with either isoflurane (2% to 3%) or sevoflurane (4% to 5%) in oxygen (± nitrous oxide).
	Medetomidine-ketamine (tortoises, 50 to 100 µg/kg–10 mg/kg; giant tortoises, 40 to 60 µg/kg–4 to 6 mg/kg; and aquatic turtles, 150 to 300 µg/kg–10 to 15 mg/kg) IM. Wait 45 min and then intubate and ventilate (2 to 4 breaths/min); maintain with either isoflurane (2% to 3%) or sevoflurane (4% to 5%) in oxygen (± nitrous oxide).[29–32]
	Lidocaine (1%) desensitization of glottis. Wait 2 to 3 min and then intubate and ventilate (2 to 4 breaths/min) with either isoflurane (5%) or sevoflurane (7%) in oxygen (± nitrous oxide); maintain with either isoflurane (2% to 3%) or sevoflurane (3% to 5%) in oxygen (± nitrous oxide).
	Ketamine (5-mg/kg boluses up to 20 mg/kg) IV. Intubate and ventilate (2 to 4 breaths/min) with either isoflurane (5%) or sevoflurane (7%) in oxygen (± nitrous oxide); maintain with either isoflurane (2% to 3%) or sevoflurane (3% to 5%) in oxygen (± nitrous oxide).

IM, intramuscularly; IO, intraosseously; IV, intravenously.
[a]The inclusion of an analgesic is mandatory for surgery and painful diagnostic procedures.

Caecilians, Frogs and Toads, Salamanders, and Newts

The most commonly used chemical immobilization agent and anesthetic in amphibians is tricaine methane sulfonate (MS-222).[45,46] This drug is dispensed as a white powder and, when dissolved in distilled water, produces a very acidic solution (pH ≥ 3.0). Consequently, it is necessary to buffer the solution back to a physiological pH (7.0 to 7.4) with 1 to 3 g/L of sodium bicarbonate ($NaHCO_3$). The pH should always be checked before immersing an animal. Buffering of the solution has the added benefit of increasing the ionized drug (the active form of the drug). When using a buffered solution of MS-222, surgical anesthesia can be provided with concentrations as low as 0.02% (0.2 g/L).[45] The induction time is around 30 min. The animal should be confined in a clear container so that it cannot escape, but can be monitored (Fig. 35.1). Once the animal is anesthetized, it is removed from the solution and placed on a clean moist surface. If the animal begins moving, it can either be reimmersed in a half-strength solution or solution added to moist towels draped over the animal. Aquatic amphibian species have much more efficient transdermal absorption than terrestrial species and thus may require a lower dosage. Similarly, larvae and tadpoles appear to require a lower dosage. Clove oil is an alternative to MS-222.[47] Ketamine produces immobilization and anesthesia, but results in prolonged recoveries. Similarly, tiletamine and zolazepam combinations produce very prolonged recoveries.

Inhalant anesthetics administered into solution are cumbersome and difficult to scavenge. A technique using a topical mixture of isoflurane and K-Y Jelly has been used to immobilize frogs.[46] A viscous isoflurane solution (1.5 mL of water plus 3.5 mL of K-Y Jelly) is produced in an empty serum container that is shaken vigorously until the contents mix. The liquid/gel is drawn into a syringe with a 16-gauge needle and then applied directly to the animal's dorsum. Dosages vary from 0.025 to 0.035 mL/g of body weight, depending on the species.[46] Lower dosages are used for frogs, newts, and salamanders, compared with toads. Once the solution is applied, the animal is placed in a small sealed container until induction occurs (5 to 15 min). When the animal has lost its withdrawal and righting reflexes, a saline-soaked gauze is used to wipe the dermis free of anesthetic solution. The animal will remain anesthetized for 45 to 80 min. These methods provide general anesthesia or can be used for intubation prior to gas anesthesia.

Nonvenomous Snakes

Small to medium-sized snakes (<20 kg) are manually restrained, their mouths are opened using a spatula, and 1 to 2 drops of a 1% lidocaine (without epinephrine) solution is applied directly into the glottal opening. A period of 2 to 3 min is allowed for the lidocaine to desensitize the mucosal surfaces before a lubricated endotracheal tube is passed through the glottal opening. Although large snakes (≥20 kg) can be manually restrained, it is preferable that an induction agent be administered first to facilitate handling and intubation. In large pythons, a tiletamine-zolazepam combination (Telazol, 3 to 4 mg/kg) is administered intramuscularly 45 min before the animal is intubated. Alter-

natively, a combination of medetomidine (30 µg/kg) and midazolam (0.3 mg/kg) may be used. These injections are given through the cloth bag restraining the snake. Ventral coccygeal vein administration of propofol is difficult even in large snakes, but can be attempted using small-gauge needles. Snakes can also be induced by placing them in an induction chamber and administering high inhalant anesthetic concentrations in oxygen. Once intubated, the snake can be connected to an anesthetic breathing system, maintained with isoflurane in oxygen, and ventilated one to six times per minute.

Venomous Snakes

The main difference between venomous and nonvenomous snake anesthesia is the importance of careful physical restraint during the perianesthetic period. Although parenteral anesthesia is never relied on to produce complete immobility, a low IM dose (3 to 4 mg/kg) of tiletamine-zolazepam 30 to 40 min before inhalation anesthesia will decrease the responsiveness of the snake and may contribute to analgesia. The authors prefer to induce anesthesia in venomous snakes in either an induction chamber or snake tube with isoflurane. Alternatively, the animal is intubated while awake while restrained in a snake tube. The snake is allowed to advance to a position just before the end of the tube. A long pair of tongue forceps or a vaginoscope is then used to open its mouth and manipulate the endotracheal tube through the glottis. Once the animal is restrained, the fangs are covered with either a syringe case or urine cup and taped in place to prevent accidental envenomation. During recovery, the endotracheal tube is removed with forceps when spontaneous respiration is present but before struggling occurs.

Lizards

Lizards may be induced with an inhalant anesthetic administered into a plastic bag, induction chamber, or mask. Breath holding, though sometimes present, is not as large a problem as some authors suggest and does not preclude its use. Gently running fingers along a lizard's chest wall will usually elicit a respiration. Some lizards may also be intubated while awake, as with chelonians and snakes. The preferred induction agent is propofol (3 to 6 mg/kg) administered into the ventral coccygeal vein. Tiletamine-zolazepam (4 to 8 mg/kg) can be given intramuscularly to facilitate handling of large lizards.

Chelonians

Some tortoises and turtles can be intubated while awake. Once intubated, they are ventilated with isoflurane in oxygen (with or without nitrous oxide). In animals in which a parenteral anesthetic is required for intubation, the authors prefer propofol (3 to 5 mg/kg) administered into the dorsal coccygeal vein (Fig. 35.5). Alternatively, small IV boluses (1 to 2 mg/kg) of ketamine may be used. If vascular access is not possible, a combination of IM ketamine and medetomidine can be used for induction.[29,31,32] The dosage is lower in land tortoises than in aquatic turtles. Atipamezole is administered intramuscularly to reverse the medetomidine and hasten recovery. Mask induction is possible with either isoflurane or sevoflurane in oxygen, but is likely to be prolonged because of breath holding and pulmonary shunting in aquatic species.

Anesthesia of sea turtles is similar to that of other chelonians.[29,48] However, they tend to be large, powerful, and sometimes more aggressive. The sea turtle glottis may be very difficult to visualize because it is hidden in the folds and spines of the pharynx. Pulmonary shunting is a problem for inhalation anesthesia in sea turtles and probably explains some of the prolonged recoveries observed in animals that appear lightly anesthetized during a procedure.[48,49] Unfortunately, there appears to be no mechanism for avoiding this problem.

Crocodilians

Crocodilian anesthesia usually requires a combination of physical restraint (Fig. 35.3) and anesthetic drugs.[4,35] Muscle relaxants have commonly been used for chemical immobilization of medium to large crocodilians. In addition to the lack of analgesia, the therapeutic index of these drugs is very low. An alternative to muscle relaxant–induced immobilization is using the combination of tiletamine and zolazepam. A recent study that also assessed medetomidine with ketamine in alligators concluded that this combination provided good reversible restraint.[16] However, the dosages used were much higher than those needed to immobilize chelonians and other reptiles. When IV access can be attained, propofol is a valuable agent for induction and maintenance of anesthesia. Dosages vary from 2 to 5 mg/kg. Once the crocodile or alligator is intubated, it can be ventilated and maintained on an inhalant anesthetic.

Fish Anesthesia

As with other veterinary patients, a solid understanding of anesthetic agents and procedures will greatly enhance the diagnostic and treatment options available to veterinarians working with fish. Although the topic of fish anesthesia may be new to most veterinarians, the concepts and procedures are relatively easy to master. With a basic understanding of fish physiology and anatomy, practitioners should be able to sedate and anesthetize a variety of fish species for both medical and surgical procedures. This discussion focuses primarily on anesthesia of teleost fish (bony fish) and contrasts differences to cartilaginous fish (sharks and rays).

Anatomy and Physiology

There are more than 24,000 species of fish. In comparison, there are only 4,000 species of mammals. Because of this tremendous diversity of species, there are many species-specific responses. Accordingly, when working with a new fish species one should anesthetize and recover a few individuals before applying a particular anesthetic protocol or technique to a large number of individuals.

Fish are vertebrates that are uniquely adapted to the aquatic environment. While they do not have lungs, they do respire and require oxygen for routine metabolic processes. Fish use their gills for respiratory gas exchange and can remove oxygen from the water and transfer carbon dioxide and other metabolic by-products back into the water. For this reason, adequate oxygen levels in the animal's aquatic environment are critical for normal respiration and safe anesthesia. During fish respiration, water enters the mouth, passes over the gill filaments, and travels out through the opercular opening. Movement of this opercular flap is a good method to grossly evaluate respirations.[50–54] The gill filaments are anatomically designed for water flow from cranial to caudal, therefore it is recommended that anesthetic-delivery systems provide water flow in a similar direction.

Depending on the procedure, the patient may remain either in its water environment or be removed for prolonged periods of time. In general, fish can be safely removed from water for periods of 1 to 4 min in order to perform routine diagnostic procedures (e.g., blood collection, biopsy, radiography, etc.).[51–54] For longer procedures (i.e., surgical intervention), the patient can remain out of water for much longer periods, but must be kept moist to prevent desiccation.[51–54] Placing the patient in a shallow water bath or on a wet foam block and intermittently dripping or spraying water over the animal can accomplish this. The gills must be kept wet for adequate oxygen exchange. If the fish is placed in a shallow water bath, the water level should be adjusted to cover the gills. If the animal is maintained on a wet foam block, water flow must be provided into the oral cavity and over the gills.

Fish are poikilothermic and their body temperature is directly influenced by their external environment. It is important to know the general water temperature ranges for different species and maintain their water anesthetic solutions in a similar temperature range.

Anesthetic Protocols

Most commonly, the anesthetic agent can be dissolved in water which is used to deliver the drug to the fish. This is a form of inhalation anesthesia since the anesthetic agent is delivered via the respiratory system. While there are some injectable anesthetic agents that are effective, difficulty with controlled delivery combined with their very different species-specific dosages makes the use of injectable agents generally more problematic.[51,53,54]

Adding an anesthetic agent to the water is a relatively simple and safe method of anesthesia. Inhalant water anesthesia allows the animal to remain in its normal environment during induction and does not require direct patient handling or knowledge of the animal's body weight. It is critical to have adequate and appropriate water for anesthetic induction, maintenance, and patient recovery. When available, it is recommended that the anesthetic water source be the animal's own environmental water (i.e., tank or pond). There are many water quality variables that have direct impact on fish physiology, and abrupt changes of water parameters can have deleterious implications.

Water quality testing should be performed prior to any anesthetic attempt. The specific tests conducted are dictated by the size of the system, the water quality history and whether it is fresh water or marine. In general, the following basic parameters should be evaluated: temperature, pH, nitrate, nitrite and ammonia.[52,54] If water from the tank is not being used, it is important that both tank water and anesthetic water are tested, and that anesthetic water quality parameters closely resemble those of the home tank. Water quality testing and maintaining appropriate parameters is more critical for longer anesthetic procedures. For short anesthetic events (i.e., less than 10 min), the equipment needs are minimal and require only an induction system and a recovery system. This "system" is usually a water filled container, the size of which will be dictated by the size of the patient. Small plastic containers or buckets work well for animals less than 1 kg, and larger plastic food coolers for larger fish. This setup is ideal for short diagnostic evaluations, including skin scrapes, gill biopsies, blood collection, body weight measurement, and diagnostic imaging. The patient is placed in a container filled with the anesthetic containing water for induction. Once the fish has become recumbent, it can be evaluated either by elevating the area of interest out of the water or by removing the whole patient to a shallow water bath. After completion of the procedure(s), the fish is placed in a container with anesthetic-free water for recovery.

As with anesthesia of other animals, appropriate oxygen supplementation is critical. Air stones can be attached to the oxygen tubing of an anesthetic machine or directly to an air tank for delivery. In general, the air stone should follow the patient through each tank system (induction, maintenance, and recovery).

For longer anesthetic procedures (e.g., more than 5 to 10 min), the patient should be removed from the induction system and placed in a container of water with a lower maintenance anesthetic concentration. For these procedures anesthetic and oxygen delivery is enhanced by an active flow of water over the gills. This can be accomplished either through the use of a gravity-fed, elevated water container or a small water pump.[51,52,54] The elevated container can easily be constructed using empty IV fluid bags and associated IV drip sets. A corner at the top of the IV bag is cut away, the bag is emptied, and the anesthetic solution poured in. An air stone is placed into the bag through the opening at the top. The IV drip set is attached to the bag and the solution directed into the patient's mouth. The flow can be adjusted using the adjustable valve on the fluid line. In general, the author uses 1-L bags with a corresponding small animal drip set for smaller patients (<200 g) and 3- to 5-L IV bags with higher flow equine drip sets for larger patients. A plastic Y piece can be attached to the end of the IV line and placed in the animal's oral cavity. The Y piece helps direct water flow directly over the gills and out through the operculum. This helps prevent water flow into the GI tract. This system is easy to create, but does require continual refilling of the bag for longer procedures.

Another option is to create a closed system with a water pump. This is much more convenient for longer procedures or if several anesthetic events are scheduled. A submersible pump is placed within the anesthetic water container and water is pumped from the tank into the patient's mouth via a flexible tube.[52] The water pump and the outflow tubing should be adjusted to allow a steady, gentle flow of water through the opercular flaps. Excessive water velocity or placement of the tube in the caudal portion of the oral cavity can cause gastric dilation and poor oxygenation. The patient should be positioned on a fenestrated platform that allows the water to drain back into the anesthetic water tank.

Perioperative Considerations

Although not required, it is generally recommended that patients be fasted 12 to 24 h prior to anesthesia. Fish do not have lungs and cannot aspirate. They can however regurgitate and digesta can become trapped in the gill arches. Fasting also helps decrease the likelihood of fecal contamination of the anesthetic and recovery water systems.

In practice, preoperative hematologic evaluation is not commonly performed in fish although the merits of a preanesthetic evaluation still apply. In many cases large numbers of animals are sedated and preanesthetic blood work may not be realistic. In addition, normal hematological blood parameters have not been documented and values for many species can be difficult to interpret.

Anesthetic Levels and Monitoring

Anesthetic monitoring is important to ensure the patient is at the appropriate anesthetic level for the procedure being conducted. As with other animals, fish pass through anesthetic stages as they become sedated and anesthetized (Table 35.4). Depending on the species, the agent, and the concentration, each stage of anesthesia may not be recognized.[1] In general, sedation is characterized by slower swimming and reduced reaction to stimuli. As the fish becomes anesthetized, it becomes ataxic, loses its righting reflex, and does not respond to stimuli. At a surgical plane of anesthesia the animal is recumbent, has decreased respiration, and does not respond to noxious stimuli (e.g., pinprick).

Fish respiration is observed by noting the rate and quality of opercular movements. As the depth of anesthesia increases, respiration rate will decrease and may eventually become nonexistent. A lack of respirations should not be cause for alarm, but the clinician should reduce the anesthetic concentration and ensure that well-oxygenated water is flowing over the gills. Gill color is also a useful method of grossly evaluating oxygenation and anesthetic depth in fish. In a critical situation, anesthetic-free water can be flushed over the gills using a large syringe. The gills should be dark pink to light red. Pale gills are an indicator of hypotension, hypoxemia, or anemia.[51,52] For longer anesthetic procedures, other anesthetic monitoring equipment including ECG, a Doppler flow detector, or ultrasonography can be used. When using these monitors in fish to evaluate heart rate, trends are more important than specific rates. Normal heart rates are not known for many species, but in general, fish have a significantly slower heart rate than similar sized mammals. The fish myocardium uses local glycogen stores rather than circulating glucose. The fish heart contracts independently of nerve impulses from the brain. It is important to note that a clinically dead fish may still have a heart beat; therefore, pulse should not be used as the sole method of anesthetic monitoring. In the author's experience, pulse oximetry has little practical application in fish.

Waterborne Anesthetics
MS-222

This anesthetic agent has several common names, but is often referred to as Tricaine-S, Finquel, or tricaine methane sulfonate. MS-222 is the most commonly used fish anesthetic agent and is the only product approved by the Food and Drug Administration

Table 35.4. Anesthetic stages of fish.[50,53,56]

Stage 0	Normal	Reacts to external stimuli Normal opercular respirations
Stage 1	Light sedation	Decreased opercular movement
		Decreased response to visual and tactile stimuli
Stage 2	Deep sedation	Only reactive to gross stimulation
Stage 3	Light anesthesia	Loss of equilibrium
		Loss of muscle tone
		Reactive only to strong tactile stimuli
Stage 4	Deep anesthesia	Total loss of reactivity and loss of reflexes
		Respiratory and heart rate diminished
Stage 5	Medullary collapse	Cardiac and respiratory arrest
		Death
		Overdose

Center for Veterinary Medicine for use in fish intended for human consumption.[50,51,54–56] The agent is supplied as a white powder that is easily soluble in water. It is an acidic compound and can cause significant pH changes when added to water. This is especially true in fresh water with a low buffering capacity.[51,52] For this reason, it is important to buffer the pH of the anesthetic water with sodium bicarbonate. Baking soda, a readily available form of sodium bicarbonate, can be added to the anesthetic water until saturation occurs (i.e., until the baking soda no longer dissolves). Adequately buffered solutions will maintain a neutral pH (7.0 to 7.5) after MS-222 has been added. MS-222 is very safe and effective in a wide variety of species and can be used for light sedation (e.g., shipments), surgical anesthesia or, at very high concentrations, for euthanasia.[50–54,56]

The desired concentration of MS-222 will depend on the desired depth of anesthesia, the water temperature, the water hardness, and the animal's species, age, and overall health.[53] In general, MS-222 is more potent and has a narrower safety margin in warmer, softer water and with young fry.[51–53] Published dosages vary widely for fish and range from 25 to 300 mg/L. Induction concentrations between 75 and 125 mg/L, and maintenance solutions of approximately 50 to 75 mg/L are usually effective.[54] Euthanasia can be achieved by placing animals in a concentration of 1000 mg/L for 5 to 10 min (Tables 35.5 and 35.6).[54]

MS-222 has no anesthetic effects in mammals, and exposure is generally considered safe for people, although there have been reports in the literature of chronic exposure to high levels of MS-222 causing reversible retinal lesions in humans.[57] For this reason, inhalation of the powder should be avoided, gloves worn, and hands washed after handling.

Clove Oil (Eugenol)

The active ingredient in clove oil is eugenol, which is available from health food stores (90% active ingredient) or from pharma-

cies as 100% eugenol.[52,57] Eugenol has become a popular anesthetic for freshwater species, including koi and trout. In New Zealand and Australia, a commercially available form of iso-eugenol is marketed under the trade name Aqui-S.[55] Eugenol oil is commonly diluted 1:10 with ethanol before being mixed with water.[51,52] It has been compared with MS-222 in a limited number of species and appears to be an effective fish anesthetic.[51,52,54,55,57–60] Eugenol has a narrower margin of safety than MS-222 and is more likely to cause respiratory failure at higher concentrations.[57] Published dosages for eugenol range from 40 to 200 mg/L, with those at the higher end being associated with longer recoveries and an increased need for manual resuscitation.[52,54,55,57–60] Fish anesthetized/immobilized with higher concentrations of eugenol appear to react more vigorously to hypodermic needle injections when compared with fish anesthetized with MS-222.[55]

Isoflurane

This technique has had limited use in fish. It is effective, but administration and safe scavenging of waste anesthetic gas is problematic. Although vaporized isoflurane can be easily bubbled into water, this method can take a long time to reach anesthetic concentrations. A much more rapid and effective method is to mix liquid isoflurane directly into the water. Since isoflurane is hydrophobic, it beads up in water. To enhance distribution into water, it can be applied by injecting the liquid isoflurane through a small-gauge needle under the water's surface. When added in this manner, small droplets of isoflurane mix in the water. Although this method of administering gaseous anesthesia is effective, a major concern is the difficulty of scavenging waste anesthetic gases. A small "fume hood" can be created by attaching a funnel to a vacuum scavenger system and inverting the funnel over the anesthetic-water mixture. Induction concentrations range from 0.4 to 0.75 mL of liquid isoflurane/L of water. Maintenance concentrations are approximately 0.25 to 0.4 mL of isoflurane/L of water.[54,58]

Other Water-Based Anesthetic Agents

Quinaldine, metomidate, and benzocaine have all been used as anesthetic immobilizing agents in fish.[51–53] Like MS-222 and eugenol, these agents are mixed with water to create an anesthetic solution that is passed over the gills of the fish. In the United States, these agents are not approved for fish intended for human consumption, are less available, and are not commonly used.

Injectable Anesthetics

Propofol

This lipid-based anesthetic emulsion has been demonstrated to be effective in several fish species.[51,61] Its major disadvantage is that it must be given intravenously. It has a rapid induction rate and provides light anesthesia for 60 to 200 min.[51,61] Similar to mammalian species, propofol produces cardiac and respiratory depression in fish. Dosages range from 3.5 to 7.5 mg/kg, and specific dose requirements will likely vary widely among species.[51,61]

Table 35.5. Tricaine methane sulfonate (MS-222) concentration dosing chart.

Gallons of Water	Liters of Water	Grams of MS-222									
		25 mg/L[a]	40 mg/L	50 mg/L	60 mg/L	70 mg/L	80 mg/L	90 mg/L	100 mg/L	125 mg/L	150 mg/L
1	3.79	0.09	0.15	0.19	0.23	0.26	0.30	0.34	0.38	0.47	0.57
2	7.57	0.19	0.30	0.38	0.45	0.53	0.61	0.68	0.76	0.95	1.14
3	11.36	0.28	0.45	0.57	0.68	0.79	0.91	1.02	1.14	1.42	1.70
4	15.14	0.38	0.61	0.76	0.91	1.06	1.21	1.36	1.51	1.89	2.27
5	18.93	0.47	0.76	0.95	1.14	1.32	1.51	1.70	1.89	2.37	2.84
6	22.71	0.57	0.91	1.14	1.36	1.59	1.82	2.04	2.27	2.84	3.41
7	26.50	0.66	1.06	1.32	1.59	1.85	2.12	2.38	2.65	3.31	3.97
8	30.28	0.76	1.21	1.51	1.82	2.12	2.42	2.73	3.03	3.79	4.54
9	34.07	0.85	1.36	1.70	2.04	2.38	2.73	3.07	3.41	4.26	5.11
10	37.85	0.95	1.51	1.89	2.27	2.65	3.03	3.41	3.79	4.73	5.68
11	41.64	1.04	1.67	2.08	2.50	2.91	3.33	3.75	4.16	5.20	6.25
12	45.42	1.14	1.82	2.27	2.73	3.18	3.63	4.09	4.54	5.68	6.81
13	49.21	1.23	1.97	2.46	2.95	3.44	3.94	4.43	4.92	6.15	7.38
14	52.99	1.32	2.12	2.65	3.18	3.71	4.24	4.77	5.30	6.62	7.95
15	56.78	1.42	2.27	2.84	3.41	3.97	4.54	5.11	5.68	7.10	8.52
16	60.56	1.51	2.42	3.03	3.63	4.24	4.84	5.45	6.06	7.57	9.08
17	64.35	1.61	2.57	3.22	3.86	4.50	5.15	5.79	6.43	8.04	9.65
18	68.13	1.70	2.73	3.41	4.09	4.77	5.45	6.13	6.81	8.52	10.22
19	71.92	1.80	2.88	3.60	4.31	5.03	5.75	6.47	7.19	8.99	10.79
20	75.70	1.89	3.03	3.79	4.54	5.30	6.06	6.81	7.57	9.46	11.36
30	113.55	2.84	4.54	5.68	6.81	7.95	9.08	10.22	11.36	14.19	17.03
40	151.40	3.79	6.06	7.57	9.08	10.60	12.11	13.63	15.14	18.93	22.71
50	189.25	4.73	7.57	9.46	11.36	13.25	15.14	17.03	18.93	23.66	28.39
100	378.50	9.46	15.14	18.93	22.71	26.50	30.28	34.07	37.85	47.31	56.78
200	757.00	18.93	30.28	37.85	45.42	52.99	60.56	68.13	75.70	94.63	113.55
300	1135.50	28.39	45.42	56.78	68.13	79.49	90.84	102.20	113.55	141.94	170.33
400	1514.00	37.85	60.56	75.70	90.84	105.98	121.12	136.26	151.40	189.25	227.10
500	1892.50	47.31	75.70	94.63	113.55	132.48	151.40	170.33	189.25	236.56	283.88
1000	3785.00	94.63	151.40	189.25	227.10	264.95	302.80	340.65	378.50	473.13	567.75
10000	37850.00	946.25	1514.00	1892.50	2271.00	2649.50	3028.00	3406.50	3785.00	4731.25	5677.50
20000	75700.00	1892.50	3028.00	3785.00	4542.00	5299.00	6056.00	6813.00	7570.00	9462.50	11355.00

[a]mg/L = ppm.

Ketamine-Medetomidine

Ketamine in combination with medetomidine is usually reserved for larger fish that cannot be manually placed in an anesthetic bath. This is common in large aquarium systems or in free-ranging open-water situations.[62] The drug combination can be delivered via a spring-loaded pole syringe if the animal is swimming in the water, or via hand injection if the animal is in a net.[52,54,62]

Teleost (bony) fish are more refractory to these agents and require fairly high dosages. Elasmobranches (sharks, rays, and skates) are more susceptible to ketamine-medetomidine effects, and this has become the regimen of choice for immobilizing large sharks.[52,62] Teleost dosages range from 1 to 7 mg/kg ketamine plus 30 to 100 µg/kg medetomidine injected intramuscularly.[52] This combination can be partially reversed with atipamezole administered at fivefold the medetomidine dose (on a milligram basis). Elasmobranch dosages range from 1 to 5 mg/kg ketamine combined with medetomidine at 50 to 100 µg/kg administered intramuscularly.[52,54,62]

Nonchemical Methods of Immobilizing Fish

In the aquaculture and fisheries industries, there are several methods of slowing or immobilizing fish that may not traditionally be considered anesthetic techniques. These include hypothermia, electroshock, and application of carbon dioxide.

Hypothermia

This is commonly used when transporting large numbers of fish. Since fish are poikilothermic, reducing their environmental temperature will slow their metabolism and reduce movement. In general, slow gradual cooling is preferred and causes less deleterious physiological changes. It should be noted that hypothermia results in immobilization only and is best reserved for transportation of fish and not used for invasive surgical procedures.[53]

Electroshock or Electroimmobilization

These methods inhibit the fish's ability to swim due to a current-induced tetany.[53] They are primarily used in freshwater animals

Table 35.6. Anesthetic agents commonly used in fish.

Agent	Method of Administration	Dose Concentration	Comments
MS-222	Supplied as a powder that is dissolved in bath water	Induction concentration: 75 to 125 mg/L Maintenance concentration: 50 to 75 mg/L	Buffer solution with sodium bicarbonate. Use a lower concentration for subadults (i.e., fry and fingerlings).
Clove oil (eugenol)	A liquid agent that is placed in bath water	40 to 100 mg/L	Eugenol is poorly soluble in water and should be dissolved in ethanol at a ratio of 1 part eugenol to 10 parts ethanol. Eugenol is commonly supplied as clove oil.
Isoflurane	Liquid isoflurane is placed in bath water	Induction concentration: 0.4 to 0.75 mL/L Maintenance concentration: 0.25 to 0.4 mL/L	Liquid isoflurane can be drawn into a syringe and injected into the water by using a 25-gauge needle.
Propofol	Intravenous	3.5 to 7.5 mg/L	Rapid onset on induction. Provides 60 to 200 min of sedation/anesthesia.
Ketamine-medetomidine	Intramuscular	Teleosts (bony fish) 1 to 7 mg/kg ketamine combined with 30 to 100 μg/kg medetomidine Elasmobranches (sharks and rays) 1 to 5 mg/kg ketamine combined with 50 to 100 μg/kg medetomidine	Atipamezole can be used to reverse medetomidine at fivefold the medetomidine dose. Not generally recommended for teleosts because of slow recovery rates. Commonly used with large sharks.

MS-222, tricaine methane sulfonate.

and typically reserved for collecting and/or sampling fish from large bodies of water (e.g., ponds or lakes). A high-voltage, direct current is applied to the water, and the fish within range that have been shocked will float to the surface. This provides enough time for fish to be processed (weighed, tagged, blood sampled, etc.) before they are recovered and returned to the water unharmed.

Carbon Dioxide

The use of carbon dioxide to induce a state of narcosis is common in many aquatic facilities. Either gaseous carbon dioxide can be bubbled into, or sodium bicarbonate dissolved in, the water. Sodium bicarbonate requires an acidic pH for adequate carbon dioxide release and thus may require the addition of acidic agents to help lower the water pH. In general, this method is reserved for transporting or culling large groups of fish and is not routinely used for individual veterinary procedures.

References

1. Pough FH, Andrews RM, Cadle JE, Crump ML, Savitzky AH, Wells KD, eds. Herpetology, 3rd ed. Upper Saddle River, NJ: Prentice Hall, 1998.
2. Schmidt-Nielsen K. Animal Physiology: Adaptation and Environment. New York: Cambridge University Press, 1997.
3. Zug GR, Vitt LJ, Caldwell JP, eds. Herpetology: An Introductory Biology of Amphibians and Reptiles, 2nd ed. New York: Academic, 2001.
4. Seymour RS, Webb GJW, Bennett AF, Bradford DF. Effect of capture on the physiology of Crocodylus porosus. In: Webb GJW, Manolis SC, Whitehead PJ, eds. Wildlife Management: Crocodiles and Alligators. Chipping Norton, Australia: Surrey Beatty and Sons, 1987:253–257.
5. Martin BJ. Evaluation of hypothermia for anesthesia in reptiles and amphibians. ILAR J 1995;37:186–190.
6. Murray MJ. Cardiology and circulation. In: Mader DR, ed. Reptile Medicine and Surgery. Philadelphia: WB Saunders, 1996:95–103.
7. Lillywhite HB. Gravity, blood circulation, and the adaptation of form and function in lower vertebrates. J Exp Zool 1996;275:217–225.
8. White FN. Circulation. In: Gans C, Dawson WR, eds. Biology of the Reptilia, vol 5: Physiology A. New York: Academic, 1976:275–334.
9. Wang T, Smits AW, Burggren WW. Pulmonary function in reptiles. In: Gans C, Gaunt AS, eds. Biology of the Reptilia, vol 19: Morphology G, Visceral Organs. St Louis: Society for the Study of Amphibians Reptiles, 1998:297–374.
10. Bienzle D, Boyd CJ. Sedative effects of ketamine and midazolam in snapping turtles (Chelydra serpentina). J Zoo Wildl Med 1992;23:201–204.
11. Harvey-Clark C. Midazolam fails to sedate painted turtles, Chrysemys picta. Bull Assoc Rept Amphib Vet 1993;3:7–8.

12. Oppenheim YV, Moon PF. Sedative effects of midazolam in red-eared slider turtles (*Trachemys scripta elegans*). J Zoo Wildl Med 1995;26:409–411.

13. Spiegel RA, Lane TJ, Larsen RE, Cardeilhac PT. Diazepam and succinylcholine chloride for restraint of the American alligator. J Am Vet Med Assoc 1984;185:1335–1336.

14. Kanui TI, Hole K. Morphine and pethidine antinoception in the crocodile. J Vet Pharmacol Ther 1992;15:101–103.

15. Machin KL. Amphibian pain and analgesia. J Zoo Wildl Med 1999;30:2–10.

16. Machin KL. Fish, amphibian, and reptile analgesia. Vet Clin North Am Exot Anim Pract 2001;4:19–34.

17. Mosley CAE, Dyson D, Smith DA. The cardiovascular dose-response effects of isoflurane alone and combined with butorphanol in the green iguana (*Iguana iguana*). Vet Anaesth Analg 2004;31:64–72.

18. Read MR. Evaluation of the use of anesthesia and analgesia in reptiles. J Am Vet Med Assoc 2004;224:547–552.

19. Benson KG, Forrest L. Characterization of the renal portal system of the common green iguana (*Iguana iguana*) by digital subtraction imaging. J Zoo Wildl Med 1999;30:235–241.

20. Holz PH. The reptilian renal-portal system: Influence on therapy. In: Fowler ME, Miller RE, eds. Zoo and Wild Animal Medicine: Current Therapy 4. Philadelphia: WB Saunders, 1999:249–251.

21. Heaton-Jones TG, Ko JC, Heaton-Jones DL. Evaluation of medetomidine-ketamine anesthesia with atipamezole reversal in American alligators (*Alligator mississippiensis*). J Zoo Wildl Med 2002;33:36–44.

22. Whitaker BR, Krum H. Medical management of sea turtles in aquaria. In: Fowler ME, Miller RE, eds. Zoo and Wild Animal Medicine: Current Therapy 4. Philadelphia: WB Saunders, 1999:217–231.

23. Arena PC, Richardson KC, Cullen LK. Anaesthesia in two species of large Australian skink. Vet Rec 1988;123:155–158.

24. Cooper JE. Ketamine hydrochloride as an anaesthetic for East African reptiles. Vet Rec 1974;95:37–41.

25. Custer RS, Bush M. Physiologic and acid-base measures of gopher snakes during ketamine or halothane-nitrous oxide anesthesia. J Am Vet Med Assoc 1980;177:870–874.

26. Glenn JL, Straight R, Snyder CC. Clinical use of ketamine hydrochloride as an anesthetic agent for snakes. Am J Vet Res 1972;33:1901–1903.

27. Harding KA. The use of ketamine anaesthesia to milk two tropical rattlesnakes (*Crotalus durissus terrificus*). Vet Rec 1977;100:289–290.

28. Schumacher J, Lillywhite HB, Norman WM, Jacobson ER. Effects of ketamine HCl on cardiopulmonary function in snakes. Copeia 1997;2:395–398.

29. Chittick EJ, Stamper MA, Beasley JF, Lewbart GA, Horne WA. Medetomidine, ketamine, and sevoflurane for anesthesia of injured loggerhead sea turtles: 13 cases (1996–2000). J Am Vet Med Assoc 2002;221:1019–1025.

30. Dennis PM, Heard DJ. Cardiopulmonary effects of a medetomidine-ketamine combination administered intravenously in gopher tortoises. J Am Vet Med Assoc 2002;220:1516–1519.

31. Lock B, Heard DJ, Dennis P. Preliminary evaluation of medetomidine/ketamine combinations for immobilization and reversal with atipamezole in three tortoise species. Bull Assoc Amphib Rept Vet 1998;8:6–9.

32. Norton TM. Medetomidine and ketamine anesthesia with atipamezole reversal in private free-ranging gopher tortoises, *Gopherus polyphemus*. In: Proceedings of the Fifth Annual Conference of the Association of Reptilian and Amphibian Veterinarians, 1998:25–26.

33. Bennett RA, Schumacher J, Hedjazi-Haring K, Newell SM. Cardiopulmonary and anesthetic effects of propofol administered intraosseously to green iguanas. J Am Vet Med Assoc 1998;212:93–98.

34. Kaufman GE, Seymour RE, Bonner BB, Court MH, Karas AZ. Use of rocuronium for endotracheal intubation of North American Gulf Coast box turtles. J Am Vet Med Assoc 2003;222:1111–1115.

35. Loveridge JP. The immobilization and anaesthesia of crocodilians. Int Zoo Yearb 1979;19:103–112.

36. Wood SC, Lenfant CJM. Respiration: Mechanics, control and gas exchange. In: Gans C, Dawson WR, eds. Biology of the Reptilia, vol 5: Physiology A. New York: Academic, 1976:225–274.

37. Diethelm G, Mader DR. The effects of FiO$_2$ on post anesthetic recovery times in the green iguana. In: Proceedings of the Association of Reptilian and Amphibian Veterinarians, 1999;169–170.

38. Bertelsen MF, Mosley C, Crawshaw GJ, Dyson D, Smith DA. Evaluation of isoflurane, sevoflurane and nitrous oxide in Dumeril's monitor (*Varanus dumerili*). In: Proceedings of the Annual Conference of the American Association of Zoo Animal Veterinarians, 2004:5–7.

39. Mosley CAE, Dyson D, Smith DA. Minimum alveolar concentration of isoflurane in green iguanas and the effect of butorphanol on minimum alveolar concentration. J Am Vet Med Assoc 2003;222:1559–1564.

40. Rooney MR, Levine G, Gaynor J, Macdonald E, Wimsatt J. Sevoflurane anesthesia in desert tortoises (*Gopherus agassizii*). J Zoo Wildl Med 1999;30:64–69.

41. Mosley CAE, Dyson D, Smith DA. The cardiac index of isoflurane in green iguanas. J Am Vet Med Assoc 2003;22:1565–1568.

42. Prezant RM, Jarchow JL. Lactated fluid therapy use in reptiles: Is there a better solution? In: Proceedings of the Association of Reptilian and Amphibian Veterinarians, 1997:83–85.

43. Kerr J, Frankel HM. Inadequacy of blood drawn by cardiac puncture as a source for respiratory gas measurements in turtle (*Pseudemys scripta*). Comp Biochem Physiol A 1972;41:913–915.

44. Diethelm G, Mader DR, Grosenbaugh DA, Muir WW. Evaluating pulse oximetry in the green iguana, *Iguana iguana*. In: Proceedings of the Association of Reptilian and Amphibian Veterinarians, 1998:11–12.

45. Downes H. Tricaine anesthesia in amphibia: A review. Bull Assoc Rept Amphib Vet 1995;5:11–16.

46. Stetter MD. Fish and amphibian anesthesia. Vet Clin North Am Exot Anim Pract 2001;4:69–82.

47. Lafortune M, Mitchell MA, Smith JA. Evaluation of medetomidine, clove oil and propofol for anesthesia of leopard frogs, *Rana pipiens*. J Herpetol Med Surg 2001;11:13–18.

48. Moon PE, Stabenau EK. Anesthetic and postanesthetic management of sea turtles. J Am Vet Med Assoc 1996;208:720–726.

49. Jenkins JR. Diagnostic and clinical techniques. In: Mader DR, ed. Reptile Medicine and Surgery. Philadelphia: WB Saunders, 1996:264–276.

50. Brown LA. Anesthesia and restraint. In: Stoskopf M, ed. Fish Medicine. Philadelphia: WB Saunders, 1993:79–90.

51. Harms CA. Fish. In: Fowler M, Miller R, eds. Zoo and Wild Animal Medicine, 5th ed. St Louis: WB Saunders, 2003:2–20.

52. Harms CA. Anesthesia in fish. In: Fowler M, Miller R, eds. Zoo and Wild Animal Medicine: Current Therapy 4. Philadelphia: WB Saunders, 1998:158–163.

53. Ross LG, Ross B. Anesthetic and Sedative Techniques for Aquatic Animals, 2nd ed. London: Blackwell Science, 1999.

54. Stetter MD. Fish and amphibian anesthesia. Vet Clin North Am Exot Anim Pract 2001;4:69–80.

55. Bowser PR. Anesthetic options for fish. In: Gleed RD, Ludders JW, eds. Recent Advances in Veterinary Anesthesia and Analgesia: Companion Animals. International Veterinary Information Service. http://www.ivis.org/advances/Anesthesia_Gleed/bowser/chapter_frm.asp?LA=1.

56. Ross LG. Restraint anesthesia and euthanasia. In: Wildgoose W, ed. BSAVA Manual of Ornamental Fish, 2nd ed. Ames, IA: Blackwell, 2001:75–83.

57. Sladky KK, Swanson CR, Stoskopf MK, Loomis MR, Lewbart GA. Comparative efficacy of tricaine methanesulfonate and clove oil for use as anesthetics in red pacu (*Piaractus brachypomus*). Am J Vet Res 2001;62:337–342.

58. Johnson EL. Anesthesia in Koi. In: Koi Health and Disease. Athens: Reade, 1997:102–108.

59. Keene JL, Noakes DL, Moccia RD, Soto CG. 1998. The efficacy of clove oil as an anaesthetic for rainbow trout, *Oncorhynchus mykiss*. Aquaculture Res 1998;29:89–101.

60. Woody CA, Nelson J, Ramstad K. Clove oil as an anesthetic for adult sockeye salmon: Field trials. J Fish Biol 2002;60:340–347.

61. Fleming GJ, Heard DJ, Floyd RF, Riggs A. Evaluation of propofol and meditomidine-ketamine for short-term immobilization of Gulf of Mexico sturgeon (*Acipenser oxyrinchus*). J Zoo Wildl Med 2002;34:153–158.

62. Snyder SB, Richard MJ, Berzins IK, Stamper MA. Immobilization of sandtiger sharks (*Odontaspsis taurus*) using medetomidine/ketamine. In: Proceedings of the International Association of Aquatic Animal Medicine, San Diego, 1998;120–121.

Section VII
ANESTHESIA AND ANALGESIA OF PATIENTS WITH SPECIFIC DISEASE

Chapter 36
Cardiovascular Disease

Ralph C. Harvey and Stephen J. Ettinger

Introduction

The anesthetic management of a patient with cardiovascular dysfunction can be very challenging, because most preanesthetic and anesthetic agents capable of depressing the central nervous system can also produce cardiovascular depression. Patients with cardiovascular dysfunction may be more prone to fluid overload and dysrhythmias. Extremes in heart rate may cause severe problems, including heart failure. Patients with cardiovascular dysfunction may lack sufficient cardiac reserve to compensate for anesthetic-induced depression. Because of the diversity of pathophysiological conditions, no single anesthetic management technique or protocol can be recommended for all animals with cardiovascular dysfunction.[1] Appropriate patient monitoring with arterial blood pressure, central venous pressure, electrocardiogram, end-tidal carbon dioxide, pulse oximetry, and other parameters is essential to reduce anesthetic and surgical risk.

Cardiovascular Physiology

The function of the myocardial cell is to contract and relax rhythmically with other myofibers so that the heart will act as a pump. The basic contractile unit of heart muscle is the sarcomere, which is composed of interdigitating protein filaments of actin and myosin. Muscle shortening begins in the myocardial muscle when the actin and myosin filaments are activated. This activation is regulated by tropomyosin and troponin. Tropomyosin prevents the interaction of actin and myosin during diastole. When tropomyosin is no longer at its blocking position, systole is initiated. The availability of ionized calcium in the area of the troponin-tropomyosin protein unit acts as an immediate catalyst for the contraction-relaxation cycle. The contraction of the heart muscle depends on the amount of free calcium ions available around the myofibril. Part of the contractile-dependent calcium originates from superficial sites on cell membranes that are in equilibrium with extracellular calcium and therefore can be affected by drugs that do not penetrate the myocardial cell.

Few clinically used drugs affect the actin and myosin proteins, but many drugs can alter the availability of calcium for activation of the contractile process.[1] Digitalis increases calcium movement to the troponin-tropomyosin protein unit and thus increases contractile strength. Barbiturates and inhalant anesthetic agents seem to disrupt calcium movements and thus cause reduced contractile strength. Myocardial intracellular acidosis also inhibits the binding of calcium to the troponin-tropomyosin unit, causing decreased myocardial contractile strength. Disease conditions or drugs that produce metabolic or respiratory acidosis may decrease contractility. Most anesthetics depress respiration and predispose patients to respiratory acidosis.

Blood pressure is the product of peripheral vascular resistance and cardiac output. Cardiac output is the product of heart rate and stroke volume. Drugs that alter any or all of these parameters may greatly affect blood pressure and tissue blood flow. Preanesthetic and anesthetic agents can alter vascular resistance (e.g., phenothiazine tranquilizers, α_2-adrenergic agonists, barbiturates, and inhalant agents), heart rate (e.g., opioids, α_2-adrenergic agonists, dissociative agents, and inhalants), and stroke volume (e.g., inhalant anesthetics). Patients that suffer from diseases causing impaired cardiac output, patients with congenital heart disease, and those suffering from hypotension, hypovolemia, anemia, and/or heartworms are at a higher anesthetic risk.

Impaired Cardiac Output

Anesthetic management of patients with impaired cardiac output depends greatly on the underlying pathology, which may require echocardiography for accurate diagnosis. General guidelines are to avoid bradycardia and tachycardia, decreased preload, and hypovolemia, as well as unnecessarily high left-atrial pressures and volume overload. The decreased tolerance of these patients for improper fluid therapy and anesthetic management emphasizes the need for adequate perioperative monitoring and support. These patients should be preoxygenated for 5 to 7 min prior to anesthetic induction. If cardiovascular function is adequate, the choice of anesthetic drugs may not be specific for these patients; however, drugs that may produce tachycardia (anticholinergics and dissociative agents) or large changes in vascular resistance should be used judiciously.

Narcotics are often used as preanesthetic medication because of their minimal effects on the myocardium, and they can be readily antagonized. Indeed, opioids are the mainstay of cardiac anesthesia. Opioids tend to maintain, and may even indirectly improve, myocardial function. They can be used in combination with acepromazine or a benzodiazepine tranquilizer for additional sedation. Use of acepromazine may be contraindicated in some forms of cardiovascular diseases (e.g., hypertrophic cardiomyopathy) but may be beneficial in others (e.g., mitral valve insufficiency) because of the potential for decreased afterload. Opioids can increase vagal afferent activity, which may decrease heart rate. If significant bradycardia occurs, atropine or glycopyrrolate should be given as needed.

If only tranquilization is needed, a low dose of acepromazine (e.g., 0.02 mg/kg) may be administered intramuscularly. Acepromazine decreases peripheral vascular resistance and very often leads to arterial hypotension and reduced preload. Acepromazine can have significant negative inotropic effects. Because of direct myocardial depression, and prominent vasodilatation and hypotension, the value of inducing sedation/tranquilization must be weighed against the potential adverse effects. Phenothiazines must be used cautiously in most cardiac patients.[2] If acepromazine is administered, patients must be monitored closely and appropriate supportive care used should adverse effects become significant.

The use of α_2-adrenergic agonists should be avoided in patients with impaired cardiac output. These drugs can produce significant dysrhythmias, including severe sinus bradycardia and sinoatrial and atrioventricular nodal blocks. Bradycardia, reduced contractility, and increased afterload are particularly disadvantageous effects of α_2-adrenergic agonists in many cardiac patients.[2,3]

Cardiomyopathy

Cardiomyopathy can be classified as hypertrophic or congestive. Hypertrophic cardiomyopathy is characterized by ventricular hypertrophy, decreased ventricular compliance, and impaired ventricular filling, which result in reduced cardiac output. Ventricular contractility (pump function) is usually not impaired.[4] Congestive (dilated) cardiomyopathy is characterized by marked ventricular dilation, increased ventricular end-diastolic and systolic volumes, and poor myocardial contractility. Often, congestive heart failure is present.[4] Since most anesthetic drugs worsen existing myocardial performance, to reduce the risk during the perianesthetic period, treatment of cardiomyopathy is warranted prior to anesthesia. Commonly employed cardiovascular medications used for treatment of congestive heart failure are listed in Table 36.1. In dogs with dilated cardiomyopathy, anesthesia is best induced with agents that have minimal direct myocardial depressant effects. Etomidate or alphaxalone would be preferable induction agents over either thiopental or propofol. The direct depressant effects of ketamine on the myocardium may be clinically significant if sympathetic nervous system efferent activity is already maximal or exhausted. The lowest possible concentra-

tion of an inhalant should be used for maintenance of anesthesia. Anesthesia is less depressing to myocardial performance when an opioid is coadministered, resulting in lower inhalant anesthetic requirements.

Pericardial Tamponade and Constrictive Pericarditis

These are associated with impaired cardiac output caused by reduced stroke volume secondary to reduced end-diastolic ventricular volume. There is limited expansion of the cardiac chambers, resulting in decreased ventricular filling such that heart rate must increase to maintain cardiac output. Pulse pressure is usually decreased, and peripheral pulses may feel abnormal. Myocardial contractility might not be impaired.[5]

Valvular Heart Disease

The heart contains four valves: mitral, tricuspid, aortic, and pulmonary. Valve changes usually can be classified as insufficiency or stenosis. Valvular heart disease is associated with impaired cardiac output and, when severe, can cause congestive heart failure. When a murmur is asculted or valvular heart disease is suspected, the preanesthetic evaluation should include thoracic radiographs and possibly an echocardiogram in addition to the routine preanesthetic screening. The value of these diagnostic tests is to facilitate anesthetic planning and intraoperative responses to abnormal monitored parameters since the management of valvular disease can vary significantly depending on which valve (valves) is (are) affected.

Although both mitral and tricuspid insufficiencies are often clinically insignificant, ventricular ejection fraction is reduced. It is useful to maintain heart rate, maintain contractility, and avoid arteriolar constriction.[6] Antimuscarinics should be used conservatively, but lower doses of atropine or glycopyrrolate are often used to inhibit anesthetic-associated bradycardia. α_2-Adrenergic agonists are contraindicated in patients with valvular insufficiency, because they can affect heart rate and peripheral vascular resistance. Opioids are a principle component of balanced anesthesia for these patients and are generally chosen based on analgesic and sedative requirements. If these patients are stable, anesthesia may be induced with ketamine and diazepam or propofol. Less stable patients may be anesthetized by induction with etomidate or high doses of opioids in combination with a benzodiazepine. To avoid pronounced vasodilatation and hypotension, lower doses of inhalants are used. Use of the inhalants helps to prevent arteriolar vasoconstriction and increased afterload. Fluid therapy should be conservative and based on continual monitoring of central venous pressure and arterial blood pressure. As with other aspects of anesthetic care, postoperative monitoring and support are individualized.

Hypertrophic Cardiomyopathy

This is the most commonly diagnosed cardiac disease of cats.[7] An inherited form of the disease has been identified in humans and in Maine coon cats. Hypertrophic cardiomyopathy (HCM) is characterized by a stiff left ventricle with poor diastolic function. As

Table 36.1. Chronic therapy for congestive heart failure

Classes	Trade Name	Mechanism of Action	Effects on Contractility	Afterload	Maintenance Dose
Nitrovasodilators					
Na nitroprusside	Nitropress	Activation of EDRF or NO. These drugs act as substrates for the formation of NO. Nitroprusside is primarily an arterial dilator, whereas nitroglycerin is a venodilator.	—	↓	2–5 µg/kg/min IV (monitor pressure) CRI suggested Protect drug from light
Nitroglycerin	Nitrostat; Nitropaste	Preload-reducing agent.	—	↓	1–5 µg/kg/min IV recommended only for acute-care situations with continuous blood pressure monitoring. Available in oral and transdermal paste formulations, but oral is rarely if ever used in animals. Pastes are considered third-line therapy. More likely to use oral hydralazine acutely. *Dog*: ¼–½ inch/kg QOD *Cat*: ⅛ inch/kg QOD
Isosorbide dinitrate	Many formulations available	Formation of NO.	—	↓	0.5–2.0 mg/kg PO, BID; also available as an ointment; uncommonly used in animals
Hydralazine	Apresoline	Hydralazine interferes with Ca^{+2} transport in smooth muscle; acts as an afterload-reducing agent.	—	↓	*Dog*: 0.5–2.0 mg/kg PO, BID *Cat*: not commonly recommended
ACE inhibitors					
Captopril	Capoten	Prevents conversion of angiotensin I to angiotensin II, which decreases blood pressure and produces some venodilation. Produces balanced vasodilation, prevents renal fluid retention, reverses cardiac fibrosis, and slows heart rate through decreased ß-adrenergic stimulation.	—	↓	This drug is rarely used in VM and is less reliable than are the other ACE I agents below. *Dog*: 0.5–2.0 PO, TID *Cat*: the same
Enalpril	Enacard		—	↓	*Dog*: 0.5 mg/kg PO, SID-BID *Cat*: 0.25–0.5 mg/kg PO, SID-QOD
Benazepril	Lotensin Foretaker		—	↓	*Dog*: 0.25–0.5 mg/kg PO, SID-BID *Cat*: 0.25–0.5 mg/kg PO, SID
Lisinopril	Zestril Prinivil	ACE I, as above for captopril		↓	*Dog*: 0.5 mg/kg PO, SID *Cat*: 0.25 mg/kg PO, SID
Diuretics					
Acetazolamide		Inhibits Na^+ from passing into the proximal tubule. The osmotic effect is at the glomerulus.	—	↓	*Dog*: 10 mg/kg q 6 h Rarely used in cardiovascular medicine
Aminophylline		Increases the vascular perfusion of the glomerulus.	↑	↓	*Dog*: 11 mg/kg PO, BID-TID *Cat*: 5 mg/kg PO, BID-TID
Spironolactone	Aldactone	Inhibits the aldosterone receptor in collecting tubule (CT). Prevention of ACE escape is the principal use of this agent now.	—	↓	*Dog*: 0.25 mg/kg SID for preventing ACE escape. Higher dosages may be considered as a diuretic. *Cat*: the same
Furosemide	Lasix	Inhibits the Na^+, K^+, and Cl^{-2} cotransporter in the thick ascending loop of Henle.	—	↓	*Dog*: 1–4 mg/kg PO, SC, IM, IV, SID-QID *Cat*: 1–2 mg/kg PO, SC, IM, IV, SID-QID

(continued)

Table 36.1. Chronic therapy for congestive heart failure (*continued*)

Classes	Trade Name	Mechanism of Action	Effects on Contractility	Afterload	Maintenance Dose
Hydrochlorothiazide	Hydrodiuril	Blocks resorption in the distal convoluted tubule by inhibiting the Na^+ and CT cotransporter.	—	↓	*Dog*: 2–4 mg/kg PO, SID-BID *Cat*: 1–2 mg/kg PO, SID-BID
Inotropes					
Digitalis	Cardoxin; Lanoxin	Inactivates the Na^+/K^+ ATPase pump, increasing Ca^{+2} intracellularly.	↑	↑	*Dog*: 0.005–0.008 mg/kg PO, BID in smaller dogs and 0.22 mg/m^2; also twice daily in larger dogs *Cat*: ¼ to ½ 0.125-mg tablet PO q 48–72 h, based on size and clinical response
T3	Tristat	Increases Ca^{+2} adenosine ATPase activity; upregulates beta-receptor activity.	↑	—	Not likely to be used and not a primary inotrope but may be part of the protocol along with traditional agents in the event of a low thyroid value
"Inodilators"					
Amrinone	Inocor	Class III phosphodiesterase enzyme inhibitors (PDEIs) prevent breakdown of cAMP, which results from the stimulation of ß-adrenergic receptors.	↑	↓	1–3 mg/kg IV slow to effect, then CRI at 10–100 µg/kg/min
Milrinone	Primacor		↑	↓	1–3 mg/kg/min IV slow, then CRI at 10–100 µg/kg/min to effect
Pimobendan	Vetmedin	Ca^{+2} sensitization and PDE inhibition.	↑	↓	*Dogs*: 0.3–0.6 mg/kg PO, SID *Cats*: not known if applicable
Beta blockers					
Metoprolol	Lopressor; Toprol XL	Upregulates damaged beta sites; reduces the adrenergic barrage; slows the cardiac rate.		↓	*Dogs*: 0.25–1.0 mg/kg PO BID-TID; begin low and titrate upwards slowly. *Cats*: very low dosages used usually for heart rate control and not CHF
Carvedilol	Coreg	Beta-blocking agent and peripheral vasodilator (blocks ß$_1$, ß$_2$, and α$_1$).	↑	↓	*Dogs*: 0.05 mg/kg PO initially once daily: slowly titrate weekly to maximum 0.3 mg/kg

ACE, angiotensin-converting enzyme; CRI, constant-rate infusion; EDRF, endothelium-derived relaxing factor; IV, intravenous; NO, nitric oxide; PO, per os (orally); and SC, subcutaneously.

This table enlists a variety of classes of medications including digitalis, "inodilators," vasodilators, ACE inhibitors, and diuretics. Dosages taken from *Textbook of Veterinary Internal Medicine*, 6th ed.[16]

ventricular wall thickness increases, end-diastolic volume and ventricular function are decreased. Congestive heart failure develops as ventricular stiffness increases, end-diastolic ventricular volume decreases, and mitral regurgitation and hypertension develop. Early HCM is often asymptomatic. Signs of progressive HCM (murmurs, arrhythmias, dyspnea, and thromboembolic disease) are consistent with the development of heart failure. Sudden death during the stresses of hospitalization, anesthesia, and medical or surgical procedures can occur with more advanced HCM.

For patients with early signs of cardiomyopathy, anesthesia can be induced by using propofol, etomidate, or a neuroleptanalgesic combination. Mask induction using one of the potent volatile inhalant anesthetics is also an acceptable technique, although the stress of induction may be detrimental to patients with impaired cardiac function. Inhalant anesthetics are most often the maintenance agents for these patients. Isoflurane is one of the preferred inhalants because of preservation of a near-normal cardiac index and minimal dysrhythmic effects in healthy animals, when compared with the effects of halothane. However, in animals with diastolic dysfunction (e.g., HCM) isoflurane may be associated with reduced preload and afterload leading to reduced end-diastolic ventricular volume and increased end-systolic ventricular to aortic pressure gradients when dynamic outflow-tract obstruction is present. Sevoflurane minimally reduces cardiac output and is associated with less vasodilation than is isoflurane at typical anesthetic doses in healthy animals. Animals may maintain a lower heart rate when anesthetized with sevoflurane than with isoflurane, although preanesthetic drugs may alter the cardiovascular responses to inhalant anesthetics. Based on the lower blood solubility and reduced pungency, sevoflurane may provide for a less stressful inhalant induction compared with either halothane or isoflurane. When a lower heart rate is desired (e.g., for cats with HCM), sevoflurane may be preferred over isoflurane.[8] Among the injectable general anesthetics, etomidate is unique in maintaining cardiac output without increasing myocardial oxygen consumption.

Congenital Heart Disease

When considering the anesthetic management of patients with congenital heart disease, the problems encountered are often similar to those in patients with congestive heart failure. The most common surgically correctable problems are patent ductus arteriosus (PDA) and persistent right aortic arch (PRAA).

PDA is usually recognized early in life before patients develop signs of heart failure. Typically, if diagnosed early, shunt blood flow is from the systemic circulation to the pulmonary artery (left-to-right shunt). However, when systemic vascular resistance decreases after induction of anesthesia, shunt flow may reverse, especially when significant pulmonary hypertension is present. Pulse oximetry is useful for rapid detection (rapid reduction in arterial hemoglobin saturation) of this reversion to a right-to-left shunt. Phenylephrine can be useful in this situation to increase systemic pressure and reestablish left-to-right flow. If the patient is normal in other respects, the anesthetic protocol is designed for the pediatric patient undergoing a thoracotomy with attention toward maintaining heart rate and cardiac output. Surgical manipulation around the heart may cause ventricular ectopic beats. These are usually transitory and do not require treatment. When the PDA is ligated, increased blood pressure may cause a reflex slowing of the heart rate. This is a normal physiological response.[8] In some instances, antimuscarinic drugs (e.g., atropine or glycopyrrolate) may be needed to counteract the sinus bradycardia. To minimize the potential for bradycardia, an anticholinergic may be administered as a preanesthetic medication. Because of the size of some patients, intraoperative hypothermia is often a problem when they undergo PDA surgery. Every effort should be made to minimize the loss of body heat.

PRAA is also usually recognized and corrected early in life. If a patient is normal in other respects, the anesthetic protocol is designed for the pediatric patient undergoing a thoracotomy. It is important to remember that a patient with PRAA may be suffering from aspiration pneumonia. As with a PDA, surgical manipulation around the heart may cause ventricular ectopic beats, and intraoperative hypothermia is of concern.

Hypotension, Hypovolemia, or Shock

Patients with hypotension and hypovolemia should be stabilized with intravenous fluids and/or whole blood prior to anesthesia. Many preanesthetic and anesthetic drugs are potentially hypotensive; therefore, these drugs can exacerbate preexisting hypotension.

Shock can be defined as an acute clinical syndrome characterized by progressive circulatory failure that leads to inadequate capillary perfusion and cellular hypoxia.[9] Shock is a complex, multisystem disorder that may be caused by a variety of insults. Shock may be classified as hypovolemic, cardiogenic, or vasculogenic. If one thinks of the cardiovascular system as a pump, fluid, and pipes to carry the fluid, then the three classifications reflect which component of the cardiovascular system is affected.

Hypovolemic shock occurs when there is an inadequate volume of fluid (blood) being pumped through the cardiovascular system. Hemorrhage, fluid loss, and trauma can all cause hypovolemic shock.

Cardiogenic shock, which occurs when the heart is no longer an effective pump, can be caused by a failure in ventricular filling (cardiac tamponade, tension pneumothorax, or collapse of the vena cava caused by inadvertent closure of the pop-off valve, resulting in airway pressure buildup) or by a failure of ventricular ejection (ruptured chordae tendineae, cardiac dysrhythmias, severe myocardial depression, or severe and prolonged increase in systemic vascular resistance).

Vasculogenic shock occurs when there are changes in venous capacitance or peripheral resistance. Numerous causes can lead to vasculogenic shock, including sepsis (vasodilation is caused by release of vasoactive substances such as histamine, prostaglandins, and bradykinin), anaphylaxis (vasodilation occurs because of histamine release), neurogenic factors (loss of vasomotor tone caused by excessive general anesthesia, trauma of the central nervous system, and spinal anesthesia), and a severe and prolonged increase in peripheral resistance.

Regardless of the underlying cause, a common pathway of circulatory failure is present in shock. Reflex mechanisms may compensate for early circulatory failure and result in recovery of a patient with mild or moderate shock. However, reflexive compensatory mechanisms may become deleterious to a patient if they are prolonged and may result in microcirculatory changes and further cellular hypoxia.

All forms of shock eventually result in decreased blood flow and hypoperfusion of the body tissues. Baroreceptors in the aorta and carotid artery and low-pressure receptors in the atria respond to the decreased cardiac output and blood pressure. This results in activation of the sympathoadrenal system. Hypothalamic sympathetic nerve centers increase release of norepinephrine from postganglionic sympathetic nerve endings and increase liberation of epinephrine and norepinephrine from the adrenal medulla into the blood. This results in splenic contraction and a release of blood into the circulation. Epinephrine and norepinephrine stimulate alpha and beta receptors. Alpha-receptor stimulation results in vasoconstriction of both arteries and veins. Beta-receptor stimulation causes vasodilation in skeletal muscle and increased force and rate of cardiac contraction. This results in a redistribution of blood flow to the heart and brain. Blood flow to the splanchnic, renal, and cutaneous vessels is markedly decreased. The catecholamines produce tachycardia, increase myocardial contractility, and stimulate hepatic glycogenolysis. Venous constriction causes decreased vascular capacity. The decreased vascular capacity improves venous return and thus cardiac output.

An important compensatory mechanism in shock is the extravascular fluid shift. Owing to vasoconstriction, there is decreased capillary blood flow and thus capillary pressure. The decreased capillary pressure allows extravascular fluid to enter the blood vessels. This is very important in expanding circulating fluid volume. Endocrine factors are also important in the compensatory mechanism of shock. Renin is released from the ischemic kidney to activate the renin-angiotensin-aldosterone system. This results in vascular constriction; renal absorption of sodium, chloride, and water; and renal excretion of potassium. Antidiuretic hormone is released because of hypovolemia, and this also promotes water retention. The overall effect is to increase extracellular fluid volume.

These compensatory mechanisms cause a significant redistribution of blood flow to the heart, brain, and adrenal glands, and may aid recovery of patients in mild to moderate shock. However, they may not be adequate in severe shock, and it may become irreversible. Irreversibility is characterized by inadequate tissue perfusion to vital organs that results in cardiac failure, disseminated intravascular coagulation, depression of the reticuloendothelial system, and peripheral vascular failure. Hypotension and decreased capillary perfusion lead to cellular hypoxia, decreased delivery of energy substrates to the cell, and increased concentration of cellular metabolites.

Glucose is first used anaerobically by the cells as an energy source with production of pyruvate and limited amounts of adenosine triphosphate (ATP). Pyruvate is then aerobically utilized to produce large amounts of ATP, or it may be released into the circulation after being reduced to lactic acid. Large amounts of oxygen are needed by cells to produce the ATP. In shock, cellular hypoxia occurs, and although ATP can be produced anaerobically, it may not be produced in adequate amounts.[9] The establishment of membrane ionic gradients depends on adequate ATP generation. Cellular edema may result if ionic gradients are not maintained. The lactic acidemia that occurs in shock results from the release of anaerobic energy in tissues unable to support adequate oxidative processes. Individual cells and then organs begin to die.

Increased cellular metabolites (lactic acid) in the capillary bed cause precapillary sphincters to relax, but postcapillary sphincters remain constricted. Blood flows into the capillary bed but is slow to leave, resulting in an increased hydrostatic pressure with net flow into the tissues and further volume deficits. Decreased perfusion of the splanchnic vasculature results in pancreatic ischemia and the release of myocardial depressant factor. Myocardial depressant factor decreases myocardial contractility.[10] Splanchnic vasoconstriction and decreased capillary perfusion depress the reticuloendothelial system in the spleen and liver. With impaired function of the reticuloendothelial system, endotoxins, bacteria, and microemboli accumulate and produce further circulatory failure. Slow-moving (stagnant) acidic blood is hypercoagulable. Clot-initiating factors are common in shock and include bacterial toxins and thromboplastin of red cells (released by hemolysis).[11] These factors result in disseminated intravascular coagulation, which results in a consumption of clotting factors, bleeding, and focal tissue infarcts due to microthrombi. Multiorgan failure (multiorgan dysfunction syndrome)

occurs, and the patient dies. Induction of anesthesia in patients with any level of shock is ill-advised.

Anemia

Anemic patients are at higher risk from an anesthetic standpoint because the oxygen-carrying capacity of the cardiovascular system is diminished. Either packed red blood cells, whole blood, or hemoglobin-based oxygen-carrying solutions should be considered if the dog or cat has a packed cell volume (PCV) of less than 25% to 30% before surgery or less than 20% after surgery. Patients with chronic anemia seem to be able to cope better with the problem than those with acute anemia. Whole blood, packed red blood cells, or a hemoglobin-based oxygen-carrying solution (e.g., Oxyglobin) should be readily available. The rate and total amount of blood administered should be tailored to the requirements of the patient. Patients with acute blood loss and hypovolemia can usually tolerate faster rates of colloid administration than can normovolemic patients that are anemic.

Anemic and/or hypoproteinemic patients should have serial PCV and total plasma protein concentration measurements during and after surgery. If an animal is anemic, supplemental oxygen may be beneficial in the preanesthetic period as well as the postoperative period to maintain maximal hemoglobin saturation. Although dissolved oxygen content is very minor compared with hemoglobin-bound oxygen content, a high inspired oxygen tension will enable more oxygen to be dissolved into the plasma and thus help counteract the decreased oxygen-carrying capacity due to low red blood cell numbers. A mask, nasal catheter, or oxygen cage can be used to deliver 40% to 100% oxygen to patients.

A pulse oximeter should be used during anesthesia and during recovery when patients are anemic. One of the periods of greatest risk for anemic patients is when anesthesia is discontinued and the fraction of inspired oxygen suddenly decreases from near 1.0 to 0.21 (room air) in the presence of anesthetic drug-related respiratory depression. In addition, as a hypothermic patient recovers, shivering will occur, dramatically increasing oxygen demands. Since approximately 5 g/dL of desaturated hemoglobin is needed for visible cyanosis to develop, anemic patients (PCV less than 15%) would not be expected to appear cyanotic even though hemoglobin oxygenation is dangerously low. Pulse oximeters are more sensitive at detecting hemoglobin desaturation in anemic patients, although a particular model's accuracy under these conditions may vary.

Hypoproteinemia

Many preanesthetic and anesthetic drugs are reversibly bound to plasma proteins, especially albumin. If plasma protein concentration is decreased, a greater fraction of highly protein-bound drug (i.e., protein binding in excess of 80%) is pharmacologically active and therefore will have an increased effect. Plasma protein, primarily albumin, is also required to maintain plasma oncotic pressure. Hypoalbuminemic patients are less tolerant of crystalloid fluid administration and more prone to volume overload and pulmonary edema. Total plasma protein concentration should be maintained above 3.5 to 4.0 g/dL. If the plasma protein concentration falls below this number, the administration of plasma or colloidal fluid substitutes should be considered.

Heartworm Disease

A positive heartworm test in itself does not contraindicate any particular anesthetic regimen or protocol. If the patient is not exhibiting clinical signs, any standard anesthetic protocol is probably satisfactory, provided patient monitoring is appropriate. One should be aware that patients with heartworms may be more prone to spontaneous and catecholamine-induced cardiac dysrhythmias while under anesthesia.[12] Additionally, pulmonary hypertension and/or pulmonary embolic disease may be present, affecting pulmonary and cardiovascular function. If a significant number of heartworms are present, cardiac output may also be decreased.

Cardiac Dysrhythmias

Ventricular dysrhythmia is relatively common in dogs and cats during anesthesia, and its incidence is increased with certain anesthetics (e.g., halothane) and diseases (e.g., splenic neoplasia). Arrhythmia is more common with inappropriate levels of inhalant anesthetics.[13–15] Ventricular tachyarrhythmia can be resolved through use of antiarrhythmics (typically lidocaine or sotalol), by providing deeper anesthesia if the patient is inadequately anesthetized, or by changing to a less arrhythmogenic anesthetic (e.g., changing from halothane to isoflurane). Catecholamine-induced arrhythmia may be more common during illness, after injury, and with other stressors.

References

1. Paddleford RR. Anesthetic considerations in patients with preexisting problems or conditions. In: Manual of Small Animal Anesthesia. New York: Churchill Livingstone, 1999:267–317.
2. Mason DE, Hubbell JAE. Anesthesia and the Heart. In: Fox PR, Sisson D, Moise NS, eds. Textbook of Canine and Feline Cardiology, 2nd ed. Philadelphia: WB Saunders, 1999:853–865.
3. Klide AM, Calderwood HW, Soma LR. Cardiopulmonary effect of xylazine in dogs. Am J Vet Res 1975;36:931–935.
4. Fox PR. Feline and canine myocardial disease. In: Fox PR, ed. Canine and Feline Cardiology. New York: Churchill Livingstone, 1988:435–493.
5. Olivier NB. Pathophysiology of cardiac failure. In: Slatter D, ed. Textbook of Small Animal Surgery, 2nd ed. Philadelphia: WB Saunders, 1993:709–723.
6. Day T. Anesthesia of patients with cardiac disease. In: Greene SA, ed. Veterinary Anesthesia and Pain Management Secrets. Philadelphia: Hanley and Belfus, 2002:157–164.
7. Fox PR. Feline cardiomyopathies. In: Ettinger SJ, Feldman EC, eds. Textbook of Veterinary Internal Medicine, 5th ed. Philadelphia: WB Saunders, 2000:896–923.
8. Hellyer PW. Anesthesia in patients with cardiopulmonary disease. In: Kirk RW, Bonagura JD, eds. Current Veterinary Therapy XI. Philadelphia: WB Saunders, 1992:655–659.
9. Green EM, Adams HR. New perspectives in circulatory shock: Pathophysiologic mediators of the mammalian response to endotoxemia and sepsis. J Am Vet Med Assoc 1992;200:1834–1841.
10. Taboada J, Hoskins JD, Morgan RV. Shock. In: Emergency Medicine and Critical Care. (The Compendium Collection.) Trenton, NJ: Veterinary Learning Systems, 1992:6–15.
11. Haskins SC. Management of septic shock. J Am Vet Med Assoc 1992;200:1915–1924.
12. Venugopalan CS, Holmes E, O'Malley NA. Comparison of arrhythmogenic doses of epinephrine in heartworm-infected and noninfected dogs. Am J Vet Res 1989;50:1872–1876.
13. Bednarski RM, Sams RA, Majors LJ, Ashcraft S. Reduction of the ventricular arrhythmogenic dose of epinephrine by ketamine administration in halothane-anesthetized cats. Am J Vet Res 1988;49:350–354.
14. Muir WW 3rd, Hubbell JA, Flaherty S. Increasing halothane concentration abolishes anesthesia-associated arrhythmias in cats and dogs. J Am Vet Med Assoc 1988;192:1730–1735.
15. Seeler DC, Dodman NH, Norman WM, Court MH. Recommended techniques in small animal anaesthesia. II. Intraoperative cardiac dysrhythmias and their treatment. Br Vet J 1987;143:97–111.
16. Ettinger SJ, Feldman EC, eds. Textbook of Veterinary Internal Medicine, 6th ed. St Louis: Elsevier, 2005.

Chapter 37
Pulmonary Disease

Robert R. Paddleford and Stephen A. Greene

Introduction

Patients with pulmonary dysfunction are often difficult to anesthetize safely. Most preanesthetic and anesthetic drugs depress respiratory function, further compromising patients with pulmonary disease and/or dysfunction. Knowledge of normal respiratory physiology and effective techniques for respiratory support is essential to provide favorable anesthetic outcomes.

Physiology of Ventilation

The primary function of the lungs is to exhale carbon dioxide generated by body metabolism and oxygenate venous blood. Alveolar ventilation can be assessed by measuring arterial carbon dioxide partial pressure ($PaCO_2$) or end-tidal carbon dioxide partial pressure ($ETCO_2$). Many factors can alter the ventilatory pattern (Table 37.1): (a) arterial carbon dioxide tension, (b) arterial pH, (c) arterial oxygen tension, (d) pulmonary stretch and upper airway receptors, (e) thermoregulation, (f) sensory input, and (g) emotional factors.[1] No conscious control is necessary to sustain ventilation.

The ventilatory control system is an integrated series of complex feedback loops made up of sensors, controllers, and effectors. The principal ventilatory receptors or sensors are (a) the peripheral carotid-body chemoreceptors (located at the bifurcations of the carotid arteries), (b) the central chemoreceptors (located near the surface on the ventrolateral aspect of the medulla oblongata), and (c) receptors sensing stretch, irritation, and proprioception in the lungs, airways, and muscles of respiration. The carotid-body chemoreceptors are responsive to oxygen and stimulate respiration when hypoxemia is present. The central chemoreceptors respond to carbon dioxide and stimulate ventilation when hypercarbia (respiratory acidosis) is present. Increased ventilation caused by metabolic acidosis may be mediated through either the central or peripheral chemoreceptors or the controllers of the ventilatory feedback loop located in the brain.[2] Automaticity of breathing is governed by specialized regions in the brain stem. The cortex controls voluntary and behavioral modifications of ventilation, and respiratory rhythm is controlled by the medulla. Control functions are integrated both centrally (brain stem) and peripherally (spinal cord). The effectors of ventilation are the muscles of respiration and include the intercostal muscles, the diaphragm, and the muscles of the upper airways.

Many preanesthetic and anesthetic agents can alter a patient's ventilatory pattern. Most preanesthetic and anesthetic agents alter ventilation by altering either the threshold or sensitivity of the respiratory centers to carbon dioxide and/or by relaxing the muscles of ventilation.[3]

Effects of Preanesthetic and Anesthetic Drugs on Ventilation

Most preanesthetic and anesthetic drugs depress respiratory function, thereby further jeopardizing a patient with respiratory dysfunction. Drugs depress or stimulate ventilation by acting directly or indirectly on one or more of the elements of the ventilatory control system.[4] Drugs used to treat respiratory disease may have significant interactions with anesthetics and anesthetic adjuncts.[5]

Atropine and glycopyrrolate decrease airway resistance by causing direct dilation of the airways. Atropine also increases respiratory dead space by dilating the larger bronchi. Both drugs will increase the viscosity of airway secretions.

Phenothiazine tranquilizers have minimal effects on ventilation at therapeutic doses, although large doses can depress ventilation. They decrease respiratory rate, but this is usually compensated for by an increase in tidal volume. Phenothiazines do not delay the central respiratory center response (threshold) to increases in arterial carbon dioxide, although the maximum ventilatory response (sensitivity) may be decreased.[3]

The α_2-adrenergic agonists (e.g., xylazine, detomidine, and medetomidine) vary in their pulmonary depressant effects and are somewhat unpredictable. Their depressant effects may range from mild to significant, depending on dose and individual patient response.[6] As with all general central nervous system (CNS) depressants, this effect is more pronounced in patients already suffering from respiratory distress caused by pneumonia, hydrothorax, or pneumothorax. When used in higher doses, α_2-adrenergic agonists may cause mucous membrane color to darken or appear cyanotic. Whereas cyanotic mucous membranes are normally interpreted as arterial hypoxemia and severe respiratory insufficiency, with α_2-adrenergic agonists the mechanism (and significance) is different. Arterial oxygen partial pressure is usually normal or near normal in these patients. The origin of the

Table 37.1. Factors affecting the ventilatory pattern

Arterial carbon dioxide tension
Arterial pH
Arterial oxygen tension
Pulmonary stretch and upper-airway receptors
Heat regulation
Sensory input
Emotional factors

increased concentration of desaturated hemoglobin in the mucous membranes is increased oxygen extraction during capillary transit rather than arterial hypoxemia. Oxygen extraction increases due to decreased tissue blood flow and increased capillary transit time. Vital organ blood flow (e.g., in the kidney, liver, and brain) may not decrease to the same extent as flow to superficial tissues (e.g., skin, mucous membranes, and skeletal muscle); therefore, the degree of darkening of the mucous membranes may not represent vital organ hypoxia. When α_2-adrenergic agonists are administered, the term *cyanosis* may not accurately reflect the true physiological status of the patient.

The benzodiazepine tranquilizers (diazepam and midazolam) usually produce minimal respiratory depression at therapeutic doses. However, both drugs have produced significant respiratory depression in isolated cases. This may be especially true when higher doses are administered intravenously.

Opioids are potentially respiratory depressant. The depression is drug and dose dependent, and may occur at doses that do not produce marked CNS depression or analgesia. The opioids directly depress the pontine and medullary centers, causing a decrease in respiratory rate and tidal volume. They also produce a delayed response (altered threshold) and a decreased response (altered sensitivity) to increases in arterial carbon dioxide.[3] The panting observed in some dogs after opioid administration (e.g., hydromorphone or oxymorphone) may be caused by an initial stimulation of the respiratory centers and/or alteration of the thermoregulation center.

The barbiturates are respiratory depressants. At anesthetizing doses, the respiratory centers of the brain are depressed. The barbiturates can depress both the respiratory rate and tidal volume, and thus minute ventilation. Barbiturates also produce a delayed response (altered threshold) and a decreased response (altered sensitivity) to increases in arterial carbon dioxide and depress the carotid-aortic chemoreceptors.

Dissociative anesthetics (ketamine and tiletamine) may have a dual effect on ventilation. They may affect ventilation at two or more anatomical sites, causing stimulation at one and depression at another. Both drugs can produce apneustic ventilation; that is, a ventilatory pattern characterized by a prolonged pause after inspiration. Although the respiratory rate may decrease, the tidal volume usually remains normal. In general, these respiratory alterations do not affect gas exchange or transport of gases to and from the lungs. However, in some patients, the dissociative agents can produce marked hypoxia and hypercarbia, especially when additional CNS-depressant drugs, such as tranquilizers,

sedatives, or opioids, are used in combination with them. Dissociative agents do not depress the pharyngeal or laryngeal reflexes, and they may be activated with stimulation. Therefore, patients may be more prone to laryngospasm, bronchospasm, and coughing. Dissociative agents increase salivation and respiratory secretions, sometimes resulting in aspiration and respiratory obstruction. For this reason, the use of an antimuscarinic in combination with these drugs may be indicated.

Propofol is an injectable anesthetic that produces respiratory depression in much the same manner as the barbiturates. The incidence of apnea with propofol is comparable to that with barbiturates, but the duration of apneic episodes may be slightly longer. Etomidate is a carboxylated imidazole that can produce mild to moderate dose-dependent respiratory depression. Apnea following administration of propofol or etomidate can usually be avoided by limiting the rate of administration to achieve tracheal intubation.

The inhalant anesthetics halothane, isoflurane, sevoflurane, and desflurane depress ventilation by decreasing tidal volume. These anesthetics typically increase respiratory rate but not adequately to compensate for the decrease in tidal volume. Potent inhalation anesthetics increase the set point at which arterial carbon dioxide initiates spontaneous ventilation (i.e., the *apneic threshold*). The degree of elevation in apneic threshold is directly related to the depth of anesthesia. Inhaled anesthetics decrease the slope of the carbon dioxide response curve. There is both a delayed response (altered threshold) and a decreased response (altered sensitivity) to increases in arterial carbon dioxide. Inhaled anesthetics also depress the ventilatory response to hypoxemia, and the interaction between hypoxemia and hypercarbia in stimulating ventilation is greatly attenuated or eliminated by even moderate concentrations of these agents.

Nitrous oxide induces minimal respiratory depression. However, because of its low potency requiring high inspired concentrations and to prevent hypoxia, this agent should be used cautiously, if at all, in patients with pulmonary dysfunction.

Anesthetic Considerations in Patients with Respiratory Dysfunction

Patients with pulmonary dysfunction may lack the ability to expand their lungs properly (extrapulmonary dysfunction) and/or may have impairment of oxygen and carbon dioxide transfer across the alveolar membranes (intrapulmonary dysfunction). Examples of extrapulmonary dysfunction include diaphragmatic hernia, pneumothorax, hydrothorax, space-occupying lesions of the thorax, flail chest, and any condition that restricts chest wall expansion. Examples of intrapulmonary dysfunction include pneumonia, pulmonary edema, intrapulmonary hemorrhage (contusions), atelectasis, interstitial disease, and upper-airway, tracheal, or bronchial obstruction.

Patients with respiratory dysfunction can be placed in one of four categories:

Category I: Dyspnea does not occur with exertion.
Category II: Dyspnea occurs with moderate exertion.

Category III: Dyspnea occurs with mild exertion.
Category IV: Dyspnea occurs at rest.

Patients in categories III and IV are at higher anesthetic risk. A thorough preanesthetic evaluation should be done on all patients with respiratory dysfunction. The thorax should be physically examined, and thoracic radiographs should be taken if the patient can tolerate handling and positioning without experiencing distress. Radiographs are valuable for arriving at a diagnosis, but the magnitude of the functional impairment is best measured with arterial blood-gas analysis. An ECG, arterial blood-gas analysis, baseline complete blood count, serum biochemistry panel, and serum electrolyte concentrations should be obtained.

Blood-gas analysis on an arterial sample obtained while the patient is breathing a low fraction of inspired oxygen (F_iO_2), such as room air ($F_iO_2 = 0.21$), and a high F_iO_2 is used by some to assess the ability of supplemental oxygen to improve arterial partial pressure of oxygen and calculate a pulmonary shunt fraction before administering anesthetic drugs. The oxygen partial pressure (PaO_2)-FiO_2 ratio is a simple way to quantify the ability to oxygenate at different levels of FiO_2. Dividing the value for PaO_2 by the decimal value of FiO_2 yields the ratio. A normal ratio is 500 (i.e., PaO_2 of 100 mm Hg divided by FiO_2 of 0.21). A PaO_2-FiO_2 ratio of 300 to 500 is consistent with mild disease, whereas a value of 200 represents significant pathology. This value is less accurate than the traditional alveolar-arterial gradients because it does not reflect the influence of PCO_2.[7] If a patient experiences cyanosis or respiratory distress when breathing a low F_iO_2, supplemental oxygen should not be withheld to obtain a measurement that can be estimated using an arterial sample collected during oxygen supplementation (e.g., alveolar-arterial gradient).

If possible, surgery and anesthesia should be delayed in patients with pneumonia, pulmonary edema, lung contusions, atelectasis, pneumothorax, and/or hydrothorax to allow time for these problems to be addressed and the condition of the patient to improve. A thoracentesis should be done in patients with moderate to severe pneumothorax or hydrothorax prior to anesthesia, and in some cases a chest tube may be needed.

Patients with respiratory dysfunction should be preoxygenated for 5 to 7 min prior to anesthetic induction.[8] A mask, nasal catheter, or oxygen chamber may be used. Supplemental oxygen should be immediately available both preoperatively and postoperatively.

Mild preanesthetic sedation may be necessary to enable the patient to be handled without causing stress and exacerbating dysfunction. Preanesthetic drugs that induce minimal respiratory depression should be considered. Several preanesthetic drugs or combinations may be used, such as the combination of acepromazine and butorphanol. Acepromazine is a phenothiazine derivative tranquilizer that produces minimal respiratory depression, especially in low doses. Butorphanol is a synthetic, opioid agonist-antagonist. Butorphanol can produce a dose-related respiratory depression similar to morphine; however, butorphanol seems to reach a ceiling beyond which higher doses do not cause significantly more depression.

After a patient has been sedated, rapid induction of anesthesia may be needed to gain quick control of the airway to enable positive pressure ventilation. Rapid anesthetic induction may be accomplished by intravenous administration of thiopental, propofol, etomidate, or ketamine. A rapid mask induction using desflurane, isoflurane, or sevoflurane may be used; however, because of the patient's inability to ventilate properly, this technique may result in delayed anesthetic induction and excessive struggling. Whichever induction technique is used, the trachea must be intubated rapidly and accurately.

Anesthesia is best maintained with an inhalant anesthetic and controlled or positive pressure ventilation. Nitrous oxide should be used with care in patients with respiratory dysfunction. It can increase the severity of a pneumothorax, and it should be discontinued if cyanosis is evident. Even if a patient with respiratory compromise seems to have adequate spontaneous ventilation, assisted or controlled ventilation is desirable unless a resolving pneumothorax is present and the patient's $PaCO_2$ and PaO_2 can be maintained at an acceptable level with spontaneous ventilation. High airway pressures from positive pressure ventilation in these patients may result in rapid development of a tension pneumothorax that requires immediate thoracentesis. Pulse oximetry, $ETCO_2$, and arterial blood-gas monitoring should be used to monitor respiratory status in these patients.

Controlled Ventilation

In spontaneously ventilating patients, the respiratory muscles increase the size of the thoracic cavity, the volume within it increases, and the pressure in the thorax falls. Thus, the intrapulmonary pressure falls, and the difference between the intrapleural pressure and alveolar pressure overcomes the elasticity of the lungs while the difference between the alveolar pressure and the pressure at the oral-pharyngeal area overcomes the airway resistance. There is a great difference between the intrapleural and alveolar pressures, and a small difference between the oral-pharyngeal pressure and airway resistance. The net effect is movement of air into the alveoli from the upper airway.

In contrast, controlled ventilation is usually *positive pressure* ventilation. Air is forced into the alveoli under pressure. Intrapleural pressure and intrapulmonary pressure increase during controlled ventilation. Controlled ventilation may be provided manually (by squeezing the rebreathing bag) or mechanically (using a ventilator).

One of three methods can be used to control a patient's ventilation and take over ventilatory effort: The patient can be hyperventilated to decrease the arterial carbon dioxide levels and decrease the stimulus for ventilation; the patient's anesthetic level can be increased (deepened); or the patient can be paralyzed by using peripherally acting muscle relaxants. Of the three methods, hyperventilating the patient (i.e., manually or mechanically increasing the patient's respiratory rate and depth) is the easiest and is usually quite effective.

Five components can be adjusted in the ventilatory cycle during controlled ventilation (Table 37.2): (a) peak airway pressure, (b) mean airway pressure, (c) length of inspiratory phase, (d) length of expiratory phase, and (e) the inspiratory-expiratory

Table 37.2. Adjustable components of the respiratory cycle during mechanical ventilation

Peak airway pressure
Mean airway pressure
Length of inspiratory phase
Length of expiratory phase
Inspiratory-expiratory ratio

ratio. Peak airway pressures are measured by a pressure manometer in the anesthesia circuit. Peak airway pressures of 15 to 20 cm water are necessary to overcome lung resistance to expansion in dogs and larger species. In cats, slightly higher pressures may be needed. Decreased lung compliance will increase the peak airway pressures needed to expand the lungs. An increase in airway resistance will increase the peak airway pressure needed to expand the lungs.

The mean airway pressure is the average pressure generated during the inspiratory and expiratory phases of positive pressure ventilation. Mean airway pressure should be kept low by minimizing the duration of positive airway pressure. Mean airway pressure most closely correlates with decreases in cardiac output.

To produce minimal cardiovascular alteration, the inspiratory phase should be shorter than the expiratory phase. Typically, the inspiratory phase should last 1 to 1.5 s. Prolonged holding of the tidal volume at peak airway pressure will not increase tidal exchange but will increase mean airway pressure and intrathoracic pressure, thereby decreasing venous return and cardiac output. The expiratory phase should begin as soon as the inspiratory phase is complete. The increased pressure within the lung must be allowed to return to 0 cm water pressure as soon as possible to prevent this preload impairment. The inspiratory-expiratory (I-E) ratio is very important during controlled or positive pressure ventilation. The inspiratory phase should be at least one-third and no more than one-half of the total ventilatory cycle. An I-E ratio of 1:2 or 1:3 will help provide an adequate period for proper cardiac filling. A 1:2 ratio will provide for a ventilatory rate of approximately 20 cycles per minute. A 1:3 or 1:4 ratio provides for a rate of 15 or 12 breaths per minute, respectively.

Although controlled or positive pressure ventilation is usually safe and effective, if it is done improperly, harmful side effects can occur.[9,10] As already described, interference with cardiac output can occur during controlled or positive pressure ventilation. During spontaneous ventilation, the intrapleural pressure at the height of inspiration is approximately a negative 8 to 10 cm water. This augments the movement of blood in the great veins into the chest (thoracic pump). However, during controlled or positive pressure ventilation, the intrapulmonary pressure increases and may reach plus 3 to 5 cm water pressure. Only during expiration is the intrapulmonary pressure the same in spontaneous ventilation and controlled ventilation. Increased alveolar pressure will also decrease pulmonary blood flow. This is why maintenance of proper peak and mean airway pressures and a proper I-E ratio is critical during ventilatory support of anesthetized patients.

Lung damage or *volutrauma* is a potential complication during positive pressure ventilation. Volutrauma (e.g., overextension or expansion of the lung tissue by excessive pressure) can range from mild trauma producing minimal alveolar hemorrhage to severe trauma producing airway rupture and a tension pneumothorax. Maintaining proper peak and mean airway pressures will help minimize pulmonary trauma.[11] A major airway blowout that occurs during positive pressure ventilation is often caused by excessive peak airway pressures and/or preexisting lung pathology. Vigilant monitoring of the anesthetic circuit's adjustable pressure limiting (e.g., pop-off) valve is crucial to preventing this type of misadventure.

Acid-base balance will be altered in accordance with changes in alveolar ventilation. Hyperventilation will cause a decreased arterial carbon dioxide level and an increased pH (alkalemia). Hyperventilation can also lead to cerebral vasoconstriction and may reduce cerebral perfusion pressure such that cerebral hypoxia occurs.[12] Hypoventilation will lead to increased arterial carbon dioxide and a decreased pH (acidemia), which may adversely increase intracranial pressure and lead to brain ischemia and/or herniation.

References

1. Benumof JL. General respiratory physiology and respiratory function during anesthesia. In: Benumof JL, ed. Anesthesia for Thoracic Surgery, 2nd ed. Philadelphia: WB Saunders, 1995:43–122.
2. Tucker A. Respiratory pathophysiology. In: Slatter D, ed. Textbook of Small Animal Surgery, 3rd ed. Philadelphia: WB Saunders, 2003:781–797.
3. Paddleford RR. Anesthetic considerations in patients with preexisting problems and conditions. In: Paddleford RR, ed. Manual of Small Animal Anesthesia. New York: Churchill Livingstone, 1988: 253–308.
4. Schatzmann URS. Clinical considerations of complications of the pulmonary system. In: Short CE, ed. Principles and Practice of Veterinary Anesthesia. Baltimore: Williams and Wilkins, 1987:208–221.
5. Boothe DM. Drugs affecting the respiratory system. In: Boothe DM, ed. Small Animal Clinical Pharmacology and Therapeutics. Philadelphia: WB Saunders, 2001:602–623.
6. Perkowski S. Respiratory system. In: Slatter D, ed. Textbook of Small Animal Surgery, 3rd ed. Philadelphia: WB Saunders, 2003: 2564–2572.
7. Clare M, Hooper K. Mechanical ventilation: Indications, goals, and prognosis. Compend Cont Educ Pract Vet 2005;27:195–207.
8. Dunlop CI. Anesthesia for patients with preexisting pneumonia and cyanosis. Vet Clin North Am Small Anim Pract 1992;22:454–455.
9. MacIntyre NR. Mechanical Ventilation. Philadelphia: WB Saunders, 2001.
10. Haskins SC, King LG. Positive pressure ventilation. In: King LG, ed. Textbook of Respiratory Disease in Dogs and Cats. Philadelphia: WB Saunders, 2004:217–229.
11. Wilson DV. Anesthesia for patients with diaphragmatic hernia and severe dyspnea. Vet Clin North Am Small Anim Pract 1992;22: 456–459.
12. Patel PM, Drummond JC. Cerebral physiology and the effects of anesthetics and techniques. In: Miller RD, ed. Miller's Anesthesia, 6th ed. Philadelphia: Elsevier, 2005:813–858.

Chapter 38
Neurological Disease

Ralph C. Harvey, Stephen A. Greene, and William B. Thomas

Introduction

Veterinary patients frequently require anesthesia for diagnostic evaluation or surgical correction of neurological disorders. Diagnostic procedures that require either general anesthesia or heavy sedation include electroencephalography (EEG), myelography, other imaging techniques, and electrodiagnostic testing. Veterinary neurosurgical anesthesia is more often required in patients with spinal cord rather than intracranial disorders. The most frequently performed neurosurgical procedure in veterinary medicine is used in the treatment of intervertebral disk disease. However, the increased use of advanced imaging techniques, such as computed tomography and magnetic resonance imaging (MRI), has led to a greater frequency of intracranial operative procedures in small animal patients where these imaging modalities are available. In patients with neurological disease, consideration of the dynamics of intracranial pressure (ICP), cerebral blood flow (CBF), and cerebrospinal fluid (CSF) production and flow is important in preventing patient morbidity or death.

Physiology

In normal awake animals, blood supply to the central nervous system (CNS) is controlled by autoregulatory mechanisms. Alteration in CBF can result from a variety of changes in arterial oxygenation, carbon dioxide partial pressure, mean arterial pressure, and venous outflow. The brain and spinal cord are protected by encasement within the bony skull and vertebral column. Increases in blood flow within the noncompliant cranial vault cause an increase in the intracranial volume.[1–3] Once increases in CBF cause the intracranial volume to exceed the limits of effective compliance, ICP increases sharply. When clinical findings suggest ICP is already increased by intracranial masses, trauma, or derangement of autoregulation, extreme care is required, because slight changes in intracranial volume greatly increase ICP.[2] Significant ICP increases may lead to cerebral ischemia and brain herniation.[1]

Autoregulation of Cerebral Blood Flow

Autoregulation of brain blood flow is usually very effective in a systemic mean arterial blood pressure range of approximately 60 to 140 mm Hg. Within this range of blood pressure, many factors—including intracranial tumors, hypercapnia, severe hypoxia, and many anesthetics—interfere with autoregulation and cause changes in ICP (Fig. 38.1).[1,4,5] Blood vessels in the brain supplying diseased or neoplastic tissues may be fully dilated and unaffected by normal autoregulation mechanisms.

The CNS depression of general anesthesia is usually accompanied by a decrease in cerebral metabolic rate and cerebral metabolic requirement for oxygen ($CMRO_2$). This decrease in oxygen requirement is thought to be protective in the possible event of relative ischemia during anesthesia and neurosurgery. There are conflicting reports on the efficacy of various anesthetics in reducing $CMRO_2$, just as there are with regard to the relative effects of the anesthetics on CBF and ICP. Isoflurane, sevoflurane, etomidate, and the barbiturates are generally recognized as contributing substantially to reduction of $CMRO_2$, affording some cerebral protection.[5]

In patients with preexisting elevated ICP, further increases can be caused by gravitational or positional interference with drainage of venous blood from the head. Obstruction by occlusion of jugular veins through surgical positioning of the head, use of a neck leash, or venous occlusion to obtain blood samples or placement of jugular vein catheters can rapidly cause dangerous increases in ICP.[6] For intracranial neurosurgery, a slight elevation of the head above the level of the heart (with the neck in a neutral position) will facilitate venous drainage, lowering ICP. Extreme elevation is avoided to minimize the risk of venous air embolization.[3]

903

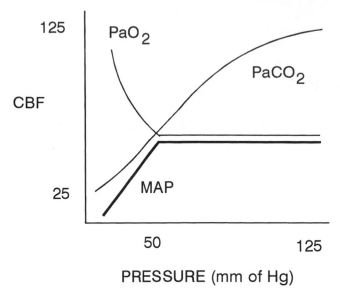

Fig. 38.1. Alterations in cerebral blood flow (CBF), in milliliters per 100 g of brain tissue per minute, caused by changes in arterial tension of oxygen (PaO_2), carbon dioxide ($PaCO_2$), and mean arterial blood pressure (MAP). Redrawn from Shapiro.[1]

Only at very low arterial oxygen tensions does the CBF change in response to oxygen partial pressure. When arterial oxygen partial pressure (PaO_2) decreases below a threshold of 50 mm Hg, CBF increases (Fig. 38.1). The relationship between arterial carbon dioxide partial pressure ($PaCO_2$) and CBF, on the other hand, is linear. CBF increases by about $2 \text{ mL} \cdot \text{min}^{-1} \cdot 100$ g^{-1} of brain tissue for every 1-mm Hg increase in arterial carbon dioxide over the range of $PaCO_2$ from 20 to 80 mm Hg.[7] Hyperventilation has been used extensively in neuroanesthesia to reduce CBF (via cerebral vasoconstriction). This maneuver decreases tissue bulk, facilitating intracranial surgery. Although quite effective, this technique is somewhat controversial in some situations, because a potential exists for the diversion of remaining blood flow preferentially to diseased tissues lacking autoregulation at the expense of normal brain tissue.[8] Deliberate hyperventilation to decrease ICP may be risky when mean arterial blood pressure is reduced to less than 50 mm Hg. The ensuing ischemia could be deleterious to normal brain tissues if a "steal" of CBF diverts remaining blood flow.[8,9] The rapid and substantial reduction in CBF and ICP achieved by hyperventilation makes it a valuable tool for the immediate reduction in brain bulk to facilitate intracranial surgery and to reduce acute brain swelling.

Although controversial, restriction of intravenous fluids to only that volume necessary to maintain adequate circulating volume and cardiac output is usually recommended in neurosurgical patients with increased ICP.[10,11] Excessive fluid volume has been associated with increased central venous pressure, decreased venous outflow, and increased risk of compounding cerebral edema. Diuretic therapy is frequently indicated in the medical management of patients with intracranial masses and elevated ICP or cerebral edema.[6] Dextrose administration is somewhat controversial and must be individualized to the situation. Hyperglycemia is associated with adverse outcome in animals with cerebral ischemia, and cerebral edema can be exacerbated by administration of isotonic dextrose. However, intravenous dextrose administration decreases the incidence of seizures in patients after metrizamide myelography and is indicated in hypoglycemic seizures or hypoglycemic coma.[1,12,13]

Glucocorticoids are effective in the treatment of some forms of cerebral edema[14] and have been shown to be effective in reducing the increased ICP that is caused by brain tumors and hydrocephalus. Glucocorticoid therapy may be considered in the management of patients with cerebral edema associated with primary or metastatic brain neoplasia. Since dexamethasone administration has been shown to reduce the rate of CSF formation in dogs, steroid administration may be of some value in the preanesthetic management of hydrocephalic patients considered at risk of further increases in ICP.[14,15] Corticosteroids are now known to be contraindicated in cases of CNS trauma.

Pharmacological Considerations

Sedatives, Tranquilizers, and Analgesics

For many years, the suspected increased seizure activity associated with administration of the phenothiazine (e.g., acepromazine) and possibly butyrophenone (e.g., droperidol) tranquilizers contraindicated their use in seizure-prone patients and in patients for diagnostic EEG.[16] A more recent retrospective study indicates that acepromazine does not potentiate seizure activity.[17] Control of seizures with benzodiazepine tranquilizers (e.g., diazepam or midazolam) is desirable in the management of seizure-prone patients but can obscure characteristic patterns in diagnostic EEGs. In addition, benzodiazepines appear to decrease CBF and ICP.[18]

Use of xylazine in dogs and cats is controversial, yet clinical evidence for or against its use in patients with neurological disease is lacking. In healthy conscious horses, xylazine (1.1 mg/kg IV) decreased CSF pressure measured at the lumbosacral space.[19] Horses anesthetized with pentobarbital and subsequently given xylazine (1.1 mg/kg IV) had no change in either lateral ventricle or lumbosacral CSF pressure.[20] Horses given detomidine (20 µg/kg IV) also had a reduction in CBF.[21] Medetomidine administered to isoflurane-anesthetized dogs had no effect on ICP measured using a fiberoptic transducer, whereas antagonism of medetomidine by using atipamezole was associated with a dramatic transient increase in ICP.[22] Dexmedetomidine, the pharmacologically active stereoisomer of medetomidine, decreased CBF in both halothane and isoflurane anesthetized dogs.[23,24] Thus, although the effects of α_2-agonists on ICP may differ in horses and dogs with head trauma or neurological disease, they appear to be rational choices to provide sedation for examination or as a preanesthetic medication. Venous congestion in the head, when positioned below the level of the heart, may be associated with an increase in ICP. Therefore, the dose of xylazine or detomidine should be titrated to prevent excessive head lowering and possible resultant increased ICP in horses or other species.

Table 38.1. Effects of anesthetics and anesthetic adjuncts on cerebral blood flow (CBF), intracranial pressure (ICP), blood pressure (BP), and cerebral perfusion pressure (CPP).

Agent	CBF	ICP	BP	CPP
Desflurane	↑	↑	↓	↓
Halothane	↑↑	↑↑	↓	↓
Isoflurane	↑	↑	↓	↓
Nitrous oxide	↔	↔	↔	↔
Sevoflurane	↑	↑	↓	↓
Atracurium	↔	↔	↔	↔
Diazepam	↓	↓ or ↔	↓	↔
Droperidol	↓	↓	↓	↔
Fentanyl	↓	↓	↓	↔
Halothane-thiopental	↔	↔	↓	↓ or ↔
Ketamine	↑↑	↑↑	↑	↓
Midazolam	↓	↔	↔	↔
Morphine[a]	↓	↔	↓ or ↔	↔
Propofol	↓↓	↓↓	↓	↔
Thiopental	↓↓	↓↓	↓	↔

[a]Indirectly, respiratory depression caused by morphine (and other opioids) may result in hypercapnia with raised CBF and ICP.

Opioids or neuroleptanalgesic combinations are sometimes used in anesthetic management of patients with increased ICP. The direct effects of opioids on CBF and ICP are minimal. However, opioids may indirectly increase CSF pressure and should be used cautiously in patients with cerebral trauma or space-occupying tumors. Increases in pressure within the cranium may aggravate the underlying condition. The elevation in CSF pressure is caused by accumulation of carbon dioxide, which in turn is caused by opioid-induced hypoventilation. If a patient is ventilated to prevent hypercapnia, the increase in CSF pressure does not occur when opioids are administered.[25] When opioids are used in these cases, the respiratory status must be assessed through arterial blood-gas analysis or end-tidal carbon dioxide levels, and when necessary, the patient should be ventilated to prevent hypercapnia. The judicious use of opioids for pain management in the postoperative period often does not cause as much respiratory depression as does pain itself.[26] Thus, opioid analgesic medication is based on the relative severity of pain in each animal.

Injectable Anesthetics

Most of these cause significant reductions in $CMRO_2$, CBF, and ICP (Table 38.1).[1–3,5,6,12] Recognition of barbiturate-induced reductions in $CMRO_2$, CBF, and ICP has contributed to the concept of *barbiturate coma* therapy for cerebral resuscitation after periods of cerebral ischemia as occurs in near-drowning and in cardiopulmonary resuscitation. The value of barbiturates as a therapy for cerebral ischemia/hypoxia is controversial at best. It is likely that barbiturates are protective if administered prior to the insult but of relatively little value if administered after clinical signs of brain ischemia have developed. Propofol or barbiturates may be of value in avoiding postoperative sequelae to sur-

gical trauma. It must be recognized, however, that barbiturate anesthesia often prolongs anesthetic recovery. In neurosurgical patients, the CNS depression associated with residual barbiturates can seriously obscure postoperative evaluation and prevent meaningful neurological evaluation.

The dissociative anesthetics represent a notable exception to the reduction in CBF, ICP, and $CMRO_2$ characteristic of most injectable anesthetics.[1–3,6,12] EEG activity also increases with dissociative anesthesia. Convulsant activity ranging from muscle twitching to seizures occurs as an infrequent adverse effect of the dissociatives. Patients with a history of seizure-related disorders and those with intracranial masses, closed-head traumatic injuries, and other conditions potentially increasing ICP should not receive dissociative anesthetics. Because benzodiazepine tranquilizers may decrease CBF and ICP, their combination with dissociative anesthetics may attenuate cerebrovascular and neurological effects of the dissociative agent.[27]

Volatile Anesthetics

Inhalant anesthetics increase CBF and alter $CMRO_2$ to varying degrees.[7,10,12,28–31] Since increased CBF and ICP are also highly influenced by carbon dioxide retention, respiratory depression associated with volatile anesthesia can be responsible for increases in ICP that are clinically significant in neurosurgical patients. There is evidence that regional changes in the distribution of CBF result from administration of the volatile anesthetics such that our understanding of cerebrovascular effects may not be accurately based on global estimates of CBF in animals.[4]

Among the volatile anesthetics clinically used in veterinary medicine, halothane dramatically blocks autoregulation, increasing CBF and ICP.[29,30] Methoxyflurane, enflurane, and isoflurane all interfere with autoregulation in a more limited extent than halothane.[3] At 1.1 minimum alveolar concentration levels of anesthesia, CBF increases almost 200% with halothane but by only about 40% with enflurane and is unchanged with isoflurane.[2,28] Higher concentrations of isoflurane cause increases in CBF. The loss of cerebral autoregulation with halothane is implicated in the greater degree of brain swelling noted during neurosurgery with this anesthetic. The increase in CBF occurs rapidly upon halothane administration and is independent of changes in arterial blood pressure, implicating halothane's direct cerebrovascular effects.

Fortunately, modest hyperventilation, reducing arterial carbon dioxide to 30–35 mm Hg, often eliminates the volatile anesthetic-induced increase in CBF.[29] Hyperventilation is rapidly effective in reducing elevated CBF and ICP or in preventing their rise in patients at risk. It is easy, rather cost free, and the safest method available. Excessive hyperventilation should be avoided because cerebral perfusion pressure may decrease, resulting in cerebral ischemia. In light of the respiratory depression of general anesthesia and the potential rise in CBF and ICP, ventilation to prevent hypercapnia should be incorporated into the anesthetic technique for animals with intracranial masses or other disorders of autoregulation. Values between 35 and 40 mm Hg of $PaCO_2$ are recommended in anesthetized patients at risk of increased morbidity associated with raised ICP.

Nitrous oxide has substantial cerebrovascular effects. Although there are conflicting reports and a minority opposing opinion, adverse effects of nitrous oxide have been well documented in animals undergoing neurosurgery.[5,31] Nitrous oxide causes the most profound increase in both CBF and ICP of all the inhalant anesthetics. Owing largely to the limited potency of nitrous oxide in veterinary patients, its use is primarily in combination with other general anesthetics. The combination of volatile anesthetic gases and nitrous oxide can produce greater increases in CBF and ICP. In rabbits, nitrous oxide administration produced a consistent increase in CBF and ICP regardless of whether it was combined with halothane, isoflurane or fentanyl-pentobarbital anesthesia.[16] Furthermore, these potentially adverse effects were not blocked by hyperventilation. In dogs, nitrous oxide increases $CMRO_2$ by 11%. In animal models of regional cerebral ischemia, the use of nitrous oxide worsens the neurological outcome.[5] The disadvantages of nitrous oxide would appear to be substantial for many neurosurgical patients.

Anesthetic Management of Specific Neurological Problems

Myelography and Intervertebral Disk Disease

For the relatively common surgical procedures to decompress cervical or thoracolumbar intervertebral disk herniation, anesthetic management should address (a) protection from possible seizures and other potential complications associated with administration of myelographic contrast agents, (b) perioperative pain relief, (c) maintenance of adequate spontaneous ventilation, and (d) management of concurrent disorders such as urinary incontinence or other factors predisposing patients to adverse recovery.

Radiographic contrast myelography is frequently performed in the immediate preoperative period to localize the lesion(s) and to identify the proper site(s) for surgical decompression. As this procedure is often performed during the same anesthetic period, patient management is designed to optimize conditions for both the diagnostic (radiographic) and the therapeutic (surgical) procedures. Dural puncture for sampling of CSF and/or for administration of myelographic contrast agent requires a depth of anesthesia at less than a surgical plane but adequate to prevent patient movement with subsequent trauma. Considerations for an anesthetic protocol suitable for spinal cord surgery are listed in Table 38.2.

Avoiding the use of potent respiratory depressants and using a light surgical plane of anesthesia will optimally maintain spontaneous ventilation during myelography. Among the less frequent complications associated with myelography are respiratory depression or respiratory arrest and cardiac arrhythmias.[32] Preoperative administration of an anticholinergic will reduce the incidence of bradycardia. Respiratory depression is probably referable to effects of the contrast agent at the level of brain stem and medullary respiratory centers. As such, respiratory effects are most likely to be associated with "high" myelograms, typically those showing contrast agent ascending to the brain and brain stem. The incidence of seizure activity and the other potential adverse side effects of myelography appears to be greatly re-

Table 38.2. Anesthetic management for intervertebral disk disease.

1. Benzodiazepine tranquilization (e.g., diazepam, 0.2 mg/kg IV)
2. Low-dose opioid (e.g., hydromorphone, 0.2 mg/kg IV or IM)
3. Anticholinergics if needed, especially before myelography (atropine, 0.04 mg/kg IM)
4. Induction with thiopental (15 mg/kg IV) or propofol (3 mg/kg IV) administered to effect
5. Avoid hyperextension of the neck in cases of cervical trauma, instability, or disk disease
6. Maintenance of protected airway during the procedure
7. Judicious fluid therapy
8. Positioning of the patient to avoid venous occlusion
9. Use of intraoperative and postoperative opioids for pain management

IM, intramuscularly; and IV, intravenously.

duced with use of newer contrast agents such as iopamidol and iohexol rather than metrizamide.[33,34] Hyperflexion of the cervical spine for cisternal CSF collection and for cervical administration of myelographic contrast can easily kink most endotracheal tubes, causing airway obstruction. Endotracheal tubes that are armored or contain spiral wire are quite resistant to kinking. Metal or other radiopaque reinforcement in the armored tubes makes them unsuitable for use in cervical and cranial radiographic studies. Close attention to adequacy of the airway and spontaneous ventilation is of paramount importance when flexing the neck.

In addition to the precautions and considerations appropriate for thoracolumbar disk disease, cervical disk disease can be associated with increased risk of cardiac arrhythmias and respiratory arrest.[3] Vagal stimulation during ventral approaches to the cervical spine may increase with retraction of the carotid sheath. Frequently, there appears to be greater postoperative pain with cervical as opposed to thoracolumbar surgical repair, possibly indicating a neuropathic component to the postoperative pain. Patient positioning for a ventral cervical approach often is dorsal recumbency with the neck extended. Patients should be observed carefully during and after positioning, because overextension may lead to respiratory arrest or cardiac arrhythmias.

Patients having lost deep-pain perception are surgical emergencies. Rapid-sequence induction, using intravenous general anesthetics rather than inhalation induction of anesthesia, is indicated if the animal has or may have a full stomach. Additional management related to the emergent nature of their distress may be indicated. The fact that these animals do not feel painful stimuli to the rear limbs suggests that these areas preferentially can be used for placement of injections and intravenous catheters without contributing additional pain to an already highly stressed patient.

Anesthesia for Horses with Cervical Vertebral Instability (Wobbler Syndrome)

The preanesthetic dose of xylazine administered to a horse with wobbler syndrome should be decreased to prevent the horse from becoming recumbent prior to induction of anesthesia. Xylazine should not be administered until the horse is moved to the induction area. Horses that are severely ataxic prior to drug administration may be anesthetized in the stall and returned there for recovery after the procedure.

Horses with wobbler syndrome may require anesthesia for myelography. For premedication, a low dose of xylazine (0.2 to 0.4 mg/kg IV) can be used. Anesthesia may be induced by using guaifenesin in combination with thiopental. Anesthesia can be maintained with halothane, isoflurane, sevoflurane, or an injectable anesthetic mixture such as guaifenesin-thiopental. Some clinicians prefer to administer guaifenesin alone until the horse becomes unsteady and then administer a bolus of thiopental (2 to 3 g/450 kg body weight). The total dose of anesthetic should be kept to a minimum so that recovery from anesthesia is optimized. As a rule of thumb, a total dose of 2 L of the guaifenesin-thiopental combination is not exceeded (5% guaifenesin with 0.3% thiopental). Horses can be expected to have an acceptable recovery when anesthesia is limited to less than 1 h. Controlled ventilation during the procedure is recommended. Assisted recovery using a tail rope or other method of assistance may be desired; however, experience and extreme caution are required because of the danger of being crushed by an ataxic horse.

Myelography or withdrawal of CSF may precipitate changes in cerebrospinal pressure, which can adversely affect function of the respiratory center in the brain stem.[35] Following administration of a contrast agent, the head should be elevated to minimize the agent's migration toward the brain. In one study, 32% of the horses with significant gait abnormalities that underwent myelography (using metrizamide as the contrast agent) had significant worsening of clinical signs after the procedure.[36] Equine myelography with iopamidol or iohexol as the contrast agent may be associated with less toxicity and fewer side effects than metrizamide.[37,38] Regardless of the contrast agent used, a sudden drop in arterial blood pressure may occur at the time of injection. Monitoring of blood pressure is recommended during the procedure. At the end of the procedure, the horse is returned to spontaneous ventilation and remains anesthetized for at least 30 min after the last injection of contrast agent. Following prolonged lateral recumbency, it is advised to allow the horse to recover with the same side down. Turning horses to the opposite side after long procedures in lateral recumbency does not improve, and may worsen, arterial oxygenation.[39,40] Recovery from anesthesia for myelography is often characterized by several hours of ataxia, which may be more severe than prior to anesthesia. Measures to observe and support recovering horses should be available. Some horses benefit from being placed in a sling for a few hours after anesthesia. To promote a smooth recovery (and possibly to decrease the incidence of postmyelogram seizure or muscle-tremor activity), a low dose of xylazine (25 to 100 mg IV) or diazepam (0.03 mg/kg intramuscularly) may be administered to adult horses. Some clinicians use phenylbutazone to minimize postmyelogram muscle-tremor activity. Because phenylbutazone is highly protein bound and may displace anesthetic from protein-binding sites, it has been recommended that phenylbutazone be administered before anesthetic agents are given. Phenylbutazone administration to horses that already are induced and/or maintained with injectable anesthetics may deepen anesthesia or prolong recovery.

Intracranial Masses and Elevated Intracranial Pressure

Patients with intracranial masses, dysfunctional CBF autoregulation, and/or increased ICP are at risk of rapid decompensation under anesthesia. Preoperative assessment should include measurement of arterial blood pressure, because many patients with elevated ICP will have an accompanying increase in systemic arterial blood pressure (Cushing's response). Systemic hypertension is an attempt to compensate and maintain adequate cerebral perfusion pressure. If mean arterial pressure is significantly elevated prior to drug administration, arterial blood pressure should not be allowed to drop to normally acceptable levels under anesthesia (e.g., a mean arterial pressure of 60 mm Hg), because cerebral ischemia can result despite an "acceptable" mean blood pressure.

Manual or mechanical positive-pressure ventilation should be immediately available and instituted at induction. Mechanical ventilation should be continued until extubation. In some cases, allowing $PaCO_2$ to rise in order to stimulate spontaneous ventilation, before the respiratory depressant effects of the anesthetics wane, may cause serious elevations in ICP and possibly herniation. Anesthetic monitoring should address the physiological variables associated with altered ICP. Venous and arterial blood pressures and airway or arterial sampling for carbon dioxide analysis should be included, if possible. Intravenous mannitol (0.5 to 1.0 g/kg IV slowly) may be useful to reduce ICP before, during, or after anesthesia. Optimal anesthetic management can substantially improve patient status and the outcome of intracranial surgical procedures. A recommended anesthetic technique is summarized in Table 38.3.

Management of Seizures in the Perianesthetic Period

Seizures are most commonly observed in animals with other signs of brain disease. Thus, animals anesthetized for diagnosis or treatment of CNS disease are more likely to exhibit seizure activity during the perianesthetic period. The animal with seizure activity should be medically treated to control standard recom

Table 38.3. Anesthetic technique for patients with elevated cerebral blood flow and/or intracranial pressure.

1. Preanesthetic critical care management and stabilization
2. Fluid therapy limited to minimize cerebral edema but adequate to support circulation
3. Avoid severe respiratory depression, jugular venous occlusion, and coughing at induction or during recovery
4. Avoid dissociative anesthetics, halothane, enflurane, and nitrous oxide
5. Thiobarbiturate or propofol induction of anesthesia preferred
6. Minimal inhalant anesthetic supplemented with opioids for maintenance
7. Modest hyperventilation to reduce cerebral blood flow and intracranial pressure
8. Postoperative critical care with support of ventilation and circulation as indicated

mendations before anesthesia is attempted. In horses, treatments for status epilepticus include use of anticonvulsants such as diazepam, midazolam, pentobarbital, phenobarbital, phenytoin, primidone, chloral hydrate, and the combination of guaifenesin with a thiobarbiturate.[41] Foals exhibiting seizure activity may be treated with diazepam (5 to 10 mg IV), phenytoin (5 to 10 mg/kg IV, intramuscularly, or orally), or phenobarbital (with plasma-level monitoring).[42] A complication associated with treatment of seizures in neonatal foals is the altered disposition of drugs. Functional hepatic microsomal enzymes and renal function in neonates is immature. Thus, concurrent medication with other drugs may cause unexpected interactions or changes in elimination, necessitating careful patient monitoring and alteration of the anticonvulsant dosage regimen.

Phenothiazine tranquilizers have been shown to augment epileptiform activity on the electroencephalogram of dogs.[43] Intrathecal injection of radiographic contrast agents is frequently associated with seizures.[44] Therefore, the use of acepromazine and other phenothiazine tranquilizers has usually been avoided in animals with preexisting seizures and in animals undergoing myelography (Table 38.4).

Horses sedated with xylazine demonstrate electroencephalographic slowing with irregular waveforms.[45] Xylazine (0.1 to 0.2 mg/kg IV) and diazepam (0.2 mg/kg IV) have both been suggested as effective injectable treatments for seizures in horses recovering from anesthesia.[46] Seizures occurring after myelography that are not controlled by injections of xylazine or diazepam may be treated by reanesthetizing the horse with guaifenesin and a thiobarbiturate. Anesthesia with an inhalation anesthetic may be necessary for up to 1 or 2 h until seizure activity wanes.

In horses, the accidental intracarotid injection of drugs such as xylazine may seriously irritate neural tissues, causing a violent reaction and seizures. Management of this potentially dangerous situation should be directed toward manual and, preferably, chemical restraint to prevent injury. Intravenous injection of thiopental alone or guaifenesin combined with thiopental is recommended as soon as accidental intracarotid injection is recognized. The preplacement of an indwelling intravenous catheter is recommended to help prevent the accidental perivascular injection of any drug. Inspired oxygen should be supplemented, and intravenous fluids should be administered. In the case of intracarotid injection of xylazine, pharmacological antagonism is not recommended. Horses given intracarotid drug injections can be sedated for 30 min by using the combination of guaifenesin and thiopental and often recover uneventfully. The accidental intracarotid injection of larger doses may have severe neurological sequelae (presumably caused by brain edema) requiring additional symptomatic treatment.

Anesthesia for Electrodiagnostic Techniques

Electrodiagnostic procedures are those that involve recording spontaneous or evoked electrical activity from tissues or organs. Although consistent with the definition, electrocardiography is usually not considered under this rubric. In veterinary medicine,

Table 38.4. Anesthetic management of seizure-prone patients.

1. Treatment or prevention of hypoglycemia
2. Use benzodiazepines for tranquilization (diazepam or midazolam, 0.2 mg/kg IV) or barbiturate sedation (phenobarbital, 2 to 5 mg/kg, IM)
3. Induction with thiopental (15 mg/kg IV) or propofol (3 mg/kg IV) administered to effect
4. Avoid enflurane for maintenance of anesthesia
5. Prevent hypoventilation and hypercapnia

IM, intramuscularly; and IV, intravenously.

clinical electrodiagnostic techniques are used to record potentials from muscle, peripheral nerves, spinal cord, brain stem, cortex, and retina. In humans, these procedures are performed without the use of general anesthetics, tranquilizers, or analgesics. With adequate instruction, most adults will tolerate some degree of discomfort or boredom to achieve good test results. Some procedures, such as nerve-conduction studies or electromyography, cause some pain, whereas others, such as visual or auditory evoked potentials, may simply require human patients to concentrate or refrain from movement. A fundamental problem encountered in the use of electrodiagnostic techniques in veterinary medicine is that of patient cooperation. Even during those procedures in which the stimulus is innocuous, artifacts caused by movement may render the technique ineffective. Therefore, many of these procedures must be performed in anesthetized or tranquilized animals. This approach is usually less stressful to the animals, insures a minimum of recording artifacts, and often gives the examiner an opportunity to collect more useful data. The obvious trade-off is nervous system function that has been chemically altered to some degree.

The effects of anesthetics on the outcome of electrodiagnostic procedures range from insignificant to dramatic. In some instances, the use of anesthetic agents altogether precludes recording certain types of potentials. The order of increasing anesthetic effects on recordings is peripheral nerve and skeletal muscle, spinal cord and retina, brain stem, and cerebral cortex. Even so, as long as the effects are understood, the benefits of the recordings may still provide valuable diagnostic data and information.

Today, intraoperative monitoring has become standard practice when a physician desires direct and prompt feedback about neural function during surgical procedures. The use of intraoperative electrodiagnostic monitoring in veterinary medicine is not widespread, but many electrodiagnostic laboratories judiciously use anesthetics for their procedures. Certainly, the precautions will vary between animal species and the physical condition of patients. An exhaustive review of anesthetic effects on these diagnostic techniques is not possible here, but some examples from the literature underscore the relevance of this information.

Electroencephalogram and Electromyography

There are two procedures in which electrical activity is recorded from spontaneously, reflexively, or volitionally active tissue. The first is the electroencephalogram (EEG), activity produced by the cerebral cortex, and the second is the electromyogram, electrical activity produced by skeletal muscle. Most other electrodiagnostic procedures require a stimulus to evoke activity from excitable tissue. The evoking stimulus may be electrical, visual, auditory, or mechanical.

The effects upon the EEG depend on the anesthetic type and depth. Anesthesia initially causes an increase in the voltage and a decrease in the frequency of cortical potentials when compared with the record of an awake alert dog. Spikes and spindles may also riddle the EEG of lightly anesthetized dogs and cats.[47,48] As anesthesia deepens, the overall voltage begins to diminish. A dose-response decrease in cerebral oxygen consumption ($CMRO_2$) accompanies the use of isoflurane in dogs and causes the EEG to become isoelectric at an end-expired concentration of 3%.[49] The same type of cortical alteration in electrical activity, sometimes referred to as *burst suppression*, has been reported in swine.[50] Isoflurane anesthesia may thereby interfere with acquisition of diagnostic information. A recommended anesthetic technique for diagnostic EEG evaluation and for procedures other than EEGs in seizure-prone patients is summarized in Table 38.4.

Dose-dependent CNS depression of EEG activity by most anesthetics is characteristic and has led to the development of EEG-based anesthetic-monitoring techniques.[51] Use of computer-analyzed *quantitative* EEG in isoflurane-anesthetized dogs has been reported.[52] Notable exceptions to the general rule that anesthetics decrease EEG activity include the dissociative anesthetics and the volatile anesthetic enflurane. Enflurane anesthesia can be accompanied by increased EEG activity extending to seizures, particularly if a patient is hyperventilated and hypocarbic.[3,12] Alterations in normal $PaCO_2$ are associated with significant changes in the quantitative EEG of dogs during halothane anesthesia.[53] Methoxyflurane and halothane anesthetics cause a progression of cerebral depression in dogs, with the latter more likely to promote burst suppression than the former.[54] Similar results in dogs have been reported for sodium pentobarbital. In dogs, barbiturate anesthesia is accompanied by reduced EEG amplitude and burst suppression.[55]

Monitoring CNS depression by using EEG during anesthesia has been the focus of study for decades. However, direct interpretation of the EEG has not proven adequately reliable or time responsive for use in operative circumstances. Processed EEG monitoring has evolved as a way to provide immediate feedback to anesthetists in regard to patients' CNS activity. Spectral edge frequency, total power, beta to delta frequency ratios, and other specific parameters derived from computer-processed EEG have been correlated to varying degrees with anesthetic depth, but interpretation can vary depending on the selection of anesthetic agents. Intraoperative EEG processing has been developed with significant improvement in reliability. For example, the bispectral index (BIS) monitor is a proprietary device that provides information related to anesthetic depth and is readily interpreted. In addition, the BIS has proven to be reliable as an indicator of anesthetic depth in people given a variety of anesthetic agents and adjuncts.[56,57] The BIS is a unitless number between 0 and 100 derived from the processed EEG.[58] People undergoing surgery are typically maintained at a depth of anesthesia that yields a BIS value between 40 and 60, which reliably prevents intraoperative awareness.[59-63]

In animals, a few reports have evaluated use of the BIS as an indicator of anesthetic depth. In dogs, isoflurane and sevoflurane anesthetic depth has been correlated to BIS.[64,65] Anesthetized cats had a nonlinear relationship of BIS with increasing multiples of sevoflurane minimum alveolar concentration.[66] The change in BIS values following stimulation in isoflurane-anesthetized cats provided a useful measure of anesthetic depth.[67] In goats anesthetized with isoflurane, BIS values significantly changed in response to intubation and noxious stimulation.[68] One study in unstimulated pigs did not demonstrate reliable correlation between isoflurane anesthetic depth and BIS, whereas others have demonstrated correlation of BIS values to anesthetic depth during surgery or with other noxious stimulation.[69-72]

Nerve-Conduction Studies

Nerve-conduction velocity has been successfully recorded in dogs while using a variety of anesthetic protocols. Because these procedures have not been done in unanesthetized animals, the effects of anesthetics on these procedures are largely unknown. Studies in dogs have been successful using thiamylal sodium and methoxyflurane for assessment of motor and sensory nerve function.[73,74]

Auditory and Visual Evoked Potentials

These may be altered by anesthetic agents, depending on the location of signal generators. Generally, cortical potentials are more likely to be affected than brain-stem potentials. In cats, administration of pentobarbital (20 mg/kg intraperitoneally) was shown to increase latency, area, and amplitude of auditory potentials.[75] In another study, brain-stem auditory evoked potentials recorded from cats were unaffected by sodium pentobarbital, ketamine, halothane, or chloralose administration.[76] Similar results were obtained from rats when ketamine or pentobarbital were used.[77] The use of ketamine in rats does, however, affect photic and field potentials recorded directly from various sensory relay nuclei when using implanted microelectrodes.[78] The use of ketamine and xylazine in cats produces only minimal changes (latency increases) in the brain-stem auditory evoked responses (BAERs) compared to xylazine alone.[79] The use of thiamylal sodium alters the BAER in dogs by increasing the latencies and decreasing the amplitudes of certain peaks.[80] The same dose of thiamylal sodium, however, completely obliterates middle-latency components of the BAER in dogs.[81] Light pentobarbital anesthesia in cats produces an increase or no change in cortical auditory evoked responses (AERs), moderate levels cause some increases in amplitude, and deep anesthesia causes all waves to disappear.[82] Although paraldehyde, ether, and ethyl chloride produce effects similar to those of pentobarbital, chloralose and chloroform are associated with an earlier and more profound period of enhancement.

In rats, the use of halothane (0.25% to 2.0%) affects AERs in a dose-related fashion.[83] These potentials are more sensitive to halothane than are visual evoked responses, especially in the auditory cortex. Pentobarbital, given to rats in sufficiently high doses to cause coma, progressively depresses and then abolishes all peaks of the auditory brain-stem potential.[84] The use of atropine and xylazine in dogs in combination with ketamine or pentobarbital produces only slight changes in the latency of BAER wave VI when compared with xylazine and atropine alone.[85] When BAER waves in dogs anesthetized with methoxyflurane are compared with those in unanesthetized dogs, all waves have significantly longer latencies.[86] In gerbils, ketamine-xylazine anesthesia induces only minor changes in the low-frequency and high-frequency components of the auditory brain-stem response.[87]

Visual evoked potentials (VEPs) have been successfully recorded in dogs and cats administered halothane, and in cats administered halothane and thiamylal sodium.[88–90] In dogs, a comparison of VEPs from dogs anesthetized with chloralose with VEPs from dogs anesthetized with halothane or halothane and thiopental did not reveal any differences in the waveform.[91]

Electroretinogram and Oscillatory Potentials

These can be recorded from small animals under a variety of anesthetic conditions.[92–94] The effects of clinical anesthetic protocols in animals is not well documented. Methoxyflurane, halothane, enflurane, ether, and chloroform anesthesia retards cone adaptation curves in monkeys.[95] Pentobarbital anesthesia in cats enables visual evoked responses to be recorded with only minor fluctuations over an 80-min period.[96] Barbiturate anesthesia has no effect on the maturation of the visual evoked response during the first 2 weeks of life.[97] Beyond 2 weeks of age, anesthesia causes an increase in the amplitude of early components while eliminating later components altogether.

Somatosensory Evoked Potentials

Somatosensory evoked potentials (abbreviated as SSEPs, SEPs, or SERs [somatosensory evoked responses]) are also affected by anesthesia. Isoflurane at 1% produces a sustained latency change in SSEP in newborn piglets.[98] Halothane administration does not affect peak latencies of lumbar spinal cord evoked potentials, but amplitudes are reduced.[99] In cats, increasing levels of pentobarbital can be used to achieve therapeutic coma levels.[100] The early brain-stem components are relatively unaffected, whereas late brain-stem and initial cortical responses show progressive latency increases. Late cortical waves are abolished at relatively low doses; central conduction is unaffected, and late waves of the visual evoked response are abolished even though a single potential survives massive doses. Components of sheep SSEPs have been shown to be differentially sensitive to barbiturate anesthesia.[101]

Motor Evoked Potentials

The effects of isoflurane on motor evoked potentials (MEPs) in rats has been examined using concentrations ranging from 0.2% to 1.5%.[102] There is a progressive increase in onset latency of the compound muscle action potentials and a decrease in the peak-to-peak amplitude and duration. Spinal cord MEPs have been reported in dogs with the use of a combination of fentanyl, droperidol, sufentanil, and nitrous oxide. Halogenated gas anesthetics raised the stimulus threshold for recording MEPs as compared with narcotic/nitrous oxide anesthesia.[103] Peripheral nerve MEPs

have been successfully recorded from dogs when using thiopental sodium, isoflurane, and oxymorphone.[104]

Considerations for Magnetic Resonance Imaging

Anesthetic concerns during MRI examination center on the potentially dangerous environment of a strong magnetic field. Ferromagnetic projectiles have had serious, even lethal, consequences in MRI suites. Anesthetic management of animals undergoing MRI exam can most simply be accomplished by means of injectable agents.[105–107] Inhalant anesthetics have been used in MRI suites by distancing the vital ferromagnetic components of the anesthesia machine from the magnetic field. Use of an extended non-rebreathing circuit, such as the Bain circuit, has been described.[108] One drawback of this technique is the higher fresh-gas flow rates required for larger animals (>50 kg). Another modification of anesthetic technique for MRI involves the use of extended rebreathing hoses with the anesthetic machine placed near the magnet, yet just beyond the critical point of magnetic attraction. For equine MRI, a large animal machine suitable for delivering inhalant anesthetics to horses can be used in this manner. There is anecdotal evidence that prolonged exposure (more than 2 h) in a 3- to 5-gauss magnetic field begins to affect vaporizer (Isotec; Datex-Ohmeda, Helsinki, Finland) output such that higher vaporizer settings are required to maintain adequate anesthesia (S. Greene, personal observation). In human patients, this effect has been reported for Fortec vaporizers (Cyprane, Keighley, U.K.).[109] Although many vaporizers are mainly constructed from nonferrous materials, many do contain components attracted or affected by magnetic fields.[110]

Anesthesia in MRI suites can be monitored by using MRI-compatible equipment to measure the electrocardiograph, blood pressure, pulse oximetry, and airway gases.[111] Less expensive alternatives include use of remotely placed monitors with specialized cabling designed to avoid interference with the magnetic field and induction of electric currents leading to burns. Simple systems can be used to measure direct arterial blood pressure, such as the aneroid manometer placed beyond the magnetic field or several feet of extension tubing placed between the transducer and patient. Some dampening and degradation of the arterial pulse wave may occur, but often direct measurement or arterial blood pressure is invaluable to assure maintenance of adequate cerebral perfusion pressure.

Because the magnetic fields vary considerably among various MRI units in clinical practice, consultation with a knowledgeable biomedical engineer is advised prior to implementing a monitoring system or novel means of anesthetic delivery.

References

1. Shapiro HH. Neurosurgical anesthesia and intracranial hypertension. In: Miller RD, ed. Anesthesia, 2nd ed. New York: Churchill Livingstone, 1986:1563–1620.
2. Stoelting RK. Pharmacology and Physiology in Anesthetic Practice. Philadelphia: JB Lippincott, 1987.

3. van Poznak A. Special consideration for veterinary neuroanesthesia. In: Short CE, ed. Principles and Practice of Veterinary Anesthesia. Baltimore: Williams and Wilkins, 1987:177–183.

4. Hansen TD, Warner DS, Vust LH, Todd MM, Trawick DC. Regional distribution of cerebral blood flow with halothane and isoflurane. Anesthesiology 69:332–337, 1988.

5. Osborn I. Choice of neuroanesthetic technique. Anesthesiology Clin North Am 5:531–540, 1987.

6. Dayrell-Hart B, Klide AM. Intracranial dysfunctions: Stupor and coma. Vet Clin North Am Small Anim Pract 19:1209–1222, 1989.

7. Grubb RL, Raichle ME, Eichling JO, Ter-Pogossian MM. The effects of changes in PaCO$_2$ on cerebral blood volume, blood flow, and vascular mean transit time. Stroke 5:530–539, 1974.

8. Cottrell JE. Deliberate hypotension. Annual Refresher Course Lectures, American Society of Anesthesiologists, sect 245, 1989:1–7.

9. Harp JR, Wollman H. Cerebral metabolic effects of hyperventilation and deliberate hypotension. Br J Anaesth 45:256–262, 1973.

10. Frost EAM. Central nervous system trauma. Anesthesiol Clin North Am 5:565–585, 1987.

11. Hirshfeld A. Fluid and electrolyte management in neurosurgical patients. Anesthesiol Clin North Am 5:491–505, 1987.

12. Gilroy BA. Neuroanesthesiology. In: Slatter D, ed. Textbook of Small Animal Surgery. Philadelphia: WB Saunders, 1985:2643–2650.

13. Gray PR, Lowrie CT, Wetmore LA. Effect of intravenous administration of dextrose or lactated Ringer's solution on seizure development in dogs after cervical myelography with metrizamide. Am J Vet Res 48:1600–1602, 1987.

14. Franklin RT. The use of glucocorticoids in treating cerebral edema. Compend Contin Educ Pract Vet 6:442–448, 1984.

15. Sato O, Hara M, Asai T, Tsugane R, Kageyama N. The effect of dexamethasone phosphate on the production rate of cerebrospinal fluid in the spinal subarachnoid space of dogs. J Neurosurg 39:480–484, 1973.

16. Gleed RD. Tranquilizers and sedative. In: Short CE, ed. Principles and Practice of Veterinary Anesthesia. Baltimore: Williams and Wilkins, 1987:16–28.

17. Tobias KM, Marioni-Henry K, Wagner RA. A retrospective study on the use of acepromazine maleate in dogs with seizures. J Am Anim Hosp Assoc 42:283–289, 2006.

18. Nugent M, Artru AA, Michnfelder JD. Cerebral metabolic, vascular and protective effects of midazolam maleate. Anesthesiology 56:172–176, 1982.

19. Moore RM, Trim CM. Effect of xylazine on cerebrospinal fluid pressure in conscious horses. Am J Vet Res 53:1558–1561, 1992.

20. Moore RM, Trim CM. Effect of hypercapnia or xylazine on lateral ventricle and lumbosacral cerebrospinal fluid pressures in pentobarbital-anesthetized horses. Vet Surg 22:151–158, 1993.

21. Short CE. Alpha-2 Agents in Animals: Sedation, Analgesia, and Anaesthesia. Santa Barbara, CA: Veterinary Practices, 1992.

22. Keegan RD, Greene SA, Bagley RS, Moore MP, Weil AB, Short CE. Effects of medetomidine administration on intracranial pressure and cardiovascular variables of isoflurane-anesthetized dogs. Am J Vet Res 56:193–198, 1995

23. Karlsson B, Forsman M, Roald O, Heier MS, Steen PA. Effect of dexmedetomidine, a selective and potent alpha 2-agonist, on cerebral blood flow and oxygen consumption during halothane anesthesia in dogs. Anesth Analg 71:125–129, 1990.

24. Zornow MH, Fleischer JE, Scheller MS, Nakakimura K, Drummond JC. Dexmedetomidine, an alpha-2 adrenergic agonist, decreases cerebral blood flow in the isoflurane-anesthetized dog. Anesth Analg 70:624–630, 1990.

25. Marsh ML, Marshall LF, Shapiro HM. Neurosurgical intensive care. Anesthesiology 47:149–163, 1977.

26. Bonica JJ, ed. The Management of Pain, 2nd ed. Philadelphia: Lea and Febiger, 1990.

27. Akeson J, Bjorkman S, Messeter K, Rosen I. Low-dose midazolam antagonizes cerebral metabolic stimulation by ketamine in the pig. Acta Anaesthesiol Scand 37:525–531, 1993.

28. Eger EI. Isoflurane (Forane): A Compendium and Reference. Madison, WI: Ohio Medical, 1984.

29. Drummond JC, Todd MM. The response of the feline cerebral circulation to PaCO$_2$ during anesthesia with isoflurane and halothane and during sedation with nitrous oxide. Anesthesiology 62:268–273, 1985.

30. Drummond JC, Todd MM, Shapiro HH. CO$_2$ responsiveness of the cerebral circulation during isoflurane anesthesia and nitrous oxide sedation in cats [Abstract]. Anesthesiology 57:A333, 1982.

31. Kaieda R, Todd MM, Warner DS. The effects of anesthetics and PaCO$_2$ on the cerebrovascular, metabolic, and electroencephalographic responses to nitrous oxide in the rabbit. Anesth Analg 68:135–143, 1989.

32. Riedesel DH. Anesthesia considerations for special diagnostic and surgical procedures. In: Short CE, ed. Principles and Practice of Veterinary Anesthesia. Baltimore: Williams and Wilkins, 1987:533–541.

33. Wheeler SJ, Davies JV. Iohexol myelography in the dog and cat: A series of one hundred cases and a comparison with metrizamide and iopamidol. J Small Anim Pract 26:247–256, 1985.

34. Cox FH. The use of iopamidol for myelography in dogs: A study of twenty-seven cases. J Small Anim Pract 27:159–165, 1986.

35. Kornegay JN, Oliver JE, Gorgacz EJ. Clinicopathologic features of brain herniation in animals. J Am Vet Med Assoc 182:1111–1116, 1983.

36. Hubbell JAE, Reed SM, Myer CW, Muir WW. Sequelae of myelography in the horse. Equine Vet J 20:438–440, 1988.

37. May SA, Wyn-Jones G, Church S. Iopamidol myelography in the horse. Equine Vet J 18:199–202, 1986.

38. Burbridge HM, Kannegieter N, Dickson LR, Goulden BE, Badcoe L. Iohexol myelography in the horse. Equine Vet J 21:347–350, 1989.

39. MacDonell WN, Hall LW, Jeffcott LB. Radiographic evidence of impaired pulmonary function in laterally recumbent anaesthetised horses. Equine Vet J 11:24–32, 1979.

40. Mason DE, Muir WW, Wade A. Arterial blood gas tensions in the horse during recovery from anesthesia [Abstract]. Vet Surg 15:461, 1986.

41. Adams R, Mayhew IG. Neurologic diseases. Vet Clin North Am Equine Pract 1:209–234, 1985.

42. Collatos C. Seizures in foals: Pathophysiology, evaluation, and treatment. Compend Contin Educ Pract Vet 12:393–399, 1990.

43. Redman HC, Wilson GL, Hogan JE. Effect of chlorpromazine combined with intermittent light stimulation in the electroencephalogram and clinical response of the Beagle dog. Am J Vet Res 34:929–936, 1973.

44. Wright JA, Clayton-Jones DG. Metrizamide myelography in sixty-eight dogs. J Small Anim Pract 22:415–435, 1981.

45. Mysinger PW, Redding RW, Vaughan JT, Purohit RC, Holladay JA. Electroencephalographic patterns of clinically normal, sedated, and tranquilized newborn foals and adult horses. Am J Vet Res 46:36–41, 1985.

46. Hodgson DS, Dunlop CI. General anesthesia for horses with specific problems. Vet Clin North Am 6:625–650, 1990.

47. Klemm WR. Subjective and quantitative analyses of the electroencephalogram of anesthetized normal dogs: Control data for clinical diagnosis. Am J Vet Res 29:1267–1277, 1968.

48. Klemm WR, Mallo GL. Clinical electroencephalography in anesthetized small animals. J Am Vet Med Assoc 148:1038–1042, 1976.

49. Newberg LA, Milde JH, Michenfelder JD. The cerebral metabolic effects of isoflurane at and above concentrations that suppress cortical electrical activity. Anesthesiology 39:23–28, 1983.

50. Rampil IJ, Weiskopf RB, Brown JG, et al. I653 and isoflurane produce similar dose-related changes in the electroencephalogram of pigs. Anesthesiology 69:298–302, 1988.

51. Goodrich JT. Electrophysiologic measurements: Intraoperative evoked potential monitoring. Anesthesiol Clin North Am 5:477–489, 1987.

52. Moore MP, Greene SA, Keegan RD, et al. Quantitative electroencephalography in dogs anesthetized with 2.0% end-tidal concentration of isoflurane. Am J Vet Res 52:551–560, 1991.

53. Smith LJ, Greene SA, Moore MP, Keegan RD. Effects of altered arterial carbon dioxide tension on quantitative EEG in halothane-anesthetized dogs. Am J Vet Res 55:467–471, 1994.

54. Prynn RB, Redding RW. Electroencephalographic continuum in dogs anesthetized with methoxyflurane and halothane. Am J Vet Res 29:1913–1928, 1968.

55. Tonuma E. Electroencephalography with barbiturate anesthesia in the dog. Can Vet J 8:181–185, 1967.

56. Sebel PS, Lang E, Rampil IJ, et al. A multicenter study of bispectral electroencephalogram analysis for monitoring anesthetic effect. Anesth Analg 84:891–899, 1997.

57. Takkallapalli R, Mehta M, DeLima L, Patel A, May W, Eichhorn J. Bispectral index: Can it predict arousal from noxious stimuli during general anesthesia? Anesth Analg 88(Suppl 2):S58, 1998.

58. Rampil IJ. A primer for EEG signal processing in anesthesia. Anesthesiology 89:980–1002, 1998.

59. Katoh T, Suzuki A, Ikeda K. Electroencephalographic derivatives as a tool for predicting the depth of sedation and anesthesia induced by sevoflurane. Anesthesiology 88:642–650, 1998.

60. Rosow C, Manberg PJ. Bispectal index monitoring. Anesthesiol Clin North Am 16:89–107, 1998.

61. Billard V, Gambus PL, Chamoun N, Stanski DR, Shafer SL. A comparison of spectral edge, delta power, and bispectral index as EEG measures of alfentanil, propofol, and midazolam drug effect. Clin Pharmacol Ther 61:45–58, 1997.

62. Sleigh J, Andrzejowski J, Steyn-Ross A, Steyn-Ross M. The bispectral index: A measure of depth of sleep? Anesth Analg 88:659–661, 1999.

63. Kearse LA, Rosow C, Zaslavsky A, Connors P, Dershwitz M, Denman W. Bispectral analysis of the EEG predicts conscious processing of information during propofol sedation hypnosis. Anesthesiology 88:25–34, 1998.

64. Greene SA, Tranquilli WJ, Benson GJ, Grimm KA. Effect of medetomidine on bispectral index measurements in dogs during anesthesia with isoflurane. Am J Vet Res 64:316–320, 2003.

65. Greene SA, Benson GJ, Tranquilli WJ, Grimm KA. Relationship of canine bispectral index to multiples of sevoflurane minimal alveolar concentration, using patch or subdermal electrodes. Comp Med 52:424–428, 2002.

66. Lamont LA, Greene SA, Grimm KA, Tranquilli WJ. Relationship of bispectral index to minimum alveolar concentration multiples of sevoflurane in cats. Am J Vet Res 65:93–98, 2004.

67. March PA, Muir WW. Use of bispectral index as a monitor of anesthetic depth in cats anesthetized with isoflurane. Am J Vet Res 64:1534–1541, 2003.

68. Antognini JF, Wang XW, Carstens E. Isoflurane anesthetic depth in goats monitored using the bispectral index of the electroencephalogram. Vet Res Commun 24:361–370, 2000.

69. Haga HA, Tevik A, Moerch H. Bispectral index as an indicator of anaesthetic depth during isoflurane anaesthesia in the pig. J Vet Anaesth 26:3–7, 1999.

70. Schmidt M, Papp-Jambor C, Marx T, Schirmer U, Reinelt H. Evaluation of bispectral index (BIS) for anaesthetic depth monitoring in pigs. Appl Cardiopulmonary Pathophysiol 9:83–86, 2000.

71. Martin-Cancho MF, Carrasco-Jimenez MS, Lima JR, Ezquerra LJ, Crisostomo V, Uson-Gargallo J. Assessment of the relationship of bispectral index values, hemodynamic changes, and recovery times associated with sevoflurane or propofol anesthesia in pigs. Am J Vet Res 65:409–416, 2004.

72. Greene SA, Benson GJ, Tranquilli WJ, Grimm KA. Effect of isoflurane, atracurium, fentanyl, and noxious stimulation on bispectral index in pigs. Comp Med 54:397–403, 2004.

73. Sims MH, Redding RW. Maturation of nerve conduction velocity and the evoked muscle potential in the dog. Am J Vet Res 41:1247–1252, 1980.

74. Sims MH, Selcer RR. Occurrence and evaluation of a reflex-evoked muscle potential (H reflex) in the normal dog. Am J Vet Res 42:975–983, 1981.

75. Guha D, Pradhan SN. Effects of mescaline, [delta9]-tetrahydrocannabinol and pentobarbital on the auditory evoked responses in the cat. Neuropharmacology 13:755–762, 1974.

76. Cohen MS, Britt RH. Effects of sodium pentobarbital, ketamine, halothane, and chloralose on brainstem auditory evoked responses. Anesth Analg 61:338–343, 1982.

77. Bobbin RP, May JG, Lemoine RL. Effect of pentobarbital and ketamine on brain stem auditory potentials. Arch Otolaryngol 105:467–470, 1983.

78. Dafney N, Rigor BM. Dose effects of ketamine on photic and acoustic field potentials. Neuropharmacology 17:851–862, 1978.

79. Sims MH, Horohow JE. Effects of xylazine and ketamine on the acoustic reflex and brain stem auditory-evoked response in the cat. Am J Vet Res 47:102–109, 1986.

80. Sims MH, Moore RE. Auditory-evoked response in the clinically normal dog: Early latency components. Am J Vet Res 45:2019–2027, 1984.

81. Sims MH, Moore RE. Auditory-evoked response in the clinically normal dog: Middle latency components. Am J Vet Res 45:2028–2033, 1984.

82. Pradhan SN, Galambos R. Some effects of anesthetics on the evoked responses in the auditory cortex of cats. J Am Vet Med Assoc 139:97–106, 1962.

83. Rabe LS, Moreno L, Rigor BM, Dafny N. Effects of halothane on evoked field potentials recorded from cortical and subcortical nuclei. Neuropharmacology 19:813–825, 1980.

84. Shapiro SM, Miller AR, Shiu GK. Brain-stem auditory evoked potentials in rats with high-dose pentobarbital. Electroencephalogr Clin Neurophysiol 58:266–276, 1984.

85. Toruriki M, Matsunami K, Uzuka Y. Relative effects of xylazine-atropine, xylazine-atropine-ketamine, and xylazine-atropine-pentobarbital combinations and time-course effects of the latter two combinations on brain stem auditory-evoked potentials in dogs. Am J Vet Res 51:97–102, 1990.

86. Myers LJ, Redding RW, Wilson S. Reference values of the brainstem auditory evoked response of methoxyflurane anesthetized and unanesthetized dogs. Vet Res Commun 9:289–294, 1985.

87. Smith DI, Mills JH. Low-frequency component of the gerbil brainstem response: Response characteristics and anesthetic effects. Hear Res 54:1–10, 1991.

88. Sims MH, Laratta LJ. Visual-evoked potentials in cats, using a light-emitting diode stimulator. Am J Vet Res 49:1876–1881, 1988.

89. Sims MH, Laratta LJ, Bubb WJ, Morgan RV. Waveform analysis and reproducibility of visual-evoked potentials in dogs. Am J Vet Res 50:1823–1828, 1989.

90. Pang XD, Bonds AB. Visual-evoked potential responses of the anesthetized cat to contrast modulation of grating patterns. Vision Res 31:1509–1516, 1991.

91. Bichsel P, Oliver JE, Coulter DB, Brown J. Recording of visual-evoked potentials in dogs with scalp electrodes. J Vet Intern Med 2:145–149, 1988.

92. Rubin LF. Clinical electroretinography in dogs. J Am Vet Med Assoc 151:1456–1469, 1967.

93. Gum GG, Gelatt KN, Samuelson DA. Maturation of the retina of the canine neonate as determined by electroretinography and histology. Am J Vet Res 45:1166–1171, 1984.

94. Sims MH, Brooks DE. Changes in oscillatory potentials in the canine electroretinogram during dark adaptation. Am J Vet Res 51:1580–1586, 1990.

95. van Norren DV, Padmos P. Influence of anesthetics, ethyl alcohol, and Freon on dark adaptation of monkey cone ERG. Invest Ophthalmol Vis Sci 16:80–83, 1977.

96. Uzuka Y, Doi S, Tokuriki M, Matsumoto H. The establishment of a clinical diagnostic method of the visual evoked potentials (VEP's) in the cat: The effects of recording electrode positions, stimulus intensity and the level of anesthesia. Jpn J Vet Sci 51:547–553, 1989.

97. Rose GH, Gruenau SP, Spencer JW. Maturation of visual electrocortical responses in unanesthetized kittens: Effects of barbiturate anesthesia. Electroencephalogr Clin Neurophysiol 33:141–158, 1972.

98. Boston JR, Davis PJ, Brandom BW, Roeber CM. Rate of change of somatosensory evoked potentials during isoflurane anesthesia in newborn piglets. Anesth Analg 70:275–283, 1990.

99. Hogan K, Gravenstein M, Sasse F. Effects of halothane dose and stimulus rate on canine spinal, far-field and near-field somatosensory evoked potentials. Electroencephalogr Clin Neurophysiol 69:277–286, 1988.

100. Sutton LN, Frewen T, Marsh R, Jaggi J, Bruce DA. The effects of deep barbiturate coma on multimodality evoked potentials. J Neurosurg 57:178–185, 1982.

101. Wilson RD, Beerwinkle KR. Somatosensory-evoked potential induced by stimulation of the caudal tibial nerve in awake and barbiturate-anesthetized sheep. Am J Vet Res 47:46–49, 1986.

102. Haghighi SS, Green KD, Oro JJ, Drake RK, Krache GR. Depressive effect of isoflurane anesthesia on motor evoked potentials. Neurosurgery 26:993–997, 1990.

103. Cook JR, Konrad PE, Tacker WA. Amplitude and latency characteristics of spinal cord motor-evoked potentials in dogs. Am J Vet Res 51:1340–1344, 1990.

104. Kraus KH, O'Brien D, Pope ER, Kraus BH. Evoked potentials induced by transcranial stimulation in dogs. Am J Vet Res 51:1732–1735, 1990.

105. Chaffin MK, Walker MA, McArthur NH, Perris EE, Matthews NS. Magnetic resonance imaging of the brain of normal neonatal foals. Vet Radiol Ultrasound 38:102–111, 1997.

106. Lukasik VM, Gillies RJ. Animal anaesthesia for in-vivo magnetic resonance. NMR Biomed 16:459–467, 2003.

107. Willis CK, Quinn RP, McDonnell WM, Gati J, Parent J, Nicolle D. Functional MRI as a tool to assess vision in dogs: The optimal anesthetic. Vet Ophthalmol 4:243–253, 2001.

108. Young AE, Brown PN, Zorab JS. Anaesthesia for children and infants undergoing magnetic resonance imaging: A prospective study. Eur J Anaesthesiol 13:400–403, 1996.

109. Kross J, Drummond JC. Successful use of a Fortec II vaporizer in the MRI suite: A case report with observations regarding magnetic field-induced vaporizer aberrancy. Can J Anaesth 38:1065–1069, 1991.

110. Zimmer C, Janssen MN, Treschan JA, Peters J. Near-miss accident during magnetic resonance imaging by a "flying sevoflurane vaporizer" due to ferromagnetism undetectable by handheld magnet. Anesthesiology 100:1329–1330, 2004.

111. Shelley K, Shelley S, Bell C. Monitoring in unusual environments. In: Lake CL, Hines RL, Blitt CD, eds. Clinical Monitoring. Philadelphia: WB Saunders, 2001:524–538.

Chapter 39
Renal Disease

Stephen A. Greene and Gregory F. Grauer

Introduction

The kidneys have three primary functions: filtration, reabsorption, and secretion. To accomplish these functions, they receive about 25% of the cardiac output. The renal tubules and collecting ducts reabsorb up to 99% of filtered solutes, indicating that the total filtration volume is much greater than daily urine production. Neurohumoral substances and physiological factors that affect reabsorption of the filtered water and sodium include aldosterone, antidiuretic hormone (ADH), arterial blood pressure, atrial natriuretic factor, catecholamines, prostaglandins, renin-angiotensin, and stress.

Renal blood flow (RBF) is regulated by extrinsic nervous and hormonal control and by intrinsic autoregulation. Renal vasculature is highly innervated by sympathetic constrictor fibers originating in the spinal cord segments between T4 and L1. The kidneys lack sympathetic dilator fibers and parasympathetic innervation. Intrinsic autoregulation of RBF is demonstrated by a constant flow when mean arterial blood pressure ranges from 80 to 180 mm Hg. When the mean arterial blood pressure is between 80 and 180 mm Hg, the kidney can control blood flow by altering resistance in the glomerular afferent arterioles. Although the exact mechanism of renal autoregulation is not known, the significance of this phenomenon relates to protection of glomerular capillaries during hypertension and preservation of renal function during hypotension. However, even within the range of blood pressure described for function of renal autoregulation, extrinsic forces (e.g., neural, hormonal, and pharmacological) and intrinsic forces (e.g., renal insufficiency/failure) may cause alterations in RBF and glomerular filtration rate (GFR). Catecholamines are the major hormonal regulators of RBF. Epinephrine and norepinephrine cause dose-dependent changes in RBF and the GFR. Low doses increase arterial blood pressure and decrease RBF with no net change in the GFR. Higher doses cause decreased RBF and GFR. The renal vascular anatomy is unique in its distribution to cortical and medullary zones. Because of this vascular dichotomy, local tissue ischemia and hypoxia may occur even though total organ blood flow is normal. Oxygen delivery to the kidney is complex, and selective regional hypoxia is a possible source of renal injury during renal hypoperfusion. Experimental evidence indicates that the medullary thick ascending limb of Henle's loop, because of its high metabolic rate associated with active transport of electrolytes, is selectively vulnerable to hypoxic injury.[1]

Anesthetic Effects on Renal Function

Effects of anesthetics on RBF can be summarized with the following generalization: All anesthetics are likely to decrease the rate of glomerular filtration. Anesthetics may directly affect RBF, or they may indirectly alter renal function via changes in cardiovascular and/or neuroendocrine activity. Most anesthetics decrease the GFR as a consequence of decreased RBF (Table 39.1). Anesthetics that cause catecholamine release (e.g., ketamine, tiletamine, and nitrous oxide) have variable effects on RBF. Inhalation anesthetics tend to decrease RBF and GFR in a dose-dependent manner. Light planes of inhalation anesthesia preserve renal autoregulation of blood flow, whereas deep planes are associated with depression of autoregulation and decreases in RBF. Although isoflurane has little effect on RBF, it decreases GFR and urine output.[2] Nitrous oxide in combination with halothane does not appear to alter autoregulation of RBF.[3] Desflurane has no effect on RBF at concentrations up to twice the minimal alveolar concentration (MAC); however, it decreases renal vascular resistance at concentrations greater than 1.75 MAC.[4]

Thiobarbiturates increase systemic vascular resistance but decrease renal vascular resistance with no net change in RBF. In contrast, ketamine increases RBF and renal vascular resistance.[5] Most anesthetics cause less disruption of renal autoregulation of blood flow at lower doses (lighter anesthetic planes). Different responses to anesthetics may occur in controlled studies of RBF compared with clinical use of anesthetics. Renal responses to anesthetics also depend on the preexisting hydration status and quantity of perioperative fluids administered, as well as preexisting renal insufficiency/failure.

Due to systemic hypotension or renal vasoconstriction, renal ischemia may occur during anesthesia. Systemic hypotension may be caused by excessive depth of inhalation anesthesia, as all potent halogenated anesthetics cause peripheral vasodilation. Inhalant anesthetics also depress myocardial contractility and cardiac output in a dose-dependent manner. Hypotension may also be induced by phenothiazine or butyrophenone tranqui-

Table 39.1. Effects of anesthetics on renal blood flow (RBF) and glomerular filtration rate (GFR)[a].

Drug	RBF	GFR
Desflurane	No change	Decrease
Enflurane	Decrease	Decrease
Etomidate	No change	No change
Halothane	Slight decrease	Decrease
Isoflurane	Slight decrease	Decrease
Ketamine	Increase	Decrease or no change
Propofol	No change	No change
Sevoflurane	Slight decrease	Decrease
Thiopental	No change	No change or slight decrease

[a]Injectable anesthetics administered as a single intravenous bolus. Halogenated inhalants administered for maintenance of anesthesia.

Table 39.2. Potential nephrotoxins in the perianesthetic period.

Aminoglycoside antibiotics
Amphotericin B
Bilirubin
Free fluoride ion
Hemoglobin
Iodinated radiographic contrast agents
Methoxyflurane
Myoglobin
Nonsteroidal anti-inflammatory agents
Oxalate

lizers. Phenothiazine and butyrophenone tranquilizers block α-adrenoceptors and dopamine receptors. α-Adrenergic blockade may induce peripheral vasodilation and hypotension. Dopamine receptor blockade by acepromazine premedication may prevent dopamine-induced increases in RBF during surgery.

Intraoperative administration of epinephrine for hemostasis will increase renal vascular resistance and may reduce RBF significantly.[6] Renal failure may occur occasionally in animals that have been given epinephrine for hemostasis during otherwise uneventful anesthesia.[7] Following the initial ischemic insult, renal perfusion may remain altered because of other mechanisms. In experimental dogs injected intrarenally with norepinephrine, saline administration restored RBF but did not correct oliguria.[8] Necropsy of animals following acute renal failure may not detect renal damage because histological evidence may not be evident until 3 or 4 days after injury.[9]

Anesthesia and the stress associated with surgery cause release of aldosterone, vasopressin, renin, and catecholamines. Thus, RBF and GFR (and therefore urine production) are generally decreased with surgery in any patient. For most patients, the effects of inhaled anesthetics on renal function are reversed at the termination of anesthesia. Some patients, however, may not regain the ability to regulate urine production for several days.[10] Postanesthetic oliguria should be evaluated as soon as is feasible.

Some drugs used in the perianesthetic period have a significant effect on urine production. α$_2$-Adrenergic agonists can dramatically increase urinary output and reduce urinary osmolality.[11] Xylazine is believed to decrease ADH concentration in mares, accounting, in part, for increased urine production.[12] Detomidine-induced diuresis has also been reported in horses.[13] Because α$_2$-adrenergic agonists can induce diuresis, they should not be used in animals that have urethral obstruction. Reports on the effects of opioids on ADH secretion are confusing. The antidiuresis following morphine administration in animals has been attributed to increased release of ADH.[14] Others suggest this is a response to stress associated with surgical stimulation.[15] Opioids

may cause urine retention when administered systemically or as an epidural injection.

Nephrotoxic drugs administered during anesthesia may cause oliguria (Table 39.2). Methoxyflurane is the only anesthetic known to cause nephrotoxicity as a consequence of biotransformation to oxalate and free fluoride ion.[16–18] Methoxyflurane anesthesia combined with flunixin meglumine precipitates renal failure in dogs.[19] Aminoglycoside antibiotics are potentially nephrotoxic and also enhance the renal toxicity of methoxyflurane.[20]

Effects of Renal Insufficiency on Anesthesia

Renal insufficiency/failure and renal azotemia in patients with renal insufficiency can alter the response to anesthetics. Azotemia may be associated with changes in the blood-brain barrier, leading to increased drug penetration into the central nervous system. Patients with renal insufficiency/failure may be acidotic, which will increase the fraction of unbound barbiturate and other injectable drugs in the plasma. Thus, lower doses of highly protein-bound injectable anesthetics may be required in acidotic patients.

Hyperkalemia may be present in animals with renal insufficiency/failure, obstructed urethra, or rupture of the urinary bladder. Acidosis may be associated with a concurrent increase in serum potassium. Patients in renal failure with hypocalcemia are at even greater risk, because hypocalcemia potentiates the myocardial toxicity of hyperkalemia. Further, administration of succinylcholine will transiently increase serum potassium concentration.[21] Succinylcholine-induced increases in potassium are potentially life threatening in animals with hyperkalemia. In contrast, elevation in serum potassium is not observed after administration of nondepolarizing neuromuscular blocking agents. It should be remembered that patients with hypermagnesemia associated with chronic renal failure may have prolonged recovery from nondepolarizing neuromuscular blocking agents.[22] In general, patients having a serum potassium concentration greater than 5.5 or 6.0 mEq/L should not be anesthetized until the hyperkalemia can be addressed. Electrocardiographic (ECG) abnormalities are commonly observed with potassium concentrations exceeding 7 mEq/L. The resting membrane potential of cardiac muscle depends on the permeability and extracellular concentration of potassium (Fig. 39.1). During hyperkalemia, the membrane's resting potential is raised (partially depolarized), and fewer sodium channels are available to participate in the action potential. As the serum potassium concentration increases, repolarization occurs more rapidly and automaticity, conductivity, contractility, and excitability are decreased. These changes produce the classic ECG appearance of a peaked T wave with a prolonged PR interval progressing to wide QRS complexes and loss of P waves. Mild chronic hyperkalemia may not require treatment prior to anesthesia. If treatment is instituted for chronic hyperkalemia, serum potassium should be lowered gradually to allow intracellular potassium time to reestablish physiological transmembrane concentration gradients. If hyperkalemia is acute or ECG abnormalities are noted, treatment should be initiated prior to induction of anesthesia. The most rapid treatment for the cardiac effects associated with hyperkalemia is 10% calcium chloride (0.1 mg/kg IV). Calcium will increase the membrane's threshold potential, resulting in increased myocardial conduction and contractility. Because increased serum potassium concentration causes the resting potential to be less negative (partially depolarized), the calcium ion–induced increase in threshold potential temporarily restores the normal gradient between resting and threshold potentials. It should be recognized that administration of calcium will not affect the serum potassium concentration, and its effects will therefore be short-lived. Regimens to decrease the serum potassium concentration by shifting potassium intracellularly include bicarbonate administration and combined infusion of glucose and insulin. Because acidemia favors extracellular movement of potassium and worsens hyperkalemia, intermittent positive pressure ventilation may be required to prevent anesthetic drug–induced hypercapnia and respiratory acidosis.

Patients with chronic renal failure may be anemic because of bone marrow suppression, chronic gastrointestinal tract blood loss, reduced red blood cell life span, and decreased erythropoietin production. In response to anemia, the cardiovascular system may become hyperdynamic in an attempt to maintain oxygen delivery. Chronic renal disease may be associated with hypertension and increased cardiac output but reduced cardiac reserve. Patients undergoing anesthesia should have a red blood cell transfusion if the hematocrit is less than 18% (cats) or 20% (dogs). Additionally, pulse oximetry can be used to rapidly detect hemoglobin desaturation and alert one to the potential for a decrease in tissue oxygen delivery.

In dogs and cats with mild renal insufficiency, a rapid intravenous induction of anesthesia may be accomplished with thiobarbiturates, propofol, etomidate, diazepam-ketamine, or diazepam-opioid combinations. Severely depressed patients can be mask induced with isoflurane or halothane. Anesthesia may be maintained with isoflurane or sevoflurane. The use of medications, including nonsteroidal anti-inflammatory drugs (NSAIDs), that are potentially nephrotoxic should be avoided (Table 39.2).

When renal function is questioned, the urinary bladder can be catheterized and urine production monitored via a closed, sterile urine-collection system. Urine production is an indirect measure of renal perfusion. Normal urine output for dogs is 0.5 to 1.0 mL $\cdot$ kg^{-1} $\cdot$ h^{-1}. In normal horses, daily urine production has been

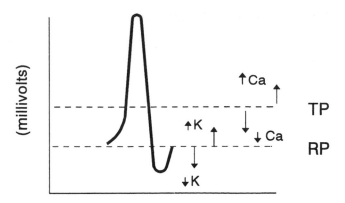

Fig. 39.1. Relationships between extracellular concentrations of potassium (K$^+$) and calcium (Ca^{2+}) and the resting potential (RP) and threshold potential (TP). An action potential is generated when there is sufficient depolarization to reach the TP. Increased extracellular potassium will result in raised (less negative) RP, whereas increased extracellular calcium will result in raised TP.

estimated to be about 15 L; horses that are denied feed and water for 24 h produce about 6 L.[23] Empty intravenous fluid bags can be saved for the purpose of collecting urine from catheterized patients.

If the urinary tract is not obstructed or the patient is anuric, intravenous fluids should be administered during anesthesia at the rate of 20 mL/kg for the first hour. A rate of 10 mL $\cdot$ kg^{-1} $\cdot$ h^{-1} is used thereafter. Lower fluid rates should be used if the patient has mild hypoproteinemia or cardiovascular disease. The choice of intravenous fluid is based on the animal's electrolyte and acid-base status. In general, animals with mild to moderate renal insufficiency/failure that are well prepared for surgery or anesthesia are given lactated Ringer's solution. Arterial blood pressure must be measured to detect systemic hypotension and decreased renal perfusion pressure. The mean arterial blood pressure should be maintained above 70 to 80 mm Hg. The central venous pressure (CVP) can be measured via a jugular catheter to evaluate the rate of intravenous fluid administration. Normal CVP should be between 3 and 5 cm of water. If the CVP rises more than 10 cm of water, the fluid administration should be slowed or stopped. If the CVP falls in response to the fluids being stopped, they may be resumed at a slower rate. An elevated CVP of more than 10 cm of water indicates inadequate myocardial function or volume overload. Myocardial function may be improved by infusion of dopamine (1 to 3 µg $\cdot$ kg^{-1} $\cdot$ min^{-1}). Low doses of dopamine will also improve RBF either through increased cardiac output, dopaminergic diuretic effects, or both. Doses of dopamine above approximately 10 µg $\cdot$ kg^{-1} $\cdot$ min^{-1} may cause α-adrenergic renal vasoconstriction and decreased RBF. Improvement in renal perfusion in cats given dopamine is less well documented, but may involve α-adrenoceptor stimulation rather than dopamine receptor agonism.[24] Putative renal dopamine receptors (DA1) in cats appear to differ from those identified in kidneys of other species.[25] Other DA1 agonists, such as fenoldopam, may prove useful in improving RBF and diuresis in this species.

Tests of Renal Function

Measurements of the GFR and renal tubular function, such as urine specific gravity and blood urea nitrogen (BUN), are not specific for renal disease. Serum creatinine is a more specific indicator of the GFR than BUN because it is influenced by fewer extrarenal variables. It is important to keep in mind that greater than 75% nephron loss is necessary for most patients to become persistently azotemic. Thus, patients with mild renal insufficiency may not have elevated serum creatinine. Persistent proteinuria and/or cellular or granular cylinduria may indicate renal damage prior to the onset of renal azotemia.

In addition to BUN, serum creatinine concentrations, and urinalysis, patients with renal insufficiency should be evaluated to determine acid-base balance, electrolyte concentrations (especially potassium), exercise intolerance, hematocrit, hydration, and urine production.

Postoperative Oliguria

Postoperative oliguria (<0.5 mL $\cdot$ kg^{-1} $\cdot$ h^{-1}) should be investigated. If the animal does not have congestive heart failure or pulmonary edema, a fluid challenge of 5 mL/kg isotonic sodium chloride may be given. If urine production increases, the animal was hypovolemic and fluids should be continued. If not, dopamine may be infused at a rate of 1 to 3 µg $\cdot$ kg^{-1} $\cdot$ min^{-1}. Dopamine improves renal function when used at low doses by increasing RBF, GFR, urine output, and sodium excretion, and by decreasing renal vascular resistance.[26] At moderate doses (approximately 5 to 10 µg $\cdot$ kg^{-1} $\cdot$ min^{-1}), dopamine activates ß-adrenoceptors in addition to DA1 receptors, which may dilate renal arterial beds and increase cardiac output. As previously mentioned, dopamine doses above approximately 10 µg $\cdot$ kg^{-1} $\cdot$ min^{-1} can cause α-adrenoceptor stimulation, vasoconstriction, and decreased RBF even though systemic arterial blood pressure may increase. Dopamine may also be beneficial because it inhibits intrarenal norepinephrine release and has an antialdosterone effect.[1] Recall that, in patients medicated with acepromazine, low-dose dopamine may be ineffective at increasing RBF, because of dopaminergic receptor blockade.

The use of diuretics in the perioperative period is controversial. In a study of human patients, acute renal failure treated with diuretics such as mannitol and furosemide was not resolved.[27] In a dog model of uranyl nitrate–induced acute renal failure, a combination of furosemide and dopamine was effective in restoring RBF and creatinine clearance, whereas either drug alone was not.[28] In a more recent study, greater diuresis, natriuresis, and calciuresis and less kaliuresis occurred in normal dogs given a constant rate infusion of furosemide (0.66 mg/kg IV loading dose followed by 0.66 mg/kg/h) when compared with intermittent bolus administration.[29] Furosemide is used to promote diuresis in patients with pulmonary edema but should not be used when a patient is known to be hypovolemic. In hypovolemia, furosemide may increase nephrotoxicity of other drugs by increasing their contact time in the renal tubules.[30] Mannitol, an osmotic diuretic, can be given (0.25 to 0.5 g/kg slowly IV) to prevent pulmonary edema or hyponatremia if the kidneys do not respond to fluid administration and the patient becomes volume overloaded.

Urethral Obstruction

Patients with urethral obstruction may become hyperkalemic, azotemic, acidotic, and hyperphosphatemic. Cats may also develop hyperglycemia, hypocalcemia, and hyponatremia. Hyponatremia is associated with leakage of urine into the peritoneal cavity.[31] Any metabolic abnormalities should be evaluated and addressed prior to anesthesia, if possible. Hyperkalemia is the primary concern in most cases of urethral obstruction, and a preanesthetic electrocardiogram assessment is warranted. Treatment of hyperkalemia has been discussed in preceding paragraphs.

In small animals with urethral obstruction, fine-needle centesis of the urinary bladder may be performed prior to anesthesia, although bladder injury is a potential concern. Rupture of the urinary bladder during induction of anesthesia in a horse has been described.[32] Perineal urethrostomy may be performed in stallions with urethral blockage by using standing restraint and epidural anesthesia. If general anesthesia is required while the bladder is distended, every attempt should be made to assist the horse into sternal or lateral recumbency during induction.

Anesthesia may be induced by using injectable or inhalation anesthetics. In many animals, distension of the urinary bladder is associated with increased heart rate. Cats that are chamber induced should not be induced with halothane due to its arrhythmic effects. Chamber induction with isoflurane or sevoflurane is preferred for small animals. Intravenous ketamine with a benzodiazepine has been used in obstructed cats even though active metabolites of the drug are excreted by the kidney. The rationale is that, once the obstruction is relieved, excretion of the anesthetic will proceed normally. However, cats with a long-term urethral obstruction may develop metabolic disturbances and renal insufficiency such that elimination of drugs is slowed even after the obstruction has been removed. Thus, if dissociative anesthesia is used, low doses of ketamine (1 to 2 mg/kg IV) can be used in combination with diazepam (0.2 mg/kg IV). With low doses, anesthetic action will be reduced after redistribution of the drug into body tissues. More commonly, injectable anesthetic induction in cats with renal disease is performed by administering propofol (2 to 5 mg/kg IV) or etomidate (1.0 mg/kg IV) slowly to effect.

Ruptured Urinary Bladder

Rupture of the urinary bladder is a surgical emergency. Animals may become hyperkalemic, hyponatremic, hypochloremic, and acidotic after urinary bladder rupture.[33] Intravenous fluids, such as 0.9% sodium chloride, should be given to aid in correcting electrolyte imbalances. Potassium enters the abdominal cavity from the ruptured bladder and is reabsorbed into the circulation, causing an increased serum potassium concentration. An electrocardiogram should be evaluated prior to induction of anesthesia to determine whether cardiac arrhythmias or evidence of hyperkalemia are present. Acute hyperkalemia (serum [K$^+$] > 5.5

mEq/L) should be treated prior to anesthesia. Anesthesia may be induced by face-mask administration of isoflurane or sevoflurane. Young foals (weighing < 200 kg) may be nasotracheally intubated while awake and then induced rapidly with an inhaled anesthetic. In larger foals, xylazine (1.1 mg/kg IV) or diazepam (0.1 mg/kg IV) in combination with ketamine (2.2 mg/kg IV) can be used for induction.[34] Isoflurane and sevoflurane are preferred over halothane because they possess less myocardial depressant action and potentiation of catecholamine-induced cardiac arrhythmias.[35] Administration of dextrose-containing solutions with or without insulin may be desired to counter hyperkalemia. Positive-pressure ventilation may be used to prevent anesthetic-associated hypercapnia and accompanying respiratory acidosis. Appropriate monitoring should be used, including end-tidal carbon dioxide, pulse oximetry, arterial blood-gas analysis, arterial blood pressure, and electrocardiogram assessment.

References

1. Brezis M, Rosen S. Hypoxia of the renal medulla: Its implications for disease. N Engl J Med 332:647, 1995.
2. Gelman S, Fowler KC, Smith LR. Regional blood flow during isoflurane and halothane anesthesia. Anesth Analg 63:57, 1984.
3. Leighton KM, Macleod BA, Burce C. Renal blood flow: Differences in autoregulation during anesthesia with halothane, methoxyflurane, or alphaprodine in the dog. Anesth Analg 57:389, 1978.
4. Merin RG, Bernard JM, Doursout MF, Cohen M, Chelly JE. Comparison of the effects of isoflurane and desflurane on cardiovascular dynamics and regional blood flow in the chronically instrumented dog. Anesthesiology 74:568, 1991.
5. Priano LL. Alteration of renal hemodynamics by thiopental, diazepam, and ketamine in conscious dogs. Anesth Analg 61:853, 1982.
6. Moss J, Glick D. The autonomic nervous system. In: Miller RD, ed. Anesthesia, 6th ed. Philadelphia: Elsevier, 2005:617.
7. Trim C. Anesthesia and the kidney. Compend Contin Educ 1:843, 1979.
8. Levinsky NG. Pathophysiology of acute renal failure. N Engl J Med 296:1453, 1977.
9. Boba A, Landmesser CM. Renal complications after anesthesia and operation. Anesthesiology 22:782, 1961.
10. Hayes MA, Goldenberg IS. Renal effects of anesthesia and operation mediated by endocrines. Anesthesiology 24:487, 1963.
11. Thurmon JC, Steffey EP, Zinkl JG, Woliner M, Howland D Jr. Xylazine causes transient dose-related hyperglycemia and increased urine volumes in mares. Am J Vet Res 45:224, 1984.
12. Greene SA, Thurmon JC, Benson GJ, Tranquilli WJ. Antidiuretic hormone prevents xylazine induced diuresis in mares [Abstract]. Vet Surg 15:459, 1986.
13. Gasthuys F, Terpstra P, van den Hende C, DeMoor A. Hyperglycaemia and diuresis during sedation with detomidine in the horse. Zentralbl Veterinarmed 334:641, 1987.
14. Papper S, Papper EM. The effects of pre-anesthetic, anesthetic, and post-operative drugs on renal function. Clin Pharmacol Ther 5:205, 1964.
15. Philbin DM, Coggins CH. Plasma antidiuretic hormone levels in cardiac surgical patients during morphine and halothane anesthesia. Anesthesiology 49:95, 1978.
16. Crandell WB, Pappas SG, MacDonald A. Nephrotoxicity associated with methoxyflurane anesthesia. Anesthesiology 27:591, 1966.
17. Benson GJ, Brock KA. Halothane-associated hepatitis and methoxyflurane-related nephropathy: a review. J Vet Pharmacol Ther 3:187, 1980.
18. Brunson DB, Stowe CM, McGrath CJ. Serum and urine inorganic fluoride concentrations and urine oxalate concentrations following methoxyflurane anesthesia in the dog. Am J Vet Res 40:197, 1979.
19. Mathews K, Doherty T, Dyson D, Wilcock B. Renal failure in dogs associated with flunixin meglumine and methoxyflurane anesthesia [Abstract]. Vet Surg 16:323, 1987.
20. Kuzucu EY. Methoxyflurane, tetracycline, and renal failure. J Am Med Assoc 211:1162, 1970.
21. Miller RD, Way WL, Hamilton WK, Layzer RB. Succinylcholine-induced hyperkalemia in patients with renal failure? Anesthesiology 36:138, 1972.
22. Ghonheim MM, Long JP. The interaction between magnesium and other neuromuscular blocking agents. Anesthesiology 32:23, 1970.
23. Rumbaugh GE, Carlson GP, Harrold D. Urinary production in the healthy horse and in horses deprived of feed and water. Am J Vet Res 43:735, 1982.
24. Clark KL, Robertson MJ, Drew GM. Do renal tubular dopamine receptors mediate dopamine-induced diuresis in the anesthetized cat? J Cardiovasc Pharmacol 17:267, 1991.
25. Flournoy WS, Wohl JS, Albrecht-Schmitt TJ, Schwartz DD. Pharmacologic identification of putative D1 dopamine receptors in feline kidneys. J Vet Pharmacol Ther 26:283, 2003.
26. Schwartz LB, Bissell MG, Murphy M, Gewertz BL. Renal effects of dopamine in vascular surgical patients. J Vasc Surg 8:367, 1988.
27. Cantarovich F, Fernandez JC, Locatelli A, Perez Loredo J, Christhot J. Furosemide in high doses in the treatment of acute renal failure. Postgrad Med J 47:13, 1978.
28. Lindner A, Cutler RE, Goodman WG. Synergism of dopamine plus furosemide in preventing acute renal failure in the dog. Kidney Int 16:158, 1979.
29. Adin DB, Taylor AW, Hill RC, Scott KC, Martin FG. Intermittent bolus injection versus continuous infusion of furosemide in normal adult greyhound dogs. J Vet Intern Med 17:632, 2003.
30. Stoelting RK. Pharmacology and Physiology in Anesthetic Practice. Philadelphia: JB Lippincott, 1987.
31. Lees GE, Rogers KS, Wold AM. Diseases of the lower urinary tract. In: Sherding RG, ed. The Cat: Diseases and Clinical Management. New York: Churchill Livingstone, 1989.
32. Pankowski RL, Fubini SL. Urinary bladder rupture in a two-year-old horse: Sequel to a surgically repaired neonatal injury. J Am Vet Med Assoc 191:560, 1987.
33. Finco DR. Kidney function. In: Kaneko JJ, ed. Clinical Biochemistry of Domestic Animals, 3rd ed. New York: Academic, 1980.
34. Tranquilli WJ, Thurmon JC. Management of anesthesia in the foal. Vet Clin North Am Equine Pract 6:651, 1990.
35. Eger EI III. Isoflurane: A review. Anesthesiology 55:559, 1981.

Chapter 40
Hepatic Disease

Stephen A. Greene and Steven L. Marks

Hepatic Blood Supply

About 20% of cardiac output is continually being delivered to the liver. Of this, the hepatic artery supplies 30% of the blood flow and 90% of the oxygen, and the remainder is supplied by blood flowing through the portal vein. Anesthetics may affect hepatic blood flow by altering vascular tone in the hepatic artery, the portal vein, or both (Table 40.1). Methoxyflurane decreases both portal vein and hepatic arterial blood flow. Halothane decreases portal vein blood flow but has only a slight effect, if any, on hepatic arterial blood flow. Isoflurane decreases portal vein blood flow but increases hepatic artery blood flow with a net overall increase in flow. Nitrous oxide has no direct effect on liver perfusion. Sevoflurane and desflurane maintain hepatic artery and portal vein resistance and are associated with decreased portal vein and total hepatic blood flow.[1] Hypercarbia has also been associated with decreased hepatic perfusion during anesthesia. Decreased blood flow may occur in cirrhotic livers or patients with portocaval shunt syndrome. Detrimental effects of decreased blood flow are likely to be more significant when an animal is hypotensive. Significant decreases in blood flow may be associated with decreased hepatic extraction and, ultimately, elimination of drugs.[2]

Hepatic Insufficiency

Clinical signs of hepatic insufficiency include ascites, depression, seizures, jaundice, hepatic encephalopathy, anorexia, and weight loss. Horses with colic have an increased incidence of concurrent hepatic disease.[3] Tests of substrate metabolism may give an indication of hepatic function. Low values for albumin, urea nitrogen, glucose, and cholesterol are associated with poor hepatic function. Coagulation defects such as prolonged prothrombin time, prolonged partial thromboplastin time, and in-

creased fibrinogen values may also indicate decreased hepatic function. Bilirubin is formed by metabolism of degraded hemoglobin by macrophages and carried by albumin to the liver for conjugation to a diglucuronide. In the horse, fasting for more than 24 h causes fatty acids to compete with bilirubin for hepatic metabolism. In this way, hyperbilirubinemia frequently causes icterus in anorexic horses. In dogs and cats, hyperbilirubinemia may be due to prehepatic, hepatic, or posthepatic causes.

Blood ammonia concentration and retention of dyes such as sulfobromophthalein (BSP) or indocyanine green (ICG) indicate liver dysfunction as evidenced by the liver's inability to eliminate these substances in a normal manner. The dyes, like bile acids, are more sensitive indicators of liver dysfunction than is a change in bilirubin concentration.[4] Bile acids are produced by the liver and excreted in the bile. They undergo a process termed *enterohepatic circulation*. Following biliary excretion, bile acids are reabsorbed by the ileum and enter the portal circulation. Bile acids are then removed by the hepatocytes, leaving only a low concentration to enter the systemic circulation during normal circumstances. Fasting does not affect bile acid concentration. Normal fasting bile acid concentrations are below 5 mmol/L for cats, below 10 mmol/L for dogs, and below 15 mmol/L for horses.

Postprandial blood samples will demonstrate an elevation in bile acid concentration caused by gallbladder contraction. Within 2 h, as a result of gallbladder emptying, the liver can remove most of the bile acids presented to it. Thus, a marked increase in postprandial bile acid concentration indicates decreased hepatic function or the presence of a portocaval vascular shunt. Normal 2-h postprandial concentrations of bile acids are below 15 mmol/L in cats and below 25 mmol/L in dogs. Because horses lack a gallbladder, postprandial elevations in bile acid concentrations are not expected. Use of bile acid concentrations to aid in assessment of hepatic disease in horses is best when combined with other tests of hepatobiliary function.[5] Tests of cell membrane integrity (i.e., alanine aminotransferase, γ-glutamyltransferase, sorbitol dehydrogenase, and lactate dehydrogenase) and serum alkaline phosphatase indicate hepatocellular damage but may not reflect altered hepatic function.

Pharmacological Considerations for Patients with Hepatic Disease

Tranquilizers/Sedatives

The use of acepromazine, droperidol, and α_2-adrenergic agonists should be avoided in patients with moderate to severe liver dis-

Table 40.1. Effect of inhaled anesthetics on hepatic blood flow

Agent	Portal Vein	Hepatic Artery
Desflurane	Decrease	No change
Halothane	Decrease	Decrease or no change
Isoflurane	Decrease	Increase
Nitrous oxide	No direct effects	
Sevoflurane	Decrease	No change
Methoxyflurane	Decrease	Decrease

ease. Hypotension may occur after administration of phenothiazine (acepromazine) or butyrophenone (droperidol) tranquilizers because of peripheral vasodilation mediated by α-adrenergic blockade. Phenothiazine administration has also been associated with thrombocytopathy and may exacerbate coagulopathy associated with hepatopathy. Dysrhythmias such as bradycardia or atrioventricular block and alterations of plasma glucose concentration may occur after administration of xylazine or detomidine. Diazepam is generally considered safe when used in intravenous doses of less than 0.2 mg/kg because it causes minimal changes in cardiovascular function. However, in animals with severe liver dysfunction, the duration of action of benzodiazepines may be significantly prolonged because of decreased hepatic biotransformation. Diazepam may not consistently tranquilize healthy young animals but frequently produces tranquilization in animals with liver disease. When diazepam is administered intravenously, it should be injected slowly to decrease vessel irritation and prevent hypotension associated with the propylene-glycol carrier. Use of benzodiazepines in animals exhibiting signs of hepatic encephalopathy is controversial.

Opioids

These can be used in patients with liver disease. Morphine and meperidine can cause release of histamine, which may cause hypotension and a decrease in total hepatic blood flow. Morphine also constricts the sphincter of Oddi in people, yet the significance in obstructive biliary disease in animals is unknown. Opioid side effects should be treated if they appear to affect cardiac or respiratory function. Opioid-induced bradycardia may decrease cardiac output and should be prevented by administration of an anticholinergic agent. Respiratory depression from opioids may lead to decreased oxygen delivery to all body tissues, including the liver. Careful dose titration of the opioid antagonist naloxone can relieve depression of respiration while maintaining some of the analgesic and sedative effects of the opioid agonist. Butorphanol and buprenorphine are associated with less respiratory depression than other opioid agonists and may be reasonable choices for patients with hepatic disease when maximal opioid analgesia is not required. Fentanyl, delivered by continuous-rate intravenous infusion, enables rapid individual patient dose titration and is an effective and reasonably safe method for providing opioid analgesia to patients when liver function is unknown.

Thiobarbiturates

These should be used in low doses or their use avoided in patients with liver disease. A single, intubating dose of thiobarbiturate is not necessarily contraindicated because it will be redistributed from the brain to less well perfused tissues, terminating the anesthetic effect. However, liver disease may affect the duration and depth of thiobarbiturate-induced anesthesia because of increased sensitivity of the central nervous system or hypoalbuminemia and decreased protein binding of the anesthetic. Anesthesia should not be maintained by redosing thiobarbiturates in patients with liver disease.

Methohexital is a methylated oxybarbiturate, and although it is more rapidly metabolized than thiobarbiturates, it is associated with excitation and possible seizures during the recovery period. For this reason, methohexital should be avoided in patients with hepatic encephalopathy.

Propofol and Etomidate

Propofol is an alkylphenolic compound used for induction of anesthesia that is supplied in a lecithin emulsion, giving it a milky white appearance. Redistribution and metabolism of propofol after a single injection are extremely rapid. The total body clearance of propofol exceeds hepatic blood flow, indicating sites other than the liver (e.g., lung) may play a role in its elimination. Propofol is about 90% excreted by the kidneys as glucuronate-conjugated metabolites.[6] Because of its dependence on glucuronidation for biotransformation, cats appear to have a more prolonged duration of propofol-induced sedation and hypnosis compared with dogs, especially following large or repeated doses. Indications for use of propofol are similar to those for the thiobarbiturates. The major advantage of propofol over a thiobarbiturate is the rapid rate of propofol elimination. In dogs, the incidence of apnea immediately after injection seems to be greater than that associated with thiobarbiturates.

Etomidate is an imidazole compound used for induction of anesthesia. It is supplied as a weak base in a propylene-glycol vehicle. As with other drugs formulated with propylene glycol, it can be irritating when injected intravenously.[7] Etomidate does not decrease hepatic perfusion. It has a short duration of action, primarily because of rapid redistribution from the brain to muscle tissue. Etomidate is metabolized by the hepatic microsomal enzyme system, as well as by plasma esterases. The total body clearance rate for etomidate is five times as fast as for thiopental, although clinically the duration of action is similar after a single dose.[4] Etomidate has been shown to cause adrenocortical suppression with repeated administration.[8] The importance of etomidate-associated inhibition of steroidogenesis after single-bolus administration in patients with hepatic disease is unknown. In both humans and dogs, etomidate continuous-rate intravenous infusion has been associated with hemolysis.[9,10] Hemolysis appears to be caused by the propylene-glycol vehicle in which etomidate is formulated. In dogs, red blood cell counts during and 10 min after termination of a 60-min infusion of etomidate were not significantly different from preinfusion values.[10] All dogs in the aforementioned study appeared normal after recovery from anesthesia maintained with etomidate. Thus, the clinical significance of etomidate-induced or propylene-glycol-induced hemolysis in dogs is not clear. Etomidate appears to be a reasonable drug choice for induction of anesthesia in patients with cardiac and/or hepatic disease.

Dissociative Anesthetics

Dissociative anesthetics such as tiletamine (Telazol) or ketamine are generally acceptable for induction of anesthesia in patients with hepatic disease. Intravenous administration is preferred in order to minimize the dose required for tracheal intubation. In dogs, these drugs are largely metabolized by the liver, so maintenance of anesthesia should be with an inhalant. Dissociative anesthetics may induce seizures in dogs or cats. In cats, ketamine is metabolized to a lesser extent by the liver to form norketamine, which has about 10% of the activity of ketamine.

Zolazepam, the benzodiazepine tranquilizer in Telazol, has been suspected of causing the prolonged recovery after intramuscular injection in cats. Flumazenil has been used intravenously (0.1 mg/kg) to antagonize midazolam in cats anesthetized with a combination of ketamine and midazolam.[11] Zolazepam's effect in cats is similarly antagonized by flumazenil, providing an alternative to the apparently slow hepatic metabolism of the benzodiazepines in this species.

Inhalation Anesthetics

Inhalation anesthetics are the best choices for maintenance of anesthesia in patients with severe liver disease. Halothane decreases hepatic blood flow and is metabolized up to 20% by the liver.[12] Halothane anesthesia in ponies is associated with decreased bile acid excretion and increased conjugated bilirubin excretion.[13] It is recommended that halothane be avoided, if possible, in patients with liver disease. However, the presence of hepatic disease does not necessarily result in increased hepatotoxicity when a patient is subsequently exposed to an unpredictable hepatotoxin such as halothane.[14] Halothane has been implicated in causing liver disease in people and possibly in animals. This is a problem in about one of every 6000 to 10,000 people and is probably genetically related.[15,16] Halothane is metabolized to trichloroacetic acid, which may undergo reductive metabolism to produce hepatotoxins during hypoxic conditions. Studies indicate that the trifluoroacetate metabolite of halothane combines with a hepatic protein, resulting in the formation of a hapten.[17–19] The trifluoroacetate hapten is subsequently attacked by serum antibodies, causing hepatitis. A clinical test for this hapten is not yet available for animals. In a study of goats hyperimmunized for production of anti–human-lymphocyte serum that were subsequently exposed to 3, 6, or 9 h of halothane anesthesia, seven (24%) of 29 showed evidence of hepatic necrosis.[20] A rat model of halothane-induced hepatopathy showed that hepatic hypoxia was required to produce symptoms.[21] To ensure adequate blood pressure, flow, and oxygen delivery during anesthesia, precautions should be taken when using halothane (or any other anesthetic!). In preventing the occurrence of postanesthetic hepatopathy, prevention of hepatic hypoxia during inhalation anesthesia is probably more important than choice of anesthetic.

Methoxyflurane decreases hepatic blood flow, and up to 50%

of an inhaled dose is metabolized by the liver.[22] In addition, oxalate and free fluoride-ion metabolites of methoxyflurane are potential renal toxins. Of the volatile anesthetics, methoxyflurane is associated with the highest metabolite production of fluoride ion.

Isoflurane increases hepatic artery blood flow in humans, whereas halothane preserves hepatic arterial flow at 1 MAC but decreases it at 2 MAC.[23] Less than 1% of inhaled isoflurane is metabolized. It has not been associated with hepatic or renal toxicity.[24] Cardiovascular function during isoflurane anesthesia is less depressed than with halothane or methoxyflurane. The higher cardiac output associated with isoflurane anesthesia is likely to maintain better hepatic perfusion and oxygen delivery than is halothane. Thus, isoflurane appears to be a good choice for maintenance of anesthesia in patients with hepatic disease.

Biotransformation of sevoflurane (3% to 5%) is less than halothane but more than isoflurane or desflurane.[25] Production of the trifluoroacetic acid hapten is extremely low and unlikely to induce an immune response such as the well-documented halothane hepatopathy. Free fluoride–ion production after exposure to sevoflurane is comparable to that from desflurane.[25] Sevoflurane reduces portal vein flow and oxygen delivery more than isoflurane. Hepatic artery flow increases in pigs concurrently receiving nitrous oxide and sevoflurane. Other studies have shown no change in hepatic artery flow associated with clinically useful concentrations of sevoflurane. Animal models therefore demonstrate that sevoflurane maintains good hepatic blood flow and liver oxygenation when administered at concentrations less than 2 MAC.[25]

The effects of desflurane on hepatic blood flow are similar to those of halothane (Table 40.1). Desflurane differs from isoflurane structurally only by substitution of a fluorine atom for a chlorine atom. The substitution of a fluorine atom for other halogens generally makes a molecule more stable in terms of biotransformation. Indeed, desflurane metabolism to free fluoride ion is less than that of isoflurane.[26] Because of its low metabolism, low blood solubility (enabling rapid induction and recovery from anesthesia), and cardiovascular stability (maintaining hepatic perfusion), desflurane would appear to be a good anesthetic for patients with hepatic disease.

Nitrous oxide has been used in patients with hepatic disease in an effort to decrease the amount of volatile anesthetic required for anesthesia. There are no reports of direct hepatic injury caused by exposure to nitrous oxide as used in clinical practice. There is evidence of hepatic injury (centrilobular necrosis) caused by nitrous oxide in the hypoxic rat model.[27] It is unknown whether this mechanism of hepatic injury in hypoxic rats is the same as for halothane.

Muscle Relaxants

Nondepolarizing muscle relaxants such as pancuronium and vecuronium are metabolized by the liver. Effects of these relaxants may be prolonged in patients with hepatic disease. Concurrent administration of aminoglycoside antibiotics with nondepolarizing muscle relaxants may also prolong neuromuscular blockade.[28] This is likely to be a problem in large animals such as horses, for which prolonged recumbency may adversely affect recovery to standing. Atracurium is a nondepolarizing muscle relaxant whose metabolism is independent of hepatic function. Atracurium undergoes plasma degradation via a metabolic pathway termed *Hofmann elimination* that depends primarily on plasma pH and temperature.[29] For patients with hepatic disease requiring neuromuscular blockade, atracurium seems to be a good choice.

Succinylcholine is a depolarizing muscle relaxant that is degraded by plasma cholinesterase. Cholinesterases are produced by the liver. Organophosphate compounds have cholinesterase-inhibiting activity and may potentiate the action of succinylcholine.[30] The phenothiazine tranquilizers (e.g., acepromazine) may inhibit cholinesterase activity, so succinylcholine should be used cautiously in patients medicated with acepromazine. The use of both acepromazine and succinylcholine should be avoided in patients with hepatic disease.

Centrally acting muscle relaxants such as guaifenesin (glyceryl guaiacolate) or mephenesin are metabolized by the liver.[31,32] Although the margin of safety for use of guaifenesin is wide, side effects following administration of large doses include moderate hypotension, decreased tidal volume, and concentration-dependent hemolysis. Toxic effects may be caused by the metabolite catechol, which causes seizures, opisthotonos, prolonged incoordination, and respiratory paralysis. Increased incidence in side effects or occurrence of toxic effects may be observed when guaifenesin is administered to animals with hepatic disease.

General Guidelines for Patients with Hepatic Disease

Hepatic disease affects several vital body functions, with significant impact on anesthetic considerations (Table 40.2). Most injectable anesthetics are metabolized by the liver, so elimination may be significantly slowed in animals that are hypothermic. Use of heated circulating water blankets and administration of warm intravenous or irrigation fluids is advised. The advent of force air-warming systems (e.g., Bair Hugger) has dramatically reduced intraoperative and postoperative hypothermia.

Glucose metabolism is frequently affected by hepatic disease. Homeostasis of glucose can be maintained with loss of up to 80% of functional liver mass. Nevertheless, patients with severe hepatic disease that are stressed by anesthesia and surgery may become hypoglycemic. Hypoglycemia is present in 35% of dogs with portocaval shunts.[33] For this reason, blood glucose concentration is routinely determined and glucose administered in combination with isotonic crystalloids when indicated. If not corrected, hypoglycemia may delay recovery from anesthesia.

Excessive weight of ascitic fluid may impede lung expansion and pulmonary function. Ascitic fluid should be removed prior to anesthesia. Rapid removal of a large quantity of fluid may cause a fluid shift from the vascular space to the abdominal cavity as the formation of ascites continues. This can cause serious hypovolemia and cardiovascular compromise. Hypoalbuminemia is often present in patients with liver disease. When the albumin concentration is less than 1.5 g/dL, the plasma oncotic pressure is decreased such that pulmonary edema may occur following in-

Table 40.2. General guidelines for patients with hepatic disease

Evaluate coagulation profile prior to surgery
Use rapidly eliminated agents when appropriate (e.g., inhalant anesthetics and propofol)
Monitor hydration status
Monitor blood glucose, plasma albumin, and total protein concentrations
Monitor and maintain arterial blood pressure greater than 60 mmHg
Maintain eucapnia using appropriate ventilatory support
Be prepared to treat seizures with diazepam
Be aware of potential thromboembolic complications

travenous fluid administration with crystalloids. Arterial blood pressure may be difficult to maintain when plasma oncotic pressure is significantly decreased. Replacement of albumin and plasma proteins is indicated in these cases. If matched plasma from a donor animal is not available, dextran 70 (up to 20 mL/kg) or Hetastarch (10 to 20 mL/kg) may be administered. Although dextran will aid in reestablishing plasma oncotic pressure, its duration of effect is not as great as that of plasma. Human albumin solution (2.5 to 5.0 mL/kg intravenously) has been used in dogs and cats, as well.

Seizures caused by hepatic encephalopathy may require treatment. Diazepam or phenobarbital is commonly used to control seizures, but both drugs are metabolized by the liver, and significantly altered pharmacokinetics may result in prolonged duration of action. Avoid the use of anesthetics that may induce seizure activity, such as enflurane, ketamine, tiletamine (Telazol), or methohexital. There may be increased cerebral sensitivity to γ-aminobutyric acid (GABA) in some patients with hepatic disease. This increased sensitivity to GABAergic inhibition within the central nervous system may enhance the depressant effects of the barbiturates and benzodiazepine tranquilizers.

When there is concern about an animal's ability to metabolize anesthetics because of hepatic disease, use of local anesthesia may be considered as an adjunct to general anesthesia or as a substitute when appropriate. Although animals that are not depressed usually require tranquilization for effective use of local anesthesia, those with hepatic disease are likely to be depressed and therefore may require less tranquilization or sedation. Local anesthetics of the ester class (e.g., procaine and tetracaine) are metabolized by plasma cholinesterases produced by the liver, whereas the amide class (lidocaine, mepivacaine, and bupivacaine) is directly metabolized by the liver. For this reason, the generalized effects of local anesthetics may be prolonged and the toxic effects more apparent in patients with severe hepatic disease. This is unlikely to be a major deterrent for their clinical use, however.

Because of the liver's role in production of coagulation factors, the coagulation profile (one-stage prothrombin time and activated partial thromboplastin time) should be evaluated before surgery in patients with hepatic disease. If coagulopathy exists, fresh-frozen plasma or whole blood should be available and administered. Additionally, some hepatic neoplasms are associated with significant abdominal hemorrhage and thrombocytopenia. A complete blood count with an estimate of the platelet concentration should be performed as part of the diagnostic workup.

Little is known about the influence of specific anesthetic techniques on coagulation in animals. In dogs, platelet aggregation was significantly decreased after administration of acepromazine and atropine but returned to normal during subsequent halothane anesthesia and surgery.[34] Coagulation deficiencies such as thrombocytopenia, thrombocytopathy, increased prothrombin time, increased activated partial thromboplastin time, hypofibrinogenemia, increased fibrin degradation products, and decreased antithrombin have been observed in dogs with gastric dilation–volvulus.[35] In dogs undergoing colonic anastomosis, there was less intraoperative bleeding and more advanced healing (detected histologically) 1 and 7 days after surgery following administration of epidural bupivacaine and general anesthesia when compared with general anesthesia alone.[36] Much work remains to be done to identify anesthetic techniques having the least effect on normal coagulation and healing during the convalescent period.

Portosystemic Shunt

Dogs with this congenital vascular anomaly are usually gaunt and small for their breed and age. Anesthetic management of dogs with portocaval shunt should be based on presenting clinical signs and physical status (Table 40.3). Signs of hepatic encephalopathy and hypokalemia may be present. Hypokalemia in animals with portocaval shunt may be caused by gastrointestinal (vomiting and diarrhea) or urinary loss (diuresis). Hypokalemia ($[K+] < 3.5$ mEq/L) should be corrected gradually prior to anesthesia. Intravenous potassium administration should not exceed the rate of $0.5 \text{ mEq} \cdot \text{kg}^{-1} \cdot \text{h}^{-1}$.

Chronic hepatic dysfunction may be associated with increased GABAergic sensitivity and permeability of the blood-brain barrier. The effect of anesthetics and anesthetic adjuncts may be greater than expected and unpredictable. Diazepam has been used as a preanesthetic medication in dogs with portocaval shunt. However, reduced dosage requirements for benzodiazepines in cases of hepatic disease have been reported.[37,38] Further, cases of fatal hepatic toxicosis associated with benzodiazepine administration have been observed in cats. Antagonists of the benzodiazepine receptor, such as flumazenil, have ameliorated signs of encephalopathy in a woman and in animal models of portocaval shunt.[37–39] The value of flumazenil in the perioperative management of dogs with portocaval shunt is controversial and remains to be determined.

Animals with portocaval shunt may have hepatic insufficiency. When termination of action is highly dependent on drug hepatic metabolism (e.g., ketamine, acepromazine, xylazine, and diazepam), the use of such drugs should be avoided. Drugs that are highly protein bound (e.g., barbiturates) will be more active in animals with hypoalbuminemia. Drugs such as methohexital and ketamine that may induce seizure activity are contraindicated in animals with hepatic encephalopathy. Of the inhaled anesthetics, methoxyflurane undergoes the greatest metabolism by the liver. Thus, elimination of methoxyflurane may be prolonged in ani-

Table 40.3. Problems associated with portocaval shunt

Problem	Significance
Weight loss	May affect drug dose or disposition
Hypoalbuminemia	May affect drug dose, disposition, or plasma oncotic pressure
Hepatic shunt	Loss of hepatic metabolism of drugs
Low bile salts	Increase in absorption of intestinal endotoxin
Portal hypertension	May require second surgery and central venous pressure monitoring

mals with portocaval shunt. The use of halothane may cause hepatopathy in animals with poor hepatic perfusion and oxygenation, and therefore should be avoided in patients with portocaval shunt. Isoflurane, sevoflurane, or desflurane are suitable anesthetics for patients with this condition. Mask induction and maintenance with an inhalant are reasonable for animals with portosystemic shunts displaying advanced signs of hepatic dysfunction. Opioids may be used as analgesic supplements prior to or following anesthesia for surgical correction of the shunt.

Arterial blood pressure should be monitored during portocaval shunt surgery. Hypoalbuminemia and hypothermia predispose patients to hypotension that may be exacerbated by isoflurane-induced peripheral vasodilation. Judicious use of plasma, dextran 70 (10 to 20 mL/kg given over 1 h) or hetastarch to aid in maintenance of plasma oncotic pressure may be indicated. At high concentrations of isoflurane, myocardial contractility and cardiac output are also decreased. Hypotensive patients with portocaval shunt may fail to respond to catecholamine infusions such as dobutamine or dopamine. Surgical retraction of the liver or compression of the caudal vena cava may further decrease venous return, cardiac output, and arterial blood pressure.

Intraoperative management of patients for correction of portocaval shunt is often uneventful until the shunt is ligated. In normal dogs, portal pressure is reported to be between 8 and 13 cm H_2O, whereas portal pressure in dogs with portocaval shunt is usually lower.[40] Following surgical correction of the shunt, portal venous pressure should not be more than 9 to 10 cm H_2O above baseline measurement, or a maximum of 20 to 23 cm H_2O. Intraoperative measurement of central venous pressure is useful for estimating portal resistance and for predicting the development of postoperative portal hypertension.[41] A decrease in central venous pressure after ligation of a single portocaval shunt indicates decreased blood transit from the intestine to the vena cava. Central venous pressure should not decrease by more than 1 cm H_2O from baseline measurement at 3 min after ligation to avoid postoperative portal hypertension.[42]

Animals with portocaval shunts or intestinal ischemia may have increased absorption of endotoxin. Medical management of these patients includes fluid administration (e.g., 0.9% or 0.45% sodium chloride combined with 2.5% dextrose), potassium supplementation, dietary management, and appropriate antibiotic therapy to reduce toxin production from enteric bacteria.[43]

References

1. Merin RG, Bernard JM, Doursout MF, Cohen M, Chelly JE. Comparison of the effects of isoflurane and desflurane on cardiovascular dynamics and regional blood flow in the chronically instrumented dog. Anesthesiology 74:568, 1991.

2. Rowland M, Tozer TN. Clinical pharmacokinetics, 2nd ed. Philadelphia: Lea and Febiger, 1989.

3. Moore JN, Traver DS, Coffman JR. Large bowel obstruction and chronic active hepatitis in a horse. Vet Med Small Anim Clin 71: 1457, 1976.

4. Meyer DJ, Embert HC, Rich LJ. Veterinary laboratory medicine: Interpretation and diagnosis. Philadelphia: WB Saunders, 1992.

5. West HJ. Evaluation of total plasma bile acid concentrations for the diagnosis of hepatobiliary disease in horses. Res Vet Sci 46:264, 1989.

6. White PF. What's new in intravenous anesthetics? Anesthesiol Clin North Am 6:297, 1988.

7. Muir WW, Mason DE. Side effects of etomidate in dogs. J Am Vet Med Assoc 194:1430, 1989.

8. Kruse-Elliot KT, Swanson CR, Aucoin DP. Effects of etomidate on adrenocortical function in canine surgical patients. Am J Vet Res 48:1098, 1987.

9. Nebauer AE, Doenicke A, Hoernecke R, Angster R, Mayer M. Does etomidate cause haemolysis? Br J Anaesth 69:58, 1992.

10. Ko JCH, Thurmon JC, Benson GJ, Tranquilli WJ, Hoffmann WE. Acute haemolysis associated with etomidate-propylene glycol infusion in dogs. J Vet Anaesth 20:92, 1993.

11. Ilkiw JE. Other potentially useful new injectable anesthetic agents. Vet Clin North Am 22:281, 1992.

12. Cousins MJ, Sharp JH, Gourlay GK. Hepatotoxicity and halothane metabolism in an animal model with application for human toxicity. Anaesth Intensive Care 7:9, 1979.

13. Engelking LR, Dodman NH, Hartman G, Valdez H, Spivak W. Effects of halothane anesthesia on equine liver function. Am J Vet Res 44:607, 1984.

14. Martin JL Jr, Njoku DB. Metabolism and toxicity of modern inhaled anesthetics. In: Miller RD, ed. Miller's Anesthesia, 6th ed. Philadelphia: Elsevier, 2005:231.

15. Cahalan MK. Post-operative hepatic dysfunction. American Society of Anesthesiologists Annual Refresher Course Lectures 133:1, 1982.

16. Benson GJ, Brock KA. Halothane-associated hepatitis and methoxyflurane-related nephropathy: A review. J Vet Pharmacol Ther 3:187, 1980.

17. Bird GL, Williams R. Detection of antibodies to a halothane metabolite hapten in sera from patients with halothane-associated hepatitis. J Hepatol 9:366, 1989.

18. Kenna JG, Satoh H, Christ DD, Pohl LR. Metabolic basis for a drug hypersensitivity: Antibodies in sera from patients with halothane hepatitis recognize liver neoantigens that contain the trifluoroacetyl group derived from halothane. J Pharmacol Exp Ther 245:1103, 1988.

19. Pohl LR, Thomassen D, Pumford NR, et al. Hapten carrier conjugates associated with halothane hepatitis. Adv Exp Med Biol 283: 111, 1991.

20. O'Brien TD, Raffe MR, Cox VS, Stevens DL, O'Leary TP. Hepatic necrosis following halothane anesthesia in goats. J Am Vet Med Assoc 189:1591, 1986.

21. Cousins MK. Mechanisms and evaluation of hepatotoxicity. American Society of Anesthesiologists Refresher Course Lectures 204:1, 1984.

22. Halsey MJ, Sawyer DC, Eger EI. Hepatic metabolism of halothane, methoxyflurane, cyclopropane, ethrane, and forane in miniature swine. Anesthesiology 35:43, 1971.

23. Gelman S, Fowler KC, Smith LR. Regional blood flow during isoflurane and halothane anesthesia. Anesth Analg 63:557, 1984.

24. Eger EI. Isoflurane: A review. Anesthesiology 55:559, 1981.

25. Frink EJ Jr. The hepatic effects of sevoflurane. Anesth Analg 81(Suppl 6):46S, 1995.

26. Koblin DD. Characteristics and implications of desflurane metabolism and toxicity. Anesth Analg 75:S10, 1992.

27. Fassoulaki A, Eger EI II, Johnson BH, et al. Nitrous oxide, too, is hepatotoxic in rats. Anesth Analg 63:1076, 1984.

28. Forsyth SF, Ilkiw JE, Hildebrand SV. Effect of gentamicin administration on the neuromuscular blockade induced by atracurium in cats. Am J Vet Res 51:1675, 1990.

29. Hughes R, Chapple DJ. The pharmacology of atracurium: A new competitive neuromuscular blocking agent. Br J Anaesth 53:31, 1981.

30. Himes JA, Edds GT, Kirkham WW, Neal FC. Potentiation of succinylcholine by organophosphate compounds in horses. J Am Vet Med Assoc 151:54, 1967.

31. Funk KA. Glyceryl guaiacolate: A centrally acting muscle relaxant. Equine Vet J 2:173, 1970.

32. Davis LE, Wolff WA. Pharmacokinetics and metabolism of glyceryl guaiacolate in ponies. Am J Vet Res 31:469, 1970.

33. Armstrong PJ. Problem: Hypoglycemia. In: Proceedings of the Fourth Annual Veterinary Medical Forum ACVIM, 1986:103.

34. Barr SC, Ludders JW, Looney AL, Gleed RD. Platelet aggregation in dogs after sedation with acepromazine and atropine and during subsequent general anesthesia and surgery. Am J Vet Res 53:2067, 1992.

35. Millis DL, Hauptman JG. Coagulation abnormalities and gastric necrosis in canine gastric dilatation–volvulus. Vet Surg 22:93, 1993.

36. Blass CE, Kirby BM, Waldron DR, Turk MA, Crawford MP. The effect of epidural and general anesthesia on the healing of colonic anastomoses. Vet Surg 16:75, 1987.

37. Ferenci P, Grimm G, Meryn S, Gangl A. Successful loading-term treatment of portal-systemic encephalopathy by the benzodiazepine antagonist flumazenil. Gastroenterology 96:240, 1989.

38. Bassett ML, Mullen KD, Skolnik P, Jones EA. Amelioration of hepatic encephalopathy by pharmacologic antagonists of the GABA$_A$-benzodiazepine receptor complex in a rabbit model of fulminant hepatic failure. Gastroenterology 93:1069, 1987.

39. Baraldi M, Zeneroli ML, Ventura E, et al. Supersensitivity of benzodiazepine receptors in hepatic encephalopathy due to fulminant hepatic failure in the rat: Reversal by a benzodiazepine antagonist. Clin Sci 67:167, 1984.

40. Tobias, KM. Portosystemic shunts and other hepatic vascular anomalies. In: Slatter D, ed. Textbook of Small Animal Surgery. Philadelphia: Saunders, 2003:727.

41. Swalec KM, Smeak DD, Brown J. Effects of mechanical and pharmacologic manipulations on portal pressure, central venous pressure, and heart rate in dogs. Am J Vet Res 52:1327, 1991.

42. Swalec KM, Smeak DD. Partial versus complete attenuation of single portosystemic shunts. Vet Surg 19:406, 1990.

43. Fossum TW. Surgery of the liver. In: Fossum TW, ed. Small Animal Surgery. St. Louis: CV Mosby, 2002:457.

Chapter 41

Gastrointestinal Disease

Stephen A. Greene and Steven L. Marks

Conditions Associated with the Oral Cavity and Pharynx

Animals with trauma or space-occupying masses of the head and neck frequently require general anesthesia. These patients are often difficult to intubate to secure and maintain a patent airway. Fractures of the mandible, maxilla, or temporomandibular joint may not permit examination to determine the range of jaw motion. Masticatory myositis may prevent opening of the mouth even while the patient is anesthetized. General anesthesia without a secure airway may result in aspiration, which can be fatal. Anesthetic management of these conditions should be initiated by preparing for placement of a tracheostomy tube. In dogs, a combination of intramuscular (IM) acepromazine (0.05 mg/kg) and intravenous (IV) hydromorphone (0.2 mg/kg) will induce a neuroleptanalgesic state with sufficient muscle relaxation to enable examination of the mouth and jaw. If the animal's laryngeal function or its ability to open its mouth is questionable, IV fentanyl (0.005 mg/kg) should be substituted for hydromorphone because there is a small, but real, risk of vomiting associated with hydromorphone administration. Owing to opioid-induced bradycardia, premedication with an anticholinergic agent is recommended. In dogs weighing over 18 kg, a maximum dose of 4 mg of hydromorphone is suggested to prevent excessive respiratory depression. In cats, a low dose of ketamine (4 mg/kg IM) combined with acepromazine (0.05 mg/kg) usually enables examination of the oral cavity.

IM or subcutaneous (SC) administration of xylazine in dogs or cats may cause emesis (Table 41.1). Dogs and cats with oral or pharyngeal masses are at high risk for aspiration pneumonia, so the use of xylazine, medetomidine, morphine, and other drugs that commonly induce emesis should be avoided. Xylazine administration in large animals is not associated with emesis and may be used to sedate horses (0.5 to 1.0 mg/kg IV) or cattle (0.1 mg/kg IM) for oral examination.

Removal of Esophageal Foreign Bodies

General anesthesia may be required for removal of esophageal foreign bodies in a variety of species. In a horse that has a foreign object lodged in the esophagus (i.e., choke), passage of a nasogastric tube or endoscope is facilitated by sedation with xylazine (0.5 mg/kg) or detomidine (10 to 20 µg/kg). If the foreign body cannot be retrieved or dislodged, the horse is anesthetized. Relaxation of the striated muscular coat of the esophagus may aid in removal of the obstruction. Skeletal muscle relaxation is enhanced at deeper planes of anesthesia. Muscle relaxation may also be improved by induction of anesthesia with guaifenesin (5% solution in 5% dextrose combined with 0.3% thiopental given to effect) or by administration of a neuromuscular blocker. In horses and cats, the proximal two-thirds of the esophagus has a striated muscle layer, whereas in dogs, the entire esophagus contains striated muscle.[1] General anesthesia is required for endoscopic foreign-body removal in dogs and cats. In anesthetized dogs and horses, skeletal muscle relaxation of the esophagus may be improved with a short-acting muscle relaxant (e.g., atracurium, 0.2 mg/kg IV). Administration of atracurium must be accompanied by tracheal intubation and support of ventilation. In some species, esophageal stricture can be a sequelae to esophageal foreign bodies. These patients require general anesthesia in order to perform balloon dilation or bougienage.

Anesthesia for Dogs with Gastric Dilation-Volvulus

It has been estimated that there are between 40,000 and 60,000 cases of canine gastric dilation-volvulus per year in the United States.[2] The condition is associated with multiple system problems (Table 41.2) resulting in a high mortality rate (40% to 60%).[2] Stomach distention severely restricts ventilation and decreases cardiac function. Metabolic alkalosis may develop from gastric sequestration of hydrogen ions. Later in the course of the disease, metabolic acidosis may occur from decreased cardiac output and poor ventilation, resulting in tissue hypoxia and lactate production. Consequently, cardiac arrhythmias such as sinus tachycardia, atrial fibrillation, ventricular tachycardia, or ventricular premature contractions are frequently observed. Because the metabolic status is difficult to predict, it is suggested that serum electrolytes, blood pH, and plasma bicarbonate concentration be measured prior to anesthesia. In one study, hypokalemia was

Table 41.1. Gastrointestinal effects of drugs used during anesthesia.

Drug	Effect
Acepromazine	Antiemetic
Atropine	Decreased motility
Cholinesterase inhibitors	Increased motility
Detomidine	Decreased motility
Diazepam	Appetite stimulant
Halothane	Decreased mucosal blood flow
Morphine	Emetic and gastrointestinal stimulant
Xylazine	Decreased motility; emetic

Table 41.2. Problems associated with gastric dilation-volvulus.

Problem	Significance
Acidosis/alkalosis	Measure pH
Cardiac arrhythmias	Attempt correction prior to anesthesia
Gastric necrosis	May cause arrhythmias
Hypokalemia/hyperkalemia	Measure K+
Impaired venous return	Correct by decompressing stomach Treat shock
Respiratory impairment	Correct by decompressing stomach Ventilate
Peritonitis	Begin antibiotics; poor prognosis
Shock	Correct underlying problems

present in 33% of the dogs with gastric dilation-volvulus.[3] Electrolyte abnormalities, acid-base imbalance, and gastric distension should be corrected as soon as possible. The derangements in acid-base balance frequently precipitate shock if left untreated. Restoration of circulating plasma volume should be initiated using high doses of isotonic saline solution (90 mL/kg IV) or hypertonic saline solution (7%, 4 mL/kg IV). In dogs with experimentally induced gastric dilation-volvulus and shock, a combination of 7% hypertonic saline in 6% dextran 70 (5 mL/kg IV) was superior to isotonic saline (60 ml/kg IV) for resuscitation.[4] It is suggested that fluids be administered through one or two large-bore IV catheters.

Cardiac arrhythmias should be identified and treated prior to induction of anesthesia. In many cases, cardiac arrhythmias may not require antiarrhythmic agents and may respond to fluid therapy and correction of acid-base and/or electrolyte abnormalities. If antiarrhythmic therapy is necessary, lidocaine (2 to 4 mg/kg slow IV bolus followed by 25 to 100 $\mu g \cdot kg^{-1} \cdot min^{-1}$) and procainamide (0.5 to 2.0 mg/kg IV, and then 20 to 40 $\mu g \cdot kg^{-1} \cdot min^{-1}$) separately or in combination have been used for treating premature ventricular contractions or ventricular tachycardia. Quinidine (6 to 8 mg/kg IM, every 6 h) has also been recommended for treatment of arrhythmias in dogs with gastric dilation-volvulus. Postoperative treatment of cardiac arrhythmias may also be necessary. A continuous lidocaine infusion may be prepared by adding 25 mL of 2% lidocaine to each 500 mL of IV fluid administered at a rate of 50 to 100 $\mu g \cdot kg^{-1} \cdot min^{-1}$.

Administration of oxygen via face mask should begin before induction of anesthesia. The use of large doses of arrhythmogenic anesthetic agents such as thiobarbiturates or halothane should be avoided. The use of α_2-agonists should be avoided in these cases because they may cause aerophagia and depressed cardiac output.[5] In addition, xylazine causes decreased gastroesophageal sphincter pressure and may allow increased gastric reflux.[6] α_2-Agonists decrease intestinal motility in dogs and may prolong recovery of normal gastrointestinal function following correction of gastric distension.[7] Neuroleptanalgesic combinations such as diazepam (0.2 mg/kg IV) and hydromorphone (0.1 mg/kg IV) are good choices for induction of anesthesia in dogs with unstable cardiovascular function. Opioids may decrease intestinal motility, but this effect is usually of minor clinical significance.[8] Propofol or diazepam-ketamine has also been suggested

as a good choice for induction of anesthesia. For maintenance of anesthesia, isoflurane or sevoflurane would be excellent inhalants. Nitrous oxide is contraindicated prior to gastric decompression because it will equilibrate with gas in the stomach, increasing the intragastric volume and pressure.

Succinylcholine initially causes contraction of skeletal muscle. The distended stomach is predisposed to rupture if succinylcholine is administered prior to relief of excessive gastric pressure. If a neuromuscular blocking agent is used in the anesthetic management of gastric dilation-volvulus, it should be a nondepolarizing drug such as pancuronium or atracurium.

Of the dogs that die of gastric dilation-volvulus, 50% die on the day of surgery.[9] Death is usually associated with septic shock or peritonitis secondary to gastric necrosis or perforation.[10] Reperfusion injury has also been implicated as a factor associated with the high mortality from this condition.[11] Iron-chelating drugs such as deferoxamine have been evaluated for their ability to decrease injury in anoxic tissues that are subsequently reperfused.

Anesthetic Management of Horses with Acute Abdominal Distress

Acute abdominal distress in horses is often characterized by severe pain. Pain elicits a variety of responses that include release of catecholamines and corticosteroids.[12] The stress response and sympathetic stimulation resulting from pain are detrimental to an animal's well-being. It is often difficult to perform diagnostic procedures or examine a horse in severe pain. Judicious use of analgesics in horses with acute abdominal distress is essential.

Because of their strong analgesic and sedative effects, the α_2-agonists have been used extensively in horses with acute abdominal pain. Depending on the amount of xylazine, detomidine, or romifidine administered in the preoperative period, the induction dose of anesthetic may need to be decreased. Cardiovascular depression associated with α_2-agonists will often persist longer than either sedation or analgesia. Even though the sedative effects of these drugs may have waned, the anesthetic requirement will be decreased. At a comparable dose, detomidine is more potent than xylazine and has a longer analgesic and sedative action.[13-15] High doses of detomidine (i.e., 0.02 mg/kg IV) decrease cardiac output by 50%.[16] The duration of cardiovascular side effects may limit the use of detomidine and romifidine as premedicants for horses undergoing surgery to correct intestinal problems.

Xylazine is a suitable alternative to detomidine in compromised horses. However, the usual 1.1 mg/kg IV dose of xylazine is often decreased to prevent excessive cardiovascular depression. Xylazine prolongs gastrointestinal transit time in a variety of species.[17] In horses, xylazine (0.55 mg/kg IV) has been shown to decrease the motility index of circular and longitudinal muscle layers for 30 min.[18] In ponies, xylazine (1.1 mg/kg IV) increased intestinal vascular resistance, motility, and oxygen consumption.[19] In a study of cecal and right ventral colon myoelectric activity in ponies, xylazine (0.5 mg/kg IV) and/or butorphanol (0.04 mg/kg IV) resulted in decreased coordinated spike bursts for 20 min or longer.[20] It should be appreciated that the results of these studies were derived from horses or ponies with healthy gastrointestinal function. Clinically, it appears that these effects are rarely a disadvantage to using xylazine for preanesthetic medication in horses with colic. Furthermore, a study comparing myoelectric activity in equine intestine following three anesthetic regimens found no prolonged effect associated with (a) xylazine and ketamine, (b) thiopental and halothane, or (c) thiopental in guaifenesin and halothane.[21] The conclusion was that the particular regimen of general anesthesia is relatively unimportant in the development of motility disturbances in horses after anesthesia.

Excessive cardiovascular depression is avoided in compromised patients by decreasing the preanesthetic dose of xylazine (0.1 to 0.5 mg/kg IV) and the subsequent administration of diazepam (0.02 to 0.04 mg/kg IV) or guaifenesin (55 to 80 mg/kg IV) when inducing anesthesia with ketamine (1 to 2 mg/kg IV). Induction may be accomplished with ketamine as a bolus or in combination with guaifenesin (1 to 2 g ketamine/1 L 5% guaifenesin). An alternative induction regimen is to combine thiopental (2 to 4 mg/kg) with guaifenesin, given to effect. Induction of anesthesia when using thiopental and guaifenesin does not depend on preanesthetic heavy sedation and muscle relaxation to prevent rigidity or excitement as does induction with ketamine.

Anesthesia may be maintained with either halothane or isoflurane (1.5% to 2.5%) in oxygen. Halothane has been associated with a 62% decrease in intestinal blood flow in ponies anesthetized at 1 minimal alveolar concentration (MAC).[22] However, clinically significant deleterious effects of halothane on recovery from colic surgery have not been demonstrated. Horses anesthetized with isoflurane have higher cardiac outputs than horses anesthetized with a similar MAC of halothane.[23] Isoflurane anesthesia in horses undergoing surgery for colic is associated with a higher heart rate and lower arterial CO_2 concentration as compared with halothane.[24] Horses anesthetized with isoflurane recover more rapidly than those anesthetized with halothane.[24,25] Thus, there are several advantages to using isoflurane over halothane for horses undergoing surgery for colic.

Damaged intestinal tissue may release toxins into the systemic circulation, which can lead to cardiovascular dysfunction and decreased tissue perfusion. Release of eicosanoids (leukotrienes, prostacyclins, prostaglandins, and thromboxanes) has been associated with colonic volvulus in ponies.[26] Administration of flunixin meglumine may counteract the deleterious effects of toxins released during abdominal surgery. In addition, generation of free radicals in the equine intestine following anoxia and subsequent reoxygenation has been demonstrated in vitro.[27] Such studies may be the basis for the empirical intraoperative treatment of certain cases of equine colic with free-radical quenchers such as dimethylsulfoxide (DMSO).

Opioid agonists such as oxymorphone, morphine, and meperidine can be safely used in horses experiencing pain.[28] These drugs frequently induce undesirable excitement in horses that are pain free, unless preceded with a suitable sedative or tranquilizer (e.g., xylazine or acepromazine). Use of an opioid agonist-antagonist such as butorphanol may be advantageous because this drug provides analgesia but has a "ceiling" on respiratory depression.[29] However, numerous other pain medications also are suitable for use in horses, including nonsteroidal anti-inflammatory drugs, local anesthetic agents, and α_2-adrenoceptor agonists.[30]

In addition to pain control, support of the respiratory and cardiovascular systems is paramount in managing anesthesia for colic surgery. The bulk and weight of the gastrointestinal tract filled with ingesta and/or gas impair venous return to the heart and consequently decrease cardiac output. Diaphragmatic excursion and pulmonary function are impaired by a full stomach during anesthesia. These effects decrease tissue perfusion and oxygenation, creating metabolic acidosis and complicating the anesthetic management of horses. Evaluation of acid-base status will aid in determining adequacy of ventilation. Respiratory acidosis (pH < 7.2) can be avoided by use of controlled ventilation. Aggressive fluid therapy with lactated Ringer's solution will aid in correcting mild to moderate metabolic acidosis if normovolemia is reestablished.[31] It is not uncommon for a horse to require 30 L or more of isotonic IV fluids during colic surgery.

Monitoring arterial blood pressure is recommended in all species to provide some indirect information concerning cardiac output and tissue perfusion. Low tissue perfusion has been implicated in the occurrence of postanesthetic myositis.[32] Maintenance of a mean arterial blood pressure above 70 mm Hg may be achieved by fluid administration, by adjusting anesthetic depth, and by careful infusion of dobutamine (3 to 5 $\mu g \cdot kg^{-1} \cdot min^{-1}$ IV) or another sympathomimetic drug. Improved cardiac output will result when IV fluids are administered to hemoconcentrated patients. A decreased packed cell volume will decrease blood viscosity and improve cardiac output. Hypertonic saline (7% at 4 mL/kg IV) has been recommended for use in hypovolemic horses to expand plasma volume rapidly.[33] One advantage of hypertonic saline administration over isotonic crystalloid solutions is that a small volume is required. Correction of an extracellular volume deficit via administration of a small volume of hypertonic saline is accomplished more rapidly than with the administration of a large volume of isotonic fluid. However, the beneficial effects of hypertonic saline administration are short-lived and should be preserved with subsequent isotonic crystalloid therapy during anesthesia.

Cardiac arrhythmias may occur during anesthesia for surgical correction of an intestinal disorder. Bradycardia caused by increased vagal tone elicited from intestinal manipulation has been observed. Anticholinergic agents are occasionally used in horses for treatment of vagally induced bradycardia. However, high doses of these drugs may decrease gastrointestinal motility for up to 12 h in horses.[34] Horses treated with anticholinergics are more likely to develop postanesthetic colic if they have been fed within 4 to 6 h of anesthesia.[35] Perhaps a more important concern during anesthesia is the effect of atropine administration on cardiac arrhythmogenicity. Administration of atropine to halothane-anesthetized horses was associated with an increased incidence of tachycardia after administration of epinephrine or dobutamine.[36,37] However, horses given low doses of atropine in combination with detomidine, guaifenesin, diazepam, ketamine, and halothane anesthesia were not predisposed to adverse cardiovascular effects when dobutamine was administered for control of arterial blood pressure.[38]

Displaced Abomasum

This is a frequent problem in adult dairy cattle and occasionally in other ruminants such as llamas. In adult cattle, a standing laparotomy is the standard surgical approach. Regional anesthesia for standing laparotomy may be accomplished by a number of techniques, including the distal paravertebral block, the proximal paravertebral block, and the line block. For small ruminants such as goats, sheep, or llamas, general anesthesia will provide a more immobilized patient on which to perform surgery.

Particular anesthetic concerns for animals with displaced abomasum include disturbances in acid-base balance and electrolyte abnormalities. Similar to the pathogenesis of gastric dilation-volvulus in dogs, displaced abomasum in ruminants may initially present with metabolic alkalosis caused by abomasal sequestration of hydrogen chloride. Hypokalemia is a common concurrent finding because potassium is excreted by the kidneys in an attempt to retain hydrogen ions in response to metabolic alkalosis. As the disease progresses, metabolic acidosis occurs because of poor tissue perfusion and lactate accumulation. Shock, followed by death, is expected in untreated animals. Dehydration, poor circulatory volume, and electrolyte abnormalities must be corrected. Serum chloride less than 79 mEq/L and heart rate greater than 100 beats/min are associated with a poor prognosis.[39]

Disorders of the Pancreas

Acute pancreatitis in dogs and cats is frequently associated with vomiting, anorexia, and abdominal pain. However, the diagnosis of acute pancreatitis is often difficult to make antemortem. Classic laboratory findings associated with pancreatitis (increased amylase and lipase activity) may not be observed. Conversely, increased pancreatic enzyme activity is not specific for pancreatitis. Intestinal foreign bodies are frequently associated with increased lipase activity. Exploratory laparotomy in healthy dogs (without signs of pancreatitis), in which abdominal tissues were examined but not surgically altered, was associated with a threefold increase in serum lipase activity.[40] Morphine administration may cause elevation of amylase and lipase activity by increasing smooth muscle contraction in the pancreatic duct (sphincter of Oddi).[41] In addition, many dogs with pancreatitis have concurrent disease, such as diabetes mellitus, hyperadrenocorticism, renal failure, neoplasia, congestive heart failure, or autoimmune disorders.[42] Acute pancreatitis has been induced by drugs, including corticosteroids, nonsteroidal anti-inflammatory agents, organophosphates, thiazide diuretics, sulfonamides, tetracycline, azothioprine, furosemide, and estrogen.[43] Thus, it is likely that animals with acute pancreatitis are often anesthetized for reasons unrelated to diagnosis or treatment of pancreatitis. However, in some situations, such as acute necrotizing pancreatitis or pancreatic phlegmon, surgical therapy may be indicated. Endoscopic, surgical, or laparoscopic techniques can be used to place enterostomy tubes for enteral nutrition. Iatrogenic pancreatitis may also occur after abdominal surgery. Humans occasionally develop acute pancreatitis after renal transplantation, gastrectomy, and biliary tract surgery.[44] The "incidental" finding of acute pancreatitis is not uncommon at the necropsy of many patients with an unknown cause of death.

Medical management of acute pancreatitis basically consists of maintaining adequate fluid therapy and nothing per os. The use of plasma and analgesics has also been advocated for management of pancreatitis. Establishing normal pancreatic circulation is paramount for tissue healing. Preanesthetic preparation of patients with pancreatitis is accomplished by withholding oral intake of food and water and administering IV fluids to correct hydration and/or electrolyte imbalances.

The choice of anesthetics for use in a patient with pancreatitis is often based on other complicating factors identified for the patient. Intravenously administered α_2-adrenergic agents have a hyperglycemic effect owing to inhibition of insulin release by the beta cells in the islets of Langerhans of the pancreas. This effect has been observed with epinephrine and with the potent sedative-analgesics such as detomidine and xylazine.[45–49] While α_2-adrenergic agonist–induced hyperglycemia is avoided by pretreatment with α_2-adrenergic antagonists, sedative and analgesic effects are similarly prevented.[45–51] It is unknown whether the α_2-adrenergic effects on the pancreas are of clinical significance in patients with pancreatitis. However, a conservative approach to anesthetic management of these patients generally avoids use of these drugs. Opioid analgesics (hydromorphone, buprenorphine, or butorphanol) are a suitable alternative to provide sedation and analgesia prior to induction of anesthesia. Morphine causes spasm of the sphincter of Oddi at the termination of the common biliary and pancreatic duct in 1% to 3% of the human population and may be associated with complications in animals with pancreatitis.[41] Other opioids cause less spasm of this sphincter and are useful when indicated for treatment of pain associated with pancreatitis. In humans, because of better pain relief with fewer side effects, epidural administration of morphine is preferred for treatment of pain associated with pancreatitis.[52]

There is no clear best choice for induction of anesthesia for patients with pancreatitis. Halothane would not be the anesthetic of choice in patients with concurrent liver disease or those with cardiac dysrhythmias. Maintenance of anesthesia with isoflurane or sevoflurane is preferred in such cases. During surgery, the anesthetist should attempt to provide vigilant monitoring of anesthetic depth, prevention of hypotension, and maintenance of adequate vascular volume.

Obesity

Obese patients often have underlying physiological problems in addition to the condition for which anesthesia is required. Evaluation of obese animals for presence of pancreatitis, diabetes mellitus, hepatic insufficiency, or cardiac disease should be included in the diagnostic workup. An obese animal's veins may be more difficult to locate and catheterize. Drug dose should be adjusted to a patient's lean weight to avoid overdosing with anesthetic drugs. Obese animals anesthetized with halothane will also have a longer recovery time than other patients because of significant sequestration of the anesthetic in fat. Isoflurane and sevoflurane are more desirable inhalation anesthetics for obese animals because of their minimal biotransformation and low tissue solubility.

Preoperative hypoxemia (Pickwickian syndrome) due to hypoventilation is a common feature of obesity in humans and is markedly worsened by anesthesia. Obesity decreases the ventilatory capacity of patients during anesthesia, owing to decreased chest wall compliance. Hypoventilation may occur because of limited diaphragmatic excursion from the increased weight of the abdominal contents. The increased mass of the pharyngeal tissues and tongue may lead to upper-airway obstruction after premedication with tranquilizers or during induction of anesthesia. Obese patients given sedatives or tranquilizers prior to anesthesia should be continuously observed for airway obstruction. Rapid control of the airway at induction and positive-pressure ventilation during anesthesia are recommended. During recovery from anesthesia, obese patients should be kept intubated until they will no longer tolerate the endotracheal tube. Obese animals must regain normal muscle function to maintain an adequate tidal volume and a patent airway after extubation.

References

1. Nickel R, Schummer A, Seiferle E, Sack WO. The Viscera of the Domestic Animals. New York: Springer-Verlag, 1973.
2. Canine bloat panel offers research and treatment recommendations. Friskies Res Dig 24:1, 1985.
3. Muir WW. Acid-base and electrolyte disturbances in dogs with gastric dilatation-volvulus. J Am Vet Med Assoc 181:2, 1982.
4. Allen DA, Schertel ER, Muir WW III, Valentine AK. Hypertonic saline/dextran resuscitation of dogs with experimentally induced gastric dilatation-volvulus shock. Am J Vet Res 52:92, 1991.
5. Booth NH. Non-narcotic analgesics. In: Booth NH, McDonald LE, eds. Veterinary Pharmacology and Therapeutics, 5th ed. Ames: Iowa State University Press, 1982:297.
6. Strombeck DR, Harrold D. Effects of atropine, acepromazine, meperidine, and xylazine on gastroesophageal sphincter pressure in the dog. Am J Vet Res 46:963, 1985.
7. Hsu WH, McNeel SV. Effect of yohimbine on xylazine-induced prolongation of gastrointestinal transit in dogs. J Am Vet Med Assoc 183:297, 1983.
8. McDonell WN. General anesthesia for equine gastrointestinal and obstetric procedures. Vet Clin North Am Large Anim Pract 3:163, 1981.
9. Betts CW, Wingfield WE, Green RW. A retrospective study of gastric dilatation-torsion in the dog. J Small Anim Pract 15:727, 1974.
10. Matthiesen DT. The gastric dilatation-volvulus complex: Medical and surgical considerations. J Am Anim Hosp Assoc 19:925, 1983.
11. Lantz GC, Badylak SF, Hiles MC, Arkin TE. Treatment of reperfusion injury in dogs with experimentally induced gastric dilatation-volvulus. Am J Vet Res 53:1594, 1992.
12. Yeager MP. Outcome of pain management. Anesthesiol Clin North Am 7:241, 1989.
13. Baller LS, Hendrickson DA. Management of equine orthopedic pain. Vet Clin Equine 18:117, 2002.
14. Saarinen H. Preanesthetic use of detomidine in horses: Some clinical observations. Acta Vet Scand 82:157, 1986.
15. Clarke KW, Taylor PM. Detomidine: A new sedative for horses. Equine Vet J 18:366, 1986.
16. Wagner AE, Muir WW, Hinchcliff KW. Cardiovascular effects of xylazine and detomidine in horses. Am J Vet Res 52:651, 1991.
17. Greene SA, Thurmon JC. Xylazine: A review of its pharmacology and use in veterinary medicine. J Vet Pharmacol Ther 11:295, 1988.
18. Clark SE, Thompson SA, Becht JL, Moore JN. Effects of xylazine on cecal mechanical activity and cecal blood flow in healthy horses. Am J Vet Res 49:720, 1989.
19. Stick JA, Chou CC, Derksen FJ, Arden WA. Effects of xylazine on equine intestinal vascular resistance, motility, compliance, and oxygen consumption. Am J Vet Res 48:198, 1987.
20. Rutkowski JA, Ross MW, Cullen K. Effects of xylazine and/or butorphanol or neostigmine on myoelectric activity of the cecum and right ventral colon in female ponies. Am J Vet Res 50:1096, 1989.
21. Lester GD, Bolton JR, Cullen LK, Thurgate SM. Effects of general anesthesia on myoelectric activity of the intestine in horses. Am J Vet Res 53:1553, 1992.
22. Manohar M, Goetz TE. Cerebral, renal, adrenal, intestinal, and pancreatic circulation in conscious ponies and during 1.0, 1.5, and 2.0 minimal alveolar concentrations of halothane-O_2 anesthesia. Am J Vet Res 46:2492, 1985.
23. Steffey EP, Howland D. Comparison of circulatory and respiratory effects of isoflurane and halothane anesthesia in horses. Am J Vet Res 40:821, 1980.
24. Harvey RC, Gleed RD, Matthews NS, Tyner CL, Erb HN, Short CE. Isoflurane anesthesia for equine colic surgery. Vet Surg 16:184, 1987.
25. Matthews NS, Miller SM, Hartsfield SM, Slater MP. Comparison of recoveries from halothane vs isoflurane anesthesia in horses. J Am Vet Med Assoc 201:559, 1992.
26. Stick JA, Arden WA, Robinson RA, Shobe EM, Roth RA. Thromboxane and prostacyclin production in ponies with colonic volvulus. Am J Vet Res 53:563, 1992.
27. Johnston JK, Freeman DE, Gillette D, Soma LR. Effects of superoxide dismutase on injury induced by anoxia and reoxygenation in equine small intestine in vitro. Am J Vet Res 52:2050, 1991.
28. Muir WW. Drugs used to produce standing chemical restraint in horses. Vet Clin North Am Large Anim Pract 3:17, 1981.
29. Nagashima H, Karamanian A, Malovany R, et al. Respiratory and circulatory effects of intravenous butorphanol and morphine. Clin Pharmacol Ther 19:738, 1976.

30. Malone E, Graham L. Management of gastrointestinal pain. Vet Clin North Am Equine Pract 18:133, 2002.

31. Hartsfield SM, Thurmon JC, Corbin JE, Benson GJ, Aiken T. Effects of sodium acetate, bicarbonate and lactate on acid-base status in anaesthetized dogs. J Vet Pharmacol Ther 4:51, 1981.

32. Lindsay WA, Robinson GM, Brunson DB, Majors LJ. Induction of equine postanesthetic myositis after halothane-induced hypotension. Am J Vet Res 50:404, 1989.

33. Schmall LM, Muir WW, Robertson JT. Hemodynamic effects of small volume hypertonic saline in experimentally induced hemorrhagic shock. Equine Vet J 22:273, 1990.

34. Ducharme NG, Fubini SL. Gastrointestinal complications associated with the use of atropine in horses. J Am Vet Med Assoc 182:229, 1983.

35. Short CE. Special considerations for equine anesthesia. In: Short CE, ed. Principles and Practice of Veterinary Anesthesia. Baltimore: Williams and Wilkins, 1987:271.

36. Lees P, Travernor WD. Influence of halothane and catecholamines on heart rate and rhythm in the horse. Br J Pharmacol 39:149, 1970.

37. Light GW, Hellyer PW, Swanson CR. Parasympathetic influence on the arrhythmogenicity of graded dobutamine infusions in halothane-anesthetized horses. Am J Vet Res 53:1154, 1992.

38. Weil AB, Keegan RD, Greene SA. Effect of low-dose atropine administration on dobutamine dose requirement in horses anesthetized with detomidine and halothane. Am J Vet Res 58:1436, 1997.

39. Benson GJ. Anesthetic management of ruminants and swine with selected pathophysiologic alterations. Vet Clin North Am Food Anim Pract 2:677, 1986.

40. Bellah JR, Bell G. Serum amylase and lipase activities after exploratory laparotomy in dogs. Am J Vet Res 50:1638, 1989.

41. Stoelting RK. Opioid agonists and antagonists. In: Stoelting RK, ed. Pharmacology and Physiology in Anesthetic Practice. Philadelphia: JB Lippincott, 1987:79.

42. Cook AK, Breitschwerdt EB, Levine JF, Bunch SE, Linn LO. Risk factors associated with acute pancreatitis in dogs: 101 cases (1985–1990). J Am Vet Med Assoc 203:673, 1993.

43. Bunch SE. The exocrine pancreas. In: Nelson RW, Couto CG, eds. Small Animal Internal Medicine, 3rd ed. St Louis: CV Mosby, 2003:552.

44. Estabrook SG, Levine EG, Bernstein LH. Gastrointestinal crises in intensive care. Anesthesiol Clin North Am 9:367, 1991.

45. Thurmon JC, Neff-Davis C, Davis LE, Stoker RA, Benson GJ, Lock TF. Xylazine hydrochloride–induced hyperglycemia and hypoinsulinemia in thoroughbred horses. J Vet Pharmacol Ther 5:241, 1982.

46. Thurmon JC, Nelson DR, Hartsfield SM, Rumore CA. Effects of xylazine hydrochloride on urine in cattle. Aust Vet J 54:178, 1978.

47. Trim CM, Hanson RR. Effects of xylazine on renal function and plasma glucose in ponies. Vet Rec 118:65, 1986.

48. Benson GJ, et al. Effect of xylazine hydrochloride upon plasma glucose and serum insulin concentrations in adult pointer dogs. J Am Anim Hosp Assoc 20:791, 1984.

49. Gasthuys F, Terpstra P, van den Hende C, De Moor A. Hyperglycaemia and diuresis during sedation with detomidine in the horse. Zentralbl Veterinarmed A 34:641, 1987.

50. Greene SA, Thurmon JC, Tranquilli WJ, Benson GJ. Yohimbine prevents xylazine-induced hypoinsulinemia and hyperglycemia in mares. Am J Vet Res 48:676, 1987.

51. Hsu WH. Yohimbine increases plasma insulin concentrations and reverses xylazine-induced hypoinsulinemia in dogs. Am J Vet Res 49:242, 1988.

52. Mulholland MW, Debas HT, Bonica JJ. Diseases of the liver, biliary system, and pancreas. In: Bonica JJ, ed. The Management of Pain, 2nd ed. Philadelphia: Lea and Febiger, 1990:1214.

Chapter 42
Endocrine Disease

Ralph C. Harvey and Michael Schaer

Introduction

Endocrine disease is more often a factor influencing anesthetic management than a disease directly requiring anesthesia for medical or surgical intervention. Patients with endocrine disease–induced derangements of homeostasis require that anesthetic management be designed to take into account the appropriate physiological support, perioperative monitoring, and selection of medications to reduce the risks associated with sedation, anesthesia, and analgesia. Recognition of physiological derangements typical of specific endocrine diseases provides the framework for customizing anesthesia for individual patients. Endocrinopathies often increase the requirements for intervention, particularly for physiological support.

Diabetes Mellitus

Insulin is essential for normal cellular function. The effects of insulin on normal cellular function include (a) inhibition of glycogenolysis, (b) inhibition of gluconeogenesis, (c) inhibition of lipolysis, (d) stimulation of glucose uptake into cells, (e) stimulation of potassium transport into cells, and (f) suppression of ketogenesis.[1]

Carbohydrate, protein, and fat metabolism are all affected with an insulin deficiency. Glucose uptake is decreased, especially in fat and muscle. Also, control of hepatic gluconeogenesis is lost, with the resultant hyperglycemia leading to osmotic diuresis. Muscle tissue undergoes catabolic metabolism for energy, and protein synthesis is inhibited, resulting in muscle wasting. Acetyl coenzyme A and ketone bodies are produced for energy. Lipolysis is inhibited with a resultant accumulation of ketone bodies causing osmotic diuresis and metabolic acidosis. Prolonged hyperglycemia and ketonemia can lead to (a) metabolic acidosis,

(b) dehydration, (c) circulatory collapse, (d) renal failure, and/or (e) coma and death.[1]

Diabetes mellitus should be suspected in any patient with the following clinical signs: (a) a recent history of polyuria, polydipsia, weight loss, or rapid onset of cataracts; (b) dehydration, weakness, collapse, mental dullness, hepatomegaly and/or muscle wasting; and/or (c) increased rate and depth of respiration and breath with a sweet acetone odor. Diabetes mellitus occurs more frequently in female dogs and male cats. These clinical signs should alert the clinician to the possibility of diabetes mellitus.

The presence of glucose with or without ketones in the urine, along with resting blood glucose of greater than 250 mg/dL with hyperketonemia, is a common finding. Electrolyte and renal function tests may be altered (especially hypokalemia) and serum alkaline phosphatase may be increased due to hepatic fatty infiltration. Severe metabolic acidosis (a pH of less than 7.1) should be treated with sufficient sodium bicarbonate to return pH to 7.2.

A patient with diabetes mellitus should be stabilized and regulated prior to anesthesia. The anesthetic protocol is probably not as critical as the adjunct support during and after anesthesia and surgery. The key to the anesthetic management of a diabetic is to use preanesthetic and anesthetic agents that will result in the shortest anesthetic recovery time with the least amount of drug hangover. Drugs that can be antagonized (narcotics, α_2-agonists, and benzodiazepine tranquilizers) or are readily eliminated from the patient (propofol, etomidate, and inhalant anesthetics) should be considered. The goal is to get the patient awake as soon as possible so that the patient can resume its normal feeding schedule.

The procedure should be scheduled early in the morning after the administration of the patient's normal dose of insulin or one-half of the usual dose.[2] Preoperative and serial intraoperative and postoperative blood glucose levels should be determined. Ideally, the blood glucose should be maintained between 150 and 250 mg/dL. During the procedure, 2.5% to 5% dextrose in a balanced electrolyte solution should be administered to prevent hypoglycemia.[3] An intraoperative fluid rate of 11 to 15 mL $\cdot$ kg^{-1} $\cdot$ h^{-1} is usually adequate. Depending on the blood glucose values, measured hourly, the dextrose drip may need to be continued following the procedure. Avoid blood glucose extremes and lower any marked elevations of blood glucose to a rate not to exceed 75 to 100 mg/dL per hour. As soon as a postoperative patient starts eating, it is probably not necessary to continue the dextrose in the intravenous fluids. Close monitoring of the patient should be continued, because the stress of anesthesia and surgery may cause a diabetic to decompensate. A return home and resumption of the normal regulation pattern is desired as soon as possible. The use of corticosteroids may also cause decompensation and should be avoided unless absolutely necessary.

Diabetes Insipidus

If anesthesia is needed before correction of electrolyte abnormalities, it becomes essential to continue with diuresis. Oral water deprivation can be very deleterious for cerebral function and blood pressure, so water should not be withdrawn from these patients. Generous intravenous fluid therapy is indicated to avoid hypertonic encephalopathy. Serum sodium concentration should be monitored, and appropriate fluids administered to prevent it from rising to more than 160 mEq/L. The fluid of choice is 5% dextrose in water as needed, or half-strength (0.45%) saline with 2.5% dextrose may be used if a more isotonic solute is desired. Metabolism of the dextrose provides free water and thereby reduces plasma sodium. Chronic hypernatremia should be corrected slowly, at rate not to exceed 12 mEq for first 24-h period, with correction achieved over 72 h. Rapid-onset hypernatremia (occurring within less than 24 h) can be carefully treated more rapidly.

Hypoglycemia from Insulinoma

Monitoring and supplementation of blood glucose are required in patients with an insulinoma. Acute hypoglycemia must be recognized and treated effectively with dextrose. If there is no response to intravenous dextrose, a glucagon infusion may be useful. In postoperative patients, there is a risk of acute pancreatitis after surgical removal of the insulinoma. These patients may be maintained non per os for 1 to 2 days after surgery to help reduce the risk of acute pancreatitis. Continued monitoring of blood glucose is necessary to recognize potential hyperglycemia and hypoglycemia in the perioperative period. These patients may become insulin dependent.

Hyperparathyroidism

Preoperative management requires decreasing the serum calcium before anesthesia and surgery. It is important to evaluate renal status and stabilize or treat accordingly. After parathyroid (or thyroid) removal, there is risk of acute hypoparathyroidism. These animals require repeated monitoring for hypocalcemia during the first 48 h after surgery and appropriate management.

Hypoparathyroidism

Hypoparathyroidism occurs less often than hyperparathyroidism and is often diagnosed in patients after surgery to remove either the thyroid or parathyroid glands. Close monitoring of blood calcium is indicated. Rarely, preparturient eclampsia is present in bitches requiring Caesarean section. Treat hypocalcemia with

calcium gluconate until signs abate and serum calcium is at safe level, greater than 7 mg/dL.

Hypoadrenocorticism (Addison's Disease)

Hypoadrenocorticism is a deficiency in aldosterone and/or glucocorticoids that results from adrenal cortex dysfunction. As with diabetics, patients with hypoadrenocorticism should be stabilized and regulated prior to anesthesia and surgery when possible.

Hypoadrenocorticism can be caused either by diseases, destruction of the adrenal glands, or by decreased corticotropin (adrenocorticotropic hormone [ACTH]) secretion. Primary idiopathic hypoadrenocorticism is the most common cause of hypoadrenocorticism in dogs and may be immune mediated. Other diseases that may destroy the adrenal glands include systemic mycosis, metastatic tumors, hemorrhagic infarction, amyloidosis of the cortices, canine distemper, and glucocorticoid therapy for certain disorders that might cause a selective deficiency of cortisol caused by negative feedback inhibition of the hypothalamic-pituitary-adrenal axis.[4]

Decreased ACTH secretion can cause secondary hypoadrenocorticism. Adrenocorticotropic hormone directly stimulates glucocorticoid secretion and is secreted by the anterior pituitary gland. Decreased ACTH secretion may develop with diseases or tumors of the pituitary gland or with decreased secretion of corticotropin-releasing factor (CRF) owing to hypothalamic lesions. Prolonged negative feedback from exogenous corticosteroid therapy can cause glucocorticoid deficiency while maintaining adequate mineralocorticoid secretion.

The clinical signs of hypoadrenocorticism will depend on the particular adrenal hormone (aldosterone or glucocorticoids) most affected by the disease. The primary function of aldosterone is to stimulate absorption of sodium in the distal renal tubules and promote potassium excretion. Aldosterone deficiency produces hyponatremia and hyperkalemia. Hyponatremia with concurrent water loss can produce lethargy, nausea, impaired cardiac output, hypovolemia, hypotension, and/or impaired renal perfusion. Hyperkalemia will produce muscle weakness, decreased cardiac conduction, and excitability and bradycardia.

Glucocorticoid deficiency can result in significant physiological abnormalities. Cortisol stimulates gluconeogenesis, increases blood glucose, enhances extravascular fluid movement to the intravascular compartment, stabilizes lysosomal membranes, and counteracts the effects of stress. Cortisol depletion impairs renal excretion of water and energy metabolism, decreases stress tolerance, and can cause anorexia, vomiting, and/or diarrhea. Cortisol depletion rarely produces electrolyte imbalances.[4]

Hypoadrenocorticism should be suspected in any dog with a history of anorexia, vomiting, diarrhea, and lethargy when clinical findings are muscle weakness, dehydration, and bradycardia. Electrolyte imbalance may be suggestive of hypoadrenocorticism. Serum sodium levels are often less than 135 mEq/L, and serum potassium levels may be greater than 5.5 mEq/L. The sodium-potassium ratio may be less than 25:1 (normal is 33:1).

Hypoadrenocorticism is confirmed by measuring serum cortisol. Determination of plasma cortisol levels is the most accurate method of diagnosing hypoadrenocorticism, and resting plasma cortisol is often less than 10 µg/mL. Plasma cortisol will not significantly increase in response to exogenous ACTH administration in hypoadrenocorticism patients. Prednisolone replacement therapy must be withheld for 1 to 2 days before testing, but dexamethasone can be used without causing interference with the radioimmunoassay for cortisol.[4]

Diagnostic testing that may be helpful in confirming the diagnosis of hypoadrenocorticism includes the complete blood count (CBC), blood urea nitrogen (BUN), and electrocardiogram (ECG). The CBC reflects dehydration, and decreased cortisol will sometimes cause eosinophilia and lymphocytosis. BUN may be elevated by prerenal uremia or renal failure. The ECG may show evidence of hyperkalemia. In severe hyperkalemic cardiotoxicity, therapy may be warranted with calcium gluconate, sodium bicarbonate, insulin, and dexamethasone.

The anesthetic protocol used in the patient with hypoadrenocorticism is not as critical as the medical management prior to anesthesia. A patient with hypoadrenocorticism must be stabilized. The treatment objectives are (a) to correct the dehydration and treat hypovolemic shock if present, (b) to return renal function to normal, (c) to correct electrolyte imbalances, and (d) to supply glucocorticoids.[5] In an Addisonian crisis, priorities are the patient's pH, hypotension, ECG complexes and rhythm, and the correction of hyponatremia, hyperkalemia, and any hypoglycemia.

Addisonian patients have decreased stress tolerance. The key to their perioperative management is to provide adequate intravenous fluid volume replacement and to provide exogenous glucocorticoids. A balanced electrolyte solution should be administered intraoperatively at a rate of 15 to 22 mL · kg^{-1} · h^{-1}. The rate may be adjusted depending on the patient's physiological status. The fluid rate may be decreased postoperatively to approximately 90 mL · kg^{-1} · day^{-1}. Again, this rate can be adjusted depending on a patient's physiological status.

Glucocorticoids should be given concomitantly with initiation of the anesthetic regimen. Preoperatively, 2 to 4 mg/kg of dexamethasone can be given intravenously or subcutaneously. Intraoperatively, a rapid-acting glucocorticoid such as prednisolone sodium succinate (Solu-Delta-Cortef) at a dose of 11 to 22 mg/kg should be administered intravenously and repeated as necessary. Postoperatively, additional glucocorticoids are given as needed. Patients with hypoadrenocorticism should be closely monitored for signs of hypotension and shock.

Hyperadrenocorticism (Cushing's Syndrome)

Although a common endocrine disease, hyperadrenocorticism is less problematic for successful anesthetic care than is hypoadrenocorticism. Patients with an excess of adrenal hormones will be predisposed to infection and poor wound healing. Most cats with hypoadrenocorticism are also diabetic. There is increased risk of pulmonary thrombosis and of thrombosis at other sites during the perioperative period.

Blood pressure monitoring and support are important for patients with hypoadrenocorticism because they are prone to hypertension. Preanesthetic evaluation should include baseline arterial blood pressure measurement. Patients with underlying hypertension should have blood pressure supported, if necessary, to prevent anesthetic-associated hypotension. Chronic hypertension predisposes patients to failures of autoregulatory control of tissue perfusion at reduced blood pressures that would be better tolerated by normotensive patients.

Pulmonary alveolar calcification is occasionally recognized on thoracic radiography with hypoadrenocorticism. This might cause hypoxemia from impaired perfusion, but is usually an incidental finding. A more commonly encountered problem related to the respiratory depression is impaired intraoperative ventilation. Many patients with hypoadrenocorticism have a large pendulous abdomen, which can impair ventilation during anesthesia. Monitoring ventilation with end-tidal carbon dioxide, pulse oximetry, and/or arterial blood-gas analysis is warranted.

When hyperadrenocorticism has been successfully treated, patients should have some functional adrenocortical reserve and thereby still be able to withstand the stresses of anesthesia and surgery. Adrenocortical reserve is indicated by a post-ACTH stimulation value of 3 to 10 µg/dL. Otherwise, these patients should be managed as having an iatrogenic adrenocortical insufficiency requiring glucocorticoid supplementation. Newer methods for medical management of pituitary gland–dependent and adrenal gland–dependent hyperadrenocorticism hold promise for more effective treatment and superior retention of adequate adrenocortical function.

Pheochromocytoma

Patients with pheochromocytoma are usually considered to be at very high anesthetic risk. The best approach to anesthetizing a patient with a pheochromocytoma is the preoperative monitoring and management of arterial blood pressures and cardiac function. Cardiac arrhythmias, particularly tachyarrhythmias, require diligent ECG monitoring. Stabilization of patients can require prolonged medical management, most often using phenoxybenzamine, a long-acting α-adrenergic antagonist, prior to anesthesia and surgery to lower and control arterial blood pressure adequately. Extreme hemodynamic instability is commonly a problem in these patients, especially if prior stabilization is inadequate. Even with prior stabilization, close attention to blood pressure and cardiac monitoring are imperative.

Surges in blood pressure and tachyarrhythmias are treated as they occur. Propranolol or esmolol may be useful in controlling tachyarrhythmias, but it is important to provide effective α-adrenergic blockade before initiating ß-adrenergic blockade. For any adrenal gland surgery, there is very significant potential for intraoperative blood loss. This is particularly true for tumors involving the right adrenal gland because of proximity to the posterior vena cava. Cross-matched blood should be available, along with colloidal fluids, for immediate volume resuscitation.

After removal of the affected adrenal gland, acute and dramatic drops in endogenous catecholamine levels may occur. This may be manifested as sudden and profound hypotension and bradycardia, especially in the presence of α-adrenergic and ß-adrenergic blockade. Intravenous inotropic (e.g., dobutamine) and pressor (e.g., ephedrine or phenylephrine) support should be immediately available to treat hypotension rapidly.

Hypothyroidism

Untreated and inadequately treated hypothyroid patients have reduced metabolic rates and may more slowly recover from sedation or anesthesia. Any anesthetic drug should be used in low doses and ideally should require minimal or no metabolism or can be readily antagonized. Opioids, low doses of tranquilizers, propofol, and inhalants are the preferred preanesthetic and anesthetic drugs.

Hypothyroid patients are often obese and may suffer from anemia. Obesity may cause ventilatory problems under anesthesia that are caused by the excess amounts of abdominal and intrathoracic fat. Assisted or controlled ventilation may be necessary in these patients to keep them adequately ventilated. Moderate anemia may occur in hypothyroid patients. If the anemia is significant, blood transfusion should be considered prior to anesthesia and surgery.[6] In severe cases of hypothyroidism (myxedema hypothyroidism), hypothermia and bradycardia may complicate anesthesia. These should be corrected slowly. Support with corticosteroids, levothyroxine, and respiratory support may be necessary.

Hyperthyroidism

Patients with thyroid adenomas, adenomatous hyperplasia, or adenocarcinomas may exhibit evidence of hyperthyroidism. Several factors may place these patients at higher anesthetic risk.[7] A thyroid tumor may place mechanical pressure on the trachea, causing a partial obstruction and interfering with respiration. The surgical site may be highly vascular, and this can lead to excessive bleeding.

Hyperthyroid patients may rarely develop a *thyroid storm* during the procedure as a result of excessive thyroid hormone production. This is precipitated by catecholamine release and is characterized by an increased heart rate, increased blood pressure, cardiac dysrhythmias, elevated body temperature, and shock. Hyperthyroid patients often have increased metabolic rates, making them more prone to developing hypoxemia. Oxygen and glucose demand and carbon dioxide production are increased. Hyperthyroid patients may be more prone to heart failure. They have an increased heart rate and myocardial oxygen consumption.

Because of their increased metabolic rate, hyperthyroid patients may rapidly metabolize anesthetic drugs. Adequate oxygenation must be provided because of the increased oxygen consumption and demands of the patient. Intubation may be difficult if the tumor is compressing the trachea. Preanesthetic and anesthetic agents that decrease catecholamine response and myocardial irritability are preferred. Low doses of acepromazine or an

α_2-agonist can be used as a preanesthetic in hyperthyroid patients. Acepromazine decreases myocardial irritability, and it blocks α-adrenergic receptors and thus may help counteract hypertension. An opioid can be combined with acepromazine because opioids generally slow heart rate and decrease myocardial oxygen consumption.

Anesthesia may be induced with low-dose thiopental, propofol, etomidate, or an inhalant by mask using isoflurane or sevoflurane. Inhalant induction alone may be stressful in some patients, worsening the overall cardiovascular status. Cardiovascular and respiratory parameters should be monitored closely and ventilation controlled when necessary. A 2.5% to 5% dextrose drip can be administered to meet increased glucose demands.

Cats with thyrotoxic cardiomyopathy, and particularly those with hyperthyroidism and concurrent hypertrophic cardiomyopathy, should be managed so as to reduce heart rate and optimize ventricular filling.[8,9] The use of dissociative anesthetics and anticholinergics is avoided to help insure that a lower heart rate is maintained. Sevoflurane (or even halothane) is preferred over isoflurane so as to reduce heart rate and myocardial work. The use of acepromazine is avoided to prevent the reduction in preload and ventricular filling. By maintaining preload, ventricular filling, and diastolic interval, both myocardial blood flow and ventricular function are improved. Preanesthetic medication with an opioid such as buprenorphine and a benzodiazepine such as midazolam is followed by inhalant induction with sevoflurane. Intravenous induction with etomidate, propofol, or thiopental is acceptable in less severe cases.

References

1. Nelson RW. Disorders of the endocrine pancreas. In: Ettinger SJ, ed. Textbook of Veterinary Internal Medicine. Philadelphia: WB Saunders, 1989:1676–1720.
2. Schaer M. Surgery in the diabetic pet. Vet Clin North Am Small Anim Pract 1995;25:651–660.
3. Paddleford RR. Anesthetic considerations in patients with preexisting problems or conditions. In: Manual of Small Animal Anesthesia. New York: Churchill Livingstone, 1988:253–308.
4. Feldman EC. Adrenal gland disease. In: Ettinger SJ, ed. Textbook of Veterinary Internal Medicine. Philadelphia: WB Saunders, 1989: 1721–1776.
5. Peterson ME. Pathophysiological changes in the endocrine system. In: Short CE, ed. Principles and Practice of Veterinary Anesthesia. Baltimore: Williams and Wilkins, 1987:251–260.
6. Peterson ME, Ferguson DC. Thyroid disease. In: Ettinger SJ, ed. Textbook of Veterinary Internal Medicine. Philadelphia: WB Saunders, 1989:1632–1675.
7. Trim CM. Anesthesia and the endocrine system. In: Slatter D, ed. Textbook of Small Animal Surgery, 2nd ed. Philadelphia: WB Saunders, 1993:2290–2294.
8. Bednarski RM. Anesthetic concerns for patients with cardiomyopathy. Vet Clin North Am Small Anim Pract 1992;22:460–465.
9. Lamont L, Bulmer B, Sisson D, Grimm KA, Tranquilli WJ. Doppler echocardiographic effects of medetomidine on dynamic left ventricular outflow tract obstruction in cats. J Am Vet Med Assoc 2002;221: 1276–1281.

Chapter 43
Airway Disease

Stephen A. Greene and Ralph C. Harvey

Introduction

Airway obstruction may be associated with trauma, congenital anatomic abnormalities, aspiration of foreign material, or laryngospasm. Specific management of airway obstruction in the perianesthetic period is determined by the severity of the obstruction and the underlying factors associated with its cause.

Respiratory Depression in the Perianesthetic Period

When possible, the use of potent respiratory-depressant medications should be avoided in patients with respiratory disease. When sedative/analgesics with respiratory-depressant effects (e.g., opioids) are used for premedication, the patient's respiration should be closely monitored (e.g., pulse oximetry, end-tidal CO_2, and arterial blood gas analysis). Mixed agonist-antagonist opioids such as butorphanol minimize respiratory depression. Butorphanol is described as having a "ceiling effect" on respiratory depression and analgesia.[1] This terminology implies that the dose-response curve for butorphanol will plateau at some point, thus imparting no further respiratory depression/analgesia as the dose is increased. Naloxone can be used to antagonize respiratory depression associated with opioid analgesics but will also antagonize analgesia.[2] Analgesia may be preserved to some extent by titrating naloxone "to effect" when reversing opioid-induced respiratory depression. However, *rapid* intravenous administration of naloxone has been associated with development of cardiac dysrhythmias and even sudden death.[3,4] Administration of a mixed–agonist-antagonist opioid such as butorphanol may effectively antagonize severe respiratory depression while maintaining some analgesic action.[5] Incremental dosing of butorphanol (0.05 mg/kg at a time) for antagonism of full-agonist opioids is advised to prevent sudden arousal and dysphoria.

Regional analgesia is gaining in popularity for improving postoperative analgesia. This technique causes less respiratory depression than do parenteral opioids. Following thoracotomy, analgesia may be enhanced by intrapleural injection of bupivacaine (1.5 mg/kg).[6] For control of pain associated with procedures involving the hind limbs (and possibly procedures more rostral), epidural analgesia is a useful adjunct to general anesthesia. Epidural analgesia prior to surgery will decrease general anesthetic requirement.[7] Inhalation anesthetics are associated with dose-dependent respiratory depression. Therefore, use of epidural analgesia as an adjunct to inhalation anesthesia may decrease respiratory and cardiovascular depression. Epidural analgesia in dogs is often accomplished using morphine (0.1 mg/kg) in sterile water or isotonic saline solution in sufficient quantity to yield 1 mL per 5 kg of body weight.[8]

Airway Trauma

Trauma to the head and neck can cause progressive respiratory distress. Airway occlusion may result from collapse or obstruction of the nasal or oral passages accompanied by tissue swelling, hemorrhage, and aspiration of tissues, blood, or foreign materials. Head trauma and secondary cerebral edema can decrease ventilation via neurological mechanisms independent of physical obstructions. Additional respiratory depression must be avoided to prevent associated increases in intracranial pressure and neurological morbidity. In a retrospective study of 85 dogs undergoing cervical spinal decompressive surgery, respiratory arrest was a significant factor in three (42%) of seven that died of complications arising during surgery.[9]

The airway and laryngeal function should be examined during a light plane of general anesthesia or while the animal is sedated. Care must be taken to avoid excessive depression from anesthetics with resultant inhibition of respiration or laryngeal activity. A clinical investigation found that observation of laryngeal function during light anesthesia with propofol or thiopental was superior to anesthesia induced with the combination of diazepam and ketamine.[10]

Surgical procedures on the nasal airway, pharynx, larynx, or trachea can be followed by obstructive postoperative swelling. Delicate surgical technique combined with perioperative anti-inflammatory doses of corticosteroids minimize this potential. Administration of pediatric strength phenylephrine nose drops in each nostril will counteract nasal passage hyperemia, improving ventilation and often stimulating increased swallowing.

Animals with thick or copious secretions in the respiratory tract have increased risk for airway obstruction. Endotracheal intubation restricts the diameter of the trachea and increases the likelihood of airway obstruction from viscid secretions. Parti-

937

cular attention should be given to patients with small endotracheal tubes (e.g., internal diameter < 5 mm). Decreased compliance detected by difficult positive-pressure ventilation (by squeezing the rebreathing bag) in a patient with abnormal respiratory tract secretions should prompt the anesthetist to inspect the airway. Suction of secretions from the endotracheal tube may be required periodically during anesthesia. In some cases, the best solution may be to reintubate the trachea with a different endotracheal tube. Pharyngeal suction prior to anesthetic recovery from nasal, pharyngeal, or oral surgery decreases risk of aspiration of blood and debris. When regurgitated material or blood has accumulated in the pharynx, the risk of aspiration can be reduced further by gently withdrawing the endotracheal tube with the cuff partially inflated. After delivery to the pharynx, matter can be removed by suction.

Administration of oxygen should continue throughout recovery when there is risk of postoperative airway obstruction or significant respiratory depression. If obstruction develops, supplementary oxygenation increases the time available for institution of airway control. Rapid-sequence induction of anesthesia with an injectable anesthetic may be necessary to regain control of the upper airway via an endotracheal tube. After reestablishment of a secure airway, it may be possible to resolve the underlying problems and then successfully recover the patient from anesthesia. In brachycephalic animals, resection of an elongated soft palate may be necessary to prevent airway obstruction associated with tissue swelling that has developed during the procedure. In severe cases of obstruction, an emergency tracheostomy may be necessary.

Brachycephalic Airway Syndrome

Anatomical abnormalities of the upper airway in brachycephalic dogs can severely compromise their ability to ventilate adequately. The primary defects of stenotic nares, elongated soft palate, and hypoplastic trachea are exacerbated in extreme cases with eversion of laryngeal saccules and redundant pharyngeal tissues. Dogs with arytenoid cartilage, laryngeal, or tracheal collapse present similar anesthetic challenges. Reduction of the cross-sectional area of the trachea greatly increases resistance to airflow and the work of breathing. In addition, vagal tone is frequently high in brachycephalic dogs. Vagal stimulation associated with pharyngeal manipulation (difficult intubation) or vagotonic drugs can contribute to significant bradycardia and further airway narrowing. Preanesthetic administration of anticholinergic agents is indicated in these cases. The anesthetist's goals are to avoid deep sedation, especially in animals that are not continuously monitored; to intubate the trachea by using a rapid intravenous induction technique when practical; and to maintain tracheal intubation until the dog demonstrates adequate recovery from anesthesia. Anesthesia induction should be preceded by having the dog breathe oxygen through a face mask. Respiratory support during anesthesia may be required, especially in overweight animals. Obesity further impairs ventilatory function by decreasing tidal volume and functional residual capacity of the lung.

Recovery from anesthesia is judged to be adequate when a dog

strongly objects to the presence of the endotracheal tube. Reversal of the effect of opioids by naloxone administration may aid in rapid return of a dog's ability to maintain its airway. However, painful or distressed animals may experience more respiratory difficulty following extubation, so the benefits of opioid reversal should be carefully weighed against the potential complications of the increased pain and stress that may accompany reversal. Because of the presence of redundant tissue in the pharynx, most brachycephalic breeds (e.g., bulldog and shar-pei) benefit from having the anesthetist hold the dog's tongue and/or extend its neck immediately after extubation of the trachea. A source of 100% oxygen, an endotracheal tube, a laryngoscope, and an intravenous anesthetic-induction drug such as propofol should be immediately available. Ventilatory function of brachycephalic dogs should be closely monitored for at least 1 h following recovery from anesthesia.

Laryngeal Abnormalities

Abnormal laryngeal anatomy due to congenital malformation or acquired disease may affect respiration, especially during sedation. Tracheal intubation may be hindered by masses protruding into the glottis or by strands of tissue that cross the glottis. Smaller-diameter endotracheal tubes may be placed to solve this problem in some instances. However, an excessively narrow endotracheal lumen may severely affect ventilation, leading to hypercapnia or hypoxia.

Laryngospasm during the perianesthetic period occurs most frequently in cats, swine, rabbits, and primates, but has also been observed in dogs and horses. Laryngospasm may occur after irritation of laryngeal tissues by secretions or blood. Spasm of the larynx may be caused by touching the larynx during a light plane of anesthesia. Topical application of a local anesthetic such as lidocaine is recommended prior to tracheal intubation in these species to minimize tactile stimulation–induced laryngospasm. Neuromuscular blocking agents such as atracurium may be useful for preventing laryngospasm during tracheal intubation, although their use in domestic veterinary species is seldom needed. Extubation of the trachea can also trigger laryngospasm in susceptible animals. In one case, a Vietnamese potbellied pig apparently developed laryngospasm 4 h after tracheal extubation in spite of an uneventful recovery from inhalation anesthesia. Treatment of laryngospasm that occurs during tracheal extubation (or later) includes reintubation using anesthetics and neuromuscular blocking agents, if necessary. Nasotracheal intubation is an effective means of reestablishing a patent airway in some species, such as horses. Oxygen should be administered and the patient should be evaluated for subsequent development of pulmonary edema over the next 1 to 4 h. Pulmonary edema may accompany laryngospasm with clinical signs of dyspnea and tachypnea and production of pink frothy material in the airway becoming apparent during recovery from anesthesia.[11] Dogs with upper-airway obstruction can develop life-threatening pulmonary edema.[12] Factors associated with generation of pulmonary edema following airway obstruction are listed in Table 43.1. The extreme negative pressure produced by an animal with airway

Table 43.1. Factors associated with development of pulmonary edema following acute airway obstruction

Severe negative intrathoracic pressure
Decreased interstitial hydrostatic pressure
Catecholamine release
Vasoconstriction
Increased vascular hydrostatic pressure
Hypoxia
Increased permeability of pulmonary vasculature
Net accumulation of interstitial fluid
Inadequate lymphatic removal of interstitial fluid

obstruction when attempting to inspire causes decreased interstitial hydrostatic pressure in the lung. Simultaneous release of catecholamines causing increased vascular hydrostatic pressure may cause a net accumulation of interstitial fluid. Hypoxia associated with an acutely obstructed airway may promote fluid movement into the interstitial spaces by increasing permeability of pulmonary vasculature. Pulmonary edema formation after airway obstruction is probably multifactorial, so treatment is symptomatic. Oxygen supplementation to maintain an SpO_2 greater than 90%, diuretics, and corticosteroids are used to treat pulmonary edema. Emergency tracheostomy may be required to establish a patent airway rapidly. Tracheal intubation and positive-pressure ventilation are routinely used in human patients with pulmonary edema, for whom the syndrome is rarely fatal.[13,14]

Horses may develop airway obstruction during tracheal extubation after anesthesia. Potential causes include laryngospasm, paralysis of the arytenoid cartilages, and mechanical obstruction. Epiglottic retroversion has been described as a cause of upper-airway obstruction in horses.[15] Syncope as a consequence of complete upper-airway obstruction caused by a subepiglottic cyst has also been reported.[16] Laryngospasm is associated with cessation of airflow, whereas paralysis of the arytenoid cartilages is characterized by stridor and decreased airflow. Laryngospasm may result from laryngeal irritation during anesthesia and/or extubation. Paralysis of the arytenoid cartilages has been associated with poor function of the recurrent laryngeal nerve. In horses, the recurrent laryngeal nerve may be susceptible to damage by hyperextension of the neck for a prolonged period during anesthesia.[17] Postanesthetic paralysis of the arytenoid cartilages has also been observed following 2- to 4-h procedures in which a horse's trachea was intubated with an excessively large (in retrospect) endotracheal tube. Mechanical obstruction of the airway may occur during recovery from anesthesia if a horse becomes cast or positioned such that the neck is improperly flexed. Pulmonary edema following transient mechanical airway obstruction in a horse has been reported.[18] Horses anesthetized with the head lower than the body may be at risk for accumulation of fluid in laryngeal tissues. These horses may develop airway obstruction by an edematous glottis after tracheal extubation. Many anesthetists prefer to recover horses at risk for upper-airway obstruction with a nasotracheal tube in place until the horse is standing. Treatment of a horse with postanesthetic airway obstruction is initiated by placement of a nasal or oral endotracheal tube. If one of these techniques is not successful, an emergency tracheostomy is indicated. Supportive treatment includes administration of oxygen, diuretics, corticosteroids, antibiotics, and analgesics.

Mishaps Involving the Airway

Unfortunately, mishaps or accidents involving management of the airway during anesthesia increase morbidity and mortality among animal patients. It is therefore imperative that anesthetists become familiar with the anesthetic machine, ventilator, and intubating equipment available to prevent such mishaps. Vigilance in preventing excessive pressure buildup within an anesthetic circuit is required. The function of the "pop-off" valve should be continuously monitored. Sudden or unexplained increases in circuit or airway pressure should be immediately investigated. Equipment failure should be ruled out while anesthesia is maintained using a different delivery system. An unusual cause of increased inspiratory plateau pressure has been attributed to a leak in the bellows of a mechanical ventilator that allowed the driving gas of the bellows to enter the breathing circuit.[19] Increased airway pressure may also occur from development of tension pneumothorax.

Venipuncture has also been associated with airway obstruction caused by iatrogenic trauma to vital structures in the neck. Injury of the recurrent laryngeal nerve may cause temporary paralysis of the arytenoid cartilage in horses. Aspiration pneumonia secondary to choke caused by a periesophageal hematoma following jugular venipuncture has been reported in a llama.[20]

Airway obstruction has occurred in intubated patients following administration of nitrous oxide, which may diffuse into the air-filled endotracheal tube cuff, causing increased cuff pressure and endotracheal tube collapse.[21] Overexpansion of the endotracheal tube cuff when administering nitrous oxide may be prevented by filling the cuff with an appropriate nitrous oxide–oxygen mixture (i.e., gas aspirated from the breathing circuit) rather than with air. Nitrous oxide may also diffuse into small bubbles of air found in some endotracheal tubes as a manufacturing defect. Expansion of these air bubbles with nitrous oxide has caused airway obstruction in guarded endotracheal tubes (those with a spiral wire used to prevent kinking of the tube).[22] Prior to use, endotracheal tubes should be examined for material defects such as presence of air bubbles that contraindicate administration of nitrous oxide.

Inadvertent displacement of the endotracheal tube may cause airway obstruction. Subtle changes in position of the endotracheal tube may occur during radiography or surgical positioning. Flexion of the neck of anesthetized dogs has resulted in caudal displacement, endobronchial placement, or total occlusion of the endotracheal tube.[23]

References

1. Nagashima H, Karamanian A, Malovany R, et al. Respiratory and circulatory effects of intravenous butorphanol and morphine. Clin Pharmacol Ther 19:738–745, 1976.

2. Copland VS, Haskins SC, Patz J. Naloxone reversal of oxymorphone effects in dogs. Am J Vet Res 50:1854–1858, 1989.

3. Michealis LL, Hickey PR, Clark TA, et al. Ventricular irritability associated with the use of naloxone hydrochloride. Ann Thorac Surg 18:608–614, 1974.

4. Andree RA. Sudden death following naloxone administration. Anesth Analg 59:782–784, 1980.

5. McCrackin MA, Harvey RC, Sackman JE, et al. Butorphanol tartrate for partial reversal of oxymorphone-induced postoperative respiratory depression in the dog. Vet Surg 23:67–74, 1994.

6. Thompson SE, Johnson JM. Analgesia in dogs after intercostal thoracotomy: Comparison of morphine, selective intercostal nerve block, and intrapleural regional analgesia with bupivacaine. Vet Surg 20:73–77, 1991.

7. Valverde A, Dyson DH, Cockshutt JR, et al. Comparison of the hemodynamic effects of halothane alone and halothane combined with epidurally administered morphine for anesthesia in ventilated dogs. Am J Vet Res 52:505–509, 1991.

8. Valverde A, Dyson DH, McDonell WN, Pascoe PJ. Use of epidural morphine in the dog for pain relief. Vet Comp Orthop Traumatol 2:55–58, 1989.

9. Clark DM. An analysis of intraoperative and early postoperative mortality associated with cervical spinal decompressive surgery in the dog. J Am Anim Hosp Assoc 22:739–744, 1986.

10. Gross ME, Dodam JR, Pope ER, et al. A comparison of thiopental, propofol, and diazepam-ketamine anesthesia for evaluation of laryngeal function in dogs premedicated with butorphanol-glycopyrrolate. J Am Anim Hosp Assoc 38:503–506, 2002.

11. Glasser SA, Siler JN. Delayed onset of laryngospasm-induced pulmonary edema in an adult outpatient. Anesthesiology 62:370–371, 1985.

12. Kerr LY. Pulmonary edema secondary to upper airway obstruction in the dog: A review of nine cases. J Am Anim Hosp Assoc 25:207–212, 1989.

13. Tobin MJ. Advances in mechanical ventilation. N Engl J Med 344:1986–1996, 2001.

14. Haskins SC, King LG. Positive pressure ventilation. In: King LG, ed. Textbook of Respiratory Disease of Dogs and Cats. Philadelphia: WB Saunders, 2004:217–229.

15. Parente EJ, Martin BB, Tulleners EP. Epiglottic retroversion as a cause of upper airway obstruction in two horses. Equine Vet J 30:270–272, 1998.

16. Hay WP, Baskett A, Abdy MJ. Complete upper airway obstruction and syncope caused by a subepiglottic cyst in a horse. Equine Vet J 29:75–76, 1997.

17. Abrahamsen EJ, Bohanon TC, Bednarski RM, et al. Bilateral arytenoid cartilage paralysis after inhalation anesthesia in a horse. J Am Vet Med Assoc 197:1363–1365, 1990.

18. Kollias-Baker CA, Pipers FS, Heard D, Seeherman H. Pulmonary edema associated with transient airway obstruction in three horses. J Am Vet Med Assoc 202:1116–1118, 1993.

19. Klein LV, Wilson DV. An unusual cause of increasing airway pressure during anesthesia. Vet Surg 18:239–241, 1989.

20. Weldon AD, Beck KA. Identifying a periesophageal hematoma as the cause of choke in a llama. Vet Med 88:1009–1011, 1993.

21. Komatsu H, Mitsuhata H, Hasegawa J, Matsumoto S. Decreased pressure of endotracheal tube cuff in general anesthesia without nitrous oxide [in Japanese]. Masui 42:831–834, 1993.

22. Populaire C, Robard S, Souron R. An armoured endotracheal tube obstruction in a child. Can J Anaesth 36:331–332, 1989.

23. Quandt JE, Robinson EP, Walter PA, Raffe MR. Endotracheal tube displacement during cervical manipulation in the dog. Vet Surg 22:235–239, 1993.

Section VIII
ANESTHESIA AND ANALGESIA FOR SELECTED PATIENTS AND PROCEDURES

Chapter 44
Ocular Patients

Marjorie E. Gross and Elizabeth A. Giuliano

General Considerations

Development of an appropriate anesthetic protocol for any ocular patient should include not only drug selection, but also a perioperative management plan to provide an optimal postoperative outcome. This requires knowledge of not only the patient's physical status and the ophthalmic procedure to be performed, but also familiarity with ocular physiology and current medications administered for ophthalmic purposes.

Ocular and periocular structures are often neglected during anesthesia induction. Positioning of hands and equipment relative to the eyes should be noted during induction, especially when dealing with severely compromised globes with the potential to rupture. Mask induction may not be an option if the mask rubs or presses on the eye, and a patient's struggling during induction with a face mask may increase intraocular pressure (IOP) or potentiate eye rupture. Similarly, nasotracheal intubation in awake foals requires heavy restraint and is accompanied by coughing and gagging, which may increase IOP and further compromise the globe. Providing analgesia is particularly important in ophthalmic patients with substantial discomfort from their primary ophthalmic disease. These patients may be more inclined to struggle when restrained, which may result in increased IOP and additional damage to the globe during induction.

Horses with a nonvisual eye should be approached from the visual side. If approach from the nonvisual side is necessary, it should be accompanied by words of reassurance and gentle hand contact, which should be maintained until induction is complete. Movement of equine patients to lateral recumbency after induction should include careful control of the head to prevent additional trauma to the eyes. It has been suggested that ventral positioning of the head relative to the body during transport causes venous stasis and increased IOP. These effects may be responsible for intraocular hemorrhage observed shortly after induction in horses with traumatized eyes.[1] Supporting the head to keep it level with the body is recommended to avoid such an occurrence.

Protection of the dependent, nonaffected eye should also be considered during positioning of patients. Corneal protection of the eye not operated on in unilateral procedures may be afforded by application of corneal lubrication with or without a temporary tarsorrhaphy. Positioning of the patient's head and application of any topical ophthalmic preparations should be coordinated between the anesthesiology personnel and ophthalmologist to ensure the best possible surgical outcome when both eyes are to be operated on. Collapse of the anterior chamber of the dependent eye, possibly resulting from increased aqueous outflow caused by physical pressure on the globe, has been reported in birds positioned in lateral recumbency. The anterior chamber was reestablished within a few minutes of repositioning.[2] Resting the periocular region of the dependent eye on a soft padded eye ring or "doughnut" may help protect the eye from corneal abrasion and external globe compression that may result in hypotony.

Laryngeal stimulation should be minimized and endotracheal intubation accomplished as smoothly as possible to avoid any possible increases in IOP.[1] Lidocaine applied topically to the larynx, or administered intravenously (1.0 mg/kg), may be helpful in suppressing the cough reflex.[3] In people, the anesthesia-related practices most likely to increase IOP significantly (i.e., at least 10 to 20 mm Hg) are laryngoscopy and endotracheal intubation.[4–6] Although the mechanism is not clear, it has been suggested that it is related to sympathetic cardiovascular responses to laryngeal stimulation. The occurrence of increases in IOP during endotracheal intubation has not been clearly established in veterinary patients.

Positioning for the ophthalmic procedure may render ocular patients less accessible for anesthetic monitoring, and maintaining their appropriate level of anesthesia may become very difficult. Eye reflexes, jaw tone, and oral mucous membranes will not be assessable, although the ophthalmologist may be able to provide information about eye position and movements. Once the head has been surgically draped, the airway also becomes inaccessible. A guarded (i.e., wire reinforced) endotracheal tube is recommended to prevent unobservable kinking and occlusion of the airway during surgical positioning. Capnography may be useful for detection of an obstructed airway or inadvertent disconnection from the anesthetic delivery system. Similarly, pulse oximetry may help detect desaturation should the endotracheal tube become kinked or the delivery system disconnected. However, the pulse oximeter may have to be placed somewhere other than on the tongue, which would put it in close proximity to the surgical field, where movement by the ophthalmologist may interfere with its function.

Monitoring heart rate (HR) and arterial blood pressure (BP) becomes essential in ocular patients when other types of monitoring are limited and are particularly important when including neuromuscular blocking agents (NMBs) in the anesthetic protocol. Preventing movement during ophthalmic procedures and facilitation of eye positioning may be accomplished by using NMBs to paralyze patients, but the inability of patients to indicate inadequate anesthesia with movement makes monitoring all the more crucial. Increased BP or HR may indicate an inadequate plane of anesthesia or the need for additional analgesics. Conversely, precipitous decreases in HR or BP may indicate too deep a plane of anesthesia or initiation of the oculocardiac reflex (OCR). Increased respiration rate may also be indicative of inadequate anesthesia, but such a response may not be evident in mechanically ventilated or paralyzed patients.

Tear production decreases during general anesthesia in people, dogs, horses, and possibly other species.[7–10] Tear production in dogs decreases from baseline values within 10 to 15 min after subcutaneous administration of atropine and continues to decline after induction of general anesthesia with halothane or methoxyflurane. Indeed, within 30 to 60 min of onset of general anesthesia, tear production in dogs can approach negligible amounts regardless of whether atropine was administered before surgery. In a comparison of preanesthetic and postanesthetic Schirmer tear test values in dogs, significant decreases in tear production were evident for up to 24 h after the anesthetic procedure. Anticholinergic administration before or during anesthesia further decreased the postanesthetic Schirmer tear test values.[11] Based on drug-retention studies in humans, it has been suggested that canine eyes be lubricated every 90 min during general anesthesia.[7] A study comparing the effects of sedative and opioid combinations on tear production in dogs determined that acepromazine-oxymorphone, diazepam-butorphanol, and xylazine-butorphanol significantly decreased tear production (80%, 68%, and 33% of baseline, respectively).[12] Xylazine alone did not significantly decrease tear production. Butorphanol alone did significantly decrease tear production, but when xylazine and butorphanol were combined, the decrease in tear production was greater than that observed with butorphanol alone. This suggests that xylazine and butorphanol act synergistically to decrease tear production in dogs.

Transient lens opacification may occur in rodents, such as mice, rats, and hamsters, during prolonged sedation or anesthesia. The opacification is believed to be caused by lack of blinking and subsequent evaporation of fluids from the shallow anterior chamber, which then resolves upon awakening.[13]

In horses undergoing general anesthesia, tear production is reduced much less dramatically than in dogs. Normal tear production was restored within 3 h in horses undergoing halothane anesthesia.[9] Although this may suggest that ocular lubrication may not be necessary to prevent corneal drying in horses, it is recommended that ocular lubrication be instilled in the eyes of all patients undergoing anesthesia. A flash fire involving ophthalmic ointment during anesthesia with nitrous oxide and oxygen has been reported,[14] but a later study concluded that ophthalmic ointments do not offer a significant fire hazard.[15] If intraocular surgery is planned or globe rupture has occurred, application of topical ophthalmic medications or lubrication should be restricted to aqueous-based formulations. Petroleum-based ointments that gain access to intraocular structures may cause severe uveitis and further compromise vision and ocular comfort. Taping the palpebrae closed or a partial temporary tarsorrhaphy are additional techniques for protecting the globe and keeping it moist.[1]

A smooth anesthetic recovery, including appropriate analgesia and prevention of self-trauma, is the primary postoperative management goal. For patients who have undergone intraocular surgery, periods of excitement, incoordination, coughing, gagging, or retching are particularly undesirable. Recovery should be in a quiet, dimly lit enclosure where external stimuli will be kept to a minimum. Patients can be kept comfortable and quiet by appropriate analgesia and sedation, although minimal physical restraint or words of reassurance while holding some small patients may be more effective. Elizabethan collars for small patients and padded helmets or protective eyecups for large patients may help protect their eyes, but may not be readily tolerated by some. Recovery cages or stalls should have extraneous structures, such as feed-bowl rings, removed to prevent eye trauma during recovery.

Physiological Considerations

Ocular Physiology

Selection of an anesthetic protocol for intraocular surgery should include consideration of the effects on IOP, pupil size, and globe position.[1]

Intraocular Pressure

Success of an ophthalmic procedure may depend on control of IOP before, during, and after the procedure. The overall effect of most anesthetics is to decrease IOP.[15] This reduction may be attributable to a combination of factors, including depression of diencephalic centers regulating IOP, increased aqueous outflow, decreased venous and arterial BPs, and relaxation of extraocular musculature.[16] Many of the factors affecting IOP are listed in Table 44.1.

IOP is determined by aqueous humor dynamics, intraocular (choroidal) blood volume, central venous pressure, and extraocular muscle tone.[16] Normal range of IOP has been reported for dogs (10 to 26 mm Hg), cats (12 to 32 mm Hg), and horses

Table 44.1. Factors altering intraocular pressure.

Altering Factors	Change in IOP	Comments
Blockade of aqueous outflow	↑	Caused by any position or maneuver that increases CVP
Acute increase in arterial pressure	↑	Causes only a transient increase in IOP
Hypoventilation, airway obstruction, hypercapnia, choroidal vessel dilatation	↑	
Hyperventilation, hypocapnia	↓	
Endotracheal intubation	↑	Topical or IV lidocaine may prevent coughing, gagging, straining
Eyeball pressure	↑	Caused by face mask, orbital tumors, surgical traction, eyeball position, retrobulbar injection
Anesthetic drugs		
Barbiturates	↓	May depress central control of IOP or promote aqueous outflow
Propofol	↓	May prevent intubation-associated increase in IOP; may suppress depolarizing NMB-induced increase in IOP
Etomidate	↑	May be predominantly due to etomidate-induced myoclonus
Ketamine	↑ or ↓	Contradictory; effect may depend on premedication
α_2-Agonists	↓	Induces bradycardia, may promote OCR; may induce vomiting; may suppress sympathetic input and aqueous production
Benzodiazepines	↓	May be in response to central relaxation of ocular muscles
Acepromazine	↓	Decreases arterial blood pressure, suppresses retching and vomiting
Opioids	↓	IOP may increase with opioid-induced vomiting or retching
Neuromuscular blockers		
Depolarizing		
Succinylcholine	↑	Transient increase in IOP
Nondepolarizing	↓	Decrease or no effect
Pancuronium		
Vecuronium		
Atracurium		
Other drugs		
Methazolamide	↓	Carbonic anhydrase inhibitor; decreases formation of aqueous humor
Hypertonic solutions (mannitol)	↓	Increases plasma osmotic pressure, decrease aqueous humor formation
Phenylephrine	↑ or ↓	Effect is dosage dependent
Epinephrine	↑ or ↓	Effect is dosage dependent

CVP, central venous pressure; IOP, intraocular pressure; IV, intravenous; NMB, neuromuscular blocking agent; and OCR, oculocardiac reflex. Modified from Thurmon et al.,[3] p. 814.

(mean, 23.5 to 28.6 mm Hg).[17–19] For intraocular surgery, a low normal IOP is desirable.[5] Lens or vitreous prolapse, expulsive choroidal hemorrhage, and subsequent retinal detachment are possible sequelae to increased IOP during or after intraocular surgery or in patients with penetrating eye wounds.[5]

Normal IOP depends on the delicate balance between aqueous inflow (production) and aqueous outflow (filtration).[1,16] Obstruction of outflow, which may dramatically increase IOP, may be induced by coughing, retching, vomiting, excessive restraint of the head and neck, or any maneuver or position that increases central venous pressure.[5] Indeed, coughing may increase IOP by as much as 40 mm Hg.[20]

Aqueous humor is produced primarily by the ciliary body. It flows from the posterior chamber anteriorly through the pupil into the anterior chamber. Most of the aqueous humor exits the anterior chamber via the filtration angle of the eye, following a pattern of flow referred to as *conventional outflow*.[1] In conven-

tional outflow, aqueous humor enters the venous vascular system via the scleral venous plexus (analogous to Schlemm's canal in humans), drains into the vortex veins, passes through the orbital vasculature, and ultimately enters the episcleral venous system. The small percentage of aqueous humor that exits the anterior chamber via diffusion through iris stroma and ciliary body musculature is referred to as uveoscleral or *unconventional outflow*. In unconventional outflow, aqueous humor flows caudally to enter the suprachoroidal space and ultimately, the scleral and choroidal vasculature.[1]

Intraocular (choroidal) blood volume is determined by arterial inflow, venous outflow, and tone of the intraocular vasculature.[6] Autoregulation of choroidal blood flow minimizes the effects of arterial BP on choroidal blood volume and IOP. Sudden increases in systolic arterial BP may cause a transient increase in choroidal blood volume and IOP, but a temporary increase in outflow will adjust IOP back to normal. Sudden increases in choroidal blood volume may also displace the vitreous forward into the anterior chamber during intraocular surgery or in patients with penetrating eye wounds. Marked IOP reductions may occur when systolic arterial pressure decreases below 90 mm Hg and choroidal blood volume decreases.[5]

A more direct, definitive relationship exists between central venous pressure and IOP.[16] Increases in central venous pressure can increase IOP and choroidal blood volume by diminishing aqueous-humor outflow into the venous system.[5] To maintain normal central venous pressure and IOP in humans, a slightly head-up position is preferred for patients undergoing intraocular surgery.[6]

Choroidal blood volume and consequently IOP increase in response to increases in $PaCO_2$ and decreases in PaO_2.[21] Hypercapnia and hypoxemia induce vasodilatation, which increases intraocular blood volume accompanied by an increase in IOP. Conversely, respiratory alkalosis and hyperbaric oxygen conditions induce vasoconstriction and decreased aqueous-humor formation through reduced carbonic anhydrase activity, which decrease choroidal blood volume and IOP.[21] In anesthetized dogs, inspired concentrations of 5% CO_2 caused a mean increase in IOP of 35.2%. Concentrations of 10% to 15% CO_2 increased IOP even higher.[21] There is no apparent correlation between increased $PaCO_2$ and IOP in anesthetized horses.[22] Unlike other species, horses have a greater dependence on unconventional outflow of aqueous humor, which may result in a more constant IOP during hypercapnia.

Vitreous has been described as a hydrogel consisting of a loose fibrillar network of collagen that supports the lens anteriorly and the retina posteriorly.[1] Although the vitreous volume is fairly constant, it may be decreased by administration of hyperosmotic agents, such as mannitol or glycerin. As indicated previously, vitreous may be displaced by changes in intraocular blood volume, but also by extraocular and orbicularis oculi muscle contractions. Muscle contractions and vitreous displacement that occur during an intraocular surgery, or with a penetrating eye wound, may cause expulsion of intraocular contents. Closure of the palpebrae may increase IOP anywhere from 10 to 50 mm Hg, depending on whether the closure is normal or forceful.[6]

Pupil Size

In mammals, iris musculature that controls pupil size is smooth muscle and is controlled primarily by the autonomic nervous system.[23] Parasympathetic stimulation of the iris constrictor muscle results in miosis (pupil constriction), and sympathetic stimulation of the iris dilator muscle results in mydriasis (pupillary dilation). In contrast, avian species have striated pupillary muscles, which are unresponsive to topically applied parasympatholytic or sympathomimetic agents.[24]

Pupils are inaccessible for anesthesia monitoring during ophthalmic surgery. Although the ophthalmologist may be able to provide information about pupil size during the procedure, pupil size as an indicator of anesthetic depth is not reliable.[25,26] Pupil size is of greatest concern in cataract-removal surgery, which requires the pupil to be widely dilated and the eye immobilized. Most anesthetic or sedative agents, with the exception of keta-

mine, will cause miosis.[1] Opioids have variable effects on pupil size among species[27,28] and may adversely affect the mydriasis required for cataract surgery.[29] An intramuscular combination of hydromorphone-acepromazine caused significant miosis in dogs at 10 and 25 min after injection.[30] Administration of opioid antagonists (i.e., naloxone) may reverse miosis when it occurs.[31] Prostaglandins, histamines, and other mediators of inflammation may cause miosis by a direct effect on the iris constrictor muscle.[26,32] Consequently, antiprostaglandins and antihistamines may be administered prior to intraocular surgery. Sympathomimetic, cholinergic, and anticholinergic drugs applied topically to the eye will affect pupil size. It has been suggested that mydriasis is more difficult to achieve after the onset of sedation or anesthesia,[29] whereas mydriasis achieved prior to anesthetic induction or sedation is usually unaffected by the miotic properties of anesthetic and sedative drugs.[1]

Globe Position

Globe motion during general anesthesia is not unusual, and position of the globe may vary among species and stages of anesthesia. However, motion is undesirable during corneal and intraocular surgery. Excessive manual traction to maintain a stable globe position may cause expulsion of intraocular contents or initiation of the OCR. In addition, eye reflexes that may be maintained during anesthesia in some species may also interfere with procedures. Paralysis with NMBs or retrobulbar regional anesthesia during general anesthesia should eliminate ocular reflexes and enable positioning of the globe without excessive manual traction, reducing the potential for expulsion of globe contents or initiation of the OCR.

Cardiovascular Physiology

Ocular patients are often elderly, with all the attendant problems associated with aging, such as loss of physiological reserve, preexisting disease, and chronic medication administration. The depth of anesthesia required for adequate depression of ocular reflexes and globe motion to facilitate intraocular surgery often results in pronounced hypotension and may represent additional risk for elderly patients.[3] Prolonged hypotension may predispose large animal patients to postanesthetic myopathy.[33] Balanced anesthesia combined with adjunctive anesthetic techniques, such as regional anesthesia or neuromuscular blockade, may allow a decrease in depth of inhalation anesthesia and a closer approximation of normal cardiovascular function.[3]

Oculocardiac Reflex

The OCR is a trigeminovagal (cranial nerves V and X) reflex that may be induced by pressure or traction on the eyeball, ocular trauma or pain, or orbital hematoma. Initiation of the reflex manifests as cardiac arrhythmias, which may include bradycardia, nodal rhythms, ectopic beats, ventricular fibrillation, or asystole.[16] The afferent pathway of the reflex follows ciliary nerves to the ciliary ganglion and then along the ophthalmic division of the trigeminal nerve. The afferent pathway terminates in the main trigeminal sensory nucleus in the floor of the fourth ventricle. The efferent pathway starts in the fibers of the vagal cardiac depressor nerve, resulting in negative inotropic and conduction effects. Although OCR may occur most commonly during ocular surgery, it may also occur during nonocular surgery when pressure is placed on the eyeball.[16] It has been suggested that the more acute the onset, and the more sustained the pressure or traction, the more likely OCR is to occur. In people, OCR occurs most frequently during strabismus surgery in children and may be related to the degree of traction necessary to expose the medial rectus muscle during surgery.[16] Hypercapnia significantly increases the incidence of bradycardia in these patients.

Atropine administration to prevent or treat the OCR is controversial in humans.[16] Cardiac dysrhythmias may occur after atropine administration, especially in the presence of halothane, and may persist longer than the OCR response. In children, intravenous (IV) atropine or glycopyrrolate were more effective in preventing OCR than was intramuscular premedication with atropine, with glycopyrrolate producing less of a tachycardic effect than atropine.[34]

Bradycardia is the most common manifestation of OCR, although other dysrhythmias are possible, as already mentioned. Treatment of OCR should begin with discontinuing stimulation. The OCR ceases when stimulation ceases, so communication with the surgeon to discontinue procedural stimulation is vital if an OCR is suspected. Fortunately, it is possible for the OCR to fatigue with repeated, prolonged stimulation.[16] If bradycardia persists, treatment with atropine (0.02 mg/kg IV), or injection of lidocaine into the eye muscles to prevent transmission along the afferent limb of the reflex, may be effective.[3] Precautions against initiation of the OCR should include assuring an adequate depth of anesthesia, maintaining normocarbia, and gentleness of surgical manipulation.[16]

Ophthalmic Medications

Eyedrops are concentrated medications that may cause systemic side effects, especially when administered to very small patients. Systemic effects may be minimized by diluting topical medications and limiting their frequency of application.[4,16]

Cholinergic Agents

Glaucoma may be treated with cholinergic agents that decrease IOP primarily by increasing aqueous outflow. Direct-acting cholinergic agents are similar in structure to acetylcholine and produce effects similar to acetylcholine when absorbed systemically. Indirect-acting cholinergic agents are anticholinesterases. These facilitate the buildup of acetylcholine by slowing its enzymatic hydrolysis. Pilocarpine is a topical, direct-acting cholinergic agent commonly used in the treatment of glaucoma and may produce bradycardia or atrioventricular block if absorbed systemically.[1] These dysrhythmias may be similar to, and difficult to distinguish from, those produced by the OCR.[35] As mentioned in the section on neuromuscular blocking agents, to prevent prolongation of depolarizing neuromuscular blockade, anticholinesterase administration should be discontinued 2 to 4 weeks prior to succinylcholine administration.[35]

Adrenergic Agents

Adrenergic agonists and antagonists are both used to treat glaucoma. Although the exact mechanisms for decreasing IOP are not clear, it is believed that the agonists primarily increase aqueous-humor outflow, whereas the antagonists primarily decrease aqueous humor production.[1] Adrenergic agonists, such as epinephrine or dipivefrin, may predispose patients to catecholamine-induced cardiac dysrhythmias. Topical application of adrenergic agonists has been associated with increased HR and BP in people.[36]

Phenylephrine is an adrenergic agonist that is used to produce mydriasis prior to cataract surgery or in patients with uveitis. Subconjunctival phenylephrine has been associated with hypertension and pulmonary edema in a horse during anesthetic recovery.[33] In dogs undergoing cataract surgery, topical treatment with phenylephrine has been associated with arterial hypertension.[37] Topical application of 10% phenylephrine increased arterial BP and reflex bradycardia in normal dogs.[38] It has been suggested that the susceptibility of patients to the adverse effects of topically applied phenylephrine during anesthesia depends on several factors, including individual variability, frequency of application, concentration of the solution, and the anesthetic regimen.[39] Acepromazine may be useful in counteracting the hypertension produced by phenylephrine.[37,39]

Timolol, a nonselective ß-adrenergic antagonist that is commonly used to treat glaucoma, has been associated with more adverse systemic effects in people than have any other topically applied glaucoma medications.[40] Systemic effects in people may include bradycardia, hypotension, congestive heart failure, and exacerbation of asthma and myasthenia gravis.[16] Profound bradycardia has been observed in dogs after topical administration. Significant decreases in HR and BP have been observed in anesthetized dogs within 30 min of topical timolol administration.[41] Decreased IOP in both the ipsilateral and the contralateral eyes further substantiated systemic absorption of the drug. Timolol administration is contraindicated in animals with heart block, cardiac failure, or obstructive pulmonary disease.[41]

Carbonic Anhydrase Inhibitors

These inhibitors, such as methazolamide, decrease IOP by decreasing aqueous-humor production.[42] Carbonic anhydrase is found in other tissues besides the eyes, most notably the red blood cells and kidneys.[42,43] Administration of systemic carbonic anhydrase inhibitors impacts ion exchange in the kidneys, resulting in the retention of chloride and the excretion of bicarbonate and potassium. Treated patients may have metabolic acidosis and electrolyte imbalances, most notably hypokalemia and hyperchloremia. Some carbonic anhydrase inhibitors cause profound potassium excretion, as evidenced by the presence of hypokalemia despite metabolic acidosis that would typically be accompanied by hyperkalemia.[43]

Acidosis and electrolyte imbalances may disrupt cardiovascular and neurological function. Hyperventilation would typically occur during metabolic acidosis as a compensatory mechanism, but hypoventilation during anesthesia may exacerbate the metabolic acidosis by inducing respiratory acidosis.[44] Acidosis may increase the potential for cardiac dysrhythmias during anesthesia.

Ideally, metabolic acidosis and electrolyte imbalance would be corrected prior to anesthesia, and ventilatory support would be provided to prevent significant respiratory acidosis.

Osmotic Agents

Examples of osmotic agents for treatment of glaucoma include mannitol and glycerin. These agents are usually used to produce a rapid decrease in IOP in patients with acute or subacute glaucoma, and are usually administered immediately prior to surgery. Increased central venous pressure, increased serum osmolality, and pulmonary edema have been reported in dogs treated with mannitol.[45,46] The increase in osmolality may last for several hours. Although clinical pulmonary edema was not evident, histological evidence of pulmonary edema has been reported for dogs that received mannitol during methoxyflurane anesthesia.[47] It was suggested that pulmonary edema was less likely in patients being mechanically ventilated when compared with patients breathing spontaneously. Osmotic agents are not recommended in patients with preexisting cardiac or pulmonary disease, renal dysfunction, or dehydration.[1]

Corticosteroids

Prolonged topical eye or systemic administration of corticosteroids may depress adrenocortical function.[48,49] The need for corticosteroid supplementation in these patients prior to the stress of surgery and anesthesia has not been clearly determined. If hypoadrenocorticism is present, corticosteroids may be administered prior to anesthesia and surgery.[50,51] It should be remembered that the coadministration of corticosteroids and NSAIDs may exacerbate the toxicity of both classes of drugs.

Anesthetic Drugs

Inhalation Agents

Inhaled anesthetics reduce IOP proportional to the depth of anesthesia in human patients during controlled ventilation and normocapnia. Reductions of 14% to 50% have been noted.[16] Methoxyflurane has historically been the inhalation anesthetic preferred by ophthalmologists. It was believed to provide greater extraocular muscle relaxation, as well as a hypotonic and centrally rotated eye.[50,52] Additionally, the slower recovery from anesthesia was preferred for ocular patients. Methoxyflurane is no longer commonly used in veterinary patients. It has been replaced with halothane, isoflurane, and sevoflurane, which provide rapid induction and recovery. Rapid recovery, however, potentially increases the risk of iatrogenic trauma or intraocular bleeding. Appropriate preoperative or postoperative medication should be used to provide a slower, calmer recovery.

In human adults, halothane decreases IOP, but in a manner that is not dose dependent and has a ceiling effect.[53] Isoflurane effects on IOP are similar to those of halothane.[53] Halothane sensitizes the heart to catecholamines,[54] which may become problematic in ocular patients that receive topical adrenergic drugs. It is not unusual for ophthalmic surgeons to administer intraocular epinephrine to dilate the pupil and control intraocular bleeding during surgery. Epinephrine may be readily absorbed through oc-

ular vasculature and produce systemic effects, such as cardiac tachydysrhythmias or premature ventricular beats, which may be exacerbated by halothane. In dogs and cats, the dysrhythmogenic dose of epinephrine is much higher when used with isoflurane,[54] possibly making it the preferred inhalation agent when used with exogenously administered catecholamines. It has been suggested that extraocular muscle relaxation and position of the globe are superior with isoflurane, but the information is anecdotal.[33]

Although there is little information on the ocular effects of sevoflurane in veterinary patients, it is presumed to have effects on the eye similar to those of halothane and isoflurane. In humans undergoing nonophthalmic surgery, IOP was decreased equally in those patients receiving sevoflurane when compared with those receiving propofol.[55] In patients undergoing elective ophthalmic surgery, IOP did not increase during sevoflurane and remifentanil anesthesia in response to tracheal intubation or laryngeal mask airway insertion.[56]

Nitrous oxide (N_2O) administration is contraindicated when intraocular gas or air injection is intended for a closed eye.[35,57] Air is sometimes injected into the anterior chamber of the eye to prevent synechia formation after corneal laceration or staphyloma repair. N_2O may diffuse into the intraocular air bubble, causing it to expand faster than the air can diffuse out, thereby increasing IOP. Sulfur hexafluoride (SF_6) may be injected into the vitreous space in retinal reattachment surgery and may expand to undesirable dimensions in conjunction with N_2O administration, resulting in increased IOP. It is recommended that if intraocular gas injection is intended in a closed eye, that N_2O be discontinued at least 15 to 20 min prior to injection. For repeat anesthetic episodes, it is also recommended that N_2O not be administered for at least 5 days after intraocular air injections and for 10 days after SF_6 injection.[35,57]

Injectable Anesthetic Agents and Adjuncts
Anticholinergic Agents

Administration of atropine or glycopyrrolate to canine ophthalmic patients is controversial.[50,58,59] One potential benefit is preventing the OCR, but anticholinergic administration may be undesirable in the presence of preexisting tachycardia. Conversely, anticholinergic administration may be appropriate in patients with preexisting bradycardia, or with concurrent administration of injectable drugs that may induce bradycardia (i.e., opioids and α_2-agonists). Cannulation of the parotid duct may be more difficult during parotid duct transposition surgery if anticholinergics are administered preoperatively.[60] The potential for colic in horses contraindicates the routine administration of anticholinergics.

Topically applied atropine produces cycloplegia, which decreases aqueous filtration, and mydriasis, which predisposes patients to filtration angle closure. Both of these effects will increase IOP in dogs and people with glaucoma, but the effects of systemically administered anticholinergics on pupil size and IOP are not clear. In people, systemically administered atropine or glycopyrrolate has no effect on IOP in normal patients, and atropine has no effect on IOP in people with glaucoma.[59,61] Atropine administered with neostigmine to reverse nondepolarizing neuromuscular blockade does not seem to increase IOP.[16]

Glycopyrrolate administered parenterally had no effect on pupil size or IOP in normal dogs, but the effects of atropine under similar circumstances was not investigated.[61] In a retrospective study of glaucomatous dogs, anticholinergic administration did not adversely affect IOP, but only 30% of the dogs in the study had received anticholinergic treatment.[61] It has been suggested that glycopyrrolate may have a lesser effect on pupil size and IOP than does atropine. This effect may be due to poor cellular penetration of end organs by quaternary ammonium compounds, such as glycopyrrolate, when compared with the tertiary amines, such as atropine. Consequently, the use of glycopyrrolate may be preferred in glaucoma patients requiring anticholinergic treatment.[59]

Barbiturates and Propofol

Thiopental and pentobarbital decrease IOP.[5,6] The mechanism for reduction is believed to be depression of the areas of the central nervous system (diencephalon) influencing IOP, and facilitation of aqueous outflow.[16] Thiopental decreases IOP in both normal and glaucomatous eyes.

Although chemically dissimilar, propofol has clinical properties similar to those of thiobarbiturates.[62] Studies in humans indicate that propofol decreases IOP and may negate the increase in IOP associated with intubation or the administration of depolarizing NMBs.[62] The effect of propofol on IOP in children is similar to that of thiopental during induction of general anesthesia.[63]

Etomidate

Although etomidate decreases IOP, etomidate-associated myoclonus may actually increase IOP.[3,16] It is recommended that etomidate not be used alone for induction, but rather in conjunction with a benzodiazepine muscle relaxant (i.e., diazepam or midazolam) in patients with penetrating eye wounds.

Dissociative Anesthetics

The effects of the dissociative anesthetics in ophthalmic patients are contradictory, both for human and veterinary patients. In people, early studies indicate that ketamine increases IOP, but ketamine does not affect IOP when administered after diazepam and meperidine. When administered intramuscularly, ketamine may even lower IOP in children.[5]

Ketamine induces extraocular muscle contractions, which may increase IOP in some species.[50,64] In horses, but not in dogs, prior administration of xylazine attenuates the increase in IOP.[64,65] In patients with the potential for globe rupture, such as a penetrating eye wound or deep corneal ulcer, the extraocular muscle contractions and increases in IOP are undesirable, suggesting that the use of ketamine should be avoided in patients when rupture of the globe is a concern.

Ketamine causes nystagmus, which may persist even when combined with xylazine, making ketamine unacceptable as the sole anesthetic for ophthalmic procedures.[50,65] The palpebrae remain open, the pupils dilate, and the palpebrae and corneal reflexes persist after ketamine administration.[25,66] Ocular reflexes also persist after administration of the anesthetic combination of tiletamine, a dissociative anesthetic, and the benzodiazepine zolazepam. Ketamine does not appear to decrease tear production in cats,[67] but the palpebrae remain open, which allows corneal drying and necessitates application of an ocular lubricant. Recoveries from ketamine administration can be very prolonged and uncoordinated, predisposing patients to ocular trauma.[50]

α_2-Adrenergic Agonists

Intramuscularly administered xylazine causes dogs and cats to vomit. Vomiting is less likely when xylazine is administered IV, but the potential still exists.[68] Consequently, xylazine should be used cautiously in patients with penetrating eye wounds.

Xylazine produces mydriasis in some species, possibly by inhibiting central parasympathetic tone to the iris or through stimulation of α_2-adrenoceptors located in the iris.[69] In cats, rabbits, and monkeys, it has been reported that xylazine decreases IOP by depressing sympathetic function and decreasing aqueous production.[70] In horses, two studies determined that IOP could be decreased by 23% with the administration of 0.3 mg/kg xylazine IV and by 27% with the administration of 1.0 mg/kg xylazine IV.[71,72]

Systemically administered xylazine may cause acute reversible lens opacity in rats and mice.[73] Topical application of xylazine produces cataract formation in the treated eye, whereas the contralateral eye remains unaffected. The mechanism for this effect is unknown. As mentioned previously, xylazine does not reduce tear production in dogs, but the combination of xylazine and butorphanol apparently works synergistically to decrease tear production significantly.[12] Xylazine does not decrease tear production in horses.[9]

Medetomidine is a more selective α_2-adrenergic agonist. Topical administration of medetomidine decreased IOP in cats and rabbits, while producing mydriasis, suggesting that there are α_2 receptors in the eye that are involved in the regulation of IOP.[74–76] In contrast, IV administration of medetomidine resulted in miosis in normal dogs, without a decrease in IOP.[77]

IOP was not affected by systemically administered medetomidine in dogs that had received tropicamide (an anticholinergic and cycloplegic agent) topically. The pupil size in these dogs increased after tropicamide administration and continued to increase slightly after medetomidine administration, although it was not determined whether the continued increase was exclusively caused by the medetomidine.[78] Lens opacification has not been reported after medetomidine administration. Medetomidine may be administered as a continuous-rate infusion (CRI) in ocular patients to provide profound sedation and moderate analgesia postoperatively. The effects of systemically administered α_2-agonists on IOP should be taken into consideration when tonometry is anticipated.

Benzodiazepines

Both midazolam and diazepam decrease IOP in dogs and cats after IV administration.[6,79,80] The IOP decrease may be related to the centrally acting muscle-relaxant properties of the benzodiazepines. One study suggests that diazepam may negate the increase in IOP that occurs after ketamine administration.[5]

Phenothiazines

Acepromazine is a sedative with antiemetic properties that may prevent vomiting and gagging in ophthalmic patients who have undergone intraocular surgery or have a ruptured eye. In horses, acepromazine has decreased IOP as much as 20%.[72] The longer action of acepromazine may be useful in providing a slower, quieter anesthetic recovery, thereby reducing the potential for postoperative trauma.

Analgesia

Ocular and periocular structures are richly innervated and highly sensitive. Symptoms of ocular pain include blepharospasm, photophobia, ocular discharge, rubbing of the eyes, and avoidance behavior. A variety of topical and systemic drug therapies are currently available to address pain management adequately in ophthalmic patients.

Opioids

Opioid selection for ocular patients should include consideration of quality of analgesia and appropriate duration of action. Opioids may be administered as a periodic injection or as a CRI.

Morphine decreases IOP, and other opioids are assumed to have the potential for a similar effect.[6] Emesis, and the associated increase in IOP, is a possible side effect of opioid administration. This may suggest that opioid administration should be delayed until the patient is anesthetized. Bradycardia, which may predispose patients to the OCR, occurs with some opioids and may necessitate administration of an anticholinergic. As mentioned previously, the effects of opioids on pupil size are variable among species.[27,28] Morphine produces miosis in dogs, rabbits, and people, and mydriasis in cats, rats, mice, and monkeys.[27,28]

Nonsteroidal Anti-inflammatory Drugs

Nonsteroidal anti-inflammatory drugs (NSAIDs) can inhibit both isoforms of the cyclooxygenase enzyme: COX-1 and COX-2. Although there is significant overlap in COX isoform functions, COX-1 is important for normal physiological function of the gastrointestinal tract, renal system, platelets, and blood flow to specific tissues.[79] Cyclooxygenase 2 is produced in part by macrophages and inflammatory cells that have been stimulated by cytokines and other inflammatory mediators, and is considered to be associated with the production of inflammation and pain.[80] Most of the currently used NSAIDs in veterinary medicine inhibit both COX-1 and COX-2.[80,81] Other possible anti-inflammatory actions of NSAIDs include suppression of polymorphonuclear cell locomotion and chemotaxis through inhibition of leukotriene synthesis, decreased expression of inflammatory cytokines and mast cell degranulation, free-radical scavenging, and local anti-inflammatory effects caused by the accumulation of NSAIDs as organic acids at the site of inflammation.[79,82–84] The responsiveness of the feline cornea to chemical stimuli of polymodal nociceptors was diminished by NSAIDs, suggesting that corneal pain may be inhibited by NSAIDs.[85] This effect may be due not only to inhibition of cyclooxygenase activity, but also to a direct effect of NSAIDs on the excitability of polymodal nerve endings.

Both systemic and topical administration of NSAIDs are widely used in ocular patients, with flunixin being the most popular. NSAIDs effectively prevent intraoperative miosis, and control postoperative pain and inflammation after intraocular procedures, as well as controlling uveitis and alleviating pain from various other ocular conditions or disease processes.[86]

NSAIDs have been associated with decreased platelet aggregation, gastrointestinal ulceration and bleeding, and renal and hepatic damage.[87] Topical NSAID administration is associated with irritation of the conjunctiva, corneal cytopathy, decreased aqueous outflow, and its systemic absorption through nasal mucosa.[88,89] The use of NSAIDs in acutely inflamed canine eyes may increase IOP, possibly due to decreased aqueous outflow.[89] Corneal complications reported with topical use of NSAIDs in humans may be attributable to the solution's vehicle, solubilizer, or preservative, rather than the active drug itself.[79]

Coordination of systemic and topical NSAID application is essential to prevent excessive administration and toxicity. The NSAIDs should be used cautiously in geriatric patients, who often have preexisting renal and gastrointestinal disease.

Intravenous Lidocaine

In a preliminary study of dogs undergoing intraocular surgery, it was determined that lidocaine administered IV as a loading dose (1.0 mg/kg) followed by CRI (0.025 mg/kg/min) may provide preemptive analgesia similar to morphine administered IV as a loading dose (0.15 mg/kg) followed by CRI (0.1 mg/kg/h).[87] The exact mechanism for the analgesic effects of IV lidocaine in these patients has not been established, although inhibition of A-δ fiber and C-fiber discharges from sensory neurons of the eye may be involved.

Local and Regional Anesthesia

Local or regional anesthesia may be adequate for less invasive procedures or may be included as part of a balanced general anesthetic regimen. Topical anesthesia for diagnostic and therapeutic procedures in veterinary ocular patients usually requires accompanying sedation to gain cooperation of the patient. Topical anesthesia and sedation may be the preferred technique in ruminants and horses in which a standing procedure is anticipated or in other patients in which general anesthesia would be accompanied by unacceptable risk.

Local anesthetics applied topically are readily absorbed through mucous membranes.[1] Systemic toxicosis is possible, though unlikely, but administration to small patients should be judicious.[90,91] Topical anesthetics can be irritating and cause transient conjunctival hyperemia, as well as damage corneal epithelium, delay corneal wound healing, and mask signs of disease or discomfort.[1] It is recommended, therefore, that topical anesthetics be reserved for diagnostic rather than therapeutic purposes. Tear production and blink reflex will be reduced after topical anesthetic administration, necessitating the application of ocular lubricant to protect the cornea after completion of the procedure.[1]

Topical administration of 1% morphine sulfate solution appears to provide local analgesia in dogs with corneal ulcers.[92] The antinociceptive effect is possibly a result of interaction with μ opioid receptors, which have been identified in small numbers in normal canine corneas, and δ opioid receptors, which have been identified in the corneal epithelium and stroma of dogs. In contrast with the local anesthetics, this local analgesic effect is produced without delaying corneal wound healing or causing any discernible tissue damage.[92]

Administration of local anesthetic to the surface of an open wound is referred to as a *splash block*. Splash blocks may be used for intraoperative and postoperative analgesia in ocular patients (i.e., after enucleation). Bupivacaine (0.5%) is commonly used for this technique because of its longer action. The maximum dose should not exceed 2.0 mg/kg to avoid potential toxicosis. Epinephrine may be added to the bupivacaine (1:200,000) to reduce bleeding and delay systemic absorption. In a recent study assessing the duration of effect of topical local anesthetic administration, it was determined that two applications of 1 drop of 0.5% proparacaine, with a 1-min interval between drops, resulted in 25 min of reduced corneal sensation in dogs.[93]

Regional anesthetic techniques commonly used for ocular patients include auriculopalpebral nerve block, supraorbital nerve block, and retrobulbar injection. Techniques for these nerve blocks are described elsewhere in this text.[94]

The auriculopalpebral nerve, which is a terminal branch of the facial nerve (cranial nerve VII), provides motor innervation to the orbicularis oculi muscle. Blockade of the auriculopalpebral nerve eliminates forceful blepharospasms, thereby facilitating ocular examination or minor surgical or diagnostic procedures.[1] In horses, auriculopalpebral block has no adverse effects on tear production or IOP.[74,95]

The supraorbital nerve, which is a termination of the ophthalmic branch of the trigeminal nerve (cranial nerve V), provides sensory innervation to most of the superior palpebra. Blockade of this nerve is commonly performed in sedated horses for placement of a subpalpebral lavage tube, repair of a palpebral laceration, or other similar minor procedures.[1] Other sensory nerves that are less commonly blocked include the infratrochlear, zygomatic, and lacrimal nerves.

Retrobulbar or peribulbar injection can be performed as an adjunct to sedation or general anesthesia. Retrobulbar injection of local anesthetic will block the optic (cranial nerve II), oculomotor (III), trochlear (IV), ophthalmic and maxillary divisions of the trigeminal (V), and the abducens (VI) nerves. Blockade of these nerves causes desensitization of the globe and palpebrae, akinesia of the globe, transient vision loss, pupil dilation, and decreased IOP.[1] The Peterson eye block is a well-known example of a retrobulbar technique used in cattle for regional anesthesia. During general anesthesia, retrobulbar injection has also been performed in horses to eliminate ocular movement without the accompanying disadvantages of deeper planes of anesthesia.[33,96] Potential complications of retrobulbar injection include retrobulbar hemorrhage, trauma to the optic nerve or globe, intrathecal injection of local anesthetic, and death.[90] Retrobulbar injection has been advocated to prevent the OCR, but performance of the technique itself has the potential to elicit the OCR.[1,16] Large volumes of local anesthetic or orbital hemorrhage may cause either proptosis of the globe or displacement of the vitreous if the globe has been penetrated.[1]

Neuromuscular Blocking Agents

Paralysis of extraocular muscles relaxes the eye, allowing the globe to roll centrally and proptose slightly. These effects greatly facilitate positioning of the globe for ophthalmic surgery,[97,98] eliminating the need for significant surgical manipulation to obtain proper globe positioning and decreasing the potential for initiating the OCR.[58]

Depolarizing NMBs, such as succinylcholine, increase IOP just prior to paralysis in horses and people.[5,6,99] This effect may be due to an increase in choroidal vascular dilatation, or initial contraction of extraocular and orbital musculature. The increase in IOP subsides after approximately 8 min.[100] Although the increase in IOP would indicate that the use of succinylcholine should be avoided in patients with severely compromised eyes that are at risk for rupture, administration in patients with intact globes would seem reasonable as long as enough time was allowed for the increase in IOP to subside prior to incision.

Nondepolarizing NMBs do not appear to increase IOP.[35] Studies have indicated that vecuronium and pancuronium decrease IOP, whereas atracurium has no effect on IOP in people and dogs.[101–105]

As mentioned previously, indirect-acting cholinergic drugs are anticholinesterases that are used for treating glaucoma. Because anticholinesterases inhibit or inactivate the plasma pseudocholinesterases responsible for the metabolism of succinylcholine, they may cause prolonged paralysis.[106] It has been recommended that indirect-acting cholinergic drugs be discontinued 2 to 4 weeks prior to neuromuscular blockade with succinylcholine, although normal levels of plasma pseudocholinesterase activity may not be totally restored for 4 to 6 weeks.[35]

The effects of depolarizing NMBs are not reversible, whereas those of the nondepolarizing NMBs are reversible with anticholinesterases, such as neostigmine and edrophonium. Anticholinesterases are not associated with increases in IOP.[3] An anticholinergic (e.g., atropine or glycopyrrolate) is commonly administered prior to the anticholinesterase to prevent profound bradycardia in small animals and ruminants. Although the use of anticholinergics is usually avoided in horses, anticholinesterases may still be used for nondepolarizing NMB reversal, but should be administered very slowly while the HR is monitored. Alternatively, the use of nondepolarizing NMBs with a briefer action, such as atracurium, may be more desirable to avoid the need for reversal.[3] Neuromuscular paralysis reversal should be complete to prevent hypoventilation, struggling during recovery, self-trauma, and increases in IOP.

As mentioned previously, birds have striated rather than smooth iris musculature and may require paralysis to produce mydriasis. Topically applied parasympatholytic or sympathomimetic agents are ineffective in birds.[1] Intracameral injection of *d*-tubocurarine has produced mydriasis in pigeons.[107] Apnea and salivation occurred in raptors after intracameral injection of muscle relaxants.[24] Topically applied vecuronium was found to produce the most consistent and greatest pupillary dilation in three species of psittacines with the fewest systemic side effects when compared with *d*-tubocurarine and pancuronium.[108] However, the differences in systemic side effects among the three psittacine species indicate that vecuronium should be used cautiously when applied bilaterally.

The use of sequential nondepolarizing and depolarizing NMBs is controversial.[3] In humans, a small amount of nondepolarizing NMB is administered first to block the initial muscle contractions of the depolarizing NMB. The depolarizing NMB is then administered to produce immobilization and allow intubation. Although this technique prevents coughing and gagging, and muscle fasciculations are not evident, IOP still increases during intubation.[16]

Increases in IOP may occur with increases in $PaCO_2$, necessitating mechanical ventilation, which may be facilitated by the administration of NMBs. It has been suggested, however, that hyperventilation may fail to decrease IOP because of the increases in intrathoracic and central venous pressure accompanying the use of mechanical ventilation.[105]

Electroretinography and Anesthesia

Electroretinography (ERG) is used primarily as a diagnostic test for progressive retinal atrophy or other degenerative retinal disorders, and to assess retinal integrity in dogs for which ophthalmoscopic evaluation of the fundus is not possible prior to cataract surgery.[109] Complete ocular akinesia is preferred during the ERG, which requires general anesthesia, and possibly neuromuscular blockade. The ERG requires dark adaptation of the patient and is performed in the dark, which makes anesthetic monitoring a challenge. There has been no standard generated for the ERG in unanesthetized patients.[109] Halothane and isoflurane depress the ERG in dogs, but the results are considered useful as long as the ERG for the patient and the control animal are generated under identical anesthesia conditions.[1,110,111] No single anesthetic protocol has been established for the performance of ERGs, although propofol induction with isoflurane maintenance has been used successfully in dogs.[112] Sedation and a cooperative patient may prove adequate for a semiquantitative ERG as is typically performed for preoperative screening of cataract patients.[1]

References

1. Collins BK, Gross ME, Moore CP, et al. Physiologic, pharmacologic, and practical considerations for anesthesia of domestic animals with eye disease. J Am Vet Med Assoc 1995;207:220–230.
2. Karpinski LG, Clubb SL. Clinical aspects of ophthalmology in caged birds. In: Kirk RW, ed. Current Veterinary Therapy IX: Small Animal Practice. Philadelphia: WB Saunders, 1986:616–621.
3. Thurmon JC, Tranquilli WJ, Benson GJ. Anesthesia for special patients: Ocular patients. In: Thurmon JC, Tranquilli WJ, Benson GJ, eds. Lumb and Jones' Veterinary Anesthesia, 3rd ed. Philadelphia: Williams and Wilkins, 1996:812–818.
4. Donlon JV Jr. Anesthesia for ophthalmic surgery. In: Barash P, ed. ASA Refresher Course Lectures, vol 16. Philadelphia: JB Lippincott, 1988:81.
5. Cunningham AJ, Barry P. Intraocular pressure: Physiology and implications for anaesthetic management. Can Anaesth Soc J 1986;33:195–208.
6. Murphy DF. Anesthesia and intraocular pressure. Anesth Analg 1985;64:520–530.
7. Vestre WA, Brightman AH, Helper LC, et al. Decreased tear production associated with general anesthesia in the dog. J Am Vet Med Assoc 1979;174:1006–1007.
8. Ludders JW, Heavner JE. Effect of atropine on tear formation in anesthetized dogs. J Am Vet Med Assoc 1979;175:585–586.
9. Brightman AH, Manning JP, Benson GJ, et al. Decreased tear production associated with general anesthesia in the horse. J Am Vet Med Assoc 1983;182:243–244.
10. Krupin T, Cross DA, Becker B. Decreased basal tear production associated with general anesthesia. Arch Ophthalmol 1977;95:107–108.
11. Herring IP, Pickett JP, Champagne ES, et al. Evaluation of aqueous tear production in dogs following general anesthesia. J Am Anim Hosp Assoc 2000;36:427–430.
12. Dodam JR, Branson KR, Martin DD. Effects of intramuscular sedative and opioid combinations on tear production in dogs. Vet Ophthalmol 1998;1:57–59.
13. Bellhorn RW. Ophthalmologic disorders of exotic and laboratory animals. Vet Clin North Am Small Anim Pract 1973;3:345–356.
14. Datta TD. Flash fire hazard with eye ointment. Anesth Analg 1984;63:700–701.
15. Carpel EF, Rice SW, Lang M, et al. Fire risks with ophthalmic ointments. Am J Ophthalmol 1985;100:477–478.
16. Donlon JV. Anesthesia for eye, ear, nose, and throat surgery. In: Miller RD, ed. Anesthesia, 5th ed. Philadelphia: Churchill Livingstone, 2000:2173–2198.
17. Miller PE, Pickett JP. Comparison of the human and canine Schiotz tonometry conversion tables in clinically normal dogs. J Am Vet Med Assoc 1992;201:1021–1025.
18. Miller PE, Pickett JP. Comparison of the human and canine Schiotz tonometry conversion tables in clinically normal cats. J Am Vet Med Assoc 1992;201:1017–1020.
19. Miller PE, Pickett JP, Majors LJ. Evaluation of two applanation tonometers in horses. Am J Vet Res 1990;51:935–937.
20. Macri FJ. Vascular pressure relationship and intraocular pressure. Arch Ophthalmol 1961;65:571–574.
21. Duncalf D, Weitzner SW. The influence of ventilation and hypercapnia on intraocular pressure during anesthesia. Anesth Analg 1963;42:232–246.
22. Cullen LK, Steffey EP, Bailey CS, et al. Effect of high $PaCO_2$ and time on cerebrospinal fluid and intraocular pressure in halothane anesthetized horses. Am J Vet Res 1990;51:300–304.
23. Collins BK, O'Brien D. Autonomic dysfunction of the eye. Semin Vet Med Surg (Small Anim) 1990;5:24–36.
24. Murphy CJ. Raptor ophthalmology. Compend Contin Educ Pract Vet 1987;9:241–260.
25. Haskins SC. General guidelines for judging anesthetic depth. Vet Clin North Am Small Anim Pract 1992;22:432–434.
26. Thompson HS. The pupil. In: Hart WM, ed. Adler's Physiology of the Eye, 9th ed. St Louis: CV Mosby, 1992:412–441.
27. Lynch TJ, Tiseo PJ, Adler MW. Morphine-induced pupillary fluctuation: Physiological evidence against selective action on the Edinger-Westphal nucleus. J Ocul Pharmacol 1990;6:165–174.
28. Lee HK, Wang SC. Mechanism of morphine-induced miosis in the dog. J Pharmacol Exp Ther 1975;192:415–431.
29. Kaswan RL, Quandt JE, Moore PA. Narcotics, miosis, and cataract surgery [Letter]. J Am Vet Med Assoc 1992;201:1819–1820.

30. Stephan DD, Vestre WA, Stiles J, et al. Changes in intraocular pressure and pupil size following intramuscular administration of hydromorphone hydrochloride and acepromazine in clinically normal dogs. Vet Ophthalmol 2003;6:73–76.

31. Sharpe LG, Pickworth WB. Opposite pupillary size effects in the cat and dog after microinjections of morphine, normorphine and clonidine in the Edinger-Westphal nucleus. Brain Res Bull 1985;15:329–333.

32. Yoshitomi T, Ito Y. Effects of indomethacin and prostaglandins on the dog iris sphincter and dilator muscles. Invest Ophthalmol Vis Sci 1988;29:127–132.

33. Hodgson DS, Dunlop CI. General anesthesia for horses with specific problems. Vet Clin North Am Equine Pract 1990;6:625–650.

34. Mirakhur RK, Jones CJ, Dundee JW, et al. IM or IV atropine or glycopyrrolate for prevention of oculocardiac reflex in children during squint surgery. Br J Anaesth 1982;54:1059–1063.

35. Wolf GL, Goldfarb H. Complications of ophthalmologic anesthesia. Semin Anesth 1990;9:108–118.

36. Farrell TA. Minimizing the systemic effects of glaucoma medications. Geriatrics 1991;46:61–73.

37. Pascoe PJ, Ilkiw JE, Stiles J, et al. Arterial hypertension associated with topical ocular use of phenylephrine in dogs. J Am Vet Med Assoc 1994;205:1562–1564.

38. Herring IP, Jacobson JD, Pickett JP. Cardiovascular effects of topical ophthalmic 10% phenylephrine in dogs. Vet Ophthalmol 2004;4:41–46.

39. Slatter D. Use of phenylephrine in dogs [Letter]. J Am Vet Med Assoc 1995;206:428–429.

40. Van Buskirk EM, Fraunfelder FT. Ocular beta blockers and systemic effects. Am J Ophthalmol 1984;98:623–624.

41. Svec AL, Strosberg AM. Therapeutic and systemic side-effects of ocular ß-adrenergic antagonists in anesthetized dogs. Invest Ophthalmol Vis Sci 1986;27:401–405.

42. Maren TH. Carbonic anhydrase: Chemistry, physiology, and inhibition. Physiol Rev 1967;47:595–781.

43. Rose RJ, Carter J. Some physiological and biochemical effects of acetazolamide in the dog. J Vet Pharmacol Ther 1979;2:215–221.

44. Ludders JW. Anesthesia for ophthalmic surgery. In: Slatter D, ed. Textbook of Small Animal Surgery, 2nd ed. Philadelphia: WB Saunders, 1993:2276–2278.

45. Brock KA, Thurmon JC. Pulmonary edema associated with mannitol administration. Can Pract 1979;6:31–33.

46. Gilroy BA. Intraocular and cardiopulmonary effects of low-dose mannitol in the dog. Vet Surg 1986;15:342–344.

47. Brock KA, Thurmon JC, Benson GJ, et al. Selected hemodynamic and renal effects of intravenous infusions of hypertonic mannitol in dogs anesthetized with methoxyflurane in oxygen. J Am Anim Hosp Assoc 1985;21:207–214.

48. Glaze MB, Crawford MA, Nachreiner TF, et al. Ophthalmic corticosteroid therapy: Systemic effects in the dog. J Am Vet Med Assoc 1988;192:73–75.

49. Roberts SM, Lavach JD, Macy DW, et al. Effect of ophthalmic prednisolone acetate on the canine adrenal gland and hepatic function. Am J Vet Res 1984;45:1711–1714.

50. Brunson DB. Anesthesia in ophthalmic surgery. Vet Clin North Am Small Anim Pract 1980;10:481–495.

51. Crispin SM. Anaesthesia for ophthalmic surgery. Proc Assoc Vet Anaesth Great Br Ir 1981;9:170–183.

52. Whitley RD, McLaughlin SA, Whitley EM, et al. Cataract removal in dogs: The surgical techniques. Vet Med 1993;88:859–866.

53. Mirakhur RK, Elliott P, Shepherd WFI, et al. Comparison of the effects of isoflurane and halothane on intraocular pressure. Acta Anaesthesiol Scand 1990;34:282–285.

54. Bednarski RM, Majors LJ. Ketamine and the arrhythmogenic dose of epinephrine in cats anesthetized with halothane and isoflurane. Am J Vet Res 1986;47:2122–2125.

55. Sator-Katzenschlager S, Deusch E, Dolezal S, et al. Sevoflurane and propofol decrease intraocular pressure equally during non-ophthalmic surgery and recovery. Br J Anaesth 2002;89:764–766.

56. Eltzschig HK, Darsow R, Schroeder TH, et al. Effect of tracheal intubation or Laryngeal Mask Airway(tm) insertion on intraocular pressure using balanced anesthesia with sevoflurane and remifentanil. J Clin Anesth 2001;13:264–267.

57. Wolf GL, Capuano C, Hartung J. Effect of nitrous oxide on gas bubble volume in the anterior chamber. Arch Ophthalmol 1985;103:418–419.

58. Clutton RE, Boyd C, Richards DLS, et al. Significance of the oculocardiac reflex during ophthalmic surgery in the dog. J Small Anim Pract 1988;29:573–579.

59. Cozanitis DA, Dundee JW, Buchanan TAS, et al. Atropine versus glycopyrrolate: A study of intraocular pressure and pupil size in man. Anesthesia 1979;34:236–238.

60. Jensen HE. Keratitis sicca and parotid duct transposition. Compend Contin Educ Pract Vet 1979;1:721–726.

61. Frischmeyer KJ, Miller PE, Bellay Y, et al. Parenteral anticholinergics in dogs with normal and elevated intraocular pressure. Vet Surg 1993;22:230–234.

62. Langley MS, Heel RC. Propofol: A review of its pharmacodynamic and pharmacokinetic properties and use as an intravenous anesthetic. Drugs 1988;35:334–372.

63. Deramoudt V, Gaudon M, Malledant Y, et al. Effect of propofol on IOP in strabismus surgery in children. Ann Fr Anesth Reanim 1990;9:1–5.

64. Gelatt KN, Gwin RM, Peiffer RL, et al. Tonography in the normal and glaucomatous beagle. Am J Vet Res 1977;38:515–520.

65. Trim CM, Colbern GT, Martin CL. Effect of xylazine and ketamine on intraocular pressure in horses. Vet Rec 1985;117:442–443.

66. Bennett K, ed. Compendium of Veterinary Products, 1st ed. Port Huron, MI: North American Compendiums, 1991:397.

67. Arnett BD, Brightman AH, Musselman EE. Effect of atropine sulfate on tear production in the cat when used with ketamine hydrochloride and acetylpromazine maleate. J Am Vet Med Assoc 1984;185:214–215.

68. Short CE, ed. Alpha₂-Agents in Animals. Santa Barbara, CA: Veterinary Practice, 1992:3-20, 43-56, 59-70.

69. Hsu WH, Lee P, Betts DM. Xylazine induced mydriasis in rats and its antagonism by α-adrenergic agents. J Vet Pharmacol Ther 1981;4:97–101.

70. Burke JA, Potter DE. The ocular effects of xylazine in rabbits, cats, and monkeys. J Ocul Pharmacol 1986;2:9–12.

71. van der Woerdt A, Gilger BC, Wilkie DA, et al. Effect of auriculopalpebral nerve block and intravenous administration of xylazine on intraocular pressure and corneal thickness in horses. Am J Vet Res 1995;56:155–158.

72. McClure JR, Gelatt KN, Gum GG, et al. The effect of parenteral acepromazine and xylazine on intraocular pressure in the horse. Vet Med Small Anim Clin 1976;71:1727–1730.

73. Calderone L., Grimes P, Shalev M. Acute reversible cataract induction by xylazine and by ketamine-xylazine anesthesia in rats and mice. Exp Eye Res 1986;42:331–337.

74. Jin Y, Wilson S, Elco EE, et al. Ocular hypotension effects of medetomidine and its analogs. J Ocul Pharmacol 1991;7:285–296.

75. Ogidigben MJ, Potter DE. Comparative effects of alpha-2 and DA2 agonists on intraocular pressure in pigmented and nonpigmented rabbits. J Ocul Pharmacol 1993;9:187–199.

76. Potter DE, Ogidigben MJ. Medetomidine-induced alterations of intraocular pressure and contraction of the nictitating membrane. Invest Ophthalmol Vis Sci 1991;32:2799–2805.

77. Verbruggen A-MJ, Akkerdaas LC, Hellebrekers LJ, et al. The effect of intravenous medetomidine on pupil size and intraocular pressure in normotensive dogs. Vet Q 2000;22:179–180.

78. Wallin-Hakanson N, Wallin-Hakanson B. The effects of topical tropicamide and systemic medetomidine, followed by atipamezole reversal, on pupil size and intraocular pressure in normal dogs. Vet Ophthalmol 2001;4:3–6.

79. Gaynes BI, Fiscella R. Topical nonsteroidal anti-inflammatory drugs for ophthalmic use: A safety review. Drug Saf 2002;25:233–250.

80. Johnston SA, Budsberg SC. Non-steroidal anti-inflammatory drugs and corticosteroids for the management of canine osteoarthritis. Vet Clin North Am Small Anim Pract 1997;27:841–862.

81. Papich MG. Principles of analgesic drug therapy. Semin Vet Med Surg Small Anim 1997;12:80–93.

82. Perianin A, Roch-Arveiller M, Giround JP, et al. In vivo effects of indomethacin and flurbiprofen on the locomotion of neutrophils elicited by immune and non-immune inflammation in the rat. Eur J Pharmacol 1985;106:327–333.

83. Leonardi A, Busato F, Fregona I, et al. Anti-inflammatory and antiallergic effects of ketorolac tromethamine in the conjunctival provocation model. Br J Ophthalmol 2000;84:1228–1232.

84. Flach AJ. Cyclo-oxygenase inhibitors in ophthalmology. Surv Ophthalmol 1992;36:259–284.

85. Chen X, Gallar J, Belmonte C. Reduction by anti-inflammatory drugs of the response of corneal sensory nerve fibers to chemical irritation. Invest Ophthalmol Vis Sci 1997;38:1944–1953.

86. Giuliano EA. Nonsteroidal anti-inflammatory drugs in veterinary ophthalmology. Vet Clin North Am Small Anim Pract 2004;34:707–723.

87. Smith LJ, Bentley E, Shih A, et al. Systemic lidocaine infusion as an analgesic for intraocular surgery in dogs: A pilot study. Vet Anaesth Analg 2004;31:53–63.

88. Schalnus R. Topical nonsteroidal anti-inflammatory therapy in ophthalmology. Ophthalmologica 2003;217:89–98.

89. Millichamp NJ, Dziezyc J, Olsen JW. Effect of flurbiprofen on facility of aqueous outflow in the eyes of dogs. Am J Vet Res 1991;52:1448–1451.

90. Gelatt KN. Veterinary Ophthalmic Pharmacology and Therapeutics, 2nd ed. Bonner Springs, KS: VM, 1978:9–28.

91. Havener WH. Ocular Pharmacology, 5th ed. St Louis: CV Mosby, 1983:72–119.

92. Stiles J, Honda CN, Krohne SG, et al. Effect of topical administration of 1% morphine sulfate solution on signs of pain and corneal wound healing in dogs. Am J Vet Res 2003;64:813–818.

93. Herring IP, Bobofchak MA, Landry MP, et al. Duration of effect and effect of multiple doses of topical ophthalmic 0.5% proparacaine hydrochloride in clinically normal dogs. Am J Vet Res 2005;66:77–80.

94. Skarda RT. Local and regional anesthetic and analgesic techniques. In: Thurmon JC, Tranquilli WJ, Benson GJ, eds. Lumb and Jones' Veterinary Anesthesia, 3rd ed. Philadelphia: Williams and Wilkins, 1996:426–514.

95. Marts BS, Bryan GM, Prieur DJ. Schirmer tear test measurement and lysozyme concentration of equine tears. J Equine Med Surg 1977;1:427–430.

96. Raffe MR, Bistner SI, Crimi AJ, et al. Retrobulbar block in combination with general anesthesia for equine ophthalmic surgery. Vet Surg 1986;15:139–141.

97. Young SS, Barnett KC, Taylor PM. Anaesthetic regimes for cataract removal in the dog. J Small Anim Pract 1991;32:236–240.

98. Donaldson LL, Holland M, Koch SA. Atracurium as an adjunct to halothane-oxygen anesthesia in a llama undergoing intraocular surgery: A case report. Vet Surg 1992;21:76–79.

99. Benson GJ, Manning JP, Hartsfield SM, et al. Intraocular tension of the horse: Effects of succinylcholine and halothane anesthesia. Am J Vet Res 1981;42:1831–1832.

100. Varghese C, Chopra SK, Daniel R, et al. Intraocular pressure profile during general anesthesia. Ophthalmic Surg 1990;21:856–859.

101. Mirakhur RK, Shepherd WFI, Lavery GG, et al. The effects of vecuronium on intra-ocular pressure. Anaesthesia 1987;42:944–949.

102. George R, Nursingh A, Downing JW, et al. Non-depolarizing neuromuscular blockers and the eye: A study of intraocular pressure: Pancuronium versus alcuronium. Br J Anaesth 1979;51:789–792.

103. Maharaj RJ, Humphrey D, Kaplan N, et al. Effects of atracurium on intraocular pressure. Br J Anaesth 1984;56:459–463.

104. Jantzen J-PAH, Earnshaw G, Hackett GH, et al. A study of the effects of neuromuscular blocking drugs on intraocular pressure. Anaesthesist 1987;36:223–227.

105. McMurphy RM, Davidson HJ, Hodgson DS. Effects of atracurium on intraocular pressure, eye position, and blood pressure in eucapnic and hypocapnic isoflurane-anesthetized dogs. Am J Vet Res 2004;65:179–182.

106. Adams HR. Cholinergic pharmacology: Autonomic drugs. In: Veterinary Pharmacology and Therapeutics, 8th ed. Ames: Iowa State University Press, 2001:117–136.

107. Verschueren CP, Lumeij JT. Mydriasis in pigeons (Columbia livia domestica) with d-tubocurarine: Topical instillation versus intracameral injection. J Vet Pharmacol Ther 1991;14:206–208.

108. Ramer JC, Paul-Murphy J, Brunson D, et al. Effects of mydriatic agents in cockatoos, African gray parrots, and blue-fronted Amazon parrots. J Am Vet Assoc 1996;208:227–230.

109. Acland GM. Diagnosis and differentiation of retinal diseases in small animals by electroretinography. Semin Vet Med Surg (Small Anim) 1988;3:15–27.

110. Acland G, Forte S, Aguirre G. Halothane effect on the canine electroretinogram. Trans Am Coll Vet Ophthalmol 1981;12:66–83.

111. Loew ER. The use of acepromazine and oxymorphone in routine clinical electroretinography. Trans Am Coll Vet Ophthalmol 1984;15:122–137.

112. Narfstrom K, Katz ML, Bragadottir R, et al. Functional and structural recovery of the retina after gene therapy in the RPE65 null mutation dog. Invest Ophthalmol Vis Sci 2003;44:1663–1672.

Chapter 45

Anesthetic Management of Cesarean Section Patients

Marc R. Raffe and Rachael E. Carpenter

Introduction

The ideal anesthetic protocol for cesarean section would provide ample analgesia, muscle relaxation, and sedation or narcosis for optimal operating conditions and safety without unduly endangering either mother or fetus. By their very nature, anesthetics, analgesics, tranquilizers, and sedatives cross the blood-brain barrier. Because the physicochemical properties that allow drugs to cross the blood-brain barrier also enable their placental transfer, it is not possible to selectively anesthetize the mother. Agents that affect the maternal central nervous system will also produce fetal effects, which effects are generally characterized by depression and decreased viability. In many cases, cesarean section is an emergency procedure. Due to the emergent nature of surgical fetal extraction, the physical condition of the mother and fetus is less than optimal because veterinary assistance has been delayed. Thus, the veterinarian is faced with the dilemma of having to anesthetize the mother, who may already be compromised, without adversely affecting the fetus.

Selection of an anesthetic protocol for cesarean section should be based on safety of the mother and fetus, patient comfort, and veteri-

narian's familiarity with the anesthetic technique. Factors in decision making regarding anesthesia protocol include considerations of the physiological alterations induced by pregnancy and labor, the pharmacology of selected drugs and their direct and indirect effects on the fetus and neonate, the benefits and risks of the techniques chosen, and the risk of procedure-related complications associated with anesthetic management. Regardless of the technique used, a major goal associated with drug selection should be to minimize fetal depression. This may be achieved by surgical expediency, which decreases maternal recumbency time and fetal drug absorption. This goal is of major importance in the larger species. With prolonged uterine isolation prior to fetal delivery, placental perfusion decreases, resulting in fetal hypoxemia, acidosis, and distress.

Physiological Alterations Induced by Pregnancy

Metabolic demands of gestation and parturition are met by altered physiological function (Table 45.1). Most of the data describing physiological alterations of pregnancy have been obtained from data collected in humans and ewes. Although little work has been done in other species, the changes should be comparable, if not greater, in magnitude. Birth weight expressed as percentage of maternal weight for people, sheep, dogs, and cats is 5.7%, 11.4%, 16.1%, and 13.2%, respectively.[1] This suggests that the physiological burden and therefore physiological alterations may actually be greater in animals than in women.

Cardiovascular

During pregnancy, maternal blood volume increases by approximately 40%; plasma volume increases more than red cell mass, resulting in decreased hemoglobin concentration and packed cell volume.[2] Increased heart rate and stroke volume cause cardiac output to increase 30% to 50% above normal.[3,4] Plasma estrogens decrease peripheral vascular resistance, resulting in an increase in cardiac output while systolic and diastolic blood pressures remain unchanged. During labor and the immediate postpartum period, cardiac output increases an additional 10% to 25% as a result of blood being extruded from the contracting uterus.[5] Cardiac output during labor is also influenced by body position, pain, and apprehension.[2] During labor, systolic pressure increases by 10 to 30 mm Hg. Although central venous pressure does not change during pregnancy, because of increased venous capacity, it increases slightly (4 to 6 cm of water) during labor and has been reported to increase by 50 cm of water during

Table 45.1. Physiological alterations induced by pregnancy.

Variable	
Heart rate	↑
Cardiac output	↑
Blood volume	↑
Plasma volume	↑
Packed cell volume, hemoglobin, and plasma protein	↓
Arterial blood pressure	o
Central venous pressure	o, ↑ During labor
Minute volume of ventilation	↑
Oxygen consumption	↑
pH_a and PaO_2	o
$PaCO_2$	↓
Total lung and vital capacity	o
Functional residual capacity	↓
Gastric emptying time and intragastric pressure	↑
Gastric motility and pH of gastric secretions	↓
Gastric chloride ion and enzyme concentration	↑
SGOT, LDH, and BSP retention time	↑
Plasma cholinesterase	↓
Renal plasma flow and glomerular filtration rate	↑
Blood urea nitrogen and creatinine	↓
Sodium ion and water balance	o

o, no change. BSP, sulfobromophthalein sodium; LDH, lactate dehydrogenase; PaO_2, arterial oxygen partial pressure; $PaCO_2$, arterial carbon dioxide partial pressure; pH_a, arterial pH; SGOT, serum glutamic-oxaloacetic transaminase.

painful fetal extraction.[6] The posterior vena cava and aorta can be compressed by the enlarged uterus and its contents during dorsal recumbency. This can cause decreased venous return and cardiac output with resultant decreased uterine and renal blood flow. Although this does not appear to be as serious a problem in dogs and cats, time spent restrained or positioned in dorsal recumbency should be kept to a minimum.[7,8]

Because cardiac work is increased during pregnancy and parturition, cardiac reserve is decreased. Patients with previously well-compensated heart disease may suffer pulmonary congestion and heart failure caused by additional cardiac workload associated with gestation and the increased hemodynamic demand secondary to parturition-associated pain. In such patients, pain and anxiety control is a key component of successful management. However, care must be taken to avoid additional cardiac depression and decompensation induced by excessive doses of sedatives or anesthetics. The use of ecbolic agents during or after parturition can adversely affect cardiovascular function. Oxytocin in large or repeated doses induces peripheral vasodilation and hypotension, which can adversely affect both mother and fetus through decreased tissue perfusion. Ergot derivatives induce vasoconstriction and hypertension.[9]

Pulmonary

During pregnancy, increased serum progesterone concentration enhances respiratory center sensitivity to arterial partial pressure

(tension) of carbon dioxide ($PaCO_2$). As a result of increased ventilatory minute volume, $PaCO_2$ progressively decreases during gestation and is near 30 mm Hg at parturition. Because of long-term renal compensation, respiratory alkalosis does not affect arterial pH. Ventilation may be further increased during labor by pain, apprehension, and anxiety. Oxygen consumption increases by 20% owing to the developing fetus, placenta, uterine muscle, and mammary tissue. Arterial oxygen tension remains unchanged.[2]

Pregnancy also affects the mechanics of ventilation. Airway conductance is increased and total pulmonary resistance is decreased by progesterone-induced relaxation of bronchial smooth muscle. Lung compliance is unaffected. Functional residual capacity (FRC) is decreased by anterior displacement of the diaphragm and abdominal organs by the gravid uterus. In addition, during labor, FRC decreases further because of increased pulmonary blood volume subsequent to intermittent uterine contraction. Because of the decrease in FRC, airway closure at end exhalation develops in approximately one-third of human parturients during tidal ventilation.[2] Total lung capacity and vital capacity are unaltered. Because FRC is decreased, hypoventilation induces hypoxemia and hypercapnia more readily in pregnant than nonpregnant patients. Hypoxemia is exacerbated by increased oxygen consumption during labor. Oxygen administration prior to anesthetic induction increases oxygen reserve by facilitating pulmonary denitrogenation. Preoxygenation is advisable if a patient is tolerant.

Induction of anesthesia with inhalation agents is more rapid in pregnant than nonpregnant patients. Equilibration rate between inspired and alveolar anesthetic partial pressure is accelerated by increased alveolar ventilation and decreased FRC. Additionally, increased progesterone and endorphin levels in the central nervous system decrease anesthetic requirements. Minimum alveolar anesthetic concentration values are reduced in pregnant compared with nonpregnant ewes. Thus, anesthetic induction may be extremely rapid, requiring as little as one-fourth to one-fifth the time required for nonpregnant patients.[10] Care must be taken to prevent volatile-agent overdose in pregnant patients.

Gastrointestinal

A number of functional changes in gastrointestinal tract physiology occur with gestation and parturition. Physical displacement of the stomach by the gravid uterus, decreased gastric motility, and increased serum progesterone delay gastric emptying during gestation and are manifest during the last trimester. Acid, chloride, and enzyme concentrations in gastric secretions are increased associated with altered hormone physiology during gestation. Lower esophageal sphincter tone is decreased, and intragastric pressure is increased. Pain and anxiety during labor have been shown to decrease gastric motility further.[2]

As a result of altered gastric function, the risk of regurgitation (both active and passive) and aspiration is greater in parturients. Because increased gastric acidity and decreased gastric muscular tone may be present, metoclopramide and an H_2 antagonist drug (cimetidine, ranitidine, or famotidine) may be administered as part of the preanesthetic protocol.[11] Frequently, patients presented for cesarean section have been fed or the time of the last feeding is unknown. Parturients should be regarded as having a full stomach, and anesthesia techniques should be selected that produce rapid airway management and control to prevent aspiration of foreign material. Incidence of vomiting is increased by hypotension, hypoxia, and toxic reactions to local anesthetics. Smooth induction of general anesthesia and prevention of hypotension during epidural anesthesia will decrease the incidence of vomiting. Because silent regurgitation can occur when intragastric pressure is high, a cuffed endotracheal tube is preferred for airway management. Passive regurgitation can be induced by positive-pressure ventilation with a face mask or by manipulation of abdominal viscera. Atropine administration may increase gastroesophageal sphincter tone, thereby helping to prevent regurgitation, but may also inhibit the actions of metoclopramide that increase gastric motility and emptying by sensitizing gastric smooth muscle to acetylcholine.[6,11]

Liver and Kidney

Pregnancy induces minor alterations in hepatic function. Plasma protein concentration decreases slightly, but total plasma protein is increased because of the increase in blood volume. Bilirubin concentration is unaltered. Serum enzyme concentrations (serum alanine aminotransferase [SALT] and alkaline phosphatase) are slightly increased, and sulfobromophthalein sodium retention is increased. Plasma cholinesterase concentration decreases. Despite these alterations, overall liver function is generally well maintained.[2]

Decreased plasma cholinesterase may lead to prolonged action of succinylcholine in pregnant patients, particularly if they have been exposed recently to organophosphate parasiticides (e.g., anthelmintic, flea collars, or dips). Normal or slightly elevated blood urea nitrogen or creatinine levels may indicate renal pathology or compromise in parturient patients. It would appear wise in such patients to avoid the use of drugs with known nephrotoxic potential, such as methoxyflurane, aminoglycoside antibiotics, and nonsteroidal anti-inflammatory drugs.

Renal plasma flow and glomerular filtration rate are increased by approximately 60% in pregnant patients, so blood urea nitrogen and creatinine concentrations are lower than in nonpregnant patients.[6] Sodium and water balance are unaffected.

Uterine Blood Flow

Maintaining stable uteroplacental circulation is important to fetal and maternal homeostasis and neonatal survival. Uterine blood flow is directly proportional to systemic perfusion pressure and inversely proportional to vascular resistance created in myometrial blood vessels. Placental perfusion is mainly dependent on uteroplacental perfusion pressure; however, placental vessels have rudimentary mechanisms for changing vascular resistance. Obstetric anesthesia may decrease uterine blood flow and thereby contribute to reduced fetal viability. In addition, uterine vascular resistance is indirectly increased by uterine contractions and hypertonia (oxytocic response). Placental hypotension is induced by hypovolemia, anesthetic-induced cardiovascular depression, or sympathetic blockade producing reduced uterine perfusion pressure. Uterine vasoconstriction is induced by endogenous sympathetic discharge or by exogenous sympathomimetic drugs having α_1-adrenergic effects (epinephrine, norepinephrine, methoxamine, phenylephrine, or metaraminol).[2,12,13] Hypotension induced by adjunctive drugs and increased uterine tone induced by ecbolics should be avoided.

Summary

Parturients are at greater anesthetic risk than are healthy nonparturient patients because of pregnancy-associated physiological alterations. Cardiac reserve diminishes during pregnancy, and high-risk patients can suffer acute cardiac decompensation or failure. Pregnant patients are prone to hypoventilation, hypoxia, and hypercapnia because of altered pulmonary function. Inhalation and local anesthetic requirement is decreased, thus increasing the likelihood of a relative overdose and excessive depression. Finally, emesis or regurgitation and aspiration can occur if induction is not immediately followed by rapid airway control.

Pharmacological Alterations Induced by Pregnancy

Pregnancy-associated alterations in physiological function affect the uptake, distribution, and disposition of anesthetic agents and adjuncts. The concentration of free (nonionized, unbound) drug in maternal plasma depends on uptake from the drug administration site, protein binding, distribution to maternal tissues, placental transfer, biotransformation by maternal liver, excretion, and fetal distribution and metabolism. The effects of pregnancy on several anesthetic agents have been studied. The rate of barbiturate biotransformation appears to be decreased in pregnancy.[14] Also, succinylcholine and procaine metabolism are decreased because of decreased plasma cholinesterase concentration; however, this effect is not clinically significant in most cases.[14] Increases in renal blood flow and glomerular filtration associated with pregnancy should favor renal excretion of drugs. Inhalation anesthetic dose (minimum alveolar anesthetic concentration) is reduced for all agents.

The placenta is highly permeable to anesthetic drugs. The physiochemical properties that make a molecule a good anesthetic drug also enable rapid transfer across the uteroplacental interface. Anesthetic drugs administered to the mother cross the placenta and induce fetal effects proportionate to those observed in the mother. Placental transfer of drugs can occur by several mechanisms; by far, the most important is simple diffusion.

Diffusion across the placenta is determined by molecular weight, the degree to which the drug is bound to maternal plasma proteins, lipid solubility, and degree of ionization. Drugs with low molecular weight (MW < 500 daltons), a low degree of protein binding, high lipid solubility, and poor ionization diffuse rapidly across the placenta. Drugs with high MW (>1000 daltons) that are highly protein bound, have low lipid solubility, and are highly ionized cross the placenta slowly. Most anesthetics and anesthetic adjuncts diffuse quickly across the placental barrier because of their low molecular weight, high lipid solubility, low degree of ionization, and low percentage of protein binding. The muscle relaxant drugs are an exception because they are highly ionized and of low lipid solubility. Although they can be recovered from fetal blood, they are generally regarded as having minimal placental transfer and negligible fetal effect.[14,15] The placenta does not appear to metabolize anesthetics or anesthetic adjuncts.

Physiochemical properties and physiological/pharmacokinetic events that occur within the fetus and dam also affect placental drug transfer.[14] The degree to which a drug is ionized is determined by its pK_a and pH of the patient's body fluids. Drugs that are weak acids will be less ionized as pH decreases.[15] For example, thiopental is a weak acid with a pK_a of 7.6. In acidemic patients (pH < 7.4), a greater proportion of the administered dose is in the nonionized form. As the ionized form of the drug decreases, the dose fraction that is protein bound is reduced, thus effectively increasing the effect on a milligram basis. As a result, it is well recognized that acidemia decreases the required anesthetic dose of thiopental and other barbiturates. Weakly basic drugs such as opioids and local anesthetics are more highly ionized at pH values less than their pK_a.[16] Thus, their effect on the mother and fetus is less on a milligram-dose basis.

Distribution of drug between mother and fetus is also influenced by their respective blood pH. Normally, the fetal pH is 0.1 pH unit less than that of the mother. Thus, weakly basic drugs such as opiates and local anesthetics are found in higher concentration in fetal tissues and plasma than in those of the mother because of ion trapping. The lower fetal pH decreases the concentration of nonionized drug, maintaining the maternal-fetal concentration gradient and increasing nonionized drug transfer across the placenta to the fetus.[17]

Fetal drug concentration is altered by fetal redistribution, metabolism, and protein binding. The drug concentration in the umbilical vein is greater than drug exposure to the fetal organs (brain, heart, and other vital organs). As much as 85% of umbilical venous blood initially passes through the fetal liver, where drug may be sequestered or metabolized. In addition, umbilical venous blood containing drug enters the inferior vena cava via the ductus venosus and mixes with drug-free blood returning from the lower extremities and pelvic viscera (Fig. 45.1). Therefore, the fetal circulation buffers vital fetal tissues from sudden high drug concentrations. Binding of drug to fetal proteins may reduce bioavailability.[14,15] Fetal drug metabolism is not efficient because the fetal microsomal enzyme system is not as active as in later life. Drug concentration and effects in the fetus can be considerably greater and last longer than in the mother. Fetal drug toxicity can be enhanced by fetal or maternal metabolism to more toxic metabolites and by drug interaction.[17]

The administration of a fixed dose of drugs with rapidly decreasing plasma concentration (e.g., thiopental, propofol, or succinylcholine) briefly exposes the fetus and placenta to a high maternal blood drug concentration. This is in contrast to the sustained maternal blood levels of drugs administered by continuous infusion or inhalation, which result in continuous placental transfer of drug to the fetus.[14,17]

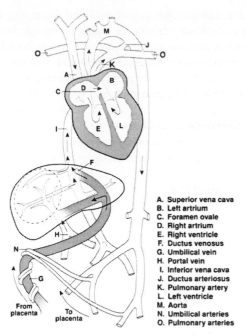

A. Superior vena cava
B. Left atrium
C. Foramen ovale
D. Right atrium
E. Right ventricle
F. Ductus venosus
G. Umbilical vein
H. Portal vein
I. Inferior vena cava
J. Ductus arteriosus
K. Pulmonary artery
L. Left ventricle
M. Aorta
N. Umbilical arteries
O. Pulmonary arteries

Fig. 45.1. The direction of blood flow in the fetal vascular system is indicated by *arrows*. The darkened vascular segments represent the umbilical blood and its path of flow into the liver and inferior vena cava via the ductus venosus. Blood flow through the foramen ovale and ductus arteriosus provides a direct path to the arterial system, bypassing the lungs. In neonates, the ductus arteriosus and foramen ovale closes shortly after birth. This functional closure results in blood flowing through the neonate's lungs, where it is arterialized as in the adult. The time required for anatomical closure of the foramen ovale in the foal may be as much as 12 months. Two months may be required for permanent closure of the foramen ovale.

Anesthetic Drugs and Cesarean Section

Anesthetic drugs should be carefully chosen and properly administered to avoid excessive maternal depression and to maximize neonatal vigor and viability. As noted above in the pharmacology section, the specific characteristics that make a drug an excellent anesthetic agent are also those that facilitate transplacental transfer and neonatal depression in short order. Therefore, it is prudent to consider that no agent should be used unless distinctly indicated. A brief overview of anesthetic drug classes in periparturient anesthesia follows.

Anticholinergic Agents

Anticholinergic drugs, such as atropine or glycopyrrolate, should be administered to most parturient patients to decrease salivation and inhibit excessive vagal tone that may occur when traction is applied to the uterus.[18,19] Many parturients have recently eaten, increasing the likelihood of regurgitation, which is enhanced by hypoxia or hypotension. The influence of anticholinergics upon emesis is controversial.[6,19] In women, atropine has not been shown to decrease the incidence of emesis at parturition.[19]

Glycopyrrolate increases gastric pH, thus decreasing severity of Mendelson's syndrome should regurgitation and aspiration of vomitus occur.[20] Additionally, because glycopyrrolate does not readily cross the placenta, it does not affect the fetus to the same extent as atropine. Therefore, it may be a more appropriate anticholinergic for use in these patients.

Tranquilizers and Sedatives

Because of their long duration of action, there are no indications for the routine use of these agents in parturient patients.[6,16,17] They should be restricted to markedly apprehensive or excited parturients and only in doses sufficient to induce a calming effect. Acepromazine can induce significant maternal and fetal depression even at relatively low doses. Diazepam and midazolam can induce neonatal depression characterized by absence of vocalization and by lethargy, hypotonus, apnea, and hypothermia immediately following birth.[21–23] It has been suggested that these effects are dose related and can be minimized by administering low doses (<0.14 mg/kg intravenously [IV]) although no safe dose has been established in domestic animals.[23] Residual benzodiazepine-induced lethargy and muscle relaxation in either the mother or neonate can be antagonized with flumazenil, a specific benzodiazepine antagonist administered to effect.[24]

Xylazine rapidly crosses the placenta and induces both maternal and fetal respiratory and circulatory depression. When used in conjunction with ketamine, significant and potentially life-threatening cardiopulmonary changes result in decreased tissue perfusion in healthy dogs.[25] The use of xylazine or xylazine-ketamine combinations probably should be avoided in small animal patients presented for cesarean section. On the other hand, xylazine-ketamine combinations have often been used in mares suffering from dystocia. Little information is available regarding use of detomidine or medetomidine in companion animal cesarean section anesthesia. Their structural and pharmacological similarities to xylazine suggest that similar precautions be observed with their use.

Opioids

These rapidly cross the placenta and can cause neonatal respiratory and neurobehavioral depression.[17,26,27] In addition, fetal elimination may require 2 to 6 days. It appears equianalgesic doses of opioids induce equal degrees of depression. Therefore, the choice of an opioid is based on the duration of desired action. The most commonly used opioids are fentanyl, meperidine, oxymorphone, and hydromorphone, in order of increasing duration of action.[17] Recently, agents having opiate agonist and antagonist activity have been used for obstetric analgesia. These agents include butorphanol and buprenorphine. They reportedly induce less respiratory depression than do pure opiate agonists. Butorphanol provides fairly predictable mild to moderate levels of sedation in some species in addition to its analgesic qualities.

One of the advantages of opioid agonists is that direct antagonists are available to reverse their action. Of the antagonist agents, naloxone (0.04 mg/kg IV) appears to be the most effective. It is a pure antagonist without agonist action. Nalorphine and levallorphan, two other antagonist agents, have opiate activ-

ity of their own and can increase respiratory depression induced by other nonopiate agents (e.g., barbiturates, phenothiazines, and inhalation agents). Because all opioid antagonists rapidly cross the placenta, maternal administration before delivery has been advocated to reverse opioid-induced neonatal depression. This technique deprives the mother of analgesia at the time when it is needed most. Therefore, these agents should be administered directly to neonates. Finally, because the action of naloxone is shorter than that of most opioid agonists, renarcotization may occur when naloxone is metabolized and excreted. Thus, both mother and neonates should be carefully monitored for recurring signs of narcosis after opioid reversal with naloxone.[17] Should this occur, additional naloxone can be given.

Sedative-Hypnotics

Thiopental given IV produces rapid induction of basal narcosis for intubation and inhalation anesthesia. The pharmacological effects of thiopental on cardiovascular and respiratory function include increased heart rate, decreased arterial pressure, and changes in peripheral vascular resistance. Cerebral blood flow, oxygen consumption, perfusion pressure, and intracranial pressure decrease with thiopental administration. Apnea is common on induction. Recovery from thiopental is generally rapid because of redistribution and metabolism. Metabolism occurs primarily in the liver. Although thiopental rapidly crosses the placenta, it is also rapidly cleared from the neonatal circulation. Fetal metabolism may contribute to its rapid clearance in utero. Barbiturates can cause neonatal respiratory depression, sleepiness, and decreased activity. Suckling activity is decreased and has been reported to be depressed for 4 days in neonates.[17] These effects are reduced when thiopental is administered in lower doses (<4 mg/kg).[17]

The administration of propofol IV produces rapid induction of basal narcosis for intubation and inhalation anesthesia. The pharmacological effects of propofol on cardiovascular and respiratory function are nearly identical to, but slightly greater than, those of thiopental: Arterial pressure and vascular resistance decrease. Cerebral blood flow, oxygen consumption, perfusion pressure, and intracranial pressure decrease as with thiopental. Apnea is common on induction. Recovery from propofol is prompt and smooth owing to rapid redistribution and metabolism. Metabolism occurs primarily in the liver, but extrahepatic metabolism also occurs. Because of its extensive distribution and rapid metabolism, recovery is very rapid in some species. Although propofol rapidly crosses the placenta, it is rapidly cleared from the neonatal circulation.

Several recent studies have compared the use of propofol in companion animal cesarean section anesthesia with more traditional general anesthesia techniques. In dogs, propofol followed by isoflurane anesthesia resulted in newborn survival rates comparable to epidural anesthesia and superior to general anesthesia induced with thiopental.[28] Cohort retrospective studies by Moon and coworkers[22,23] indicated that administration of propofol IV followed by isoflurane increased puppy vigor, vocalization, and survival following surgery. Their findings were similar to those in the previously reported study by Funkquist et al.[28] Constant-rate infusion of propofol as a sole anesthetic agent in pregnant ewes demonstrated maternal hemodynamics superior to those of isoflurane anesthesia.[29] The uterine blood-flow profile was similar in both techniques. Propofol-sevoflurane anesthesia in pregnant goats demonstrated that fetal physiology was maintained following propofol administration, but hemodynamic indices decreased after exposure to sevoflurane.[30] These studies support the inclusion of propofol in a balanced general anesthesia protocol for cesarean section. In dogs and cats, the induction dose of propofol is 4 to 8 mg/kg IV. Supplemental doses are 0.5 to 2.0 mg/kg IV. Longer-term constant-rate infusions of propofol to maintain anesthesia may result in some fetal depression, however. The induction dose in sheep and goats is 3 to 5 mg/kg IV.

Etomidate is a short-acting nonbarbiturate hypnotic. In dosages suitable for anesthetic induction, etomidate induces rapid anesthesia with no significant cardiovascular effects in dogs.[31,32] Cerebral blood flow, oxygen consumption, perfusion pressure, and intracranial pressure decrease as with thiopental. Apnea is common on induction. Etomidate is rapidly redistributed and metabolized by hepatic microsomal enzymes and by plasma esterases. Fetal tissue perfusion is well maintained, as shown by more rapid initiation of neonatal spontaneous breathing and greater fetal vitality at delivery than with thiopental.[33] The induction dose of etomidate in non-premedicated dogs and cats is 1.0 to 3.0 mg/kg IV.[34] Based on its rapid elimination profile in cats, etomidate may be suitable for repeated administration IV in low doses in this species.[35] However, repeated administration of etomidate may also cause acute hemolysis, as has been reported in dogs.[36] Etomidate frequently causes pain on IV injection in non-premedicated patients. In addition, myoclonus or involuntary movements can occur upon injection, but can be prevented by premedication with benzodiazepines and/or opioids.

Saffan is a combination of two progesterone-like steroids (alphaxalone, 9 mg/mL, and alphadolone, 3 mg/mL). This agent can be administered intravenously or intramuscularly to cats. Anesthetic induction is smooth and rapid. Cardiovascular depression is proportionate to dose and similar to that of equivalent doses of thiopental or methohexital. Saffan induces less respiratory depression than barbiturates and is compatible with the commonly used preanesthetics, muscle relaxants, and inhalation anesthetics.[37] It has been shown to cross the placenta. Its use in dogs is not recommended because the solubilizing agent (cremaphore) causes severe histamine release. However, it has been used to induce anesthesia in dogs pretreated with antihistamines.[38] Alphaxan-CD has recently been introduced in Australia as a short-acting anesthetic for use in dogs and cats. In this formulation, alphaxalone is solubilized in a cyclodextran carrier void of histamine-releasing properties. It has proved to be an effective short-acting anesthetic with minimal cardiopulmonary depression and few adverse effects. Because of these properties, its use for anesthesia in cesarean section surgery appears promising.

Dissociatives

Ketamine has been used in general anesthesia for cesarean section. In women, doses of less than 1 mg/kg induced minimal neonatal depression.[19,24] Alternatively, thiopental (2 to 3 mg/kg)

and ketamine (0.5 mg/kg) have been coadministered to induce anesthesia in parturient women. A more recent publication indicates that low doses of ketamine (3 to 5 mg/kg IV in dogs, 2 to 4 mg/kg IV in cats, and 2 mg/kg IV in horses) may be used for anesthetic induction.[39] Because effective induction doses for these agents are higher in companion animals than humans, neonatal depression is more likely to be associated with their use. A retrospective cohort study in dogs indicated that ketamine use leads to increased puppy risk associated with respiratory depression, apnea, decreased vocalization, and increased mortality at birth.[22,23] For these reasons, ketamine should be used cautiously in this species. No data for comparative fetal viability are available in other species.

Little information is available regarding the use of tiletamine-zolazepam in cesarean section. Based on pharmacological profile, characteristics of this proprietary drug mixture are qualitatively similar to other dissociative-benzodiazepine tranquilizer mixtures. In vivo characteristics of these agents suggest that caution be used in companion animal cesarean section anesthesia, because of their rapid and extensive transplacental transfer and absence of specific antagonist agents.

Neuroleptanalgesia

The combination of opioid and tranquilizer class drugs can induce anesthetic effectively in depressed, exhausted parturients. As noted above, both opioids and tranquilizers extensively cross the uteroplacental interface and may cause significant fetal depression. These agents are usually used as an anesthetic supplement following fetal removal, although they have been successfully used for induction and maintenance prior to fetal extraction. If fetal depression is noted after administration of these agents, oral sublingual administration of naloxone (1 to 2 drops) rapidly reverses opioid effects in neonates. Continuous monitoring for neonatal renarcotization is warranted.[39]

Inhalation Agents

Inhalation anesthetics may be used to induce anesthesia in calm or depressed dams. These agents readily cross the placenta with rapid fetal and maternal equilibration. Thus, the degree of neonatal depression is proportional to the depth of anesthesia induced in the mother. Deep levels of maternal anesthesia cause maternal hypotension, decreased uterine blood flow, and fetal acidosis. Isoflurane, sevoflurane, or desflurane are preferred because induction and recovery of mother and neonate are more rapid. Nitrous oxide can be used to potentiate their effect, thus decreasing the total amount of volatile agent administered. If nitrous oxide is administered at 60% or less, fetal depression is minimal and neonatal diffusion hypoxia does not occur upon delivery.[17–19]

Skeletal Muscle Relaxants

These cross the placenta to a very limited degree and have little effect on neonates when used in reasonable clinical doses; thus, these drugs are very useful in balanced anesthesia techniques for cesarean section to facilitate rapid airway management and provide surgical site relaxation.[15,18,19] Because of its rapid onset of action and relatively brief duration, succinylcholine is a traditional choice when combined with an ultra–short-acting barbiturate or propofol for induction of anesthesia and airway control. Mivacurium has also been used because of its rapid onset of effect and relatively brief (15 to 20 min) duration of action. Atracurium and vecuronium provide an intermediate (20 to 35 min) duration of action.[39] Their characteristics make them attractive alternatives in longer procedures. The use of long-acting muscle relaxants, such as pancuronium (45 min), is generally avoided because of their length of action when compared with procedure time.[17]

Guaifenesin has been used to relax skeletal muscle in horses, cattle, and small ruminants. Although limited in reports, clinical impressions indicate that transplacental transfer is minimal based on vigor of the newborn after delivery.

Local Anesthetics

These are frequently used in combination with other agents or as the sole anesthetic agent for regional techniques. Esters of paraaminobenzoic acid (procaine or tetracaine) are metabolized by maternal and fetal pseudocholinesterase. Thus, there is little accumulation of these agents in the fetus. Amide derivatives (e.g., lidocaine, mepivacaine, bupivacaine, etidocaine, and ropivacaine) are metabolized by hepatic microsomal enzymes. After absorption from the injection site, blood levels decrease slowly but can reach significance in the fetus. Neonatal blood concentrations in excess of 3 μg/mL of lidocaine or mepivacaine can cause neonatal depression at delivery. These concentrations rarely occur after epidural administration but can occur with excessive volumes of drug used for local infiltration.[17]

Sympathetic blockade resulting in maternal hypotension and decreased uteroplacental perfusion may occur after epidural injection. This can be controlled by judicious administration of IV fluids to offset increased capacity of the vascular tree.[17] In addition to IV fluids, vasopressors can be used to treat maternal hypotension caused by sympathetic blockade. Because ephedrine acts centrally and has minimal arterial vasoconstrictor properties while increasing venous tone and thereby preload, it can be used to treat maternal hypotension, thus restoring uterine blood flow. Mephentermine acts in a similar manner. Other agents with α-adrenergic activity increase maternal blood pressure by increasing systemic vascular resistance. This may cause uterine blood flow to decrease, and fetal deterioration often occurs. In addition, these agents can stimulate hypertonic uterine contractions, further decreasing uteroplacental perfusion.[17,19]

Anesthetic Techniques for Cesarean Section

General Anesthesia

Cesarean section anesthesia can be accomplished either by regional or general anesthesia. Advantages of general anesthesia include speed and ease of induction, reliability, reproducibility, and control. General anesthesia provides optimum operating conditions with relaxed immobile patients. Tracheal intubation ensures control of the maternal airway, thereby preventing aspiration of vomitus or regurgitated rumen contents. In addition, it provides a route for maternal oxygen administration, thereby improving fetal oxygenation. When general anesthesia is administered properly, maternal cardiopulmonary function is well maintained.[19,39]

General anesthesia may be more appropriate than regional anesthesia in selected clinical situations. These include maternal hypovolemia, prolonged dystocia in which the mother is exhausted and the fetus is severely stressed, maternal cardiac disease or failure, morbid obesity, cases in which the mother is so aggressive or fractious as to preclude regional anesthesia, and brachycephalic dogs with upper airway obstruction. Finally, most veterinarians are more confident of their ability to induce general anesthesia safely than to use regional anesthesia techniques.

General anesthesia does have certain disadvantages. It will likely produce greater neonatal depression than will regional anesthesia. Inadequate anesthetic plane causes maternal catecholamine release, which may result in hypertension and decreased uteroplacental perfusion, leading to both maternal and fetal stress and deterioration of cardiopulmonary function.[12,13,26] Loss of airway protective reflexes following anesthetic induction may produce aspiration and airway management challenges when the trachea is not properly intubated. Aspiration and inability to intubate the trachea successfully are the leading causes of maternal mortality associated with cesarean section in women.[19,39] Fortunately, dogs, cats, and horses are relatively easy to intubate because of their anatomical features. However, ruminants and swine are relatively difficult to intubate, and this presents problems for most veterinarians in rural practice.

Dystocia in mares is an emergency in which duration has a profound effect on the survival of foals.[40] Foals are normally delivered within 20 to 30 min after chorioallantoic membrane rupture. Few foals survive when the duration is increased to 40 min, and none are likely to survive when the duration is 90 min or longer.[41,42] In a recent article, the time from chorioallantoic rupture to delivery was significantly different in surviving foals (71.7 ± 34.3 min) when compared with nonsurviving foals (85.3 ± 37.4 min).[40] This makes dystocia in mares more of an emergency than it is for most species, where as little as 15 min can mean the difference between a live and dead foal. Importantly, the method of resolving a dystocia has an impact on the time from chorioallantoic rupture to birth. Four procedures can be attempted: assisted vaginal delivery (AVD), in which the mare is awake and manually assisted to some degree; controlled vaginal delivery (CVD), where the mare is anesthetized and the clinician is in control of delivering an intact foal; fetotomy, where the dead fetus is reduced to more than one part and removed vaginally in the awake or anesthetized mare; and cesarean section, where the fetus is removed through a uterine incision by celiotomy.[43] It has been suggested that CVD, followed rapidly by cesarean section if initial attempts are unsuccessful, is the best choice for dystocia resolution.[40]

Physical examination, anesthetic induction, and delivery should be accomplished in the shortest period possible when there is the chance of delivering a live foal.[40] Time-consuming methods of anesthetic induction in mares should be abandoned in favor of methods that provide reliable sedation and smooth controlled induction with favorable recoveries. Sedation can be achieved rapidly with xylazine (0.8 mg/kg IV) followed by induction with ketamine (2.2 mg/kg IV) and diazepam (Valium, 0.08 mg/kg IV). Anesthesia is then maintained with isoflurane or halothane in 100% oxygen.[40] While CVD is attempted, the ventral abdomen is clipped and prepped so that, if needed, cesarean section may be accomplished rapidly. In one report this approach to dystocia resulted in 94% of the CVD mares and 89% of the cesarean section mares surviving to discharge with a 42% delivery of live foals. Nearly 30% of foals survived to discharge.[40] In these scenarios, specific choice of anesthetic agent is probably less important than the time to induction and delivery of the foal.

Much of the previously published recommendations for anesthesia of term mares has been extrapolated from work done in other species and may not be relevant. Goals for delivering anesthesia are no different than for other species, but with a greater emphasis placed on rapid completion of the procedure. Laboring mares are typically agitated and distressed prior to anesthetic induction, and good sedation is therefore important to ensure a smooth and safe induction. Xylazine and detomidine will provide sufficient sedation and can be reversed in neonates after delivery. Detomidine may cause less increase in uterine tone than xylazine and has been suggested by some as the sedative of choice in mares.[44] When butorphanol is combined with xylazine or detomidine, reliable restraint and analgesia occur. The dose of xylazine or detomidine can be lowered when combined with butorphanol, minimizing potential side effects of the α_2-agonists.

There is little work regarding use of tiletamine-zolazepam in mares presenting for dystocia, but based on pharmacological profile, it should be similar to other dissociative-benzodiazepine tranquilizer anesthetic combinations. It has been suggested that because of the potential for ion trapping, the use of benzodiazepines should be avoided in mares presenting for cesarean section,[45] but there is no evidence to support that this occurs excessively in foals. Ketamine is rapidly cleared from maternal and fetal circulation, causes minimal cardiovascular depression, and provides for a smooth induction, making it suitable for induction in pregnant mares. Thiopental is also rapidly cleared from fetal circulation and would be acceptable for inducing anesthesia, though induction may be rough when used alone. Recent work done in pony mares has found that maintenance of anesthesia with propofol or a combination of guaifenesin, ketamine, and detomidine (GKD) preserved cardiovascular function in both the mare and fetus.[46,47] This suggests that GKD could be suitable for anesthetic induction of term mares. Guaifenesin is a centrally acting muscle relaxant that crosses in minimal amounts to the fetal circulation. In the field where equipment is not readily available for delivering inhalation anesthesia, a mixture of guaifenesin-ketamine-xylazine has been infused to effect for up to 1 h to maintain an adequate level of central nervous system depression.[48]

Studies have been done comparing the effects of isoflurane and halothane in pregnant mares, and no marked differences between the two have been demonstrated.[49] Less soluble agents (such as isoflurane and sevoflurane) would have the advantage of being more rapidly cleared from foals after delivery as compared with the more soluble agent halothane.[45]

Monitoring and support of an anesthetized pregnant mare are no different than for any anesthetized horse. Care should be taken to avoid maternal hypoxia in order to maintain fetal oxygenation until delivery. Mechanical ventilation should be considered to help offset the ventilation-perfusion mismatching that occurs. When using positive-pressure ventilation (PPV) to improve oxygenation of mares, arterial blood gases should be assessed shortly after initiating PPV to ensure that the desired increase in PaO_2 is actually occurring. PPV in a mare with severe abdominal distension has the potential to drastically decrease cardiac output to all tissues, including maternal circulation to the foal. Arterial blood pressure should be monitored directly and ideally kept above 70 mm Hg by adjusting anesthetic depth and rate of fluid delivery, and by administering inotropes and vasopressors, as needed.

Mares recovering from dystocia or cesarean section may have a difficult time regaining the strength needed to stand. Special attention should be given to the condition of the recovery stall, and the floor should be cleaned of all obstetric lubricant and dried. Mares should be placed on a well-padded surface in the recovery stall and may be rope assisted during recovery when necessary.

A spectrum of techniques for induction of general anesthesia for cesarean section in dogs and cats have been reported to be satisfactory (Table 45.2).[50] All reported techniques have common strategies for successful patient management which include the following points. Induction of anesthesia must be smooth and rapid. Excitement and struggling associated with excessive restraint and poor technique must be avoided. Intubation should be accomplished quickly and ventilation supported to ensure adequate oxygenation.

Maternal oxygen administration can significantly increase fetal oxygen content. Administration of oxygen to the mother is not associated with a significant decrease in uterine blood flow or fetal acidosis.[17] Fetal red blood cells have a lower 2,3-diphosphoglycerate concentration than do adult red blood cells. Thus, fetal hemoglobin can carry more oxygen at low oxygen tensions than can adult hemoglobin. Physiologically, this is important because it ensures a higher level of hemoglobin saturation at the normally low oxygen partial pressures (PO_2 of umbilical vein, 30 mm Hg) to which the fetus is exposed.[20,51] Inspired oxygen concentrations of 50% or more during general anesthesia result in more vigorous neonates because of improved oxygenation.[17] Therefore, oxygen administration is indicated regardless of the anesthetic protocol.

Tidal and minute ventilation must be critically evaluated during the anesthetic period to avoid either hypoventilation or hyperventilation. The total effect of carbon dioxide on the fetus is not clear, but passive hyperventilation of the dam causes hypocapnia with decreased uterine artery blood flow. This decreased placental perfusion causes fetal hypoxia, hypercapnia, and acidosis. With adequate arterial oxygenation, a modest increase in $PaCO_2$ is well tolerated by the fetus.[17] Adequacy of ventilation and oxygenation may be assessed by observing rate of respiration, excursion of the chest wall and/or reservoir bag, and color of mucous membranes; by implementation of pulse oximetry; and by determination of $PaCO_2$ and PaO_2.

Table 45.2. Selected anesthesia techniques for elective and emergency cesarean section anesthesia in common domestic species.

Species	Drug or Technique		
	Elective Cesarean Section	**Emergency Cesarean Section**	**Comments**

Dog	1. Lumbosacral epidural
	2. Anticholinergic
	  Propofol, 4–8 mg/kg
	  Isoflurane or sevoflurane
	  Post–removal pain meds
	3. Anticholinergic
	  Fentanyl, 3 µg/kg
	  Propofol, 4–8 mg/kg
	  Isoflurane or sevoflurane
		1. Lumbosacral epidural
		2. Sevoflurane or isoflurane mask
		  induction
		3. Anticholinergic
		  Fentanyl, 3 µg/kg
		  Propofol, 4–8 mg/kg
		  Isoflurane or sevoflurane
		4. Anticholinergic
		  Fentanyl, 3 µg/kg
		  Propofol, 4–8 mg/kg
		  Line block
		  Atracurium, 0.2 mg/kg
			1. May require assistant to restrain
			  epidural patients
			2. Give oxygen to all patients as soon
			  as possible
			3. Monitor heart rate and redo anti-
			  cholinergic if needed
			4. Minimal inhalant agent dose until all
			  fetuses are removed
			5. May need to reverse fentanyl with
			  sublingual naloxone if fetus is
			  depressed

Cat	1. Propofol, 4–8 mg/kg
	  Laryngeal anesthesia
	  Sevoflurane or isoflurane
	  Additional analgesia following
	    fetal removal
	2. Fentanyl, 3–5 µg/kg
	  Propofol, 4 mg/kg
	  Laryngeal anesthesia
	  Sevoflurane or isoflurane
	  Additional analgesia following
	    fetal removal
		1. Ketamine, 3 mg/kg
		  Fentanyl, 3–5 µg/kg
		  Lumbosacral epidural
		2. Ketamine, 3 mg/kg
		  Fentanyl, 3–5 µg/kg
		  Propofol, 2–4 mg/kg
		  Sevoflurane or isoflurane
		  Additional analgesia following
		    fetal removal
			1. May require assistant to restrain
			  epidural patients
			2. Give oxygen to all patients as soon
			  as possible
			3. Minimal inhalant agent dose until all
			  fetuses are removed
			4. May need to reverse fentanyl with
			  sublingual naloxone if fetus is
			  depressed

Horse	1. GGE to effect
	  Ketamine, 2 mg/kg
	  Isoflurane or sevoflurane
	  Caudal epidural for pain
	    management
	2. GGE to effect
	  Thiopental, 4–6 mg/kg
	  Isoflurane or sevoflurane
	  Caudal epidural for pain management
		1. GGE to effect
		  Ketamine, 2 mg/kg
		  Isoflurane or sevoflurane
		  Caudal epidural for pain management
			1. Standing restraint not performed
			  in horses for cesarean section
			  anesthesia
			2. Postoperative pain management
			  similar to that for colic patients

Cattle	1. Xylazine, 10 mg
	  Paravertebral block
	2. Xylazine, 10 mg
	  Inverted "L" block
	3. Incisional line block
	4. Xylazine, 10 mg
	  GGE to recumbency
	  Isoflurane or sevoflurane
	    following intubation
		1. Xylazine, 10 mg
		  Paravertebral block
		2. Xylazine, 10 mg
		  Inverted "L" block
		3. Incisional line block
		4. Xylazine, 10 mg
		  GGE to recumbency
		  Isoflurane/sevoflurane
		    following intubation
			1. Avoid recumbency with regional
			  techniques
			2. Can reverse xylazine in newborns if
			  depression is noted
			3. Supplemental analgesia in postoper-
			  ative period as warranted
			4. Caudal epidural to reduce post-
			  parturient "straining"

Sheep/Goat	1. Lumbosacral epidural
	  Sedation
	2. Incisional line block
	  Sedation
	3. Propofol, 4–6 mg/kg
	  Isoflurane or sevoflurane
		1. Lumbosacral epidural
		  Sedation
		2. Incisional line block
		  Sedation
		3. Propofol, 4–6 mg/kg
		  Isoflurane or sevoflurane
			1. Sheep have a high pain sensitivity
			2. Variable and inconsistent response
			  to opioids for pain management
			3. α_2 Agents are frequently selected
			  for supplemental analgesia

(continued)

Table 45.2. Selected anesthesia techniques for elective and emergency cesarean section anesthesia in common domestic species (*continued*).

Species	Drug or Technique		
	Elective Cesarean Section	**Emergency Cesarean Section**	**Comments**
Pig	1. Lumbosacral epidural Sedation 2. Incisional line block Sedation 3. Propofol, 4–6 mg/kg Isoflurane or sevoflurane	1. Lumbosacral epidural Sedation 2. Incisional line block Sedation 3. Propofol, 4–6 mg/kg Isoflurane or sevoflurane	1. Will need sedation in addition to regional analgesia in elective section 2. Good response to opioid analgesic agents following fetal removal 3. NSAIDs are frequently used for pain management
Llama	1. GGE to effect 2. Propofol, 2–4 mg/kg 3. Isoflurane or sevoflurane	1. GGE to effect 2. Isoflurane or sevoflurane	1. Limited reports in literature 2. Pain management following fetal removal as per other procedures

GGE, guaifenesin glycerate ester; NSAIDs, nonsteroidal anti-inflammatory drugs.

Regional Anesthesia

This is a well-established technique for cesarean section.[16] There is an increased sensitivity and distribution to local anesthetic agents during gestation and parturition. As a result, the dose of local anesthetic for epidural or spinal anesthesia can be reduced by approximately one-third in pregnant patients as compared with nonparturients. Regional anesthesia (epidural or subarachnoid) has the advantages of technique simplicity, minimal exposure of the fetus to drugs, less intraoperative bleeding and, because the mother remains awake, minimal risk of aspiration.[52] In addition, muscle relaxation and analgesia are optimal. Caudal spinal anatomy in the lumbosacral region varies by species. The spinal cord terminates at the level of the sixth lumbar vertebra in dogs, reducing the risk of subarachnoid (true spinal) injection of the anesthetic agent. The spinal cord terminates variably between L7 and midsacrum in cats, making subarachnoid injection a greater possibility.[53] In swine and ruminants, the spinal cord terminates at the midsacrum, making subarachnoid injection a possibility at the lumbosacral junction.

Epidural anesthesia has been successfully used in dogs and cats for cesarean section anesthesia. Traditionally, a short-acting local anesthetic (2% lidocaine) is administered at a dose of 1 mL per 3.25 to 4.5 kg of body weight in the epidural space to provide surgical site anesthesia. In recent years, epidurally administered drugs, including lidocaine and bupivacaine in a 1:1 volumetric mixture, have provided extended duration of surgical anesthesia and pain management in the early recovery period. This may be supplemented with epidural opioids and α_2-adrenergic agonists to extend the postoperative analgesic period.

Spinal techniques work well in sows, sheep, and goats. The technique is well established and not difficult. When using this technique, it is sometimes necessary to restrain a sow's head and forelimbs. If pigs are sedated and restrained in lateral recumbency with the head extended, the soft palate may occlude the airway and the patient may suffocate. This has been observed in sows and gilts undergoing cesarean section with spinal anesthesia without additional sedatives or tranquilizers. Because cesarean section in swine is often viewed as a last-ditch effort by producers, it is often delayed until the sow's condition has deteriorated severely. Thus, a high percentage of sows presented for cesarean section are hypovolemic and hypotensive. Fluids can be readily administered to sows via indwelling catheters placed into the ear veins prior to anesthetic administration. This will restore circulating volume and offset hypotension induced by spinal techniques.

Spinal anesthesia often induces recumbency, which may not be desirable in large ruminants. If the veterinarian prefers, standing cesarean section in cattle may be performed using either a proximal or distal paralumbar block. In cows that are in poor condition, exhausted, or in shock, the distal technique is preferred because it does not induce a scoliosis-like position and the cow is more likely to remain standing throughout the procedure.

Disadvantages of epidural or subarachnoid anesthesia include hypotension secondary to sympathetic blockade. Hypotension induced by epidural anesthesia can be managed with IV fluid and catecholamine administration. Lactated Ringer's solution or 0.9% or 0.45% sodium chloride mixed with equal volumes of 5% dextrose solution can be administered at approximately 20 mL/kg over 15 to 20 min to maintain arterial blood pressure. When hypotension is severe, ephedrine may be administered (0.15 mg/kg IV). Hypotension and visceral manipulation during the procedure can cause nausea and vomiting.[54] Because the dam remains conscious, the forelimbs and head often move. This precludes the use of a spinal technique in highly excited or fractious patients and in mares, because they become hysterical when they are unable to stand.

Local Anesthesia

Local infiltration or field block may be used, but these techniques have several disadvantages when compared with regional techniques. Infiltration requires larger amounts of anesthetic agent, which are absorbed and can create fetal depression. In addition, muscle relaxation and analgesia are not as profound or as uniform when compared with regional anesthesia. In many cases, field block is supplemented with heavy sedation or tranquilization to calm and stabilize a dam; these agents further contribute to maternal and fetal depression. For these reasons, field block is often abandoned for either general or epidural anesthesia.

Care of Newborns

Following delivery, the newborn's head is cleared of membranes and the oropharynx of fluid. The umbilical vessels should be milked toward the fetus to empty them of blood, clamped approximately 2 to 5 cm from the body wall, and severed from the placenta. Neonates can then be gently rubbed with a towel to dry them and stimulate breathing. It may also be helpful to swing neonates gently in a head-down position to help clear the respiratory tree of fluid. Vigorous motion should be avoided because amniotic fluid is readily absorbed in the lungs and contributes to distribution of pulmonary surfactant in the alveoli. The head and neck should be supported to avoid whiplash and prevent injury.

Flow-by oxygen administration in the vicinity of the muzzle is helpful to increase heart rate and oxygen delivery to tissues in distressed, exhausted neonates. Reversal of opioids by sublingual administration of 1 to 2 drops naloxone is warranted in cases where opioids were administered as part of the general anesthesia technique. An oral dose of 2.5% dextrose (0.1 to 0.5 mL) is helpful to improve energy substrates required for initial breathing effort in stressed neonates. Finally, maintaining warmth is vital because hypothermia can occur rapidly after birth.

A small IV catheter may be used to intubate and support oxygen delivery in neonates that will not initiate breathing, and their breathing can be artificially supported by using a syringe and three-way valve attached to an oxygen source. As a final measure, doxapram can be used to stimulate breathing in neonates. In pups, a dosage of 1 to 5 mg (approximately 1 to 5 drops from a 20- to 22-gauge needle) is topically administered to the oral mucosa or injected intramuscularly or subcutaneously. In kittens, the dosage is 1 to 2 mg (1 to 2 drops).[50] Airways must be clear before doxapram administration. External thoracic compressions may be warranted if heart rate is slow and does not respond to support measures. A rapid physical examination checking for genetic defects (cleft palate, chest deformity, or abdominal wall fusion) is also important to determine whether viability is present.

When general anesthesia is used in ruminants or horses, an alternate method of managing neonates may be used to good advantage. After uterine incision, the fetal head is delivered through the incision, the oropharynx is cleared of fluid, and the trachea is intubated with a cuffed tube. The fetus can then be delivered and the umbilicus severed. Because the uteroplacental and umbilical circulation is preserved until the airway is secured, hypoxia is prevented. Once the fetus is delivered, ventilation can be supported, if necessary, via a bag valve mask resuscitator.

After completion of surgery and recovery from anesthesia, the young can be introduced to their mother. If introduction is delayed, the neonates should be exposed briefly to the mother to provide colostrum and then kept in a warm environment until anesthesia recovery is complete to avoid accidental crushing. If regional anesthesia was used, they can be placed with their mother as soon as the surgery is complete.

Perioperative Pain Management

This represents a challenge in cesarean section patients because of concerns regarding transfer of anesthetic and analgesic drugs into milk and its impact on neonates. This area has been extensively studied in people and in food-producing species. Most of the current information is from humans and cattle; however, because of the similarity of the lactation process in all mammals, the information may be extrapolated to other species.

The phenothiazine tranquilizer chlorpromazine does not appear to transfer to milk at levels that cause fetal depression.[55] No corollary evidence is available for acepromazine, but similarity in molecular structure coupled with clinical experience supports a similar effect on newborns. The benzodiazepine class tranquilizer diazepam significantly crosses into milk and may cause lethargy, sedation, and weight loss in newborns.[56] Other class members, including clonazepam and alprazolam, induce drowsiness, hypotonia, and apnea in newborns after nursing episodes. The effect of lorazepam and midazolam are unknown; however, based on the effects attributed to other class members, they should be used with caution in lactating mothers. Xylazine transiently increases in milk and then decreases to nondetectable levels by 12 h after administration.[57] Detomidine (80 µg/kg) can be detected at a low level in milk after administration but is nondetectable by 23 h later.[58]

Codeine, propoxyphene, and morphine are well tolerated by newborns when used in maternal pain management, even when repeat doses are administered over several days.[59] Meperidine (pethidine) has been reported to cause decreased suckling behavior and sedation when used in serial doses.[59,60] Fentanyl (100 µg) and sufentanil (10 to 50 µg) are not detectable in breast milk after epidural administration in humans.[61]

Thiopental has been detected in colostrum and breast milk after a single bolus induction dose (5 mg/kg) in women.[62] Long-acting barbiturates such as phenobarbital are contraindicated because of their extensive presence in milk.[55] Propofol is detectable in colostrum and milk after a single-dose administration.[63] However, little clinical effect is noted based on excellent newborn vitality immediately after delivery.[22,23] The residual presence of inhalation anesthetic agents in milk is not known; however, clinical experience suggests that prolonged neonatal sedation following clinical recovery of dams is not common.

Local anesthetic drugs (e.g., lidocaine and bupivacaine) and first-generation bupivacaine metabolites are excreted in milk after their epidural administration in humans. Although these agents are detectable in milk, their influence on neonates is negligible based on maximum Apgar (activity, pulse, grimace, appearance, and respiration) scores at delivery.[64]

Nonsteroidal anti-inflammatory drugs appear to reach only limited levels in milk after maternal administration. In humans, acetaminophen and aspirin are considered compatible with breast feeding.[59] Studies evaluating carprofen in cattle indicated that milk levels were below detectable limits (<0.022 μg/mL) after a single-dose administration. After experimental induction of mastitis, carprofen was detected at low levels (0.16 μg/mL) for 12 h following single-bolus administration and decreased to undetectable levels (<0.022 μg/mL) by 24 h.[65] Following a single dose of ketoprofen (3.3 mg/kg) in cattle, nonquantifiable concentrations of ketoprofen were detected in milk for only 2 h.[66] Similar results have been reported in lactating goats.[67]

With the possible exception of the nonsteroidal anti-inflammatory drugs and their potential for inhibiting newborn organ maturation, it appears that most commonly used analgesic drug classes may be safely administered during the lactation period without adverse effects on newborns.

References

1. Dawes GS. Foetal and Neonatal Physiology. Chicago: Year Book, 1968:15.
2. Shnider SM. The physiology of pregnancy. In: Annual Refresher Course Lectures. Park Ridge, IL: American Society of Anesthesiologists, 1978:1251–1258.
3. Kerr MG. Cardiovascular dynamics in pregnancy and labour. Br Med Bull 24:19–24, 1968.
4. Ueland K, Parer JT. Effects of estrogens on the cardiovascular system of the ewe. Am J Obstet Gynecol 96:400–406, 1966.
5. Ueland K, Hansen JM. Maternal cardiovascular dynamics. II. Posture and uterine contractions. Am J Obstet Gynecol 103:1–7, 1969.
6. James EM III. Physiologic changes during pregnancy. In: Annual Refresher Course Lectures. Park Ridge, IL: American Society of Anesthesiologists, 1980:1251–1255.
7. Marx CE. Physiology of pregnancy: High risk implications. In: Annual Refresher Course Lectures. Park Ridge, IL, American Society of Anesthesiologists, 1979:1251–1254.
8. Kerr MC, Scott DB. Inferior vena caval occlusion in late pregnancy. Clin Anesth 10:17–22, 1973.
9. Lipton B, Hershey SC, Baez S. Compatibility of oxytocics with anesthetic agents. J Am Med Assoc 179:410–416, 1962.
10. Palahniuk RJ, Shnider SM, Eger EI III, Lopez-Manzanara P. Pregnancy decreases the requirements of inhaled anesthetic agents. Anesthesiology 41:82–83, 1974.
11. Paddleford RR. Anesthesia for cesarean section in the dog. Vet Clin North Am Small Anim Pract 22:481–484, 1992.
12. Wright RC, Shnider SM, Levinsan G, et al. The effect of maternal stress on plasma catecholamines and uterine blood flow in the ewe [Abstract]. In: Annual Meeting of the Society of Obstetric Anesthesia and Perinatology, 1978:17–20.
13. Morishema HO, Yeh M-N, James LS. The effects of maternal pain and hyperexcitability upon the fetus: Possible benefits of maternal sedation [Abstract]. In: Scientific Session of American Society of Anesthesiologists Annual Meeting, Atlanta, Georgia, 1977.
14. Alper MH. Perinatal pharmacology. In: Annual Refresher Course Lectures. Park Ridge, IL: American Society of Anesthesiologists, 1979:1261–1267.
15. Einster M. Perinatal pharmacology. In: Annual Refresher Course Lectures. Park Ridge, IL: American Society of Anesthesiologists, 1980:1261–1264.
16. Collins VI. Principles of Anesthesiology, 2nd ed. Philadelphia: Lea and Febiger, 1976:199.
17. Gutsche B. Perinatal pharmacology. In: Annual Refresher Course Lectures. Park Ridge, IL: American Society of Anesthesiologists, 1978:1291–1299.
18. Gibbs CP. Anesthesia for cesarean section: General. In: Annual Refresher Course Lectures. Park Ridge, IL: American Society of Anesthesiologists, 1981:2181–2185.
19. Datta S, Alper MH. Anesthesia for cesarean section. Anesthesiology 53:142–160, 1980.
20. Goodger WJ, Levy W. Anesthetic management of the cesarean section. Vet Clin North Am 3:85–99, 1973.
21. Moon PF, Erb HN, Ludders JW, Gleed RD, Pascoe PJ. Perioperative management and mortality rates of dogs undergoing cesarean section in the United States and Canada. J Am Vet Med Assoc 213:365–369, 1998.
22. Moon PF, Erb HN, Ludders JW, Gleed RD, Pascoe PJ. Perioperative risk factors for puppies delivered by cesarean section in the United States and Canada. J Am An Hosp Assoc 36:359–368, 2000.
23. Moon-Massat PF, Erb HN. Perioperative factors associated with puppy vigor after delivery by cesarean section. J Am An Hosp Assoc 38:90–96, 2002.
24. Tranquilli WJ, Lemke K, Williams LL, et al. Flumazenil efficacy in reversing diazepam or midazolam overdose in dogs. J Vet Anaesth 19:65–68, 1992.
25. McDonnell W, Van Corder I. Cardiopulmonary effects of xylazine/ketamine in dogs [Abstract]. In: Annual Scientific Meeting American College of Veterinary Anesthesiologists, Las Vegas, Nevada, 1982.
26. Palahniuk RJ. Obstetric anesthesia in the healthy parturient. In: Annual Refresher Course Lectures. Park Ridge, IL: American Society of Anesthesiologists, 1979:1271–1274.
27. Hodgkinson R, Bhatt M, Wang CN. Double-blind comparison of the neurobehaviour of neonates following the administration of different doses of meperidine to the mother. Can Anaesth Soc J 25:405–411, 1978.
28. Funkquist PM, Nyman GC, Lofgren AJ, Fahlbrink EM. Use of propofol-isoflurane as an anesthetic regimen for cesarean section in dogs. J Am Vet Med Assoc 211:313–317, 1997.
29. Gaynor JS, Wertz EM, Alvis M, Turner AS. A comparison of the haemodynamic effects of propofol and isoflurane in pregnant ewes. J Vet Pharmacol Ther 21:69–73, 1998.
30. Setoyama K, Shinzato T, Kazuhiro M, Makato F, Sakamoto H. Effects of propofol-sevoflurane anesthesia on the maternal and fetal hemodynamics, blood gases, and uterine activity in pregnant goats. J Vet Med Sci 65:1075–1081, 2003.
31. Nagel ML, Muir WW, Nguyen K. Comparison of the cardiopulmonary effects of etomidate and thiamylal in dogs. Am J Vet Res 40:193–196, 1979.
32. Muir WW, Swanson CR. Principles, techniques, and complications of feline anesthesia and chemical restraint. In: Sherding R, ed. The Cat: Diseases and Clinical Management. New York: Churchill Livingstone, 1989:81–116.
33. Downing JW, Buley RJR, Brock-Utney JG, Houlton PC. Etomidate for induction of anesthesia at caesarean section: Comparison with thiopentone. Br J Anaesth 51:135–140, 1979.
34. Tranquilli WJ. Anesthesia for cesarean section in the cat. Vet Clin North Am Small Anim Pract 22:484–486, 1992.
35. Wertz EM, Benson GJ, Thurmon JC, Tranquilli WJ, Davis LE, Koritz GD. Pharmacokinetics of etomidate in cats. Am J Vet Res 5:281–285, 1990.

36. Ko JCH, Thurmon JC, Benson GJ, Tranquilli WJ. Acute hemolysis with etomidate-propylene glycol infusion in the dog. J Vet Anaesth 20:92–94, 1993.

37. Hall LW. Althesin in the large animal. Postgrad Med J 48(Suppl 2):55–58, 1972.

38. Corbet HR. The use of Saffan in the dog. Aust Vet Pract 7:184–188, 1977.

39. Greene SA. Veterinary Anesthesia and Pain Management Secrets. Philadelphia: Hanley and Belfus, 2002:229–231.

40. Byron CR, Embertson RM, Bernard WV, Hance SR, Bramlage LR, Hopper SA. Dystocia in a referral hospital setting: Approach and results. Equine Vet J 35:82–85, 2002.

41. Youngquist RS. Equine obstetrics. In: Morrow DA, ed. Current Therapy in Theriogenology, 2nd ed. Philadelphia: WB Saunders, 1986:693–699.

42. Freeman DE, Hungerford LL, Schaeffer D, et al. Caesarean section and other methods for assisted delivery: Comparison of effects on mare mortality and complications. Equine Vet J 31:203–207, 1999.

43. Embertson RM. Dystocia and caesarian sections: The importance of duration and good judgement. Equine Vet J 31:179–180, 1999.

44. Taylor PM. Anaesthesia for pregnant animals. Equine Vet J 24:1–6, 1997.

45. Wilson DV. Anesthesia and sedation for late-term mares. Vet Clin North Am Equine Pract 10:219–236, 1994.

46. Taylor PM, Luna SPL, White KL, Bloomfield M, Fowden AL. Intravenous anaesthesia using detomidine, ketamine and guaiphenesin for laparotomy in pregnant pony mares. Vet Anaesth Analg 28:119–125, 2001.

47. Taylor PM, White KL, Fowden AL, Giussani DA, Bloomfield M, Sear JW. Propofol anaesthesia for surgery in late gestation pony mares. Vet Anaesth Analg 28:177–187, 2001.

48. Lin HC, Wallace RL, Harrison IW, Thurmon JC. A case report on the use of guaifenesin-ketamine-xylazine anesthesia for equine dystocia. Cornell Vet J 84:61–66, 1994.

49. Daunt DA, Steffey EP, Pascoe JR, Willits N, Daels PF. Actions of isoflurane and halothane in pregnant mares. J Am Vet Med Assoc 201:1367–1374, 1992.

50. Hellyer PW. Anesthesia for cesarian section: Anesthetic considerations for surgery. In: Slatter D, ed. Slatter's Textbook of Small Animal Surgery, 2nd ed. Philadelphia: WB Saunders, 1991:2300–2303.

51. Guyton AC. Textbook of Medical Physiology, 4th ed. Philadelphia: WB Saunders, 1971:78.

52. Ratra CK, Badola RP, Bhargava KP. A study of factors concerned with emesis during spinal anaesthesia. Br J Anaesth 44:1208–1211, 1972.

53. Hall LW, Taylor PM. Anaesthesia of the Cat. London: Baillière Tindall 1994:124.

54. Dow TJB, Brock-Utney JG, Rubin J, Welman S, Dimopoulos GE, Moshal MG. The effect of atropine on the lower esophageal sphincter in late pregnancy. Obstet Gynecol 51:426–430, 1978.

55. Knowles JA. Effects on the infant of drug therapy in nursing mothers. Drug Ther 3:57–59, 1973.

56. Iqbal MM, Sobhan T, Ryals T. Effects of commonly used benzodiazepines on the fetus, the neonate, and the nursing patient. Psychiatr Serv 53:39–49, 2002.

57. Delehant TM, Denhart JW, Lloyd WE, Powell JD. Pharmacokinetics of xylazine, 2,6-dimethylaniline, and tolazoline in tissues from yearling cattle and milk from mature dairy cows after sedation with xylazine hydrochloride and reversal with tolazoline hydrochloride. Vet Ther 4:128–134, 2003.

58. Salonen JS, Vaha-Vahe T, Vainio O, Vakkuri O. Single dose pharmacokinetics of detomidine in the horse and cow. J Vet Pharmacol Ther 12:65–72, 1989.

59. Bar-Oz B, Bukowstein M, Benyamini L, et al. Use of antibiotic and analgesic drugs during lactation. Drug Saf 26:925–935, 2003.

60. Wittels B, Glosten B, Faure EA, et al. Postcesarean analgesia with both epidural morphine and intravenous patient-controlled analgesia: Neurobehavioral outcomes among nursing neonates. Anesth Analg 85:600–606, 1997.

61. Madej TH, Strunin L. Comparison of epidural fentanyl with sufentanil: Analgesia and side effects after a single bolus dose during elective cesarean section. Anaesthesia 42:1156–1161, 1987.

62. Andersen LW, Qvist T, Hertz J, Mogensen F. Concentrations of thiopentone in mature breast milk and colostrum following an induction dose. Acta Anaesthesiol Scand 31:30–32, 1987.

63. Schmitt JP, Schwoerer D, Diemunsch P, Gauthier-Lafaye J. Passage of propofol in the colostrum: Preliminary data. Ann Fr Anesth Reanim 6:267–268, 1987.

64. Ortega D, Viviand X, Loree AM, Gamerre M, Martin C, Bruguerolle B. Excretion of lidocaine and bupivacaine in breast milk following epidural anesthesia for cesarean delivery. Acta Anaesthesiol Scand 43:394–397, 1999.

65. Lohuis JA, van Werven T, Brand A, et al. Pharmacodynamics and pharmacokinetics of carprofen, a nonsteroidal anti-inflammatory drug, in healthy cows and cows with Escherichia coli endotoxin-induced mastitis. J Vet Pharmacol Ther 14:219–229, 1991.

66. De Graves FJ, Riddell MG, Schumacher J. Ketoprofen concentrations in plasma and milk after intravenous administration in dairy cattle. Am J Vet Res 57:1031–1033, 1996.

67. Musser JM, Anderson KL, Tyczkowska KL. Pharmacokinetic parameters and milk concentrations of ketoprofen after administration as a single intravenous bolus dose to lactating goats. J Vet Pharmacol Ther 21:358–363, 1998.

Chapter 46
Trauma and Critical Patients

Gwendolyn L. Carroll and David D. Martin

Introduction

Proper care of trauma or critical patients requires advanced planning, an ordered protocol, and efficient use of time and resources. When a team approach is taken in the emergency room, with each member of the team given preassigned duties, rapid evaluation and treatment are possible. Airway, breathing, circulation, and neurological status should be immediately assessed upon a patient's arrival, and circulation, ventilation, and neurological function should be reassessed frequently during the initial treatment period. Respiratory rate and effort, heart rate and rhythm, blood pressure, pulse quality, capillary refill, central nervous system (CNS) function, and pain should be evaluated to determine the patient's status and prognosis.[1] Severely traumatized or critical patients are subject to a variety of complications that may manifest in the first few days following presentation. These complications may not be directly related to the initial insult, but reflect overall tissue destruction, immune suppression, and metabolic imbalances. These complications may be septic, nonseptic, or both in origin.[2,3]

Critically ill patients should always be considered likely candidates for developing some form of *shock*, a state of generalized inadequate tissue perfusion. Hypotension usually accompanies shock, but during early compensation, shock can occur with normal blood pressure. Shock may result from blood loss, poor cardiac function, sepsis, or interruption of tissue blood flow. The probability of recovery from shock is related to the magnitude of the oxygen debt that occurs. After an overwhelming injury or infection, the sequelae to oxygen debt may not be reversible. Inadequate resuscitation, another major insult (e.g., anesthesia and surgery), or several small insults during this time often result in death.

When anesthetizing critically ill patients, the primary goal is to optimize tissue perfusion and oxygen delivery to all vital organ systems while inducing unconsciousness, an appropriate degree of analgesia, and muscle relaxation. The ultimate goal of therapy should be optimal physiological function rather than restoration of measured hemodynamic parameters to normal. Values generally considered normal for healthy anesthetized patients are associated with higher rates of mortality in high-risk patients. In prospective studies of human trauma patients, survivability is associated with cardiac indexes 50% higher and blood volumes 110% to 120% higher than normal at the end of surgery.[4] These values are necessary to meet the increased metabolic demand of fever and tissue repair in posttrauma and postoperative patients (Table 46.1).

Traumatized or critically ill patients are often near cardiopulmonary collapse or arrest. Causes of acute circulatory failure in these patients include severe myocardial ischemia, malignant dysrhythmias, hypoxemia associated with severe lung damage or airway obstruction, hemorrhagic shock, acid-base or electrolyte abnormalities, profound vagal tone such as is associated with the oculocardiac reflex, and electrocution. When cardiovascular collapse occurs during attempts to stabilize severely traumatized or critically ill patients, cardiopulmonary resuscitation should be instituted immediately.

Shock

Septic Shock

As a general rule, anesthesia should not be undertaken until a patient's vital organ functions have been assessed and stabilized. If the patient is in shock, the etiology should be determined and corrective measures initiated before anesthesia. Anaphylactic shock and neurogenic shock are characterized by relative hypovolemia and hypotension caused by acute increases in vascular capacitance. Hypovolemic shock and neurogenic shock are typically observed in acutely traumatized patients, whereas septic shock and the systemic inflammatory response syndrome (SIRS) develop after the initial insult. SIRS is a global activation of the

Table 46.1. Cardiovascular resuscitation goals for animals with systemic inflammatory response syndrome.

Variable	Goal
Mixed venous oxygen tension, PvO$_2$ (mm Hg)	>40
Pulmonary artery pressure (mm Hg)	>25/10
Pulmonary wedge pressure (mm Hg)	218
Systemic vascular resistance (dyne $\times$ s/cm^{-5} $\times$ m^2)	>1450
Pulmonary vascular resistance (dyne $\times$ s/cm^{-5} $\times$ m^2)	45–250
Oxygen extraction (%)	22–30
Cardiac index (L/min $\times$ m^2)	>4.5
Oxygen delivery (mL/min $\times$ m^2)	>600
Oxygen consumption (mL/min $\times$ m^2)	>170

PvO$_2$, mixed venous oxygen tension.
From Hardie.[5]

Table 46.2. Proposed definitions of systemic inflammatory response syndrome in dogs and cats.

Proposed for dogs, the presence of two or more of the following clinical conditions:
    Body temperature > 40°C or < 38°C
    Heart rate > 120 beats/min in calm, resting dogs
    Hyperventilation of PaCO$_2$ < 30 mm Hg
    White blood cell count > 18,000/mL or < 5000/mL or > 5% immature (band) forms
Proposed for cats, the presence of two or more of the following clinical conditions:
    Body temperature > 40°C or < 38°C
    Heart rate > 140 beats/min in calm, resting cats
    Respiratory rate > 20 breaths/min or PaCO$_2$ < 28 mm Hg
    White blood cell count > 18,000/mL or < 5000/mL or > 5% immature (band) forms

PaCO$_2$, arterial carbon dioxide partial pressure.
From Hardie.[5]

immune system and release of many cytokines, resulting in a generalized increase in vascular permeability, neutrophil infiltration, and capillary microemboli. Early signs of SIRS and septic shock include brick-red mucous membranes, tachycardia, high cardiac output (in euvolemic patients), normal or low blood pressure, and low vascular resistance. Classifications of SIRS for dogs and cats based on the presence of various key clinical signs have been proposed and are listed in Table 46.2.[5] Clinically, in cats, the signs of late-stage sepsis are more commonly recognized than are those of early hyperdynamic sepsis.[6] Cats often differ from dogs in that a cat's signs of late shock include bradycardia, hypotension, and hypoglycemia.

In cats, lung function is often impaired early in SIRS because of rapid fluid accumulation. In dogs, the order of organ dysfunction is commonly gastrointestinal tract, followed by liver, kidney, and then lung. Patients suffering from noncardiogenic pulmonary edema may have this condition exacerbated by rapid crystalloid fluid administration. Persistent microcirculatory perfusion fail-

ure may lead to sludging of blood and increased immune cell and platelet aggregation. Along with the release of inflammatory mediators, these conditions result in poorly regulated coagulation and propagation of the inflammatory response. Toxic oxygen free radicals can cause further cellular damage, persistent edema, and increased oxygen diffusion distance between cells and capillaries. If oxygen delivery to tissues is chronically impaired, the systemic inflammatory state can lead to multiple organ dysfunction syndrome (MODS), traditionally defined as *irreversible shock*.

Successful management of animals with septic shock or SIRS depends on anticipation, not reaction.[3] Appropriate antibiotic administration, aggressive cardiovascular support, and monitoring of the susceptible organs must be undertaken early. An algorithm depicting SIRS management is presented in Fig. 46.1.[3] Therapeutic agents and doses used in the treatment of various metabolic derangements associated with SIRS are listed in Table 46.3.

Hemorrhagic Shock

Clinical signs of hemorrhagic shock most commonly encountered in acutely traumatized patients include pallor, cyanosis, disorientation, tachycardia, cold extremities, cardiac dysrhythmias, pump failure, tachypnea, hypotension, oliguria, disseminated intravascular coagulation, and progressive metabolic acidosis.[1] With acute blood loss, normal homeostatic reflexes vigorously defend blood pressure in an attempt to maintain vital organ function. As hemorrhage ensues, plasma renin levels elevate, the antidiuretic hormone level increases, and the sympathetic nervous system activates to produce tachycardia and arteriolar vasoconstriction. These mechanisms can maintain blood pressure until about 40% of normal blood volume is lost (more loss than is clinically acceptable).[1] Thus, an animal can be severely hypovolemic but normotensive. Once blood loss exceeds 40% of blood volume, compensatory organ mechanisms fail over time, and shock becomes irreversible. Prolonged poor tissue perfusion causes tissue ischemia, loss of cell membrane integrity, and cell death.[1] If the trauma involves crushing of tissues or severe burns, shock is accompanied by increased capillary permeability and rapid translocation of fluids. In addition, toxic factors from exogenous

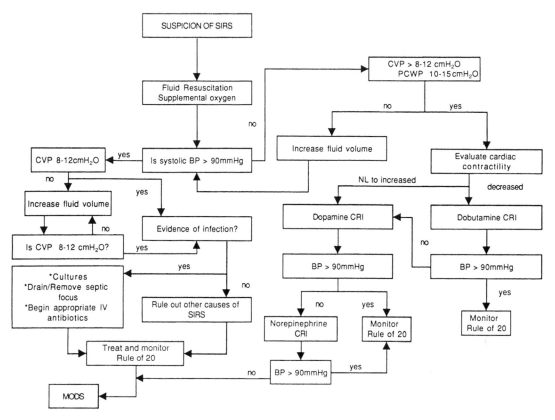

Fig. 46.1. Algorithm depicting SIRS patient management. BP, blood pressure (implies systolic); CRI, continuous-rate infusion; CVP, central venous pressure; IV, intravenous; MODS, multiple organ–dysfunction syndrome; NL, normal; PCWP, pulmonary capillary wedge pressure; and SIRS, systemic inflammatory response syndrome. From Purvis and Kirby.[3]

sources (e.g., microbial toxins) and endogenous sources (e.g., fat emboli, potassium-ion release, lysosomal enzymes, and myocardial depressant factor) are simultaneously released, causing further organ malfunction.[7]

The primary treatment of hemorrhagic shock is aggressive fluid therapy. Large-bore intravenous catheters should be placed in each cephalic vein and/or jugular veins, and warm, crystalloid solutions, blood, and/or hemoglobin-based oxygen-carrying solutions infused. If necessary, fluids can also be administered rapidly into the intraosseous space of the tibia or femur. When rapid infusion of large volumes of crystalloids decreases the concentration of serum total solids to below 3.5 to 4.0 g/dL, simultaneous colloid solution administration is advantageous in maintaining intravascular volume.[8]

Albumin is an excellent plasma expander, but is expensive and can induce immune responses. Hetastarch compares favorably to albumin and has an extremely low toxicity in people and animals.[9] The dose of hetastarch is up to 20 mL/kg/day in dogs. In cats, a smaller volume and slower rate of administration are recommended. All colloids can affect coagulation, but rapid hemodilution with larger volumes of crystalloids can, as well. In dogs administered less than 30 mL/kg hetastarch, clotting time, clot retraction, platelet count, and whole clot lysis are not significantly affected.[10,11] Hetastarch does, however, decrease all three components of the factor VIII–related complex. After a single

hetastarch dose, plasma expansion can last 24 to 48 h.[9] Plasma administration decreases the continual decline of plasma protein level, but it is difficult to increase total protein significantly by plasma administration alone. The use of fresh-frozen plasma is best reserved for patients that are deficient in coagulation factors.

Hypertonic saline may be beneficial in the early treatment of hypovolemic and hemorrhagic shock.[12] Intravenous administration of small volumes (4 to 6 mL/kg) of 7.5% hypertonic saline has beneficial cardiovascular effects in hypovolemic dogs and cats.[13–15] Increases in pressure and cardiac output appear to be mediated primarily by rapid increases in plasma volume.[14] A second potential benefit of hypertonic saline administration is minimization of the risk of cerebral edema in patients with head trauma.[16,17] Hypertonic saline (7.2% sodium chloride [formulations vary]; 4 mL/kg intravenously [IV]) may be administered over 15 min in acute hypovolemic episodes. The addition of a colloid to hypertonic saline appears to prolong its effects. It is important to remember that hypertonic saline shifts fluid from the extravascular space to the intravascular space. Total body water does not significantly increase unless additional crystalloid fluids are given soon after the hypertonic saline. Contraindications for hypertonic saline administration include hypernatremia, cardiogenic shock, renal failure, hyperosmolarity, uncontrolled hemorrhage, and thrombocytopenia (if in dextran). Hypertonic solutions may produce hyperchloremic nonrespiratory acidosis and hypokalemia.

Table 46.3. Therapeutic agents used to treat metabolic derangements associated with systemic inflammatory response syndrome.

Metabolic Derangement	Dose Regimen	Use and/or Frequency
Hypovolemia		
Hypertonic crystalloids		
7.5% NaCl solution (70 mL 23.4% NaCl in 180 mL 0.9% NaCl or 6% dextran 70)	4 mL/kg IV	Once
Colloids		
Plasma	Maximum: 20 mL/kg/24 h IV	As needed
Hetastarch 120	Maximum: 20 mL/kg/first 24 h, and then 10 mL/kg/24 h IV (slow infusion)	As needed
Dextran 70	Maximum: 20 mL/kg/first 24 h, and then 10 mL/kg/24 h IV (slow infusion)	As needed
3% Albumin (12 mL 25% human albumin in 488 mL lactated Ringer's solution)	20 mL/kg IV	Resuscitation
Isotonic crystalloids		
Lactated Ringer's solution	90–270 mL/kg IV	Resuscitation
	10–20 mL/kg/h IV	To meet ongoing needs
Altered clotting function		
Heparin (low dosage)	75–100 U/kg SC	Every 6–8 h
Heparin-activated plasma (incubate 5–10 U/kg heparin with 1 U fresh plasma for 30 min)	10 mL/kg IV	Every 3 h, based on clotting function
Metabolic dysfunction		
KCl	0.125–0.25 mEq/kg/h IV; do not exceed 0.5 mEq/kg/h	As needed
Glucose	50–500 mg/kg/h IV	As needed
NaHCO$_3$	Base excess $\times$ 0.3 $\times$ body weight in kg = mEq needed to correct deficit, IV (slow infusion)	As needed (pH 7.1 or less)
Gastrointestinal tract dysfunction		
Cimetidine	5–10 mg/kg IV, IM, PO	Every 6–8 h
Ranitidine	2 mg/kg IV, IM, PO	Every 8–12 h
Omeprazole	0.7 mg/kg PO	Every 24 h
Misoprostol	3 µg/kg PO	Every 24 h
Sucralfate	250 mg (cats) PO	Every 8–12 h
	500 mg (dogs < 20 kg) PO	Every 8–12 h
	1 g (dogs > 20 kg) PO	Every 8–12 h
Kaolin-pectin	1–2 mL/kg PO	Every 6–8 h
Metoclopramide	0.2–0.5 mg/kg SC	Every 6–8 h
Renal dysfunction		
Mannitol	0.25–1 g/kg IV	Once (slow bolus)
Furosemide	1–2 mg/kg IV	If no effect, repeat in 2 h and increase dose by 1 mg/kg
Dopamine	1–3 µg/kg/min IV	As needed until urine production consistently > 2 mL/kg/h

IM, intramuscularly; IV, intravenously; PO, per os (orally); SC, subcutaneously; U, units.
From Hardie.[5]

Massive blood loss will eventually require transfusion of whole blood or packed red blood cells to replace oxygen-transport capacity. Hemoglobin-based oxygen-carrying solutions (e.g., Oxyglobin [bovine hemoglobin glutamer 200]) can serve to increase oxygen capacity; however, the effects are usually brief, requiring additional blood-product transfusion. Trend monitoring of hematocrit (or hemoglobin concentration), total solids, central venous pressure, and urine output is helpful in guiding resuscitation. The use of whole blood should be reserved for patients that need cells and plasma. If the packed cell volume (PCV) is less

Table 46.4. Vasoconstrictor and mixed inotropic-vasoconstrictor drugs.

Drug (Trade Name)	Catecholamine Receptor Activation				Drug Dose and Infusion Schemes
	α_1	α_2	β_1	β_2	
Phenylephrine (Neo-Synephrine)	+++	+	− Little at high dose	−	Bolus: 0.15 mg/kg IV Infusion: 0.5–1.0 µg/kg/min
Methoxamine (Vasoxyl)	++	+	−	−	Bolus: 0.1–0.8 mg/kg IV (cardiac arrest) Bolus: 0.01–0.04 mg/kg IV (vasopressor)
Ephedrine	+	+	+	+	Bolus: 0.1–0.25 mg/kg IM; 0.03–0.07 mg/kg IV
	Direct and indirect (NE release) effects				
Metaraminol (Aramine)	+	+	+	+	Bolus: 30–100 µg/kg IM Infusion: 20–50 µg/kg/min
	Similar to ephedrine effects initially[a]				
Mephenteramine (Wyamine)	+	+	+	+	Bolus: 0.2–0.6 mg/kg IM
	Similar to ephedrine effects				
Norepinephrine (Levophed)	+++	+++	+	Little	Infusion: 0.01–0.03 µg/kg/min up to a maximum 0.1 µg/ kg/min to effect

IM, intramuscularly; IV, intravenously; NE, norepinephrine; +, positive effect; −, no effect.
[a]Metaraminol replaces NE in storage vesicles in the nerve terminal. It has only one-tenth the potency of NE at α receptors and may eventually produce a hypotensive effect.

that 20% and the protein level is normal, transfuse cells. The rule of thumb is that 2.2 mL of blood/kg body weight increases the recipient's PCV by 1%; however, this depends somewhat on the hematocrit of the donor blood.

Oxyglobin is a hemoglobin-based oxygen-carrying solution that increases plasma and total hemoglobin concentration. Its elimination half-life is 30 to 40 h, but its effective action may be much shorter. Some blood tests that use colorimetric changes will be altered after the administration of Oxyglobin, because of the change in plasma color. The recommended dose in dogs is approximately 15 mL/kg IV (the label dose is up to 30 mL/kg) at a rate of 5 mL/kg/h (the label rate is 10 mL/kg/h). Patients should be carefully monitored during and after Oxyglobin administration because of its effects on vascular resistance and right atrial pressure. A more conservative dosing strategy considers trends in monitored total hemoglobin concentration (i.e., maintain 8 to 10 g/dL total hemoglobin). In cats, smaller volumes and slower administration should be used. To avoid volume overload when administering larger doses of Oxyglobin, it is recommended that central venous or right atrial pressure be monitored.

Spinal Shock

This is a common sequela to spinal cord injury or blunt trauma, which can disrupt sympathetic nervous system outflow. The patient's extremities will feel warm (peripheral vasodilation), and even though hypotension is present, heart rate is slow because of sympathetic denervation. These patients are relatively hypovolemic; that is, intravascular capacity greatly exceeds intravascular volume. Organ perfusion may or may not be adequate, and vascular resistance is drastically reduced. These patients are more susceptible to hypothermia because they cannot constrict peripheral vasculature. Fluids should be administered to increase vascular volume. If arterial pressure is low and the pulse cannot be pal-

pated, mixed inotropic-pressor–type drugs should be given to increase blood flow to vital organs. Intravenous ephedrine, mephentermine, or metaraminol are good choices in these patients (Table 46.4).[18] Since resistance and flow are inversely related, the usefulness of pressors alone is limited. Use of vasopressors may compound compromised visceral perfusion and increase cardiac workload.[6] If there is any question as to adequacy of contractility, pressors should not be used before inotropes. Not all inotropic or vasoconstrictor drugs produce equivalent hemodynamic effects. Hemodynamic responses to norepinephrine, epinephrine, and isoproterenol are illustrated in Fig. 46.2. These differences are medi-

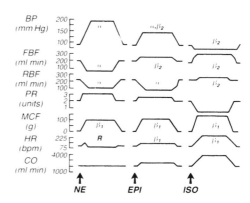

Fig. 46.2. Differences in cardiovascular effects of intravenously administered norepinephrine (NE), epinephrine (EPI), and isoproterenol (ISO). Schematics represent relative effects on blood pressure (BP), femoral blood flow (FBF), renal blood flow (RBF), peripheral vascular resistance (PR), myocardial contractile force (MCF), heart rate (HR), and cardiac output (CO). Primary responses are noted as either α-, β_1-, or β_2-receptor mediated; and R, reflex mediated. Differences in cardiovascular effects of these catecholamines are caused by variation in α and β selectivity for each agonist and dose.

ated by variations in adrenergic receptor activation and dose. Indirect-acting agents such as ephedrine enhance release of endogenous norepinephrine from sympathetic neuronal terminals and also induce direct vasoconstrictive effects.

Cardiogenic Shock

This type of shock occurs when the ability of the heart to maintain cardiac output is insufficient to meet the body's demand. The circulatory compromise is caused entirely by cardiac dysfunction. Once overwhelming cardiac disease progresses and a patient can no longer compensate, signs of failure appear. If therapy does not improve systemic perfusion and the patient's ability to meet metabolic needs, the patient will die. The diagnosis and treatment of cardiogenic shock are beyond the scope of this chapter, but have been reviewed.[19]

Patient Monitoring and Pharmacological Support

Measurement of perfusion is challenging in veterinary patients. Lactate can be used as a surrogate measure for perfusion. In low-flow situations, tissue hypoxia results in increased anaerobic metabolism and subsequent increased lactate production. Studies suggest that trends in lactate concentration are more helpful in predicting outcome than is measuring cardiac output.[20,21] The magnitude of the elevation is positively correlated with the magnitude of the underlying problem and negatively correlated with prognosis. The normal lactate concentration should be determined for each laboratory, but is generally less than 1.5 mM/L.

In traumatized or critically ill patients, either a continuous or intermittent electrocardiogram should be monitored with a rhythm printout obtained immediately prior to anesthesia or if abnormalities are noted. Antiarrhythmic drugs that may be useful during management of traumatized or critically ill patients include lidocaine, procainamide, and esmolol. Lidocaine can be used to treat ventricular arrhythmias (dogs: 1 to 4 mg/kg IV bolus, followed by 40 to 80 µg/kg/min IV infusion).[22] Lidocaine should be used more cautiously in cats (0.25 to 1.0 mg/kg IV over 5 min).[22] Refractory ventricular arrhythmias may require treatment with procainamide (1 to 10 mg/kg IV, followed by 20 to 50 µg/kg/min IV infusion).[22] Since procainamide may cause profound hypotension, it should be administered in smaller doses, which are repeated when necessary. Esmolol (0.5 mg/kg slow IV, followed by 50 to 200 µg/kg/min IV infusion) is a β blocker with a very short half-life (a half-life of elimination of about 10 min) that may be used in the treatment of supraventricular tachycardias and ventricular arrhythmias. Esmolol significantly decreases contractility and should not be routinely used unless hemodynamic monitoring is available.[23,24]

Several drugs commonly recommended for resuscitation and stabilization have been reevaluated since their introduction. Because of the potential complications of sodium bicarbonate, its use in resuscitation and intensive care units is continuously scrutinized. It has been used in advanced cardiac life support for 40 years, but its nonselective use has become controversial over the last 15 to 20 years.[25] In the treatment of arrest, it has gone from

being a first-line drug in the first American Heart Association's Standards for Cardiopulmonary Resuscitation and Advanced Cardiac Life Support to current recommendations that its use may be indicated in cases of protracted arrest or long resuscitative efforts with preexisting metabolic acidosis.[25] Reasons include lack of clinical studies of buffer therapy, knowledge that normal pH can be maintained by compression and hyperventilation, and the potential ill effects of bicarbonate therapy.[26]

If sodium bicarbonate is used, it is reasonable that the time interval to its administration be based on the rate of metabolic acidosis development, rather than the duration of resuscitative efforts.[25] In dogs, serum-base deficits increase by 1.1 to 1.5 mEq/L for every minute of circulatory arrest; the arterial lactate concentration increases by 0.3 mmol/L/min (with epinephrine administration) and 0.6 mmol/L/min (without epinephrine administration) of arrest and cardiopulmonary resuscitation.[25]

The role of bicarbonate therapy for metabolic acidosis caused by diminished oxygen delivery to tissues in critically ill or traumatized patients is also controversial.[27] Successful treatment of the underlying excessive intracellular production of hydrogen ions will often resolve the acidosis. It is not clear whether buffering the blood, extracellular fluid, and intracellular fluid actually slows the production of metabolic acid or simply facilitates its removal. Most current recommendations advise avoiding bicarbonate therapy for lactic acidosis unless acidosis is so severe that physiological functions are dangerously impaired. Little existing experimental data support the use of bicarbonate for the treatment of acidosis.[27] Additionally, bicarbonate administration is not without risk. Its potential adverse effects include negative inotropy, paradoxical cerebrospinal fluid acidosis, hypercarbia, alkalosis, vasodilation, hyperosmolarity, electrolyte disturbance (e.g., hypokalemia and hypocalcemia), shifting of the oxyhemaglobin-dissociation curve (i.e., decreased oxygen delivery because of increased affinity of hemoglobin for oxygen), and volume overload caused by sodium.[28] The standard formula used to calculate bicarbonate replacement is milliequivalents of bicarbonate = base deficit $\times$ 0.3 $\times$ body weight (kg). This formula is used for correcting metabolic acidosis in the extracellular fluid compartment. Total-body base-deficit correction may require a greater dose and intravascular correction a smaller dose. To avoid a vascular alkalosis, the dose should not be administered faster than it can be redistributed from the vascular space to the interstitial space. If administered too quickly, severe hypotension and death may result. A more conservative approach is to calculate the deficit, but administer only one-third of the dose at a time. Allow enough time for equilibration and recheck a blood gas. There are alternative alkalinizing agents such as tromethamine (THAM) and Carbicarb (a mixture of sodium carbonate and sodium bicarbonate), but these alternative agents have not proven to be superior.

Dopamine has been used as a sympathomimetic and dopaminergic drug since the 1960s. The potential for protective effects of low-dose dopamine on renal and splanchnic perfusion has led to the widespread use of this drug in critically ill patients (Table 46.5). Although low-dose dopamine may increase urine production, it neither prevents nor improves acute renal failure. Even

Table 46.5. Positive inotropic drugs.

Drug (Trade Name)	Catecholamine Receptor Activation					Noncatecholamine Mechanism	Drug Dose and Infusion Schemes
	α_1	α_2	β_1	β_2	Dopamine		
Epinephrine (Adrenalin)	+++	+++	++	++	−	No	0.01–0.03 µg/kg/min (vasopressor) 0.1–0.2 mg/kg IV (cardiac arrest)
Isoproterenol (Isuprel)	−	−	+++	+++	−	No	0.01–0.1 µg/kg/min; used primarily to increase heart rate; may cause hypotension
Dobutamine (Dubutrex)	Little	Little	+++	++	−	No[a]	2–10 µg/kg/min
	Direct and minimal indirect effects						
Dopamine (Intropin)	++ (High dose)	+	++ (Low dose)	+ (Low dose)	+++	No[a,b]	2–5 µg/kg/min; "renal dose" 5–10 µg/kg/min; β effects 10–20 µg/kg/min; vasoconstriction
	Direct and indirect actions						
Dopexamine	−	−	Little	+++	++	No[a]	1–10 µg/kg/min
Ephedrine	+	+	+	+	−	No[b]	0.1–0.25 mg/kg/min IM 0.03–0.07 mg/kg IV
	Both direct and indirect effects						
Milrinone	−	−	−	−	−	Yes	50–75 µg/kg IV bolus; oral administration possible
	Phosphodiesterase inhibitor, ↑ cAMP in heart, peripheral vasodilator, ↑ inotropy additive to other types						

cAMP, cyclic adenosine monophosphate; IM, intramuscularly; IV, intravenously; +, positive effect; −, no effect; ↑, increased.
[a]Blocks reuptake of norepinephrine.
[b]Promotes release of norepinephrine from nerve terminal.

though low-dose dopamine does increase diuresis, it may actually increase the risk of acute renal failure in normovolemic and hypovolemic patients.[29] Similarly, there is no evidence that low-dose dopamine has beneficial effects on splanchnic function or decreased progression to MODS in sepsis.[29] Because of its effects on gastrointestinal motility, and respiratory, endocrine, and immunologic function, the use of low-dose dopamine is no longer routinely advised.[29] At higher doses, dopamine has been used as a pressor in septic patients, with the thought that β_1 activity, in addition to α_1-adrenergic–mediated pressor effects, would improve contractility and minimize the effect of increasing afterload on cardiac output. Because of the aforementioned potential adverse effects, its use as a pressor is likewise being further questioned.[29]

Additional controversy exists regarding the presence of dopaminergic receptors in the feline kidney. Putative DA_1-like receptors have been discovered in the cortex of the feline kidney.[30] DA_1 receptor pharmacology in the feline kidney appears to be similar to that of humans. There is a much smaller population of receptors in the feline renal cortex than in the renal cortex of rats, dogs, or people. It has been hypothesized that the smaller population of DA_1 receptors could account for the higher dose requirement to induce diuresis and natriuresis in cats when compared with other species.[30] However, as indicated for dogs, diuresis does not necessarily equate with improved renal function. Dopamine may be useful as an inotropic sympathomimetic agent in cats that have decreased cardiac output secondary to anesthetic drug administration.

Management of Selected Traumatized Patients

Head Trauma

The hallmark of severe closed head injury is loss of consciousness associated with increased intracranial pressure and brain ischemia. Severe lacerations of the head may be associated with severe blood loss and shock. If airway obstruction is evident, a tracheostomy may be necessary to ensure airway patency. Time is of the essence, because intracranial hemorrhage or hypertension can have devastating effects if undiagnosed or untreated for even a short period. In general, severe closed head injury resulting in stupor or coma has a poor prognosis.

Anesthetic agents that increase cerebral blood flow (e.g., halothane, nitrous oxide, and ketamine) are not recommended for use in these patients. Because barbiturates produce rapid induction, decrease cerebral metabolic requirement for oxygen ($CMRO_2$), and decrease cerebral blood flow, they may be reasonable agents for patients with severe head injury.[31] Following acute brain injury, large doses of glucocorticosteroids (1 to 3 mg/kg dexamethasone) may be helpful in controlling cerebral edema, although this use is now quite controversial.[32] Intubation and modest hyperventilation (arterial carbon dioxide partial pressure [$PaCO_2$] values of 28 to 32 mm Hg) may protect against dangerous increases in cerebral blood flow and pressure. Care should be exercised not to negatively impact arterial blood pressure and cardiac output with positive-pressure ventilation. If the $PaCO_2$ is allowed to decrease below 25 mm Hg, there is a danger that the affected area of the brain may become ischemic because of excessive constriction of cerebral arterioles. The use of hyperosmotic solutions may help to minimize intracranial pressure caused by tissue edema. Mannitol is an ideal drug for preventing or treating increased intracranial pressure and cerebral edema associated with global ischemia or neoplasia. However, it is *not* recommended for immediate use in patients with suspected intracranial hemorrhage (head trauma). Hemorrhage or leaking of hyperosmotic solutions into perivascular neural tissue would increase interstitial fluid volume and intracranial pressure.

Cervical trauma may injure the innervation to respiratory muscles (phrenic and intercostal nerves) such that oxygen therapy, tracheal intubation, and mechanical ventilation may be necessary. Spinal injury may also cause autonomic dysfunction, resulting in gastric bloat, bradycardia, and electrolyte imbalances. Thermoregulation may also be seriously impaired.

Thoracic and Abdominal Trauma

Penetrating trauma of the thorax and abdomen is usually obvious. Blunt trauma presents a greater diagnostic challenge, because external examination may reveal no obvious abnormalities. A chest radiograph is essential following any type of thoracic trauma. Lung contusions, broken ribs, and flail chest are common. Pulmonary contusions may not become apparent until 12 to 24 h after injury. Radiographic findings might not correlate with functional deficits; therefore, arterial blood-gas analysis is essential for evaluating patient status. Severe hypoxemia often results from extensive lung contusions, and ventilatory support or oxygen therapy may be required. Low inspiratory pressures (<12 cm of water) should be used if intermittent positive-pressure ventilation (IPPV) is deemed necessary in patients that have a pneumothorax or bullae. Any accessible gas should be removed prior to anesthesia or if respiratory difficulty develops. Intermittent thoracocentesis may be adequate, but an indwelling chest drain should be considered if respiratory difficulty continues to develop. Pulmonary lesions tend to worsen within 24 to 36 h after injury.[33] Lung contusions will usually resolve in 2 to 5 days.[1] Medical management of pulmonary contusions includes oxygen, corticosteroid, analgesic, and antibiotic administration, and diuretic therapy when pulmonary edema is present. When contusions are severe, anesthesia, intubation, and low-pressure mechanical ventilation may be necessary.[33]

In small animals, thoracic and abdominal injuries are commonly associated with blunt trauma rather than with penetrating objects. Common cardiac injuries include tamponade, contusion, and rupture. Patients with pericardial effusion and cardiac tamponade will manifest jugular vein distension, muffled heart sounds, and hypotension (Beck's triad) in addition to tachycardia and reduced pulse pressure. The administration of intravenous fluid and inotropic drugs (Table 46.5), and immediate pericardial drainage (pericardiocentesis), may be necessary to maintain an adequate cardiac output. It is best to avoid controlled IPPV in patients that have tamponade. An infusion of fentanyl (0.8 µg/kg/min IV) and midazolam (8 µg/kg/min IV) with orotracheal intubation and oxygen support, rather than an inhalant, may be used for anesthetic maintenance until the pericardium can be opened and cardiac output improved. Patients with myocardial contusions will often develop ventricular dysrhythmias, which appear to be most common 24 to 72 h after trauma. Arrhythmias require correct diagnosis and appropriate therapy with antiarrhythmic agents prior to and during the surgical period. Myocardial rupture usually causes death at the scene of the accident.

In the urban environment, the incidence of abdominal injury has been reported at 13% of all dog and cat trauma cases treated.[34] Blunt abdominal trauma can damage several vital organs by rupturing spleen and/or liver, or kidney and urinary bladder, or perforating the bowel or large abdominal vessels. In cases with a history of severe abdominal trauma, common sequelae are hypovolemic shock caused by organ or vessel rupture and/or septic shock resulting from septicemia. Abdominal ultrasound and radiographs should be used to evaluate abdominal injuries. Abdominal vascular injuries can be assessed by diagnostic peritoneal lavage. Although not organ specific, this technique is helpful in diagnosing unstable patients with a history of severe abdominal injury. Abdominal compression may reduce hemorrhage, but can also reduce vital tissue perfusion. Urinary catheterization will help to evaluate urinary tract injury and renal function.

Thermal/Burn Trauma

Although treatment of severely burned patients is uncommon, several factors important to intensive care management should be kept in mind. As is true with any trauma patient, initial treatment involves attention to airway, breathing, and circulation. If a patient is apneic or in stridor, or if the face is burned or the history indicates inhalation of steam, smoke, or toxic fumes, the trachea should be intubated immediately after sedation and induction.[1] Inhalation of carbon monoxide can cause severe tissue hypoxia even though mucous membranes and arterial oxygen partial pressure (PaO_2) may be near normal. Blood oxygen content can be drastically reduced because carbon monoxide has 200 times more affinity for hemoglobin than does oxygen. Since the majority of oxygen is carried on hemoglobin, and not in solution in the plasma (as measured with arterial blood gas), oxygen delivery to the tissues may be severely impaired. After intubation, the animal should be placed in an oxygen cage or ventilated mechanically with oxygen. After the airway has been secured, the burn patient will require large volumes of fluid. Fluid loss because of increased capillary permeability, protein loss into the interstitial tissues, and evaporative losses can be extensive, especially within the first 12 to 24 h after injury.[1] It has been suggested that only crystalloid solutions be administered during this time, because colloid solutions would likely rapidly extravasate. Volume replacement should be closely monitored by measuring urine output and hemodynamic parameters regularly. Burn patients are hypermetabolic and will often have increased temperatures, increased catabolism, and increased oxygen requirements. Tachypnea and tachycardia are common, and parenteral nutrition is usually necessary to overcome metabolic losses.

Providing anesthesia for burned and crushed patients presents some unique problems, but selection of anesthetics is not critical if done on a rational patient-by-patient basis. To enhance preoperative and postoperative analgesia, the use of opioids (e.g., fentanyl patches placed on an area of nonburned skin) should be considered with any technique. Transdermal or topical medications should not be applied to damaged epithelial surfaces, because the pharmacokinetics of the drug may be significantly altered. If there are no contraindications, ketamine may provide some degree of somatic analgesia. Ketamine may be given as a low-dose infusion (0.5 mg/kg IV, followed by 2 to 10 µg/kg/min IV) as an adjunct to opioid analgesia.

Burn patients may not respond normally to muscle relaxants.[35] For example, within 24 h of injury, succinylcholine administration is associated with a rapid increase in serum potassium concentration, which can cause cardiac arrest (see Chapter 15). In contrast, burn patients may demonstrate increased resistance to nondepolarizing muscle relaxants (e.g., pancuronium and atracurium).

The principles of treatment for patients with electrical burns are similar to those for patients with thermal burns. If the burn is located in the oral cavity, severe swelling of pharyngeal tissues may complicate efforts to intubate. The extent of burn is often misleading. Small cutaneous lesions may overlie extensive areas of devitalized tissue and muscle. Accordingly, these patients should be carefully observed for myoglobinemia and renal failure, as well as neurological deficits and pulmonary edema.[1]

Anesthetic Management of Trauma and Critically Ill Patients

Most classes of anesthetic agents may be used in trauma and critically ill patients; however, the dosage requirement is usually reduced. Release of endogenous enkephalins, endorphins, and other amino peptides to reduce pain and stress may produce mild sedation and analgesia, reducing the dose requirement of anesthetic agents. Anesthetic management includes protection of the airway, provision for ventilatory support, and appropriate monitoring of the patient's condition. Premedicants may be advantageous to reduce anxiety and pain, and to offset anesthetic drug-induced adverse effects.

Premedication

During the preoperative period, vagal influences on cardiopulmonary function and excess secretions can be controlled by atropine or glycopyrrolate administration. Antimuscarinics are not routinely recommended for use in critically ill patients, though, because they often increase heart rate and myocardial oxygen consumption while decreasing the threshold for cardiac dysrhythmias.[36] Because the stomach may be full, measures to prevent regurgitation and aspiration before induction need to be considered. Aspiration of acidic gastric contents (pH < 2.5) will usually lead to pneumonitis and increased morbidity and mortality. When the risk of aspiration is high, several steps can be taken to minimize its occurrence and consequences, including glycopyrrolate administration to increase the pH of gastric contents, positioning of the animal to reduce gastric pressure, immediate intubation of the unconscious patient by using cricoid pressure and immediate inflation of the cuff, and the availability of suction to clear the pharynx of gastric reflux.[32,37]

When stabilization is necessary prior to surgery, analgesics and/or sedatives can be given to help alleviate pain, fear, and apprehension. Some clinicians apply partial (cats and small dogs) or full (large dogs) fentanyl patches (Duragesic; 25-, 50-, 75-, or 100-µg/h release rate) that provide continual release for transcutaneous absorption of fentanyl over several days. In cats, partial exposure to a 25-µg/h release patch results in lower plasma fentanyl concentrations (1.14 ± 0.86 vs. 1.78 ± 0.92 ng/mL for a full 25-µg/h patch).[38] All patients should be observed for either inadequate analgesia and signs of overdose. To allow time for efficacious blood fentanyl concentrations to develop, 12 to 24 h are required in most patients. Anesthetic induction and maintenance dose requirements may be lessened in patients who have had fentanyl patches applied long enough for effective blood concentrations to be achieved; however, anesthetic management is not usually altered unless obvious sedation is present before anesthetic induction. If an analgesic is needed for immediate pain relief, either butorphanol (0.2 mg/kg IV) or a µ-agonist such as oxymorphone (0.05 mg/kg IV) may be given in small incremental doses. When further CNS depression is desirable, diazepam (0.2 mg/kg IV) or midazolam (0.2 mg/kg IV or intramuscularly [IM]) can be combined with the opioid. Benzodiazepines are not usually administered alone because they can induce unpredictable behavior in both dogs and cats. In depressed dogs, however, lower doses have been associated with rapid and profound CNS depression.[39] If neurological status needs to be serially assessed, a fentanyl constant-rate infusion (1 to 4 µg/kg IV loading dose, followed by 2 to 6 µg/kg/h IV) may be used. By 30 min after discontinuation of the constant-rate infusion, the sedative effects have usually abated. If shock, severe blood loss, and clotting are not of concern, acepromazine (0.01 to 0.05 mg/kg, up to 1 mg maximum) can be combined with butorphanol or oxymorphone to induce neuroleptanalgesia. If there is no contraindication to its use, medetomidine (1 to 3 µg/kg/h) can also be used for additional sedation and analgesia. In critically ill cats, both oxymorphone and buprenorphine have proven to be useful and relatively safe analgesics.

Induction

Barbiturates may decrease myocardial contractility, depress baroreceptor reflexes, enhance respiratory depressants, and are poor analgesics.[40] When given intravenously for anesthesia, they can cause venodilation and usually decrease venous return, cardiac output, and blood pressure. In the presence of moderate blood loss, however, thiopental has been shown to increase renal blood flow.[41] The degree of myocardial depression induced is a function of dose and rate of injection, which together determine peak blood concentration following intravenous injection.[42] Barbiturates are highly bound to proteins, and their pharmacokinetics can be influenced by a patient's acid-base status, albumin concentration, and concurrent drug administration.[36] Trauma patients are often acidotic and hypoproteinemic, so the induction dose requirement may be greatly decreased and should be anticipated by clinicians. Because barbiturates can be arrhythmogenic, they should be used cautiously in patients with preexisting arrhythmias. In severely hypovolemic patients or when severe cardiac disease and/or preexisting arrhythmias are present, other agents or induction combinations may prove safer. If barbiturates are used, simultaneous administration of adjuvant drugs such as diazepam (0.2 mg/kg) or lidocaine (2.0 mg/kg) will decrease the barbiturate requirement and the incidence of arrhythmias.[43] Propofol induces similar hemodynamic depressive effects to those of thiopental. Accordingly, propofol is not recommended as a primary induction agent in trauma patients unless cardiovascular stability has been restored.

Unlike injectable agents, inhalation agents are readily excreted via the lung should an adverse response (other than cardiac or respiratory arrest) result. Inhalation agents are equally hypotensive compared with barbiturates and are safer than some injectable induction agents only because homeostatic mechanisms have longer to compensate for the depressant effects of the anesthetic during induction. The disadvantage of inhalant anesthetic induction is that higher concentrations must be used for intubation than would be required for maintenance. Halothane, enflurane, isoflurane, and sevoflurane all induce dose-dependent cardiopulmonary depression. Isoflurane and sevoflurane are the least depressant to cardiac output at equipotent (e.g., 1.5 minimum alveolar concentration [MAC]) concentrations. If the traumatized or critically ill dog or cat is alert or likely to struggle, has a full stomach, or has severe pulmonary dysfunction, induction with an inhalation agent alone is not recommended. Intravenous inductions in traumatized or critically ill patients may be preferred so that the airway may be controlled rapidly. Mask inductions are strictly contraindicated in patients that are vomiting or have been recently fed.

When planning anesthesia for trauma patients, there is a tendency to choose an anesthetic that is an adrenergic stimulant or is associated with minimal hypotensive effects. However, there are limited data to suggest the superiority of stimulant drugs for maintenance of anesthesia during severe hypovolemic shock or in patients with severe CNS injury.[1] For example, in hypovolemic pigs, ketamine's overall cardiovascular effects are similar to those of thiopental.[44]

Ketamine is one of the few anesthetic agents with indirect cardiovascular stimulant properties. In healthy patients, it increases blood pressure, heart rate, and cardiac output secondary to increased sympathetic activity.[45] However, ketamine induces a direct myocardial depressant effect in patients whose sympathetic system is maximally stressed by hemorrhagic shock.[44] This is often the case in severely traumatized or critically ill patients. In patients with hypertrophic or restrictive cardiomyopathy (e.g., cats with idiopathic cardiomyopathy and normal left ventricular contractility), ketamine is contraindicated because it may induce tachycardia and decrease preload.[36] In patients with mitral regurgitation, ketamine is contraindicated because it may increase the regurgitant fraction through increased afterload. In contrast, in large-breed or giant-breed dogs suffering cardiogenic shock and myocardial failure as defined by poor contractility (dilated cardiomyopathy), ketamine may be a good choice for inducing anesthesia. When given alone, ketamine does not provide good muscle relaxation, and spontaneous movement is common. Because of their propensity to increase intracranial pressure, dis-

sociatives are not recommended for patients with severe closed head injury or open eye injury (e.g., corneal laceration).

Benzodiazepines enhance muscle relaxation and sedation when combined with ketamine, barbiturates, or opioids. Small intravenous doses of ketamine (5.5 mg/kg) combined with diazepam (0.27 mg/kg) titrated to effect can be administered to some high-risk patients if there are no contraindications to the use of ketamine. Lower intravenous doses of diazepam (0.2 mg/kg) and ketamine (2 to 3 mg/kg) may be given in rapid sequence to induce anesthesia in either traumatized or critically ill dogs or cats. If a patient is not sufficiently depressed after diazepam-ketamine administration, additional ketamine or delivery of low concentrations of sevoflurane or isoflurane by face mask will complete the induction. Isoflurane and sevoflurane are less arrhythmogenic and act faster than halothane and thus are the preferred agents in any trauma patient exhibiting arrhythmias or suspected of having myocardial injury.[46,47]

Induction of anesthesia with opioids usually necessitates concomitant use of an adjunctive tranquilizer-sedative or inhalation agent. Because most opioid agonists can depress respiration and slow heart rate, intravenous administration should be preceded by preoxygenation, and an antimuscarinic should be available for rapid administration in the event that severe bradycardia is induced. In dogs, intravenously administered meperidine and morphine can be associated with a dose-dependent histamine release, which can cause severe hypotension. Cautious, slow administration is acceptable if blood pressure is monitored. In contrast, intravenous administration of oxymorphone, hydromorphone, or fentanyl has not been associated with histamine release and has proven relatively safe in critically ill patients. A µ opioid receptor agonist may be combined with a benzodiazepine for induction in critically ill patients. Oxymorphone or hydromorphone is commonly given intravenously in small increments (0.05 mg/kg) along with diazepam (0.2 mg/kg) until intubation is possible. Alternatively, intravenous midazolam (0.2 mg/kg) and fentanyl (5 to 10 µg/kg) may be used. Because opioids and benzodiazepines given together do not cause myocardial depression or vasodilation, they make a good induction combination in patients in hypovolemic, cardiogenic, or septic shock, and in dehydrated patients. Nevertheless, because opioid inductions are slower than those achieved with barbiturates, nonbarbiturate hypnotics, or dissociatives, they are *not* recommended if rapid intubation of the airway is a necessity for patient survival.

For arrhythmic patients and patients with severe cardiac disease, etomidate is perhaps the safest drug for inducing anesthesia while maintaining cerebral and hemodynamic homeostasis. In doses of 0.5 to 2.0 mg/kg, etomidate produces minimal hemodynamic alterations and cardiac depression in animals.[48–50] Adrenal cortical suppression may follow anesthesia induction, but this suppression is of limited concern when etomidate is administered as a single bolus to a hemodynamically unstable patient.[1] Etomidate is a rational selection for anesthesia induction in patients in compensated or decompensated (congestive) heart failure, whether caused by acquired chronic atrioventricular valvular disease or myocardial failure (dilated cardiomyopathy). To minimize side effects such as retching and myoclonus, etomidate injection should follow the administration of a benzodiazepine and/or an opioid. With repeated use of etomidate in cats, hemolysis caused by the propylene glycol vehicle has been observed.

Anesthetic Maintenance

Along with proper monitoring, the first priority during maintenance of anesthesia is adequate oxygenation, which may require controlled ventilation of the lungs for normal gas exchange. Blood oxygen saturation can be easily monitored by pulse oximetry using a buccal mucosa, vulva or prepuce, tongue, toe, or ear site. Ventilation is monitored by using capnometry or capnography. Preservation of hemodynamic stability, which is also essential, is achieved by providing adequate intravascular volume, which can be monitored by placing central venous and arterial pressure catheters, by using inotropic agents if necessary (Table 46.5), and by maintaining proper anesthetic dose and ventilator settings.[18]

Opioids such as oxymorphone (0.1 mg/kg IV), hydromorphone (0.1 to 0.2 mg/kg IV), or fentanyl (0.005 mg/kg IV) combined with ketamine can be administered in small aliquots along with diazepam or midazolam to maintain brief periods of anesthesia. Administration of ketamine should be repeated at an approximate dosage of 1 to 2 mg/kg IV every 20 to 30 min or as necessary to maintain anesthesia. Administration of diazepam or midazolam can also be repeated (0.2 mg/kg IV) every 30 to 60 min or as necessary to relax muscles adequately. Recovery can be prolonged with repeated injections of benzodiazepines. Anesthesia should be limited to less than 2 h. Long recoveries may be problematic in cats because they metabolize benzodiazepines more slowly than do dogs. Flumazenil may be administered to antagonize benzodiazepines once the effects of the ketamine have worn off. Similarly, tiletamine plus zolazepam (Telazol) may be useful when given in low doses for minimal restraint. These injectable regimens are often supplemented with low concentrations of sevoflurane or isoflurane if anesthesia must be extended. For airway examinations or diagnostic procedures that are not painful, propofol may be used as an infusion (0.04 mg/kg/h IV) in patients in stable hemodynamic condition. Since propofol is relatively noncumulative in dogs, recoveries are similar to those from an induction dose. Recoveries are longer in cats than in dogs when infusion lasts longer than 30 min (probably because of decreased glucuronide conjugation). Cats are comparatively intolerant of phenols, which are linked to oxidative injury of feline hemoglobin. The safety of consecutive-day propofol administration (a propofol bolus and 0.2 to 0.3 mg/kg/min IV for 30 min) has been evaluated in cats.[51] After 3 days, recovery times were prolonged, and there was a significant increase in Heinz bodies; by day 5, cats did not appear to feel well, were anorexic, and had diarrhea. Accordingly, propofol should not be administered continuously nor repeatedly at short intervals in cats.

When administered to hypovolemic animals, nitrous oxide does not appear to offer any hemodynamic advantage over halothane.[52] Because trauma patients frequently have pulmonary contusions with increased venous admixture, nitrous oxide is not routinely recommended, and it is contraindicated if blunt tho-racic trauma is suspected or either pneumothorax or hemothorax is present. Similarly, the use of nitrous oxide should be avoided in patients with a distended abdomen or diaphragmatic hernia that has caused respiratory compromise. Nitrous oxide is a known stimulant of cerebral metabolism and causes increased cerebral blood flow and intracranial pressure.[53] Therefore, it is not recommended for trauma patients with severe head or open eye injury.

Isoflurane and sevoflurane are equally hypotensive but do not sensitize the myocardium to the arrhythmogenic effects of catecholamines to the same extent as halothane.[54] Sevoflurane is less soluble than isoflurane and provides a potentially faster and smoother induction and recovery than isoflurane. When an inhalant anesthetic agent is used, myocardial depression and hypotension can be minimized by using as low a concentration as possible. In people, it is common to administer a muscle relaxant to help prevent patient movement when using low inhalant concentrations. Unfortunately, some human patients have recalled surgical events under these conditions.[1] Preanesthetic or intraoperative administration of an opioid or benzodiazepine tranquilizer with or without a muscle relaxant can help assure adequate CNS depression during low-dose inhalation anesthesia. In hypovolemic anesthetized patients, fentanyl, oxymorphone, butorphanol, or diazepam are preferred for reduction in inhalant requirement. Continuous-rate intravenous infusions of fentanyl, fentanyl-midazolam, ketamine, or lidocaine may be used to decrease the inhalant requirement. Acepromazine is not a good choice in these circumstances because it may increase vascular capacity, reducing blood pressure. In hypovolemic patients, compensatory vasoconstriction is often present preoperatively due to increased catecholamine activity. When anesthesia is induced, compensatory mechanisms may be blocked or fail, resulting in profound hypotension and reduced preload and cardiac output, especially if acepromazine has been administered. On the other hand, if adequate volume replacement has been achieved prior to acepromazine administration and inotropic support is available as needed, decreasing arterial resistance (α-adrenergic blockade) may improve perfusion (e.g., to kidneys and intestines).

Regional Anesthesia

Performing epidural or intrathecal blocks is contraindicated in patients that are septic or have a bleeding diathesis. Epidural or spinal blocks are contraindicated in hypovolemic patients because of the potential for profound sympathetic blockade induced by these techniques when using local anesthetics. Epidural administration of opioids (0.1 mg/kg of preservative-free morphine) or low doses of α_2-adrenergic agonists (e.g., 1 to 3 μg/kg medetomidine) may prove to be effective alternatives to local anesthetics in providing regional analgesia with minimal sympathetic blockade.[55,56] In severely depressed patients, or in patients administered neuroleptanalgesia, superficial lacerations and wounds of the extremities can be managed with infiltration of local anesthetic or by performing peripheral nerve blocks. Local anesthetics may not be as effective when deposited in infected tissue because of ongoing inflammation and pH alterations.

Adjunctive regional therapy using a local anesthetic improves analgesia while lowering the inhalation agent requirement. Intercostal nerve blocks (0.5 to 1.0 mL per site in dogs) with 2% lidocaine or 0.5% bupivacaine can be performed to control postoperative thoracotomy pain, as well as pain associated with fractured ribs. Interpleural administration of local anesthetics is also effective as an adjunct for thoracotomy and cranial abdominal pain associated with pancreatitis or with diaphragmatic hernia repair. With regional techniques, care should be taken to avoid exceeding the toxic local anesthetic dose for a given species. The maximum dose of bupivacaine is approximately 2 mg/kg in dogs and 1 mg/kg in cats. The maximum dose may be diluted, if necessary, for more complete coverage.

Intraoperative Support

Documentation of the medical history of each patient evaluated should include previous drug administration, because concomitant drug therapy must be considered when anesthetizing a patient. Adverse cardiovascular drug interactions are increasingly being reported. Examples of commonly administered cardiovascular drugs will be illustrated here, but a more complete discussion is available elsewhere.[57] Many cardiovascular drugs are metabolized in the liver through the several different isoforms of the cytochrome oxidase system. Drugs may either induce the isoforms, thereby decreasing the plasma concentrations of certain drugs, or inhibit the isoforms, thereby increasing the plasma concentrations of drugs. One of the first known interactions resulted from the decreased rate of hepatic metabolism of lidocaine when cimetidine was concurrently administered, leading to potential lidocaine toxicity. Cimetidine also increases plasma concentrations of quinidine, verapamil, and propranolol. Ranitidine inhibits fewer isoforms and is less likely to cause such interactions. Cimetidine also increases plasma concentrations of procainamide by inhibiting clearance by the kidneys. The likelihood of lidocaine toxicity increases when a β-adrenergic antagonist is administered with lidocaine. During the coadministration of agents that depress sinoatrial nodal function, lidocaine may cause sinoatrial arrest.[57] β-Adrenergic stimulants, such as dobutamine, decrease potassium concentrations and should be administered cautiously to patients receiving potassium-losing diuretics. Coadministration of captopril with hydralazine or procainamide may precipitate neutropenia because of impaired immune status. Nonsteroidal antiinflammatory drugs may attenuate the antihypertensive effects of β blockers.[57] Many companion animals are administered herbal formulations that may interact with anesthetic, cardiovascular, tricyclic antidepressant, and monoamine oxidase–inhibitor drugs. The aforementioned interactions are representative of the many potential adverse interactions possible.

Perioperative Fluid Support

Several choices of fluids are available for use in traumatized patients undergoing anesthesia and surgery. With hemorrhage, there is contraction of extracellular volume as the intravascular compartment deficit is replaced with interstitial fluid. Administration of a physiological salt solution such as lactated Ringer's restores this depletion and also expands intravascular volume to help maintain cardiac output. In general, patients should be administered 20 to 40 mL/kg intravenously prior to anesthetic induction. An exception is when patients are severely anemic or hypoproteinemic, have poor myocardial contractility, or have advanced valvular heart disease. Patients in hypovolemic shock can be given up to 1 blood volume (60 to 90 mL/kg) of isotonic electrolyte solution in the first hour. Many more animals have experienced problems after anesthetic drug injection, when compensatory mechanisms failed and underlying hypovolemia was unmasked, than have developed problems when crystalloid fluids were administered unnecessarily at these rates.[36] During anesthesia, hypotension caused by volume depletion often responds to replacement of one-quarter of the blood volume in 15 min as an intravenous fluid challenge. Replacement solutions should be isotonic, but not all isotonic solutions are optimal. Although 5% dextrose in water and lactated Ringer's with 2.5% dextrose are isotonic, once glucose is metabolized the remaining fluid is hypotonic and contains either all (5% dextrose) or half (2.5% dextrose) free water, which rapidly leaves the vascular compartment and may contribute to microvascular edema.[17] In general, even optimal isotonic physiological salt solutions remain in the intravascular space for only 30 to 60 min before redistributing throughout the entire extracellular space.[58]

Plasma expanders such as colloid solutions maintain intravascular volume for 2 to 5 h, but may have associated complications (Table 46.3). Dextran solutions can cause bleeding disorders and allergic reactions, and must be stored at stable temperatures (25°C) to prevent precipitate formation.[59,60] Protein solutions can impair pulmonary function if they extravasate into damaged lung.[61] Hydroxyethyl starch (6% solution in 0.9% sodium chloride) is a glucose polymer that has proven useful as a volume expander when the dose is limited to less than 20 mL/kg in dogs and 12 to 15 mL/kg in cats.[62] Because colloid solutions can be hypertonic, they must be administered slowly to avoid rapid fluid shifts and volume overload.[16]

When extreme blood loss occurs, red cells must eventually be infused. Fresh whole blood (less than 6 h old) is preferable. After 1 day of storage, only 12% of the original platelets remain in human whole blood. Similar reductions may occur in stored blood of domestic animals. Regardless of its age, whole blood is preferred over packed red blood cells.[1] Fresh-frozen plasma should be reserved for specific coagulation disorders.[63] In acute trauma, the large majority of clotting disorders are secondary to large-volume fluid replacement that causes dilutional thrombocytopenia. If possible, surgery and anesthesia should be delayed until the PCV can be increased to above 20% and platelet abnormalities addressed. When ongoing losses and replacement occur simultaneously, the best method of assessing adequate blood volume replacement is to assess urine output (1 to 2 mL $\cdot$ kg^{-1} $\cdot$ h^{-1} is optimal), serial hematocrits, and total protein. Some questions remain with regard to optimum fluid management of severely traumatized patients in the perioperative period, including (a) the best methods of using non-erythrocyte-containing fluids in trauma resuscitation, (b) feasibility of systemic oxygen delivery (DO_2) and consumption-oriented resuscitation in high-risk surgical patients, and (c) the effects of fluid therapy on cerebral hemodynamics.[64]

With regard to nonblood fluid resuscitation, if membrane permeability is normal, fluids containing colloids (albumin, dextran, and hydroxyethyl starch) expand plasma volume (PV) rather than interstitial fluid volume (IFV) or intracellular volume (ICV). Each gram of intravascular colloid can draw and hold approximately 20 mL of water (e.g., 16 to 17 mL of water per gram of hydroxyethyl starch) in the vascular space. To estimate the effects of fluid infusion on PV, the following formula can be used: $PV = volume\ infused \times (PV/V_d)$, where V_d = distribution volume. In mature animals, total body water accounts for 60% of the total body weight. The ICV is 40%, the extracellular volume (ECV) is 20%, the IFV is 16%, and the PV is 4% of total body weight. If an acute blood loss of 500 mL is to be replaced using the preceding formula and 5% dextrose, which contains no sodium, the remaining water after glucose metabolism, distributes throughout the total body water. For a 70-kg dog where plasma volume of 500 mL is to be replaced, the volume of 5% dextrose infused is 500 mL = volume infused $\times$ (3 L/42 L), or approximately 7 L. In contrast, 500 mL of blood loss can be replaced with lactated Ringer's solution (LRS), for which the V_d is equal to the ECV or only 20% of the body weight (3 L/14 L) with just 2.3 L of LRS. If hyperosmotic fluids such as hypertonic saline (HS) are used, blood volume increases primarily by endogenous fluid PV expansion. These fluids come from the IFV initially and are transient in their duration of effect on PV. The immediate effect of 7.5% HS is to increase plasma volume by 2 to 4 mL for each milliliter infused. Thus, 500 mL of PV may be replaced with only 150 to 200 mL of HS. However, following equilibration, 7.5% saline increases PV by only approximately 1.0 mL for each milliliter infused. Small volumes of hyperosmotic solutions transiently restore hemodynamic function during shock, but because improved PV and flow decrease rather rapidly following resuscitation with hypertonic fluids, ongoing attention to maintenance of intravascular volume is necessary.[64] To prolong the initial improvement seen with hyperosmotic solutions beyond 30 to 60 min, continued infusion with a hypertonic solution, blood (if PCV is below 20%), or conventional fluids, or the addition of colloids, should be considered. One suggested protocol for volume resuscitation combines bolusing a synthetic colloid solution (1 to 5 mL/kg) with a replacement crystalloid solution (15 mL/kg). The dose of colloid solution should not exceed 20 mL/kg in dogs and 12 to 15 mL/kg in cats within the first 24 h. Rapid fluid loading is often associated with dilutional thrombocytopenia, hypoglycemia, and/or hypokalemia, and fluids should be supplemented to maintain serum levels within normal ranges.[5]

Studies in dogs have documented that HS may have a negative inotropic effect, whereas hyperosmotic dextrose produces a positive inotropic action.[65] Rapid (<30 s) administration of 2 to 4 mL of HS is also associated with an acute transient period of hypotension.[65] Infusion over a 3- to 4-min period will diminish this initial response. HS likely exerts its beneficial effect in treating hemorrhagic or endotoxic shock by rapidly increasing preload, whereas hyperosmotic dextrose solutions exert their beneficial effects by transiently increasing both preload and contractility.[65]

In high-risk traumatized patients who survive, it has been doc-umented that average blood flow and DO_2 are greater than in those patients that did not survive.[66] Survival is correlated with a DO_2 that is at least 600 mL $O_2 \cdot min^{-1} \cdot m^{-2}$ (Table 46.1). When DO_2 is maintained at this level, complications are also reduced. To implement DO_2 goal-oriented fluid resuscitation, cardiac output, hemoglobin content, and oxygen-hemoglobin saturation must be continually monitored. In many traumatized patients, improvement of overall systemic DO_2 may be less critical than the immediate restoration of adequate oxygen delivery to selected vital organ systems.

With respect to the effects of fluid therapy on cerebral hemodynamics, it appears that, in some subsets of traumatized patients (severe head injury), initial fluid therapy with 7.5% saline in 6% dextran improves patient survival (32%) when compared with those treated with conventional LRS (16%).[64] Concerns over adverse neurological sequelae with hypertonic solutions have not proven valid, with the exception of hyperosmotic resuscitation in canine experimental models of uncontrolled hemorrhage where hyperosmotic solutions actually increase bleeding tendency.[67]

Commonly, trauma cases will present with nonrespiratory acidosis caused by shock and generalized stress. Ventilation of the lungs to induce a mild respiratory alkalosis will help normalize blood pH for the short term. With time, improved tissue perfusion and renal and hepatic function should resolve the problem. Treatment of metabolic acidosis with bicarbonate or other buffers should be carefully considered. More important measures in treating metabolic acidosis are fluid resuscitation, adequate ventilation, and rewarming. It is possible for patients with normal liver function to develop metabolic alkalosis 6 to 24 h after large-volume replacement with LRS.

Inotropic Support

Drugs commonly used to enhance myocardial contractility and increase cardiac output are listed in Tables 46.4 and 46.5.[18] Ephedrine has proven an effective alternative to dopamine or dobutamine when administered during inhalation anesthesia to enhance cardiac output.[68] A 0.1-mg/kg intravenous dose of ephedrine transiently increases arterial pressure, cardiac index, stroke volume, arterial oxygen content (CaO_2), and oxygen delivery in dogs anesthetized with isoflurane (1.5 MAC). A intravenous dose of 0.25 mg/kg causes a greater and prolonged increase in arterial pressure while actually decreasing heart rate.[68] This presumably results from a reflex bradycardia associated with an acute increase in arterial pressure. The higher dose of ephedrine also increases hemoglobin concentration and CaO_2, resulting in a 20% to 35% increase in oxygen delivery for at least 1 h. Increased hemoglobin concentration likely results from contraction of the spleen and increased circulating red blood cells. Splenic contraction results from either ephedrine's direct α-agonist effects or enhanced norepinephrine release. Because ephedrine can be administered as a convenient intravenous bolus with an onset of less than a minute, it is a useful for inotropic support of anesthetized patients. Dopamine and dobutamine have short half-lives and require constant infusion (Table 46.5). Close monitoring for development of arrhythmias is necessary, and, with dopamine, to avoid intense α receptor–mediated vasoconstriction. In refractive cases, inotropic doses of dopamine and dobutamine may be supplemented with the coadministration of ephedrine to reduce vascular compliance and improve preload and stroke volume.[69]

In septic shock, vasopressin has been used for unresponsive hypotension. During anesthesia, vasopressin has also been used to support blood pressure. It is a peptide hormone stored in the posterior pituitary and synthesized in the supraoptic and periventricular nuclei of the hypothalamus. The release of vasopressin can result from an increased plasma osmolarity, decreased blood volume or pressure, nausea, pain, endotoxemia, cytokines, and other stimuli. Either low secretion or excessive secretion leading to depletion causes a deficiency in vasopressin. Vasopressin may be effective in situations where severe refractory hypotension no longer responds to adrenergic agonists. Intravenous infusion of 0.25 to 1.0 mU/kg/min increases blood pressure and urine flow in many patients. Vassopressor therapy has been reviewed elsewhere.[70]

Temperature, Oxygen, and Renal Support

Hypothermia should be treated vigorously because it is associated with reduced kidney function, poor platelet function, impaired glucose utilization, shivering and increased oxygen consumption by nonvital tissues, and decreased metabolism of anesthetics.[1] Bradyarrhythmias that do not respond to anticholinergics and spontaneous fibrillation may occur in hypothermic patients. Warming fluids and blood before administration helps maintain body temperature, reduces blood viscosity, and improves tissue blood flow. Warm-water blankets and heat lamps may help prevent further heat loss, but may not effectively rewarm patients because of inadequate body-surface-area contact and poor skin blood flow. Forced-air blankets will increase body temperature, but slowly. Maintenance of body temperature and rewarming may be easier when animals are anesthetized, because of high skin blood flow following inhibition of vasomotor control by anesthetics. Intense vasoconstriction after recovery from anesthesia may slow surface-rewarming efforts.

To prevent acute oliguric renal failure in severely traumatized patients, every effort should be made to maintain normal renal function. Unfortunately, there is no way to predict the degree of hypoperfusion that will result in renal failure in a given patient. Myoglobinemia must be treated by vigorous diuresis after muscle damage or electrocution. Once fluid volume and blood pressure have been normalized, furosemide (1 mg/kg) and dopamine (2 to 5 μg/kg/min) have been used together to increase renal blood flow and water and solute excretion, but renal therapy strategy remains somewhat controversial. Maintaining a functional renal system is essential for a favorable outcome following massive tissue damage.[1]

Questions regarding perioperative renal function and renal physiology in critically ill patients remain.[71] It is common for severely traumatized, critically ill patients to produce inadequate urine output. These patients are often given a "renal dose" of dopamine in an attempt to improve urine production and prevent oliguria. Dopaminergic receptors (DA_1 and DA_2) increase glomerular filtration rate (GFR) and inhibit proximal tubular re-

absorption of sodium. This combination of effects increases sodium excretion in euvolemic patients, but this action is diminished with prolonged infusion. Furthermore, in critically ill patients, dopamine's natriuretic action is not always apparent, because antinatriuretic factors (antidiuretic hormone and aldosterone) may be elevated to induce sodium conservation. With lower-than-normal levels of GFR, low doses of dopamine become less effective. This lack of response may be caused by exhaustion of the renal reserve system, where low renal blood flow may have already caused a shift of blood flow to the inner cortex in an adaptive response to loss of nephron renal function. Hence, dopamine's actions produce little additional urine. Despite these problems, dopamine can increase urine output in oliguric patients and in patients that are adequately hydrated. Several studies have also shown that dopamine improves urine output in patients that have not responded to fluid expansion or furosemide alone. By increasing renal flow, dopamine may improve delivery of furosemide to its site of action in the nephron.[71]

It is unclear whether dopamine is advantageous in the treatment of oliguric renal failure. Dopamine appears to be no better than saline in protecting renal function. In fact, dopamine-induced natriuresis may cause intravascular volume depletion, making the kidney even more susceptible to ongoing ischemic injury. Questions remain as to the clinical implication of increasing renal perfusion when there is decreased systemic blood volume. The routine administration of dopamine in severely traumatized patients should be carefully considered in the perioperative period.[71]

Urine flow, regardless of the quantity, indicates there is blood flow to the kidney, because, without it, urine production would cease. Numerous studies have shown, however, that there is no correlation between the urine volume produced and histological evidence of acute tubular necrosis, GFR, creatinine clearance, blood urea nitrogen levels, and creatinine levels in burn patients, trauma patients, or shock states.[71,72] The control of blood flow to the kidney, the fraction filtered, and the volume returned to the systemic circulation are all regulated by a variety of mechanisms in an attempt to preserve filtration function during compromised circulation. These compensatory mechanisms have limits, and excessive vasoconstriction may eventually decrease filtration. This shift from compensation to decompensation may be prevented or exacerbated by pharmacological manipulations. The cortical-to-medullary redistribution of renal blood flow is designed to protect vulnerable medullary oxygen supply and demand balance at the expense of urine formation. Reduced GFR may reduce medullary tubular workload and oxygen consumption. Oliguria may be viewed in some circumstances (e.g., anesthesia) as a sign of normal protective compensatory mechanisms at work. Thus, an acute reduction in urine output could be either the result of acute renal failure or the consequence of normal compensatory mechanisms induced to prevent oliguria.[71]

Traditionally, inadequate urine production or oliguria has been defined as a urine output of less than $0.5 \text{ mL} \cdot \text{kg}^{-1} \cdot \text{h}^{-1}$. Oliguria may, however, reflect a variety of factors independent of inadequate glomerular filtration. Thus, normal hourly urine output does not rule out impending renal failure any more than lower-than-normal hourly urine output predicts renal failure. Reduced urine output during the anesthetic period in euvolemic patients is usually of little consequence to long-term renal function. It is more likely to be the result of compensatory renal mechanisms than a consequence of acute tubular damage or necrosis.[71]

Recovery

In postoperative patients, bowel and bladder function, pulmonary function, and skin integrity should be addressed. Patients that cannot turn themselves should be turned every 2 to 4 h. Bandages should be kept clean and dry; dried blood and soap should be removed. Eyes should be lubricated. Oxygen should be supplemented as needed. The environment should be quiet. Patients that are hospitalized for extended periods have special needs for appropriate social interaction.

References

1. Priano LL. Trauma. In: Barash PG, Cullen BF, Stoelting RK, eds. Clinical Anesthesia. Philadelphia: JB Lippincott, 1989:1365–1377.
2. Drobatz KJ, Powell S. Global approach to the trauma patient. In: Proceedings of the Fourth International Veterinary Emergency and Critical Care Symposium, San Antonio, TX, September 29 to October 2, 1994:32–36.
3. Purvis D, Kirby R. Systemic inflammatory response syndrome: Septic shock. Vet Clin North Am Small Anim Pract 24:1225–1247, 1994.
4. Shoemaker WC. Resuscitation of the trauma patient: Restoration of hemodynamic functions using clinical algorithms. Ann Emerg Med 15:1437–1444, 1986.
5. Hardie EM. Life-threatening bacterial infection. Compend Contin Educ 17:763–777, 1995.
6. Brady CA, Otto CM. Systemic inflammatory response syndrome, sepsis, and multiple organ dysfunction. Vet Clin North Am Small Anim Pract 31:1147–1162, 2001.
7. Stamp G. Metabolic responses to trauma. In: Zaslow I, ed. Trauma and Critical Care. Philadelphia: Lea and Febiger, 1984:25–63.
8. Gallagher TJ, Banner MJ, Barnes PA. Large volume crystalloid resuscitation does not increase extravascular lung water. Anesth Analg 64:323–326, 1985.
9. Smiley LE. The use of hetastarch for plasma expansion. Probl Vet Med 4:652–667, 1992.
10. Garzon AA, Cheng C, Lerner B, Lichtenstein S, Karlson KE. Hydroxyethyl starch (hes) and bleeding: An experimental investigation of its effects on hemostasis. J Trauma 7:757–766, 1967.
11. Karlson KE, Garson AA, Shafton GW, Chu CJ. Increased blood loss associated with administration of certain plasma expanders: Dextran 75, dextran 40, and hydroxyethyl starch. Surgery 62:670–678, 1967.
12. Layon J, Duncan D, Gallagher TJ, Banner MJ. Hypertonic saline as a resuscitation solution in hemorrhagic shock. Anesth Analg 66:154–158, 1987.
13. Bitterman H, Triolo J, Lefer AM. Use of hypertonic saline in the treatment of hemorrhagic shock. Circ Shock 21:271–283, 1987.
14. Lopes OU, Velasco IT, Guertzenstein PG, et al. Hypertonic sodium restores mean circulatory filling pressure in severely hypovolemic dogs. In: Proceedings Supplement 1, Hypertension, Inter-American Society, 1986:I195.
15. Muir WW III, Sally J. Small volume resuscitation with hypertonic saline solution in hypovolemic cats. Am J Vet Res 50:1883–1888, 1989.
16. Garvey MS. Fluid and electrolyte balance in critical patients. Vet Clin North Am Small Anim Pract 19:1021–1058, 1989.
17. Layon AJ, Kirby RR. Fluids and electrolytes in the critically ill. In: Civetta JM, Taylor RM, Kirby RR, eds. Critical Care. Philadelphia: JB Lippincott, 1988:451–474.
18. Schwinn DA. Cardiovascular pharmacology. In: IARS 1994 Review Course Lectures, Supplement to Anesthesia and Analgesia, Orlando, FL, March 5–9, 1994:154–164.
19. Cote E. Cardiogenic shock and cardiac arrest. Vet Clin North Am Small Anim Pract 31:1129–1145, 2001.
20. Mizock BA, Falk JL. Lactic acidosis in critical illness. Crit Care Med 20:80–93, 1992.
21. Bakker J, Coffernils M, Leon M, Gris P, Vincent JL. Blood lactate levels are superior to oxygen-derived variables in predicting outcome in septic shock. Chest 99:956–962, 1991.
22. Muir WW, Sams RA. Pharmacology and pharmacokinetics of antiarrhythmic drugs. In Fox PR, ed. Canine and Feline Cardiology. New York: Churchill Livingstone, 1988:309–334.
23. Plumb DC. Drug monographs. In: Veterinary Drug Handbook, 3rd ed. Ames: Iowa State University Press, 1999:1–652.
24. Hamlin RL. Current uses and hazards of ventricular antiarrhythmic therapy. In: Kirk RW, Bonagura JD, eds. Current Veterinary Therapy XI. Philadelphia: WB Saunders, 1992:694–699.
25. Bar-Joseph G, Abramson NS, Jansen-McWilliams L, et al. Clinical use of sodium bicarbonate during cardiopulmonary resuscitation: Is it used sensibly? Resuscitation 54:47–55, 2002.
26. Dybvik T, Strand T, Steen PA. Buffer therapy during out-of-hospital cardiopulmonary resuscitation. Resuscitation 29:89–95, 1995.
27. Ammari A, Schulze K. Uses and abuses of sodium bicarbonate in the neonatal intensive care unit. Curr Opin Pediatr 14:151–156, 2002.
28. Hartsfield SM. Sodium bicarbonate and bicarbonate precursors for treatment of metabolic acidosis. J Am Vet Med Assoc 179:914–916, 1981.
29. Debaveye YA, Berghe GH. Is there still a place for dopamine in the modern intensive care unit? Anesth Analg 98:461–468, 2004.
30. Flournoy WS, Wohl JS, Albrecht-Schmitt TJ, Schwartz DD. Pharmacologic identification of putative D_1 dopamine receptors in feline kidneys. J Vet Pharmacol Ther 2003;26:283–290.
31. Rockoff MA, Shapiro HM. Barbiturates following cardiac arrest: Possible benefit or Pandora's box? Anesthesiology 49:385–387, 1978.
32. Evans T. Anesthesia and monitoring for trauma and critical care patients. In: Slatter DH, ed. Textbook of Small Animal Surgery, 1985:2702–2711.
33. Hackner SG. Emergency management of traumatic pulmonary contusions. Compend Contin Educ 17:677–686, 1995.
34. Kolata RJ, Kraut NJ, Johnston DE. Patterns of trauma in urban dogs and cats: A study of 1,000 cases. J Am Vet Med Assoc 164:499–502, 1974.
35. Martyn J. Clinical pharmacology and drug therapy in the burned patient. Anesthesiology 65:67–75, 1986.
36. Bednarski RM. Anesthesia and pain control. Vet Clin North Am Small Anim Pract 19:1223–1238, 1989.
37. Salem MR, Wong AY, Mani M, Bennett EJ, Toyama T. Premedicant drugs and gastric juice pH and volume in pediatric patients. Anesthesiology 44:216–219, 1976.
38. Davidson CD, Pettifer GR, Henry JD. Plasma fentanyl concentrations and analgesic effects during full or partial exposure to trans-

dermal fentanyl patches in cats. J Am Vet Med Assoc 2004;224: 700–705.

39. Haskins SC, Farver TB, Patz BA. Cardiovascular changes in dogs given diazepam and diazepam-ketamine. Am J Vet Res 47:795–798, 1986.

40. Bernards C, Marvone B, Priano L. Effect of anesthetic induction agents on baroreceptor function [Abstract]. Anesthesiology 63:A31, 1985.

41. Priano LL. Renal hemodynamic alterations following administration of thiopental, diazepam, or ketamine in conscious hypovolemic dogs. Adv Shock Res 9:173–188, 1983.

42. Roberts JG. Intravenous anesthetic agents. In: Prys-Roberts C, ed. The Circulation in Anesthesia: Applied Physiology and Pharmacology. London: Blackwell Scientific, 1980:311–327.

43. Rawlings CA, Kolata RJ. Cardiopulmonary effects of thiopental/lidocaine combination during anesthetic induction in the dog. Am J Vet Res 44:144–149, 1983.

44. Weiskopf RB, Bogetz MS, Roizen MF, Reid IA. Cardiovascular and metabolic sequelae of inducing anesthesia with ketamine or thiopental in hypovolemic swine. Anesthesiology 60:214–219, 1984.

45. Haskins SC, Farver TB, Patz JD. Ketamine in dogs. Am J Vet Res 46:1855–1860, 1985.

46. Harvey RC, Short CE. The use of isoflurane for safe anesthesia in animals with traumatic myocarditis or other myocardial sensitivity [Abstract]. Canine Pract 10:18, 1983.

47. Hubble JAE, Muir WW, Bednarski RM, Bednarski LS. Change of inhalation anesthetic agents for management of ventricular premature depolarizations in anesthetized cats and dogs. J Am Vet Med Assoc 185:643–646, 1984.

48. Robertson S. Advantages of etomidate use as an anesthetic agent. Vet Clin North Am Small Anim Pract 22:277–280, 1992.

49. Gooding JM, Corssen G. Effect of etomidate on the cardiovascular system. Anesth Analg 56:717–719, 1977.

50. Pascoe PJ, Ilkiw JE, Haskins SC, Patz JD. Cardiopulmonary effects of etomidate in hypovolemic dogs. Am J Vet Res 53:2178–2182, 1992.

51. Andress JL, Day TK, Day DG. The effects of consecutive day propofol anesthesia on feline red blood cells. Vet Surg 24:277–282, 1995.

52. Weiskopf RB, Bogetz MS. Cardiovascular action of nitrous oxide and halothane in hypovolemic swine. Anesthesiology 63:509–516, 1985.

53. Sakabe T, Kuramoto T, Inone S, Takeshita H. Cerebral effects of nitrous oxide in the dog. Anesthesiology 48:195–200, 1978.

54. Joas TA, Stevens WC. Comparison of the arrhythmic doses of epinephrine during Forane, halothane, and fluroxene anesthesia in dogs. Anesthesiology 35:48–53, 1971.

55. Tung AS, Yaksh TL. The antinociceptive effects of epidural opiates in the cat: Studies on the pharmacology and the effects of lipophilicity in spinal analgesia. Pain 12:343–356, 1982.

56. Valverde A, Dyson DH, McDonell WN. Epidural morphine reduces halothane MAC in the dog. Can J Anaesth 36:629–632, 1989.

57. Opie LH. Adverse cardiovascular drug interactions. Curr Probl Cardiol 25:621–676, 2000.

58. Cervera LA, Moss G. Crystalloid distribution following hemorrhage and hemodilution. J Trauma 14:506–520, 1974.

59. Giesecke AH Jr. Anesthesia for trauma surgery. In: Miller RD, ed. Anesthesia. New York: Churchill Livingstone, 1981:1247–1264.

60. Giesecke AH, Jenkins MT. Fluid therapy. Clin Anesth 11:57–69, 1976.

61. Holcraft JW, Trunkey DD, Carpenter MA. Sepsis in the baboon: Factors affecting resuscitation and pulmonary edema in animals resuscitated with Ringer's lactate versus Plasmanate. J Trauma 17: 600–610, 1977.

62. Munoz E, Raciti A, Dove DB, et al. Effect of hydroxyethyl starch versus albumin on hemodynamic and respiratory function in patients in shock. Crit Care Med 8:255–263, 1980.

63. Baldini M, Costea N, Dameshek W. The viability of stored human platelets. Blood 16:1669–1692, 1960.

64. Prough DS. Controversies in perioperative fluid management. In: IARS 1994 Review Course Lectures, Supplement to Anesthesia and Analgesia, Orlando, FL, March 5–9, 1994:16–24.

65. Constable PD, Muir WW, Binkley PF. Hypertonic saline is a negative inotropic agent in normovolemic dogs. Am J Physiol 267: H667–H677, 1994.

66. Kovacic J. Management of life-threatening trauma. Vet Clin North Am Small Anim Pract 24:1057–1094, 1994.

67. Gross D, Landau EH, Klin B, Krausz MM. Treatment of uncontrolled hemorrhagic shock with hypertonic saline solution. Surg Gynecol Obstet 170:106–112, 1990.

68. Wagner AE, Dunlop CI, Chapman PL. Effects of ephedrine on cardiovascular function and oxygen delivery in isoflurane-anesthetized dogs. Am J Vet Res 54:1917–1922, 1993.

69. Raffe M. Anesthetic management of the unstable trauma patient. In: Proceedings of the Fourth International Veterinary Emergency and Critical Care Symposium, San Antonio, TX, 1994:281–287.

70. Palmer J. When fluids are not enough: Inopressor therapy. In: Proceedings of the Eighth International Veterinary Emergency and Critical Care Symposium, San Antonio, TX, 2002:669–673.

71. Aronson S. Controversies: Should anesthesiologists worry about the kidney? In: IARS 1995 Review Course Lectures, Supplement to Analgesia and Anesthesia, Honolulu, HI, March 10–14, 1995:68–73.

72. Kellen M, Aronson S, Roizen-Thisted R. Predictive and diagnostic tests of acute renal failure: A review. Anesth Analg 78:134–142, 1994.

Chapter 47
Neonatal and Geriatric Patients

Glenn R. Pettifer and Tamara L. Grubb

Introduction

In the practice of veterinary anesthesia, neonatal and geriatric animals are a significant proportion of the patient population. Attention to the unique physiology and particular requirements of individuals within either of these age groups will contribute to the provision of safe, effective anesthesia and analgesia.

Physiology of Neonatal and Pediatric Animals

Neonatal and pediatric veterinary patients may be presented for either elective or emergency anesthesia. Much of our knowledge of the delivery of anesthesia to neonatal animals is based on our experience with young to middle-aged animals or is extrapolated from information obtained from human neonates.

Although the process of maturation and aging varies greatly between individual animals, species, and breeds, the neonatal and pediatric phases of life can be roughly defined. In dogs and cats, the neonatal period extends for the first 6 weeks of life and the pediatric period for the first 12 weeks.[1–3] Foals and calves are generally considered to be physiologically mature by 4 to 6 weeks of age.[4]

Compared with young and middle-aged adults, neonatal and pediatric patients have a limited organ reserve, a decreased ability to respond to a physiological challenge or change, and increased "sensitivity" to anesthetic drugs that is manifest as exaggerated or prolonged effects after the administration of drug dosages that are appropriate for young adults. This results in an increased risk of perianesthetic complications in neonates, necessitating judicious administration of anesthetics and vigilant monitoring.

The unique physiology of neonates results in differences in pharmacokinetics and pharmacodynamics that contribute to altered sensitivity to drugs. These differences include the following:

1. Hypoalbuminemia, which results in a greater free, active portion of protein-bound drugs. This may have a profound impact on the activity of highly protein-bound drugs like barbiturates, ketamine, etomidate, and the nonsteroidal anti-inflammatory drugs (NSAIDs).

2. Increased permeability of the neonatal blood-brain barrier, which enables a larger percentage of drug to reach the brain.

3. An increased percentage of body-water content, which alters the volume of distribution. In foals, extracellular fluid volume is 43% of body weight, compared with 22% body weight in adult horses.[5] The larger extracellular fluid volume results in a greater apparent volume of distribution of drugs that are highly ionized in plasma or relatively polar (e.g., NSAIDs).

4. A circulating fluid volume that is fixed and relatively centralized, making the neonatal patient more susceptible to hypovolemia. This reduced circulating volume also allows for greater delivery of anesthetic agents to the highly perfused tissues, including the brain.

5. Low body-fat percentage, resulting in a smaller adipose tissue compartment for drug redistribution.[6] In foals, for example, total body fat is 2% to 3%, compared with 5% in adult horses.[7]

6. Immature hepatic metabolism for the first 3 to 4 weeks (perhaps up to 12 weeks) of life.[8–10] Drug metabolism may be prolonged, extending the duration of effect of drugs or their active metabolites.

7. Immature glomerular filtration rate (GFR). In small animals, GFR does not mature until 2 to 3 weeks of age. Tubular secretion does not mature until 4 to 8 weeks of age.[8,11,12] As a result of this immaturity in renal function, the effects of drugs dependent on renal excretion for termination of activity are prolonged. For example, the half-life of diazepam is increased in neonates due to decreased renal excretion.[9] Although the kidneys mature more rapidly in foals and calves (the GFR is mature by 2 to 4 days of life and tubular secretion by 2 weeks of life),[4,8] immature renal function may be prolonged in unhealthy animals.

8. A high metabolic rate with a concomitant higher rate of oxygen consumption. This necessitates a need for a rate of alveolar ventilation that is much greater than that of adults. Because of this increase in alveolar ventilation, anesthetic induction with inhalant anesthetics may occur more rapidly.

In addition to physiological differences that result in alterations in the pharmacokinetics and pharmacodynamics of anesthetics, neonatal physiology alone can contribute to increased anesthetic risk (Table 47.1). These physiological differences include:

Table 47.1. Physiological characteristics of neonates.

Cardiovascular system
Low myocardial contractile mass
Low ventricular compliance
High cardiac index
Low cardiac reserve
Cardiac output rate dependent
Poor vasomotor control
Respiratory system
High oxygen consumption
High minute volume
Nervous system
Immature sympathetic nervous system
Poor vasomotor control
Renal and hepatic systems
Immature hepatic microsomal enzyme system
Immature renal function
Body composition
Limited thermoregulation
Low body fat and muscle mass
Low protein binding of drugs
High body-water content
Large extracellular fluid compartment

1. Compared with the adult heart, the neonatal heart has less contractile tissue per gram of myocardial tissue, and ventricular compliance is limited.[13] Stroke volume and cardiac reserve are limited in pediatric patients, and cardiac output is dependent on heart rate. Furthermore, the resting cardiac index is much higher in neonates than adults and is very close to maximal cardiac output, making the cardiac reserve minimal. An adult can increase cardiac output by 300%, whereas the neonate can only increase output by 30%.[14]

2. The sympathetic nervous system is not fully developed in neonates, and sympathetic stimulation results in only minimal increases in rate and contractility, further impairing the ability to increase cardiac output.[12] Sympathetic immaturity also manifests itself in poor vasomotor control and an incomplete or inadequate hypotension-induced baroresponse.

3. Fetal circulation may persist in some patients. For example, normal healthy foals have a right-to-left shunt for the first 3 days, and the duration of the shunt is often extended in unhealthy foals.[15]

4. In the first 1 to 3 days (foals and calves) or 1 to 2 weeks of life (puppies and kittens), neonatal kidneys may be less efficient than adult kidneys at eliminating fluid loads and regulating electrolytes, so judicious use of appropriate intravenous fluids is necessary.[6,8] Rapid or excessive fluid administration may result in pulmonary edema.

5. Pulmonary reserve is minimal, increasing the possibility of hypoxia during apnea or airway obstruction. The neonatal rib cage is compliant, resulting in less efficient ventilation and greater work of breathing. This predisposes young patients to hypoxia and ventilatory fatigue, especially in the event of airway obstruction (e.g., endotracheal tube plugged with mucus) or respiratory disease.

6. Minute ventilation is high in neonates, raising the alveolar ventilation to a functional residual capacity ratio above that of adults. Closing volume is high in the neonate and occurs within the lower range of the tidal volume.

7. In small animals, the hematocrit decreases by more than a third in the first 28 days of life;[16,17] thus, even minor hemorrhage can greatly affect oxygen delivery to tissues.

8. Neonates are more susceptible to hypothermia because of their immature thermoregulatory system, high body surface to mass ratio, and limited ability to vasoconstrict to conserve heat.

Physiology of Geriatric Animals

The effect of age per se on perioperative morbidity and mortality is related to the decreased physiological reserve of the various organ systems that occur with aging. Aging is a progressive physiological process that results in unavoidable alterations in organ system function. Within organ systems, reductions in functional reserve manifest as a decreased capacity for adaptation, a predisposition to the failure of homeostasis, and a reduced ability to respond to external stress. The effects of disease, stress, lack of exercise, genetics, malnutrition, and environment may hasten changes associated with aging. The time course of the aging process varies between organ systems within the same individual and between individuals. Assessment of the influence of aging on anatomical and physiological function in animals is further complicated by the marked variations in life span and life expectancy within and between species. There is little correlation between chronological and physiological age. For the purposes of this discussion, geriatric animals are considered to be those that have attained 75% of their expected life span.[18]

Pathophysiological changes associated with aging in organ systems influence anesthetic management (Table 47.2). Cardiovascular changes are multifactorial, reflecting not only age-related degeneration but also age-related disease. In the absence of a particular cardiovascular disease, the major anatomical changes in aging hearts are primarily an increase in the severity of myocardial fibrosis, valvular fibrocalcification, and ventricular wall thickening. Variable degrees of myocardial fiber atrophy result in decreased pump function and cardiac output. The heart rate may be affected if the pacemaker cells are involved. Fibrosis of the endocardium and valves leads to decreased compliance. Valvular incompetence may accompany valvular fibrocalcification. The vascular tree gradually loses elasticity, resulting in a decrease in distensibility, increased resistance to left ventricular output, and progressive hypertrophy of the ventricle. As ventricular hypertrophy and decreased chamber elasticity progress, the aging heart is more dependent on atrial contraction for diastolic ventricular filling. Thus, the atrial kick and normal sinus rhythm become more important in the maintenance of appropriate cardiac output.[19,20]

In geriatric animals, the maximal chronotropic response during physiological stress decreases. In addition, despite higher endogenous levels of norepinephrine, the response to stress is decreased. This appears to be due to receptor attrition and reduced affinity for

Table 47.2. Changes in the anatomy and function of major organ systems in geriatric animals.

Cardiovascular system
Decreased arterial compliance
Decreased myocardial compliance
Decreased maximal heart rate
Decreased maximal cardiac output
Blunted ß-receptor responsiveness
Pulmonary system
Reduced gas-exchange efficiency
Reduced vital capacity
Increased work of breathing
Decreased thoracic compliance
Decreased lung elasticity
Increased degree of airway closure
Nervous system
Increased sympathetic nervous system activity
Downregulation of ß receptors
Decreased parasympathetic nervous system activity
Reduced central neurotransmitter activity
Increased sympathetic nervous system outflow
Renal and hepatic systems
Decreased drug clearance
Decreased glomerular filtration rate
Difficulty handling water-and-salt loads
   Decreased urine concentrating ability and decreased ability to
     conserve sodium
Decreased perfusion and system blood flow
Decreased tissue mass
Body composition
Decreased skeletal muscle mass
Increased lipid fraction

agonist molecules. Whereas young adults increase cardiac output primarily through increased heart rate, geriatric animals increase cardiac output by increasing stroke volume in association with an increase in end-diastolic volume. Thus, geriatric animals depend more on preload than do younger animals and are not as tolerant of volume depletion in the perianesthetic period. This said, fit individuals maintain high levels of cardiac output and oxygen consumption, and reductions in cardiac index occur in direct proportion to reductions in skeletal muscle mass and metabolic rate associated with reductions in lean-tissue mass.[19–21]

Pulmonary changes associated with aging include a decrease in ventilatory volumes and a reduction in the efficiency of gas exchange. Vital capacity, total lung capacity, and maximum breathing capacity decrease as the intercostal and diaphragmatic muscle masses reduce and the thorax becomes more rigid and less compliant. Functional alveoli and elasticity progressively decrease. As pulmonary elasticity decreases as result of decreases in lung elastin, the ratio of residual volume and of functional residual capacity to total lung capacity increase. Closing volume is increased, resulting in air trapping and an increase in ventilation-perfusion mismatch. As a result, PaO_2 decreases with age.[22]

In the central nervous system, aging is associated with a reduction in brain size that occurs with the loss of neurons. Cerebro-

spinal fluid volume increases to maintain normal intracranial pressure. Despite this loss in brain tissue, functional and anatomical redundancy within the nervous system provides for the maintenance of functioning at levels that approximate those observed at somatic maturity. With the loss of brain tissue, cerebral blood flow decreases, but cerebral autoregulation of blood flow is well maintained. In addition to the loss of functional neurons in aging individuals, generalized depletions of dopamine, norepinephrine, tyrosine, and serotonin occur. Receptor affinity for neurotransmitters may be reduced. Compared with the neuronal plasticity observed in the young, this process is slower and less complete in geriatric individuals. As a result of these functional and anatomical changes in the central nervous system, geriatric individuals have a decreased requirement for anesthetic agents. The minimum alveolar concentration for inhalant anesthetics decreases linearly with age, and the requirement for local anesthetics, opioids, barbiturates, benzodiazepines, and other intravenous drugs is likely similarly reduced.[19,23,24]

With aging, there is a primary loss of cortical kidney mass and functional nephron units. Total renal blood flow decreases with age, with the majority of the loss occurring in the renal cortex. In humans, one-half of the glomeruli present in the young adult atrophy or are nonfunctional by the age of 80. Glomerular filtration rate decreases, partly in response to a reduction in renal plasma flow. Geriatric individuals are less responsive to antidiuretic hormone and have an impaired ability to conserve sodium or concentrate urine. A reduction in renal blood flow makes the geriatric animal more susceptible to renal failure in the face of renal ischemia. Since geriatric patients cannot maximally retain sodium or water under conditions of volume depletion, the ability to correct fluid, electrolyte, and acid-base disturbances or to tolerate hemodynamic insults is reduced. Because geriatric patients have difficulty excreting a salt-and-water load, vigorous fluid and electrolyte therapy may result in excessive intravascular and extravascular volume, with the possible sequelae of congestive heart failure and peripheral edema. Those anesthetic drugs eliminated primarily by renal excretion have a greater elimination half-time in geriatric animals, necessitating a reduction in doses when these drugs are administered.[25,26]

Hepatic clearance of drugs decreases with age as the mass of the liver decreases. In geriatric people, the liver mass, and consequently hepatic blood flow, may be decreased by 40% to 50%. Microsomal and nonmicrosomal enzyme function appears to be well maintained, although the reduction in hepatic mass significantly impairs overall hepatic function. Consequently, the metabolism of lipid-soluble drugs, particularly anesthetics, is decreased. Combined with decreased glomerular filtration and renal excretory capacity, the reduction in hepatic clearance of drugs results in an increase in the half-life and duration of effect of drugs that depend on these routes of elimination.[19,25–27]

Aging results in changes in body composition that include a decrease in skeletal muscle, an increase in body fat as a percentage of total body weight, and a loss of intracellular water. A loss in total body water occurs as a result of decreased intracellular water and a reduction in plasma volume, although fit geriatric individuals maintain plasma volume well. Intravenous injection of anesthetic drugs into a contracted volume of distribution results in an increased plasma concentration that may be responsible for the observation that geriatric animals are more sensitive to anesthetics. Increased adipose tissue is associated with an increase in the fraction of a single dose of a lipid-soluble drug redistributed to adipose tissue, further delaying elimination from the body.

Reductions in serum albumin concentrations in association with aging can lead to reduced protein binding of drugs. In addition, structural changes in the serum protein that occur with aging may decrease binding to the available protein. Theoretically, the administration of highly protein-bound drugs to animals with reduced serum proteins may lead to an exaggerated clinical effect.[28]

A decrease in basal resting metabolic rate with age results in a reduction in the production of body heat. Consequently, geriatric individuals are less able to maintain core body temperature. This is particularly important in anesthetized animals placed in cold environments. Anesthetized geriatric animals tend to be more hypothermic than younger animals in the operative and postoperative periods, and rewarming occurs at a slower rate. Because shivering during recovery increases oxygen consumption by 200% to 300%, perianesthetic hypothermia alone may place severe demands on the cardiopulmonary system. If these demands are not met, arterial hypoxemia may ensue.[19]

Anesthesia

Preparation for Anesthesia

A thorough physical examination, including careful auscultation of the heart, is an essential component of preanesthetic assessment. In geriatric people, exercise tolerance is one of the most important predictors of perioperative outcome, and this is likely an important predictor of outcome in the anesthesia of geriatric animals. Significant, preexisting abnormalities should be corrected prior to the induction of anesthesia. Left untreated, these abnormalities are likely to be exacerbated by anesthesia. Neonatal, pediatric, or geriatric animals with limited physiological reserves are less able to respond to altered homeostasis. Hydration status should be assessed and fluid requirements carefully calculated. Fluid deficits should be corrected prior to anesthesia.

In neonates, standard preanesthetic blood work should include a minimum of hematocrit, total and fractionated protein, and blood glucose. Other blood work should be performed as indicated. In geriatrics, the preanesthetic assessment should include a complete blood count, serum chemistry profile, electrocardiogram, and urinalysis.

Neonates that are still suckling should not be held off food prior to anesthesia. Pediatric animals that are eating solid food should be denied food for only 3 to 4 h prior to anesthesia and should not be denied water at any time.

Premedication and Pain Management

Because of the immaturity of the neonatal nervous system, it has been a commonly held thesis that neonates are incapable of experiencing pain. However, we now know that neonatal humans and animals do indeed experience pain.[29,30] In addition, evidence suggests that pain experienced at an extremely young age may lead to dynamic changes in the nociceptive pathway, resulting in chronic pain conditions later in life.[31] Like many pathologies, pain is easier to prevent than to treat. Regardless of age, every patient anesthetized for a painful procedure should receive appropriate analgesic therapy. As with other drugs, dosages of the analgesic drugs should be conservative, and patients should be closely monitored for signs of adverse side effects. Opioids are potent analgesics whose effects are reversible, making them an excellent choice for analgesia in neonates with immature metabolism or geriatrics with reduced hepatic function. The addition of local anesthetic techniques to anesthetic protocols for neonatal or geriatric animals is particularly appropriate. The inclusion of such techniques provides for additional analgesia and an associated reduction in the requirement for general anesthetics that may have more profound side effects. NSAIDs may be an option in older pediatric patients, but this class of drugs should be reserved for patients with mature, competent renal function.

The routine use of anticholinergics is not necessary, but, because neonates depend on adequate heart rate for maintenance of cardiac output, anticholinergics may be used to treat sinus bradycardia. Anticholinergics should also be considered in breeds with high vagal tone (e.g., brachycephalic breeds) and for surgical procedures that are likely to stimulate a vagal reflex (e.g., many ocular procedures). Geriatric animals may be less able to compensate for a slow heart rate than younger adult animals.

Sedation may not be necessary in quiet or debilitated patients. However, sedatives alleviate stress in anxious patients and decrease the dosage of drugs needed for induction and maintenance of anesthesia. The side effects of sedatives should be weighed against the side effects of having to use a larger dose of anesthetic drug. The opioids often provide adequate sedation and have the added advantage of providing analgesia. μ-Agonist opioids such as morphine, hydromorphone, and oxymorphone provide the most profound analgesia but also may cause greater cardiovascular and respiratory depression.[32] Partial agonists (buprenorphine) and agonist-antagonists (butorphanol) provide only mild to moderate analgesia but also cause minimal cardiovascular and respiratory depression. Selection of an appropriate opioid is best made based on the particular analgesic requirements and the health status of the patient and the intended procedure.

Benzodiazepines are also useful sedatives/anxiolytics in neonatal or geriatric animals. Although they do not provide analgesia, they are reversible and produce little to no cardiovascular and respiratory depression. Benzodiazepines do not provide consistent or deep sedation and may need to be combined with other sedatives in very active or anxious neonatal or geriatric animals. The judicious use of low doses of α_2-adrenergic agonists may also be considered for use in neonatal or geriatric animals. However, drugs in this class produce profound cardiovascular side effects (bradycardia, atrioventricular conduction block, and increased peripheral vascular resistance), and their use in either neonatal or geriatric animals should be confined to those cases where the benefit of their use outweighs the negative side effects associated with their administration. Low dosages of xylazine have been shown to be safe and effective in foals as young as 10 days of age.[33] Acepromazine may also be used for sedation of neonates or geriatrics, but the cardiovascular effects, including hypotension, may be poorly tolerated in both geriatric and neonatal animals. The vasodilation caused by acepromazine can also contribute to the development of hypothermia. Acepromazine is not reversible and alone does not provide analgesia.

Induction

Anesthesia can be induced by using a variety of injectable anesthetic drugs or by mask delivery of inhaled anesthetics, when necessary. Etomidate or propofol may be excellent choices in neonates and geriatrics. Both agents are rapidly eliminated from the body by a variety of routes so that termination of activity does not depend on the functioning of a single organ system.[34] Propofol does produce respiratory and cardiovascular depression and should be titrated to achieve the desired depth of anesthesia. The administration of oxygen by face mask for approximately 5 min prior to the induction of anesthesia with propofol will reduce the risk of complications associated with propofol-induced apnea in either neonatal or geriatric animals. Preinduction sedation of animals, particularly with a sedative/analgesic drug, will reduce the dose of etomidate or propofol needed for induction. Ketamine, in combination with a benzodiazepine, is also a choice for the induction of anesthesia in either neonates or geriatric animals. Ketamine causes only mild respiratory depression and may actually improve cardiovascular function through stimulation of the sympathetic nervous system.[35] Although of benefit to geriatric animals, this response may be less in neonates because of their immature sympathetic nervous system. Ketamine requires either hepatic metabolism or renal clearance for termination of activity; thus, the effects of ketamine may be prolonged in patients with either immature or failing hepatic and renal systems.[35] Barbiturates may be used in low dosages for the induction of anesthesia in neonatal, pediatric, or geriatric animals, keeping in mind that drugs of this class are highly protein bound, and their termination of activity depends on both redistribution and hepatic metabolism. The response to barbiturates can be both pronounced and prolonged in either neonates or geriatrics with reduced plasma protein concentrations and/or immature or failing hepatic or renal function.

Inhaled anesthetics may be used for induction, as well as maintenance of anesthesia. This method is recommended only in sedated or debilitated patients because the prolonged excitement phase that occurs during induction can be more physiologically detrimental than a judicious dose of an injectable anesthetic. Environmental pollution and personnel exposure are also concerns during mask inductions with inhaled anesthetics. Induction in foals and calves with an inhaled anesthetic following nasotracheal intubation often results in rapid, excitement-free anesthesia simply because bypassing the nasal passages eliminates the ability to smell anesthetic gas.[36,37] Because anesthesia can be induced with an inhaled anesthetic very rapidly in depressed neonatal and geriatric animals, excessive anesthetic depth may be reached very rapidly. Careful monitoring is a must.

Maintenance

Inhaled anesthetics that are minimally metabolized and easily cleared in animals with either immature or reduced hepatic or renal function should be used for maintenance of anesthesia. However, it should be remembered that inhaled anesthetics cause dose-dependent hypotension, hypoventilation, impaired cardiac contractility, and hypothermia. Because of these side effects, inhaled anesthetics must be very carefully titrated, and vigilant monitoring should be employed to avoid excessive anesthetic depth. The concurrent administration of analgesics and sedatives will reduce the inhaled anesthetic requirement while decreasing the magnitude of their unwanted side effects.

Support

Along with a carefully chosen anesthetic protocol and conservative drug dosing, meticulous physiological support and vigilant monitoring are imperative during the anesthesia of neonatal, pediatric, or geriatric animals. Compared with adults, fluid requirements are greater in neonates (60 to 180 mL/kg/day)[38] because of their higher body-surface area, immature renal function (decreased ability to concentrate urine), higher percentage of body water, and higher respiratory rates leading to greater fluid losses.[9] Conversely, overhydration should be avoided, because renal clearance may be limited and excessive dilution of serum protein can occur more readily in animals with preexisting hypoalbuminemia. Neonates have minimal stores of hepatic glycogen and are prone to hypoglycemia, so the use of dextrose-containing fluids should be considered.

In geriatric patients that have difficulty excreting a salt-and-water load, aggressive fluid and electrolyte therapy may result in excessive intravascular and extravascular volume, with the possible sequelae of congestive heart failure and peripheral edema. Thus, fluid therapy in the perianesthetic period of geriatric animals should be targeted at correcting specific deficits and maintaining adequate perfusion and oxygen delivery without delivering excessive electrolyte loads or fluid volumes.

Both neonatal and geriatric animals are highly susceptible to hypothermia, so every effort should be made to maintain normal body temperature. Hypothermia increases the incidence of adverse myocardial outcomes in high-risk patients, increases the incidence of surgical wound infection, adversely affects antibody- and cell-mediated immune defenses, changes the kinetics and action of various anesthetic and paralyzing agents, increases thermal discomfort, and is associated with delayed postanesthetic recovery.[39] The attempt of the body to rewarm itself is not benign, because shivering may cause a tremendous increase in oxygen consumption (200% to 300%), and this increased oxygen demand may not be met by an increase in oxygen delivery, particularly if anesthetic-induced hypoventilation occurs.

Diligent monitoring is crucial during the entire anesthetic period and well into recovery. Some commonly monitored indices are different in neonates than in adults, and anesthetists should be familiar with the normal physiological indices for each species and age group of individuals that are being anesthetized. Generally, neonatal and pediatric animals have a higher heart rate but lower blood pressure than adults. The normal heart rate in conscious neonatal dogs and cats is approximately 200 beats per minute, and the respiratory rate is approximately 15 to 35 breaths per minute. Mean arterial blood pressure in 1-month-old puppies

Table 47.3. Drugs commonly used in geriatric small animals.[a]

	Dose (mg/kg)	
Drug	Dog	Cat
Anticholinergics		
Atropine[b]	0.01–0.02	0.01–0.02
Glycopyrrolate[b]	0.005–0.01	0.005–0.01
Sedatives and analgesics		
Midazolam[b]	0.1–0.3	0.1–0.3
Diazepam[c]	0.2–0.4	0.2–0.4
Oxymorphone	0.1–0.2	0.1–0.2
Hydromorphone	0.1–0.2	0.1–0.2
Butorphanol	0.2–0.4	0.2–0.4
Buprenorphine	0.005–0.02	0.005–0.02
Induction		
Propofol	4–6	4–6
Ketamine-midazolam	3–5 and 0.1–0.2	3–5 and 0.1–0.2
Hydromorphone-diazepam	0.1 and 0.2	0.1 and 0.2
Etomidate	0.5–1.5	0.5–1.5

[a]Endeavor always to use the minimum effective dose of all drugs to achieve surgical or diagnostic objectives.
[b]Intramuscular or intravenous administration is appropriate.
[c]Diazepam is not recommended for intramuscular use and should be given slowly when administered intravenously.

is only 49 mm Hg.[40] The average heart rate in foals 1 to 2 days of age ranges from 70 to 90[41] beats per minute, and the normal respiratory rate is 30 to 40 breaths per minute.[42]

Summary of Protocols

Suggested protocols for neonatal animals include an opioid premedicant with an additional sedative or tranquilizer, if required. Anesthesia can be induced with the intravenous administration of propofol or ketamine-benzodiazepine combinations. In severely compromised animals, anesthesia may be induced with an inhaled anesthetic delivered by face mask.[43,44] For neonatal horses and cattle, suggested protocols include sedation with low-dose xylazine plus butorphanol followed either by intravenous administration of propofol or valium-ketamine or by nasal intubation and subsequent induction with an inhalant anesthesic.[4,37] For all species, anesthesia is maintained with an inhalant and local blockade employed when possible to augment analgesia.

No one ideal anesthetic protocol exists for all geriatric patients. An understanding of the pathophysiological changes and the alterations in pharmacodynamics and pharmacokinetics that arise in conjunction with aging is necessary when choosing an anesthetic protocol for any geriatric animal. Particular attention to decreased dosage requirements and the titration of anesthetics to achieve the central nervous system depression necessary for a specific surgical procedure is advocated (Table 47.3). Whenever possible, local and regional anesthetic techniques should be employed to reduce the dosage of concomitantly administered inhaled or injectable anesthetics. Appropriate anesthetic manage-

ment of geriatric animals is centered around thorough evaluation and assessment; preoperative correction of identified abnormalities; vigilant, aggressive perianesthetic monitoring; careful titration of anesthetic drugs; and appropriate perianesthetic support.

References

1. Robinson EP. Anaesthesia of pediatric patients. Compend Contin Educ Pract Vet 1983;5:1004–1011.
2. Breazile JE. Neurologic and behavioral development in the puppy. Vet Clin North Am Small Animal Pract 1978;8:31–45.
3. Fox MW. Canine Pediatrics. Springfield, IL: Charles C Thomas, 1966.
4. Tranquilli WJ, Thurmon JC. Management of anesthesia in the foal. Vet Clin North Am Equine Pract 1990;6:651–663.
5. Kami G, Merritt AM, Duelly P. Preliminary studies of plasma and extracellular fluid volume in neonatal ponies. Equine Vet J 1984;16:356–358.
6. Baggot JD. Drug therapy in the neonatal animal. In: Baggot JD, ed. Principles of Drug Disposition in Domestic Animals: The Basis of Veterinary Clinical Pharmacology. Philadelphia: WB Saunders, 1992:21–236.
7. Webb AI, Weaver BMQ. Body composition of the horse. Equine Vet J 1979;11:39–47.
8. Baggot JD, Short CR. Drug disposition in the neonatal animal, with particular reference to the foal. Equine Vet J 1987;19:169–171.
9. Boothe DM, Tannert K. Special considerations for drug and fluid therapy in the pediatric patient. Compend Contin Educ Pract Vet 1992;14:313–329.
10. Short CR. Drug disposition in neonatal animals. J Am Vet Med Assoc 1984;184:1161–1163.
11. Thurmon JC, Tranquilli WJ, Benson GJ, Martin DD. Anesthesia for special patients: Neonatal and geriatric patients. In: Thurmon JC, Tranquilli WJ, Benson GJ, eds. Lumb & Jones Veterinary Anesthesia, 3rd ed. Baltimore: Williams and Wilkins, 1996:844–848.
12. Meyer RE. Anesthesia for neonatal and geriatric patients. In: Short CE, ed. Principles and Practices of Veterinary Anesthesia. Baltimore: Williams and Wilkins, 1987:330–337.
13. Friedman WF. The intrinsic physiologic properties of the developing heart. Prog Cardiovasc Dis 1972;15:87–111.
14. Friedman WF, George BL. Treatment of congestive heart failure by altering loading conditions of the heart. J Pediatr 1985;106:697–706.
15. Thomas WP, Madigan JE, Backus KQ, Powell WE. Systemic and pulmonary haemodynamics in normal neonatal foals. J Reprod Fertil 1987;35:623–628.
16. Earl FL, Melveger BE, Wilson RL. The hemogram and bone marrow profile of normal neonatal and weanling beagle dogs. Lab Anim Sci 1973;23:690–695.
17. Meyers-Wallen VN, Haskins ME, Patterson DF. Hematologic values in healthy neonatal, weanling and juvenile kittens. Am J Vet Res 1984;45:1322-1327.
18. Hoskins J. Geriatrics and Gerontology of the Dog and Cat, 2nd ed. St Louis: WB Saunders, 2004:71–84.
19. Muravchick S. Anesthesia for the elderly. In: Miller RD, ed. Anesthesia, 5th ed. Philadelphia: Churchill Livingstone, 2000:2140–2156.
20. Wei JY. Age and the cardiovascular system. N Engl J Med 1992;327:1735–1739.
21. Lakatta EG. Diminished beta-adrenergic modulation of cardiovascular function in advanced age. Cardiol Clin 1986;4:185–200.

22. Wahba WM. Influence of aging on lung function: Clinical significance of changes from age twenty. Anesth Analg 1983;62:764–776.

23. Stevens WD, Dolan WM, Gibbons RT, et al. Minimum alveolar concentrations (MAC) of isoflurane with and without nitrous oxide in patients of various ages. Anesthesiology 1975;42:197–200.

24. Gregory GA, Eger EI, Munson ES. The relationship between age and halothane requirement in man. Anesthesiology 1969;30:488–491.

25. Beck LH. The aging kidney: Defending a delicate balance of fluid and electrolytes. Geriatrics 2000;55:26–28, 31–32.

26. Evers BM, Townsend CM, Thompson JC. Organ physiology of aging. Surg Clin North Am 1994;74:23–39.

27. Geokas MC, Haverback BJ. The aging gastrointestinal tract. Am J Surg 1969;117:881–892.

28. Homer TD, Stanski DR. The effect of increasing age on thiopental disposition and anesthetic requirement. Anesthesiology 1985;62:714–724.

29. Anand KJS, Sippel WG, Aynsley-Green A. Randomised trial of fentanyl anaesthesia in preterm babies undergoing surgery: Effects on the stress response. Lancet 1987;1:243–248.

30. Luks AM, Zwass MS, Brown RC, Lau M, Chari G, Fisher DM. Opioid-induced analgesia in neonatal dogs: Pharmacodynamic differences between morphine and fentanyl. Pharmacol Exp Ther 1998;284:136–141.

31. Buskila D, Neumann L, Zmora E, Feldman M, Bolotin A, Press J. Pain sensitivity in prematurely born adolescents. Arch Pediatr Adolesc Med 2003;157:1079–1082.

32. Bragg P, Zwass MS, Lau M, Fisher DM. Opioid pharmacodynamics in neonatal dogs: Differences between morphine and fentanyl. J Appl Physiol 1995;79:1519–1524.

33. Carter SW, Robertson SA, Steel CA, Jourdenais DA. Cardiopulmonary effects of xylazine sedation in the foal. Equine Vet J 1990;22:384–388.

34. Saint-Maurice C. Propofol in pediatric anesthesia. Cah Anesthesiol 1991;39:411–420.

35. Wright M. Pharmacologic effects of ketamine and its use in veterinary medicine. J Am Vet Med Assoc 1982;180:1462–1471.

36. Webb AI. Nasal intubation in foals. J Am Vet Med Assoc 1984;185:48–51.

37. Quandt JE, Robinson EP. Nasotracheal intubation in calves. J Am Vet Med Assoc 1996;209:967–968.

38. Mosier JE. Canine pediatrics: The neonate. AAHA Sci Present 1981;48:339–347.

39. Doufas AG. Consequences of inadvertent perioperative hypothermia. Best Pract Res Clin Anaesthesiol 2003;17:535–549.

40. McMicheal M, Dhupa N. Pediatric critical care medicine: Physiologic considerations. Compend Contin Educ Pract Vet 2000;22:206–214.

41. Rossdale PD. Clinical studies in the newborn thoroughbred foal. II. Heart rate, auscultation and electrocardiogram. Br Vet J 1967;123:521–532.

42. Rossdale PD. Some parameters of respiratory function in normal and abnormal newborn foals with specific reference to levels of P_aO_2 during air and oxygen inhalation. Res Vet Sci 1970;11:270–276.

43. Grandy JL, Dunlop CI. Anesthesia of pups and kittens. J Am Vet Med Assoc 1991:1244–1249.

44. Fagella AM, Aronsohn MG. Evaluation of anesthetic protocols for neutering 6- to 14-week-old pups. J Am Vet Med Assoc 1993;205:308–314.

Chapter 48
Dental Patients

Rachael E. Carpenter and Sandra Manfra Marretta

Introduction

Although sedation and local blocks alone have been advocated by some authors for dental procedures,[1] most procedures are best accomplished under inhalant anesthesia. Quite recently, several individuals have advocated anesthesia-free teeth cleaning. Proponents feel that more clients will pursue teeth cleaning if anesthesia is not used, because of the decreased cost and alleviated fears of anesthetic death or complications.[2] Many of the people performing and teaching these procedures are nonveterinarians, and a recent decision in a case brought before the Veterinary Medical Board in California has ruled that the procedure amounts to "the practice of veterinary medicine without a license."[3] The American College of Veterinary Dentistry has stated that thorough oral exams and dental radiographs are not possible in an unanesthetized patient and are needed to uncover any hidden dental disease that may be present.[4]

General Preparation and Monitoring

As with any anesthetic procedure, appropriate premedications and induction agents should be selected based on the requirements of the individual. An intravenous catheter should be placed to enable administration of fluids and for emergency access, if needed. All dental patients should be intubated with a cuffed endotracheal tube immediately after induction to prevent aspiration of water or cleaning solutions during dental procedures. Gauze sponges may be inserted in the pharyngeal area to further prevent aspiration. Packing the pharyngeal area too tightly can impede venous return and result in swelling of the tongue.[5] If pharyngeal packing is used, a systematic method of ensuring that gauze is removed after the procedure prior to recovery from anesthesia is necessary. Dentistry in cats has been associated with tracheal rupture, likely from overinflation of the cuff contributing to tracheal trauma when the patient is turned from side to side to enable access to both sides of the mouth.[6] In all instances and species, it is best to disconnect the breathing circuit from the endotracheal tube (after turning off the oxygen flow to minimize waste gas exposure) before repositioning the patient.

Following induction, heart and respiratory rates are assessed, and pulse oximetry, capnography, and blood pressure monitoring should be considered. Because vasodilation during inhalant anesthesia can exacerbate heat loss, hypothermia is a real threat to patients' overall well-being. Anesthetics further reduce the body's ability to respond to hypothermia. If a patient's attempt to regain body temperature is accompanied by severe shivering, increases in both myocardial work and systemic hypoxia are likely and undesirable. This may be especially important in geriatric animals with significant loss in functional cardiopulmonary reserve. Generally, it is safer to maintain a core body temperature during anesthesia than to try to regain body heat after anesthesia and surgery.

Pain Management

A balanced anesthetic plan for dental patients should include preemptive, intraoperative, and postoperative analgesics (Table 48.1). Pain associated with the procedure should be estimated prior to induction of anesthesia.[7] Depending on the degree and magnitude of oral surgery performed, most pain will occur in the first 24 to 74 h postoperatively.[8] Some residual discomfort might last longer. Individual patients should be frequently reassessed and treated, as needed. Behaviors indicative of pain (willingness to eat and drink, grooming behaviors, and activity level) may be best observed by the owners in the home environment. Analgesics commonly used in managing pain are the local anesthetics, opioids, α_2-agonists and nonsteroidal anti-inflammatory drugs (NSAIDs). Opioids and α_2-agonists can be used in the immediate preoperative and postoperative periods while the patient is in the hospital. Injectable or oral NSAIDs and longer-acting opioid preparations may be used during prolonged convalescence and for take-home medications.

Local and Regional Blocks

Local and regional anesthetic techniques are commonly used in the analgesic management of dental patients. Infraorbital, maxillary, mental, and mandibular inferior alveolar nerve blocks may be used before extractions. Caution should be used when blocking the inferior alveolar branch of the mandibular nerve, because inadvertent blocking of the lingual nerve may result in desensitization of the tongue and potential self-mutilation upon recovery. The lingual nerve is best avoided by keeping the needle close to the bone of the ventral mandible when performing the intraoral approach to the inferior alveolar branch of the mandibular nerve.[5]

Table 48.1. Common dental techniques and anesthetic/analgesic requirements

Dental Technique	Sedation/Anesthesia Requirement	Analgesic Requirement
Dental radiographs	Heavy sedation or general anesthesia	None
Gingivectomy/gingival biopsy	Heavy sedation or general anesthesia	Topical, infiltration or local blocks, and systemic analgesics for mild to moderate pain
Dental prophylaxis	General anesthesia	None
Minor extractions (minimal elevation required), deep subgingival scaling, and/or root planning and curettage	General anesthesia	Infiltration technique, local blocks, and systemic analgesics for mild pain
Surgical extractions (major elevation and bone removal required)	General anesthesia	Regional nerve blocks (e.g., infraorbital nerve block), and systemic analgesics for moderate to severe pain
Root canal therapy	General anesthesia	Regional nerve blocks, and systemic analgesics for moderate pain
Mandibulectomy/maxillectomy	General anesthesia	Regional nerve blocks, and systemic analgesics for severe pain
Jaw fracture	General anesthesia	Regional nerve blocks, systemic analgesics for moderate to severe pain (depending on type of fracture)

For analgesia of the maxillary teeth, care should also be taken to avoid insertion of the needle into the infraorbital canal when performing infraorbital blocks in cats and brachycephalic breed dogs. The canal is extremely short in these animals, and insertion of the needle into it may cause ocular damage. As an alternative, infiltration anesthesia can be used where local anesthetic is injected directly into the periodontal ligament and surrounding tissues. It is most effective when performed in areas with thin cortical bone (maxillary teeth and mandibular incisors) and when a small number of teeth need to be desensitized.[5,9]

When using either lidocaine or bupivacaine, it is important to calculate the total dose of local anesthetic that can be safely used to avoid toxicity (Table 48.2). Generally, toxic doses of lidocaine are 10 mg/kg in dogs and 6 mg/kg in cats. The toxic doses of bupivacaine are lower and are approximately 3 mg/kg in dogs and 2 mg/kg in cats. Recent reports have examined the usefulness of opioids in extending the analgesia from local anesthetic in regional anesthetic techniques in humans. Both 0.075 mg/kg (0.035 mg/lb) morphine and 0.003 mg/kg (0.0015 mg/lb) buprenorphine have been shown to double the analgesic duration in humans when combined with either lidocaine or bupivacaine.[10,11] Mu-opioid receptors have been located in human dental pulp, suggesting that local administration of opioids may be beneficial for dental procedures.[12] One study in humans found that pain scores were lowered for up to 24 h when morphine was added to the local anesthetics compared with patients that received local anesthetics alone.[13] Little data are available regarding the use of opioids with local analgesics for dental blocks in veterinary patients, but it may prove to be a useful local application of this class of analgesics.

Take-Home Pain Medications

One challenging aspect of pain management for veterinary dental patients involves medication that can be sent home for managing lingering pain (Table 48.3). At present, oral NSAIDs ap-

Table 48.2. Recommended local anesthetic doses for dental blocks

Local Anesthetic	Dog	Cat
Bupivacaine	Up to 2.0 mg/kg	Up to 1.0 mg/kg
Lidocaine	Up to 6.0 mg/kg	Up to 3.0 mg/kg
Mepivacaine	Up to 6.0 mg/kg	Up to 3.0 mg/kg

pear to be the most commonly recommended dispensable medications for short-term treatment of dental pain.[14] When using NSAIDS, appropriate patient selection is important to reduce the risk associated with the use of this class of drugs. If additional analgesics are needed, oral opioids (such as butorphanol tablets, codeine tablets, and morphine tablets) are available that may be combined with the NSAIDs.[15] In recent years, an opioid-like oral agent, tramadol, has demonstrated good analgesic activity for mild to moderate pain.[16] Tramadol is not scheduled and has been shown to be useful for management of postoperative pain in dogs.[17] In addition, a handful of commercially available opioid/NSAID preparations combine an opioid with acetaminophen (e.g., codeine or oxycodone plus acetaminophen) that could be used in dogs to relieve dental pain but not in cats.

Cats may be more difficult for owners to medicate at home, but recent studies have shown that the parenteral form of buprenorphine is well absorbed when administered transmucosally to cats.[18] In this same study, owners were surveyed as to their preferred method of administering medications to cats. Cat owners overwhelmingly chose oral medications as their preferred technique for home administration. The oral administration of buprenorphine and meloxicam (or other NSAID) may provide an effective method of controlling moderate to severe pain in cats after invasive dental manipulation (Table 48.3).

Table 48.3. Dispensable oral medications for dental patients

Drug	Dogs	Cats
NSAID		
Acetaminophen	15 mg/kg PO TID	*Toxic to cats*
Aspirin	10–25 mg/kg PO BID	10–20 mg/kg PO q 48–72 h
Carprofen	2 mg/kg PO BID or 4.4 mg/kg PO SID	1–2 mg/kg PO SID (1–2 doses only)
Ketoprofen	2 mg/kg PO loading dose, then 1 mg/kg SID (max. 5 days)	1 mg/kg PO loading dose, then 0.05 mg/kg SID (max. 3–5 days)
Etodolac	10–15 mg/kg PO SID	—
Meloxicam	0.2 mg/kg PO loading dose, then 0.1 mg/kg PO SID	0.1 mg/kg loading dose, then 0.025 mg/kg PO SID (3–4 days)
Opioid		
Buprenorphine	—	0.010–0.040 mg/kg transmucosally BID to q.i.d.
Butorphanol	0.2–1.0 mg/kg PO q 1–4 h	0.2–1.0 mg/kg PO q 1–4 h
Codeine	1–2.0 mg/kg PO q 6–8 h	0.1–1.0 mg/kg PO q 4–8 h
Morphine	0.3–1.0 mg/kg PO q 4–8 h	—
Tramadol	2–10 mg/kg/day PO divided BID or TID	2–10 mg/kg/day PO divided BID or TID

NSAID, nonsteroidal anti-inflammatory drug.

References

1. Boyd JC. SafeSmile. http://www.pacificpetcare.com/safesmile.html (accessed January 24, 2005).
2. Houndstooth. Non-anesthetic Dog and Cat Teeth Cleaning. http://home1.gte.net/midilaw/houndstooth.htm (accessed January 24, 2005).
3. California Department of Consumer Affairs. Administrative Law Judge Backs Veterinary Board on Pet Teeth-Cleaning. http://www.dca.ca.gov/press_releases/2004/1028_vmb.htm (accessed January 24, 2005).
4. Lyon K, Holmstrom S, eds. American College of Veterinary Dentistry Position Statement on Companion Animal Dental Scaling without Anesthesia. 2004. http://www.avdc.org/Dental_Scaling_Without_Anesthesia.pdf (accessed January 19, 2005).
5. Gorrel C. Anesthesia and analgesia. In: Gorrel C., ed. Veterinary Dentistry for the General Practitioner. Edinburgh: WB Saunders, 2004:11–22.
6. Hardie EM, Spodnick GJ, Gilson SD, et al. Tracheal rupture in cats: 16 cases (1983–1998). J Am Vet Med Assoc 1999;214:508–512.
7. Mathews KA. Pain assessment and general approach to management. Vet Clin North Am Small Anim Pract 2000;30:729–756.
8. Lantz GC. Regional anesthesia for dentistry and oral surgery. J Vet Dent 2003;20:181–186.
9. Bellows J. Local and regional anesthesia and pain control. In: Bellows J, ed. Small Animal Dental Equipment, Materials and Techniques. Ames, IA: Blackwell, 2004:105–114.
10. Candido KD, Winnie AP, Ghaleb AH, et al. Buprenorphine added to the local anesthetic for axillary brachial plexus block prolongs postoperative analgesia. Reg Anesth Pain Med 2002;27:162–167.
11. Bazin JE, Massoni C, Bruelle P, et al. The addition of opioids to local anesthetics in brachial plexus block: The comparative effects of morphine, buprenorphine and sufentanil. Anaesthesia 1997;52:858–862.
12. Jaber L, Swaim WD, Dionne RA. Immunohistochemical localization of mu-opioid receptors in human dental pulp. J Endod 2003;29:108–110.
13. Likar R, Sittl R, Gragger K, et al. Peripheral morphine analgesia in dental surgery. Pain 1998;76:145–150.
14. Tranquilli WJ, Grimm KA, Lamont LA, eds. Pain Management for the Small Animal Practitioner, 2nd ed. Jackson, WY: Teton New Media, 2004.
15. Pascoe PJ. Opioid analgesics. Vet Clin North Am Small Anim Pract 2000;30:757–772.
16. KuKanich B, Papich MG. Pharmacokinetics of tramadol and the metabolite O-desmethyltramadol in dogs. J Vet Pharmacol Ther 2004;27:239–246.
17. Mastrocinque S, Fantoni DT. A comparison of preoperative tramadol and morphine for the control of early postoperative pain in canine ovariohysterectomy. Vet Anaesth Analg 2003;30:220–228.
18. Robertson SA, Taylor PM, Sear JW. Systemic uptake of buprenorphine by cats after oral mucosal administration. Vet Rec 2003;152:675–678.

Chapter 49
Cancer Patients

Duncan X. Lascelles and James S. Gaynor

Introduction

We know very little about cancer pain in animals, and very few studies have been published evaluating cancer pain and its alleviation.[1–4] Given the lack of veterinary clinical studies, the information in this chapter cannot be based solely on peer-reviewed investigations. Rather, it is based on the experience of veterinary clinicians involved in the treatment of cancer patients. Considered extrapolations from human medicine and from veterinary research in other chronically painful conditions, such as osteoarthritis, are relied on, as well.

This chapter reviews the assessment and treatment of chronic cancer pain in dogs and cats. The control of perioperative pain in cancer patients is very important and readers are encouraged to refer to appropriate texts and other chapters in this text for information on perioperative pain control.[5,6]

General Approach to Cancer-Pain Management

Barriers to effective cancer-pain control in animals include

- Lack of appreciation that many cancers are associated with significant pain
- Inability to assess pain accurately in cancer patients
- Lack of knowledge of drugs, drug therapy, and other pain-relieving techniques
- Lack of communication with clients and lack of involvement of clients in the assessment and treatment phases
- Underuse of nursing staff for assessment and reevaluation of pain in cancer patients

There are four main steps in overcoming these barriers and assuring that chronic pain management is optimized in veterinary patients:

- Assure that veterinarians have the appropriate education and training about the importance of alleviating pain, assessment of pain, available drugs and potential complications, and interventional techniques.
- Educate the client about realistic expectations surrounding pain control and quality of life and convey the idea that most patients' pain can be managed. This involves letting the client know that owner involvement in evaluating the pet and providing feedback on therapy is crucial to success. The veterinarian and owner should both participate in developing effective strategies to alleviate pain. The clients' involvement also helps decrease their feelings of helplessness.
- Thoroughly assess the pet's pain at the start and throughout the course of therapy, not just when it becomes severe.
- Have good support from the veterinary practice or institution for the use of opioids and other controlled substances.

Although pharmacological treatment is the mainstay of cancer-pain treatment, adjunctive nondrug therapies such as acupuncture may play an important role in the management of patients' chronic cancer pain. It must also be remembered that surgery and radiation therapy have very important roles in the management of cancer pain through treatment or palliation of the disease.

A basic approach to cancer-pain management can be summarized:

1. Assess the pain. Ask for the owner's perceptions of the pet's pain or of any compromise in its quality of life.
2. Believe the owner. The owner sees the pet every day in its own environment and knows when alterations in behavior occur. Owners can rarely suggest diagnoses but do know when something is wrong and when their pet is in pain. The veterinarian should become familiar with the owner's terminology when explaining the pet's abnormal behaviors to establish a baseline of communication for further assessment in the home environment once therapy has been initiated.
3. Choose appropriate therapy depending on the stage of the disease. Anything other than mild pain should be treated with

more than one class of analgesic or with an analgesic drug combined with nondrug adjunctive therapy. Also consider concurrent problems and drug therapy; be aware of potential drug interactions and toxicity.

4. Deliver the therapy in a logical, coordinated manner and explain carefully to the owner about any possible side effects.

5. Empower the clients to participate actively in their pet's treatment; ask for feedback and updates on how the therapy is working.

The Importance of Alleviating Pain

The alleviation of pain is important from physiological and biological standpoints, as well as from an ethical perspective.[7] Pain can induce a stress response in patients that is associated with elevations in andrenocorticotropic hormone, cortisol, antidiuretic hormone, catecholamines, aldosterone, renin, angiotensin II, and glucose, along with decreases in insulin and testosterone.[8] A prolonged stress response can decrease the rate of healing. In addition, the stress response can adversely affect the cardiovascular and pulmonary systems, fluid homeostasis, and gastrointestinal (GI) tract function.[8]

Veterinarians have an ethical obligation to treat animal pain. Most undertreatment of chronic pain is probably a result of lack of adequate knowledge and resources rather than a lack of concern. Outward show of concern for the pet and family is important for demonstrating a bond-centered approach to cancer therapy and pain management. Most owners who are willing to undergo the emotional stress and financial commitment to cancer therapy have already shown they have a strong attachment to their pet. It is important for the veterinarian to foster good communication surrounding primary therapy and pain treatment and at the same time demonstrate empathy for the owner. In cancer patients especially, pain prevention and treatment are not the only aspects that impact animal welfare, and veterinarians must evaluate all aspects of welfare when making treatment decisions. To help in an evaluation of welfare, *five freedoms*, initially proposed by the Brambell committee in reference to farmed animals, have been suggested as a rubric for the evaluation of welfare.[9] These may equally be applied to the context of companion animals:[7]

- Freedom from hunger and thirst
- Freedom from physical and thermal discomfort
- Freedom from pain, injury, and disease
- Freedom to express normal behavior
- Freedom from fear and distress

The approach to the treatment of cancer patients should be one that considers all aspects of welfare. For each freedom, the severity, incidence, and duration of perturbation should be considered. For example, for pain, the longer the pain lasts, such as in long-standing painful cancers, the more welfare is compromised.

It is of significant interest that the provision of analgesics significantly reduces the tumor-promoting effects of undergoing and recovering from surgery.[10] Surgery is well known to suppress several immune functions, including natural killer (NK) cell ac-

tivity in animals and people, probably as a result of substances released, such as catecholamines and prostaglandins. This suppression of NK cell activity can enhance metastasis.[11–13] The reduction of the tumor-promoting effects of surgery by analgesics seems to be due to the alleviation of pain-induced reduced NK cell function, but unrecognized factors other than immune cells probably also play a role.[10] Thus, the provision of adequate perioperative pain management in oncological surgery may protect clinical patients against metastatic sequelae. It may also be that the treatment of the chronic pain may somewhat protect against metastasis and possibly the local extension of cancer. This is an, as yet, unproven but interesting hypothesis.

Assessment of Cancer Pain

Assessment of pain in animals can be very difficult and frustrating. The tolerance of pain in a veterinary patient probably varies greatly from individual to individual, as it does in humans. Coupled with the innate ability of dogs and, particularly, cats to mask significant disease and probably pain, this makes it very difficult to assess pain. Often veterinarians need to rely on human experience to help define pain in animals. The mainstay of pain assessment in cats and dogs with cancer is likely to be changes in behavior. Table 49.1 outlines behaviors that are indicative of pain. The main point to remember is that any change in behavior can be associated with pain. Veterinarians should also allow technicians and other staff members to be involved in the assessment. Technicians and other staff members are usually better able to evaluate pain and quality of life in animals because they spend more time with the patients in the hospital. Thus, they are more likely to be able to converse in a relaxed and informal way with pet owners.

The best and most important people to assess their animal's behavior are the owners. The veterinary surgeon must work closely and communicate effectively with the owner to be able to capture this information. Often owners need education as to what signs to look for, or education that certain behaviors may be indicative of pain. Once very specific changes in behavior can be identified and recorded, these can be used to monitor the effectiveness of analgesic therapy. This approach has proved very sensitive in the evaluation of chronic pain caused by osteoarthritis.[14] In cases where pain does not cause a specific behavioral change, but rather a vague change in an animal's behavior, the owner is still the best person to assess the pet's pain or—as the combination of pain and other welfare considerations is often described—*well-being* or *quality of life*. Capturing this information can also be a very sensitive indicator of the effectiveness and appropriateness of therapy. Physiological variables, such as heart rate, respiratory rate, temperature, and pupil size, have been shown to be unreliable measures of acute perioperative pain in dogs and are therefore unlikely to be useful in chronic pain states.[15]

Principles of Alleviation of Cancer Pain

Drugs are the mainstay of cancer-pain management, although nondrug adjunctive therapies are becoming recognized as in-

Table 49.1. Outline of behaviors that may be seen with cancer-associated or cancer therapy–associated pain in cats and dogs.

Behavior	Notes
Activity	Less activity than normal.
	Very specific activities may be changed: decreased jumping; less playing; less venturing outside; and less willing to go on walks (dogs).
	Stiff gait, altered gait, or lameness can be associated with generalized pain, but are more often associated with the appendicular or axial musculoskeletal system.
	Slow to rise and get moving after rest (osteoarthritis, which is often concurrently present).
Appetite	Often decreased with cancer pain.
Attitude	Any change in behavior can be associated with cancer pain: aggressiveness, dullness, shyness, "clinginess," and increased dependence.
Facial expression	Cats: head hung low, squinted eyes.
	Dogs: sad expression, head carried low.
Grooming	Failure to groom, caused by either a painful oral lesion or generalized pain
Response to palpation	This is one of the best ways to diagnose and monitor pain. Pain can be elicited by palpation of the affected area or by manipulation of the affected area, which exacerbates low-grade pain to produce transient severe pain. This is manifested as an aversion response from the animal, i.e., the animal attempts to escape the procedure, or yowls, cries, hisses, or bites. Pain is inferred when this occurs.
Respiration	This may be elevated with severe cancer pain.
Self-traumatization	Licking at an area (e.g., a joint with osteoarthritis, bone with primary bone cancer, or abdomen with intra-abdominal cancer) can indicate pain.
	Scratching can indicate pain (e.g., scratching at cutaneous tumors or scratching and biting at the flank with prostatic or colonic neoplasia).
	Self-traumatization can also indicate the presence of neuropathic pain, or referred pain.
Urinary and bowel elimination	Cats: failure to use litter box.
	Dogs: urinating and defecating inside.
Vocalization	Vocalization is rare in response to chronic pain in dogs and cats, but owners of dogs will often report frequent odd noises (whining and grunting) associated with cancer pain. Occasionally, cats will hiss, utter spontaneous plaintive meows, or purr in association with cancer pain. This may be in response to the intermittent severe spontaneous pain associated with neuropathic pain.

creasingly important. The World Health Organization (WHO) has outlined a general approach to the management of cancer pain, based on the use of the following groups of analgesics:[16]

- Nonopioid analgesics (e.g., nonsteroidal anti-inflammatory drugs and acetaminophen)
- Weak opioid drugs (e.g., codeine)
- Strong opioid drugs (e.g., morphine)
- Adjuvant drugs (e.g., corticosteroids, tricyclic antidepressants, anticonvulsants, *N*-methyl-D-aspartate [NMDA] antagonists)

The general approach of the WHO ladder is a three-step hierarchy (see Fig. 49.1). Within the same category of drugs, there can be different side effects for individuals. Therefore, if possible, it may be best to substitute drugs within a category before switching therapies. It is always best to try to keep dosage scheduling as simple as possible. The more complicated the regimen is, the more likely is owner noncompliance. Drugs should be dosed on a regular basis, not just as needed, as pain becomes moderate to severe. Continuous analgesia will facilitate maintaining patient comfort. Additional doses of analgesics can then be administered as pain is intermittently more severe. Adjuvant drugs can be administered to help with specific types of pain and anxiety.

There are two potential problems with the use of the WHO analgesic ladder in veterinary medicine. First, there is very little information from human medicine, and virtually none from veterinary medicine, on which drugs are most effective for a particular type of cancer pain. It may well be that *third tier* drugs are the most effective for a particular condition and therefore best used initially.

The second problem is that such an approach may not be best suited for patients that present with severe pain. Many veterinary cancer patients present at an advanced stage of disease and thus are already in severe pain. Once pain has been present for a period, changes may have occurred in the central nervous system (CNS) that alter the way pain signals are processed. This alteration in processing (*central sensitization*) makes traditional analgesics less effective and requires that multiple classes of drugs be used concurrently to minimize pain. This is known as *multimodal pain therapy*. Once pain is minimized, and central changes are partially reversed, the administration of various classes of analgesic drugs initially used can be decreased. This approach has been termed the *analgesic reverse pyramid* approach.[17] It is currently unknown which of these two approaches (the WHO ladder or the reverse pyramid) is most appropriate and, indeed, one approach may be best at one disease stage and the other later on. The most important aspect in the treatment of cancer pain is that, in the majority of situations, *multimodal therapy* (i.e., concurrent

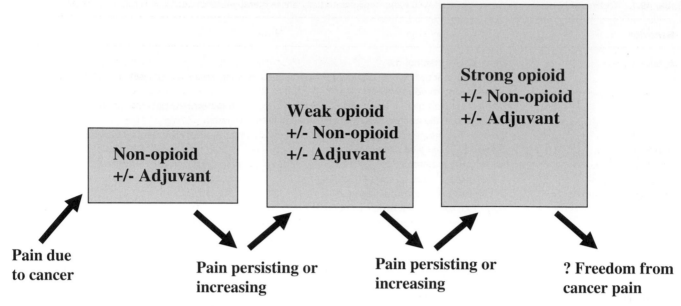

Fig. 49.1. Diagram showing the World Health Organization *analgesic ladder* for the treatment of cancer pain. The three standard analgesics making up this ladder are nonsteroidal anti-inflammatory drugs, opioids (such as codeine), and full μ opioid agonists (such as morphine). Alternatives are substituted as necessary. This simple approach is likely to be superseded by a more complex approach based on the mechanism of pain associated with particular cancer types. The three-step WHO ladder approach is not always suitable for veterinary patients, who often initially present with relatively advanced disease and significant pain.

use of more than one class of drug) is required for successful alleviation of the pain. The drugs that can be used for chronic cancer-pain management are outlined in Tables 49.2 (dogs) and 49.3 (cats).

Nonsteroidal Anti-inflammatory Drugs (NSAIDs)

The cyclooxygenase (COX) enzyme exists in (at least) two different forms. This relatively recent finding led to the rather simple designation of one COX enzyme producing *essential prostaglandins* (e.g., those involved in maintaining mucosal integrity of the stomach) on a minute-to-minute basis, and another that is activated by tissue trauma and produces *inflammatory* or *pain-mediating prostaglandins*. However, it is not as simple as COX-1 being good and COX-2 bad, because COX-2 has been shown to be expressed constitutively in certain tissues such as the canine kidney (although data are conflicting) and the canine CNS.[18-20] It is not fully understood what role, if any, COX-2 plays in canine GI mucosa. Simplistic theory would suggest that selective or preferential COX-2 inhibitors (e.g., carprofen, deracoxib, meloxicam, and firocoxib) might be associated with fewer GI side effects than would a nonselective drug. Although clinical experience with COX-2 selective drugs in human patients suggests that fewer side effects occur with these agents (such as celecoxib or rofecoxib) than with nonselective NSAIDs (such as ibuprofen or aspirin), widespread clinical experience is required before a similar statement can be made with respect to COX-2 selective drug use in dogs. Prostaglandins produced by COX-2 are involved in the healing of injured GI tract, and the safety of

COX-2 selective drugs in patients with inflammatory bowel disease or subclinical GI erosion or ulceration is unknown. Theory would also suggest that COX-2 selective drugs are not any safer for the kidney than are the nonselective drugs. Again, widespread clinical experience in dogs is required to substantiate this, although the COX-2 selective drugs used in humans have been found to be associated with a similar incidence of renal toxicity as traditional NSAIDs.[21] The relevance of this discussion to cancer treatment is that veterinarians need to be very aware of the possible side effects of NSAIDs and communicate this to owners. Very often, because of preexisting disease or concurrent therapy, cancer patients are at greater risk for toxic side effects from NSAIDs.

More recently, research has shown COX-2 plays a significant role in the development and progression of cancer. The production of prostaglandin E_2 by COX-2 has been linked to the promotion of tumorigenesis.[22] COX-2 overexpression in cells will inhibit apoptosis, allowing neoplastic cells to continue to live. Other mechanisms by which COX-2 contributes to tumor development include facilitating the adhesion and increasing the invasiveness of cancer cells, increased cell growth, suppression of the immune system, and enhanced angiogenesis.[23]

COX-2 overexpression has been demonstrated in a number of premalignant and malignant conditions, including colon cancer, non-small-cell lung cancer, breast cancer, bladder cancer, pancreatic cancer, prostate cancer, and head-and-neck cancer in people.[24-30] Overexpression of COX-2 in tumors has been linked with a poor prognosis and more aggressive cancer. As a result of these findings, selective COX-2 inhibitors are being used in chemotherapy protocols against these cancers.[31,32] NSAIDs are

Table 49.2. Suggested doses of analgesics that may be used for the alleviation of chronic cancer pain in dogs[a].

Drug	Dose for Dogs	Comments
Acetaminophen (paracetamol)	10–15 mg/kg PO q 8 h for 5 days Long-term therapy: up to 10 mg/kg every 12 h	This seems to be associated with fewer GI side effects than are regular NSAIDs, and not noted to be associated with renal toxicity. Toxicity has, however, not been evaluated clinically in dogs. It has been combined with regular NSAIDs (e.g., meloxicam or carprofen) in severe cancer pain, but this combination has not been evaluated for toxicity, and increased toxicity is likely to be seen.
Acetaminophen (paracetamol) (300 mg) + codeine (30 or 60 mg)	Dose based on 10–15 mg/kg of acetaminophen	The acetaminophen dose corresponds to 2 mg/kg codeine. Sedation may be a side effect.
Amantadine	3.0–5.0 mg/kg PO q 24 h	This is an NMDA antagonist (although originally marketed as an antiviral agent) that seems to produce a significant level of analgesia when given in combination with an NSAID. Loose stools and excess GI gas can be seen at higher doses for a few days. It should not be combined with drugs such as selegiline or sertraline until more is known about interactions among these drugs.
Amitriptyline	0.5–2.0 mg/kg PO q 24 h	This augments the descending serotonergic system, which is one of the body's endogenous analgesic mechanisms. It is not a "strong" analgesic, but, like amantadine, tramadol, and codeine, is useful when combined with an NSAID or paracetamol. It has not been evaluated for clinical toxicity in dogs.
Aspirin	10 mg/kg PO q 12 h	This causes significantly more GI ulceration than approved NSAIDs. *Caution*: Do not administer near the time of surgery because platelet function is inhibited.
Butorphanol	0.2–0.5 mg/kg PO up to q 8 h	This may produce sedation at higher doses. It is not a very predictable analgesic and is best used in combination with other analgesics, e.g., NSAIDs.
Codeine	0.5–2.0 mg/kg PO q 24 h	Sedation can be seen at the higher doses.
Carprofen	2 mg/kg PO q 12 h or 4 mg/kg PO q 24 h	—
Deracoxib	1–2 mg/kg PO q 24 h long term	This is one of the most specific COX-2 inhibitors approved for use in dogs with osteoarthritis (USA).
Etodolac	5–15 mg/kg PO q 24 h	(Available only in the USA.)
Fentanyl, transdermal	2–5 µg/kg/h	This can be very useful for the short-term control of cancer pain. For long-term therapy, its usefulness is limited by the need to change the patch every 4 to 5 days and the expense involved.
Gabapentin	3–10 mg/kg PO q 24 h	This has not been evaluated in dogs as an analgesic; it is most frequently used as an antiseizure drug and is rapidly metabolized in dogs. It can be useful for neuropathic pain, such as after limb amputation or for nerve-root tumor pain, or cancers that seem to have a significant component of neuropathic pain (osteosarcoma). Its best effects are seen when used in combination with other analgesics, such as NSAIDs or acetaminophen (paracetamol).
Glucosamine and chondroitin sulfate	13–15 mg/kg chondroitin sulfate PO q 24 h	This can be used in a variety of cancer pain because of its mild anti-inflammatory and analgesic effects. It is best used in combination with an NSAID or other analgesic.
Meloxicam	0.2 mg/kg PO day 1, and then 0.1 mg/kg q 24 h	—
Morphine, liquid	0.2–0.5 mg/kg PO q 6–8 h	This can be useful for dosing smaller dogs when morphine tablets are not suitable. Sedation and (particularly) constipation are side effects that are seen as the dose is increased. Oral morphine may not be as effective in dogs as it is in humans.

(continued)

Table 49.2. Suggested doses of analgesics that may be used for the alleviation of chronic cancer pain in dogs[a] (*continued*).

Drug	Dose for Dogs	Comments
Morphine, sustained release	0.5–3.0 mg/kg PO q 8–12 h	Doses higher than 0.5–1.0 mg/kg are often associated with unacceptable constipation according to owners, so the suggested use is 0.5 mg/kg several times a day. However, recent evidence indicates the "first pass" effect for oral morphine is very high in dogs, and analgesic tissue levels may be very difficult to attain.
Pamidronate (one of the bisphosphonate class of drugs)	1–1.5 mg/kg slowly IV, probably once a month (although this has not been defined yet)	This drug inhibits osteoclast activity and thus provides analgesia in patients with a primary or metastatic bone tumor that is causing osteolysis.
Piroxicam	0.3 mg/kg PO q 48 h	Despite its widespread use as a mild chemotherapeutic agent for epithelial tumors, the incidence of side effects in dogs is not known but appears to be quite high at 0.3 mg/kg q 24 h, so suggested use is 0.3 mg/kg q 48 h.
Prednisolone	0.25–1.0 mg/kg PO q 12–24 h. Taper to q 48 h, if possible, after 14 days	Do *not* use this concurrently with NSAIDs. It can be particularly useful in providing analgesia when there is a significant inflammatory component associated with the tumor.
Tepoxalin	10–20 mg/kg PO on day 1, followed by 10 mg/kg daily	This NSAID is a "dual inhibitor" that inhibits both cyclooxygenase and lipoxygenase enzymes. It is likely to be particularly useful in cancer pain where there is a significant inflammatory component.
Tramadol	4–5 mg/kg PO q 6–12 h	This has not been evaluated for efficacy or toxicity in dogs but appears to be a useful adjunctive analgesic (when combined with other analgesics, such as acetaminophen or the NSAIDs) for the treatment of cancer pain in dogs. If sedation is seen, the dose should be reduced.

[a]None of the drugs have been evaluated for efficacy in the treatment of cancer pain. None of these drugs are approved or licensed for use in chronic cancer pain. Some drugs are approved for use in osteoarthritis, and doses are extrapolated from recommended doses for the treatment of osteoarthritis. The doses listed come from the authors' experience and from the experience of others working in the area of clinical cancer-pain control. GI, gastrointestinal; IV, intravenously; NMDA, *N*-methyl-D-aspartate; NSAID, nonsteroidal anti-inflammatory drug; and PO, per os (orally).

Table 49.3. Suggested doses of analgesics that may be used for the alleviation of chronic cancer pain in cats.[a,b]

Drug	Cat Dose (mg/kg)	Comments
Acetaminophen (paracetamol)	Contraindicated	It is contraindicated because small doses rapidly cause death in cats.
Amantadine	3.0 mg/kg PO q 24 h	This has not been evaluated for toxicity but is well tolerated by dogs and people, with occasional side effects of agitation and GI irritation. It may be a useful addition to NSAIDs in the treatment of chronic cancer-pain conditions. The 100-mg capsules need to be recompounded for cats, or capsules compounded from the powder drug.
Amitriptyline	0.5–2.0 mg/kg PO q 24 h	This appears to be well tolerated for up to 12 months of daily administration in cats. Occasionally drowsiness is seen (<10%). This drug may be a useful addition to NSAIDs for treatment of chronic pain conditions.[74,81]
Aspirin	10 mg/kg PO q 48 h	This can cause significant GI ulceration.

(*continued*)

Table 49.3. Suggested doses of analgesics that may be used for the alleviation of chronic cancer pain in cats[a,b] (*continued*).

Drug	Cat Dose (mg/kg)	Comments
Buprenorphine	0.02 mg/kg sublingual q 6–7 h	Recent information from the University of Florida, using a research model, suggests that this provides good analgesia when administered sublingually (20 µg/kg; injectable formulation) and provides good analgesia predictably for 6–7 h (buprenorphine IV provides analgesia for the same period when administered at the same dose). The sublingual route is not resented by cats and may be a good way to provide postoperative analgesia at home. Feedback from owners indicates that, after 2–3 days at this dose, anorexia develops. Smaller doses (5–10 µg/kg) may be more appropriate for long-term administration, especially in combination with other drugs.[57]
Butorphanol	0.2–1.0 mg/kg PO q 6 h	One study suggests that using this PO after surgery may be beneficial. It is generally considered to be a poor analgesic in cats except for visceral pain, but the authors have found it to be useful as part of a multimodal approach to cancer-pain therapy.[82]
Glucosamine/chondroitin sulfate combinations	Ca. 15 mg/kg chondroitin sulfate PO q 12 to 24 h	This combination appears to produce mild anti-inflammatory and analgesic effects in cats more predictably than in dogs. It can be used in conjunction with NSAIDs, opioids, and amantadine.
Ketoprofen	1 mg/kg PO q 24 h; maximum 5 days	This is probably well tolerated as pulse therapy for chronic pain, with a few days rest between treatments. It has also been used by some at 1 mg/kg every 3 days long term or at 0.5 mg/kg every other day long term. A safe long-term dosing regimen has not been established.
Meloxicam	0.1 mg/kg PO on day 1, followed by 0.05 mg/kg PO daily for 4 days, and then 0.025 mg/kg to 0.05 mg/kg every other day	This is particularly well received by cats because of its formulation as a honey syrup. The drop formulation makes it very easy to decrease the dose gradually and accurately. A safe long-term dosing regimen has not been established.[83]
Morphine (oral liquid)	0.2–0.5 mg/kg PO TID–QID	This is best compounded into a palatable flavored syrup, but cats usually strongly resent this medication. Morphine may not be as effective in cats as it is in dogs.
Piroxicam	1 mg/cat PO daily for a maximum of 7 days If longer-term medication is considered, suggested use is dosing every other day, but see the note at right	This can be compounded into a palatable liquid, but recent information suggests that the active drug decreases significantly over a 10-day period after compounding in an aqueous solution. In the authors' experience, significant drops in PCV (presumably caused by GI hemorrhage) occur in up to 30% of cats after 2–3 weeks of drug therapy.
Prednisolone	0.25–0.5 mg/kg PO q 24 h	This can be particularly effective in cancers associated with significant inflammation (such as squamous cell carcinoma of the oral cavity in cats). Do *not* combine it with concurrent NSAID administration.
Tolfenamic acid	4 mg/kg PO q 24 h for 3 days maximum	—
Tramadol	1–2 mg/kg once or twice daily	This has not been evaluated for toxicity in cats and has not yet been used extensively by the authors for treatment of cancer pain in cats. However, early results are encouraging, but toxicity appears to be seen more readily in cats than dogs.
Transdermal fentanyl patch	2–5 µg/kg/h	A 25-µg/h patch can be applied to average-size cats (7.7–11.0 lb; 3.5–5.0 kg). In smaller cats, other methods of providing analgesia should be sought because it is not recommended to cut patches in half, and covering half of the patch produces unpredictable results. The decay in plasma levels following patch removal is slow.[84,85]

[a]None of these drugs have been evaluated for efficacy in the treatment of cancer pain. None are approved or licensed for use in the treatment of chronic cancer pain. Some are approved for treatment of inflammatory or painful conditions in cats in certain countries, and doses for the control of cancer pain are extrapolated from these. The doses listed come from the authors' experience and from the experience of others working in the area of clinical cancer-pain control. GI, gastrointestinal; IV, intravenously; NSAID, nonsteroidal anti-inflammatory drug; PCV, packed cell volume; and PO, per os (orally).

[b]Adapted from Lascelles[86] and from Tranquilli et al.[87]

also being used to protect against cancer in people genetically at risks for certain cancers, such as colon cancer, although it seems that some NSAIDs may be more effective than others.[33–35] Basic research has also shown that COX-2 inhibitors may enhance the effects of radiation of tumors.[36]

Significant research has recently been directed toward examining the role of COX-2 in dogs with cancer. In dogs, COX-2 is overexpressed in a number of carcinomas, including bladder and renal, mammary, intestinal, cutaneous (squamous cell), and nasal, and, in some sarcomas, such as osteosarcoma.[37–40] A number of investigators have examined the anticancer properties of NSAIDs (to date, mainly only those of piroxicam) in canine tumors. Administration of piroxicam causes regression of, and slows the progression of, rectal tubulopapillary polyps.[41] Piroxicam has also been shown to have anticancer effects in canine transitional cell carcinoma and canine oral squamous cell carcinoma.[42–47] In multicentric lymphoma, there was no apparent benefit to adding piroxicam to doxorubicin.[48]

NSAIDs have been the mainstay of therapy for chronic pain, especially in osteoarthritis. The choice among available NSAIDs can be bewildering, but a few key points follow:

• On a population basis, all NSAIDs appear equally effective in relieving pain associated with osteoarthritis, but for a given patient one drug may be more effective than another. This is probably even truer for cancer pain, where the mechanisms of pain may be very different from one patient to another.

• GI side effects associated with NSAID use appear to be more common with drugs that preferentially block COX-1 over COX-2, although COX-2–inhibiting drugs have the potential to exacerbate GI injury when there is preexisting pathology. This results from inhibition of the beneficial role that the COX-2 enzyme may play in GI healing.

• There is no difference in renal toxicity between COX-1 selective drugs and COX-2 selective drugs. Both COX-1 and COX-2 are constitutively expressed in the kidney.

• Liver toxicity with NSAIDs is an idiosyncratic event that can happen with any NSAID.

Monitoring

If the NSAID chosen is effective and does not cause significant adverse effects, it should be continued. If not, therapy may be changed to another NSAID, provided the animal did not experience a serious side effect (e.g., GI bleeding, azotemia, or hepatopathy). If serious toxicity occurs, the patient should be carefully evaluated and the benefits of continued NSAID therapy weighed against the potential for further adverse events. Changing therapy to another class of drugs (e.g., opioids) may be the safest strategy if the patient's tolerance for NSAIDs is low. If another NSAID is chosen, the patient should be monitored closely for toxicity. This consists of two aspects:

• Informing the owner of the potential for further toxicity and what signs to watch for (lethargy, anorexia, depression, vomiting, melena, and increased water ingestion).

• Regular blood work (and urinalysis) to evaluate renal function (urea, creatinine, and urine specific gravity) and liver function (alkaline phosphatase and alanine aminotransferase and, if these enzymes are raised, bile acids). A baseline should be obtained when NSAID therapy is initiated and parameters monitored regularly thereafter. The reevaluation is done more frequently if multiple drugs are used, because there is no information on clinical toxicity associated with combinations of analgesics administered chronically.

NSAIDs in Cats

Cats have generally longer, but variable and inconsistent, rates of biotransformation and excretion of NSAIDs when compared with other species. All of the kinetic studies performed in cats have been on single doses, and no studies have yet examined the metabolism of chronically administered NSAIDs.[49–52] However, given that most of the NSAIDs have a relatively long half-life in cats, chronic dosing at the dosing level and frequency described for dogs is likely to be more dangerous for cats than for dogs.

No NSAIDs have been licensed for chronic administration (>5 days) in cats. A number of available NSAIDs can probably be used relatively safely (Table 49.3); however, no NSAID has been fully evaluated for safe use in cats. The key to safe chronic NSAID administration in cats is to individualize the dose by using the smallest effective dose or extend the dosing interval relative to other species. Since half-lives can be longer and more variable, some cats may metabolize drug at a rapid rate, requiring more frequent dosing, whereas other cats may accumulate drug to toxic levels unless the dosing interval is increased or the dose is reduced. Cats are more prone to toxicity associated with NSAIDs than are dogs; therefore, blood and urine should probably be analyzed even more frequently than recommended for dogs.

Analgesics for Cancer-Pain Relief

If pain relief with NSAIDs is inadequate, oral opioid medications, such as morphine or tramadol, can be administered. Transdermal fentanyl patches can also be used. Fentanyl, morphine, or tramadol can be used for dogs that cannot be given NSAIDs, although adverse effects may be more common. Acetaminophen has been used in conjunction with NSAIDs (except in cats), although safety data on combined use are lacking. Other agents that are used to treat chronic pain include amantadine (an NMDA antagonist); anticonvulsants, such as gabapentin; and tricyclic antidepressants, such as amitriptyline. These can all be combined with NSAIDs.

Acetaminophen

Acetaminophen (paracetamol) is a nonacid NSAID, though many pharmacologists do not consider it an NSAID because it probably acts by different mechanisms than do most currently marketed NSAIDs. Although its mechanism of action is poorly understood, it has been suggested that it acts on a variant of the cyclooxygenase enzyme (COX-3), which is present in CNS tissues of dogs.[53,54] With any chronic pain, there are always CNS changes, so centrally acting analgesics can be very effective for what seems a peripheral problem, such as many cancers.

Although highly toxic in cats, even in small quantities, acetaminophen can be effectively used to control pain in dogs. No studies of toxicity in dogs have been done, but, if toxicity is seen, it will probably affect the liver, and thus the drug should be used cautiously in dogs with liver dysfunction. It can be used on its own or in combination with codeine and is initially dosed at about 10 to 15 mg/kg PO bid. The authors often use it as the first line of analgesic therapy in dogs with renal compromise where NSAIDs cannot be used, or in dogs that appear to be otherwise intolerant to NSAIDs (e.g., vomiting or GI ulceration).

Opioids

Many veterinarians may be unfamiliar with the use of opioids outside the perioperative period, but opioids can be a very effective part of a multimodal approach (i.e., the use of NSAIDs or adjunctive analgesics with concurrent use of opioids). Adverse effects of opioids can include behavior changes, diarrhea, vomiting, occasionally sedation, and constipation with long-term use. It is very often the constipation, and occasionally the sedation seen, which owners seem to object to most, especially with the administration of oral morphine. The opioids that have been used clinically most often to alleviate chronic cancer pain are oral morphine, transdermal fentanyl, oral butorphanol, transmucosal buprenorphine, and oral codeine. None of these drugs has been fully evaluated for clinical toxicity when administered long term, nor for efficacy against chronic cancer pain. It is important to realize that dosing must be done on an individual basis, and adjustment of the dose to produce analgesia without undesirable side effects requires excellent communication with clients. Recent studies have indicated that certain preparations of prolonged-release oral morphine and oral methadone may not reach effective plasma concentrations in dogs when dosed at the currently recommended levels.[55,56] Much work has to be done to better evaluate the efficacy and safety of long-term oral opioids in dogs.

Opioid Use in Cats

There is currently no information on the long-term use of oral opioids for chronic pain in cats. Interestingly, there seems to be significant individual variation in the level of analgesia obtained with certain opioids, especially morphine and butorphanol, in the acute setting. Buprenorphine appears to produce predictable analgesia when given sublingually in cats.[57] Compared with humans, the sublingual route appears to result in near 100% bioavailability in cats; this may be a result of differences in ionization in the alkaline environment (pH 8 to 9) of the cat mouth compared with that of humans (pH 6.5 to 7.0). Sublingual administration of buprenorphine is well accepted by cats, with no resentment or salivation, so there is no need to compound the injectable solution. The small volume required makes administration simple. Based on clinical feedback from owners, this is a very acceptable technique for them to perform at home. However, inappetance can occur after several days of treatment. Slightly lower doses can usually overcome this problem. When administered concurrently with other drugs, longer dosing intervals appear to be all that is required to minimize the potential for toxicity.[57]

NMDA Antagonists

Since NMDA receptor appears to be important for the induction and maintenance of central sensitization, the use of NMDA receptor antagonists would appear to offer benefit in the treatment of pain where central sensitization has become established.[58–61]

Ketamine, tiletamine, dextromethorphan, and amantadine possess NMDA-antagonist properties, among other actions. Ketamine is not useful for the management of chronic pain in the injectable formulation that is currently available. However, intraoperative microdose ketamine appears to provide beneficial effects for a variety of surgical procedures, including limb amputations, and may decrease the incidence of chronic pain following surgery. Other recent publications suggest a benefit of using ketamine perioperatively (an intravenous bolus [0.5 mg/kg] followed by a continuous intravenous infusion [10.0 µg/kg/min] prior to and during surgery), particularly in patients that have pain caused by neoplasia prior to surgery.[62,63] A lower continuous intravenous infusion rate (2.0 µg/kg/min) may be beneficial for the first 24 h postoperatively and an even lower rate (1.0 µg/kg/min) for the next 24 h. In the absence of an infusion pump, ketamine can be mixed in a bag of crystalloid fluids for administration during anesthesia.

Dextromethorphan has received attention as an orally administered NMDA receptor antagonist for use in human patients suffering from chronic pain. Although it appears effective in some people, dogs do not make the active metabolite after oral administration of dextromethorphan, probably negating its use as an analgesic in dogs.[64]

Amantadine has been used for the treatment of neuropathic pain in humans.[65,66] It does not appear to have the undesirable CNS adverse effects associated with ketamine administration. Amantadine has been used in dogs as an adjunctive drug for the alleviation of chronic pain, particularly in osteoarthritis and cancer. It is used as an adjunct to NSAIDs, and it appears to augment pain relief with a low incidence of adverse effects (mainly agitation and diarrhea over the first few days of administration). It usually takes about 5 to 7 days to be effective and is usually used long term. Suggested doses for dogs and cats are listed in Tables 49.2 and 49.3. Amantadine should probably not be used in patients with congestive heart failure, nor in patients on selegiline, sertraline, or tricyclic antidepressants.

Combination Analgesics

Tramadol is a synthetic derivative of codeine and is classified as an opioidergic/monoaminergic drug.[67,68] It has been found to be effective in the alleviation of pain associated with osteoarthritis in humans, as part of a multimodal approach.[69–72] Studies establishing dosing regimens and effectiveness in veterinary species are limited. Tramadol and its metabolite have agonist action at the µ opioid receptor and also facilitate the descending serotonergic system, which is part of the body's endogenous analgesic system. Tramadol has been used in many parts of the world to treat perioperative pain in animals and is occasionally used to treat chronic pain. The doses listed in Tables 49.2 and 49.3 are for the regular (not prolonged release) form of the drug. It has not been evaluated for toxicity in dogs or cats.

Anticonvulsants

Gabapentin is a structural analogue of γ-aminobutyric acid (GABA) and was introduced as an antiepileptic drug, although its GABAergic actions appear minimal. It is thought to act by modulating the α_2-delta subunit of calcium channels, thereby decreasing calcium influx and so neurotransmitter release. It appears to be useful for treating neuropathic pain and central sensitization in some patients, although effectiveness in humans (and probably veterinary patients) is unpredictable. It is metabolized rapidly in dogs and is most often used for its anticonvulsive properties. It appears to have some analgesic properties at low doses administered two or three times daily.

Tricyclic Antidepressants

The tricyclic antidepressant amitriptyline appears to be effective in cats for pain alleviation in interstitial cystitis, and many practitioners have anecdotally reported efficacy in other chronically painful conditions in cats and dogs.[73,74] Amitriptyline has been used daily for periods of up to 1 year for interstitial cystitis, and few side effects have been reported. There are no other studies of its possible analgesic effects in dogs or cats. It should probably not be used concurrently with amantadine until more is known about drug interactions.

Steroids

These have a mild analgesic action, are anti-inflammatory, and can produce a state of euphoria. Steroids are often used to palliate cancer and cancer pain in cats and dogs. They should not be used concurrently with NSAIDs because of the increased risk of serious adverse effects.

Bisphosphonates

Bone pain induced by primary or metastatic bone tumors is thought to be caused mainly by osteoclast activity; therefore, drugs that block osteoclast activity should markedly reduce bone pain.[75,76] Bisphosphonates inhibit osteoclast activity and can thus produce analgesia. There is very little information on their use in dogs for palliation of bone pain, but drugs such as pamidronate are being used, and early anecdotal reports suggest effectiveness in approximately 40% of cases.[1]

Other Cancer Pain–Relieving Modalities

Local or whole body radiation can enhance analgesic drug effectiveness by reducing metastatic or primary-tumor bulk.[77] Radiation dose should be balanced between the amount necessary to kill tumor cells and that which would affect normal cells. Mucositis of the oral cavity and pharynx can develop after radiation to the neck, head, or oral cavities, resulting in impaired ability to eat and drink. Therapies to treat mucositis include analgesics, sucralfate, 2% viscous lidocaine, and green-tea rinses. Intravenous administration of strontium 89 has also been shown to provide analgesia related to bony metastases in approximately 50% of humans, but its use is uncommon in veterinary patients.

Acupuncture can be used as a pain-relieving modality, often when conventional therapy does not work. It is also useful in conjunction with other therapy to allow lower doses of drugs to be used that may have significant side effects. While some practitioners have difficulty accepting acupuncture because of traditional Chinese medical explanations that may be scientifically untenable, it is important to remember that there are documented physiological theories and evidence for its clinical effects in animals.[78,79]

In general, acupuncture analgesia is extremely useful for treatment of pelvic, radius/ulna, and femoral bone pain, as well as cutaneous discomfort secondary to radiation therapy. Acupuncture may also help alleviate nausea associated with chemotherapy and some analgesics, as well as promote general well-being. Acupuncture can be provided through simple needle placement or by needle placement combined with electrical stimulation (of high or low frequency, although most types of pain respond to low-frequency stimulation).[80]

Nutraceutical products may contain a variety of compounds, but the main ones are glucosamine and chondroitin sulfate. These are often recommended for osteoarthritis therapy, and there is evidence that they provide mild anti-inflammatory and analgesic effects. They may be of benefit in the alleviation of chronic cancer pain, but only when used as part of a multimodal approach. Interestingly, based on the authors' experience, the analgesic effect appears to be more predictable in cats than in dogs.

References

1. Fan TM, de Lorimier LP, Charney SC, et al. Evaluation of intravenous pamidronate administration in 33 cancer-bearing dogs with primary or secondary bone involvement. J Vet Intern Med 2005; 19:74–80.
2. Ramirez O III, Dodge RK, Page RL, et al. Palliative radiotherapy of appendicular osteosarcoma in 95 dogs. Vet Radiol Ultrasound 1999;40:517–522.
3. Bateman KE, Catton PA, Pennock PW, et al. 0-7-21 radiation therapy for the palliation of advanced cancer in dogs. J Vet Intern Med 1994;8:394–399.
4. Karai L, Brown DC, Mannes AJ, et al. Deletion of vanilloid receptor 1–expressing primary afferent neurons for pain control. J Clin Invest 2004;113:1344–1352.
5. Flecknell PA, Waterman-Pearson AE. Pain Management in Animals. London: WB Saunders, 2000:184.
6. Gaynor JS, Muir WW. Handbook of Veterinary Pain Management, 1st ed. St Louis: CV Mosby, 2002:452.
7. Lascelles BD, Main DC. Surgical trauma and chronically painful conditions: Within our comfort level but beyond theirs? J Am Vet Med Assoc 2002;221:215–222.
8. Hamill RJ. The physiologic and metabolic response to pain and stress. In: Hamill RJ, Rowlingson JC, eds. Handbook of Critical Care Pain Management. New York: McGraw-Hill, 1994:39–52.
9. Brambell FWR. Report of the Technical Committee to Enquire into the Welfare of Animals Kept Under Intensive Husbandry Systems [Cmnd 2836]. London: HM Stationery Office, 1965.
10. Page GG, Blakely WP, Ben-Eliyahu S. Evidence that postoperative pain is a mediator of the tumor-promoting effects of surgery in rats. Pain 2001;90:191–199.
11. Sandoval BA, Robinson AV, Sulaiman TT, et al. Open versus laparoscopic surgery: A comparison of natural antitumoral cellular immu-

nity in a small animal model. Am Surg 1996;62:625–630; Discussion, 630–631.

12. Kutza J, Gratz I, Afshar M, et al. The effects of general anaesthesia and surgery on basal and interferon stimulated natural killer cell activity of humans. Anaesth Analg 1997;85:918–923.

13. Page GG, Ben-Eliyahu S, Liebeskind JC. The role of LGL/NK cells in surgery-induced promotion of metastasis and its attenuation by morphine. Brain Behav Immun 1994;8:241–250.

14. Gingerich DA, Strobel JD. Use of client-specific outcome measures to assess treatment effects in geriatric, arthritic dogs: Controlled clinical evaluation of a nutraceutical. Vet Ther 2003;4:56–66.

15. Conzemius MG, Hill CM, Sammarco JL, et al. Correlation between subjective and objective measures used to determine severity of postoperative pain in dogs. J Am Vet Med Assoc 1997;210:1619–1622.

16. Committee WHO. Cancer Pain Relief, 2nd ed. In. Geneva: World Health Organization, 1996.

17. Lascelles BD. Relief of chronic cancer pain. In: Dobson JM, Lascelles BD, eds. BSAVA Manual of Small Animal Oncology. Cheltenham, UK: BSAVA, 2003:137–151.

18. Khan KN, Venturini CM, Bunch RT, et al. Interspecies differences in renal localization of cyclooxygenase isoforms: Implications in nonsteroidal antiinflammatory drug–related nephrotoxicity. Toxicol Pathol 1998;26:612–620.

19. Wilson JE, Chandrasekharan NV, Westover KD, et al. Determination of expression of cyclooxygenase-1 and -2 isozymes in canine tissues and their differential sensitivity to nonsteroidal anti-inflammatory drugs. Am J Vet Res 2004;65:810–818.

20. Ostrom RS, Gregorian C, Drenan RM, et al. Key role for constitutive cyclooxygenase-2 of MDCK cells in basal signaling and response to released ATP. Am J Physiol Cell Physiol 2001;281:C524–C531.

21. Rossat J, Maillard M, Nussberger J, et al. Renal effects of selective cyclooxygenase-2 inhibition in normotensive salt-depleted subjects. Clin Pharmacol Ther 1999;66:76–84.

22. Zweifel BS, Davis TW, Ornberg RL, et al. Direct evidence for a role of cyclooxygenase 2–derived prostaglandin E_2 in human head and neck xenograft tumors. Cancer Res 2002;62:6706–6711.

23. Raegg C, Dormond O. Suppression of tumor angiogenesis by nonsteroidal anti-inflammatory drugs: A new function for old drugs. Sci World J 2001;1:808–811.

24. Koki A, Khan NK, Woerner BM, et al. Cyclooxygenase-2 in human pathological disease. Adv Exp Med Biol 2002;507:177–184.

25. Kulkarni S, Rader JS, Zhang F, et al. Cyclooxygenase-2 is overexpressed in human cervical cancer. Clin Cancer Res 2001;7:429–434.

26. Soslow RA, Dannenberg AJ, Rush D, et al. COX-2 is expressed in human pulmonary, colonic, and mammary tumors. Cancer 2000;89:2637–2645.

27. Buckman SY, Gresham A, Hale P, et al. COX-2 expression is induced by UVB exposure in human skin: Implications for the development of skin cancer. Carcinogenesis 1998;19:723–729.

28. Chan G, Boyle JO, Yang EK, et al. Cyclooxygenase-2 expression is up-regulated in squamous cell carcinoma of the head and neck. Cancer Res 1999;59:991–994.

29. Tucker ON, Dannenberg AJ, Yang EK, et al. Cyclooxygenase-2 expression is up-regulated in human pancreatic cancer. Cancer Res 1999;59:987–990.

30. Yoshimura R, Sano H, Masuda C, et al. Expression of cyclooxygenase-2 in prostate carcinoma. Cancer 2000;89:589–596.

31. Howe LR, Subbaramaiah K, Patel J, et al. Celecoxib, a selective cyclooxygenase 2 inhibitor, protects against human epidermal growth factor receptor 2 (HER-2)/neu–induced breast cancer. Cancer Res 2002;62:5405–5407.

32. Koki AT, Masferrer JL. Celecoxib: A specific COX-2 inhibitor with anticancer properties. Cancer Control 2002;9:28–35.

33. Burke CA, Bauer WM, Lashner B. Chemoprevention of colorectal cancer: Slow, steady progress. Cleve Clin J Med 2003;70:346–350.

34. Ricchi P, Zarrilli R, Di Palma A, et al. Nonsteroidal anti-inflammatory drugs in colorectal cancer: From prevention to therapy. Br J Cancer 2003;88:803–807.

35. Friis S, Sorensen HT, McLaughlin JK, et al. A population-based cohort study of the risk of colorectal and other cancers among users of low-dose aspirin. Br J Cancer 2003;88:684–688.

36. Kishi K, Petersen S, Petersen C, et al. Preferential enhancement of tumor radioresponse by a cyclooxygenase-2 inhibitor. Cancer Res 2000;60:1326–1331.

37. Khan KN, Stanfield KM, Trajkovic D, et al. Expression of cyclooxygenase-2 in canine renal cell carcinoma. Vet Pathol 2001;38:116–119.

38. Dore M, Lanthier I, Sirois J. Cyclooxygenase-2 expression in canine mammary tumors. Vet Pathol 2003;40:207–212.

39. McEntee MF, Cates JM, Neilsen N. Cyclooxygenase-2 expression in spontaneous intestinal neoplasia of domestic dogs. Vet Pathol 2002;39:428–436.

40. Pestili de Almeida EM, Piche C, Sirois J, et al. Expression of cyclo-oxygenase-2 in naturally occurring squamous cell carcinomas in dogs. J Histochem Cytochem 2001;49:867–875.

41. Knottenbelt CM, Simpson JW, Tasker S, et al. Preliminary clinical observations on the use of piroxicam in the management of rectal tubulopapillary polyps. J Small Anim Pract 2000;41:393–397.

42. Knapp DW, Richardson RC, Bottoms GD, et al. Phase I trial of piroxicam in 62 dogs bearing naturally occurring tumors. Cancer Chemother Pharmacol 1992;29:214–218.

43. Knapp D, Richardson R, TCK C, et al. Piroxicam therapy in 34 dogs with transitional cell carcinoma of the urinary bladder. J Vet Intern Med 1994;8:273–278.

44. Knapp DW, Chan TC, Kuczek T, et al. Evaluation of in vitro cytotoxicity of nonsteroidal anti-inflammatory drugs against canine tumor cells. Am J Vet Res 1995;56:801–805.

45. Knapp DW, Glickman NW, Widmer WR, et al. Cisplatin versus cisplatin combined with piroxicam in a canine model of human invasive urinary bladder cancer. Cancer Chemother Pharmacol 2000;46:221–226.

46. Mohammed SI, Bennett PF, Craig BA, et al. Effects of the cyclooxygenase inhibitor, piroxicam, on tumor response, apoptosis, and angiogenesis in a canine model of human invasive urinary bladder cancer. Cancer Res 2002;62:356–358.

47. Schmidt BR, Glickman NW, DeNicola DB, et al. Evaluation of piroxicam for the treatment of oral squamous cell carcinoma in dogs. J Am Vet Med Assoc 2001;218:1783–1786.

48. Mutsaers AJ, Glickman NW, DeNicola DB, et al. Evaluation of treatment with doxorubicin and piroxicam or doxorubicin alone for multicentric lymphoma in dogs. J Am Vet Med Assoc 2002;220:1813–1817.

49. Lees P, Taylor PM. Pharmacodynamics and pharmacokinetics of flunixin in the cat. Br Vet J 1991;147:298–305.

50. Parton K, Balmer TV, Boyle J, et al. The pharmacokinetics and effects of intravenously administered carprofen and salicylate on gastrointestinal mucosa and selected biochemical measurements in healthy cats. J Vet Pharmacol Ther 2000;23:73–79.

51. Taylor PM, Delatour P, Landoni FM, ct al. Pharmacodynamics and enantioselective pharmacokinetics of carprofen in the cat. Res Vet Sci 1996;60:144–151.

52. Taylor PM, Winnard JG, Jefferies R, et al. Flunixin in the cat: A pharmacodynamic, pharmacokinetic and toxicological study. Br Vet J 1994;150:253–262.

53. Schwab JM, Schluesener HJ, Laufer S. COX-3: Just another COX or the solitary elusive target of paracetamol? Lancet 2003;361:981–982.

54. Chandrasekharan NV, Dai H, Roos KL, et al. COX-3, a cyclooxygenase-1 variant inhibited by acetaminophen and other analgesic/antipyretic drugs: Cloning, structure, and expression. Proc Natl Acad Sci USA 2002;99:13,926–13,931.

55. Kukanich B, Lascelles BD, Aman AM, et al. The effects of inhibiting cytochrome P450 3A, p-glycoprotein, and gastric acid secretion on the oral bioavailability of methadone in dogs. J Vet Pharmacol Ther 2005;28:461–466.

56. Kukanich B, Lascelles BD, Papich MG. Pharmacokinetics of morphine and plasma concentrations of morphine-6-glucuronide following morphine administration to dogs. J Vet Pharmacol Ther 2005;28: 371–376.

57. Lascelles BD, Robertson SA, Taylor PM, et al. Comparison of the pharmacokinetics and thermal antinociceptive pharmacodynamics of 20 mcg/kg buprenorphine administered sublingually or intravenously in cats [Abstract]. Vet Anaesth Analg 2003;30:109.

58. Woolf CJ, Thompson SWN. The induction and maintenance of central sensitization is dependent on N-methyl-D-aspartic acid receptor activation: Implication for the treatment of post-injury pain hypersensitivity states. Pain 1991;44:293–299.

59. Julius D, Basbaum AI. Molecular mechanisms of nociception. Nature 2001;413:203–210.

60. Graven-Nielsen T, Arendt-Nielsen L. Peripheral and central sensitization in musculoskeletal pain disorders: An experimental approach. Curr Rheumatol Rep 2002;4:313–321.

61. Fisher K, Coderre TJ, Hagen NA. Targeting the N-methyl-D-aspartate receptor for chronic pain management: Preclinical animal studies, recent clinical experience and future research directions. J Pain Symptom Manage 2000;20:358–373.

62. Wagner AE, Walton JA, Hellyer PW, et al. Use of low doses of ketamine administered by constant rate infusion as an adjunct for postoperative analgesia in dogs. J Am Vet Med Assoc 2002;221:72–75.

63. Slingsby LS, Waterman-Pearson AE. The post-operative analgesic effects of ketamine after canine ovariohysterectomy: A comparison between pre- or post-operative administration. Res Vet Sci 2000; 69:147–152.

64. Kukanich B, Papich MG. Plasma profile and pharmacokinetics of dextromethorphan after intravenous and oral administration in healthy dogs. J Vet Pharmacol Ther 2004;27:337–341.

65. Pud D, Eisenberg E, Spitzer A, et al. The NMDA receptor antagonist amantadine reduces surgical neuropathic pain in cancer patients: A double blind, randomized, placebo controlled trial. Pain 1998;75:349–354.

66. Eisenberg E, Pud D. Can patients with chronic neuropathic pain be cured by acute administration of the NMDA receptor antagonist amantadine? Pain 1998;74:337–339.

67. Dayer P, Desmeules J, Collart L. Pharmacology of tramadol [in French]. Drugs 1997;53(Suppl 2):18–24.

68. Oliva P, Aurilio C, Massimo F, et al. The antinociceptive effect of tramadol in the formalin test is mediated by the serotonergic component. Eur J Pharmacol 2002;445:179–185.

69. Katz WA. Pharmacology and clinical experience with tramadol in osteoarthritis. Drugs 1996;52(Suppl 3):39–47.

70. Reig E. Tramadol in musculoskeletal pain: A survey. Clin Rheumatol 2002;21(Suppl 1):S9–S11; Discussion, S11–S12.

71. Adler L, McDonald C, O'Brien C, et al. A comparison of once-daily tramadol with normal release tramadol in the treatment of pain in osteoarthritis. J Rheumatol 2002;29:2196–2199.

72. Schnitzer TJ. Non-NSAID pharmacologic treatment options for the management of chronic pain. Am J Med 1998;105:45S–52S.

73. Buffington CAT. Visceral pain in humans: Lessons from animals. Curr Pain Headache Rep 2001;5:44–51.

74. Buffington CAT, Chew DJ, Woodworth BE. Feline interstitial cystitis. J Am Vet Med Assoc 1999;215:682–687.

75. Luger NM, Honore P, Sabino MA, et al. Osteoprotegerin diminishes advanced bone cancer pain. Cancer Res 2001;61:4038–4047.

76. Honore P, Luger NM, Sabino MA, et al. Osteoprotegerin blocks bone cancer–induced skeletal destruction, skeletal pain and pain-related neurochemical reorganization of the spinal cord. Nat Med 2000;6:521–528.

77. Friedland J. Local and systemic radiation for palliation of metastatic disease. Urol Clin North Am 1999;26:391–402.

78. Janssens LA, Rogers PA, Schoen AM. Acupuncture analgesia: A review. Vet Rec 1988;122:355–358.

79. Wright M, McGrath CJ. Physiologic and analgesic effects of acupuncture in the dog. J Am Vet Med Assoc 1981;178:502–507.

80. Ulett GA, Han S, Han JS. Electroacupuncture: Mechanisms and clinical application. Biol Psychiatry 1998;44:129–138.

81. Buffington T, Pacak K. Increased plasma norepinephrine concentrations in cats with interstitial cystitis [Abstract]. Urology 2001;57(6 Suppl 1):102.

82. Carroll GL, Howe LB, Slater MR, et al. Evaluation of analgesia provided by postoperative administration of butorphanol to cats undergoing onychectomy. J Am Vet Med Assoc 1998;213:246–250.

83. Lascelles BDX. Clinical efficacy of meloxicam ("Metacam") in cats with locomotor disorders. J Small Anim Pract 2001;42:587–593.

84. Franks JN, Boothe HW, Taylor L, et al. Evaluation of transdermal fentanyl patches for analgesia in cats undergoing onychectomy. J Am Vet Med Assoc 2000;217:1013–1020.

85. Glerum LE, Egger CM, Allen SW, et al. Analgesic effect of the transdermal fentanyl patch during and after feline ovariohysterectomy. Vet Surg. 2001;30:351–358.

86. Lascelles BDX. Drug therapy for acute and chronic pain in the cat. Int J Pharm Compounding 2002;6:338–343.

87. Tranquilli WJ, Grimm KA, Lamont LA. Pain Management for the Small Animal Practitioner, 2nd ed. Jackson, WY: Teton NewMedia, 2004.

Chapter 50
Orthopedic Patients

Elizabeth M. Hardie and Victoria M. Lukasik

Introduction

Veterinarians are asked to assess and treat orthopedic pain almost daily. In many cases, surgical correction of the orthopedic disease is not an option, and a treatment plan for managing ongoing chronic pain must be devised. If surgery is indicated, a plan for both anesthesia and perioperative analgesia must be designed. If trauma is the cause of the orthopedic injury, the anesthetic plan includes assessment and management of shock and injuries to other body systems. Aggressive treatment of pain associated with acute orthopedic injuries will help prevent progression to chronic pain. Once chronic pain is present, sensitization of the central nervous system may make pain control more difficult. Drug combinations, using multiple classes of drugs, are often required to obtain adequate pain relief.

Patient Evaluation

Documenting a patient's history helps to determine the chronicity of the orthopedic injury. Acute pain is more likely with traumatic or recent injury and a good response to normal doses of analgesics would be expected. If injury is more chronic, anatomical and biochemical changes in pain processing may be present, indicating a more complex approach to pain management may be required. Selection of appropriate anesthetic and analgesic drugs is influenced by general health status and the type of pain present.

The physical exam should include all body systems. Examination of the cardiovascular system should include evaluation of mucous membrane (MM) color, capillary refill time (CRT), heart rate, pulse rate, pulse quality, cardiac auscultation over all four heart valves, and blood pressure. Evaluation of the respiratory system should include rate and depth of ventilation, as well as auscultation of all lung lobes, larynx, and trachea. Evaluation of the neurological system is particularly important in trauma and older patients. Mentation should be noted, along with any other neurological deficits.

A basic laboratory evaluation is performed on all orthopedic patients undergoing anesthesia and surgery. Testing in young, healthy patients should include determination of packed cell volume (PCV), total plasma solids, blood urea nitrogen, and blood glucose. This minimal laboratory evaluation is designed to aid in the recognition of disease processes not related to the surgical problem. More complete testing is performed on trauma patients, patients with any type of localized or systemic disease, and in apparently healthy older patients. Additional testing may include a complete blood count (CBC), serum chemistry profile, electrolyte analysis, endocrine testing, electrocardiogram, and determination of blood gas or infectious disease profile. Thoracic radiographs should be performed on trauma patients to rule out pneumothorax, pulmonary contusion, or diaphragmatic hernia.

Patient Preparation

If physical exam or laboratory values for PCV, total plasma solids, or blood urea nitrogen indicate preexisting dehydration, the patient should have fluid deficits replaced intravenously. An adequate amount of the appropriate fluid (e.g., isotonic, hypertonic, hypotonic, or colloid) should be administered prior to induction of anesthesia. Recommended preanesthetic PCVs for dogs and cats are at least 30% to 34% and 25% to 29%, respectively. PCV will likely decrease after anesthetic induction, because of the vasodilatory effects of the anesthetic drugs, depressed compensatory reflexes, intravenous (IV) fluid administration, and surgical blood loss.[1] If the PCV is less than 25%, bovine hemoglobin glutamer 200 (Oxyglobin; Biopure, Cambridge, MA), whole blood, or packed red blood cells should be administered prior to the administration of any anesthetic drugs. Cardiac arrhythmias should be evaluated and treated, if necessary, prior to anesthesia and surgery. Hypothermia can be corrected by providing an external heat source, pain is managed with analgesic drugs, and acid-base or electrolyte abnormalities are addressed.

Food should be withheld for at least 8 h before anesthesia, but water can remain available until 2 h prior to administration of preanesthetic drugs.[2] This regimen will help avoid regurgitation of foodstuff, decrease gastric acidity, and minimize dehydration.

Premedication

Drugs are given prior to induction of anesthesia in order to produce mild sedation, decrease anxiety, provide analgesia, improve muscle relaxation, decrease salivary and respiratory secretions, and suppress vomiting and regurgitation. Additional reasons to use preanesthetic drugs include possibly reducing unwanted anesthetic effects by decreasing doses of induction and maintenance drugs, providing smooth anesthesia induction and recovery, and contributing to postoperative analgesia. Moderate dosing is usually preferable to the administration of a large dose of a single drug. Commonly used classes of preanesthetic drugs include antimuscarinics, benzodiazepines, opioid analgesics, phenothiazine tranquilizers, α_2-adrenergic agonists, and dissociatives.

The antimuscarinics, atropine and glycopyrrolate, can be used to decrease salivary secretions and to treat vagally mediated bradycardia associated with anesthetic and anesthetic-adjunctive drugs. Antimuscarinic administration should be avoided in patients with tachyarrhythmias and in patients with glaucoma or keratoconjunctivitis sicca. Antimuscarinics decrease tear formation and relax the iris sphincter muscle, causing mydriasis. Antimuscarinics may also increase the viscosity of respiratory secretions and should be used with caution in patients with pulmonary infections. However, muscarinic receptor block may facilitate bronchodilation and may improve some indices of respiratory function when conditions such as asthma are present.

Atropine is a small, unionized molecule that crosses the blood–brain and placental barriers. Though rare, overdose may cause seizures or altered mentation. The effect of atropine lasts approximately 1 h. Glycopyrrolate is a large, ionized molecule that does not cross the blood-brain barrier or placenta in significant quantities. It is less likely to induce tachyarrhythmias than is atropine, and overdose will usually not cause central nervous system toxicity. Vagal inhibition induced by glycopyrrolate lasts 2 to 3 h, and secretions are decreased up to 7 h.

The benzodiazepines, diazepam and midazolam, which are often used in compromised or geriatric patients, have minimal effect on cardiovascular function and have no useful analgesic activity. Both drugs are reversible with the benzodiazepine receptor antagonist flumazenil. Diazepam is supplied in a propylene-glycol vehicle, and uptake of diazepam after intramuscular (IM) or subcutaneous (SC) injection is slower and unpredictable. Diazepam should be administered slowly intravenously because the propylene glycol can cause pain, hemolysis, thrombophlebitis, and cardiotoxicity if administered rapidly.[3] Diazepam cannot be physically mixed with water-soluble drugs without risk of precipitate formation. It also begins to adsorb into plastic within a few minutes of contact, resulting in the appearance of decreased potency. In contrast, midazolam is in an aqueous vehicle and can be administered SC or IM with rapid and complete uptake and minimal pain on injection.

The addition of an opioid analgesic to premedication combinations in orthopedic patients will enhance sedation, enable a decrease in maintenance drugs, and contribute to, but not replace, postoperative analgesia. Opioids commonly used in IM or SC preanesthetic drug combinations for patients with orthopedic pain include oxymorphone, hydromorphone, morphine, and buprenorphine. Oxymorphone, hydromorphone, and morphine are full μ-receptor agonists and may be most effective for patients experiencing, or anticipated to experience, moderate to severe perioperative pain. They provide excellent analgesia and may have useful sedative properties. The μ opioid agonists may precipitate panting, which is seldom problematic.

Buprenorphine is usually classified as a partial μ, δ, and ORL-1 (nociceptin) opioid receptor agonist and a κ opioid receptor antagonist.[4,5] Buprenorphine binds with high affinity to all opioid receptors, providing a longer analgesic effect (approximately 6 to 8 h). Buprenorphine may be effective in the treatment of mild to moderate pain, but is usually a less effective analgesic than the pure μ agonists for severe pain. Butorphanol is usually classified as a partial μ antagonist and a κ and δ agonist.[6] Butorphanol has a brief analgesic action, particularly in dogs, and is usually only effective against mild pain. Both butorphanol and buprenorphine can antagonize μ receptor–mediated actions of oxymorphone, hydromorphone, or morphine. However, the net effect of combinations of opioids on analgesia may be a function of dose or route of administration. Butorphanol has better sedative properties than buprenorphine. It is the authors' opinion that butorphanol is inappropriate for managing the pain intensity experienced by most orthopedic patients. These patients would be better served by choosing an opioid with greater analgesic efficacy.

Arguably, the most commonly used phenothiazine tranquilizer in veterinary medicine is acepromazine. Its onset of action is 30 to 60 min after SC or IM injection. Acepromazine has no inherent analgesic effects, but may potentiate opioid analgesia. Acepromazine has α_1-adrenergic antagonist properties and may cause vasodilation and hypotension. Tranquilization can be overridden by stress or excitement and should not be solely relied on for chemical restraint. Acepromazine predisposes patients to hypothermia, may potentiate organophosphate toxicity and anesthetic hypoventilation, and can increase vagal tone, resulting in bradycardia.[7] It may also cause splenic sequestration of circulating erythrocytes, resulting in rapid decreases of PCV by up to 50% within 30 min of administration.[7]

The use of epinephrine to treat hypotension or cardiac arrest is relatively contraindicated when acepromazine overdose has occurred. α-Adrenergic blockade along with ß$_2$-adrenergic agonism results in paradoxical vasodilation and additional cardiovascular collapse (i.e., *epinephrine reversal*).[7] The most effective treatment for phenothiazine overdose is aggressive IV fluid administration and vasoconstrictors with minimal ß$_2$-adrenergic agonist activity, such as phenylephrine, ephedrine, or norepinephrine. After fights, trauma, or other stressful incidents, patients that have increased amounts of circulating endogenous catecholamines may also experience cardiovascular collapse because of epinephrine reversal and are not good candidates for phenothiazine administration. Acepromazine should be used with caution in patients with cardiac dysfunction, decreased cardiac reserve, hepatic dysfunction, or general debilitation, and in pediatric and geriatric patients. It has been considered by many as contraindicated in patients with a history of seizure activity. It should not be used in patients exhibiting signs of shock, trauma, hypovolemia, or organophosphate toxicity. Clinically used doses of acepromazine are not consistent with the label dose and generally are approximately one-tenth the recommended label dose.

α_2-Adrenergic agonists (e.g., medetomidine and xylazine) may be used in preanesthetic drug combinations. Unlike phenothiazines, α_2-adrenergic agonists have both profound sedative and mild analgesic properties, with sedation lasting longer than analgesia. All available α_2-adrenergic agonists are reversible with the selective α_2-adrenergic antagonist atipamezole. The α_2-adrenergic agonists cause decreased insulin release, hyperglycemia, diuresis, and potentially vomiting. The sedative effects can be overridden by pain, excitement, or stress. α_2-Adrenergic agonists may alter thermoregulation and, after high-dose administration, may make it difficult to raise peripheral veins for catheterization. Patients given α_2-adrenergic agonists may experience bradycardia, second-degree atrioventricular heart block, muscle twitching (jactitations), prolonged sedation, and pale or bluish mucous membranes. The effects on arterial blood pressure depend on route of administration, dose, and species, but are generally biphasic with an initial period of vasoconstriction and hypertension lasting 20 to 40 min, followed by a longer period of vasodilation and hypotension. α_2-Adrenergic agonists are absolutely contraindicated in patients with shock, hypotension, severe anemia, exercise intolerance, cardiac disease, increased afterload, or uncontrolled arterial hemorrhage. They are generally contraindicated in patients with respiratory disease or pulmonary dysfunction, hepatic disease, renal disease, debilitation, or stress caused by heat, cold, fatigue, or extremely high altitude. The onset of action of xylazine can be from 3 to 15 min, with sedation lasting 1 to 2 h and analgesia lasting 15 to 30 min.[8] Medetomidine is more specific for the α_2 receptor compared with xylazine, and sedation lasts approximately 2 to 4 h, with analgesia lasting a considerably shorter time. Following IM injection of an α_2-adrenergic agonist, anesthesia should not be induced for approximately 20 min to allow maximal sedative and anesthetic sparing effects to occur. Higher doses of medetomidine usually do not increase sedation, but prolong the effect. Clinically useful doses of medetomidine are considerably less than the labeled doses, especially if combined with an opioid analgesic or benzodiazepine agonist.

Dissociative anesthetic combinations given in low doses have been used as immobilization to facilitate catheterization or induction of anesthesia. The proprietary combination of the dissociative tiletamine and benzodiazepine zolazepam (Telazol) can be used to premedicate dogs and cats. This drug combination may provide enough sedation to decrease the dose of subsequent anesthetics by 50% or more. Patients receiving this drug combination may experience vomiting, salivation, excess respiratory secretions, muscle twitching or rigidity, dysphoria, and pain at the injection site. Dogs may vocalize or experience erratic or prolonged recoveries. Telazol provides only mild somatic analgesia and should not be used alone for procedures that precipitate moderate to severe pain (i.e., orthopedic procedures).

There are many potential preanesthetic protocols. In general, the combination of an opioid analgesic with a sedative-tranquilizer produces the most reliable and predictable results. The addition of

glycopyrrolate (0.01 mg/kg) SC, IM, or IV, or atropine (0.04 mg/kg) SC or IM or 0.01 mg/kg IV, may be appropriate, especially with protocols known to precipitate profound bradycardia.

General Anesthesia for Orthopedic Procedures

Preanesthetic Management

General anesthesia is a reversible process that induces immobilization, muscle relaxation, unconsciousness, and freedom from pain. It is important to have all necessary drugs and equipment ready in advance. This includes the appropriate breathing circuit, correct-size endotracheal tube and reservoir bag, changing CO_2 absorbent if necessary, checking the anesthesia machine and breathing circuit for leaks, and ensuring an adequate oxygen and anesthetic supply. Being prepared for any complication before drug administration is the key to successful anesthetic administration.

Placement of an IV catheter is recommended for all patients undergoing general anesthesia. Use the largest bore possible to enable rapid infusion of fluids and drugs in an emergency. Fluids may be bolused to dehydrated patients at this time. Other support prior to anesthetic induction includes preoxygenating patients via facemask for 1 to 2 min. This creates an increased oxygen partial pressure in the functional residual capacity, allowing more time for intubation before hemoglobin desaturation occurs. The application of sterile eye ointment will aid in keeping the cornea moist during anesthesia. It is best to avoid the use of triple-antibiotic eye ointments in feline patients because there have been some recent reports of anaphylactic reactions.[9] The operating room and prep tables should be padded appropriately, and an external heat source should be supplied. Checking MM color, CRT, heart rate, and respiratory rate prior to anesthesia enables the recognition of unwanted side effects from preanesthetic drugs.

Induction

Induction of general anesthesia in orthopedic patients is best accomplished using injectable drugs. Injectable inductions are preferred because they allow a more rapid loss of consciousness, less patient struggling, earlier control of the airway, and less danger of injury to the patient and staff. Popular drugs for IV induction include propofol (2 to 4 mg/kg IV), thiopental (5 to 15 mg/kg IV), and the combination of diazepam and ketamine. Induction doses will vary with the general health and age of the patient. Administration of preanesthetics can considerably reduce induction dose requirements. Ketamine causes a central release of catecholamines resulting in tachycardia, increased cardiac output, and increased blood pressure. However, in catecholamine-depleted patients, ketamine may act as a direct myocardial depressant and decrease cardiac output.

Immediately after anesthetic induction, an endotracheal tube is placed and the cuff inflated. Avoid overinflation of the endotracheal tube cuff to avoid tracheal crush injury or tracheal rupture. The patient's respiratory rate, heart rate and rhythm, MM color, CRT, and other parameters are checked immediately after induction and at intervals of 5 min or less. In animals with lung injury caused by trauma, pneumothorax can occur as a consequence of positive-pressure ventilation during anesthesia. When a pneumothorax is anticipated or is present, placement of a chest-drainage catheter shortly after induction allows management of what might be an anesthetic emergency during the surgical procedure. If not needed, the catheter is removed prior to recovery.

Anesthesia Maintenance

Orthopedic procedures are usually longer than 30 to 45 min, and inhalant anesthetics are preferred to injectable drugs for procedures of this duration. Isoflurane, halothane, sevoflurane, or desflurane can be used. All inhalant anesthetics cause some degree of vasodilation, hypotension, myocardial depression, and respiratory depression, necessitating appropriate anesthetic monitoring and intraoperative adjustments. Other effects may include postoperative nausea, vomiting, ileus, and cardiac arrhythmias.

Analgesic and Adjunctive Techniques

Orthopedic pain is typically classified as severe, and patients with orthopedic injuries are at risk of becoming chronic pain patients. Aggressive pain management at the time of initial injury or surgery helps to prevent progression to chronic pain.[10] In particular, patients undergoing procedures that involve severing large portions of muscles and large nerves, such as leg or tail amputation, require local anesthetic blockade of nociceptive impulses to the spinal cord. Chronic pain patients undergoing surgery to correct orthopedic disease may already have sensitized central nervous systems, thus requiring adjunctive techniques to manage their pain. Techniques used to provide additional analgesia for orthopedic patients include preoperative administration of nonsteroidal anti-inflammatory drugs (NSAIDs) if no contraindication to their use is present, ongoing provision of opioid analgesics by using transdermal patches, IV administration of opioid analgesics given as repeated bolus injections or as a continuous infusion, local anesthetic techniques, and epidural administration of analgesic drugs. Ketamine IV continuous-rate infusions (CRIs) with opioids and/or lidocaine have been described. Adjunctive analgesic techniques will decrease overall anesthetic requirement hopefully lessening the incidence and severity of unwanted side effects. Ongoing administration of sedatives, such as midazolam by CRI, may also allow for a reduction in the concentration of inhaled anesthetic gases.

Risks associated with preoperative NSAID administration include increased bleeding and exacerbation of renal disease.[11,12] Preoperative NSAID administration should therefore be limited to well-hydrated healthy patients, with normal coagulation and hemostasis parameters, that are at minimal risk of developing hypotension during the surgical procedure. IV fluids should be administered and blood pressure monitored in all patients given a preoperative NSAID.

Ongoing administration of opioid analgesics throughout the surgical procedure provides additional intraoperative and postoperative analgesia. Fentanyl can be administered as an IV CRI throughout surgery. A loading dose of 5 to 20 µg/kg is given slowly, followed by 0.3 to 0.7 µg/kg/min. Fentanyl patches are not generally relied on for intraoperative and immediate postoperative opioid delivery, but if used for this purpose, the patch should be placed on the animal at least 12 h before the start of surgery. The location of the patch is selected so that the patch will not come into direct contact with a heating pad during surgery, because heat can increase the absorption of fentanyl. Longer-acting opioids, such as oxymorphone or hydromorphone, can be administered in repeated IV bolus doses of 0.05 to 0.1 mg/kg, as needed. The effects of buprenorphine last 6 to 8 h; thus, repeated administration during surgery is usually not necessary if buprenorphine is given as a premedication.

Local anesthetic blocks are often used to inhibit nociceptive input to the central nervous system during surgical manipulations. Blockade of the infraorbital or maxillary nerve can be used when performing procedures that involve the maxilla. The mandibular nerve can be blocked when procedures involve the mandible. The foot can be desensitized by several techniques: ring block, blocks of the radial, median, and ulnar sensory nerves, and IV regional anesthesia (i.e., Bier block). The front limb can be desensitized from the elbow distally by performing a brachial plexus block. When amputating a body part, nerves are blocked with long-acting local anesthetics (e.g., bupivacaine) prior to being severed.

Lumbosacral epidural administration of opioids can be used for both forelimb amputations, which are at risk of causing chronic ghost pain, and for rear-limb procedures. Morphine alone is used for forelimb procedures, because it is water soluble and will travel cranially. Opioids are typically combined with long-acting local anesthetics to provide sensory blockade for hindlimb, pelvic, and tail procedures.

IV infusions of midazolam can increase muscle relaxation and decrease the amount of inhalant anesthetic drug necessary to maintain surgical anesthesia. The loading dose of midazolam is approximately 0.1 mg/kg IV followed by a CRI of 0.5 to 1.5 µg/kg/min IV. Midazolam has fewer cardiovascular depressant effects when compared with inhalant anesthetics. Patients with unstable cardiovascular function may benefit from decreased inhalant anesthetic doses.

Monitoring

Merril C. Sosman once stated, "You see only what you look for. You recognize only what you know."[13] Patient monitoring requires the use of one's eyes, ears, and hands in addition to electronic monitors. Monitoring heart rate, pulse, MM color, CRT, chest excursions, reservoir-bag movement, depth of anesthesia, and pulse quality is easily accomplished and gives vital clues as to how well patients are maintaining normal physiology. Electronic monitors that can be used to evaluate patient physiology under anesthesia include Doppler ultrasound, oscillometric and direct arterial blood pressure monitors, electrocardiogram monitors, pulse oximeters, thermometers, respiratory gas monitors, and blood chemistry analyzers.

The three most common unwanted side effects of anesthetic drugs are hypotension, hypothermia, and hypoventilation. Hypotension is present when mean arterial blood pressure in dogs falls below 70 mm Hg, or when systolic arterial blood pressure falls below 90 mm Hg in dogs and 100 mm Hg in cats.[14] The most common causes of hypotension in orthopedic patients are relative or absolute hypovolemia and drug effects. Therapies for hypotension include decreasing the depth of anesthesia, increasing the administration rate of IV fluids from maintenance levels (10 to 20 mL/kg/h) to as much as 90 mL/kg/h (for limited periods), and supporting circulation by the administration of inotropic drugs and vasopressors. Dopamine may be administered as a constant rate infusion at 2 to 5 µg/kg/min or dobutamine at 5 to 20 µg/kg/min. Alternatively, ephedrine may be given as an IV bolus of 0.1 to 0.25 mg/kg.

Temperature is easily monitored using a handheld thermometer or integrated temperature probe attached to a multiparameter monitor. Due to muscle relaxation, rectal temperature may be as low as 1°C (2°F) less than core body temperature. Hypothermia can be slowed or reversed by providing an external heat source. Desirable heat sources include circulating hot-water blankets, hot-water bottles, forced hot-air blankets, and resistive heating units with temperature control probes. Care should be taken to avoid thermal burns when placing plastic or metallic objects near the heat source and patient. Patients can also be warmed by administering warmed IV or lavage fluids, wrapping the extremities in an insulator-like bubble wrap, avoiding evaporative cooling by not prepping with alcohol, and keeping ambient temperatures warm. Dangerous methods of warming patients include the use of electric heating pads and infrared lamps, because of the increased risk of thermal injury. Hyperthermia is treated by removing heat sources, cooling the patient with alcohol or cool-water baths, and the administration of cool IV fluids. It is important to rule out malignant hyperthermia in patients that may be predisposed to this syndrome. It is not uncommon for Nordic breeds to become hyperthermic under anesthesia without the severe electrolyte imbalance that occurs with malignant hyperthermia syndrome. Cats may develop hyperthermia in response to higher doses of some opioids.[15]

Adequacy of ventilation may be assessed by observing movement of the reservoir bag for adequate inspiratory volume or, better, by monitoring end-tidal carbon dioxide (ETCO$_2$). Capnometers or capnographs are more useful than pulse oximetry for early detection of hypoventilation because arterial carbon dioxide, and therefore ETCO$_2$, will elevate due to hypoventilation before hemoglobin will desaturate, especially in patients breathing 100% oxygen. Additionally, pulse oximeters do not assess blood pressure and become inaccurate in the presence of hypotension, vasoconstriction, anemia, and pigmented tissues. Pulse-oximeter probes may compress vascular beds in small patients and may need to be moved periodically.

Supportive Care

It is vital to patients undergoing long periods of orthopedic repair that physiological parameters are maintained as close to normal as possible during the perianesthetic period. This mandates good supportive care for all patients undergoing surgery. As stated previously, supportive care includes the use of IV fluids to aid circulating blood volume to vital organs, provision of an external heat source to prevent hypothermia, assisted or mechanical ventilation in those patients with inadequate spontaneous ventilation,

proper patient positioning in natural anatomical alignment, and correction of specific physiologic derangements.

IV fluids will replace fluid losses and fill the increased vascular space that results from vasodilation induced by anesthetic drugs. Indications for fluid therapy include hypotension, decreased oxygen delivery, hypovolemia, dehydration, electrolyte disorders, metabolic disorders, and acid-base disturbances. Fluid selection is based on an individual patient's needs. Isotonic crystalloids are used to replace fluid from dehydration (e.g., preanesthetic fasting), hypovolemia, vasodilation, and hypotension, for normovolemic hemodilution, and to maintain plasma volume and promote renal blood flow and urine production. Approximately 4 L of isotonic crystalloid are needed to increase plasma volume by 1 L.[1] Isotonic crystalloids should be administered by a constant infusion because they are redistributed into the interstitial space within 30 to 60 min. They are recommended for all anesthesia patients at maintenance rates of 10 to 20 mL/kg/h and should be warmed to body temperature before administration. In hypotensive patients, boluses of 10 to 20 mL/kg can be administered in an attempt to increase blood pressure; however, boluses should not exceed a total volume of 90 mL/kg/h or decrease the PCV below 25%. Examples of isotonic crystalloids are Normosol-R, Isolyte-S, Plasmalyte 148, 0.9% NaCl, and lactated Ringer's solution.

Colloids are indicated in hypovolemia, hypotension, hypoalbuminemia, and for isovolemic hemodilution. They are distributed only within the plasma; therefore, it takes only 1 L of colloid to increase plasma volume by 1 L. The effect of most colloids lasts between 3 and 24 h. Examples of colloid fluids include dextran 40, dextran 70, hydroxyethyl starch, gelatin, albumin, plasma, and Oxyglobin. Synthetic colloids such as dextrans and hydroxyethyl starch may affect coagulation and should be administered judiciously in animals with the potential for ongoing hemorrhage. Polymerized hemoglobin solutions (i.e., Oxyglobin) can be used to replace intraoperative blood loss without delay for crossmatching, but have been associated with systemic hypertension and increased free-radical production.[16,17] Rapid administration of large doses of colloids in cats can lead to pulmonary edema and pleural effusion. Perhaps the best use of colloids is to administer lower doses (5 mL/kg) to reduce the amount of crystalloid fluids needed to maintain blood pressure and oxygen delivery.

Blood-replacement products should be considered if intraoperative hemorrhage is greater than 10% of total blood volume or PCV falls below 20%. Blood volume in dogs is approximately 8% to 10% body weight and in cats is 6% of body weight.[1] Estimating blood loss can be difficult. A commonly used rule of thumb is that one soaked 3 × 3-inch gauze holds 10 mL and ten soaked Q-tips hold 1 mL. Evaluating the PCV of fluid in the suction bottle can also guide an estimate of blood loss. The blood on drapes, surgeon gown and gloves, table, and floor must also be taken into account. If there is a question as to when critical blood loss is occurring, measure the patient's PCV intraoperatively and treat accordingly. For an accurate measurement, take blood for the PCV directly from a peripheral vein and do not dilute the sample with excess heparin or EDTA.

Proper patient positioning and padding is important, especially during long procedures, in arthritic patients and patients with intervertebral disk disease. Patients should be positioned to maintain normal anatomical alignment, and large muscle groups should be well padded. It is important to avoid unnecessary stress on joints and to roll patients with the spine aligned. When rolling patients, the endotracheal tube should be disconnected to avoid tracheal mucosal damage caused by twisting of the tube. Occasionally, the tube can be occluded if it is twisted.

Recovery

Pain can have severe detrimental effects within the postoperative period. Effects include delayed or poor wound healing, increased incidence of infection or sepsis, increased incidence of tumor metastasis, cardiovascular stress or compromise, increased metabolism with a negative energy balance, increased tissue catabolism, and a prolonged convalescence.[18] Therefore, it is essential to provide adequate pain relief to all orthopedic patients even though they may not show outward signs of pain or distress.

Some techniques for providing postoperative analgesia require preoperative and intraoperative planning. Fentanyl patches are best placed before surgery, because therapeutic levels of fentanyl will not be present until 8 to 12 h after placement. Provision of a wound infusion catheter for ongoing administration of local anesthetics into the wound requires placement of the catheter during surgery (Box 50.1). Single intra-articular injections of local anesthetics, morphine, and/or ketamine are performed at the conclusion of the surgical procedure. Placement of an epidural catheter for management of severely painful patients is best performed while the animal is still anesthetized.

Patients that awaken and are dysphoric may risk reinjuring the surgical site. They may need a tranquilizer to calm them and to potentiate analgesic drugs. Acceptable postoperative tranquilizers include diazepam, midazolam, medetomidine, or acepromazine at low doses. Most orthopedic patients require systemic opioid analgesics for at least 24 h after surgery (Table 50.1). Typical regimens include IV CRI of morphine, hydromorphone, or fentanyl, or periodic IV injections of oxymorphone, hydromorphone, or buprenorphine. The IV CRI of a mixture of morphine (3.3 µg/kg/min), lidocaine (50 µg/kg/min), and ketamine (10 µg/kg/min) provides excellent analgesia in dogs.[19] Wound infusion catheters can also provide excellent analgesia for cats and dogs undergoing major surgery.

Continuing to provide adequate padding, an external heat source, and a quiet environment are all essential for a smooth and uneventful recovery. Physiological monitoring should be continued during the postoperative period until patients are awake, aware, responsive, and resting quietly. Physical therapy is begun in the immediate postoperative period to reduce swelling and pain and to maintain range of motion in the joints operated on.

Patients are transitioned to oral analgesic drugs for discharge to the owner's care. Orthopedic patients are typically given analgesics for at least 1 week after surgery, and often for much longer periods. If analgesic requirements suddenly change, or are prolonged, the surgery site should be reassessed to rule out reinjury,

Box 50.1

Wound infusion catheters are sold commercially (ON-Q Soaker Catheter; I-flow, Lake Forest, CA) . Commercially available catheters are associated with less liability. Homemade medical devices carry additional risks and liabilities for veterinarians. In an emergency, a homemade catheter can be made from the following materials:

1	Five French 16- to 22-inch red rubber catheters
1	Insulin syringe with a 27- to 28-gauge needle
1	Empty sterile 3-mL syringe
1	Cigarette lighter
1	Sterile mosquito forceps
1	Sterile scissors
1	Injection cap
6	4 × 4-inch gauze sponges
1	Syringe loaded with slightly more than 1 mg/kg 0.25% bupivacaine (0.5 mg/kg for cats)

This catheter may be made in advance and then sterilized, or made up while you are gowned and gloved for surgery. Using sterile technique, cut the end off the red rubber catheter, removing its side holes. Clamp the cut tip within the jaws of the mosquito forceps and apply (or if you are gloved in, have your assistant hold the lighter) flame to the jaws of the forceps to heat them to a temperature that melts and seals the end of the catheter. Take care to avoid flaming the catheter, because the rubber will singe and turn black. One trick is to begin gently rocking the hemostat to cause the tubing to swing back and forth; when sufficiently heated, it will break off easily. In most instances, the tip will be effectively sealed. Once heating is complete, remove the forceps and attempt to inject some air into the catheter with the empty sterile syringe. If it is sealed correctly, the syringe plunger will bounce back after you attempt to push in some air. Next, place the catheter on a stack of five 4 × 4-inch gauze sponges and poke holes in it with the insulin syringe's needle. Beginning 0.5 cm back from the sealed tip, and spacing the holes no more than 0.5 cm apart, stab all the way through the center of the catheter so the needle enters the sponges underneath (the sponges keep the needle from puncturing through your tray drape). Work your way up the catheter, rotating it as you go to each new spot to avoid having all the holes in a row. Create a section of punctures long enough to cover the entire wound, plug the luer end of the catheter with the injection cap, and prime the system with bupivacaine. When properly made, the catheter will leak droplets of anesthetic along the entire working surface. Place the catheter in the deepest layer of the wound and make sure to position a portion of it over any transected large nerves. Don't anchor it firmly with any sutures. If the closed wound will be wider than 1 inch on either side of the catheter, it may help to place two or more, running in parallel to each other, to help distribute the anesthetic over a larger surface area. The catheter(s) should exit from the most dorsal part of a wound on the side of the body or from one end of a long horizontal incision. Close the wound and administer the local anesthetic. If using 0.25% bupivacaine, administer 2 mg/kg or less, repeat the injection at 6- to 8-h intervals for as long as needed (usually 1 to 3 days), and then pull the catheter. In cats, give 0.5 mg/kg every 6 to 8 h, with a total daily dose < 2 mg/kg. Intermittent administration should be performed by injecting through an injection cap attached to the luer adapter. An in-line bacterial filter (e.g., Acrodisc; Pall BioPharmaceuticals, East Hills, NY) further reduces the risk of contamination.

Table 50.1. Analgesic drugs used in dogs and cats[a].

Drug	Dose for Dogs (mg/kg)	Dose for Cats (mg/kg)
Acetaminophen	10–15 PO q 8 h for 5 days	Toxic
	Long-term therapy: ≤10 q 8 h	
Acetaminophen (300 mg) + codeine (60 mg)	Acute pain: 5–10 of acetaminophen (=1–2 of codeine) q 8	Toxic
Amantadine	3 PO q 24	3 PO q 24
Aspirin	10 PO q 12 h, *not near surgery*	10 PO q 48–72 h, *not near surgery*
Bupivacaine 0.5% solution	Up to 2, at site q 4–6 h	Up to 1, at site q 4–6 h
	Maximum is 6 on day 1, 4/day thereafter	Maximum is 2/day
Bupivacaine (preservative-free 0.25% solution)	1 mL/5 kg epidural q 4–6 h	Epidural not recommended
Buprenorphine	0.01–0.03 IM, IV, SC q 6–8 h	0.01–0.03 IM, IV, SC q 6–8 h
		0.01–0.03 PO q 6–12 h
Butorphanol	Not recommended	0.2–0.4 IV, IM SC q 2–4 h
		0.5–1.0 PO q 6–8 h
Carprofen	2 PO, SC, IV q 12 h or 4 PO, SC, IV q 24 h	1–4 PO, SC, or IV once
Deracoxib	3–4 q 24 h	Not recommended
	1–2 q 24 for chronic use	
Etodolac	5–15 PO q 24 h	Not recommended
Fentanyl, injectable	2–5 µg/kg/h IV	2–5 µg/kg/h IV
Fentanyl, transdermal	Patch to provide 2–5 µg/kg/h	25-µg patch; in small cats, cover half the patch
Gabapentin	1.25–10.0 PO q 24	1.25–10.0 PO q 24
Glucosamine and chondroitin sulfate	13–15 chondroitin sulfate PO q 24–48 h	15–20 chondroitin sulfate PO q 24–48 h
Hydromorphone or oxymorphone	0.05–0.2 IV, IM, SC q 2–4 h or 0.05 mg/kg/h IV	0.02–0.05 IV, IM, SC q 2–4 h
Ketamine (to prevent central sensitization)	0.5–2.0 IV bolus, then 1–2 mg/kg/h	0.5–2.0 IV bolus, then 1–2 mg/kg/h
Ketoprofen	1–2 IV, SC q 24 h for 3 days, or 1 PO q 24 h for 5 days	0.5–1.0 IV, SC q 24 h for 3 days, or 0.5–1.0 PO q 24 h for 3 days
Lidocaine 1%–2% solution	Up to 7, at site q 1–2 h or 1–2 mg/kg/h CRI IV or into wound	Up to 2, at site, q 1–2 h; IV not recommended; or 0.5 mg/kg/h into wound
Lidocaine 5% topical patch (Lidoderm)	Applied to affected area of skin per label directions	Safety is unclear in cats
Medetomidine (adjunct to opioid)	0.001–0.005 IV, IM	0.001–0.005 IV, IM
Meloxicam	Acute pain:	Acute pain:
	≤0.2 PO IV SC once, then ≤0.1 q 24 h	≤0.1 PO IV SC once, then ≤0.05 PO q 24 h for 3 days
	Long-term therapy: ≤0.1 q 24 h	Long-term therapy: ≤0.02 q 48–72 h
Methadone	0.5–2.2 SC, IM, 0.1–0.5 IV	0.1–0.5 SC, IM, 0.05–0.1 IV
Morphine	0.05–1.0 IV q 1–4 h	0.02–0.1 IV, q 1–4 h
	0.1–0.5/h IV infusion	
	0.2–2.0 IM, SC q 2–4 h	0.2–0.5 SC, IM q 3–4 h
	0.5–1.0 PO q 6–8 h	0.2–0.5 PO q 6–8 h (in capsule)
Morphine (preservative free)	0.1 epidural q 8 h	0.1 epidural q 8 h
	0.05 spinal q 8 h	0.05 spinal q 8 h
Naproxen	2 PO q 48 h	Toxic
Piroxicam	0.3 PO q 48 h	Controversial
Polysulfated glycosaminoglycan	5 IM weekly	No established dose, dog dose used by some
Prednisolone	0.5–1.0 PO q 12–24 h, taper to q 48 h	2 PO q 12–24 h, taper to q 48 h
Tepoxalin	10 PO q 24 h	Not recommended
Tramadol	2–5 PO q 8–12 h	No established dose, dog dose used by some
Xylazine (adjunct)	0.05–0.1 IV	0.05–0.1 IV

[a]All drugs are available in the United States. Not all drugs are approved for use in dogs and cats. CRI, continuous-rate infusion; IM, intramuscular; IV, intravenous; PO, per os (oral); and SC, subcutaneous.

infection, or other surgical complications. Tramadol-NSAID combinations, opioid-NSAID combinations, and NSAIDs alone can all be acceptable choices for longer-term analgesic therapy (Table 50.1). Transmucosal buprenorphine can be used in cats (Table 50.1). To maintain patients on individualized, optimal analgesic protocols, it is important to evaluate analgesic needs and patient well-being often.

Long-Term Patient Management

Management of chronic orthopedic pain requires a partnership between the veterinarian and the owner. The goal of long-term pain management is to provide good quality of life. The owner can be relied on to evaluate how well the animal is functioning within its normal daily activities. Weight control and routine controlled exercise, including physical rehabilitation, are essential elements in the management of orthopedic disease and require an ongoing commitment from the owner. Pharmacological approaches to chronic pain management involve a "stepladder" approach. After establishing a baseline pain-control regimen, additional drugs are added in to obtain better analgesia or to manage progressively worsening pain. The owner must assess efficacy at each step, using assessments that have been individualized for the specific patient (can climb the three porch stairs, can get up on the green couch, etc.). Nonpharmacological approaches to treatment of chronic pain, such as rehabilitation therapy, acupuncture, or therapeutic massage, require a large time commitment. Enrollment of the owner as a key element of the treatment and assessment team helps to ensure optimal pain management.

In most instances, NSAIDs are the first-line drugs for the treatment of orthopedic pain. Baseline serum chemistry and CBC should be determined and urinalysis should be performed when chronic dosing is anticipated or preexisting disease(s) are present. Renal disease, liver disease, hyperadrenocorticism, ongoing corticosteroid therapy, and evidence of gastrointestinal bleeding or occult blood loss are contraindications to initiating NSAID therapy. If there are no contraindications, an NSAID is chosen and a trial period is initiated. If the animal tolerates the NSAID without adverse effects, efficacy is evaluated by the owner. On a population basis, there is no difference in efficacy between different NSAIDS, but in individual patients efficacy can vary greatly.[20] Adverse events associated with NSAID therapy include inappetance, vomiting and diarrhea, acute idiosyncratic liver toxicity, perforating duodenal ulcer, gastrointestinal hemorrhage, and renal disease. Owners should be adequately informed of potential complications, and the owner information handouts provided by pharmaceutical manufactures should be given to owners when drugs are dispensed.

NSAIDs may be used intermittently in the early stages of orthopedic pain, particularly if a period of sustained activity is anticipated. Once an animal is dependent on NSAIDs to maintain normal daily movements, adjunctive drugs should be considered. Tramadol and acetaminophen or acetaminophen with codeine (dogs only) may be added at this stage.[21] If there are contraindications to normal NSAID use, the adjunctive and opioid drugs become the preferred treatment. Nondrug therapy (e.g., weight control, ongoing rehabilitation medical therapy and exercise, use of diets or dietary supplements containing anti-inflammatory compounds, and acupuncture) is used to slow the progression of pain and disability. As pain progresses, more potent opioids, such as oral morphine, are initiated.[22] If managed well, comfortable and active lives can often be reestablished.

References

1. Moon PF. Fluid therapy and blood transfusion. In: Seymour C, Gleed RD, eds. Manual of Small Animal Anaesthesia and Analgesia. Cheltenham: British Small Animal Veterinary Association, 1999:119–137.
2. Thurmon JC, Tranquilli WJ, Benson GJ. Considerations for general anesthesia. In: Thurmon JC, Tranquilli WJ, Benson GJ, eds. Lumb and Jones' Veterinary Anesthesia, 3rd ed. Philadelphia: Williams and Wilkins, 1996:5–349.
3. Plumb DC. Diazepam. In: Plumb DC, ed. Veterinary Drug Handbook. Ames: Iowa State University Press, 2002:245–249.
4. Miller W, Hussain F, Shan S, Hachicha M, Kyle D, Valenzano KJ. In vitro pharmacological profile of buprenorphine at mu, kappa, delta and ORL-1 opioid receptors. Soc Neurosci Abstr 2001;27:101.
5. Plumb DC. Buprenorphine. In: Plumb DC, ed. Veterinary Drug Handbook. Ames: Iowa State University Press, 2002:107–109.
6. Plumb DC. Butorphanol tartrate. In: Plumb DC, ed. Veterinary Drug Handbook. Ames: Iowa State University Press, 2002:111–114.
7. Plumb DC. Acepromazine. In: Plumb DC, ed. Veterinary Drug Handbook. Ames: Iowa State University Press, 2002:2–5.
8. Plumb DC. Xylazine HCl. In: Plumb DC, ed. Veterinary Drug Handbook. Ames: Iowa State University Press, 2002:841–884.
9. Plunkett SJ. Anaphylaxis to ophthalmic medication in a cat. Vet Emerg Crit Care 2000;10:169–171.
10. Katz J, Jackson M, Kavanagh BP, Sandler AN. Acute pain after thoracic surgery predicts long-term post-thoracotomy pain. Clin J Pain 1996;12:50–55.
11. Lemke KA, Runyon CL, Horney BS. Effects of preoperative administration of ketoprofen on whole blood platelet aggregation, buccal mucosal bleeding time, and hematologic indices in dogs undergoing elective ovariohysterectomy. J Am Vet Med Assoc 2002;220:1818–1822.
12. Lobetti RG, Joubert KE. Effect of administration of nonsteroidal anti-inflammatory drugs before surgery on renal function in clinically normal dogs. Am J Vet Res 2000;6:1501–1507.
13. Muir WW, Hubbell JAE, Skarda RT, Bednarski RM. Patient monitoring during anesthesia. In: Muir WW, Hubbell JAE, Skarda RT, Bednarski RM, eds. Handbook of Veterinary Anesthesia, 2nd ed. St Louis: CV Mosby, 2000:250–283.
14. Johnson C. Patient monitoring. In: Seymour C, Gleed RD, eds. Manual of Small Animal Anaesthesia and Analgesia. Cheltenham: British Small Animal Veterinary Association, 1999:43–55.
15. Wallenstein MC. Temperature response to morphine in paralyzed cats. Eur J Pharmacol 1978;49:331–333.
16. Oxyglobin Solution package insert. Cambridge: Biopure, 2000.
17. Olson JS, Foley EW, Rogge C, Tsai AL, Doyle MP, Lemon DD. No scavenging and the hypertensive effect of hemoglobin-based blood substitutes. Free Radic Biol Med 2004;36:685–697.
18. Hellerbrekers LJ. Pain in animals. In: Hellerbrekers LJ, ed. Animal Pain. Utrecht, The Netherlands: Van der Wees, 2000:11.
19. Muir WW III, Wiese AJ, March PA. Effects of morphine, lidocaine, ketamine, and morphine-lidocaine-ketamine drug combination on minimum alveolar concentration in dogs anesthetized with isoflurane. Am J Vet Res 2003;64:1155–1160.

20. Gibofsky A, Williams GW, McKenna F, Fort JG. Comparing the efficacy of cyclooxygenase 2–specific inhibitors in treating osteoarthritis: Appropriate trial design considerations and results of a randomized, placebo-controlled trial. Arthritis Rheum 2003;48:3102–3111.

21. Emkey R, Rosenthal N, Wu SC, Jordan D, Kamin M, for the CAPSS-114 Study Group. Efficacy and safety of tramadol/acetaminophen tablets (Ultracet) as add-on therapy for osteoarthritis pain in subjects receiving a COX-2 nonsteroidal antiinflammatory drug: A multicenter, randomized, double-blind, placebo-controlled trial. J Rheumatol 2004;31:150–156.

22. Dohoo SE, Tasker RA. Pharmacokinetics of oral morphine sulfate in dogs: A comparison of sustained release and conventional formulations. Can J Vet Res 1997;61:251–255.

Chapter 51
Horses with Colic

Cynthia M. Trim and James N. Moore

Introduction

Diseases of the gastrointestinal tract are the most common causes of colic that necessitates surgical correction. Intestinal displacement or obstruction causes abnormalities in fluid and electrolyte balance and renal function that predispose horses to risks of anesthetic overdose and circulatory failure during anesthesia. A serious consequence of intestinal hypoperfusion is endotoxemia that induces adverse changes in cellular and cardiovascular system function. Increased intra-abdominal pressure from intestinal distension causes lung collapse, hypercarbia, and hypoxemia in anesthetized horses. Ventilation is further compromised by pneumothorax in horses with concurrent diaphragmatic rupture.

Preanesthetic evaluation of each horse with colic is an essential component of case preparation to determine the horse's fluid requirements before induction of anesthesia, to anticipate and plan for the most probable complications, and to assess the need to adjust anesthetic dose rates. Administration of anesthesia must incorporate flexibility and particular attention to physiological monitoring devices to ensure timely and appropriate actions designed to maintain physiological parameters within acceptable ranges.

Impact of Endotoxemia on Physiological Status

In equine veterinary practice, endotoxemia has been associated with the diseases characterized by intestinal inflammation or ischemia. Based on several clinical studies, approximately 30% to 40% of horses presented to university hospitals with clinical signs of colic have endotoxins in their circulation.[1-4] Consequently, endotoxemia is a common complicating factor in horses being anesthetized for emergency abdominal surgery.

Endotoxin, which is a structural component of the outer cell wall of Gram-negative bacteria, is comprised of a hydrophilic region and a hydrophobic region.[5] The presence of the two regions accounts for the formation of micellar aggregates when endotox-ins enter biological fluids, such as plasma or peritoneal fluid. The hydrophilic region of endotoxin consists of an inner core, an outer core, and the O-specific polysaccharides. The polysaccharides account for serotype specificity of endotoxins among different bacterial strains. The hydrophobic region, which includes a unique fatty acid–rich portion termed *lipid A*, is responsible for the majority of the deleterious effects caused by endotoxins.[6,7] Because the core and lipid A regions of endotoxins have been well conserved, these portions are used in vaccines designed to generate antibodies to neutralize endotoxins from different Gram-negative species.

A horse's intestinal tract normally contains endotoxins as they are released from Gram-negative bacteria when they die or multiply rapidly. These endotoxins are retained within the intestinal lumen by the intestinal mucosal barrier, which is composed of epithelial cells, their secretions, and resident bacteria.[5] Some disease processes, such as intestinal ischemia or inflammation, damage this mucosal barrier, allowing endotoxins to enter the systemic circulation. Endotoxins also cross ischemic or inflamed intestine and enter the peritoneal cavity, where they stimulate the synthesis of inflammatory mediators. In at least one clinical study of horses with colic, endotoxins and inflammatory mediators were detected more commonly in peritoneal fluid than in plasma samples obtained from these horses.[8]

When endotoxins enter the circulation, they form aggregates, which interact with a plasma protein named *lipopolysaccharide (LPS)-binding protein*. LPS-binding protein is an acute-phase protein synthesized by hepatocytes.[9] LPS-binding protein transfers individual endotoxin molecules from the endotoxin aggregates to a cell surface receptor called *CD14* on mononuclear phagocytes. CD14 is a pathogen pattern recognition receptor that identifies endotoxin as part of a pathogen. CD14 exists either as a membrane-bound form or as a soluble form in biological fluids. Soluble CD14 interacts with endotoxin and LPS-binding protein, and then with cells, such as endothelial cells, that lack membrane-bound CD14. This interaction renders the endothelial cells responsive to endotoxins.[10]

Interaction among endotoxin, LPS-binding protein, and CD14 increases the sensitivity of cells to endotoxin. Although CD14 plays an important role in the cellular response to endotoxins, this receptor lacks a transmembrane component and thus cannot by itself activate the cell in response to endotoxin. In the late 1990s, biologists discovered a family of 10 receptor proteins, called *Toll-like receptors*, that also are pathogen pattern recognition receptors. Unlike CD14, the Toll-like receptors have transmembrane and intracellular components, allowing them to communicate between the exterior and interior aspects of the cell.[11] Toll-like receptor 4 is responsible for delivery of the endotoxin signal to the interior of the cell and is assisted in this function by an associated protein called *MD-2*.[12] Stimulation of Toll-like receptor 4 results in activation of genes encoding for inflammatory mediators such as tumor necrosis factor α (TNF-α) and cyclooxygenase 2, as well as those encoding for anti-inflammatory mediators such as interleukin 10.[13]

Serum concentrations of TNF-α increase shortly after in vivo administration of endotoxin and correlate with hypotension, hemoconcentration, metabolic acidosis, and disseminated intravascular coagulation.[14] TNF-α initiates these responses by increasing the synthesis of other inflammatory mediators (including the interleukins, eicosanoids, and tissue factor), stimulating the acute-phase response and fever. Several clinical studies in horses have revealed correlations between increases in serum concentrations of TNF-α and prognosis for survival.[15,16] Increased concentrations of TNF-α also have been documented in peritoneal fluid from horses with naturally occurring intestinal diseases.[8]

Arachidonic acid, a 20-carbon fatty acid in cell membrane phospholipids, is metabolized by cyclooxygenase to vasoactive substances such as thromboxane A_2 and prostaglandins I_2, E_2, and $F_2\alpha$. There is considerable information regarding the cyclooxygenase metabolites of arachidonic acid, which mediate many of the early hemodynamic effects of endotoxemia.[17]

Tissue factor, otherwise known as thromboplastin or procoagulant activity, is a glycoprotein that is synthesized primarily by monocytes and macrophages. Because tissue factor remains associated with the surface of these cells, it is exposed to coagulation factor VII in plasma. As a result, cells that synthesize tissue factor in response to endotoxin may become a focus for the formation of microthrombi. Tissue factor activity increases in equine monocytes exposed to endotoxin in vitro, in horses with experimentally induced endotoxemia, and in horses with naturally occurring diseases characterized by colic.[18,19] In a clinical study of horses with colic, the severity of the increase in tissue factor activity correlated inversely with prognosis.[19]

In addition to the synthesis of proinflammatory mediators in response to endotoxins, there is considerable evidence that the synthesis and release of anti-inflammatory mediators also is increased. The most widely studied of these anti-inflammatory mediators is *interleukin 10*, a cytokine that deactivates mononuclear phagocytes and inhibits the synthesis of proinflammatory cytokines.[20] The results of studies in other species indicate that neutralization of interleukin 10 increases both production of TNF-α and lethality. There also is evidence indicating that susceptibility to infectious agents increases if the synthesis and release of anti-inflammatory mediators becomes the predominant response.[21]

Preparation for Anesthesia

Preparation for anesthesia includes all the procedures implemented for elective anesthesia, such as checking the anesthetic and monitoring equipment, assembling anesthetic and emergency drugs, and preanesthetic evaluation of the patient. Preparation of the patient should include treatment of hypovolemia, critical electrolyte abnormalities, and severe metabolic acidosis. Preanesthetic fluid therapy commonly includes infusion of at least 20 mL/kg of balanced electrolyte solution to expand circulatory blood volume. Horses with evidence of impaired cardiovascular function, such as weak pulses and prolonged capillary refill, given hypertonic (7.5%) saline before anesthesia, 2 to 4 mL/kg over 10 min, are less likely to develop hypotension immediately after induction of anesthesia. It is important to infuse balanced electrolyte in the following 1 to 2 h after hypertonic saline administration to prevent dehydration. Hypocalcemia can be treated with 23% intravenous (IV) calcium borogluconate, 0.5 mL/kg.

In addition to the aforementioned approaches to preparing patients for anesthesia and surgery, three additional therapeutic approaches should be considered when endotoxemia is suspected: (a) minimizing the movement of endotoxin into the circulation, (b) interfering with the interaction between endotoxins and the inflammatory cells, and (c) preventing the synthesis, release, or action of inflammatory mediators.

For horses with intestinal ischemia, the decision for surgery must be made as early as possible to remove the affected intestine and, hopefully, reduce the transmural movement of endotoxin across the damaged mucosa. Although the vast majority of horses with endotoxemia are not bacteremic, some clinicians elect to include *antimicrobial agents* in the treatment of horses undergoing emergency abdominal surgery. Based on recent experimental studies with isolated equine leukocytes, killing of *Escherichia coli* bacteria with ß-lactam antimicrobial agents significantly increases both the release of endotoxin and cellular synthesis of TNF-α when compared with the effects elicited by amikacin or the combination of amikacin and ampicillin. Consequently, it may be advantageous to administer polymyxin B or serum containing antiendotoxin antibodies to neutralize endotoxin when ß-lactam antimicrobials are used.[22]

Currently, two approaches are used in an effort to neutralize endotoxin before it activates inflammatory cells. The first of these involves administration of antibodies directed against the conserved core and lipid A regions of endotoxin. Serum or plasma products enriched in these antibodies are commercially available and have been used in clinical and experimental trials with conflicting results. In some studies, *antiendotoxin antibodies* have been of benefit in experimental endotoxemia and in horses with colic.[23–25] The results of other studies have failed to identify the same positive effects.[26–28] A common treatment regimen involves administration of 1.5 mL/kg IV of the antiendotoxin serum diluted at least twofold and preferably 10- to 20-fold in balanced IV fluids. Controlled clinical trials with strict entrance criteria are needed to compare the efficacy of antiendotoxin antibodies and nonspecific immunoglobulins. In such trials, the treatments would have to be instituted as early as possible in the course of the disease to give this method of treatment an opportunity to be successful.

Alternatively, *polymyxin B*, an antibiotic that binds tightly with lipid A, may be used to prevent endotoxin from interacting with the horse's inflammatory cells.[26,29] Although many clinicians initially expressed concern about the known toxic side effects of this drug, it appears that the concentrations needed to bind endotoxin are far less than those that cause the toxic effects. As a result, polymyxin B has been evaluated in several experimental studies and currently is being used in clinical cases. Based on the results of those studies, polymyxin B is used at 1000 to 5000 units/kg two to three times daily.[26,30] It also has been recommended that particular attention be paid to maintaining fluid-replacement therapy and periodic monitoring of serum creatinine concentration.[30]

A mainstay in the treatment of endotoxemia is the administration of drugs that interfere with the synthesis of inflammatory mediators. Currently, the most common types of drugs used for this purpose are the *nonsteroidal anti-inflammatory drugs* (NSAIDs). NSAIDs exert their beneficial effects by inhibiting cyclooxygenase, the enzyme responsible for generation of prostaglandins and thromboxanes.[31] These arachidonic acid metabolites have been associated with many of the early hemodynamic responses to endotoxin. Of the two primary cyclooxygenase isoforms, it appears that the inducible isoform (cyclooxygenase 2 [COX-2]) is responsible for the increased synthesis of prostanoids in response to inflammatory stimuli, such as endotoxin.[32] The constitutive isoform (COX-1) is more responsible for maintaining mucosal and renal blood flow.[33] The results of studies comparing nonselective NSAIDs indicate that flunixin meglumine and ketoprofen are most effective at preventing endotoxin-induced synthesis of prostaglandins and thromboxane and clinical signs of endotoxemia. With the toxic side effects of NSAIDs (gastrointestinal ulceration and renal papillary necrosis) being of concern, a study was performed to determine whether a reduced dosage of flunixin meglumine (0.25 mg/kg) might be effective in an experimental model of endotoxemia.[34] As a result of that study, use of this reduced dosage of flunixin meglumine has become standard practice in many clinical settings. However, no clinical studies have been performed to test whether this form of treatment is efficacious or how long it should be continued after surgery. With the development of new selective COX-2 inhibitors, it will be interesting to compare their effectiveness in endotoxemic horses with naturally occurring gastrointestinal diseases.

Pentoxifylline is another drug that has been used in the treatment of endotoxemic horses. Although it reduced endotoxin-induced production of cytokines, thromboxane, and expression of tissue factor in studies in vitro, its beneficial effects in endotoxemic horses in vivo appear very limited.[35] Additionally, only slight benefits of either drug alone were detected when pentoxifylline and flunixin meglumine were used in combination in a study of experimental endotoxemia.[36] However, because of its reported ability to increase the erythrocyte deformability and, as a result, improve microvascular blood flow, pentoxifylline is used widely in horses with laminitis.[37]

Horses with colic that have clinical signs consistent with endotoxemia (i.e., alterations in mucous membrane color and capillary refill time, decreased gastrointestinal sounds, increased heart and respiratory rates, and evidence of dehydration) are candidates for treatment. Although the primary goal should be to identify the underlying cause of endotoxemia, treatment usually must be started before a definitive diagnosis can be made. In these situations, it is reasonable to administer flunixin meglumine and either polymyxin B or antiendotoxin serum diluted in balanced IV fluids. Many clinicians also treat horses with pentoxifylline in an attempt to prevent acute laminitis.

Anesthetic Protocols

There is no universal choice of anesthetic agents for induction and maintenance of anesthesia in horses with colic. This author's preference for premedication of adult horses is a combination of xylazine (up to 1.1 mg/kg IV), butorphanol (0.02 mg/kg IV), and diazepam (0.05 mg/kg IV), with ketamine (up to 2.2 mg/kg IV) for induction of anesthesia. Anesthesia is maintained with isoflurane or sevoflurane in oxygen with controlled ventilation. Premedication may be considerably decreased or omitted if sedatives or opioids have been recently administered during the preoperative evaluation period. Romifidine or detomidine are other sedatives that can be used as substitutes for xylazine. Small doses of detomidine (0.004 mg/kg) can be used with reduced doses of xylazine (up to 0.8 mg/kg) to increase the analgesia and sedation over that usually provided by xylazine alone. Xylazine, romifidine, and detomidine produce dose-dependent decreases in intestinal motility; therefore, doses administered should be as low as possible.

Horses with colic may become hypotensive for a variety of reasons during anesthesia, including hypovolemia, acidosis, endotoxemia, effects of anesthetic drugs, increased intra-abdominal pressure, and aortocaval syndrome. *Guaifenesin* decreases mean arterial pressure in proportion to the dose administered and, therefore, lower-than-usual dose rates for guaifenesin should be used for horses with colic when guaifenesin is included in the anesthetic protocol. Guaifenesin is a useful muscle-relaxing drug for induction of anesthesia in excited or violent horses because it may facilitate tracheal intubation and transportation of the horse to the surgery room. Unfortunately, even when blood pressure is satisfactory immediately after induction of anesthesia when the horse is in lateral recumbency, arterial pressure frequently decreases dramatically when the horse is turned onto its back for hoisting or positioning on the surgery table. Horses that need immediate induction of anesthesia because abdominal distension is causing life-threatening hypoventilation and cardiovascular collapse can be supported by infusion of dobutamine and nasal insufflation of oxygen throughout induction. Rapid intubation and controlled ventilation with oxygen are advisable before transportation to the surgery room.

There are pronounced differences in cardiovascular function in horses maintained under anesthesia with halothane or isoflurane. *Isoflurane* anesthesia causes less depression of the cardiovascular system than does halothane, thereby allowing cardiac output, arterial oxygen tension, and muscle blood flow to remain higher during controlled ventilation.[38–41] After anesthesia is discontinued, the duration of recumbency is largely determined by the adjunct anesthetic agents administered, the temperament of the horse, and the features of the environment used for recovery (e.g., pads, lighting, and sound). However, elimination of isoflurane is more rapid than halothane, and this decreases the duration of ataxia after standing. *Sevoflurane* is eliminated even more rapidly than isoflurane, and that may result in a better quality of recovery, a factor that may be a persuasive argument for using sevoflurane for anesthesia in sick horses.[42,43] All inhalation agents cause vasodilation and progressive decreases in arterial blood pressure with increasing depth of anesthesia. This may result in a worsening of hypotension in dehydrated, endotoxemic horses. Various anesthetic manipulations may be necessary to maintain mean arterial blood pressure above 70 mm Hg.

Inclusion of an *opioid* in anesthetic protocols has long been recommended for balanced anesthesia in humans. Inclusion of the opioid is to provide analgesia and contribute to the central nervous system depression provided by the combination of drugs used for induction and maintenance of anesthesia. A dilemma in equine anesthesia is that some opioids induce central nervous system stimulation, characterized primarily by increased locomotor activity, an untoward effect limiting the choice of opioids that can be used in horses. Intuitively, inclusion of an opioid in anesthetic management seems to be a logical step to providing analgesia. Analgesia by opioid use has been demonstrated in conscious horses by using a variety of experimental models. However, studies of several opioids have failed to confirm that these agents consistently reduce inhalation anesthetic requirements in horses.[44–46]

Butorphanol is licensed for use in horses and provides significant sedation. As a result, butorphanol is often used for premedication and to facilitate a smooth induction of anesthesia. The effect of this opioid lasts about 1 h, so repeated injections or continuous infusion must be given for continued effect. One published study has confirmed that infusion of butorphanol at 0.024 mg/kg/h in healthy awake horses maintains constant blood butorphanol concentrations.[47] Butorphanol can be administered conveniently during anesthesia by adding it to 0.9% saline to achieve a concentration of 1 mg/mL. The solution is then administered with a syringe pump that enables the infusion rate to be closely regulated. Although butorphanol does not significantly reduce an animal's requirement for an inhalant agent, our clinical impression is that its inclusion in the anesthetic regimen adds positively to the overall anesthetic effect.

Although *morphine* has been used intraoperatively as an analgesic in horses under anesthesia,[48] the results of another investigation failed to identify any reduction in inhalation agent requirement when a low dose of morphine was administered.[46] Furthermore, efforts to provide additional analgesia by using higher doses of morphine resulted in excitement during recovery from anesthesia.[46] Morphine also causes significant depression of intestinal motility, thereby further reducing the advisability of its systemic use in horses with colic.

Continuous infusion of *lidocaine* (loading dose 2.5 mg/kg, followed by an infusion of 0.05 mg/kg/min) has been reported to decrease the isoflurane requirement by 25% in healthy horses anesthetized for elective surgery.[49] Thus, one purpose for administering lidocaine during anesthesia is to reduce the dose-dependent vasodilation that occurs with inhalation anesthetics and to maintain a higher arterial blood pressure.[50] A second reason for administering lidocaine is its potential to provide analgesia and decrease postoperative hyperesthesia induced by surgery. In a recent study in which lidocaine was administered as a continuous infusion,[49] no significant differences in mean arterial pressure, arterial blood gases, or plasma concentrations of cortisol and nonesterified fatty acids were identified between horses administered lidocaine and horses not administered lidocaine. There is some evidence in other species that systemic administration of lidocaine may have analgesic activity and prevent induction of central hyperalgesia. As evidence of this, the results of a recently published investigation of human patients undergoing major abdominal surgery determined that patients who received lidocaine during anesthesia needed less morphine during the first 72 h after surgery.[51]

A third potential benefit to the administration of lidocaine may be the ability to modulate the inflammatory response.[52] In rabbits, for example, lidocaine given intravenously immediately after an endotoxin bolus prevented the adverse hemodynamic and cytokine responses to endotoxemia.[53] In rats, systemic or topically applied lidocaine reversed the secretory change in the intestinal wall induced by intestinal obstruction.[54]

Endotoxemia and postoperative ileus are both serious consequences of colic in horses. In a survey of 54 horses undergoing anesthesia and surgery for colic, endotoxin was detected in the circulation during anesthesia in 20 horses (37%), and endotoxemia developed after the start of surgery in 9 of the 20 horses.[55] The incidence of postoperative ileus has been reported to be as high as 20% and imposes considerable morbidity and hospitalization costs.[56] The effects of lidocaine on intestinal function have been studied in clinical colic patients by using a loading dose of lidocaine (0.65 mg/kg IV), followed by infusion of the drug (0.025 mg/kg/min) through anesthesia and then at twice that rate after anesthesia.[57] The control horses received an equal volume of saline, and the investigators were blinded as to the treatment. Of the horses, 64% had large colon disease and 28.6% required small intestinal resections. Measured intraoperative serum lidocaine concentrations were from 0.39 to 2.72 µg/mL (mean, 1.06 µg/mL). No differences were obtained between horses given lidocaine and control horses for presence of gastrointestinal sounds on auscultation, time to passage of first feces, duodenal or jejunal wall thickness, or maximum duodenal and jejunal cross-sectional area as judged by percutaneous ultrasonography. Significant differences were measured between the groups for minimum jejunal cross-sectional area and diameter. The authors concluded these small changes were not sufficient to assess the influence of lidocaine on postoperative ileus. Another study of risk factors associated with postoperative ileus in horses identified increased odds for ileus in horses that had a small intestinal lesion, high preoperative hematocrit, and anesthesia duration exceeding 3 h for lesions not involving small intestine.[56]

Significant difficulties arise in interpreting data from clinical studies when a variety of treatments are used. Evaluation of the impact of treatments on postoperative events should take into account use of *hypertonic saline* because hypertonic saline has been shown to modulate inflammatory responses in patients in shock. Recent studies using a model of intestinal ischemia and reperfusion in laboratory animals have demonstrated that hypertonic saline decreases mucosal injury and decreases ileus.[58] Other investigations have demonstrated that hypertonic saline dramatically improves survival rate in animal models of hemorrhagic shock and sepsis.[59]

Hypoventilation and Hypoxemia During Anesthesia

Hypoventilation is a common complication in horses during anesthesia for colic surgery. Controlled ventilation is advisable to avoid the adverse consequences of severe hypercarbia. Ventilation with a tidal volume of 10 mL/kg at a respiratory rate of 10 breaths per minute will result in normocarbia in horses undergoing elective procedures. Peak inspiratory pressure in these animals is usually about 20 to 24 cm H_2O. Higher pressures will be needed to deliver an adequate tidal volume in horses with abdominal distension. Pressures exceeding 40 cm H_2O may cause alveolar rupture, however, and, until the abdomen has been opened and the colon decompressed, adequate ventilation may not be achieved even at these pressures in some horses with colonic distention. The risk of pulmonary damage in these horses can be reduced by limiting the peak inspiratory pressure to 40 cm H_2O and permitting some degree of hypercarbia to occur. Although elevations in $PaCO_2$ can be confirmed by blood-gas analysis, capnography may or may not provide an accurate estimate of $PaCO_2$ in these patients. The difference between end-tidal CO_2 and $PaCO_2$ in colic horses is greater than in healthy horses, and $PaCO_2$ during controlled ventilation has been reported to be 10 to 13 mm Hg higher than end-tidal CO_2.[60,61] In fact, the difference between end-tidal CO_2 and $PaCO_2$ may be as high as 25 mm Hg in some animals and is greater during spontaneous ventilation. One way of dealing with this problem is to use blood-gas analysis at the beginning of anesthesia to determine whether a large difference exists and then use capnography as a guide for the remainder of the anesthetic period. Ventilation of horses for colic surgery to end-tidal CO_2 values of 30 to 40 mm Hg in the absence of blood-gas analysis will maintain $PaCO_2$ values close to the normal range in the majority of horses.

Lung collapse may be sufficient to result in hypoxemia (PaO_2 < 60 mm Hg). Occasionally, opening the abdomen and decompression of the intestines will enable a sufficient increase in ventilation to expand the lung and improve oxygenation. More frequently, however, PaO_2 does not increase until after anesthesia. Maneuvers such as changing the ventilatory pattern or imposing positive end-expiratory pressure (PEEP) are not often successful in increasing PaO_2. Horses with hypoxemia often survive anesthesia, rendering the impact of hypoxemia on morbidity speculative. Interestingly, in a survey of 600 horses anesthetized for colic surgery, hypoxemia was present in 17%, and the survival rates for these horses and horses with normal oxygenation were not different (C.M. Trim, unpublished data).

Cardiovascular Performance During Anesthesia

Decreased cardiovascular performance commonly occurs in horses during anesthesia for colic surgery. Consequently, one of the first priorities is to maintain mean arterial pressure above 70 mm Hg. Horses that have insufficient fluid therapy before anesthesia will need rapid volume expansion to counter vasodilation caused by inhalation anesthetics. A balanced electrolyte solution, such as acetated or lactated Ringer's solution, should be infused at 10 mL/kg/h in horses with a normal fluid balance and at an increased rate in horses that are volume depleted. Hypertonic (7.5%) saline (4 mL/kg IV) can be administered over 10 min as a rapid infusion to counteract hypovolemia. Increases in cardiac output and mean arterial blood pressure have been measured for 1 h after infusion of hypertonic saline in horses subjected to endotoxemia[62] or hemorrhage.[63]

Vasoactive drugs, such as dobutamine, dopamine, and ephedrine, are used to increase cardiac output and blood pressure during anesthesia. Dobutamine (0.5 to 5.0 µg/kg/min) is frequently effective in correcting anesthetic-induced hypotension. Potential adverse effects of dobutamine treatment are bradycardia and tachycardia. Dobutamine infusion may induce bradycardia, with or without second-degree heart block, that is sufficient to decrease arterial blood pressure further. Management of second-degree heart block includes decreasing the dose rate of the dobutamine and administering ephedrine, atropine (0.005 to 0.01 mg/kg), or dopamine to increase the heart rate and blood pressure. Endotoxemia may alter the sensitivity of cardiac ß receptors such that administration of dobutamine has less effect on cardiac output and causes tachycardia. Techniques to increase arterial blood pressure then must focus on efforts to expand blood volume and decrease the concentration of anesthetic delivered. Dopamine (3.0 to 6.0 µg/kg/min) is used to increase renal blood flow in horses with increased serum creatinine concentrations, to increase cardiac output, and to increase heart rate in horses with advanced atrioventricular heart block. Ephedrine is most effective in animals with excessive vasodilation, because ephedrine-induced venoconstriction increases venous return to the heart. Ephedrine (0.06 mg/kg IV bolus) has been reported to increase cardiac output and mean arterial blood pressure in anesthetized horses for 30 to 40 min.[64] Arterial pressure in anesthetized horses with colic also can be increased by an infusion of a 23% solution of calcium gluconate (100 to 200 mL per adult horse) given over 15 min. Significant increases in cardiac output and mean arterial pressure have been measured in healthy anesthetized horses during infusion of calcium gluconate.[40] An infusion rate of 0.1 mg/kg/min effectively improved cardiac function in horses anesthetized with isoflurane, whereas a higher dose rate of 0.4 mg/kg/min was necessary to improve cardiac function in horses anesthetized with halothane. Preanesthetic determination of serum electrolyte concentrations will identify some horses with colic that are hypocalcemic, and treatment of these horses with calcium gluconate before anesthesia is warranted. Of concern is the potential adverse impact of exogenously administered calcium in critically ill horses with cardiovascular failure, endotoxemia, or hypoxemia.

Assessment of cardiovascular system function must include interpretation of mean arterial pressure with systolic-diastolic pressure difference, arterial pressure waveform, capillary refill time (CRT), and mucous membrane color to arrive at an estimate of cardiac output. A low systolic pressure, dramatic fluctuations in systolic pressure with the ventilator cycle, flattened arterial waveform, and prolonged CRT are indicators of low cardiac output. Further, increases in arterial pressure after vasoconstriction, such as that induced by onset of surgery, may be accompanied by any change in cardiac output, including a decrease resulting from an excessive increase in afterload.[65]

Hypotension that is primarily caused by vasodilation and that is unresponsive to both fluid loading and catecholamines may be countered by decreasing the inspired concentration of the inhalation agent. Under such circumstances, administration of sedatives, opioids, or injectable anesthetics will be necessary to maintain the desired lack of response to surgery. Continuous infusions of either lidocaine, ketamine, or a mixture of guaifenesin-ketamine-xylazine have been used to provide sufficient additional analgesia to reduce the inspired inhalent concentration. Collectively, any of these treatments may result in an increase in mean arterial pressure, because of a reduction in anesthetic agent–induced vasodilation.[49,50] Inclusion of a morphine epidural nerve block may provide additional analgesia. Definitive studies that include measurement of cardiac output are needed to ascertain the effects of different treatments on overall cardiovascular performance. It is unclear whether these treatments allow a decreased inhalation agent requirement by providing sedation or analgesia or both.

Cardiac dysrhythmias are an occasional complication in horses anesthetized for colic surgery. The concurrent presence of atrial fibrillation and gastrointestinal disease can result in hypotension that is difficult to treat. If the usual therapies to improve cardiovascular function fail to produce an adequate mean arterial pressure, administration of *quinidine* (up to 10 mg/kg in divided IV boluses) is the recommended treatment. Premature ventricular depolarizations also develop in a small number of horses as a consequence of endotoxemia. Treatment is not always necessary, but lidocaine can be used to decrease the frequency of abnormal beats when arterial blood pressure is decreased by the dysrhythmias.

Recovery from Anesthesia

Controlled ventilation can be continued up to the time the horse is disconnected from the anesthesia machine, where a demand valve should be available to continue ventilation in the recovery stall. Sometimes reducing the depth of anesthesia before the end of surgery to ensure rapid return of spontaneous ventilation is not feasible, especially when horses must be hoisted from the surgery table or if the time required to transport a horse from the surgery room to the recovery stall is long. Although oxygenation is maintained for some minutes when a horse becomes apneic after being disconnected from the anesthesia machine, PaO_2 values will decrease dramatically in horses breathing room air spontaneously early in the recovery period. This author's preference is to control ventilation with a demand valve and oxygen for the first 10 min of recovery and then to allow the horse to breathe spontaneously with oxygen insufflated at a rate of 15 L/min into the nose or endotracheal tube. The nasogastric tube is removed for recovery from anesthesia.

Some anesthesiologists prefer to leave the endotracheal tube in place while a horse recovers from anesthesia, whereas others prefer to remove it once the horse can swallow. However, if regurgitation around the nasogastric tube has occurred during anesthesia or if the nasal mucosa is congested and swollen, the endotracheal tube should remain in place until the horse is sternal or stands.

The usual methods to discourage horses from attempting to stand too early, such as positioning the horse on pads or an air cushion in a warm, quiet recovery room with dim lighting, should also be applied to horses after colic surgery. Often supplemental sedation is provided in the form of xylazine (0.2 mg/kg IV) given approximately 5 min after the inhalant is discontinued. Assistance to a standing position using ropes tied to the halter and tail should be considered when factors that contribute to ataxia are present, such as horses that are more than 20 years of age, rectal temperature less than 35.5°C (96°F), hypotension during anesthesia, clinical evidence of endotoxemia, and an anesthesia time that exceeds 3 h.

Analgesia is continued into the postoperative period by using nonsteroidal anti-inflammatory agents and continuous infusions of butorphanol and lidocaine. The results of one published investigation of butorphanol administration by continuous IV infusion documented a significant delay in the time to passage of feces when compared with values for horses that were not given butorphanol (median times of 15 and 4 h, respectively).[47] Preliminary evaluation of a transdermal fentanyl patch (Duragesic) to provide analgesia in horses has identified evidence of analgesia for conditions involving visceral pain.[66] One investigation of the pharmacokinetics of transdermally applied fentanyl described rapid absorption and blood concentrations exceeding 1 ng/mL by 3 h after application of two 10-mg transdermal fentanyl patches to healthy adult horses.[67] Serum concentrations of this magnitude were sustained for 32 h, thus offering a convenient method of supplying a constant level of analgesic drug.

References

1. Steverink PJGM, Sturk A, Rutten VPMG, Wagenaar-Hilbers JPA, Klein WR, van der Velden MA. Endotoxin, interleukin-6 and tumor necrosis factor concentrations in equine acute abdominal disease: Relation to clinical outcome. J Endotoxin Res 1995;2:289–299.
2. King JN, Gerring EL. Detection of endotoxin in cases of equine colic. Vet Rec 1988;123:269–271.
3. Fessler JF, Bottoms GD, Coppoc GL, Gimarc S, Latshaw HS, Noble JK. Plasma endotoxin concentrations in experimental and clinical equine subjects. Equine Vet J Suppl 1989;7:24–28.
4. Barton MH, Morris DD, Norton N, Prasse KW. Hemostatic and fibrinolytic indices in neonatal foals with presumed septicemia. J Vet Intern Med 1998;12:26–35.
5. Raetz CR, Whitfield C. Lipopolysaccharide endotoxins. Annu Rev Biochem 2002;71:635–700.
6. Moore JN. Endotoxemia: Definition, characterization, and host defenses. Compend Contin Educ 1981;3:355–359.

7. Moore JN, Morris DD. Endotoxemia and septicemia in horses: Experimental and clinical correlates. J Am Vet Med Assoc 1992; 200:1903–1914.

8. Barton MH, Collatos C. Tumor necrosis factor and interleukin-6 activity and endotoxin concentration in peritoneal fluid and blood of horses with acute abdominal disease. J Vet Intern Med 1999;13: 457–464.

9. Wurfel MM, Wright SD. Lipopolysaccharide-binding protein and soluble CD14 transfer lipopolysaccharide to phospholipid bilayers: Preferential interaction with particular classes of lipid. J Immunol 1997;158:3925–3934.

10. Tobias PS, Ulevitch RJ. Lipopolysaccharide binding protein and CD14 in LPS dependent macrophage activation. Immunobiology 1993;187:227–232.

11. Wright SD. Toll, a new piece in the puzzle of innate immunity. J Exp Med 1999;189:605–609.

12. Shimazu R, Akashi S, Ogata H, et al. MD-2, a molecule that confers lipopolysaccharide responsiveness on Toll-like receptor 4. J Exp Med 1999;189:1777–1782.

13. Nakao S, Ogtata Y, Shimizu E, Yamazaki M, Furuyama S, Sugiya H. Tumor necrosis factor alpha (TNF-alpha)–induced prostaglandin E2 release is mediated by the activation of cyclooxygenase-2 (COX-2) transcription via NFkappaB in human gingival fibroblasts. Mol Cell Biochem 2002;238:11–18.

14. Morris DD, Crowe N, Moore JN. Correlation of clinical and laboratory data with serum tumor necrosis factor activity in horses with experimentally induced endotoxemia. Am J Vet Res 1990;51: 1935–1940.

15. Morris DD, Moore JN, Crowe N. Serum tumor necrosis factor activity in horses with colic attributable to gastrointestinal tract disease. Am J Vet Res 1991;52:1565–1569.

16. MacKay RJ. Association between serum cytotoxicity and selected clinical variables in 240 horses admitted to a veterinary hospital. Am J Vet Res 1992;53:748–752.

17. Moore JN, Hardee MM, Hardee GE. Modulation of arachidonic acid metabolism in endotoxemic horses: Comparison of flunixin meglumine, phenylbutazone and a selective thromboxane synthetase inhibitor. Am J Vet Res 1986;47:110–113.

18. Henry MM, Moore JN. Endotoxin-induced procoagulant activity in equine peripheral blood monocytes. Circ Shock 1988;26:297–309.

19. Henry MM, Moore JN. Clinical relevance of monocyte procoagulant activity in horses with colic. J Am Vet Med Assoc 1991;198: 843–848.

20. Hawkins DL, MacKay RJ, MacKay SL, Moldawer LL. Human interleukin 10 suppresses production of inflammatory mediators by LPS-stimulated equine peritoneal macrophages. Vet Immunol Immunopathol 1998;66:1–10.

21. Bone RC. Sir Isaac Newton, sepsis, SIRS, and CARS. Crit Care Med 1996;24:1125–1128.

22. Bentley AP, Barton MH, Lee MD, Norton NA, Moore JN. Antimicrobial-induced endotoxin and cytokine activity in an in vitro model of septicemia in foals. Am J Vet Res 2002;63:660–668.

23. Garner HE, Sprouse RF, Green EM. Active and passive immunization for blockade of endotoxemia. In: Milne FJ, ed. Proceedings of the Annual Convention of the American Association of Equine Practitioners, Lexington, KY, 1986.

24. Garner HE, Sprouse RF, Lager K. Cross-protection of ponies from sublethal Escherichia coli endotoxemia by Salmonella typhimurium antiserum. Equine Pract 1988;10:10–17.

25. Spier SJ, Lavoie JP, Cullor JS, Smith BP, Snyder JR, Sischo WM. Protection against clinical endotoxemia in horses by using plasma

26. Durando MM, MacKay RJ, Linda S, Skelley LA. Effects of polymyxin B and Salmonella typhimurium antiserum on horses given endotoxin intravenously. Am J Vet Res 1994;55:921–927.

27. Morris DD, Whitlock RH, Corbeil LB. Endotoxemia in horses: Protection provided by antiserum to core lipopolysaccharide. Am J Vet Res 1986;47:544–550.

28. Morris DD, Whitlock RH. Therapy of suspected septicemia in neonatal foals using plasma-containing antibodies to core lipopolysaccharide (LPS). J Vet Intern Med 1987;1:175–182.

29. Parviainen AK, Barton MH, Norton NN. Evaluation of polymyxin B in an ex vivo model of endotoxemia in horses. Am J Vet Res 2001;62:72–76.

30. Barton MH. Use of polymyxin B for treatment of endotoxemia in horses. Compend Contin Educ 2000;11:1056–1059.

31. Daels PF, Stabenfeldt GH, Hughes JP, Odensvik K, Kindahl H. Effects of flunixin meglumine on endotoxin-induced prostaglandin F2 alpha secretion during early pregnancy in mares. Am J Vet Res 1991;52:276–281.

32. Hocherl K, Dreher F, Kurtz A, Bucher M. Cyclooxygenase-2 inhibition attenuates lipopolysaccharide-induced cardiovascular failure. Hypertension 2002;40:947–953.

33. Penglis PS, James MJ, Cleland LG. Cyclooxygenase inhibitors: Any reservations? Intern Med J 2001;31:37–41.

34. Semrad SD, Hardee GE, Hardee MM, Moore JN. Low dose flunixin meglumine: Effects on eicosanoid production and clinical signs induced by experimental endotoxaemia in horses. Equine Vet J 1987;19:201–206.

35. Barton MH, Moore JN, Norton N. Effects of pentoxifylline infusion on response of horses to in vivo challenge exposure with endotoxin. Am J Vet Res 1997;58:1300–1307.

36. Baskett A, Barton MH, Norton N, Anders B, Moore JN. Effect of pentoxifylline, flunixin meglumine, and their combination on a model of endotoxemia in horses. Am J Vet Res 1997;58:1291–1299.

37. Mollitt DL, Poulos ND. The role of pentoxifylline in endotoxin-induced alterations of red cell deformability and whole blood viscosity in the neonate. J Pediatr Surg 1991;26:572–574.

38. Steffey EP, Howland D Jr. Comparison of circulatory and respiratory effects of isoflurane and halothane anesthesia in horses. Am J Vet Res 1980;41:821–825.

39. Whitehair KJ, Steffey EP, Woliner MJ, Willits NH. Effects of inhalation anesthetic agents on response of horses to three hours of hypoxemia. Am J Vet Res 1996;57:351–360.

40. Grubb TL, Benson GJ, Foreman JH, et al. Hemodynamic effects of ionized calcium in horses anesthetized with halothane or isoflurane. Am J Vet Res 1999;60:1430–1435.

41. Sertyn D, Coppens P, Mottart E, et al. Measurement of muscular microcirculation by laser Doppler flowmetry in isoflurane and halothane anaesthetized horses. Vet Rec 1987;121:324–326.

42. Carroll GL, Hooper RN, Rains CB, et al. Maintenance of anaesthesia with sevoflurane and oxygen in mechanically-ventilated horses subjected to exploratory laparotomy treated with intra- and post operative anaesthetic adjuncts. Equine Vet J 1998;30:402–407.

43. Matthews NS, Hartsfield SM, Mercer D, Beleau MH, MacKenthun A. Recovery from sevoflurane anesthesia in horses: Comparison to isoflurane and effect of postmedication with xylazine. Vet Surg 1998;27:480–485.

44. Pascoe PJ, Steffey EP, Black WD, Claxton JM, Jacobs JR, Woliner MJ. Evaluation of the effect of alfentanil on the minimum alveolar concentration of halothane in horses. Am J Vet Res 1993;54:1327–1332.

containing antibody to an Rc mutant E. coli (J5). Circ Shock 1989;28:235–248.

45. Doherty TJ, Geiser DR, Rohrbach BW. Effect of acepromazine and butorphanol on halothane minimum alveolar concentration in ponies. Equine Vet J 1997;29:374–376.

46. Steffey EP, Eisele JH, Baggot D. Interactions of morphine and isoflurane in horses. Am J Vet Res 2003;64:166–175.

47. Sellon DC, Monroe VL, Roberts MC, Papich MG. Pharmacokinetics and adverse effects of butorphanol administered by single intravenous or continuous intravenous infusion in horses. Am J Vet Res 2001;62:183–189.

48. Mircica E, Clutton RE, Kyles KW, Blissett KJ. Problems associated with perioperative morphine: A retrospective analysis. Vet Anaesth Analg 2003;30:147–155.

49. Dzikiti TB, Hellebrekers LJ, van Dijk P. Effects of intravenous lidocaine on isoflurane concentration, physiologic parameters, metabolic parameters and stress-related hormones in horses undergoing surgery. J Vet Med A Physiol Pathol Clin Med 2003;50:190–195.

50. Doherty TJ, Frazier DL. Effect of intravenous lidocaine on halothane minimum alveolar concentration in ponies. Equine Vet J 1998;30:300–303.

51. Koppert W, Weigand M, Neumann F, et al. Perioperative intravenous lidocaine has preventive effects on postoperative pain and morphine consumption after major abdominal surgery. Anesth Analg 2004;98: 1050–1055.

52. Hollmann MW, Durieux ME. Local anesthetics and the inflammatory response: A new therapeutic indication? Anesthesiology 2000;93:858–875.

53. Taniguchi T, Shibata K, Yamamoto K, Mizukoshi Y, Kobayashi T. Effects of lidocaine administration on hemodynamics and cytokine responses to endotoxemia in rabbits. Crit Care Med 2000;28: 755–759.

54. Nellgard P, Jonsson A, Bojo L, Tarnow P, Cassuto J. Small bowel obstruction and the effects of lidocaine, atropine, and hexamethonium on inflammation and fluid losses. Acta Anaesthesiol Scand 1996;40:287–292.

55. Trim CM, Barton MH, Quandt JE. Plasma endotoxin concentrations in anesthetized horses with colic. Vet Surg 1997;26:163.

56. Cohen ND, Lester GD, Sanchez LC, Merritt AM, Roussel AJ Jr. Evaluation of risk factors associated with development of postoperative ileus in horses. J Am Vet Med Assoc 2004;225:1070–1078.

57. Brianceau P, Chevalier H, Karas A, et al. Intravenous lidocaine and small intestinal size, abdominal fluid, and outcome after colic surgery in horses. J Vet Intern Med 2002;16:736–741.

58. Attuwaybi B, Kozar RA, Gates KS, et al. Hypertonic saline prevents inflammation, injury, and impaired intestinal transit after gut ischemia/reperfusion by inducing heme oxygenase 1 enzyme. J Trauma 2004;56:749–759.

59. Coimbra R, Hoyt DB, Junger WG, et al. Hypertonic saline resuscitation decreases susceptibility to sepsis after hemorrhagic shock. J Trauma 1997;42:602–606.

60. Trim CM. Monitoring during anaesthesia: Techniques and interpretation. Equine Vet Educ 1998;10:207–218.

61. Koenig J, McDonell W, Valverde A. Accuracy of pulse oximetry in healthy and compromised horses during spontaneous and controlled ventilation. Can J Vet Res 2003;67:169–174.

62. Bertone JJ, Gossett KA, Shoemaker KE, Bertone AL, Schneiter HL. Effect of hypertonic vs isotonic saline solution on responses to sublethal *Escherichia coli* endotoxemia in horses. Am J Vet Res 1990;51:999–1007.

63. Schmall LM, Muir WW, Robertson JT. Haemodynamic effects of small volume hypertonic saline in experimentally induced haemorrhagic shock. Equine Vet J 1990;22:273–277.

64. Grandy JL, Hodgson DS, Dunlop CJ, Chapman PL, Heath RB. Cardiopulmonary effects of ephedrine in halothane-anesthetized horses. 1989;12:389–396.

65. Wagner AE, Dunlop CI, Wertz EM, Chapman PL. Evaluation of five common induction protocols by comparison of hemodynamic responses to surgical manipulation in halothane-anesthetized horses. J Am Vet Med Assoc 1996;208:252–257.

66. Wegner K, Franklin RP, Long MT, Robertson SA. How to use fentanyl transdermal patches for analgesia in horses. Proc Am Assoc Equine Pract 2002;48:291–294.

67. Maxwell LK, Thomasy SM, Slovis N, Kollias-Baker C. Pharmacokinetics of fentanyl following intravenous and transdermal administration in horses. Equine Vet J 2003;35:484–490.

Chapter 52
Selected Diagnostic Procedures

Janyce L. Cornick-Seahorn, Jennifer Grimm, and Steven L. Marks

Introduction

Several minimally invasive advanced diagnostic and therapeutic procedures have become more commonly used over the last decade because of increased availability of the technology and expertise in application and interpretation. General anesthesia or sedation is usually required to assure patient immobility during these procedures. Animals vary greatly in physical status and underlying disease processes. Thus, the saying "There is no *one* ideal anesthetic protocol" applies aptly to these patients. Because many of the procedures discussed in this chapter may be considered to be elective, minimally invasive, and of short duration, an anesthetic protocol that will provide a rapid recovery is desirable. Perianesthetic considerations are presented for selected minimally invasive diagnostic techniques, including laryngoscopy, bronchoscopy, bone marrow aspiration, thoracic drain placement, and esophagostomy tube placement; for advanced imaging techniques, including computed tomography (CT), magnetic resonance imaging (MRI), and ultrasonography; and for radiation therapy. With a few exceptions, these procedures are not considered lifesaving, but rather diagnostic, and should be planned to minimize the potential adverse effects of general anesthesia or sedation.

The approach to anesthetic management should be kept simple, with the following principles in mind:

1. Identify and correct (when possible) underlying patient problems to minimize anesthetic risk.

2. Formulate an anesthetic protocol that will work in the existing environment and that can be readily adapted to each individual patient and its unique disease process(es).
3. Apply effective and adequate monitoring tools that will alert the anesthetist to potential problems so that quick and effective correction can be instituted.
4. Provide appropriate supportive therapy (as guided by underlying patient disease and information provided by monitoring devices).

Laryngoscopy and Bronchoscopy

Laryngoscopy is used in evaluating laryngeal disease—specifically, laryngeal paralysis. Sedation is required to facilitate relaxation of the jaw, but must be carefully selected to have a minimal effect on laryngeal function. It can be challenging to keep patients adequately sedated without affecting laryngeal function. A neuroleptanalgesic combination of an opioid and benzodiazepine (Table 52.1) is adequate for most patients. These drugs have the advantage of preserving laryngeal function and being reversible if respiratory distress develops. Challenge with doxapram (1.0 mg/kg intravenously [IV]) to increase respiratory activity may be used if evaluation is hindered by drug-induced respiratory depression.

Bronchoscopy is performed in dogs and cats for evaluation of airway disease and to perform bronchoalveolar lavage. Many of the patients presented for laryngoscopy and bronchoscopy are at increased risk for development of hypoxemia. Preoxygenation should accompany both procedures, and the anesthetist should always be prepared to take control of the airway by intubation and application of ventilatory support. During the bronchoscopy, oxygen may be delivered to smaller patients via an endoscope (working channel). Larger patients may be intubated and connected to oxygen by a breathing system; a Y-piece aperture may be used to pass the endoscope into the trachea. An opioid-benzodiazepine combination for sedation, followed by administration of low-dose propofol to effect, is commonly used to facilitate bronchoscopy (Table 52.1).

Thoracic Drain Placement

Thoracostomy tube placement may be required to manage pleural space disorders, such as pneumothorax, pyothorax, and chylothorax. These patients are often high risk, especially animals

Table 52.1. Suggested anesthetic doses for protocols for diagnostic procedures[a]

Premedication: opioid-benzodiazepine combination	
Opioids (IV, IM, or SC; IV administration of morphine is not recommended)	
Butorphanol	0.2–0.4 mg/kg
Buprenorphine	0.01–0.04 mg/kg
Morphine	0.4–1.0 mg/kg
Hydromorphone	0.1–0.2 mg/kg
Oxymorphone	0.05–0.1 mg/kg
Benzodiazepines (diazepam: IV only; midazolam: IV, IM, or SC)	
Diazepam	0.1–0.4 mg/kg
Midazolam	0.1–0.3 mg/kg
Antagonists	
Naloxone (opioid)	0.001 mg/kg
Flumazenil (benzodiazepine)	0.01–0.02 mg/kg
Induction	
Propofol	2–6 mg/kg IV
Etomidate	0.5–2.0 mg/kg IV
Ketamine	2–5 mg/kg[b] IV, IM
Maintenance	
Inhalation anesthesia: isoflurane or sevoflurane	
Propofol CRI	0.4 mg/kg/min
Propofol IB	0.5–2.0 mg/kg

CRI, continuous-rate infusion; IB, intermittent bolus; IM, intramuscular; IV, intravenous; and SC, subcutaneous.
[a]These protocols pertain to dogs and cats.
[b]Ketamine for induction is administered IV at 5 mg/kg combined with a benzodiazepine at 0.25 mg/kg and given to effect. For feline immobilization, 2 mg/kg IM is used with a benzodiazepine-opioid combination.

with pneumothorax and concurrent pulmonary contusions. In dogs, thoracic drain placement can often be performed using sedation in combination with a local anesthetic technique, such as infiltration or intercostal nerve block (see Chapter 20). To assure airway control, oxygen delivery, and provision of ventilatory support throughout the procedure in patients with respiratory distress or with hypoxemia, general anesthesia may also be used and may be superior. For cats, general anesthesia is preferred. Reversible agents with mild cardiopulmonary effects, such as the combination of a benzodiazepine with butorphanol or buprenorphine (Table 52.1), provide adequate sedation for most patients. For general anesthesia, a rapid-sequence induction to gain control of the airway is recommended. Propofol, benzodiazepine-ketamine combination, or etomidate (Table 52.1) are good induction choices, providing for relatively rapid recoveries.

Bone Marrow Aspiration

This is performed to evaluate bone marrow disease and to stage certain cancer patients. Protocol selection should be based on the individual patient; depending on the level of an animal's activity, bone marrow aspiration may be performed in dogs with local in-

filtration alone or in combination with sedation. Uncooperative dogs and the majority of cats may require general anesthesia. The aforementioned protocols for thoracostomy tube placement are appropriate.

Esophagostomy Tube Placement

This is used to provide enteral nutrition for both dogs and cats. General anesthesia is required to protect the airway in case of regurgitation and the endotracheal tube facilitates placement of the esophageal tube. The aforementioned protocols for thoracostomy tube placement are applicable for this procedure.

For the procedures listed earlier, identification of an individual animal's underlying disease, anticipation of and planning for potential complications, and close monitoring throughout the anesthetic period will help to assure a successful outcome, regardless of the anesthetic agents used.

Computed Tomography and Magnetic Resonance Imaging

General Considerations

CT and MRI were first introduced in 1972 and 1980, respectively. Routine clinical use of CT and MRI technology has evolved recently as availability of equipment and expertise in interpretation have increased. Anesthetic management for CT and MRI presents a unique challenge in that there is no painful stimulation during the anesthetic period; thus, response to a noxious stimulus does not provide a method for assessing anesthetic depth. The majority of scans are performed with the patient in dorsal recumbency; this position has the most significant detrimental effects on ventilation and perfusion matching. And patient access is usually limited during both CT and MRI. Depending on unit configuration, patients placed in a magnet are often difficult to access, so subjective evaluation, such as assessment of pulse quality and mucous membrane color, may not be feasible. With CT, although patient access is not problematic, exposure of the anesthetist to radiation is an issue, and direct patient assessment while the scan is being performed is discouraged.

Contrast Agents for CT and MRI

An additional consideration is the common use of contrast for both MRI and CT. While reaction to contrast administration appears to be relatively uncommon in animals, anesthetists must be aware of this potential complication. Intravenous iodinated contrast is often given to patients during a CT scan. These contrast agents consist of meglumine and/or sodium salts of iothalamate or diatrizoate (Table 52.2) and are ionic and hyperosmolar, which contributes to their side effects. Adverse reactions to these contrast agents include hypotension, tachycardia, and depressed ST segments and prolonged Q-T intervals on the electrocardiogram (ECG).[1] One case of cardiac arrest has been reported in a dog after intravenous (IV) administration of iodinated contrast media.[2] Adverse reactions are usually seen in the first 5 to 10 min following administration and are potentiated by dehydration; thus, normal hydration status is essential prior to the CT contrast

Table 52.2. Properties of contrast agents used for diagnostic imaging

Ionic, hyperosmolar iodinated contrast media

Brand Name	Cation	Anion	mg I/mL	Osmolality (mOsm/kg H$_2$O)	Viscosity at 37°C
Conray	Meglumine	Iothalamate	282	1400	4
Conray 400	Sodium	Iothalamate	400	2300	4.5
Hypaque 76	Meglumine 66% Sodium 10%	Diatrizoate	370	2016	9
Hypaque 50%	Sodium	Diatrizoate	300	1515	2.34
Hypaque 60%	Meglumine	Diatrizoate	282	1415	4.12
Renografin 76	Meglumine 66% Sodium 10%	Diatrizoate	370	1940	8.4
Renografin 60	Meglumine 52% Sodium 8%	Diatrizoate	290	1450	4

Nonionic, low-osmolar iodinated contrast media

Brand Name	Generic Name	mg I/mL	Osmolality (mOsm/kg H$_2$O)	Viscosity at 37°C
Omnipaque	Iohexol	140	322	1.5
		180	408	2
		240	520	3.4
		300	672	6.3
		350	844	10.4
Isovue	Iopamidol	150	342	1.5
		200	413	2
		300	616	4.7
		370	796	9.4
Visipaque	Iodixanol	270	290	6.3
		320	290	11.8
Ultravist	Iopromide	300	607	4.9
		370	774	10
Optiray	Ioversol	160	355	1.9
		240	502	3
		300	651	5.5
		320	702	5.8
		350	792	9
Imagopaque	Iopentol	150	310	1.7
		200	410	2.8
		250	520	3.9
		300	640	6.5
		350	810	12

administration. Humans are at risk for serious reactions if they have any of the following preexisting conditions: diabetes mellitus, renal insufficiency, congestive heart failure, hypovolemia, multiple myeloma, hypertension, or combined hepatic and renal failure.[1] No specific treatment is necessary following a mild reaction to the contrast media; however, fluid administration rate should be increased for treatment of mild hypotension and tachycardia. If an anaphylactic reaction does occur, administration of epinephrine, diphenhydramine, and/or corticosteroids is indicated. Fluid administration rate for patients with underlying renal disease should be increased to 20 mL/kg during the first 30 min of anesthesia to promote contrast clearance and to maintain adequate renal perfusion.

All contrast agents used in MRI contain a paramagnetic element: gadolinium. These contrast agents present a lower osmotic burden to the patient, and smaller volumes are required compared with CT contrast agents. There have been no reported cases of adverse reactions to MRI contrast agents in animals, but allergy-type symptoms, hypotension, hypertension, vasodilation, tachycardia, nausea, vomiting, and headache have been reported in humans. An increased administration rate of IV fluids should be used to treat hypotension and tachycardia.[3]

MRI Safety Considerations

MRI safety is an important concern in anesthesia monitoring because ferromagnetic objects are attracted toward the magnet; therefore, projectile-related accidents can occur. Traditional anesthetic equipment and monitors may be unsafe, may be damaged, may malfunction, or may interfere with image generation when used in the MRI suite. The MRI consists of a strong static magnetic field, gradient magnetic fields, and radiofrequency (RF) fields. Any ferromagnetic object has the potential to be drawn into the bore of the magnet, causing injury to the patient or personnel in the room. The influence of the MRI scanner on equipment depends on the strength of the magnet, proximity to the magnet bore, the amount of ferromagnetic material present, and the design of the circuitry.[4] Also, the RF fields and the applied magnetic gradient fields in the room can affect the function and accuracy of the monitoring equipment, or, conversely, the monitoring equipment can alter the quality of the images obtained. Ferromagnetic equipment within the room should be replaced with nonferromagnetic or minimally ferromagnetic metal, such as stainless steel, brass, or aluminum. Alternatively, ferromagnetic equipment may be securely anchored to a wall or the floor as far away from the bore of the magnet as possible. Monitoring equipment may be adapted by placing the devices outside of the room and using long connecting wires. If possible, oxygen tanks should be located outside of the MRI suite, or tanks made of aluminum should be used.

Several companies sell MRI-compatible anesthesia and monitoring equipment. Keep in mind the definitions of MRI safe and MRI compatible. *MRI safe* means that the device, when used in the MR environment, has been demonstrated to present no additional risk to the patient or other individual, but may affect the quality of the diagnostic information. *MRI compatible* means that a device is MR safe and, when used in the MR environment, has been demonstrated neither to significantly affect the quality of the diagnostic information nor to have its operations affected by the MR unit.[4] Some companies market their product as MRI compatible, but the instruction manuals must be carefully read because there have been several reports of "MRI compatible" monitoring equipment being propelled into the bore of the magnet.[5,6] Instructions for such potentially hazardous equipment state that the item must be placed a certain distance away from the magnet.[6,7] Ideally, equipment should be checked by a biomedical engineer responsible for the area before it is brought into the vicinity of the MRI scanner. Some companies that supply MRI-compatible or MRI-safe anesthetic equipment and monitors are listed in Table 52.3.

Special consideration should also be given to patients with any type of metallic implants, such as hemoclips, patent ductus arteriosus (PDA) occlusion coils, or pacemakers. Ferromagnetic hemoclips can dislodge and migrate, causing internal damage. An electrical current can be induced in PDA coils, causing thermal damage, and pacemaker leads or generators can dislodge. The magnetic field may cause the pacemaker generator to malfunction or readjust. An electrical current in the lead wire may produce enough heat to cause injury. If a metallic implant is located in the region that is being imaged, severe image artifacts often occur, resulting in a nondiagnostic study.

Table 52.3. Companies that manufacture MRI-compatible, MRI-safe anesthesia equipment

Smiths Medical PM, Veterinary Division (Surgivet)	www.surgivet.com/index.asp
DRE Medical	www.dreveterinary.com
In vivo	www.invivoresearch.com
Medrad	www.medrad.com
Datex	www.datex-ohmeda.com
Nonin	www.nonin.com

One other safety issue that may occur in the MRI suite is magnetic quenching. If the liquid helium that surrounds and cools the superconducting solenoid of the magnet rapidly escapes, it can displace the oxygen in the room, causing hypoxia to the patient and personnel present. Ideally, oxygen sensors should be placed in MRI suites.

Ultrasonography

This has been used in veterinary medicine since the late 1970s and has become a routine diagnostic procedure for animals. Most animals tolerate ultrasonographic evaluation without sedation or anesthesia, but sedation may be necessary in fractious, aggressive, or painful animals. Ultrasound-guided organ or tissue biopsies are becoming more common as a method for collecting samples less invasively. Small animals usually tolerate the procedure well with sedation and local anesthetic infiltration, but general anesthesia may be more effective in some individuals. Local anesthetic infiltration alone or with mild sedation, combined with proper restraint, is effective for collecting biopsy samples in standing horses, cows, and other large animal species.

Radiation Therapy

External beam radiation is used to treat many types of neoplasia in small animals. Treatment usually consists of multiple small doses of radiation daily for a curative intent or larger, less frequent doses for pain palliation. Treatment times per dose last anywhere from about 1 min up to 7 or 8 min. Therefore, patients must remain motionless and be precisely positioned for radiation therapy. Since most animals receive their radiation doses daily and remain in the hospital for up to 4 weeks or go home nightly, a profound sedation or general anesthetic protocol should be used that is easily administered and has a quick recovery time. During treatment, personnel cannot be present in the therapy room to directly monitor the animal because of radiation safety. Remote monitors or cameras focused on the patient and in-room monitors should be used to assess the patient.

Patient Preparation

The procedures presented in this chapter, though essential to the well-being of the individual patient, are largely elective. Ade-

Table 52.4. Disease processes that may be present in patients presented for computed tomography (CT), magnetic resonance imaging (MRI), and ultrasonography

Organ or Organ System: Examples
Skull: orbital, nasal, sinus, and oral tumors
Brain: tumors, cerebrovascular bleeding (stroke), and hydrocephalus
Spinal cord: tumors, intervertebral disk disease, and trauma
Musculoskeletal: soft tissue and skeletal tumors, and ligament and cartilage damage
Thorax: intrathoracic masses, effusions, and pneumonia
Cardiac: masses, murmurs, and arrhythmias
Abdomen: abnormalities associated with the liver, pancreas, adrenal glands, spleen, kidneys, ureters, and bladder

This list is not exhaustive but is based on the literature and personal experience of the authors. As a general rule, CT is superior for skeletal imaging, whereas MRI is superior for soft tissue imaging. Movement artifact can be problematic for abdominal and thoracic MRI, depending on the speed and sophistication of the scanner. CT may provide superior images for body cavity structures.

quate preanesthetic patient assessment, including physical examination and laboratory evaluation (complete blood count, chemistry panel, and urinalysis), is essential for successful outcome. Fortunately, since the aforementioned techniques may be considered to be advanced techniques, a thorough workup has already been performed in many of the presenting patients. For marrow and organ biopsy, a coagulation profile should also be evaluated. Table 52.4 provides some examples of disorders that may exist in patients presented for MRI, CT, and ultrasound procedures. Readers are directed to Chapters 36 to 51, which address anesthetic management of system-specific diseases, for additional anesthetic management considerations.

Protocol Selection

When formulating an anesthetic plan, reversibility, familiarity (comfort zone), and maintenance of homeostasis by provision of adequate supportive care and monitoring should be addressed. Since the technique itself will vary minimally among patients, an anesthetic plan that will meet the needs of the majority of patients and will be compatible with the facility is desirable. The drugs used should be short-acting and/or reversible; some options are listed in Table 52.1. For premedication, an opioid alone or combined with a benzodiazepine has relatively mild cardiopulmonary effects and will provide sedation and reduce induction and maintenance requirements. These drugs can be reversed with an opioid antagonist, such as naloxone, and the benzodiazepine antagonist flumazenil, if necessary (Table 52.1). Acepromazine premedication may be beneficial for healthy animals that are difficult to restrain or aggressive, if there are no patient contraindications. Acepromazine facilitates a smooth but somewhat prolonged recovery, so benefits should be weighed against this disadvantage. Intramuscular ketamine (2 to 4 mg/kg),

with an opioid-benzodiazepine combination, may be beneficial in fractious cats to provide sedation and immobilization. Induction options include propofol, etomidate, ketamine, and inhalation agents. Propofol is probably most frequently used because of its short duration of action, but can be detrimental in animals with underlying hypotension that remains uncorrected prior to induction. Etomidate may provide a better alternative in cardiovascular-compromised patients. Ketamine with a benzodiazepine represents an alternative method of induction, but recovery may be prolonged (compared with etomidate, propofol, and inhalation agents). Contraindications for ketamine use, such as a history of seizures and the presence of increased intracranial pressure, are particularly germane to patients undergoing MRI and/or CT. Induction with an inhalation agent via face mask may be used if rapid control of the airway is not an issue, if the patient is tractable, and if the induction room is well ventilated. However, this method is recommended only when other options present unacceptable patient risk. A major disadvantage to mask induction is waste-gas pollution and subsequent exposure of personnel. Anesthesia for MRI and CT is most commonly maintained with an inhalation agent. Isoflurane and sevoflurane both facilitate a rapid recovery. Anesthesia machines and ventilators that are MRI compatible or MRI safe are available, and some suppliers are listed in Table 52.3. If an MRI-compatible anesthesia machine is not available or if a traditional machine cannot be configured from outside the MRI room, anesthesia can be maintained with propofol by using a constant rate infusion or intermittent bolus technique (Table 52.1). Maintenance with propofol should always include intubation, supplemental oxygen, and a method for ventilatory support.

Monitoring

General Considerations

Considering the diversity of patient signalment, physical status, and organ system abnormalities, and irregardless of the relatively short duration of the procedures, one or more monitoring devices should be applied to every individual patient to help assure its well-being. Monitoring techniques could include continuous ECG, pulse oximetry, capnography, blood pressure monitoring, and measurement of end-tidal anesthetic gas concentration (ET_{agent}). Application should be tailored to the individual and to the procedure. For example, pulse oximetry is especially important for assessing patients at risk for developing hypoxemia, such as during bronchoscopy and thoracostomy tube placement. Capnography is useful for intubated patients at risk of hypoventilating (thoracostomy tube placement). Readers are referred to Chapter 19 for a detailed description of the information afforded by these devices.

Monitoring for MRI and CT

Considering the challenge of patient accessibility and the diversity of patient presentation, several monitoring tools should be applied to maximize patient safety. Essential monitoring devices include capnography, pulse oximetry, and continuous ECG. Capnography ($ETCO_2$) and pulse oximetry (SpO_2) provide continuous, noninvasive methods of assessing adequacy of ventilation, perfusion, and oxygenation, and also provide an assessment of respiratory rate and pulse rate, respectively. The capnographic waveform provides an early warning to the anesthetist that a problem is developing. Noninvasive or invasive blood pressure monitoring and ET_{agent} monitoring are also recommended. Anesthetic agents compromise cardiovascular homeostasis and, in the absence of a surgical stimulus, hypotension should be anticipated, especially if underlying cardiovascular abnormalities are present. Use of blood pressure monitoring will alert the anesthetist to the development of hypotension so that supportive measures can be instituted (increase in fluid administration rate, administration of an inotrope, or decrease in anesthetic depth). ET_{agent} reflects an agent's alveolar partial pressure and thus closely approximates arterial and brain anesthetic partial pressures (once equilibration is reached). The minimum alveolar concentration (MAC) has been reported for inhalant agents commonly used for a variety of animals. Although many factors, such as premedications administered, will affect patient inhalation agent requirements, maintaining an ET_{agent} concentration of 1.2 to 1.4 MAC is considered to be appropriate for most animals. Some suppliers that offer MRI-compatible monitoring equipment are listed in Table 52.3. Additional information regarding MRI-compatible equipment has been published.[5,6]

Monitoring patients undergoing MRI can be difficult for many reasons in addition to patient inaccessibility. Some scanners are extremely loud during image acquisition, making direct cardiopulmonary auscultation impossible. The gradient magnetic fields and RF fields are capable of generating electrical currents in metal wires, so ECG leads can burn a patient's skin. Burns caused by ECG leads during MRI have been cited in the literature on human patients[8] and have been reported to occur during animal imaging. Electrical current induction can occur within a loop of wire in a pulse oximetry unit, which can severely burn patients. To avoid patient injury, it is important that MRI-compatible lead connections be used. Additionally, the MRI may interfere with ECG waveforms, making it difficult to evaluate the rhythm trace.

Patients anesthetized for MRI and CT require intravenous fluid administration to maintain adequate perfusion and the application of monitoring devices to identify and address alterations in homeostasis proactively. Availability of mechanical ventilation to provide intermittent positive-pressure ventilation (IPPV) is important during diagnostic imaging. Application of IPPV in combination with capnography will enhance patient management by assuring ventilatory homeostasis. Increased intracranial pressure caused by trauma or brain tumor is a common presenting sign in patients undergoing CT and MR imaging. Maintaining these patients in a mildly hypocapneic state (e.g., $PaCO_2$ = 30 mm Hg) will improve anesthetic outcome by minimizing the detrimental effects of increased $PaCO_2$ on intracranial pressure.[9]

Summary

Anesthetic management of patients presented for advanced diagnostic and therapeutic techniques should include thorough preoperative patient assessment, a protocol that addresses patient needs, and application of effective monitoring tools and supportive therapy throughout the anesthetic period.

References

1. Walter PA, Feeney DA, Johnston GR. Diagnosis and treatment of adverse reactions to radiopaque contrast agents. In: Kirk RW, ed. Current Veterinary Therapy X: Small Animal Practice. Philadelphia: WB Saunders, 1989:47–52.
2. Herrtage ME, Dennis R. Contrast media and their use in small animal radiology. J Small Anim Pract 1987;28:1105–1114.
3. Shellock FG, Kanal E. Safety of magnetic resonance imaging contrast agents. J Magn Reson Imaging 1999;10;477–484.
4. Shellock FG. Magnetic resonance safety update 2002: Implants and devices. J Magn Reson Imaging 2002;16:485–526.
5. Keens SJ, Laurence AS. Magnet safe is not the same as magnet compatible in the MR scanner. Anaesthesia 2004;59:516–517.
6. Farling P, McBrien ME, Winder RJ. Magnetic resonance compatible equipment: Read the small print. Anaesthesia 2003;58:84–85.
7. Laurence AS. Magnetic resonance compatible equipment: Apply common sense. Anaesthesia 2003;58:615.
8. Keens SJ, Laurence AS. Burns caused by ECG monitoring during MRI imaging. Anaesthesia 1996;51:1188–1189.
9. Drummond JC, Todd MM, Shapiro HH. CO_2 responsiveness of the cerebral circulation during isoflurane anesthesia and nitrous oxide sedation in cats. Anesthesiology 1985;62:268–273.

Chapter 53
Anesthetic Emergencies and Procedures

A. Thomas Evans and Deborah V. Wilson

Introduction

In many veterinary practices, after the induction of anesthesia, no one is assigned the task of anesthetist to monitor anesthesia and be vigilant for untoward events that might result in accidental morbidity and mortality. As with most unwanted events, the anticipation of possible complications and having a plan of action already prepared will facilitate successful resolution of the problem. Since the onset of general anesthesia upsets the physiological equilibrium of patients and can bring them closer to harmful outcomes, preparation to manage these problems is even more critical. Monitors that display vital parameters such as oxygen saturation of hemoglobin, end-tidal carbon dioxide, blood pressure, and heart rhythm are available to facilitate early detection of critical events such as bradycardia, changes in oxygen availability, and hypoventilation. Veterinarians who vigilantly monitor have a better opportunity to respond quickly to a harmful trend before a disaster occurs.

Anesthetic Risk

The risk of death from disease or related surgery is usually greater than the risk of death from anesthesia. However, anesthesia involves the controlled administration of potentially toxic drugs and thus carries a risk of organ dysfunction and damage, delayed recovery, and death. Mistakes are not necessarily reversible, and death can occur suddenly and often without warning when patients are not appropriately monitored. The goal of anesthetists should be to manage the risks associated with anesthesia and the perioperative period, affording patients the best chance of a successful outcome. *Risk management* is a term developed by the insurance industry and adopted by the health care industry to describe processes used to prevent injury, litigation, and financial loss.[1,2] The real aim of this process is to use analysis of adverse events to prevent similar injuries to subsequent patients. Risk management starts with an unbiased and nonjudgmental review and analysis of all "critical events" causing real or potential patient harm. The next step is formation or modification of standard operating procedures. For example, in aviation, accident investigation begins with discovery of the facts by an independent board (National Transportation Safety Board) and then analysis and publication of the findings. There is also an anonymous reporting system (Aviation Safety Reporting System) that involves the documentation and analysis of events that were considered hazardous by the participants but did not lead to an accident. These aviation review procedures provide a model for the improvement of anesthesia safety in both human and veterinary medicine. A commitment to the highest-quality patient care will ultimately lead to the routine performance of such analyses by medical providers.

Species-Related Risk

Advances in medical technology and pharmacology, as well as the increase in training of anesthesiologists, veterinarians, and licensed technicians, have done much to decrease the inherent risks associated with anesthesia. The risk of anesthetic-related death in people is estimated at between 1:10,000 and 1:200,000.[3–5] The rate of anesthetic-related death among dogs and cats anesthetized in private practice has been assessed at 0.1%.[6] Horses present an inherently greater challenge during anesthesia because of unique anatomical, physiological, and behavioral factors. Several studies suggest an anesthetic-related mortality rate of between 0.08% and 0.9% in healthy horses.[7,8] Postanesthetic lameness caused by myopathies and neuropathies reportedly occurs in 6.4% of anesthetized horses.[9] Emergency cases, including colics, are associated with an apparent mortality rate of 31.4%.[10] Another retrospective analysis of cases from a single facility using a fairly standardized anesthetic protocol found an incidence of anesthetic-related mortality of 0.12% (L.

Bidwell, personal communication, 2004). In this study of 21 deaths from among 17,961 equine anesthetics, the incidence of cardiac arrest was 0.06% (10 deaths), that of long-bone fractures was 0.04% (8 deaths), and that of myoneuropathies 0.02% (3 deaths). When interpreting studies of comparative anesthetic-related morbidity and mortality, it should be remembered the definitions of the anesthetic period may vary and often include additional surgical and disease risk factors.

High-Risk Patients

Based on clinical experience, the small animal patients that are associated with a high risk of adverse outcome from anesthesia and surgery include geriatric (especially hyperthyroid) cats; post-trauma cases with pulmonary pathology, hemothorax, or pneumothorax or pulmonary hemorrhage; and cases of acute head trauma and severe intra-abdominal hemorrhage. Patients requiring a high level of care and commitment to achieve a good outcome include neonates; those with low body weight or morbid obesity; and patients undergoing portosystemic shunt occlusion or cardiac, intracranial, or intraocular surgery.

The procedures or conditions associated with high risk of adverse outcome in equine patients include advanced age, heavily muscled young horses, extreme emaciation, ethmoidal hematoma, or guttural pouch mycosis with severe hemorrhage, septic shock, and intra-abdominal hemorrhage. Periparturient mares also have a greater risk of adverse outcome.[11,12]

Cardiovascular Emergencies

Hemorrhage and Fluid Loss

Blood loss during surgery may be insidious or obvious. Body fluids may also be lost during surgery to transudation, sequestration, or evaporation. Extravasation of fluid to a nonfunctioning or sequestered edema space is commonly referred to as *loss to the third space*, the first and second spaces being the intracellular and extracellular spaces. These losses may reduce circulating blood volume significantly. Regardless of cause or route of loss, a decrease in circulating blood volume is not well tolerated by anesthetized patients.

Quantifying blood loss is important but can be difficult, so the severity of hemorrhage is often assessed by its impact on the patient. Severe blood loss causes tachycardia, reduced arterial pressure, pale mucous membranes, decreased pulse pressure, and decreased area under the arterial pulse wave.[13,14] Packed cell volume decreases only during resuscitation or fluid shift into the vascular space, but base deficit increases as changes in bicarbonate, and venous pH correlate with blood volume lost.[15] All of the aforementioned changes have been reported in anesthetized horses, with one difference: Tachycardia in response to blood loss is not usually observed in horses that are under anesthesia.[16] Physiological responses to blood loss may be blunted or masked by anesthetic and anesthetic adjunctive drugs (e.g., α_2-agonists), further emphasizing the need for appropriate monitoring for early detection and correction of hypovolemia.

Shed blood can be replaced with crystalloids, colloids such as plasma, hemoglobin-based oxygen-carrying solutions, dextrans, whole blood, or a combination of these solutions (Table 53.1). In most situations, hypertonic solutions do not seem to have a distinct advantage over isotonic crystalloid solutions.[17] Crystalloid solutions such as lactated Ringer's or Plasmalyte are usually administered at threefold the volume of shed blood, as a rough guideline for resuscitation. The main advantage of crystalloid solutions is their low cost. Colloid solutions such as whole blood, plasma, hydroxyethyl starch, and hemoglobin-based oxygen carriers can be used as a substitute for crystalloids.[18] Hemoglobin-based oxygen-carrying solutions (e.g., Oxyglobin) are relatively

Table 53.1. Management of complications associated with anesthesia.

Complication	Treatment	Trade Name	Dosage	Side Effects
Excitement, delirium	Acepromazine	PromAce	0.05–0.2 mg/kg IV, IM	Prolonged recovery
	Medetomidine	Domitor	1–2 μg/kg IV	Bradycardia
	Diazepam	Valium	0.25–0.5 mg/kg IV	Hypothermia
	Midazolam	Versed	0.05–0.2 mg/kg IV, IM	
Hypoventilation	Oxygen	—	—	Respiratory depression
	Ventilation	—	—	Additional hypoventilation if too aggressive ventilation
				Resisting mask
Laryngospasm	Topical lidocaine	Xylocaine 2%	—	
	Lidocaine jelly	—		
	Lidocaine IV		1–2 mg/kg IV	
Hypoxemia	Oxygen		—	
	Tracheostomy	Portex[a]		Subcutaneous emphysema
	Ventilation			Hyperventilation
Pneumothorax	Oxygen			
	Chest tubes	Sherwood[b]	—	Infection
	Thora-Seal III			
	Ventilation			Hyperventilation

(continued)

Table 53.1. Management of complications associated with anesthesia (*continued*).

Complication	Treatment	Trade Name	Dosage	Side Effects
Cardiac dysrhythmias				
Tachycardia	LRS	—	10–20 mL/kg per hour	Bradycardia
	Esmolol	Brevibloc	0.01–0.1 mg/kg IV	Bradycardia
	Propranolol	Inderal	0.05–0.1 mg/kg IV	Hypotension
	Increase anesthesia	—	—	Bradycardia
Bradycardia	Atropine	—	0.02 mg/kg IV	Tachycardia
	Glycopyrrolate	Robinul V	0.005 mg/kg IV	
Ventricular dysrhythmias	Lidocaine	Xylocaine	Dogs: 0.5 mg/kg IV	Bradycardia
			Cats: 0.2 mg/kg IV	Convulsions
	Procainamide	Pronestyl	10–20 mg/kg IM	Hypotension
			10–20 mg/kg IV per hour	
	Amiodarone	Cordarone	5 mg/kg IV	Liver toxicity
				Hypothyroidism
Hypotension	Fluids (LRS)	—	10–20 mL/kg IV	
	Dopamine	Intropin	3–5 µg/kg per minute	Dysrhythmias
	Dobutamine	Dobutrex	3–5 µg/kg per minute	Tachycardia
				Hypertension
Blood or fluid loss	Fluids (LRS)		40–90 mL/kg IV per hour	Pulmonary edema
	Blood		20–40 mL/kg IV	Allergic reaction
	Hydroxyethyl starch 6%	Hetastarch	10–20 mL/kg IV per day	Circulatory overload
	Hemoglobin glutamer 200	Oxyglobin	10–30 mL/kg IV	Circulatory overload
Hypothermia	Warmed fluids		5–10 mL/kg IV per hour	Overhydration
	Water-heating pad	Gaymar[d]		
	Forced air warming	Bair Hugger[c]		Hyperthermia
Hypoglycemia	Dextrose 5%	—	1–2 mL/kg IV	Hyperosmolality
Metabolic acidosis	Sodium bicarbonate	—	1–2 mEq/kg IV every 10 min	Metabolic alkalosis
				Hypokalemia
				Hyperosmolality
Hyperkalemia	Sodium bicarbonate	—	0.5–1.0 mEq/kg IV	As above
	Sodium chloride 0.9%	—	10–40 mL/kg per hour	
	Calcium chloride	—	10 mg/kg IV	Tachycardia
Hyperpyrexia	Oxygen			
	Fluids (LRS)		5–10 mL/kg IV	
	Tranquilizers	PromAce	0.05–0.1 mg/kg IM	
	Dantrolene sodium		2–4 mg/kg IV	
Prolonged recovery	Doxapram	Dopram V	1–2 mg/kg IV	Excitement
	Yohimbine	Yobine	0.5 mg/kg IV	
Postoperative pain	Morphine sulfate		0.1–1.0 mg/kg IM	Respiratory depression
	Buprenorphine	Buprenex	0.01 mg/kg IV, IM	Slow recovery
	Butorphanol	Torbugesic	0.2–0.4 mg/kg IM	Slow recovery
	Meloxicam	Metacam	0.2 mg/kg SC	Vomiting

IM, intramuscularly; IV, intravenously; LRS, lactated Ringer's solution; SC, subcutaneously.
[a]Shiley, Irvine, CA.
[b]Sherwood Medical, St. Louis, MO.
[c]Arizant Healthcare, Eden Prairie, MN.
[d]Gaymar, Orchard Park, NY.

expensive but have a long shelf life, and do not require cross-matching.[19] The use of colloids has the advantage of sustaining colloid osmotic pressure while preserving plasma volume but has the disadvantage of being more expensive than crystalloid solutions.

Acute hemorrhage of greater than 20% of the blood volume or a decline in pack cell volume to less than 20% because of the combined effects of blood loss and crystalloid fluid administration can be treated with an appropriate mass of red blood cells by either transfusion of whole blood, packed red cells, or 10 to 30 mL/kg of a hemoglobin-based oxygen carrier.[20,21] Hemoglobin-based oxygen-carrying solutions or red blood cells are preferred because of the need for restoring adequate hemoglobin concentrations to carry oxygen to the tissues. Smaller amounts of ● surgical hemorrhage, not associated with severe decreases in the hemoglobin concentration, can be replaced with crystalloids (e.g., lactated Ringer's) or colloids rather than blood.

Cardiac Dysrhythmia

Most dysrhythmias are caused by preexisting medical conditions, administration of premedications, anesthesia induction and maintenance agents, and surgical stimulation. Dysrhythmias require treatment if they reduce cardiac output, cause sustained tachycardia, or are likely to initiate dangerous ventricular dysrhythmias.

Canine gastric dilation/volvulus or multiple trauma often precipitates dysrhythmias that may require treatment prior to induction of anesthesia.[22,23] Dysrhythmias following gastric dilation/volvulus presumably have their origin in acid-base imbalance, electrolyte disturbance, myocardial ischemia, circulating cardiac stimulatory substances, and/or autonomic nervous system imbalance. Treatment involves correcting physiological abnormalities and administering lidocaine or procainamide. It is absolutely imperative that ventricular premature contractions (VPCs) be differentiated from ventricular escape beats before administration of antiarrhythmic drugs, because suppression of an escape rhythm can cause immediate asystole and death. If the sinus rate is low, an intravenous atropine injection of 0.02 mg/kg may increase the sinus rate and invoke overdrive suppression, which may inhibit the dysrhythmia. VPCs and ventricular tachycardia resulting from a traumatized myocardium are commonly treated with lidocaine or procainamide. If possible, surgery should be delayed 2 to 4 days or until the dysrhythmias have subsided.

Several of the popular drugs used as preanesthetic medication can predispose patients to conduction abnormalities. Atropine or glycopyrrolate can cause sinus tachycardia and increase myocardial work and oxygen consumption. Phenothiazine tranquilizers reportedly predispose the heart to sinus bradycardia, sinus arrest, and, occasionally, first-degree and second-degree heart block, although it has also been shown to protect against VPCs. Xylazine causes bradycardia and second-degree atrioventricular blockade and decreases the epinephrine threshold for VPCs. The μ-receptor agonist opioids morphine, hydromorphone, fentanyl, and oxymorphone will also precipitate a slowing of heart rate via increased vagal efferent activity. The anesthesia induction agents thiopental and ketamine have been reported to increase the likelihood of dysrhythmia formation after epinephrine administration during halothane anesthesia.[24,25] This multidrug interaction has also been described for thiopental and isoflurane.[24]

Other factors responsible for the development of the dysrhythmias during the surgical period include altered arterial carbon dioxide partial pressure ($PaCO_2$), altered PaO_2, altered pH, and autonomic reflexes from surgical manipulation, as well as central nervous system disturbances and cardiac disease. Because most perioperative dysrhythmias do not seriously affect cardiac output, treatment can be discrete. Changing to a different inhalation anesthetic, using intermittent positive-pressure ventilation, or increasing the depth of anesthesia may eliminate the dysrhythmia.[26,27] Other treatments for controlling ventricular dysrhythmias include correcting blood-gas abnormalities or administering

a small quantity of intravenous lidocaine (0.5 mg/kg) or procainamide (1.0 mg/kg).

Allergic Reactions

Allergic reactions involving anesthetics are uncommon but could occur after sensitization to a drug. Allergic or anaphylactic reactions are mediated by the immune system. They are more commonly associated with repeated exposure to an allergen, but cross-reactivity may be seen with some preexisting allergies (e.g., allergies to eggs and to egg proteins in propofol). Anaphylactic reactions following thiopental administration have been reported.[28,29] Intravenous injection of the intravenous contrast agent diatrizoic acid (Hypaque; Amersham Health, Princeton, NJ) has caused tachypnea, bronchoconstriction, and mucoid diarrhea in dogs. Allergic reactions are treated with intravenous fluids, antihistamines, and corticosteroids. Epinephrine should be administered in severe reactions accompanied by severe bronchoconstriction or cardiovascular collapse. Many unexpected responses to anesthetic and anesthetic adjunctive drugs have been labeled as "allergies" by veterinarians; however, proper diagnosis is crucial because it may have serious ramifications for future anesthetic delivery.

Cardiac Arrest

Successful treatment of cardiac arrest requires early diagnosis. The brain is the organ most susceptible to hypoxia or ischemia, because serious brain injury develops after only 4 or 5 min of cardiac arrest. The brain injury can be multifactorial, including the rapid loss of high-energy phosphate compounds during ischemia, cell structural damage during reperfusion, progressive brain hypoperfusion especially in certain areas, and suppression of protein synthesis in selectively vulnerable neurons.[30] Once the diagnosis of cardiac arrest has been confirmed, all efforts must be toward developing effective blood flow and reestablishing a heartbeat. Cardiopulmonary resuscitation (CPR) with external cardiac massage appears to be ineffective in protecting the brain from injury and should be only part of the initial resuscitation protocol. If unsuccessful, time should not be wasted with external CPR in lieu of more effective internal techniques.[31]

Cardiac arrest is diagnosed when some or all the signs listed in Table 53.2 are present. When the heartbeat or peripheral pulse cannot be palpated, the systolic blood pressure is generally less than 50 mm Hg. In this circumstance, the heart may actually have a weak beat, but cardiac output is probably very low and true cardiac arrest imminent. A nonpalpable weak heartbeat along with a regular rhythm has been termed *pulseless electrical activity* (PEA), formerly known as electrical mechanical dissociation. This type of functional cardiac arrest occurs with anesthesia overdose and from many other causes, such as hypovolemia, acute cardiogenic decompensation, severe acidosis, or hypoxemia. It is important to look for correctable causes of PEA during the first moments of resuscitation to improve the odds of success. Other forms of cardiac arrest include asystole and ventricular fibrillation. The three types of cardiac arrest can be

Table 53.2. Signs of cardiac arrest.

1. No palpable heart beat
2. No palpable pulse
3. Apnea
4. Lack of surgical hemorrhage
5. Cyanosis
6. No muscle tone
7. Dilated pupils (later)

differentiated with an electrocardiogram (ECG) or by direct observation of the heart during thoracic surgery or internal CPR.

Cardiopulmonary Resuscitation

When any or all of the signs listed in Table 53.2 are present, the traditional *ABCD* protocol for treatment of cardiac arrest must be started immediately. *A* refers to *airway* and reminds the resuscitator that a patent airway is a necessity. Endotracheal intubation is the best method of insuring a patent airway. The goal of *B*, *breathing*, is to supply high concentrations of oxygen to the alveoli and to eliminate carbon dioxide. Intermittent positive-pressure ventilation is usually instituted in intubated patients, although, when breathing room air and using chest compressions only (no artificial ventilation), dogs have maintained adequate gas exchange and oxygen saturation greater than 90% for longer than 4 min.[32] The real value of artificial breathing has been questioned for routine resuscitation in people.[33] The current recommendations for a breathing rate of 10 to 24 breaths/min may be too high.[34] Assuming there is enough blood flow to provide a reading, the pulse oximeter can be useful as a guide to determine respiratory rate. Simply ventilate at a rate that maintains hemoglobin saturation at 90% or higher.

C refers to *cardiac massage*, which can be either external (thoracic) or internal. External thoracic massage is thought to produce cardiac output by one or a combination of two methods. The *thoracic pump theory* holds that blood moves out of the thoracic cavity during the compression half of the CPR cycle because of a buildup of internal thoracic pressure (Fig. 53.1). This mechanism is thought to occur primarily in animals with a body weight greater than 15 to 20 kg. Evidence for the thoracic pump theory includes the phenomenon of cough CPR in humans and artificial cough CPR in dogs.[35,36] The *cardiac pump theory* explains blood flow in smaller animals or animals with a narrow side-to-side thoracic width and refers to actual mechanical compression of the myocardium by the thoracic wall during CPR systole (Fig. 53.2). Blood flow in some patients may be produced by a combination of the cardiac and thoracic pump mechanisms. Whatever the reason for forward blood flow, it appears that external thoracic massage is not very protective of the brain, because CPR performed for more than 3 or 4 min is often associated with significant neurological injury.[37] Because traditional external thoracic massage is apparently ineffective in many patients, various maneuvers have been proposed to improve blood flow during CPR. For example, *interposed abdominal compression* (IAC)[38] involves manually compressing the abdomen in counterpoint to

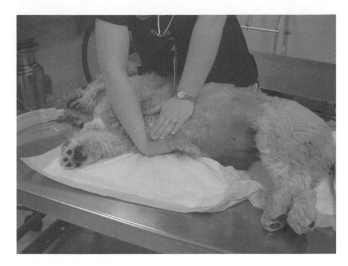

Fig. 53.1. External thoracic massage administered to a larger dog that probably derives blood flow primarily from the thoracic pump mechanism. The resuscitator, standing at the dog's back, is applying thoracic compressions over interspace 4 or 5 at the level of the costochondral junction. In larger dogs, the thoracic compressions may not mechanically contact the heart, so all blood flow is derived from increased intrathoracic pressure. The right hand is supplying a counterforce for thoracic compressions with the palm of the left hand. The compression rate for this dog should be from 80 to 100 beats/min.

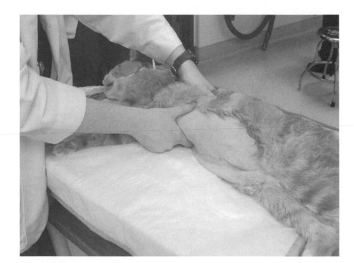

Fig. 53.2. External thoracic massage administered to a cat with blood flow derived from the cardiac pump. The thoracic walls contact the heart with each compression. Note that only the thumb and fingers of the right hand compress the thorax, while the left hand stabilizes the cat. The compression rate should be from 100 to 120 beats/min.

the rhythm of the chest compression. The physiological reason for improvement of blood flow is that compression of the abdominal aorta responds like an intra-aortic balloon pump and that pressure on the abdominal veins primes the right heart and pulmonary vasculature in preparation for the next thoracic compression.[39] This method of augmenting external CPR has been associated with improved survival in people and vital organ perfusion in dogs.[40,41] Utilization of IAC-CPR in over 100 dog CPR labs as part of a clinical anesthesia rotation demonstrated that venous return and arterial blood pressure improved for about 1 min, after which hemodynamics began to fail again (A. T. Evans, personal observation). Another way of improving blood flow during CPR is to simultaneously ventilate at the time of thoracic compression. Simultaneous ventilation-compression (SVC) CPR has improved carotid blood flow during resuscitation of animals.[42] Opposing evidence has also been presented that shows that the mitral valve of dogs may actually close in response to rhythmic increases in intrathoracic pressure.[43] Despite this evidence to the contrary, SVC-CPR probably improves blood flow during CPR of large dogs when the thoracic pump is the primary mechanism in generating blood flow.

Open thoracic or internal CPR is more effective at perfusing the heart and brain during the critical beginning minutes of CPR.[44–46] Higher blood pressure and cardiac output can be achieved with internal CPR. Most veterinary practices are well equipped to perform internal CPR because controlled ventilation and thoracotomy can be performed. The limiting factor in its employment is often the surgical inexperience of the attending veterinarian or the "do not resuscitate" wishes of the animal owner. Although it can be a difficult subject to broach, it is desirable to ascertain prior to the procedure the owner's wishes concerning CPR, in writing, in the event that cardiac arrest should occur during anesthesia and surgery. Valuable time may be lost trying to contact owners. Whichever method of CPR is chosen, there are some guidelines for CPR technique that, when followed, can improve success. The animal should be in right lateral recumbency with the resuscitator standing at its back (Fig. 53.1). The thoracic or cardiac compression rate should be 80 (large dogs) to 120 (cats) per minute.[47,48] A longer compression time will augment forward blood flow when using the thoracic pump mechanism.

The recommendations for D, *definitive* or *drug therapy*, start with the immediate use of epinephrine. Epinephrine should be administered early, preferably into a central vein or alternatively into a peripheral vein, intrabronchially, or directly into the chamber of the left ventricle.[49] For intrabronchial administration, use a flexible catheter wedged into a distal bronchus.[50] For intracardiac placement, use a long, 22-gauge needle inserted at the left thoracic fourth or fifth interspace and costochondral junction. For intravenous administration, a dose of 0.05 to 0.1 mg/kg is used, whereas bronchial administration requires 0.05 to 0.1 mg/kg diluted to a 2- to 3-mL volume with saline. The dose for intracardiac epinephrine is 0.025 to 0.05 mg/kg. Even though intracardiac epinephrine seems appealing as a way of efficiently delivering the drug to the heart, the technical difficulty of positioning the needle in the chamber of the left ventricle when the heart cannot be palpated, along with the potential for myocardial or coronary vascular injury, makes this technique the least advantageous. Since the goal of CPR is to revive the heart as soon as possible, early administration of epinephrine is crucial, and it should be given immediately after diagnosis of cardiac arrest.

The use of vasopressin in asystolic cardiac arrest has been recommended as a new standard of care in people.[51] The interest in

vasopressin as treatment for cardiac arrest was due to an observation in the early 1990s that endogenous vasopressin levels were greater in survivors of cardiac arrest than in patients that died.[52] The resuscitation success from the injection of vasopressin compared with epinephrine may be because the heart continues to consume oxygen after epinephrine injection (especially with tachycardia that often follows successful epinephrine-assisted resuscitation), whereas vasopressin augments coronary blood flow through an increase in systemic vascular resistance and increased diastolic perfusion pressure without an accompanying tachycardia.[53,54] In people, epinephrine may be potentially detrimental in early asystolic cardiac arrest because exogenous epinephrine could be expected to potentiate hypoxemia and advancing acidosis, which could further impair the pressor effects of epinephrine.[51] Tracheal administration of vasopressin (1.2 units/kg) in anesthetized dogs has resulted in systolic, diastolic, and mean blood pressure increases that last longer than 1 h.[55] Although research into the effects of vasopressin in treating cardiac arrest in dogs is scarce, an intravenous dose of 0.8 units/kg has been suggested for treatment of shock-refractory ventricular fibrillation, pulseless ventricular tachycardia, asystole, and PEA.[56]

Lidocaine is used after resuscitation if ventricular dysrhythmias are compromising cardiac output. The use of lidocaine during ventricular fibrillation to improve the results of electrical defibrillation is being reevaluated.[57] Lidocaine is usually given as an intravenous bolus at a dose of 0.5 mg/kg. Amiodarone has also been recommended for shock-refractory ventricular tachycardia or fibrillation in people.[58] Because of its vasodilatory effects on the coronary circulation, amiodarone (5 mg/kg intravenously) is best administered in combination with epinephrine.[59] Metabolic acidosis from hypoxia and ischemia, and respiratory alkalosis caused by iatrogenic hyperventilation during treatment of cardiac arrest, commonly occur during resuscitation.[60] The immediate use of bicarbonate is controversial, because metabolic acidosis is slow to develop during CPR and is somewhat neutralized by an ensuing respiratory alkalosis. Respiratory alkalosis is caused by external thoracic compression and controlled ventilation during CPR. Sodium bicarbonate (1 mEq/kg) administered after 10 min of resuscitation will improve the chance of return of spontaneous circulation and may play a role in mitigating postresuscitation cerebral acidosis.[61,62] However, bicarbonate administration can result in production of carbon dioxide as metabolic acid is neutralized. Careful monitoring of $PaCO_2$ can be a guide to adequate ventilation postresuscitation to avoid paradoxical cerebral acidosis.

Atropine or glycopyrrolate are important drugs to administer during CPR because reflex bradycardia may have contributed to the initial cardiac arrest. In addition, bradycardia often occurs after a heartbeat has been established. Atropine at 0.02 to 0.04 mg/kg or glycopyrrolate at a dose of 0.01 mg/kg intravenously will enhance the automaticity and conduction of both sinoatrial and atrioventricular nodes.[63]

In dogs and cats, pulseless electrical activity is apparently more common than ventricular fibrillation.[64] Asystole, observed as a flatline ECG, is the next most common form of cardiac arrest, with ventricular fibrillation the least common. It is fortu-

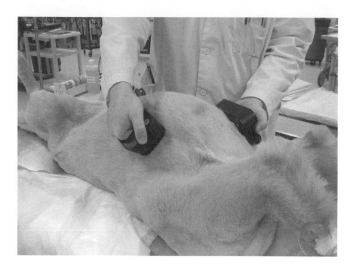

Fig. 53.3. Placement of direct-current paddles for defibrillation of the heart during cardiac arrest. An area under the paddles has been shaved and electrode jelly applied to the paddles. Administer a shock of approximately 3 to 5 joules (watts/second) per kilogram of body weight. Sequential discharges of increasing energy of 50% at each shock may be more effective at converting fibrillation.

itous that ventricular fibrillation is the least common expression of cardiac arrest, because most veterinary practices do not have access to a direct-current defibrillator. If a direct-current defibrillator is available, clip the hair from a small area from each side of the thorax. After applying electrode gel to each paddle, firmly apply the paddles to the thorax (Fig. 53.3) and administer a shock of approximately 3 to 5 joules (watts/seconds) per kilogram of body weight. Sequential discharges of increasing energy may be more effective at converting fibrillation.[56] Internal defibrillation requires a smaller electrical discharge: a total of 10 to 50 joules. Alcohol should not be used for ECG lead placement during CPR because alcohol is highly flammable and may be ignited by a defibrillator.

Internal Cardiopulmonary Resuscitation

After administration of epinephrine, and after attention to airway (A) and breathing (B) of the CPR protocol, begin external thoracic massage. It seems reasonable to start external CPR even though success rates are low with this method. Some animals respond positively to one or two doses of epinephrine and 1 or 2 min of external CPR. These appear to be primarily animals in PEA or asystole. If there is no response after 2 min, one should quickly begin the more productive internal CPR technique.[65] Unfortunately, many practitioners may not feel confident about performing a thoracotomy when they have little or no previous experience with this procedure. There is little to lose, however, when a patient is in cardiac arrest and has not responded to initial resuscitation attempts. Emergency thoracotomy can be accomplished quickly in an arrested animal. Clip the hair from the left thorax at the fifth interspace. Spray or wipe the area with an antiseptic solution and incise the skin starting 1 inch from the spine to within 1 inch of the sternum. With surgical scissors, con-

tinue incision through the various tissue layers, avoiding the internal thoracic artery near the sternum. Bluntly penetrate the pleura, extend the incision, and spread the ribs. If the abdomen is open during surgery, a transdiaphragmatic approach has been used (especially during diaphragmatic hernia surgery) to reach the heart in a timely manner. Reach into the thorax and begin cardiac massage at a rate of 80 to 120 compressions per minute. Depending on its size, the heart can be massaged with fingers, one hand, or two hands.[66] Epinephrine can now be easily administered into the left ventricle as required. If the resuscitation is successful and mental alertness improves, the patient can be anesthetized to complete closure of the thoracic incision. The thorax should be flushed with warm, sterile physiological saline and closed in a routine manner. Infection is rare after emergency thoracotomy in people and, from clinical experience, uncommon in dogs.[67,68] An algorithm for patients with confirmed cardiac arrest is presented in Fig. 53.4.

Postresuscitation Care

Once there is a return of spontaneous circulation, attention must be directed toward limiting the neurological injury and other sequelae produced by the cardiac arrest. Intensive care must be provided to address blood-gas abnormalities, respiratory insufficiency, hypotension, cardiac dysrhythmias, and temperature. Clinical trials in people have demonstrated neurological benefit of mild therapeutic hypothermia (32°C to 34°C) in survivors of out-of-hospital cardiac arrest.[69] Mild hypothermia should be instituted as soon as possible after resuscitation and maintained for at least 12 h. Cooling methods that may work in smaller animals involve surface cooling of the head and neck, as well as circulation of cool air over the patient's body. Tympanic membrane temperature can be used as a proxy for brain temperature. Application of mild hypothermia may improve the rather dismal success rate of cardiac and brain resuscitation in animals.

After successful CPR, the use of intravenous antibiotics has been recommended to counter the potential septicemia that can follow ischemic insult of the integrity of the lining of the gastrointestinal tract. Administration of osmotic diuretics such as mannitol (0.5 to 1.0 g/kg intravenously) after resuscitation has also been recommended to counter cerebral edema secondary to ischemia.

Perivascular Injection

Among all of the injectable anesthetics in use today, the perivascular injection of thiopental has likely caused more local tissue damage than all other anesthetics put together, primarily because of its very alkaline pH. It is, however, unusual for a perivascular slough to occur if the concentration of thiopental is 2.5% or less. If thiopental is inadvertently injected, perivascular treatment should consist of infiltration of the area with saline to dilute the thiopental, lidocaine to vasodilate capillaries and increase absorption, and corticosteroids to decrease the inflammatory response. Propofol, ketamine, and etomidate normally do not cause tissue sloughing if accidentally injected perivascularly. In horses or cattle, glycerol guiacolate is irritating and will likely cause a tissue

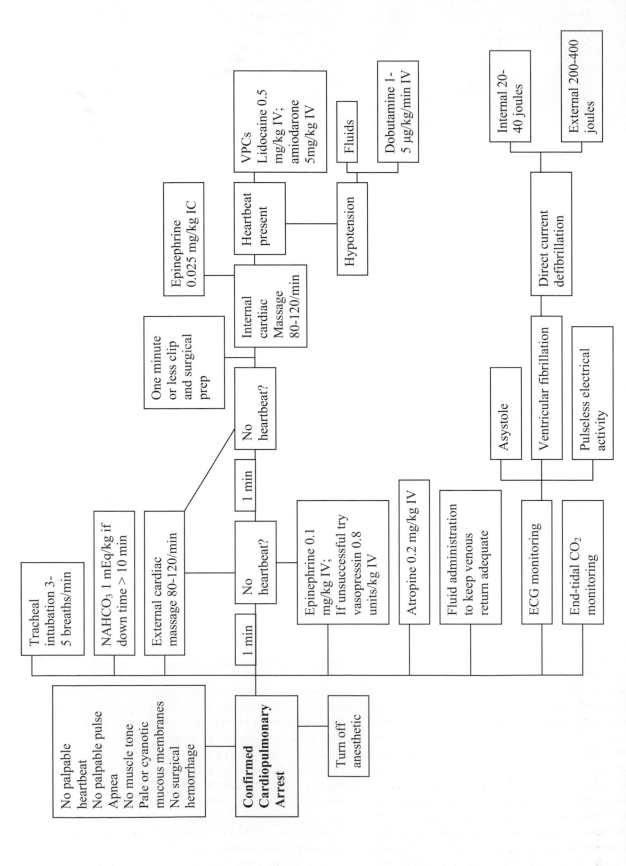

Fig. 53.4. An algorithm for cardiopulmonary resuscitation (CPR). This simplified protocol for CPR is used to resuscitate animals that might be able to survive cardiac arrest. Because early restoration of brain perfusion is the most important goal, a quick decision for internal cardiac massage is required. ECG, electrocardiogram; IC, intracardiac; IV, intravenously; NaHCO₃, sodium bicarbonate; and VPCs, ventricular premature contractions.

slough if a large volume is injected or infused outside the intended vessel. Many catecholamine solutions including dopamine can lead to tissue necrosis after perivascular injection. Intense α_1-receptor–mediated vasoconstriction is likely the cause.

Respiratory Insufficiency

Respiratory depression is defined by an increase in $PaCO_2$, and not by a decrease in respiratory rate alone. It is common for respiratory rate to decrease with a decrease in the level of activity and awareness (e.g., sleep), but tidal volume typically increases to compensate, resulting in no net change in $PaCO_2$. During anesthesia, respiratory insufficiency is common because many factors alter the chemoreceptor responsiveness to carbon dioxide, leading to elevated $PaCO_2$. Causes include the administration of opioids and other sedatives prior to anesthesia, the relative overdose of induction agents, positioning for surgery, respiratory depressant effects of inhalants, surgical trauma, recovery from bronchial alveolar lavage, and excessive use of opioids during recovery. The use of opioids with or without tranquilizers prior to induction of anesthesia to provide sedation and analgesia often results in a patient being well sedated but with depressed ventilatory drive. High doses of μ-receptor agonists such as oxymorphone, hydromorphone, and morphine are more likely to produce respiratory depression than is the κ-receptor agonist butorphanol. In addition, the decreased responsiveness to increased carbon dioxide tensions during halothane, isoflurane, or sevoflurane anesthesia tends to cause hypoventilation, although surgical stimulation often overrides some anesthetic-induced loss in respiratory drive.[70,71] In addition to the depressant effects of inhalants on responsiveness to increased $PaCO_2$, subanesthetic doses depress the peripheral chemoreceptors such that hypoxia does not stimulate a ventilation response.[72,73] Hypoxia often occurs during recovery from anesthesia after diagnostic bronchial alveolar lavage (BAL). Although BAL with volumes of up to 4 L have only transient effects in healthy dogs, BAL can lead to increased morbidity and mortality in dogs and cats with severe respiratory disease.[74–76] During BAL, supplemental oxygen can be administered by insufflation with a small rubber tube placed in the trachea alongside the bronchoscope (Fig. 53.5). After the procedure, oxygen should be administered by endotracheal tube, mask, or chamber until the pulse-oximeter readings remain at 90% saturation or higher while room air is breathed. Airway obstruction may also occur after ear-ablation surgery. Soft tissue swelling in the posterior pharynx may be severe enough to require a tracheostomy for relief.

Apnea is common during routine anesthesia. It occurs during induction after the administration of thiobarbiturates or propofol, during maintenance of anesthesia with ketamine, when controlled ventilation is discontinued, and as a consequence of deeper-inhalation anesthesia. Apnea occurring at induction is generally transient and is treated by low-frequency intermittent ventilation that is adequate to maintain hemoglobin-oxygen saturation at greater than 90%. Apnea occurring later during anesthesia, especially in spontaneously breathing animals, must be quickly recognized and treated with decreasing anesthetic concentrations and/or high-frequency positive-pressure ventilation. Apnea late in

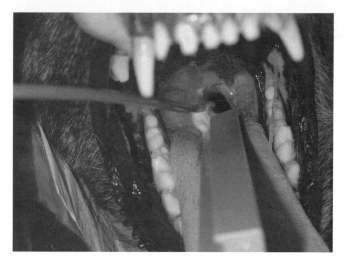

Fig. 53.5. Placement of a red rubber tube into the trachea for insufflation of oxygen during bronchial alveolar lavage. The red rubber tube via an extension is connected to the oxygen line that normally connects the anesthesia machine with the circle.

anesthesia is usually caused by excessive depression of the respiratory centers of the brain secondary to high anesthetic concentrations, or because of decompensation associated with severe neurological disease such as hydrocephalus or intracranial neoplasia.

Generally, apnea during induction of anesthesia with thiobarbiturates or propofol is caused by a relative overdose or a fast bolus injection.[77] Ketamine and diazepam in a 1:1 mixture by volume is commonly used for anesthesia in cats. Apnea often occurs, especially when anesthesia is maintained with supplemental isoflurane. This combination of drugs, each of which is a respiratory depressant alone, can induce a persistent respiratory depression. If, in response to respiratory depression, assisted or controlled ventilation is employed, $PaCO_2$ will often be reduced below the arterial or alveolar PCO_2 level at which cats will remain apneic (apneic threshold). Decreased functional residual capacity (FRC) during anesthesia can increase hypoxia by lowering alveolar ventilation-perfusion ratios (V_A/Q) and expanding atelectatic areas. This occurs because the FRC is close to or less than the closing volume (CV) of the lung. The CV is the volume of the lung at which small airways begin to close. When the tidal volume is less than the CV, small airways remain closed throughout the breathing cycle, and atelectasis increases. If the CV of some airways remains within the tidal volume range, then there is some air exchange during inspiration and expiration, though not the normal amount. This partial ventilation decreases the V_A/Q. These lung changes are prevalent in older animals and during anesthesia. Intermittent positive-pressure breathing and positive end-expiratory pressure (PEEP) can be used to diminish the hypoxia that occurs from changes in FRC.

Equipment Malfunction

Routine equipment maintenance and leak tests should be used to reduce the chances of anesthesia-machine malfunctions. Com-

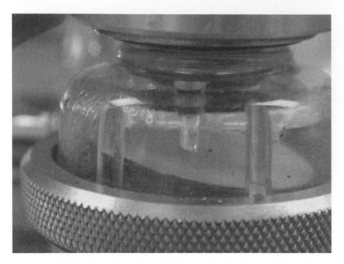

Fig. 53.6. Because of condensation of humidified exhaled gases on the dome and valve, this exhalation check valve has become lodged in the open position, enabling rebreathing of expired gases. An end-tidal carbon dioxide monitor would detect this equipment problem.

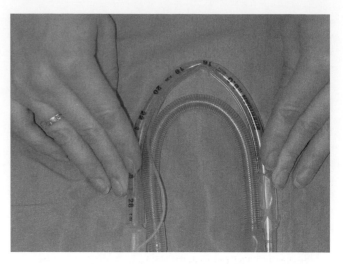

Fig. 53.7. The use of a wire-reinforced endotracheal tube will prevent kinking of the tube and obstruction of oxygen flow to patients. The protected endotracheal tube should be used when extreme flexion of the animal's head and neck or of the endotracheal tube is anticipated.

mon equipment malfunctions include "channeling" of gas flow through the carbon dioxide–absorbent canister, "sticking" of the exhalation check valve in the open position, interruption of oxygen supply, and kinking of the endotracheal tube. All of these equipment malfunctions can be rapidly detected with the routine use of a capnograph and pulse oximeter during inhalant or injectable anesthesia. *Channeling* occurs when gas flow through the carbon dioxide–absorbent canister is uneven, resulting in early termination of carbon dioxide absorption. If the pathway is through the center of the canister, there is not likely to be any observable change in color of the carbon dioxide absorbent, although the end-tidal carbon dioxide monitor should indicate increased rebreathing of exhaled gases (i.e., elevation of inspired carbon dioxide). Another cause of increased rebreathing of exhaled gases involves a malfunction of the exhalation check valve. The accumulation of moisture from humidified exhaled gases condensing on the cooler anesthesia machine parts can cause the check valve to remain in the open position (Fig. 53.6). In this situation, patients will rebreathe more exhaled gas and higher levels of carbon dioxide. The oxygen supply to a patient can be mistakenly interrupted when the oxygen lines have been pressurized before the oxygen cylinder has been turned off. When the oxygen flowmeter is turned on again, oxygen flow is initially present, giving the impression the oxygen cylinder is open, but will cease when the oxygen in the lines is exhausted. This is more likely to occur when switching from a central supply of oxygen to smaller oxygen cylinders mounted onto the anesthetic machine. The endotracheal tube can kink during extreme flexion of the animal's neck during positioning for cerebral spinal fluid tap, cervical spine radiographs, or ophthalmologic procedures. One should always determine patency of the endotracheal tube after extreme flexion of the head and neck. Use of a wire-reinforced endotracheal tube can reduce the incidence of obstruction (Fig. 53.7). If any problem is suspected

with the anesthesia machine, the patient should be disconnected from the machine and temporarily ventilated with room air until the problem is solved.

Delayed Recovery

Occasionally, an animal will fail to recover normally from anesthesia. Common causes of this problem include hypothermia, hypoglycemia, and heavy narcotization. Hypoglycemia has been shown to decrease the minimum alveolar concentration of halothane in rats.[78] Hypoglycemia can be clinically silent in anesthetized patients, which emphasizes the importance of glucose monitoring in susceptible patients. During anesthesia, signs of sympathetic overactivity or ventricular arrhythmias may be the only detectable evidence of life-threatening hypoglycemia.[79] Patients at high risk of developing hypoglycemia in the perianesthetic period include neonates, very small patients, fasting diabetics treated with their usual insulin dose, and dogs with glucocorticoid deficiency.[80]

Occasionally, coma or blindness can follow anesthetic-related insult to the central nervous system. If persistent neurological deficit follows an apparently uneventful anesthetic procedure, likely causes include hypoxia, severe hypotension, undiagnosed hydrocephalus, other preexisting neurological dysfunction, or an idiosyncratic drug-related response. In these cases, the exact etiology may be harder to determine. Treatment of these patients is primarily supportive, and the prognosis has to be guarded. In cases of anesthesia-related cortical blindness, vision may return as long as 2 weeks later, so cautious optimism is appropriate.

Reports of poor or delayed recoveries from anesthesia abound in popular canine and feline breed journals, and many breed societies relay stories of anesthetic-related problems. There are indeed situations where breed-specific anatomical or physiological peculiarities may complicate anesthetic management. Also, genetic differences in specific populations of a species or breed can perhaps increase the risk of performing anesthesia in some individual animals. Nevertheless, most animals presented with non-specific warnings about delayed recovery from anesthesia respond normally to the careful dosing of commonly used anesthetic agents. Inappropriate dosage of anesthetic or inadequate patient monitoring is more likely the common culprit in many cases of reported "anesthetic sensitivity."

Gastroesophageal Reflux and Regurgitation

Reflux of gastric contents into the esophagus has occurred if esophageal pH decreases below 4 (reflux of gastric acid) or above 7.5 (reflux of bile). This reflux is clinically silent and usually acidic.[81,82] The lower esophageal sphincter is considered to be the primary barrier to the development of this reflux.[83] Lower esophageal sphincter pressure in dogs is decreased with the use of isoflurane, atropine, acepromazine, and xylazine.[84,85] The effects of many other anesthetic agents on sphincter function have not been determined. Gastroesophageal reflux (GER) reportedly occurs during anesthesia in approximately 17% of dogs receiving thiopental, halothane, and other agents; in 50% of dogs receiving propofol; and in up to 60% of dogs receiving preanesthetic morphine.[81,82,86,87] A 5% incidence of GER has been reported in a population of anesthetized people, which suggests that anesthetic-induced GER occurs less frequently in people than in dogs, even though opioids are commonly used in both species.[88] In some cases, the refluxate is of sufficient volume to reach the pharynx and even drain from the mouth (regurgitation). The incidence of regurgitation is currently estimated at around 0.1% in animals anesthetized at the Michigan State University Veterinary Teaching Hospital.[89] This material may be aspirated into the lungs, leading to pneumonitis, or may cause local irritation of the esophagus as a prelude to development of ulcerative esophagitis and stricture formation.[83,88,90,91]

Hypothermia

This occurs commonly in anesthetized patients because of depressed thermoregulation, excessive heat loss relative to metabolic production, and mixing of core and peripheral blood by indiscriminant vasodilation. Heat is lost to the environment through convection, conduction, radiation, and evaporation, and occurs more rapidly when body surface is larger relative to body mass. Many anesthetic drugs, including opioids, the inhalant anesthetics, and α_2-agonists, interfere with thermoregulation and contribute to prolonged postoperative hypothermia.[92–94] Inhalation anesthetics lower the threshold for response to hypothermia in people to about 34.5°C, and presumably this occurs in animals, as well.[92] The rate of core temperature decrease in horses under halothane anesthesia has been shown to be 0.37°C/h, which is reduced to 0.19°C/h with the application of a forced-air warmer to help maintain patient body temperature.[95] Anesthetized dogs have been shown to have a decrease in rectal temperature of 1.9°C/h in the first hour of anesthesia.[96]

Hypothermia has been associated with pain, suppressed phagocytic activity including decreased migration of polymorphonuclear cells, reduced superoxide anion production, and reduced bacterial killing, and thus may contribute to systemic suppression of immune reactivity in the perioperative period.[97] In a retrospective study of dogs, mild decreases (1°C) in body temperature during surgery were not related to increased risk of incisional infections.[98] Accidental surgical hypothermia can be limited by increasing the ambient temperature, but this is seldom feasible. Circulating warm-water pads, especially applied to the legs, have been shown to help preserve body heat in dogs.[99] Forced-air warming systems currently are the most efficient and effective means of preserving or increasing body heat in anesthetized patients. This warming technique has been shown to delay or reduce the rate of heat loss in horses, dogs, and parrots.[95,100] Humidification and warming of inhaled gas has been shown to be ineffective as a sole means of maintaining core temperature in dogs or cats.[96,101,102] The use of uncovered electrical heating pads or "hot-water gloves" is discouraged because of potential for thermal injury.[103,104]

Hyperthermia

Drug-induced hyperthermia is rare in the practice of veterinary anesthesia. However, μ-receptor opioid agonists such as hydromorphone and fentanyl have been associated with moderate hyperthermia in some cats. The most commonly used drugs in human practice that can cause hyperthermia include antipsychotic agents, serotonin antagonists, sympathomimetic agents, inhalation anesthetics, and agents with anticholinergic properties.[105] The resultant hyperthermia is frequently accompanied by intense skeletal muscle rigidity (contracture), rhabdomyolysis, and hyperkalemia. Neuroleptic malignant syndrome is a rare but potentially lethal reaction to antipsychotic drugs, including phenothiazines and lithium.[96] Dopaminergic antagonism, a direct myotoxicity, altered thermoregulation, or extrapyramidal hyperactivity are postulated to contribute to the development of this syndrome. It is very possible that this syndrome could even occur in phenothiazine-treated animals placed in a very warm environment.

Malignant hyperthermia is an inherited membrane-linked abnormality (ryanodine receptor mutation) that has been documented in several species, including pigs, dogs, cats, and horses.[106–109] Susceptible patients should be anesthetized with barbiturates, propofol, opiates, and tranquilizers, and may be pretreated with dantrolene. Avoidance of known triggering agents—such as potent inhalation anesthetics, depolarizing muscle relaxants and stress—is advised.

Accidental iatrogenic hyperthermia can develop during warm ambient temperatures, in animals with thick hair coats, and with the use of forced-air warming systems. It is important to monitor body temperature in patients where active heating strategies are being used. Some smaller patients when treated with forced-air warming on the highest setting (43°C) heat up rapidly. In most situations, iatrogenic hyperthermia subsides rapidly after the heat source is removed.

Injuries

A number of other conditions can lead to injury during anesthesia:

Swollen feet: Limbs can be secured by ties placed so tight that they reduce venous drainage.

Corneal ulcers: Anesthetics reduce or eliminate the palpebral and corneal reflex and reduce tear formation. Chemical irritants, physical trauma, or drying can lead to ulceration. Artificial tears are important in preventing these problems.

Tracheal mucosal injury: Overinflation of the cuff or moving the cuff while it is inflated can cause mucosal injury, tracheal rupture, or tracheal chondromalacia. Tracheal rupture is an uncommon sequela to intubation in cats and can usually be treated medically.[110] When changing patient positions, the endotracheal tube should be disconnected from the Y adapter, and the patient's head and neck supported to prevent sliding or movement of the endotracheal tube cuff. To prevent pressure-induced mucosal necrosis, it is wise to inflate the cuff of the endotracheal tube only sufficiently to seal a leak at 10 to 20 cm H_2O. It is not recommended to simply put "some air" in the cuff without checking its pressure.

Joint pain: Older animals with arthritic joints that are placed on their backs for surgery may have joint pain for days following anesthesia.

Pulmonary barotrauma: Overinflation of the lungs will damage the pulmonary structures significantly if pressures exceed 30 cm H_2O.[111–113] Inadvertently leaving the adjustable pressure-limiting valve (pop-off valve) closed or using the oxygen flush when the patient is on a Bain's system can create pulmonary overpressurization. One simple way to provide protection for the patient if the pop-off valve inadvertently remains in the closed position is to place a commercially available PEEP valve in the breathing circuit (Fig. 53.8).

Epidural Analgesia and Regional Nerve Block

The use of the epidural route for delivery of opioids and local anesthetics is becoming increasingly popular, especially with prolonged drug delivery by epidural catheter.[114–118] There are reports of epidural catheters having been placed and left in dogs for 7 days and in horses for up to 20 days, with the main complication being catheter dislodgement and local tissue response.[116–118] Meticulous attention to aseptic technique is essential when drugs or catheters are placed in the epidural space. Epidural abscessation and discospondylitis have been reported following epidural injection.[119] Other complications reported following epidural injection in dogs include urinary retention, prolonged cerebrospinal fluid levels of morphine, myotonus, and pruritus.[114,120–122] Subarachnoid injection of preservative-free morphine in a dog caused such severe pruritus and myoclonus that the dog had to be anesthetized for several hours until the reaction resolved.[121] The authors have observed one horse with severe pruritus of the hind feet after epidural injection of xylazine and local anesthetic. Sedation with detomidine was sufficient to calm

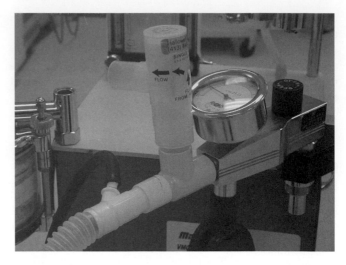

Fig. 53.8. A 20-cm water positive end-expiratory pressure (PEEP) valve can serve as an emergency release valve in case the adjustable pressure-limiting valve (pop-off valve) is accidentally closed and pressure begins to build in the anesthesia system. The PEEP valve can be used with circle and Bain's anesthesia delivery systems.

this horse. It appears from anecdotal reports that when a local anesthetic is combined with xylazine for epidural injection in horses, hind-limb ataxia and weakness are more likely to occur.

Regional nerve block has some risk of causing local anesthetic toxicity, although combining local anesthetics with epinephrine (5 µg/mL) will dramatically reduce this risk. Direct needle trauma to the nerve being blocked can cause a prolonged or permanent neural deficit. Local hemorrhage may result in hematoma formation, but this is generally self-limiting.

Electrolyte Abnormalities

Hyperkalemia is one electrolyte abnormality that can be associated with acute death.[123,124] The causes of rapid-onset hyperkalemia during anesthesia and surgery include transfusion of old stored blood, chronic heparin therapy (dogs), uroperitoneum (especially foals and cats), iatrogenic administration (potassium penicillin or potassium chloride), and hyperkalemic periodic paralysis (HPP). Horses that are homozygous or heterozygous for HPP should be closely monitored. Diet change or the stress of fasting, anesthesia, and pain may lead to an attack in the perianesthetic period. Signs of an HPP attack are obvious even in anesthetized horses as hyperkalemia produces very characteristic ECG changes.[125] Arrhythmias caused by hyperkalemia can lead to cardiac arrest and may not respond to conventional antiarrhythmic therapies, but do respond to the rapid treatment of hyperkalemia.[125,126] Aggressive lowering of serum potassium by using acetazolamide, furosemide, dextrose, and sodium bicarbonate, and the reversal of hyperkalemic effects on cell membrane potential by calcium administration can help resolve an HPP crisis if it occurs during anesthesia.[125,126]

Hypokalemia caused by hemodilution and decreased intake is the most common cause of postoperative arrhythmias in people.

Arrhythmias (ventricular ectopy) associated with this electrolyte disturbance are not commonly observed in other animals. Hypocalcemia is an insidious electrolyte disturbance that can also be a problem for anesthetized patients. Hypocalcemia can lead to muscle weakness, which can be particularly problematic for horses trying to stand while recovering from anesthesia.

References

1. Davies JM. On-site risk management. Can J Anaesth 1991;38:1029–1030.
2. Armstrong JN, Davies JM. A systematic method for the investigation of anaesthetic incidents. Can J Anaesth 1991;38:1033–1035.
3. Eichorn JH. Documenting improved anesthesia outcome. J Clin Anesth 1991;3:351–353.
4. Cohen MM, Duncan PG, Tate RB. Does anesthesia contribute to operative mortality? J Am Med Assoc 1988;260:2859–2863.
5. Lagasse RS. Anesthesia safety: Model or myth? Anesthesiology 2002;97:1609–1617.
6. Dyson DH, Maxie MG, Schnurr D. Morbidity and mortality associated with anesthetic management in small animal veterinary practice in Ontario. J Am Anim Hosp Assoc 1998;34:325–335.
7. Johnston GM, Taylor PM, Holmes MA, Wood JLN. Confidential enquiry of perioperative equine fatalities (CEPEF-1): Preliminary results. Equine Vet J 1995;27:193–200.
8. Mee AM, Cripps PJ, Jones RS. A retrospective study of mortality associated with general anaesthesia in horses: Elective procedures. Vet Rec 1998;142:275–276.
9. Richey MT, Holland MS, McGrath CJ, et al. Equine post-anesthetic lameness: A retrospective study. Vet Surg 1990;19:392–397.
10. Mee AM, Cripps PJ, Jones RS. A retrospective study of mortality associated with general anaesthesia in horses: Emergency procedures. Vet Rec 1998;142:307–309.
11. Freeman DE, Hungerford LL, Schaeffer D, et al. Caesarean section and other methods for assisted delivery: Comparison of effects on mare mortality and complications. Equine Vet J 1999;31:203–207.
12. Bidwell LA, Bramlage LR, Rood WA. Fatality rates associated with equine general anesthesia. In: Proceedings of the American Association of Equine Practitioners, Denver, CO, 2004:21–28.
13. Schmall LM, Muir WW, Robertson JT. Haemodynamic effects of small volume hypertonic saline in experimentally induced haemorrhagic shock. Equine Vet J 1990;22:273–277.
14. Skillman JJ, Olson JE, Lyons JH, Moore FD. The hemodynamic effect of acute blood loss in normal man, with observations on the effect of the Valsalva maneuver and breath holding. Ann Surg 1967;166:713–738.
15. Waisman Y, Eichacker PQ, Banks SM, Hoffman WD, MacVittie TJ, Natanson C. Acute hemorrhage in dogs: Construction and validation of models to quantify blood loss. J Appl Physiol 1993;74:510–519.
16. Wilson DV, Shance PU, Rondenay Y. The cardiopulmonary effects of severe blood loss in anesthetized horses. Vet Anaesth Analg 2003;30:80–86.
17. Prough DS, Johnston WE. Fluid resuscitation in septic shock: No solution yet. Anesth Analg 1989;69:699–704.
18. Friedman Z, Berkenstadt H, Preisman S, Perel A. A comparison of lactated ringer's solution to hydroxyethyl starch 6% in a model of severe hemorrhagic shock and continuous bleeding in dogs. Anesth Analg 2003;96:39–45.
19. Callan MB, Rentko VT. Clinical application of a hemoglobin-based oxygen-carrying solution. Vet Clin North Am Small Anim Pract 2003;33:1277–1293.
20. Driessen B, Fahr JS, Lurie F, Griffey SM, Gunther RA. Effects of haemoglobin-based oxygen carrier hemoglobin glutamer-200 (bovine) on intestinal perfusion and oxygenation in a canine hypovolaemia model. Br J Anaesth 2001;86:682–692.
21. Driessen B, Jahr FS, Lurie F, Golkaryeh MS, Gunther RA. Arterial oxygenation and oxygen delivery after hemoglobin-based oxygen carrier infusion in canine hypovolemic shock: A dose-response study. Crit Care Med 2003:31:1771–1779.
22. Muir WW III, Lipowitz AJ. Cardiac dysrhythmias associated with gastric dilatation-volvulus in the dog. J Am Vet Med Assoc 1978;172:683–689.
23. Macintire DK, Snider TG III. Cardiac arrhythmias associated with multiple trauma in dogs. J Am Vet Med Assoc 1984;184:541–545.
24. Atlee JL, Roberts FL. Thiopental and epinephrine-induced dysrhythmias in dogs anesthetized with enflurane or isoflurane. Anesth Analg 1986;65:437–443.
25. Hikasa Y, Okabe C, Takase K, Ogasawara S. Ventricular arrhythmogenic dose of adrenaline during sevoflurane, isoflurane, and halothane anaesthesia either with or without ketamine or thiopentone in cats. Res Vet Sci 1996;60:134–137.
26. Hubbell JAE, Muir WW III, Bednarski RM, Bednarski LS. Change of inhalation anesthetic agents for management of ventricular premature depolarizations in anesthetized cats and dogs. J Am Vet Med Assoc 1984;185:643–646.
27. Muir WW III, Hubbell JAE, Flaherty S. Increasing halothane concentration abolishes anesthesia-associated arrhythmias in cats and dogs. J Am Vet Med Assoc 1988;192:1730–1735.
28. Burren VS, Mason KV. Suspected anaphylaxis to thiopentone in a dog. Aust Vet J 1986;63:384–385.
29. Mason TA. Anaphylactic response to thiopentone in a dog. Vet Rec 1976;98:136.
30. White BC, Sullivan JM, DeGracia DJ, et al. Brain ischemia and reperfusion: Molecular mechanisms of neuronal injury. J Neurol Sci 2000;179:1–33.
31. Wingfield WE, Van Pelt DR. Respiratory and cardiopulmonary arrest in dogs and cats: 265 cases (1986–1991). J Am Vet Med Assoc 1992;200:1993–1996.
32. Chandra NC, Gruben KG, Tsitlik JE, et al. Observations of ventilation during resuscitation in a canine model. Circulation 1994;90:3070–3075.
33. Kern K. Cardiopulmonary resuscitation without ventilation. Crit Care Med 2000;28(Suppl):N186–N189.
34. Cole SG, Otto CM, Hughes D. Cardiopulmonary cerebral resuscitation in small animals: A clinical practice review (Part 1). J Vet Emerg Crit Care 2002;12:261–271.
35. Criley JM, Blaufuss AN, Kissel GL. Cough-induced cardiac compression: Self-administered form of cardiopulmonary resuscitation. J Am Med Assoc 1976;236:1246–1250.
36. Niemann JT, Roshorough JP, Niskanen, Alferness C, Criley JM. Mechanical "cough" cardiopulmonary resuscitation during cardiac arrest in dogs. Am J Cardiol 1985;55:199–204.
37. Kern KB, Ewy GA, Sanders AB, Voorhees WD, Babbs CF, Tacker WA. Neurologic outcome following successful cardiopulmonary resuscitation in dogs. Resuscitation 1986;14:149–155.
38. Ralston SH, Babbs CF, Niebauer MJ. Cardiopulmonary resuscitation with interposed abdominal compression in dogs. Anesth Analg 1982;61:645–651.

39. Babbs CF. Interposed abdominal compression CPR: A comprehensive evidence based review. Resuscitation 2003;59:71–82.

40. Sack JB, Kesselbrenner MB, Bregman D. Survival from in-hospital cardiac arrest with interposed abdominal counterpulsation during cardiopulmonary resuscitation. J Am Med Assoc 1992;267:379–385.

41. Hoekstra OS, van Lambalgen AA, Groeneveld AB, van den Bos GC, Thijs LG. Abdominal compressions increase vital organ perfusion during CPR in dogs: Relation with efficacy of thoracic compressions. Ann Emerg Med 1995;25:375–385.

42. Chandra N, Weisfeldt ML, Tsitlik J, Vaghaiwalla F, Snyder L. Augmentation of carotid flow during cardiopulmonary resuscitation by ventilation at high airway pressure simultaneous with chest compression. Am J Cardiol 1981;48:1053–1063.

43. Halperin HR, Weiss JL, Buerci AD, et al. Cyclic elevation of intrathoracic pressure can close the mitral valve during cardiac arrest in dogs. Circulation 1988;78:754–760.

44. Sanders AB, Kern KB, Ewy GA, Atlas M, Bailey L. Improved resuscitation from cardiac arrest with open-chest massage. Ann Emerg Med 1984;13:672–675.

45. Kern KB, Sanders AB, Ewy GA. Open-chest cardiac massage after closed-chest compression in a canine model: When to intervene. Resuscitation 1987;15:51–57.

46. Kern KB, Sanders AB, Janas W, et al. Limitations of open-chest cardiac massage after prolonged, untreated cardiac arrest in dogs. Ann Emerg Med 1991;20:761–767.

47. Feneley MP, Maier GW, Kern KB, et al. Influence of compression rate on initial success of resuscitation and 24 hour survival after prolonged manual cardiopulmonary resuscitation in dogs. Circulation 1988;77:240–250.

48. Henik RA. Basic life support and external cardiac compression in dogs and cats. J Am Vet Med Assoc 1992;200:1925–1931.

49. Van Pelt DT, Wingfield WE. Controversial issues in drug treatment during cardiopulmonary resuscitation. J Am Vet Med Assoc 1992;200:1938–1944.

50. Mazkereth R, Paret G, Ezra D, et al. Epinephrine blood concentrations after peripheral bronchial versus endotracheal administration of epinephrine in dogs. Crit Care Med 1992;20:1582–1587.

51. McIntyre KM. Vasopressin in asystolic cardiac arrest. N Engl J Med 2004;350:179–181.

52. Lindner KH, Strohmenger HU, Ensinger H, Hetzel WD, Ahnefeld FW, Georgieff M. Stress hormone response during and after cardiopulmonary resuscitation. Anesthesiology 1992;77:662–668.

53. Paradis NA, Wenzel V, Southall J. Pressor drugs in the treatment of cardiac arrest. Cardiol Clin 2002;20:61–78.

54. Mayr VD, Wenzel V, Voelckel WG, et al. Developing a vasopressor combination in a pig model of adult asphyxial cardiac arrest. Circulation 2001;104:1651–1656.

55. Efrati O, Barak A, Ben-Abraham R, et al. Hemodynamic effects of tracheal administration of vasopressin in dogs. Resuscitation 2001;50:227–232.

56. Cole SG, Otto CM, Hughes D. Cardiopulmonary cerebral resuscitation in small animals: A clinical practice review. Part II. J Vet Emerg Crit Care 2003;13:13–23.

57. Echt DS, Black JN, Barbey JT. Evaluation of antiarrhythmic drugs on defibrillation energy requirements in dogs. Circulation 1989;79:1106–1117.

58. American Heart Association. Guidelines 2000 for cardiopulmonary resuscitation and emergency cardiovascular care. Circulation 2000;102(Suppl):I112–I128.

59. Paiva EF, Perondi MB, Dern DB, et al. Effect of amiodarone on haemodynamics during cardiopulmonary resuscitation in a canine model of resistant ventricular fibrillation. Resuscitation 2003;58:203–208.

60. Sanders AB, Ewy GA, Taft TV. Resuscitation and arterial blood gas abnormalities during prolonged cardiopulmonary resuscitation. Ann Emerg Med 1984;13:676–679.

61. Leong EC, Bendall JC, Boyd AC, Einstein R. Sodium bicarbonate improves the chance of resuscitation after 10 minutes of cardiac arrest in dogs. Resuscitation 2001;51:309–315.

62. Liu X, Nozari A, Rubertsson S, Wiklund L. Buffer administration during CPR promotes cerebral reperfusion after return of spontaneous circulation and mitigates post-resuscitation cerebral acidosis. Resuscitation 2002;55:45–55.

63. Vincent R. Drugs in modern resuscitation. Br J Anaesth 1997;79:188–197.

64. Rush JE, Wingfield WE. Recognition and frequency of dysrhythmias during cardiopulmonary arrest. J Am Vet Med Assoc 1992;200:1932–1937.

65. Haskins SC. Internal cardiac compression. J Am Vet Med Assoc 1992;200:1945–1946.

66. Barnett WM, Alifimoff JK, Paris PM, Stewart RD, Safar P. Comparison of open-chest cardiac massage techniques in dogs. Ann Emerg Med 1986;15:408–411.

67. Altemeier WA, Todd J. Studies on the incidence of infection following open-chest cardiac massage for cardiac arrest. Ann Surg 1963;158:596–607.

68. Bircher M, Safar P. Manual open-chest cardiopulmonary resuscitation. Ann Emerg Med 1984;13:770–773.

69. Hypothermia After Cardiac Arrest Study Group. Mild therapeutic hypothermia to improve the neurologic outcome after cardiac arrest. N Engl J Med 2002;346:549–556.

70. Eger EL. Desflurane (Suprane): A Compendium and Reference. Nutley, NJ: Anaquest, 1993.

71. Dunlop CI, Steffey EP, Miller MF, Woliner MJ. Temporal effects of halothane and isoflurane in laterally recumbent ventilated male horses. Am J Vet Res 1987;48:1250–1255.

72. Weiskopf RB, Raymond LW, Severinghaus JW. Effects of halothane on canine respiratory responses to hypoxia with and without hypercarbia. Anesthesiology 1974;41:350–360.

73. Hirshman CA, McCullough RE, Cohen PJ. Depression of hypoxic ventilatory response by halothane, enflurane and isoflurane in dogs. Br J Anaesth 1977;49:957–963.

74. Muggenburg BA, Mauderly JL, Pickrell JA, et al. Pathophysiologic sequelae of bronchopulmonary lavage in the dog. Am Rev Respir Dis 1972;106:219–232.

75. Hawkins EC, DeNicola DB, Plier ML. Cytological analysis of bronchoalveolar lavage fluid in the diagnosis of spontaneous respiratory tract disease in dogs: A retrospective study. J Vet Intern Med 1995;9:386–392.

76. Hawkins EC. Bronchoalveolar lavage. In: King LG, ed. Respiratory Disease in Dogs and Cats. St Louis: WB Saunders, 2004:118–128.

77. Goodman NW, Black AM, Carter JA. Some ventilatory effects of propofol as sole anesthetic agent. Br J Anaesth 1987;59:1497–1503.

78. Ishizawa Y, Ohta S, Shimonaka H, Dohi S. Effects of blood glucose changes and physostigmine on anesthetic requirements of halothane in rats. Anesthesiology 1997;87:354–360.

79. Chelliah YR. Ventricular arrhythmias associated with hypoglycaemia. Anaesth Intensive Care 2000;28:698–700.

80. Lane IF, Matwichuk CL, Carpenter LG, Behrend EN. Profound postanesthetic hypoglycemia attributable to glucocorticoid deficiency in 2 dogs. Can Vet J 1999;40:497–500.

81. Galatos AD, Raptopoulos D. Gastro-oesophageal reflux during anaesthesia in the dog: The effect of preoperative fasting and premedication. Vet Rec 1995;137:479–483.

82. Galatos AD, Raptopoulos D. Gastro-oesophageal reflux during anaesthesia in the dog: The effects of age, positioning and type of surgical procedure. Vet Rec 1995;137:513–516.

83. Behar J. The role of the lower esophageal sphincter in reflux prevention. J Clin Gastroenterol 1986;8:2–4.

84. Hashim MA, Waterman AE, Pearson H. A comparison of the effects of halothane and isoflurane in combination with nitrous oxide on lower oesophageal sphincter pressure and barrier pressure in anaesthetized dogs. Vet Rec 1995;23:658–661.

85. Strombeck DR, Harrold D. Effects of atropine, acepromazine, meperidine, and xylazine on gastro-esophageal sphincter pressure in the dog. Am J Vet Res 1985;46:963–965.

86. Raptopoulos D, Galatos AD. Gastro-esophageal reflux during anaesthesia induced with either thiopentone or propofol in the dog. J Vet Anaesth 1997;24:20–22.

87. Wilson DV, Evans AT. Anesthetic-induced gastro-esophageal reflux in dogs: Effect of pre-anesthetic morphine [Abstract]. In: Eighth World Congress of Veterinary Anesthesia Scientific Proceedings, Knoxville, TN, 2003.

88. Martin C, Auffray JP, Ragni J, et al. Measurement of lower oesophageal pH during induction of anaesthesia: Use of oesophageal probe. Acta Anaesthesiol Scand 1992;36:226–229.

89. Wilson DV, Walshaw R. Postanesthetic esophageal dysfunction in 13 dogs. J Am Anim Hosp Assoc 2004;40:455–460.

90. Fransson BA, Bagley RS, Gay JM, et al. Pneumonia after intracranial surgery in dogs. Vet Surg 2001;30:432–439.

91. Ng A, Smith G. Gastroesophageal reflux and aspiration of gastric contents in anesthetic practice. Anesth Analg 2001;93:494–513.

92. Sessler DI, Olofsson CI, Rubinstein EH, Beebe JJ. The thermoregulatory threshold in humans during halothane anesthesia. Anesthesiology 1988;68:836–842.

93. Vainio O. Introduction to the clinical pharmacology of medetomidine. Acta Vet Scand Suppl 1989;85:85–88.

94. Barnhart MD, Hubbell JA, Muir WW, Sams RA, Bednarski RM. Pharmacokinetics, pharmacodynamics, and analgesic effects of morphine after rectal, intramuscular, and intravenous administration in dogs. Am J Vet Res 2000;61:24–28.

95. Tomasic M. Temporal changes in core body temperature in anesthetized adult horses. Am J Vet Res 1999;60:556–562.

96. Tan C, Govendir M, Zaki S, Miyake Y, Packiarajah P, Malik R. Evaluation of four warming procedures to minimise heat loss induced by anaesthesia and surgery in dogs. Aust Vet J 2004;82:65–68.

97. Beilin B, Shavit Y, Razumovsky J, Wolloch Y, Zeidel A, Bessler H. Effects of mild perioperative hypothermia on cellular immune responses. Anesthesiology 1998;89:1133–1140.

98. Beal MW, Brown DC, Shofer FS. The effects of perioperative hypothermia and the duration of anesthesia on postoperative wound infection rate in clean wounds: A retrospective study. Vet Surg 2000;29:123–127.

99. Cabell LW, Perkowski SZ, Gregor T, Smith GK. The effects of active peripheral skin warming on perioperative hypothermia in dogs. Vet Surg 1997;26:79–85.

100. Rembert FS, Smith JA, Hosgood G, Marks SL, Tully TN. Comparison of traditional thermal support devices with the forced-air warmer system in anesthetized Hispaniolan Amazon parrots (*Amazona ventralis*). J Avian Med Surg 2001;15:187–193.

101. Haskins SC, Patz JD. Effect of inspired-air warming and humidification in the prevention of hypothermia during general anesthesia in cats. Am J Vet Res 1980;41:1669–1673.

102. Raffe MR, Martin FB. Effect of inspired air heat and humidification on anesthetic-induced hypothermia in dogs. Am J Vet Res 1983;44:455–458.

103. Swaim SF, Lee AH, Hughes KS. Heating pads and thermal burns in small animals. J Am Anim Hosp Assoc 1989;25:156–162.

104. Dunlop CI, Daunt DA, Haskins SC. Thermal burns in four dogs during anesthesia. Vet Surg 1989;18:242–246.

105. Hadad E, Weinbroum AA, Ben-Abraham R. Drug-induced hyperthermia and muscle rigidity: A practical approach. Eur J Emerg Med 2003;10:149–154.

106. Bellah JR, Robertson SR, Buergelt CD, McGavin AD. Suspected malignant hyperthermia after halothane anesthesia in a cat. Vet Surg 1989;18:483–488.

107. Bagshaw RJ, Cox RH, Knight DH, Detweiler DK. Malignant hyperthermia in a greyhound. J Am Vet Med Assoc 1978;172:61–62.

108. Waldron-Mease EW, Klein LV, Rosenberg H, Leitch M. Malignant hyperthermia in a halothane-anesthetized horse. J Am Vet Med Assoc 1981;179:896–898.

109. Gronert GA. Malignant hyperthermia. Anesthesiology 1980;53:395–423.

110. Mitchell SL, McCarthy R, Rudloff E, Pernell RT. Tracheal rupture associated with intubation in cats: 20 cases (1996–1998). J Am Vet Med Assoc 2000;216:1592–1595.

111. Manning MM, Brunson DB. Barotrauma in a cat. J Am Vet Med Assoc 1994;205:62–64.

112. Singh JM, Stewart TE. High-frequency mechanical ventilation principles and practices in the era of lung-protective ventilation strategies. Respir Care Clin North Am 2002;8:247–260.

113. Anzueto A, Frutos-Vivar F, Esteban A, et al. Incidence, risk factors and outcome of barotrauma in mechanically ventilated patients. Intensive Care Med 2004;30:612–619.

114. Cousins MJ, Mather LM. Intrathecal and epidural administration of opioids. Anesthesiology 1984;61:276–310.

115. Troncy E, Junot S, Keroack S, et al. Results of preemptive epidural administration of morphine with or without bupivacaine in dogs and cats undergoing surgery: 265 cases (1997–1999). J Am Vet Med Assoc 2002;221:666–72.

116. Martin CA, Kerr CL, Pearce SG, Lansdowne JL, Boure LP. Outcome of epidural catheterization for delivery of analgesics in horses: 43 cases (1998–2001). J Am Vet Med Assoc 2003;222:1394–1398.

117. Sysel AM, Pleasant RS, Jacobson JD, et al. Systemic and local effects associated with long-term epidural catheterization and morphine-detomidine administration in horses. Vet Surg 1997;26:141–149.

118. Swalander DB, Crowe DT Jr, Hittenmiller DH, Jahn PJ. Complications associated with the use of indwelling epidural catheters in dogs: 81 cases (1996–1999). J Am Vet Med Assoc 2000;216:368–370.

119. Remedios AM, Wagner R, Caulkett NA, Duke T. Epidural abscess and discospondylitis in a dog after administration of a lumbosacral epidural analgesic. Can Vet J 1996;37:106–107.

120. Herperger LJ. Postoperative urinary retention in a dog following morphine with bupivacaine epidural analgesia. Can Vet J 1998;39:650–652.

121. Kona-Boun JJ, Pibarot P, Quesnel A. Myoclonus and urinary retention following subarachnoid morphine injection in a dog. Vet Anaesth Analg 2003;30:257–264.

122. Valverde A, Conlon PD, Dyson DH, Burger JP. Cisternal CSF and serum concentrations of morphine following epidural administration in the dog. J Vet Pharmacol Ther 1992;15:91–95.

123. Richardson DW, Kohn CW. Uroperitoneum in the foal. J Am Vet Med Assoc 1983;182:267–271.

124. Waldridge BM, Lin HC, Purohit RC. Anesthetic management of horses with hyperkalemic periodic paralysis. Comp Contin Educ Pract Vet 1996;18:1030–1039.

125. Bailey JE, Pablo L, Hubbell JAE. Hyperkalemic periodic paralysis episode during halothane anesthesia in a horse. J Am Vet Med Assoc 1996;208:1859–1865.

126. Cornick JL, Seahorn TL, Hartsfield SM. Hyperthermia during isoflurane anesthesia in a horse with suspected hyperkalemic periodic paralysis. Equine Vet J 1994;26:511–514.

Appendix

Standard Values and Equivalents*

Metric Weights

1 gram (1 g) = weight of 1 cc water at 4°C

1,000 g = 1 kilogram (kg)

0.1 g = 1 decigram (dg)

0.01 g = 1 centigram (cg)

0.001 g = 1 milligram (mg)

0.001 mg = 1 microgram (μg)

Metric Volumes

1 liter (L) = 1 cubic decimeter or 1,000 cubic centimeters (cc)

0.001 liter = 1 milliliter (mL)

Solution Equivalents

1 part in	10 =	10.00	% (1 mL contains	100	mg)
1 part in	50 =	2.00	% (1 mL contains	20	mg)
1 part in	100 =	1.00	% (1 mL contains	10	mg)
1 part in	200 =	0.50	% (1 mL contains	5	mg)
1 part in	500 =	0.20	% (1 mL contains	2	mg)
1 part in	1,000 =	0.10	% (1 mL contains	1	mg)
1 part in	1,500 =	0.066	% (1 mL contains	0.66	mg)
1 part in	2,600 =	0.038	% (1 mL contains	0.38	mg)
1 part in	5,000 =	0.02	% (1 mL contains	0.20	mg)
1 part in	50,000 =	0.002	% (1 mL contains	0.02	mg)

The number of milligrams in 1 milliliter of any solution of known percentage strength is obtained by moving the decimal one place to the right.

Apothecaries' or Troy Weight

(Used in Prescriptions)

1 pound (lb)	= 12 ounces	= 5,760 grains
1 ounce	= 8 drams	= 480 grains
1 dram	= 60 grains	

Apothecaries' Volume

1 pint	= 16 fluid ounces	
1 fluid ounce	= 8 fluid dram	= 480 minims
1 fluid dram	= 60 minims	

*Systeme International (SI) units and conversions are shown later in this appendix.

Avoirdupois or Imperial Weight
(Used in commerce in the United States and in the British Pharmacopeia)

Grain	= same as Troy grain	
Ounce (oz)	=	437.5 grains
Pound (lb)	= 16 oz	= 7,000 grains
Ton	= 2,000 lb	

Imperial Volume

		Apothecaries' System
Minims	=	0.96
Fluidrachm (fl dr)	= 60 minims	= 0.96 fl
Fluidounce (fl oz)	= 8 drachms	= 0.96 fl
Pint	= 20 fluid ounces	= 1.2 ounces
Gallon	= 8 pints	= 1.2 gallons

Approximate Equivalent Weights

1 kilogram	= 2.2 Avoirdupois/Imperial pounds
1 kilogram	= 2.6 Apothecary or Troy pounds
1 gram	= 15 (15.4) grains
1 milligram	= 1/60 (1/64) grain
1 ounce	= 30 grams
(Avoirdupois or Imperial	= 28.350 grams)
(Apothecary or Troy	= 31.1035 grams)
1 dram	= 4 grams
1 grain	= 60 milligrams

Approximate Equivalent Volumes

1 liter	= 1 quart
1 milliliter or cubic centimeter	= 15 minims
1 pint	= 500 cubic centimeters
1 fluid ounce	= 30 cubic centimeters
(Avoirdupois or Imperial	= 28.412 cubic centimeters)
(Apothecary or Troy	= 29.574 cubic centimeters)
1 fluid dram	= 4 cubic centimeters

Equivalents of Centigrade and Fahrenheit Thermometric Scales

Centigrade Degree	Fahrenheit Degree	Centigrade Degree	Fahrenheit Degree
−17	+ 1.4	14	57.2
−16	3.2	15	59.0
−15	5.0	16	60.8
−14	6.8	17	62.6
−13	8.6	18	64.4
−12	10.4	19	66.2
−11	12.2	20	68.0
−10	14.0	21	69.8
− 9	15.8	22	71.6
− 8	17.6	23	73.4
− 7	19.4	24	75.2
− 6	21.2	25	77.0
− 5	23.0	26	78.8
− 4	24.8	27	80.6
− 3	26.6	28	82.4
− 2	28.4	29	84.2
− 1	30.2	30	86.0
0	32.0	31	87.8
+ 1	33.8	32	89.6
2	35.6	33	91.4
3	37.4	34	93.2
4	39.2	35	95.0
5	41.0	36	96.8
6	42.8	37	98.6
7	44.6	38	100.4
8	46.4	39	102.2
9	48.2	40	104.0
10	50.0	41	105.8
11	51.8	42	107.6
12	53.6	43	109.4
13	55.4	44	111.2
		45	113.0

Gas Densities

(Weight of Unit Volume)

22.4 liters of any gas are equal to its molecular weight in grams at a pressure of 760 mm of mercury (Hg) and 0°C.

Molecular Weights

Air	= 29 g
Oxygen	= 32 g
Nitrous oxide	= 44 g
Carbon dioxide	= 44 g
Ether	= 74 g

Special Symbols*

– A *dash* above any symbol indicates a mean value.
· A *dot* above any symbol indicates a time derivative.

For Gases

Primary Symbols
(Large Capital Letters)

V = gas volume
$\dot{V}$ = gas volume per unit time
P = gas pressure
$\bar{P}$ = mean gas pressure
F = fractional concentration in dry gas phase
f = respiratory frequency (breaths per unit time)
D = diffusing capacity
R = respiratory exchange ratio

Examples

V_A = volume of alveolar gas
$\dot{V}_{O_2}$ = oxygen consumption/min
$P_{A}O_2$ = alveolar oxygen pressure
$P_{A}O_2$ = arterial partial pressure of oxygen
$P_{C}O_2$ = mean capillary oxygen pressure
$F_{I}O_2$ = fractional concentration of oxygen in inspired gas
DO_2 = diffusing capacity for (O_2 [mL O_2/min/mm/Hg])
R = $\dot{V}CO_2/\dot{V}O_2$

Secondary Symbols
(Small Capital Letters)

I = inspired gas
E = expired gas
A = alveolar gas
T = tidal gas
D = dead space gas
B = barometric
ATPS = ambient temperature and pressure saturated with water vapor
BTPS = body temperature and pressure saturated with water vapor
STPD = 0°C, 760 mm Hg, dry

Examples

$F_{I}CO_2$ = fractional concentration of carbon dioxide in inspired gas
V_E = volume of expired gas
$\dot{V}_A$ = alveolar ventilation per minute
V_T = tidal volume
V_D = volume of dead-space gas
P_B = barometric pressure
V_D/V_T = ratio of physiological dead space to tidal volume

For Blood

Primary Symbols
(Large Capital Letters)

Q = volume of blood
$\dot{Q}$ = volume flow of blood per unit time
C = concentration of gas in blood
S = percent saturation of hemoglobin with oxygen or carbon dioxide
$\dot{V}/\dot{Q}$ = ventilation-perfusion ratio

Examples

Qc = volume of blood in pulmonary capillaries
$\dot{Q}c$ = blood flow through pulmonary capillaries/min
$C_{a}O_2$ = milliliters of oxygen in 100 mL of arterial blood
$S_{\bar{V}}O_2$ = saturation of hemoglobin with oxygen in mixed venous blood

Secondary Symbols
(Lowercase Letters)

a = arterial blood
v = venous blood
c = capillary blood

Examples

$P_{a}CO_2$ = partial pressure of carbon dioxide in arterial blood
$P_{\bar{v}}O_2$ = partial pressure of oxygen in mixed venous blood
$P_{c}CO_2$ = partial pressure of carbon dioxide in pulmonary capillary blood

*Adapted from Julius H. Comroe Jr. et al., *The Lung* (based on report in *Fed Proc* 9:602–605, 1950). Copyright © 1962 (second edition) Chicago: Year Book Medical Publishers. Used with permission.

For Lung Volumes

VC	= vital capacity	= maximal volume that can be expired after maximal inspiration
IC	= inspiratory capacity	= maximal volume that can be inspired from resting expiratory level
IRV	= inspiratory reserve volume	= maximal volume that can be inspired from end-tidal inspiration
ERV	= expiratory reserve volume	= maximal volume that can be expired from resting expiratory level
FRC	= functional residual capacity	= volume of gas in lungs at resting expiratory level
RV	= residual volume	= volume of gas in lungs at end of maximal expiration
TLC	= total lung capacity	= volume of gas in lungs at end of maximal inspiration

Systeme International*

The following information on SI units and factors for conversion between SI and older conventional units is provided for the convenience of readers.

Basic SI Units

Physical Quantity	Name	Symbol
Length	meter	m
Mass	kilogram	kg
Time	second*	s
Electric current	ampere	A
Thermodynamic temperature	kelvin	K
Luminous intensity	candela	cd
Amount of substance	mole	mol

*Minute (min), hour (h), and day (d) will remain in use although they are not official SI units.

Prefixes for SI Units

Factor	Name	Symbol	Factor	Name	Symbol
10^{18}	exa-	E	10^{-18}	atto-	a
10^{15}	peta-	P	10^{-15}	femto-	f
10^{12}	tera-	T	10^{-12}	pico-	p
10^{9}	giga-	G	10^{-9}	nano-	n
10^{6}	mega-	M	10^{-6}	micro-	µ
10^{3}	kilo-	k	10^{-3}	milli-	m
10^{2}	hecto-	h	10^{-2}	centi-	c
10^{1}	deca-	da	10^{-1}	deci-	d

Derived SI Units

Quantity	SI Unit	Symbol	Expression in Terms of SI Base Units or Derived Units
Frequency	Hertz	Hz	$1\ Hz = 1\ cycle/s\ (1\ s^{-1})$
Force	Newton	N	$1\ N = 1\ kg \cdot m/s^2\ (1\ kg \cdot m\text{\textsc{ps}}^{-2})$
Work, energy, quantity of heat	Joule	J	$1\ J = 1\ N \cdot m$
Power	Watt	W	$1\ W = 1\ J/s\ (1\ J \cdot s^{-1})$
Quantity of electricity	Coulomb	C	$1\ C = 1\ A \cdot s$
Electric potential, potential difference, tension, electromotive force	Volt	V	$1\ V = 1\ W/A\ (1\ W \cdot A^{-1})$
Electric capacitance	Farad	F	$1\ F = 1\ A \cdot s/V\ (1\ A \cdot s \cdot V^{-1})$
Electric resistance	Ohm	Ω	$1\ \Omega = 1\ V/A\ (1\ V \cdot A^{-1})$
Flux of magnetic induction, magnetic flux	Weber	Wb	$1\ Wb = 1\ V \cdot s$
Magnetic flux density, magnetic induction	Tesla	T	$1\ T = 1\ Wb/m^2\ (1\ Wb \cdot m^{-2})$
Inductance	Henry	H	$1\ H = 1\ V \cdot s/A\ (1\ V \cdot s \cdot A^{-1})$
Pressure	Pascal	Pa	$1\ Pa = 1\ N/m^2\ (1\ N \cdot m^2)$ $= 1\ kg/m \cdot s^2\ (1\ kg \cdot m^{-1} \cdot s^{-2})$

The liter ($10^{-3}\ m^{-3} = dm^3$), though not official, will remain in use as a unit of volume as also will the dyne (dyn) as a unit of force ($1\ dyn = 10^{-5}\ N$).

SI Unit Conversions

SI Unit	Old Unit	Conversion Factors Old to SI (Exact)	SI to Old (Approx.)
kPa	mm Hg*	0.133	7.5
kPa	1 standard atmosphere† (approx. 1 Bar)	101.3	0.01
kPa	cm H_2O	0.0981	10
kPa	lbs/square inch	6.89	0.145

*For example, a systolic blood pressure of 120 mm Hg = 16 kPa and a diastolic blood pressure of 80 mm Hg = 11 kPa.
†= 760 mm Hg.

Blood Chemistry Units and Conversion Factors

Measurement (Approx.)	SI Unit	Old Unit	Conversion Factors	
			Old to SI (Exact)	SI to Old (Approx.)
Blood acid-base				
PCO_2	kPa	mm Hg	0.133	7.5
PO_2	kPa	mm Hg	0.133	7.5
Standard bicarbonate	mmol/liter	mEq/liter	Numerically equivalent	
Base excess	mmol/liter	mEq/liter	Numerically equivalent	
Glucose	mmol/liter	mg/100 mL	0.0555	18
Plasma				
Sodium	mmol/liter	mEq/liter	Numerically equivalent	
Potassium	mmol/liter	mEq/liter	Numerically equivalent	
Magnesium	mmol/liter	mEq/liter	0.5	2
Chloride	mmol/liter	mEq/liter	Numerically equivalent	
Phosphate (inorganic)	mmol/liter	mEq/liter	0.323	3.0
Creatinine	µmol/1liter	mg/100 mL	88.4	0.01
Urea	mmol/liter	mg/100 mL	0.166	6.0
Serum				
Calcium	mmol/liter	mg/100 mL	0.25	4.0
Iron	µmol/liter	µg/100 mol	0.179	5.6
Bilirubin	µmol/liter	mg/100 mL	17.1	0.06
Cholesterol	mmol/liter	mg/100 mL	0.0259	39
Total proteins	g/liter	g/100 mL	10.0	0.1
Albumin	g/liter	g/100 mL	10.0	0.1
Globulin	g/liter	g/100 mL	10.0	0.1

Biochemical Content of Other Body Fluids

Measurement	SI Unit	Old Unit	Conversion Factors	
			Old to SI (Exact)	SI to Old (Approx.)
Urine				
Calcium	mmol/24 h	mg/24 h	0.025	40
Creatinine	mmol/24 h	mg/24 h	0.00884	113
Potassium	mmol/liter	mEq/liter	Numerically equivalent	
Sodium	mmol/liter	mEq/liter	Numerically equivalent	
Cerebrospinal fluid				
Protein	g/liter	mg/100 mL	0.01	100
Glucose	mmol/liter	mg/100 mL	0.0555	18

Hematology

Measurement	SI Unit	Old Unit	Conversion Factors Old to SI	Conversion Factors SI to Old
Hemoglobin (Hb)	g/dL	g/100 mL		Numerically equivalent
Packed cell volume	No unit*	Percent	0.01	100
Mean cell Hb concentration	g/dL	Percent		Numerically equivalent
Mean cell Hb	pg	pg		Numerically equivalent
Red cell count	Cells/liter	Cells/mm^3	10^6	10^{-6}
White cell count	Cells/liter	Cell/mm^3	10^6	10^{-6}
Reticulocytes	Percent	Percent		Numerically equivalent
Platelets	Cell/liter	Cell/mm^3	10^6	10^{-6}

*Expressed as decimal fraction; for example, the normal adult male value is 0.40 to 0.54.

pH and Nanomoles Per Liter of Hydrogen-Ion Activity

pH	nmol/Liter
6.80	158
6.90	126
7.00	100
7.10	79
7.20	63
7.25	56
7.30	50
7.35	45
7.40	40
7.45	36
7.50	32
7.55	28
7.60	25
7.70	20

Index